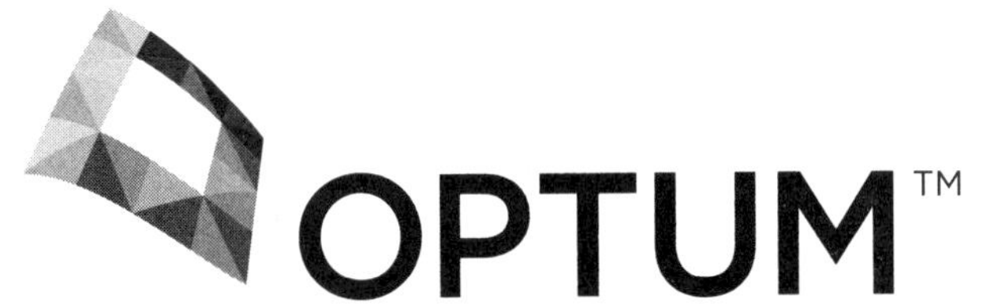

Current Procedural Coding Expert

2015

Our Commitment to Accuracy
Optum is committed to producing accurate and reliable materials.

To report corrections, please visit www.optumcoding.com/accuracy or email accuracy@optum.com. You can also reach customer service by calling 1.800.464.3649, option 1.

Made in the USA

ISBN 978-1-60151-897-2

Acknowledgments
Julie Van, CPC, CPC-P, CEMC, *Product Manager*
Karen Schmidt, BSN, *Technical Director*
Stacy Perry, *Manager, Desktop Publishing*
Lisa Singley, *Project Manager*
Karen H. Kachur, RN, CPC, *Clinical/Technical Editor*
Anita Schmidt, BS, RHIT, *Clinical/Technical Editor*
Elizabeth Leibold, RHIT, *Clinical/Technical Editor*
Karen Krawzik, RHIT, CCS, AHIMA-Approved ICD-10-CM/PCS Trainer, *Clinical/Technical Editor*
Tracy Betzler, *Senior Desktop Publishing Specialist*
Hope M. Dunn, *Senior Desktop Publishing Specialist*
Katie Russell, *Desktop Publishing Specialist*
Kate Holden, *Editor*

About the Contributors

Karen H. Kachur, RN, CPC
Ms. Kachur is a clinical/technical editor for Optum with expertise in CPT/HCPCS and ICD-9-CM coding, in addition to physician billing, compliance, and fraud and abuse. Prior to joining Optum, she worked for many years as a staff RN in a variety of clinical settings, including medicine, surgery, intensive care, and psychiatry. In addition to her clinical background, Ms. Kachur served as assistant director of a hospital utilization management and quality assurance department and has extensive experience as a nurse reviewer for Blue Cross/Blue Shield. She is an active member of the American Academy of Professional Coders.

Elizabeth Leibold, RHIT
Ms. Leibold has expertise in hospital outpatient coding and compliance. Her experience includes conducting coding audits and providing staff education to both tenured and new coding staff. She has a background in professional component coding, with CPT expertise in interventional procedures. Most recently Ms. Leibold was responsible for outpatient coding audits and compliance for a health information management services company. She is an active member of the American Health Information Management Association (AHIMA).

Karen Krawzik, RHIT, CCS, AHIMA-Approved ICD-10-CM/PCS Trainer
Ms. Krawzik has expertise in ICD-10-CM, ICD-9-CM, and CPT/HCPCS coding. Her coding experience includes inpatient, ambulatory surgery, and ancillary and emergency room records. She has served as a DRG analyst and auditor of commercial and government payer claims, and as a contract administrator. Most recently she was responsible for the conversion of the ICD-9-CM code set to ICD-10 and for analyzing audit results, identifying issues and trends, and developing remediation plans. Ms. Krawzik is credentialed by the American Health Information Management Association (AHIMA) as a Certified Coding Specialist (CCS) and is an AHIMA-approved ICD-10-CM/PCS trainer. She is an active member of AHIMA and the Missouri Health Information Management Association.

Anita Schmidt, BS, RHIT
Ms. Schmidt has expertise in Level I Adult and Pediatric Trauma hospital coding, specializing in ICD-9-CM, DRG, and CPT coding. Her experience includes analyzing medical record documentation and assigning ICD-9-CM codes and DRGs, as well as CPT codes for same-day surgery cases. She has conducted coding training and auditing, including DRG validation, conducted electronic health record training, and worked with clinical documentation specialists to identify documentation needs and potential areas for physician education. Ms. Schmidt is an active member of the American Health Information Management Association (AHIMA) and the Minnesota Health Information Management Association (MNHIMA).

Contents

Introduction

Welcome to Optum's *Current Procedural Coding Expert*, an exciting Medicare coding and reimbursement tool and definitive procedure coding source that combines the work of the Centers for Medicare and Medicaid Services, American Medical Association, and Optum experts with the technical components you need for proper reimbursement and coding accuracy.

This approach to CPT® Medicare coding utilizes innovative and intuitive ways of communicating the information you need to code claims accurately and efficiently. *Includes* and *Excludes* notes, similar to those found in your ICD-9-CM manuals, help determine what services are related to the codes you are reporting. Icons help you crosswalk the code you are reporting to laboratory and radiology procedures necessary for proper reimbursement. CMS-mandated icons and relative value units (RVUs) help you determine which codes are most appropriate for the service you are reporting. In addition, icons denoting codes that apply to Physician Quality Reporting System (PQRS) quality indicators are included along with their denominators. Add to that additional information identifying age and sex edits, ambulatory surgery center (ASC) and ambulatory payment classification (APC) indicators, and Medicare coverage and payment rule citations, and *Current Procedural Coding Expert* provides the best in Medicare procedure reporting.

Current Procedural Coding Expert includes the information needed to submit claims to federal contractors and most commercial payers, and is correct at the time of printing. However, CMS, federal contractors, and commercial payers may change payment rules at any time throughout the year. *Current Procedural Coding Expert* includes effective codes that will not be published in the AMA's Physicians' Current Procedural Terminology (CPT) book until the following year. Commercial payers will announce changes through monthly news or information posted on their websites. CMS will post changes in policy on its website at http://www.cms.gov/transmittals. National and local coverage determinations (NCDs and LCDs) provide universal and individual contractor guidelines for specific services. The existence of a procedure code does not imply coverage under any given insurance plan.

Current Procedural Coding Expert is based on the AMA's Physicians' Current Procedural Terminology coding system, which is copyrighted and owned by the physician organization. CPT is the nation's official, Health Information Portability and Accountability Act (HIPAA) compliant code set for procedures and services provided by physicians, ambulatory surgery centers (ASCs), and hospital outpatient services, as well as laboratories, imaging centers, physical therapy clinics, urgent care centers, and others.

In the 2015 update, the AMA made official changes to the following codes but did not identify them with a change icon or in appendix B. These codes were either first in a series under which other codes were indented, or were previously indented under another code that was deleted. When the nonindented, main code was deleted, its descriptor was incorporated into that of each previously indented code under it, and the semicolon was changed to a comma. Conversely, when a single indented code was deleted, and the code under which it was deleted became an individual stand-alone code, the semicolon was changed to a comma.

33474	Valvotomy, pulmonary valve, open heart, with cardiopulmonary bypass
36468	Single or multiple injections of sclerosing solutions, spider veins (telangiectasia), limb or trunk
61610	Transection or ligation, carotid artery in cavernous sinus, with repair by anastomosis or graft (List separately in addition to code for primary procedure)
61870	Craniectomy for implantation of neurostimulator electrodes, cerebellar, cortical
74290	Cholecystography, oral contrast
82075	Alcohol (ethanol), breath
83070	Hemosiderin, qualitative
83633	Lactose, urine, qualitative
83864	Mucopolysaccharides, acid, quantitative
84126	Porphyrins, feces, quantitative
87003	Animal inoculation, small animal, with observation and dissection
88348	Electron microscopy, diagnostic

Getting Started with *Current Procedural Coding Expert*

Current Procedural Coding Expert is an exciting tool combining the most current material at publication time from the AMA's *CPT 2015*, CMS's online manual system, the Correct Coding Initiative (CCI), CMS fee schedules, official Medicare guidelines for reimbursement and coverage, and Optum's own coding expertise.

Note: The AMA releases code changes quarterly. *Current Procedural Coding Expert* contains the most current information from the AMA, including new, changed, and deleted codes that are released on its website for future inclusion in the CPT book. Some of these changes will not appear in the AMA's CPT book until the following year.

Another feature of *Current Procedural Coding Expert* that differs from the official CPT book is the addition of appendix H, "Glossary." The glossary includes the definition of terms used throughout the manual.

Material is presented in a logical fashion for those billing Medicare, Medicaid, and many private payers. The format, based on customer comments, better addresses what customers tell us they need in a comprehensive Medicare procedure coding guide.

Designed to be easy to use and full of information, this product is an excellent companion to your AMA CPT manual and to Medicare, Optum, or other resources.

General Conventions

Sources of information in this book can be determined by color:

- Information compiled by Optum experts from official sources and based on coding knowledge is in blue ink.
- Medicare-derived information is in red ink.
- Codes, descriptions, and evaluation and management (E/M) guidelines from the American Medical Association are in black ink.

Guidelines

Coding guidelines have been incorporated into more specific section notes, code notes, icons, and the glossary. Section notes are listed under a range of codes and apply to all the codes in that range. Code notes are found under individual codes and apply to the single code. Definitions of coding terms are listed in the glossary and can be found in appendix H.

Resequencing of CPT Codes

The American Medical Association (AMA) uses a numbering methodology of resequencing, which is the practice of displaying codes outside of their numerical order according to the description relationship. According to the AMA, there are instances in which a new code is needed within an existing grouping of codes but an unused code number is not available. In these situations, the AMA will resequence the codes. In other words, it will assign a code that is not in numeric sequence with the related codes. However, the code and description will appear in the CPT manual with the other related codes.

Introduction

An example of resequencing from *Current Procedural Coding Expert* follows:

	21555	**Excision, tumor, soft tissue of neck or anterior thorax, subcutaneous; less than 3 cm**
#	**21552**	**3 cm or greater**
	21556	**Excision, tumor, soft tissue of neck or anterior thorax, subfascial (eg, intramuscular); less than 5 cm**
#	**21554**	**5 cm or greater**

Note that codes 21552 and 21554 are out of numeric sequence. However, as they are indented codes, they are in the correct place.

In *Current Procedural Coding Expert* the resequenced codes are listed twice. They appear in their resequenced position as shown above as well as in their original numeric position with a note indicating that the code is out of numerical sequence and where it can be found. (See example below.)

51797 Resequenced code. See code following 51729.

This differs from the AMA CPT book, in which the coder is directed to a code range that contains the resequenced code and description, rather than to a specific location.

Resequenced codes will appear in brackets in the headers, section notes, and code ranges. For example:

82286-82308 [82652]Chemistry: Bradykinin-Calcitonin
Code [82652] is included in section 82286-82308 Chemistry: Bradykinin-Calcitonin in its resequenced position.

Excludes Evaluation and management services (~99201-99499 [99224, 99225, 99226, 99485, 99486, 99490])

This shows that codes 99224–99226, 99485–99486, and 99490 are resequenced in this range of codes.

Appendix D identifies all CPT codes that are resequenced. Optum will display the resequenced coding as assigned by the AMA in its CPT products so that the user may understand the code description relationships.

Each particular group of CPT codes in *Current Procedural Coding Expert* is organized in a more intuitive fashion for Medicare billing, being grouped by the Medicare rules and regulations that govern payment of these particular procedures and services, as in this example:

95199-95199 Allergy Immunotherapy

CMS 100-2,15,20.2 Physician Expense for Allergy Treatment
CMS 100-3,110.9 Antigens Prepared for Sublingual Administration
CMS 100-4,12,200 Allergy Testing and Immunotherapy

Icons

● **New Codes**
Codes that have been added since the last edition of the book was printed.

△ **Revised Codes**
Codes that have been revised since the last edition of the book was printed.

Resequenced Codes
Codes that are out of numeric order but apply to the appropriate category.

❍ **Reinstated Code**
Codes that have been reinstated since the last edition of the book was printed.

Red Color Bar—Not Covered by Medicare
Services and procedures identified by this color bar are never covered benefits under Medicare. Services and procedures that are not covered may be billed directly to the patient at the time of the service.

Yellow Color Bar—Unlisted Procedure
Unlisted CPT codes report procedures that have not been assigned a specific code number. An unlisted code delays payment due to the extra time necessary for review.

Blue Color Bar—Resequenced Codes
Resequenced codes are codes that are out of numeric sequence—they are indicated with a blue color bar. They are listed twice, in their resequenced position as well as in their original numeric position with a note that the code is out of numerical sequence and where the resequenced code and description can be found.

INCLUDES **Includes notes**
Includes notes identify procedures and services that would be bundled in the procedure code. These are derived from AMA, CMS, CCI, and Optum coding guidelines. This is not meant to be an all-inclusive list.

EXCLUDES **Excludes notes**
Excludes notes may lead the user to other codes. They may identify services that are not bundled and may be separately reported, OR may lead the user to another more appropriate code. These are derived from AMA, CMS CCI, and Optum coding guidelines.

Code Also This note identifies an additional code that should be reported with the service and may relate to another CPT code or an appropriate HCPCS device code(s) that should be reported along with the CPT code when appropriate.

Code First Found under add-on codes, this note identifies codes for primary procedures that should be reported first, with the add-on code reported as a secondary code.

Do Not Report Indicates when a service is not separately reportable.

Laboratory/Pathology Crosswalk
This icon denotes CPT codes in the laboratory and pathology section of CPT that may be reported separately with the primary CPT code.

Radiology Crosswalk
This icon denotes codes in the radiology section that may be used with the primary CPT code being reported.

TC **Technical Component Only**
Codes with this icon represent only the technical component (staff and equipment costs) of a procedure or service. Do not use either modifier 26 (physician component) or TC (technical component) with these codes.

26 **Professional Component**
Only codes with this icon represent the physician's work or professional component of a procedure or service. Do not use either modifier 26 (physician component) or TC (technical component) with these codes.

50 **Bilateral Procedure**
This icon identifies codes that can be reported bilaterally when the same surgeon provides the service for the same patient on the same date. Medicare allows payment for both procedures at 150 percent of the usual amount for one procedure. The modifier does not apply to bilateral procedures inclusive to one code.

80 **Assist-at-Surgery Allowed**
Services noted by this icon are allowed an assistant at surgery with a Medicare payment equal to 16 percent of the allowed amount for the global surgery for that procedure. No documentation is required.

80 **Assist-at-Surgery Allowed with Documentation**
Services noted by this icon are allowed an assistant at surgery with a Medicare payment equal to 16 percent of the allowed amount for the global surgery for that procedure. Documentation is required.

\+ **Add-on Codes**
This icon identifies procedures reported in addition to the primary procedure. The icon "+" denotes add-on codes. An add-on code is neither a stand-alone code nor subject to multiple procedure rules since it describes work in addition to the primary procedure.

Modifier 51 Exempt
Codes identified by this icon indicate that the procedure should not be reported with modifier 51 (Multiple procedures).

Optum Modifier 51 Exempt
Codes identified by this Optum icon indicate that the procedure should not be reported with modifier 51 (Multiple procedures). Any code with this icon is backed by official AMA guidelines but was not identified by the AMA with their modifier 51 exempt icon.

Correct Coding Initiative (CCI)
Current Procedural Coding Expert identifies those codes with corresponding CCI edits. The CCI edits define correct coding practices that serve as the basis of the national Medicare policy for paying claims. The code noted is the major service/procedure. The code may represent a column 1 code within the column 1/column 2 correct coding edits table or a code pair that is mutually exclusive of each other.

CLIA Waived Test
This symbol is used to distinguish those laboratory tests that can be performed using test systems that are waived from regulatory oversight established by the Clinical Laboratory Improvement Amendments of 1988 (CLIA). The applicable CPT code for a CLIA waived test may be reported by providers who perform the testing but do not hold a CLIA license.

Modifier 63 Exempt
This icon identifies procedures performed on infants that weigh less than 4 kg. Due to the complexity of performing procedures on infants less than 4 kg, modifier 63 may be added to the surgery codes to inform the payers of the special circumstances involved.

A2–Z3 **ASC Payment Indicators**
This icon identifies ASC status payment indicators. They indicate how the ASC payment rate was derived and/or how the procedure, item, or service is treated under the revised ASC payment system. For more information about these indicators and how they affect billing, consult Optum's *Outpatient Billing Editor*.

- A2 Surgical procedure on ASC list in calendar year (CY) 2007; payment based on OPPS relative payment weight.
- F4 Corneal tissue acquisition; hepatitis B vaccine; paid at reasonable cost.
- G2 Non-office-based surgical procedure added in CY 2008 or later; payment based on outpatient prospective payment system (OPPS) relative payment weight.
- H2 Brachytherapy source paid separately when provided integral to a surgical procedure on ASC list; payment based on OPPS rate.
- J7 OPPS pass-through device paid separately when provided integral to a surgical procedure on ASC list; payment contractor-priced.
- J8 Device-intensive procedure; paid at adjusted rate.
- K2 Drugs and biologicals paid separately when provided integral to a surgical procedure on ASC list; payment based on OPPS rate.
- K7 Unclassified drugs and biologicals; payment contractor-priced.
- L1 Influenza vaccine; pneumococcal vaccine. Packaged item/service; no separate payment made.
- L6 New technology intraocular lens (NTIOL); special payment.
- N1 Packaged service/item; no separate payment made.
- P2 Office-based surgical procedure added to ASC list in CY 2008 or later with Medicare physician fee schedule (MPFS) nonfacility practice expense (PE) RVUs; payment based on OPPS relative payment weight.
- P3 Office-based surgical procedure added to ASC list in CY 2008 or later with MPFS nonfacility PE RVUs; payment based on MPFS nonfacility PE RVUs.
- R2 Office-based surgical procedure added to ASC list in CY 2008 or later without MPFS nonfacility PE RVUs; payment based on OPPS relative payment weight.
- Z2 Radiology or diagnostic service paid separately when provided integral to a surgical procedure on ASC list; payment based on OPPS relative payment weight.
- Z3 Radiology or diagnostic service paid separately when provided integral to a surgical procedure on ASC list; payment based on MPFS nonfacility PE RVUs.

Moderate Sedation
This icon identifies procedures that include moderate sedation. Moderate sedation codes should not be reported separately with these procedures.

Age Edit
This icon denotes codes intended for use with a specific age group, such as neonate, newborn, pediatric, and adult. Carefully review the code description to ensure the code you report most appropriately reflects the patient's age.

Maternity
This icon identifies procedures that by definition should be used only for maternity patients generally between 12 and 55 years of age.

♀ **Female Only**
This icon identifies procedures that some payers may consider for females only.

♂ **Male Only**
This icon identifies procedures that some payers may consider for males only.

Facility RVU
This icon precedes the facility RVU from CMS's 2014 physician fee schedule (PFS). It can be found under the code description.

Nonfacility RVU
This icon precedes the nonfacility RVU from CMS's 2014 PFS. It can be found under the code description.

Global Days The global period is the time following surgery during which routine care by the physician is considered postoperative and included in the surgical fee. Office visits or other routine care related to the original surgery cannot be separately reported if provided during the global period. Global days are sometimes referred to as "follow-up days," or FUDs. The statuses are:

- 000 No follow-up care included in this procedure
- 010 Normal postoperative care is included in this procedure for ten days
- 090 Normal postoperative care is included in the procedure for 90 days
- MMM Maternity codes; usual global period does not apply
- XXX The global concept does not apply to the code
- YYY The carrier is to determine whether the global concept applies and establishes postoperative period, if appropriate, at time of pricing
- ZZZ The code is related to another service and is always included in the global period of the other service

CMS: This notation indicates that there is a specific CMS guideline pertaining to this code in the CMS Online Manual System which includes the internet-only manual (IOM) *National Coverage Determinations Manual* (NCD). These CMS sources present the rules for submitting these services to the federal government or its contractors and are included in the appendix G of this book.

AMA: This indicates discussion of the code in the American Medical Association's *CPT Assistant* newsletter. Use the citation to find the correct issue.

〃 **Drug Not Approved by FDA**
The AMA CPT Editorial Panel is publishing new vaccine product codes prior to Food and Drug Administration approval. This symbol indicates which of these codes are pending FDA approval at press time.

[PQ] **Physician Quality Reporting System (PQRS)**
This icon denotes CPT codes that specifically address one or more of the CMS-determined quality measures. See appendix K for a list of denominators that apply to those codes.

[A]–[Y] **OPPS Status Indicators (OPSI)**
Status indicators identify how individual CPT codes are paid or not paid under the latest available hospital outpatient prospective payment system (OPPS). The same status indicator is assigned to all the codes within an ambulatory payment classification (APC). Consult your payer or other resource to learn which CPT codes fall within various APCs.

- [A] Services furnished to a hospital outpatient that are paid under a fee schedule or payment system other than OPPS
- [B] Codes that are not recognized by OPPS when submitted on an outpatient hospital Part B bill type (12x and 13x).
- [C] Inpatient procedures
- [D] Discontinued codes
- [E] Items, codes, and services:
  - For which pricing information is not available
  - Not covered by any Medicare outpatient benefit category
  - Statutorily excluded by Medicare
  - Not reasonable and necessary
- [F] Corneal tissue acquisition; certain CRNA services and hepatitis B vaccines
- [G] Pass-through drugs and biologicals
- [H] Pass-through device categories
- [J1] Hospital Part B services paid through a comprehensive APC
- [K] Nonpass-through drugs and nonimplantable biologicals, including therapeutic radiopharmaceuticals
- [L] Influenza vaccine; pneumococcal pneumonia vaccine
- [M] Items and services not billable to the FI/MAC
- [N] Items and services packaged into APC rates
- [P] Partial hospitalization
- [Q1] STV-packaged codes
- [Q2] T-packaged codes
- [Q3] Codes that may be paid through a composite APC
- [R] Blood and blood products
- [S] Procedure or service, not discounted when multiple
- [T] Procedure or service, multiple procedure reduction applies
- [U] Brachytherapy sources
- [V] Clinic or emergency department visit
- [Y] Nonimplantable durable medical equipment

Appendixes

Appendix A: Modifiers—This appendix identifies the modifiers. A modifier is a two-position alpha or numeric code that is appended to a CPT or HCPCS code to clarify the services being billed. Modifiers provide a means by which a service can be altered without changing the procedure code. They add more information, such as anatomical site, to the code. In addition, they help eliminate the appearance of duplicate billing and unbundling. Modifiers are used to increase the accuracy in reimbursement and coding consistency, ease editing, and capture payment data.

Appendix B: New, Changed, and Deleted Codes—This is a list of new, changed, and deleted CPT codes for the current year.

Appendix C: Crosswalk of Deleted Codes—This appendix is a cross-reference from a deleted CPT code to an active code when one is available. The deleted code cross-reference will also appear under the deleted code description in the tabular section of the book.

Appendix D: Resequenced Codes—This appendix contains a list of codes that are not in numeric order in the book. AMA resequenced some of the code numbers to relocate codes in the same category but not in numeric sequence.

Appendix E: Add-on, Modifier 51 Exempt, Optum Modifier 51 Exempt, Modifier 63 Exempt, and Moderate Sedation Codes—This list includes add-on codes that cannot be reported alone, codes that are exempt from modifier 51, codes that should not be reported with modifier 63, and codes that include moderate sedation.

Appendix F: Place of Service and Type of Service—This appendix contains lists of place-of-service codes that should be used on professional claims and type-of-service codes used by the Medicare Common Working File.

Appendix G: Pub. 100 References—This appendix contains a verbatim printout of the Medicare Internet Only Manual references that pertain to specific codes. The reference, when available, is listed after the header in the CPT section. For example:

60600–60605 Carotid Body Procedures

CMS 100-3, 20.18, Carotid Body Resection/Carotid Body Denervation

Since appendix G contains this reference from the *Medicare Claims Processing Manual*, Pub. 100-3 chapter 20, section 20.18, there is no need to search the Medicare website for the applicable reference.

Appendix H: Glossary—This appendix contains general terms and definitions as well as those that would apply to or be helpful for billing and reimbursement.

Appendix I: Listing of Sensory, Motor, and Mixed Nerves—This appendix lists a summary of each sensory, motor, and mixed nerve with its appropriate nerve conduction study code.

Appendix J: Vascular Families—Appendix J contains a table of vascular families starting with the aorta. Additional information can be found in the interventional radiology illustrations located behind the index.

Appendix K: Physician Quality Reporting System (PQRS)—Lists the numerators and denominators applicable to Medicare PQRS.

Appendix L: Medically Unlikely Edits—This appendix contains the published medically unlikely edits (MUEs). These edits establish maximum daily allowable units of service. The edits will be applied to the services provided to the same patient, for the same CPT code, on the same date of service when billed by the same provider. Included are the physician and facility edits.

Appendix M: Inpatient-Only Procedures—This appendix identifies services with the status indicator C. Medicare will not pay an OPPS hospital or ASC when these procedures are performed on a Medicare patient as an outpatient. Physicians should refer to this list when scheduling Medicare patients for surgical procedures. CMS will update this list quarterly.

Appendix N: Multianalyte Assays with Algorithmic Analyses —This appendix lists the administrative codes for multianalyte assays with algorithmic analyses. The AMA will update this list three times a year.

For more information about ongoing development of the CPT coding system, consult the AMA website at URL http://www.ama-assn.org/.

Note: All data current as of November 8, 2014.

Anatomical Illustrations

Body Planes and Movements

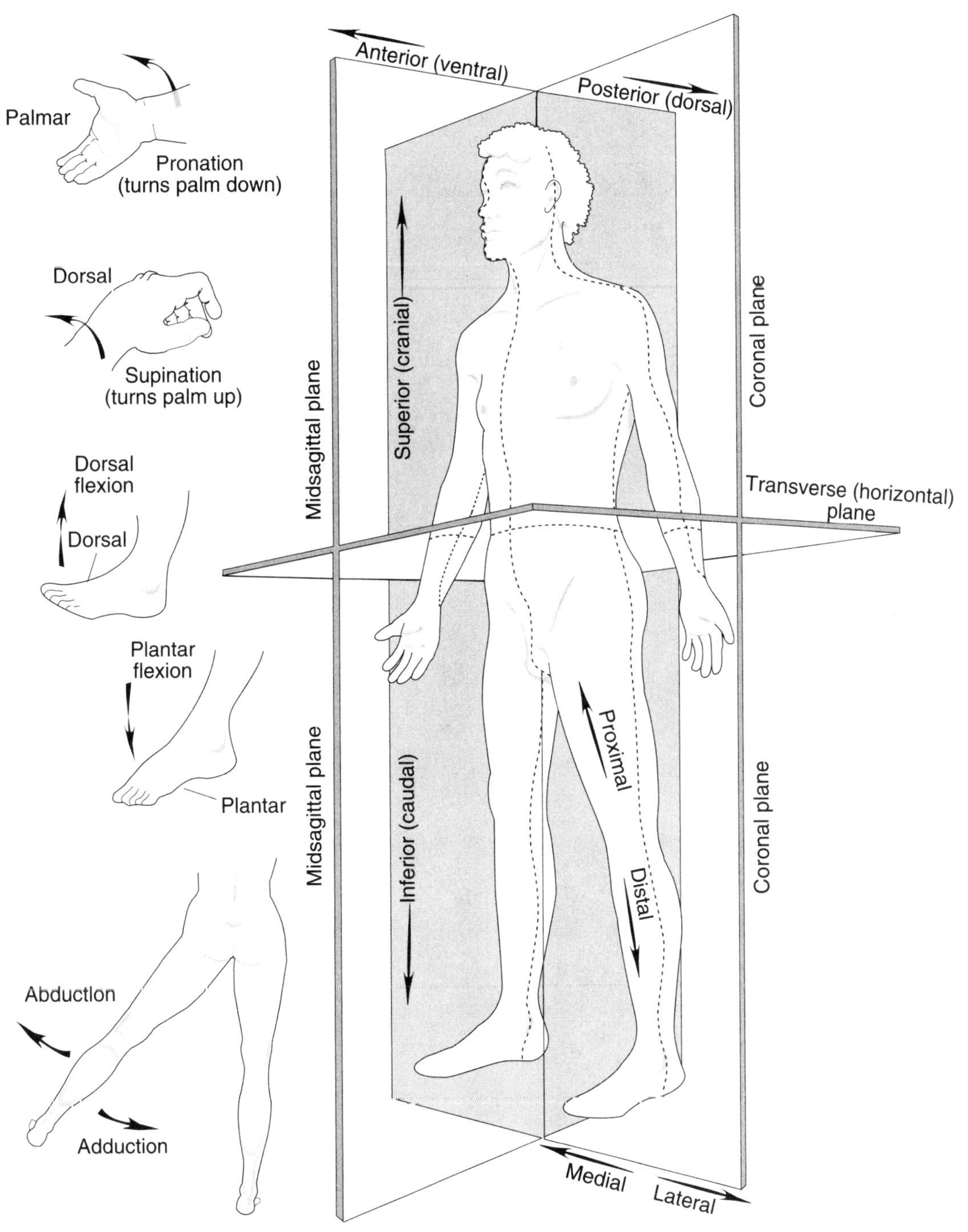

Musculoskeletal System

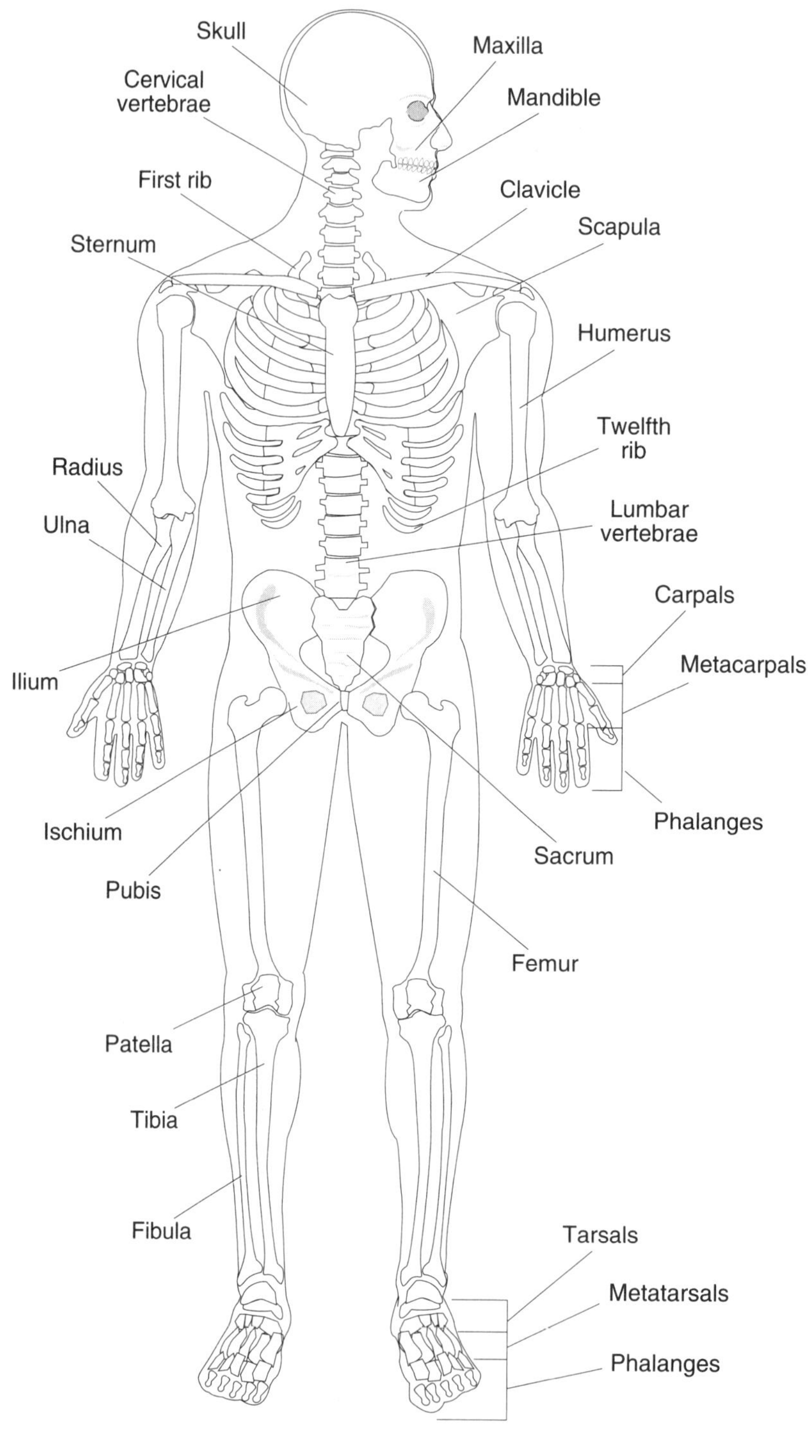

Musculoskeletal System

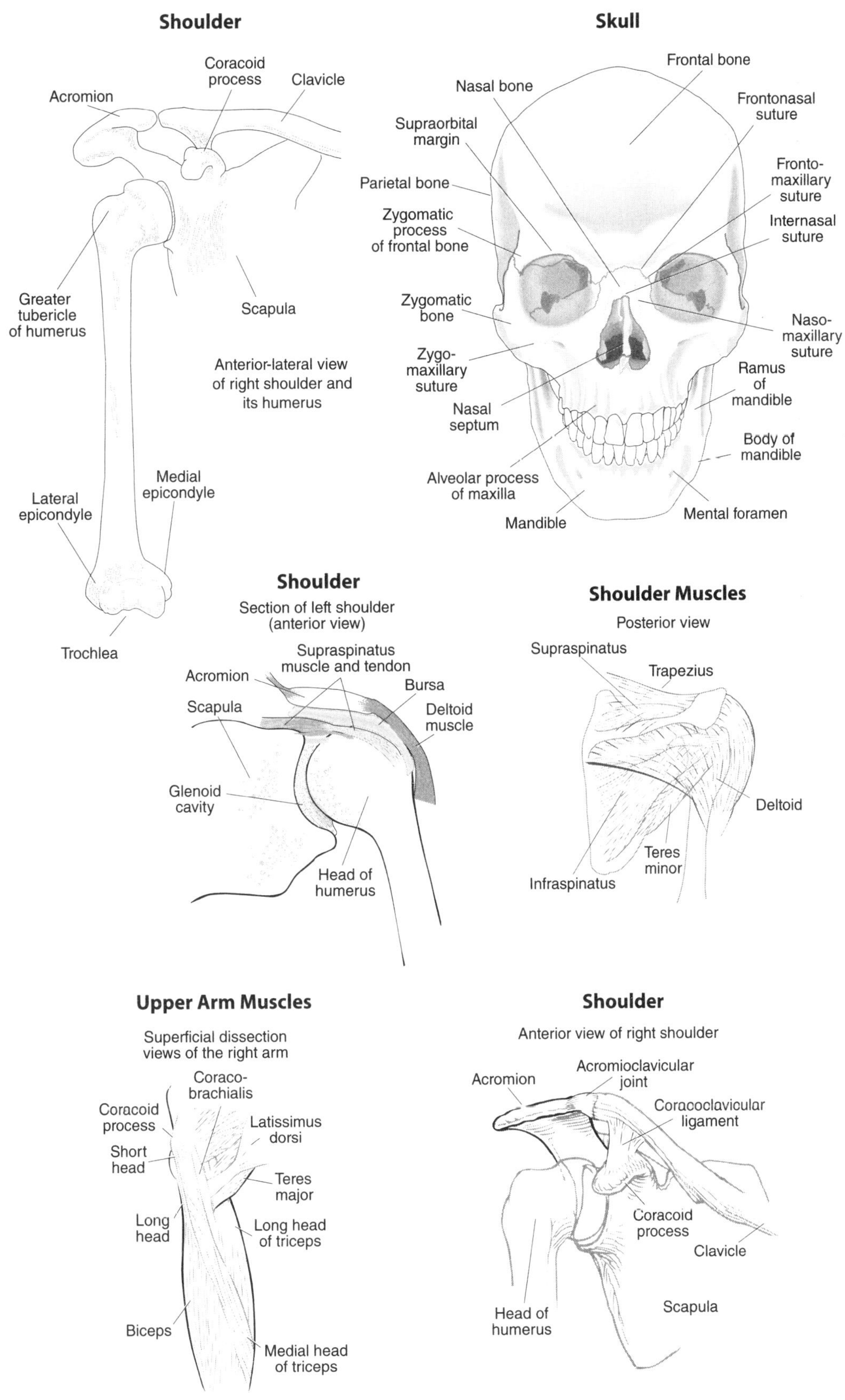

Musculoskeletal System

Elbow

Anterior view of right arm and elbow

Humerus
Coronoid fossa
Radial fossa
Lateral epicondyle
Medial epicondyle
Capitulum
Trochlea
Radius
Ulna

Elbow

Anterior view of right elbow

Humerus
Joint capsule
Lateral epicondyle
Medial epicondyle
Radial collateral ligament
Ulnar collateral ligament
Radius
Ulna

Lateral view of right elbow joint

Body of humerus
Head of radius
Joint capsule
Radial collateral ligament
Annular ligament of radius

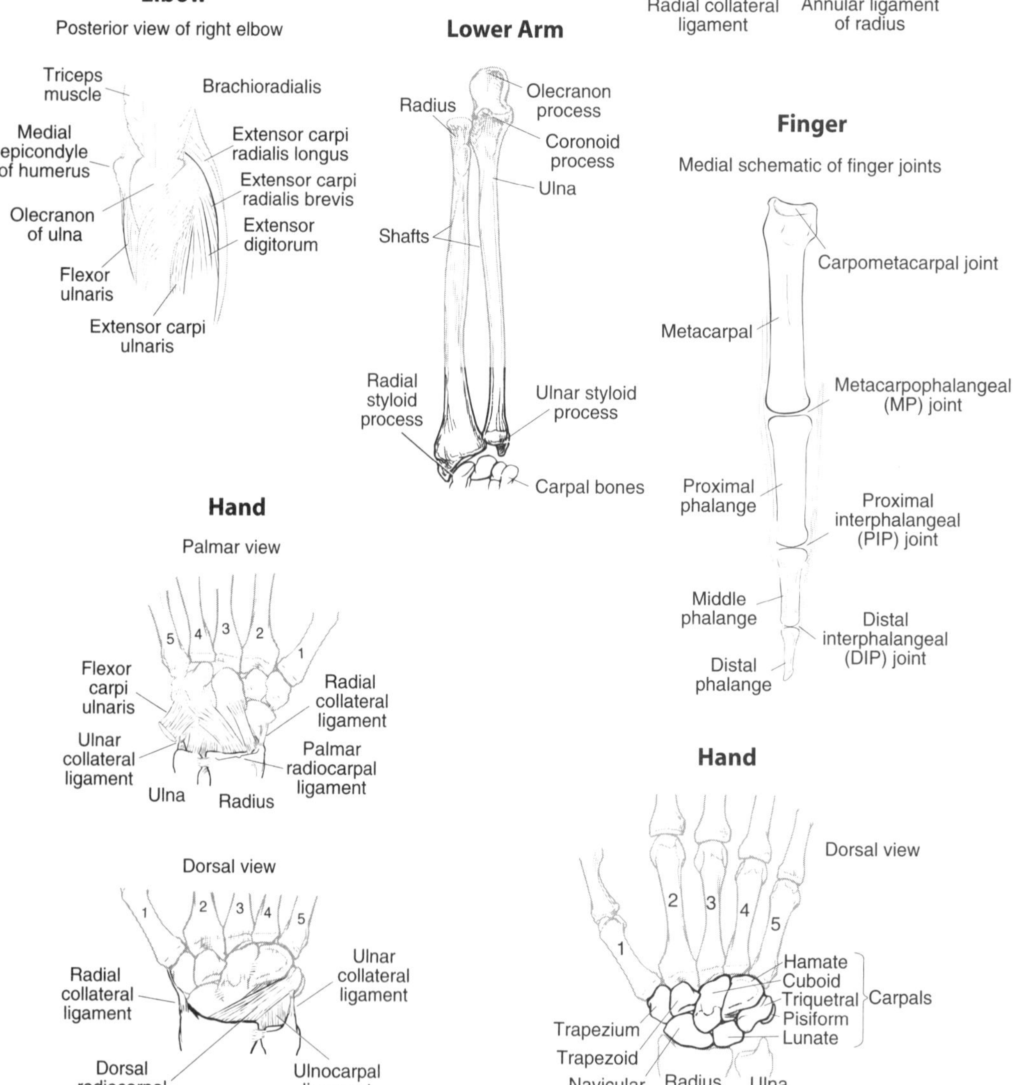

Musculoskeletal System

Ankle

Lateral and posterior views of right ankle

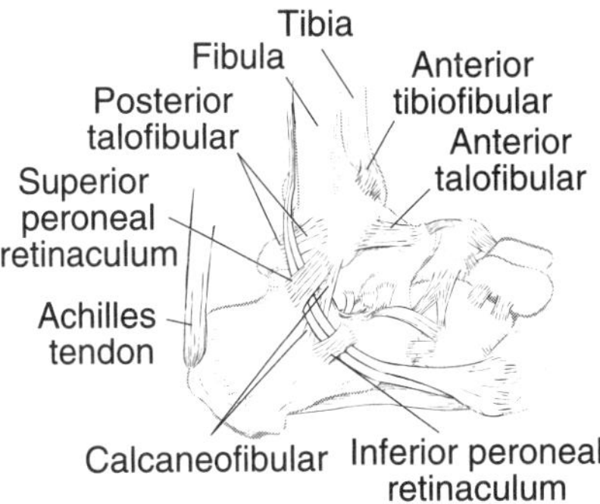

Achilles tendon not shown

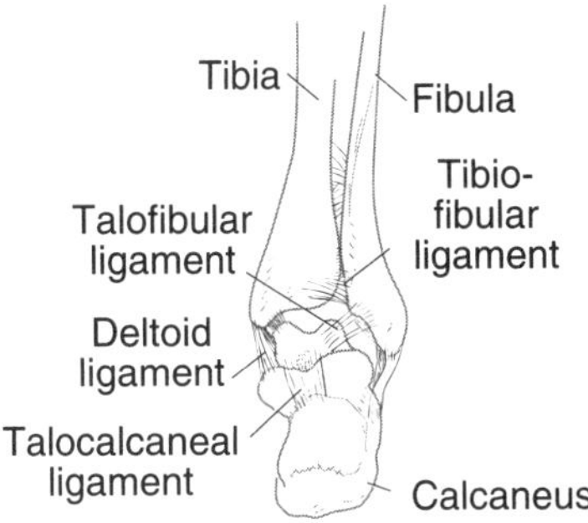

Foot

Select extensors of the foot

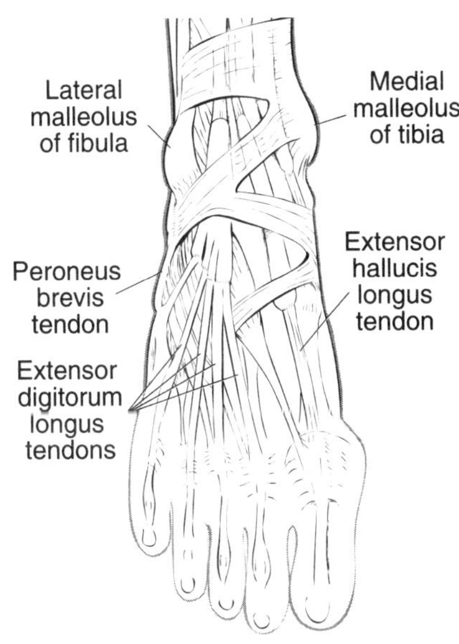

Foot

Tarsals, excluding talus and calcaneus (dark), superior view

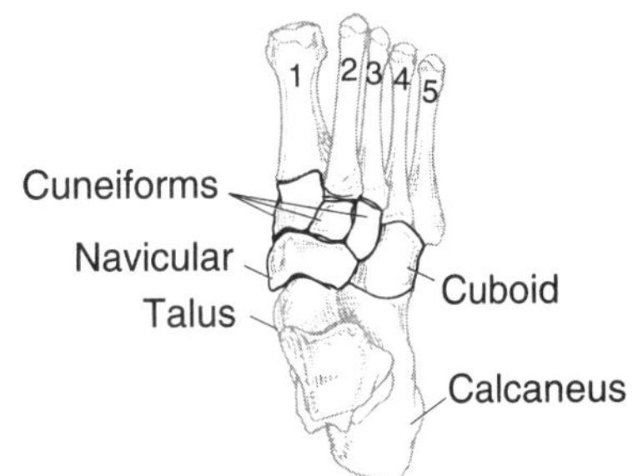

Foot

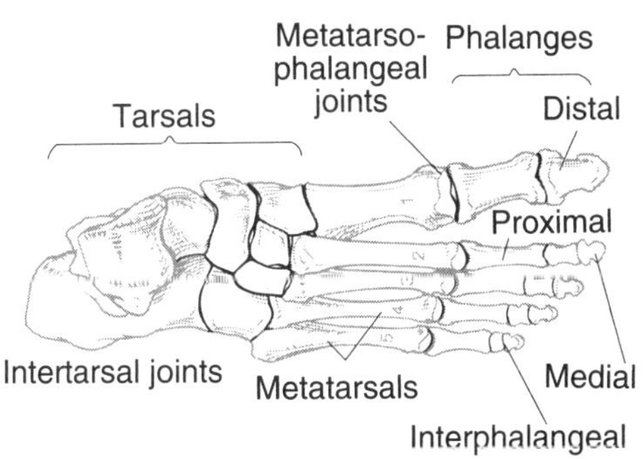

Musculoskeletal System

Leg

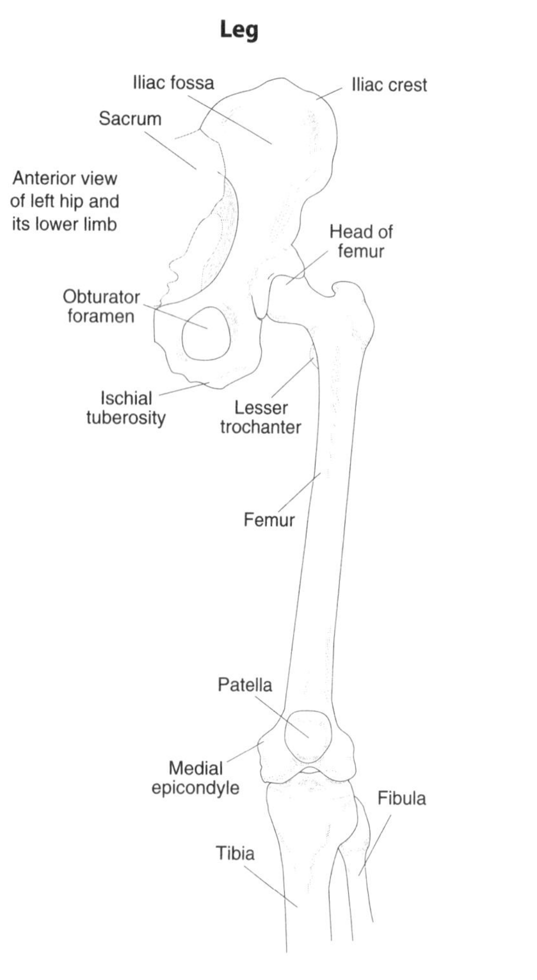

Hip

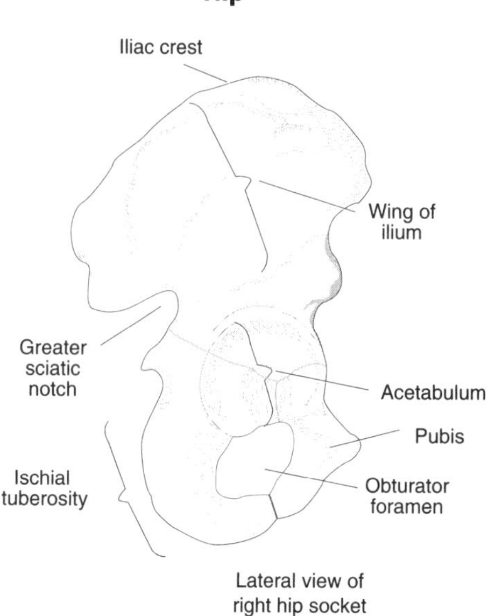

Knee

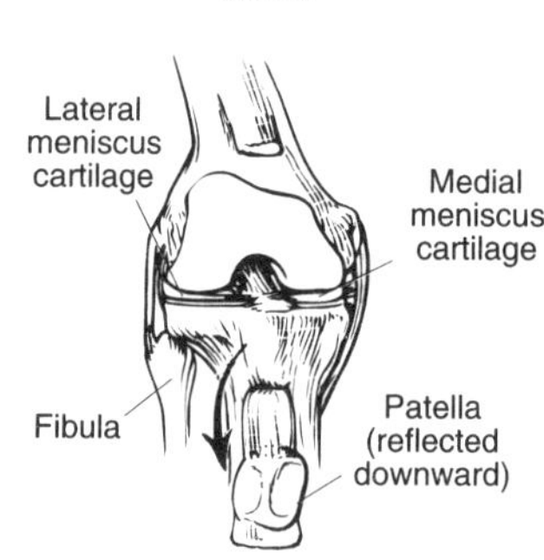

Anterior view of right knee

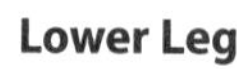

Lower Leg

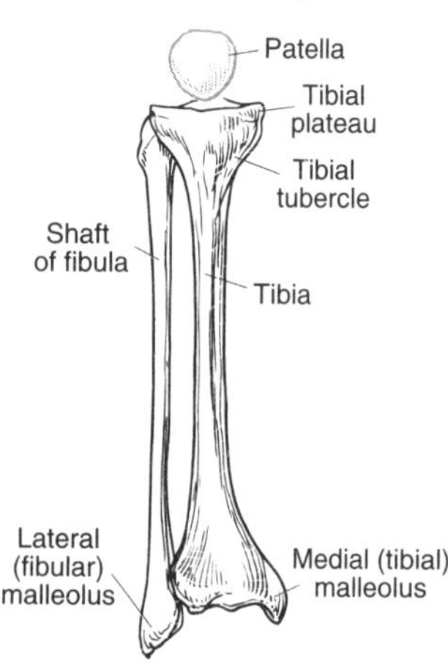

Knee

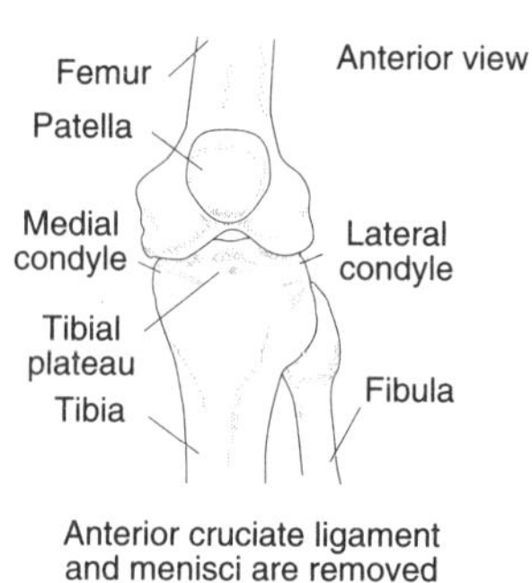

Anterior cruciate ligament and menisci are removed

Assessment of Burn Surface Area

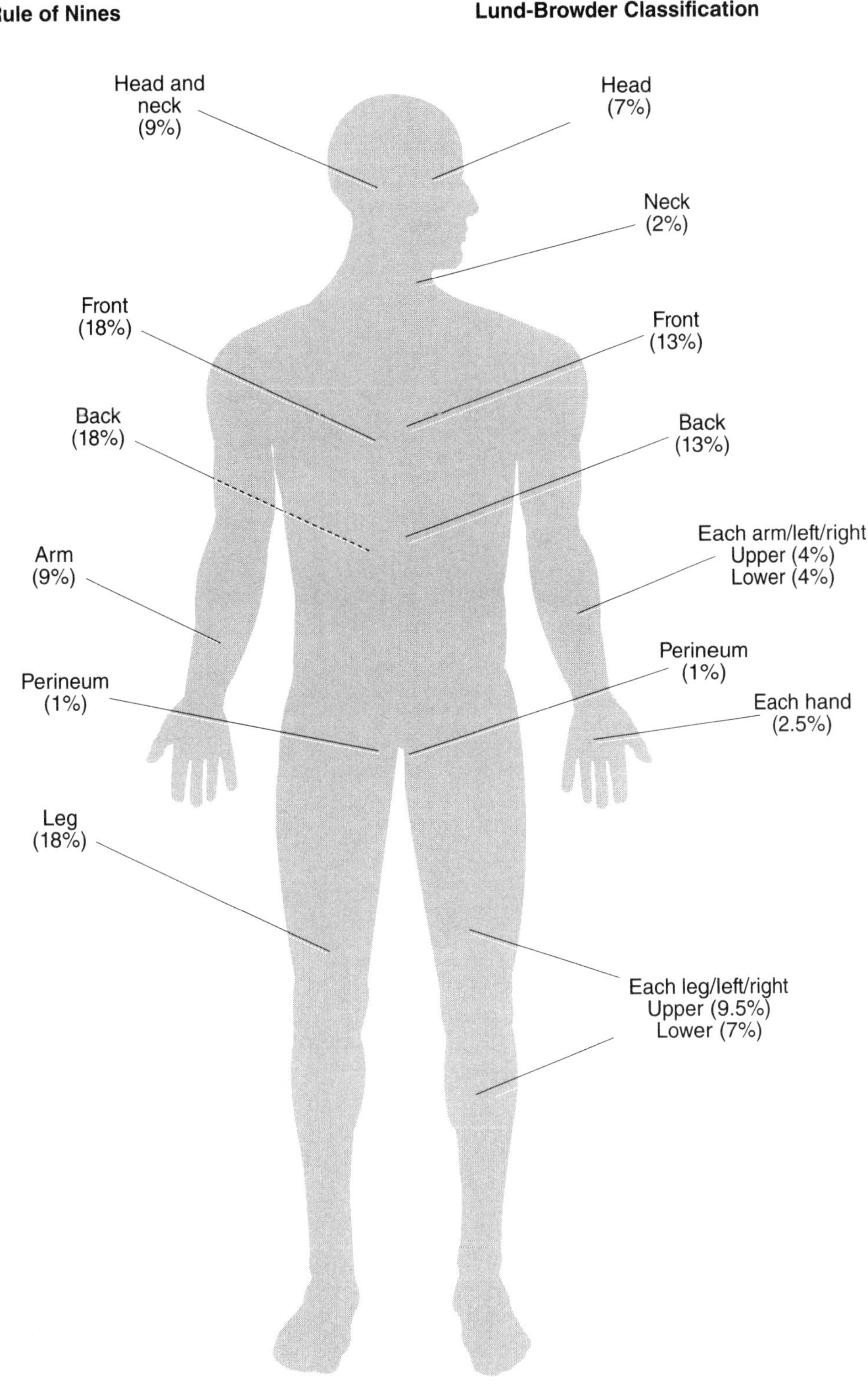

Digestive system

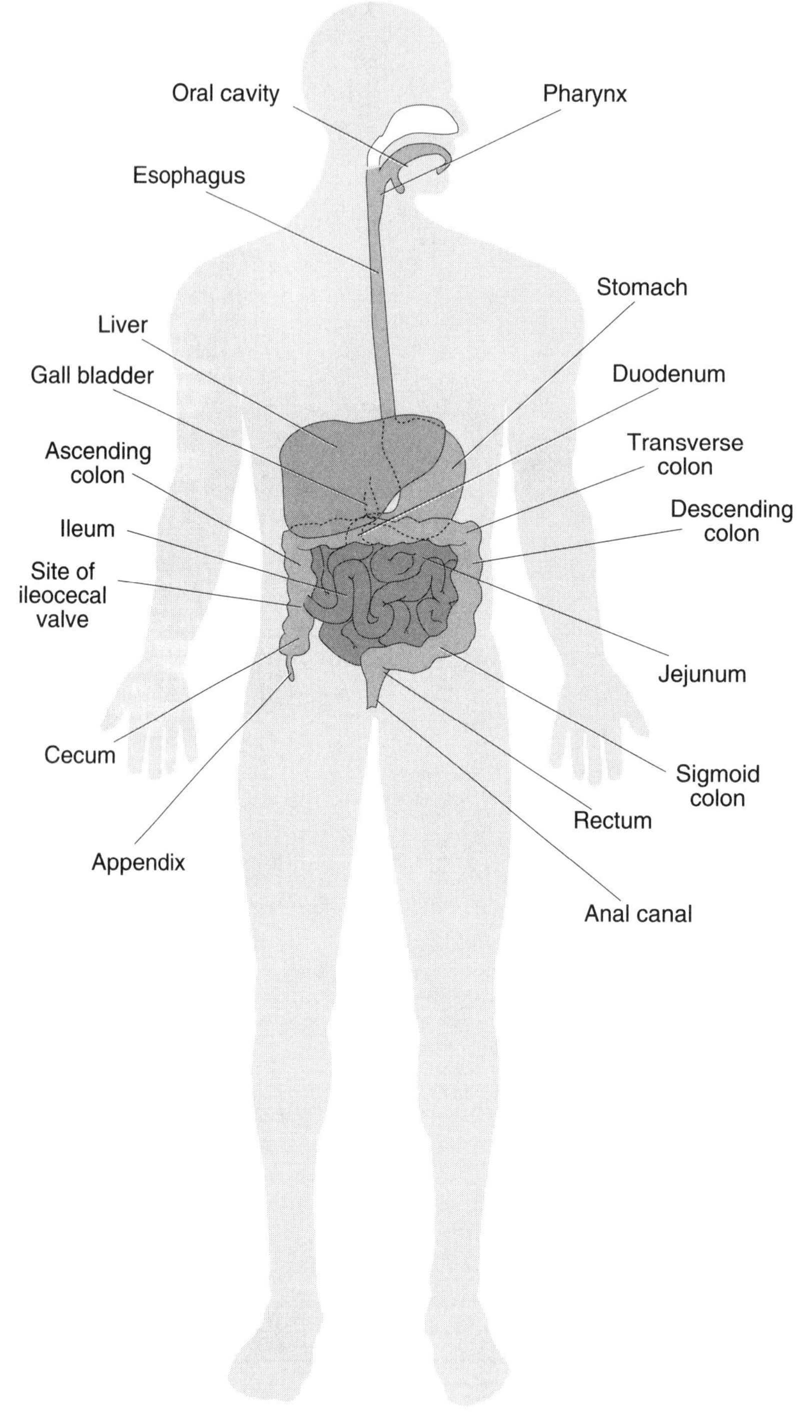

Digestive System

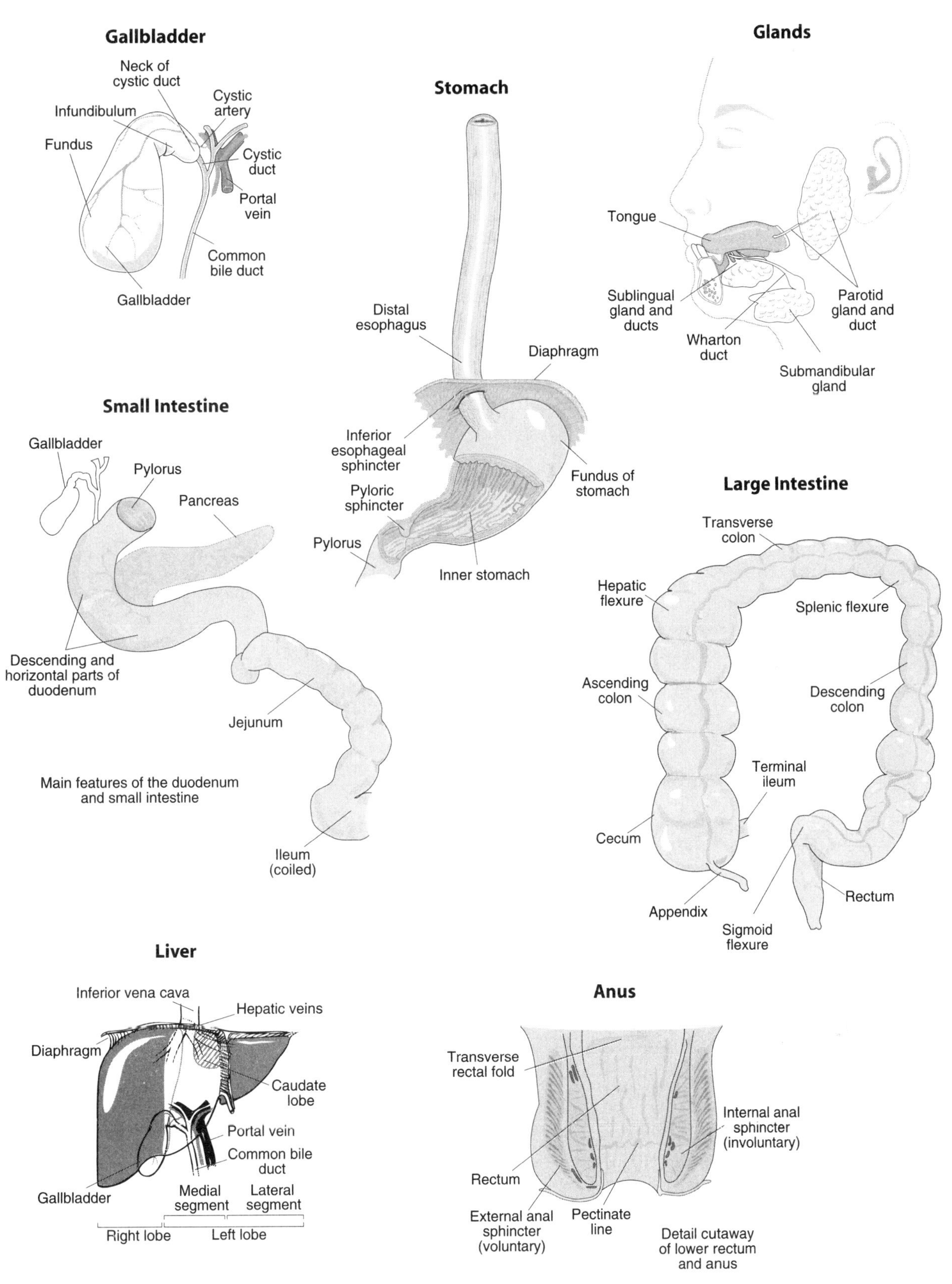

Arterial System

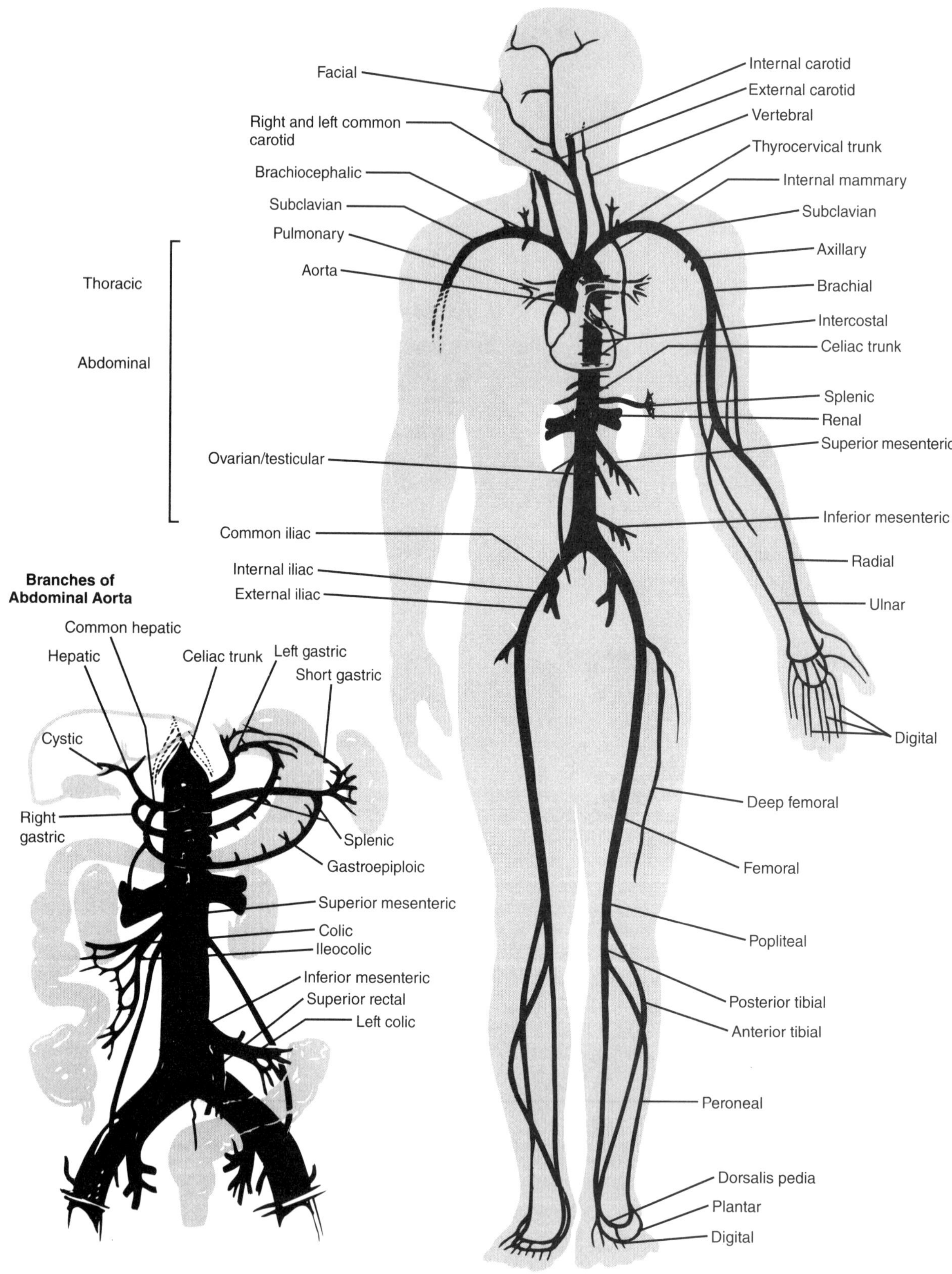

Arterial System

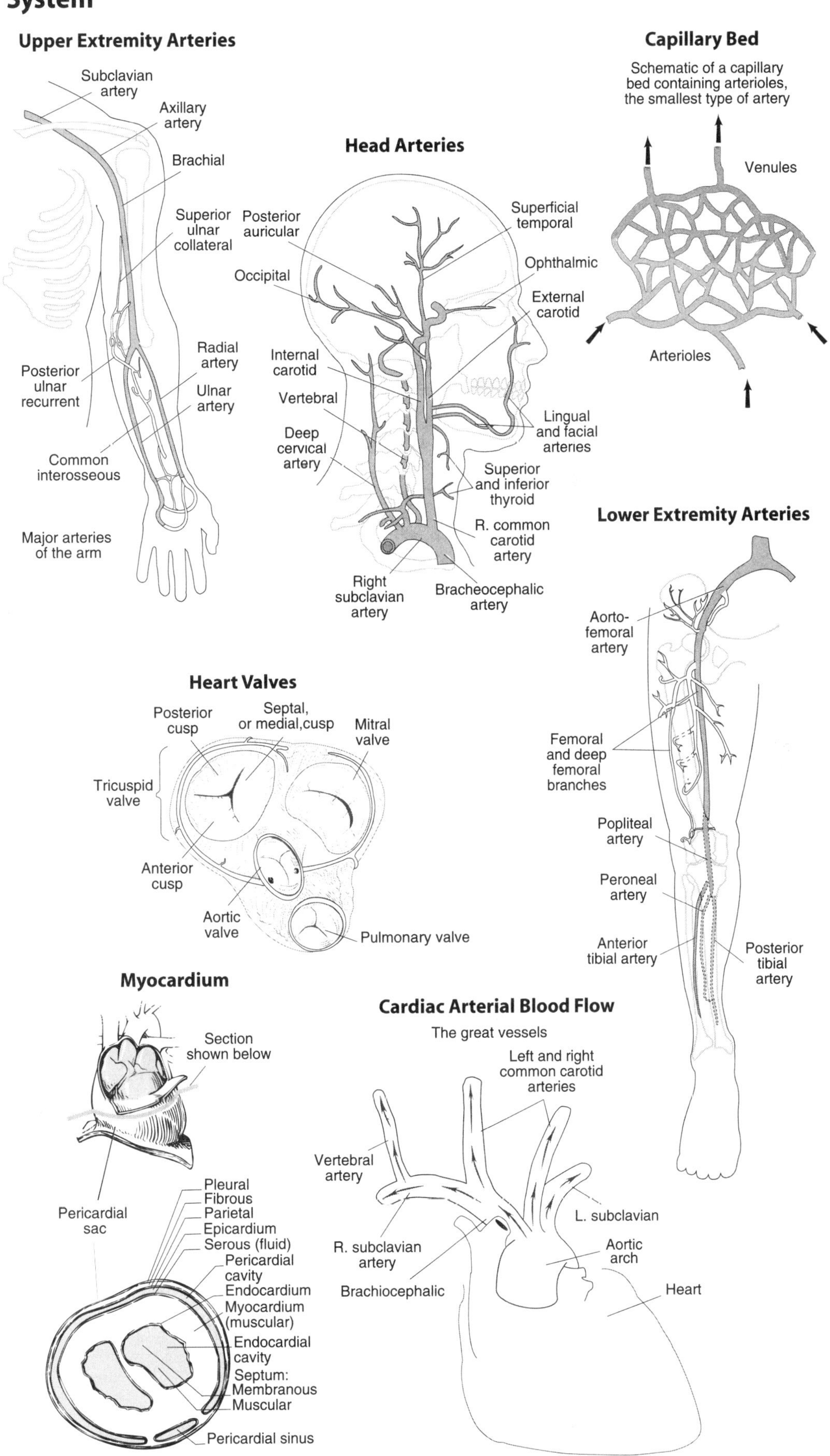

Venous System

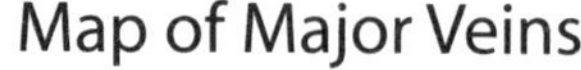

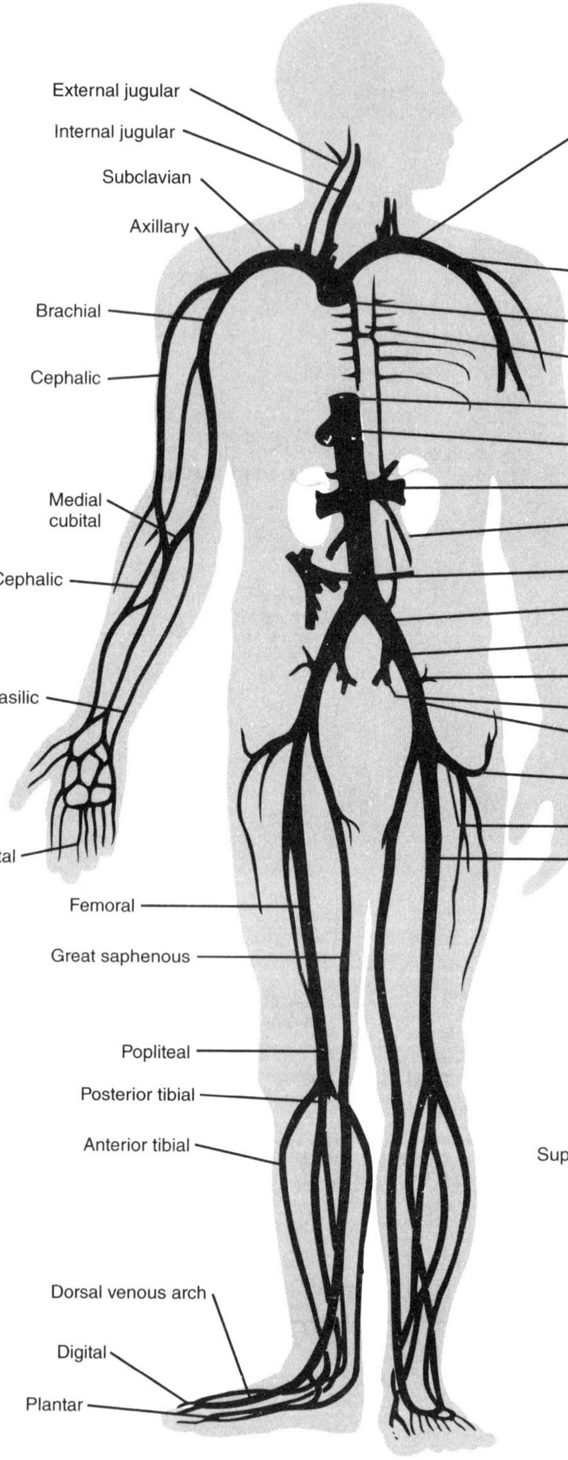

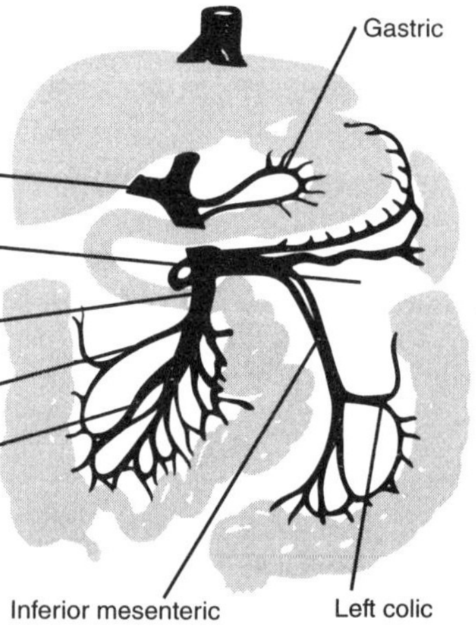

Venous System

Upper Extremity Veins

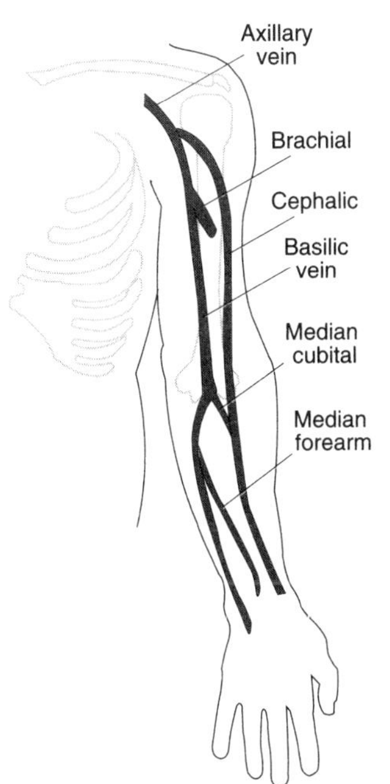

Venae Comitantes

Artery

Venae comitantes

Heart Veins

Superior vena cava vein

Anterior cardiac veins

Great cardiac vein

Coronary sinus

Small cardiac vein

Middle cardiac vein

Head Veins

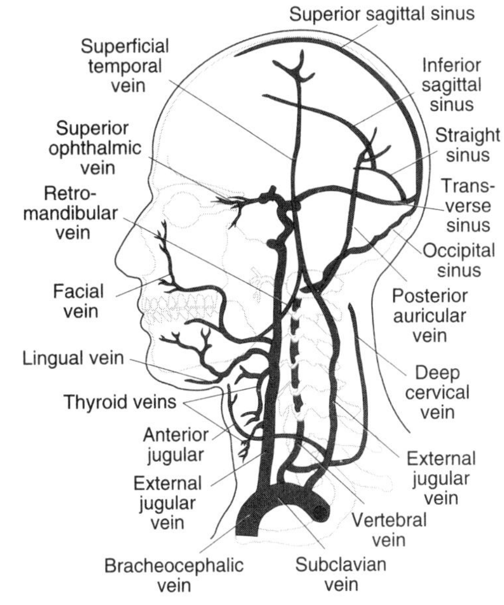

Venous Blood Flow

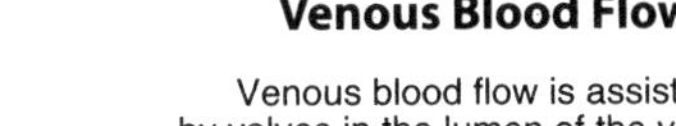

Venous blood flow is assisted by valves in the lumen of the vessels

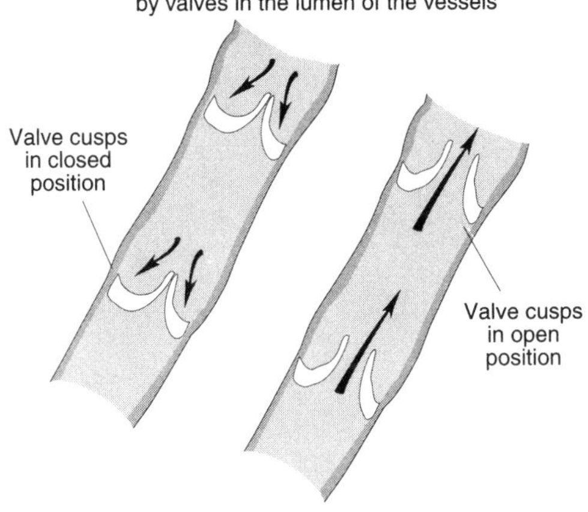

Cardiac Venous Blood Flow

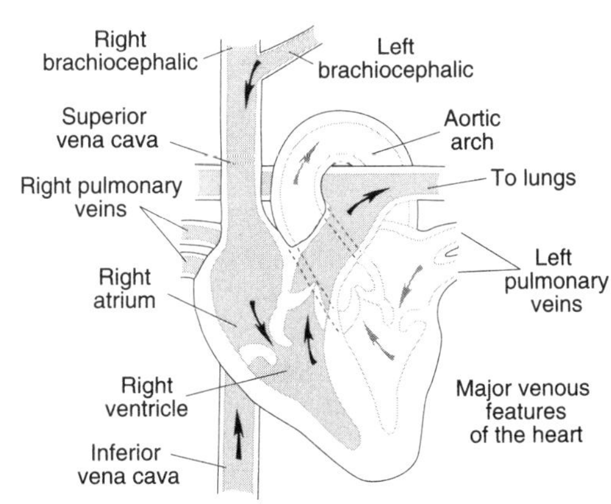

Abdominal Veins

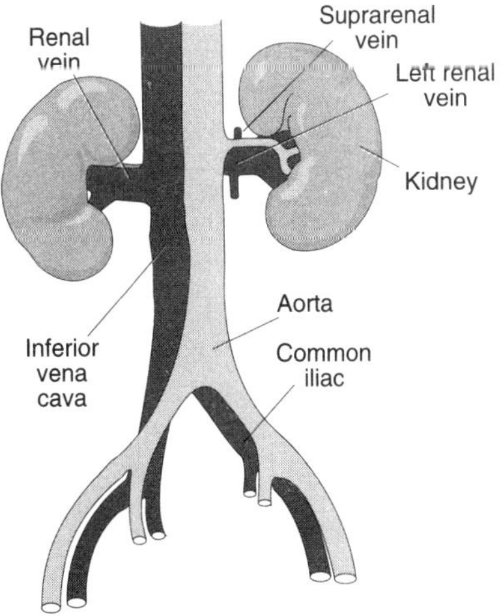

Nervous System

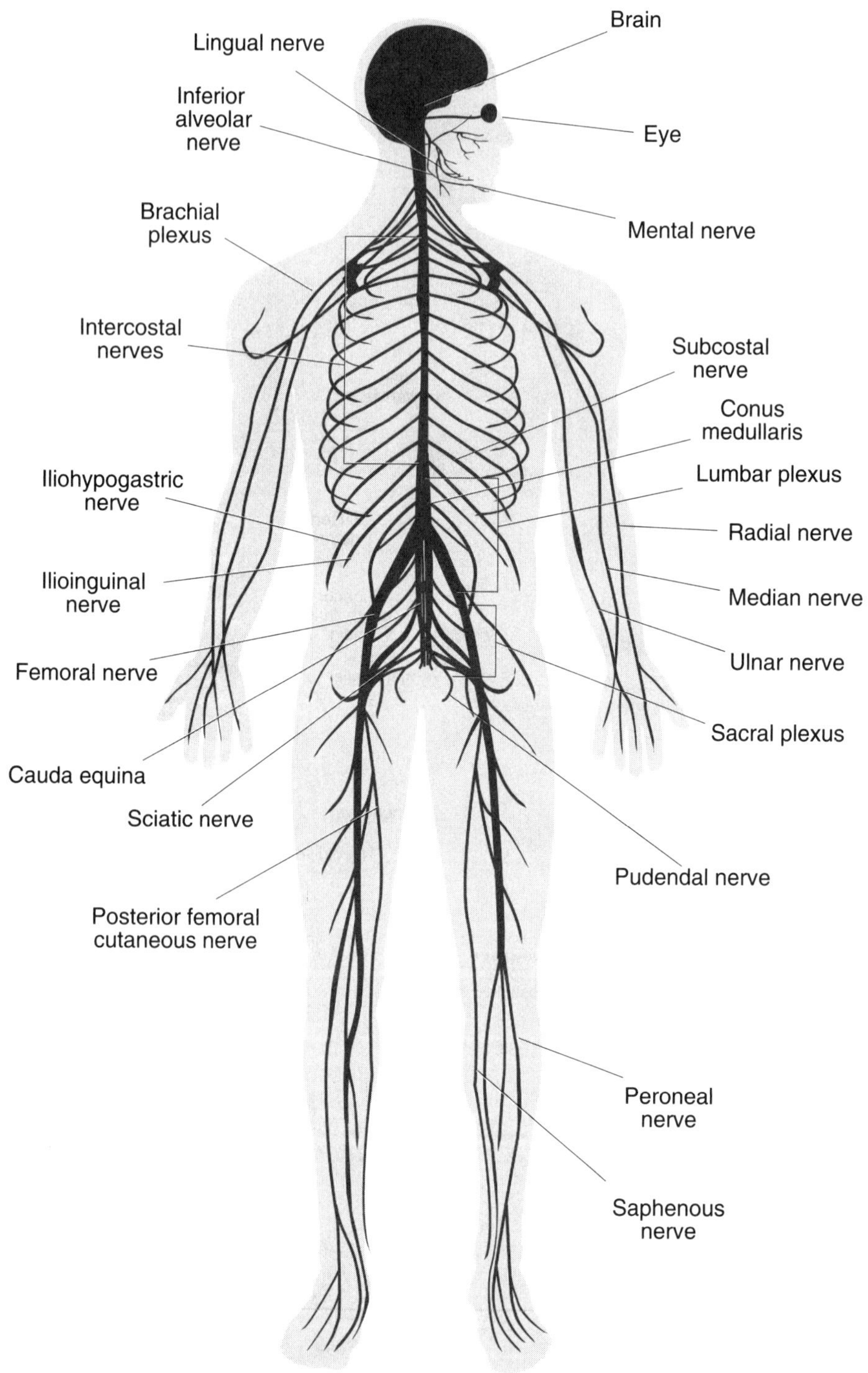

Nervous System

Brain

Corpus callosum
Cerebrum
Hypothalamus
Optic chiasm
Hypophysis
Mamillary body
Peduncle
Medulla oblangata
Interventricular foramen
Fornix
Third ventricle
Pineal body
Corpora quadrigemina
Cerebral aqueduct
Vermis
Fourth ventricle
Median aperture
Spinal cord
Pons

Cranial Nerves

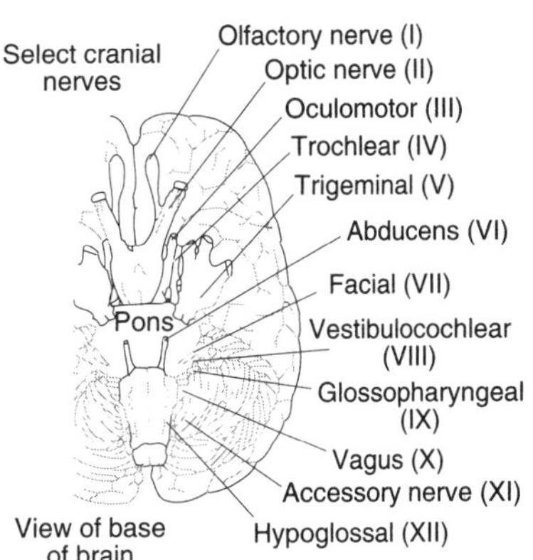

Spinal Cord

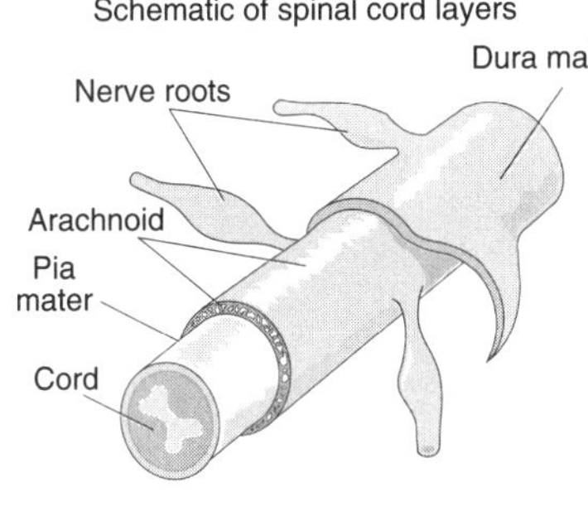

Spinal Column

Cranial Layers

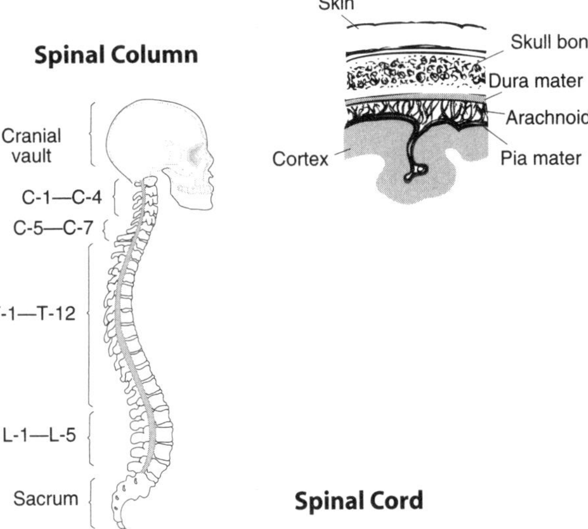

Spinal Cord

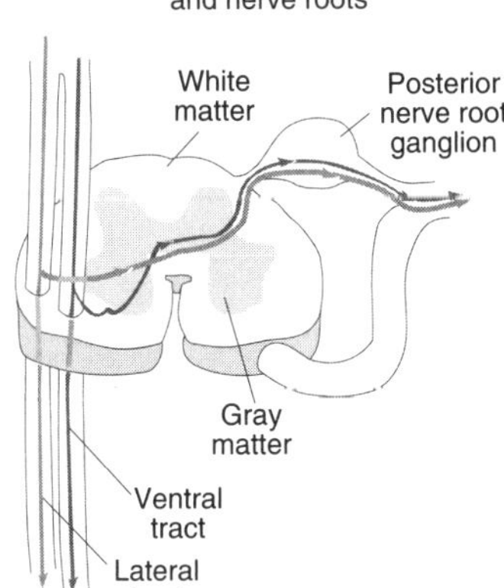

Spinal Cord

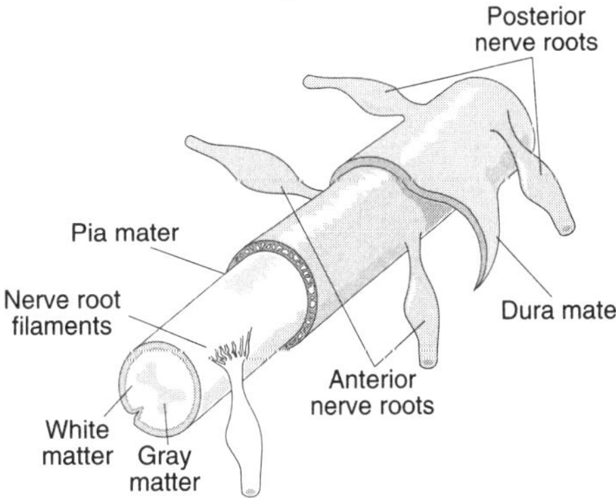

Lymphatic System

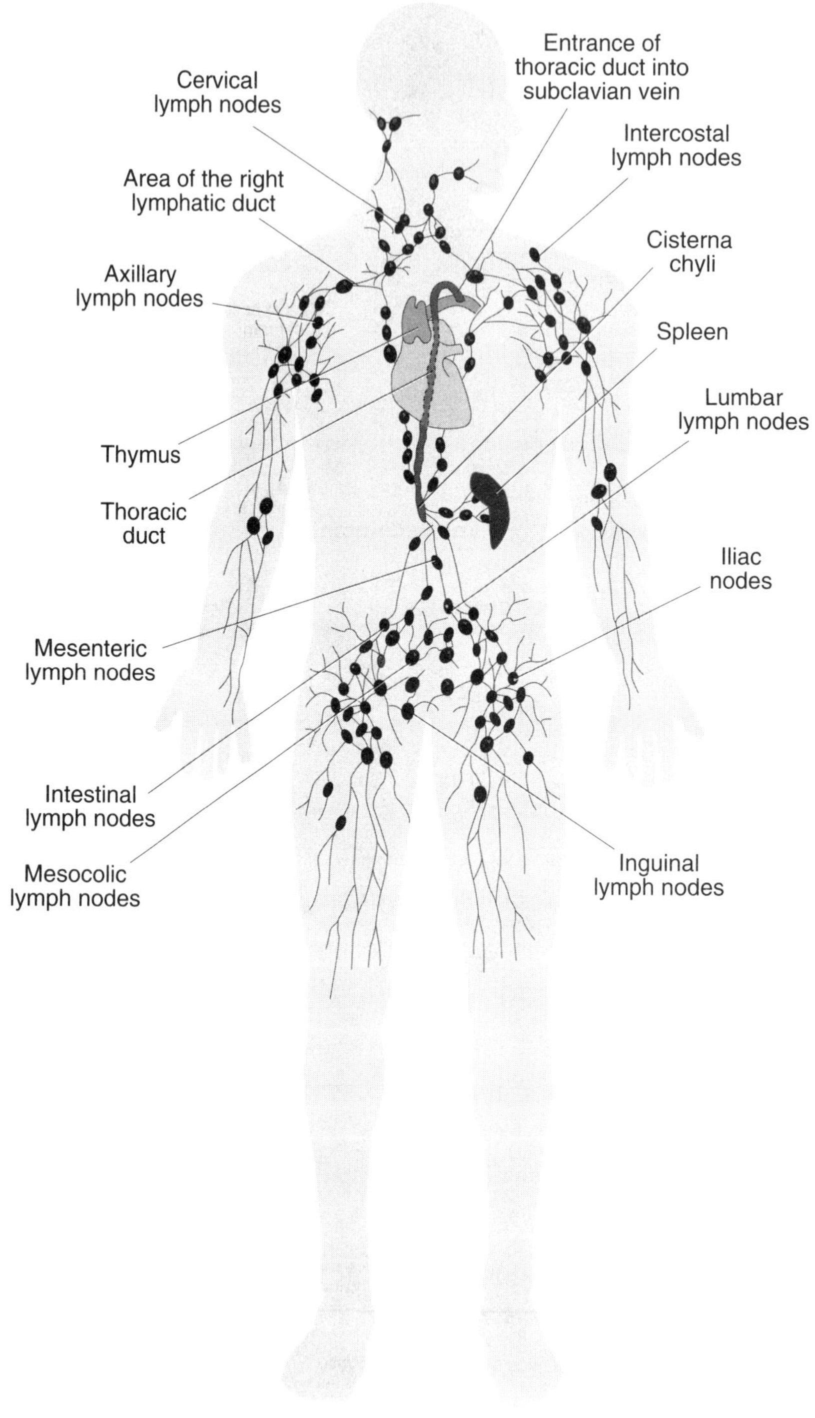

Lymphatic System

Axillary Lymph Nodes

Sternum
Clavicle
Deltoid
Brachialis
Parasternal nodes
Lateral nodes
Subscapular nodes
Pectoral nodes
Axillary lymph nodes
Central lymph nodes
Latissimus dorsi muscle
Rectus abdominis

Lymphatic Capillaries

Schematic of lymphatic capillaries
Tissue cells
Valves
Endothelial cells

Fluids and particles can enter the capillary through overlapping valves

Lymphatic Drainage

Lymphatic drainage of the colon follows blood supply

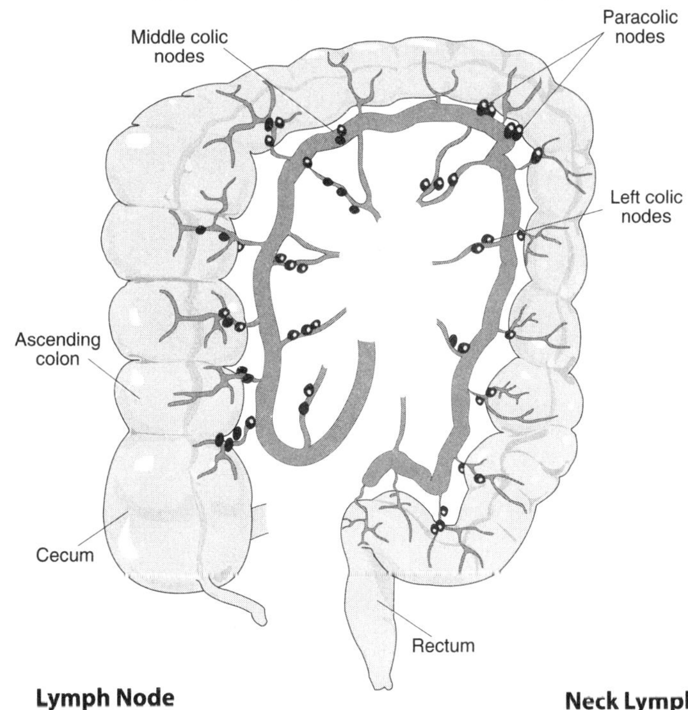

Lymph Node

Schematic of lymph node

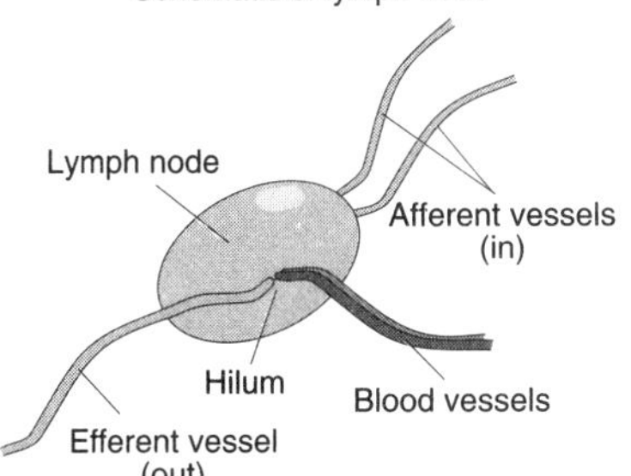

Neck Lymph Nodes

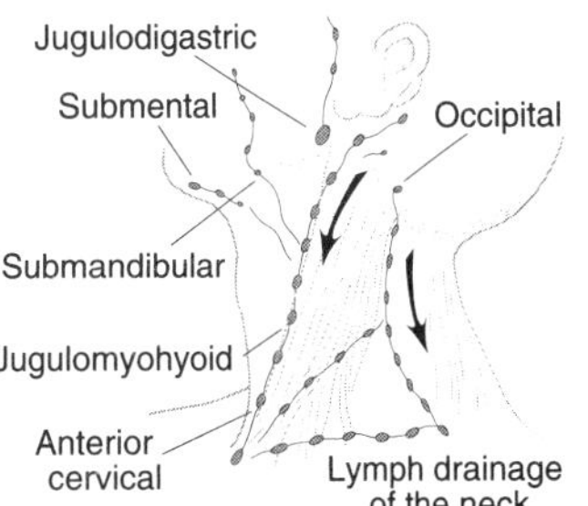

Endocrine System

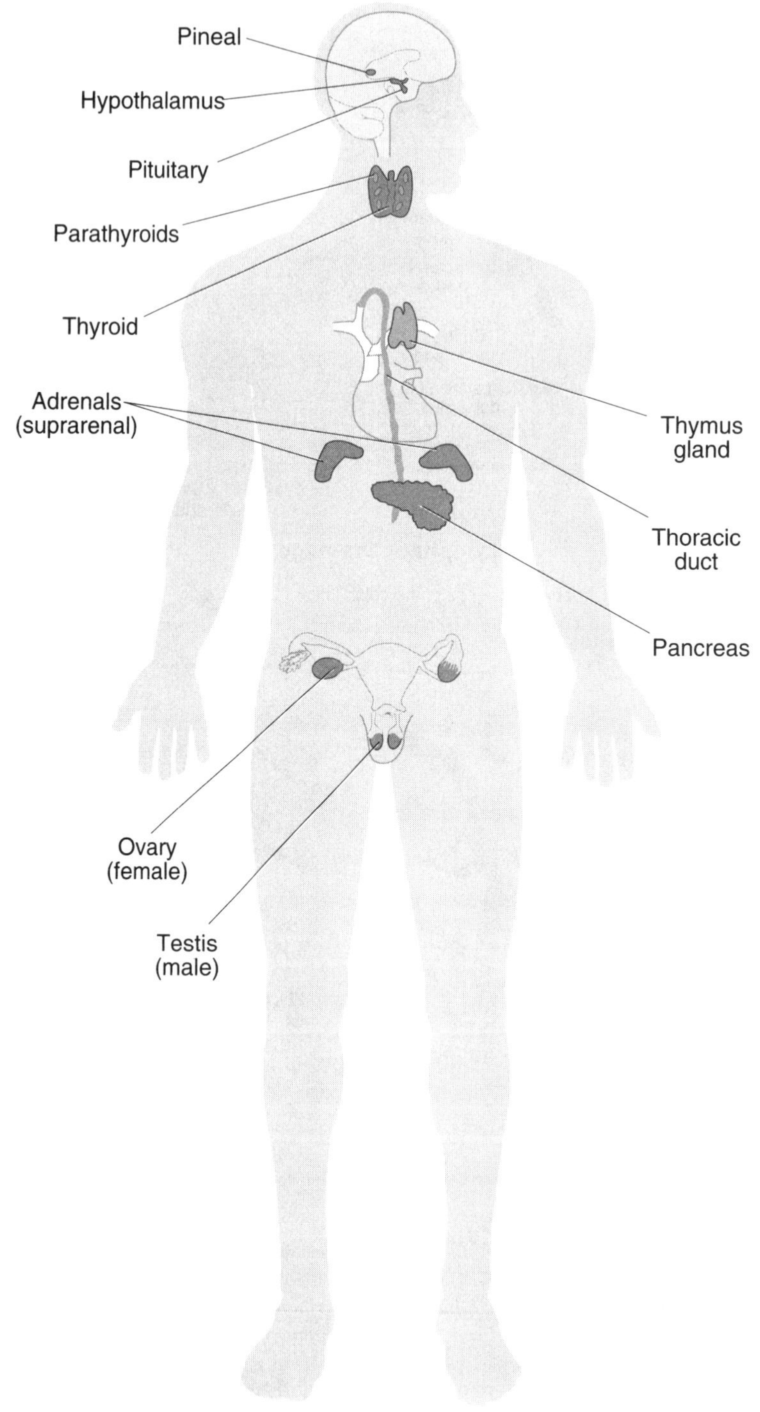

Endocrine System

Thyroid Glands

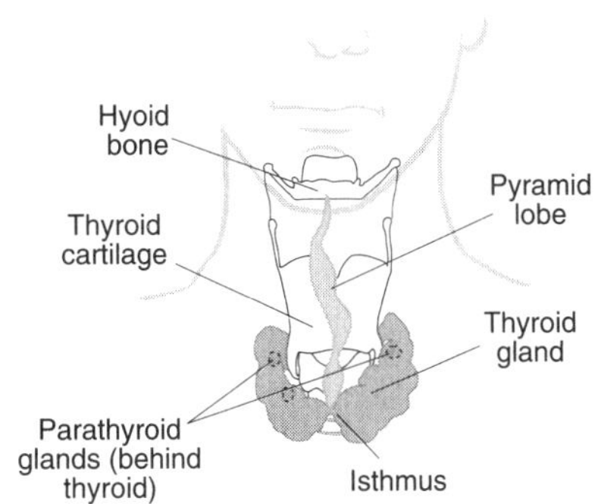

Pituitary Glands

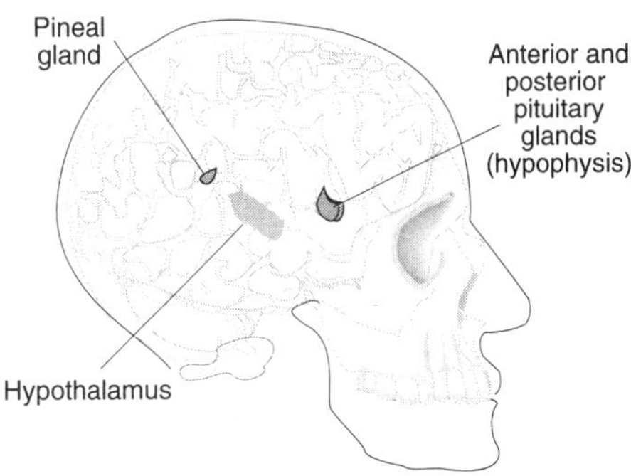

The pituitary gland and its controller, the hypothalamus, control body growth and stimulate and regulate other glands

Thyroid

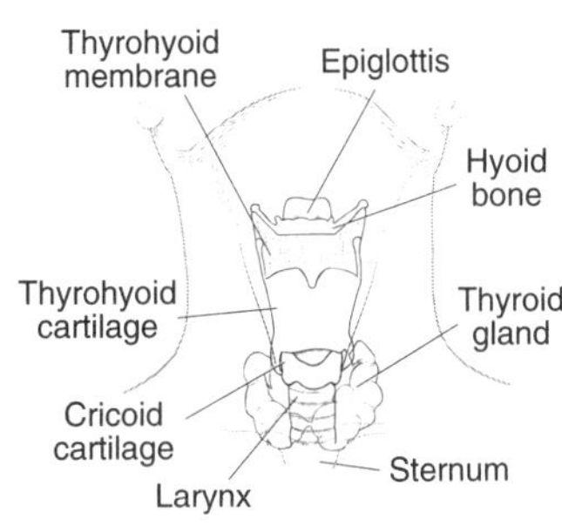

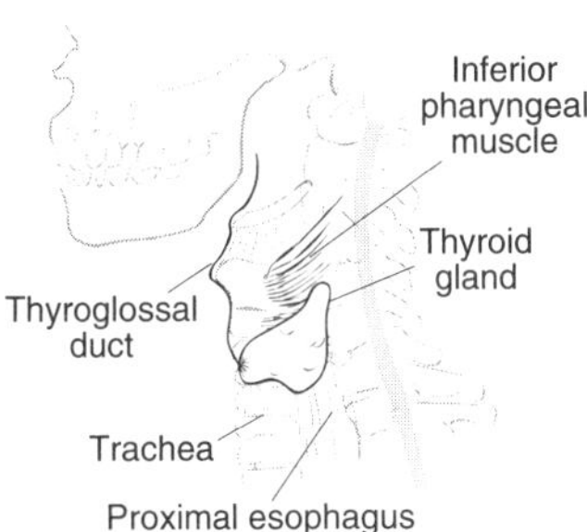

Thyroid

Superior view

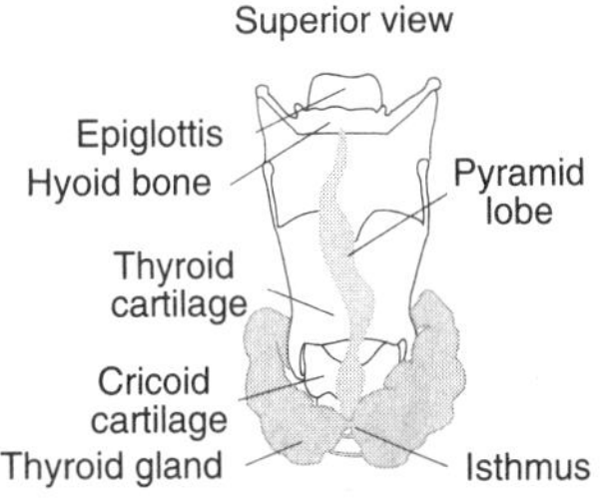

Posterior view

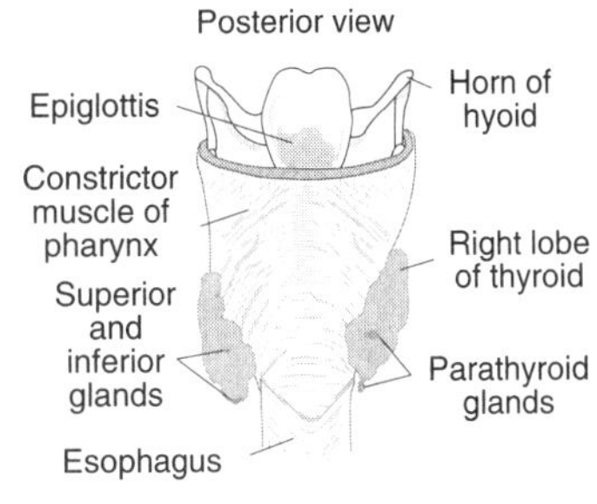

Placenta

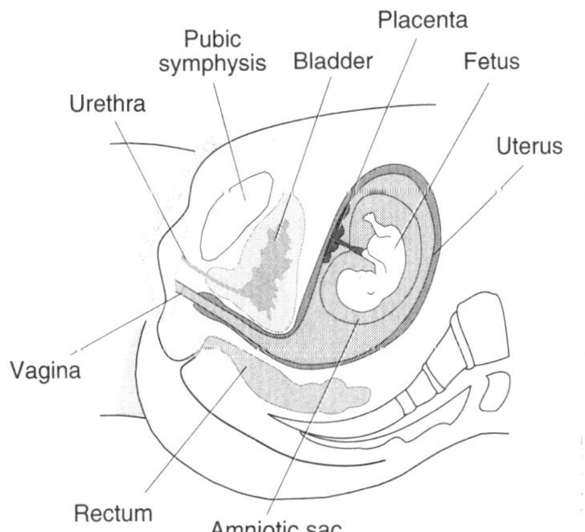

The placenta is considered part of the endocrine system, secreting chorionic gonadotropin, estrogen, progesterone, and somatomammotropin

Genitourinary System

Kidney

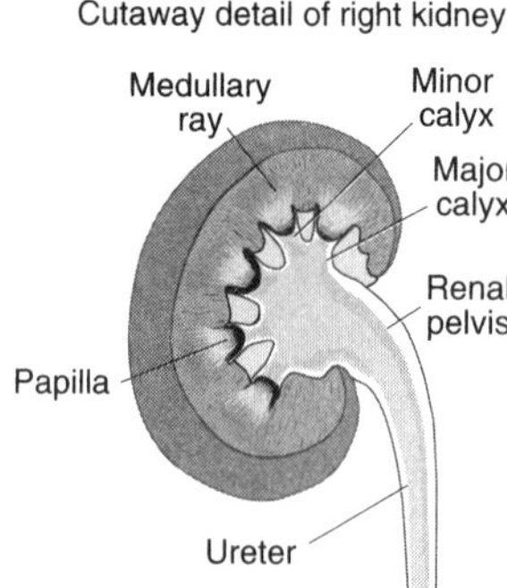

Nephron

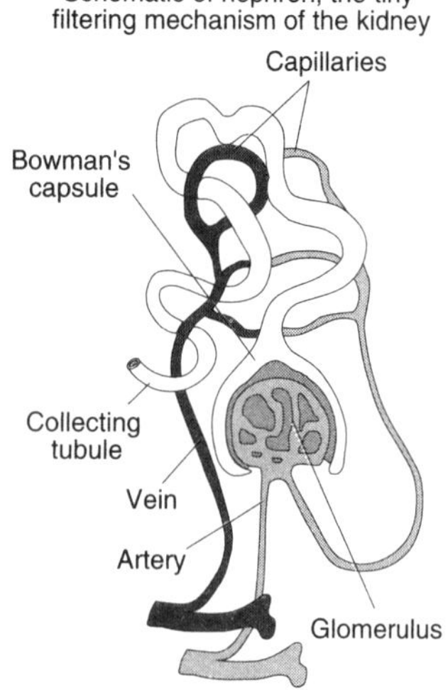

Urinary

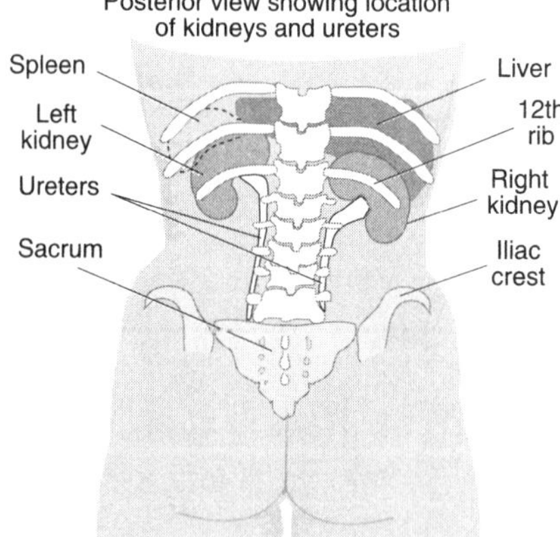

Male Urinary

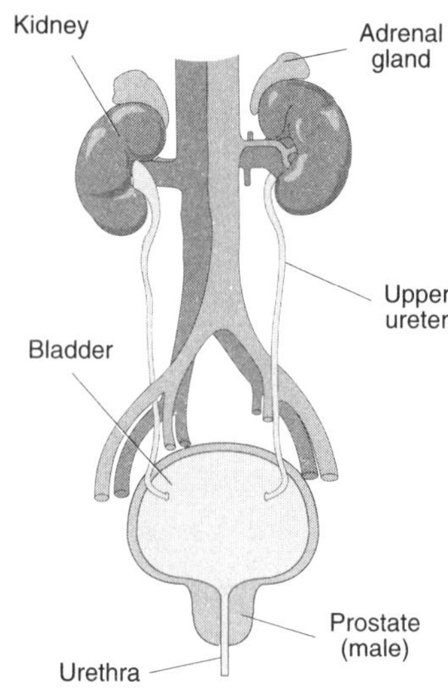

Male Genitourinary

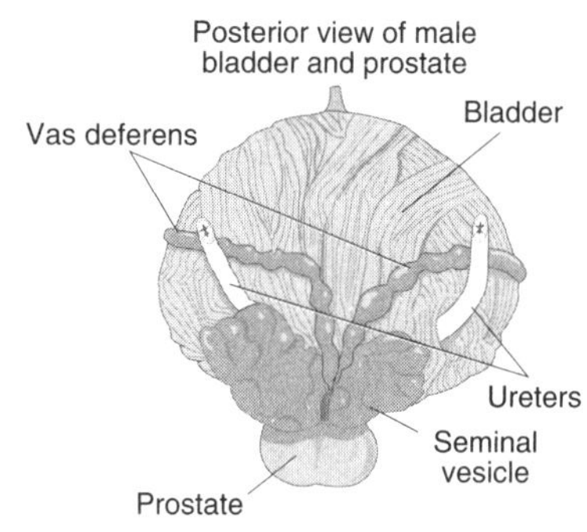

Male Reproductive

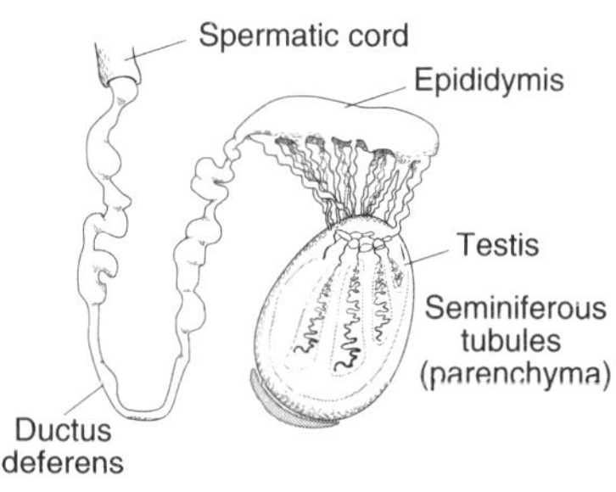

Genitourinary System

Female Genitourinary

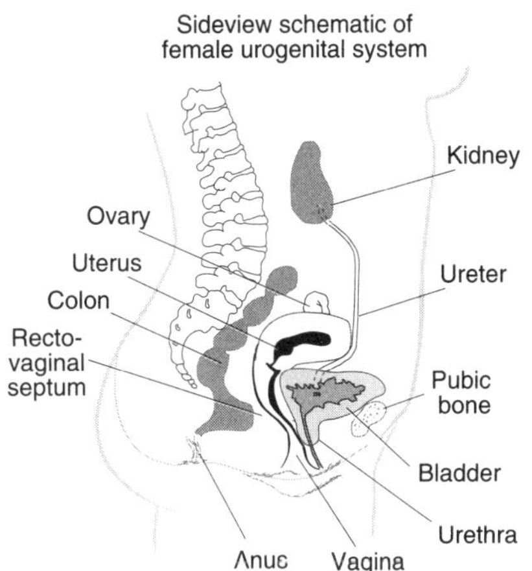

Female Rectoperineal

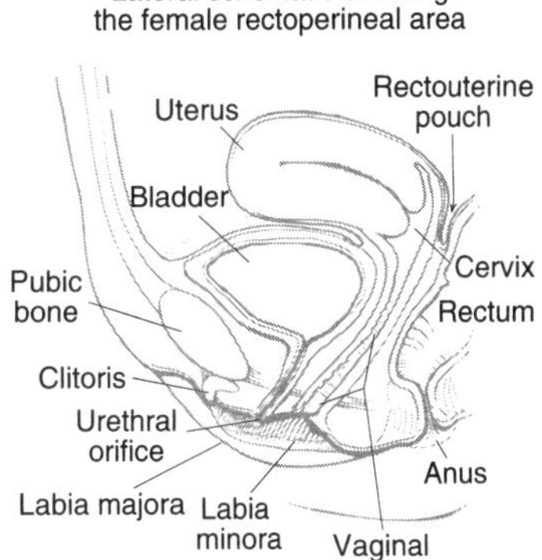

Female Bladder

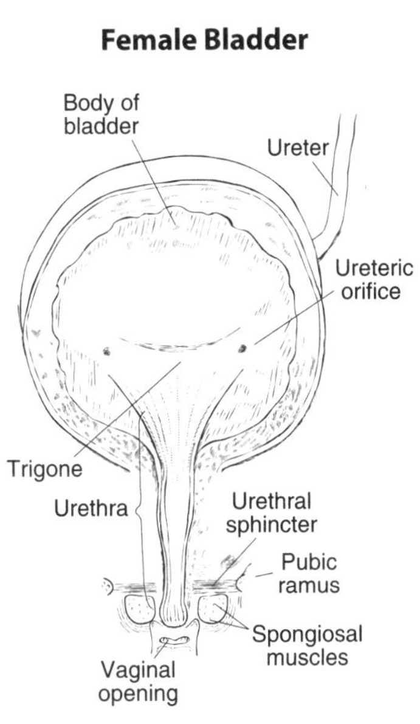

Female Reproductive

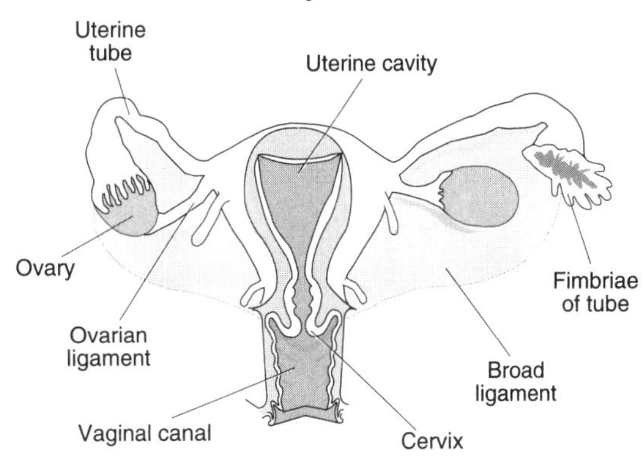

Female Reproductive

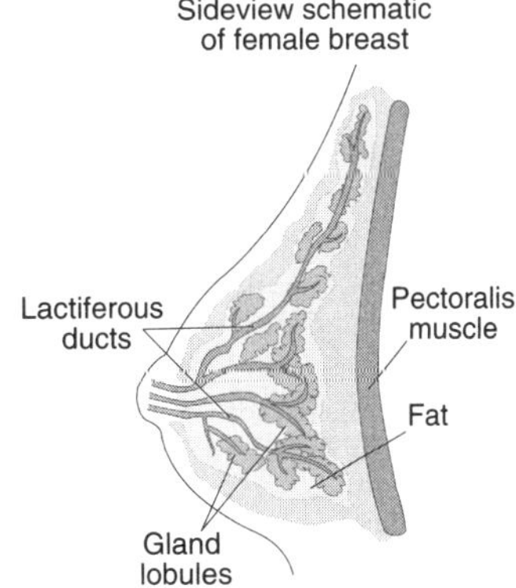

Respiratory System

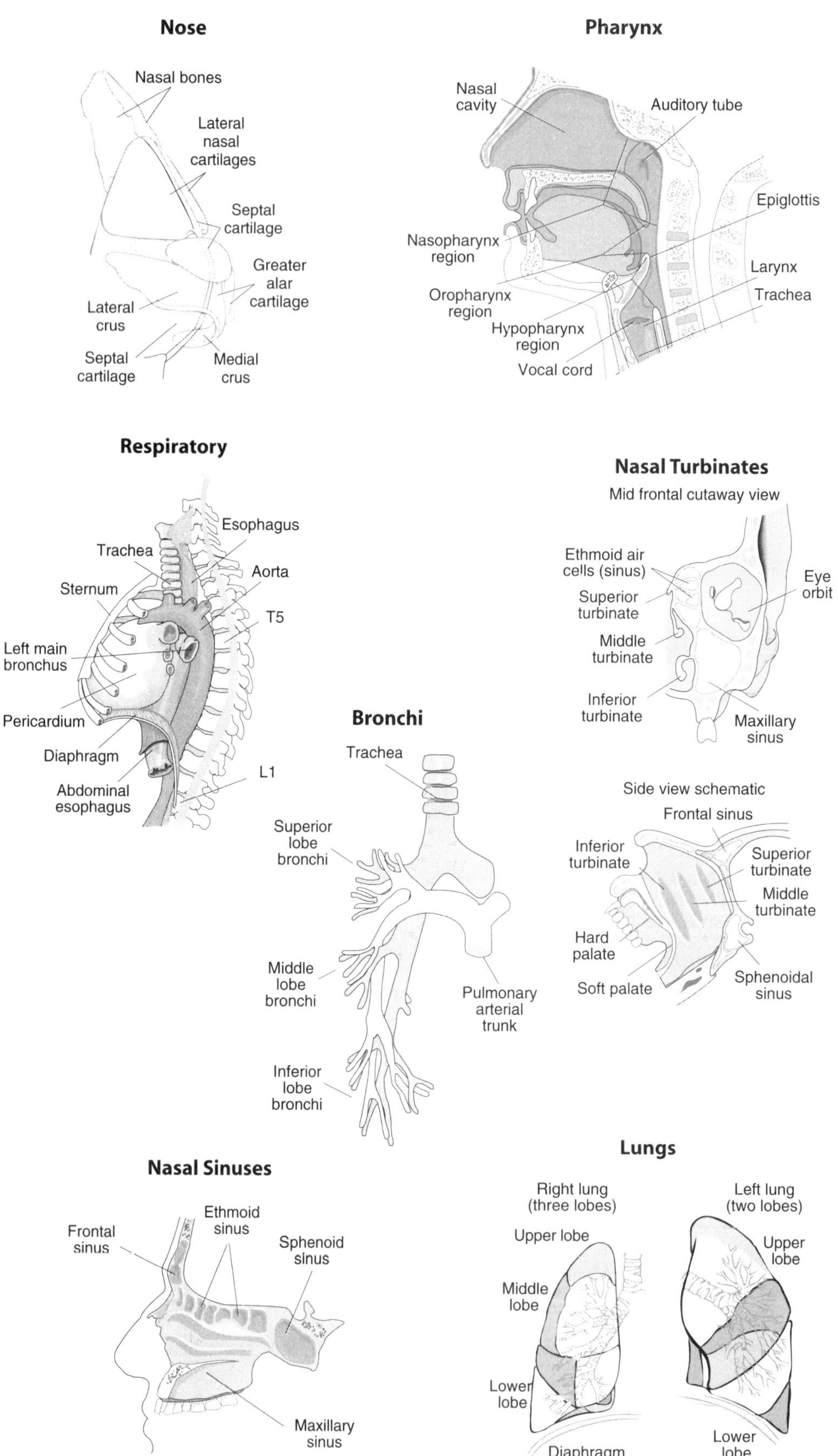

Eye

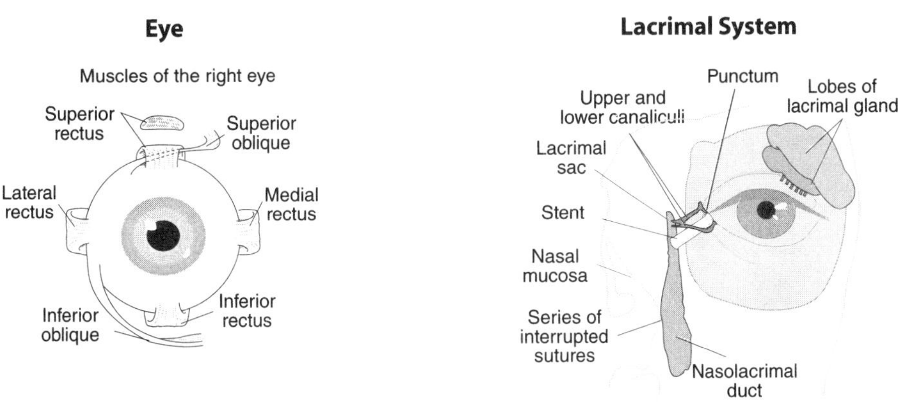

Eye

Anterior and posterior chambers of the eye

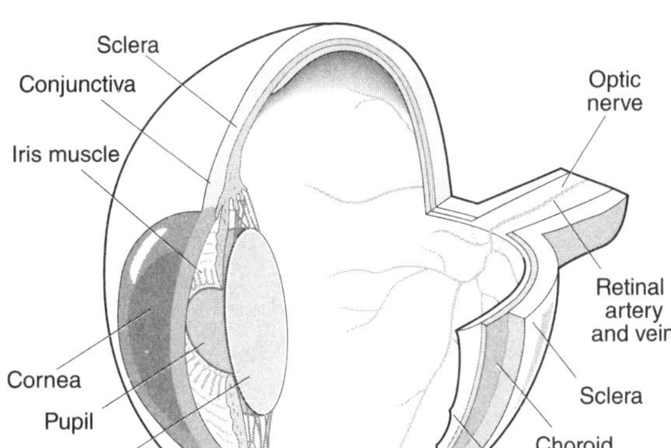

Ear

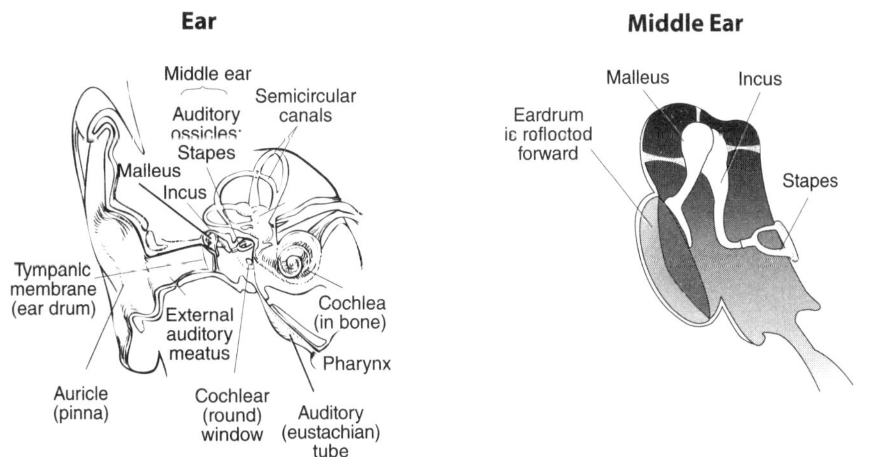

Normal Aortic Arch and Branch Anatomy—Transfemoral Approach

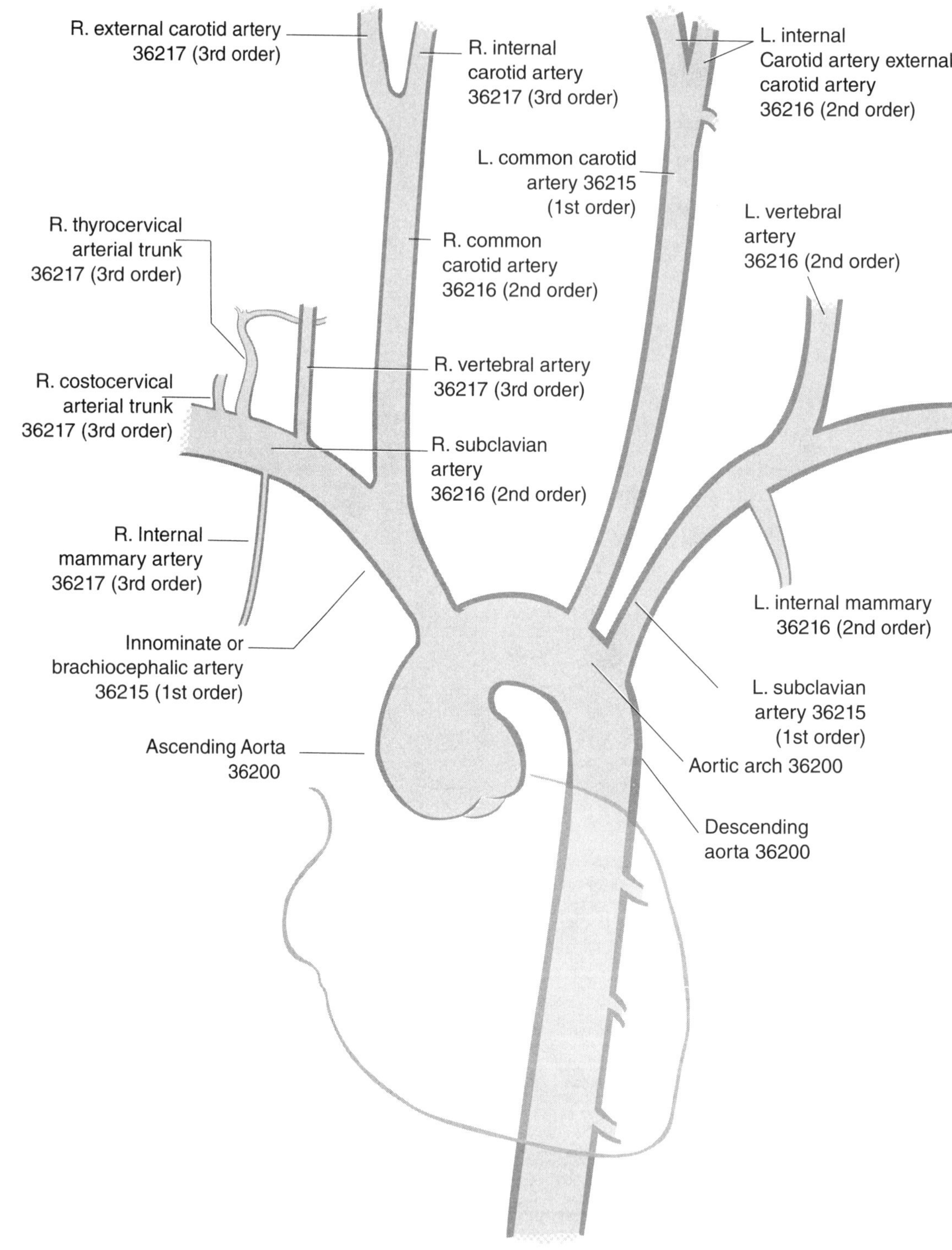

Superior and Inferior Mesenteric Arteries and Branches

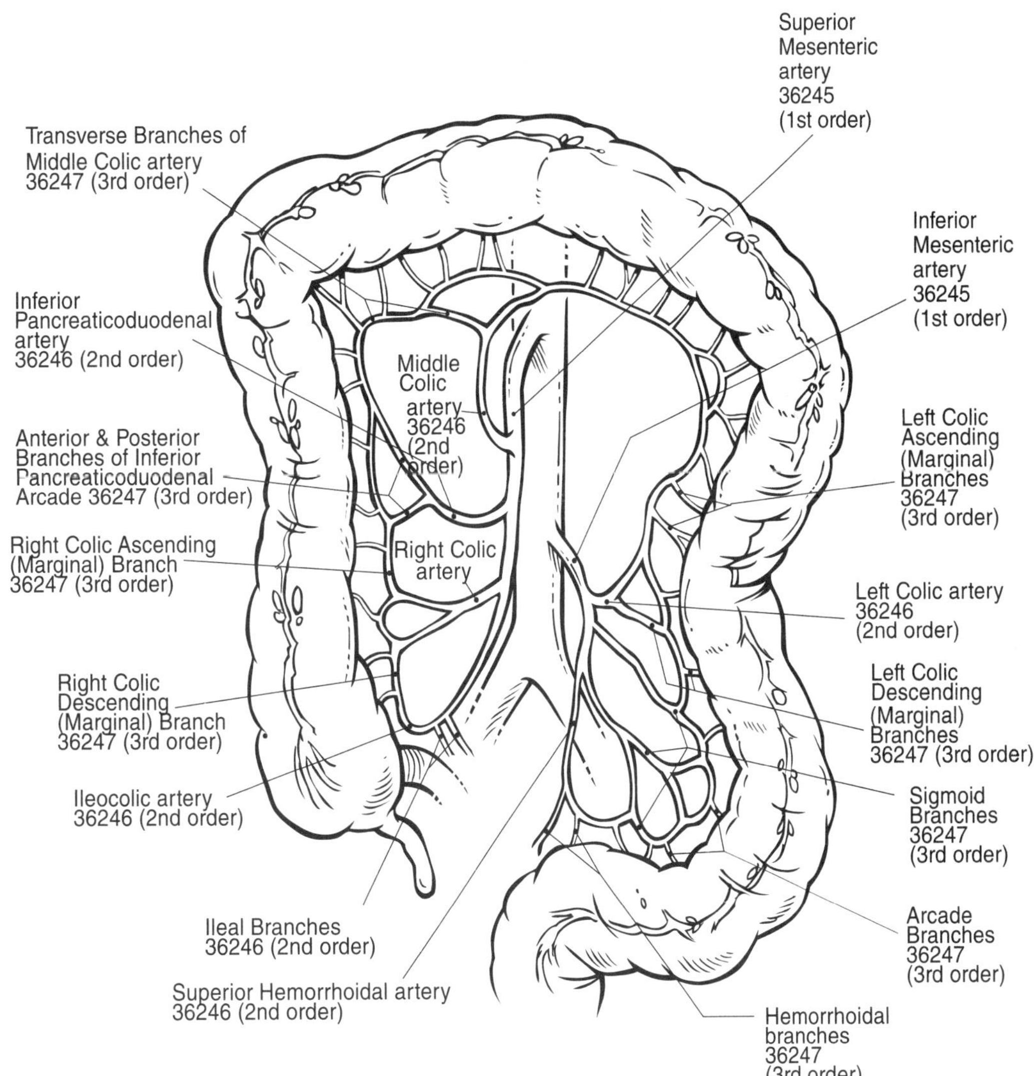

Portal System

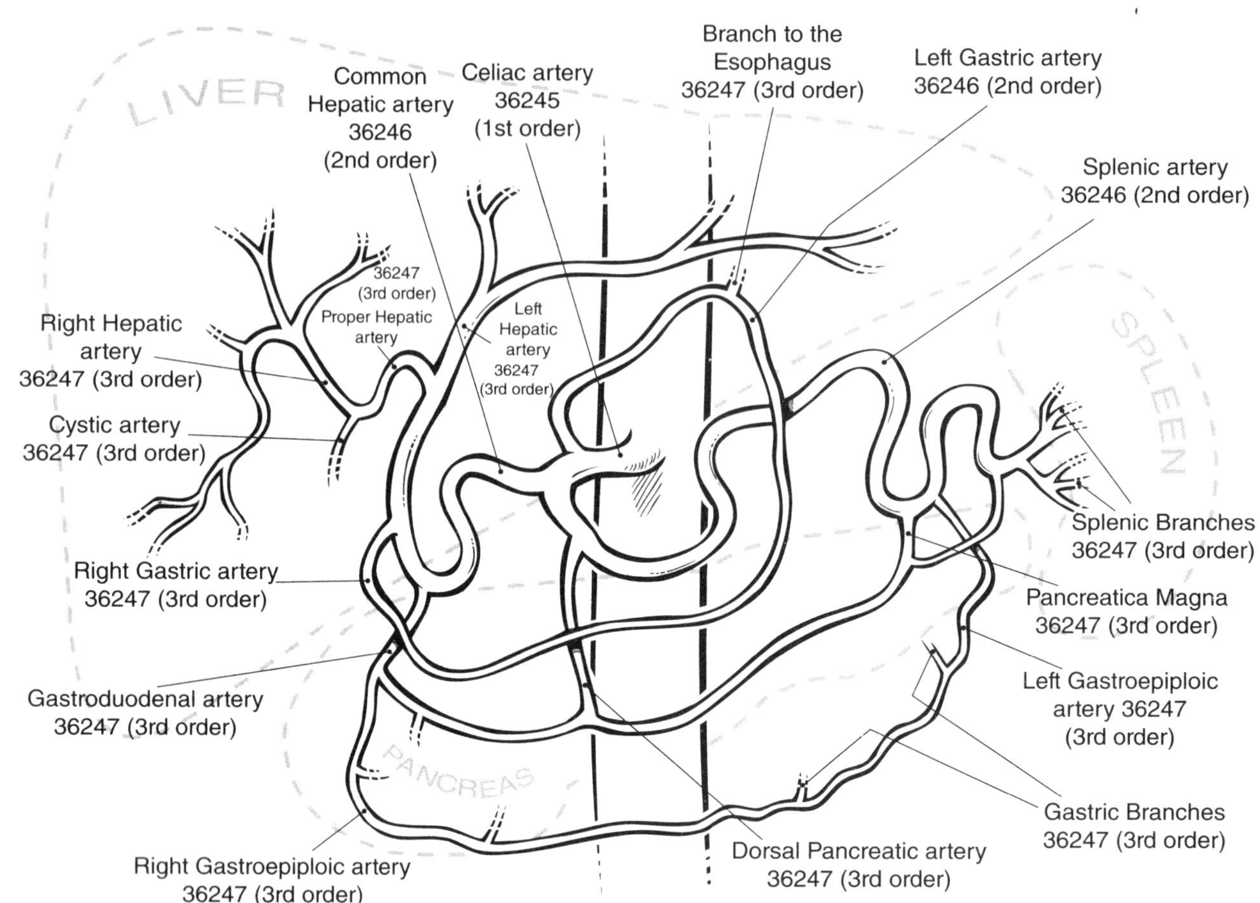

Renal Artery Anatomy—Femoral Approach

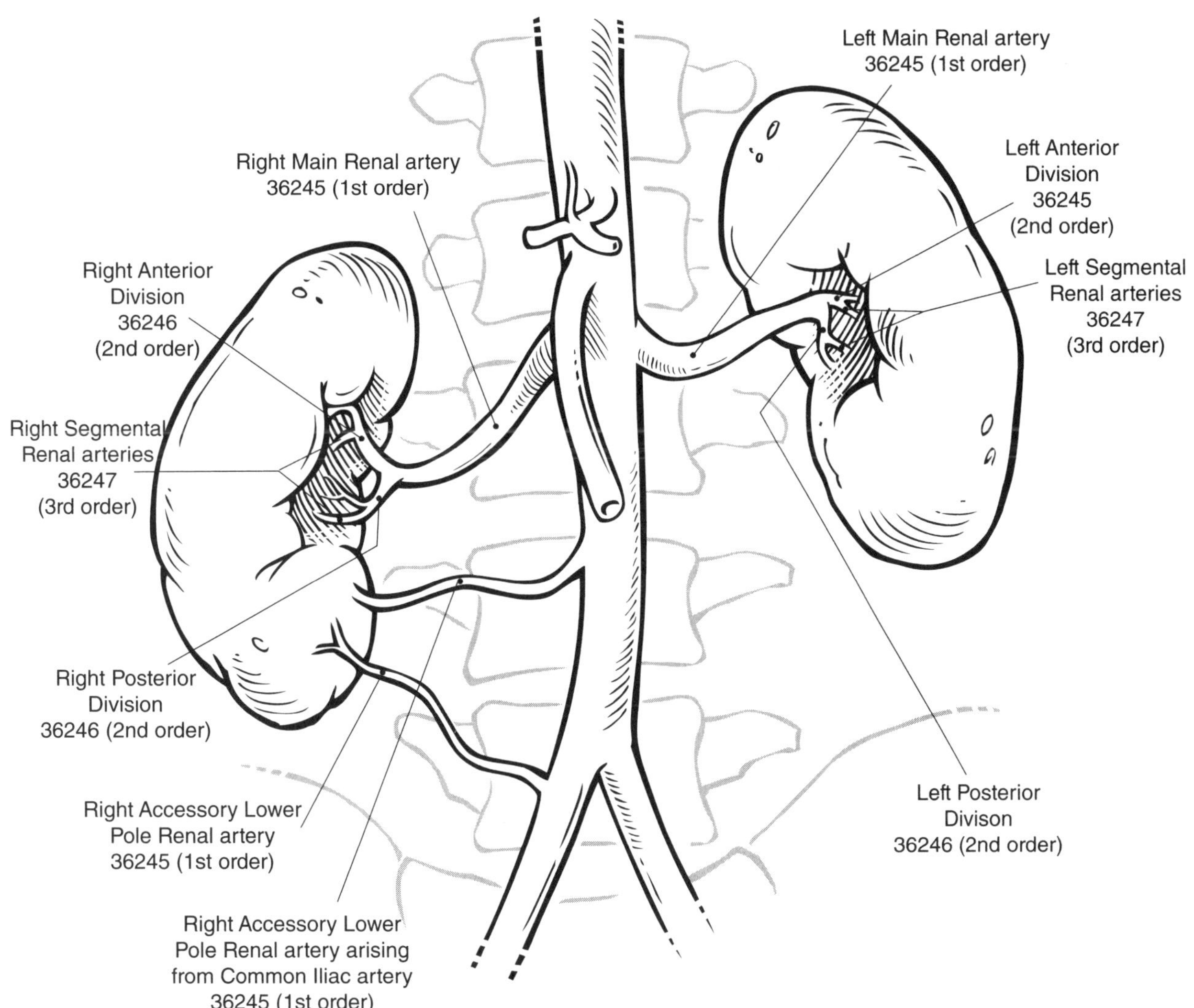

Upper Extremity Arterial Anatomy—Transfemoral or Contralateral Approach

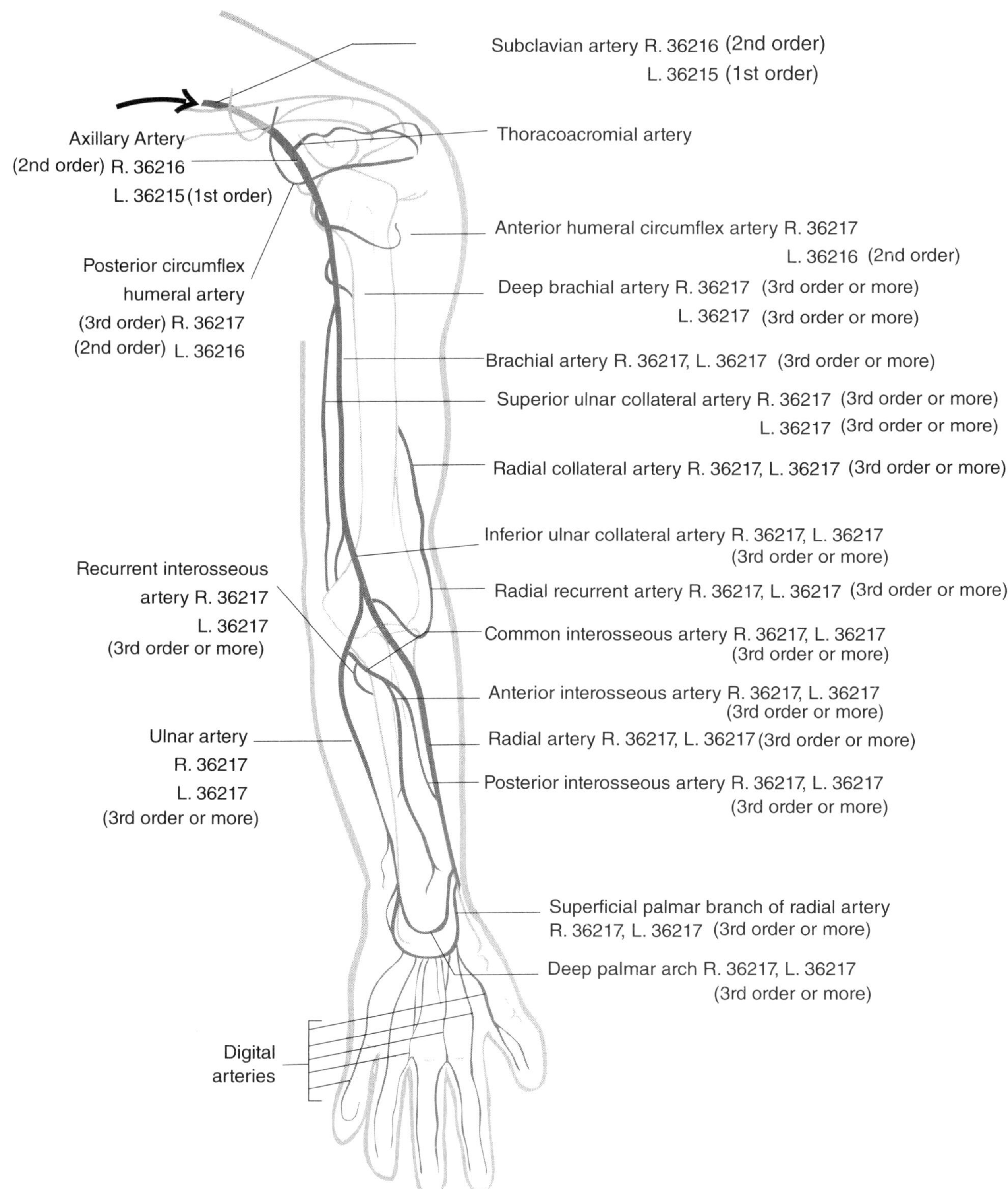

Lower Extremity Arterial Anatomy—Contralateral, Axillary or Brachial Approach

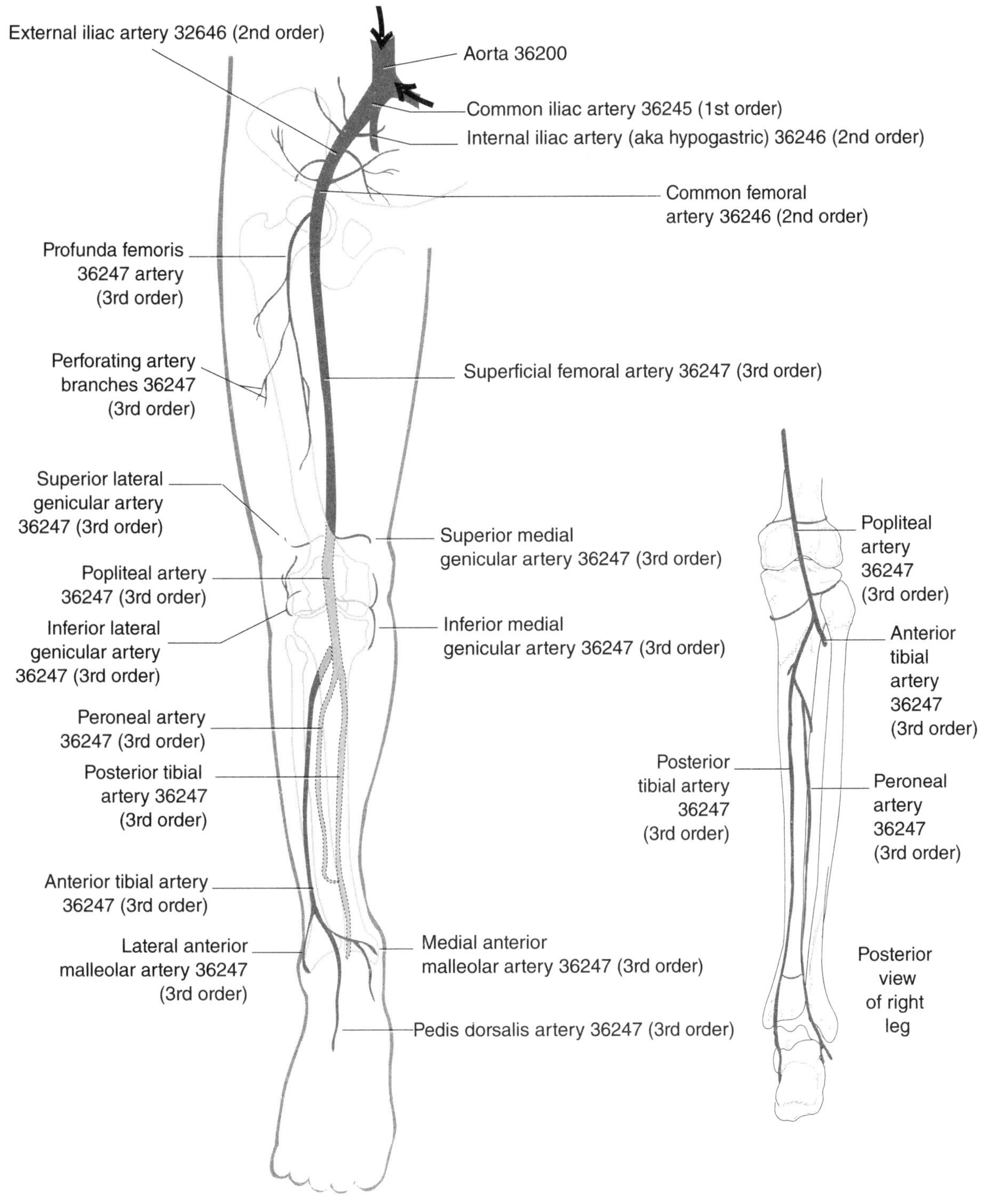

Portal System

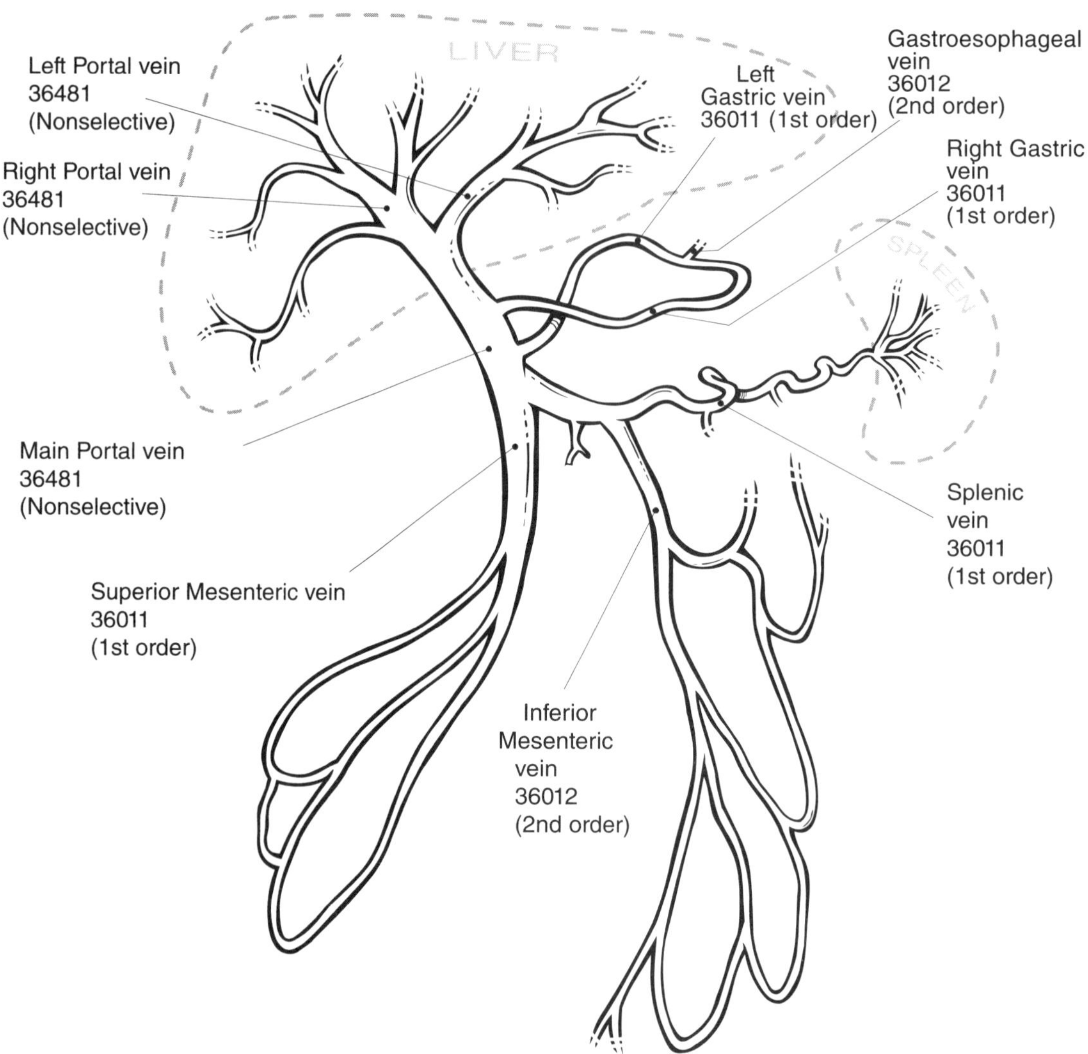

Coronary Arteries Anterior View

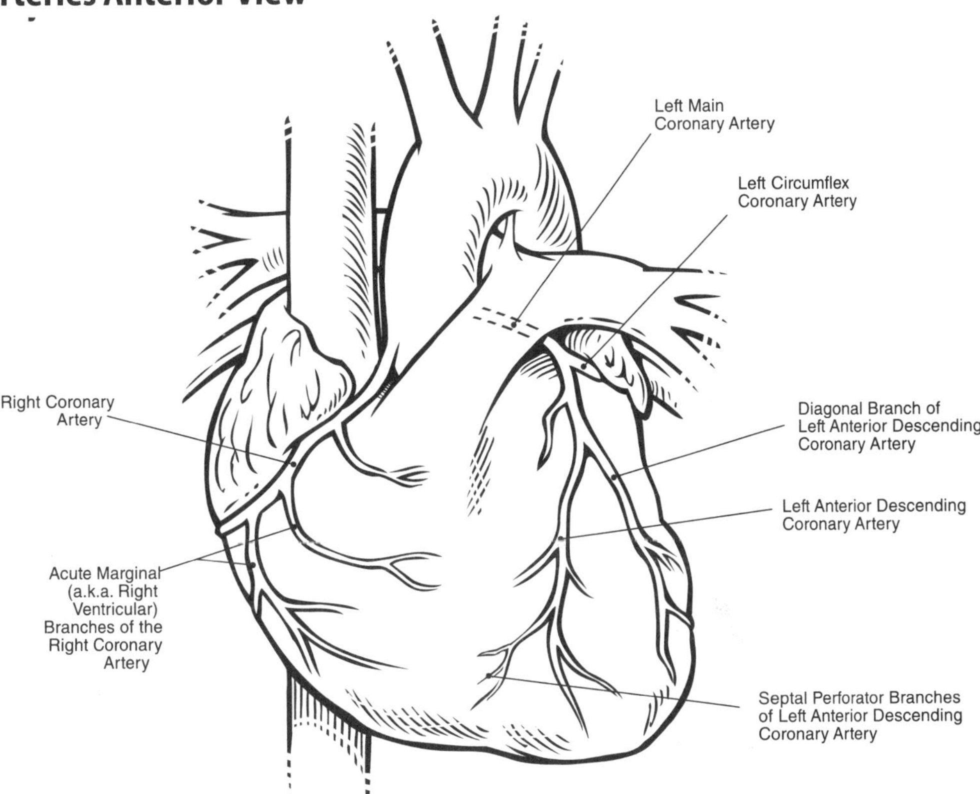

Left Heart Catheterization

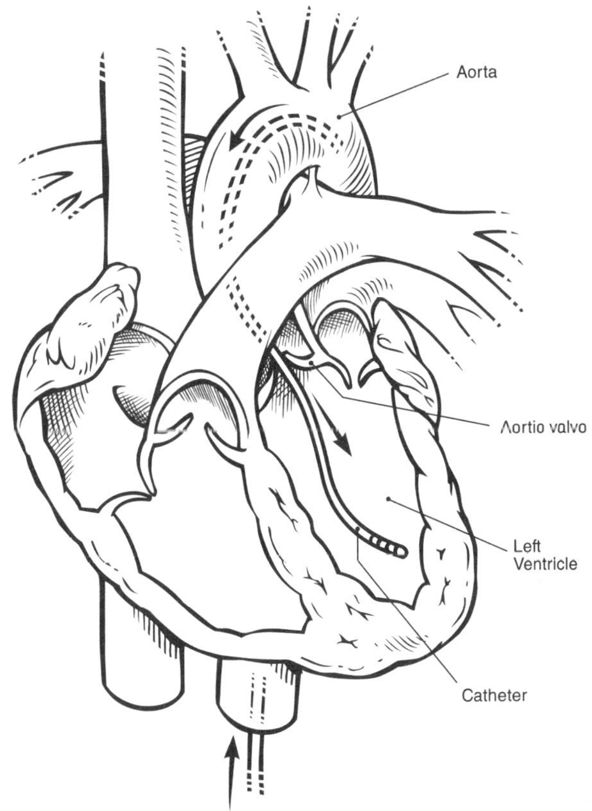

Heart Conduction System

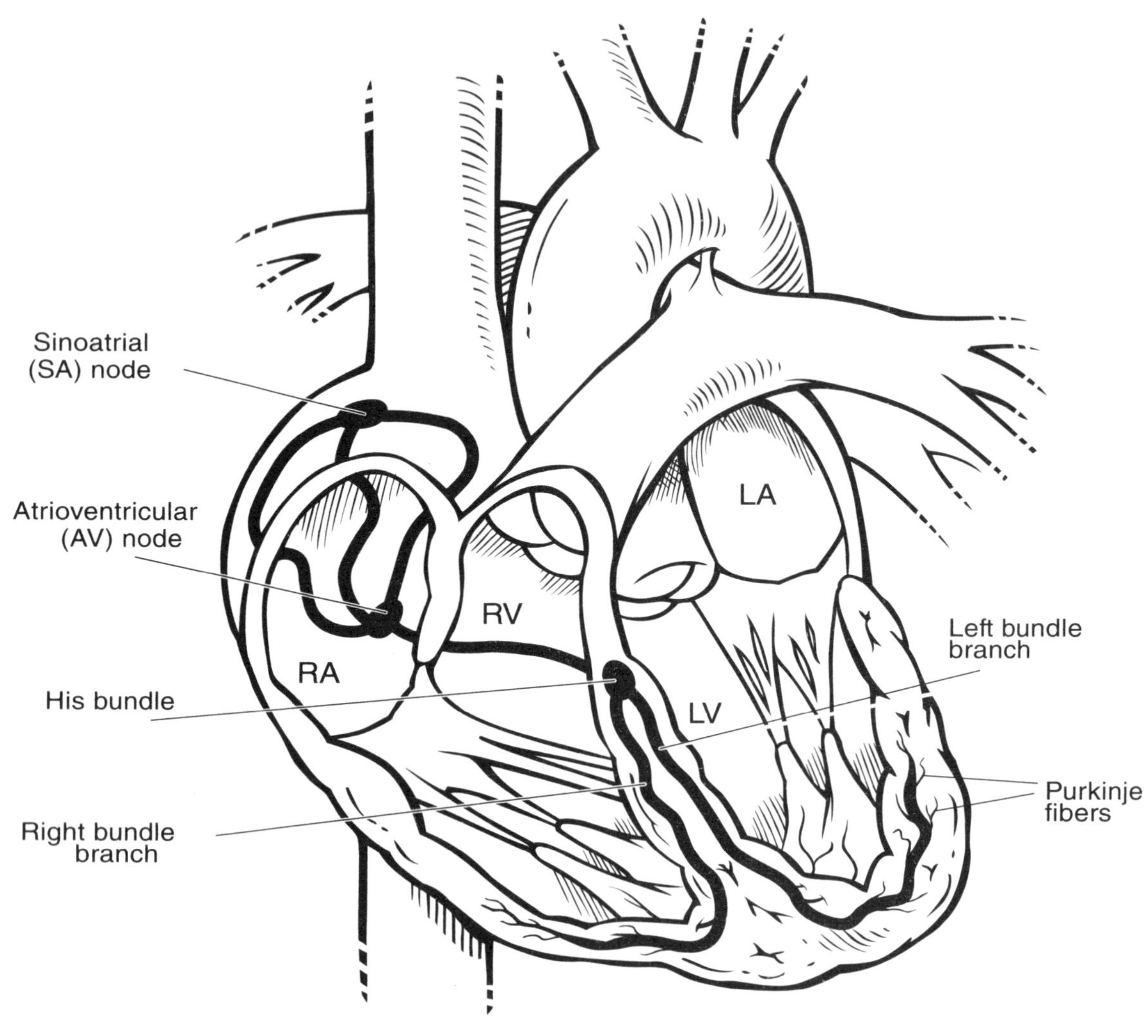

0-Numeric

A

 [Resequenced]

D

 [Resequenced]

E

G

I

Index
Infusion — Insertion

J

M

T

V

W

X

Y

Z

00100-00126 Anesthesia for Cleft Lip, Ear, ECT, Eyelid, and Salivary Gland Procedures

CMS 100-4,4,10.4 Packaging Rules Under OPPS
CMS 100-4,4,20.6 Modifier Use Under OPPS
CMS 100-4,4,20.6.4 Modifiers for Discontinued Services
CMS 100-4,12,50 Anesthesia Services
CMS 100-4,12,140.2 Payment for CRNA Services
CMS 100-4,12,140.3.2 Anesthesia Time and Units

00100 Anesthesia for procedures on salivary glands, including biopsy
N 0.00 0.00 FUD XXX

00102 Anesthesia for procedures involving plastic repair of cleft lip
N 0.00 0.00 FUD XXX

00103 Anesthesia for reconstructive procedures of eyelid (eg, blepharoplasty, ptosis surgery)
N 0.00 0.00 FUD XXX

00104 Anesthesia for electroconvulsive therapy
N 0.00 0.00 FUD XXX

00120 Anesthesia for procedures on external, middle, and inner ear including biopsy; not otherwise specified
N 0.00 0.00 FUD XXX

00124 otoscopy
N 0.00 0.00 FUD XXX

00126 tympanotomy
N 0.00 0.00 FUD XXX

00140-00148 Anesthesia for Eye Procedures

CMS 100-3,230.1 NCD for Treatment of Kidney Stones
CMS 100-4,4,10.4 Packaging Rules Under OPPS
CMS 100-4,4,20.6 Modifier Use Under OPPS
CMS 100-4,4,20.6.4 Modifiers for Discontinued Services
CMS 100-4,12,50 Anesthesia Services
CMS 100-4,12,140.3.2 Anesthesia Time and Units

00140 Anesthesia for procedures on eye; not otherwise specified
N 0.00 0.00 FUD XXX

00142 lens surgery
N 0.00 0.00 FUD XXX

00144 corneal transplant
N 0.00 0.00 FUD XXX

00145 vitreoretinal surgery
N 0.00 0.00 FUD XXX

00147 iridectomy
N 0.00 0.00 FUD XXX

00148 ophthalmoscopy
N 0.00 0.00 FUD XXX

00160-00326 Anesthesia for Face and Head Procedures

CMS 100-4,4,10.4 Packaging Rules Under OPPS
CMS 100-4,4,20.6 Modifier Use Under OPPS
CMS 100-4,12,50 Anesthesia Services
CMS 100-4,12,140.2 Payment for CRNA Services
CMS 100-4,12,140.3.2 Anesthesia Time and Units

00160 Anesthesia for procedures on nose and accessory sinuses; not otherwise specified
N 0.00 0.00 FUD XXX

00162 radical surgery
N 0.00 0.00 FUD XXX

00164 biopsy, soft tissue
N 0.00 0.00 FUD XXX

00170 Anesthesia for intraoral procedures, including biopsy; not otherwise specified
N 0.00 0.00 FUD XXX

00172 repair of cleft palate
N 0.00 0.00 FUD XXX

00174 excision of retropharyngeal tumor
N 0.00 0.00 FUD XXX

00176 radical surgery
C 0.00 0.00 FUD XXX

00190 Anesthesia for procedures on facial bones or skull; not otherwise specified
N 0.00 0.00 FUD XXX

00192 radical surgery (including prognathism)
C 0.00 0.00 FUD XXX

00210 Anesthesia for intracranial procedures; not otherwise specified
N 0.00 0.00 FUD XXX

00211 craniotomy or craniectomy for evacuation of hematoma
C 0.00 0.00 FUD XXX

00212 subdural taps
N 0.00 0.00 FUD XXX

00214 burr holes, including ventriculography
C 0.00 0.00 FUD XXX

00215 cranioplasty or elevation of depressed skull fracture, extradural (simple or compound)
C 0.00 0.00 FUD XXX

00216 vascular procedures
N 0.00 0.00 FUD XXX

00218 procedures in sitting position
N 0.00 0.00 FUD XXX

00220 cerebrospinal fluid shunting procedures
N 0.00 0.00 FUD XXX

00222 electrocoagulation of intracranial nerve
N 0.00 0.00 FUD XXX

00300 Anesthesia for all procedures on the integumentary system, muscles and nerves of head, neck, and posterior trunk, not otherwise specified
N 0.00 0.00 FUD XXX

00320 Anesthesia for all procedures on esophagus, thyroid, larynx, trachea and lymphatic system of neck; not otherwise specified, age 1 year or older
N 0.00 0.00 FUD XXX

00322 needle biopsy of thyroid
EXCLUDES *Cervical spine and spinal cord procedures (00600, 00604, 00670)*
N 0.00 0.00 FUD XXX

00326 Anesthesia for all procedures on the larynx and trachea in children younger than 1 year of age A
Do not report with (99100)
N 0.00 0.00 FUD XXX

00350-00352 Anesthesia for Neck Vessel Procedures

CMS 100-4,4,10.4 Packaging Rules Under OPPS
CMS 100-4,4,20.6 Modifier Use Under OPPS
CMS 100-4,4,20.6.4 Modifiers for Discontinued Services
CMS 100-4,12,50 Anesthesia Services
CMS 100-4,12,140.2 Payment for CRNA Services
CMS 100-4,12,140.3.2 Anesthesia Time and Units

EXCLUDES *Arteriography (01916)*

00350 Anesthesia for procedures on major vessels of neck; not otherwise specified
N 0.00 0.00 FUD XXX

00352 simple ligation
N 0.00 0.00 FUD XXX

00400-00529 Anesthesia for Chest/Pectoral Girdle Procedures

CMS 100-4,4,10.4 Packaging Rules Under OPPS
CMS 100-4,4,20.6 Modifier Use Under OPPS
CMS 100-4,4,20.6.4 Modifiers for Discontinued Services
CMS 100-4,12,50 Anesthesia Services
CMS 100-4,12,140.2 Payment for CRNA Services
CMS 100-4,12,140.3.2 Anesthesia Time and Units

00400 **Anesthesia for procedures on the integumentary system on the extremities, anterior trunk and perineum; not otherwise specified**
N PQ 0.00 0.00 FUD XXX

00402 **reconstructive procedures on breast (eg, reduction or augmentation mammoplasty, muscle flaps)**
N PQ 0.00 0.00 FUD XXX

00404 **radical or modified radical procedures on breast**
N PQ 0.00 0.00 FUD XXX

00406 **radical or modified radical procedures on breast with internal mammary node dissection**
N PQ 0.00 0.00 FUD XXX

00410 **electrical conversion of arrhythmias**
N PQ 0.00 0.00 FUD XXX

00450 **Anesthesia for procedures on clavicle and scapula; not otherwise specified**
N PQ 0.00 0.00 FUD XXX

~~**00452** **radical surgery**~~

00454 **biopsy of clavicle**
N PQ 0.00 0.00 FUD XXX

00470 **Anesthesia for partial rib resection; not otherwise specified**
N PQ 0.00 0.00 FUD XXX

00472 **thoracoplasty (any type)**
N PQ 0.00 0.00 FUD XXX

00474 **radical procedures (eg, pectus excavatum)**
C PQ 0.00 0.00 FUD XXX

00500 **Anesthesia for all procedures on esophagus**
N PQ 0.00 0.00 FUD XXX

00520 **Anesthesia for closed chest procedures; (including bronchoscopy) not otherwise specified**
N PQ 0.00 0.00 FUD XXX

00522 **needle biopsy of pleura**
N PQ 0.00 0.00 FUD XXX

00524 **pneumocentesis**
C PQ 0.00 0.00 FUD XXX

00528 **mediastinoscopy and diagnostic thoracoscopy not utilizing 1 lung ventilation**
EXCLUDES *Tracheobronchial reconstruction (00539)*
N PQ 0.00 0.00 FUD XXX

00529 **mediastinoscopy and diagnostic thoracoscopy utilizing 1 lung ventilation**
N PQ 0.00 0.00 FUD XXX

00530 Anesthesia for Cardiac Pacemaker Procedure

CMS 100-4,4,10.4 Packaging Rules Under OPPS
CMS 100-4,4,20.6 Modifier Use Under OPPS
CMS 100-4,4,20.6.4 Modifiers for Discontinued Services
CMS 100-4,12,50 Anesthesia Services
CMS 100-4,12,140.2 Payment for CRNA Services
CMS 100-4,12,140.3.2 Anesthesia Time and Units

00530 **Anesthesia for permanent transvenous pacemaker insertion**
N PQ 0.00 0.00 FUD XXX

00532-00550 Anesthesia for Heart and Lung Procedures

CMS 100-4,4,10.4 Packaging Rules Under OPPS
CMS 100-4,4,20.6 Modifier Use Under OPPS
CMS 100-4,12,50 Anesthesia Services
CMS 100-4,12,140.2 Payment for CRNA Services
CMS 100-4,12,140.3.2 Anesthesia Time and Units

00532 **Anesthesia for access to central venous circulation**
N PQ 0.00 0.00 FUD XXX

00534 **Anesthesia for transvenous insertion or replacement of pacing cardioverter-defibrillator**
EXCLUDES *Transthoracic approach (00560)*
N PQ 0.00 0.00 FUD XXX

00537 **Anesthesia for cardiac electrophysiologic procedures including radiofrequency ablation**
N PQ 0.00 0.00 FUD XXX

00539 **Anesthesia for tracheobronchial reconstruction**
N PQ 0.00 0.00 FUD XXX

00540 **Anesthesia for thoracotomy procedures involving lungs, pleura, diaphragm, and mediastinum (including surgical thoracoscopy); not otherwise specified**
EXCLUDES *Thoracic spine and spinal cord procedures via anterior transthoracic approach (00625-00626)*
C PQ 0.00 0.00 FUD XXX

00541 **utilizing 1 lung ventilation**
EXCLUDES *Thoracic spine and spinal cord procedures via anterior transthoracic approach (00625-00626)*
N PQ 0.00 0.00 FUD XXX

00542 **decortication**
C PQ 0.00 0.00 FUD XXX

00546 **pulmonary resection with thoracoplasty**
C PQ 0.00 0.00 FUD XXX

00548 **intrathoracic procedures on the trachea and bronchi**
N PQ 0.00 0.00 FUD XXX

00550 **Anesthesia for sternal debridement**
N PQ 0.00 0.00 FUD XXX

00560-00580 Anesthesia for Open Heart Procedures

CMS 100-3,160.9 Electroencephalographic (EEG) Monitoring During Open-Heart Surgery
CMS 100-4,12,50 Anesthesia Services
CMS 100-4,12,140.2 Payment for CRNA Services
CMS 100-4,12,140.3.2 Anesthesia Time and Units

00560 **Anesthesia for procedures on heart, pericardial sac, and great vessels of chest; without pump oxygenator**
C PQ 0.00 0.00 FUD XXX

00561 **with pump oxygenator, younger than 1 year of age** A
Do not report with (99100, 99116, 99135)
C PQ 0.00 0.00 FUD XXX

00562 **with pump oxygenator, age 1 year or older, for all non-coronary bypass procedures (eg, valve procedures) or for re-operation for coronary bypass more than 1 month after original operation** A
C PQ 0.00 0.00 FUD XXX

00563 **with pump oxygenator with hypothermic circulatory arrest**
N PQ 0.00 0.00 FUD XXX

00566 **Anesthesia for direct coronary artery bypass grafting; without pump oxygenator**
N PQ 0.00 0.00 FUD XXX

00567 **with pump oxygenator**
C PQ 0.00 0.00 FUD XXX

00580 Anesthesia for heart transplant or heart/lung transplant
C PQ 0.00 0.00 FUD XXX

00600-00670 Anesthesia for Spinal Procedures

CMS 100-4,4,10.4 Packaging Rules Under OPPS
CMS 100-4,4,20.6 Modifier Use Under OPPS
CMS 100-4,4,20.6.4 Modifiers for Discontinued Services
CMS 100-4,12,50 Anesthesia Services
CMS 100-4,12,140.2 Payment for CRNA Services
CMS 100-4,12,140.3.2 Anesthesia Time and Units

00600 Anesthesia for procedures on cervical spine and cord; not otherwise specified
EXCLUDES *Percutaneous image-guided spine and spinal cord anesthesia services (01935-01936)*
N PQ 0.00 0.00 FUD XXX

00604 procedures with patient in the sitting position
C PQ 0.00 0.00 FUD XXX

00620 Anesthesia for procedures on thoracic spine and cord, not otherwise specified
N PQ 0.00 0.00 FUD XXX

~~**00622** thoracolumbar sympathectomy~~

00625 Anesthesia for procedures on the thoracic spine and cord, via an anterior transthoracic approach; not utilizing 1 lung ventilation
EXCLUDES *Anesthesia services for thoracotomy procedures other than spine (00540-00541)*
N PQ 0.00 0.00 FUD XXX

00626 utilizing 1 lung ventilation
EXCLUDES *Anesthesia services for thoracotomy procedures other than spine (00540-00541)*
N PQ 0.00 0.00 FUD XXX

00630 Anesthesia for procedures in lumbar region; not otherwise specified
N PQ 0.00 0.00 FUD XXX

00632 lumbar sympathectomy
C PQ 0.00 0.00 FUD XXX

~~**00634** chemonucleolysis~~

00635 diagnostic or therapeutic lumbar puncture
N PQ 0.00 0.00 FUD XXX

00640 Anesthesia for manipulation of the spine or for closed procedures on the cervical, thoracic or lumbar spine
N PQ 0.00 0.00 FUD XXX

00670 Anesthesia for extensive spine and spinal cord procedures (eg, spinal instrumentation or vascular procedures)
C PQ 0.00 0.00 FUD XXX

00700-00882 Anesthesia for Abdominal Procedures

CMS 100-4,4,10.4 Packaging Rules Under OPPS
CMS 100-4,4,20.6 Modifier Use Under OPPS
CMS 100-4,4,20.6.4 Modifiers for Discontinued Services
CMS 100-4,12,50 Anesthesia Services
CMS 100-4,12,140.2 Payment for CRNA Services
CMS 100-4,12,140.3.2 Anesthesia Time and Units

00700 Anesthesia for procedures on upper anterior abdominal wall; not otherwise specified
N PQ 0.00 0.00 FUD XXX

00702 percutaneous liver biopsy
N PQ 0.00 0.00 FUD XXX

00730 Anesthesia for procedures on upper posterior abdominal wall
N PQ 0.00 0.00 FUD XXX

00740 Anesthesia for upper gastrointestinal endoscopic procedures, endoscope introduced proximal to duodenum
N PQ 0.00 0.00 FUD XXX

00750 Anesthesia for hernia repairs in upper abdomen; not otherwise specified
N PQ 0.00 0.00 FUD XXX

00752 lumbar and ventral (incisional) hernias and/or wound dehiscence
N PQ 0.00 0.00 FUD XXX

00754 omphalocele
N PQ 0.00 0.00 FUD XXX

00756 transabdominal repair of diaphragmatic hernia
N PQ 0.00 0.00 FUD XXX

00770 Anesthesia for all procedures on major abdominal blood vessels
N PQ 0.00 0.00 FUD XXX

00790 Anesthesia for intraperitoneal procedures in upper abdomen including laparoscopy; not otherwise specified
N PQ 0.00 0.00 FUD XXX

00792 partial hepatectomy or management of liver hemorrhage (excluding liver biopsy)
C PQ 0.00 0.00 FUD XXX

00794 pancreatectomy, partial or total (eg, Whipple procedure)
C PQ 0.00 0.00 FUD XXX

00796 liver transplant (recipient)
EXCLUDES *Physiological support during liver harvest (01990)*
C PQ 0.00 0.00 FUD XXX

00797 gastric restrictive procedure for morbid obesity
N PQ 0.00 0.00 FUD XXX

00800 Anesthesia for procedures on lower anterior abdominal wall; not otherwise specified
N PQ 0.00 0.00 FUD XXX

00802 panniculectomy
C PQ 0.00 0.00 FUD XXX

00810 Anesthesia for lower intestinal endoscopic procedures, endoscope introduced distal to duodenum
N PQ 0.00 0.00 FUD XXX

00820 Anesthesia for procedures on lower posterior abdominal wall
N PQ 0.00 0.00 FUD XXX

00830 Anesthesia for hernia repairs in lower abdomen; not otherwise specified
EXCLUDES *Anesthesia for hernia repairs on infants one year old or less (00834, 00836)*
N PQ 0.00 0.00 FUD XXX

00832 ventral and incisional hernias
EXCLUDES *Anesthesia for hernia repairs on infants one year old or less (00834, 00836)*
N PQ 0.00 0.00 FUD XXX

00834 Anesthesia for hernia repairs in the lower abdomen not otherwise specified, younger than 1 year of age A
Do not report with (99100)
N PQ 0.00 0.00 FUD XXX

00836 Anesthesia for hernia repairs in the lower abdomen not otherwise specified, infants younger than 37 weeks gestational age at birth and younger than 50 weeks gestational age at time of surgery A
Do not report with (99100)
N PQ 0.00 0.00 FUD XXX

00840 Anesthesia for intraperitoneal procedures in lower abdomen including laparoscopy; not otherwise specified
N PQ 0.00 0.00 FUD XXX

00842 amniocentesis M ♀
N PQ 0.00 0.00 FUD XXX

00844 abdominoperineal resection
C PQ 0.00 0.00 FUD XXX

00846 radical hysterectomy ♀
C PQ 0.00 0.00 FUD XXX

00848 pelvic exenteration
C PQ 0.00 0.00 FUD XXX

00851 tubal ligation/transection ♀
N PQ 0.00 0.00 FUD XXX

00860 Anesthesia for extraperitoneal procedures in lower abdomen, including urinary tract; not otherwise specified
N PQ 0.00 0.00 FUD XXX

00862 renal procedures, including upper one-third of ureter, or donor nephrectomy
N PQ 0.00 0.00 FUD XXX

00864 total cystectomy
C PQ 0.00 0.00 FUD XXX

00865 radical prostatectomy (suprapubic, retropubic) ♂
C PQ 0.00 0.00 FUD XXX

00866 adrenalectomy
C PQ 0.00 0.00 FUD XXX

00868 renal transplant (recipient)
EXCLUDES *Anesthesia for donor nephrectomy (00862)*
Physiological support during kidney harvest (01990)
C PQ 0.00 0.00 FUD XXX

00870 cystolithotomy
N PQ 0.00 0.00 FUD XXX

00872 Anesthesia for lithotripsy, extracorporeal shock wave; with water bath
N PQ 0.00 0.00 FUD XXX

00873 without water bath
N PQ 0.00 0.00 FUD XXX

00880 Anesthesia for procedures on major lower abdominal vessels; not otherwise specified
N PQ 0.00 0.00 FUD XXX

00882 inferior vena cava ligation
C PQ 0.00 0.00 FUD XXX

00902-00952 Anesthesia for Genitourinary Procedures

CMS 100-4,4,10.4 Packaging Rules Under OPPS
CMS 100-4,4,20.6 Modifier Use Under OPPS
CMS 100-4,4,20.6.4 Modifiers for Discontinued Services
CMS 100-4,12,50 Anesthesia Services
CMS 100-4,12,140.2 Payment for CRNA Services
CMS 100-4,12,140.3.2 Anesthesia Time and Units

EXCLUDES *Perineal procedures on skin, muscles, and nerves (00300, 00400)*

00902 Anesthesia for; anorectal procedure
N PQ 0.00 0.00 FUD XXX

00904 radical perineal procedure
C PQ 0.00 0.00 FUD XXX

00906 vulvectomy ♀
N PQ 0.00 0.00 FUD XXX

00908 perineal prostatectomy ♂
C PQ 0.00 0.00 FUD XXX

00910 Anesthesia for transurethral procedures (including urethrocystoscopy); not otherwise specified
N PQ 0.00 0.00 FUD XXX

00912 transurethral resection of bladder tumor(s)
N PQ 0.00 0.00 FUD XXX

00914 transurethral resection of prostate ♂
N PQ 0.00 0.00 FUD XXX

00916 post-transurethral resection bleeding
N PQ 0.00 0.00 FUD XXX

00918 with fragmentation, manipulation and/or removal of ureteral calculus
N PQ 0.00 0.00 FUD XXX

00920 Anesthesia for procedures on male genitalia (including open urethral procedures); not otherwise specified ♂
N PQ 0.00 0.00 FUD XXX

00921 vasectomy, unilateral or bilateral ♂
N PQ 0.00 0.00 FUD XXX

00922 seminal vesicles ♂
N PQ 0.00 0.00 FUD XXX

00924 undescended testis, unilateral or bilateral ♂
N PQ 0.00 0.00 FUD XXX

00926 radical orchiectomy, inguinal ♂
N PQ 0.00 0.00 FUD XXX

00928 radical orchiectomy, abdominal ♂
N PQ 0.00 0.00 FUD XXX

00930 orchiopexy, unilateral or bilateral ♂
N PQ 0.00 0.00 FUD XXX

00932 complete amputation of penis ♂
C PQ 0.00 0.00 FUD XXX

00934 radical amputation of penis with bilateral inguinal lymphadenectomy ♂
C PQ 0.00 0.00 FUD XXX

00936 radical amputation of penis with bilateral inguinal and iliac lymphadenectomy ♂
C PQ 0.00 0.00 FUD XXX

00938 insertion of penile prosthesis (perineal approach) ♂
N PQ 0.00 0.00 FUD XXX

00940 Anesthesia for vaginal procedures (including biopsy of labia, vagina, cervix or endometrium); not otherwise specified ♀
N PQ 0.00 0.00 FUD XXX

00942 colpotomy, vaginectomy, colporrhaphy, and open urethral procedures ♀
N PQ 0.00 0.00 FUD XXX

00944 vaginal hysterectomy ♀
C PQ 0.00 0.00 FUD XXX

00948 cervical cerclage ♀
N PQ 0.00 0.00 FUD XXX

00950 culdoscopy ♀
N PQ 0.00 0.00 FUD XXX

00952 hysteroscopy and/or hysterosalpingography ♀
N PQ 0.00 0.00 FUD XXX

01112-01522 Anesthesia for Lower Extremity Procedures

CMS 100-4,4,10.4 Packaging Rules Under OPPS
CMS 100-4,4,20.6 Modifier Use Under OPPS
CMS 100-4,4,20.6.4 Modifiers for Discontinued Services
CMS 100-4,12,50 Anesthesia Services
CMS 100-4,12,140.2 Payment for CRNA Services
CMS 100-4,12,140.3.2 Anesthesia Time and Units

01112 Anesthesia for bone marrow aspiration and/or biopsy, anterior or posterior iliac crest
N PQ 0.00 0.00 FUD XXX

01120 Anesthesia for procedures on bony pelvis
N PQ 0.00 0.00 FUD XXX

01130 Anesthesia for body cast application or revision
N PQ 0.00 0.00 FUD XXX

01140 Anesthesia for interpelviabdominal (hindquarter) amputation
C PQ 0.00 0.00 FUD XXX

01150 Anesthesia for radical procedures for tumor of pelvis, except hindquarter amputation
C CCI PQ 0.00 0.00 FUD XXX

01160 Anesthesia for closed procedures involving symphysis pubis or sacroiliac joint
N CCI PQ 0.00 0.00 FUD XXX

01170 Anesthesia for open procedures involving symphysis pubis or sacroiliac joint
N CCI PQ 0.00 0.00 FUD XXX

01173 Anesthesia for open repair of fracture disruption of pelvis or column fracture involving acetabulum
N CCI PQ 0.00 0.00 FUD XXX

01180 Anesthesia for obturator neurectomy; extrapelvic
N CCI PQ 0.00 0.00 FUD XXX

01190 intrapelvic
N CCI PQ 0.00 0.00 FUD XXX

01200 Anesthesia for all closed procedures involving hip joint
N CCI PQ 0.00 0.00 FUD XXX

01202 Anesthesia for arthroscopic procedures of hip joint
N CCI PQ 0.00 0.00 FUD XXX

01210 Anesthesia for open procedures involving hip joint; not otherwise specified
N CCI PQ 0.00 0.00 FUD XXX

01212 hip disarticulation
C CCI PQ 0.00 0.00 FUD XXX

01214 total hip arthroplasty
C CCI PQ 0.00 0.00 FUD XXX

01215 revision of total hip arthroplasty
N CCI PQ 0.00 0.00 FUD XXX

01220 Anesthesia for all closed procedures involving upper two-thirds of femur
N CCI PQ 0.00 0.00 FUD XXX

01230 Anesthesia for open procedures involving upper two-thirds of femur; not otherwise specified
N CCI PQ 0.00 0.00 FUD XXX

01232 amputation
C CCI PQ 0.00 0.00 FUD XXX

01234 radical resection
C CCI PQ 0.00 0.00 FUD XXX

01250 Anesthesia for all procedures on nerves, muscles, tendons, fascia, and bursae of upper leg
N CCI PQ 0.00 0.00 FUD XXX

01260 Anesthesia for all procedures involving veins of upper leg, including exploration
N CCI PQ 0.00 0.00 FUD XXX

01270 Anesthesia for procedures involving arteries of upper leg, including bypass graft; not otherwise specified
N CCI PQ 0.00 0.00 FUD XXX

01272 femoral artery ligation
C CCI PQ 0.00 0.00 FUD XXX

01274 femoral artery embolectomy
C CCI PQ 0.00 0.00 FUD XXX

01320 Anesthesia for all procedures on nerves, muscles, tendons, fascia, and bursae of knee and/or popliteal area
N CCI PQ 0.00 0.00 FUD XXX

01340 Anesthesia for all closed procedures on lower one-third of femur
N CCI PQ 0.00 0.00 FUD XXX

01360 Anesthesia for all open procedures on lower one-third of femur
N CCI PQ 0.00 0.00 FUD XXX

01380 Anesthesia for all closed procedures on knee joint
N CCI PQ 0.00 0.00 FUD XXX

01382 Anesthesia for diagnostic arthroscopic procedures of knee joint
N CCI PQ 0.00 0.00 FUD XXX

01390 Anesthesia for all closed procedures on upper ends of tibia, fibula, and/or patella
N CCI PQ 0.00 0.00 FUD XXX

01392 Anesthesia for all open procedures on upper ends of tibia, fibula, and/or patella
N CCI PQ 0.00 0.00 FUD XXX

01400 Anesthesia for open or surgical arthroscopic procedures on knee joint; not otherwise specified
N CCI PQ 0.00 0.00 FUD XXX

01402 total knee arthroplasty
C CCI PQ 0.00 0.00 FUD XXX

01404 disarticulation at knee
C CCI PQ 0.00 0.00 FUD XXX

01420 Anesthesia for all cast applications, removal, or repair involving knee joint
N CCI PQ 0.00 0.00 FUD XXX

01430 Anesthesia for procedures on veins of knee and popliteal area; not otherwise specified
N CCI PQ 0.00 0.00 FUD XXX

01432 arteriovenous fistula
N CCI PQ 0.00 0.00 FUD XXX

01440 Anesthesia for procedures on arteries of knee and popliteal area; not otherwise specified
N CCI PQ 0.00 0.00 FUD XXX

01442 popliteal thromboendarterectomy, with or without patch graft
C CCI PQ 0.00 0.00 FUD XXX

01444 popliteal excision and graft or repair for occlusion or aneurysm
C CCI PQ 0.00 0.00 FUD XXX

01462 Anesthesia for all closed procedures on lower leg, ankle, and foot
N CCI PQ 0.00 0.00 FUD XXX

01464 Anesthesia for arthroscopic procedures of ankle and/or foot
N CCI PQ 0.00 0.00 FUD XXX

01470 Anesthesia for procedures on nerves, muscles, tendons, and fascia of lower leg, ankle, and foot; not otherwise specified
N CCI PQ 0.00 0.00 FUD XXX

01472 repair of ruptured Achilles tendon, with or without graft
N CCI PQ 0.00 0.00 FUD XXX

01474 gastrocnemius recession (eg, Strayer procedure)
N CCI PQ 0.00 0.00 FUD XXX

01480 Anesthesia for open procedures on bones of lower leg, ankle, and foot; not otherwise specified
N CCI PQ 0.00 0.00 FUD XXX

01482 radical resection (including below knee amputation)
N CCI PQ 0.00 0.00 FUD XXX

01484 osteotomy or osteoplasty of tibia and/or fibula
N CCI PQ 0.00 0.00 FUD XXX

01486 total ankle replacement
C CCI PQ 0.00 0.00 FUD XXX

01490 Anesthesia for lower leg cast application, removal, or repair
N CCI PQ 0.00 0.00 FUD XXX

01500 Anesthesia for procedures on arteries of lower leg, including bypass graft; not otherwise specified
N CCI PQ 0.00 0.00 FUD XXX

01502 embolectomy, direct or with catheter
C CCI PQ 0.00 0.00 FUD XXX

01520 Anesthesia for procedures on veins of lower leg; not otherwise specified
N PQ 0.00 0.00 FUD XXX

01522 venous thrombectomy, direct or with catheter
N PQ 0.00 0.00 FUD XXX

01610-01682 Anesthesia for Shoulder Procedures

CMS 100-4,12,50 Anesthesia Services
CMS 100-4,12,140.2 Payment for CRNA Services
CMS 100-4,12,140.3.2 Anesthesia Time and Units

INCLUDES Acromioclavicular joint
Humeral head and neck
Shoulder joint
Sternoclavicular joint

01610 Anesthesia for all procedures on nerves, muscles, tendons, fascia, and bursae of shoulder and axilla
N PQ 0.00 0.00 FUD XXX

01620 Anesthesia for all closed procedures on humeral head and neck, sternoclavicular joint, acromioclavicular joint, and shoulder joint
N PQ 0.00 0.00 FUD XXX

01622 Anesthesia for diagnostic arthroscopic procedures of shoulder joint
N PQ 0.00 0.00 FUD XXX

01630 Anesthesia for open or surgical arthroscopic procedures on humeral head and neck, sternoclavicular joint, acromioclavicular joint, and shoulder joint; not otherwise specified
N PQ 0.00 0.00 FUD XXX

01634 shoulder disarticulation
C PQ 0.00 0.00 FUD XXX

01636 interthoracoscapular (forequarter) amputation
C PQ 0.00 0.00 FUD XXX

01638 total shoulder replacement
C PQ 0.00 0.00 FUD XXX

01650 Anesthesia for procedures on arteries of shoulder and axilla; not otherwise specified
N PQ 0.00 0.00 FUD XXX

01652 axillary-brachial aneurysm
C PQ 0.00 0.00 FUD XXX

01654 bypass graft
C PQ 0.00 0.00 FUD XXX

01656 axillary-femoral bypass graft
C PQ 0.00 0.00 FUD XXX

01670 Anesthesia for all procedures on veins of shoulder and axilla
N PQ 0.00 0.00 FUD XXX

01680 Anesthesia for shoulder cast application, removal or repair; not otherwise specified
N PQ 0.00 0.00 FUD XXX

01682 shoulder spica
N PQ 0.00 0.00 FUD XXX

01710-01860 Anesthesia for Upper Extremity Procedures

CMS 100-4,12,50 Anesthesia Services
CMS 100-4,12,140.2 Payment for CRNA Services
CMS 100-4,12,140.3.2 Anesthesia Time and Units

01710 Anesthesia for procedures on nerves, muscles, tendons, fascia, and bursae of upper arm and elbow; not otherwise specified
N PQ 0.00 0.00 FUD XXX

01712 tenotomy, elbow to shoulder, open
N PQ 0.00 0.00 FUD XXX

01714 tenoplasty, elbow to shoulder
N PQ 0.00 0.00 FUD XXX

01716 tenodesis, rupture of long tendon of biceps
N PQ 0.00 0.00 FUD XXX

01730 Anesthesia for all closed procedures on humerus and elbow
N PQ 0.00 0.00 FUD XXX

01732 Anesthesia for diagnostic arthroscopic procedures of elbow joint
N PQ 0.00 0.00 FUD XXX

01740 Anesthesia for open or surgical arthroscopic procedures of the elbow; not otherwise specified
N PQ 0.00 0.00 FUD XXX

01742 osteotomy of humerus
N PQ 0.00 0.00 FUD XXX

01744 repair of nonunion or malunion of humerus
N PQ 0.00 0.00 FUD XXX

01756 radical procedures
C PQ 0.00 0.00 FUD XXX

01758 excision of cyst or tumor of humerus
N PQ 0.00 0.00 FUD XXX

01760 total elbow replacement
N PQ 0.00 0.00 FUD XXX

01770 Anesthesia for procedures on arteries of upper arm and elbow; not otherwise specified
N PQ 0.00 0.00 FUD XXX

01772 embolectomy
N PQ 0.00 0.00 FUD XXX

01780 Anesthesia for procedures on veins of upper arm and elbow; not otherwise specified
N PQ 0.00 0.00 FUD XXX

01782 phleborrhaphy
N PQ 0.00 0.00 FUD XXX

01810 Anesthesia for all procedures on nerves, muscles, tendons, fascia, and bursae of forearm, wrist, and hand
N PQ 0.00 0.00 FUD XXX

01820 Anesthesia for all closed procedures on radius, ulna, wrist, or hand bones
N PQ 0.00 0.00 FUD XXX

01829 Anesthesia for diagnostic arthroscopic procedures on the wrist
N PQ 0.00 0.00 FUD XXX

01830 Anesthesia for open or surgical arthroscopic/endoscopic procedures on distal radius, distal ulna, wrist, or hand joints; not otherwise specified
N PQ 0.00 0.00 FUD XXX

01832 total wrist replacement
N PQ 0.00 0.00 FUD XXX

01840 Anesthesia for procedures on arteries of forearm, wrist, and hand; not otherwise specified
N PQ 0.00 0.00 FUD XXX

01842 embolectomy
N PQ 0.00 0.00 FUD XXX

01844 Anesthesia for vascular shunt, or shunt revision, any type (eg, dialysis)
N PQ 0.00 0.00 FUD XXX

01850 Anesthesia for procedures on veins of forearm, wrist, and hand; not otherwise specified
N PQ 0.00 0.00 FUD XXX

01852 phleborrhaphy
N PQ 0.00 0.00 FUD XXX

01860 Anesthesia for forearm, wrist, or hand cast application, removal, or repair
N PQ 0.00 0.00 FUD XXX

01916-01936 Anesthesia for Interventional Radiology Procedures

CMS 100-4,12,50 Anesthesia Services
CMS 100-4,12,140.2 Payment for CRNA Services
CMS 100-4,12,140.3.2 Anesthesia Time and Units

01916 **Anesthesia for diagnostic arteriography/venography**
Do not report with (01924-01926, 01930-01933)
N 0.00 0.00 FUD XXX

01920 **Anesthesia for cardiac catheterization including coronary angiography and ventriculography (not to include Swan-Ganz catheter)**
N 0.00 0.00 FUD XXX

01922 **Anesthesia for non-invasive imaging or radiation therapy**
N 0.00 0.00 FUD XXX

01924 **Anesthesia for therapeutic interventional radiological procedures involving the arterial system; not otherwise specified**
N PQ 0.00 0.00 FUD XXX

01925 **carotid or coronary**
N PQ 0.00 0.00 FUD XXX

01926 **intracranial, intracardiac, or aortic**
N PQ 0.00 0.00 FUD XXX

01930 **Anesthesia for therapeutic interventional radiological procedures involving the venous/lymphatic system (not to include access to the central circulation); not otherwise specified**
N PQ 0.00 0.00 FUD XXX

01931 **intrahepatic or portal circulation (eg, transvenous intrahepatic portosystemic shunt[s] [TIPS])**
N PQ 0.00 0.00 FUD XXX

01932 **intrathoracic or jugular**
N PQ 0.00 0.00 FUD XXX

01933 **intracranial**
N PQ 0.00 0.00 FUD XXX

01935 **Anesthesia for percutaneous image guided procedures on the spine and spinal cord; diagnostic**
N PQ 0.00 0.00 FUD XXX

01936 **therapeutic**
N PQ 0.00 0.00 FUD XXX

01951-01953 Anesthesia for Burn Procedures

CMS 100-4,3,20.1.2.8 Special Payments for Burn Cases
CMS 100-4,12,50 Anesthesia Services
CMS 100-4,12,140.2 Payment for CRNA Services
CMS 100-4,12,140.3.2 Anesthesia Time and Units

01951 **Anesthesia for second- and third-degree burn excision or debridement with or without skin grafting, any site, for total body surface area (TBSA) treated during anesthesia and surgery; less than 4% total body surface area**
N PQ 0.00 0.00 FUD XXX

01952 **between 4% and 9% of total body surface area**
N PQ 0.00 0.00 FUD XXX

+ **01953** **each additional 9% total body surface area or part thereof (List separately in addition to code for primary procedure)**
Code first (01952)
N PQ 0.00 0.00 FUD XXX

01958-01969 Anesthesia for Obstetric Procedures

CMS 100-4,12,50 Anesthesia Services
CMS 100-4,12,140.2 Payment for CRNA Services
CMS 100-4,12,140.3.2 Anesthesia Time and Units

01958 **Anesthesia for external cephalic version procedure** M♀
N 0.00 0.00 FUD XXX

01960 **Anesthesia for vaginal delivery only** M♀
N 0.00 0.00 FUD XXX

01961 **Anesthesia for cesarean delivery only** M♀
N PQ 0.00 0.00 FUD XXX

01962 **Anesthesia for urgent hysterectomy following delivery** M♀
N PQ 0.00 0.00 FUD XXX

01963 **Anesthesia for cesarean hysterectomy without any labor analgesia/anesthesia care** M♀
N PQ 0.00 0.00 FUD XXX

01965 **Anesthesia for incomplete or missed abortion procedures** M♀
N PQ 0.00 0.00 FUD XXX

01966 **Anesthesia for induced abortion procedures** M♀
N PQ 0.00 0.00 FUD XXX

01967 **Neuraxial labor analgesia/anesthesia for planned vaginal delivery (this includes any repeat subarachnoid needle placement and drug injection and/or any necessary replacement of an epidural catheter during labor)** M♀
N 0.00 0.00 FUD XXX

+ **01968** **Anesthesia for cesarean delivery following neuraxial labor analgesia/anesthesia (List separately in addition to code for primary procedure performed)** M♀
Code first (01967)
N PQ 0.00 0.00 FUD XXX

+ **01969** **Anesthesia for cesarean hysterectomy following neuraxial labor analgesia/anesthesia (List separately in addition to code for primary procedure performed)** M♀
Code first (01967)
N PQ 0.00 0.00 FUD XXX

01990-01999 Anesthesia Miscellaneous

CMS 100-4,12,50 Anesthesia Services
CMS 100-4,12,140.2 Payment for CRNA Services
CMS 100-4,12,140.3.2 Anesthesia Time and Units

01990 **Physiological support for harvesting of organ(s) from brain-dead patient**
C 0.00 0.00 FUD XXX

01991 **Anesthesia for diagnostic or therapeutic nerve blocks and injections (when block or injection is performed by a different physician or other qualified health care professional); other than the prone position**
EXCLUDES *Bier block for pain management (64999)*
Pain management via intra-arterial or IV therapy (96373-96374)
Regional or local anesthesia of arms or legs for surgical procedure
Do not report with (99143-99150)
N 0.00 0.00 FUD XXX

01992 **prone position**
EXCLUDES *Bier block for pain management (64999)*
Pain management via intra-arterial or IV therapy (96373-96374)
Regional or local anesthesia of arms or legs for surgical procedure
Do not report with (99143-99150)
N 0.00 0.00 FUD XXX

01996 Daily hospital management of epidural or subarachnoid continuous drug administration

INCLUDES Continuous epidural or subarachnoid drug services performed after insertion of an epidural or subarachnoid catheter

N 0.00 0.00 FUD XXX

01999 Unlisted anesthesia procedure(s)

N 0.00 0.00 FUD XXX

10021-10022 Fine Needle Aspiration

CMS 100-4,13,80.1 Supervision and Interpretation Codes
CMS 100-4,13,80.2 S&I Multiple Procedure Reduction

EXCLUDES *Percutaneous localization clip placement during breast biopsy (19081-19086)*
Percutaneous needle biopsy of:
Abdominal or retroperitoneal mass (49180)
Bone (20220, 20225)
Bone marrow (38220-38221)
Breast (19081-19086)
Epididymis (54800)
Kidney (50200)
Liver (47000)
Lung or mediastinum (32405)
Lymph node (38505)
Muscle (20206)
Nucleus pulposus, paravertebral tissue, intervertebral disc (62267)
Pancreas (48102)
Pleura (32400)
Prostate (55700, 55706)
Salivary gland (42400)
Spinal cord (62269)
Testis (54500)
Thyroid (60100)
Soft tissue percutaneous fluid drainage by catheter using image guidance (10030)

10021 Fine needle aspiration; without imaging guidance
88172-88173
P2 T 80 ⚑ 2.03 4.20 FUD XXX

10022 with imaging guidance
76942, 77002, 77012, 77021
88172-88173
G2 T 80 ⚑ 1.88 3.94 FUD XXX

10030-10180 Treatment of Fluid-filled Lesions: Skin and Subcutaneous Tissues

CMS 100-4,12,30 Correct Coding Policy
CMS 100-4,13,80.1 Physician Presence
CMS 100-4,13,80.2 S&I Multiple Procedure Reduction

EXCLUDES *Excision benign lesion (11400-11471)*

⊙ **10030 Image-guided fluid collection drainage by catheter (eg, abscess, hematoma, seroma, lymphocele, cyst), soft tissue (eg, extremity, abdominal wall, neck), percutaneous**
EXCLUDES *Percutaneous drainage with imaging guidance of:*
Peritoneal or retroperitoneal collections (49406)
Visceral collections (49405)
Transvaginal or transrectal drainage with imaging guidance of:
Peritoneal or retroperitoneal collections (49407)
Code also every instance of fluid collection drained using a separate catheter (10030)
Do not report with (75989, 76942, 77002-77003, 77012, 77021)
P2 I 80 4.45 22.07 FUD XXX

10040 Acne surgery (eg, marsupialization, opening or removal of multiple milia, comedones, cysts, pustules)
P2 T ⚑ 2.49 2.84 FUD 010

10060 Incision and drainage of abscess (eg, carbuncle, suppurative hidradenitis, cutaneous or subcutaneous abscess, cyst, furuncle, or paronychia); simple or single
P3 T ⚑ 2.72 3.25 FUD 010

10061 complicated or multiple
P2 T ⚑ 5.07 5.78 FUD 010

10080 Incision and drainage of pilonidal cyst; simple
P2 T ⚑ 2.93 5.02 FUD 010

10081 complicated
EXCLUDES *Excision of pilonidal cyst (11770-11772)*
P3 T ⚑ 4.91 7.61 FUD 010

10120 Incision and removal of foreign body, subcutaneous tissues; simple
P3 T ⚑ 2.93 4.26 FUD 010

10121 complicated
EXCLUDES *Debridement associated with a fracture or dislocation (11010-11012)*
Exploration penetrating wound (20100-20103)
A2 T ⚑ 5.29 7.72 FUD 010

Hematoma may be decompressed with a hemostat

Drain may be placed to allow further drainage

10140 Incision and drainage of hematoma, seroma or fluid collection
76942, 77012, 77021
P3 T ⚑ 3.36 4.57 FUD 010

10160 Puncture aspiration of abscess, hematoma, bulla, or cyst
76942, 77012, 77021
P3 T ⚑ 2.72 3.65 FUD 010

10180 Incision and drainage, complex, postoperative wound infection
EXCLUDES *Wound dehiscence (12020-12021, 13160)*
A2 T ⚑ 5.08 6.94 FUD 010

11000-11012 Removal of Foreign Substances and Infected/Devitalized Tissue

CMS 100-4,12,40.1 Global Surgery Package
CMS 100-4,12,40.2 Billing Requirements for Global Surgeries

EXCLUDES *Debridement of:*
Burns (16000-16030)
Deeper tissue (11042-11047 [11045, 11046])
Nails (11720-11721)
Skin only (97597-97598)
Wounds (11042-11047 [11045, 11046])
Dermabrasions (15780-15783)
Pressure ulcer excision (15920-15999)

11000 Debridement of extensive eczematous or infected skin; up to 10% of body surface
EXCLUDES *Necrotizing soft tissue infection of:*
Abdominal wall (11005-11006)
External genitalia and perineum (11004, 11006)
P3 T ⚑ 0.82 1.53 FUD 000

\+ **11001 each additional 10% of the body surface, or part thereof (List separately in addition to code for primary procedure)**
EXCLUDES *Necrotizing soft tissue infection of:*
Abdominal wall (11005-11006)
External genitalia and perineum (11004, 11006)
Code first (11000)
N1 N 0.41 0.60 FUD ZZZ

11004 **Debridement of skin, subcutaneous tissue, muscle and fascia for necrotizing soft tissue infection; external genitalia and perineum**

EXCLUDES *Skin grafts or flaps (14000-14350, 15040-15770)*

C 16.60 16.60 FUD 000

11005 **abdominal wall, with or without fascial closure**

EXCLUDES *Skin grafts or flaps (14000-14350, 15040-15770)*

C 80 22.36 22.36 FUD 000

11006 **external genitalia, perineum and abdominal wall, with or without fascial closure**

EXCLUDES *Orchiectomy (54520)*
Skin grafts or flaps (14000-14350, 15040-15770)
Testicular transplant (54680)

C 20.12 20.12 FUD 000

+ **11008** **Removal of prosthetic material or mesh, abdominal wall for infection (eg, for chronic or recurrent mesh infection or necrotizing soft tissue infection) (List separately in addition to code for primary procedure)**

EXCLUDES *Insertion of mesh (49568)*
Skin grafts or flaps (14000-14350, 15040-15770)

Code first (10180, 11004-11006)
Do not report with (11000-11001, 11010-11044 [11045, 11046])

C 80 7.84 7.84 FUD ZZZ

11010 **Debridement including removal of foreign material at the site of an open fracture and/or an open dislocation (eg, excisional debridement); skin and subcutaneous tissues**

A2 T 7.93 13.72 FUD 010

11011 **skin, subcutaneous tissue, muscle fascia, and muscle**

A2 T 8.61 15.17 FUD 000

11012 **skin, subcutaneous tissue, muscle fascia, muscle, and bone**

A2 T 12.16 20.05 FUD 000

11042-11047 [11045, 11046] Removal of Infected/Devitalized Tissue

CMS 100-2,15,260 Covered ASC Procedures
CMS 100-4,12,40.1 Global Surgery Definition
CMS 100-4,12,40.2 Billing Requirements for Global Surgeries
CMS 100-4,14,10 ASC Procedures

INCLUDES Debridement reported by the size and depth
Debridement reported for multiple wounds by adding the total surface area of wounds of the same depth
Injuries, wounds, chronic ulcers, infections

EXCLUDES *Debridement of:*
Burn (16020-16030)
Dermis/epidermis only (97597-97598)
Eczematous or infected skin (11000-11001)
Nails (11720-11721)
Necrotizing soft tissue infection of external genitalia, perineum, or abdominal wall (11004-11006)
Dermabrasions (15780-15783)
Excision of pressure ulcers (15920-15999)

Code also each additional single wound of different depths
Code also modifier 59 for additional wound debridement
Code also multiple wound groups of different depths
Do not report with active care and management of same wound (97597-97602)

11042 **Debridement, subcutaneous tissue (includes epidermis and dermis, if performed); first 20 sq cm or less**

A2 T P0 1.76 3.27 FUD 000

+ # **11045** **each additional 20 sq cm, or part thereof (List separately in addition to code for primary procedure)**

Code first (11042)

N1 N 80 0.79 1.20 FUD ZZZ

11043 **Debridement, muscle and/or fascia (includes epidermis, dermis, and subcutaneous tissue, if performed); first 20 sq cm or less**

A2 T P0 4.50 6.49 FUD 000

+ # **11046** **each additional 20 sq cm, or part thereof (List separately in addition to code for primary procedure)**

Code first (11043)

N1 N 80 1.61 2.08 FUD ZZZ

11044 **Debridement, bone (includes epidermis, dermis, subcutaneous tissue, muscle and/or fascia, if performed); first 20 sq cm or less**

A2 T P0 6.71 9.00 FUD 000

11045 *Resequenced code. See code following 11042.*

11046 *Resequenced code. See code following 11043.*

+ **11047** **each additional 20 sq cm, or part thereof (List separately in addition to code for primary procedure)**

Code first (11044)

N1 N 80 2.88 3.55 FUD ZZZ

11055-11057 Excision Benign Hypertrophic Skin Lesions

CMS 100-2,15,290 Routine Foot Care

EXCLUDES *Destruction (17000-17004)*

11055 **Paring or cutting of benign hyperkeratotic lesion (eg, corn or callus); single lesion**

P3 T P0 0.46 1.33 FUD 000

11056 **2 to 4 lesions**

P3 T P0 0.65 1.63 FUD 000

11057 **more than 4 lesions**

P3 T P0 0.85 1.84 FUD 000

11100-11101 Surgical Biopsy Skin and Mucous Membranes

CMS 100-4,12,30 Correct Coding Policy

INCLUDES Attaining tissue for pathologic exam

EXCLUDES *Biopsy of:*
Conjunctiva (68100)
Eyelid ([67810])

Do not report with related procedures

11100 **Biopsy of skin, subcutaneous tissue and/or mucous membrane (including simple closure), unless otherwise listed; single lesion**

P3 T P0 1.39 2.86 FUD 000

+ **11101** **each separate/additional lesion (List separately in addition to code for primary procedure)**

Code first (11100)

N1 N 0.70 0.91 FUD ZZZ

11200-11201 Skin Tag Removal - All Techniques

CMS 100-4,12,30 Correct Coding Policy
CMS 100-4,12,40.1 Global Surgery Package Definition
CMS 100-4,12,40.2 Billing Requirements for Global Surgeries

INCLUDES Chemical destruction
Electrocauterization
Electrosurgical destruction
Ligature strangulation
Local anesthesia when used
Removal with or without local anesthesia
Sharp excision or scissoring

EXCLUDES *Extensive or complicated secondary wound closure (13160)*

11200 **Removal of skin tags, multiple fibrocutaneous tags, any area; up to and including 15 lesions**

P2 T 2.07 2.46 FUD 010

+ **11201** **each additional 10 lesions, or part thereof (List separately in addition to code for primary procedure)**

Code first (11200)

N1 N 0.48 0.54 FUD ZZZ

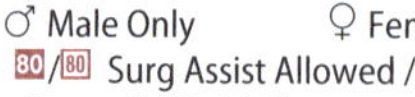

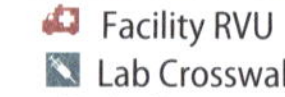

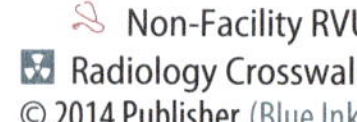

11300-11313 Skin Lesion Removal: Shaving

CMS 100-4,12,40.1 Global Surgery Package Definition
CMS 100-4,12,40.2 Global Surgery Billing Requirements
CMS 100-4,12,50 Local anesthesia

INCLUDES Local anesthesia
Partial thickness excision by horizontal slicing
Wound cauterization

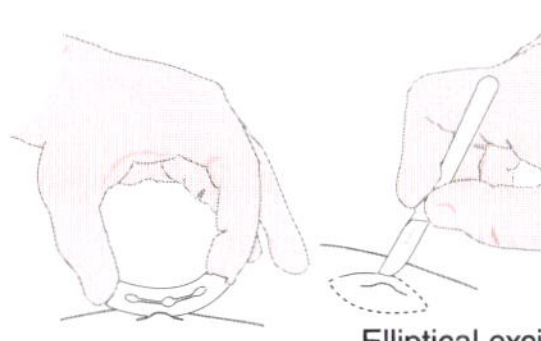

Shave excision of an elevated lesion; technique also used to biopsy

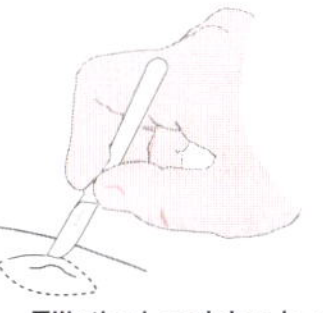

Elliptical excision is often used when tissue removal is larger than 4 mm or when deep pathology is suspected

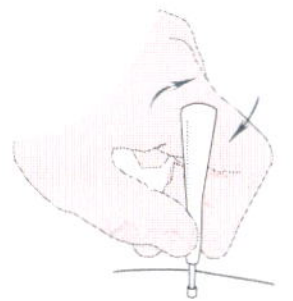

A punch biopsy cuts a core of tissue as the tool is twisted downward

11300 **Shaving of epidermal or dermal lesion, single lesion, trunk, arms or legs; lesion diameter 0.5 cm or less**
P2 T 80 1.00 2.68 FUD 000

11301 **lesion diameter 0.6 to 1.0 cm**
P2 T 80 1.52 3.30 FUD 000

11302 **lesion diameter 1.1 to 2.0 cm**
P2 T 80 1.78 3.89 FUD 000

11303 **lesion diameter over 2.0 cm**
P2 T 80 2.12 4.32 FUD 000

11305 **Shaving of epidermal or dermal lesion, single lesion, scalp, neck, hands, feet, genitalia; lesion diameter 0.5 cm or less**
P2 T 80 1.11 2.74 FUD 000

11306 **lesion diameter 0.6 to 1.0 cm**
P2 T 80 1.48 3.37 FUD 000

11307 **lesion diameter 1.1 to 2.0 cm**
P2 T 80 1.90 3.98 FUD 000

11308 **lesion diameter over 2.0 cm**
P2 T 80 2.10 4.19 FUD 000

11310 **Shaving of epidermal or dermal lesion, single lesion, face, ears, eyelids, nose, lips, mucous membrane; lesion diameter 0.5 cm or less**
P2 T 80 1.35 3.14 FUD 000

11311 **lesion diameter 0.6 to 1.0 cm**
P2 T 80 1.86 3.08 FUD 000

11312 **lesion diameter 1.1 to 2.0 cm**
P2 T 80 2.24 4.45 FUD 000

11313 **lesion diameter over 2.0 cm**
P2 T 80 2.87 5.17 FUD 000

11400-11446 Skin Lesion Removal: Benign

CMS 100-2,16,120 Cosmetic Procedures
CMS 100-4,12,40.1 Global Surgery Package Definition
CMS 100-4,12,40.2 Billing Requirements for Global Surgeries
CMS 100-4,12,50 Local anesthesia

INCLUDES Biopsy on same lesion
Full thickness removal including margins
Lesion measurement before excision at largest diameter plus margin
Local anesthesia
Simple, nonlayered closure

EXCLUDES *Biopsy of eyelid ([67810])*
Destruction of eyelid lesion (67850)
Excision and reconstruction of eyelid (67961-67975)
Excision of chalazion (67800-67808)
Eyelid procedures involving more than skin (67800 and subsequent codes)
Shave removal (11300-11313)

Code also complex closure (13100-13153)
Code also each separate lesion
Code also intermediate closure (12031-12057)
Code also modifier 22 if excision is complicated or unusual
Code also reconstruction (15002-15261, 15570-15770)

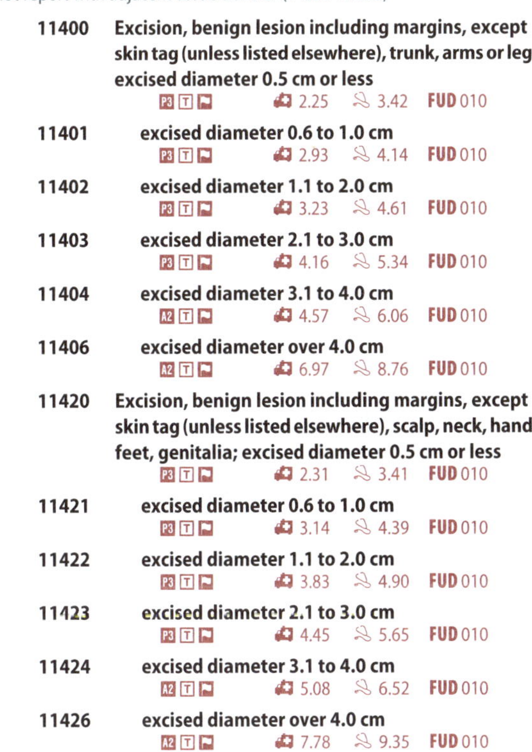

Do not report with adjacent tissue transfer (14000-14302)

11400 **Excision, benign lesion including margins, except skin tag (unless listed elsewhere), trunk, arms or legs; excised diameter 0.5 cm or less**
P3 T 2.25 3.42 FUD 010

11401 **excised diameter 0.6 to 1.0 cm**
P3 T 2.93 4.14 FUD 010

11402 **excised diameter 1.1 to 2.0 cm**
P3 T 3.23 4.61 FUD 010

11403 **excised diameter 2.1 to 3.0 cm**
P3 T 4.16 5.34 FUD 010

11404 **excised diameter 3.1 to 4.0 cm**
A2 T 4.57 6.06 FUD 010

11406 **excised diameter over 4.0 cm**
A2 T 6.97 8.76 FUD 010

11420 **Excision, benign lesion including margins, except skin tag (unless listed elsewhere), scalp, neck, hands, feet, genitalia; excised diameter 0.5 cm or less**
P3 T 2.31 3.41 FUD 010

11421 **excised diameter 0.6 to 1.0 cm**
P3 T 3.14 4.39 FUD 010

11422 **excised diameter 1.1 to 2.0 cm**
P3 T 3.83 4.90 FUD 010

11423 **excised diameter 2.1 to 3.0 cm**
P3 T 4.45 5.65 FUD 010

11424 **excised diameter 3.1 to 4.0 cm**
A2 T 5.08 6.52 FUD 010

11426 **excised diameter over 4.0 cm**
A2 T 7.78 9.35 FUD 010

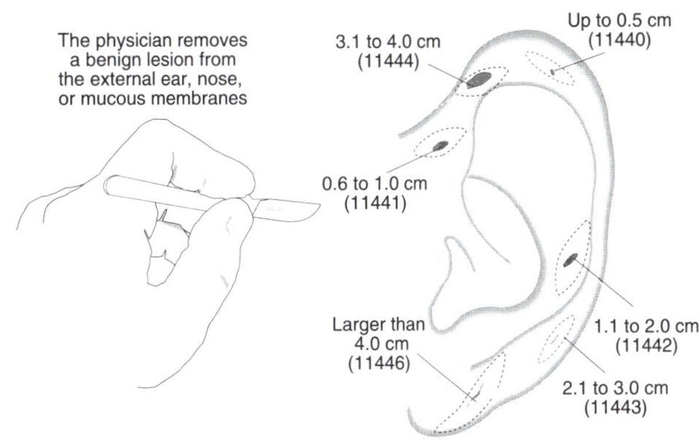

The physician removes a benign lesion from the external ear, nose, or mucous membranes

11440 **Excision, other benign lesion including margins, except skin tag (unless listed elsewhere), face, ears, eyelids, nose, lips, mucous membrane; excised diameter 0.5 cm or less**
P3 T 2.93 3.78 FUD 010

11441 **excised diameter 0.6 to 1.0 cm**
P3 T 3.72 4.70 FUD 010

11442 **excised diameter 1.1 to 2.0 cm**
P3 T 4.13 5.26 FUD 010

11443 **excised diameter 2.1 to 3.0 cm**
P3 T 5.05 6.27 FUD 010

11444 **excised diameter 3.1 to 4.0 cm**
A2 T 6.46 7.92 FUD 010

11446 **excised diameter over 4.0 cm**
A2 T 9.29 11.01 FUD 010

11450-11471 Treatment of Hidradenitis: Excision and Repair

CMS 100-2,15,260 Covered ASC Procedures
CMS 100-4,14,10 General ASC Services

Code also closure by skin graft or flap (14000-14350, 15040-15770)

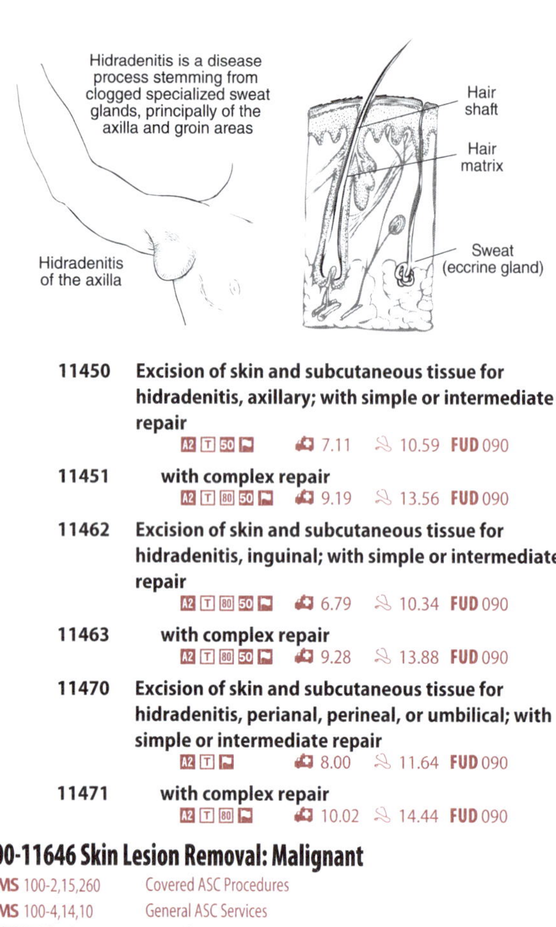

11450 **Excision of skin and subcutaneous tissue for hidradenitis, axillary; with simple or intermediate repair**
A2 T 50 — 7.11 — 10.59 FUD 090

11451 **with complex repair**
A2 T 80 50 — 9.19 — 13.56 FUD 090

11462 **Excision of skin and subcutaneous tissue for hidradenitis, inguinal; with simple or intermediate repair**
A2 T 80 50 — 6.79 — 10.34 FUD 090

11463 **with complex repair**
A2 T 80 50 — 9.28 — 13.88 FUD 090

11470 **Excision of skin and subcutaneous tissue for hidradenitis, perianal, perineal, or umbilical; with simple or intermediate repair**
A2 T — 8.00 — 11.64 FUD 090

11471 **with complex repair**
A2 T 80 — 10.02 — 14.44 FUD 090

11600-11646 Skin Lesion Removal: Malignant

CMS 100-2,15,260 Covered ASC Procedures
CMS 100-4,14,10 General ASC Services

INCLUDES Biopsy on same lesion
Excision of additional margin at same operative session
Full thickness removal including margins
Lesion measurement before excision at largest diameter plus margin
Local anesthesia
Simple, nonlayered closure

EXCLUDES *Destruction (17260-17286)*
Excision of additional margin at subsequent operative session (11600-11646)

Code also complex closure (13100-13153)
Code also each separate lesion
Code also intermediate closure (12031-12057)
Code also modifier 58 if re-excision is performed during postoperative period
Code also reconstruction (15002-15261, 15570-15770)
Do not report with adjacent tissue transfer. Report only adjacent tissue transfer code. (14000-14302)

11600 **Excision, malignant lesion including margins, trunk, arms, or legs; excised diameter 0.5 cm or less**
P3 T PQ — 3.40 — 5.38 FUD 010

11601 **excised diameter 0.6 to 1.0 cm**
P3 T PQ — 4.22 — 6.36 FUD 010

11602 **excised diameter 1.1 to 2.0 cm**
P3 T PQ — 4.63 — 6.90 FUD 010

11603 **excised diameter 2.1 to 3.0 cm**
P3 T PQ — 5.53 — 7.87 FUD 010

11604 **excised diameter 3.1 to 4.0 cm**
A2 T PQ — 6.12 — 8.79 FUD 010

11606 **excised diameter over 4.0 cm**
A2 T PQ — 9.11 — 12.60 FUD 010

11620 **Excision, malignant lesion including margins, scalp, neck, hands, feet, genitalia; excised diameter 0.5 cm or less**
P3 T PQ — 3.45 — 5.44 FUD 010

11621 **excised diameter 0.6 to 1.0 cm**
P3 T PQ — 4.24 — 6.40 FUD 010

11622 **excised diameter 1.1 to 2.0 cm**
P3 T PQ — 4.86 — 7.14 FUD 010

11623 **excised diameter 2.1 to 3.0 cm**
P3 T PQ — 6.03 — 8.40 FUD 010

11624 **excised diameter 3.1 to 4.0 cm**
A2 T PQ — 6.84 — 9.48 FUD 010

11626 **excised diameter over 4.0 cm**
A2 T PQ — 8.41 — 11.47 FUD 010

11640 **Excision, malignant lesion including margins, face, ears, eyelids, nose, lips; excised diameter 0.5 cm or less**
EXCLUDES *Eyelid excision involving more than skin (67800 and subsequent codes)*
P3 T PQ — 3.56 — 5.60 FUD 010

11641 **excised diameter 0.6 to 1.0 cm**
EXCLUDES *Eyelid excision involving more than skin (67800 and subsequent codes)*
P3 T PQ — 4.44 — 6.64 FUD 010

11642 **excised diameter 1.1 to 2.0 cm**
EXCLUDES *Eyelid excision involving more than skin (67800 and subsequent codes)*
P3 T PQ — 5.22 — 7.56 FUD 010

11643 **excised diameter 2.1 to 3.0 cm**
EXCLUDES *Eyelid excision involving more than skin (67800 and subsequent codes)*
P3 T PQ — 6.58 — 8.98 FUD 010

11644 **excised diameter 3.1 to 4.0 cm**
EXCLUDES *Eyelid excision involving more than skin (67800 and subsequent codes)*
A2 T PQ — 8.15 — 11.08 FUD 010

11646 **excised diameter over 4.0 cm**
EXCLUDES *Eyelid excision involving more than skin (67800 and subsequent codes)*
A2 T PQ — 11.33 — 14.51 FUD 010

11719-11765 Nails and Supporting Structures

CMS 100-2,15,290 Foot Care

EXCLUDES *Drainage of paronychia or onychia (10060-10061)*

11719 **Trimming of nondystrophic nails, any number**
P3 T PQ — 0.22 — 0.39 FUD 000

11720 **Debridement of nail(s) by any method(s); 1 to 5**
P3 T PQ — 0.43 — 0.91 FUD 000

11721 **6 or more**
P3 T PQ — 0.71 — 1.26 FUD 000

11730 **Avulsion of nail plate, partial or complete, simple; single**
P3 T PQ — 1.46 — 2.78 FUD 000

\+ **11732** **each additional nail plate (List separately in addition to code for primary procedure)**
Code first (11730)
NI N — 0.58 — 1.00 FUD ZZZ

11740 **Evacuation of subungual hematoma**
P2 T PQ — 0.93 — 1.39 FUD 000

11750 **Excision of nail and nail matrix, partial or complete (eg, ingrown or deformed nail), for permanent removal;**
EXCLUDES *Skin graft (15050)*
P3 T — 4.94 — 6.30 FUD 010

11752 **with amputation of tuft of distal phalanx**
EXCLUDES *Skin graft (15050)*
P3 T — 7.40 — 9.06 FUD 010

11755 **Biopsy of nail unit (eg, plate, bed, matrix, hyponychium, proximal and lateral nail folds) (separate procedure)**
P3 T 80 PQ — 2.24 — 3.76 FUD 000

11760 **Repair of nail bed**
G2 T — 3.80 — 6.53 FUD 010

11762 **Reconstruction of nail bed with graft**
P3 T — 5.29 — 7.95 FUD 010

11765 **Wedge excision of skin of nail fold (eg, for ingrown toenail)**
INCLUDES Cotting's operation
P2 T 2.65 4.66 FUD 010

11770-11772 Treatment Pilonidal Cyst: Excision

CMS 100-2,15,260 Covered ASC Procedures

EXCLUDES *Incision of pilonidal cyst (10080-10081)*

11770 **Excision of pilonidal cyst or sinus; simple**
A2 T 5.23 7.79 FUD 010

11771 **extensive**
A2 T 12.28 16.05 FUD 090

11772 **complicated**
A2 T 16.27 19.49 FUD 090

11900-11901 Treatment of Lesions: Injection

CMS 100-4,17,20.5.7 Injection Services

EXCLUDES *Injection of veins (36470-36471)*
Intralesional chemotherapy (96405, 96406)

Do not report for injection of local anesthesia performed preoperatively

11900 **Injection, intralesional; up to and including 7 lesions**
P3 T 0.89 1.54 FUD 000

11901 **more than 7 lesions**
P3 T 1.39 1.95 FUD 000

11920-11971 Tattoos, Tissue Expanders, and Dermal Fillers

CMS 100-2,16,10 Exclusions from Coverage
CMS 100-2,16,120 Cosmetic Procedures
CMS 100-2,16,180 Services Related to Noncovered Procedures

11920 **Tattooing, intradermal introduction of insoluble opaque pigments to correct color defects of skin, including micropigmentation; 6.0 sq cm or less**
P3 T 80 3.30 4.82 FUD 000

11921 **6.1 to 20.0 sq cm**
P3 T 80 3.88 5.60 FUD 000

+ 11922 **each additional 20.0 sq cm, or part thereof (List separately in addition to code for primary procedure)**
Code first (11921)
N1 N 80 0.86 1.73 FUD ZZZ

11950 **Subcutaneous injection of filling material (eg, collagen); 1 cc or less**
P3 T 80 1.52 2.14 FUD 000

11951 **1.1 to 5.0 cc**
P3 T 80 2.18 2.92 FUD 000

11952 **5.1 to 10.0 cc**
P3 T 80 2.88 3.84 FUD 000

11954 **over 10.0 cc**
P3 T 80 3.32 4.48 FUD 000

11960 **Insertion of tissue expander(s) for other than breast, including subsequent expansion**
EXCLUDES *Breast reconstruction with tissue expander(s) (19357)*
A2 T 26.53 26.53 FUD 090

11970 **Replacement of tissue expander with permanent prosthesis**
A2 T 50 17.50 17.50 FUD 090

11971 **Removal of tissue expander(s) without insertion of prosthesis**
A2 Q2 80 50 9.12 13.28 FUD 090

11976-11983 Drug Implantation

CMS 100-2,15,50 Drugs and Biologicals
CMS 100-2,16,20 General Exclusions

11976 **Removal, implantable contraceptive capsules** ♀
P3 Q2 80 2.78 4.10 FUD 000

11980 **Subcutaneous hormone pellet implantation (implantation of estradiol and/or testosterone pellets beneath the skin)**
P3 X 2.29 2.92 FUD 000

11981 **Insertion, non-biodegradable drug delivery implant**
P2 X 80 2.33 3.87 FUD XXX

11982 **Removal, non-biodegradable drug delivery implant**
P2 X 80 2.79 4.38 FUD XXX

11983 **Removal with reinsertion, non-biodegradable drug delivery implant**
P2 X 80 4.85 6.10 FUD XXX

12001-12021 Suturing of Superficial Wounds

CMS 100-2,15,260 Covered ASC Procedures
CMS 100-4,14,10 ASC Procedures

INCLUDES Administration of local anesthesia
Cauterization without closure
Simple:
Exploration nerves, blood vessels, tendons
Vessel ligation, in wound
Simple repair that involves:
Routine debridement and decontamination
Simple one layer closure
Superficial tissues
Sutures, staples, tissue adhesives
Total length of several repairs in same code category

EXCLUDES *Adhesive strips only, see appropriate evaluation and management service*
Complex repair nerves, blood vessels, tendons (see appropriate anatomical section)
Debridement:
Performed separately, no closure (11042-11047 [11045, 11046])
That requires:
Comprehensive cleaning
Removal of significant tissue
Removal soft tissue and/or bone, no fracture/dislocation (11042-11047 [11045, 11046])
Removal soft tissue and/or bone with open fracture/dislocation (11010-11012)
Deep tissue repair (12031-13153)
Major exploration (20100-20103)
Repair of nerves, blood vessels, tendons (See appropriate anatomical section. These repairs include simple and intermediate closure. Report complex closure with modifier 59.)
Secondary closure/dehiscence (13160)

Code also modifier 59 added to the less complicated procedure code if reporting more than one classification of wound repair

12001 **Simple repair of superficial wounds of scalp, neck, axillae, external genitalia, trunk and/or extremities (including hands and feet); 2.5 cm or less**
P2 T 1.29 2.52 FUD 000

12002 **2.6 cm to 7.5 cm**
P2 T 1.70 3.06 FUD 000

12004 **7.6 cm to 12.5 cm**
P2 T 2.12 3.61 FUD 000

12005 **12.6 cm to 20.0 cm**
A2 T 2.87 4.70 FUD 000

12006 **20.1 cm to 30.0 cm**
A2 T 3.48 5.65 FUD 000

12007 **over 30.0 cm**
A2 T 4.32 6.56 FUD 000

12011 **Simple repair of superficial wounds of face, ears, eyelids, nose, lips and/or mucous membranes; 2.5 cm or less**
P2 T 1.61 3.08 FUD 000

12013 **2.6 cm to 5.0 cm**
P2 T 1.80 3.37 FUD 000

12014 **5.1 cm to 7.5 cm**
P2 T 2.29 3.98 FUD 000

12015 **7.6 cm to 12.5 cm**
G2 T 2.85 4.86 FUD 000

Integumentary System

11765 — 12015

12016 12.6 cm to 20.0 cm
A2 T 3.87 6.01 FUD 000

12017 20.1 cm to 30.0 cm
A2 T 80 4.43 4.43 FUD 000

12018 over 30.0 cm
A2 T 80 5.01 5.01 FUD 000

12020 Treatment of superficial wound dehiscence; simple closure
EXCLUDES *Secondary closure major/complex wound or dehiscence (13160)*
A2 T 5.43 8.05 FUD 010

12021 **with packing**
EXCLUDES *Secondary closure major/complex wound or dehiscence (13160)*
A2 T 4.02 4.71 FUD 010

12031-12057 Suturing of Intermediate Wounds

CMS 100-4,14,10 General ASC Services

INCLUDES Administration of local anesthesia
Intermediate repair that involves:
Closure of contaminated single layer wound
Layer closure (e.g., subcutaneous tissue, superficial fascia)
Removal foreign material (e.g. gravel, glass)
Routine debridement and decontamination
Simple:
Exploration nerves, blood vessels, tendons in wound
Vessel ligation, in wound
Total length of several repairs in same code category

EXCLUDES *Debridement:*
Performed separately, no closure (11042-11047 [11045, 11046])
That requires:
Removal soft tissue and/or bone, no fracture/dislocation (11042-11047 [11045, 11046])
Removal soft tissue/bone due to open fracture/dislocation (11010-11012)
Major exploration (20100-20103)
Repair of nerves, blood vessels, tendons (See appropriate anatomical section. These repairs include simple and intermediate closure. Report complex closure with modifier 59.)
Secondary closure major/complex wound or dehiscence (13160)
Wound repair involving more than layer closure

Code also modifier 59 added to the less complicated procedure code if reporting more than one classification of wound repair

12031 Repair, intermediate, wounds of scalp, axillae, trunk and/or extremities (excluding hands and feet); 2.5 cm or less
P2 T 4.34 6.60 FUD 010

12032 2.6 cm to 7.5 cm
P2 T 5.51 8.41 FUD 010

12034 7.6 cm to 12.5 cm
A2 T 5.88 8.70 FUD 010

12035 12.6 cm to 20.0 cm
A2 T 6.91 10.80 FUD 010

12036 20.1 cm to 30.0 cm
A2 T 8.02 11.91 FUD 010

12037 over 30.0 cm
A2 T 80 9.38 13.41 FUD 010

12041 Repair, intermediate, wounds of neck, hands, feet and/or external genitalia; 2.5 cm or less
P2 T 4.44 6.73 FUD 010

12042 2.6 cm to 7.5 cm
P2 T 5.67 8.03 FUD 010

12044 7.6 cm to 12.5 cm
A2 T 6.14 10.04 FUD 010

12045 12.6 cm to 20.0 cm
A2 T 7.70 11.25 FUD 010

12046 20.1 cm to 30.0 cm
A2 T 80 8.74 13.39 FUD 010

12047 over 30.0 cm
A2 T 80 9.74 14.72 FUD 010

12051 Repair, intermediate, wounds of face, ears, eyelids, nose, lips and/or mucous membranes; 2.5 cm or less
P2 T 4.87 7.20 FUD 010

12052 2.6 cm to 5.0 cm
P2 T 5.77 8.19 FUD 010

12053 5.1 cm to 7.5 cm
P2 T 6.20 9.64 FUD 010

12054 7.6 cm to 12.5 cm
A2 T 6.53 10.30 FUD 010

12055 12.6 cm to 20.0 cm
A2 T 8.67 13.36 FUD 010

12056 20.1 cm to 30.0 cm
A2 T 80 10.77 15.39 FUD 010

12057 over 30.0 cm
A2 T 80 10.86 15.75 FUD 010

13100-13160 Suturing of Complicated Wounds

CMS 100-4,14,10 General ASC Services

INCLUDES Creation of a limited defect for repair
Debridement complicated wounds/avulsions
More complicated than layered closure
Simple:
Exploration nerves, vessels, tendons in wound
Vessel ligation in wound
Total length of several repairs in same code category
Undermining, stents, retention sutures

EXCLUDES *Complex/secondary wound closure or dehiscence*
Debridement of open fracture/dislocation (15002-15005)
Excision:
Benign lesions (11400-11446)
Malignant lesions (11600-11646)
Extensive exploration (20100-20103)
Repair of nerves, blood vessel, tendons (See appropriate anatomical section. These repairs include simple and intermediate closure. Report complex closure with modifier 59.)
Surgical preparation of a wound bed (15002-15005)

Code also modifier 59 added to the less complicated procedure code if reporting more than one classification of wound repair

13100 Repair, complex, trunk; 1.1 cm to 2.5 cm
EXCLUDES *Complex repair 1.0 cm or less (12001, 12031)*
A2 T 5.86 9.32 FUD 010

13101 2.6 cm to 7.5 cm
A2 T 7.21 11.02 FUD 010

\+ 13102 **each additional 5 cm or less (List separately in addition to code for primary procedure)**
Code first (13101)
N1 N 2.14 3.42 FUD ZZZ

13120 Repair, complex, scalp, arms, and/or legs; 1.1 cm to 2.5 cm
EXCLUDES *Complex repair 1.0 cm or less (12001, 12031)*
A2 T 6.72 9.75 FUD 010

13121 2.6 cm to 7.5 cm
A2 T 7.61 11.89 FUD 010

\+ 13122 **each additional 5 cm or less (List separately in addition to code for primary procedure)**
Code first (13121)
N1 N 2.46 3.75 FUD ZZZ

13131 Repair, complex, forehead, cheeks, chin, mouth, neck, axillae, genitalia, hands and/or feet; 1.1 cm to 2.5 cm
EXCLUDES *Complex repair 1.0 cm or less (12001, 12011, 12031, 12041, 12051)*
A2 T 7.14 10.75 FUD 010

13132 2.6 cm to 7.5 cm
A2 T 8.96 13.27 FUD 010

\+ 13133 **each additional 5 cm or less (List separately in addition to code for primary procedure)**
Code first (13132)
N1 N 3.76 5.01 FUD ZZZ

13151 **Repair, complex, eyelids, nose, ears and/or lips; 1.1 cm to 2.5 cm**
EXCLUDES *Complex repair 1.0 cm or less (12011, 12051)*
A2 T ⚑ 8.19 11.79 FUD 010

13152 **2.6 cm to 7.5 cm**
A2 T ⚑ 9.93 14.14 FUD 010

\+ **13153** **each additional 5 cm or less (List separately in addition to code for primary procedure)**
Code first (13152)
N1 N ⚑ 4.07 5.46 FUD ZZZ

13160 **Secondary closure of surgical wound or dehiscence, extensive or complicated**
EXCLUDES *Packing or simple secondary wound closure (12020-12021)*
A2 T ⚑ 23.13 23.13 FUD 090

14000-14350 Reposition Contiguous Tissue

CMS 100-2,16,120 Cosmetic Procedures
CMS 100-4,14,10 Part B ASC Payment

INCLUDES Excision of lesion with repair by adjacent tissue transfer or tissue rearrangement
Size of defect includes primary (due to excision) and secondary (due to flap design)
Z-plasty, W-plasty, VY-plasty, rotation flap, advancement flap, double pedicle flap, random island flap

EXCLUDES *Closure of wounds by undermining surrounding tissue without additional incisions (13100-13160)*
Full thickness closure of:
Eyelid (67930-67935, 67961-67975)
Lip (40650-40654)

Code also skin graft necessary to repair secondary defect (15040-15731)

Example of common Z-plasty. Lesion is removed with oval-shaped incision

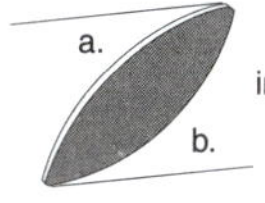

Two additional incisions (a. and b.) intersect the area

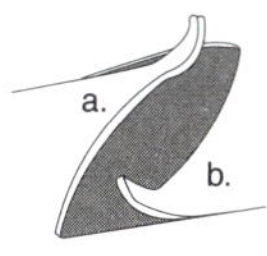

Skin of each incision is reflected back

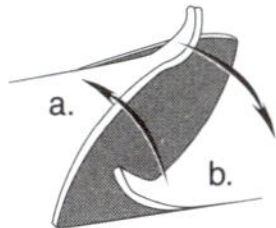

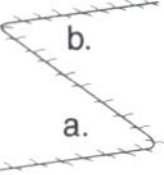

The flaps are then transposed and the repair is closed

An adjacent flap, or other rearrangement flap, is performed to repair a defect of 10 sq cm or less (14000); a larger defect (up to 30 sq cm) is coded 14001

14000 **Adjacent tissue transfer or rearrangement, trunk; defect 10 sq cm or less**
INCLUDES Burrow's operation
Do not report with (11400-11446, 11600-11646)
A2 T ⚑ PQ 14.30 17.48 FUD 090

14001 **defect 10.1 sq cm to 30.0 sq cm**
Do not report with (11400-11446, 11600-11646)
A2 T ⚑ PQ 18.59 22.43 FUD 090

14020 **Adjacent tissue transfer or rearrangement, scalp, arms and/or legs; defect 10 sq cm or less**
Do not report with (11400-11446, 11600-11646)
A2 T ⚑ PQ 16.20 19.59 FUD 090

14021 **defect 10.1 sq cm to 30.0 sq cm**
Do not report with (11400-11446, 11600-11646)
A2 T ⚑ PQ 20.45 24.45 FUD 090

14040 **Adjacent tissue transfer or rearrangement, forehead, cheeks, chin, mouth, neck, axillae, genitalia, hands and/or feet; defect 10 sq cm or less**
INCLUDES Krimer's palatoplasty
Do not report with (11400-11446, 11600-11646)
A2 T ⚑ PQ 18.04 21.44 FUD 090

14041 **defect 10.1 sq cm to 30.0 sq cm**
Do not report with (11400-11446, 11600-11646)
A2 T ⚑ PQ 22.12 26.45 FUD 090

14060 **Adjacent tissue transfer or rearrangement, eyelids, nose, ears and/or lips; defect 10 sq cm or less**
INCLUDES Denonvillier's operation
EXCLUDES *Eyelid, full thickness (67961-67966)*
Do not report with (11400-11446, 11600-11646)
A2 T ⚑ PQ 19.22 21.90 FUD 090

14061 **defect 10.1 sq cm to 30.0 sq cm**
EXCLUDES *Eyelid, full thickness (67961 and subsequent codes)*
Do not report with (11400-11446, 11600-11646)
A2 T ⚑ PQ 23.66 28.43 FUD 090

14301 **Adjacent tissue transfer or rearrangement, any area; defect 30.1 sq cm to 60.0 sq cm**
Do not report with (11400-11446, 11600-11646)
G2 T 80 PQ 25.22 30.36 FUD 090

\+ **14302** **each additional 30.0 sq cm, or part thereof (List separately in addition to code for primary procedure)**
Do not report with (11400-11446, 11600-11646)
Code first (14301)
N1 N 80 PQ 6.37 6.37 FUD ZZZ

14350 **Filleted finger or toe flap, including preparation of recipient site**
A2 T 80 ⚑ 20.29 20.29 FUD 090

15002-15005 Development of Base for Tissue Grafting

CMS 100-4,3,20.1.2.8 Special Payments for Burn Cases
CMS 100-4,14,10 Part B ASC Payment

INCLUDES Add together the surface area of multiple wounds in the same anatomical locations as indicated in the code descriptor groups, such as face and scalp. Do not add together multiple wounds at different anatomical site groups such as trunk and face
Ankle or wrist if code description describes leg or arm
Cleaning and preparing a viable wound surface for grafting or negative pressure wound therapy used to heal the wound primarily
Code selection based on the defect size and location
Percentage applies to children younger than age 10
Removal of nonviable tissue in nonchronic wounds for primary healing
Square centimeters applies to children and adults age 10 or older

EXCLUDES *Chronic wound management on wounds left to heal by secondary intention (11042-11047 [11045, 11046], 97597-97598)*
Necrotizing soft tissue infections for specific anatomical locations (11004-11008)

15002 **Surgical preparation or creation of recipient site by excision of open wounds, burn eschar, or scar (including subcutaneous tissues), or incisional release of scar contracture, trunk, arms, legs; first 100 sq cm or 1% of body area of infants and children**
EXCLUDES *Linear scar revision (13100-13153)*
A2 T 80 6.51 9.79 FUD 000

\+ **15003** **each additional 100 sq cm, or part thereof, or each additional 1% of body area of infants and children (List separately in addition to code for primary procedure)**
Code first (15002)
N1 N 80 1.31 2.14 FUD ZZZ

15004 **Surgical preparation or creation of recipient site by excision of open wounds, burn eschar, or scar (including subcutaneous tissues), or incisional release of scar contracture, face, scalp, eyelids, mouth, neck, ears, orbits, genitalia, hands, feet and/or multiple digits; first 100 sq cm or 1% of body area of infants and children**
A2 T 80 7.81 11.36 FUD 000

+ 15005 **each additional 100 sq cm, or part thereof, or each additional 1% of body area of infants and children (List separately in addition to code for primary procedure)**
Code first (15004)
N1 N 80 2.63 3.55 FUD ZZZ

15040 Obtain Autograft

CMS 100-4,3,20.1.2.8 Special Payments for Burn Cases

INCLUDES Ankle or wrist if code description describes leg or arm
Percentage applies to children younger than age 10
Square centimeters applies to children and adults age 10 or older

15040 **Harvest of skin for tissue cultured skin autograft, 100 sq cm or less**
A2 T 3.65 7.23 FUD 000

15050 Pinch Graft

INCLUDES Autologous skin graft harvest and application
Current graft removal
Fixation and anchoring skin graft
Simple cleaning

Code also graft or flap necessary to repair donor site
Do not report with (97602)

15050 **Pinch graft, single or multiple, to cover small ulcer, tip of digit, or other minimal open area (except on face), up to defect size 2 cm diameter**
A2 T 12.72 15.97 FUD 090

15100-15261 Skin Grafts and Replacements

CMS 100-4,3,20.1.2.8 Special Payments for Burn Cases
CMS 100-4,14,10 Part B ASC Payment

INCLUDES Add together the surface area of multiple wounds in the same anatomical locations as indicated in the code description groups, such as face and scalp. Do not add together multiple wounds at different anatomical site groups such as trunk and face.
Ankle or wrist if code description describes leg or arm
Autologous skin graft harvest and application
Code selection based on recipient site location and size and type of graft
Current graft removal
Fixation and anchoring skin graft
Percentage applies to children younger than age 10
Simple cleaning
Simple tissue debridement
Square centimeters applies to children and adults age 10 or older

EXCLUDES *Debridement without immediate primary closure, when wound is grossly contaminated and extensive cleaning is needed, or when necrotic or contaminated tissue is removed (11042-11044 [11045, 11046, 11047], 97597-97598)*

Code also graft or flap necessary to repair donor site
Code also primary procedure requiring skin graft for definitive closure
Do not report with (97602)

15100 **Split-thickness autograft, trunk, arms, legs; first 100 sq cm or less, or 1% of body area of infants and children (except 15050)**
A2 T 20.50 24.31 FUD 090

+ 15101 **each additional 100 sq cm, or each additional 1% of body area of infants and children, or part thereof (List separately in addition to code for primary procedure)**
Code first (15100)
N1 N 3.18 5.23 FUD ZZZ

15110 **Epidermal autograft, trunk, arms, legs; first 100 sq cm or less, or 1% of body area of infants and children**
A2 T 21.51 24.52 FUD 090

+ 15111 **each additional 100 sq cm, or each additional 1% of body area of infants and children, or part thereof (List separately in addition to code for primary procedure)**
Code first (15110)
N1 N 2.93 3.24 FUD ZZZ

15115 **Epidermal autograft, face, scalp, eyelids, mouth, neck, ears, orbits, genitalia, hands, feet, and/or multiple digits; first 100 sq cm or less, or 1% of body area of infants and children**
A2 T 21.66 24.64 FUD 090

+ 15116 **each additional 100 sq cm, or each additional 1% of body area of infants and children, or part thereof (List separately in addition to code for primary procedure)**
Code first (15115)
N1 N 3.88 4.30 FUD ZZZ

15120 **Split-thickness autograft, face, scalp, eyelids, mouth, neck, ears, orbits, genitalia, hands, feet, and/or multiple digits; first 100 sq cm or less, or 1% of body area of infants and children (except 15050)**
EXCLUDES *Other eyelid repair (67961-67975)*
A2 T 20.06 24.16 FUD 090

+ 15121 **each additional 100 sq cm, or each additional 1% of body area of infants and children, or part thereof (List separately in addition to code for primary procedure)**
EXCLUDES *Other eyelid repair (67961-67975)*
Code first (15120)
N1 N 3.78 5.84 FUD ZZZ

15130 **Dermal autograft, trunk, arms, legs; first 100 sq cm or less, or 1% of body area of infants and children**
A2 T 16.26 19.21 FUD 090

+ 15131 **each additional 100 sq cm, or each additional 1% of body area of infants and children, or part thereof (List separately in addition to code for primary procedure)**
Code first (15130)
N1 N 2.68 2.90 FUD ZZZ

15135 **Dermal autograft, face, scalp, eyelids, mouth, neck, ears, orbits, genitalia, hands, feet, and/or multiple digits; first 100 sq cm or less, or 1% of body area of infants and children**
A2 T 21.41 24.27 FUD 090

+ 15136 **each additional 100 sq cm, or each additional 1% of body area of infants and children, or part thereof (List separately in addition to code for primary procedure)**
Code first (15135)
N1 N 2.45 2.63 FUD ZZZ

15150 **Tissue cultured skin autograft, trunk, arms, legs; first 25 sq cm or less**
A2 T 17.89 19.54 FUD 090

+ 15151 **additional 1 sq cm to 75 sq cm (List separately in addition to code for primary procedure)**
EXCLUDES *Grafts over 75 sq cm (15152)*
Code first (15150)
Do not report more than one time per session
N1 N 3.13 3.38 FUD ZZZ

+ 15152 **each additional 100 sq cm, or each additional 1% of body area of infants and children, or part thereof (List separately in addition to code for primary procedure)**
Code first (15151)
N1 N 4.04 4.31 FUD ZZZ

15155 **Tissue cultured skin autograft, face, scalp, eyelids, mouth, neck, ears, orbits, genitalia, hands, feet, and/or multiple digits; first 25 sq cm or less**
A2 T 18.42 19.91 FUD 090

+ **15156** **additional 1 sq cm to 75 sq cm (List separately in addition to code for primary procedure)**
EXCLUDES *Grafts over 75 sq cm (15157)*
Code first (15155)
Do not report more than one time per session
N1 N 4.31 4.57 FUD ZZZ

+ **15157** **each additional 100 sq cm, or each additional 1% of body area of infants and children, or part thereof (List separately in addition to code for primary procedure)**
Code first (15156)
N1 N 4.36 4.66 FUD ZZZ

15200 **Full thickness graft, free, including direct closure of donor site, trunk; 20 sq cm or less**
A2 T 19.23 23.45 FUD 090

+ **15201** **each additional 20 sq cm, or part thereof (List separately in addition to code for primary procedure)**
Code first (15200)
N1 N 2.30 4.19 FUD ZZZ

15220 **Full thickness graft, free, including direct closure of donor site, scalp, arms, and/or legs; 20 sq cm or less**
A2 T 17.56 21.70 FUD 090

+ **15221** **each additional 20 sq cm, or part thereof (List separately in addition to code for primary procedure)**
Code first (15220)
N1 N 2.07 3.86 FUD ZZZ

15240 **Full thickness graft, free, including direct closure of donor site, forehead, cheeks, chin, mouth, neck, axillae, genitalia, hands, and/or feet; 20 sq cm or less**
EXCLUDES *Fingertip graft (15050)*
Syndactyly repair fingers (26560-26562)
A2 T 22.85 26.29 FUD 090

+ **15241** **each additional 20 sq cm, or part thereof (List separately in addition to code for primary procedure)**
Code first (15240)
N1 N 3.23 5.23 FUD ZZZ

15260 **Full thickness graft, free, including direct closure of donor site, nose, ears, eyelids, and/or lips; 20 sq cm or less**
EXCLUDES *Other eyelid repair (67961-67975)*
A2 T 24.52 28.51 FUD 090

+ **15261** **each additional 20 sq cm, or part thereof (List separately in addition to code for primary procedure)**
EXCLUDES *Other eyelid repair (67961-67975)*
Code first (15260)
N1 N 4.04 6.09 FUD ZZZ

15271-15278 Skin Substitute Graft Application

INCLUDES Add together the surface area of multiple wounds in the same anatomical locations as indicated in the code description groups, such as face and scalp. Do not add together multiple wounds at different anatomical site groups such as trunk and face.
Ankle or wrist if code description describes leg or arm
Code selection based on defect site location and size
Fixation and anchoring skin graft
Graft types include:
- Biological material used for scaffolding for growing skin
- Nonautologous human skin such as:
  - Acellular
  - Allograft
  - Cellular
  - Dermal
  - Epidermal
  - Homograft
- Nonhuman grafts

Percentage applies to children younger than age 10
Removing current graft
Simple cleaning
Simple tissue debridement
Square centimeters applies to children and adults age 10 or older

Code also biologic implant for soft tissue reinforcement (15777)
Code also primary procedure requiring skin graft for definitive closure
Code also supply of skin substitute product
Do not report for application of nongraft dressing
Do not report for injected skin substitutes
Do not report with (97602)

15271 **Application of skin substitute graft to trunk, arms, legs, total wound surface area up to 100 sq cm; first 25 sq cm or less wound surface area**
EXCLUDES *Total wound area greater than or equal to 100 sq cm (15273-15274)*
Do not report with (15273-15274)
G2 T 2.47 4.00 FUD 000

+ **15272** **each additional 25 sq cm wound surface area, or part thereof (List separately in addition to code for primary procedure)**
EXCLUDES *Total wound area greater than or equal to 100 sq cm (15273-15274)*
Code first (15271)
Do not report with (15273-15274)
N1 N 0.49 0.75 FUD ZZZ

15273 **Application of skin substitute graft to trunk, arms, legs, total wound surface area greater than or equal to 100 sq cm; first 100 sq cm wound surface area, or 1% of body area of infants and children**
EXCLUDES *Total wound surface area up to 100 cm (15271-15272)*
Do not report with (15271-15272)
G2 T 5.79 8.35 FUD 000

+ **15274** **each additional 100 sq cm wound surface area, or part thereof, or each additional 1% of body area of infants and children, or part thereof (List separately in addition to code for primary procedure)**
EXCLUDES *Total wound surface area up to 100 cm (15271-15272)*
Code first (15273)
N1 N 1.26 1.95 FUD ZZZ

15275 **Application of skin substitute graft to face, scalp, eyelids, mouth, neck, ears, orbits, genitalia, hands, feet, and/or multiple digits, total wound surface area up to 100 sq cm; first 25 sq cm or less wound surface area**
EXCLUDES *Total wound area greater than or equal to 100 sq cm (15277-15278)*
Do not report with (15277-15278)
G2 T 2.87 4.32 FUD 000

+ **15276** **each additional 25 sq cm wound surface area, or part thereof (List separately in addition to code for primary procedure)**
EXCLUDES *Total wound area greater than or equal to 100 sq cm (15277-15278)*
Code first (15275)
Do not report with (15277-15278)
N1 N 0.72 0.97 FUD ZZZ

15277 **Application of skin substitute graft to face, scalp, eyelids, mouth, neck, ears, orbits, genitalia, hands, feet, and/or multiple digits, total wound surface area greater than or equal to 100 sq cm; first 100 sq cm wound surface area, or 1% of body area of infants and children**
EXCLUDES *Total surface area up to 100 sq cm (15275-15276)*
Do not report with (15275-15276)
G2 T 6.32 8.93 FUD 000

+ **15278** **each additional 100 sq cm wound surface area, or part thereof, or each additional 1% of body area of infants and children, or part thereof (List separately in addition to code for primary procedure)**
EXCLUDES *Total surface area up to 100 sq cm (15275-15276)*
Code first (15277)
Do not report with (15275-15276)
N1 N 1.57 2.33 FUD ZZZ

15570-15731 Wound Reconstruction: Skin Flaps

CMS 100-4,3,20.1.2.8 Special Payments for Burn Cases

INCLUDES Ankle or wrist if code description describes leg or arm
Code based on recipient site when the flap is attached in the transfer or to a final site and is based on donor site when a tube is created for transfer later or when the flap is delayed prior to transfer
Fixation and anchoring skin graft
Simple tissue debridement
Tube formation for later transfer

EXCLUDES *Contiguous tissue transfer flaps (14000-14302)*
Debridement without immediate primary closure (11042-11047 [11045, 11046], 97597-97598)
Excision of:
Benign lesion (11400-11471)
Burn eschar or scar (15002-15005)
Malignant lesion (11600-11646)
Microvascular repair (15756-15758)
Primary procedure such as radical mastectomy, extensive tumor removal, orbitectomy (see appropriate anatomical site)

Code also application of extensive immobilization apparatus
Code also repair of donor site with skin grafts or flaps

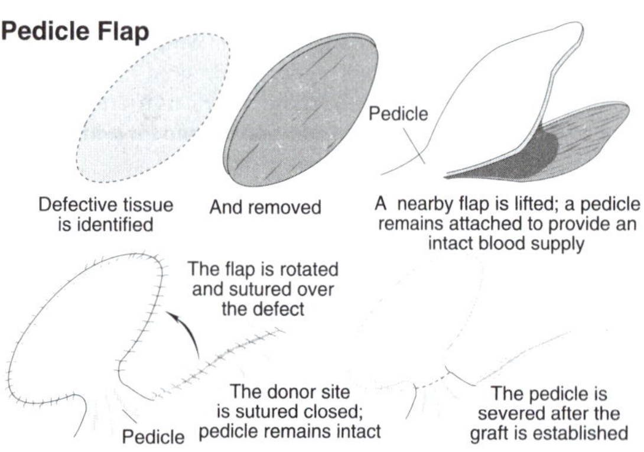

15570 **Formation of direct or tubed pedicle, with or without transfer; trunk**
INCLUDES Flaps without a vascular pedicle
A2 T 21.16 25.90 FUD 090

15572 **scalp, arms, or legs**
INCLUDES Flaps without a vascular pedicle
A2 T 21.31 25.06 FUD 090

15574 **forehead, cheeks, chin, mouth, neck, axillae, genitalia, hands or feet**
INCLUDES Flaps without a vascular pedicle
A2 T 22.00 25.90 FUD 090

15576 **eyelids, nose, ears, lips, or intraoral**
INCLUDES Flaps without a vascular pedicle
A2 T 19.32 22.92 FUD 090

15600 **Delay of flap or sectioning of flap (division and inset); at trunk**
A2 T 80 5.87 9.00 FUD 090

15610 **at scalp, arms, or legs**
A2 T 80 6.84 9.95 FUD 090

15620 **at forehead, cheeks, chin, neck, axillae, genitalia, hands, or feet**
A2 T 9.30 12.38 FUD 090

15630 **at eyelids, nose, ears, or lips**
A2 T 9.87 12.91 FUD 090

15650 **Transfer, intermediate, of any pedicle flap (eg, abdomen to wrist, Walking tube), any location**
EXCLUDES *Defatting, revision, or rearranging of transferred pedicle flap or skin graft (13100-14302)*
Eyelids, ears, lips, and nose - refer to anatomical area
A2 T 80 10.96 14.28 FUD 090

15731 **Forehead flap with preservation of vascular pedicle (eg, axial pattern flap, paramedian forehead flap)**
EXCLUDES *Muscle, myocutaneous, or fasciocutaneous flap of the head or neck (15732)*
A2 T 80 29.04 32.18 FUD 090

15732-15738 Wound Reconstruction: Muscle Flaps

INCLUDES Code based on donor site

EXCLUDES *Contiguous tissue transfer flaps (14000-14302)*
Microvascular repair (15756-15758)

Code also application of extensive immobilization apparatus
Code also repair of donor site with skin grafts or flaps

15732 **Muscle, myocutaneous, or fasciocutaneous flap; head and neck (eg, temporalis, masseter muscle, sternocleidomastoid, levator scapulae)**
EXCLUDES *Forehead flap with preservation of vascular pedicle (15731)*
A2 T 32.66 37.02 FUD 090

15734 **trunk**
A2 T 80 PQ 37.90 42.66 FUD 090

15736 **upper extremity**
A2 T 32.88 37.57 FUD 090

15738 **lower extremity**
A2 T 80 PQ 35.68 40.11 FUD 090

15740-15758 Wound Reconstruction: Other

CMS 100-4,3,20.1.2.8 Special Payments for Burn Cases
CMS 104-4,12,30 Correct Coding Policy

INCLUDES Fixation and anchoring skin graft
Routine dressing
Simple tissue debridement

EXCLUDES *Adjacent tissue transfer (14000-14302)*
Excision of:
Benign lesion (11400-11471)
Burn eschar or scar (15002-15005)
Malignant lesion (11600-11646)
Flaps without addition of a vascular pedicle (15570-15576)
Primary procedure such as radical mastectomy, extensive tumor removal, orbitectomy (see appropriate anatomical section)
Skin graft for repair of donor site (15050-15278)

Code also repair of donor site with skin grafts or flaps (14000-14350, 15050-15278)

15740 **Flap; island pedicle requiring identification and dissection of an anatomically named axial vessel**
EXCLUDES *V-Y subcutaneous flaps, random island flaps, and other flaps from adjacent areas (14000-14302)*
A2 T 24.31 28.66 FUD 090

15750 **neurovascular pedicle**
EXCLUDES *V-Y subcutaneous flaps, random island flaps, and other flaps from adjacent areas (14000-14302)*
A2 T 80 26.16 26.16 FUD 090

15756 **Free muscle or myocutaneous flap with microvascular anastomosis**
INCLUDES Includes operating microscope (69990)
C 80 67.22 67.22 FUD 090

15757 **Free skin flap with microvascular anastomosis**
INCLUDES Includes operating microscope (69990)
C 80 66.33 66.33 FUD 090

15758 **Free fascial flap with microvascular anastomosis**
INCLUDES Includes operating microscope (69990)
C 80 66.37 66.37 FUD 090

15760-15770 Grafts Comprising Multiple Tissue Types

CMS 100-4,3,20.1.2.8 Special Payments for Burn Cases

INCLUDES Fixation and anchoring skin graft
Routine dressing
Simple tissue debridement

EXCLUDES *Adjacent tissue transfer (14000-14302)*
Excision of:
Benign lesion (11400-11471)
Burn eschar or scar (15002-15005)
Malignant lesion (11600-11646)
Flaps without addition of vascular pedicle (15570-15576)
Microvascular repair (15756-15758)
Primary procedure such as extensive tumor removal (see appropriate anatomical site)
Repair of donor site with skin grafts or flaps (14000-14350, 15050-15278)
Skin graft (15050-15278)

15760 **Graft; composite (eg, full thickness of external ear or nasal ala), including primary closure, donor area**
A2 T 20.34 24.20 FUD 090

15770 **derma-fat-fascia**
A2 T 80 19.41 19.41 FUD 090

15775-15839 Plastic, Reconstructive, and Aesthetic Surgery

CMS 100-2,16,10 Exclusions from Coverage
CMS 100-2,16,120 Cosmetic Procedures
CMS 100-2,16,180 Services Related to Noncovered Procedures

Hair shaft within follicle
Epidermis
Sebaceous gland attached to hair follicle
Ecrine sweat gland with duct open directly to surface
Typical male pattern hair loss
Apocrine sweat gland connected by duct to a hair follicle

15775 **Punch graft for hair transplant; 1 to 15 punch grafts**
EXCLUDES *Strip transplant (15220)*
A2 T 80 6.15 8.27 FUD 000

15776 **more than 15 punch grafts**
EXCLUDES *Strip transplant (15220)*
A2 T 80 9.68 13.52 FUD 000

+ **15777** **Implantation of biologic implant (eg, acellular dermal matrix) for soft tissue reinforcement (ie, breast, trunk) (List separately in addition to code for primary procedure)**
EXCLUDES *Application of skin substitute to an external wound (15271-15278)*
Mesh implantation for:
Open repair of ventral or incisional hernia (49568)
Repair of devitalized soft tissue infection (49568)
Repair of pelvic floor (57267)
Repair anorectal fistula with plug (46707)
Soft tissue reinforcement with biologic implants other than in the breast or trunk (17999)
Code also supply of biologic implant
Code first primary procedure
N1 N 50 6.12 6.12 FUD ZZZ

15780 **Dermabrasion; total face (eg, for acne scarring, fine wrinkling, rhytids, general keratosis)**
P3 T 80 17.93 23.56 FUD 090

15781 **segmental, face**
P3 T 12.29 15.54 FUD 090

15782 **regional, other than face**
P2 T 80 12.63 17.82 FUD 090

15783 **superficial, any site (eg, tattoo removal)**
P2 T 80 10.54 13.49 FUD 090

15786 **Abrasion; single lesion (eg, keratosis, scar)**
P2 T 3.96 6.98 FUD 010

+ **15787** **each additional 4 lesions or less (List separately in addition to code for primary procedure)**
Code first (15786)
N1 N 0.51 1.39 FUD ZZZ

15788 **Chemical peel, facial; epidermal**
P2 T 7.11 12.93 FUD 090

15789 **dermal**
P2 T 11.56 15.09 FUD 090

15792 **Chemical peel, nonfacial; epidermal**
P2 T 80 7.35 12.09 FUD 090

15793 **dermal**
P2 T 80 10.31 13.68 FUD 090

15819 **Cervicoplasty**
G2 T 80 21.05 21.05 FUD 090

15820 **Blepharoplasty, lower eyelid;**
A2 T 80 50 15.16 16.68 FUD 090

15821 **with extensive herniated fat pad**
A2 T 80 50 16.08 17.79 FUD 090

15822 **Blepharoplasty, upper eyelid;**
A2 T 50 11.38 12.88 FUD 090

15823 **with excessive skin weighting down lid**
A2 T 50 16.09 17.81 FUD 090

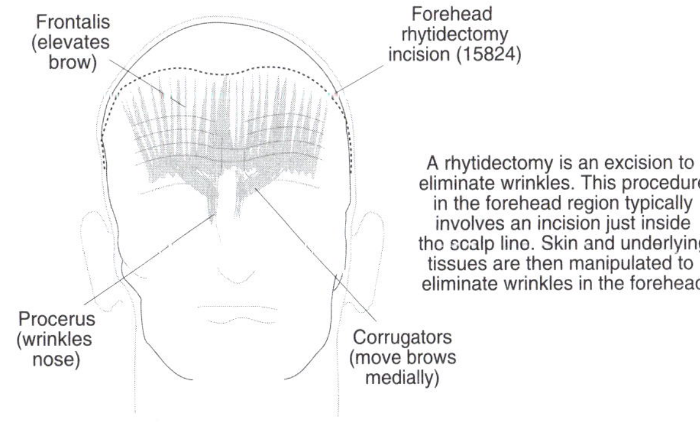

15824 **Rhytidectomy; forehead**
EXCLUDES *Repair of brow ptosis (67900)*
A2 T 80 50 0.00 0.00 FUD 000

15825	neck with platysmal tightening (platysmal flap, P-flap) A2 T 80 50 0.00 0.00 FUD 000
15826	glabellar frown lines A2 T 80 50 0.00 0.00 FUD 000
15828	cheek, chin, and neck A2 T 80 50 0.00 0.00 FUD 000
15829	superficial musculoaponeurotic system (SMAS) flap A2 T 80 50 0.00 0.00 FUD 000

15830 **Excision, excessive skin and subcutaneous tissue (includes lipectomy); abdomen, infraumbilical panniculectomy**

EXCLUDES *Other abdominoplasty (17999)*

Code also (15847)

Do not report with (12031-12032, 12034-12037, 13100-13102, 14000-14001, 14302)

A2 T 80 33.61 33.61 FUD 090

15832 **thigh** A2 T 80 50 26.33 26.33 FUD 090

15833 **leg** A2 T 80 50 25.11 25.11 FUD 090

15834 **hip** A2 T 80 50 25.61 25.61 FUD 090

15835 **buttock** A2 T 80 27.04 27.04 FUD 090

15836 **arm** A2 T 80 50 21.85 21.85 FUD 090

15837 **forearm or hand** G2 T 80 18.66 22.49 FUD 090

15838 **submental fat pad** G2 T 80 16.35 16.35 FUD 090

15839 **other area** A2 T 80 21.12 25.10 FUD 090

15840-15845 Reanimation of the Paralyzed Face

CMS 100-2,15,260 Covered ASC Procedures

CMS 100-4,12,40.7 Bilateral Procedures

INCLUDES Routine dressing and supplies

EXCLUDES *Intravenous fluorescein evaluation of blood flow in graft or flap (15860)*

Nerve:

Decompression (69720, 69725, 69955)

Pedicle transfer (64905, 64907)

Suture (64831-64876, 69740, 69745)

Code also repair of donor site with skin grafts or flaps

15840 **Graft for facial nerve paralysis; free fascia graft (including obtaining fascia)** A2 T 29.31 29.31 FUD 090

15841 **free muscle graft (including obtaining graft)** A2 T 80 46.01 46.01 FUD 090

15842 **free muscle flap by microsurgical technique**

INCLUDES Operating microscope (69990)

G2 T 80 75.99 75.99 FUD 090

15845 **regional muscle transfer** A2 T 80 29.25 29.25 FUD 090

15847 Removal of Excess Abdominal Tissue Add-on

\+ 15847 **Excision, excessive skin and subcutaneous tissue (includes lipectomy), abdomen (eg, abdominoplasty) (includes umbilical transposition and fascial plication) (List separately in addition to code for primary procedure)**

EXCLUDES *Abdominal wall hernia repair (49491-49587)*

Other abdominoplasty (17999)

Code first (15830)

N1 N 80 0.00 0.00 FUD YYY

15850-15852 Suture Removal/Dressing Change: Anesthesia Required

CMS 100-4,12,40.1 Global Surgery Package Definition

CMS 100-4,12,50 Anesthesia Services

15850 **Removal of sutures under anesthesia (other than local), same surgeon** G2 T 1.13 2.44 FUD XXX

15851 **Removal of sutures under anesthesia (other than local), other surgeon** P3 T 1.33 2.78 FUD 000

15852 **Dressing change (for other than burns) under anesthesia (other than local)**

EXCLUDES *Dressing change for burns (16020-16030)*

R2 X 1.34 1.34 FUD 000

15860 Injection for Vascular Flow Determination

15860 **Intravenous injection of agent (eg, fluorescein) to test vascular flow in flap or graft** G2 X 80 3.20 3.20 FUD 000

15876-15879 Liposuction

CMS 100-2,16,10 Exclusions from Coverage

CMS 100-2,16,120 Cosmetic Procedures

CMS 100-2,16,180 Services Related to Noncovered Procedures

CMS 100-4,12,20.4.3 Payment for Assistant at Surgery

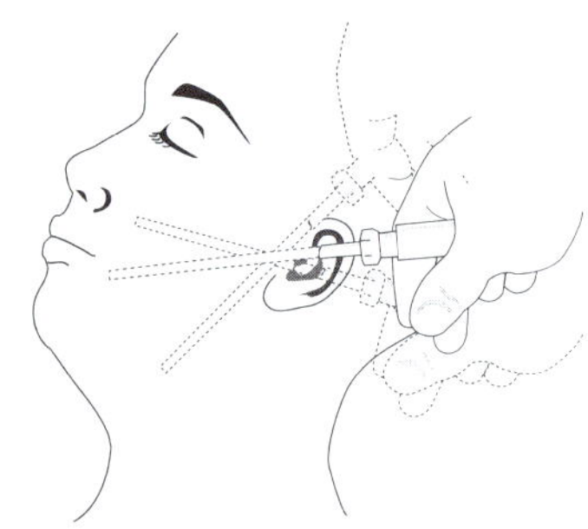

15876 **Suction assisted lipectomy; head and neck** A2 T 80 0.00 0.00 FUD 000

15877 **trunk** A2 T 80 0.00 0.00 FUD 000

15878 **upper extremity** A2 T 80 50 0.00 0.00 FUD 000

15879 **lower extremity** A2 T 80 50 0.00 0.00 FUD 000

15920-15999 Treatment of Decubitus Ulcers

CMS 100-3,270.4 Treatment of Decubitus

CMS 100-4,12,20.4.3 Payment for Assistant at Surgery

CMS 100-4,12,40.6 Multiple procedures

CMS 100-4,12,40.8 Co-surgery and team surgery

Code also free skin graft to repair ulcer or donor site

15920 **Excision, coccygeal pressure ulcer, with coccygectomy; with primary suture** A2 T 80 17.30 17.30 FUD 090

15922 **with flap closure** A2 T 80 22.47 22.47 FUD 090

15931 **Excision, sacral pressure ulcer, with primary suture;** A2 T 19.49 19.49 FUD 090

15933 **with ostectomy** A2 T 80 24.32 24.32 FUD 090

15934 **Excision, sacral pressure ulcer, with skin flap closure;** A2 T 26.35 26.35 FUD 090

15935 **with ostectomy**
A2 T 80 ☐ 31.21 31.21 FUD 090

15936 **Excision, sacral pressure ulcer, in preparation for muscle or myocutaneous flap or skin graft closure;**
Code also any defect repair with:
Muscle or myocutaneous flap (15734 and/or 15738)
Split skin graft (15100 and/or 15101)
A2 T ☐ 25.59 25.59 FUD 090

15937 **with ostectomy**
Code also any defect repair with:
Muscle or myocutaneous flap (15734 and/or 15738)
Split skin graft (15100 and/or 15101)
A2 T ☐ 29.82 29.82 FUD 090

15940 **Excision, ischial pressure ulcer, with primary suture;**
A2 T ☐ 19.99 19.99 FUD 090

15941 **with ostectomy (ischiectomy)**
A2 T 80 ☐ 25.86 25.86 FUD 090

15944 **Excision, ischial pressure ulcer, with skin flap closure;**
A2 T 80 ☐ 25.47 25.47 FUD 090

15945 **with ostectomy**
A2 T 80 ☐ 28.05 28.05 FUD 090

15946 **Excision, ischial pressure ulcer, with ostectomy, in preparation for muscle or myocutaneous flap or skin graft closure**
Code also any defect repair with:
Muscle or myocutaneous flap (15734 and/or 15738)
Split skin graft (15100 and/or 15101)
A2 T ☐ 47.09 47.09 FUD 090

15950 **Excision, trochanteric pressure ulcer, with primary suture;**
A2 T ☐ 16.86 16.86 FUD 090

15951 **with ostectomy**
A2 T 80 ☐ 25.28 25.28 FUD 090

15952 **Excision, trochanteric pressure ulcer, with skin flap closure;**
A2 T 80 ☐ 26.24 26.24 FUD 090

15953 **with ostectomy**
A2 T ☐ 28.64 28.64 FUD 090

15956 **Excision, trochanteric pressure ulcer, in preparation for muscle or myocutaneous flap or skin graft closure;**
Code also any defect repair with:
Muscle or myocutaneous flap (15734 and/or 15738)
Split skin graft (15100 and/or 15101)
A2 T ☐ 33.30 33.30 FUD 090

15958 **with ostectomy**
Code also any defect repair with:
Muscle or myocutaneous flap (15734 and/or 15738)
Split skin graft (15100 and/or 15101)
A2 T ☐ 33.73 33.73 FUD 090

15999 **Unlisted procedure, excision pressure ulcer**
T 80 0.00 0.00 FUD YYY

16000-16036 Burn Care

CMS 100-4,3,20.1.2.8 Special Payments for Burn Cases

INCLUDES Local care of burn surface only

EXCLUDES *Application of skin grafts including all services described in the following codes (15100-15777)*
Evaluation and management services
Flaps (15570-15650)

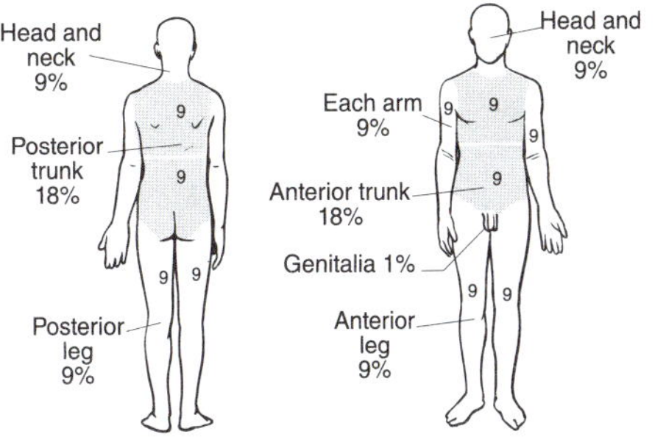

16000 **Initial treatment, first degree burn, when no more than local treatment is required**
P2 T ☐ 1.32 1.95 FUD 000

16020 **Dressings and/or debridement of partial-thickness burns, initial or subsequent; small (less than 5% total body surface area)**
INCLUDES Wound coverage other than skin graft
P3 T ☐ 1.55 2.30 FUD 000

16025 **medium (eg, whole face or whole extremity, or 5% to 10% total body surface area)**
INCLUDES Wound coverage other than skin graft
A2 T ☐ 3.21 4.17 FUD 000

16030 **large (eg, more than 1 extremity, or greater than 10% total body surface area)**
INCLUDES Wound coverage other than skin graft
A2 T ☐ 3.88 5.28 FUD 000

16035 **Escharotomy; initial incision**
EXCLUDES *Debridement or scraping of burn (16020-16030)*
G2 T ☐ 5.70 5.70 FUD 000

\+ 16036 **each additional incision (List separately in addition to code for primary procedure)**
EXCLUDES *Debridement or scraping of burn (16020-16030)*
Code first (16035)
C 2.35 2.35 FUD ZZZ

17000-17004 Destruction Any Method: Premalignant Lesion

CMS 100-2,16,10 Exclusions from Coverage
CMS 100-2,16,120 Cosmetic Procedures
CMS 100-2,16,180 Services Related to Noncovered Procedures
CMS 100-3,140.5 Laser Procedures
CMS 100-4,12,40.6 Multiple procedures

EXCLUDES *Cryotherapy acne (17340)*
Destruction of:
Benign lesions other than cutaneous vascular proliferative lesions (17110-17111)
Cutaneous vascular proliferative lesions (17106-17108)
Malignant lesions (17260-17286)
Plantar warts (17110-17111)
Destruction of lesion of:
Anus (46900-46917, 46924)
Conjunctiva (68135)
Eyelid (67850)
Penis (54050-54057, 54065)
Vagina (57061, 57065)
Vestibule of mouth (40820)
Vulva (56501, 56515)
Destruction or excision of skin tags (11200-11201)
Localized chemotherapy treatment see appropriate office visit service code
Paring or excision of benign hyperkeratotic lesion (11055-11057)
Shaving skin lesions (11300-11313)
Treatment of inflammatory skin disease via laser (96920-96922)

17000 **Destruction (eg, laser surgery, electrosurgery, cryosurgery, chemosurgery, surgical curettement), premalignant lesions (eg, actinic keratoses); first lesion**
P2 T 1.49 2.10 FUD 010

\+ **17003** **second through 14 lesions, each (List separately in addition to code for first lesion)**
Code first (17000)
N1 N 0.07 0.28 FUD ZZZ

⊘ **17004** **Destruction (eg, laser surgery, electrosurgery, cryosurgery, chemosurgery, surgical curettement), premalignant lesions (eg, actinic keratoses), 15 or more lesions**
Do not report with (17000-17003)
P3 T 2.82 4.17 FUD 010

17106-17250 Destruction Any Method: Vascular Proliferative Lesion

CMS 100-2,16,10 Exclusions from Coverage
CMS 100-2,16,120 Cosmetic Procedures
CMS 100-2,16,180 Services Related to Noncovered Procedures

EXCLUDES *Destruction of lesion of:*
Anus (46900-46917, 46924)
Conjunctiva (68135)
Eyelid (67850)
Penis (54050-54057, 54065)
Vagina (57061, 57065)
Vestibule of mouth (40820)
Vulva (56501, 56515)
Treatment of inflammatory skin disease via laser (96920-96922)

17106 **Destruction of cutaneous vascular proliferative lesions (eg, laser technique); less than 10 sq cm**
P2 T 7.73 9.46 FUD 090

17107 **10.0 to 50.0 sq cm**
P2 T 9.93 12.24 FUD 090

17108 **over 50.0 sq cm**
P2 T 80 14.86 17.82 FUD 090

17110 **Destruction (eg, laser surgery, electrosurgery, cryosurgery, chemosurgery, surgical curettement), of benign lesions other than skin tags or cutaneous vascular proliferative lesions; up to 14 lesions**
P2 T 1.95 3.05 FUD 010

17111 **15 or more lesions**
P2 T 2.40 3.62 FUD 010

17250 **Chemical cauterization of granulation tissue (proud flesh, sinus or fistula)**
Do not report with excision/removal codes for the same lesion
P3 T 1.06 2.22 FUD 000

17260-17286 Destruction, Any Method: Malignant Lesion

CMS 100-3,140.5 Laser Procedures
CMS 100-4,12,30 Correct Coding Policy

EXCLUDES *Destruction of lesion of:*
Anus (46900-46917, 46924)
Conjunctiva (68135)
Eyelid (67850)
Penis (54050-54057, 54065)
Vestibule of mouth (40820)
Vulva (56501-56515)
Localized chemotherapy treatment see appropriate office visit service code
Shaving skin lesion (11300-11313)
Treatment of inflammatory skin disease via laser (96920-96922)

17260 **Destruction, malignant lesion (eg, laser surgery, electrosurgery, cryosurgery, chemosurgery, surgical curettement), trunk, arms or legs; lesion diameter 0.5 cm or less**
P3 T 1.96 2.61 FUD 010

17261 **lesion diameter 0.6 to 1.0 cm**
P2 T 2.59 3.98 FUD 010

17262 **lesion diameter 1.1 to 2.0 cm**
P2 T 3.29 4.85 FUD 010

17263 **lesion diameter 2.1 to 3.0 cm**
P2 T 3.65 5.30 FUD 010

17264 **lesion diameter 3.1 to 4.0 cm**
P2 T 3.91 5.70 FUD 010

17266 **lesion diameter over 4.0 cm**
P3 T 4.58 6.47 FUD 010

17270 **Destruction, malignant lesion (eg, laser surgery, electrosurgery, cryosurgery, chemosurgery, surgical curettement), scalp, neck, hands, feet, genitalia; lesion diameter 0.5 cm or less**
P2 T 2.83 4.17 FUD 010

17271 **lesion diameter 0.6 to 1.0 cm**
P2 T 3.15 4.54 FUD 010

17272 **lesion diameter 1.1 to 2.0 cm**
P2 T 3.62 5.17 FUD 010

17273 **lesion diameter 2.1 to 3.0 cm**
P3 T 4.11 5.78 FUD 010

17274 **lesion diameter 3.1 to 4.0 cm**
P3 T 4.99 6.83 FUD 010

17276 **lesion diameter over 4.0 cm**
P3 T 6.03 7.94 FUD 010

17280 **Destruction, malignant lesion (eg, laser surgery, electrosurgery, cryosurgery, chemosurgery, surgical curettement), face, ears, eyelids, nose, lips, mucous membrane; lesion diameter 0.5 cm or less**
P2 T 2.57 3.91 FUD 010

17281 **lesion diameter 0.6 to 1.0 cm**
P3 T 3.54 4.94 FUD 010

17282 **lesion diameter 1.1 to 2.0 cm**
P3 T 4.09 5.68 FUD 010

17283 **lesion diameter 2.1 to 3.0 cm**
P3 T 5.09 6.81 FUD 010

17284 **lesion diameter 3.1 to 4.0 cm**
P3 T 5.95 7.79 FUD 010

17286 **lesion diameter over 4.0 cm**
P2 T 8.03 10.05 FUD 010

17311-17315 Mohs Surgery

CMS 100-4,12,40.1 Global Surgery Package Definition

INCLUDES The following surgical/pathology services performed by the same physician or other qualified health care provider:
Evaluation of skin margins by surgeon
Pathology exam on Mohs surgery specimen (88302-88309)
Routine frozen section stain (88314)
Tumor removal, mapping, preparation, and examination of lesion

EXCLUDES *Frozen section if no prior diagnosis determination has been performed (88331)*

Code also any special histochemical stain on a frozen section, nonroutine (with modifier 59) (88311-88314, 88342)
Code also biopsy (with modifier 59) if no prior diagnosis determination has been performed, if biopsy is indeterminate, or performed more than 90 days preoperatively (11100-11101)
Code also complex repair (13100-13160)
Code also flaps or grafts (14000-14350, 15050-15770)
Code also intermediate repair (12031-12057)
Code also simple repair (12001-12021)

17311 **Mohs micrographic technique, including removal of all gross tumor, surgical excision of tissue specimens, mapping, color coding of specimens, microscopic examination of specimens by the surgeon, and histopathologic preparation including routine stain(s) (eg, hematoxylin and eosin, toluidine blue), head, neck, hands, feet, genitalia, or any location with surgery directly involving muscle, cartilage, bone, tendon, major nerves, or vessels; first stage, up to 5 tissue blocks**
P2 T P0 10.72 18.32 FUD 000

+ **17312** **each additional stage after the first stage, up to 5 tissue blocks (List separately in addition to code for primary procedure)**
Code first (17311)
N1 N 5.69 10.74 FUD ZZZ

17313 **Mohs micrographic technique, including removal of all gross tumor, surgical excision of tissue specimens, mapping, color coding of specimens, microscopic examination of specimens by the surgeon, and histopathologic preparation including routine stain(s) (eg, hematoxylin and eosin, toluidine blue), of the trunk, arms, or legs; first stage, up to 5 tissue blocks**
P2 T P0 9.62 17.13 FUD 000

+ **17314** **each additional stage after the first stage, up to 5 tissue blocks (List separately in addition to code for primary procedure)**
Code first (17313)
N1 N 5.28 10.30 FUD ZZZ

+ **17315** **Mohs micrographic technique, including removal of all gross tumor, surgical excision of tissue specimens, mapping, color coding of specimens, microscopic examination of specimens by the surgeon, and histopathologic preparation including routine stain(s) (eg, hematoxylin and eosin, toluidine blue), each additional block after the first 5 tissue blocks, any stage (List separately in addition to code for primary procedure)**
Code first (17311-17314)
N1 N 1.49 2.21 FUD ZZZ

17340-17999 Treatment for Active Acne and Permanent Hair Removal

17340 **Cryotherapy (CO2 slush, liquid N2) for acne**
P3 T 1.40 1.47 FUD 010

17360 **Chemical exfoliation for acne (eg, acne paste, acid)**
P3 T 2.81 3.61 FUD 010

17380 **Electrolysis epilation, each 30 minutes**
EXCLUDES *Actinotherapy (96900)*
R2 T 80 0.00 0.00 FUD 000

17999 **Unlisted procedure, skin, mucous membrane and subcutaneous tissue**
T 80 0.00 0.00 FUD YYY

19000-19030 Treatment of Breast Abscess and Cyst with Injection, Aspiration, Incision

19000 **Puncture aspiration of cyst of breast;**
76942, 77021
P3 T 1.26 3.16 FUD 000

+ **19001** **each additional cyst (List separately in addition to code for primary procedure)**
Code first (19000)
76942, 77021
N1 N 0.62 0.76 FUD ZZZ

19020 **Mastotomy with exploration or drainage of abscess, deep**
A2 T 50 8.62 13.20 FUD 090

19030 **Injection procedure only for mammary ductogram or galactogram**
77053-77054
N1 N 50 2.22 4.60 FUD 000

19081-19086 Breast Biopsy with Imaging Guidance

CMS 100-2,15,260 Covered ASC Procedures
CMS 100-3,220.13 Percutaneous Image-guided Breast Biopsy
CMS 100-4,13,80.1 Supervision and Interpretation Codes
CMS 100-4,13,80.2 Physician Presence

INCLUDES Breast biopsy with placement of localization devices

EXCLUDES *Biopsy of breast without imaging guidance (19100-19101)*
Lesion removal without concentration on surgical margins (19110-19126)
Open biopsy after placement of localization device (19101, 19281-19288)
Partial mastectomy (19301-19302)
Placement of localization devices only (19281-19288)
Total mastectomy (19303-19307)

Code also additional biopsies performed with different imaging modalities
Do not report for same lesion with (19281-19288, 76098, 76942, 77002, 77021)

19081 **Biopsy, breast, with placement of breast localization device(s) (eg, clip, metallic pellet), when performed, and imaging of the biopsy specimen, when performed, percutaneous; first lesion, including stereotactic guidance**
G2 T 80 50 5.23 19.04 FUD 000

+ **19082** **each additional lesion, including stereotactic guidance (List separately in addition to code for primary procedure)**
Code first (19081)
N1 N 80 2.49 15.38 FUD ZZZ

19083 **Biopsy, breast, with placement of breast localization device(s) (eg, clip, metallic pellet), when performed, and imaging of the biopsy specimen, when performed, percutaneous; first lesion, including ultrasound guidance**
G2 T 80 50 4.90 18.91 FUD 000

+ **19084** **each additional lesion, including ultrasound guidance (List separately in addition to code for primary procedure)**
Code first (19083)
N1 N 80 2.34 15.17 FUD ZZZ

19085 **Biopsy, breast, with placement of breast localization device(s) (eg, clip, metallic pellet), when performed, and imaging of the biopsy specimen, when performed, percutaneous; first lesion, including magnetic resonance guidance**
G2 T 80 50 5.72 28.62 FUD 000

+ **19086** **each additional lesion, including magnetic resonance guidance (List separately in addition to code for primary procedure)**
Code first (19085)
N1 N 80 2.55 22.81 FUD ZZZ

19100-19101 Breast Biopsy Without Imaging Guidance

EXCLUDES *Biopsy of breast with imaging guidance (19081-19086)*
Lesion removal without concentration on surgical margins (19110-19126)
Partial mastectomy (19301-19302)
Total mastectomy (19303-19307)

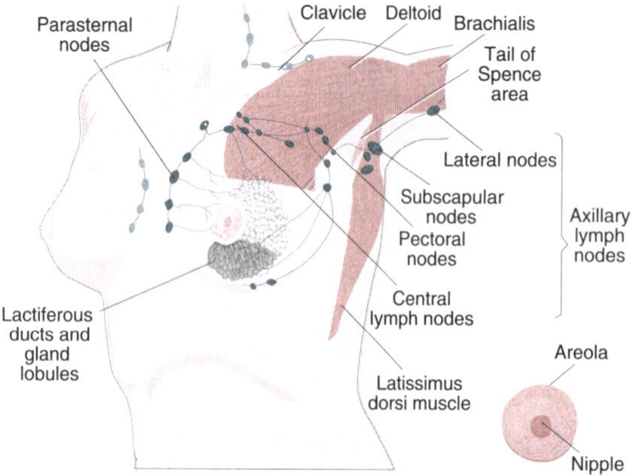

19100 Biopsy of breast; percutaneous, needle core, not using imaging guidance (separate procedure)
EXCLUDES *Fine needle aspiration:*
With imaging guidance (10022)
Without imaging guidance (10021)
A2 T 50 PQ 1.98 4.22 FUD 000

19101 open, incisional
Code also placement of localization device with imaging guidance (19281-19288)
A2 T 50 PQ 6.25 9.53 FUD 010

19105 Treatment of Fibroadenoma: Cryoablation

CMS 100-4,13,80.1 Supervision and Interpretation Codes
CMS 100-4,13,80.2 Physician Presence
INCLUDES Adjacent lesions treated with one cryoprobe
Ultrasound guidance

19105 Ablation, cryosurgical, of fibroadenoma, including ultrasound guidance, each fibroadenoma
Do not report with (76940, 76942)
P2 T 50 5.46 53.96 FUD 000

19110-19126 Excisional Procedures: Breast

CMS 100-4,12,40.7 Bilateral Procedures
INCLUDES Open removal of breast mass without concentration on surgical margins

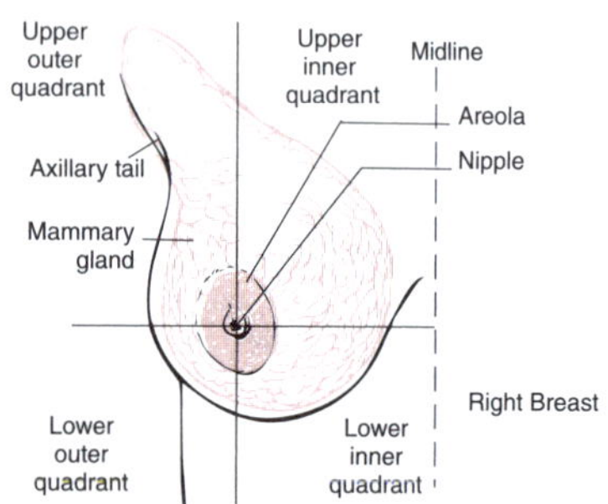

19110 Nipple exploration, with or without excision of a solitary lactiferous duct or a papilloma lactiferous duct
A2 T 50 9.64 13.59 FUD 090

19112 Excision of lactiferous duct fistula
A2 T 80 50 8.81 12.88 FUD 090

19120 Excision of cyst, fibroadenoma, or other benign or malignant tumor, aberrant breast tissue, duct lesion, nipple or areolar lesion (except 19300), open, male or female, 1 or more lesions
A2 T 50 11.68 13.87 FUD 090

19125 Excision of breast lesion identified by preoperative placement of radiological marker, open; single lesion
A2 T 50 PQ 12.97 15.38 FUD 090

+ **19126 each additional lesion separately identified by a preoperative radiological marker (List separately in addition to code for primary procedure)**
Code first (19125)
N1 N 4.60 4.60 FUD ZZZ

19260-19272 Excisional Procedures: Chest Wall

CMS 100-4,12,20.4.3 Payment for Assistant at Surgery
Do not report with (32100, 32503-32504, 32551, 32554-32555)

19260 Excision of chest wall tumor including ribs
T 80 PQ 34.37 34.37 FUD 090

19271 Excision of chest wall tumor involving ribs, with plastic reconstruction; without mediastinal lymphadenectomy
C 80 PQ 46.21 46.21 FUD 090

19272 with mediastinal lymphadenectomy
C 80 PQ 51.63 51.63 FUD 090

19281-19288 Placement of Localization Markers

CMS 100-4,12,40.7 Bilateral Procedures
CMS 100-4,13,80.1 Supervision and Interpretation Codes
CMS 100-4,13,80.2 Physician Presence
INCLUDES Placement of localization devices only
EXCLUDES *Biopsy of breast without imaging guidance (19100-19101)*
Localization device placement with biopsy of breast (19081-19086)
Code also radiography of surgical specimen (76098)
Code also open incisional breast biopsy when performed after localization device placement (19101)
Do not report for same lesion with (19081-19086, 76942, 77002, 77021)

19281 Placement of breast localization device(s) (eg, clip, metallic pellet, wire/needle, radioactive seeds), percutaneous; first lesion, including mammographic guidance
N1 Q2 80 50 2.93 6.86 FUD 000

+ **19282 each additional lesion, including mammographic guidance (List separately in addition to code for primary procedure)**
Code first (19281)
N1 N 80 1.40 4.76 FUD ZZZ

19283 Placement of breast localization device(s) (eg, clip, metallic pellet, wire/needle, radioactive seeds), percutaneous; first lesion, including stereotactic guidance
N1 Q2 80 50 2.96 7.79 FUD 000

+ **19284 each additional lesion, including stereotactic guidance (List separately in addition to code for primary procedure)**
Code first (19283)
N1 N 80 1.41 5.71 FUD ZZZ

19285 Placement of breast localization device(s) (eg, clip, metallic pellet, wire/needle, radioactive seeds), percutaneous; first lesion, including ultrasound guidance
N1 Q2 80 50 2.51 13.18 FUD 000

+ **19286 each additional lesion, including ultrasound guidance (List separately in addition to code for primary procedure)**
Code first (19285)
N1 N 80 1.21 11.05 FUD ZZZ

19287 Placement of breast localization device(s) (eg clip, metallic pellet, wire/needle, radioactive seeds), percutaneous; first lesion, including magnetic resonance guidance
N1 Q2 80 50 4.08 24.42 FUD 000

+ **19288** each additional lesion, including magnetic resonance guidance (List separately in addition to code for primary procedure)
Code first (19287)
N1 N 80 1.81 19.44 FUD ZZZ

19296-19298 Insertion Radiotherapy Afterloading Catheters

19296 Placement of radiotherapy afterloading expandable catheter (single or multichannel) into the breast for interstitial radioelement application following partial mastectomy, includes imaging guidance; on date separate from partial mastectomy
Code also (C1728)
G2 T 80 50 5.97 111.03 FUD 000

+ **19297** concurrent with partial mastectomy (List separately in addition to code for primary procedure)
Code also (C1728)
Code first (19301-19302)
G2 T 80 2.68 2.68 FUD ZZZ

⊙ **19298** Placement of radiotherapy afterloading brachytherapy catheters (multiple tube and button type) into the breast for interstitial radioelement application following (at the time of or subsequent to) partial mastectomy, includes imaging guidance
Code also (C1728)
G2 T 80 50 9.26 29.37 FUD 000

19300-19307 Mastectomies: Partial, Simple, Radical

CMS 100-4,12,20.4.3 Payment for Assistant at Surgery
CMS 100-4,12,40.7 Bilateral Procedures
EXCLUDES *Insertion of prosthesis (19340, 19342)*

19300 Mastectomy for gynecomastia ♂
A2 T 50 11.64 14.68 FUD 090

19301 Mastectomy, partial (eg, lumpectomy, tylectomy, quadrantectomy, segmentectomy);
EXCLUDES *Insertion of radiotherapy afterloading balloon or brachytherapy catheters (19296-19298)*
A2 T 80 50 PQ 18.46 18.46 FUD 090

19302 with axillary lymphadenectomy
EXCLUDES *Insertion of radiotherapy afterloading balloon or brachytherapy catheters (19296-19298)*
A2 T 80 50 PQ 25.42 25.42 FUD 090

19303 Mastectomy, simple, complete
EXCLUDES *Gynecomastia (19300)*
A2 T 80 50 PQ 28.59 28.59 FUD 090

19304 Mastectomy, subcutaneous
A2 T 80 50 PQ 16.15 16.15 FUD 090

19305 Mastectomy, radical, including pectoral muscles, axillary lymph nodes
C 80 50 PQ 32.01 32.01 FUD 090

19306 Mastectomy, radical, including pectoral muscles, axillary and internal mammary lymph nodes (Urban type operation)
C 80 50 PQ 33.92 33.92 FUD 090

19307 Mastectomy, modified radical, including axillary lymph nodes, with or without pectoralis minor muscle, but excluding pectoralis major muscle
T 80 50 PQ 33.84 33.84 FUD 090

19316-19499 Plastic, Reconstructive, and Aesthetic Breast Procedures

CMS 100-2,16,120 Cosmetic Procedures
CMS 100-2,16,180 Services Related to Noncovered Procedures
CMS 100-3,140.2 Breast Reconstruction Following Mastectomy
CMS 100-4,12,40.7 Bilateral Procedures
Code also biologic implant for tissue reinforcement (15777)

19316 Mastopexy
A2 T 80 50 PQ 22.12 22.12 FUD 090

19318 Reduction mammaplasty ♀
INCLUDES Aries-Pitanguy mammaplasty
Biesenberger mammaplasty
A2 T 80 50 PQ 31.87 31.87 FUD 090

19324 Mammaplasty, augmentation; without prosthetic implant
A2 T 80 50 PQ 13.85 13.85 FUD 090

19325 with prosthetic implant
EXCLUDES *Flap or graft (15100-15650)*
Code also (C1789, L8600)
G2 T 80 50 PQ 18.55 18.55 FUD 090

19328 Removal of intact mammary implant
A2 Q2 50 PQ 14.23 14.23 FUD 090

19330 Removal of mammary implant material
A2 Q2 50 PQ 18.20 18.20 FUD 090

19340 Immediate insertion of breast prosthesis following mastopexy, mastectomy or in reconstruction
EXCLUDES *Supply of prosthetic implant (99070, L8030, L8039, L8600)*
A2 T 50 28.95 28.95 FUD 090

19342 Delayed insertion of breast prosthesis following mastopexy, mastectomy or in reconstruction
EXCLUDES *Preparation of moulage for custom breast implant (19396)*
Code also (C1789, L8600)
G2 T 80 50 PQ 26.59 26.59 FUD 090

19350 Nipple/areola reconstruction
A2 T 50 PQ 19.38 23.46 FUD 090

19355 Correction of inverted nipples
A2 T 80 50 PQ 16.13 19.73 FUD 090

19357 Breast reconstruction, immediate or delayed, with tissue expander, including subsequent expansion
G2 T 80 50 PQ 43.26 43.26 FUD 090

19361 Breast reconstruction with latissimus dorsi flap, without prosthetic implant
EXCLUDES *Implant of prosthesis (19340)*
C 80 50 PQ 45.59 45.59 FUD 090

19364 Breast reconstruction with free flap
INCLUDES Closure of donor site
Harvesting of skin graft
Inset shaping of flap into breast
Microvascular repair
Operating microscope (69990)
C 80 50 PQ 79.89 79.89 FUD 090

19366 Breast reconstruction with other technique
EXCLUDES *Operating microscope (69990)*
Code also implant of prosthesis if appropriate (19340, 19342)
A2 T 80 50 PQ 40.45 40.45 FUD 090

19367 Breast reconstruction with transverse rectus abdominis myocutaneous flap (TRAM), single pedicle, including closure of donor site;
C 80 50 PQ 51.89 51.89 FUD 090

19368 with microvascular anastomosis (supercharging)
INCLUDES Operating microscope (69990)
C 80 50 PQ 63.86 63.86 FUD 090

19369 Breast reconstruction with transverse rectus abdominis myocutaneous flap (TRAM), double pedicle, including closure of donor site
C 80 50 PQ 59.25 59.25 FUD 090

Integumentary System

19287 — 19369

19370 **Open periprosthetic capsulotomy, breast**
A2 T 50 PQ 19.73 19.73 FUD 090

19371 **Periprosthetic capsulectomy, breast**
A2 T 50 PQ 22.59 22.59 FUD 090

19380 **Revision of reconstructed breast**
A2 T 50 PQ 22.25 22.25 FUD 090

19396 **Preparation of moulage for custom breast implant**
G2 T 80 50 4.26 8.27 FUD 000

19499 **Unlisted procedure, breast**
T 80 50 0.00 0.00 FUD YYY

20005 Incisional Treatment Soft Tissue Abscess

EXCLUDES *Superficial incision and drainage (10040-10160)*

20005 Incision and drainage of soft tissue abscess, subfascial (ie, involves the soft tissue below the deep fascia)
62 T ▪ 6.68 8.74 FUD 010

20100-20103 Exploratory Surgery of Traumatic Wound

INCLUDES Debridement
Expanded dissection of wound for exploration
Extraction of foreign material
Open examination
Tying or coagulation of small vessels

EXCLUDES *Cutaneous/subcutaneous incision and drainage procedures (10060-10061)*
Laparotomy (49000-49010)
Repair of major vessels of:
Abdomen (35221, 35251, 35281)
Chest (35211, 35216, 35241, 35246, 35271, 35276)
Extremity (35206-35207, 35226, 35236, 35256, 35266, 35286)
Neck (35201, 35231, 35261)
Thoracotomy (32100-32160)

20100 Exploration of penetrating wound (separate procedure); neck
T 80 50 ▪ 17.31 17.31 FUD 010

20101 chest
T ▪ 5.91 12.67 FUD 010

20102 abdomen/flank/back
T ▪ 7.27 13.83 FUD 010

20103 extremity
62 T 80 ▪ 9.98 16.43 FUD 010

20150 Epiphyseal Bar Resection

EXCLUDES *Bone marrow aspiration (38220)*

20150 Excision of epiphyseal bar, with or without autogenous soft tissue graft obtained through same fascial incision
62 T 80 50 ▪ 26.10 26.10 FUD 090

20200-20206 Muscle Biopsy

EXCLUDES *Removal of muscle tumor (see appropriate anatomic section)*

20200 Biopsy, muscle; superficial
A2 T ▪ PQ 2.72 5.82 FUD 000

20205 deep
A2 T ▪ PQ 4.42 8.10 FUD 000

20206 Biopsy, muscle, percutaneous needle
INCLUDES Fluoroscopic guidance (77002)
EXCLUDES *Fine needle aspiration (10021-10022)*
76942, 77012, 77021
88172-88173
A2 T ▪ PQ 1.71 6.61 FUD 000

20220-20225 Percutaneous Bone Biopsy

CMS 100-3,150.3 Bone (Mineral) Density Studies

EXCLUDES *Bone marrow biopsy (38221)*

20220 Biopsy, bone, trocar, or needle; superficial (eg, ilium, sternum, spinous process, ribs)
77002, 77012, 77021
A2 T ▪ PQ 2.09 4.74 FUD 000

20225 deep (eg, vertebral body, femur)
Do not report at same level as (22510-22515, 0200T-0201T)
77002, 77012, 77021
A2 T ▪ PQ 3.18 14.82 FUD 000

20240-20251 Open Bone Biopsy

CMS 100-3,150.3 Bone (Mineral) Density Studies

EXCLUDES *Sequestrectomy or incision and drainage of bone abscess of:*
Calcaneus (28120)
Carpal bone (25145)
Clavicle (23170)
Humeral head (23174)
Humerus (24134)
Olecranon process (24138)
Radius (24136, 25145)
Scapula (23172)
Skull (61501)
Talus (28120)
Ulna (24138, 24145)

20240 Biopsy, bone, open; superficial (eg, ilium, sternum, spinous process, ribs, trochanter of femur)
A2 T ▪ PQ 6.28 6.28 FUD 010

20245 deep (eg, humerus, ischium, femur)
A2 T ▪ PQ 17.75 17.75 FUD 010

20250 Biopsy, vertebral body, open; thoracic
A2 T ▪ PQ 11.06 11.06 FUD 010

20251 lumbar or cervical
A2 T 80 ▪ PQ 12.04 12.04 FUD 010

20500-20501 Injection Fistula/Sinus Tract

CMS 100-4,13,80.1 Supervision and Interpretation Codes
CMS 100-4,13,80.2 Physician Presence

EXCLUDES *Arthrography injection of:*
Ankle (27648)
Elbow (24220)
Hip (27093, 27095)
Knee (27370)
Sacroiliac joint (27096)
Shoulder (23350)
Temporomandibular joint (TMJ) (21116)
Wrist (25246)

20500 Injection of sinus tract; therapeutic (separate procedure)
76080
P3 T ▪ 2.41 2.96 FUD 010

20501 diagnostic (sinogram)
EXCLUDES *Contrast injection or injections for radiological evaluation of existing gastrostomy, duodenostomy, jejunostomy, gastro-jejunostomy, or cecostomy (or other colonic) tube from percutaneous approach (49465)*
76080
N1 N ▪ 1.10 3.31 FUD 000

20520-20525 Foreign Body Removal

CMS 100-4,12,30 Correct Coding Policy

20520 Removal of foreign body in muscle or tendon sheath; simple
P3 T ▪ 4.18 5.75 FUD 010

20525 deep or complicated
A2 T ▪ 7.09 13.51 FUD 010

20526-20553 Therapeutic Injections: Tendons, Trigger Points

CMS 100-3,150.7 Prolotherapy, Joint Sclerotherapy, and Ligamentous Injections with Sclerosing Agents
CMS 100-4,12,30 Correct Coding Policy
CMS 100-4,13,80.1 Supervision and Interpretation Codes
CMS 100-4,13,80.2 Physician Presence

EXCLUDES *Platelet rich plasma (PRP) injections (0232T)*

20526 Injection, therapeutic (eg, local anesthetic, corticosteroid), carpal tunnel
P3 T 50 ▪ 1.62 2.15 FUD 000

20527 **Injection, enzyme (eg, collagenase), palmar fascial cord (ie, Dupuytren's contracture)**
EXCLUDES *Post injection palmar fascial cord manipulation (26341)*
P3 T 50 1.86 2.34 FUD 000

20550 **Injection(s); single tendon sheath, or ligament, aponeurosis (eg, plantar "fascia")**
EXCLUDES *Morton's neuroma (64455, 64632)*
Do not report with (0232T)
76942, 77002, 77021
P3 T 50 1.19 1.65 FUD 000

20551 **single tendon origin/insertion**
EXCLUDES *Platelet rich plasma injection (0232T)*
Do not report with (0232T)
76942, 77002, 77021
P3 T 1.22 1.71 FUD 000

20552 **single or multiple trigger point(s), 1 or 2 muscle(s)**
76942, 77002, 77021
P3 T 1.09 1.56 FUD 000

20553 **single or multiple trigger point(s), 3 or more muscle(s)**
76942, 77002, 77021
P3 T 1.23 1.80 FUD 000

20555 Placement of Catheters/Needles for Brachytherapy

Do not report with (0232T)

20555 **Placement of needles or catheters into muscle and/or soft tissue for subsequent interstitial radioelement application (at the time of or subsequent to the procedure)**
EXCLUDES *Interstitial radioelement:*
Devices placed into the breast (19296-19298)
Placement of needle, catheters, or devices into muscle or soft tissue of the head and neck (41019)
Placement of needles or catheters into pelvic organs or genitalia (55920)
Placement of needles or catheters into prostate (55875)
Radioelement application (77776-77778, 77785-77787)
76942, 77002, 77012, 77021
R2 T 80 9.53 9.53 FUD 000

20600-20611 Aspiration and/or Injection of Joint

CMS 100-3,150.6 Vitamin B12 Injections to Strengthen Tendons, Ligaments of Foot
CMS 100-3,150.7 Prolotherapy, Joint Sclerotherapy, and Ligamentous Injections with Sclerosing Agents
CMS 100-4,12,30 Correct Coding Policy
CMS 100-4,13,80.1 Supervision and Interpretation Codes
CMS 100-4,13,80.2 Physician Presence

▲ **20600** **Arthrocentesis, aspiration and/or injection, small joint or bursa (eg, fingers, toes); without ultrasound guidance**
Do not report with (76942)
77002, 77012, 77021
P3 T 50 1.02 1.35 FUD 000

● **20604** **with ultrasound guidance, with permanent recording and reporting**
Do not report with (76942)
77002, 77012, 77021

▲ **20605** **intermediate joint or bursa (eg, temporomandibular, acromioclavicular, wrist, elbow or ankle, olecranon bursa)**
Do not report with (76942)
77002, 77012, 77021
P3 T 50 1.07 1.41 FUD 000

● **20606** **with ultrasound guidance, with permanent recording and reporting**
Do not report with (76942)
77002, 77012, 77021

▲ **20610** **without ultrasound guidance**
Do not report with (27370, 76942)
77002, 77012, 77021
P3 T 50 1.32 1.70 FUD 000

● **20611** **with ultrasound guidance, with permanent recording and reporting**
Do not report with (27370, 76942)
77002, 77012, 77021

20612-20615 Aspiration and/or Injection of Cyst

CMS 100-4,12,30 Correct Coding Policy

20612 **Aspiration and/or injection of ganglion cyst(s) any location**
Code also modifier 59 for multiple major joint aspirations or injections
P3 T 1.19 1.70 FUD 000

20615 **Aspiration and injection for treatment of bone cyst**
P3 T 4.65 6.88 FUD 010

20650-20697 Procedures Related to Bony Fixation

CMS 100-4,12,30 Correct Coding Policy

20650 **Insertion of wire or pin with application of skeletal traction, including removal (separate procedure)**
A2 T 4.41 5.78 FUD 010

20660 **Application of cranial tongs, caliper, or stereotactic frame, including removal (separate procedure)**
Q2 6.93 6.93 FUD 000

20661 **Application of halo, including removal; cranial**
C 14.33 14.33 FUD 090

20662 **pelvic**
A2 T 80 12.49 12.49 FUD 090

20663 **femoral**
A2 T 80 50 12.83 12.83 FUD 090

20664 **Application of halo, including removal, cranial, 6 or more pins placed, for thin skull osteology (eg, pediatric patients, hydrocephalus, osteogenesis imperfecta)**
C 24.68 24.68 FUD 090

20665 **Removal of tongs or halo applied by another individual**
G2 Q2 80 2.57 2.97 FUD 010

20670 **Removal of implant; superficial (eg, buried wire, pin or rod) (separate procedure)**
A2 Q2 4.20 10.67 FUD 010

20680 **deep (eg, buried wire, pin, screw, metal band, nail, rod or plate)**
A2 Q2 80 12.15 17.55 FUD 090

20690 **Application of a uniplane (pins or wires in 1 plane), unilateral, external fixation system**
A2 T 16.92 16.92 FUD 090

20692 **Application of a multiplane (pins or wires in more than 1 plane), unilateral, external fixation system (eg, Ilizarov, Monticelli type)**
A2 T 80 31.96 31.96 FUD 090

20693 **Adjustment or revision of external fixation system requiring anesthesia (eg, new pin[s] or wire[s] and/or new ring[s] or bar[s])**
A2 T 12.83 12.83 FUD 090

20694 **Removal, under anesthesia, of external fixation system**
A2 Q2 9.63 12.02 FUD 090

20696 **Application of multiplane (pins or wires in more than 1 plane), unilateral, external fixation with stereotactic computer-assisted adjustment (eg, spatial frame), including imaging; initial and subsequent alignment(s), assessment(s), and computation(s) of adjustment schedule(s)**
Do not report with (20692, 20697)
G2 T 80 — 32.28 — 32.28 FUD 090

⊘ 20697 **exchange (ie, removal and replacement) of strut, each**
Do not report with (20692, 20696)
P2 T TC 80 — 51.93 — 51.93 FUD 000

20802-20838 Reimplantation Procedures

CMS 100-4,12,30 Correct Coding Policy
CMS 100-4,12,40.1 Global Surgery Package Definition

EXCLUDES *Repair of incomplete amputation (see individual repair codes for bone(s), ligament(s), tendon(s), nerve(s), or blood vessel(s) and append modifier 52)*

20802 **Replantation, arm (includes surgical neck of humerus through elbow joint), complete amputation**
C 80 50 — 66.35 — 66.35 FUD 090

20805 **Replantation, forearm (includes radius and ulna to radial carpal joint), complete amputation**
C 80 50 — 87.57 — 87.57 FUD 090

20808 **Replantation, hand (includes hand through metacarpophalangeal joints), complete amputation**
C 80 50 — 113.61 — 113.61 FUD 090

20816 **Replantation, digit, excluding thumb (includes metacarpophalangeal joint to insertion of flexor sublimis tendon), complete amputation**
C 80 — 56.88 — 56.88 FUD 090

20822 **Replantation, digit, excluding thumb (includes distal tip to sublimis tendon insertion), complete amputation**
G2 T 80 — 52.20 — 52.20 FUD 090

20824 **Replantation, thumb (includes carpometacarpal joint to MP joint), complete amputation**
C 80 50 — 61.18 — 61.18 FUD 090

20827 **Replantation, thumb (includes distal tip to MP joint), complete amputation**
C 80 50 — 52.09 — 52.09 FUD 090

20838 **Replantation, foot, complete amputation**
C 80 50 — 74.59 — 74.59 FUD 090

20900-20926 Bone and Tissue Autografts

CMS 100-4,12,30 Correct Coding Policy

EXCLUDES *Acquisition of autogenous bone graft, cartilage, tendon, fascia lata through distinct incision unless included in the code description*
Bone graft procedures on the spine (20930-20938)

20900 **Bone graft, any donor area; minor or small (eg, dowel or button)**
A2 T 80 — 5.49 — 11.88 FUD 000

20902 **major or large**
A2 T 80 — 8.22 — 8.22 FUD 000

20910 **Cartilage graft; costochondral**
EXCLUDES *Graft with ear cartilage (21235)*
A2 T 80 — 11.74 — 11.74 FUD 090

20912 **nasal septum**
EXCLUDES *Graft with ear cartilage (21235)*
A2 T 80 — 13.81 — 13.81 FUD 090

20920 **Fascia lata graft; by stripper**
A2 T — 11.31 — 11.31 FUD 090

20922 **by incision and area exposure, complex or sheet**
A2 T 80 — 14.28 — 17.43 FUD 090

20924 **Tendon graft, from a distance (eg, palmaris, toe extensor, plantaris)**
A2 T 80 — 14.39 — 14.39 FUD 090

20926 **Tissue grafts, other (eg, paratenon, fat, dermis)**
Do not report with (0232T)
A2 T — 12.53 — 12.53 FUD 090

20930-20938 Bone Allograft and Autograft of Spine

CMS 100-4,12,40.1 Global Surgery Package Definition

EXCLUDES *Bone marrow aspiration for bone grafting (38220)*

+ 20930 **Allograft, morselized, or placement of osteopromotive material, for spine surgery only (List separately in addition to code for primary procedure)**
Code first (22319, 22532-22533, 22548-22558, 22590-22612, 22630, 22633-22634, 22800-22812)
N1 N — 0.00 — 0.00 FUD XXX

+ 20931 **Allograft, structural, for spine surgery only (List separately in addition to code for primary procedure)**
Code first (22319, 22532-22533, 22548-22558, 22590-22612, 22630, 22633-22634, 22800-22812)
N1 N — 3.23 — 3.23 FUD ZZZ

+ 20936 **Autograft for spine surgery only (includes harvesting the graft); local (eg, ribs, spinous process, or laminar fragments) obtained from same incision (List separately in addition to code for primary procedure)**
Code first (22319, 22532-22533, 22548-22558, 22590-22612, 22630, 22633-22634, 22800-22812)
C — 0.00 — 0.00 FUD XXX

+ 20937 **morselized (through separate skin or fascial incision) (List separately in addition to code for primary procedure)**
Code first (22319, 22532-22533, 22548-22558, 22590-22612, 22630, 22633-22634, 22800-22812)
C 80 — 4.82 — 4.82 FUD ZZZ

+ 20938 **structural, bicortical or tricortical (through separate skin or fascial incision) (List separately in addition to code for primary procedure)**
Code first (22319, 22532-22533, 22548-22558, 22590-22612, 22630, 22633-22634, 22800-22812)
C 80 — 5.28 — 5.28 FUD ZZZ

20950 Measurement of Intracompartmental Pressure

CMS 100-4,12,20.4.3 Payment for Assistant at Surgery
CMS 100-4,12,30 Correct Coding Policy

20950 **Monitoring of interstitial fluid pressure (includes insertion of device, eg, wick catheter technique, needle manometer technique) in detection of muscle compartment syndrome**
G2 T 80 — 2.60 — 7.06 FUD 000

20955-20973 Bone and Osteocutaneous Grafts

CMS 100-4,12,20.4.3 Payment for Assistant at Surgery
CMS 100-4,12,30 Correct Coding Policy

INCLUDES Operating microscope (69990)

20955 **Bone graft with microvascular anastomosis; fibula**
C 80 — 72.26 — 72.26 FUD 090

20956 **iliac crest**
C 80 — 75.82 — 75.82 FUD 090

20957 **metatarsal**
C 80 — 65.63 — 65.63 FUD 090

20962 **other than fibula, iliac crest, or metatarsal**
C 80 — 62.90 — 62.90 FUD 090

20969 **Free osteocutaneous flap with microvascular anastomosis; other than iliac crest, metatarsal, or great toe**
C 80 — 80.10 — 80.10 FUD 090

20970 iliac crest
C 80 ⚑ 82.04 82.04 FUD 090

20972 metatarsal
G2 T 80 ⚑ 63.11 63.11 FUD 090

20973 great toe with web space
EXCLUDES *Wrap-around repair (26551)*
R2 T 80 50 ⚑ 80.77 80.77 FUD 090

20974-20979 Osteogenic Stimulation

CMS 100-3,150.2 Osteogenic Stimulation
CMS 100-4,12,20.4.3 Payment for Assistant at Surgery
CMS 100-4,12,30 Correct Coding Policy

⊘ 20974 **Electrical stimulation to aid bone healing; noninvasive (nonoperative)**
A ⚑ 1.41 2.13 FUD 000

⊘ 20975 **invasive (operative)**
N1 N 80 ⚑ 5.05 5.05 FUD 000

20979 **Low intensity ultrasound stimulation to aid bone healing, noninvasive (nonoperative)**
P3 X ⚑ 0.94 1.50 FUD 000

20982-20999 General Musculoskeletal Procedures

CMS 100-4,12,20.4.3 Payment for Assistant at Surgery
CMS 100-4,12,30 Correct Coding Policy
CMS 100-4,12,40.7 Bilateral Procedures

⊙ ▲ 20982 **Ablation therapy for reduction or eradication of 1 or more bone tumors (eg, metastasis) including adjacent soft tissue when involved by tumor extension, percutaneous, including imaging guidance when performed; radiofrequency**
Do not report with (76940, 77002, 77013, 77022)
G2 T 50 ⚑ 10.93 103.83 FUD 000

⊙ ● 20983 **cryoablation**
Do not report with (76940, 77002, 77013, 77022)

\+ 20985 **Computer-assisted surgical navigational procedure for musculoskeletal procedures, image-less (List separately in addition to code for primary procedure)**
EXCLUDES *Image guidance derived from intraoperative and preoperative obtained images (0054T-0055T)*
Code first primary procedure
Do not report with (61781-61783)
N1 N 80 4.23 4.23 FUD ZZZ

20999 **Unlisted procedure, musculoskeletal system, general**
T 80 0.00 0.00 FUD YYY

21010 Temporomandibular Joint Arthrotomy

21010 **Arthrotomy, temporomandibular joint**
EXCLUDES *Excision of foreign body from dentoalveolar site (41805-41806)*
Soft tissue (subfascial) abscess drainage (20005)
Superficial abscess and hematoma drainage (10060-10061)
A2 T 80 50 ⚑ 21.41 21.41 FUD 090

21011-21016 Excision Soft Tissue Tumors Face and Scalp

CMS 100-4,12,30 Correct Coding Policy
CMS 100-4,14,10 General ASC Services

INCLUDES Any necessary elevation of tissue planes or dissection
Measurement of tumor and necessary margin at greatest diameter prior to excision
Simple and intermediate repairs
Types of excisions:
Fascial or subfascial soft tissue tumors: simple and marginal resection of tumors found either in or below the deep fascia, not including bone or excision of a substantial amount of normal tissue; primarily benign and intramuscular tumors
Radical resection soft tissue tumor: wide resection of tumor involving substantial margins of normal tissue and may include tissue removal from one or more layers; most often malignant or aggressive benign
Subcutaneous: simple and marginal resection of tumors in the subcutaneous tissue above the deep fascia; most often benign

EXCLUDES *Complex repair*
Excision of benign cutaneous lesions (eg, sebaceous cyst) (11420-11426)
Radical resection of cutaneous tumors (eg, melanoma) (11620-11646)
Significant exploration of vessels or neuroplasty

21011 **Excision, tumor, soft tissue of face or scalp, subcutaneous; less than 2 cm**
P3 T 80 7.29 9.74 FUD 090

21012 **2 cm or greater**
R2 T 80 9.53 9.53 FUD 090

21013 **Excision, tumor, soft tissue of face and scalp, subfascial (eg, subgaleal, intramuscular); less than 2 cm**
P3 T 80 11.32 14.55 FUD 090

21014 **2 cm or greater**
R2 T 80 14.74 14.74 FUD 090

21015 **Radical resection of tumor (eg, sarcoma), soft tissue of face or scalp; less than 2 cm**
EXCLUDES *Removal of cranial tumor for osteomyelitis (61501)*
G2 T ⚑ 20.35 20.35 FUD 090

21016 **2 cm or greater**
G2 T 80 29.67 29.67 FUD 090

21025-21070 Procedures of Cranial and Facial Bones

INCLUDES Any necessary elevation of tissue planes or dissection
Measurement of tumor and necessary margins prior to excision
Radical resection of bone tumor involves resection of the tumor (may include entire bone) and wide margins of normal tissue primarily for malignant or aggressive benign tumors
Simple and intermediate repairs

EXCLUDES *Complex repair*
Radical resection of cutaneous tumors (e.g., melanoma) (11620-11646)
Significant exploration of vessels, neuroplasty, reconstruction, or complex bone repair

Do not report excision of soft tissue codes when adjacent soft tissue is removed during the bone tumor resection (21011-21016)

21025 **Excision of bone (eg, for osteomyelitis or bone abscess); mandible**
A2 T ⚑ 21.59 25.52 FUD 090

21026 **facial bone(s)**
A2 T ⚑ 14.32 17.66 FUD 090

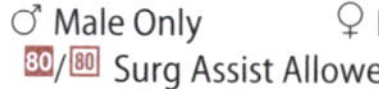
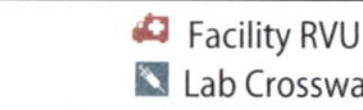

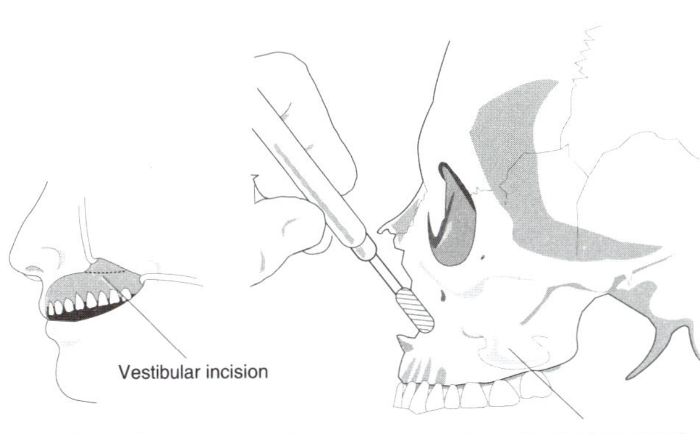

Burs, files, and osteotomes used to remove bone Area of benign bone growth

21029 **Removal by contouring of benign tumor of facial bone (eg, fibrous dysplasia)**
A2 T 80 | 18.66 | 22.29 | FUD 090

21030 **Excision of benign tumor or cyst of maxilla or zygoma by enucleation and curettage**
P3 T 50 | 12.05 | 14.90 | FUD 090

21031 **Excision of torus mandibularis**
P3 T 50 | 8.42 | 11.22 | FUD 090

21032 **Excision of maxillary torus palatinus**
P3 T | 8.34 | 11.42 | FUD 090

21034 **Excision of malignant tumor of maxilla or zygoma**
A2 T 80 | 33.35 | 37.76 | FUD 090

21040 **Excision of benign tumor or cyst of mandible, by enucleation and/or curettage**
INCLUDES Removal of benign tumor or cyst without osteotomy
EXCLUDES *Removal of benign tumor or cyst with osteotomy (21046-21047)*
A2 T | 12.07 | 15.01 | FUD 090

21044 **Excision of malignant tumor of mandible;**
A2 T 80 | 25.33 | 25.33 | FUD 090

21045 **radical resection**
Code also bone graft procedure (21215)
C 80 | 35.22 | 35.22 | FUD 090

21046 **Excision of benign tumor or cyst of mandible; requiring intra-oral osteotomy (eg, locally aggressive or destructive lesion[s])**
A2 T 80 | 31.90 | 31.90 | FUD 090

21047 **requiring extra-oral osteotomy and partial mandibulectomy (eg, locally aggressive or destructive lesion[s])**
A2 T 80 | 37.51 | 37.51 | FUD 090

21048 **Excision of benign tumor or cyst of maxilla; requiring intra-oral osteotomy (eg, locally aggressive or destructive lesion[s])**
R2 T 80 | 32.77 | 32.77 | FUD 090

21049 **requiring extra-oral osteotomy and partial maxillectomy (eg, locally aggressive or destructive lesion[s])**
T 80 | 34.97 | 34.97 | FUD 090

21050 **Condylectomy, temporomandibular joint (separate procedure)**
A2 T 80 50 | 24.81 | 24.81 | FUD 090

21060 **Meniscectomy, partial or complete, temporomandibular joint (separate procedure)**
A2 T 80 50 | 23.80 | 23.80 | FUD 090

21070 **Coronoidectomy (separate procedure)**
A2 T 80 50 | 17.62 | 17.62 | FUD 090

21073 Temporomandibular Joint Manipulation with Anesthesia

CMS 100-3,150.1 Manipulation

21073 **Manipulation of temporomandibular joint(s) (TMJ), therapeutic, requiring an anesthesia service (ie, general or monitored anesthesia care)**
EXCLUDES *Closed treatment of TMJ dislocation (21480, 21485)*
Manipulation of TMJ without general or MAC anesthesia (97140, 98925-98929, 98943)
P3 T 80 50 | 7.40 | 11.18 | FUD 090

21076-21089 Medical Impressions for Fabrication Maxillofacial Prosthesis

CMS 100-4,12,30 Correct Coding Policy
INCLUDES Design, preparation, and professional services rendered by a physician or other qualified health care professional
EXCLUDES *Application or removal of caliper or tongs (20660, 20665)*
Professional services rendered for outside laboratory designed and prepared prosthesis

21076 **Impression and custom preparation; surgical obturator prosthesis**
P3 T 80 | 23.97 | 28.57 | FUD 010

21077 **orbital prosthesis**
P3 T 80 50 | 60.63 | 71.77 | FUD 090

21079 **interim obturator prosthesis**
P3 T | 40.00 | 48.18 | FUD 090

21080 **definitive obturator prosthesis**
P3 T | 44.65 | 54.16 | FUD 090

21081 **mandibular resection prosthesis**
P3 T 80 | 41.05 | 50.04 | FUD 090

21082 **palatal augmentation prosthesis**
P3 T 80 | 38.68 | 47.48 | FUD 090

21083 **palatal lift prosthesis**
P3 T 80 | 34.87 | 44.20 | FUD 090

21084 **speech aid prosthesis**
P3 T 80 | 41.49 | 51.57 | FUD 090

21085 **oral surgical splint**
P2 T 80 | 18.41 | 23.86 | FUD 010

21086 **auricular prosthesis**
P3 T 80 50 | 44.72 | 53.46 | FUD 090

21087 **nasal prosthesis**
P3 T 80 | 44.72 | 53.46 | FUD 090

21088 **facial prosthesis**
R2 T 80 | 0.00 | 0.00 | FUD 090

21089 **Unlisted maxillofacial prosthetic procedure**
T | 0.00 | 0.00 | FUD YYY

21100-21110 Application Fixation Device

CMS 100-4,12,40.1 Global Surgery Package Definition

21100 **Application of halo type appliance for maxillofacial fixation, includes removal (separate procedure)**
A2 T 80 | 10.88 | 20.20 | FUD 090

21110 **Application of interdental fixation device for conditions other than fracture or dislocation, includes removal**
EXCLUDES *Removal of interdental fixation by another individual (20670-20680)*
P2 02 | 19.27 | 22.96 | FUD 090

21116 Injection for TMJ Arthrogram

CMS 100-4,13,80.1 Supervision and Interpretation Codes
CMS 100-4,13,80.2 Physician Presence

21116 **Injection procedure for temporomandibular joint arthrography**
70332
NI N 50 | 1.23 | 4.05 | FUD 000

21120-21299 Repair/Reconstruction Craniofacial Bones

CMS 100-2,16,10 Exclusions from Coverage
CMS 100-2,16,120 Cosmetic Procedures
CMS 100-2,16,180 Services Related to Noncovered Procedures
CMS 100-4,12,40.1 Global Surgery Package Definition

EXCLUDES *Cranioplasty (21179-21180, 62120, 62140-62147)*

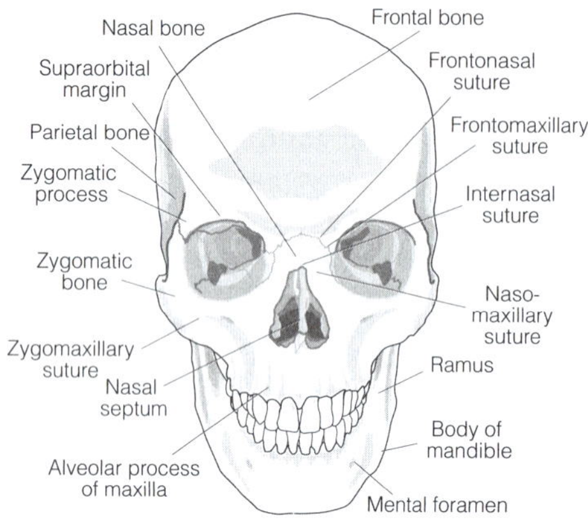

21120 **Genioplasty; augmentation (autograft, allograft, prosthetic material)**
A2 T 15.17 18.99 FUD 090

21121 **sliding osteotomy, single piece**
A2 T 80 18.14 21.80 FUD 090

21122 **sliding osteotomies, 2 or more osteotomies (eg, wedge excision or bone wedge reversal for asymmetrical chin)**
A2 T 80 19.82 19.82 FUD 090

21123 **sliding, augmentation with interpositional bone grafts (includes obtaining autografts)**
A2 T 80 25.07 25.07 FUD 090

21125 **Augmentation, mandibular body or angle; prosthetic material**
A2 T 80 23.18 87.18 FUD 090

21127 **with bone graft, onlay or interpositional (includes obtaining autograft)**
A2 T 80 24.81 120.88 FUD 090

21137 **Reduction forehead; contouring only**
G2 T 80 21.72 21.72 FUD 090

21138 **contouring and application of prosthetic material or bone graft (includes obtaining autograft)**
G2 T 80 26.19 26.19 FUD 090

21139 **contouring and setback of anterior frontal sinus wall**
G2 T 80 30.74 30.74 FUD 090

21141 **Reconstruction midface, LeFort I; single piece, segment movement in any direction (eg, for Long Face Syndrome), without bone graft**
C 80 39.36 39.36 FUD 090

21142 **2 pieces, segment movement in any direction, without bone graft**
C 80 40.49 40.49 FUD 090

21143 **3 or more pieces, segment movement in any direction, without bone graft**
C 80 41.04 41.04 FUD 090

21145 **single piece, segment movement in any direction, requiring bone grafts (includes obtaining autografts)**
C 80 43.38 43.38 FUD 090

21146 **2 pieces, segment movement in any direction, requiring bone grafts (includes obtaining autografts) (eg, ungrafted unilateral alveolar cleft)**
C 80 50.07 50.07 FUD 090

21147 **3 or more pieces, segment movement in any direction, requiring bone grafts (includes obtaining autografts) (eg, ungrafted bilateral alveolar cleft or multiple osteotomies)**
C 80 43.47 43.47 FUD 090

21150 **Reconstruction midface, LeFort II; anterior intrusion (eg, Treacher-Collins Syndrome)**
G2 T 80 51.72 51.72 FUD 090

21151 **any direction, requiring bone grafts (includes obtaining autografts)**
C 80 58.52 58.52 FUD 090

21154 **Reconstruction midface, LeFort III (extracranial), any type, requiring bone grafts (includes obtaining autografts); without LeFort I**
C 80 63.72 63.72 FUD 090

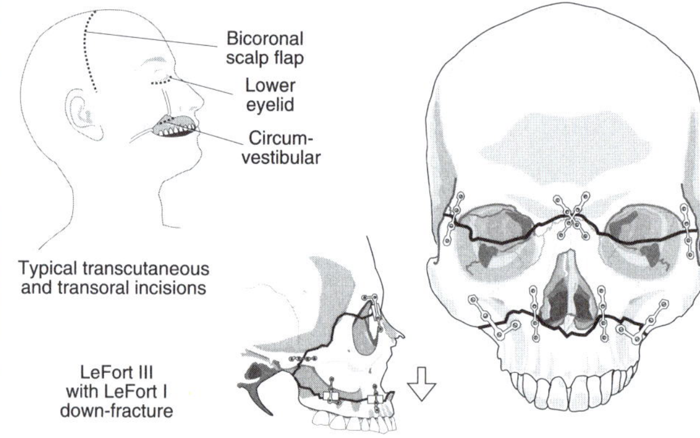

21155 **with LeFort I**
C 80 64.43 64.43 FUD 090

21159 **Reconstruction midface, LeFort III (extra and intracranial) with forehead advancement (eg, mono bloc), requiring bone grafts (includes obtaining autografts); without LeFort I**
C 80 71.69 71.69 FUD 090

21160 **with LeFort I**
C 80 75.22 75.22 FUD 090

21172 **Reconstruction superior-lateral orbital rim and lower forehead, advancement or alteration, with or without grafts (includes obtaining autografts)**
EXCLUDES *Frontal or parietal craniotomy for craniosynostosis (61556)*
T 80 53.78 53.78 FUD 090

21175 **Reconstruction, bifrontal, superior-lateral orbital rims and lower forehead, advancement or alteration (eg, plagiocephaly, trigonocephaly, brachycephaly), with or without grafts (includes obtaining autografts)**
EXCLUDES *Bifrontal craniotomy for craniosynostosis (61557)*
T 80 61.45 61.45 FUD 090

21179 **Reconstruction, entire or majority of forehead and/or supraorbital rims; with grafts (allograft or prosthetic material)**
EXCLUDES *Extensive craniotomy for numerous suture craniosynostosis (61558-61559)*
C 80 44.74 44.74 FUD 090

21180 with autograft (includes obtaining grafts)
EXCLUDES *Extensive craniotomy for numerous suture craniosynostosis (61558-61559)*
C 80 44.08 44.08 FUD 090

21181 Reconstruction by contouring of benign tumor of cranial bones (eg, fibrous dysplasia), extracranial
A2 T 80 20.72 20.72 FUD 090

21182 Reconstruction of orbital walls, rims, forehead, nasoethmoid complex following intra- and extracranial excision of benign tumor of cranial bone (eg, fibrous dysplasia), with multiple autografts (includes obtaining grafts); total area of bone grafting less than 40 sq cm
EXCLUDES *Removal of benign tumor of the skull (61563-61564)*
C 80 55.15 55.15 FUD 090

21183 total area of bone grafting greater than 40 sq cm but less than 80 sq cm
EXCLUDES *Removal of benign tumor of the skull (61563-61564)*
C 80 68.53 68.53 FUD 090

21184 total area of bone grafting greater than 80 sq cm
EXCLUDES *Removal of benign tumor of the skull (61563-61564)*
C 80 63.70 63.70 FUD 090

21188 Reconstruction midface, osteotomies (other than LeFort type) and bone grafts (includes obtaining autografts)
C 80 45.12 45.12 FUD 090

21193 Reconstruction of mandibular rami, horizontal, vertical, C, or L osteotomy; without bone graft
T 80 37.29 37.29 FUD 090

21194 with bone graft (includes obtaining graft)
C 80 39.25 39.25 FUD 090

21195 Reconstruction of mandibular rami and/or body, sagittal split; without internal rigid fixation
T 80 38.32 38.32 FUD 090

21196 with internal rigid fixation
C 80 42.49 42.49 FUD 090

21198 Osteotomy, mandible, segmental;
EXCLUDES *Total maxillary osteotomy (21141-21160)*
G2 T 80 33.40 33.40 FUD 090

21199 with genioglossus advancement
EXCLUDES *Total maxillary osteotomy (21141-21160)*
G2 T 80 30.20 30.20 FUD 090

21206 Osteotomy, maxilla, segmental (eg, Wassmund or Schuchard)
A2 T 80 34.58 34.58 FUD 090

21208 Osteoplasty, facial bones; augmentation (autograft, allograft, or prosthetic implant)
A2 T 80 24.71 54.45 FUD 090

21209 reduction
A2 T 80 18.28 23.81 FUD 090

21210 Graft, bone; nasal, maxillary or malar areas (includes obtaining graft)
EXCLUDES *Cleft palate procedures (42200-42225)*
A2 T 24.70 65.55 FUD 090

21215 mandible (includes obtaining graft)
A2 T 26.49 117.96 FUD 090

21230 rib cartilage, autogenous, to face, chin, nose or ear (includes obtaining graft)
EXCLUDES *Augmentation of facial bones (21208)*
A2 T 80 21.17 21.17 FUD 090

21235 ear cartilage, autogenous, to nose or ear (includes obtaining graft)
EXCLUDES *Augmentation of facial bones (21208)*
A2 T 16.28 20.71 FUD 090

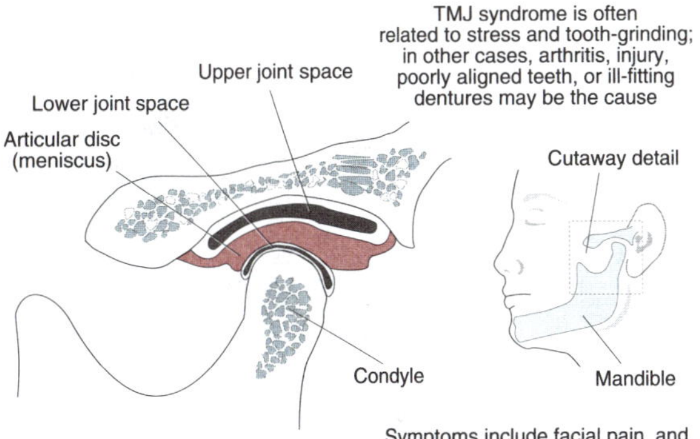

Upper joint space
Lower joint space
Articular disc (meniscus)
TMJ syndrome is often related to stress and tooth-grinding; in other cases, arthritis, injury, poorly aligned teeth, or ill-fitting dentures may be the cause
Cutaway detail
Condyle
Mandible
Cutaway view of temporomandibular joint (TMJ)
Symptoms include facial pain and chewing problems; TMJ syndrome occurs more frequently in women

21240 Arthroplasty, temporomandibular joint, with or without autograft (includes obtaining graft)
A2 T 80 50 31.69 31.69 FUD 090

21242 Arthroplasty, temporomandibular joint, with allograft
A2 T 80 50 29.06 29.06 FUD 090

21243 Arthroplasty, temporomandibular joint, with prosthetic joint replacement
A2 T 80 50 48.14 48.14 FUD 090

21244 Reconstruction of mandible, extraoral, with transosteal bone plate (eg, mandibular staple bone plate)
A2 T 80 30.73 30.73 FUD 090

21245 Reconstruction of mandible or maxilla, subperiosteal implant; partial
A2 T 80 25.50 31.86 FUD 090

21246 complete
A2 T 80 23.61 23.61 FUD 090

21247 Reconstruction of mandibular condyle with bone and cartilage autografts (includes obtaining grafts) (eg, for hemifacial microsomia)
C 80 50 45.57 45.57 FUD 090

21248 Reconstruction of mandible or maxilla, endosteal implant (eg, blade, cylinder); partial
EXCLUDES *Midface reconstruction (21141-21160)*
A2 T 25.90 31.71 FUD 090

21249 complete
EXCLUDES *Midface reconstruction (21141-21160)*
A2 T 80 36.95 43.52 FUD 090

21255 Reconstruction of zygomatic arch and glenoid fossa with bone and cartilage (includes obtaining autografts)
C 80 50 39.79 39.79 FUD 090

21256 Reconstruction of orbit with osteotomies (extracranial) and with bone grafts (includes obtaining autografts) (eg, micro-ophthalmia)
T 80 50 35.31 35.31 FUD 090

21260 Periorbital osteotomies for orbital hypertelorism, with bone grafts; extracranial approach
G2 T 80 38.42 38.42 FUD 090

21261 combined intra- and extracranial approach
T 80 62.46 62.46 FUD 090

Musculoskeletal System

21180 — 21261

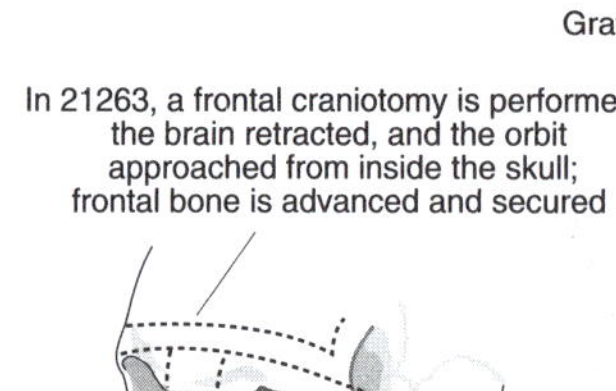

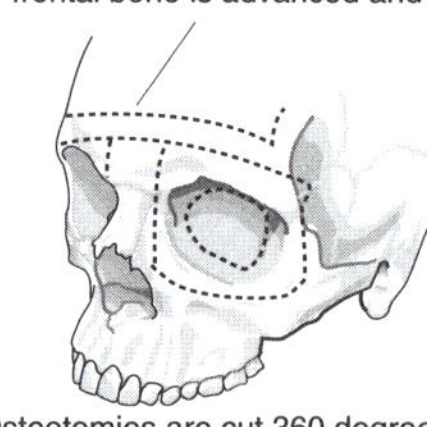

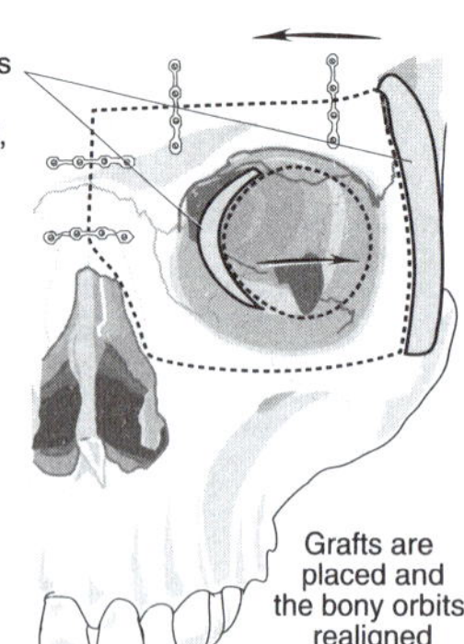

21263 **with forehead advancement**
T 80 — 53.89 — 53.89 FUD 090

21267 **Orbital repositioning, periorbital osteotomies, unilateral, with bone grafts; extracranial approach**
A2 T 80 50 — 47.65 — 47.65 FUD 090

21268 **combined intra- and extracranial approach**
C 80 50 — 51.44 — 51.44 FUD 090

21270 **Malar augmentation, prosthetic material**
EXCLUDES *Bone graft (21210)*
A2 T 80 50 — 21.02 — 27.52 FUD 090

21275 **Secondary revision of orbitocraniofacial reconstruction**
A2 T 80 — 24.21 — 24.21 FUD 090

21280 **Medial canthopexy (separate procedure)**
EXCLUDES *Reconstruction of canthus (67950)*
A2 T 80 50 — 16.87 — 16.87 FUD 090

21282 **Lateral canthopexy**
A2 T 50 — 11.09 — 11.09 FUD 090

21295 **Reduction of masseter muscle and bone (eg, for treatment of benign masseteric hypertrophy); extraoral approach**
A2 T 80 50 — 5.85 — 5.85 FUD 090

21296 **intraoral approach**
A2 T 80 50 — 13.24 — 13.24 FUD 090

21299 **Unlisted craniofacial and maxillofacial procedure**
T 80 — 0.00 — 0.00 FUD YYY

21310-21499 Care of Fractures/Dislocations of the Cranial and Facial Bones

CMS 100-4,12,40.1 Global Surgery Package Definition
CMS 100-4,14,10 General ASC Services

EXCLUDES *Closed treatment of skull fracture, report with appropriate evaluation and management service*
Open treatment of skull fracture (62000-62010)

21310 **Closed treatment of nasal bone fracture without manipulation**
A2 T — 0.80 — 3.71 FUD 000

21315 **Closed treatment of nasal bone fracture; without stabilization**
A2 T — 4.37 — 7.92 FUD 010

21320 **with stabilization**
A2 T — 3.88 — 7.33 FUD 010

21325 **Open treatment of nasal fracture; uncomplicated**
A2 T 80 — 13.45 — 13.45 FUD 090

21330 **complicated, with internal and/or external skeletal fixation**
A2 T 80 — 16.07 — 16.07 FUD 090

21335 **with concomitant open treatment of fractured septum**
A2 T — 20.90 — 20.90 FUD 090

21336 **Open treatment of nasal septal fracture, with or without stabilization**
A2 T 80 — 18.47 — 18.47 FUD 090

21337 **Closed treatment of nasal septal fracture, with or without stabilization**
A2 T 80 — 8.48 — 11.56 FUD 090

21338 **Open treatment of nasoethmoid fracture; without external fixation**
A2 T 80 — 20.55 — 20.55 FUD 090

21339 **with external fixation**
A2 T 80 — 22.18 — 22.18 FUD 090

21340 **Percutaneous treatment of nasoethmoid complex fracture, with splint, wire or headcap fixation, including repair of canthal ligaments and/or the nasolacrimal apparatus**
A2 T 80 — 21.54 — 21.54 FUD 090

21343 **Open treatment of depressed frontal sinus fracture**
C 80 — 34.95 — 34.95 FUD 090

21344 **Open treatment of complicated (eg, comminuted or involving posterior wall) frontal sinus fracture, via coronal or multiple approaches**
C 80 — 44.68 — 44.68 FUD 090

21345 **Closed treatment of nasomaxillary complex fracture (LeFort II type), with interdental wire fixation or fixation of denture or splint**
A2 T 80 — 17.88 — 22.15 FUD 090

21346 **Open treatment of nasomaxillary complex fracture (LeFort II type); with wiring and/or local fixation**
T PQ — 26.07 — 26.07 FUD 090

21347 **requiring multiple open approaches**
C 80 PQ — 31.66 — 31.66 FUD 090

21348 **with bone grafting (includes obtaining graft)**
C 80 PQ — 33.88 — 33.88 FUD 090

21355 **Percutaneous treatment of fracture of malar area, including zygomatic arch and malar tripod, with manipulation**
A2 T 80 50 — 9.23 — 12.31 FUD 010

21356 **Open treatment of depressed zygomatic arch fracture (eg, Gillies approach)**
A2 T 80 50 — 10.82 — 14.26 FUD 010

21360 **Open treatment of depressed malar fracture, including zygomatic arch and malar tripod**
G2 T 80 50 — 15.34 — 15.34 FUD 090

21365 **Open treatment of complicated (eg, comminuted or involving cranial nerve foramina) fracture(s) of malar area, including zygomatic arch and malar tripod; with internal fixation and multiple surgical approaches**
T 80 50 — 32.16 — 32.16 FUD 090

21366 **with bone grafting (includes obtaining graft)**
C 80 50 — 34.20 — 34.20 FUD 090

21385 **Open treatment of orbital floor blowout fracture; transantral approach (Caldwell-Luc type operation)**
T 80 50 — 19.62 — 19.62 FUD 090

21386 **periorbital approach**
T 80 50 — 20.13 — 20.13 FUD 090

21387 **combined approach**
T 80 50 — 21.11 — 21.11 FUD 090

21390 **periorbital approach, with alloplastic or other implant**
G2 T 80 50 — 23.21 — 23.21 FUD 090

21395 **periorbital approach with bone graft (includes obtaining graft)**
T 80 50 — 28.26 — 28.26 FUD 090

21400 **Closed treatment of fracture of orbit, except blowout; without manipulation**
A2 T 80 50 4.46 5.49 FUD 090

21401 **with manipulation**
A2 T 80 50 8.88 14.07 FUD 090

21406 **Open treatment of fracture of orbit, except blowout; without implant**
G2 T 80 50 14.74 14.74 FUD 090

21407 **with implant**
G2 T 80 50 18.85 18.85 FUD 090

21408 **with bone grafting (includes obtaining graft)**
T 80 50 26.07 26.07 FUD 090

21421 **Closed treatment of palatal or maxillary fracture (LeFort I type), with interdental wire fixation or fixation of denture or splint**
A2 T 80 18.59 21.93 FUD 090

21422 **Open treatment of palatal or maxillary fracture (LeFort I type);**
C 80 PQ 19.15 19.15 FUD 090

21423 **complicated (comminuted or involving cranial nerve foramina), multiple approaches**
C 80 PQ 23.82 23.82 FUD 090

21431 **Closed treatment of craniofacial separation (LeFort III type) using interdental wire fixation of denture or splint**
C 80 20.74 20.74 FUD 090

21432 **Open treatment of craniofacial separation (LeFort III type); with wiring and/or internal fixation**
C 80 PQ 18.90 18.90 FUD 090

21433 **complicated (eg, comminuted or involving cranial nerve foramina), multiple surgical approaches**
C 80 PQ 50.54 50.54 FUD 090

21435 **complicated, utilizing internal and/or external fixation techniques (eg, head cap, halo device, and/or intermaxillary fixation)**
EXCLUDES *Removal of internal or external fixation (20670)*
C 80 PQ 36.34 36.34 FUD 090

21436 **complicated, multiple surgical approaches, internal fixation, with bone grafting (includes obtaining graft)**
C 80 PQ 59.28 59.28 FUD 090

21440 **Closed treatment of mandibular or maxillary alveolar ridge fracture (separate procedure)**
P3 T 80 13.61 16.71 FUD 090

21445 **Open treatment of mandibular or maxillary alveolar ridge fracture (separate procedure)**
A2 T 80 17.99 22.08 FUD 090

21450 **Closed treatment of mandibular fracture; without manipulation**
A2 T 80 14.08 17.50 FUD 090

21451 **with manipulation**
A2 T 80 18.39 21.88 FUD 090

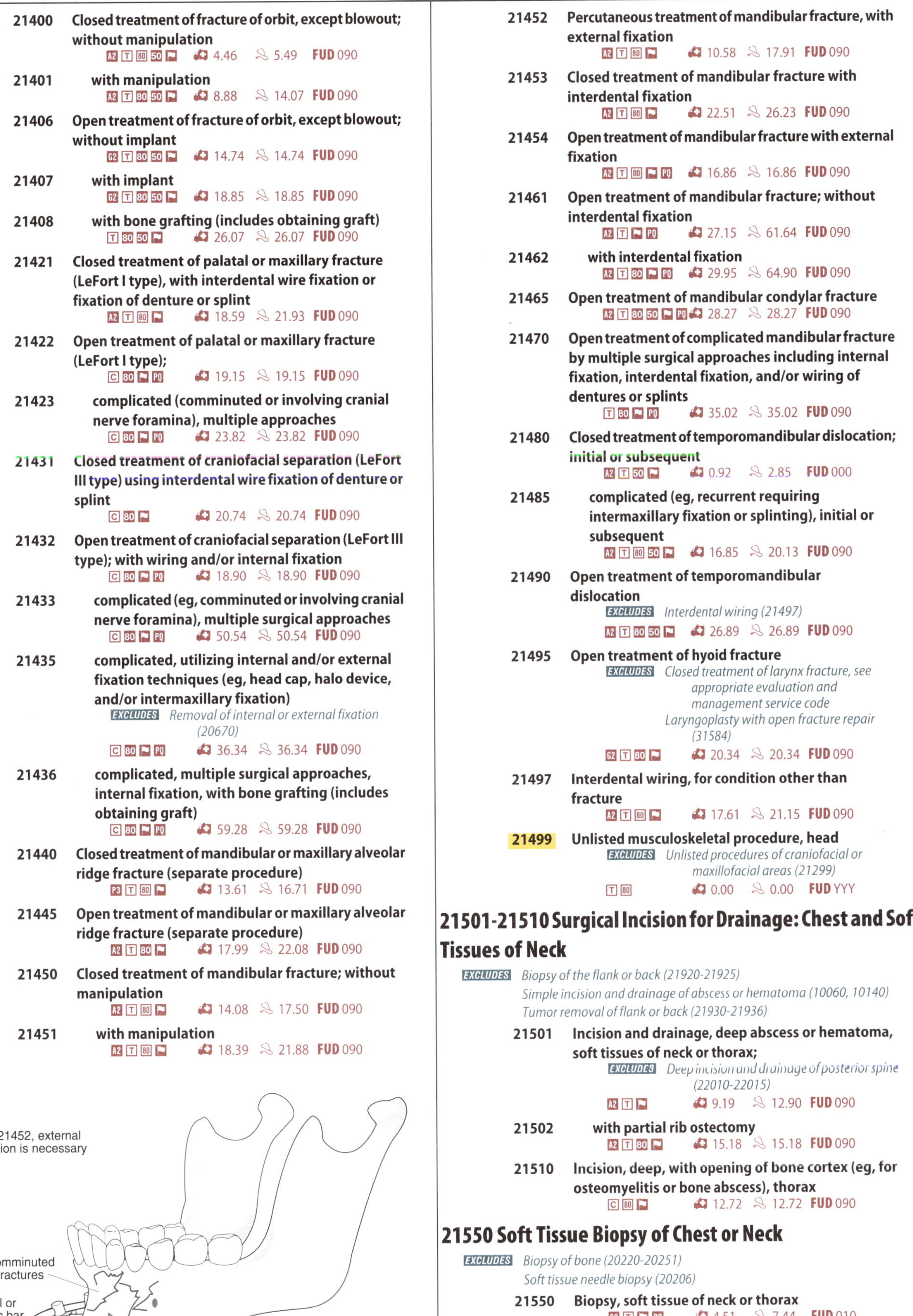

21452 **Percutaneous treatment of mandibular fracture, with external fixation**
A2 T 80 10.58 17.91 FUD 090

21453 **Closed treatment of mandibular fracture with interdental fixation**
A2 T 80 22.51 26.23 FUD 090

21454 **Open treatment of mandibular fracture with external fixation**
A2 T 80 PQ 16.86 16.86 FUD 090

21461 **Open treatment of mandibular fracture; without interdental fixation**
A2 T PQ 27.15 61.64 FUD 090

21462 **with interdental fixation**
A2 T 80 PQ 29.95 64.90 FUD 090

21465 **Open treatment of mandibular condylar fracture**
A2 T 80 50 PQ 28.27 28.27 FUD 090

21470 **Open treatment of complicated mandibular fracture by multiple surgical approaches including internal fixation, interdental fixation, and/or wiring of dentures or splints**
T 80 PQ 35.02 35.02 FUD 090

21480 **Closed treatment of temporomandibular dislocation; initial or subsequent**
A2 T 50 0.92 2.85 FUD 000

21485 **complicated (eg, recurrent requiring intermaxillary fixation or splinting), initial or subsequent**
A2 T 80 50 16.85 20.13 FUD 090

21490 **Open treatment of temporomandibular dislocation**
EXCLUDES *Interdental wiring (21497)*
A2 T 80 50 26.89 26.89 FUD 090

21495 **Open treatment of hyoid fracture**
EXCLUDES *Closed treatment of larynx fracture, see appropriate evaluation and management service code*
Laryngoplasty with open fracture repair (31584)
G2 T 80 20.34 20.34 FUD 090

21497 **Interdental wiring, for condition other than fracture**
A2 T 80 17.61 21.15 FUD 090

21499 **Unlisted musculoskeletal procedure, head**
EXCLUDES *Unlisted procedures of craniofacial or maxillofacial areas (21299)*
T 80 0.00 0.00 FUD YYY

21501-21510 Surgical Incision for Drainage: Chest and Soft Tissues of Neck

EXCLUDES *Biopsy of the flank or back (21920-21925)*
Simple incision and drainage of abscess or hematoma (10060, 10140)
Tumor removal of flank or back (21930-21936)

21501 **Incision and drainage, deep abscess or hematoma, soft tissues of neck or thorax;**
EXCLUDES *Deep incision and drainage of posterior spine (22010-22015)*
A2 T 9.19 12.90 FUD 090

21502 **with partial rib ostectomy**
A2 T 80 15.18 15.18 FUD 090

21510 **Incision, deep, with opening of bone cortex (eg, for osteomyelitis or bone abscess), thorax**
C 80 12.72 12.72 FUD 090

21550 Soft Tissue Biopsy of Chest or Neck

EXCLUDES *Biopsy of bone (20220-20251)*
Soft tissue needle biopsy (20206)

21550 **Biopsy, soft tissue of neck or thorax**
G2 T PQ 4.51 7.44 FUD 010

21552-21558 [21552, 21554] Excision Soft Tissue Tumors Chest and Neck

INCLUDES Any necessary elevation of tissue planes or dissection
Measurement of tumor and necessary margin at greatest diameter prior to excision
Resection without removal of significant normal tissue
Simple and intermediate repairs
Types of excisions:
Fascial or subfascial soft tissue tumors: simple and marginal resection of tumors found either in or below the deep fascia, not involving bone or excision of a substantial amount of normal tissue; primarily benign and intramuscular tumors
Radical resection soft tissue tumor: wide resection of tumor, involving substantial margins of normal tissue and may involve tissue removal from one or more layers; most often malignant or aggressive benign
Subcutaneous: simple and marginal resection of tumors in the subcutaneous tissue above the deep fascia; most often benign

EXCLUDES *Complex repair*
Excision of benign cutaneous lesions (eg, sebaceous cyst) (11400-11426)
Radical resection of cutaneous tumors (eg, melanoma) (11600-11626)
Significant exploration of the vessels or neuroplasty

21552 Resequenced code. See code following 21555.

21554 Resequenced code. See code following 21556.

21555 Excision, tumor, soft tissue of neck or anterior thorax, subcutaneous; less than 3 cm
G2 T 8.73 11.75 FUD 090

\# **21552 3 cm or greater**
G2 T 80 12.64 12.64 FUD 090

21556 Excision, tumor, soft tissue of neck or anterior thorax, subfascial (eg, intramuscular); less than 5 cm
G2 T 15.22 15.22 FUD 090

\# **21554 5 cm or greater**
G2 T 80 20.76 20.76 FUD 090

21557 Radical resection of tumor (eg, sarcoma), soft tissue of neck or anterior thorax; less than 5 cm
G2 T 80 27.49 27.49 FUD 090

21558 5 cm or greater
G2 T 80 38.51 38.51 FUD 090

21600-21632 Bony Resection Chest and Neck

21600 Excision of rib, partial
EXCLUDES *Extensive debridement (11044, 11047)*
Extensive tumor removal (19260)
A2 T 80 16.06 16.06 FUD 090

21610 Costotransversectomy (separate procedure)
A2 T 80 34.16 34.16 FUD 090

21615 Excision first and/or cervical rib;
C 80 50 18.16 18.16 FUD 090

21616 with sympathectomy
C 80 50 24.42 24.42 FUD 090

21620 Ostectomy of sternum, partial
C 80 14.57 14.57 FUD 090

21627 Sternal debridement
EXCLUDES *Debridement with sternotomy closure (21750)*
C 80 PQ 15.54 15.54 FUD 090

21630 Radical resection of sternum;
C 80 34.92 34.92 FUD 090

21632 with mediastinal lymphadenectomy
C 80 PQ 34.92 34.92 FUD 090

21685-21750 Repair/Reconstruction Chest and Soft Tissues Neck

EXCLUDES *Biopsy of chest or neck (21550)*
Repair of simple wounds (12001-12007)
Tumor removal of chest or neck (21556-21558 [21552, 21554])

21685 Hyoid myotomy and suspension
G2 T 80 28.80 28.80 FUD 090

21700 Division of scalenus anticus; without resection of cervical rib
A2 T 80 50 10.67 10.67 FUD 090

21705 with resection of cervical rib
C 80 50 15.95 15.95 FUD 090

21720 Division of sternocleidomastoid for torticollis, open operation; without cast application
EXCLUDES *Transection of spinal accessory and cervical nerves (63191, 64722)*
A2 T 80 13.84 13.84 FUD 090

21725 with cast application
EXCLUDES *Transection of spinal accessory and cervical nerves (63191, 64722)*
A2 T 80 13.45 13.45 FUD 090

21740 Reconstructive repair of pectus excavatum or carinatum; open
C 80 PQ 29.25 29.25 FUD 090

21742 minimally invasive approach (Nuss procedure), without thoracoscopy
T 80 0.00 0.00 FUD 090

21743 minimally invasive approach (Nuss procedure), with thoracoscopy
T 80 0.00 0.00 FUD 090

21750 Closure of median sternotomy separation with or without debridement (separate procedure)
C 80 PQ 19.81 19.81 FUD 090

21800-21825 Fracture Care: Ribs and Sternum

EXCLUDES *Closed treatment uncomplicated rib fractures*

~~**21800 Closed treatment of rib fracture, uncomplicated, each**~~
To report, see Evaluation and Management Codes

21805 Open treatment of rib fracture without fixation, each
EXCLUDES *External rib fixation (21899)*
A2 T 80 PQ 7.81 7.81 FUD 090

~~**21810 Treatment of rib fracture requiring external fixation (flail chest)**~~
To report, see 21899

● **21811 Open treatment of rib fracture(s) with internal fixation, includes thoracoscopic visualization when performed, unilateral; 1-3 ribs**

● **21812 4-6 ribs**

● **21813 7 or more ribs**

21820 Closed treatment of sternum fracture
A2 T 4.15 4.05 FUD 090

21825 Open treatment of sternum fracture with or without skeletal fixation
EXCLUDES *Treatment of sternoclavicular dislocation (23520-23532)*
C 80 PQ 15.70 15.70 FUD 090

21899 Unlisted Procedures of Chest or Neck

21899 Unlisted procedure, neck or thorax
T 80 0.00 0.00 FUD YYY

21920-21925 Biopsy Soft Tissue of Back and Flank

EXCLUDES *Soft tissue needle biopsy (20206)*

21920 Biopsy, soft tissue of back or flank; superficial
P3 T PQ 4.62 7.31 FUD 010

21925 deep
A2 T PQ 10.05 12.58 FUD 090

21930-21936 Excision Soft Tissue Tumors Back or Flank

INCLUDES Any necessary elevation of tissue planes or dissection
Measurement of tumor and necessary margin at greatest diameter prior to excision
Simple and intermediate repairs
Types of excision:
Fascial or subfascial soft tissue tumors: simple and marginal resection of tumors found either in or below the deep fascia, not involving bone or excision of a substantial amount of normal tissue; most often benign and intramuscular tumors
Radical resection soft tissue tumor: wide resection of tumor, involving substantial margins of normal tissue and may include tissue removal from one or more layers; most often malignant or aggressive benign
Subcutaneous: simple and marginal resection of tumors in the subcutaneous tissue above the deep fascia; most often benign

EXCLUDES *Complex repair*
Excision of benign cutaneous lesions (eg, sebaceous cyst) (11400-11406)
Radical resection of cutaneous tumors (eg, melanoma) (11600-11606)
Significant exploration of the vessels or neuroplasty

21930 **Excision, tumor, soft tissue of back or flank, subcutaneous; less than 3 cm**
62 T 10.37 13.34 FUD 090

21931 **3 cm or greater**
62 T 80 13.34 13.34 FUD 090

21932 **Excision, tumor, soft tissue of back or flank, subfascial (eg, intramuscular); less than 5 cm**
62 T 80 18.77 18.77 FUD 090

21933 **5 cm or greater**
62 T 80 20.91 20.91 FUD 090

21935 **Radical resection of tumor (eg, sarcoma), soft tissue of back or flank; less than 5 cm**
62 T 29.30 29.30 FUD 090

21936 **5 cm or greater**
62 T 80 40.26 40.26 FUD 090

22010-22015 Incision for Drainage of Deep Spinal Abscess

EXCLUDES *Incision and drainage of hematoma (10060, 10140)*
Injection:
Chemonucleolysis (62292)
Discography (62290-62291)
Facet joint (64490-64495, [64633, 64634, 64635, 64636])
Myelography (62284)
Needle/trocar biopsy (20220-20225)

22010 **Incision and drainage, open, of deep abscess (subfascial), posterior spine; cervical, thoracic, or cervicothoracic**
C 80 27.10 27.10 FUD 090

22015 **lumbar, sacral, or lumbosacral**
Do not report with (10180, 22010, 22850, 22852)
C 25.65 25.65 FUD 090

22100-22103 Partial Resection Vertebral Component

EXCLUDES *Back or flank biopsy (21920-21925)*
Bone biopsy (20220-20251)
Injection:
Chemonucleolysis (62292)
Discography (62290-62291)
Facet joint (64490-64495, [64633, 64634, 64635, 64636])
Myelography (62284)
Removal of tumor flank or back (21930)
Soft tissue needle biopsy (20206)

22100 **Partial excision of posterior vertebral component (eg, spinous process, lamina or facet) for intrinsic bony lesion, single vertebral segment; cervical**
T 80 24.98 24.98 FUD 090

22101 **thoracic**
T 80 25.40 25.40 FUD 090

22102 **lumbar**
EXCLUDES *Insertion of posterior spinous process distraction devices (0171T-0172T)*
62 T 80 23.34 23.34 FUD 090

\+ **22103** **each additional segment (List separately in addition to code for primary procedure)**
Code first (22100-22102)
N1 N 80 4.09 4.09 FUD ZZZ

22110-22116 Partial Resection Vertebral Component without Decompression

EXCLUDES *Back or flank biopsy (21920-21925)*
Bone biopsy (20220-20251)
Bone grafting procedures (20930-20938)
Harvest bone graft (20931, 20938)
Injection:
Chemonucleolysis (62292)
Discography (62290-62291)
Facet joint (64490-64495, [64633, 64634, 64635, 64636])
Myelography (62284)
Osteotomy (22210-22226)
Removal of tumor flank or back (21930)
Restoration after vertebral body resection (22585, 63082 or 63086 or 63088 or 63091)
Spinal restoration with graft:
Cervical (20931 or 20938, 22554, 63081)
Lumbar (20931 or 20938, 22558, 63087 or 63090)
Thoracic (20931 or 20938, 22556, 63085 or 63087)
Spinal restoration with prosthesis:
Cervical (20931 or 20938, 22554, 22851, 63081)
Lumbar (20931 or 20938, 22558, 22851, 63087 or 63090)
Thoracic (20931 or 20938, 22556, 22851, 63085 or 63087)
Vertebral corpectomy (63081-63091)

22110 **Partial excision of vertebral body, for intrinsic bony lesion, without decompression of spinal cord or nerve root(s), single vertebral segment; cervical**
C 80 30.97 30.97 FUD 090

22112 **thoracic**
C 80 30.58 30.58 FUD 090

22114 **lumbar**
C 80 28.41 28.41 FUD 090

\+ **22116** **each additional vertebral segment (List separately in addition to code for primary procedure)**
Code first (22110-22114)
C 80 4.02 4.02 FUD ZZZ

22206-22216 Spinal Osteotomy: Posterior/Posterolateral Approach

CMS 100-4,12,40.8 Co-surgery and team surgery

EXCLUDES *Decompression of the spinal cord and/or nerve roots (63001-63308)*
Injection:
Chemonucleolysis (62292)
Discography (62290-62292)
Facet joint (64490-64495, [64633, 64634, 64635, 64636])
Myelography (62284)
Repair of vertebral fracture by the anterior approach, see appropriate arthrodesis, bone graft, instrumentation codes, and (63081-63091)

Code also arthrodesis (22590-22632)
Code also bone grafting procedures (20930-20938)
Code also spinal instrumentation (22840-22855)

22206 **Osteotomy of spine, posterior or posterolateral approach, 3 columns, 1 vertebral segment (eg, pedicle/vertebral body subtraction); thoracic**
Do not report with (22207)
Do not report with the following codes if performed at same level (22210-22226, 22830, 63001-63048, 63055-63066, 63075-63091, 63101-63103)
C 80 67.56 67.56 FUD 090

Musculoskeletal System

21930 — 22206

22207 **lumbar**

Do not report with (22206)

Do not report with the following codes if performed at the same level (22210-22226, 22830, 63001-63048, 63055-63066, 63075-63091, 63101-63103)

C 80 68.54 68.54 FUD 090

+ 22208 **each additional vertebral segment (List separately in addition to code for primary procedure)**

Code first (22206 or 22207)

Do not report with the following codes if performed at the same level (22210-22226, 22830, 63001-63048, 63055-63066, 63075-63091, 63101-63103)

C 80 16.90 16.90 FUD ZZZ

22210 **Osteotomy of spine, posterior or posterolateral approach, 1 vertebral segment; cervical**

C 80 50.63 50.63 FUD 090

22212 **thoracic**

C 80 42.09 42.09 FUD 090

22214 **lumbar**

C 80 42.40 42.40 FUD 090

+ 22216 **each additional vertebral segment (List separately in addition to primary procedure)**

Code first (22210-22214)

C 80 10.45 10.45 FUD ZZZ

22220-22226 Spinal Osteotomy: Anterior Approach

CMS 100-4,12,40.8 Co-surgery and team surgery

EXCLUDES *Corpectomy (63081-63091)*

Decompression of the spinal cord and/or nerve roots (63001-63308)

Injection:

Chemonucleolysis (62292)

Discography (62290-62291)

Facet joint (64490-64495, [64633], [64634], [64635], [64636])

Myelography (62284)

Needle/trocar biopsy (20220-20225)

Repair of vertebral fracture by the anterior approach, see appropriate arthrodesis, bone graft, instrumentation codes, and (63081-63091)

Code also arthrodesis (22590-22632)

Code also bone grafting procedures (20930-20938)

Code also spinal instrumentation (22840-22855)

22220 **Osteotomy of spine, including discectomy, anterior approach, single vertebral segment; cervical**

C 80 46.23 46.23 FUD 090

22222 **thoracic**

T 80 44.70 44.70 FUD 090

22224 **lumbar**

C 80 45.43 45.43 FUD 090

+ 22226 **each additional vertebral segment (List separately in addition to code for primary procedure)**

Code first (22220-22224)

C 80 10.49 10.49 FUD ZZZ

22305-22315 Closed Treatment Vertebral Fractures

EXCLUDES *Injection:*

Chemonucleolysis (62292)

Discography (62290-62291)

Facet joint (64490-64495, [64633], [64634], [64635], [64636])

Myelography (62284)

Code also arthrodesis (22590-22632)

Code also bone grafting procedures (20930-20938)

Code also spinal instrumentation (22840-22855)

22305 **Closed treatment of vertebral process fracture(s)**

A2 T PQ 4.92 5.42 FUD 090

22310 **Closed treatment of vertebral body fracture(s), without manipulation, requiring and including casting or bracing**

Do not report at same level as (22510-22515)

A2 T PQ 8.05 8.73 FUD 090

22315 **Closed treatment of vertebral fracture(s) and/or dislocation(s) requiring casting or bracing, with and including casting and/or bracing by manipulation or traction**

EXCLUDES *Spinal manipulation (97140)*

Do not report at the same level as (22510-22515)

A2 T PQ 22.06 25.12 FUD 090

22318-22319 Open Treatment Odontoid Fracture: Anterior Approach

EXCLUDES *Injection:*

Chemonucleolysis (62292)

Discography (62290-62291)

Facet joint (64490-64495, [64633, 64634, 64635, 64636])

Myelography (62284)

Needle/trocar biopsy (20220-20225)

Code also arthrodesis (22590-22632)

Code also bone grafting procedures (20930-20938)

Code also spinal instrumentation (22840-22855)

22318 **Open treatment and/or reduction of odontoid fracture(s) and or dislocation(s) (including os odontoideum), anterior approach, including placement of internal fixation; without grafting**

C 80 PQ 46.64 46.64 FUD 090

22319 **with grafting**

C 80 PQ 52.06 52.06 FUD 090

22325-22328 Open Treatment Vertebral Fractures: Posterior Approach

EXCLUDES *Corpectomy (63081-63091)*

Injection:

Chemonucleolysis (62292)

Discography (62290-62291)

Facet joint (64490-64495, [64633], [64634], [64635], [64636])

Myelography (62284)

Needle/trocar biopsy (20220-20225)

Spine decompression (63001-63091)

Vertebral fracture care by arthrodesis (22548-22632)

Vertebral fracture care frontal approach (63081-63091)

Code also arthrodesis (22548-22632)

Code also bone grafting procedures (20930-20938)

Code also spinal instrumentation (22840-22855)

22325 **Open treatment and/or reduction of vertebral fracture(s) and/or dislocation(s), posterior approach, 1 fractured vertebra or dislocated segment; lumbar**

Do not report at the same level as (22511-22512, 22514-22515)

C 80 PQ 41.18 41.18 FUD 090

22326 **cervical**

Do not report at the same level as (22510, 22512)

C 80 PQ 42.50 42.50 FUD 090

22327 thoracic
Do not report at the same level as (22510, 22512-22513, 22515)
C 80 PQ 42.49 42.49 FUD 090

+ 22328 each additional fractured vertebra or dislocated segment (List separately in addition to code for primary procedure)
Code first (22325-22327)
C 80 8.12 8.12 FUD ZZZ

22505 Spinal Manipulation with Anesthesia

EXCLUDES *Manipulation not requiring anesthesia (97140)*

22505 Manipulation of spine requiring anesthesia, any region
A2 T 3.50 3.50 FUD 010

22510-22525 Percutaneous Vertebroplasty/Kyphoplasty

INCLUDES Bone biopsy when applicable

EXCLUDES *Sacroplasty/augmentation (0200T-0201T)*

Do not report sacral procedures more than one time per encounter
Do not report with (20225, 22310, 22315, 22325, 22327)

⊙ ● 22510 Percutaneous vertebroplasty (bone biopsy included when performed), 1 vertebral body, unilateral or bilateral injection, inclusive of all imaging guidance; cervicothoracic

⊙ ● 22511 lumbosacral

+ ⊙ ● 22512 each additional cervicothoracic or lumbosacral vertebral body (List separately in addition to code for primary procedure)
Code first (22510-22511)

⊙ ● 22513 Percutaneous vertebral augmentation, including cavity creation (fracture reduction and bone biopsy included when performed) using mechanical device (eg, kyphoplasty), 1 vertebral body, unilateral or bilateral cannulation, inclusive of all imaging guidance; thoracic

⊙ ● 22514 lumbar

+ ⊙ ● 22515 each additional thoracic or lumbar vertebral body (List separately in addition to code for primary procedure)
Code first (22513-22514)

~~22520~~ ~~Percutaneous vertebroplasty (bone biopsy included when performed), 1 vertebral body, unilateral or bilateral injection; thoracic~~
To report, see 22510

~~22521~~ ~~lumbar~~
To report, see 22511

~~22522~~ ~~each additional thoracic or lumbar vertebral body (List separately in addition to code for primary procedure)~~
To report, see 22512

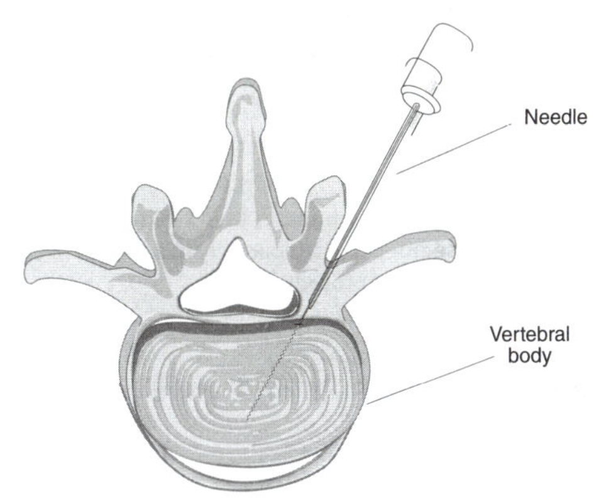

~~22523~~ ~~Percutaneous vertebral augmentation, including cavity creation (fracture reduction and bone biopsy included when performed) using mechanical device, 1 vertebral body, unilateral or bilateral cannulation (eg, kyphoplasty); thoracic~~
To report, see 22513

~~22524~~ ~~lumbar~~
To report, see 22514

~~22525~~ ~~each additional thoracic or lumbar vertebral body (List separately in addition to code for primary procedure)~~
To report, see 22515

22526-22527 Percutaneous Annuloplasty

EXCLUDES *Needle/trocar biopsy (20220-20225)*
Injection:
Chemonucleolysis (62292)
Discography (62290-62291)
Facet joint (64490-64495, [64633], [64634], [64635], [64636])
Myelography (62284)
Procedure performed by other methods (22899)

Do not report with (77002, 77003)

⊙ 22526 Percutaneous intradiscal electrothermal annuloplasty, unilateral or bilateral including fluoroscopic guidance; single level
INCLUDES Contrast injection during fluoroscopic guidance/localization (77003)
EXCLUDES *Percutaneous intradiscal annuloplasty other than electrothermal (22899)*
E 9.79 66.55 FUD 010

+ ⊙ 22527 1 or more additional levels (List separately in addition to code for primary procedure)
INCLUDES Contrast injection during fluoroscopic guidance/localization (77003)
EXCLUDES *Percutaneous intradiscal annuloplasty other than electrothermal (22899)*
Code first (22526)
E 4.42 55.27 FUD ZZZ

22532-22534 Spinal Fusion: Lateral Extracavitary Approach

CMS 100-3,150.2 Osteogenic Stimulation

EXCLUDES *Corpectomy (63101-63103)*
Exploration of spinal fusion (22830)
Fracture care (22305-22328)
Injection:
Chemonucleolysis (62292)
Discography (62290-62291)
Facet joint (64490-64495, [64633], [64634], [64635], [64636])
Myelography (62284)
Laminectomy (63001-63017)
Needle/trocar biopsy (20220-20225)
Osteotomy (22206-22226)

Code also bone grafting procedures (20930-20938)

Code also spinal instrumentation (22840-22855)

22532 Arthrodesis, lateral extracavitary technique, including minimal discectomy to prepare interspace (other than for decompression); thoracic
C 80 ▶ 51.24 51.24 FUD 090

22533 lumbar
C 80 ▶ 47.99 47.99 FUD 090

+ **22534 thoracic or lumbar, each additional vertebral segment (List separately in addition to code for primary procedure)**
Code first (22532-22533)
C 80 ▶ 10.42 10.42 FUD ZZZ

22548-22634 Spinal Fusion: Anterior and Posterior Approach

CMS 100-3,150.2 Osteogenic Stimulation

EXCLUDES *Corpectomy (63081-63091)*
Exploration of spinal fusion (22830)
Fracture care (22305-22328)
Facet joint arthrodesis (0219T-0222T)
Injection:
Chemonucleolysis (62292)
Discography (62290-62291)
Facet joint (64490-64495, [64633], [64634], [64635], [64636])
Myelography (62284)
Laminectomy (63001-63017)
Needle/trocar biopsy (20220-20225)
Osteotomy (22206-22226)

Code also bone grafting procedures (20930-20938)
Code also spinal instrumentation (22840-22855)

22548 Arthrodesis, anterior transoral or extraoral technique, clivus-C1-C2 (atlas-axis), with or without excision of odontoid process
EXCLUDES *Laminectomy or laminotomy with disc removal (63020-63042)*
C 80 ▶ 55.93 55.93 FUD 090

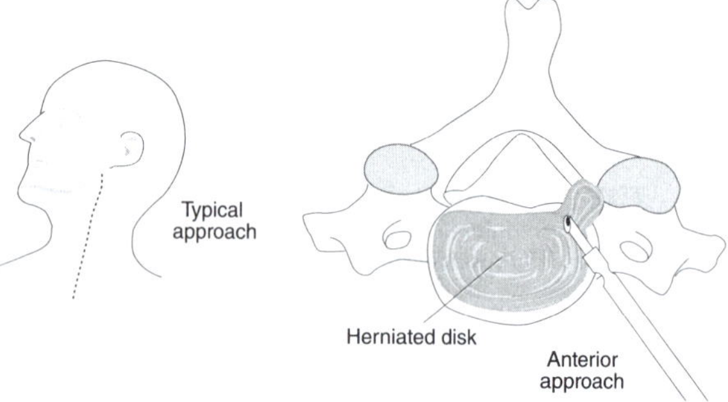

22551 Arthrodesis, anterior interbody, including disc space preparation, discectomy, osteophytectomy and decompression of spinal cord and/or nerve roots; cervical below C2
INCLUDES Operating microscope (69990)
T 80 49.09 49.09 FUD 090

+ **22552 cervical below C2, each additional interspace (List separately in addition to code for separate procedure)**
INCLUDES Operating microscope (69990)
Code first (22551)
C 80 11.33 11.33 FUD ZZZ

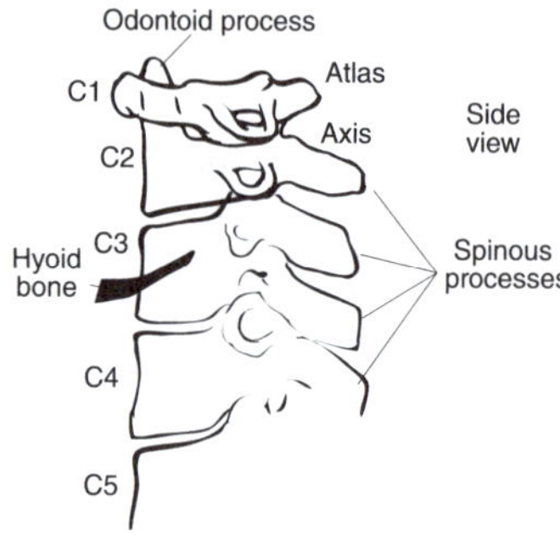

22554 Arthrodesis, anterior interbody technique, including minimal discectomy to prepare interspace (other than for decompression); cervical below C2
EXCLUDES *Anterior discectomy and interbody fusion during the same operative session (regardless if performed by multiple surgeons) (22551)*
Do not report with anterior discectomy (even by separate individual) (63075)
T 80 ▶ PQ 36.35 36.35 FUD 090

22556 thoracic
C 80 ▶ 47.76 47.76 FUD 090

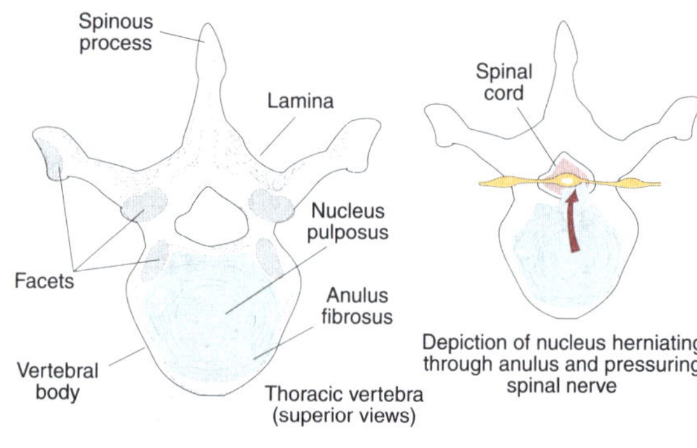

22558 lumbar
EXCLUDES *Arthrodesis using pre-sacral interbody technique (22586, 0195T)*
C 80 ▶ PQ 44.13 44.13 FUD 090

+ **22585 each additional interspace (List separately in addition to code for primary procedure)**
EXCLUDES *Anterior discectomy and interbody fusion during the same operative session (regardless if performed by multiple surgeons) (22552)*
Code first (22554-22558)
Do not report with anterior discectomy (even by another individual) (63075)
C 80 ▶ 9.63 9.63 FUD ZZZ

22586 Arthrodesis, pre-sacral interbody technique, including disc space preparation, discectomy, with posterior instrumentation, with image guidance, includes bone graft when performed, L5-S1 interspace
Do not report with (20930-20938, 22840, 22848, 72275, 77002-77003, 77011-77012)
C 80 53.76 53.76 FUD 090

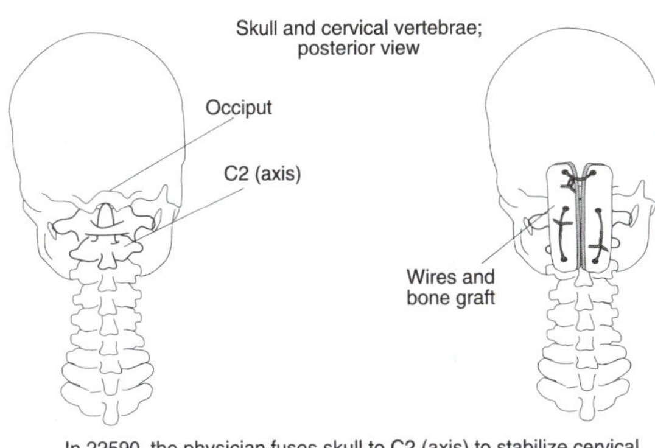

In 22590, the physician fuses skull to C2 (axis) to stabilize cervical vertebrae; anchor holes are drilled in the occiput of the skull

22590 **Arthrodesis, posterior technique, craniocervical (occiput-C2)**
EXCLUDES *Posterior intrafacet implant insertion (0219T-0222T)*
C 80 ⚑ 45.13 45.13 **FUD** 090

22595 **Arthrodesis, posterior technique, atlas-axis (C1-C2)**
EXCLUDES *Posterior intrafacet implant insertion (0219T-0222T)*
C 80 ⚑ 42.97 42.97 **FUD** 090

22600 **Arthrodesis, posterior or posterolateral technique, single level; cervical below C2 segment**
EXCLUDES *Posterior intrafacet implant insertion (0219T-0222T)*
C 80 ⚑ PQ 36.84 36.84 **FUD** 090

22610 **thoracic (with lateral transverse technique, when performed)**
EXCLUDES *Posterior intrafacet implant insertion (0219T-0222T)*
C 80 ⚑ 36.06 36.06 **FUD** 090

22612 **lumbar (with lateral transverse technique, when performed)**
EXCLUDES *Combined technique at the same interspace and segment (22633)*
Posterior intrafacet implant insertion (0219T-0222T)
Do not report with the following code when performed at the same interspace and segment (22630)
T 80 ⚑ PQ 45.68 45.68 **FUD** 090

+ **22614** **each additional vertebral segment (List separately in addition to code for primary procedure)**
INCLUDES Additional level fusion arthrodesis posterior or posterolateral interbody
EXCLUDES *Additional level interbody arthrodesis combined posterolateral or posterior with posterior interbody arthrodesis (22634)*
Additional level posterior interbody arthrodesis (22632)
Posterior intrafacet implant insertion (0219T-0222T)
Code first (22600, 22610, 22612, 22630, 22633)
N 80 ⚑ 11.25 11.25 **FUD** ZZZ

22630 **Arthrodesis, posterior interbody technique, including laminectomy and/or discectomy to prepare interspace (other than for decompression), single interspace; lumbar**
EXCLUDES *Combined technique at the same interspace and segment (22633)*
Do not report with the following code at the same interspace and segment (22612)
C 80 ⚑ PQ 44.37 44.37 **FUD** 090

+ **22632** **each additional interspace (List separately in addition to code for primary procedure)**
INCLUDES Includes posterior interbody fusion arthrodesis, additional level
EXCLUDES *Additional level combined technique (22634)*
Additional level posterior or posterolateral fusion (22614)
Code first (22612, 22630, 22633)
C 80 ⚑ 9.17 9.17 **FUD** ZZZ

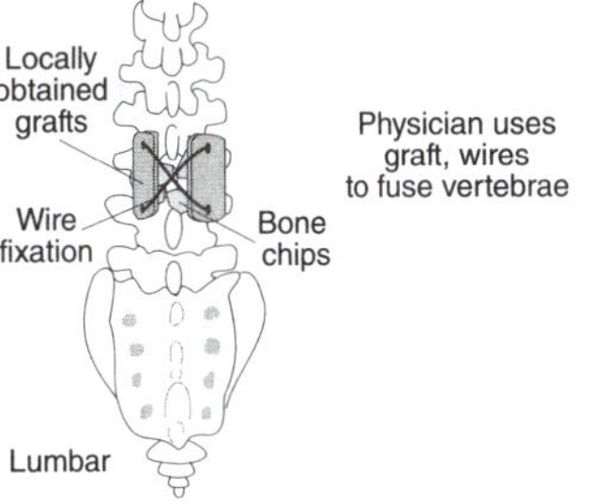

Using a posterior or posterolateral technique the vertebral interbody is fused

22633 **Arthrodesis, combined posterior or posterolateral technique with posterior interbody technique including laminectomy and/or discectomy sufficient to prepare interspace (other than for decompression), single interspace and segment; lumbar**
Do not report same level (22612, 22630)
C 80 52.86 52.86 **FUD** 090

+ **22634** **each additional interspace and segment (List separately in addition to code for primary procedure)**
Code first (22633)
C 80 14.27 14.27 **FUD** ZZZ

22800-22819 Procedures to Correct Anomalous Spinal Vertebrae

EXCLUDES *Facet injection (64490-64495, [64633, 64634, 64635, 64636])*
Code also bone grafting procedures (20930-20938)
Code also spinal instrumentation (22840-22855)

22800 **Arthrodesis, posterior, for spinal deformity, with or without cast; up to 6 vertebral segments**
C 80 ⚑ PQ 38.89 38.89 **FUD** 090

22802 **7 to 12 vertebral segments**
C 80 ⚑ PQ 60.13 60.13 **FUD** 090

22804 **13 or more vertebral segments**
C 80 ⚑ PQ 69.20 69.20 **FUD** 090

22808 **Arthrodesis, anterior, for spinal deformity, with or without cast; 2 to 3 vertebral segments**
INCLUDES Smith-Robinson arthrodesis
C 80 ⚑ 52.28 52.28 **FUD** 090

22810 **4 to 7 vertebral segments**
C 80 ⚑ 58.56 58.56 **FUD** 090

22812 **8 or more vertebral segments**
C 80 ⚑ 64.34 64.34 **FUD** 090

22818 **Kyphectomy, circumferential exposure of spine and resection of vertebral segment(s) (including body and posterior elements); single or 2 segments**
EXCLUDES *Arthrodesis (22800-22804)*
C 80 ⚑ 62.30 62.30 **FUD** 090

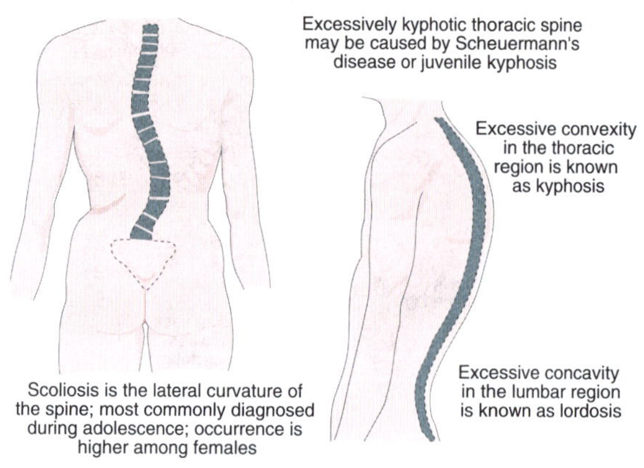

22819 **3 or more segments**

EXCLUDES *Arthrodesis (22800-22804)*

C 80 ▪ Facility RVU 78.31 Non-Facility RVU 78.31 **FUD** 090

22830 Surgical Exploration Previous Spinal Fusion

CMS 100-3,150.2 Osteogenic Stimulation

EXCLUDES *Arthrodesis (22532-22819)*
Bone grafting procedures (20930-20938)
Facet injection (64490-64495, [64633, 64634, 64635, 64636])
Spinal decompression (63001-63103)

Code also spinal instrumentation (22840-22855)

22830 **Exploration of spinal fusion**

Do not report with (22850, 22852, 22855)

C 80 ▪ Facility RVU 23.23 Non-Facility RVU 23.23 **FUD** 090

22840-22848 Posterior, Anterior, Pelvic Spinal Instrumentation

INCLUDES Removal or revision of previously placed spinal instrumentation during same session as insertion of new instrumentation at levels including all or part of previously instrumented segments

EXCLUDES *Arthrodesis (22532-22534, 22548-22812)*
Bone grafting procedures (20930-20938)
Exploration of spinal fusion (22830)
Fracture treatment (22325-22328)

Do not report removal or reinsertion in addition to insertion of the new instrumentation (22849, 22850, 22852, 22855)

\+ **22840** **Posterior non-segmental instrumentation (eg, Harrington rod technique, pedicle fixation across 1 interspace, atlantoaxial transarticular screw fixation, sublaminar wiring at C1, facet screw fixation) (List separately in addition to code for primary procedure)**

EXCLUDES *Insertion of posterior spinous process distraction devices (0171T-0172T)*

Code first (22100-22102, 22110-22114, 22206-22207, 22210-22214, 22220-22224, 22305-22327, 22532-22533, 22548-22558, 22590-22612, 22630, 22633-22634, 22800-22812, 63001-63030, 63040-63042, 63045-63047, 63050-63056, 63064, 63075, 63077, 63081, 63085, 63087, 63090, 63101-63102, 63170-63290, 63300-63307)

C 80 ▪ Facility RVU 21.94 Non-Facility RVU 21.94 **FUD** ZZZ

\+ **22841** **Internal spinal fixation by wiring of spinous processes (List separately in addition to code for primary procedure)**

Code first (22100-22102, 22110-22114, 22206-22207, 22210-22214, 22220-22224, 22305-22327, 22532-22533, 22548-22558, 22590-22612, 22630, 22633-22634, 22800-22812, 63001-63030, 63040-63042, 63045-63047, 63050-63056, 63064, 63075, 63077, 63081, 63085, 63087, 63090, 63101-63102, 63170-63290, 63300-63307)

C Facility RVU 0.00 Non-Facility RVU 0.00 **FUD** XXX

Example of rod hook; may be attached at top and bottom only, or also at segments

Rod

Segment

\+ **22842** **Posterior segmental instrumentation (eg, pedicle fixation, dual rods with multiple hooks and sublaminar wires); 3 to 6 vertebral segments (List separately in addition to code for primary procedure)**

Code first (22100-22102, 22110-22114, 22206-22207, 22210-22214, 22220-22224, 22305-22327, 22532-22533, 22548-22558, 22590-22612, 22630, 22633-22634, 22800-22812, 63001-63030, 63040-63042, 63045-63047, 63050-63056, 63064, 63075, 63077, 63081, 63085, 63087, 63090, 63101-63102, 63170-63290, 63300-63307)

C 80 ▪ Facility RVU 21.96 Non-Facility RVU 21.96 **FUD** ZZZ

\+ **22843** **7 to 12 vertebral segments (List separately in addition to code for primary procedure)**

Code first (22100-22102, 22110-22114, 22206-22207, 22210-22214, 22220-22224, 22305-22327, 22532-22533, 22548-22558, 22590-22612, 22630, 22633-22634, 22800-22812, 63001-63030, 63040-63042, 63045-63047, 63050-63056, 63064, 63075, 63077, 63081, 63085, 63087, 63090, 63101-63102, 63170-63290, 63300-63307)

C 80 ▪ Facility RVU 23.36 Non-Facility RVU 23.36 **FUD** ZZZ

\+ **22844** **13 or more vertebral segments (List separately in addition to code for primary procedure)**

Code first (22100-22102, 22110-22114, 22206-22207, 22210-22214, 22220-22224, 22305-22327, 22532-22533, 22548-22558, 22590-22612, 22630, 22633-22634, 22800-22812, 63001-63030, 63040-63042, 63045-63047, 63050-63056, 63064, 63075, 63077, 63081, 63085, 63087, 63090, 63101-63102, 63170-63290, 63300-63307)

C 80 ▪ Facility RVU 28.12 Non-Facility RVU 28.12 **FUD** ZZZ

\+ **22845** **Anterior instrumentation; 2 to 3 vertebral segments (List separately in addition to code for primary procedure)**

INCLUDES Dwyer instrumentation technique

Code first (22100-22102, 22110-22114, 22206-22207, 22210-22214, 22220-22224, 22305-22327, 22532-22533, 22548-22558, 22590-22612, 22630, 22633-22634, 22800-22812, 63001-63030, 63040-63042, 63045-63047, 63050-63056, 63064, 63075, 63077, 63081, 63085, 63087, 63090, 63101-63102, 63170-63290, 63300-63307)

C 80 ▪ Facility RVU 21.18 Non-Facility RVU 21.18 **FUD** ZZZ

\+ **22846** **4 to 7 vertebral segments (List separately in addition to code for primary procedure)**

INCLUDES Dwyer instrumentation technique

Code first (22100-22102, 22110-22114, 22206-22207, 22210-22214, 22220-22224, 22305-22327, 22532-22533, 22548-22558, 22590-22612, 22630, 22633-22634, 22800-22812, 63001-63030, 63040-63042, 63045-63047, 63050-63056, 63064, 63075, 63077, 63081, 63085, 63087, 63090, 63101-63102, 63170-63290, 63300-63307)

C 80 ▪ Facility RVU 21.98 Non-Facility RVU 21.98 **FUD** ZZZ

\+ 22847 **8 or more vertebral segments (List separately in addition to code for primary procedure)**

INCLUDES Dwyer instrumentation technique

Code first (22100-22102, 22110-22114, 22206-22207, 22210-22214, 22220-22224, 22305-22327, 22532-22533, 22548-22558, 22590-22612, 22630, 22633-22634, 22800-22812, 63001-63030, 63040-63042, 63045-63047, 63050-63056, 63064, 63075, 63077, 63081, 63085, 63087, 63090, 63101-63102, 63170-63290, 63300-63307)

C 80 25.27 25.27 FUD ZZZ

\+ 22848 **Pelvic fixation (attachment of caudal end of instrumentation to pelvic bony structures) other than sacrum (List separately in addition to code for primary procedure)**

Code first (22100-22102, 22110-22114, 22206-22207, 22210-22214, 22220-22224, 22305-22327, 22532-22533, 22548-22558, 22590-22612, 22630, 22633-22634, 22800-22812, 63001-63030, 63040-63042, 63045-63047, 63050-63056, 63064, 63075, 63077, 63081, 63085, 63087, 63090, 63101-63102, 63170-63290, 63300-63307)

C 80 10.29 10.29 FUD ZZZ

22849-22855 Miscellaneous Spinal Instrumentation

EXCLUDES *Arthrodesis (22532-22534, 22548-22812)*
Bone grafting procedures (20930-20938)
Exploration of spinal fusion (22830)
Facet injection (64490-64495, [64633], [64634], [64635], [64636])
Fracture treatment (22325-22328)

Do not report with insertion of the new instrumentation (22840-22848)

22849 **Reinsertion of spinal fixation device**

Do not report with removal of instrumentation at the same level (22850, 22852, 22855)

C 80 37.30 37.30 FUD 090

22850 **Removal of posterior nonsegmental instrumentation (eg, Harrington rod)**

C 80 20.69 20.69 FUD 090

\+ 22851 **Application of intervertebral biomechanical device(s) (eg, synthetic cage(s), methylmethacrylate) to vertebral defect or interspace (List separately in addition to code for primary procedure)**

EXCLUDES *Application of intervertebral bone device/graft (20930-20938)*
Insertion of posterior spinous process distraction devices (0171T-0172T)

Code first (22100-22102, 22110-22114, 22206-22207, 22210-22214, 22220-22224, 22305-22327, 22532-22533, 22548-22558, 22590-22612, 22630, 22633-22634, 22800-22812, 63001-63030, 63040-63042, 63045-63047, 63050-63056, 63064, 63075, 63077, 63081, 63085, 63087, 63090, 63101-63102, 63170-63290, 63300-63307)

N 80 11.75 11.75 FUD ZZZ

22852 **Removal of posterior segmental instrumentation**

C 80 19.78 19.78 FUD 090

22855 **Removal of anterior instrumentation**

C 80 32.02 32.02 FUD 090

22856-22899 Artificial Disc Replacement

CMS 100-3,150.10 Lumbar Artificial Disc Replacement (LADR)

INCLUDES Fluoroscopy (76000-76001)

EXCLUDES *Facet injection (64490-64495, [64633], [64634], [64635], [64636])*
Spinal decompression (63001-63048)

▲ 22856 **Total disc arthroplasty (artificial disc), anterior approach, including discectomy with end plate preparation (includes osteophytectomy for nerve root or spinal cord decompression and microdissection); single interspace, cervical**

INCLUDES Operating microscope (69990)

EXCLUDES *Cervical total disc arthroplasty, 3 or more levels (0375T)*

Code also ([22858]) when one additional cervical interspace involved

Do not report at same level as (22554, 22845, 22851, 63075, 0375T)

T 80 47.49 47.49 FUD 090

\+ #● 22858 **second level, cervical (List separately in addition to code for primary procedure)**

Code first (22856)

Do not report at the same level as (0375T)

22857 **Total disc arthroplasty (artificial disc), anterior approach, including discectomy to prepare interspace (other than for decompression), single interspace, lumbar**

INCLUDES Operating microscope (69990)

EXCLUDES *Arthroplasty more than one interspace (0163T)*

Do not report at same level (22558, 22845, 22851, 49010)

C 80 52.34 52.34 FUD 090

22858 Resequenced code. See code following 22856.

22861 **Revision including replacement of total disc arthroplasty (artificial disc), anterior approach, single interspace; cervical**

INCLUDES Operating microscope (69990)

EXCLUDES *Revision of additional cervical arthroplasty (0098T)*
Removal of artificial disc (22864)

Do not report at same level (22845, 22851, 22864, 63075)

C 80 63.15 63.15 FUD 090

22862 **lumbar**

EXCLUDES *Arthroplasty revision more than one interspace (0165T)*

Do not report at same level (22558, 22845, 22851, 22864, 49010)

C 80 61.06 61.06 FUD 090

22864 **Removal of total disc arthroplasty (artificial disc), anterior approach, single interspace; cervical**

INCLUDES Operating microscope (69990)

EXCLUDES *Cervical total disc arthroplasty with additional interspace removal (0095T)*

Do not report with (22861)

C 80 56.80 56.80 FUD 090

22865 **lumbar**

EXCLUDES *Arthroplasty more than one level (0164T)*

Do not report with (49010)

C 80 58.75 58.75 FUD 090

22899 **Unlisted procedure, spine**

T 80 0.00 0.00 FUD YYY

22900-22999 Musculoskeletal Procedures of Abdomen

INCLUDES Any necessary elevation of tissue planes or dissection
Measurement of tumor and necessary margin at greatest diameter prior to excision
Simple and intermediate repairs
Types of excision:
Fascial or subfascial soft tissue tumors: simple and marginal resection of tumors found either in or below the deep fascia, not involving bone or excision of a substantial amount of normal tissue; primarily benign and intramuscular tumors
Radical resection soft tissue tumor: wide resection of tumor involving substantial margins of normal tissue and may include tissue removal from one or more layers; most often malignant or aggressive benign
Subcutaneous: simple and marginal resection of tumors in the subcutaneous tissue above the deep fascia; most often benign

EXCLUDES *Complex repair*
Excision of benign cutaneous lesions (eg, sebaceous cyst) (11400-11406)
Radical resection of cutaneous tumors (eg, melanoma) (11600-11606)
Significant exploration of the vessels or neuroplasty

22900 **Excision, tumor, soft tissue of abdominal wall, subfascial (eg, intramuscular); less than 5 cm**
G2 T 80 ⚑ 15.99 15.99 FUD 090

22901 **5 cm or greater**
G2 T 80 18.80 18.80 FUD 090

22902 **Excision, tumor, soft tissue of abdominal wall, subcutaneous; less than 3 cm**
G2 T 80 9.19 12.17 FUD 090

22903 **3 cm or greater**
G2 T 80 12.29 12.29 FUD 090

22904 **Radical resection of tumor (eg, sarcoma), soft tissue of abdominal wall; less than 5 cm**
G2 T 80 29.85 29.85 FUD 090

22905 **5 cm or greater**
G2 T 80 38.03 38.03 FUD 090

22999 **Unlisted procedure, abdomen, musculoskeletal system**
T 80 0.00 0.00 FUD YYY

23000-23044 Surgical Incision Shoulder: Drainage, Foreign Body Removal, Contracture Release

23000 **Removal of subdeltoid calcareous deposits, open**
EXCLUDES *Arthroscopic removal calcium deposits of bursa (29999)*
A2 T 80 50 ⚑ 10.53 16.43 FUD 090

23020 **Capsular contracture release (eg, Sever type procedure)**
EXCLUDES *Simple incision and drainage (10040-10160)*
A2 T 80 50 ⚑ 19.64 19.64 FUD 090

23030 **Incision and drainage, shoulder area; deep abscess or hematoma**
A2 T ⚑ 7.27 12.43 FUD 010

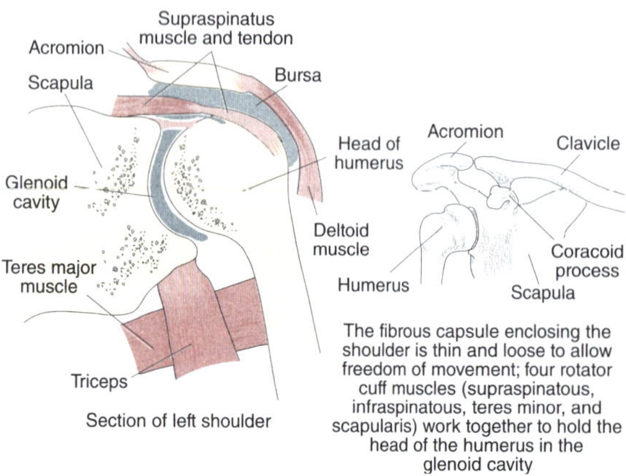

Section of left shoulder

The fibrous capsule enclosing the shoulder is thin and loose to allow freedom of movement; four rotator cuff muscles (supraspinatous, infraspinatous, teres minor, and scapularis) work together to hold the head of the humerus in the glenoid cavity

23031 **infected bursa**
A2 T 50 ⚑ 6.24 11.96 FUD 010

23035 **Incision, bone cortex (eg, osteomyelitis or bone abscess), shoulder area**
A2 T 80 50 ⚑ 19.48 19.48 FUD 090

23040 **Arthrotomy, glenohumeral joint, including exploration, drainage, or removal of foreign body**
A2 T 80 50 ⚑ 20.48 20.48 FUD 090

23044 **Arthrotomy, acromioclavicular, sternoclavicular joint, including exploration, drainage, or removal of foreign body**
A2 T 50 ⚑ 16.15 16.15 FUD 090

23065-23066 Shoulder Biopsy

EXCLUDES *Soft tissue needle biopsy (20206)*

23065 **Biopsy, soft tissue of shoulder area; superficial**
P3 T 50 ⚑ PQ 4.77 6.11 FUD 010

23066 **deep**
A2 T 50 ⚑ PQ 10.10 15.64 FUD 090

23071-23078 [23071, 23073] Excision Soft Tissue Tumors of Shoulder

INCLUDES Any necessary elevation of tissue planes or dissection
Measurement of tumor and necessary margin at greatest diameter prior to excision
Simple and intermediate repairs
Types of Excision:
Fascial or subfascial soft tissue tumors: simple and marginal resection of tumors found either in or below the deep fascia, not involving bone or excision of a substantial amount of normal tissue; primarily benign and intramuscular tumors
Radical resection soft tissue tumor: wide resection of tumor, involving substantial margins of normal tissue and may involve tissue removal from one or more layers; most often malignant or aggressive benign
Subcutaneous: simple and marginal resection of tumors in the subcutaneous tissue above the deep fascia; most often benign

EXCLUDES *Complex repair*
Excision of benign cutaneous lesions (eg, sebaceous cyst) (11400-11406)
Radical resection of cutaneous tumors (eg, melanoma) (11600-11606)
Significant exploration of the vessels or neuroplasty

23071 ***Resequenced code. See code following 23075.***

23073 ***Resequenced code. See code following 23076.***

23075 **Excision, tumor, soft tissue of shoulder area, subcutaneous; less than 3 cm**
G2 T 50 ⚑ 9.26 13.19 FUD 090

\# **23071** **3 cm or greater**
G2 T 80 50 11.89 11.89 FUD 090

23076 **Excision, tumor, soft tissue of shoulder area, subfascial (eg, intramuscular); less than 5 cm**
G2 T 50 ⚑ 15.32 15.32 FUD 090

\# **23073** **5 cm or greater**
G2 T 80 50 19.67 19.67 FUD 090

23077 **Radical resection of tumor (eg, sarcoma), soft tissue of shoulder area; less than 5 cm**
G2 T 80 50 ⚑ 32.64 32.64 FUD 090

23078 **5 cm or greater**
G2 T 80 50 41.21 41.21 FUD 090

23100-23195 Bone and Joint Procedures of Shoulder

INCLUDES Acromioclavicular joint
Clavicle
Head and neck of humerus
Scapula
Shoulder joint
Sternoclavicular joint

23100 **Arthrotomy, glenohumeral joint, including biopsy**
A2 T 80 50 ⚑ PQ 14.21 14.21 FUD 090

23101 Arthrotomy, acromioclavicular joint or sternoclavicular joint, including biopsy and/or excision of torn cartilage
A2 T 50 PQ 12.95 12.95 FUD 090

23105 Arthrotomy; glenohumeral joint, with synovectomy, with or without biopsy
A2 T 80 50 18.17 18.17 FUD 090

23106 sternoclavicular joint, with synovectomy, with or without biopsy
A2 T 50 14.09 14.09 FUD 090

23107 Arthrotomy, glenohumeral joint, with joint exploration, with or without removal of loose or foreign body
A2 T 80 50 18.84 18.84 FUD 090

23120 Clavicullectomy; partial
INCLUDES Mumford operation
EXCLUDES *Arthroscopic claviculectomy (29824)*
A2 T 80 50 16.66 16.66 FUD 090

23125 total
A2 T 80 50 20.16 20.16 FUD 090

23130 Acromioplasty or acromionectomy, partial, with or without coracoacromial ligament release
A2 T 50 17.31 17.31 FUD 090

23140 Excision or curettage of bone cyst or benign tumor of clavicle or scapula;
A2 T 50 15.06 15.06 FUD 090

23145 with autograft (includes obtaining graft)
A2 T 80 50 19.77 19.77 FUD 090

23146 with allograft
A2 T 80 50 17.64 17.64 FUD 090

23150 Excision or curettage of bone cyst or benign tumor of proximal humerus;
A2 T 80 50 18.78 18.78 FUD 090

23155 with autograft (includes obtaining graft)
A2 T 80 50 22.57 22.57 FUD 090

23156 with allograft
A2 T 80 50 19.28 19.28 FUD 090

23170 Sequestrectomy (eg, for osteomyelitis or bone abscess), clavicle
A2 T 50 15.92 15.92 FUD 090

23172 Sequestrectomy (eg, for osteomyelitis or bone abscess), scapula
A2 T 80 50 16.11 16.11 FUD 090

23174 Sequestrectomy (eg, for osteomyelitis or bone abscess), humeral head to surgical neck
A2 T 80 50 21.55 21.55 FUD 090

23180 Partial excision (craterization, saucerization, or diaphysectomy) bone (eg, osteomyelitis), clavicle
A2 T 50 18.96 18.96 FUD 090

23182 Partial excision (craterization, saucerization, or diaphysectomy) bone (eg, osteomyelitis), scapula
A2 T 80 50 18.81 18.81 FUD 090

23184 Partial excision (craterization, saucerization, or diaphysectomy) bone (eg, osteomyelitis), proximal humerus
A2 T 80 50 20.91 20.91 FUD 090

23190 Ostectomy of scapula, partial (eg, superior medial angle)
A2 T 80 50 16.22 16.22 FUD 090

23195 Resection, humeral head
EXCLUDES *Arthroplasty with replacement with implant (23470)*
A2 T 80 50 21.49 21.49 FUD 090

23200-23220 Radical Resection of Bone Tumors of Shoulder

INCLUDES Any necessary elevation of tissue planes or dissection
Measurement of tumor and necessary margin at greatest diameter prior to excision
Radical resection of cutaneous tumors (e.g., melanoma)
Resection of the tumor (may include entire bone) and wide margins of normal tissues primarily for malignant or aggressive benign tumors
Simple and intermediate repairs

EXCLUDES *Complex repair*
Significant exploration of vessels, neuroplasty, reconstruction, or complex bone repair

Do not report excision of soft tissue codes when adjacent soft tissue is removed during the bone tumor resection (23076-23078 [23071, 23073])

23200 Radical resection of tumor; clavicle
C 80 50 43.33 43.33 FUD 090

23210 scapula
C 80 50 50.96 50.96 FUD 090

23220 Radical resection of tumor, proximal humerus
C 80 50 55.90 55.90 FUD 090

23330-23335 Removal Implant/Foreign Body from Shoulder

EXCLUDES *Bursal arthrocentesis or needling (20610)*
K-wire or pin insertion (20650)
K-wire or pin removal (20670, 20680)

23330 Removal of foreign body, shoulder; subcutaneous
A2 T 80 50 4.30 6.80 FUD 010

23333 deep (subfascial or intramuscular)
G2 T 80 50 13.01 13.01 FUD 090

23334 Removal of prosthesis, includes debridement and synovectomy when performed; humeral or glenoid component
EXCLUDES *Foreign body removal (23330, 23333)*
Hardware removal other than prosthesis (20680)
Do not report with prosthesis removal and replacement in same shoulder (eg, glenoid and/or humeral components) (23470-23472)
G2 T 50 30.71 30.71 FUD 090

23335 humeral and glenoid components (eg, total shoulder)
EXCLUDES *Foreign body removal (23330, 23333)*
Hardware removal other than prosthesis (20680)
Do not report with prosthesis removal and replacement in same shoulder (eg, glenoid and/or humeral components) (23470-23472)
C 50 36.62 36.62 FUD 090

23350 Injection for Shoulder Arthrogram

23350 Injection procedure for shoulder arthrography or enhanced CT/MRI shoulder arthrography
EXCLUDES *Shoulder biopsy (29805-29826)*
73040, 73201-73202, 73222-73223, 77002
N1 N 50 1.48 3.66 FUD 000

23395-23491 Repair/Reconstruction of Shoulder

23395 Muscle transfer, any type, shoulder or upper arm; single
A2 T 80 36.74 36.74 FUD 090

23397 multiple
A2 T 80 32.57 32.57 FUD 090

23400 Scapulopexy (eg, Sprengels deformity or for paralysis)
A2 T 80 50 27.68 27.68 FUD 090

23405 Tenotomy, shoulder area; single tendon
A2 T 80 17.93 17.93 FUD 090

23406 multiple tendons through same incision
A2 T 80 22.01 22.01 FUD 090

23410 Repair of ruptured musculotendinous cuff (eg, rotator cuff) open; acute
EXCLUDES *Arthroscopic repair (29827)*
A2 T 80 50 23.43 23.43 FUD 090

23412 chronic
EXCLUDES *Arthroscopic repair (29827)*
A2 T 80 50 24.33 24.33 FUD 090

23415 Coracoacromial ligament release, with or without acromioplasty
EXCLUDES *Arthroscopic repair (29826)*
A2 T 50 19.82 19.82 FUD 090

23420 Reconstruction of complete shoulder (rotator) cuff avulsion, chronic (includes acromioplasty)
A2 T 80 50 27.65 27.65 FUD 090

23430 Tenodesis of long tendon of biceps
EXCLUDES *Arthroscopic biceps tenodesis (29828)*
A2 T 80 50 21.33 21.33 FUD 090

23440 Resection or transplantation of long tendon of biceps
A2 T 80 50 21.57 21.57 FUD 090

23450 Capsulorrhaphy, anterior; Putti-Platt procedure or Magnuson type operation
EXCLUDES *Arthroscopic thermal capsulorrhaphy (29999)*
A2 T 80 50 27.04 27.04 FUD 090

23455 with labral repair (eg, Bankart procedure)
EXCLUDES *Arthroscopic repair (29806)*
A2 T 80 50 28.63 28.63 FUD 090

23460 Capsulorrhaphy, anterior, any type; with bone block
INCLUDES Bristow procedure
A2 T 80 50 31.09 31.09 FUD 090

23462 with coracoid process transfer
EXCLUDES *Open thermal capsulorrhaphy (23929)*
A2 T 80 50 30.61 30.61 FUD 090

23465 Capsulorrhaphy, glenohumeral joint, posterior, with or without bone block
EXCLUDES *Sternoclavicular and acromioclavicular joint repair (23530, 23550)*
A2 T 80 50 31.89 31.89 FUD 090

23466 Capsulorrhaphy, glenohumeral joint, any type multi-directional instability
A2 T 80 50 32.02 32.02 FUD 090

23470 Arthroplasty, glenohumeral joint; hemiarthroplasty
T 80 50 34.50 34.50 FUD 090

23472 total shoulder (glenoid and proximal humeral replacement (eg, total shoulder))
EXCLUDES *Proximal humerus osteotomy (24400)*
Removal of total shoulder components (23334-23335)
C 80 50 41.85 41.85 FUD 090

23473 Revision of total shoulder arthroplasty, including allograft when performed; humeral or glenoid component
Do not report with removal of prosthesis only (glenoid and/or humeral component) (23334-23335)
T 80 50 46.67 46.67 FUD 090

23474 humeral and glenoid component
Do not report with removal of prosthesis only (glenoid and/or humeral component) (23334-23335)
C 80 50 50.45 50.45 FUD 090

23480 Osteotomy, clavicle, with or without internal fixation;
A2 T 50 23.37 23.37 FUD 090

23485 with bone graft for nonunion or malunion (includes obtaining graft and/or necessary fixation)
A2 T 80 50 27.27 27.27 FUD 090

23490 Prophylactic treatment (nailing, pinning, plating or wiring) with or without methylmethacrylate; clavicle
A2 T 80 50 24.57 24.57 FUD 090

23491 proximal humerus
A2 T 80 50 28.92 28.92 FUD 090

23500-23680 Treatment of Shoulder Fracture/Dislocation

23500 Closed treatment of clavicular fracture; without manipulation
A2 T 50 6.29 6.19 FUD 090

23505 with manipulation
A2 T 50 9.44 9.98 FUD 090

23515 Open treatment of clavicular fracture, includes internal fixation, when performed
A2 T 80 50 20.56 20.56 FUD 090

23520 Closed treatment of sternoclavicular dislocation; without manipulation
A2 T 80 50 6.61 6.51 FUD 090

23525 with manipulation
A2 T 80 50 10.03 10.83 FUD 090

23530 Open treatment of sternoclavicular dislocation, acute or chronic;
A2 T 80 50 16.27 16.27 FUD 090

23532 with fascial graft (includes obtaining graft)
A2 T 80 50 17.73 17.73 FUD 090

23540 Closed treatment of acromioclavicular dislocation; without manipulation
A2 T 50 6.44 6.34 FUD 090

23545 with manipulation
A2 T 80 50 8.77 9.63 FUD 090

23550 Open treatment of acromioclavicular dislocation, acute or chronic;
A2 T 80 50 16.30 16.30 FUD 090

23552 with fascial graft (includes obtaining graft)
A2 T 80 50 18.66 18.66 FUD 090

23570 Closed treatment of scapular fracture; without manipulation
A2 T 50 6.74 6.54 FUD 090

23575 with manipulation, with or without skeletal traction (with or without shoulder joint involvement)
A2 T 80 50 10.61 11.30 FUD 090

23585 Open treatment of scapular fracture (body, glenoid or acromion) includes internal fixation, when performed
A2 T 80 50 28.01 28.01 FUD 090

23600 Closed treatment of proximal humeral (surgical or anatomical neck) fracture; without manipulation
P2 T 50 8.71 9.22 FUD 090

23605 with manipulation, with or without skeletal traction
A2 T 50 12.07 13.15 FUD 090

23615 Open treatment of proximal humeral (surgical or anatomical neck) fracture, includes internal fixation, when performed, includes repair of tuberosity(s), when performed;
A2 T 80 50 25.26 25.26 FUD 090

23616 with proximal humeral prosthetic replacement
A2 T 80 50 35.51 35.51 FUD 090

23620 Closed treatment of greater humeral tuberosity fracture; without manipulation
P2 T 50 7.25 7.61 FUD 090

23625 with manipulation
A2 T 50 10.03 10.75 FUD 090

23630 Open treatment of greater humeral tuberosity fracture, includes internal fixation, when performed
A2 T 80 50 ⚑ 22.32 22.32 FUD 090

23650 Closed treatment of shoulder dislocation, with manipulation; without anesthesia
A2 T 50 ⚑ 8.16 8.87 FUD 090

23655 requiring anesthesia
A2 T 50 ⚑ 11.32 11.32 FUD 090

23660 Open treatment of acute shoulder dislocation
EXCLUDES *Chronic dislocation repair (23450-23466)*
A2 T 80 50 ⚑ 16.61 16.61 FUD 090

23665 Closed treatment of shoulder dislocation, with fracture of greater humeral tuberosity, with manipulation
A2 T 50 ⚑ 11.24 12.05 FUD 090

23670 Open treatment of shoulder dislocation, with fracture of greater humeral tuberosity, includes internal fixation, when performed
A2 T 80 50 ⚑ 25.05 25.05 FUD 090

23675 Closed treatment of shoulder dislocation, with surgical or anatomical neck fracture, with manipulation
A2 T 50 ⚑ 14.20 15.56 FUD 090

23680 Open treatment of shoulder dislocation, with surgical or anatomical neck fracture, includes internal fixation, when performed
A2 T 80 50 ⚑ 26.51 26.51 FUD 090

23700-23929 Other/Unlisted Shoulder Procedures

23700 Manipulation under anesthesia, shoulder joint, including application of fixation apparatus (dislocation excluded)
A2 T 50 ⚑ 5.56 5.56 FUD 010

23800 Arthrodesis, glenohumeral joint;
A2 T 80 50 ⚑ 29.27 29.27 FUD 090

23802 with autogenous graft (includes obtaining graft)
A2 T 80 50 ⚑ 36.62 36.62 FUD 090

23900 Interthoracoscapular amputation (forequarter)
C 80 ⚑ 39.66 39.66 FUD 090

23920 Disarticulation of shoulder;
C 80 50 ⚑ 32.15 32.15 FUD 090

23921 secondary closure or scar revision
A2 T 50 ⚑ 13.50 13.50 FUD 090

23929 Unlisted procedure, shoulder
T 80 0.00 0.00 FUD YYY

23930-24006 Surgical Incision Elbow/Upper Arm

EXCLUDES *Simple incision and drainage procedures (10040-10160)*

23930 Incision and drainage, upper arm or elbow area; deep abscess or hematoma
A2 T 50 ⚑ 6.12 9.93 FUD 010

23931 bursa
A2 T 50 ⚑ 4.56 8.13 FUD 010

23935 Incision, deep, with opening of bone cortex (eg, for osteomyelitis or bone abscess), humerus or elbow
A2 T 80 50 ⚑ 14.47 14.47 FUD 090

24000 Arthrotomy, elbow, including exploration, drainage, or removal of foreign body
A2 T 80 50 ⚑ 13.56 13.56 FUD 090

24006 Arthrotomy of the elbow, with capsular excision for capsular release (separate procedure)
A2 T 80 50 ⚑ 20.26 20.26 FUD 090

24065-24066 Biopsy of Elbow/Upper Arm

24065 Biopsy, soft tissue of upper arm or elbow area; superficial
EXCLUDES *Soft tissue needle biopsy (20206)*
P3 T 50 ⚑ PQ 4.77 7.21 FUD 010

24066 deep (subfascial or intramuscular)
EXCLUDES *Soft tissue needle biopsy (20206)*
A2 T 50 ⚑ PQ 11.70 17.39 FUD 090

24071-24079 [24071, 24073] Excision Soft Tissue Tumors Elbow/Upper Arm

INCLUDES Any necessary elevation of tissue planes or dissection
Measurement of tumor and necessary margin at greatest diameter prior to excision
Types of excision:
Fascial or subfascial soft tissue tumors: simple and marginal resection of tumors found either in or below the deep fascia, not involving bone or excision of a substantial amount of normal tissue; primarily benign and intramuscular tumors
Radical resection of soft tissue tumor: wide resection of tumor involving substantial margins of normal tissue and may involve tissue removal from one or more layers; most often malignant or aggressive benign
Subcutaneous: simple and marginal resection of tumors found in the subcutaneous tissue above the deep fascia; most often benign

EXCLUDES *Complex repair*
Excision of benign cutaneous lesion (eg, sebaceous cyst) (11400-11406)
Radical resection of cutaneous tumors (eg, melanoma) (11600-11606)
Significant exploration of vessels or neuroplasty

24071 Resequenced code. See code following 24075

24073 Resequenced code. See code following 24076.

24075 Excision, tumor, soft tissue of upper arm or elbow area, subcutaneous; less than 3 cm
G2 T 50 ⚑ 9.35 13.79 FUD 090

24071 3 cm or greater
G2 T 80 50 11.53 11.53 FUD 090

24076 Excision, tumor, soft tissue of upper arm or elbow area, subfascial (eg, intramuscular); less than 5 cm
G2 T 50 ⚑ 15.44 15.44 FUD 090

24073 5 cm or greater
G2 T 80 50 19.65 19.65 FUD 090

24077 Radical resection of tumor (eg, sarcoma), soft tissue of upper arm or elbow area; less than 5 cm
G2 T 50 ⚑ 29.57 29.57 FUD 090

24079 5 cm or greater
G2 T 80 50 37.87 37.87 FUD 090

24100-24149 Bone/Joint Procedures Upper Arm/Elbow

24100 Arthrotomy, elbow; with synovial biopsy only
A2 T 80 50 ⚑ PQ 11.86 11.86 FUD 090

24101 with joint exploration, with or without biopsy, with or without removal of loose or foreign body
A2 T 80 50 ⚑ PQ 14.19 14.19 FUD 090

24102 with synovectomy
A2 T 80 50 ⚑ 17.52 17.52 FUD 090

24105 Excision, olecranon bursa
A2 T 50 ⚑ 9.90 9.90 FUD 090

24110 Excision or curettage of bone cyst or benign tumor, humerus;
A2 T 50 ⚑ 16.70 16.70 FUD 090

24115 with autograft (includes obtaining graft)
A2 T 80 50 ⚑ 20.98 20.98 FUD 090

24116 with allograft
A2 T 80 50 ⚑ 24.55 24.55 FUD 090

24120 Excision or curettage of bone cyst or benign tumor of head or neck of radius or olecranon process;
A2 T 80 50 ⚑ 15.02 15.02 FUD 090

Musculoskeletal System

23630 — 24120

24125 **with autograft (includes obtaining graft)**
A2 T 80 50 17.62 17.62 FUD 090

24126 **with allograft**
A2 T 80 50 18.45 18.45 FUD 090

24130 **Excision, radial head**
EXCLUDES *Radial head arthroplasty with implant (24366)*
A2 T 50 14.41 14.41 FUD 090

24134 **Sequestrectomy (eg, for osteomyelitis or bone abscess), shaft or distal humerus**
A2 T 80 50 21.25 21.25 FUD 090

24136 **Sequestrectomy (eg, for osteomyelitis or bone abscess), radial head or neck**
A2 T 50 18.11 18.11 FUD 090

24138 **Sequestrectomy (eg, for osteomyelitis or bone abscess), olecranon process**
A2 T 80 50 19.15 19.15 FUD 090

24140 **Partial excision (craterization, saucerization, or diaphysectomy) bone (eg, osteomyelitis), humerus**
A2 T 80 50 19.89 19.89 FUD 090

24145 **Partial excision (craterization, saucerization, or diaphysectomy) bone (eg, osteomyelitis), radial head or neck**
A2 T 50 16.82 16.82 FUD 090

24147 **Partial excision (craterization, saucerization, or diaphysectomy) bone (eg, osteomyelitis), olecranon process**
A2 T 50 17.67 17.67 FUD 090

24149 **Radical resection of capsule, soft tissue, and heterotopic bone, elbow, with contracture release (separate procedure)**
EXCLUDES *Capsular and soft tissue release (24006)*
G2 T 80 50 33.43 33.43 FUD 090

24150-24152 Radical Resection Bone Tumor Upper Arm

INCLUDES Any necessary elevation of tissue planes or dissection
Measurement of tumor and necessary margin at greatest diameter prior to excision
Resection of the tumor (may include entire bone) and wide margins of normal tissue primarily for malignant or aggressive benign tumors
Simple and intermediate repairs

EXCLUDES *Complex repair*
Significant exploration of vessels, neuroplasty, reconstruction, or complex bone repair

Do not report excision of soft tissue codes when adjacent soft tissue is removed during the bone tumor resection (24076-24079 [24071, 24073])

24150 **Radical resection of tumor, shaft or distal humerus**
T 80 50 44.50 44.50 FUD 090

24152 **Radical resection of tumor, radial head or neck**
G2 T 80 50 39.32 39.32 FUD 090

24155 Elbow Arthrectomy

24155 **Resection of elbow joint (arthrectomy)**
A2 T 80 50 24.32 24.32 FUD 090

24160-24201 Removal Implant/Foreign Body from Elbow/Upper Arm

EXCLUDES *Bursal or joint arthrocentesis or needling (20605)*
K-wire or pin insertion (20650)
K-wire or pin removal (20670, 20680)

24160 **Removal of prosthesis, includes debridement and synovectomy when performed; humeral and ulnar components**
EXCLUDES *Foreign body removal (24200-24201)*
Hardware removal other than prosthesis (20680)
Do not report with prosthesis removal and replacement in same elbow (eg, humeral and/or ulnar component(s)) (24370-24371)
A2 Q2 50 35.99 35.99 FUD 090

24164 **radial head**
EXCLUDES *Foreign body removal (24200-24201)*
Hardware removal other than prosthesis (20680)
A2 Q2 50 20.76 20.76 FUD 090

24200 **Removal of foreign body, upper arm or elbow area; subcutaneous**
P3 T 80 50 3.96 5.80 FUD 010

24201 **deep (subfascial or intramuscular)**
A2 T 50 10.48 15.81 FUD 090

24220 Injection for Elbow Arthrogram

24220 **Injection procedure for elbow arthrography**
EXCLUDES *Injection tennis elbow (20550)*
73085
N1 N 80 50 1.97 4.50 FUD 000

24300-24498 Repair/Reconstruction of Elbow/Upper Arm

24300 **Manipulation, elbow, under anesthesia**
EXCLUDES *External fixation (20690, 20692)*
G2 T 50 11.67 11.67 FUD 090

24301 **Muscle or tendon transfer, any type, upper arm or elbow, single (excluding 24320-24331)**
A2 T 80 21.44 21.44 FUD 090

24305 **Tendon lengthening, upper arm or elbow, each tendon**
A2 T 80 16.38 16.38 FUD 090

24310 **Tenotomy, open, elbow to shoulder, each tendon**
A2 T 80 13.52 13.52 FUD 090

24320 **Tenoplasty, with muscle transfer, with or without free graft, elbow to shoulder, single (Seddon-Brookes type procedure)**
A2 T 80 22.23 22.23 FUD 090

24330 **Flexor-plasty, elbow (eg, Steindler type advancement);**
A2 T 80 50 20.41 20.41 FUD 090

24331 **with extensor advancement**
A2 T 80 50 22.39 22.39 FUD 090

24332 **Tenolysis, triceps**
G2 T 50 17.40 17.40 FUD 090

24340 **Tenodesis of biceps tendon at elbow (separate procedure)**
A2 T 80 50 17.50 17.50 FUD 090

24341 **Repair, tendon or muscle, upper arm or elbow, each tendon or muscle, primary or secondary (excludes rotator cuff)**
A2 T 80 50 21.27 21.27 FUD 090

24342 **Reinsertion of ruptured biceps or triceps tendon, distal, with or without tendon graft**
A2 T 80 50 22.14 22.14 FUD 090

24343 **Repair lateral collateral ligament, elbow, with local tissue**
G2 T 80 50 20.06 20.06 FUD 090

24344 Reconstruction lateral collateral ligament, elbow, with tendon graft (includes harvesting of graft)
G2 T 80 50 ⚑ 31.30 31.30 FUD 090

24345 Repair medial collateral ligament, elbow, with local tissue
A2 T 80 50 ⚑ 19.95 19.95 FUD 090

24346 Reconstruction medial collateral ligament, elbow, with tendon graft (includes harvesting of graft)
G2 T 80 50 ⚑ 31.30 31.30 FUD 090

24357 Tenotomy, elbow, lateral or medial (eg, epicondylitis, tennis elbow, golfer's elbow); percutaneous
Do not report with (29837-29838)
G2 T 80 50 12.51 12.51 FUD 090

24358 debridement, soft tissue and/or bone, open
Do not report with (29837-29838)
G2 T 80 50 14.86 14.86 FUD 090

24359 debridement, soft tissue and/or bone, open with tendon repair or reattachment
Do not report with (29837-29838)
G2 T 80 50 18.78 18.78 FUD 090

24360 Arthroplasty, elbow; with membrane (eg, fascial)
A2 T 80 50 ⚑ 25.60 25.60 FUD 090

24361 with distal humeral prosthetic replacement
Code also (C1776)
J8 T 80 50 ⚑ 28.69 28.69 FUD 090

24362 with implant and fascia lata ligament reconstruction
A2 T 80 50 ⚑ 30.25 30.25 FUD 090

24363 with distal humerus and proximal ulnar prosthetic replacement (eg, total elbow)
EXCLUDES *Total elbow implant revision (24370-24371)*
Code also (C1776)
J8 T 80 50 ⚑ 41.69 41.69 FUD 090

24365 Arthroplasty, radial head;
A2 T 80 50 ⚑ 18.17 18.17 FUD 090

24366 with implant
Code also (C1776)
J8 T 80 50 ⚑ 19.39 19.39 FUD 090

24370 Revision of total elbow arthroplasty, including allograft when performed; humeral or ulnar component
Do not report with prosthesis removal without replacement (eg, humeral and/or ulnar component/s) (24160)
J8 T 80 50 44.13 44.13 FUD 090

24371 humeral and ulnar component
Do not report with prosthesis removal without replacement (eg, humeral and/or ulnar component/s) (24160)
J8 T 80 50 50.97 50.97 FUD 090

24400 Osteotomy, humerus, with or without internal fixation
A2 T 80 50 ⚑ 23.31 23.31 FUD 090

24410 Multiple osteotomies with realignment on intramedullary rod, humeral shaft (Sofield type procedure)
A2 T 80 50 ⚑ 30.14 30.14 FUD 090

24420 Osteoplasty, humerus (eg, shortening or lengthening) (excluding 64876)
A2 T 80 50 ⚑ 28.30 28.30 FUD 090

24430 Repair of nonunion or malunion, humerus; without graft (eg, compression technique)
A2 T 80 50 ⚑ 30.22 30.22 FUD 090

24435 with iliac or other autograft (includes obtaining graft)
A2 T 80 50 ⚑ 30.77 30.77 FUD 090

24470 Hemiepiphyseal arrest (eg, cubitus varus or valgus, distal humerus)
A2 T 80 50 ⚑ 16.69 16.69 FUD 090

24495 Decompression fasciotomy, forearm, with brachial artery exploration
A2 T 80 50 ⚑ 18.48 18.48 FUD 090

24498 Prophylactic treatment (nailing, pinning, plating or wiring), with or without methylmethacrylate, humeral shaft
A2 T 80 50 ⚑ 24.74 24.74 FUD 090

24500-24685 Treatment of Fracture/Dislocation of Elbow/Upper Arm

INCLUDES Treatment for either closed or open fractures or dislocations

24500 Closed treatment of humeral shaft fracture; without manipulation
A2 T 50 ⚑ 9.20 10.09 FUD 090

24505 with manipulation, with or without skeletal traction
A2 T 50 ⚑ 12.80 14.12 FUD 090

24515 Open treatment of humeral shaft fracture with plate/screws, with or without cerclage
A2 T 80 50 ⚑ 24.99 24.99 FUD 090

24516 Treatment of humeral shaft fracture, with insertion of intramedullary implant, with or without cerclage and/or locking screws
A2 T 80 50 ⚑ 24.55 24.55 FUD 090

24530 Closed treatment of supracondylar or transcondylar humeral fracture, with or without intercondylar extension; without manipulation
A2 T 50 ⚑ 9.72 10.72 FUD 090

24535 with manipulation, with or without skin or skeletal traction
A2 T 50 ⚑ 16.14 17.44 FUD 090

24538 Percutaneous skeletal fixation of supracondylar or transcondylar humeral fracture, with or without intercondylar extension
A2 T 50 ⚑ 21.12 21.12 FUD 090

24545 Open treatment of humeral supracondylar or transcondylar fracture, includes internal fixation, when performed; without intercondylar extension
A2 T 80 50 ⚑ 26.54 26.54 FUD 090

24546 with intercondylar extension
A2 T 80 50 ⚑ 29.71 29.71 FUD 090

24560 Closed treatment of humeral epicondylar fracture, medial or lateral; without manipulation
A2 T 50 ⚑ 8.16 9.08 FUD 090

24565 with manipulation
A2 T 50 ⚑ 13.84 15.06 FUD 090

24566 Percutaneous skeletal fixation of humeral epicondylar fracture, medial or lateral, with manipulation
A2 T 50 ⚑ 20.38 20.38 FUD 090

24575 Open treatment of humeral epicondylar fracture, medial or lateral, includes internal fixation, when performed
A2 T 80 50 ⚑ 20.91 20.91 FUD 090

24576 Closed treatment of humeral condylar fracture, medial or lateral; without manipulation
A2 T 50 ⚑ 8.63 9.57 FUD 090

24577 with manipulation
A2 T 50 ⚑ 14.23 15.51 FUD 090

24579 Open treatment of humeral condylar fracture, medial or lateral, includes internal fixation, when performed
EXCLUDES *Closed treatment without manipulation (24530, 24560, 24576, 24650, 24670)*
Repair with manipulation (24535, 24565, 24577, 24675)
A2 T 80 50 ⚑ 23.80 23.80 FUD 090

24582 Percutaneous skeletal fixation of humeral condylar fracture, medial or lateral, with manipulation
A2 T 50 — 22.96 — 22.96 FUD 090

24586 Open treatment of periarticular fracture and/or dislocation of the elbow (fracture distal humerus and proximal ulna and/or proximal radius);
A2 T 80 50 — 30.98 — 30.98 FUD 090

24587 with implant arthroplasty
EXCLUDES *Distal humerus arthroplasty with implant (24361)*
A2 T 80 50 — 30.90 — 30.90 FUD 090

24600 Treatment of closed elbow dislocation; without anesthesia
A2 T 50 — 9.50 — 10.34 FUD 090

24605 requiring anesthesia
A2 T 50 — 13.31 — 13.31 FUD 090

24615 Open treatment of acute or chronic elbow dislocation
A2 T 80 50 — 20.25 — 20.25 FUD 090

24620 Closed treatment of Monteggia type of fracture dislocation at elbow (fracture proximal end of ulna with dislocation of radial head), with manipulation
A2 T 80 50 — 15.73 — 15.73 FUD 090

24635 Open treatment of Monteggia type of fracture dislocation at elbow (fracture proximal end of ulna with dislocation of radial head), includes internal fixation, when performed
A2 T 80 50 — 19.16 — 19.16 FUD 090

24640 Closed treatment of radial head subluxation in child, nursemaid elbow, with manipulation A
P3 T 80 50 — 2.69 — 3.94 FUD 010

24650 Closed treatment of radial head or neck fracture; without manipulation
P2 T 50 — 6.79 — 7.38 FUD 090

24655 with manipulation
A2 T 50 — 11.32 — 12.40 FUD 090

24665 Open treatment of radial head or neck fracture, includes internal fixation or radial head excision, when performed;
A2 T 80 50 — 18.53 — 18.53 FUD 090

24666 with radial head prosthetic replacement
A2 T 80 50 — 20.86 — 20.86 FUD 090

24670 Closed treatment of ulnar fracture, proximal end (eg, olecranon or coronoid process[es]); without manipulation
A2 T 50 — 7.43 — 8.21 FUD 090

24675 with manipulation
A2 T 50 — 11.75 — 12.86 FUD 090

24685 Open treatment of ulnar fracture, proximal end (eg, olecranon or coronoid process[es]), includes internal fixation, when performed
Do not report with (24100-24102)
A2 T 80 50 — 18.62 — 18.62 FUD 090

24800-24999 Other/Unlisted Elbow/Upper Arm Procedures

24800 Arthrodesis, elbow joint; local
A2 T 80 50 — 23.61 — 23.61 FUD 090

24802 with autogenous graft (includes obtaining graft)
A2 T 80 50 — 28.55 — 28.55 FUD 090

24900 Amputation, arm through humerus; with primary closure
C 80 50 — 20.93 — 20.93 FUD 090

24920 open, circular (guillotine)
C 80 50 — 20.84 — 20.84 FUD 090

24925 secondary closure or scar revision
A2 T 80 50 — 16.07 — 16.07 FUD 090

24930 re-amputation
C 80 50 — 22.04 — 22.04 FUD 090

24931 with implant
C 80 50 — 22.08 — 22.08 FUD 090

24935 Stump elongation, upper extremity
T 80 50 — 29.81 — 29.81 FUD 090

24940 Cineplasty, upper extremity, complete procedure
C 80 50 — 0.00 — 0.00 FUD 090

24999 Unlisted procedure, humerus or elbow
T 80 50 — 0.00 — 0.00 FUD YYY

25000-25001 Incision Tendon Sheath of Wrist

25000 Incision, extensor tendon sheath, wrist (eg, deQuervains disease)
EXCLUDES *Carpal tunnel release (64721)*
A2 T 50 — 9.48 — 9.48 FUD 090

25001 Incision, flexor tendon sheath, wrist (eg, flexor carpi radialis)
G2 T 50 — 9.69 — 9.69 FUD 090

25020-25025 Decompression Fasciotomy Forearm/Wrist

25020 Decompression fasciotomy, forearm and/or wrist, flexor OR extensor compartment; without debridement of nonviable muscle and/or nerve
EXCLUDES *Brachial artery exploration (24495)*
Superficial incision and drainage (10060-10160)
A2 T 50 — 16.21 — 16.21 FUD 090

25023 with debridement of nonviable muscle and/or nerve
EXCLUDES *Debridement (11000-11044 [11045, 11046])*
Decompression fasciotomy with exploration brachial artery exploration (24495)
Superficial incision and drainage (10060-10160)
A2 T 80 50 — 31.35 — 31.35 FUD 090

25024 Decompression fasciotomy, forearm and/or wrist, flexor AND extensor compartment; without debridement of nonviable muscle and/or nerve
A2 T 50 — 22.10 — 22.10 FUD 090

25025 with debridement of nonviable muscle and/or nerve
A2 T 80 50 — 34.62 — 34.62 FUD 090

25028-25040 Incision for Drainage/Foreign Body Removal

25028 Incision and drainage, forearm and/or wrist; deep abscess or hematoma
A2 T 50 — 14.77 — 14.77 FUD 090

25031 bursa
A2 T 80 50 — 10.31 — 10.31 FUD 090

25035 Incision, deep, bone cortex, forearm and/or wrist (eg, osteomyelitis or bone abscess)
A2 T 80 50 — 16.49 — 16.49 FUD 090

25040 Arthrotomy, radiocarpal or midcarpal joint, with exploration, drainage, or removal of foreign body
A2 T 80 50 — 15.95 — 15.95 FUD 090

25065-25066 Biopsy Forearm/Wrist

EXCLUDES *Soft tissue needle biopsy (20206)*

25065 Biopsy, soft tissue of forearm and/or wrist; superficial
P3 T 50 PQ — 4.65 — 7.12 FUD 010

25066 deep (subfascial or intramuscular)
A2 T 50 PQ — 10.11 — 10.11 FUD 090

25071-25078 [25071, 25073] Excision Soft Tissue Tumors Forearm/Wrist

INCLUDES Any necessary elevation of tissue planes or dissection
Measurement of tumor and necessary margin at greatest diameter prior to excision
Simple and intermediate repairs
Types of excision:
Fascial or subfascial soft tissue tumors: simple and marginal resection of tumors found either in or below the deep fascia, not involving bone or excision of a substantial amount of normal tissue; primarily benign and intramuscular tumors
Radical resection soft tissue tumor: wide resection of tumor involving substantial margins of normal tissue and may include tissue removal from one or more layers; most often malignant or aggressive benign
Subcutaneous: simple and marginal resection of tumors in the subcutaneous tissue above the deep fascia; most often benign

EXCLUDES *Complex repair*
Excision of benign cutaneous lesions (eg, sebaceous cyst) (11312-11403)
Radical resection of cutaneous tumors (eg, melanoma) (11600-11606)
Significant exploration of vessels or neuroplasty

25071 Resequenced code. See code following 25075.

25073 Resequenced code. See code following 25076.

25075 **Excision, tumor, soft tissue of forearm and/or wrist area, subcutaneous; less than 3 cm**
G2 T 50 CCI 8.98 13.47 FUD 090

\# **25071** **3 cm or greater**
G2 T 80 50 12.07 12.07 FUD 090

25076 **Excision, tumor, soft tissue of forearm and/or wrist area, subfascial (eg, intramuscular); less than 3 cm**
G2 T 50 CCI 14.68 14.68 FUD 090

\# **25073** **3 cm or greater**
G2 T 80 50 15.07 15.07 FUD 090

25077 **Radical resection of tumor (eg, sarcoma), soft tissue of forearm and/or wrist area; less than 3 cm**
G2 T 50 CCI 25.20 25.20 FUD 090

25078 **3 cm or greater**
G2 T 80 50 33.37 33.37 FUD 090

25085-25240 Procedures of Bones/Joints Lower Arm/Wrist

25085 **Capsulotomy, wrist (eg, contracture)**
A2 T 80 50 CCI 12.77 12.77 FUD 090

25100 **Arthrotomy, wrist joint; with biopsy**
A2 T 80 50 CCI PQ 9.80 9.80 FUD 090

25101 **with joint exploration, with or without biopsy, with or without removal of loose or foreign body**
A2 T 80 50 CCI PQ 11.44 11.44 FUD 090

25105 **with synovectomy**
A2 T 80 50 CCI 13.69 13.69 FUD 090

25107 **Arthrotomy, distal radioulnar joint including repair of triangular cartilage, complex**
A2 T 80 50 CCI 17.46 17.46 FUD 090

25109 **Excision of tendon, forearm and/or wrist, flexor or extensor, each**
G2 T 50 15.27 15.27 FUD 090

25110 **Excision, lesion of tendon sheath, forearm and/or wrist**
A2 T 50 CCI 9.63 9.63 FUD 090

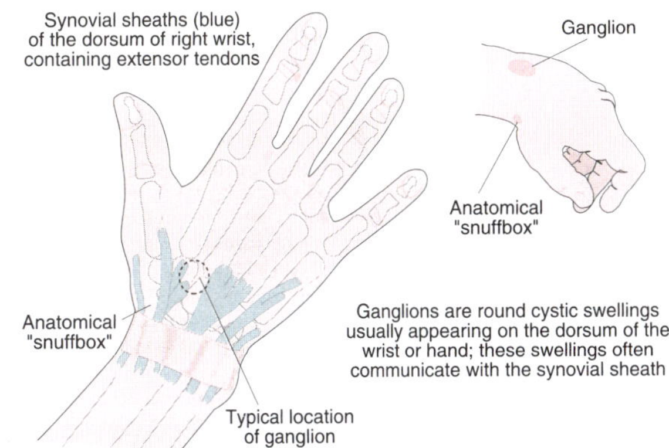

25111 **Excision of ganglion, wrist (dorsal or volar); primary**
EXCLUDES *Excision of ganglion hand or finger (26160)*
A2 T 50 CCI 9.05 9.05 FUD 090

25112 **recurrent**
EXCLUDES *Excision of ganglion hand or finger (26160)*
A2 T 50 CCI 10.95 10.95 FUD 090

25115 **Radical excision of bursa, synovia of wrist, or forearm tendon sheaths (eg, tenosynovitis, fungus, Tbc, or other granulomas, rheumatoid arthritis); flexors**
EXCLUDES *Finger synovectomy (26145)*
A2 T 50 CCI 21.53 21.53 FUD 090

25116 **extensors, with or without transposition of dorsal retinaculum**
EXCLUDES *Finger synovectomy (26145)*
A2 T 80 50 CCI 17.00 17.00 FUD 090

25118 **Synovectomy, extensor tendon sheath, wrist, single compartment;**
EXCLUDES *Finger synovectomy (26145)*
A2 T 50 CCI 10.77 10.77 FUD 090

25119 **with resection of distal ulna**
EXCLUDES *Finger synovectomy (26145)*
A2 T 80 50 CCI 14.11 14.11 FUD 090

25120 **Excision or curettage of bone cyst or benign tumor of radius or ulna (excluding head or neck of radius and olecranon process);**
EXCLUDES *Removal of bone cyst or tumor of radial head, neck, or olecranon process (24120-24126)*
A2 T 80 50 CCI 14.11 14.11 FUD 090

25125 **with autograft (includes obtaining graft)**
A2 T 80 50 CCI 16.83 16.83 FUD 090

25126 **with allograft**
A2 T 80 50 CCI 16.95 16.95 FUD 090

25130 **Excision or curettage of bone cyst or benign tumor of carpal bones;**
A2 T 80 50 CCI 12.68 12.68 FUD 090

25135 **with autograft (includes obtaining graft)**
A2 T 80 50 CCI 15.83 15.83 FUD 090

25136 **with allograft**
A2 T 80 50 CCI 13.99 13.99 FUD 090

25145 **Sequestrectomy (eg, for osteomyelitis or bone abscess), forearm and/or wrist**
A2 T 80 50 CCI 14.66 14.66 FUD 090

25150 **Partial excision (craterization, saucerization, or diaphysectomy) of bone (eg, for osteomyelitis); ulna**
A2 T 50 CCI 16.02 16.02 FUD 090

25151 **radius**
EXCLUDES *Partial removal of radial head, neck, or olecranon process (24145, 24147)*
A2 T 80 50 CCI 16.59 16.59 FUD 090

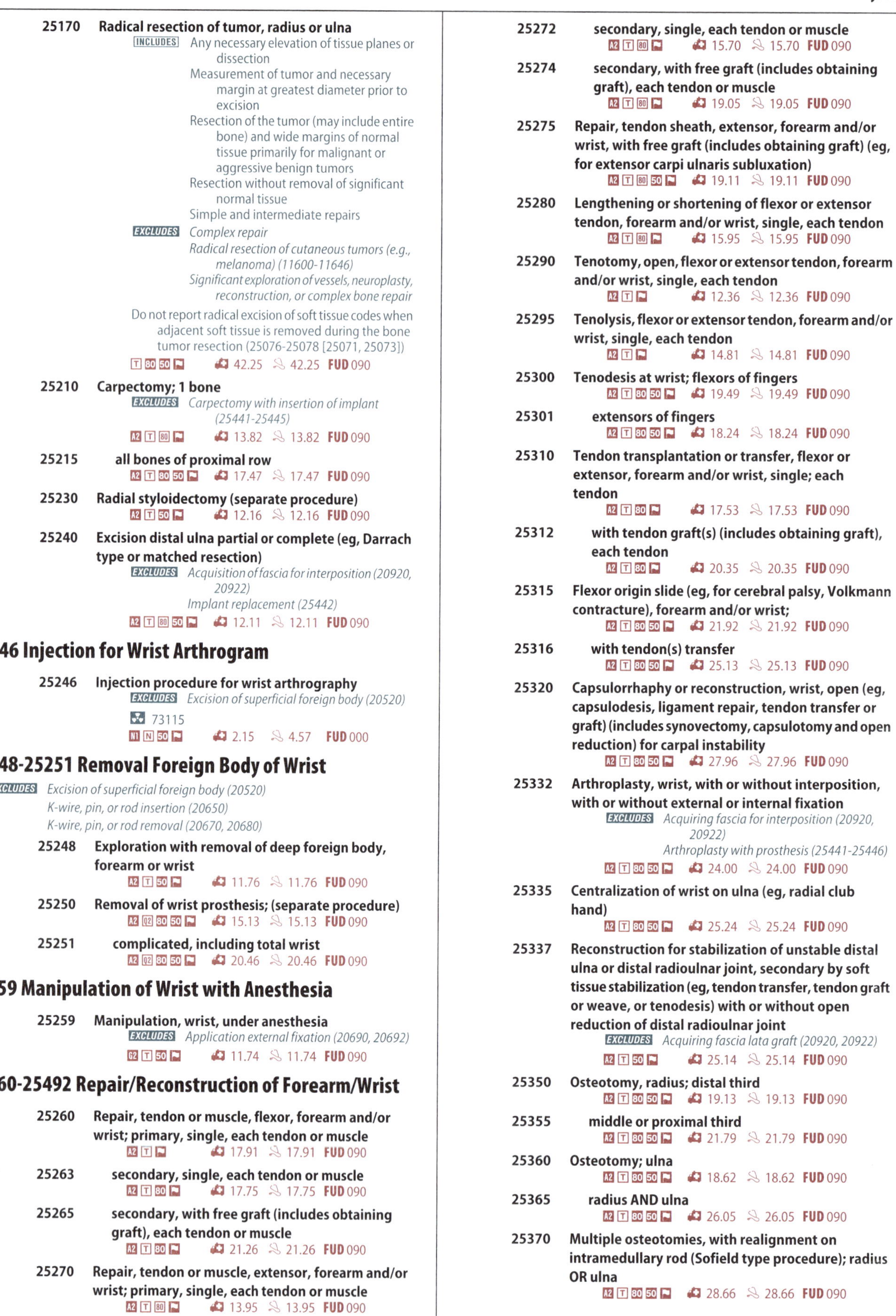

25170 **Radical resection of tumor, radius or ulna**
INCLUDES Any necessary elevation of tissue planes or dissection
Measurement of tumor and necessary margin at greatest diameter prior to excision
Resection of the tumor (may include entire bone) and wide margins of normal tissue primarily for malignant or aggressive benign tumors
Resection without removal of significant normal tissue
Simple and intermediate repairs
EXCLUDES *Complex repair*
Radical resection of cutaneous tumors (e.g., melanoma) (11600-11646)
Significant exploration of vessels, neuroplasty, reconstruction, or complex bone repair
Do not report radical excision of soft tissue codes when adjacent soft tissue is removed during the bone tumor resection (25076-25078 [25071, 25073])
T 80 50 42.25 42.25 FUD 090

25210 **Carpectomy; 1 bone**
EXCLUDES *Carpectomy with insertion of implant (25441-25445)*
A2 T 80 13.82 13.82 FUD 090

25215 **all bones of proximal row**
A2 T 80 50 17.47 17.47 FUD 090

25230 **Radial styloidectomy (separate procedure)**
A2 T 50 12.16 12.16 FUD 090

25240 **Excision distal ulna partial or complete (eg, Darrach type or matched resection)**
EXCLUDES *Acquisition of fascia for interposition (20920, 20922)*
Implant replacement (25442)
A2 T 80 50 12.11 12.11 FUD 090

25246 Injection for Wrist Arthrogram

25246 **Injection procedure for wrist arthrography**
EXCLUDES *Excision of superficial foreign body (20520)*
73115
N1 N 50 2.15 4.57 FUD 000

25248-25251 Removal Foreign Body of Wrist

EXCLUDES *Excision of superficial foreign body (20520)*
K-wire, pin, or rod insertion (20650)
K-wire, pin, or rod removal (20670, 20680)

25248 **Exploration with removal of deep foreign body, forearm or wrist**
A2 T 50 11.76 11.76 FUD 090

25250 **Removal of wrist prosthesis; (separate procedure)**
A2 Q2 80 50 15.13 15.13 FUD 090

25251 **complicated, including total wrist**
A2 Q2 80 50 20.46 20.46 FUD 090

25259 Manipulation of Wrist with Anesthesia

25259 **Manipulation, wrist, under anesthesia**
EXCLUDES *Application external fixation (20690, 20692)*
G2 T 50 11.74 11.74 FUD 090

25260-25492 Repair/Reconstruction of Forearm/Wrist

25260 **Repair, tendon or muscle, flexor, forearm and/or wrist; primary, single, each tendon or muscle**
A2 T 17.91 17.91 FUD 090

25263 **secondary, single, each tendon or muscle**
A2 T 80 17.75 17.75 FUD 090

25265 **secondary, with free graft (includes obtaining graft), each tendon or muscle**
A2 T 80 21.26 21.26 FUD 090

25270 **Repair, tendon or muscle, extensor, forearm and/or wrist; primary, single, each tendon or muscle**
A2 T 80 13.95 13.95 FUD 090

25272 **secondary, single, each tendon or muscle**
A2 T 80 15.70 15.70 FUD 090

25274 **secondary, with free graft (includes obtaining graft), each tendon or muscle**
A2 T 80 19.05 19.05 FUD 090

25275 **Repair, tendon sheath, extensor, forearm and/or wrist, with free graft (includes obtaining graft) (eg, for extensor carpi ulnaris subluxation)**
A2 T 80 50 19.11 19.11 FUD 090

25280 **Lengthening or shortening of flexor or extensor tendon, forearm and/or wrist, single, each tendon**
A2 T 80 15.95 15.95 FUD 090

25290 **Tenotomy, open, flexor or extensor tendon, forearm and/or wrist, single, each tendon**
A2 T 12.36 12.36 FUD 090

25295 **Tenolysis, flexor or extensor tendon, forearm and/or wrist, single, each tendon**
A2 T 14.81 14.81 FUD 090

25300 **Tenodesis at wrist; flexors of fingers**
A2 T 80 50 19.49 19.49 FUD 090

25301 **extensors of fingers**
A2 T 80 50 18.24 18.24 FUD 090

25310 **Tendon transplantation or transfer, flexor or extensor, forearm and/or wrist, single; each tendon**
A2 T 80 17.53 17.53 FUD 090

25312 **with tendon graft(s) (includes obtaining graft), each tendon**
A2 T 80 20.35 20.35 FUD 090

25315 **Flexor origin slide (eg, for cerebral palsy, Volkmann contracture), forearm and/or wrist;**
A2 T 80 50 21.92 21.92 FUD 090

25316 **with tendon(s) transfer**
A2 T 80 50 25.13 25.13 FUD 090

25320 **Capsulorrhaphy or reconstruction, wrist, open (eg, capsulodesis, ligament repair, tendon transfer or graft) (includes synovectomy, capsulotomy and open reduction) for carpal instability**
A2 T 80 50 27.96 27.96 FUD 090

25332 **Arthroplasty, wrist, with or without interposition, with or without external or internal fixation**
EXCLUDES *Acquiring fascia for interposition (20920, 20922)*
Arthroplasty with prosthesis (25441-25446)
A2 T 80 50 24.00 24.00 FUD 090

25335 **Centralization of wrist on ulna (eg, radial club hand)**
A2 T 80 50 25.24 25.24 FUD 090

25337 **Reconstruction for stabilization of unstable distal ulna or distal radioulnar joint, secondary by soft tissue stabilization (eg, tendon transfer, tendon graft or weave, or tenodesis) with or without open reduction of distal radioulnar joint**
EXCLUDES *Acquiring fascia lata graft (20920, 20922)*
A2 T 50 25.14 25.14 FUD 090

25350 **Osteotomy, radius; distal third**
A2 T 80 50 19.13 19.13 FUD 090

25355 **middle or proximal third**
A2 T 80 50 21.79 21.79 FUD 090

25360 **Osteotomy; ulna**
A2 T 80 50 18.62 18.62 FUD 090

25365 **radius AND ulna**
A2 T 80 50 26.05 26.05 FUD 090

25370 **Multiple osteotomies, with realignment on intramedullary rod (Sofield type procedure); radius OR ulna**
A2 T 80 50 28.66 28.66 FUD 090

25375 radius AND ulna
A2 T 80 50 25.49 25.49 FUD 090

25390 Osteoplasty, radius OR ulna; shortening
A2 T 80 50 21.82 21.82 FUD 090

25391 lengthening with autograft
A2 T 80 50 28.39 28.39 FUD 090

25392 Osteoplasty, radius AND ulna; shortening (excluding 64876)
A2 T 80 50 28.90 28.90 FUD 090

25393 lengthening with autograft
A2 T 80 50 32.24 32.24 FUD 090

25394 Osteoplasty, carpal bone, shortening
G2 T 80 50 22.31 22.31 FUD 090

25400 Repair of nonunion or malunion, radius OR ulna; without graft (eg, compression technique)
A2 T 80 50 22.82 22.82 FUD 090

25405 with autograft (includes obtaining graft)
A2 T 80 50 29.50 29.50 FUD 090

25415 Repair of nonunion or malunion, radius AND ulna; without graft (eg, compression technique)
A2 T 80 50 27.55 27.55 FUD 090

25420 with autograft (includes obtaining graft)
A2 T 80 50 33.31 33.31 FUD 090

25425 Repair of defect with autograft; radius OR ulna
A2 T 80 50 27.42 27.42 FUD 090

25426 radius AND ulna
A2 T 80 50 32.04 32.04 FUD 090

25430 Insertion of vascular pedicle into carpal bone (eg, Hori procedure)
G2 T 50 20.11 20.11 FUD 090

25431 Repair of nonunion of carpal bone (excluding carpal scaphoid (navicular)) (includes obtaining graft and necessary fixation), each bone
G2 T 80 50 22.45 22.45 FUD 090

25440 Repair of nonunion, scaphoid carpal (navicular) bone, with or without radial styloidectomy (includes obtaining graft and necessary fixation)
A2 T 80 50 21.82 21.82 FUD 090

25441 Arthroplasty with prosthetic replacement; distal radius
Code also (C1776)
J8 T 80 50 26.15 26.15 FUD 090

25442 distal ulna
Code also (C1776)
J8 T 80 50 22.36 22.36 FUD 090

25443 scaphoid carpal (navicular)
A2 T 80 50 22.21 22.21 FUD 090

25444 lunate
A2 T 80 50 22.12 22.12 FUD 090

25445 trapezium
A2 T 50 20.45 20.45 FUD 090

25446 distal radius and partial or entire carpus (total wrist)
Code also (C1776)
J8 T 80 50 33.32 33.32 FUD 090

25447 Arthroplasty, interposition, intercarpal or carpometacarpal joints
EXCLUDES *Wrist arthroplasty (25332)*
A2 T 80 50 23.48 23.48 FUD 090

25449 Revision of arthroplasty, including removal of implant, wrist joint
A2 T 80 50 29.62 29.62 FUD 090

25450 Epiphyseal arrest by epiphysiodesis or stapling; distal radius OR ulna
A2 T 50 17.48 17.48 FUD 090

25455 distal radius AND ulna
A2 T 50 19.43 19.43 FUD 090

25490 Prophylactic treatment (nailing, pinning, plating or wiring) with or without methylmethacrylate; radius
A2 T 80 50 19.80 19.80 FUD 090

25491 ulna
A2 T 80 50 21.02 21.02 FUD 090

25492 radius AND ulna
A2 T 80 50 25.72 25.72 FUD 090

25500-25695 Treatment of Fracture/Dislocation of Forearm/Wrist

Code also external fixation (20690)

25500 Closed treatment of radial shaft fracture; without manipulation
P2 T 50 7.07 7.68 FUD 090

25505 with manipulation
A2 T 50 13.03 14.20 FUD 090

25515 Open treatment of radial shaft fracture, includes internal fixation, when performed
A2 T 80 50 19.03 19.03 FUD 090

25520 Closed treatment of radial shaft fracture and closed treatment of dislocation of distal radioulnar joint (Galeazzi fracture/dislocation)
A2 T 50 15.23 16.04 FUD 090

25525 Open treatment of radial shaft fracture, includes internal fixation, when performed, and closed treatment of distal radioulnar joint dislocation (Galeazzi fracture/ dislocation), includes percutaneous skeletal fixation, when performed
A2 T 80 50 22.35 22.35 FUD 090

25526 Open treatment of radial shaft fracture, includes internal fixation, when performed, and open treatment of distal radioulnar joint dislocation (Galeazzi fracture/ dislocation), includes internal fixation, when performed, includes repair of triangular fibrocartilage complex
A2 T 80 50 27.18 27.18 FUD 090

25530 Closed treatment of ulnar shaft fracture; without manipulation
P2 T 50 6.69 7.38 FUD 090

25535 with manipulation
A2 T 50 12.82 13.82 FUD 090

25545 Open treatment of ulnar shaft fracture, includes internal fixation, when performed
A2 T 80 50 17.70 17.70 FUD 090

25560 Closed treatment of radial and ulnar shaft fractures; without manipulation
P2 T 50 7.12 7.87 FUD 090

25565 with manipulation
A2 T 50 13.34 14.70 FUD 090

25574 Open treatment of radial AND ulnar shaft fractures, with internal fixation, when performed; of radius OR ulna
A2 T 80 50 19.14 19.14 FUD 090

25575 of radius AND ulna
A2 T 80 50 25.64 25.64 FUD 090

25600 Closed treatment of distal radial fracture (eg, Colles or Smith type) or epiphyseal separation, includes closed treatment of fracture of ulnar styloid, when performed; without manipulation
Do not report with (25650)
P2 T 50 PQ 8.76 9.25 FUD 090

25605 with manipulation
Do not report with (25650)
A2 T 50 PQ 14.63 15.53 FUD 090

25606 **Percutaneous skeletal fixation of distal radial fracture or epiphyseal separation**
EXCLUDES *Open repair of ulnar styloid fracture (25652)*
Percutaneous repair of ulnar styloid fracture (25651)
Do not report with (25650)
A2 T 50 PQ 18.80 18.80 FUD 090

25607 **Open treatment of distal radial extra-articular fracture or epiphyseal separation, with internal fixation**
EXCLUDES *Open repair of ulnar styloid fracture (25652)*
Percutaneous repair of ulnar styloid fracture (25651)
Do not report with (25650)
A2 T 80 50 PQ 20.89 20.89 FUD 090

25608 **Open treatment of distal radial intra-articular fracture or epiphyseal separation; with internal fixation of 2 fragments**
EXCLUDES *Open repair of ulnar styloid fracture (25652)*
Percutaneous repair of ulnar styloid fracture (25651)
Do not report with (25609, 25650)
A2 T 80 50 PQ 23.43 23.43 FUD 090

25609 **with internal fixation of 3 or more fragments**
EXCLUDES *Open repair of ulnar styloid fracture (25652)*
Percutaneous repair of ulnar styloid fracture (25651)
Do not report with (25650)
A2 T 80 50 PQ 29.80 29.80 FUD 090

25622 **Closed treatment of carpal scaphoid (navicular) fracture; without manipulation**
P2 T 50 7.84 8.58 FUD 090

25624 **with manipulation**
A2 T 80 50 12.25 13.43 FUD 090

25628 **Open treatment of carpal scaphoid (navicular) fracture, includes internal fixation, when performed**
A2 T 80 50 20.46 20.46 FUD 090

25630 **Closed treatment of carpal bone fracture (excluding carpal scaphoid [navicular]); without manipulation, each bone**
P2 T 50 7.93 8.62 FUD 090

25635 **with manipulation, each bone**
A2 T 80 50 11.19 12.56 FUD 090

25645 **Open treatment of carpal bone fracture (other than carpal scaphoid [navicular]), each bone**
A2 T 80 50 16.16 16.16 FUD 090

25650 **Closed treatment of ulnar styloid fracture**
Do not report with (25600, 25605, 25607-25609)
P2 T 50 8.53 9.07 FUD 090

25651 **Percutaneous skeletal fixation of ulnar styloid fracture**
G2 T 80 50 PQ 13.75 13.75 FUD 090

25652 **Open treatment of ulnar styloid fracture**
G2 T 50 17.67 17.67 FUD 090

25660 **Closed treatment of radiocarpal or intercarpal dislocation, 1 or more bones, with manipulation**
A2 T 80 50 11.47 11.47 FUD 090

25670 **Open treatment of radiocarpal or intercarpal dislocation, 1 or more bones**
A2 T 80 50 17.21 17.21 FUD 090

25671 **Percutaneous skeletal fixation of distal radioulnar dislocation**
A2 T 50 15.02 15.02 FUD 090

25675 **Closed treatment of distal radioulnar dislocation with manipulation**
A2 T 80 50 11.30 12.35 FUD 090

25676 **Open treatment of distal radioulnar dislocation, acute or chronic**
A2 T 80 50 17.85 17.85 FUD 090

25680 **Closed treatment of trans-scaphoperilunar type of fracture dislocation, with manipulation**
A2 T 80 50 13.41 13.41 FUD 090

25685 **Open treatment of trans-scaphoperilunar type of fracture dislocation**
A2 T 80 50 20.90 20.90 FUD 090

25690 **Closed treatment of lunate dislocation, with manipulation**
A2 T 80 50 13.62 13.62 FUD 090

25695 **Open treatment of lunate dislocation**
A2 T 80 50 17.99 17.99 FUD 090

25800-25830 Wrist Fusion

25800 **Arthrodesis, wrist; complete, without bone graft (includes radiocarpal and/or intercarpal and/or carpometacarpal joints)**
A2 T 80 50 20.79 20.79 FUD 090

25805 **with sliding graft**
A2 T 80 50 24.03 24.03 FUD 090

25810 **with iliac or other autograft (includes obtaining graft)**
A2 T 80 50 24.66 24.66 FUD 090

25820 **limited, without bone graft (eg, intercarpal or radiocarpal)**
A2 T 80 50 17.42 17.42 FUD 090

25825 **with autograft (includes obtaining graft)**
A2 T 80 50 21.48 21.48 FUD 090

25830 **Arthrodesis, distal radioulnar joint with segmental resection of ulna, with or without bone graft (eg, Sauve-Kapandji procedure)**
A2 T 80 50 26.95 26.95 FUD 090

25900-25999 Amputation Through Forearm/Wrist

25900 **Amputation, forearm, through radius and ulna;**
C 80 50 20.13 20.13 FUD 090

25905 **open, circular (guillotine)**
C 80 50 18.08 18.08 FUD 090

25907 **secondary closure or scar revision**
A2 T 80 50 17.40 17.40 FUD 090

25909 **re-amputation**
T 80 50 19.48 19.48 FUD 090

25915 **Krukenberg procedure**
C 80 50 29.72 29.72 FUD 090

25920 **Disarticulation through wrist;**
C 80 50 19.78 19.78 FUD 090

25922 **secondary closure or scar revision**
A2 T 80 50 14.03 14.03 FUD 090

25924 **re-amputation**
C 80 50 17.44 17.44 FUD 090

25927 **Transmetacarpal amputation;**
C 80 50 22.98 22.98 FUD 090

25929 **secondary closure or scar revision**
A2 T 80 50 16.94 16.94 FUD 090

25931 **re-amputation**
G2 T 50 19.06 19.06 FUD 090

25999 **Unlisted procedure, forearm or wrist**
T 80 50 0.00 0.00 FUD YYY

26010-26037 Incision Hand/Fingers

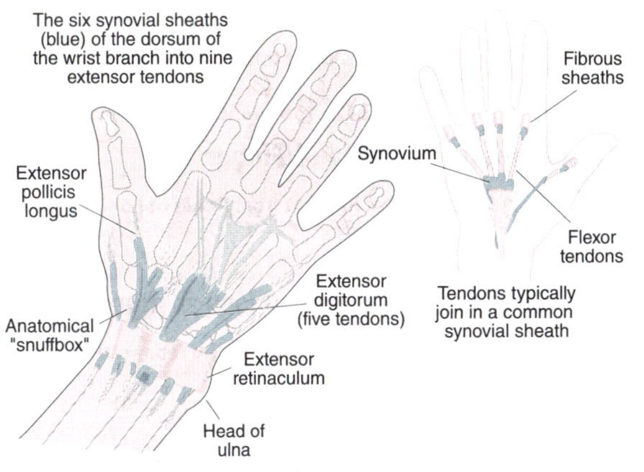

26010 Drainage of finger abscess; simple
P2 T CCI 3.92 7.41 FUD 010

26011 complicated (eg, felon)
A2 T CCI 5.24 10.92 FUD 010

26020 Drainage of tendon sheath, digit and/or palm, each
A2 T CCI 12.26 12.26 FUD 090

26025 Drainage of palmar bursa; single, bursa
A2 T 80 50 CCI 11.91 11.91 FUD 090

26030 multiple bursa
A2 T 80 50 CCI 13.98 13.98 FUD 090

26034 Incision, bone cortex, hand or finger (eg, osteomyelitis or bone abscess)
A2 T CCI 15.17 15.17 FUD 090

26035 Decompression fingers and/or hand, injection injury (eg, grease gun)
G2 T 80 CCI 24.62 24.62 FUD 090

26037 Decompressive fasciotomy, hand (excludes 26035)
EXCLUDES *Injection injury (26035)*
G2 T 80 50 CCI 16.12 16.12 FUD 090

26040-26045 Incision Palmar Fascia

EXCLUDES *Enzyme injection fasciotomy (20527, 26341)*
Fasciectomy (26121, 26123, 26125)

26040 Fasciotomy, palmar (eg, Dupuytren's contracture); percutaneous
A2 T 50 CCI 8.76 8.76 FUD 090

26045 open, partial
A2 T 50 CCI 13.27 13.27 FUD 090

26055-26080 Incision Tendon/Joint of Fingers/Hand

26055 Tendon sheath incision (eg, for trigger finger)
A2 T CCI 8.75 15.63 FUD 090

26060 Tenotomy, percutaneous, single, each digit
EXCLUDES *Arthrocentesis (20610)*
A2 T 80 CCI 7.49 7.49 FUD 090

26070 Arthrotomy, with exploration, drainage, or removal of loose or foreign body; carpometacarpal joint
A2 T 50 CCI 8.89 8.89 FUD 090

26075 metacarpophalangeal joint, each
A2 T 50 CCI 9.32 9.32 FUD 090

26080 interphalangeal joint, each
A2 T CCI 11.03 11.03 FUD 090

26100-26110 Arthrotomy with Biopsy of Joint Hand/Fingers

26100 Arthrotomy with biopsy; carpometacarpal joint, each
A2 T 80 50 CCI PQ 9.47 9.47 FUD 090

26105 metacarpophalangeal joint, each
A2 T 80 50 CCI PQ 9.45 9.45 FUD 090

26110 interphalangeal joint, each
A2 T CCI PQ 9.07 9.07 FUD 090

26111-26118 [26111, 26113] Excision Soft Tissue Tumors Fingers and Hand

INCLUDES Any necessary elevation of tissue planes or dissection
Measurement of tumor and necessary margin at greatest diameter prior to excision
Simple and intermediate repairs
Type of excisions:
Fascial or subfascial soft tissue tumors: simple and marginal resection of tumors found either in or below the deep fascia, not involving bone or excision of a substantial amount of normal tissue; primarily benign and intramuscular tumors
Tumors of fingers and toes involving joint capsules, tendons and tendon sheaths
Radical resection soft tissue tumor: wide resection of tumor, involving substantial margins of normal tissue and may include tissue removal from one or more layers; most often malignant or aggressive benign
Tumors of fingers and toes adjacent to joints, tendons and tendon sheaths
Subcutaneous: simple and marginal resection of tumors found in the subcutaneous tissue above the deep fascia; most often benign

EXCLUDES *Complex repair*
Excision of benign cutaneous lesions (eg, sebaceous cyst) (11420-11426)
Radical resection of cutaneous tumors (eg, melanoma) (11620-11626)
Significant exploration of the vessels or neuroplasty

26111 Resequenced code. See code following 26115.

26113 Resequenced code. See code following 26116.

26115 Excision, tumor or vascular malformation, soft tissue of hand or finger, subcutaneous; less than 1.5 cm
G2 T CCI 9.41 14.14 FUD 090

 # 26111 1.5 cm or greater
G2 T 80 11.82 11.82 FUD 090

26116 Excision, tumor, soft tissue, or vascular malformation, of hand or finger, subfascial (eg, intramuscular); less than 1.5 cm
G2 T CCI 14.92 14.92 FUD 090

 # 26113 1.5 cm or greater
G2 T 80 15.55 15.55 FUD 090

26117 Radical resection of tumor (eg, sarcoma), soft tissue of hand or finger; less than 3 cm
G2 T CCI 21.21 21.21 FUD 090

26118 3 cm or greater
G2 T 80 30.03 30.03 FUD 090

26121-26236 Procedures of Bones, Fascia, Joints and Tendons Hands and Fingers

26121 Fasciectomy, palm only, with or without Z-plasty, other local tissue rearrangement, or skin grafting (includes obtaining graft)
EXCLUDES *Enzyme injection fasciotomy (20527, 26341)*
Fasciotomy (26040, 26045)
A2 T 50 CCI 16.92 16.92 FUD 090

26123 Fasciectomy, partial palmar with release of single digit including proximal interphalangeal joint, with or without Z-plasty, other local tissue rearrangement, or skin grafting (includes obtaining graft);
EXCLUDES *Enzyme injection fasciotomy (20527, 26341)*
Fasciotomy (26040, 26045)
A2 T 50 CCI 23.62 23.62 FUD 090

\+ **26125** **each additional digit (List separately in addition to code for primary procedure)**
EXCLUDES *Enzyme injection fasciotomy (20527, 26341)*
Fasciotomy (26040, 26045)
Code first (26123)
N1 N 7.84 7.84 FUD ZZZ

26130 **Synovectomy, carpometacarpal joint**
A2 T 50 13.06 13.06 FUD 090

26135 **Synovectomy, metacarpophalangeal joint including intrinsic release and extensor hood reconstruction, each digit**
A2 T 80 15.60 15.60 FUD 090

26140 **Synovectomy, proximal interphalangeal joint, including extensor reconstruction, each interphalangeal joint**
A2 T 14.27 14.27 FUD 090

26145 **Synovectomy, tendon sheath, radical (tenosynovectomy), flexor tendon, palm and/or finger, each tendon**
EXCLUDES *Wrist synovectomy (25115-25116)*
A2 T 14.48 14.48 FUD 090

26160 **Excision of lesion of tendon sheath or joint capsule (eg, cyst, mucous cyst, or ganglion), hand or finger**
EXCLUDES *Trigger finger (26055)*
Wrist ganglion removal (25111-25112)
A2 T 9.41 16.07 FUD 090

26170 **Excision of tendon, palm, flexor or extensor, single, each tendon**
Do not report with (26390, 26415)
A2 T 80 11.49 11.49 FUD 090

26180 **Excision of tendon, finger, flexor or extensor, each tendon**
Do not report with (26390, 26415)
A2 T 80 12.52 12.52 FUD 090

26185 **Sesamoidectomy, thumb or finger (separate procedure)**
A2 T 80 50 15.62 15.62 FUD 090

26200 **Excision or curettage of bone cyst or benign tumor of metacarpal;**
A2 T 80 12.75 12.75 FUD 090

26205 **with autograft (includes obtaining graft)**
A2 T 17.10 17.10 FUD 090

26210 **Excision or curettage of bone cyst or benign tumor of proximal, middle, or distal phalanx of finger;**
A2 T 12.49 12.49 FUD 090

26215 **with autograft (includes obtaining graft)**
A2 T 15.99 15.99 FUD 090

26230 **Partial excision (craterization, saucerization, or diaphysectomy) bone (eg, osteomyelitis); metacarpal**
A2 T 80 14.14 14.14 FUD 090

26235 **proximal or middle phalanx of finger**
A2 T 80 13.96 13.96 FUD 090

26236 **distal phalanx of finger**
A2 T 12.48 12.48 FUD 090

26250-26262 Radical Resection Bone Tumor of Hand/Finger

INCLUDES Any necessary elevation of tissue planes or dissection
Measurement of tumor and necessary margin at greatest diameter prior to excision
Resection of the tumor (may include entire bone) and wide margins of normal tissue primarily for malignant or aggressive benign tumors
Simple and intermediate repairs

EXCLUDES *Complex repair*
Significant exploration of vessels, neuroplasty, reconstruction, or complex bone repair

Do not report radical excision of soft tissue codes when adjacent soft tissue is removed during the bone tumor resection (26116-26118 [26111, 26113])

26250 **Radical resection of tumor, metacarpal**
A2 T 80 31.15 31.15 FUD 090

26260 **Radical resection of tumor, proximal or middle phalanx of finger**
A2 T 80 23.26 23.26 FUD 090

26262 **Radical resection of tumor, distal phalanx of finger**
A2 T 80 18.16 18.16 FUD 090

26320 Implant Removal Hand/Finger

26320 **Removal of implant from finger or hand**
EXCLUDES *Excision of foreign body (20520, 20525)*
A2 Q2 9.78 9.78 FUD 090

26340-26548 Repair/Reconstruction of Fingers and Hand

26340 **Manipulation, finger joint, under anesthesia, each joint**
EXCLUDES *Application external fixation (20690, 20692)*
G2 T 50 9.40 9.40 FUD 090

26341 **Manipulation, palmar fascial cord (ie, Dupuytren's cord), post enzyme injection (eg, collagenase), single cord**
EXCLUDES *Enzyme injection fasciotomy (20527)*
Code also custom orthotic fabrication and/or fitting
P3 T 50 2.09 2.75 FUD 010

26350 **Repair or advancement, flexor tendon, not in zone 2 digital flexor tendon sheath (eg, no man's land); primary or secondary without free graft, each tendon**
A2 T 19.78 19.78 FUD 090

26352 **secondary with free graft (includes obtaining graft), each tendon**
A2 T 80 22.82 22.82 FUD 090

26356 **Repair or advancement, flexor tendon, in zone 2 digital flexor tendon sheath (eg, no man's land); primary, without free graft, each tendon**
A2 T 30.56 30.56 FUD 090

26357 **secondary, without free graft, each tendon**
A2 T 80 24.34 24.34 FUD 090

26358 **secondary, with free graft (includes obtaining graft), each tendon**
A2 T 80 25.69 25.69 FUD 090

26370 **Repair or advancement of profundus tendon, with intact superficialis tendon; primary, each tendon**
A2 T 80 21.15 21.15 FUD 090

26372 **secondary with free graft (includes obtaining graft), each tendon**
A2 T 80 24.76 24.76 FUD 090

26373 **secondary without free graft, each tendon**
A2 T 80 23.74 23.74 FUD 090

26390 **Excision flexor tendon, with implantation of synthetic rod for delayed tendon graft, hand or finger, each rod**
A2 T 80 23.44 23.44 FUD 090

26392 **Removal of synthetic rod and insertion of flexor tendon graft, hand or finger (includes obtaining graft), each rod**
A2 T 80 27.28 27.28 FUD 090

26410 **Repair, extensor tendon, hand, primary or secondary; without free graft, each tendon**
A2 T 15.70 15.70 FUD 090

26412 **with free graft (includes obtaining graft), each tendon**
A2 T 80 18.94 18.94 FUD 090

26415 **Excision of extensor tendon, with implantation of synthetic rod for delayed tendon graft, hand or finger, each rod**
A2 T 80 22.28 22.28 FUD 090

26416 Removal of synthetic rod and insertion of extensor tendon graft (includes obtaining graft), hand or finger, each rod
A2 T 21.30 21.30 FUD 090

26418 Repair, extensor tendon, finger, primary or secondary; without free graft, each tendon
A2 T 16.05 16.05 FUD 090

26420 with free graft (includes obtaining graft) each tendon
A2 T 80 19.83 19.83 FUD 090

26426 Repair of extensor tendon, central slip, secondary (eg, boutonniere deformity); using local tissue(s), including lateral band(s), each finger
A2 T 14.19 14.19 FUD 090

26428 with free graft (includes obtaining graft), each finger
A2 T 80 21.16 21.16 FUD 090

26432 Closed treatment of distal extensor tendon insertion, with or without percutaneous pinning (eg, mallet finger)
A2 T 13.84 13.84 FUD 090

26433 Repair of extensor tendon, distal insertion, primary or secondary; without graft (eg, mallet finger)
EXCLUDES *Trigger finger (26055)*
A2 T 14.76 14.76 FUD 090

26434 with free graft (includes obtaining graft)
EXCLUDES *Trigger finger (26055)*
A2 T 80 18.08 18.08 FUD 090

26437 Realignment of extensor tendon, hand, each tendon
A2 T 17.29 17.29 FUD 090

26440 Tenolysis, flexor tendon; palm OR finger, each tendon
A2 T 17.16 17.16 FUD 090

26442 palm AND finger, each tendon
A2 T 26.91 26.91 FUD 090

26445 Tenolysis, extensor tendon, hand OR finger, each tendon
A2 T 15.98 15.98 FUD 090

26449 Tenolysis, complex, extensor tendon, finger, including forearm, each tendon
A2 T 80 19.63 19.63 FUD 090

26450 Tenotomy, flexor, palm, open, each tendon
A2 T 80 11.33 11.33 FUD 090

26455 Tenotomy, flexor, finger, open, each tendon
A2 T 80 11.24 11.24 FUD 090

26460 Tenotomy, extensor, hand or finger, open, each tendon
A2 T 10.97 10.97 FUD 090

26471 Tenodesis; of proximal interphalangeal joint, each joint
A2 T 80 17.12 17.12 FUD 090

26474 of distal joint, each joint
A2 T 80 16.76 16.76 FUD 090

26476 Lengthening of tendon, extensor, hand or finger, each tendon
A2 T 16.27 16.27 FUD 090

26477 Shortening of tendon, extensor, hand or finger, each tendon
A2 T 16.22 16.22 FUD 090

26478 Lengthening of tendon, flexor, hand or finger, each tendon
A2 T 80 17.31 17.31 FUD 090

26479 Shortening of tendon, flexor, hand or finger, each tendon
A2 T 80 17.25 17.25 FUD 090

26480 Transfer or transplant of tendon, carpometacarpal area or dorsum of hand; without free graft, each tendon
A2 T 80 20.95 20.95 FUD 090

26483 with free tendon graft (includes obtaining graft), each tendon
A2 T 80 23.53 23.53 FUD 090

26485 Transfer or transplant of tendon, palmar; without free tendon graft, each tendon
A2 T 80 22.43 22.43 FUD 090

26489 with free tendon graft (includes obtaining graft), each tendon
A2 T 80 26.02 26.02 FUD 090

26490 Opponensplasty; superficialis tendon transfer type, each tendon
EXCLUDES *Thumb fusion (26820)*
A2 T 80 22.17 22.17 FUD 090

26492 tendon transfer with graft (includes obtaining graft), each tendon
EXCLUDES *Thumb fusion (26820)*
A2 T 80 24.65 24.65 FUD 090

26494 hypothenar muscle transfer
EXCLUDES *Thumb fusion (26820)*
A2 T 80 22.37 22.37 FUD 090

26496 other methods
EXCLUDES *Thumb fusion (26820)*
A2 T 80 23.48 23.48 FUD 090

26497 Transfer of tendon to restore intrinsic function; ring and small finger
A2 T 80 24.25 24.25 FUD 090

26498 all 4 fingers
A2 T 80 32.13 32.13 FUD 090

26499 Correction claw finger, other methods
A2 T 80 23.25 23.25 FUD 090

26500 Reconstruction of tendon pulley, each tendon; with local tissues (separate procedure)
A2 T 80 17.37 17.37 FUD 090

26502 with tendon or fascial graft (includes obtaining graft) (separate procedure)
A2 T 80 19.72 19.72 FUD 090

26508 Release of thenar muscle(s) (eg, thumb contracture)
A2 T 80 50 17.82 17.82 FUD 090

26510 Cross intrinsic transfer, each tendon
A2 T 80 16.64 16.64 FUD 090

26516 Capsulodesis, metacarpophalangeal joint; single digit
A2 T 80 50 19.51 19.51 FUD 090

26517 2 digits
A2 T 80 50 23.11 23.11 FUD 090

26518 3 or 4 digits
A2 T 80 50 23.34 23.34 FUD 090

26520 Capsulectomy or capsulotomy; metacarpophalangeal joint, each joint
EXCLUDES *Carpometacarpal joint arthroplasty (25447)*
A2 T 18.07 18.07 FUD 090

26525 interphalangeal joint, each joint
EXCLUDES *Carpometacarpal joint arthroplasty (25447)*
A2 T 18.05 18.05 FUD 090

26530 Arthroplasty, metacarpophalangeal joint; each joint
EXCLUDES *Carpometacarpal joint arthroplasty (25447)*
A2 T 80 15.20 15.20 FUD 090

26531 with prosthetic implant, each joint
EXCLUDES *Carpometacarpal joint arthroplasty (25447)*
A2 T 80 17.65 17.65 FUD 090

26535 **Arthroplasty, interphalangeal joint; each joint**
EXCLUDES *Carpometacarpal joint arthroplasty (25447)*
A2 T 11.85 11.85 FUD 090

26536 **with prosthetic implant, each joint**
EXCLUDES *Carpometacarpal joint arthroplasty (25447)*
A2 T 80 19.83 19.83 FUD 090

26540 **Repair of collateral ligament, metacarpophalangeal or interphalangeal joint**
A2 T 80 18.33 18.33 FUD 090

26541 **Reconstruction, collateral ligament, metacarpophalangeal joint, single; with tendon or fascial graft (includes obtaining graft)**
A2 T 80 22.31 22.31 FUD 090

26542 **with local tissue (eg, adductor advancement)**
A2 T 80 18.99 18.99 FUD 090

26545 **Reconstruction, collateral ligament, interphalangeal joint, single, including graft, each joint**
A2 T 80 19.30 19.30 FUD 090

26546 **Repair non-union, metacarpal or phalanx (includes obtaining bone graft with or without external or internal fixation)**
A2 T 80 50 27.70 27.70 FUD 090

26548 **Repair and reconstruction, finger, volar plate, interphalangeal joint**
A2 T 80 21.30 21.30 FUD 090

26550-26556 Reconstruction Procedures with Finger and Toe Transplants

26550 **Pollicization of a digit**
A2 T 80 50 46.37 46.37 FUD 090

26551 **Transfer, toe-to-hand with microvascular anastomosis; great toe wrap-around with bone graft**
INCLUDES Operating microscope (69990)
EXCLUDES *Big toe with web space (20973)*
C 80 50 83.96 83.96 FUD 090

26553 **other than great toe, single**
INCLUDES Operating microscope (69990)
C 80 50 87.26 87.26 FUD 090

26554 **other than great toe, double**
INCLUDES Operating microscope (69990)
C 80 50 90.84 90.84 FUD 090

26555 **Transfer, finger to another position without microvascular anastomosis**
A2 T 80 38.71 38.71 FUD 090

26556 **Transfer, free toe joint, with microvascular anastomosis**
INCLUDES Operating microscope (69990)
EXCLUDES *Big toe to hand transfer (20973)*
C 80 77.91 77.91 FUD 090

26560-26596 Repair of Other Deformities of the Fingers/Hand

26560 **Repair of syndactyly (web finger) each web space; with skin flaps**
A2 T 80 15.95 15.95 FUD 090

26561 **with skin flaps and grafts**
A2 T 80 26.54 26.54 FUD 090

26562 **complex (eg, involving bone, nails)**
A2 T 80 35.97 35.97 FUD 090

26565 **metacarpal, each**
A2 T 80 19.01 19.01 FUD 090

26567 **phalanx of finger, each**
A2 T 80 18.98 18.98 FUD 090

26568 **Osteoplasty, lengthening, metacarpal or phalanx**
A2 T 80 25.19 25.19 FUD 090

26580 **Repair cleft hand**
INCLUDES Barsky's procedure
A2 T 80 50 43.02 43.02 FUD 090

26587 **Reconstruction of polydactylous digit, soft tissue and bone**
EXCLUDES *Soft tissue removal only (11200)*
A2 T 80 26.77 26.77 FUD 090

26590 **Repair macrodactylia, each digit**
A2 T 80 39.72 39.72 FUD 090

26591 **Repair, intrinsic muscles of hand, each muscle**
A2 T 80 12.11 12.11 FUD 090

26593 **Release, intrinsic muscles of hand, each muscle**
A2 T 16.61 16.61 FUD 090

26596 **Excision of constricting ring of finger, with multiple Z-plasties**
EXCLUDES *Graft repair or scar contracture release (11042, 14040-14041, 15120, 15240)*
A2 T 80 21.49 21.49 FUD 090

26600-26785 Treatment of Fracture/Dislocation of Fingers and Hand

INCLUDES Closed, percutaneous, and open treatment of fractures or dislocations

26600 **Closed treatment of metacarpal fracture, single; without manipulation, each bone**
P2 T 7.83 8.30 FUD 090

26605 **with manipulation, each bone**
A2 T 8.28 9.07 FUD 090

26607 **Closed treatment of metacarpal fracture, with manipulation, with external fixation, each bone**
A2 T 80 12.91 12.91 FUD 090

26608 **Percutaneous skeletal fixation of metacarpal fracture, each bone**
A2 T 80 PQ 13.50 13.50 FUD 090

26615 **Open treatment of metacarpal fracture, single, includes internal fixation, when performed, each bone**
A2 T 16.30 16.30 FUD 090

26641 **Closed treatment of carpometacarpal dislocation, thumb, with manipulation**
P2 T 80 50 9.63 10.49 FUD 090

26645 **Closed treatment of carpometacarpal fracture dislocation, thumb (Bennett fracture), with manipulation**
A2 T 80 50 11.07 12.04 FUD 090

26650 **Percutaneous skeletal fixation of carpometacarpal fracture dislocation, thumb (Bennett fracture), with manipulation**
A2 T 50 PQ 13.51 13.51 FUD 090

26665 **Open treatment of carpometacarpal fracture dislocation, thumb (Bennett fracture), includes internal fixation, when performed**
A2 T 50 17.84 17.84 FUD 090

26670 **Closed treatment of carpometacarpal dislocation, other than thumb, with manipulation, each joint; without anesthesia**
P2 T 80 8.73 9.58 FUD 090

26675 **requiring anesthesia**
A2 T 80 11.81 12.82 FUD 090

26676 **Percutaneous skeletal fixation of carpometacarpal dislocation, other than thumb, with manipulation, each joint**
A2 T PQ 14.16 14.16 FUD 090

26685 **Open treatment of carpometacarpal dislocation, other than thumb; includes internal fixation, when performed, each joint**
A2 T 16.45 16.45 FUD 090

26686 **complex, multiple, or delayed reduction**
A2 T 80 17.71 17.71 FUD 090

26700 Closed treatment of metacarpophalangeal dislocation, single, with manipulation; without anesthesia
P2 T CCI 8.66 9.22 FUD 090

26705 requiring anesthesia
A2 T 80 CCI 10.72 11.68 FUD 090

26706 Percutaneous skeletal fixation of metacarpophalangeal dislocation, single, with manipulation
A2 T CCI PQ 12.45 12.45 FUD 090

26715 Open treatment of metacarpophalangeal dislocation, single, includes internal fixation, when performed
A2 T 80 CCI 16.26 16.26 FUD 090

26720 Closed treatment of phalangeal shaft fracture, proximal or middle phalanx, finger or thumb; without manipulation, each
P2 T CCI 5.22 5.61 FUD 090

26725 with manipulation, with or without skin or skeletal traction, each
P2 T CCI 8.61 9.51 FUD 090

26727 Percutaneous skeletal fixation of unstable phalangeal shaft fracture, proximal or middle phalanx, finger or thumb, with manipulation, each
A2 T CCI PQ 13.26 13.26 FUD 090

26735 Open treatment of phalangeal shaft fracture, proximal or middle phalanx, finger or thumb, includes internal fixation, when performed, each
A2 T CCI 16.91 16.91 FUD 090

26740 Closed treatment of articular fracture, involving metacarpophalangeal or interphalangeal joint; without manipulation, each
P2 T CCI 6.06 6.45 FUD 090

26742 with manipulation, each
A2 T CCI 9.47 10.40 FUD 090

26746 Open treatment of articular fracture, involving metacarpophalangeal or interphalangeal joint, includes internal fixation, when performed, each
A2 T CCI 21.03 21.03 FUD 090

26750 Closed treatment of distal phalangeal fracture, finger or thumb; without manipulation, each
P2 T CCI 5.23 5.22 FUD 090

26755 with manipulation, each
G2 T CCI 7.76 8.89 FUD 090

26756 Percutaneous skeletal fixation of distal phalangeal fracture, finger or thumb, each
A2 T 80 CCI 11.79 11.79 FUD 090

26765 Open treatment of distal phalangeal fracture, finger or thumb, includes internal fixation, when performed, each
A2 T CCI 14.21 14.21 FUD 090

26770 Closed treatment of interphalangeal joint dislocation, single, with manipulation; without anesthesia
G2 T CCI 7.26 7.82 FUD 090

26775 requiring anesthesia
P2 S CCI 9.76 10.76 FUD 090

26776 Percutaneous skeletal fixation of interphalangeal joint dislocation, single, with manipulation
A2 T CCI 12.50 12.50 FUD 090

26785 Open treatment of interphalangeal joint dislocation, includes internal fixation, when performed, single
A2 T CCI 15.49 15.49 FUD 090

26820-26863 Fusion of Joint(s) of Fingers or Hand

26820 Fusion in opposition, thumb, with autogenous graft (includes obtaining graft)
A2 T 80 50 CCI 22.04 22.04 FUD 090

26841 Arthrodesis, carpometacarpal joint, thumb, with or without internal fixation;
A2 T 80 50 CCI 20.33 20.33 FUD 090

26842 with autograft (includes obtaining graft)
A2 T 80 50 CCI 22.03 22.03 FUD 090

26843 Arthrodesis, carpometacarpal joint, digit, other than thumb, each;
A2 T 80 CCI 20.65 20.65 FUD 090

26844 with autograft (includes obtaining graft)
A2 T 80 CCI 22.85 22.85 FUD 090

26850 Arthrodesis, metacarpophalangeal joint, with or without internal fixation;
A2 T 80 CCI 19.28 19.28 FUD 090

26852 with autograft (includes obtaining graft)
A2 T 80 CCI 22.15 22.15 FUD 090

26860 Arthrodesis, interphalangeal joint, with or without internal fixation;
A2 T CCI 15.63 15.63 FUD 090

+ 26861 each additional interphalangeal joint (List separately in addition to code for primary procedure)
Code first (26860)
N1 N CCI 2.97 2.97 FUD ZZZ

26862 with autograft (includes obtaining graft)
A2 T 80 CCI 20.17 20.17 FUD 090

+ 26863 with autograft (includes obtaining graft), each additional joint (List separately in addition to code for primary procedure)
Code first (26862)
N1 N 80 CCI 6.57 6.57 FUD ZZZ

26910-26989 Amputations and Unlisted Procedures Finger/Hand

26910 Amputation, metacarpal, with finger or thumb (ray amputation), single, with or without interosseous transfer
EXCLUDES *Repositioning (26550, 26555)*
Transmetacarpal amputation of hand (25927)
A2 T CCI 20.06 20.06 FUD 090

26951 Amputation, finger or thumb, primary or secondary, any joint or phalanx, single, including neurectomies; with direct closure
EXCLUDES *Repair necessitating flaps or grafts (15050-15758)*
Transmetacarpal amputation of hand (25927)
A2 T CCI 18.22 18.22 FUD 090

26952 with local advancement flaps (V-Y, hood)
EXCLUDES *Repair necessitating flaps or grafts (15050-15758)*
Transmetacarpal amputation of hand (25927)
A2 T CCI 18.03 18.03 FUD 090

26989 Unlisted procedure, hands or fingers
T 0.00 0.00 FUD YYY

26990-26992 Incision for Drainage of Pelvis or Hip

EXCLUDES *Simple incision and drainage procedures (10040-10160)*

26990 Incision and drainage, pelvis or hip joint area; deep abscess or hematoma
A2 T CCI 17.70 17.70 FUD 090

26991 infected bursa
A2 T 80 CCI 14.89 19.92 FUD 090

26992 Incision, bone cortex, pelvis and/or hip joint (eg, osteomyelitis or bone abscess)
C 80 CCI 27.46 27.46 FUD 090

27000-27006 Tenotomy Procedures of Hip

27000 **Tenotomy, adductor of hip, percutaneous (separate procedure)**
A2 T 50 — 11.97 — 11.97 FUD 090

27001 **Tenotomy, adductor of hip, open**
A2 T 80 50 — 15.41 — 15.41 FUD 090

27003 **Tenotomy, adductor, subcutaneous, open, with obturator neurectomy**
A2 T 80 50 — 16.93 — 16.93 FUD 090

27005 **Tenotomy, hip flexor(s), open (separate procedure)**
C 80 50 — 20.71 — 20.71 FUD 090

27006 **Tenotomy, abductors and/or extensor(s) of hip, open (separate procedure)**
T 80 50 — 20.96 — 20.96 FUD 090

27025-27036 Surgical Incision of Hip

CMS 100-3,160.1 Induced Lesions of Nerve Tracts

27025 **Fasciotomy, hip or thigh, any type**
C 80 50 — 26.16 — 26.16 FUD 090

27027 **Decompression fasciotomy(ies), pelvic (buttock) compartment(s) (eg, gluteus medius-minimus, gluteus maximus, iliopsoas, and/or tensor fascia lata muscle), unilateral**
T 80 50 — 24.18 — 24.18 FUD 090

27030 **Arthrotomy, hip, with drainage (eg, infection)**
C 80 50 — 26.18 — 26.18 FUD 090

27033 **Arthrotomy, hip, including exploration or removal of loose or foreign body**
A2 T 80 50 — 27.81 — 27.81 FUD 090

27035 **Denervation, hip joint, intrapelvic or extrapelvic intra-articular branches of sciatic, femoral, or obturator nerves**
EXCLUDES *Transection of obturator nerve (64763, 64766)*
A2 T 80 50 — 33.60 — 33.60 FUD 090

27036 **Capsulectomy or capsulotomy, hip, with or without excision of heterotopic bone, with release of hip flexor muscles (ie, gluteus medius, gluteus minimus, tensor fascia latae, rectus femoris, sartorius, iliopsoas)**
C 80 50 — 28.87 — 28.87 FUD 090

27040-27041 Biopsy of Hip/Pelvis

EXCLUDES *Soft tissue needle biopsy (20206)*

27040 **Biopsy, soft tissue of pelvis and hip area; superficial**
A2 T 50 P0 — 5.74 — 9.75 FUD 010

27041 **deep, subfascial or intramuscular**
A2 T 50 P0 — 19.63 — 19.63 FUD 090

27043-27059 [27043, 27045, 27059] Excision Soft Tissue Tumors Hip/ Pelvis

INCLUDES Any necessary elevation of tissue planes or dissection
Measurement of tumor and necessary margin at greatest diameter prior to excision
Simple and intermediate repairs
Types of excision:
Fascial or subfascial soft tissue tumors: simple and marginal resection of tumors found either in or below the deep fascia, not involving bone or excision of a substantial amount of normal tissue; primarily benign and intramuscular tumors
Radical resection of soft tissue tumor: wide resection of tumor involving substantial margins of normal tissue and may involve tissue removal from one or more layers; mostly malignant or aggressive benign,
Subcutaneous: simple and marginal resection of tumors found in the subcutaneous tissue above the deep fascia; most often benign

EXCLUDES *Complex repair*
Excision of benign cutaneous lesions (eg, sebaceous cyst) (11400-11406)
Radical resection of cutaneous tumors (eg, melanoma) (11600-11606)
Significant exploration of vessels, neuroplasty, reconstruction, or complex bone repair

27043 ***Resequenced code. See code following 27047.***

27045 ***Resequenced code. See code following 27048.***

27047 **Excision, tumor, soft tissue of pelvis and hip area, subcutaneous; less than 3 cm**
G2 T 50 — 10.32 — 13.21 FUD 090

\# **27043** **3 cm or greater**
G2 T 50 — 13.30 — 13.30 FUD 090

27048 **Excision, tumor, soft tissue of pelvis and hip area, subfascial (eg, intramuscular); less than 5 cm**
G2 T 80 50 — 17.35 — 17.35 FUD 090

\# **27045** **5 cm or greater**
G2 T 80 50 — 21.32 — 21.32 FUD 090

27049 **Radical resection of tumor (eg, sarcoma), soft tissue of pelvis and hip area; less than 5 cm**
G2 T 80 50 — 38.99 — 38.99 FUD 090

\# **27059** **5 cm or greater**
G2 T 80 50 — 51.62 — 51.62 FUD 090

27050-27071 Procedures of Bones and Joints of Hip and Pelvis

27050 **Arthrotomy, with biopsy; sacroiliac joint**
A2 T 80 50 P0 — 11.39 — 11.39 FUD 090

27052 **hip joint**
A2 T 80 50 P0 — 16.43 — 16.43 FUD 090

27054 **Arthrotomy with synovectomy, hip joint**
C 80 50 — 19.53 — 19.53 FUD 090

27057 **Decompression fasciotomy(ies), pelvic (buttock) compartment(s) (eg, gluteus medius-minimus, gluteus maximus, iliopsoas, and/or tensor fascia lata muscle) with debridement of nonviable muscle, unilateral**
T 80 50 — 27.14 — 27.14 FUD 090

27059 ***Resequenced code. See code following 27049.***

27060 **Excision; ischial bursa**
A2 T 50 — 13.21 — 13.21 FUD 090

27062 **trochanteric bursa or calcification**
EXCLUDES *Arthrocentesis (20610)*
A2 T 50 — 12.95 — 12.95 FUD 090

27065 **Excision of bone cyst or benign tumor, wing of ilium, symphysis pubis, or greater trochanter of femur; superficial, includes autograft, when performed**
A2 T 80 50 — 14.59 — 14.59 FUD 090

27066 **deep (subfascial), includes autograft, when performed**
A2 T 80 50 — 23.17 — 23.17 FUD 090

27067 with autograft requiring separate incision
A2 T 80 50 29.49 29.49 FUD 090

27070 Partial excision, wing of ilium, symphysis pubis, or greater trochanter of femur, (craterization, saucerization) (eg, osteomyelitis or bone abscess); superficial
C 80 50 24.26 24.26 FUD 090

27071 deep (subfascial or intramuscular)
C 80 50 26.15 26.15 FUD 090

27075-27078 Radical Resection Bone Tumor of Hip/Pelvis

INCLUDES Any necessary elevation of tissue planes or dissection
Measurement of tumor and necessary margin at greatest diameter prior to excision
Resection of the tumor (may include entire bone) and wide margins of normal tissue primarily for malignant or aggressive benign tumors
Simple and intermediate repairs

EXCLUDES *Complex repair*
Significant exploration of vessels, neuroplasty, reconstruction, or complex bone repair

Do not report radical excision of soft tissue codes when adjacent soft tissue is removed during the bone tumor resection (27048-27049 [27043, 27045, 27059])

27075 Radical resection of tumor; wing of ilium, 1 pubic or ischial ramus or symphysis pubis
C 80 60.15 60.15 FUD 090

27076 ilium, including acetabulum, both pubic rami, or ischium and acetabulum
C 80 72.33 72.33 FUD 090

27077 innominate bone, total
C 80 81.32 81.32 FUD 090

27078 ischial tuberosity and greater trochanter of femur
C 80 50 59.30 59.30 FUD 090

27080 Excision of Coccyx

EXCLUDES *Surgical excision of decubitus ulcers (15920, 15922, 15931-15958)*

27080 Coccygectomy, primary
A2 T 80 14.56 14.56 FUD 090

27086-27091 Removal Foreign Body or Hip Prosthesis

27086 Removal of foreign body, pelvis or hip; subcutaneous tissue
A2 T 80 50 4.70 8.23 FUD 010

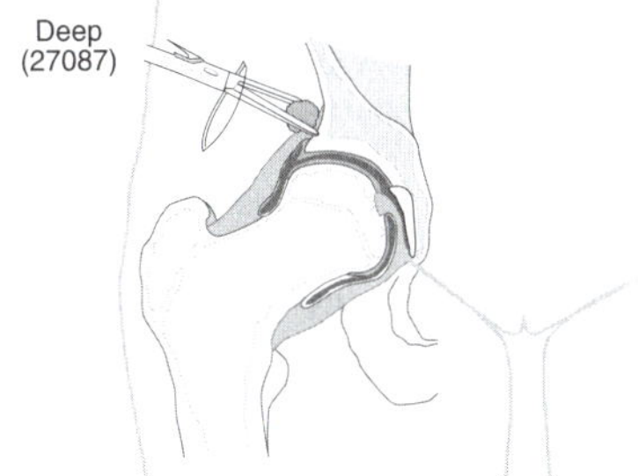

A foreign body is removed from the pelvis or hip

27087 deep (subfascial or intramuscular)
A2 T 80 50 17.89 17.89 FUD 090

27090 Removal of hip prosthesis; (separate procedure)
C 80 50 23.63 23.63 FUD 090

27091 complicated, including total hip prosthesis, methylmethacrylate with or without insertion of spacer
C 80 50 45.83 45.83 FUD 090

27093-27096 Injection for Arthrogram Hip/Sacroiliac Joint

27093 Injection procedure for hip arthrography; without anesthesia
73525
N1 N 50 2.02 5.26 FUD 000

27095 with anesthesia
73525
N1 N 50 2.36 6.72 FUD 000

27096 Injection procedure for sacroiliac joint, anesthetic/steroid, with image guidance (fluoroscopy or CT) including arthrography when performed
INCLUDES Confirmation of intra-articular needle placement with CT or fluoroscopy
EXCLUDES *Procedure performed without fluoroscopy or CT guidance (20552)*
Do not report with (77002-77003)
B 50 2.43 4.61 FUD 000

27097-27187 Revision/Reconstruction Hip and Pelvis

INCLUDES Closed, open and percutaneous treatment of fractures and dislocations

27097 Release or recession, hamstring, proximal
A2 T 80 50 19.40 19.40 FUD 090

27098 Transfer, adductor to ischium
A2 T 80 50 19.74 19.74 FUD 090

27100 Transfer external oblique muscle to greater trochanter including fascial or tendon extension (graft)
INCLUDES Eggers procedure
A2 T 80 50 23.32 23.32 FUD 090

27105 Transfer paraspinal muscle to hip (includes fascial or tendon extension graft)
A2 T 80 50 24.66 24.66 FUD 090

27110 Transfer iliopsoas; to greater trochanter of femur
A2 T 80 50 27.61 27.61 FUD 090

27111 to femoral neck
A2 T 80 50 25.60 25.60 FUD 090

27120 Acetabuloplasty; (eg, Whitman, Colonna, Haygroves, or cup type)
C 80 50 37.13 37.13 FUD 090

27122 resection, femoral head (eg, Girdlestone procedure)
C 80 50 31.42 31.42 FUD 090

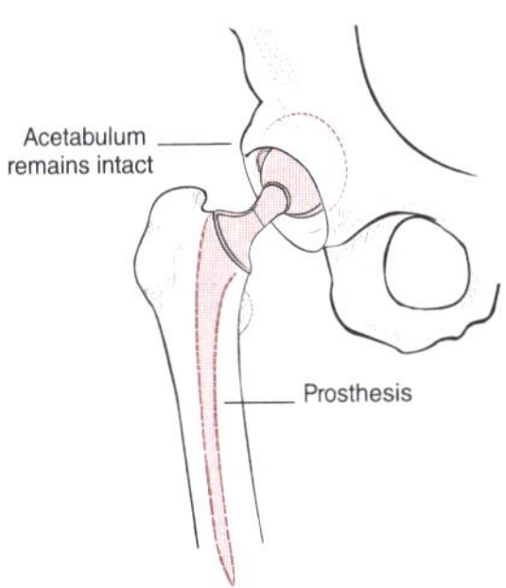

27125 Hemiarthroplasty, hip, partial (eg, femoral stem prosthesis, bipolar arthroplasty)
EXCLUDES *Hip replacement following hip fracture (27236)*
C 80 50 PQ 32.43 32.43 FUD 090

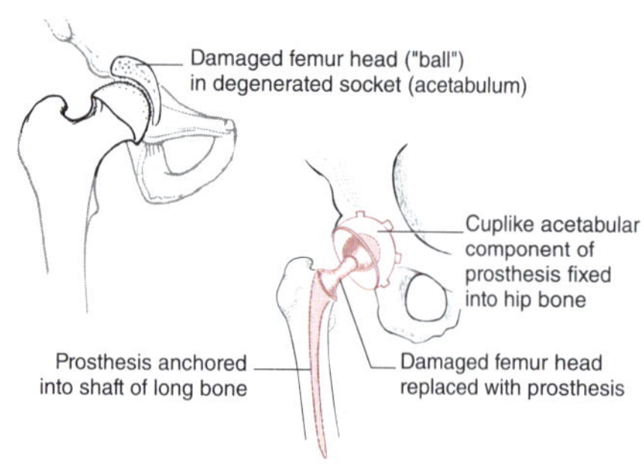

27130 **Arthroplasty, acetabular and proximal femoral prosthetic replacement (total hip arthroplasty), with or without autograft or allograft**
C 80 50 PQ 38.94 38.94 FUD 090

27132 **Conversion of previous hip surgery to total hip arthroplasty, with or without autograft or allograft**
C 80 50 PQ 48.11 48.11 FUD 090

27134 **Revision of total hip arthroplasty; both components, with or without autograft or allograft**
C 80 50 PQ 55.08 55.08 FUD 090

27137 **acetabular component only, with or without autograft or allograft**
C 80 50 PQ 42.28 42.28 FUD 090

27138 **femoral component only, with or without allograft**
C 80 50 PQ 43.96 43.96 FUD 090

27140 **Osteotomy and transfer of greater trochanter of femur (separate procedure)**
C 80 50 25.50 25.50 FUD 090

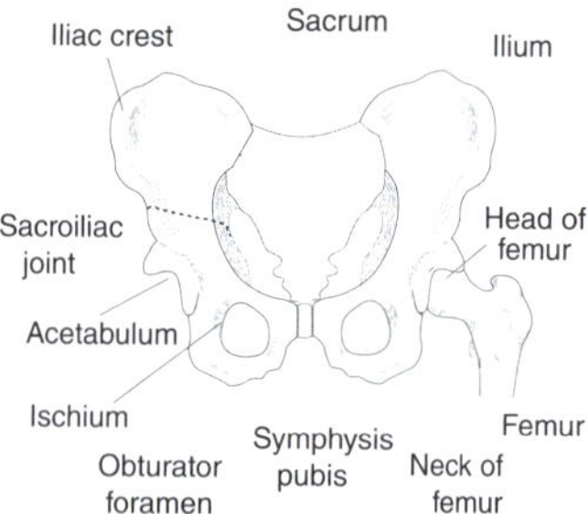

27146 **Osteotomy, iliac, acetabular or innominate bone;**
INCLUDES Salter osteotomy
C 80 50 36.72 36.72 FUD 090

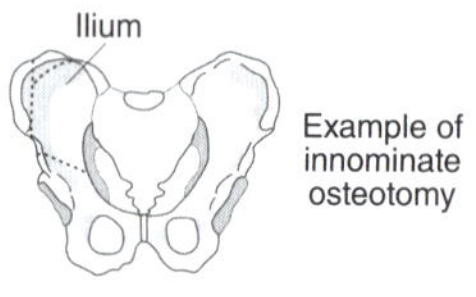

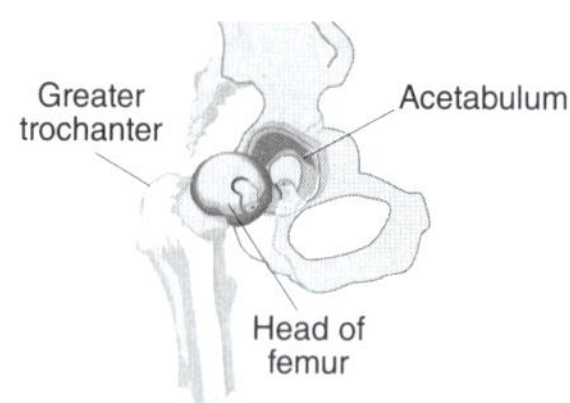

Femoral head is reduced into the acetabulum

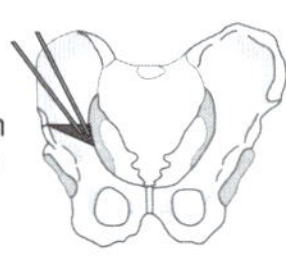

27147 **with open reduction of hip**
INCLUDES Pemberton osteotomy
C 80 50 42.02 42.02 FUD 090

27151 **with femoral osteotomy**
C 80 50 45.51 45.51 FUD 090

27156 **with femoral osteotomy and with open reduction of hip**
INCLUDES Chiari osteotomy
C 80 50 49.07 49.07 FUD 090

27158 **Osteotomy, pelvis, bilateral (eg, congenital malformation)**
C 80 40.07 40.07 FUD 090

27161 **Osteotomy, femoral neck (separate procedure)**
C 80 50 34.79 34.79 FUD 090

27165 **Osteotomy, intertrochanteric or subtrochanteric including internal or external fixation and/or cast**
C 80 50 39.43 39.43 FUD 090

27170 **Bone graft, femoral head, neck, intertrochanteric or subtrochanteric area (includes obtaining bone graft)**
C 80 50 33.67 33.67 FUD 090

27175 **Treatment of slipped femoral epiphysis; by traction, without reduction**
C 80 50 16.83 16.83 FUD 090

27176 **by single or multiple pinning, in situ**
C 80 50 26.18 26.18 FUD 090

27177 **Open treatment of slipped femoral epiphysis; single or multiple pinning or bone graft (includes obtaining graft)**
C 80 50 31.78 31.78 FUD 090

27178 **closed manipulation with single or multiple pinning**
C 80 50 26.18 26.18 FUD 090

27179 **osteoplasty of femoral neck (Heyman type procedure)**
T 80 50 27.83 27.83 FUD 090

27181 **osteotomy and internal fixation**
C 80 50 29.13 29.13 FUD 090

27185 **Epiphyseal arrest by epiphysiodesis or stapling, greater trochanter of femur**
C 50 16.78 16.78 FUD 090

27187 Prophylactic treatment (nailing, pinning, plating or wiring) with or without methylmethacrylate, femoral neck and proximal femur
C 80 50 — 28.35 — 28.35 FUD 090

27193-27269 Treatment of Fracture/Dislocation Hip/Pelvis

27193 Closed treatment of pelvic ring fracture, dislocation, diastasis or subluxation; without manipulation
A2 T — 13.58 — 13.40 FUD 090

27194 with manipulation, requiring more than local anesthesia
A2 T 80 — 19.98 — 19.98 FUD 090

27200 Closed treatment of coccygeal fracture
P2 T — 5.31 — 5.10 FUD 090

27202 Open treatment of coccygeal fracture
A2 T 80 — 15.18 — 15.18 FUD 090

27215 Open treatment of iliac spine(s), tuberosity avulsion, or iliac wing fracture(s), unilateral, for pelvic bone fracture patterns that do not disrupt the pelvic ring, includes internal fixation, when performed
E — 17.19 — 17.19 FUD 090

27216 Percutaneous skeletal fixation of posterior pelvic bone fracture and/or dislocation, for fracture patterns that disrupt the pelvic ring, unilateral (includes ipsilateral ilium, sacroiliac joint and/or sacrum)
EXCLUDES *Sacroiliac joint arthrodesis without fracture and/or dislocation, percutaneous or minimally invasive (27279)*
E — 25.51 — 25.51 FUD 090

27217 Open treatment of anterior pelvic bone fracture and/or dislocation for fracture patterns that disrupt the pelvic ring, unilateral, includes internal fixation, when performed (includes pubic symphysis and/or ipsilateral superior/inferior rami)
E — 23.94 — 23.94 FUD 090

27218 Open treatment of posterior pelvic bone fracture and/or dislocation, for fracture patterns that disrupt the pelvic ring, unilateral, includes internal fixation, when performed (includes ipsilateral ilium, sacroiliac joint and/or sacrum)
EXCLUDES *Sacroiliac joint arthrodesis without fracture and/or dislocation, percutaneous or minimally invasive (27279)*
E — 33.06 — 33.06 FUD 090

27220 Closed treatment of acetabulum (hip socket) fracture(s); without manipulation
G2 T 50 — 14.96 — 15.09 FUD 090

27222 with manipulation, with or without skeletal traction
C 50 — 27.83 — 27.83 FUD 090

27226 Open treatment of posterior or anterior acetabular wall fracture, with internal fixation
C 80 50 — 30.29 — 30.29 FUD 090

27227 Open treatment of acetabular fracture(s) involving anterior or posterior (one) column, or a fracture running transversely across the acetabulum, with internal fixation
C 80 50 — 47.60 — 47.60 FUD 090

27228 Open treatment of acetabular fracture(s) involving anterior and posterior (two) columns, includes T-fracture and both column fracture with complete articular detachment, or single column or transverse fracture with associated acetabular wall fracture, with internal fixation
C 80 50 — 54.23 — 54.23 FUD 090

27230 Closed treatment of femoral fracture, proximal end, neck; without manipulation
A2 T 50 PQ — 13.40 — 13.49 FUD 090

27232 with manipulation, with or without skeletal traction
C 50 PQ — 21.74 — 21.74 FUD 090

27235 Percutaneous skeletal fixation of femoral fracture, proximal end, neck
T 50 PQ — 25.96 — 25.96 FUD 090

27236 Open treatment of femoral fracture, proximal end, neck, internal fixation or prosthetic replacement
C 80 50 PQ — 34.26 — 34.26 FUD 090

27238 Closed treatment of intertrochanteric, peritrochanteric, or subtrochanteric femoral fracture; without manipulation
A2 T 50 PQ — 13.07 — 13.07 FUD 090

27240 with manipulation, with or without skin or skeletal traction
C 50 PQ — 27.30 — 27.30 FUD 090

27244 Treatment of intertrochanteric, peritrochanteric, or subtrochanteric femoral fracture; with plate/screw type implant, with or without cerclage
C 80 50 PQ — 35.22 — 35.22 FUD 090

27245 with intramedullary implant, with or without interlocking screws and/or cerclage
C 80 50 PQ — 35.23 — 35.23 FUD 090

27246 Closed treatment of greater trochanteric fracture, without manipulation
A2 T 50 PQ — 10.98 — 10.92 FUD 090

27248 Open treatment of greater trochanteric fracture, includes internal fixation, when performed
C 80 50 PQ — 21.25 — 21.25 FUD 090

27250 Closed treatment of hip dislocation, traumatic; without anesthesia
A2 T 50 — 5.26 — 5.26 FUD 000

27252 requiring anesthesia
A2 T 50 — 21.67 — 21.67 FUD 090

27253 Open treatment of hip dislocation, traumatic, without internal fixation
C 80 50 — 26.92 — 26.92 FUD 090

27254 Open treatment of hip dislocation, traumatic, with acetabular wall and femoral head fracture, with or without internal or external fixation
EXCLUDES *Acetabular fracture treatment (27226-27227)*
C 80 50 — 36.24 — 36.24 FUD 090

27256 Treatment of spontaneous hip dislocation (developmental, including congenital or pathological), by abduction, splint or traction; without anesthesia, without manipulation
G2 T 80 50 — 6.74 — 8.54 FUD 010

27257 with manipulation, requiring anesthesia
A2 T 80 50 — 10.30 — 10.30 FUD 010

27258 Open treatment of spontaneous hip dislocation (developmental, including congenital or pathological), replacement of femoral head in acetabulum (including tenotomy, etc);
INCLUDES Lorenz's operation
C 80 50 — 31.69 — 31.69 FUD 090

27259 with femoral shaft shortening
C 80 50 — 44.37 — 44.37 FUD 090

27265 Closed treatment of post hip arthroplasty dislocation; without anesthesia
A2 T 50 — 11.38 — 11.38 FUD 090

27266 requiring regional or general anesthesia
A2 T 50 — 16.54 — 16.54 FUD 090

27267 Closed treatment of femoral fracture, proximal end, head; without manipulation
G2 T 80 50 — 12.44 — 12.44 FUD 090

27268 with manipulation
C 80 50 — 15.30 — 15.30 FUD 090

27269 Open treatment of femoral fracture, proximal end, head, includes internal fixation, when performed

Do not report with (27033, 27253)

C 80 50 PQ 35.62 35.62 FUD 090

27275 Hip Manipulation with Anesthesia

27275 Manipulation, hip joint, requiring general anesthesia

A2 T 5.16 5.16 FUD 010

27279-27286 Arthrodesis of Hip and Pelvis

● 27279 Arthrodesis, sacroiliac joint, percutaneous or minimally invasive (indirect visualization), with image guidance, includes obtaining bone graft when performed, and placement of transfixing device

▲ 27280 Arthrodesis, open, sacroiliac joint, including obtaining bone graft, including instrumentation, when performed

EXCLUDES *Sacroiliac joint arthrodesis without fracture and/or dislocation, percutaneous or minimally invasive (27279)*

C 80 50 29.74 29.74 FUD 090

27282 Arthrodesis, symphysis pubis (including obtaining graft)

C 80 24.33 24.33 FUD 090

27284 Arthrodesis, hip joint (including obtaining graft);

C 80 50 46.34 46.34 FUD 090

27286 with subtrochanteric osteotomy

C 80 50 47.29 47.29 FUD 090

27290-27299 Amputations and Unlisted Procedures of Hip and Pelvis

27290 Interpelviabdominal amputation (hindquarter amputation)

INCLUDES Pean's amputation

C 80 46.46 46.46 FUD 090

27295 Disarticulation of hip

C 80 50 36.21 36.21 FUD 090

27299 Unlisted procedure, pelvis or hip joint

T 80 50 0.00 0.00 FUD YYY

27301-27310 Incisional Procedures Femur or Knee

EXCLUDES *Superficial incision and drainage (10040-10160)*

27301 Incision and drainage, deep abscess, bursa, or hematoma, thigh or knee region

A2 T 50 14.09 18.63 FUD 090

27303 Incision, deep, with opening of bone cortex, femur or knee (eg, osteomyelitis or bone abscess)

C 80 50 18.19 18.19 FUD 090

27305 Fasciotomy, iliotibial (tenotomy), open

EXCLUDES *Ober-Yount (gluteal-iliotibial) fasciotomy (27025)*

A2 T 80 50 13.77 13.77 FUD 090

27306 Tenotomy, percutaneous, adductor or hamstring; single tendon (separate procedure)

A2 T 80 50 10.52 10.52 FUD 090

27307 multiple tendons

A2 T 80 50 13.63 13.63 FUD 090

27310 Arthrotomy, knee, with exploration, drainage, or removal of foreign body (eg, infection)

A2 T 80 50 20.84 20.84 FUD 090

27323-27324 Biopsy Femur or Knee

EXCLUDES *Soft tissue needle biopsy (20206)*

27323 Biopsy, soft tissue of thigh or knee area; superficial

A2 T 50 PQ 5.07 7.65 FUD 010

27324 deep (subfascial or intramuscular)

A2 T 50 PQ 11.23 11.23 FUD 090

27325-27326 Neurectomy

27325 Neurectomy, hamstring muscle

A2 T 80 50 15.83 15.83 FUD 090

27326 Neurectomy, popliteal (gastrocnemius)

A2 T 80 50 14.58 14.58 FUD 090

27327-27329 [27337, 27339] Excision Soft Tissue Tumors Femur/ Knee

INCLUDES Any necessary elevation of tissue planes or dissection
Measurement of tumor and necessary margin at greatest diameter prior to excision
Simple and intermediate repairs
Types of Excision:
Fascial or subfascial soft tissue tumors: simple and marginal resection of tumors found either in or below the deep fascia, not including bone or excision of a substantial amount of normal tissue; primarily benign and intramuscular tumors
Radical resection of soft tissue tumor: wide resection of tumor involving substantial margins of normal tissue and may involve tissue removal from one or more layers; most often malignant or aggressive benign
Subcutaneous: simple and marginal resection of tumors in the subcutaneous tissue above the deep fascia; most often benign

EXCLUDES *Complex repair*
Excision of benign cutaneous lesions (eg, sebaceous cyst) (11400-11406)
Radical resection of cutaneous tumors (eg, melanoma) (11600-11606)
Significant exploration of vessels or neuroplasty

27327 Excision, tumor, soft tissue of thigh or knee area, subcutaneous; less than 3 cm

G2 T 50 8.91 12.96 FUD 090

\# 27337 3 cm or greater

G2 T 80 50 11.87 11.87 FUD 090

27328 Excision, tumor, soft tissue of thigh or knee area, subfascial (eg, intramuscular); less than 5 cm

G2 T 50 17.62 17.62 FUD 090

\# 27339 5 cm or greater

G2 T 80 50 21.35 21.35 FUD 090

27329 Resequenced code. See code following 27360.

27330-27360 Resection Procedures Thigh/Knee

27330 Arthrotomy, knee; with synovial biopsy only

A2 T 50 PQ 11.86 11.86 FUD 090

27331 including joint exploration, biopsy, or removal of loose or foreign bodies

A2 T 80 50 PQ 13.53 13.53 FUD 090

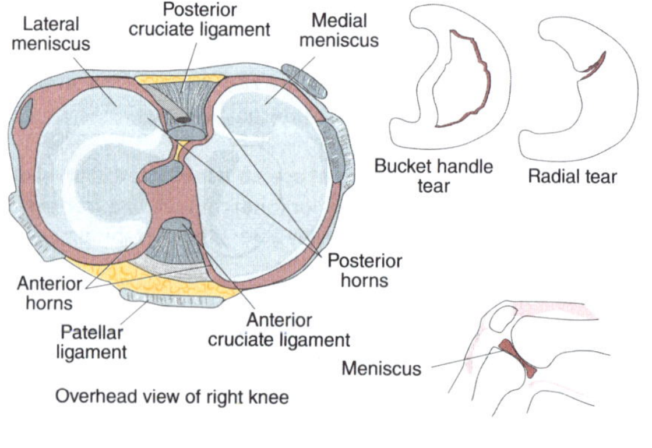

27332 Arthrotomy, with excision of semilunar cartilage (meniscectomy) knee; medial OR lateral

A2 T 80 50 18.22 18.22 FUD 090

27333 medial AND lateral

A2 T 80 50 16.64 16.64 FUD 090

27334 **Arthrotomy, with synovectomy, knee; anterior OR posterior**
A2 T 80 50 19.49 19.49 FUD 090

27335 **anterior AND posterior including popliteal area**
A2 T 80 50 21.79 21.79 FUD 090

27337 ***Resequenced code. See code following 27327.***

27339 ***Resequenced code. See code following 27328.***

27340 **Excision, prepatellar bursa**
A2 T 50 10.54 10.54 FUD 090

27345 **Excision of synovial cyst of popliteal space (eg, Baker's cyst)**
A2 T 80 50 13.67 13.67 FUD 090

27347 **Excision of lesion of meniscus or capsule (eg, cyst, ganglion), knee**
A2 T 80 50 15.04 15.04 FUD 090

27350 **Patellectomy or hemipatellectomy**
A2 T 80 50 18.61 18.61 FUD 090

27355 **Excision or curettage of bone cyst or benign tumor of femur;**
A2 T 80 50 17.17 17.17 FUD 090

27356 **with allograft**
A2 T 80 50 21.02 21.02 FUD 090

27357 **with autograft (includes obtaining graft)**
A2 T 80 50 23.19 23.19 FUD 090

\+ 27358 **with internal fixation (List in addition to code for primary procedure)**
Code first (27355-27357)
N1 N 80 7.99 7.99 FUD ZZZ

27360 **Partial excision (craterization, saucerization, or diaphysectomy) bone, femur, proximal tibia and/or fibula (eg, osteomyelitis or bone abscess)**
A2 T 80 50 24.29 24.29 FUD 090

27329-27365 [27329] Radical Resection Tumor Knee/Thigh

INCLUDES Any necessary elevation of tissue planes or dissection
Measurement of tumor and necessary margin at greatest diameter prior to excision
Radical resection of bone tumor: resection of the tumor (may include entire bone) and wide margins of normal tissue primarily for malignant or aggressive benign tumors
Radical resection of soft tissue tumor: wide resection of tumor involving substantial margins of normal tissue that may include tissue removal from one or more layers; most often malignant or aggressive benign
Simple and intermediate repairs

EXCLUDES *Complex repair*
Radical resection of cutaneous tumors (eg, melanoma) (11600-11606)
Significant exploration of vessels, neuroplasty, reconstruction, or complex bone repair

Do not report radical excision of soft tissue codes when adjacent soft tissue is removed during the bone tumor resection

\# 27329 **Radical resection of tumor (eg, sarcoma), soft tissue of thigh or knee area; less than 5 cm**
G2 T 80 50 29.65 29.65 FUD 090

27364 **5 cm or greater**
G2 T 80 50 44.70 44.70 FUD 090

27365 **Radical resection of tumor, femur or knee**
EXCLUDES *Soft tissue tumor excision thigh or knee area ([27329], 27364)*
C 80 50 59.31 59.31 FUD 090

27370 Injection for Arthrogram of Knee

EXCLUDES *Knee lavage/drainage via arthroscope (29871)*

Do not report with (20610-20611, 29871)

▲ 27370 **Injection of contrast for knee arthrography**
73580
N1 N 50 1.49 4.53 FUD 000

27372 Foreign Body Removal Femur or Knee

EXCLUDES *Arthroscopic procedures (29870-29887)*
Removal of knee prosthesis (27488)

27372 **Removal of foreign body, deep, thigh region or knee area**
A2 T 80 50 11.52 17.20 FUD 090

27380-27499 Repair/Reconstruction of Femur or Knee

27380 **Suture of infrapatellar tendon; primary**
A2 T 80 50 16.92 16.92 FUD 090

27381 **secondary reconstruction, including fascial or tendon graft**
A2 T 80 50 22.79 22.79 FUD 090

27385 **Suture of quadriceps or hamstring muscle rupture; primary**
A2 T 80 50 16.36 16.36 FUD 090

27386 **secondary reconstruction, including fascial or tendon graft**
A2 T 80 50 23.67 23.67 FUD 090

27390 **Tenotomy, open, hamstring, knee to hip; single tendon**
A2 T 80 50 12.72 12.72 FUD 090

27391 **multiple tendons, 1 leg**
A2 T 80 16.39 16.39 FUD 090

27392 **multiple tendons, bilateral**
A2 T 80 20.25 20.25 FUD 090

27393 **Lengthening of hamstring tendon; single tendon**
A2 T 80 50 14.48 14.48 FUD 090

27394 **multiple tendons, 1 leg**
A2 T 80 18.56 18.56 FUD 090

27395 **multiple tendons, bilateral**
A2 T 80 25.01 25.01 FUD 090

27396 **Transplant or transfer (with muscle redirection or rerouting), thigh (eg, extensor to flexor); single tendon**
A2 T 80 50 17.51 17.51 FUD 090

27397 **multiple tendons**
A2 T 80 50 26.09 26.09 FUD 090

27400 **Transfer, tendon or muscle, hamstrings to femur (eg, Egger's type procedure)**
A2 T 80 50 19.75 19.75 FUD 090

27403 **Arthrotomy with meniscus repair, knee**
EXCLUDES *Arthroscopic treatment (29882)*
A2 T 80 50 18.24 18.24 FUD 090

27405 **Repair, primary, torn ligament and/or capsule, knee; collateral**
A2 T 80 50 19.28 19.28 FUD 090

27407 **cruciate**
EXCLUDES *Reconstruction (27427)*
A2 T 80 50 22.55 22.55 FUD 090

27409 **collateral and cruciate ligaments**
EXCLUDES *Reconstruction (27427-27429)*
A2 T 80 50 27.51 27.51 FUD 090

27412 **Autologous chondrocyte implantation, knee**
EXCLUDES *Obtaining chondrocytes (29870)*
Do not report with (20926, 27331, 27570)
T 80 50 47.31 47.31 FUD 090

27415 **Osteochondral allograft, knee, open**
EXCLUDES *Arthroscopic procedure (29867)*
Do not report with (27416)
G2 T 80 50 39.26 39.26 FUD 090

27416 Osteochondral autograft(s), knee, open (eg, mosaicplasty) (includes harvesting of autograft[s])

EXCLUDES *Surgical arthroscopy of the knee with osteochondral autograft(s) (29866)*

Do not report with the following procedures in the same compartment (29874, 29877, 29879, 29885-29887)

Do not report with the following procedures performed at the same surgical session (27415, 29870-29871, 29875, 29884)

G2 T 80 50 27.97 27.97 FUD 090

27418 Anterior tibial tubercleplasty (eg, Maquet type procedure)

A2 T 80 50 23.70 23.70 FUD 090

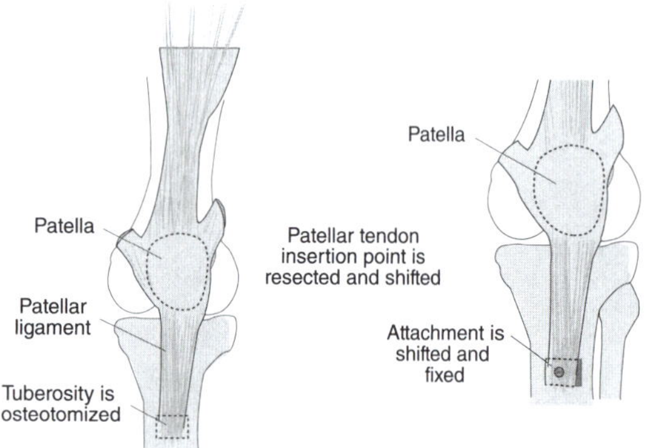

27420 Reconstruction of dislocating patella; (eg, Hauser type procedure)

A2 T 80 50 20.95 20.95 FUD 090

27422 with extensor realignment and/or muscle advancement or release (eg, Campbell, Goldwaite type procedure)

A2 T 80 50 21.20 21.20 FUD 090

27424 with patellectomy

A2 T 80 50 21.27 21.27 FUD 090

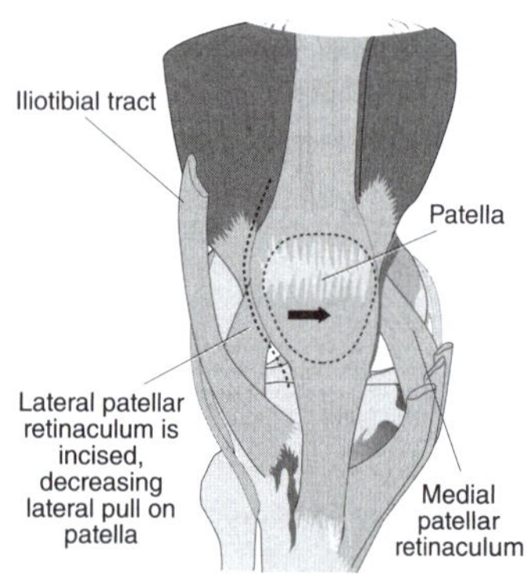

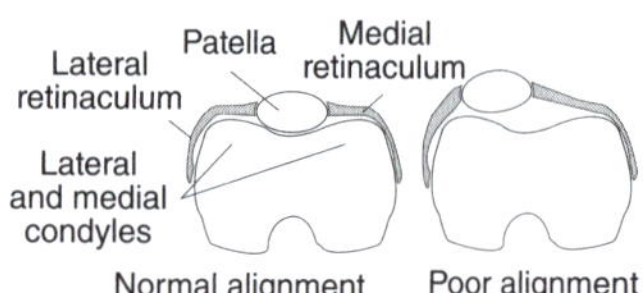

27425 Lateral retinacular release, open

EXCLUDES *Arthroscopic release (29873)*

A2 T 50 12.70 12.70 FUD 090

27427 Ligamentous reconstruction (augmentation), knee; extra-articular

EXCLUDES *Primary repair of ligament(s) (27405, 27407, 27409)*

A2 T 80 50 20.38 20.38 FUD 090

27428 intra-articular (open)

EXCLUDES *Primary repair of ligament(s) (27405, 27407, 27409)*

A2 T 80 50 31.77 31.77 FUD 090

27429 intra-articular (open) and extra-articular

EXCLUDES *Primary repair of ligament(s) (27405, 27407, 27409)*

A2 T 80 50 35.73 35.73 FUD 090

27430 Quadricepsplasty (eg, Bennett or Thompson type)

A2 T 80 50 21.12 21.12 FUD 090

27435 Capsulotomy, posterior capsular release, knee

A2 T 80 50 23.09 23.09 FUD 090

27437 Arthroplasty, patella; without prosthesis

A2 T 50 18.79 18.79 FUD 090

27438 with prosthesis

A2 T 80 50 24.05 24.05 FUD 090

27440 Arthroplasty, knee, tibial plateau;

G2 T 80 50 PQ 22.71 22.71 FUD 090

27441 with debridement and partial synovectomy

A2 T 80 50 PQ 23.47 23.47 FUD 090

27442 Arthroplasty, femoral condyles or tibial plateau(s), knee;

A2 T 80 50 PQ 24.85 24.85 FUD 090

27443 with debridement and partial synovectomy

A2 T 80 50 PQ 23.26 23.26 FUD 090

27445 Arthroplasty, knee, hinge prosthesis (eg, Walldius type)

EXCLUDES *Removal knee prosthesis (27488)*
Revision knee arthroplasty (27487)

C 80 50 PQ 35.86 35.86 FUD 090

27446 Arthroplasty, knee, condyle and plateau; medial OR lateral compartment

EXCLUDES *Removal knee prosthesis (27488)*
Revision knee arthroplasty (27487)

Code also (C1776)

J8 T 80 50 PQ 33.28 33.28 FUD 090

27447 medial AND lateral compartments with or without patella resurfacing (total knee arthroplasty)

EXCLUDES *Removal knee prosthesis (27488)*
Revision knee arthroplasty (27487)

C 80 50 PQ 38.92 38.92 FUD 090

27448 Osteotomy, femur, shaft or supracondylar; without fixation

C 80 50 23.05 23.05 FUD 090

27450 with fixation

C 80 50 28.94 28.94 FUD 090

27454 Osteotomy, multiple, with realignment on intramedullary rod, femoral shaft (eg, Sofield type procedure)

C 80 50 37.12 37.12 FUD 090

27455 Osteotomy, proximal tibia, including fibular excision or osteotomy (includes correction of genu varus [bowleg] or genu valgus [knock-knee]); before epiphyseal closure

C 80 50 26.86 26.86 FUD 090

27457 after epiphyseal closure

C 80 50 27.33 27.33 FUD 090

27465 Osteoplasty, femur; shortening (excluding 64876)

C 80 50 35.82 35.82 FUD 090

27466 lengthening

C 80 50 33.68 33.68 FUD 090

27468 combined, lengthening and shortening with femoral segment transfer

C 80 50 34.43 34.43 FUD 090

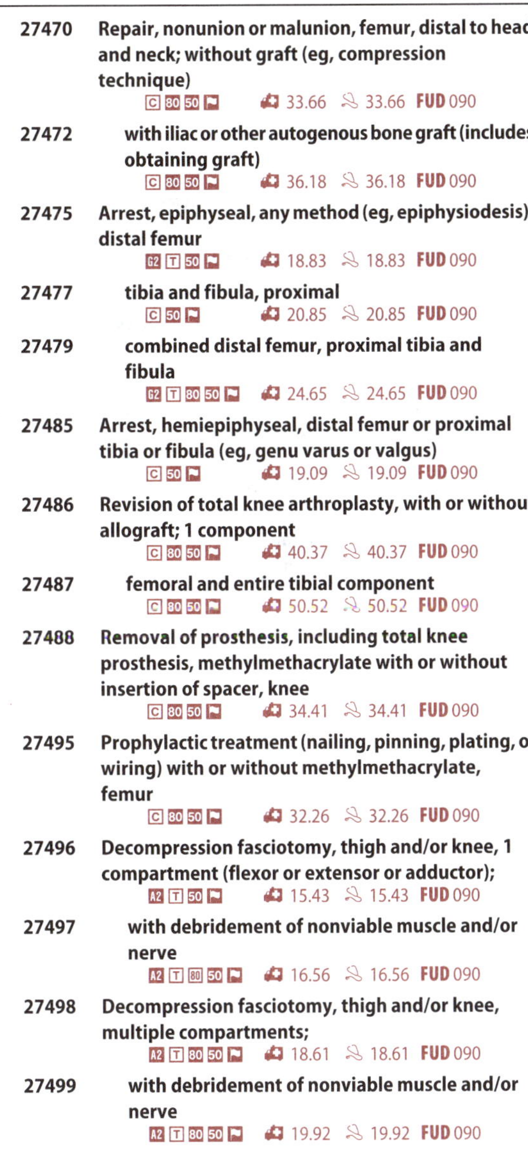

27470 Repair, nonunion or malunion, femur, distal to head and neck; without graft (eg, compression technique)
C 80 50 33.66 33.66 FUD 090

27472 with iliac or other autogenous bone graft (includes obtaining graft)
C 80 50 36.18 36.18 FUD 090

27475 Arrest, epiphyseal, any method (eg, epiphysiodesis); distal femur
G2 T 50 18.83 18.83 FUD 090

27477 tibia and fibula, proximal
C 50 20.85 20.85 FUD 090

27479 combined distal femur, proximal tibia and fibula
G2 T 80 50 24.65 24.65 FUD 090

27485 Arrest, hemiepiphyseal, distal femur or proximal tibia or fibula (eg, genu varus or valgus)
C 50 19.09 19.09 FUD 090

27486 Revision of total knee arthroplasty, with or without allograft; 1 component
C 80 50 40.37 40.37 FUD 090

27487 femoral and entire tibial component
C 80 50 50.52 50.52 FUD 090

27488 Removal of prosthesis, including total knee prosthesis, methylmethacrylate with or without insertion of spacer, knee
C 80 50 34.41 34.41 FUD 090

27495 Prophylactic treatment (nailing, pinning, plating, or wiring) with or without methylmethacrylate, femur
C 80 50 32.26 32.26 FUD 090

27496 Decompression fasciotomy, thigh and/or knee, 1 compartment (flexor or extensor or adductor);
A2 T 50 15.43 15.43 FUD 090

27497 with debridement of nonviable muscle and/or nerve
A2 T 80 50 16.56 16.56 FUD 090

27498 Decompression fasciotomy, thigh and/or knee, multiple compartments;
A2 T 80 50 18.61 18.61 FUD 090

27499 with debridement of nonviable muscle and/or nerve
A2 T 80 50 19.92 19.92 FUD 090

27500-27566 Treatment of Fracture/Dislocation of Femur/Knee

INCLUDES Closed, percutaneous, and open treatment of fractures and dislocations

27500 Closed treatment of femoral shaft fracture, without manipulation
A2 T 50 13.62 14.69 FUD 090

27501 Closed treatment of supracondylar or transcondylar femoral fracture with or without intercondylar extension, without manipulation
A2 T 80 50 14.18 14.29 FUD 090

27502 Closed treatment of femoral shaft fracture, with manipulation, with or without skin or skeletal traction
A2 T 50 22.01 22.01 FUD 090

27503 Closed treatment of supracondylar or transcondylar femoral fracture with or without intercondylar extension, with manipulation, with or without skin or skeletal traction
A2 T 80 50 22.89 22.89 FUD 090

27506 Open treatment of femoral shaft fracture, with or without external fixation, with insertion of intramedullary implant, with or without cerclage and/or locking screws
C 80 50 38.30 38.30 FUD 090

27507 Open treatment of femoral shaft fracture with plate/screws, with or without cerclage
C 80 50 27.86 27.86 FUD 090

27508 Closed treatment of femoral fracture, distal end, medial or lateral condyle, without manipulation
A2 T 50 14.08 14.94 FUD 090

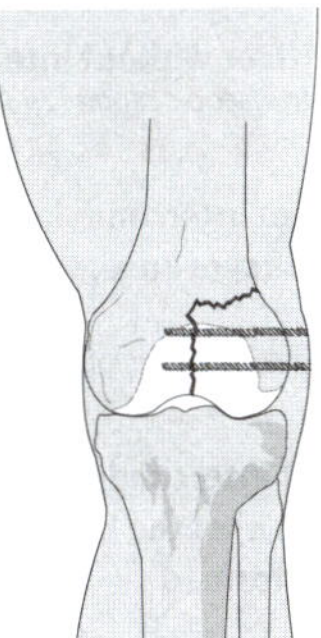

27509 Percutaneous skeletal fixation of femoral fracture, distal end, medial or lateral condyle, or supracondylar or transcondylar, with or without intercondylar extension, or distal femoral epiphyseal separation
A2 T 80 50 PQ 18.33 18.33 FUD 090

27510 Closed treatment of femoral fracture, distal end, medial or lateral condyle, with manipulation
A2 T 50 19.55 19.55 FUD 090

27511 Open treatment of femoral supracondylar or transcondylar fracture without intercondylar extension, includes internal fixation, when performed
C 80 50 28.57 28.57 FUD 090

27513 Open treatment of femoral supracondylar or transcondylar fracture with intercondylar extension, includes internal fixation, when performed
C 80 50 35.57 35.57 FUD 090

27514 Open treatment of femoral fracture, distal end, medial or lateral condyle, includes internal fixation, when performed
C 80 50 27.68 27.68 FUD 090

27516 Closed treatment of distal femoral epiphyseal separation; without manipulation
A2 T 50 13.52 14.38 FUD 090

27517 with manipulation, with or without skin or skeletal traction
A2 T 80 50 19.49 19.49 FUD 090

27519 Open treatment of distal femoral epiphyseal separation, includes internal fixation, when performed
C 80 50 25.45 25.45 FUD 090

27520 Closed treatment of patellar fracture, without manipulation
A2 T 50 8.36 9.14 FUD 090

27524 Open treatment of patellar fracture, with internal fixation and/or partial or complete patellectomy and soft tissue repair
G2 T 80 50 21.46 21.46 FUD 090

27530 Closed treatment of tibial fracture, proximal (plateau); without manipulation
EXCLUDES *Arthroscopic repair (29855-29856)*
A2 T 50 7.93 8.53 FUD 090

27532 with or without manipulation, with skeletal traction
EXCLUDES *Arthroscopic repair (29855-29856)*
A2 T 50 16.42 17.47 FUD 090

27535 Open treatment of tibial fracture, proximal (plateau); unicondylar, includes internal fixation, when performed
EXCLUDES *Arthroscopic repair (29855-29856)*
C 80 50 25.68 25.68 FUD 090

27536 bicondylar, with or without internal fixation
EXCLUDES *Arthroscopic repair (29855-29856)*
C 80 50 34.08 34.08 FUD 090

27538 Closed treatment of intercondylar spine(s) and/or tuberosity fracture(s) of knee, with or without manipulation
EXCLUDES *Arthroscopic repair (29850-29851)*
A2 T 80 50 12.58 13.42 FUD 090

27540 Open treatment of intercondylar spine(s) and/or tuberosity fracture(s) of the knee, includes internal fixation, when performed
C 80 50 23.20 23.20 FUD 090

27550 Closed treatment of knee dislocation; without anesthesia
A2 T 80 50 13.37 14.37 FUD 090

27552 requiring anesthesia
A2 T 80 50 17.81 17.81 FUD 090

27556 Open treatment of knee dislocation, includes internal fixation, when performed; without primary ligamentous repair or augmentation/reconstruction
C 80 50 24.95 24.95 FUD 090

27557 with primary ligamentous repair
C 80 50 29.95 29.95 FUD 090

27558 with primary ligamentous repair, with augmentation/reconstruction
C 80 50 34.15 34.15 FUD 090

27560 Closed treatment of patellar dislocation; without anesthesia
EXCLUDES *Recurrent dislocation (27420-27424)*
A2 T 50 9.48 10.23 FUD 090

27562 requiring anesthesia
EXCLUDES *Recurrent dislocation (27420-27424)*
A2 T 80 50 13.72 13.72 FUD 090

27566 Open treatment of patellar dislocation, with or without partial or total patellectomy
EXCLUDES *Recurrent dislocation (27420-27424)*
A2 T 80 50 25.45 25.45 FUD 090

27570 Knee Manipulation with Anesthesia

27570 Manipulation of knee joint under general anesthesia (includes application of traction or other fixation devices)
A2 T 50 4.28 4.28 FUD 010

27580 Knee Arthrodesis

27580 Arthrodesis, knee, any technique
INCLUDES Albert's operation
C 80 50 41.09 41.09 FUD 090

27590-27599 Amputations and Unlisted Procedures at Femur or Knee

27590 Amputation, thigh, through femur, any level;
C 80 50 23.32 23.32 FUD 090

27591 immediate fitting technique including first cast
C 80 50 27.72 27.72 FUD 090

27592 open, circular (guillotine)
C 80 50 19.72 19.72 FUD 090

27594 secondary closure or scar revision
A2 T 50 14.67 14.67 FUD 090

27596 re-amputation
C 50 20.95 20.95 FUD 090

27598 Disarticulation at knee
INCLUDES Batch-Spittler-McFaddin operation
Callandar knee disarticulation
Gritti amputation
C 80 50 21.00 21.00 FUD 090

27599 Unlisted procedure, femur or knee
T 80 50 0.00 0.00 FUD YYY

27600-27602 Decompression Fasciotomy of Leg

EXCLUDES *Fasciotomy with debridement (27892-27894)*
Simple incision and drainage (10140-10160)

27600 Decompression fasciotomy, leg; anterior and/or lateral compartments only
A2 T 50 11.88 11.88 FUD 090

27601 posterior compartment(s) only
A2 T 50 12.64 12.64 FUD 090

27602 anterior and/or lateral, and posterior compartment(s)
A2 T 80 50 14.37 14.37 FUD 090

27603-27612 Incisional Procedures Lower Leg and Ankle

27603 Incision and drainage, leg or ankle; deep abscess or hematoma
A2 T 50 11.09 14.97 FUD 090

27604 infected bursa
A2 T 80 50 9.48 13.16 FUD 090

27605 Tenotomy, percutaneous, Achilles tendon (separate procedure); local anesthesia
A2 T 80 50 5.31 9.68 FUD 010

27606 general anesthesia
A2 T 50 8.17 8.17 FUD 010

27607 Incision (eg, osteomyelitis or bone abscess), leg or ankle
A2 T 50 17.45 17.45 FUD 090

27610 Arthrotomy, ankle, including exploration, drainage, or removal of foreign body
A2 T 50 18.69 18.69 FUD 090

27612 Arthrotomy, posterior capsular release, ankle, with or without Achilles tendon lengthening
EXCLUDES *Lengthening or shortening tendon (27685)*
A2 T 80 50 16.14 16.14 FUD 090

27613-27614 Biopsy Lower Leg and Ankle

EXCLUDES *Needle biopsy (20206)*

27613 Biopsy, soft tissue of leg or ankle area; superficial
P3 T 50 PQ 4.65 7.14 FUD 010

27614 deep (subfascial or intramuscular)
A2 T 50 PQ 11.63 16.45 FUD 090

27615-27634 [27632, 27634] Excision Soft Tissue Tumors Lower Leg/Ankle

INCLUDES Any necessary elevation of tissue planes or dissection
Measurement of tumor and necessary margin at greatest diameter prior to excision
Resection without removal of significant normal tissue
Simple and intermediate repairs
Types of excision:
Fascial or subfascial soft tissue tumors: simple and marginal resection of most often benign and intramuscular tumors found either in or below the deep fascia, not involving bone
Resection of the tumor (may include entire bone) and wide margins of normal tissue primarily for malignant or aggressive benign tumors
Subcutaneous: simple and marginal resection of most often benign tumors found in the subcutaneous tissue above the deep fascia

EXCLUDES *Complex repair*
Excision of benign cutaneous lesions (eg, sebaceous cyst) (11400-11406)
Radical resection of cutaneous tumors (eg, melanoma) (11600-11606)
Significant exploration of vessels or neuroplasty

27615 **Radical resection of tumor (eg, sarcoma), soft tissue of leg or ankle area; less than 5 cm**
G2 T 80 50 29.26 29.26 FUD 090

27616 **5 cm or greater**
G2 T 80 50 36.20 36.20 FUD 090

27618 **Excision, tumor, soft tissue of leg or ankle area, subcutaneous; less than 3 cm**
G2 T 50 8.70 12.64 FUD 090

27632 **3 cm or greater**
G2 T 80 50 11.77 11.77 FUD 090

27619 **Excision, tumor, soft tissue of leg or ankle area, subfascial (eg, intramuscular); less than 5 cm**
G2 T 50 13.48 13.48 FUD 090

27634 **5 cm or greater**
G2 T 80 50 19.47 19.47 FUD 090

27620-27641 Bone and Joint Procedures Ankle/Leg

27620 **Arthrotomy, ankle, with joint exploration, with or without biopsy, with or without removal of loose or foreign body**
A2 T 80 50 PQ 12.99 12.99 FUD 090

27625 **Arthrotomy, with synovectomy, ankle;**
A2 T 80 50 16.57 16.57 FUD 090

27626 **including tenosynovectomy**
A2 T 80 50 17.90 17.90 FUD 090

27630 **Excision of lesion of tendon sheath or capsule (eg, cyst or ganglion), leg and/or ankle**
A2 T 50 10.51 15.99 FUD 090

27632 ***Resequenced code. See code following 27618.***

27634 ***Resequenced code. See code following 27619.***

27635 **Excision or curettage of bone cyst or benign tumor, tibia or fibula;**
A2 T 50 16.84 16.84 FUD 090

27637 **with autograft (includes obtaining graft)**
A2 T 80 50 21.48 21.48 FUD 090

27638 **with allograft**
A2 T 80 50 22.01 22.01 FUD 090

27640 **Partial excision (craterization, saucerization, or diaphysectomy), bone (eg, osteomyelitis); tibia**
EXCLUDES *Excision of exostosis (27635)*
A2 T 50 23.83 23.83 FUD 090

27641 **fibula**
EXCLUDES *Excision of exostosis (27635)*
A2 T 50 19.14 19.14 FUD 090

27645-27647 Radical Resection Bone Tumor Ankle/Leg

INCLUDES Any necessary elevation of tissue planes or dissection
Measurement of tumor and necessary margin at greatest diameter prior to excision
Resection of the tumor (may include entire bone) and wide margins of normal tissue primarily for malignant or aggressive benign tumors
Simple and intermediate repairs

EXCLUDES *Complex repair*
Significant exploration of vessels, neuroplasty, reconstruction, or complex bone repair

Do not report radical excision of soft tissue codes when adjacent soft tissue is removed during the bone tumor resection (27615-27619 [27632, 27634])

27645 **Radical resection of tumor; tibia**
C 80 50 50.96 50.96 FUD 090

27646 **fibula**
C 80 50 44.17 44.17 FUD 090

27647 **talus or calcaneus**
A2 T 80 50 29.95 29.95 FUD 090

27648 Injection for Ankle Arthrogram

EXCLUDES *Arthroscopy (29894-29898)*

27648 **Injection procedure for ankle arthrography**
73615
N1 N 80 50 1.50 4.60 FUD 000

27650-27745 Repair/Reconstruction Lower Leg/Ankle

27650 **Repair, primary, open or percutaneous, ruptured Achilles tendon;**
A2 T 80 50 18.97 18.97 FUD 090

27652 **with graft (includes obtaining graft)**
A2 T 50 19.73 19.73 FUD 090

27654 **Repair, secondary, Achilles tendon, with or without graft**
A2 T 80 50 20.27 20.27 FUD 090

27656 **Repair, fascial defect of leg**
A2 T 80 50 11.23 17.92 FUD 090

27658 **Repair, flexor tendon, leg; primary, without graft, each tendon**
A2 T 80 10.69 10.69 FUD 090

27659 **secondary, with or without graft, each tendon**
A2 T 80 13.93 13.93 FUD 090

27664 **Repair, extensor tendon, leg; primary, without graft, each tendon**
A2 T 80 10.32 10.32 FUD 090

27665 **secondary, with or without graft, each tendon**
A2 T 80 11.84 11.84 FUD 090

27675 **Repair, dislocating peroneal tendons; without fibular osteotomy**
A2 T 80 50 13.90 13.90 FUD 090

27676 **with fibular osteotomy**
A2 T 80 50 17.58 17.58 FUD 090

27680 **Tenolysis, flexor or extensor tendon, leg and/or ankle; single, each tendon**
A2 T 12.25 12.25 FUD 090

27681 **multiple tendons (through separate incision[s])**
A2 T 50 15.53 15.53 FUD 090

27685 **Lengthening or shortening of tendon, leg or ankle; single tendon (separate procedure)**
A2 T 80 50 13.33 18.98 FUD 090

27686 **multiple tendons (through same incision), each**
A2 T 50 15.79 15.79 FUD 090

27687 **Gastrocnemius recession (eg, Strayer procedure)**
A2 T 80 50 13.01 13.01 FUD 090

27690 **Transfer or transplant of single tendon (with muscle redirection or rerouting); superficial (eg, anterior tibial extensors into midfoot)**
INCLUDES Toe extensors considered a single tendon with transplant into midfoot
A2 T 80 50 18.08 18.08 FUD 090

27691 **deep (eg, anterior tibial or posterior tibial through interosseous space, flexor digitorum longus, flexor hallucis longus, or peroneal tendon to midfoot or hindfoot)**
INCLUDES Barr procedure
Toe extensors considered a single tendon with transplant into midfoot
A2 T 80 50 21.54 21.54 FUD 090

\+ **27692** **each additional tendon (List separately in addition to code for primary procedure)**
INCLUDES Toe extensors considered a single tendon with transplant into midfoot
Code first (27690-27691)
N1 N 80 3.05 3.05 FUD ZZZ

Lateral view of right ankle showing components of the collateral ligament

27695 **Repair, primary, disrupted ligament, ankle; collateral**
A2 T 50 13.71 13.71 FUD 090

27696 **both collateral ligaments**
A2 T 50 16.06 16.06 FUD 090

27698 **Repair, secondary, disrupted ligament, ankle, collateral (eg, Watson-Jones procedure)**
A2 T 80 50 18.37 18.37 FUD 090

27700 **Arthroplasty, ankle;**
A2 T 80 50 16.98 16.98 FUD 090

27702 **with implant (total ankle)**
C 80 50 PQ 27.82 27.82 FUD 090

27703 **revision, total ankle**
C 80 50 PQ 32.11 32.11 FUD 090

27704 **Removal of ankle implant**
A2 Q2 50 PQ 16.48 16.48 FUD 090

27705 **Osteotomy; tibia**
EXCLUDES *Genu varus or genu valgus repair (27455-27457)*
A2 T 80 50 21.69 21.69 FUD 090

27707 **fibula**
EXCLUDES *Genu varus or genu valgus repair (27455-27457)*
A2 T 50 11.51 11.51 FUD 090

27709 **tibia and fibula**
EXCLUDES *Genu varus or genu valgus repair (27455-27457)*
A2 T 80 50 33.45 33.45 FUD 090

27712 **multiple, with realignment on intramedullary rod (eg, Sofield type procedure)**
EXCLUDES *Genu varus or genu valgus repair (27455-27457)*
C 80 50 31.55 31.55 FUD 090

27715 **Osteoplasty, tibia and fibula, lengthening or shortening**
INCLUDES Anderson tibial lengthening
C 80 50 30.57 30.57 FUD 090

27720 **Repair of nonunion or malunion, tibia; without graft, (eg, compression technique)**
G2 T 80 50 25.03 25.03 FUD 090

27722 **with sliding graft**
T 80 50 25.36 25.36 FUD 090

27724 **with iliac or other autograft (includes obtaining graft)**
C 80 50 36.35 36.35 FUD 090

27725 **by synostosis, with fibula, any method**
C 80 50 34.83 34.83 FUD 090

27726 **Repair of fibula nonunion and/or malunion with internal fixation**
Do not report with (27707)
G2 T 50 27.75 27.75 FUD 090

27727 **Repair of congenital pseudarthrosis, tibia**
C 80 50 26.31 26.31 FUD 090

27730 **Arrest, epiphyseal (epiphysiodesis), open; distal tibia**
A2 T 50 16.66 16.66 FUD 090

27732 **distal fibula**
A2 T 50 10.90 10.90 FUD 090

27734 **distal tibia and fibula**
A2 T 50 17.60 17.60 FUD 090

27740 **Arrest, epiphyseal (epiphysiodesis), any method, combined, proximal and distal tibia and fibula;**
EXCLUDES *Epiphyseal arrest of proximal tibia and fibula (27477)*
A2 T 80 50 17.70 17.70 FUD 090

27742 **and distal femur**
EXCLUDES *Epiphyseal arrest of proximal tibia and fibula (27477)*
A2 T 80 50 19.48 19.48 FUD 090

27745 **Prophylactic treatment (nailing, pinning, plating or wiring) with or without methylmethacrylate, tibia**
A2 T 80 50 21.61 21.61 FUD 090

27750-27848 Treatment of Fracture/Dislocation Lower Leg/Ankle

INCLUDES Treatment of open or closed fracture or dislocation

27750 **Closed treatment of tibial shaft fracture (with or without fibular fracture); without manipulation**
A2 T 50 9.02 9.80 FUD 090

27752 **with manipulation, with or without skeletal traction**
A2 T 50 14.10 15.25 FUD 090

27756 **Percutaneous skeletal fixation of tibial shaft fracture (with or without fibular fracture) (eg, pins or screws)**
A2 T 80 50 PQ 16.37 16.37 FUD 090

27758 **Open treatment of tibial shaft fracture (with or without fibular fracture), with plate/screws, with or without cerclage**
A2 T 80 50 PQ 25.45 25.45 FUD 090

27759 **Treatment of tibial shaft fracture (with or without fibular fracture) by intramedullary implant, with or without interlocking screws and/or cerclage**
A2 T 80 50 PQ 28.56 28.56 FUD 090

27760 **Closed treatment of medial malleolus fracture; without manipulation**
A2 T 50 8.67 9.47 FUD 090

27762 **with manipulation, with or without skin or skeletal traction**
A2 T 50 12.43 13.57 FUD 090

27766 **Open treatment of medial malleolus fracture, includes internal fixation, when performed**
A2 T 50 PQ 17.38 17.38 FUD 090

27767 **Closed treatment of posterior malleolus fracture; without manipulation**
Do not report with (27808-27823)
P2 T 50 8.06 8.01 FUD 090

27768 **with manipulation**
Do not report with (27808-27823)
G2 T 50 12.49 12.49 FUD 090

27769 **Open treatment of posterior malleolus fracture, includes internal fixation, when performed**
Do not report with (27808-27823)
G2 T 50 PQ 20.83 20.83 FUD 090

27780 **Closed treatment of proximal fibula or shaft fracture; without manipulation**
A2 T 50 7.91 8.67 FUD 090

27781 **with manipulation**
A2 T 50 11.02 11.86 FUD 090

27784 **Open treatment of proximal fibula or shaft fracture, includes internal fixation, when performed**
A2 T 50 20.48 20.48 FUD 090

27786 **Closed treatment of distal fibular fracture (lateral malleolus); without manipulation**
A2 T 50 8.13 8.97 FUD 090

27788 **with manipulation**
A2 T 50 10.93 11.94 FUD 090

27792 **Open treatment of distal fibular fracture (lateral malleolus), includes internal fixation, when performed**
EXCLUDES *Repair of tibia and fibula shaft fracture (27750-27759)*
A2 T 50 PQ 18.66 18.66 FUD 090

27808 **Closed treatment of bimalleolar ankle fracture (eg, lateral and medial malleoli, or lateral and posterior malleoli or medial and posterior malleoli); without manipulation**
A2 T 50 8.54 9.48 FUD 090

27810 **with manipulation**
A2 T 50 12.11 13.31 FUD 090

27814 **Open treatment of bimalleolar ankle fracture (eg, lateral and medial malleoli, or lateral and posterior malleoli, or medial and posterior malleoli), includes internal fixation, when performed**
A2 T 80 50 PQ 22.08 22.08 FUD 090

27816 **Closed treatment of trimalleolar ankle fracture; without manipulation**
A2 T 50 8.12 9.03 FUD 090

27818 **with manipulation**
A2 T 50 12.40 13.78 FUD 090

27822 **Open treatment of trimalleolar ankle fracture, includes internal fixation, when performed, medial and/or lateral malleolus; without fixation of posterior lip**
A2 T 80 50 24.06 24.06 FUD 090

27823 **with fixation of posterior lip**
A2 T 80 50 27.32 27.32 FUD 090

27824 **Closed treatment of fracture of weight bearing articular portion of distal tibia (eg, pilon or tibial plafond), with or without anesthesia; without manipulation**
A2 T 50 8.66 8.90 FUD 090

27825 **with skeletal traction and/or requiring manipulation**
A2 T 80 50 14.08 15.49 FUD 090

27826 **Open treatment of fracture of weight bearing articular surface/portion of distal tibia (eg, pilon or tibial plafond), with internal fixation, when performed; of fibula only**
A2 T 80 50 23.95 23.95 FUD 090

27827 **of tibia only**
A2 T 80 50 30.98 30.98 FUD 090

27828 **of both tibia and fibula**
A2 T 80 50 37.09 37.09 FUD 090

27829 **Open treatment of distal tibiofibular joint (syndesmosis) disruption, includes internal fixation, when performed**
A2 T 80 50 19.57 19.57 FUD 090

27830 **Closed treatment of proximal tibiofibular joint dislocation; without anesthesia**
A2 T 80 50 10.03 10.75 FUD 090

27831 **requiring anesthesia**
A2 T 80 50 11.32 11.32 FUD 090

27832 **Open treatment of proximal tibiofibular joint dislocation, includes internal fixation, when performed, or with excision of proximal fibula**
A2 T 80 50 21.52 21.52 FUD 090

27840 **Closed treatment of ankle dislocation; without anesthesia**
A2 T 50 10.55 10.55 FUD 090

27842 **requiring anesthesia, with or without percutaneous skeletal fixation**
A2 T 50 14.08 14.08 FUD 090

27846 **Open treatment of ankle dislocation, with or without percutaneous skeletal fixation; without repair or internal fixation**
EXCLUDES *Arthroscopy (29894-29898)*
A2 T 80 50 20.92 20.92 FUD 090

27848 **with repair or internal or external fixation**
EXCLUDES *Arthroscopy (29894-29898)*
A2 T 80 50 23.34 23.34 FUD 090

27860 Ankle Manipulation with Anesthesia

27860 **Manipulation of ankle under general anesthesia (includes application of traction or other fixation apparatus)**
A2 T 80 50 5.07 5.07 FUD 010

27870-27871 Arthrodesis Lower Leg/Ankle

27870 **Arthrodesis, ankle, open**
EXCLUDES *Arthroscopic arthrodesis of ankle (29899)*
A2 T 80 50 29.66 29.66 FUD 090

27871 **Arthrodesis, tibiofibular joint, proximal or distal**
A2 T 80 50 19.67 19.67 FUD 090

27880-27889 Amputations of Lower Leg/Ankle

27880 **Amputation, leg, through tibia and fibula;**
INCLUDES Burgess amputation
C 80 50 26.60 26.60 FUD 090

27881 **with immediate fitting technique including application of first cast**
C 80 50 25.35 25.35 FUD 090

27882 **open, circular (guillotine)**
C 80 50 17.49 17.49 FUD 090

27884 **secondary closure or scar revision**
A2 T 50 16.63 16.63 FUD 090

27886 **re-amputation**
C 50 19.03 19.03 FUD 090

27888 **Amputation, ankle, through malleoli of tibia and fibula (eg, Syme, Pirogoff type procedures), with plastic closure and resection of nerves**
C 80 50 19.38 19.38 FUD 090

27889 Ankle disarticulation
A2 T 50 ⚑ 19.15 19.15 FUD 090

27892-27899 Decompression Fasciotomy Lower Leg

EXCLUDES *Decompression fasciotomy without debridement (27600-27602)*

27892 Decompression fasciotomy, leg; anterior and/or lateral compartments only, with debridement of nonviable muscle and/or nerve
A2 T 80 50 ⚑ 15.89 15.89 FUD 090

27893 posterior compartment(s) only, with debridement of nonviable muscle and/or nerve
A2 T 80 50 ⚑ 17.45 17.45 FUD 090

27894 anterior and/or lateral, and posterior compartment(s), with debridement of nonviable muscle and/or nerve
A2 T 80 50 ⚑ 24.57 24.57 FUD 090

27899 Unlisted procedure, leg or ankle
T 80 50 0.00 0.00 FUD YYY

28001-28008 Surgical Incision Foot/Toe

EXCLUDES *Simple incision and drainage (10060-10160)*

28001 Incision and drainage, bursa, foot
P3 T ⚑ 4.85 7.89 FUD 010

28002 Incision and drainage below fascia, with or without tendon sheath involvement, foot; single bursal space
A2 T ⚑ 9.24 12.77 FUD 010

28003 multiple areas
A2 T ⚑ 16.40 20.42 FUD 090

28005 Incision, bone cortex (eg, osteomyelitis or bone abscess), foot
A2 T ⚑ 16.68 16.68 FUD 090

28008 Fasciotomy, foot and/or toe
EXCLUDES *Plantar fascia division (28250)*
Plantar fasciectomy (28060, 28062)
A2 T 50 ⚑ 8.40 12.36 FUD 090

28010-28011 Tenotomy/Toe

EXCLUDES *Open tenotomy (28230-28234)*
Simple incision and drainage (10140-10160)

28010 Tenotomy, percutaneous, toe; single tendon
P3 T ⚑ 6.01 6.66 FUD 090

28011 multiple tendons
A2 T ⚑ 8.32 9.29 FUD 090

28020-28024 Arthrotomy Foot/Toe

EXCLUDES *Simple incision and drainage (10140-10160)*

28020 Arthrotomy, including exploration, drainage, or removal of loose or foreign body; intertarsal or tarsometatarsal joint
A2 T ⚑ 10.37 15.47 FUD 090

28022 metatarsophalangeal joint
A2 T ⚑ 9.31 13.99 FUD 090

28024 interphalangeal joint
A2 T ⚑ 8.71 13.16 FUD 090

28035 Tarsal Tunnel Release

EXCLUDES *Other nerve decompression (64722)*
Other neuroplasty (64704)

28035 Release, tarsal tunnel (posterior tibial nerve decompression)
A2 T 50 ⚑ 10.26 15.20 FUD 090

28039-28047 [28039, 28041] Excision Soft Tissue Tumors Foot/Toe

INCLUDES Any necessary elevation of tissue planes or dissection
Measurement of tumor and necessary margin at greatest diameter prior to excision
Simple and intermediate repairs
Types of excision:
- Fascial or subfascial soft tissue tumors: simple and marginal resection of tumors found either in or below the deep fascia, not involving bone or excision of a substantial amount of normal tissue; primarily benign and intramuscular tumors
  - Tumors of fingers and toes involving joint capsules, tendons and tendon sheaths
- Radical resection soft tissue tumor: wide resection of tumor, involving substantial margins of normal tissue and may involve tissue removal from one or more layers; most often malignant or aggressive benign
  - Tumors of fingers and toes adjacent to joints, tendons and tendon sheaths
- Subcutaneous: simple and marginal resection of tumors in the subcutaneous tissue above the deep fascia; most often benign

EXCLUDES *Complex repair*
Excision of benign cutaneous lesions (eg, sebaceous cyst) (11420-11426)
Radical resection of cutaneous tumors (eg, melanoma) (11620-11626)
Significant exploration of vessels, neuroplasty, or reconstruction

28039 ***Resequenced code. See code following 28043.***

28041 ***Resequenced code. See code following 28045.***

28043 Excision, tumor, soft tissue of foot or toe, subcutaneous; less than 1.5 cm
G2 T 50 ⚑ 7.51 11.42 FUD 090

\# **28039** 1.5 cm or greater
G2 T 80 50 10.05 14.66 FUD 090

28045 Excision, tumor, soft tissue of foot or toe, subfascial (eg, intramuscular); less than 1.5 cm
G2 T 80 50 ⚑ 10.01 14.23 FUD 090

\# **28041** 1.5 cm or greater
G2 T 80 50 13.19 13.19 FUD 090

28046 Radical resection of tumor (eg, sarcoma), soft tissue of foot or toe; less than 3 cm
G2 T 50 ⚑ 21.13 21.13 FUD 090

28047 3 cm or greater
G2 T 80 50 29.48 29.48 FUD 090

28050-28160 Resection Procedures Foot/Toes

28050 Arthrotomy with biopsy; intertarsal or tarsometatarsal joint
A2 T 50 ⚑ PQ 8.08 12.21 FUD 090

28052 metatarsophalangeal joint
A2 T 50 ⚑ PQ 8.07 12.58 FUD 090

28054 interphalangeal joint
A2 T 80 50 ⚑ PQ 6.75 10.74 FUD 090

28055 Neurectomy, intrinsic musculature of foot
A2 T 80 50 10.82 10.82 FUD 090

28060 Fasciectomy, plantar fascia; partial (separate procedure)
EXCLUDES *Plantar fasciotomy (28008, 28250)*
A2 T 50 ⚑ 10.20 14.81 FUD 090

28062 radical (separate procedure)
EXCLUDES *Plantar fasciotomy (28008, 28250)*
A2 T 50 ⚑ 11.68 16.79 FUD 090

28070 Synovectomy; intertarsal or tarsometatarsal joint, each
A2 T ⚑ 10.15 15.23 FUD 090

28072 metatarsophalangeal joint, each
A2 T ⚑ 9.57 14.57 FUD 090

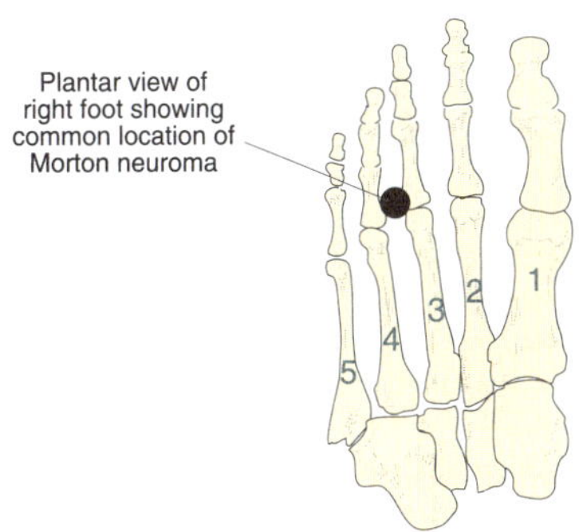

Morton neuroma is a chronic inflammation or irritation of the nerves in the web space between the heads of the metatarsals and phalanges

28080 **Excision, interdigital (Morton) neuroma, single, each**
A2 T 80 ▣ 10.47 14.96 FUD 090

28086 **Synovectomy, tendon sheath, foot; flexor**
A2 T 80 50 ▣ 10.33 15.63 FUD 090

28088 **extensor**
A2 T 80 50 ▣ 8.41 13.35 FUD 090

28090 **Excision of lesion, tendon, tendon sheath, or capsule (including synovectomy) (eg, cyst or ganglion); foot**
A2 T 50 ▣ 8.83 13.47 FUD 090

28092 **toe(s), each**
A2 T ▣ 7.70 12.10 FUD 090

28100 **Excision or curettage of bone cyst or benign tumor, talus or calcaneus;**
A2 T 80 50 ▣ 11.76 17.33 FUD 090

28102 **with iliac or other autograft (includes obtaining graft)**
A2 T 80 50 ▣ 16.34 16.34 FUD 090

28103 **with allograft**
A2 T 80 50 ▣ 11.24 11.24 FUD 090

28104 **Excision or curettage of bone cyst or benign tumor, tarsal or metatarsal, except talus or calcaneus;**
A2 T 80 ▣ 10.04 15.00 FUD 090

28106 **with iliac or other autograft (includes obtaining graft)**
A2 T 80 ▣ 12.79 12.79 FUD 090

28107 **with allograft**
A2 T 80 ▣ 10.49 15.71 FUD 090

28108 **Excision or curettage of bone cyst or benign tumor, phalanges of foot**
EXCLUDES *Hallux valgus (28290)*
A2 T ▣ 8.27 12.64 FUD 090

28110 **Ostectomy, partial excision, fifth metatarsal head (bunionette) (separate procedure)**
A2 T 50 ▣ 8.27 13.24 FUD 090

28111 **Ostectomy, complete excision; first metatarsal head**
A2 T 50 ▣ 9.42 14.24 FUD 090

28112 **other metatarsal head (second, third or fourth)**
A2 T 50 ▣ 8.99 14.03 FUD 090

28113 **fifth metatarsal head**
A2 T 80 50 ▣ 12.21 16.98 FUD 090

28114 **all metatarsal heads, with partial proximal phalangectomy, excluding first metatarsal (eg, Clayton type procedure)**
A2 T 80 50 ▣ 24.00 30.76 FUD 090

28116 **Ostectomy, excision of tarsal coalition**
A2 T 50 ▣ 16.17 21.33 FUD 090

28118 **Ostectomy, calcaneus;**
A2 T 80 50 ▣ 11.75 16.86 FUD 090

28119 **for spur, with or without plantar fascial release**
A2 T 50 ▣ 10.35 15.06 FUD 090

28120 **Partial excision (craterization, saucerization, sequestrectomy, or diaphysectomy) bone (eg, osteomyelitis or bossing); talus or calcaneus**
INCLUDES Barker operation
A2 T 50 ▣ 14.31 19.46 FUD 090

28122 **tarsal or metatarsal bone, except talus or calcaneus**
EXCLUDES *Hallux rigidus cheilectomy (28289)*
Partial removal of talus or calcaneus (28120)
A2 T 80 50 ▣ 12.63 17.16 FUD 090

28124 **phalanx of toe**
P3 T 50 ▣ 9.45 13.65 FUD 090

28126 **Resection, partial or complete, phalangeal base, each toe**
A2 T ▣ 7.14 11.37 FUD 090

28130 **Talectomy (astragalectomy)**
INCLUDES Whitman astragalectomy
EXCLUDES *Calcanectomy (28118)*
A2 T 80 50 ▣ 19.03 19.03 FUD 090

28140 **Metatarsectomy**
A2 T ▣ 12.70 17.23 FUD 090

28150 **Phalangectomy, toe, each toe**
A2 T ▣ 8.06 12.25 FUD 090

28153 **Resection, condyle(s), distal end of phalanx, each toe**
A2 T ▣ 7.59 11.83 FUD 090

28160 **Hemiphalangectomy or interphalangeal joint excision, toe, proximal end of phalanx, each**
A2 T ▣ 7.72 12.04 FUD 090

28171-28175 Radical Resection Bone Tumor Foot/Toes

INCLUDES Any necessary elevation of tissue planes or dissection
Measurement of tumor and necessary margin at greatest diameter prior to excision
Resection of the tumor (may include entire bone) and wide margins of normal tissue primarily for malignant or aggressive benign tumors
Simple and intermediate repairs

EXCLUDES *Complex repair*
Significant exploration of vessels, neuroplasty, reconstruction, or complex bone repair

Do not report radical excision of soft tissue codes when adjacent soft tissue is removed during the bone tumor resection (28045-28047 [28039, 28041])

28171 **Radical resection of tumor; tarsal (except talus or calcaneus)**
EXCLUDES *Talus or calcaneus resection (27647)*
A2 T 80 ▣ 24.42 24.42 FUD 090

28173 **metatarsal**
EXCLUDES *Talus or calcaneus resection (27647)*
A2 T ▣ 22.20 22.20 FUD 090

28175 **phalanx of toe**
EXCLUDES *Talus or calcaneus resection (27647)*
A2 T ▣ 14.02 14.02 FUD 090

28190-28193 Foreign Body Removal: Foot

28190 **Removal of foreign body, foot; subcutaneous**
P3 T 50 ▣ 3.84 7.33 FUD 010

28192 **deep**
A2 T 50 ▣ PQ 9.02 13.51 FUD 090

28193 **complicated**
A2 T 50 ▣ PQ 10.63 15.28 FUD 090

28200-28360 Repair/Reconstruction of Foot/Toe

INCLUDES Closed, open and percutaneous treatment of fractures and dislocations

28200 **Repair, tendon, flexor, foot; primary or secondary, without free graft, each tendon**
A2 T ▣ 9.12 13.92 FUD 090

28202 secondary with free graft, each tendon (includes obtaining graft)
A2 T 80 — Facility RVU 12.22 — Non-Facility RVU 17.10 — FUD 090

28208 Repair, tendon, extensor, foot; primary or secondary, each tendon
A2 T — Facility RVU 8.92 — Non-Facility RVU 13.56 — FUD 090

28210 secondary with free graft, each tendon (includes obtaining graft)
A2 T 80 — Facility RVU 11.57 — Non-Facility RVU 16.18 — FUD 090

28220 Tenolysis, flexor, foot; single tendon
P3 T 50 — Facility RVU 8.61 — Non-Facility RVU 12.82 — FUD 090

28222 multiple tendons
A2 T 50 — Facility RVU 10.05 — Non-Facility RVU 14.58 — FUD 090

28225 Tenolysis, extensor, foot; single tendon
A2 T 50 — Facility RVU 7.40 — Non-Facility RVU 11.70 — FUD 090

28226 multiple tendons
A2 T 50 — Facility RVU 10.63 — Non-Facility RVU 16.84 — FUD 090

28230 Tenotomy, open, tendon flexor; foot, single or multiple tendon(s) (separate procedure)
P3 T 50 — Facility RVU 8.13 — Non-Facility RVU 12.50 — FUD 090

28232 toe, single tendon (separate procedure)
P3 T — Facility RVU 6.99 — Non-Facility RVU 11.13 — FUD 090

28234 Tenotomy, open, extensor, foot or toe, each tendon
EXCLUDES *Tendon transfer (27690-27691)*
A2 T — Facility RVU 7.54 — Non-Facility RVU 11.68 — FUD 090

28238 Reconstruction (advancement), posterior tibial tendon with excision of accessory tarsal navicular bone (eg, Kidner type procedure)
EXCLUDES *Extensor hallucis longus transfer with big toe fusion (28760)*
Jones procedure (28760)
Subcutaneous tenotomy (28010-28011)
Transfer or transplant of tendon with muscle redirection or rerouting (27690-27692)
A2 T 80 50 — Facility RVU 14.02 — Non-Facility RVU 19.33 — FUD 090

28240 Tenotomy, lengthening, or release, abductor hallucis muscle
A2 T 50 — Facility RVU 8.30 — Non-Facility RVU 12.60 — FUD 090

28250 Division of plantar fascia and muscle (eg, Steindler stripping) (separate procedure)
A2 T 80 50 — Facility RVU 11.57 — Non-Facility RVU 16.59 — FUD 090

28260 Capsulotomy, midfoot; medial release only (separate procedure)
A2 T 80 50 — Facility RVU 14.62 — Non-Facility RVU 19.62 — FUD 090

28261 with tendon lengthening
A2 T 80 50 — Facility RVU 21.95 — Non-Facility RVU 27.71 — FUD 090

28262 extensive, including posterior talotibial capsulotomy and tendon(s) lengthening (eg, resistant clubfoot deformity)
A2 T 80 50 — Facility RVU 33.49 — Non-Facility RVU 41.70 — FUD 090

28264 Capsulotomy, midtarsal (eg, Heyman type procedure)
A2 T 80 50 — Facility RVU 20.68 — Non-Facility RVU 27.53 — FUD 090

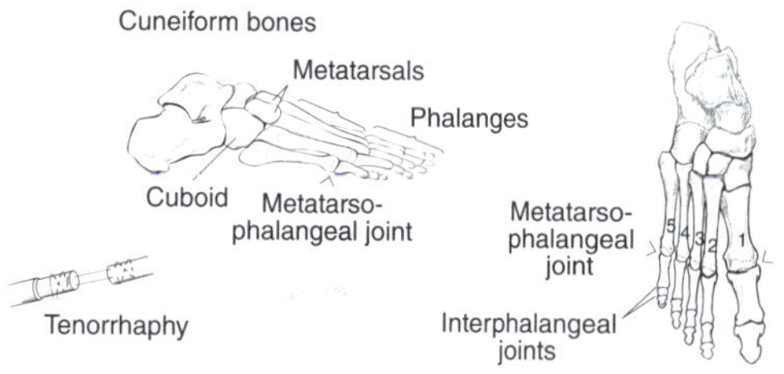

28270 Capsulotomy; metatarsophalangeal joint, with or without tenorrhaphy, each joint (separate procedure)
A2 T 50 — Facility RVU 9.57 — Non-Facility RVU 14.08 — FUD 090

28272 interphalangeal joint, each joint (separate procedure)
P3 T 50 — Facility RVU 7.28 — Non-Facility RVU 11.28 — FUD 090

28280 Syndactylization, toes (eg, webbing or Kelikian type procedure)
A2 T 80 50 — Facility RVU 10.10 — Non-Facility RVU 14.94 — FUD 090

28285 Correction, hammertoe (eg, interphalangeal fusion, partial or total phalangectomy)
A2 T 50 — Facility RVU 10.79 — Non-Facility RVU 15.28 — FUD 090

28286 Correction, cock-up fifth toe, with plastic skin closure (eg, Ruiz-Mora type procedure)
A2 T 50 — Facility RVU 8.61 — Non-Facility RVU 13.00 — FUD 090

28288 Ostectomy, partial, exostectomy or condylectomy, metatarsal head, each metatarsal head
A2 T — Facility RVU 12.31 — Non-Facility RVU 17.33 — FUD 090

28289 Hallux rigidus correction with cheilectomy, debridement and capsular release of the first metatarsophalangeal joint
A2 T 80 50 — Facility RVU 15.73 — Non-Facility RVU 21.07 — FUD 090

Correction of hallux valgus bunion by resection of joint

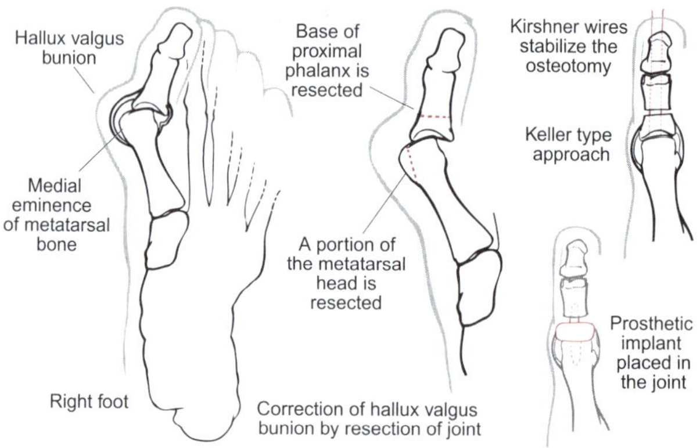

28290 Correction, hallux valgus (bunion), with or without sesamoidectomy; simple exostectomy (eg, Silver type procedure)
A2 T 50 — Facility RVU 11.29 — Non-Facility RVU 16.78 — FUD 090

28292 Keller, McBride, or Mayo type procedure
A2 T 80 50 — Facility RVU 17.25 — Non-Facility RVU 22.63 — FUD 090

28293 resection of joint with implant
A2 T 80 50 PQ — Facility RVU 20.38 — Non-Facility RVU 29.95 — FUD 090

28294 with tendon transplants (eg, Joplin type procedure)
A2 T 80 50 — Facility RVU 15.34 — Non-Facility RVU 21.50 — FUD 090

28296 with metatarsal osteotomy (eg, Mitchell, Chevron, or concentric type procedures)
A2 T 80 50 — Facility RVU 14.93 — Non-Facility RVU 20.43 — FUD 090

28297 Lapidus-type procedure
A2 T 80 50 — Facility RVU 16.78 — Non-Facility RVU 23.36 — FUD 090

28298 by phalanx osteotomy
INCLUDES Akin procedure
A2 T 80 50 — Facility RVU 14.50 — Non-Facility RVU 20.69 — FUD 090

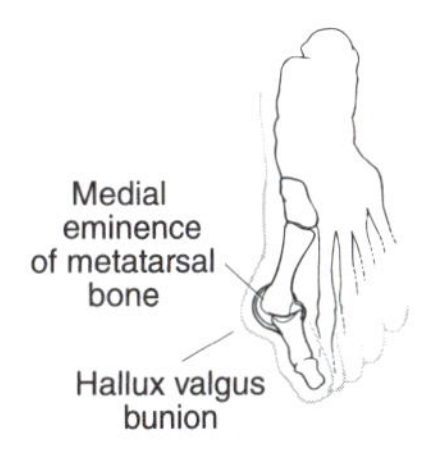

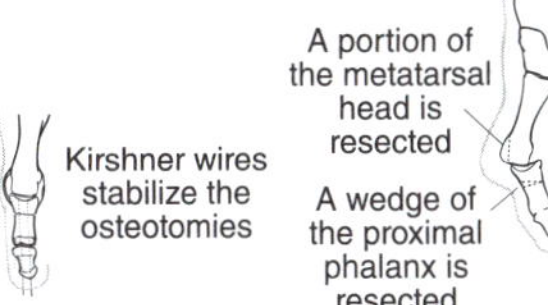

28299 by double osteotomy
A2 T 80 50 19.36 25.59 FUD 090

28300 calcaneus (eg, Dwyer or Chambers type procedure), with or without internal fixation
A2 T 80 50 18.79 18.79 FUD 090

28302 talus
A2 T 80 50 20.37 20.37 FUD 090

28304 Osteotomy, tarsal bones, other than calcaneus or talus;
A2 T 80 50 17.12 23.27 FUD 090

28305 with autograft (includes obtaining graft) (eg, Fowler type)
A2 T 80 50 18.29 18.29 FUD 090

28306 Osteotomy, with or without lengthening, shortening or angular correction, metatarsal; first metatarsal
A2 T 80 50 11.62 17.63 FUD 090

28307 first metatarsal with autograft (other than first toe)
A2 T 80 50 13.33 20.02 FUD 090

28308 other than first metatarsal, each
A2 T 80 50 10.75 16.11 FUD 090

28309 multiple (eg, Swanson type cavus foot procedure)
A2 T 80 50 25.68 25.68 FUD 090

28310 Osteotomy, shortening, angular or rotational correction; proximal phalanx, first toe (separate procedure)
A2 T 50 10.18 15.52 FUD 090

28312 other phalanges, any toe
A2 T 9.18 14.65 FUD 090

28313 Reconstruction, angular deformity of toe, soft tissue procedures only (eg, overlapping second toe, fifth toe, curly toes)
A2 T 10.35 15.25 FUD 090

28315 Sesamoidectomy, first toe (separate procedure)
A2 T 50 9.29 13.75 FUD 090

28320 Repair, nonunion or malunion; tarsal bones
A2 T 80 50 17.75 17.75 FUD 090

28322 metatarsal, with or without bone graft (includes obtaining graft)
A2 T 80 16.66 22.73 FUD 090

28340 Reconstruction, toe, macrodactyly; soft tissue resection
A2 T 11.87 16.61 FUD 090

28341 requiring bone resection
A2 T 14.15 19.29 FUD 090

28344 Reconstruction, toe(s); polydactyly
A2 T 50 8.22 12.42 FUD 090

28345 syndactyly, with or without skin graft(s), each web
A2 T 80 10.46 14.98 FUD 090

28360 Reconstruction, cleft foot
T 80 50 25.48 25.48 FUD 090

28400-28675 Treatment of Fracture/Dislocation of Foot/Toe

28400 Closed treatment of calcaneal fracture; without manipulation
A2 T 50 6.49 7.09 FUD 090

28405 with manipulation
INCLUDES Bohler reduction
A2 T 80 50 10.07 11.07 FUD 090

28406 Percutaneous skeletal fixation of calcaneal fracture, with manipulation
A2 T 80 50 PQ 15.10 15.10 FUD 090

28415 Open treatment of calcaneal fracture, includes internal fixation, when performed;
A2 T 80 50 PQ 31.78 31.78 FUD 090

28420 with primary iliac or other autogenous bone graft (includes obtaining graft)
A2 T 80 50 PQ 35.80 35.80 FUD 090

28430 Closed treatment of talus fracture; without manipulation
P2 T 50 5.96 6.70 FUD 090

28435 with manipulation
A2 T 80 50 8.32 9.29 FUD 090

28436 Percutaneous skeletal fixation of talus fracture, with manipulation
A2 T 50 PQ 12.77 12.77 FUD 090

28445 Open treatment of talus fracture, includes internal fixation, when performed
A2 T 80 50 PQ 30.39 30.39 FUD 090

28446 Open osteochondral autograft, talus (includes obtaining graft[s])
EXCLUDES *Arthroscopically aided osteochondral talus graft (29892)*
Open osteochondral allograft or repairs with industrial grafts (28899)
Do not report with (27705-27707)
G2 T 80 50 34.98 34.98 FUD 090

28450 Treatment of tarsal bone fracture (except talus and calcaneus); without manipulation, each
P2 T 5.49 6.16 FUD 090

28455 with manipulation, each
P2 T 80 7.65 8.51 FUD 090

28456 Percutaneous skeletal fixation of tarsal bone fracture (except talus and calcaneus), with manipulation, each
A2 T PQ 9.04 9.04 FUD 090

28465 Open treatment of tarsal bone fracture (except talus and calcaneus), includes internal fixation, when performed, each
A2 T PQ 17.91 17.91 FUD 090

28470 Closed treatment of metatarsal fracture; without manipulation, each
P2 T 5.87 6.28 FUD 090

28475 with manipulation, each
P2 T 6.48 7.29 FUD 090

28476 Percutaneous skeletal fixation of metatarsal fracture, with manipulation, each
A2 T 80 PQ 9.96 9.96 FUD 090

28485 Open treatment of metatarsal fracture, includes internal fixation, when performed, each
A2 T PQ 15.02 15.02 FUD 090

28490 Closed treatment of fracture great toe, phalanx or phalanges; without manipulation
P2 T 50 3.55 4.13 FUD 090

28495 with manipulation
P2 T 50 4.25 5.04 FUD 090

28496 Percutaneous skeletal fixation of fracture great toe, phalanx or phalanges, with manipulation
A2 T 50 ▸ 6.64 12.45 FUD 090

28505 Open treatment of fracture, great toe, phalanx or phalanges, includes internal fixation, when performed
A2 T 50 PQ 14.22 18.96 FUD 090

28510 Closed treatment of fracture, phalanx or phalanges, other than great toe; without manipulation, each
P2 T 3.41 3.51 FUD 090

28515 with manipulation, each
P2 T 4.04 4.57 FUD 090

28525 Open treatment of fracture, phalanx or phalanges, other than great toe, includes internal fixation, when performed, each
A2 T 80 PQ 11.49 16.33 FUD 090

28530 Closed treatment of sesamoid fracture
P2 T 80 50 2.90 3.26 FUD 090

28531 Open treatment of sesamoid fracture, with or without internal fixation
A2 T 50 PQ 5.51 10.08 FUD 090

28540 Closed treatment of tarsal bone dislocation, other than talotarsal; without anesthesia
P2 T 80 50 5.25 5.82 FUD 090

28545 requiring anesthesia
A2 T 80 50 7.43 8.37 FUD 090

28546 Percutaneous skeletal fixation of tarsal bone dislocation, other than talotarsal, with manipulation
A2 T 80 50 9.63 16.39 FUD 090

28555 Open treatment of tarsal bone dislocation, includes internal fixation, when performed
A2 T 80 50 PQ 18.92 24.82 FUD 090

28570 Closed treatment of talotarsal joint dislocation; without anesthesia
P2 T 80 50 5.19 6.15 FUD 090

28575 requiring anesthesia
A2 T 80 50 9.35 10.33 FUD 090

28576 Percutaneous skeletal fixation of talotarsal joint dislocation, with manipulation
A2 T 80 50 11.24 11.24 FUD 090

28585 Open treatment of talotarsal joint dislocation, includes internal fixation, when performed
A2 T 80 50 PQ 19.58 24.78 FUD 090

28600 Closed treatment of tarsometatarsal joint dislocation; without anesthesia
P2 T 80 5.39 6.26 FUD 090

28605 requiring anesthesia
A2 T 80 8.35 9.26 FUD 090

28606 Percutaneous skeletal fixation of tarsometatarsal joint dislocation, with manipulation
A2 T 11.40 11.40 FUD 090

28615 Open treatment of tarsometatarsal joint dislocation, includes internal fixation, when performed
A2 T 80 PQ 22.60 22.60 FUD 090

28630 Closed treatment of metatarsophalangeal joint dislocation; without anesthesia
P3 T 80 3.14 4.48 FUD 010

28635 requiring anesthesia
A2 T 80 3.79 5.00 FUD 010

28636 Percutaneous skeletal fixation of metatarsophalangeal joint dislocation, with manipulation
A2 T 4.97 7.41 FUD 010

28645 Open treatment of metatarsophalangeal joint dislocation, includes internal fixation, when performed
A2 T PQ 13.87 18.78 FUD 090

28660 Closed treatment of interphalangeal joint dislocation; without anesthesia
P2 T 2.55 3.31 FUD 010

28665 requiring anesthesia
A2 S 80 3.76 4.39 FUD 010

28666 Percutaneous skeletal fixation of interphalangeal joint dislocation, with manipulation
A2 T 5.43 5.43 FUD 010

28675 Open treatment of interphalangeal joint dislocation, includes internal fixation, when performed
A2 T PQ 11.51 16.23 FUD 090

28705-28760 Arthrodesis of Foot/Toe

28705 Arthrodesis; pantalar
A2 T 80 50 PQ 36.44 36.44 FUD 090

28715 triple
A2 T 80 50 PQ 26.82 26.82 FUD 090

28725 subtalar
INCLUDES Dunn arthrodesis
Grice arthrosis
A2 T 80 50 PQ 22.15 22.15 FUD 090

28730 Arthrodesis, midtarsal or tarsometatarsal, multiple or transverse;
INCLUDES Lambrinudi arthrodesis
A2 T 80 50 PQ 21.08 21.08 FUD 090

28735 with osteotomy (eg, flatfoot correction)
A2 T 80 50 PQ 22.45 22.45 FUD 090

28737 Arthrodesis, with tendon lengthening and advancement, midtarsal, tarsal navicular-cuneiform (eg, Miller type procedure)
A2 T 80 50 PQ 19.80 19.80 FUD 090

28740 Arthrodesis, midtarsal or tarsometatarsal, single joint
A2 T 80 18.01 24.43 FUD 090

28750 Arthrodesis, great toe; metatarsophalangeal joint
A2 T 80 50 17.05 23.41 FUD 090

28755 interphalangeal joint
A2 T 50 9.48 14.59 FUD 090

28760 Arthrodesis, with extensor hallucis longus transfer to first metatarsal neck, great toe, interphalangeal joint (eg, Jones type procedure)
EXCLUDES *Hammer toe repair or interphalangeal fusion (28285)*
A2 T 80 50 16.45 22.43 FUD 090

28800-28825 Amputation Foot/Toe

28800 Amputation, foot; midtarsal (eg, Chopart type procedure)
C 80 50 15.69 15.69 FUD 090

28805 transmetatarsal
T 80 50 21.45 21.45 FUD 090

28810 Amputation, metatarsal, with toe, single
EXCLUDES *Removal of tuft of distal phalanx (11752)*
A2 T 80 12.55 12.55 FUD 090

28820 Amputation, toe; metatarsophalangeal joint
EXCLUDES *Removal of tuft of distal phalanx (11752)*
A2 T 11.47 16.33 FUD 090

28825 interphalangeal joint
EXCLUDES *Removal of tuft of distal phalanx (11752)*
A2 T 10.74 15.57 FUD 090

28890-28899 Other/Unlisted Procedures Foot/Toe

28890 **Extracorporeal shock wave, high energy, performed by a physician or other qualified health care professional, requiring anesthesia other than local, including ultrasound guidance, involving the plantar fascia**

EXCLUDES *Extracorporeal shock wave therapy of integumentary system not otherwise specified (0299T-0300T)*
Extracorporeal shock wave therapy of musculoskeletal system not otherwise specified (0019T, 0101T, 0102T)

Do not report with treatment of same area (0299T-0300T)

P3 T 50 6.47 9.28 FUD 090

28899 **Unlisted procedure, foot or toes**
T 80 0.00 0.00 FUD YYY

29000-29086 Casting: Arm/Shoulder/Torso

CMS 100-2,15,100 Surgical Dressings, Splints, Casts, and Devices for Reductions of Fractures/Dislocations
CMS 100-4,4,240 Inpatient Part B Hospital Services Paid Under OPPS

INCLUDES Application of cast or strapping when provided as:
An initial service to stabilize the fracture or injury without restorative treatment
A replacement procedure
Removal of cast

EXCLUDES *Cast or splint material*
Evaluation and management services provided as part of the initial service when restorative treatment is not provided
Orthotic supervision and training (97760-97762)

Do not report with restorative procedures that include application and removal of the initial cast

29000 **Application of halo type body cast (see 20661-20663 for insertion)**
P2 S 80 4.78 8.50 FUD 000

29010 **Application of Risser jacket, localizer, body; only**
P2 S 80 4.30 6.94 FUD 000

29015 **including head**
P2 S 80 5.00 7.90 FUD 000

~~29020~~ **~~Application of turnbuckle jacket, body; only~~**

~~29025~~ **~~including head~~**

29035 **Application of body cast, shoulder to hips;**
P2 S 80 3.88 6.59 FUD 000

29040 **including head, Minerva type**
P2 S 80 5.33 9.90 FUD 000

29044 **including 1 thigh**
P2 S 80 4.57 7.51 FUD 000

29046 **including both thighs**
P2 S 80 4.99 7.84 FUD 000

29049 **Application, cast; figure-of-eight**
P2 S 80 2.00 2.80 FUD 000

29055 **shoulder spica**
P2 S 80 3.94 6.29 FUD 000

29058 **plaster Velpeau**
P2 S 80 2.68 3.48 FUD 000

29065 **shoulder to hand (long arm)**
P3 S 50 1.95 2.73 FUD 000

29075 **elbow to finger (short arm)**
P3 S 50 1.78 2.46 FUD 000

29085 **hand and lower forearm (gauntlet)**
P2 S 50 1.92 2.69 FUD 000

29086 **finger (eg, contracture)**
P3 S 50 1.46 2.23 FUD 000

29105-29280 Splinting and Strapping: Torso/Upper Extremities

CMS 100-2,15,100 Surgical Dressings, Splints, Casts, and Devices for Reductions of Fractures/Dislocations
CMS 100-4,4,240 Inpatient Part B Hospital Services Paid Under OPPS

INCLUDES Application of splint or strapping when provided as:
An initial service to stabilize the fracture or dislocation
A replacement procedure

EXCLUDES *Evaluation and management services provided as part of the initial service when restorative treatment is not provided*
Orthotic supervision and training (97760-97762)
Splinting and strapping material

Do not report with restorative procedures that included application and removal of the initial splint or strap

29105 **Application of long arm splint (shoulder to hand)**
P3 S 50 1.70 2.49 FUD 000

29125 **Application of short arm splint (forearm to hand); static**
P3 S 50 1.13 1.83 FUD 000

29126 **dynamic**
P3 S 50 1.39 2.17 FUD 000

29130 **Application of finger splint; static**
P3 S 50 0.82 1.17 FUD 000

29131 **dynamic**
P3 S 50 0.95 1.46 FUD 000

29200 **Strapping; thorax**
EXCLUDES *Strapping of low back (29799)*
P3 S 1.13 1.49 FUD 000

29240 **shoulder (eg, Velpeau)**
P3 S 50 1.24 1.61 FUD 000

29260 **elbow or wrist**
P3 S 50 1.05 1.44 FUD 000

29280 **hand or finger**
P2 S 50 1.02 1.42 FUD 000

29305-29450 Casting: Legs

CMS 100-2,15,100 Surgical Dressings, Splints, Casts, and Devices for Reductions of Fractures/Dislocations
CMS 100-4,4,240 Inpatient Part B Hospital Services Paid Under OPPS

INCLUDES Application of cast when provided as:
An initial service to stabilize the fracture or injury without restorative treatment
A replacement procedure
Removal of cast

EXCLUDES *Cast or splint materials*
Evaluation and management services provided as part of the initial service when restorative treatment is not provided
Orthotic supervision and training (97760-97762)

Do not report with restorative procedures that include application and removal of the initial cast

29305 **Application of hip spica cast; 1 leg**
EXCLUDES *Hip spica cast thighs only (29046)*
P2 S 80 4.53 6.99 FUD 000

29325 **1 and one-half spica or both legs**
EXCLUDES *Hip spica cast thighs only (29046)*
P2 S 80 5.09 7.74 FUD 000

29345 **Application of long leg cast (thigh to toes);**
P2 S 50 2.90 3.88 FUD 000

29355 **walker or ambulatory type**
P2 S 50 3.08 4.04 FUD 000

29358 **Application of long leg cast brace**
P2 S 50 2.98 4.56 FUD 000

29365 **Application of cylinder cast (thigh to ankle)**
P3 S 50 2.52 3.50 FUD 000

29405 **Application of short leg cast (below knee to toes);**
P3 S 50 1.71 2.32 FUD 000

29425 **walking or ambulatory type**
P3 S 50 1.62 2.23 FUD 000

29435 **Application of patellar tendon bearing (PTB) cast**
P3 S 50 ◼ 2.37 3.28 FUD 000

29440 **Adding walker to previously applied cast**
P3 S 50 ◼ 0.87 1.28 FUD 000

29445 **Application of rigid total contact leg cast**
P3 S 50 ◼ 3.02 3.87 FUD 000

29450 **Application of clubfoot cast with molding or manipulation, long or short leg**
P2 S 50 ◼ 3.21 4.05 FUD 000

29505-29584 Splinting and Strapping Ankle/Foot/Leg/Toes

CMS 100-2,15,100 Surgical Dressings, Splints, Casts, and Devices for Reductions of Fractures/Dislocations
CMS 100-4,4,240 Inpatient Part B Hospital Services Paid Under OPPS

INCLUDES Application of splinting and strapping when provided as:
An initial service to stabilize the fracture or injury without restorative treatment
A replacement procedure

EXCLUDES *Evaluation and management services provided as part of the initial service when restorative treatment is not provided*
Orthotic supervision and training (97760-97762)

Do not report with restorative procedures that include application and removal of the initial cast

29505 **Application of long leg splint (thigh to ankle or toes)**
P2 S 50 ◼ 1.43 2.36 FUD 000

29515 **Application of short leg splint (calf to foot)**
P3 S 50 ◼ 1.43 2.04 FUD 000

29520 **Strapping; hip**
P3 S 80 50 ◼ 0.99 1.35 FUD 000

29530 **knee**
P3 S 50 ◼ 1.05 1.43 FUD 000

29540 **ankle and/or foot**
Do not report with (29581, 29582)
P3 S 50 ◼ 0.74 1.05 FUD 000

29550 **toes**
P3 S 50 ◼ 0.55 0.88 FUD 000

29580 **Unna boot**
Do not report with (29581-29582)
P3 S 50 ◼ PQ 1.02 1.49 FUD 000

29581 **Application of multi-layer compression system; leg (below knee), including ankle and foot**
Do not report with (29540, 29580, 29582, 36475-36476, 36478-36479)
P3 S 80 50 PQ 0.36 1.74 FUD 000

29582 **thigh and leg, including ankle and foot, when performed**
Do not report with (29540, 29580-29581, 36475-36476, 36478-36479)
P3 S 80 50 0.45 1.98 FUD 000

29583 **upper arm and forearm**
Do not report with (29584)
P2 S 80 50 0.32 1.23 FUD 000

29584 **upper arm, forearm, hand, and fingers**
Do not report with (29583)
P2 S 80 50 0.45 1.98 FUD 000

29700-29799 Casting Services Other Than Application

INCLUDES Casts applied by treating individual

Do not report removal of casts applied by treating individual

29700 **Removal or bivalving; gauntlet, boot or body cast**
P3 S ◼ 0.97 1.76 FUD 000

29705 **full arm or full leg cast**
P3 S 50 ◼ 1.34 1.89 FUD 000

29710 **shoulder or hip spica, Minerva, or Risser jacket, etc.**
P3 S 80 50 ◼ 2.33 3.30 FUD 000

~~29715~~ ~~**turnbuckle jacket**~~

29720 **Repair of spica, body cast or jacket**
P2 S ◼ 1.25 2.39 FUD 000

29730 **Windowing of cast**
P3 S ◼ 1.29 1.84 FUD 000

29740 **Wedging of cast (except clubfoot casts)**
P3 S ◼ 1.97 2.78 FUD 000

29750 **Wedging of clubfoot cast**
P3 S 80 50 ◼ 1.90 2.45 FUD 000

29799 **Unlisted procedure, casting or strapping**
S 80 0.00 0.00 FUD YYY

29800-29999 [29914, 29915, 29916] Arthroscopic Procedures

INCLUDES Diagnostic arthroscopy with surgical arthroscopy

Code also modifier 51 if arthroscopy is performed with arthrotomy

29800 **Arthroscopy, temporomandibular joint, diagnostic, with or without synovial biopsy (separate procedure)**
A2 T 80 50 ◼ 14.86 14.86 FUD 090

29804 **Arthroscopy, temporomandibular joint, surgical**
EXCLUDES *Open surgery (21010)*
A2 T 80 50 ◼ 18.73 18.73 FUD 090

29805 **Arthroscopy, shoulder, diagnostic, with or without synovial biopsy (separate procedure)**
EXCLUDES *Open surgery (23065-23066, 23100-23101)*
A2 T 50 ◼ 13.44 13.44 FUD 090

29806 **Arthroscopy, shoulder, surgical; capsulorrhaphy**
EXCLUDES *Open surgery (23450-23466)*
Thermal capsulorrhaphy (29999)
A2 T 50 ◼ 30.33 30.33 FUD 090

29807 **repair of SLAP lesion**
A2 T 50 ◼ 29.55 29.55 FUD 090

29819 **with removal of loose body or foreign body**
EXCLUDES *Open surgery (23040-23044, 23107)*
A2 T 50 ◼ 16.71 16.71 FUD 090

29820 **synovectomy, partial**
EXCLUDES *Open surgery (23105)*
A2 T 80 50 ◼ 15.42 15.42 FUD 090

29821 **synovectomy, complete**
EXCLUDES *Open surgery (23105)*
A2 T 80 50 ◼ 16.86 16.86 FUD 090

29822 **debridement, limited**
EXCLUDES *Open surgery (see specific shoulder section)*
A2 T 80 50 ◼ 16.40 16.40 FUD 090

29823 **debridement, extensive**
EXCLUDES *Open surgery (see specific shoulder section)*
A2 T 80 50 ◼ 17.90 17.90 FUD 090

29824 **distal claviculectomy including distal articular surface (Mumford procedure)**
INCLUDES Mumford procedure
EXCLUDES *Open surgery (23120)*
A2 T 80 50 ◼ 19.33 19.33 FUD 090

29825 **with lysis and resection of adhesions, with or without manipulation**
EXCLUDES *Open surgery (see specific shoulder section)*
A2 T 80 50 ◼ 16.72 16.72 FUD 090

\+ 29826 **decompression of subacromial space with partial acromioplasty, with coracoacromial ligament (ie, arch) release, when performed (List separately in addition to code for primary procedure)**
EXCLUDES *Open surgery (23130, 23415)*
Code also modifier 51 when performed arthroscopically during the same session ([29824], [29826])
Code first (29806-29825, 29827-29828)
N1 N 80 50 ◼ 5.07 5.07 FUD ZZZ

29827 **with rotator cuff repair**
EXCLUDES *Distal clavicle excision (29824)*
Open surgery or mini open repair (23412)
Subacromial decompression (29826)
A2 T 80 50 ◼ 30.74 30.74 FUD 090

29828 **biceps tenodesis**
EXCLUDES *Tenodesis of long tendon of biceps (23430)*
Do not report with (29805, 29820, 29822)
G2 T 80 50 — 26.43 — 26.43 FUD 090

29830 **Arthroscopy, elbow, diagnostic, with or without synovial biopsy (separate procedure)**
A2 T 50 — 12.97 — 12.97 FUD 090

29834 **Arthroscopy, elbow, surgical; with removal of loose body or foreign body**
A2 T 80 50 — 13.99 — 13.99 FUD 090

29835 **synovectomy, partial**
A2 T 80 50 — 14.44 — 14.44 FUD 090

29836 **synovectomy, complete**
A2 T 80 50 — 16.47 — 16.47 FUD 090

29837 **debridement, limited**
A2 T 80 50 — 15.08 — 15.08 FUD 090

29838 **debridement, extensive**
A2 T 80 50 — 16.78 — 16.78 FUD 090

29840 **Arthroscopy, wrist, diagnostic, with or without synovial biopsy (separate procedure)**
A2 T 80 50 — 12.87 — 12.87 FUD 090

29843 **Arthroscopy, wrist, surgical; for infection, lavage and drainage**
A2 T 80 50 — 13.77 — 13.77 FUD 090

29844 **synovectomy, partial**
A2 T 80 50 — 14.18 — 14.18 FUD 090

29845 **synovectomy, complete**
A2 T 80 50 — 16.47 — 16.47 FUD 090

29846 **excision and/or repair of triangular fibrocartilage and/or joint debridement**
A2 T 80 50 — 14.82 — 14.82 FUD 090

29847 **internal fixation for fracture or instability**
A2 T 80 50 — 15.52 — 15.52 FUD 090

29848 **Endoscopy, wrist, surgical, with release of transverse carpal ligament**
EXCLUDES *Open surgery (64721)*
A2 T 50 — 14.50 — 14.50 FUD 090

29850 **Arthroscopically aided treatment of intercondylar spine(s) and/or tuberosity fracture(s) of the knee, with or without manipulation; without internal or external fixation (includes arthroscopy)**
A2 T 80 50 — 17.77 — 17.77 FUD 090

29851 **with internal or external fixation (includes arthroscopy)**
EXCLUDES *Bone graft (20900, 20902)*
A2 T 80 50 — 26.61 — 26.61 FUD 090

29855 **Arthroscopically aided treatment of tibial fracture, proximal (plateau); unicondylar, includes internal fixation, when performed (includes arthroscopy)**
A2 T 80 50 — 22.48 — 22.48 FUD 090

29856 **bicondylar, includes internal fixation, when performed (includes arthroscopy)**
EXCLUDES *Bone graft (20900, 20902)*
A2 T 80 50 — 28.47 — 28.47 FUD 090

29860 **Arthroscopy, hip, diagnostic with or without synovial biopsy (separate procedure)**
A2 T 80 50 — 19.02 — 19.02 FUD 090

29861 **Arthroscopy, hip, surgical; with removal of loose body or foreign body**
A2 T 80 50 — 20.73 — 20.73 FUD 090

29862 **with debridement/shaving of articular cartilage (chondroplasty), abrasion arthroplasty, and/or resection of labrum**
A2 T 80 50 — 23.33 — 23.33 FUD 090

29863 **with synovectomy**
A2 T 80 50 — 23.40 — 23.40 FUD 090

\# **29914** **with femoroplasty (ie, treatment of cam lesion)**
Do not report with (29862-29863)
G2 T 80 50 — 28.91 — 28.91 FUD 090

\# **29915** **with acetabuloplasty (ie, treatment of pincer lesion)**
Do not report with (29862-29863)
G2 T 80 50 — 29.50 — 29.50 FUD 090

\# **29916** **with labral repair**
EXCLUDES *Labral repair secondary to acetabuloplasty*
Do not report with (29862-29863, [29915])
G2 T 80 50 — 29.51 — 29.51 FUD 090

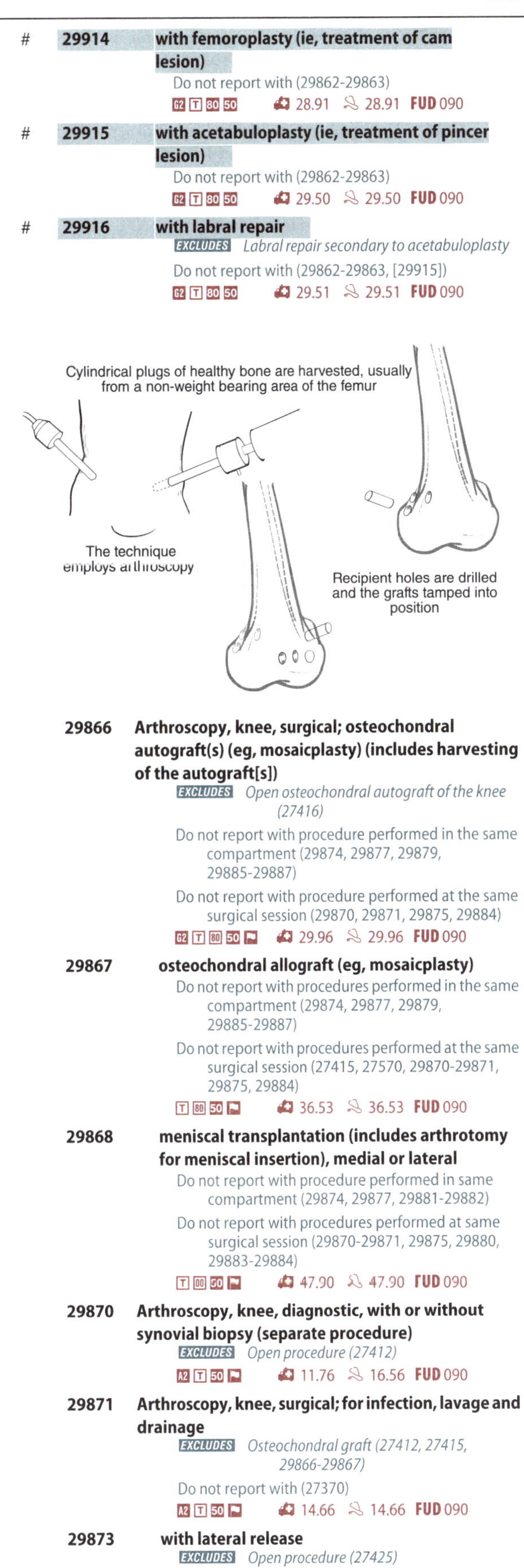

29866 **Arthroscopy, knee, surgical; osteochondral autograft(s) (eg, mosaicplasty) (includes harvesting of the autograft[s])**
EXCLUDES *Open osteochondral autograft of the knee (27416)*
Do not report with procedure performed in the same compartment (29874, 29877, 29879, 29885-29887)
Do not report with procedure performed at the same surgical session (29870, 29871, 29875, 29884)
G2 T 80 50 — 29.96 — 29.96 FUD 090

29867 **osteochondral allograft (eg, mosaicplasty)**
Do not report with procedures performed in the same compartment (29874, 29877, 29879, 29885-29887)
Do not report with procedures performed at the same surgical session (27415, 27570, 29870-29871, 29875, 29884)
T 80 50 — 36.53 — 36.53 FUD 090

29868 **meniscal transplantation (includes arthrotomy for meniscal insertion), medial or lateral**
Do not report with procedure performed in same compartment (29874, 29877, 29881-29882)
Do not report with procedures performed at same surgical session (29870-29871, 29875, 29880, 29883-29884)
T 80 50 — 47.90 — 47.90 FUD 090

29870 **Arthroscopy, knee, diagnostic, with or without synovial biopsy (separate procedure)**
EXCLUDES *Open procedure (27412)*
A2 T 50 — 11.76 — 16.56 FUD 090

29871 **Arthroscopy, knee, surgical; for infection, lavage and drainage**
EXCLUDES *Osteochondral graft (27412, 27415, 29866-29867)*
Do not report with (27370)
A2 T 50 — 14.66 — 14.66 FUD 090

29873 **with lateral release**
EXCLUDES *Open procedure (27425)*
A2 T 50 — 14.94 — 14.94 FUD 090

Musculoskeletal System
29828 — 29873

29874 for removal of loose body or foreign body (eg, osteochondritis dissecans fragmentation, chondral fragmentation)
A2 T 80 50 15.35 15.35 FUD 090

29875 synovectomy, limited (eg, plica or shelf resection) (separate procedure)
A2 T 80 50 14.13 14.13 FUD 090

29876 synovectomy, major, 2 or more compartments (eg, medial or lateral)
A2 T 50 18.75 18.75 FUD 090

29877 debridement/shaving of articular cartilage (chondroplasty)
Do not report when arthroscopic meniscectomy is also performed (29880-29881)
A2 T 80 50 17.79 17.79 FUD 090

29879 abrasion arthroplasty (includes chondroplasty where necessary) or multiple drilling or microfracture
A2 T 80 50 18.95 18.95 FUD 090

29880 with meniscectomy (medial AND lateral, including any meniscal shaving) including debridement/shaving of articular cartilage (chondroplasty), same or separate compartment(s), when performed
A2 T 80 50 16.09 16.09 FUD 090

29881 with meniscectomy (medial OR lateral, including any meniscal shaving) including debridement/shaving of articular cartilage (chondroplasty), same or separate compartment(s), when performed
A2 T 80 50 15.47 15.47 FUD 090

29882 with meniscus repair (medial OR lateral)
EXCLUDES *Meniscus transplant (29868)*
A2 T 50 20.00 20.00 FUD 090

29883 with meniscus repair (medial AND lateral)
EXCLUDES *Meniscus transplant (29868)*
A2 T 80 50 24.09 24.09 FUD 090

29884 with lysis of adhesions, with or without manipulation (separate procedure)
A2 T 80 50 17.71 17.71 FUD 090

29885 drilling for osteochondritis dissecans with bone grafting, with or without internal fixation (including debridement of base of lesion)
A2 T 80 50 21.46 21.46 FUD 090

29886 drilling for intact osteochondritis dissecans lesion
A2 T 50 18.14 18.14 FUD 090

29887 drilling for intact osteochondritis dissecans lesion with internal fixation
A2 T 80 50 21.37 21.37 FUD 090

29888 Arthroscopically aided anterior cruciate ligament repair/augmentation or reconstruction
Do not report with ligamentous reconstruction (27427-27429)
A2 T 80 50 28.29 28.29 FUD 090

29889 Arthroscopically aided posterior cruciate ligament repair/augmentation or reconstruction
Do not report with ligamentous reconstruction (27427-27429)
A2 T 80 50 34.93 34.93 FUD 090

29891 Arthroscopy, ankle, surgical, excision of osteochondral defect of talus and/or tibia, including drilling of the defect
A2 T 80 50 19.66 19.66 FUD 090

29892 Arthroscopically aided repair of large osteochondritis dissecans lesion, talar dome fracture, or tibial plafond fracture, with or without internal fixation (includes arthroscopy)
A2 T 80 50 17.80 17.80 FUD 090

29893 Endoscopic plantar fasciotomy
A2 T 50 12.22 17.45 FUD 090

29894 Arthroscopy, ankle (tibiotalar and fibulotalar joints), surgical; with removal of loose body or foreign body
A2 T 80 50 14.56 14.56 FUD 090

29895 synovectomy, partial
A2 T 80 50 13.60 13.60 FUD 090

29897 debridement, limited
A2 T 80 50 14.65 14.65 FUD 090

29898 debridement, extensive
A2 T 80 50 16.20 16.20 FUD 090

29899 with ankle arthrodesis
EXCLUDES *Open procedure (27870)*
A2 T 80 50 29.66 29.66 FUD 090

29900 Arthroscopy, metacarpophalangeal joint, diagnostic, includes synovial biopsy
Do not report with (29901-29902)
A2 T 80 50 13.37 13.37 FUD 090

29901 Arthroscopy, metacarpophalangeal joint, surgical; with debridement
A2 T 80 50 15.16 15.16 FUD 090

29902 with reduction of displaced ulnar collateral ligament (eg, Stenar lesion)
A2 T 80 50 17.34 17.34 FUD 090

29904 Arthroscopy, subtalar joint, surgical; with removal of loose body or foreign body
G2 T 80 50 18.18 18.18 FUD 090

29905 with synovectomy
G2 T 80 50 19.67 19.67 FUD 090

29906 with debridement
G2 T 80 50 20.71 20.71 FUD 090

29907 with subtalar arthrodesis
G2 T 80 50 25.01 25.01 FUD 090

29914 Resequenced code. See code following 29863.

29915 Resequenced code. See code following 29863.

29916 Resequenced code. See code before 29866.

29999 Unlisted procedure, arthroscopy
T 80 50 0.00 0.00 FUD YYY

30000-30115 I&D, Biopsy, Excision Procedures of the Nose

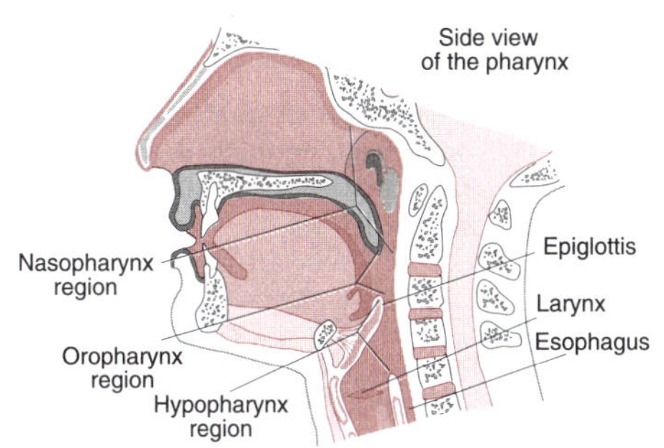

The nasopharynx is the membranous passage above the level of the soft palate; the oropharynx is the region between the soft palate and the upper edge of the epiglottis; the hypopharynx is the region of the epiglottis to the juncture of the larynx and esophagus; the three regions are collectively known as the pharynx

30000 **Drainage abscess or hematoma, nasal, internal approach**
EXCLUDES *Incision and drainage (10060, 10140)*
P2 T 80 ▣ 3.42 6.63 FUD 010

30020 **Drainage abscess or hematoma, nasal septum**
EXCLUDES *Lateral rhinotomy incision (30118, 30320)*
P2 T ▣ 3.41 6.67 FUD 010

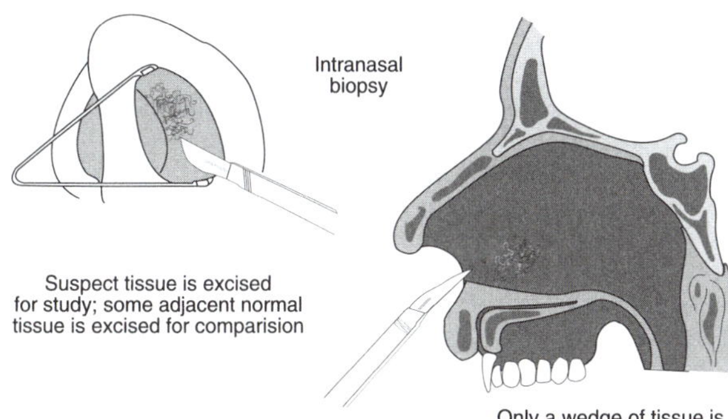

30100 **Biopsy, intranasal**
EXCLUDES *Superficial biopsy of nose (11100-11101)*
P3 T ▣ PQ 1.97 4.02 FUD 000

30110 **Excision, nasal polyp(s), simple**
P3 T 50 ▣ 3.74 6.59 FUD 010

30115 **Excision, nasal polyp(s), extensive**
A2 T 50 ▣ 12.25 12.25 FUD 090

30117-30118 Destruction Procedures Nose

CMS 100-3,140.5 Laser Procedures

30117 **Excision or destruction (eg, laser), intranasal lesion; internal approach**
A2 T ▣ 9.61 24.91 FUD 090

30118 **external approach (lateral rhinotomy)**
A2 T ▣ 21.93 21.93 FUD 090

30120-30140 Excision Procedures Nose, Turbinate

30120 **Excision or surgical planing of skin of nose for rhinophyma**
A2 T ▣ 12.44 14.70 FUD 090

30124 **Excision dermoid cyst, nose; simple, skin, subcutaneous**
A2 T ▣ 8.16 8.16 FUD 090

Middle turbinate
Superior turbinate
Inferior turbinate

30125 **complex, under bone or cartilage**
A2 T 80 ▣ 17.36 17.36 FUD 090

30130 **Excision inferior turbinate, partial or complete, any method**
EXCLUDES *Excision middle/superior turbinate(s) (30999)*
Do not report with (30801, 30802, 30930)
A2 T 50 ▣ 10.80 10.80 FUD 090

30140 **Submucous resection inferior turbinate, partial or complete, any method**
EXCLUDES *Endoscopic resection of concha bullosa of middle turbinate (31240)*
Submucous resection:
Nasal septum (30520)
Superior or middle turbinate (30999)
Do not report with (30801, 30802, 30930)
A2 T 50 ▣ 12.54 12.54 FUD 090

30150-30160 Surgical Removal: Nose

EXCLUDES *Reconstruction and/or closure (primary or delayed primary intention) (13151-13160, 14060-14302, 15120-15121, 15260-15261, 15760, 20900-20912)*

30150 **Rhinectomy; partial**
A2 T ▣ 22.02 22.02 FUD 090

30160 **total**
A2 T 80 ▣ 22.09 22.09 FUD 090

30200-30320 Turbinate Injection, Removal Foreign Substance in the Nose

30200 **Injection into turbinate(s), therapeutic**
P3 T ▣ 1.72 3.26 FUD 000

30210 **Displacement therapy (Proetz type)**
P3 T ▣ 2.85 4.28 FUD 010

30220 **Insertion, nasal septal prosthesis (button)**
A2 T ▣ 3.59 8.68 FUD 010

30300 **Removal foreign body, intranasal; office type procedure**
P2 X ▣ 3.61 6.59 FUD 010

30310 **requiring general anesthesia**
A2 T 80 ▣ 5.92 5.92 FUD 010

30320 **by lateral rhinotomy**
A2 T 80 ▣ 12.87 12.87 FUD 090

30400-30630 Reconstruction or Repair of Nose

EXCLUDES *Bone/tissue grafts (20900-20926, 21210)*

30400 **Rhinoplasty, primary; lateral and alar cartilages and/or elevation of nasal tip**
INCLUDES Carpue's operation
EXCLUDES *Reconstruction of columella (13151-13153)*
A2 T 80 ▣ 28.75 28.75 FUD 090

30410 **complete, external parts including bony pyramid, lateral and alar cartilages, and/or elevation of nasal tip**
A2 T 80 ▣ 33.75 33.75 FUD 090

30420 **including major septal repair**
A2 T ▣ 39.17 39.17 FUD 090

30430 **Rhinoplasty, secondary; minor revision (small amount of nasal tip work)**
A2 T 80 27.62 27.62 FUD 090

30435 **intermediate revision (bony work with osteotomies)**
A2 T 80 31.73 31.73 FUD 090

30450 **major revision (nasal tip work and osteotomies)**
A2 T 80 42.73 42.73 FUD 090

Cleft lip and cleft palate are described according to length of cleft and whether bilateral or unilateral

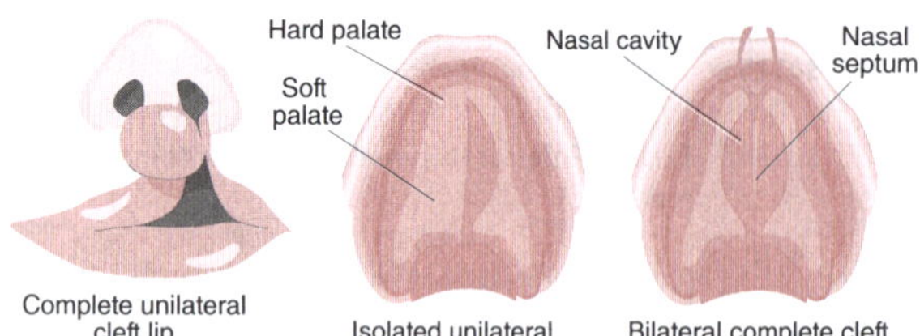

30460 **Rhinoplasty for nasal deformity secondary to congenital cleft lip and/or palate, including columellar lengthening; tip only**
A2 T 80 21.48 21.48 FUD 090

30462 **tip, septum, osteotomies**
A2 T 80 44.84 44.84 FUD 090

30465 **Repair of nasal vestibular stenosis (eg, spreader grafting, lateral nasal wall reconstruction)**
INCLUDES Bilateral procedure
Code also modifier 52 for unilateral procedure
A2 T 80 28.09 28.09 FUD 090

30520 **Septoplasty or submucous resection, with or without cartilage scoring, contouring or replacement with graft**
EXCLUDES *Turbinate resection (30140)*
A2 T 17.82 17.82 FUD 090

30540 **Repair choanal atresia; intranasal**
A2 T 80 63 19.61 19.61 FUD 090

30545 **transpalatine**
A2 T 80 63 26.20 26.20 FUD 090

30560 **Lysis intranasal synechia**
A2 T 3.94 7.70 FUD 010

30580 **Repair fistula; oromaxillary (combine with 31030 if antrotomy is included)**
A2 T 14.48 18.46 FUD 090

30600 **oronasal**
A2 T 80 12.61 16.69 FUD 090

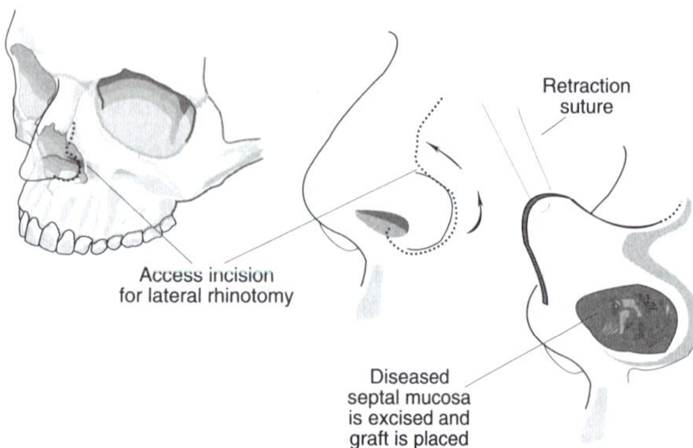

30620 **Septal or other intranasal dermatoplasty (does not include obtaining graft)**
A2 T 17.83 17.83 FUD 090

30630 **Repair nasal septal perforations**
A2 T 80 17.89 17.89 FUD 090

30801-30802 Turbinate Destruction

EXCLUDES *Cautery to stop nasal bleeding (30901-30906)*
Do not report with (30130, 30140)

30801 **Ablation, soft tissue of inferior turbinates, unilateral or bilateral, any method (eg, electrocautery, radiofrequency ablation, or tissue volume reduction); superficial**
EXCLUDES *Ablation middle/superior turbinates (30999)*
Do not report with (30802)
A2 T 3.91 6.49 FUD 010

30802 **intramural (ie, submucosal)**
A2 T 5.44 8.25 FUD 010

30901-30920 Control Nose Bleed

30901 **Control nasal hemorrhage, anterior, simple (limited cautery and/or packing) any method**
P2 T 50 1.63 2.72 FUD 000

30903 **Control nasal hemorrhage, anterior, complex (extensive cautery and/or packing) any method**
A2 T 50 2.29 5.88 FUD 000

30905 **Control nasal hemorrhage, posterior, with posterior nasal packs and/or cautery, any method; initial**
A2 T 2.91 7.31 FUD 000

30906 **subsequent**
A2 T 3.78 8.04 FUD 000

30915 **Ligation arteries; ethmoidal**
EXCLUDES *External carotid artery (37600)*
A2 T 16.50 16.50 FUD 090

30920 **internal maxillary artery, transantral**
EXCLUDES *External carotid artery (37600)*
A2 T 23.89 23.89 FUD 090

30930-30999 Other and Unlisted Procedures of Nose

30930 **Fracture nasal inferior turbinate(s), therapeutic**
EXCLUDES *Fracture of superior or middle turbinate(s) (30999)*
Do not report with (30130, 30140)
A2 T 50 3.54 3.54 FUD 010

30999 **Unlisted procedure, nose**
T 80 0.00 0.00 FUD YYY

31000-31230 Opening Sinuses

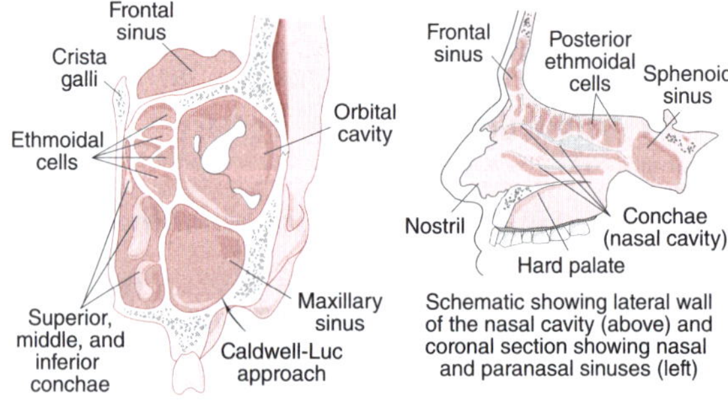

Schematic showing lateral wall of the nasal cavity (above) and coronal section showing nasal and paranasal sinuses (left)

31000 **Lavage by cannulation; maxillary sinus (antrum puncture or natural ostium)**
P3 T 50 3.00 5.20 FUD 010

31002 **sphenoid sinus**
R2 T 80 50 5.74 5.74 FUD 010

31020 **Sinusotomy, maxillary (antrotomy); intranasal**
A2 T 50 10.18 13.69 FUD 090

31030 radical (Caldwell-Luc) without removal of antrochoanal polyps
A2 T 50 — 15.00 — 19.57 FUD 090

31032 radical (Caldwell-Luc) with removal of antrochoanal polyps
A2 T 50 — 16.34 — 16.34 FUD 090

31040 Pterygomaxillary fossa surgery, any approach
EXCLUDES *Transantral ligation internal maxillary artery (30920)*
A2 T 50 — 21.82 — 21.82 FUD 090

31050 Sinusotomy, sphenoid, with or without biopsy;
A2 T 50 PQ — 13.79 — 13.79 FUD 090

31051 with mucosal stripping or removal of polyp(s)
A2 T 50 PQ — 18.36 — 18.36 FUD 090

31070 Sinusotomy frontal; external, simple (trephine operation)
INCLUDES Killian operation
EXCLUDES *Intranasal frontal sinusotomy (31276)*
A2 T 50 — 12.52 — 12.52 FUD 090

31075 transorbital, unilateral (for mucocele or osteoma, Lynch type)
A2 T 80 50 — 22.27 — 22.27 FUD 090

31080 obliterative without osteoplastic flap, brow incision (includes ablation)
INCLUDES Ridell sinusotomy
A2 T 80 50 — 29.36 — 29.36 FUD 090

31081 obliterative, without osteoplastic flap, coronal incision (includes ablation)
A2 T 80 50 — 42.22 — 42.22 FUD 090

31084 obliterative, with osteoplastic flap, brow incision
A2 T 80 50 — 32.88 — 32.88 FUD 090

31085 obliterative, with osteoplastic flap, coronal incision
A2 T 80 50 — 44.86 — 44.86 FUD 090

31086 nonobliterative, with osteoplastic flap, brow incision
A2 T 80 50 — 31.94 — 31.94 FUD 090

31087 nonobliterative, with osteoplastic flap, coronal incision
A2 T 80 50 — 30.82 — 30.82 FUD 090

31090 Sinusotomy, unilateral, 3 or more paranasal sinuses (frontal, maxillary, ethmoid, sphenoid)
A2 T 50 — 29.30 — 29.30 FUD 090

31200 Ethmoidectomy; intranasal, anterior
A2 T 50 — 16.32 — 16.32 FUD 090

31201 intranasal, total
A2 T 50 — 21.16 — 21.16 FUD 090

31205 extranasal, total
A2 T 80 50 — 25.95 — 25.95 FUD 090

31225 Maxillectomy; without orbital exenteration
C 80 50 — 53.51 — 53.51 FUD 090

31230 with orbital exenteration (en bloc)
EXCLUDES *Orbital exenteration without maxillectomy (65110-65114)*
Skin grafts (15120-15121)
C 80 50 — 59.34 — 59.34 FUD 090

31231-31235 Nasal Endoscopy, Diagnostic

CMS 100-3,100.2 Endoscopy
CMS 100-4,12,40.6 Multiple procedures
INCLUDES Complete sinus exam (e.g., nasal cavity, turbinates, sphenoethmoidal recess)

31231 Nasal endoscopy, diagnostic, unilateral or bilateral (separate procedure)
P2 T — 1.85 — 5.92 FUD 000

31233 Nasal/sinus endoscopy, diagnostic with maxillary sinusoscopy (via inferior meatus or canine fossa puncture)
Do not report for same sinus with (31295)
A2 T 80 50 — 3.95 — 7.54 FUD 000

31235 Nasal/sinus endoscopy, diagnostic with sphenoid sinusoscopy (via puncture of sphenoidal face or cannulation of ostium)
Do not report for same sinus with (31297)
A2 T 80 50 — 4.66 — 8.55 FUD 000

31237-31240 Nasal Endoscopy, Surgical

CMS 100-3,100.2 Endoscopy
INCLUDES Diagnostic nasal/sinus endoscopy
Unilateral procedure
EXCLUDES *Frontal sinus exploration (31276)*
Maxillary antrostomy (31256)
Osteomeatal complex (OMC) resection and/or partial (anterior) ethmoidectomy (31254)
Removal of maxillary sinus tissue (31267)
Total (anterior and posterior) ethmoidectomy (31255)

31237 Nasal/sinus endoscopy, surgical; with biopsy, polypectomy or debridement (separate procedure)
A2 T 50 PQ — 4.65 — 7.35 FUD 000

31238 with control of nasal hemorrhage
A2 T 80 50 — 4.86 — 7.32 FUD 000

31239 with dacryocystorhinostomy
A2 T 80 50 — 17.85 — 17.85 FUD 010

31240 with concha bullosa resection
A2 T 80 50 — 4.64 — 4.64 FUD 000

31254-31255 Nasal Endoscopy with Ethmoid Removal

CMS 100-3,100.2 Endoscopy
CMS 100-4,12,40.6 Multiple procedures
INCLUDES Diagnostic nasal/sinus endoscopy
Sinusotomy, when applicable

31254 Nasal/sinus endoscopy, surgical; with ethmoidectomy, partial (anterior)
Code also any combination of the following endoscopic procedures when performed in conjunction with partial (anterior) ethmoidectomy and/or osteomeatal complex (OMC) resection, regardless of whether polyps are removed:
Antrostomy, with or without removal of maxillary sinus tissue; either (31256 or 31267)
Frontal sinus exploration (31276)
A2 T 50 — 7.85 — 7.85 FUD 000

31255 with ethmoidectomy, total (anterior and posterior)
Code also any combination of the following endoscopic procedures when performed in conjunction with total (anterior and posterior) ethmoidectomy, regardless of whether polyps are removed:
Antrostomy, with or without removal of maxillary sinus tissue; either (31256 or 31267)
Frontal sinus exploration (31276)
Sphenoidotomy, with or without removal of tissue; either (31287 or 31288)
A2 T 50 — 11.50 — 11.50 FUD 000

31256-31267 Nasal Endoscopy with Maxillary Procedures

CMS 100-3,100.2 Endoscopy
CMS 100-4,12,40.6 Multiple procedures
INCLUDES Diagnostic nasal/sinus endoscopy
Sinusotomy, when applicable
Do not report with (31295)

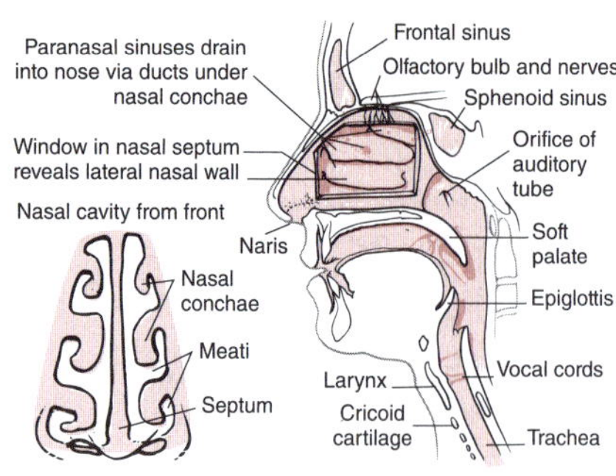

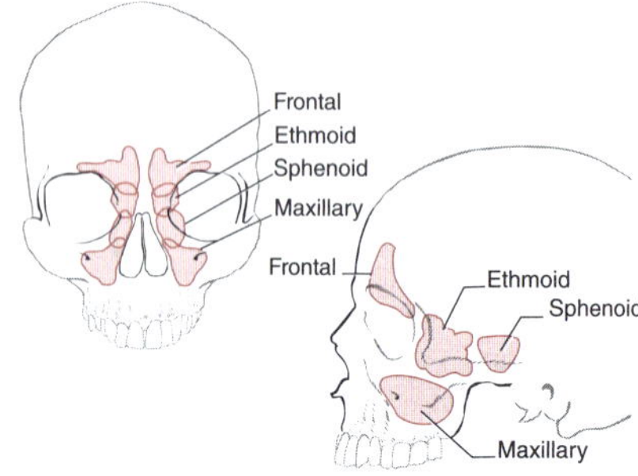

31256 **Nasal/sinus endoscopy, surgical, with maxillary antrostomy;**

Code also any combination of the following endoscopic procedures when performed in conjunction with maxillary antrostomy, regardless if polyps are removed:
- Frontal sinus exploration (31276)
- Sphenoidotomy, with or without removal of tissue; either (31287 or 31288)
- Total (anterior and posterior) ethmoidectomy (31255)

A2 T 50 ⚑ 5.68 5.68 FUD 000

31267 **with removal of tissue from maxillary sinus**

Code also any combination of the following endoscopic procedures when performed in conjunction with maxillary antrostomy with removal of maxillary sinus tissue, regardless of whether polyps are removed:
- Frontal sinus exploration (31276)
- Sphenoidotomy, with or without removal of tissue; either (31287 or 31288)
- Total (anterior and posterior) ethmoidectomy (31255)

A2 T 50 ⚑ 9.12 9.12 FUD 000

31276 Nasal Endoscopy with Frontal Sinus Examination

CMS 100-3,100.2 Endoscopy
CMS 100-4,12,40.6 Multiple procedures

INCLUDES Diagnostic nasal/sinus endoscopy
Sinusotomy, when applicable
Unilateral procedure

EXCLUDES *Unilateral endoscopy two or more sinuses (31231-31235)*

Code also any combination of the following endoscopic procedures when performed in conjunction with frontal sinus exploration, regardless of whether polyps are removed:
- Antrostomy, with or without removal of maxillary sinus tissue; either (31256 or 31267)
- Sphenoidotomy, with or without removal of tissue; either (31287 or 31288)
- Total (anterior and posterior) ethmoidectomy (31255)

Do not report with (31296)

31276 **Nasal/sinus endoscopy, surgical with frontal sinus exploration, with or without removal of tissue from frontal sinus**

A2 T 50 ⚑ 14.52 14.52 FUD 000

31287-31288 Nasal Endoscopy with Sphenoid Procedures

CMS 100-3,100.2 Endoscopy
CMS 100-4,12,40.6 Multiple procedures

Do not report with (31297)

31287 **Nasal/sinus endoscopy, surgical, with sphenoidotomy;**

A2 T 80 50 ⚑ 6.68 6.68 FUD 000

31288 **with removal of tissue from the sphenoid sinus**

A2 T 80 50 ⚑ 7.74 7.74 FUD 000

31290-31294 Nasal Endoscopy with Repair and Decompression

CMS 100-3,100.2 Endoscopy
CMS 100-4,12,40.6 Multiple procedures

INCLUDES Diagnostic nasal/sinus endoscopy
Sinusotomy, when applicable

31290 **Nasal/sinus endoscopy, surgical, with repair of cerebrospinal fluid leak; ethmoid region**

C 80 50 ⚑ 33.23 33.23 FUD 010

31291 **sphenoid region**

C 80 50 ⚑ 35.29 35.29 FUD 010

31292 **with medial or inferior orbital wall decompression**

T 80 50 ⚑ 28.67 28.67 FUD 010

31293 **with medial orbital wall and inferior orbital wall decompression**

T 80 50 ⚑ 31.11 31.11 FUD 010

31294 **with optic nerve decompression**

T 80 50 ⚑ 35.63 35.63 FUD 010

31295-31297 Nasal Endoscopy with Sinus Ostia Dilation

INCLUDES Any method of tissue displacement
Fluoroscopy, when performed

31295 **Nasal/sinus endoscopy, surgical; with dilation of maxillary sinus ostium (eg, balloon dilation), transnasal or via canine fossa**

Do not report with (31233, 31256, 31267)

P2 T 80 50 4.80 58.74 FUD 000

31296 **with dilation of frontal sinus ostium (eg, balloon dilation)**

Do not report with (31276)

P2 T 80 50 5.74 59.62 FUD 000

31297 **with dilation of sphenoid sinus ostium (eg, balloon dilation)**

Do not report with (31235, 31287, 31288)

P2 T 80 50 4.72 58.64 FUD 000

31299 Unlisted Procedures of Accessory Sinuses

31299 **Unlisted procedure, accessory sinuses**

EXCLUDES *Hypophysectomy (61546, 61548)*

T 80 0.00 0.00 FUD YYY

31300-31502 Procedures of the Larynx

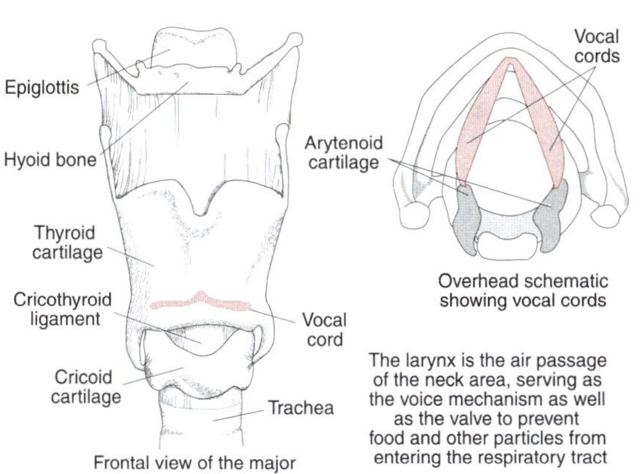

Frontal view of the major structures of the larynx

Overhead schematic showing vocal cords

The larynx is the air passage of the neck area, serving as the voice mechanism as well as the valve to prevent food and other particles from entering the respiratory tract

31300 **Laryngotomy (thyrotomy, laryngofissure); with removal of tumor or laryngocele, cordectomy**
A2 T 80 ▣ 35.95 35.95 FUD 090

31320 **diagnostic**
A2 T 80 ▣ 18.68 18.68 FUD 090

31360 **Laryngectomy; total, without radical neck dissection**
C 80 ▣ PQ 59.56 59.56 FUD 090

31365 **total, with radical neck dissection**
C 80 ▣ PQ 73.71 73.71 FUD 090

31367 **subtotal supraglottic, without radical neck dissection**
C 80 ▣ PQ 63.00 63.00 FUD 090

31368 **subtotal supraglottic, with radical neck dissection**
C 80 ▣ PQ 69.83 69.83 FUD 090

31370 **Partial laryngectomy (hemilaryngectomy); horizontal**
C 80 ▣ PQ 59.16 59.16 FUD 090

31375 **laterovertical**
C 80 ▣ PQ 56.16 56.16 FUD 090

31380 **anterovertical**
C 80 ▣ PQ 55.36 55.36 FUD 090

31382 **antero-latero-vertical**
C 80 ▣ PQ 60.77 60.77 FUD 090

31390 **Pharyngolaryngectomy, with radical neck dissection; without reconstruction**
C 80 ▣ PQ 82.04 82.04 FUD 090

31395 **with reconstruction**
C 80 ▣ PQ 85.99 85.99 FUD 090

31400 **Arytenoidectomy or arytenoidopexy, external approach**
EXCLUDES *Endoscopic arytenoidectomy (31560)*
A2 T 80 ▣ 28.40 28.40 FUD 090

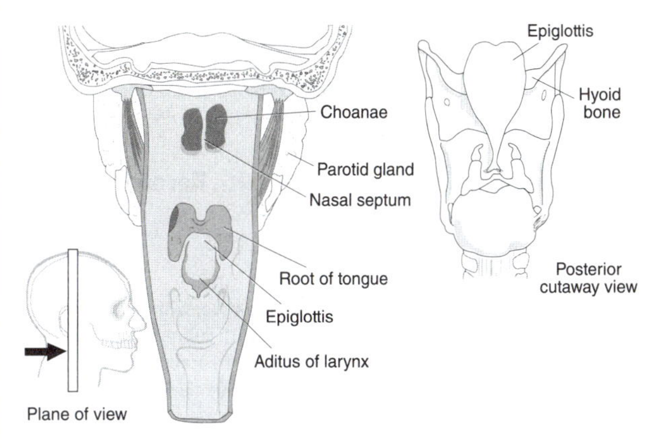

31420 **Epiglottidectomy**
A2 T 80 ▣ 23.88 23.88 FUD 090

⊘ **31500** **Intubation, endotracheal, emergency procedure**
G2 S ▣ 3.18 3.18 FUD 000

31502 **Tracheotomy tube change prior to establishment of fistula tract**
G2 S ▣ 1.01 1.01 FUD 000

31505-31541 Endoscopy of the Larynx

CMS 100-3,100.2 Endoscopy
CMS 100-4,12,40.6 Multiple procedures

31505 **Laryngoscopy, indirect; diagnostic (separate procedure)**
P3 T ▣ 1.41 2.37 FUD 000

31510 **with biopsy**
A2 T 80 ▣ PQ 3.49 5.99 FUD 000

31511 **with removal of foreign body**
A2 T ▣ 3.75 5.99 FUD 000

31512 **with removal of lesion**
A2 T 80 ▣ 3.76 5.91 FUD 000

31513 **with vocal cord injection**
A2 T 80 ▣ 3.82 3.82 FUD 000

31515 **Laryngoscopy direct, with or without tracheoscopy; for aspiration**
A2 T ▣ 3.21 5.95 FUD 000

31520 **diagnostic, newborn** A
G2 T 80 ▣ 63 4.55 4.55 FUD 000

31525 **diagnostic, except newborn**
A2 T ▣ 4.63 7.24 FUD 000

31526 **diagnostic, with operating microscope or telescope**
INCLUDES Operating microscope (69990)
A2 T ▣ 4.56 4.56 FUD 000

31527 **with insertion of obturator**
A2 T 80 ▣ 5.65 5.65 FUD 000

31528 **with dilation, initial**
A2 T 80 ▣ 4.19 4.19 FUD 000

31529 **with dilation, subsequent**
A2 T 80 ▣ 4.69 4.69 FUD 000

31530 **Laryngoscopy, direct, operative, with foreign body removal;**
A2 T ▣ 5.72 5.72 FUD 000

31531 **with operating microscope or telescope**
INCLUDES Operating microscope (69990)
A2 T 80 ▣ 6.15 6.15 FUD 000

31535 **Laryngoscopy, direct, operative, with biopsy;**
A2 T ▣ 5.48 5.48 FUD 000

31536 **with operating microscope or telescope**
INCLUDES Operating microscope (69990)
A2 T ▣ 6.10 6.10 FUD 000

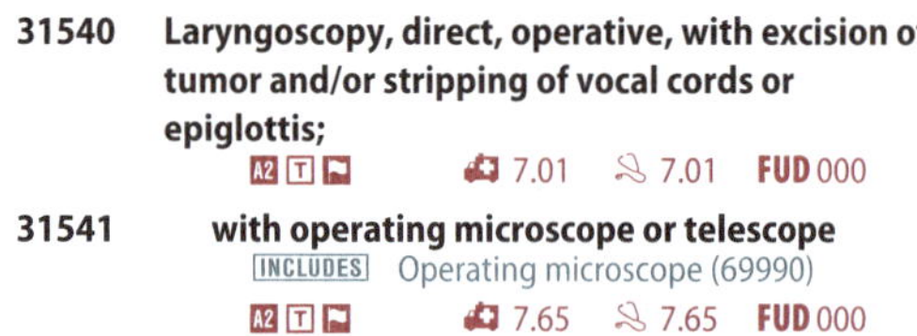

31540 **Laryngoscopy, direct, operative, with excision of tumor and/or stripping of vocal cords or epiglottis;**
A2 T ⚑ Facility RVU 7.01 Non-Facility RVU 7.01 FUD 000

31541 **with operating microscope or telescope**
INCLUDES Operating microscope (69990)
A2 T ⚑ Facility RVU 7.65 Non-Facility RVU 7.65 FUD 000

31545-31546 Endoscopy of Larynx with Reconstruction

INCLUDES Operating microscope (69990)

EXCLUDES *Vocal cord reconstruction with allograft (31599)*

Do not report with (31540, 31541)

31545 **Laryngoscopy, direct, operative, with operating microscope or telescope, with submucosal removal of non-neoplastic lesion(s) of vocal cord; reconstruction with local tissue flap(s)**
A2 T 50 ⚑ Facility RVU 10.52 Non-Facility RVU 10.52 FUD 000

31546 **reconstruction with graft(s) (includes obtaining autograft)**
Do not report with (20926)
A2 T 50 ⚑ Facility RVU 15.98 Non-Facility RVU 15.98 FUD 000

31560-31571 Endoscopy of Larynx with Arytenoid Removal, Vocal Cord Injection

CMS 100-3,100.2 Endoscopy
CMS 100-4,12,40.6 Multiple procedures

31560 **Laryngoscopy, direct, operative, with arytenoidectomy;**
A2 T 80 ⚑ Facility RVU 9.07 Non-Facility RVU 9.07 FUD 000

31561 **with operating microscope or telescope**
INCLUDES Operating microscope (69990)
A2 T 80 ⚑ Facility RVU 9.94 Non-Facility RVU 9.94 FUD 000

31570 **Laryngoscopy, direct, with injection into vocal cord(s), therapeutic;**
A2 T ⚑ Facility RVU 6.64 Non-Facility RVU 9.73 FUD 000

31571 **with operating microscope or telescope**
INCLUDES Operating microscope (69990)
A2 T ⚑ Facility RVU 7.23 Non-Facility RVU 7.23 FUD 000

31575-31579 Endoscopy of Larynx, Flexible Fiberoptic

EXCLUDES *Evaluation by flexible fiberoptic endoscope:*
Sensory assessment (92614-92615)
Swallowing (92612-92613)
Swallowing and sensory assessment (92616-92617)
Flexible fiberoptic endoscopic examination/testing by cine or video recording (92612-92617)

31575 **Laryngoscopy, flexible fiberoptic; diagnostic**
Do not report with (43197-43198)
P3 T ⚑ Facility RVU 2.18 Non-Facility RVU 3.24 FUD 000

31576 **with biopsy**
A2 T ⚑ P0 Facility RVU 3.57 Non-Facility RVU 6.41 FUD 000

31577 **with removal of foreign body**
A2 T 80 ⚑ Facility RVU 4.32 Non-Facility RVU 6.92 FUD 000

31578 **with removal of lesion**
A2 T 80 ⚑ Facility RVU 4.95 Non-Facility RVU 7.99 FUD 000

31579 **Laryngoscopy, flexible or rigid fiberoptic, with stroboscopy**
P3 T ⚑ Facility RVU 4.09 Non-Facility RVU 6.06 FUD 000

31580-31599 Larynx Reconstruction

31580 **Laryngoplasty; for laryngeal web, 2-stage, with keel insertion and removal**
A2 T 80 ⚑ Facility RVU 34.82 Non-Facility RVU 34.82 FUD 090

31582 **for laryngeal stenosis, with graft or core mold, including tracheotomy**
A2 T ⚑ Facility RVU 54.00 Non-Facility RVU 54.00 FUD 090

31584 **with open reduction of fracture**
C 80 ⚑ Facility RVU 43.10 Non-Facility RVU 43.10 FUD 090

31587 **Laryngoplasty, cricoid split**
C 80 ⚑ Facility RVU 28.73 Non-Facility RVU 28.73 FUD 090

31588 **Laryngoplasty, not otherwise specified (eg, for burns, reconstruction after partial laryngectomy)**
A2 T 80 ⚑ Facility RVU 32.64 Non-Facility RVU 32.64 FUD 090

31590 **Laryngeal reinnervation by neuromuscular pedicle**
A2 T 80 ⚑ Facility RVU 25.28 Non-Facility RVU 25.28 FUD 090

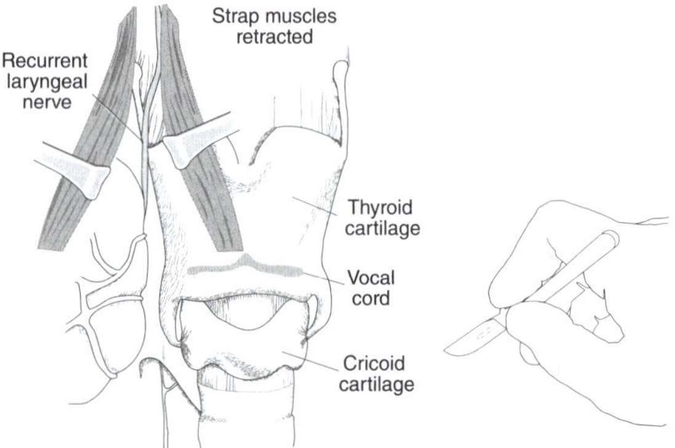

31595 **Section recurrent laryngeal nerve, therapeutic (separate procedure), unilateral**
A2 T 80 50 ⚑ Facility RVU 21.77 Non-Facility RVU 21.77 FUD 090

31599 **Unlisted procedure, larynx**
T 80 Facility RVU 0.00 Non-Facility RVU 0.00 FUD YYY

31600-31610 Stoma Creation: Trachea

EXCLUDES *Aspiration of trachea, direct vision (31515)*
Endotracheal intubation (31500)

31600 **Tracheostomy, planned (separate procedure);**
T ⚑ Facility RVU 11.41 Non-Facility RVU 11.41 FUD 000

31601 **younger than 2 years** A
T 80 ⚑ Facility RVU 7.47 Non-Facility RVU 7.47 FUD 000

31603 **Tracheostomy, emergency procedure; transtracheal**
A2 T ⚑ Facility RVU 6.48 Non-Facility RVU 6.48 FUD 000

31605 **cricothyroid membrane**
G2 T ⚑ Facility RVU 5.31 Non-Facility RVU 5.31 FUD 000

31610 **Tracheostomy, fenestration procedure with skin flaps**
T ⚑ Facility RVU 20.47 Non-Facility RVU 20.47 FUD 090

31611-31614 Procedures of the Trachea

31611 **Construction of tracheoesophageal fistula and subsequent insertion of an alaryngeal speech prosthesis (eg, voice button, Blom-Singer prosthesis)**
A2 T 80 ⚑ Facility RVU 15.45 Non-Facility RVU 15.45 FUD 090

31612 **Tracheal puncture, percutaneous with transtracheal aspiration and/or injection**
EXCLUDES *Tracheal aspiration under direct vision (31515)*
A2 T 80 ⚑ Facility RVU 1.37 Non-Facility RVU 2.37 FUD 000

31613 **Tracheostoma revision; simple, without flap rotation**
A2 T ⚑ Facility RVU 13.01 Non-Facility RVU 13.01 FUD 090

31614 **complex, with flap rotation**
A2 T ⚑ Facility RVU 21.68 Non-Facility RVU 21.68 FUD 090

31615 Endoscopy Through Tracheostomy

INCLUDES Diagnostic bronchoscopy

⊙ 31615 **Tracheobronchoscopy through established tracheostomy incision**
A2 T ⚑ Facility RVU 3.71 Non-Facility RVU 5.20 FUD 000

31620 Endobronchial Ultrasound (EBUS)

+ ⊙ 31620 **Endobronchial ultrasound (EBUS) during bronchoscopic diagnostic or therapeutic intervention(s) (List separately in addition to code for primary procedure[s])**
Code first (31622-31646)
N1 N 1.94 8.12 FUD ZZZ

31622-31651 [31651] Endoscopy of Lung

INCLUDES Diagnostic bronchoscopy with surgical bronchoscopy procedures
Fluoroscopic imaging guidance, when performed

⊙ 31622 **Bronchoscopy, rigid or flexible, including fluoroscopic guidance, when performed; diagnostic, with cell washing, when performed (separate procedure)**
A2 T 4.23 8.83 FUD 000

⊙ 31623 **with brushing or protected brushings**
A2 T 4.23 9.34 FUD 000

⊙ 31624 **with bronchial alveolar lavage**
A2 T 4.26 8.79 FUD 000

⊙ 31625 **with bronchial or endobronchial biopsy(s), single or multiple sites**
A2 T PQ 4.92 9.45 FUD 000

⊙ 31626 **with placement of fiducial markers, single or multiple**
Code also device
G2 T 80 5.95 12.56 FUD 000

+ ⊙ 31627 **with computer-assisted, image-guided navigation (List separately in addition to code for primary procedure[s])**
INCLUDES 3D reconstruction
Code first (31615, 31622-31626, 31628-31631, 31635-31636, 31638-31643)
Do not report with (76376-76377)
N1 N 80 2.73 36.56 FUD ZZZ

⊙ 31628 **with transbronchial lung biopsy(s), single lobe**
INCLUDES All biopsies taken from lobe
EXCLUDES *Transbronchial biopsies by needle aspiration (31629, 31633)*
Transbronchial biopsies of additional lobe(s) (31632)
A2 T PQ 5.47 10.64 FUD 000

⊙ 31629 **with transbronchial needle aspiration biopsy(s), trachea, main stem and/or lobar bronchus(i)**
INCLUDES All biopsies from same lobe or upper airway
EXCLUDES *Transbronchial biopsies of lung (31628, 31632)*
Transbronchial needle biopsies of another lobe(s) (31633)
A2 T PQ 5.89 16.74 FUD 000

31630 **with tracheal/bronchial dilation or closed reduction of fracture**
A2 T 5.80 5.80 FUD 000

31631 **with placement of tracheal stent(s) (includes tracheal/bronchial dilation as required)**
EXCLUDES *Bronchial stent placement (31636-31637)*
Revision bronchial or tracheal stent (31638)
A2 T 6.64 6.64 FUD 000

+ 31632 **with transbronchial lung biopsy(s), each additional lobe (List separately in addition to code for primary procedure)**
INCLUDES All biopsies of additional lobe of lung
Code first (31628)
N1 N 1.41 2.02 FUD ZZZ

+ 31633 **with transbronchial needle aspiration biopsy(s), each additional lobe (List separately in addition to code for primary procedure)**
INCLUDES All needle biopsies from another lobe or from trachea
Code first (31629)
N1 N 1.82 2.50 FUD ZZZ

⊙ 31634 **with balloon occlusion, with assessment of air leak, with administration of occlusive substance (eg, fibrin glue), if performed**
Do not report with (31647, [31651])
G2 T 80 5.78 52.66 FUD 000

⊙ 31635 **with removal of foreign body**
EXCLUDES *Removal implanted bronchial valves (31648-31649)*
A2 T 5.43 9.83 FUD 000

31636 **with placement of bronchial stent(s) (includes tracheal/bronchial dilation as required), initial bronchus**
A2 T 6.41 6.41 FUD 000

+ 31637 **each additional major bronchus stented (List separately in addition to code for primary procedure)**
Code first (31636)
N1 N 2.13 2.13 FUD ZZZ

31638 **with revision of tracheal or bronchial stent inserted at previous session (includes tracheal/bronchial dilation as required)**
A2 T 7.36 7.36 FUD 000

31640 **with excision of tumor**
A2 T 7.37 7.37 FUD 000

31641 **with destruction of tumor or relief of stenosis by any method other than excision (eg, laser therapy, cryotherapy)**
Code also any photodynamic therapy via bronchoscopy (96570-96571)
A2 T 7.46 7.46 FUD 000

31643 **with placement of catheter(s) for intracavitary radioelement application**
Code also if appropriate (77761-77763, 77785-77787)
A2 T 5.08 5.08 FUD 000

⊙ 31645 **with therapeutic aspiration of tracheobronchial tree, initial (eg, drainage of lung abscess)**
EXCLUDES *Bedside aspiration of trachea, bronchi (31725)*
A2 T 4.66 9.02 FUD 000

⊙ 31646 **with therapeutic aspiration of tracheobronchial tree, subsequent**
EXCLUDES *Bedside aspiration of trachea, bronchi (31725)*
A2 T 4.04 8.11 FUD 000

⊙ 31647 **with balloon occlusion, when performed, assessment of air leak, airway sizing, and insertion of bronchial valve(s), initial lobe**
G2 T 6.36 6.36 FUD 000

+ ⊙ # 31651 **with balloon occlusion, when performed, assessment of air leak, airway sizing, and insertion of bronchial valve(s), each additional lobe (List separately in addition to code for primary procedure[s])**
Code first (31647)
N1 N 2.29 2.29 FUD ZZZ

⊙ 31648 **with removal of bronchial valve(s), initial lobe**
EXCLUDES *Removal with reinsertion bronchial valve during same session (31647 and 31648) and ([31651])*
G2 T 6.09 6.09 FUD 000

+ ⊙ 31649 **with removal of bronchial valve(s), each additional lobe (List separately in addition to code for primary procedure)**
Code first (31648)
[G2] [Q2] Facility RVU 1.97 Non-Facility RVU 1.97 FUD ZZZ

31651 Resequenced code. See code following 31647.

31660-31661 Bronchial Thermoplasty

INCLUDES Fluoroscopic imaging guidance, when performed

⊙ 31660 **with bronchial thermoplasty, 1 lobe**
[T] Facility RVU 6.08 Non-Facility RVU 6.08 FUD 000

⊙ 31661 **with bronchial thermoplasty, 2 or more lobes**
[T] Facility RVU 6.41 Non-Facility RVU 6.41 FUD 000

31717-31899 Respiratory Procedures

EXCLUDES *Endotracheal intubation (31500)*
Tracheal aspiration under direct vision (31515)

31717 **Catheterization with bronchial brush biopsy**
[A2] [T] [flag] [PQ] Facility RVU 3.13 Non-Facility RVU 7.42 FUD 000

31720 **Catheter aspiration (separate procedure); nasotracheal**
[A2] [S] [flag] Facility RVU 1.47 Non-Facility RVU 1.47 FUD 000

⊙ 31725 **tracheobronchial with fiberscope, bedside**
[C] [flag] Facility RVU 2.64 Non-Facility RVU 2.64 FUD 000

31730 **Transtracheal (percutaneous) introduction of needle wire dilator/stent or indwelling tube for oxygen therapy**
[A2] [T] [flag] Facility RVU 4.21 Non-Facility RVU 34.26 FUD 000

31750 **Tracheoplasty; cervical**
[A2] [T] [80] [flag] Facility RVU 39.11 Non-Facility RVU 39.11 FUD 090

31755 **tracheopharyngeal fistulization, each stage**
[A2] [T] [80] [flag] Facility RVU 49.15 Non-Facility RVU 49.15 FUD 090

31760 **intrathoracic**
[C] [80] [flag] [PQ] Facility RVU 39.62 Non-Facility RVU 39.62 FUD 090

31766 **Carinal reconstruction**
[C] [80] [flag] [PQ] Facility RVU 51.43 Non-Facility RVU 51.43 FUD 090

31770 **Bronchoplasty; graft repair**
EXCLUDES *Bronchoplasty done with lobectomy (32501)*
[C] [80] [flag] [PQ] Facility RVU 38.52 Non-Facility RVU 38.52 FUD 090

31775 **excision stenosis and anastomosis**
EXCLUDES *Bronchoplasty done with lobectomy (32501)*
[C] [80] [flag] [PQ] Facility RVU 39.31 Non-Facility RVU 39.31 FUD 090

31780 **Excision tracheal stenosis and anastomosis; cervical**
[C] [80] [flag] Facility RVU 33.95 Non-Facility RVU 33.95 FUD 090

31781 **cervicothoracic**
[C] [80] [flag] Facility RVU 44.31 Non-Facility RVU 44.31 FUD 090

31785 **Excision of tracheal tumor or carcinoma; cervical**
[T] [80] [flag] Facility RVU 31.14 Non-Facility RVU 31.14 FUD 090

31786 **thoracic**
[C] [80] [flag] [PQ] Facility RVU 41.72 Non-Facility RVU 41.72 FUD 090

31800 **Suture of tracheal wound or injury; cervical**
[C] [80] [flag] Facility RVU 20.35 Non-Facility RVU 20.35 FUD 090

31805 **intrathoracic**
[C] [80] [flag] [PQ] Facility RVU 23.55 Non-Facility RVU 23.55 FUD 090

31820 **Surgical closure tracheostomy or fistula; without plastic repair**
EXCLUDES *Tracheoesophageal fistula repair (43305, 43312)*
[A2] [T] [80] [flag] Facility RVU 9.46 Non-Facility RVU 12.46 FUD 090

31825 **with plastic repair**
EXCLUDES *Tracheoesophageal fistula repair (43305, 43312)*
[A2] [T] [80] [flag] Facility RVU 13.83 Non-Facility RVU 17.29 FUD 090

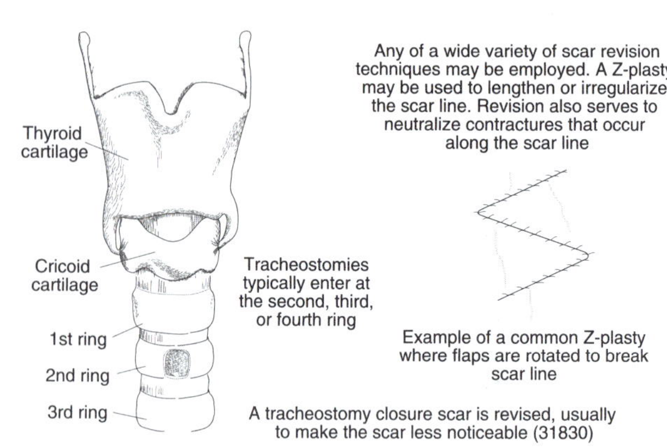

31830 **Revision of tracheostomy scar**
[A2] [T] [80] [flag] Facility RVU 9.81 Non-Facility RVU 12.66 FUD 090

31899 **Unlisted procedure, trachea, bronchi**
[T] [80] Facility RVU 0.00 Non-Facility RVU 0.00 FUD YYY

32035-32036 Procedures for Empyema

32035 **Thoracostomy; with rib resection for empyema**
[C] [80] [50] [flag] Facility RVU 20.65 Non-Facility RVU 20.65 FUD 090

32036 **with open flap drainage for empyema**
EXCLUDES *Wound exploration due to penetrating trauma without thoracotomy (20101)*
[C] [80] [50] [flag] Facility RVU 22.44 Non-Facility RVU 22.44 FUD 090

32096-32098 Open Biopsy of Chest and Pleura

INCLUDES Varying amounts of lung tissue excised for analysis
Wedge technique with tissue obtained without precise consideration of margins

EXCLUDES *Percutaneous needle biopsy of pleura, lung, and mediastinum (32400, 32405)*
Thoracoscopy with biopsy (32607-32609)
Thoracoscopy with diagnostic wedge resection resulting in anatomic lung resection (32668)
Thoracotomy with diagnostic wedge resection resulting in anatomic lung resection (32507)

32096 **Thoracotomy, with diagnostic biopsy(ies) of lung infiltrate(s) (eg, wedge, incisional), unilateral**
Code also appropriate add-on code for the more extensive procedure at the same location if diagnostic wedge resection results in the need for further surgery (32507, 32668)
Do not report more than one time per lung
Do not report with (32440-32445, 32488)
[C] [80] Facility RVU 23.32 Non-Facility RVU 23.32 FUD 090

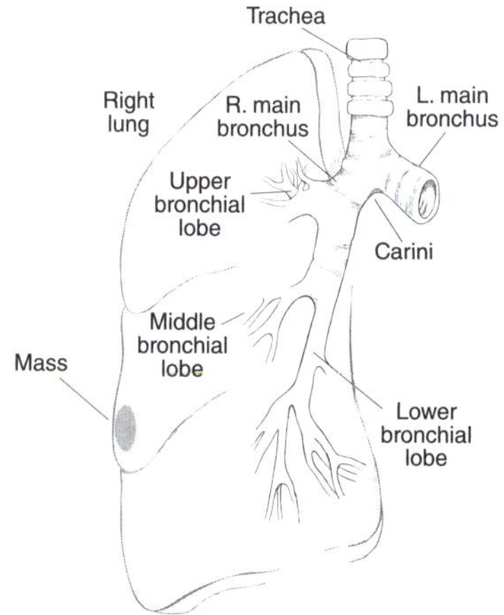

32097 **Thoracotomy, with diagnostic biopsy(ies) of lung nodule(s) or mass(es) (eg, wedge, incisional), unilateral**

Code also appropriate add-on code for the more extensive procedure in the same location if diagnostic wedge resection results in the need for further surgery (32507, 32668)

Do not report more than one time per lung

Do not report with (32440-32445, 32488)

C 80 23.33 23.33 FUD 090

32098 **Thoracotomy, with biopsy(ies) of pleura**

C 80 22.02 22.02 FUD 090

32100-32160 Open Procedures: Chest

INCLUDES Exploration of penetrating wound of chest

EXCLUDES *Lung resection (32480-32504)*

Wound exploration without thoracotomy for penetrating wound of chest (20101)

32100 **Thoracotomy; with exploration**

Do not report with (19260, 19271-19272, 32503-32504, 33955-33957, [33963, 33964])

C 80 PQ 23.58 23.58 FUD 090

32110 **with control of traumatic hemorrhage and/or repair of lung tear**

C 80 PQ 42.07 42.07 FUD 090

32120 **for postoperative complications**

C 80 PQ 25.20 25.20 FUD 090

32124 **with open intrapleural pneumonolysis**

C 80 PQ 26.85 26.85 FUD 090

32140 **with cyst(s) removal, includes pleural procedure when performed**

C 80 PQ 28.68 28.68 FUD 090

32141 **with resection-plication of bullae, includes any pleural procedure when performed**

EXCLUDES *Lung volume reduction (32491)*

C 80 PQ 44.32 44.32 FUD 090

32150 **with removal of intrapleural foreign body or fibrin deposit**

C 80 PQ 29.04 29.04 FUD 090

32151 **with removal of intrapulmonary foreign body**

C 80 28.95 28.95 FUD 090

32160 **with cardiac massage**

C 80 22.74 22.74 FUD 090

32200-32320 Open Procedures: Lung

32200 **Pneumonostomy, with open drainage of abscess or cyst**

EXCLUDES *Image-guided, percutaneous drainage (eg, abscess, cyst) of lungs/mediastinum via catheter (49405)*

75989

C 80 32.77 32.77 FUD 090

32215 **Pleural scarification for repeat pneumothorax**

C 80 50 PQ 23.12 23.12 FUD 090

32220 **Decortication, pulmonary (separate procedure); total**

C 80 50 PQ 45.88 45.88 FUD 090

32225 **partial**

C 80 50 PQ 28.77 28.77 FUD 090

32310 **Pleurectomy, parietal (separate procedure)**

C 80 PQ 26.54 26.54 FUD 090

32320 **Decortication and parietal pleurectomy**

C 80 PQ 46.20 46.20 FUD 090

32400-32405 Lung Biopsy

EXCLUDES *Open lung biopsy (32096-32097)*

Open mediastinal biopsy (39000-39010)

Thoracoscopic (VATS) biopsy of lung, pericardium, pleural or mediastinal space (32604-32609)

32400 **Biopsy, pleura; percutaneous needle**

EXCLUDES *Fine needle aspiration (10021-10022)*

76942, 77002, 77012, 77021

A2 T PQ 2.53 4.29 FUD 000

⊙ **32405** **Biopsy, lung or mediastinum, percutaneous needle**

EXCLUDES *Fine needle aspiration (10022)*

76942, 77002, 77012, 77021

A2 T PQ 3.00 12.62 FUD 000

32440-32501 Lung Resection

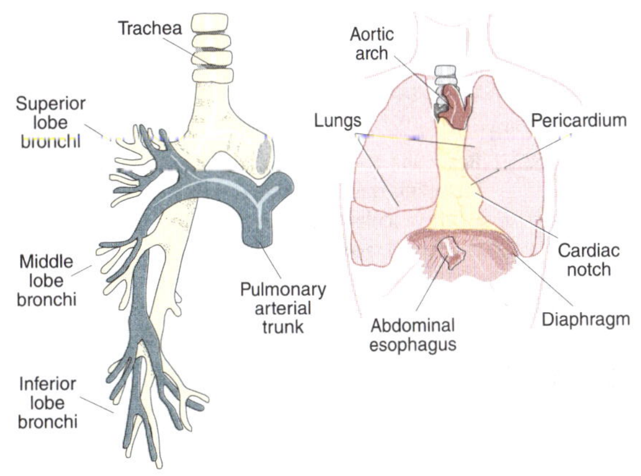

32440 **Removal of lung, pneumonectomy;**

Code also excision of chest wall tumor (19260-19272)

C 80 PQ 45.33 45.33 FUD 090

32442 **with resection of segment of trachea followed by broncho-tracheal anastomosis (sleeve pneumonectomy)**

Code also excision of chest wall tumor (19260-19272)

C 80 PQ 93.04 93.04 FUD 090

32445 **extrapleural**

Code also empyemectomy with extrapleural pneumonectomy (32540)

Code also excision of chest wall tumor (19260-19272)

C 80 PQ 102.37 102.37 FUD 090

32480 **Removal of lung, other than pneumonectomy; single lobe (lobectomy)**

EXCLUDES *Lung removal with bronchoplasty (32501)*

Code also decortication (32320)

Code also excision of chest wall tumor (19260-19272)

C 80 PQ 42.82 42.82 FUD 090

32482 **2 lobes (bilobectomy)**

EXCLUDES *Lung removal with bronchoplasty (32501)*

Code also decortication (32320)

Code also excision of chest wall tumor (19260-19272)

C 80 PQ 45.86 45.86 FUD 090

32484 **single segment (segmentectomy)**

EXCLUDES *Lung removal with bronchoplasty (32501)*

Code also decortication (32320)

Code also excision of chest wall tumor (19260-19272)

C 80 PQ 41.54 41.54 FUD 090

32486 **with circumferential resection of segment of bronchus followed by broncho-bronchial anastomosis (sleeve lobectomy)**

Code also decortication (32320)

Code also excision of chest wall tumor (19260-19272)

C 80 PQ 68.04 68.04 FUD 090

32488 **with all remaining lung following previous removal of a portion of lung (completion pneumonectomy)**

Code also decortication (32320)

Code also excision of chest wall tumor (19260-19272)

C 80 PQ 69.54 69.54 FUD 090

32491 **with resection-plication of emphysematous lung(s) (bullous or non-bullous) for lung volume reduction, sternal split or transthoracic approach, includes any pleural procedure, when performed**

C 80 50 PQ 42.56 42.56 FUD 090

\+ **32501** **Resection and repair of portion of bronchus (bronchoplasty) when performed at time of lobectomy or segmentectomy (List separately in addition to code for primary procedure)**

INCLUDES Plastic closure of bronchus, not closure of a resected end of bronchus

Code first (32480-32484)

C 80 PQ 7.11 7.11 FUD ZZZ

32503-32504 Excision of Lung Neoplasm

EXCLUDES *Lung resection performed in conjunction with chest wall resection*

Do not report with (19260, 19271-19272, 32100, 32551, 32554-32555)

32503 **Resection of apical lung tumor (eg, Pancoast tumor), including chest wall resection, rib(s) resection(s), neurovascular dissection, when performed; without chest wall reconstruction(s)**

C 80 PQ 52.56 52.56 FUD 090

32504 **with chest wall reconstruction**

C 80 PQ 59.94 59.94 FUD 090

32505-32507 Thoracotomy with Wedge Resection

INCLUDES Wedge technique with tissue obtained with precise consideration of margins and complete resection

Code also resection of chest wall tumor with lung resection when performed (19260-19272)

32505 **Thoracotomy; with therapeutic wedge resection (eg, mass, nodule), initial**

Code also a more extensive procedure of the lung when performed on the contralateral lung or different lobe with modifier 59 regardless of intraoperative pathology consultation

Do not report with (32440, 32442, 32445, 32488)

C 80 PQ 26.92 26.92 FUD 090

\+ **32506** **with therapeutic wedge resection (eg, mass or nodule), each additional resection, ipsilateral (List separately in addition to code for primary procedure)**

Code also a more extensive procedure of the lung when performed on the contralateral lung or different lobe with modifier 59

Code first (32505)

C 80 4.57 4.57 FUD ZZZ

\+ **32507** **with diagnostic wedge resection followed by anatomic lung resection (List separately in addition to code for primary procedure)**

INCLUDES Classification as a diagnostic wedge resection if intraoperative pathology consultation dictates more extensive resection in the same anatomical area

EXCLUDES *Diagnostic wedge resection by thoracoscopy (32668)*

Therapeutic wedge resection (32505-32506, 32666-32667)

Code first (32440, 32442, 32445, 32480-32488, 32503-32504)

C 80 4.57 4.57 FUD ZZZ

32540 Removal of Empyema

32540 **Extrapleural enucleation of empyema (empyemectomy)**

EXCLUDES *Lung removal code when empyemectomy is performed with lobectomy (see appropriate lung removal code)*

Code also appropriate removal of lung code when done with lobectomy (32480-32488)

C 80 50.25 50.25 FUD 090

32550-32552 Chest Tube/Catheter

⊙ **32550** **Insertion of indwelling tunneled pleural catheter with cuff**

Code also (C1729)

Do not report on same side of chest with (32554-32557)

75989

G2 T 6.48 22.19 FUD 000

⊙ **32551** **Tube thoracostomy, includes connection to drainage system (eg, water seal), when performed, open (separate procedure)**

T 50 5.13 5.13 FUD 000

32552 **Removal of indwelling tunneled pleural catheter with cuff**

G2 Q2 80 4.79 5.48 FUD 010

32553 Intrathoracic Placement Radiation Therapy Devices

EXCLUDES *Percutaneous placement of interstitial device(s) for radiation therapy guidance: intra-abdominal, intrapelvic, and/or retroperitoneal (49411)*

Code also device

⊙ **32553** **Placement of interstitial device(s) for radiation therapy guidance (eg, fiducial markers, dosimeter), percutaneous, intra-thoracic, single or multiple**

76942, 77002, 77012, 77021

G2 X 80 6.12 16.67 FUD 000

32554-32557 Pleural Aspiration and Drainage

EXCLUDES *Open tube thoracostomy (32551)*

Placement of indwelling tunneled pleural drainage catheter (cuffed) (32550)

Do not report for same side of chest with (32550-32551)

Do not report with (75989, 76942, 77002, 77012, 77021)

32554 **Thoracentesis, needle or catheter, aspiration of the pleural space; without imaging guidance**

G2 T 50 2.60 5.61 FUD 000

32555 **with imaging guidance**

G2 T 50 3.27 8.37 FUD 000

32556 **Pleural drainage, percutaneous, with insertion of indwelling catheter; without imaging guidance**

G2 T 50 3.59 15.13 FUD 000

32557 **with imaging guidance**

G2 T 50 4.79 16.13 FUD 000

32560-32562 Instillation Drug/Chemical by Chest Tube

EXCLUDES *Insertion of chest tube (32551)*

32560 **Instillation, via chest tube/catheter, agent for pleurodesis (eg, talc for recurrent or persistent pneumothorax)**

T 2.28 6.93 FUD 000

32561 **Instillation(s), via chest tube/catheter, agent for fibrinolysis (eg, fibrinolytic agent for break up of multiloculated effusion); initial day**

Do not report more than one time on the date of initial treatment

T 80 2.06 2.71 FUD 000

32562 **subsequent day**

Do not report more than one time on each day of subsequent treatment

T 80 1.84 2.44 FUD 000

32601-32674 Thoracic Surgery: Video-Assisted (VATS)

CMS 100-3,100.2 Endoscopy

CMS 100-4,12,40.6 Multiple procedures

INCLUDES Diagnostic thoracoscopy in surgical thoracoscopy

32601 **Thoracoscopy, diagnostic (separate procedure); lungs, pericardial sac, mediastinal or pleural space, without biopsy**
T 80 ⚑ 8.95 8.95 FUD 000

32604 **pericardial sac, with biopsy**
EXCLUDES *Open biopsy of pericardium (39010)*
T 80 ⚑ 13.94 13.94 FUD 000

32606 **mediastinal space, with biopsy**
T 80 ⚑ 13.39 13.39 FUD 000

32607 **Thoracoscopy; with diagnostic biopsy(ies) of lung infiltrate(s) (eg, wedge, incisional), unilateral**
Do not report more than one time per lung
Do not report with (32440-32445, 32488, 32671)
T 80 8.96 8.96 FUD 000

32608 **with diagnostic biopsy(ies) of lung nodule(s) or mass(es) (eg, wedge, incisional), unilateral**
Do not report more than one time per lung
Do not report with (32440-32445, 32488, 32671)
T 80 11.00 11.00 FUD 000

32609 **with biopsy(ies) of pleura**
T 80 7.59 7.59 FUD 000

32650 **Thoracoscopy, surgical; with pleurodesis (eg, mechanical or chemical)**
C 80 50 ⚑ 19.23 19.23 FUD 090

32651 **with partial pulmonary decortication**
C 80 50 ⚑ 31.61 31.61 FUD 090

32652 **with total pulmonary decortication, including intrapleural pneumonolysis**
C 80 50 ⚑ 48.02 48.02 FUD 090

32653 **with removal of intrapleural foreign body or fibrin deposit**
C 80 ⚑ 30.56 30.56 FUD 090

32654 **with control of traumatic hemorrhage**
C 80 50 ⚑ 33.94 33.94 FUD 090

32655 **with resection-plication of bullae, includes any pleural procedure when performed**
EXCLUDES *Thoracoscopic lung volume reduction surgery (32672)*
C 80 50 ⚑ 27.62 27.62 FUD 090

32656 **with parietal pleurectomy**
C 80 50 ⚑ 23.06 23.06 FUD 090

32658 **with removal of clot or foreign body from pericardial sac**
C 80 ⚑ 20.63 20.63 FUD 090

32659 **with creation of pericardial window or partial resection of pericardial sac for drainage**
C 80 ⚑ 21.13 21.13 FUD 090

32661 **with excision of pericardial cyst, tumor, or mass**
C 80 ⚑ 23.08 23.08 FUD 090

32662 **with excision of mediastinal cyst, tumor, or mass**
C 80 ⚑ 25.85 25.85 FUD 090

32663 **with lobectomy (single lobe)**
EXCLUDES *Thoracoscopic segmentectomy (32669)*
C 80 ⚑ PQ 40.54 40.54 FUD 090

32664 **with thoracic sympathectomy**
C 80 50 ⚑ 24.53 24.53 FUD 090

32665 **with esophagomyotomy (Heller type)**
EXCLUDES *Exploratory thoracoscopy with and without biopsy (32601-32609)*
C 80 ⚑ 35.26 35.26 FUD 090

32666 **with therapeutic wedge resection (eg, mass, nodule), initial unilateral**
Code also a more extensive procedure of the lung when performed on the contralateral lung or different lobe with modifier 59 regardless of pathology consultation
Do not report with (32440-32445, 32488, 32671)
C 80 PQ 25.17 25.17 FUD 090

+ **32667** **with therapeutic wedge resection (eg, mass or nodule), each additional resection, ipsilateral (List separately in addition to code for primary procedure)**
Code also a more extensive procedure of the lung when performed on the contralateral lung or different lobe with modifier 59 regardless of intraoperative pathology consultation
Code first (32666)
Do not report with (32440-32445, 32488, 32671)
C 80 4.58 4.58 FUD ZZZ

+ **32668** **with diagnostic wedge resection followed by anatomic lung resection (List separately in addition to code for primary procedure)**
INCLUDES Classification as a diagnostic wedge resection if intraoperative pathology consultation dictates more extensive resection in the same anatomical area
Code first (32440-32488, 32503-32504, 32663, 32669-32671)
C 80 4.58 4.58 FUD ZZZ

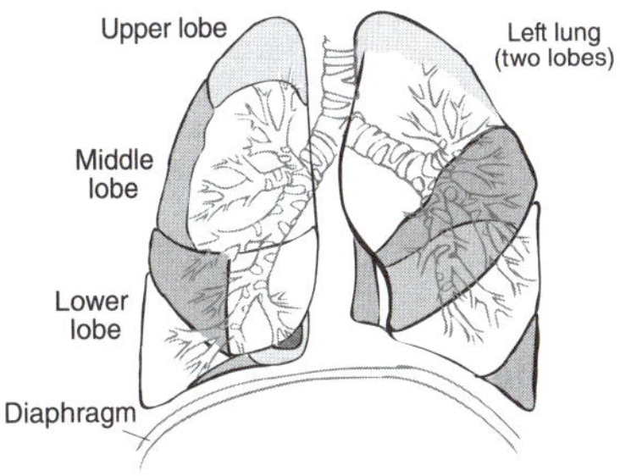

32669 **with removal of a single lung segment (segmentectomy)**
C 80 PQ 38.95 38.95 FUD 090

32670 **with removal of two lobes (bilobectomy)**
C 80 PQ 46.27 46.27 FUD 090

32671 **with removal of lung (pneumonectomy)**
C 80 PQ 51.57 51.57 FUD 090

32672 **with resection-plication for emphysematous lung (bullous or non-bullous) for lung volume reduction (LVRS), unilateral includes any pleural procedure, when performed**
C 80 PQ 44.21 44.21 FUD 090

32673 **with resection of thymus, unilateral or bilateral**
EXCLUDES *Exploratory thoracoscopy with and without biopsy (32601-32609)*
Open excision mediastinal cyst (39200)
Open excision mediastinal tumor (39220)
Open thymectomy (60520-60522)
C 80 PQ 34.92 34.92 FUD 090

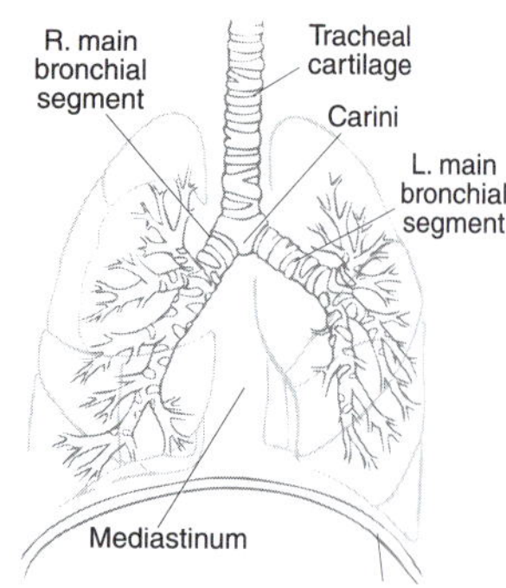

\+ **32674** **with mediastinal and regional lymphadenectomy (List separately in addition to code for primary procedure)**

INCLUDES Mediastinal lymph nodes:
- Left side:
  - Aortopulmonary window
  - Inferior pulmonary ligament
  - Paraesophageal
  - Subcarinal
- Right side:
  - Inferior pulmonary ligament
  - Paraesophageal
  - Paratracheal
  - Subcarinal

EXCLUDES *Mediastinal and regional lymphadenectomy by thoracotomy (38746)*

Code first (19260, 31760, 31766, 31786, 32096-32200, 32220-32320, 32440-32491, 32503-32505, 32601-32663, 32666, 32669-32673, 32815, 33025, 33030, 33050-33130, 39200-39220, 39560-39561, 43101, 43112, 43117-43118, 43122-43123, 43351, 60270, 60505)

C 80 Facility 6.26 Non-Facility 6.26 FUD ZZZ

32701 Target Delineation for Stereotactic Radiation Therapy

INCLUDES Collaboration between the radiation oncologist and surgeon
Correlation of tumor and contiguous body structures
Determination of borders and volume of tumor
Identification of fiducial markers
Verification of target when fiducial markers are not used

EXCLUDES *Fiducial marker insertion (31626, 32553)*
Radiation oncology services ([77295], 77331, 77370, 77373, 77435)

Do not report when performed by same physician as radiation treatment management (77427-77499)

Do not report with (77261-77799 [77295, 77424, 77425])

32701 **Thoracic target(s) delineation for stereotactic body radiation therapy (SRS/SBRT), (photon or particle beam), entire course of treatment**
B 26 80 Facility 6.40 Non-Facility 6.40 FUD XXX

32800-32820 Chest Repair and Reconstruction Procedures

32800 **Repair lung hernia through chest wall**
C 80 PQ Facility 27.27 Non-Facility 27.27 FUD 090

32810 **Closure of chest wall following open flap drainage for empyema (Clagett type procedure)**
C 80 PQ Facility 26.07 Non-Facility 26.07 FUD 090

32815 **Open closure of major bronchial fistula**
C 80 PQ Facility 81.48 Non-Facility 81.48 FUD 090

32820 **Major reconstruction, chest wall (posttraumatic)**
C 80 Facility 38.48 Non-Facility 38.48 FUD 090

32850-32856 Lung Transplant Procedures

INCLUDES Harvesting donor lung(s), cold preservation, preparation of donor lung(s), transplantation into recipient

EXCLUDES *Repairs or resection of donor lung(s) (32491, 32505-32507, 35216, 35276)*

32850 **Donor pneumonectomy(s) (including cold preservation), from cadaver donor**
C Facility 0.00 Non-Facility 0.00 FUD XXX

32851 **Lung transplant, single; without cardiopulmonary bypass**
C 80 Facility 95.43 Non-Facility 95.43 FUD 090

32852 **with cardiopulmonary bypass**
C 80 Facility 104.12 Non-Facility 104.12 FUD 090

32853 **Lung transplant, double (bilateral sequential or en bloc); without cardiopulmonary bypass**
C 80 Facility 133.15 Non-Facility 133.15 FUD 090

32854 **with cardiopulmonary bypass**
C 80 Facility 141.71 Non-Facility 141.71 FUD 090

32855 **Backbench standard preparation of cadaver donor lung allograft prior to transplantation, including dissection of allograft from surrounding soft tissues to prepare pulmonary venous/atrial cuff, pulmonary artery, and bronchus; unilateral**
C 80 Facility 0.00 Non-Facility 0.00 FUD XXX

32856 **bilateral**
EXCLUDES *Procedures on the donor lung*
C 80 Facility 0.00 Non-Facility 0.00 FUD XXX

32900-32997 Chest and Respiratory Procedures

CMS 100-4,12,40.6 Multiple procedures

32900 **Resection of ribs, extrapleural, all stages**
C 80 PQ Facility 40.63 Non-Facility 40.63 FUD 090

32905 **Thoracoplasty, Schede type or extrapleural (all stages);**
C 80 PQ Facility 38.67 Non-Facility 38.67 FUD 090

32906 **with closure of bronchopleural fistula**
EXCLUDES *Open closure of bronchial fistula (32815)*
Resection first rib for thoracic compression (21615-21616)
C 80 PQ Facility 47.81 Non-Facility 47.81 FUD 090

32940 **Pneumonolysis, extraperiosteal, including filling or packing procedures**
C 80 PQ Facility 35.74 Non-Facility 35.74 FUD 090

32960 **Pneumothorax, therapeutic, intrapleural injection of air**
G2 T Facility 2.98 Non-Facility 4.28 FUD 000

32997 **Total lung lavage (unilateral)**
EXCLUDES *Broncho-alveolar lavage by bronchoscopy (31624)*
C 50 Facility 10.21 Non-Facility 10.21 FUD 000

32998-32999 Destruction of Lung Neoplasm

32998 **Ablation therapy for reduction or eradication of 1 or more pulmonary tumor(s) including pleura or chest wall when involved by tumor extension, percutaneous, radiofrequency, unilateral**
Radiology Crosswalk 76940, 77013, 77022
G2 T 80 50 Facility 8.31 Non-Facility 83.51 FUD 000

32999 **Unlisted procedure, lungs and pleura**
T Facility 0.00 Non-Facility 0.00 FUD YYY

33010-33050 Procedures of the Pericardial Sac

EXCLUDES *Surgical thoracoscopy (video-assisted thoracic surgery [VATS]) procedures of pericardium (32601, 32604, 32658-32659, 32661)*

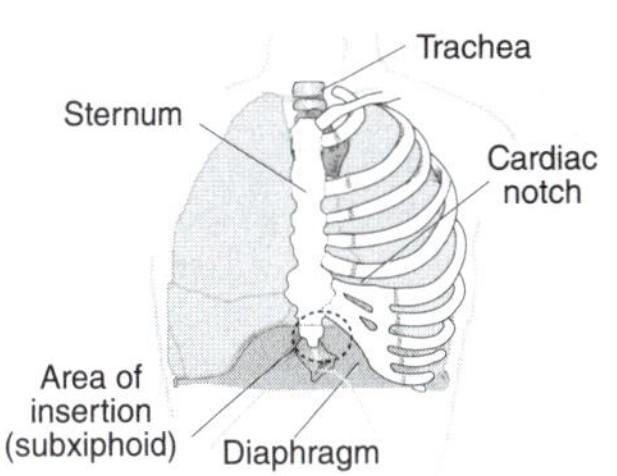

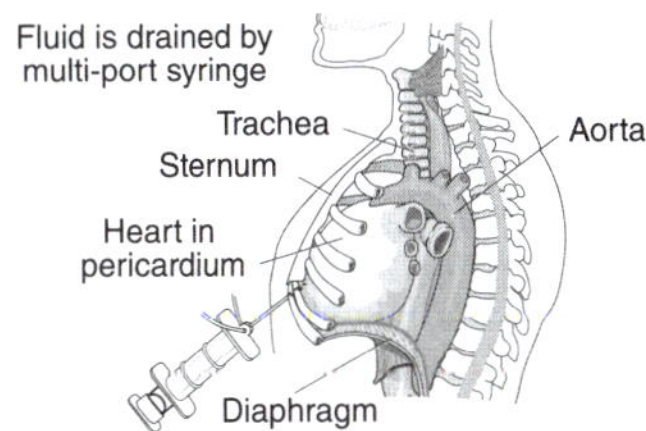

A centesis syringe is inserted into the pericardial sac, either under fluoroscopic guidance or by use of anatomical landmarks, and excess fluid is removed

⊙ **33010 Pericardiocentesis; initial**
76930
A2 T CCI 3.43 3.43 FUD 000

⊙ **33011 subsequent**
76930
A2 T 80 CCI 3.48 3.48 FUD 000

33015 Tube pericardiostomy
C CCI 14.63 14.63 FUD 090

33020 Pericardiotomy for removal of clot or foreign body (primary procedure)
C 80 CCI PQ 25.39 25.39 FUD 090

33025 Creation of pericardial window or partial resection for drainage
EXCLUDES *Surgical thoracoscopy (video-assisted thoracic surgery [VATS]) creation of pericardial window (32659)*
C 80 CCI PQ 23.18 23.18 FUD 090

33030 Pericardiectomy, subtotal or complete; without cardiopulmonary bypass
INCLUDES Delorme pericardiectomy
C 80 CCI PQ 58.16 58.16 FUD 090

33031 with cardiopulmonary bypass
C 80 CCI PQ 72.16 72.16 FUD 090

33050 Resection of pericardial cyst or tumor
EXCLUDES *Open biopsy of pericardium (39010)*
Surgical thoracoscopy (video-assisted thoracic surgery [VATS]) resection of cyst, mass, or tumor of pericardium (32661)
C 80 CCI PQ 28.95 28.95 FUD 090

33120-33130 Neoplasms of Heart

Code also removal of thrombus through a separate heart incision, when performed (33310-33315); append modifier 59 to (33315)

33120 Excision of intracardiac tumor, resection with cardiopulmonary bypass
C 80 CCI PQ 61.16 61.16 FUD 090

33130 Resection of external cardiac tumor
C 80 CCI PQ 40.39 40.39 FUD 090

33140-33141 Transmyocardial Revascularization

CMS 100-3,20.6 Transmyocardial Revascularization (TMR) for Severe Angina

33140 Transmyocardial laser revascularization, by thoracotomy; (separate procedure)
C 80 CCI PQ 45.92 45.92 FUD 090

\+ **33141 performed at the time of other open cardiac procedure(s) (List separately in addition to code for primary procedure)**
Code first (33400-33496, 33510-33536, 33542)
C 80 PQ 3.86 3.86 FUD ZZZ

33202-33203 Placement Epicardial Leads

Code also insertion of pulse generator when performed by same physician/same surgical session (33212-33213, [33221], 33240, [33230, 33231])

Epicardial electrodes are placed on the outside of the heart in an open procedure

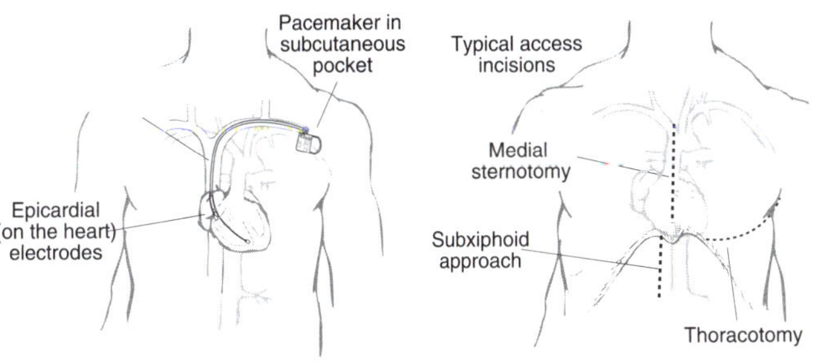

33202 Insertion of epicardial electrode(s); open incision (eg, thoracotomy, median sternotomy, subxiphoid approach)
C PQ 22.44 22.44 FUD 090

33203 endoscopic approach (eg, thoracoscopy, pericardioscopy)
C PQ 23.33 23.33 FUD 090

33206-33214 [33221] Pacemakers

CMS 100-3,20.4 Implantable Automatic Defibrillators
CMS 100-3,20.8 Cardiac Pacemakers
CMS 100-3,20.8.1 Cardiac Pacemaker Evaluation Services
CMS 100-3,20.8.2 Self-contained Pacemaker Monitors

INCLUDES Dual lead: device that paces and senses in two heart chambers
Multiple lead: device that paces and senses in three or more heart chambers
Radiological supervision and interpretation for pacemaker procedure
Single lead: device that paces and senses in one heart chamber
Skin pocket revision, when performed
If revision includes incision/drainage of a wound infection or hematoma code also (10140, 10180, 11042-11044 [11045, 11046, 11047])

EXCLUDES *Electrode repositioning:*
Left ventricle (33226)
Pacemaker (33215)
Insertion of lead for left ventricular (biventricular) pacing (33224-33225)

Do not report with codes for device evaluation (93279-93299 [93260, 93261])

⊙ **33206 Insertion of new or replacement of permanent pacemaker with transvenous electrode(s); atrial**
INCLUDES Pulse generator insertion/transvenous electrode placement
Code also removal of pacemaker pulse generator and electrodes when removal and replacement of pulse generator and electrodes is performed (33233 and 33234 or 33235)
Code also (C1779, C1785, C1786, C1898, C2619, C2620, C2621)
Do not report with (33216-33217, [33227, 33228, 33229])
J8 T CCI PQ 13.17 13.17 FUD 090

⊙ **33207** **ventricular**

INCLUDES Pulse generator insertion/transvenous electrode placement

Code also removal of pacemaker pulse generator and electrodes when removal and replacement of pulse generator and electrodes is performed (33233 and 33234 or 33235)

Code also (C1779, C1785, C1786, C1898, C2619, C2620, C2621)

Do not report with (33216-33217, [33227, 33228, 33229])

J8 T PQ 14.04 14.04 FUD 090

⊙ **33208** **atrial and ventricular**

INCLUDES Pulse generator insertion/transvenous electrode placement

Code also removal of pacemaker pulse generator and electrodes when removal and replacement of pulse generator and electrodes is performed (33233 and 33234 or 33235)

Code also (C1779, C1785, C1898, C2619, C2621)

Do not report with (33216-33217, [33227, 33228, 33229])

J8 T PQ 15.20 15.20 FUD 090

⊙ **33210** **Insertion or replacement of temporary transvenous single chamber cardiac electrode or pacemaker catheter (separate procedure)**

G2 T 5.15 5.15 FUD 000

⊙ **33211** **Insertion or replacement of temporary transvenous dual chamber pacing electrodes (separate procedure)**

Code also (C1779, C1898)

G2 T 5.29 5.29 FUD 000

⊙ **33212** **Insertion of pacemaker pulse generator only; with existing single lead**

EXCLUDES *Removal and replacement of pacemaker pulse generator ([33227, 33228, 33229])*

Code also placement of epicardial leads by same physician/same surgical session (33202-33203)

Code also (C1786, C2620, C2621)

Do not report with (33216-33217, 33233)

J8 T PQ 9.52 9.52 FUD 090

⊙ **33213** **with existing dual leads**

EXCLUDES *Removal and replacement of pacemaker pulse generator ([33227, 33228, 33229])*

Code also placement of epicardial leads by same physician/same surgical session (33202-33203)

Code also (C1785, C2619, C2621)

Do not report with (33216-33217, 33233)

J8 T PQ 9.95 9.95 FUD 090

⊙ # **33221** **with existing multiple leads**

EXCLUDES *Removal and replacement of pacemaker pulse generator ([33227, 33228, 33229])*

Code also placement of epicardial leads by same physician/same surgical session (33202-33203)

Code also (C1786, C2619, C2620, C2621)

Do not report with (33216-33217, 33233)

J8 T 10.58 10.58 FUD 090

⊙ **33214** **Upgrade of implanted pacemaker system, conversion of single chamber system to dual chamber system (includes removal of previously placed pulse generator, testing of existing lead, insertion of new lead, insertion of new pulse generator)**

Code also (C1779, C1785, C1898, C2619, C2621)

Do not report with (33216-33217, [33227, 33228, 33229])

J8 T 80 PQ 14.02 14.02 FUD 090

33215-33249 [33227, 33228, 33229, 33230, 33231, 33262, 33263, 33264] Pacemakers/Implantable Defibrillator/Electrode Insertion/Replacement/Revision/Repair

INCLUDES Dual lead: device that paces and senses in two heart chambers

Multiple lead: device that paces and senses in three or more heart chambers

Radiological supervision and interpretation for pacemaker or pacing cardioverter-defibrillator procedure

Single lead: device that paces and senses in one heart chamber

Skin pocket revision, when performed

If revision includes incision/drainage of a wound infection or hematoma code also (10140, 10180, 11042-11044 [11045, 11046, 11047])

EXCLUDES *Electrode repositioning:*

Left ventricle (33226)

Pacemaker or implantable defibrillator (33215)

Insertion of lead for left ventricular (biventricular) pacing (33224-33225)

Testing of defibrillator threshold (DFT) during insertion/replacement (93640-93641)

Do not report with codes for device evaluation (93279-93299 [93260, 93261])

▲ **33215** **Repositioning of previously implanted transvenous pacemaker or implantable defibrillator (right atrial or right ventricular) electrode**

G2 T PQ 8.82 8.82 FUD 090

⊙ ▲ **33216** **Insertion of a single transvenous electrode, permanent pacemaker or implantable defibrillator**

EXCLUDES *Insertion or replacement of a lead for a cardiac venous system (33224-33225)*

Code also (C1777, C1779, C1895, C1896, C1898, C1899)

Do not report with (33206-33208, 33212-33213, [33221], 33214, [33227, 33228, 33229], 33240, [33230, 33231], [33262, 33263, 33264], 33249)

G2 T PQ 10.89 10.89 FUD 090

⊙ ▲ **33217** **Insertion of 2 transvenous electrodes, permanent pacemaker or implantable defibrillator**

EXCLUDES *Insertion or replacement of a lead for a cardiac venous system (33224-33225)*

Code also (C1777, C1779, C1895, C1896, C1898, C1899)

Do not report with (33206-33208, 33212-33213, [33221], 33214, [33227, 33228, 33229], 33240, [33230, 33231], [33262, 33263, 33264], 33249)

G2 T PQ 10.73 10.73 FUD 090

⊙ ▲ **33218** **Repair of single transvenous electrode, permanent pacemaker or implantable defibrillator**

Code also replacement of pacemaker pulse generator, when performed ([33227, 33228, 33229])

Code also replacement of implantable defibrillator pulse generator, when performed ([33262, 33263, 33264])

G2 T PQ 11.38 11.38 FUD 090

⊙ ▲ **33220** **Repair of 2 transvenous electrodes for permanent pacemaker or implantable defibrillator**

Code also modifier 52 Reduced services, when one electrode of a two-chamber system is repaired

Code also replacement of pacemaker pulse generator, when performed ([33228, 33229])

Code also replacement of implantable defibrillator pulse generator, when performed ([33263, 33264])

G2 T PQ 11.46 11.46 FUD 090

33207 — 33220

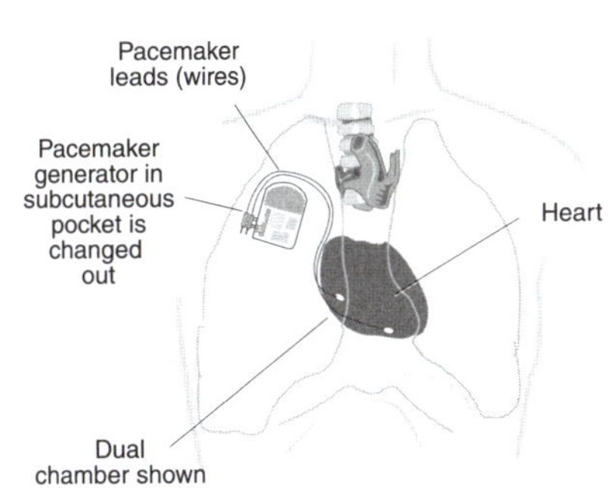

33221 Resequenced code. See code following 33213.

⊙ **33222 Relocation of skin pocket for pacemaker**

INCLUDES Formation of the new pocket
Procedures related to the existing pocket:
Accessing the pocket
Incision/drainage of any abscess or hematoma
Pocket closure

Code also removal and replacement of an existing generator

Do not report with (10140, 10180, 11042-11044 [11045, 11046, 11047], 13100-13102)

A2 T CCI PQ 9.96 9.96 FUD 090

⊙ ▲ **33223 Relocation of skin pocket for implantable defibrillator**

INCLUDES Formation of the new pocket
Procedures related to the existing pocket:
Accessing the pocket
Incision/drainage of any abscess or hematoma
Pocket closure

Code also removal and replacement of an existing generator

Do not report with (10140, 10180, 11042-11044 [11045, 11046, 11047], 13100-13102)

A2 T 80 CCI PQ 12.00 12.00 FUD 090

▲ **33224 Insertion of pacing electrode, cardiac venous system, for left ventricular pacing, with attachment to previously placed pacemaker or implantable defibrillator pulse generator (including revision of pocket, removal, insertion, and/or replacement of existing generator)**

Code also placement of epicardial electrode when appropriate (33202-33203)

Code also (C1900)

J8 T CCI PQ 14.71 14.71 FUD 000

+ ▲ **33225 Insertion of pacing electrode, cardiac venous system, for left ventricular pacing, at time of insertion of implantable defibrillator or pacemaker pulse generator (eg, for upgrade to dual chamber system) (List separately in addition to code for primary procedure)**

Code also (C1900)

Code first (33206-33208, 33212-33213, [33221], 33214, 33216-33217, 33223, 33233, [33228, 33229], 33234-33235, 33240, [33230, 33231], [33263, 33264], 33249)

Code first (33222) for relocation of pocket for pacemaker pulse generator

Code first (33223) for relocation of pocket for implantable defibrillator

J8 Q3 CCI PQ 13.34 13.34 FUD ZZZ

33226 Repositioning of previously implanted cardiac venous system (left ventricular) electrode (including removal, insertion and/or replacement of existing generator)

G2 T CCI PQ 14.12 14.12 FUD 000

33227 Resequenced code. See code following 33233.

33228 Resequenced code. See code following 33233.

33229 Resequenced code. See code before 33234.

33230 Resequenced code. See code following 33240.

33231 Resequenced code. See code before 33241.

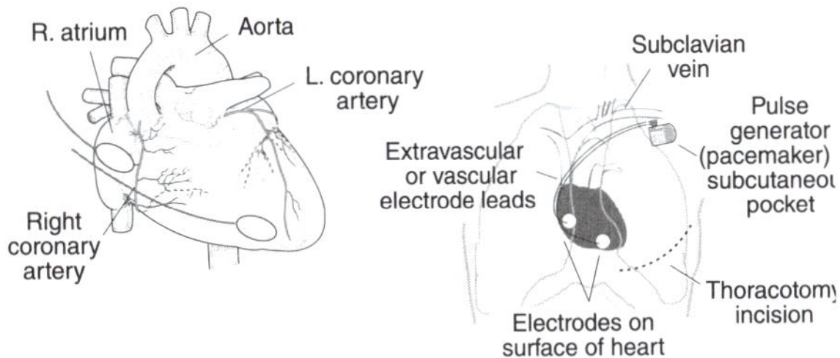

⊙ **33233 Removal of permanent pacemaker pulse generator only**

EXCLUDES *Removal and replacement of pacemaker pulse generator and transvenous electrode(s): code 33233 with (33206 or 33207 or 33208, and 33234 or 33235)*

Do not report with ([33227, 33228, 33229])

A2 Q2 CCI PQ 6.88 6.88 FUD 090

⊙ # **33227 Removal of permanent pacemaker pulse generator with replacement of pacemaker pulse generator; single lead system**

Code also (C1786, C2620)

Do not report with (33214, 33216-33217, 33233)

J8 T 10.03 10.03 FUD 090

⊙ # **33228 dual lead system**

Code also (C1785, C2619, C2621)

Do not report with (33214, 33216-33217, 33233)

J8 T 10.45 10.45 FUD 090

⊙ # **33229 multiple lead system**

Code also (C2621)

Do not report with (33214, 33216-33217, 33233)

J8 T 10.97 10.97 FUD 090

⊙ **33234 Removal of transvenous pacemaker electrode(s); single lead system, atrial or ventricular**

EXCLUDES *Removal and replacement of pacemaker pulse generator and transvenous electrode 33234 and 33233 and (33206 or 33207 or 33208)*
Thoracotomy to remove electrodes (33238)

Code also pacing electrode insertion in cardiac venous system for pacing of left ventricle during insertion of pulse generator (pacemaker or implantable defibrillator) when performed (33225)

G2 Q2 CCI PQ 14.14 14.14 FUD 090

⊙ **33235 dual lead system**

EXCLUDES *Removal and replacement of pacemaker pulse generator and transvenous electrode(s) 33235 and 33233 and (33206 or 33207 or 33208)*
Thoracotomy to remove electrodes (33238, 33243)

Code also pacing electrode insertion in cardiac venous system for pacing of left ventricle during insertion of pulse generator (pacemaker or implantable defibrillator) when performed (33225)

G2 Q2 CCI PQ 18.45 18.45 FUD 090

33236 Removal of permanent epicardial pacemaker and electrodes by thoracotomy; single lead system, atrial or ventricular

EXCLUDES *Removal of implantable defibrillator electrode(s) by thoracotomy (33243)*
Removal of transvenous electrodes by thoracotomy (33238)
Removal of transvenous pacemaker electrodes, single or dual lead system; without thoracotomy (33234, 33235)

C 80 22.81 22.81 FUD 090

33237 dual lead system

EXCLUDES *Removal of implantable defibrillator electrode(s) by thoracotomy (33243)*
Removal of transvenous electrodes by thoracotomy (33238)
Removal of transvenous pacemaker electrodes, single or dual lead system; without thoracotomy (33234, 33235)

C 80 24.29 24.29 FUD 090

33238 Removal of permanent transvenous electrode(s) by thoracotomy

EXCLUDES *Removal of implantable defibrillator electrode(s) by thoracotomy (33243)*
Removal of transvenous pacemaker electrodes, single or dual lead system; without thoracotomy (33234, 33235)

C 80 27.21 27.21 FUD 090

⊙ ▲ **33240 Insertion of implantable defibrillator pulse generator only; with existing single lead**

EXCLUDES *Removal and replacement of implantable defibrillator pulse generator ([33262, 33263, 33264])*

Code also placement of epicardial leads by same physician/same surgical session as generator insertion (33202-33203)
Code also (C1721-C1722, C1882)
Do not report with (33216-33217, [33271], [93260], [93261])

J8 T 10.83 10.83 FUD 090

⊙ #▲ **33230 with existing dual leads**

EXCLUDES *Removal and replacement of implantable defibrillator pulse generator ([33262, 33263, 33264])*

Code also placement of epicardial leads by same physician/same surgical session as generator insertion (33202-33203)
Code also (C1721, C1882)
Do not report with (33216-33217)

J8 T 11.40 11.40 FUD 090

⊙ #▲ **33231 with existing multiple leads**

EXCLUDES *Removal and replacement of implantable defibrillator pulse generator ([33262, 33263, 33264])*

Code also placement of epicardial leads by same physician/same surgical session as generator placement (33202-33203)
Code also (C1882)
Do not report with (33216-33217)

J8 T 11.76 11.76 FUD 090

⊙ ▲ **33241 Removal of implantable defibrillator pulse generator only**

Code also electrode removal by thoracotomy (33243)
Code also insertion of subcutaneous defibrillator system and removal of subcutaneous defibrillator lead, when performed ([33270] and [33272])
Code also removal of defibrillator leads and insertion of defibrillator system, when performed (33243 or 33244 and 33249)
Code also transvenous removal of electrode(s) (33244)
Do not report with (33240, [33230, 33231], [33262, 33263, 33264], [93260], [93261])

G2 Q2 6.48 6.48 FUD 090

⊙ #▲ **33262 Removal of implantable defibrillator pulse generator with replacement of implantable defibrillator pulse generator; single lead system**

EXCLUDES *Repair of implantable defibrillator pulse generator and/or leads (33218, 33220)*

Code also subcutaneous electrode removal ([33272])
Code also electrode(s) removal by thoracotomy (33243)
Code also transvenous removal of electrode(s) (33244)
Code also (C1722)
Do not report with (33216-33217, 33241, [33271], [93260], [93261])

J8 T 10.99 10.99 FUD 090

⊙ #▲ **33263 dual lead system**

EXCLUDES *Repair of implantable defibrillator pulse generator and/or leads (33218, 33220)*

Code also subcutaneous electrode removal ([33272])
Code also removal of electrodes by thoracotomy (33243)
Code also transvenous removal of electrodes (33244)
Code also (C1721, C1882)
Do not report with (33216-33217, 33241)

J8 T 11.43 11.43 FUD 090

⊙ #▲ **33264 multiple lead system**

EXCLUDES *Repair of implantable defibrillator pulse generator and/or leads (33218, 33220)*

Code also subcutaneous electrode removal ([33272])
Code also removal of electrodes by thoracotomy (33243)
Code also transvenous removal of electrodes (33244)
Code also (C1882)
Do not report with (33216-33217, 33241)

J8 T 11.91 11.91 FUD 090

▲ **33243 Removal of single or dual chamber implantable defibrillator electrode(s); by thoracotomy**

EXCLUDES *Transvenous removal of defibrillator electrode(s) (33244)*

Code also removal of defibrillator generator and insertion/replacement of defibrillator system (generator and leads), when performed (33241 and 33249)

C 80 39.66 39.66 FUD 090

⊙ ▲ **33244 by transvenous extraction**

EXCLUDES *Thoracotomy to remove electrodes (33243)*

Code also removal of defibrillator generator and insertion/replacement of defibrillator system (generator and leads), when performed (33241 and 33249)

Q2 24.80 24.80 FUD 090

⊙ ▲ **33249 Insertion or replacement of permanent implantable defibrillator system, with transvenous lead(s), single or dual chamber**

Code also removal of defibrillator generator and removal of leads (by thoracotomy or transvenous), when performed(33241 and 33243 or 33244)
Code also removal of defibrillator generator when upgrading from single to dual-chamber system (33241)
Code also (C1722, C1777, C1779, C1882, C1895, C1896, C1898, C1900)
Do not report with (33216-33217)

J8 Q3 26.40 26.40 FUD 090

33270-33273 [33270, 33271, 33272, 33273] Subcutaneous Implantable Defibrillator

Do not report with ([93260], [93261])

#● **33270 Insertion or replacement of permanent subcutaneous implantable defibrillator system, with subcutaneous electrode, including defibrillation threshold evaluation, induction of arrhythmia, evaluation of sensing for arrhythmia termination, and programming or reprogramming of sensing or therapeutic parameters, when performed**

Code also removal of defibrillator generator and subcutaneous electrode, when performed (33241 and [33272])
Do not report with ([33271], 93644)

#● **33271 Insertion of subcutaneous implantable defibrillator electrode**

Do not report with (33240, [33262], [33270])

#● **33272 Removal of subcutaneous implantable defibrillator electrode**

Code also removal defibrillator generator and insertion/replacement subcutaneous defibrillator system (generator and leads), when performed (33241 and [33270])

Code also removal of defibrillator generator with replacement, when performed ([33262])

Code also removal of defibrillator generator (without replacement), when performed (33241)

#● **33273 Repositioning of previously implanted subcutaneous implantable defibrillator electrode**

33250-33251 Surgical Ablation Arrhythmogenic Foci, Supraventricular

INCLUDES Procedures using cryotherapy, laser, microwave, radiofrequency, and ultrasound

33250 Operative ablation of supraventricular arrhythmogenic focus or pathway (eg, Wolff-Parkinson-White, atrioventricular node re-entry), tract(s) and/or focus (foci); without cardiopulmonary bypass

EXCLUDES *Pacing and mapping during surgery by other provider (93631)*

C 80 CCI PQ 42.79 42.79 FUD 090

33251 with cardiopulmonary bypass

C 80 CCI PQ 47.37 47.37 FUD 090

33254-33256 Surgical Ablation Arrhythmogenic Foci, Atrial (e.g., Maze)

INCLUDES Excision or isolation of the left atrial appendage

Procedures using cryotherapy, laser, microwave, radiofrequency, and ultrasound

Do not report with (32100, 32551, 33120, 33130, 33210-33211, 33400-33507, 33510-33523, 33533-33548, 33600-33853, 33860-33864, 33910-33920)

Do not report with any procedure involving median sternotomy or cardiopulmonary bypass

33254 Operative tissue ablation and reconstruction of atria, limited (eg, modified maze procedure)

C 80 PQ 39.74 39.74 FUD 090

33255 Operative tissue ablation and reconstruction of atria, extensive (eg, maze procedure); without cardiopulmonary bypass

C 80 PQ 48.34 48.34 FUD 090

33256 with cardiopulmonary bypass

C 80 PQ 57.12 57.12 FUD 090

33257-33259 Surgical Ablation Arrhythmogenic Foci, Atrial, with Other Heart Procedure(s)

Do not report with (32551, 33210-33211, 33254-33256, 33265-33266)

\+ **33257 Operative tissue ablation and reconstruction of atria, performed at the time of other cardiac procedure(s), limited (eg, modified maze procedure) (List separately in addition to code for primary procedure)**

Code first (33120-33130, 33250-33251, 33261, 33300-33335, 33400-33496, 33500-33507, 33510-33516, 33533-33548, 33600-33619, 33641-33697, 33702-33732, 33735-33767, 33770-33814, 33840-33877, 33910-33922, 33925-33926, 33935, 33945, 33975-33980)

C 80 16.95 16.95 FUD ZZZ

\+ **33258 Operative tissue ablation and reconstruction of atria, performed at the time of other cardiac procedure(s), extensive (eg, maze procedure), without cardiopulmonary bypass (List separately in addition to code for primary procedure)**

Code first (33130, 33250, 33300, 33310, 33320-33321, 33330, 33401, 33414-33417, 33420, 33470-33471, 33501-33503, 33510-33516, 33533-33536, 33690, 33735, 33737, 33800-33813, 33840-33852, 33915, 33925)

C 80 19.05 19.05 FUD ZZZ

\+ **33259 Operative tissue ablation and reconstruction of atria, performed at the time of other cardiac procedure(s), extensive (eg, maze procedure), with cardiopulmonary bypass (List separately in addition to code for primary procedure)**

Code first (33120, 33251, 33261, 33305, 33315, 33322, 33335, 33400, 33403-33413, 33422-33468, 33474-33478, 33496, 33500, 33504-33507, 33510-33516, 33533-33548, 33600-33688, 33692-33722, 33730, 33732, 33736, 33750-33767, 33770-33781, 33786-33788, 33814, 33853, 33860-33877, 33910, 33916-33922, 33926, 33935, 33945, 33975-33980)

C 80 24.63 24.63 FUD ZZZ

33261-33264 Surgical Ablation Arrhythmogenic Foci, Ventricular

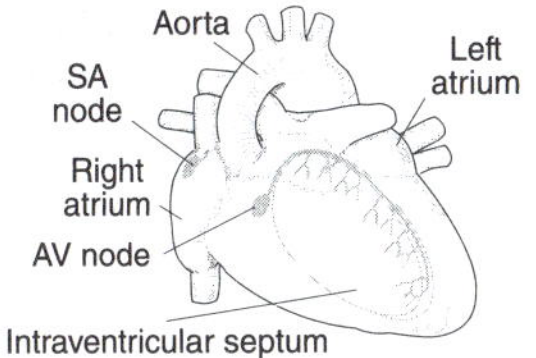

33261 Operative ablation of ventricular arrhythmogenic focus with cardiopulmonary bypass

C 80 CCI PQ 47.97 47.97 FUD 090

33262 Resequenced code. See code following 33241.

33263 Resequenced code. See code following 33241.

33264 Resequenced code. See code before 33243.

33265-33273 Surgical Ablation Arrhythmogenic Foci, Endoscopic

Do not report with (32551, 33210-33211)

33265 Endoscopy, surgical; operative tissue ablation and reconstruction of atria, limited (eg, modified maze procedure), without cardiopulmonary bypass

C 80 39.68 39.68 FUD 090

33266 operative tissue ablation and reconstruction of atria, extensive (eg, maze procedure), without cardiopulmonary bypass

C 80 53.87 53.87 FUD 090

33270 Resequenced code. See code following 33249.

33271 Resequenced code. See code following 33249.

33272 Resequenced code. See code following 33249.

33273 Resequenced code. See code following 33249.

33282-33284 Implantable Loop Recorder

CMS 100-3,20.15 Electrocardiographic Services

⊙ **33282 Implantation of patient-activated cardiac event recorder**

INCLUDES Initial programming of device

EXCLUDES *Subsequent electronic analysis and/or reprogramming of device (93285, 93291, 93298-93299)*

Code also (C1764)

6.79 6.79 FUD 090

⊙ **33284 Removal of an implantable, patient-activated cardiac event recorder**

5.99 5.99 FUD 090

33300-33315 Procedures for Injury of the Heart

INCLUDES Procedures with and without cardiopulmonary bypass

EXCLUDES *Cardiac assist services (33946-33949, 33967-33983, 33990-33993)*

33300 Repair of cardiac wound; without bypass

71.18 71.18 FUD 090

33305 with cardiopulmonary bypass

119.49 119.49 FUD 090

33310 Cardiotomy, exploratory (includes removal of foreign body, atrial or ventricular thrombus); without bypass

Do not report with other cardiac procedures unless separate incision into heart is necessary in order to remove thrombus

33.76 33.76 FUD 090

33315 with cardiopulmonary bypass

Code also excision of thrombus with cardiopulmonary bypass and append modifier 59 if separate incision is required with (33120, 33130, 33420-33430, 33460-33468, 33496, 33542, 33545, 33641-33647, 33670, 33681, 33975-33980)

Do not report with other cardiac procedures unless separate incision into heart is necessary in order to remove thrombus

55.90 55.90 FUD 090

33320-33335 Procedures for Injury of the Aorta/Great Vessels

33320 Suture repair of aorta or great vessels; without shunt or cardiopulmonary bypass

30.94 30.94 FUD 090

33321 with shunt bypass

34.76 34.76 FUD 090

33322 with cardiopulmonary bypass

40.42 40.42 FUD 090

33330 Insertion of graft, aorta or great vessels; without shunt, or cardiopulmonary bypass

41.88 41.88 FUD 090

~~**33332 with shunt bypass**~~

33335 with cardiopulmonary bypass

54.83 54.83 FUD 090

33361-33369 Transcatheter Aortic Valve Replacement

INCLUDES Access and implantation of the aortic valve (33361-33366)
- Access sheath placement
- Advancement of valve delivery system
- Arteriotomy closure
- Balloon aortic valvuloplasty
- Cardiac or open arterial approach
- Deployment of valve
- Percutaneous access
- Temporary pacemaker
- Valve repositioning when necessary
- Radiology procedures:
  - Angiography during and after procedure
  - Assessment of access site for closure
  - Documentation of completion of the intervention
  - Guidance for valve placement
  - Supervision and interpretation

EXCLUDES *Percutaneous coronary interventional procedures*
Transvascular ventricular support (33967, 33970, 33973, 33975-33976, 33990-33993, 33999)

Code also add-on codes for cardiopulmonary bypass, when appropriate (33367-33369)

Code also cardiac catheterization services for purposes other than TAVR/TAVI

Code also diagnostic coronary angiography at a different session from the interventional procedure

Code also diagnostic coronary angiography at the same time as TAVR/TAVI when:
- A previous study is available, but documentation states the patient's condition has changed since the previous study, visualization of the anatomy/pathology is inadequate, or a change occurs during the procedure warranting additional evaluation of an area outside the current target area
- No previous catheter-based coronary angiography study is available, and a full diagnostic study is performed, with the decision to perform the intervention based on that study

Code also modifier 59 when diagnostic coronary angiography procedures are performed as separate and distinct procedural services on the same day or session as TAVR/TAVI

Code also modifier 62 as all TAVI/TAVR procedures require the work of two physicians

Do not report separately when included in the TAVR/TAVI service (93452-93453, 93458-93461, 93567)

33361 Transcatheter aortic valve replacement (TAVR/TAVI) with prosthetic valve; percutaneous femoral artery approach

Code also cardiopulmonary bypass when performed (33367-33369)

39.18 39.18 FUD 000

33362 open femoral artery approach

Code also cardiopulmonary bypass when performed (33367-33369)

42.85 42.85 FUD 000

33363 open axillary artery approach

Code also cardiopulmonary bypass when performed (33367-33369)

44.35 44.35 FUD 000

33364 open iliac artery approach

Code also cardiopulmonary bypass when performed (33367-33369)

46.66 46.66 FUD 000

33365 transaortic approach (eg, median sternotomy, mediastinotomy)

Code also cardiopulmonary bypass when performed (33367-33369)

51.46 51.46 FUD 000

33366 transapical exposure (eg, left thoracotomy)

Code also cardiopulmonary bypass when performed (33367-33369)

55.69 55.69 FUD 000

\+ **33367 cardiopulmonary bypass support with percutaneous peripheral arterial and venous cannulation (eg, femoral vessels) (List separately in addition to code for primary procedure)**

Code first (33361-33366, 33418)

Do not report with (33368-33369)

17.97 17.97 FUD ZZZ

+ **33368** **cardiopulmonary bypass support with open peripheral arterial and venous cannulation (eg, femoral, iliac, axillary vessels) (List separately in addition to code for primary procedure)**
Code first (33361-33366, 33418)
Do not report with (33367, 33369)
C 80 21.78 21.78 FUD ZZZ

+ **33369** **cardiopulmonary bypass support with central arterial and venous cannulation (eg, aorta, right atrium, pulmonary artery) (List separately in addition to code for primary procedure)**
Code first (33361-33366, 33418)
Do not report with (33367-33368)
C 80 28.74 28.74 FUD ZZZ

33400-33415 Aortic Valve Procedures

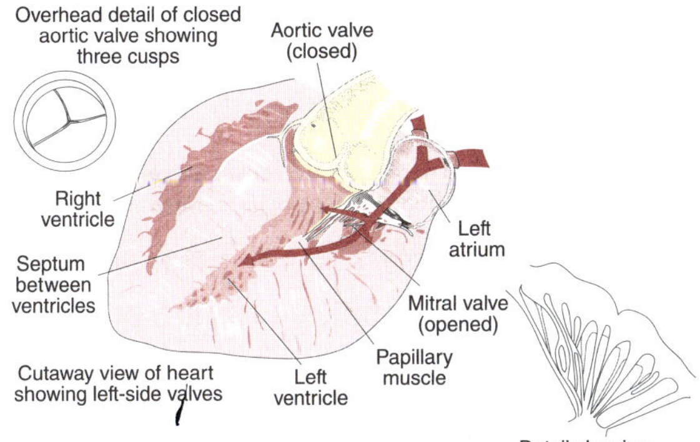

33400 **Valvuloplasty, aortic valve; open, with cardiopulmonary bypass**
C 80 PQ 66.63 66.63 FUD 090

33401 **open, with inflow occlusion**
C 80 PQ 63 41.32 41.32 FUD 090

33403 **using transventricular dilation, with cardiopulmonary bypass**
C 80 PQ 63 43.31 43.31 FUD 090

33404 **Construction of apical-aortic conduit**
C 80 PQ 50.97 50.97 FUD 090

33405 **Replacement, aortic valve, with cardiopulmonary bypass; with prosthetic valve other than homograft or stentless valve**
EXCLUDES *Valvotomy of aortic valve:*
With cardiopulmonary bypass (33403)
With inflow occlusion (33401)
C 80 PQ 66.29 66.29 FUD 090

33406 **with allograft valve (freehand)**
EXCLUDES *Valvotomy of aortic valve:*
With cardiopulmonary bypass (33403)
With inflow occlusion (33401)
C 80 PQ 84.01 84.01 FUD 090

33410 **with stentless tissue valve**
C 80 PQ 74.15 74.15 FUD 090

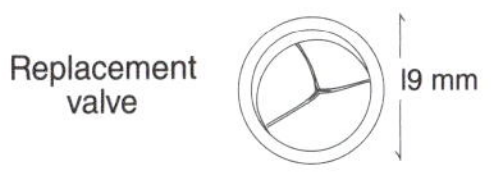

The aortic valve is replaced

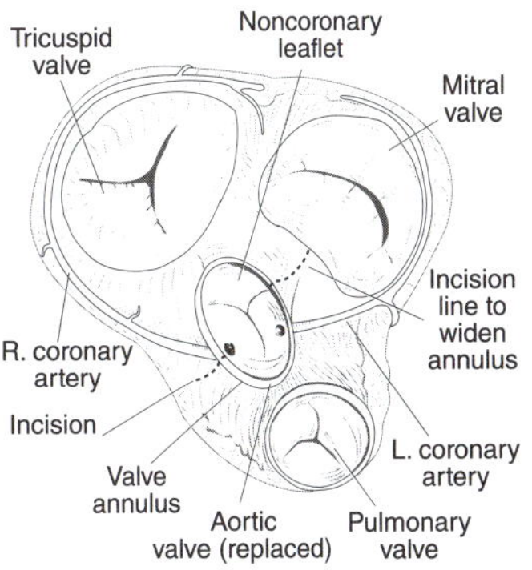

Overhead schematic of major heart valves

33411 **Replacement, aortic valve; with aortic annulus enlargement, noncoronary sinus**
C 80 PQ 98.05 98.05 FUD 090

33412 **with transventricular aortic annulus enlargement (Konno procedure)**
C 80 PQ 92.95 92.95 FUD 090

33413 **by translocation of autologous pulmonary valve with allograft replacement of pulmonary valve (Ross procedure)**
C 80 PQ 94.14 94.14 FUD 090

33414 **Repair of left ventricular outflow tract obstruction by patch enlargement of the outflow tract**
C 80 PQ 62.77 62.77 FUD 090

33415 **Resection or incision of subvalvular tissue for discrete subvalvular aortic stenosis**
C 80 PQ 59.12 59.12 FUD 090

33416 Ventriculectomy

CMS 100-3,20.26 Partial Ventriculectomy

EXCLUDES *Percutaneous transcatheter septal reduction therapy (93583)*

33416 **Ventriculomyotomy (-myectomy) for idiopathic hypertrophic subaortic stenosis (eg, asymmetric septal hypertrophy)**
C 80 PQ 59.32 59.32 FUD 090

33417 Repair of Supravalvular Stenosis by Aortoplasty

33417 **Aortoplasty (gusset) for supravalvular stenosis**
C 80 PQ 48.41 48.41 FUD 090

33418-33419 Transcatheter Mitral Valve Procedures

INCLUDES Access sheath placement
Advancement of valve delivery system
Deployment of valve
Radiology procedures:
- Angiography during and after procedure
- Documentation of completion of the intervention
- Guidance for valve placement
- Supervision and interpretation

Valve repositioning when necessary

EXCLUDES *Cardiac catheterization services for purposes other than TMVR*
Diagnostic angiography at different session from interventional procedure
Percutaneous coronary interventional procedures

Code also cardiopulmonary bypass:
Central (33369)
Open peripheral (33368)
Percutaneous peripheral (33367)

Code also diagnostic coronary angiography and cardiac catheterization procedures when:
- No previous study available and full diagnostic study performed
- Previous study inadequate or patient's clinical indication for the study changed prior to or during the procedure
- Use modifier 59 with cardiac catheterization procedures when on same day or same session as TMVR

Code also transvascular ventricular support:
- Balloon pump (33967, 33970, 33973)
- Ventricular assist device (33990-33993)

● **33418** **Transcatheter mitral valve repair, percutaneous approach, including transseptal puncture when performed; initial prosthesis**
Code also left heart catheterization when performed by transapical puncture (93462)

\+ ● **33419** **additional prosthesis(es) during same session (List separately in addition to code for primary procedure)**
EXCLUDES *Percutaneous approach through the coronary sinus for TMVR (0345T)*
Code first (33418)
Do not report more than one time per session

33420-33430 Mitral Valve Procedures

Code also removal of thrombus through a separate heart incision, when performed (33310-33315); append modifier 59 to (33315)

33420 **Valvotomy, mitral valve; closed heart**
C PQ 42.45 42.45 FUD 090

33422 **open heart, with cardiopulmonary bypass**
C 80 PQ 49.18 49.18 FUD 090

33425 **Valvuloplasty, mitral valve, with cardiopulmonary bypass;**
C 80 PQ 79.80 79.80 FUD 090

33426 **with prosthetic ring**
C 80 PQ 69.58 69.58 FUD 090

33427 **radical reconstruction, with or without ring**
C 80 PQ 71.43 71.43 FUD 090

33430 **Replacement, mitral valve, with cardiopulmonary bypass**
C 80 PQ 81.73 81.73 FUD 090

33460-33468 Tricuspid Valve Procedures

Code also removal of thrombus through a separate heart incision, when performed (33310-33315); append modifier 59 to (33315)

33460 **Valvectomy, tricuspid valve, with cardiopulmonary bypass**
C 80 PQ 71.19 71.19 FUD 090

33463 **Valvuloplasty, tricuspid valve; without ring insertion**
C 80 PQ 90.25 90.25 FUD 090

33464 **with ring insertion**
C 80 PQ 71.47 71.47 FUD 090

33465 **Replacement, tricuspid valve, with cardiopulmonary bypass**
C 80 PQ 80.53 80.53 FUD 090

33468 **Tricuspid valve repositioning and plication for Ebstein anomaly**
C 80 PQ 71.59 71.59 FUD 090

33470-33474 Pulmonary Valvotomy

INCLUDES Brock's operation

Code also the concurrent ligation/takedown of a systemic-to-pulmonary artery shunt (33924)

33470 **Valvotomy, pulmonary valve, closed heart; transventricular**
C 80 PQ 63 37.41 37.41 FUD 090

33471 **via pulmonary artery**
EXCLUDES *Percutaneous valvuloplasty of pulmonary valve (92990)*
C 80 PQ 40.35 40.35 FUD 090

33472 ~~**Valvotomy, pulmonary valve, open heart; with inflow occlusion**~~

33474 **Valvotomy, pulmonary valve, open heart, with cardiopulmonary bypass**
C 80 PQ 63.28 63.28 FUD 090

33475-33478 Other Procedures Pulmonary Valve

Code also the concurrent ligation/takedown of a systemic-to-pulmonary artery shunt (33924)

33475 **Replacement, pulmonary valve**
C 80 PQ 68.47 68.47 FUD 090

33476 **Right ventricular resection for infundibular stenosis, with or without commissurotomy**
INCLUDES Brock's operation
C 80 PQ 44.59 44.59 FUD 090

33478 **Outflow tract augmentation (gusset), with or without commissurotomy or infundibular resection**
Code also (33768) for cavopulmonary anastomosis to a second superior vena cava
C 80 PQ 45.83 45.83 FUD 090

33496 Prosthetic Valve Repair

Code also reoperation if performed (33530)
Code also removal of thrombus through a separate heart incision, when performed (33310-33315); append modifier 59 to (33315)

33496 **Repair of non-structural prosthetic valve dysfunction with cardiopulmonary bypass (separate procedure)**
C 80 PQ 48.53 48.53 FUD 090

33500-33507 Repair Aberrant Coronary Artery Anatomy

INCLUDES Angioplasty and/or endarterectomy

33500 **Repair of coronary arteriovenous or arteriocardiac chamber fistula; with cardiopulmonary bypass**
C 80 46.15 46.15 FUD 090

33501 **without cardiopulmonary bypass**
C 80 32.97 32.97 FUD 090

33502 **Repair of anomalous coronary artery from pulmonary artery origin; by ligation**
C 80 63 37.20 37.20 FUD 090

33503 **by graft, without cardiopulmonary bypass**
C 80 63 38.16 38.16 FUD 090

33504 **by graft, with cardiopulmonary bypass**
C 80 42.93 42.93 FUD 090

33505 **with construction of intrapulmonary artery tunnel (Takeuchi procedure)**
C 80 63 60.56 60.56 FUD 090

33506 **by translocation from pulmonary artery to aorta**
C 80 63 59.72 59.72 FUD 090

33507 **Repair of anomalous (eg, intramural) aortic origin of coronary artery by unroofing or translocation**
C 80 49.84 49.84 FUD 090

33508 Endoscopic Harvesting of Venous Graft

INCLUDES Diagnostic endoscopy

EXCLUDES *Harvesting of vein of upper extremity (35500)*

Code first (33510-33523)

\+ **33508** **Endoscopy, surgical, including video-assisted harvest of vein(s) for coronary artery bypass procedure (List separately in addition to code for primary procedure)**
N1 N 80 0.47 0.47 FUD ZZZ

33510-33516 Coronary Artery Bypass: Venous Grafts

INCLUDES Obtaining saphenous vein grafts
Venous bypass grafting only

EXCLUDES *Arterial bypass (33533-33536)*
Combined arterial-venous bypass (33517-33523, 33533-33536)
Obtaining vein graft:
Femoropopliteal vein (35572)
Upper extremity vein (35500)
Percutaneous ventricular assist devices (33990-33993)

Code also modifier 80 when assistant at surgery obtains grafts

33510 **Coronary artery bypass, vein only; single coronary venous graft**
C 80 PQ 56.49 56.49 FUD 090

33511 **2 coronary venous grafts**
C 80 PQ 62.03 62.03 FUD 090

33512 **3 coronary venous grafts**
C 80 PQ 70.53 70.53 FUD 090

33513 **4 coronary venous grafts**
C 80 PQ 72.57 72.57 FUD 090

33514 **5 coronary venous grafts**
C 80 PQ 76.56 76.56 FUD 090

33516 **6 or more coronary venous grafts**
C 80 PQ 79.65 79.65 FUD 090

33517-33523 Coronary Artery Bypass: Venous AND Arterial Grafts

INCLUDES Obtaining saphenous vein grafts

EXCLUDES *Obtaining arterial graft:*
Upper extremity (35600)
Obtaining vein graft:
Femoropopliteal vein graft (35572)
Upper extremity (35500)
Percutaneous ventricular assist devices (33990-33993)

Code also modifier 80 when assistant at surgery obtains grafts
Code first (33533-33536)

\+ **33517** **Coronary artery bypass, using venous graft(s) and arterial graft(s); single vein graft (List separately in addition to code for primary procedure)**
C 80 PQ 5.48 5.48 FUD ZZZ

\+ **33518** **2 venous grafts (List separately in addition to code for primary procedure)**
C 80 PQ 12.06 12.06 FUD ZZZ

\+ **33519** **3 venous grafts (List separately in addition to code for primary procedure)**
C 80 PQ 15.94 15.94 FUD ZZZ

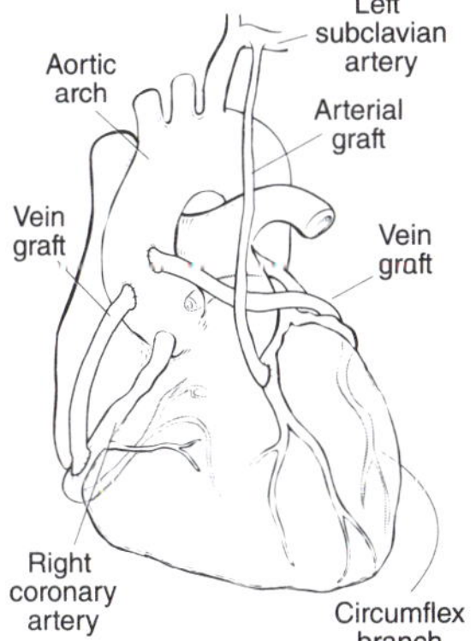

\+ **33521** **4 venous grafts (List separately in addition to code for primary procedure)**
C 80 PQ 19.15 19.15 FUD ZZZ

\+ **33522** **5 venous grafts (List separately in addition to code for primary procedure)**
C 80 PQ 21.49 21.49 FUD ZZZ

\+ **33523** **6 or more venous grafts (List separately in addition to code for primary procedure)**
C 80 PQ 24.37 24.37 FUD ZZZ

33530 Reoperative Coronary Artery Bypass Graft or Valve Procedure

EXCLUDES *Percutaneous ventricular assist devices (33990-33993)*

Code first (33400-33496, 33510-33536, 33863)

\+ **33530** **Reoperation, coronary artery bypass procedure or valve procedure, more than 1 month after original operation (List separately in addition to code for primary procedure)**
C 80 PQ 15.38 15.38 FUD ZZZ

33533-33536 Coronary Artery Bypass: Arterial Grafts

INCLUDES Obtaining arterial graft (eg, epigastric, internal mammary, gastroepiploic and others)

EXCLUDES *Obtaining arterial graft:*
Upper extremity (35600)
Obtaining venous graft:
Femoropopliteal vein (35572)
Upper extremity (35500)
Percutaneous ventricular assist devices (33990-33993)
Venous bypass (33510-33516)

Code also (33517-33523)
Code also modifier 80 when assistant at surgery obtains grafts

33533 **Coronary artery bypass, using arterial graft(s); single arterial graft**
C 80 PQ 54.60 54.60 FUD 090

33534 **2 coronary arterial grafts**
C 80 PQ 64.19 64.19 FUD 090

33535 **3 coronary arterial grafts**
C 80 PQ 71.56 71.56 FUD 090

33536 **4 or more coronary arterial grafts**
C 80 PQ 76.84 76.84 FUD 090

33542-33548 Ventricular Reconstruction

CMS 100-3,20.26 Partial Ventriculectomy

33542 **Myocardial resection (eg, ventricular aneurysmectomy)**
Code also removal of thrombus through a separate heart incision, when performed (33310-33315); append modifier 59 to (33315)
C 80 PQ 76.72 76.72 FUD 090

33545 **Repair of postinfarction ventricular septal defect, with or without myocardial resection**
Code also removal of thrombus through a separate heart incision, when performed (33310-33315); append modifier 59 to (33315)
C 80 PQ 90.27 90.27 FUD 090

33548 **Surgical ventricular restoration procedure, includes prosthetic patch, when performed (eg, ventricular remodeling, SVR, SAVER, Dor procedures)**
EXCLUDES *Batista procedure or pachopexy (33999)*
Do not report with (32551, 33210-33211, 33310, 33315)
C 80 PQ 86.85 86.85 FUD 090

33572 Endarterectomy with CABG (LAD, RCA, Cx)

\+ **33572** **Coronary endarterectomy, open, any method, of left anterior descending, circumflex, or right coronary artery performed in conjunction with coronary artery bypass graft procedure, each vessel (List separately in addition to primary procedure)**
Code first (33510-33516, 33533-33536)
C 80 PQ 6.76 6.76 FUD ZZZ

33600-33622 Repair Aberrant Heart Anatomy

33600 Closure of atrioventricular valve (mitral or tricuspid) by suture or patch
Code also the concurrent ligation/takedown of a systemic-to-pulmonary artery shunt (33924)
C 80 Facility RVU 49.61 Non-Facility RVU 49.61 FUD 090

33602 Closure of semilunar valve (aortic or pulmonary) by suture or patch
Code also the concurrent ligation/takedown of a systemic-to-pulmonary artery shunt (33924)
C 80 Facility RVU 47.83 Non-Facility RVU 47.83 FUD 090

33606 Anastomosis of pulmonary artery to aorta (Damus-Kaye-Stansel procedure)
Code also the concurrent ligation/takedown of a systemic-to-pulmonary artery shunt (33924)
C 80 Facility RVU 50.99 Non-Facility RVU 50.99 FUD 090

33608 Repair of complex cardiac anomaly other than pulmonary atresia with ventricular septal defect by construction or replacement of conduit from right or left ventricle to pulmonary artery
EXCLUDES *Unifocalization of arborization anomalies of pulmonary artery (33925, 33926)*
Code also the concurrent ligation/takedown of a systemic-to-pulmonary artery shunt (33924)
C 80 Facility RVU 51.98 Non-Facility RVU 51.98 FUD 090

33610 Repair of complex cardiac anomalies (eg, single ventricle with subaortic obstruction) by surgical enlargement of ventricular septal defect
Code also the concurrent ligation/takedown of a systemic-to-pulmonary artery shunt (33924)
C 80 63 Facility RVU 51.27 Non-Facility RVU 51.27 FUD 090

33611 Repair of double outlet right ventricle with intraventricular tunnel repair;
Code also the concurrent ligation/takedown of a systemic-to-pulmonary artery shunt (33924)
C 80 63 Facility RVU 56.99 Non-Facility RVU 56.99 FUD 090

33612 with repair of right ventricular outflow tract obstruction
Code also the concurrent ligation/takedown of a systemic-to-pulmonary artery shunt (33924)
C 80 Facility RVU 57.69 Non-Facility RVU 57.69 FUD 090

33615 Repair of complex cardiac anomalies (eg, tricuspid atresia) by closure of atrial septal defect and anastomosis of atria or vena cava to pulmonary artery (simple Fontan procedure)
Code also the concurrent ligation/takedown of a systemic-to-pulmonary artery shunt (33924)
C 80 Facility RVU 58.61 Non-Facility RVU 58.61 FUD 090

33617 Repair of complex cardiac anomalies (eg, single ventricle) by modified Fontan procedure
Code also 33768 for cavopulmonary anastomosis to a second superior vena cava
Code also the concurrent ligation/takedown of a systemic-to-pulmonary artery shunt (33924)
C 80 Facility RVU 62.53 Non-Facility RVU 62.53 FUD 090

33619 Repair of single ventricle with aortic outflow obstruction and aortic arch hypoplasia (hypoplastic left heart syndrome) (eg, Norwood procedure)
Code also the concurrent ligation/takedown of a systemic-to-pulmonary artery shunt (33924)
C 80 63 Facility RVU 82.88 Non-Facility RVU 82.88 FUD 090

33620 Application of right and left pulmonary artery bands (eg, hybrid approach stage 1)
EXCLUDES *Banding of main pulmonary artery related to septal defect (33690)*
Code also transthoracic insertion of catheter for stent placement with removal of catheter and closure when performed during same session
C 80 Facility RVU 42.62 Non-Facility RVU 42.62 FUD 090

33621 Transthoracic insertion of catheter for stent placement with catheter removal and closure (eg, hybrid approach stage 1)
Code also application of right and left pulmonary artery bands when performed during same session (33620)
Code also stent placement (37236)
C 80 Facility RVU 25.52 Non-Facility RVU 25.52 FUD 090

33622 Reconstruction of complex cardiac anomaly (eg, single ventricle or hypoplastic left heart) with palliation of single ventricle with aortic outflow obstruction and aortic arch hypoplasia, creation of cavopulmonary anastomosis, and removal of right and left pulmonary bands (eg, hybrid approach stage 2, Norwood, bidirectional Glenn, pulmonary artery debanding)
Code also anastomosis, cavopulmonary, second superior vena cava for bilateral bidirectional Glenn procedure (33768)
Code also the concurrent ligation/takedown of a systemic-to-pulmonary artery shunt (33924)
Do not report with (33619, 33767, 33822, 33840, 33845, 33851, 33853, 33917)
C 80 Facility RVU 100.42 Non-Facility RVU 100.42 FUD 090

33641-33645 Closure of Defect: Atrium

33641 Repair atrial septal defect, secundum, with cardiopulmonary bypass, with or without patch
C 80 Facility RVU 47.74 Non-Facility RVU 47.74 FUD 090

33645 Direct or patch closure, sinus venosus, with or without anomalous pulmonary venous drainage
Do not report with (33724, 33726)
C 80 Facility RVU 50.51 Non-Facility RVU 50.51 FUD 090

33647 Closure of Septal Defect: Atrium AND Ventricle

33647 Repair of atrial septal defect and ventricular septal defect, with direct or patch closure
EXCLUDES *Tricuspid atresia repair procedures (33615)*
C 80 63 Facility RVU 53.34 Non-Facility RVU 53.34 FUD 090

33660-33670 Closure of Defect: Atrioventricular Canal

33660 Repair of incomplete or partial atrioventricular canal (ostium primum atrial septal defect), with or without atrioventricular valve repair
C 80 Facility RVU 51.29 Non-Facility RVU 51.29 FUD 090

33665 Repair of intermediate or transitional atrioventricular canal, with or without atrioventricular valve repair
C 80 Facility RVU 56.20 Non-Facility RVU 56.20 FUD 090

33670 Repair of complete atrioventricular canal, with or without prosthetic valve
Code also removal of thrombus through a separate heart incision, when performed (33310-33315); append modifier 59 to (33315)
C 80 63 Facility RVU 57.95 Non-Facility RVU 57.95 FUD 090

33675-33677 Closure of Multiple Septal Defects: Ventricle

EXCLUDES *Percutaneous closure (93581)*

Do not report with (32100, 32551, 32554-32555, 33210, 33681, 33684, 33688)

33675 Closure of multiple ventricular septal defects;
C 80 Facility RVU 57.59 Non-Facility RVU 57.59 FUD 090

33676 with pulmonary valvotomy or infundibular resection (acyanotic)
C 80 Facility RVU 62.51 Non-Facility RVU 62.51 FUD 090

33677 with removal of pulmonary artery band, with or without gusset
C 80 Facility RVU 64.95 Non-Facility RVU 64.95 FUD 090

33681-33688 Closure of Septal Defect: Ventricle

EXCLUDES Repair of pulmonary vein that requires creating an atrial septal defect (33724)

33681 Closure of single ventricular septal defect, with or without patch;
EXCLUDES Code also removal of thrombus through a separate heart incision, when performed (33310-33315); append modifier 59 to (33315)
C 80 53.48 53.48 FUD 090

33684 with pulmonary valvotomy or infundibular resection (acyanotic)
Code also concurrent ligation/takedown of a systemic-to-pulmonary artery shunt if performed (33924)
C 80 55.15 55.15 FUD 090

33688 with removal of pulmonary artery band, with or without gusset
Code also the concurrent ligation/takedown of a systemic-to-pulmonary artery shunt if performed (33924)
C 80 55.06 55.06 FUD 090

33690 Reduce Pulmonary Overcirculation in Septal Defects

EXCLUDES Left and right pulmonary artery banding in a single ventricle (33620)

33690 Banding of pulmonary artery
C 80 63 34.61 34.61 FUD 090

33692-33697 Repair of Defects of Tetralogy of Fallot

Code also the concurrent ligation/takedown of a systemic-to-pulmonary artery shunt (33924).

33692 Complete repair tetralogy of Fallot without pulmonary atresia;
C 80 60.53 60.53 FUD 090

33694 with transannular patch
C 80 63 57.28 57.28 FUD 090

33697 Complete repair tetralogy of Fallot with pulmonary atresia including construction of conduit from right ventricle to pulmonary artery and closure of ventricular septal defect
C 80 60.13 60.13 FUD 090

33702-33722 Repair Anomalies Sinus of Valsalva

33702 Repair sinus of Valsalva fistula, with cardiopulmonary bypass;
C 80 45.07 45.07 FUD 090

33710 with repair of ventricular septal defect
C 80 61.55 61.55 FUD 090

33720 Repair sinus of Valsalva aneurysm, with cardiopulmonary bypass
C 80 44.93 44.93 FUD 090

33722 Closure of aortico-left ventricular tunnel
C 80 47.67 47.67 FUD 090

33724-33732 Repair Aberrant Pulmonary Venous Connection

33724 Repair of isolated partial anomalous pulmonary venous return (eg, Scimitar Syndrome)
Do not report with (32551, 33210-33211)
C 80 44.73 44.73 FUD 090

33726 Repair of pulmonary venous stenosis
Do not report with (32551, 33210-33211)
C 80 60.59 60.59 FUD 090

33730 Complete repair of anomalous pulmonary venous return (supracardiac, intracardiac, or infracardiac types)
EXCLUDES Partial anomalous pulmonary venous return (33724)
Repair of pulmonary venous stenosis (33726)
C 80 63 58.51 58.51 FUD 090

33732 Repair of cor triatriatum or supravalvular mitral ring by resection of left atrial membrane
C 80 63 50.70 50.70 FUD 090

33735-33737 Creation of Atrial Septal Defect

Code also the concurrent ligation/takedown of a systemic-to-pulmonary artery shunt (33924)

33735 Atrial septectomy or septostomy; closed heart (Blalock-Hanlon type operation)
C 80 63 37.76 37.76 FUD 090

33736 open heart with cardiopulmonary bypass
C 80 63 40.95 40.95 FUD 090

33737 open heart, with inflow occlusion
EXCLUDES Atrial septectomy/septostomy:
Blade method (92993)
Transvenous balloon method (92992)
C 80 39.21 39.21 FUD 090

33750-33767 Systemic Vessel to Pulmonary Artery Shunts

Code also the concurrent ligation/takedown of a systemic-to-pulmonary artery shunt (33924)

33750 Shunt; subclavian to pulmonary artery (Blalock-Taussig type operation)
C 80 63 39.10 39.10 FUD 090

33755 ascending aorta to pulmonary artery (Waterston type operation)
C 80 63 39.36 39.36 FUD 090

33762 descending aorta to pulmonary artery (Potts-Smith type operation)
C 80 63 39.27 39.27 FUD 090

33764 central, with prosthetic graft
C 80 37.78 37.78 FUD 090

33766 superior vena cava to pulmonary artery for flow to 1 lung (classical Glenn procedure)
C 80 40.05 40.05 FUD 090

33767 superior vena cava to pulmonary artery for flow to both lungs (bidirectional Glenn procedure)
C 80 41.70 41.70 FUD 090

33768 Cavopulmonary Anastomosis to Decrease Volume Load

Code first (33478, 33617, 33622, 33767)
Do not report with (32551, 33210-33211)

+ **33768 Anastomosis, cavopulmonary, second superior vena cava (List separately in addition to primary procedure)**
C 80 12.97 12.97 FUD ZZZ

33770-33783 Repair Aberrant Anatomy: Transposition Great Vessels

Code also the concurrent ligation/takedown of a systemic-to-pulmonary artery shunt (33924)

33770 Repair of transposition of the great arteries with ventricular septal defect and subpulmonary stenosis; without surgical enlargement of ventricular septal defect
C 80 64.82 64.82 FUD 090

33771 with surgical enlargement of ventricular septal defect
C 80 67.60 67.60 FUD 090

33774 Repair of transposition of the great arteries, atrial baffle procedure (eg, Mustard or Senning type) with cardiopulmonary bypass;
C 80 52.73 52.73 FUD 090

33775 with removal of pulmonary band
C 80 56.83 56.83 FUD 090

33776 with closure of ventricular septal defect
C 80 57.17 57.17 FUD 090

33777 with repair of subpulmonic obstruction
C 80 ⚑ 58.20 58.20 FUD 090

33778 Repair of transposition of the great arteries, aortic pulmonary artery reconstruction (eg, Jatene type);
C 80 ⚑ 63 72.49 72.49 FUD 090

33779 with removal of pulmonary band
C 80 ⚑ 64.29 64.29 FUD 090

33780 with closure of ventricular septal defect
C 80 ⚑ 69.36 69.36 FUD 090

33781 with repair of subpulmonic obstruction
C 80 ⚑ 71.82 71.82 FUD 090

33782 Aortic root translocation with ventricular septal defect and pulmonary stenosis repair (ie, Nikaidoh procedure); without coronary ostium reimplantation
Do not report with (33412-33413, 33608, 33681, 33770-33771, 33778, 33780, 33920)
C 80 95.99 95.99 FUD 090

33783 with reimplantation of 1 or both coronary ostia
C 80 107.04 107.04 FUD 090

33786-33788 Repair Aberrant Anatomy: Truncus Arteriosus

33786 Total repair, truncus arteriosus (Rastelli type operation)
Code also the concurrent ligation/takedown of a systemic-to-pulmonary artery shunt (33924)
C 80 ⚑ 63 66.93 66.93 FUD 090

33788 Reimplantation of an anomalous pulmonary artery
EXCLUDES *Pulmonary artery banding (33690)*
C 80 ⚑ 44.95 44.95 FUD 090

33800-33853 Repair Aberrant Anatomy: Aorta

33800 Aortic suspension (aortopexy) for tracheal decompression (eg, for tracheomalacia) (separate procedure)
C 80 ⚑ 26.67 26.67 FUD 090

33802 Division of aberrant vessel (vascular ring);
C 80 ⚑ 31.74 31.74 FUD 090

33803 with reanastomosis
C 80 ⚑ 35.19 35.19 FUD 090

33813 Obliteration of aortopulmonary septal defect; without cardiopulmonary bypass
C 80 ⚑ 36.00 36.00 FUD 090

33814 with cardiopulmonary bypass
C 80 ⚑ 44.39 44.39 FUD 090

33820 Repair of patent ductus arteriosus; by ligation
EXCLUDES *Percutaneous transcatheter closure patent ductus arteriosus (93582)*
C 80 ⚑ 28.40 28.40 FUD 090

33822 by division, younger than 18 years A
EXCLUDES *Percutaneous transcatheter closure patent ductus arteriosus (93582)*
C 80 ⚑ 29.97 29.97 FUD 090

33824 by division, 18 years and older
EXCLUDES *Percutaneous closure patent ductus arteriosus (93582)*
C 80 ⚑ 34.05 34.05 FUD 090

33840 Excision of coarctation of aorta, with or without associated patent ductus arteriosus; with direct anastomosis
C 80 ⚑ 37.71 37.71 FUD 090

33845 with graft
C 80 ⚑ 38.84 38.84 FUD 090

33851 repair using either left subclavian artery or prosthetic material as gusset for enlargement
C 80 ⚑ 38.73 38.73 FUD 090

33852 Repair of hypoplastic or interrupted aortic arch using autogenous or prosthetic material; without cardiopulmonary bypass
EXCLUDES *Hypoplastic left heart syndrome repair by excision of coarctation of aorta (33619)*
C 80 ⚑ 40.98 40.98 FUD 090

33853 with cardiopulmonary bypass
EXCLUDES *Hypoplastic left heart syndrome repair by excision of coarctation of aorta (33619)*
C 80 ⚑ 53.73 53.73 FUD 090

33860-33877 Aortic Graft Procedures

33860 Ascending aorta graft, with cardiopulmonary bypass, includes valve suspension, when performed
C 80 ⚑ 93.83 93.83 FUD 090

33863 Ascending aorta graft, with cardiopulmonary bypass, with aortic root replacement using valved conduit and coronary reconstruction (eg, Bentall)
Do not report with (33405-33406, 33410-33413, 33860)
C 80 ⚑ 92.01 92.01 FUD 090

33864 Ascending aorta graft, with cardiopulmonary bypass with valve suspension, with coronary reconstruction and valve-sparing aortic root remodeling (eg, David Procedure, Yacoub Procedure)
Do not report with (33400, 33860-33863)
C 80 93.84 93.84 FUD 090

33870 Transverse arch graft, with cardiopulmonary bypass
C 80 ⚑ 73.55 73.55 FUD 090

33875 Descending thoracic aorta graft, with or without bypass
C 80 ⚑ 80.39 80.39 FUD 090

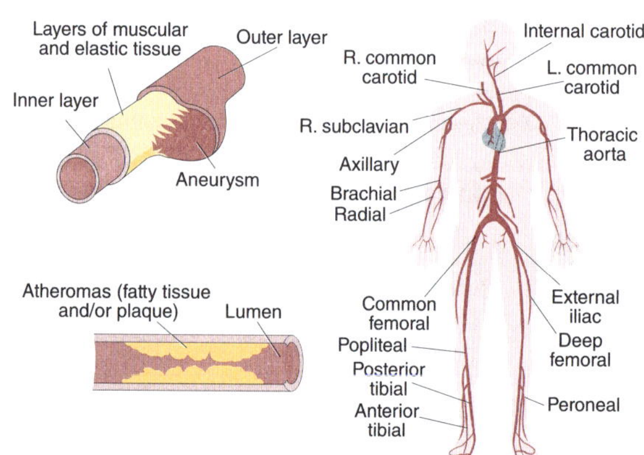

33877 Repair of thoracoabdominal aortic aneurysm with graft, with or without cardiopulmonary bypass
C 80 ⚑ PQ 106.61 106.61 FUD 090

33880-33891 Endovascular Repair Aortic Aneurysm: Thoracic

INCLUDES Balloon angioplasty
Deployment of stent
Introduction, manipulation, placement, and deployment of the device

EXCLUDES *Additional interventional procedures provided during the endovascular repair*
Carotid-carotid bypass (33891)
Guidewire and catheter insertion (36140, 36200-36218)
Open exposure of artery/subsequent closure (34812, 34820, 34833-34834)
Study, interpretation, and report of implanted wireless pressure sensor in an aneurysmal sac (93982)
Subclavian to carotid artery transposition (33889)
Substantial artery repair/replacement (35226, 35286)
Transcatheter insertion of wireless physiologic sensor in an aneurysmal sac (34806)

33880 **Endovascular repair of descending thoracic aorta (eg, aneurysm, pseudoaneurysm, dissection, penetrating ulcer, intramural hematoma, or traumatic disruption); involving coverage of left subclavian artery origin, initial endoprosthesis plus descending thoracic aortic extension(s), if required, to level of celiac artery origin**
INCLUDES Placement of distal extensions in distal thoracic aorta
EXCLUDES *Proximal extensions*
75956
C 80 PQ 52.93 52.93 FUD 090

33881 **not involving coverage of left subclavian artery origin, initial endoprosthesis plus descending thoracic aortic extension(s), if required, to level of celiac artery origin**
INCLUDES Placement of distal extensions in distal thoracic aorta
EXCLUDES *Proximal extensions*
Do not report if placement of extension includes coverage of left subclavian artery origin
75957
C 80 PQ 45.53 45.53 FUD 090

33883 **Placement of proximal extension prosthesis for endovascular repair of descending thoracic aorta (eg, aneurysm, pseudoaneurysm, dissection, penetrating ulcer, intramural hematoma, or traumatic disruption); initial extension**
Do not report if placement of extension includes coverage of left subclavian artery origin
75958
C 80 PQ 32.98 32.98 FUD 090

\+ **33884** **each additional proximal extension (List separately in addition to code for primary procedure)**
Code first (33883)
75958
C 80 12.10 12.10 FUD ZZZ

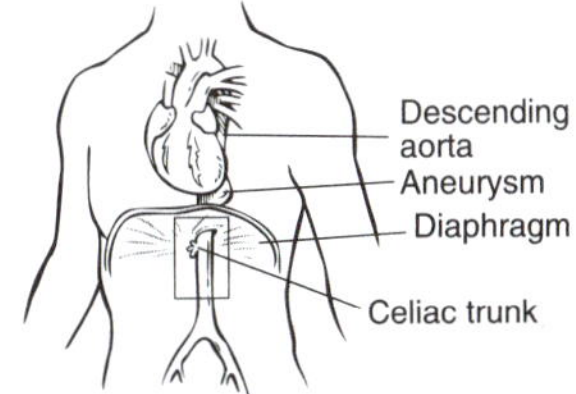

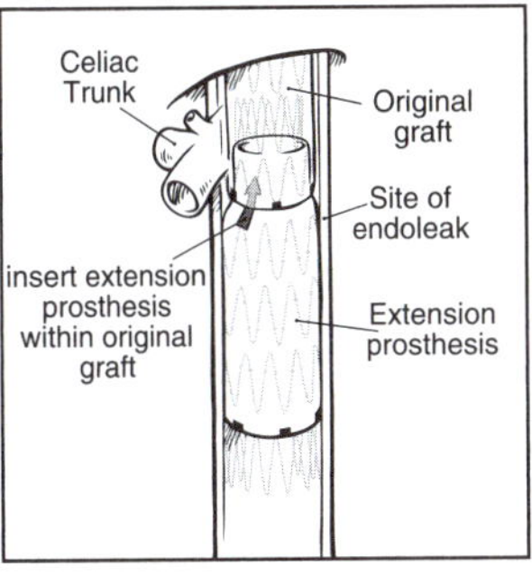

Repair of endoleak in descending thoracic aorta

33886 **Placement of distal extension prosthesis(s) delayed after endovascular repair of descending thoracic aorta**
INCLUDES All modules deployed
Do not report with (33880, 33881)
75959
C 80 PQ 28.68 28.68 FUD 090

33889 **Open subclavian to carotid artery transposition performed in conjunction with endovascular repair of descending thoracic aorta, by neck incision, unilateral**
Do not report with (35694)
C 80 50 23.53 23.53 FUD 000

33891 **Bypass graft, with other than vein, transcervical retropharyngeal carotid-carotid, performed in conjunction with endovascular repair of descending thoracic aorta, by neck incision**
Do not report with (35509, 35601)
C 80 50 PQ 28.79 28.79 FUD 000

33910-33926 Surgical Procedures of Pulmonary Artery

CMS 100-3,240.6 Transvenous (Catheter) Pulmonary Embolectomy

33910 **Pulmonary artery embolectomy; with cardiopulmonary bypass**
C 80 77.45 77.45 FUD 090

33915 **without cardiopulmonary bypass**
C 80 37.09 37.09 FUD 090

33916 **Pulmonary endarterectomy, with or without embolectomy, with cardiopulmonary bypass**
C 80 122.96 122.96 FUD 090

33917 **Repair of pulmonary artery stenosis by reconstruction with patch or graft**
Code also the concurrent ligation/takedown of a systemic-to-pulmonary artery shunt (33924)
C 80 42.07 42.07 FUD 090

33920 **Repair of pulmonary atresia with ventricular septal defect, by construction or replacement of conduit from right or left ventricle to pulmonary artery**
EXCLUDES *Repair of complicated cardiac anomalies by creating/replacing conduit from ventricle to pulmonary artery (33608)*
Code also the concurrent ligation/takedown of a systemic-to-pulmonary artery shunt (33924)
C 80 53.07 53.07 FUD 090

33922 **Transection of pulmonary artery with cardiopulmonary bypass**

Code also the concurrent ligation/takedown of a systemic-to-pulmonary artery shunt (33924)

C 80 63 40.70 40.70 FUD 090

+ **33924** **Ligation and takedown of a systemic-to-pulmonary artery shunt, performed in conjunction with a congenital heart procedure (List separately in addition to code for primary procedure)**

Code first (33470-33478, 33600-33617, 33622, 33684-33688, 33692-33697, 33735-33767, 33770-33783, 33786, 33917, 33920-33922, 33925-33926, 33935, 33945)

C 80 8.27 8.27 FUD ZZZ

33925 **Repair of pulmonary artery arborization anomalies by unifocalization; without cardiopulmonary bypass**

Code also the concurrent ligation/takedown of a systemic-to-pulmonary artery shunt (33924)

C 80 49.68 49.68 FUD 090

33926 **with cardiopulmonary bypass**

Code also the concurrent ligation/takedown of a systemic-to-pulmonary artery shunt (33924)

C 80 70.61 70.61 FUD 090

33930-33945 Heart and Heart-Lung Transplants

CMS 100-4,3,90.2 Heart Transplants

CMS 100-4,3,90.2.1 Artificial Hearts and Related Devices

INCLUDES Backbench work to prepare the donor heart and/or lungs for transplantation (33933, 33944)

Harvesting of donor organs with cold preservation (33930, 33940)

Transplantation of heart and/or lungs into recipient (33935, 33945)

EXCLUDES *Implantation/repair/replacement of artificial heart or components (0051T-0053T)*

Procedures performed on donor heart (33300, 33310, 33320, 33400, 33463, 33464, 33510, 33641, 35216, 35276, 35685)

33930 **Donor cardiectomy-pneumonectomy (including cold preservation)**

C 0.00 0.00 FUD XXX

33933 **Backbench standard preparation of cadaver donor heart/lung allograft prior to transplantation, including dissection of allograft from surrounding soft tissues to prepare aorta, superior vena cava, inferior vena cava, and trachea for implantation**

C 80 0.00 0.00 FUD XXX

33935 **Heart-lung transplant with recipient cardiectomy-pneumonectomy**

Code also the concurrent ligation/takedown of a systemic-to-pulmonary artery shunt (33924)

C 80 PO 146.10 146.10 FUD 090

33940 **Donor cardiectomy (including cold preservation)**

C 0.00 0.00 FUD XXX

33944 **Backbench standard preparation of cadaver donor heart allograft prior to transplantation, including dissection of allograft from surrounding soft tissues to prepare aorta, superior vena cava, inferior vena cava, pulmonary artery, and left atrium for implantation**

C 80 0.00 0.00 FUD XXX

33945 **Heart transplant, with or without recipient cardiectomy**

Code also the concurrent ligation/takedown of a systemic-to-pulmonary artery shunt (33924)

C 80 PO 141.55 141.55 FUD 090

33946-33989 [33962, 33963, 33964, 33965, 33966, 33969, 33984, 33985, 33986, 33987, 33988, 33989] Extracorporeal Circulatory and Respiratory Support

INCLUDES Multiple physician and nonphysician team collaboration

Veno-arterial ECMO/ECLS for heart and lung support

Veno-venous ECMO/ECLS for lung support

EXCLUDES *Overall daily management services needed to manage a patient; report the appropriate observation, hospital inpatient, or critical care E/M codes*

Code also extensive arterial repair/replacement (35266, 35286, 35371, 35665)

Do not report cannula repositioning and cannula insertion performed during same session

Do not report cannula repositioning and initiation of ECMO/ECLS on the same day

Do not report ECMO/ECLS daily management codes with ECMO/ECLS initiation codes

● **33946** **Extracorporeal membrane oxygenation (ECMO)/extracorporeal life support (ECLS) provided by physician; initiation, veno-venous**

Code also cannula insertion (33951-33956)

Do not report with (33948, 33957-33959 [33962, 33963, 33964])

63

● **33947** **initiation, veno-arterial**

Code also cannula insertion (33951-33956)

Do not report with (33949, 33957-33959 [33962, 33963, 33964])

63

● **33948** **daily management, each day, veno-venous**

Do not report with (33946)

63

● **33949** **daily management, each day, veno-arterial**

Do not report with (33947)

63

● **33951** **insertion of peripheral (arterial and/or venous) cannula(e), percutaneous, birth through 5 years of age (includes fluoroscopic guidance, when performed)** A

INCLUDES Cannula replacement in same vessel

Cannula repositioning during same episode of care

Code also ECMO/ECLS initiation or daily management (33946-33947 or 33948-33949)

Code also cannula removal if new cannula inserted in different vessel with ([33965, 33966, 33969, 33984, 33985, 33986])

● **33952** **insertion of peripheral (arterial and/or venous) cannula(e), percutaneous, 6 years and older (includes fluoroscopic guidance, when performed)** A

INCLUDES Cannula replacement in same vessel

Cannula repositioning during same episode of care

Code also ECMO/ECLS initiation or daily management (33946-33947 or 33948-33949)

Code also cannula removal if new cannula inserted in different vessel with ([33965, 33966, 33969, 33984, 33985, 33986])

● **33953** **insertion of peripheral (arterial and/or venous) cannula(e), open, birth through 5 years of age** A

INCLUDES Cannula replacement in same vessel

Cannula repositioning during same episode of care

Code also ECMO/ECLS initiation or daily management (33496-33947 or 33948-33949)

Code also cannula removal if new cannula inserted in different vessel with ([33965, 33966, 33969, 33984, 33985, 33986])

Do not report with (34812, 34820, 34834)

● 33954 **insertion of peripheral (arterial and/or venous) cannula(e), open, 6 years and older**
INCLUDES Cannula replacement in same vessel
Cannula repositioning during same episode of care
Code also ECMO/ECLS initiation or daily management (33946-33947 or 33948-33949)
Code also cannula removal if new cannula inserted in different vessel with ([33965, 33966, 33969, 33984, 33985, 33986])
Do not report with (34812, 34820, 34834)

● 33955 **insertion of central cannula(e) by sternotomy or thoracotomy, birth through 5 years of age**
INCLUDES Cannula replacement in same vessel
Cannula repositioning during same episode of care
Code also ECMO/ECLS initiation or daily management (33946-33947 or 33948-33949)
Code also cannula removal if new cannula inserted in different vessel with ([33965, 33966, 33969, 33984, 33985, 33986])
Do not report with (32100, 39010)

● 33956 **insertion of central cannula(e) by sternotomy or thoracotomy, 6 years and older**
INCLUDES Cannula replacement in same vessel
Cannula repositioning during same episode of care
Code also ECMO/ECLS initiation or daily management (33946-33947 or 33948-33949)
Code also cannula removal if new cannula inserted in different vessel with ([33965, 33966, 33969, 33984, 33985, 33986])
Do not report with (32100, 39010)

● 33957 **reposition peripheral (arterial and/or venous) cannula(e), percutaneous, birth through 5 years of age (includes fluoroscopic guidance, when performed)**
INCLUDES Fluoroscopic guidance
Do not report when cannula insertion performed during same session
Do not report with (33946-33947, 34812, 34820, 34834)

● 33958 **reposition peripheral (arterial and/or venous) cannula(e), percutaneous, 6 years and older (includes fluoroscopic guidance, when performed)**
INCLUDES Fluoroscopic guidance
Do not report when cannula insertion performed during same session
Do not report with (33946-33947, 34812, 34820, 34834)

● 33959 **reposition peripheral (arterial and/or venous) cannula(e), open, birth through 5 years of age (includes fluoroscopic guidance, when performed)**
INCLUDES Fluoroscopic guidance
Do not report when cannula insertion performed during same session
Do not report with (33946-33947, 34812, 34820, 34834)

#● 33962 **reposition peripheral (arterial and/or venous) cannula(e), open, 6 years and older (includes fluoroscopic guidance, when performed)**
INCLUDES Fluoroscopic guidance
Do not report when cannula insertion performed during same session
Do not report with (33946-33947, 34812, 34820, 34834)

#● 33963 **reposition of central cannula(e) by sternotomy or thoracotomy, birth through 5 years of age (includes fluoroscopic guidance, when performed)**
INCLUDES Fluoroscopic guidance
Do not report when cannula insertion performed during same session
Do not report with (32100, 33946-33947, 39010)

#● 33964 **reposition central cannula(e) by sternotomy or thoracotomy, 6 years and older (includes fluoroscopic guidance, when performed)**
INCLUDES Fluoroscopic guidance
Do not report when cannula insertion performed during same session
Do not report with (32100, 33946-33947, 39010)

#● 33965 **removal of peripheral (arterial and/or venous) cannula(e), percutaneous, birth through 5 years of age**
Code also new cannula insertion into different vessel (33951-33956)
Code also extensive arterial repair/replacement, when performed (35266, 35286, 35371, 35665)

#● 33966 **removal of peripheral (arterial and/or venous) cannula(e), percutaneous, 6 years and older**
Code also new cannula insertion into different vessel (33951-33956)
Code also extensive arterial repair/replacement, when performed (35266, 35286, 35371, 35665)

#● 33969 **removal of peripheral (arterial and/or venous) cannula(e), open, birth through 5 years of age**
Code also new cannula insertion into different vessel (33951-33956)
Code also extensive arterial repair/replacement, when performed (35266, 35286, 35371, 35665)
Do not report with (34812, 34820, 34834, 35201, 35206, 35211, 35216, 35226)

#● 33984 **removal of peripheral (arterial and/or venous) cannula(e), open, 6 years and older**
Code also new cannula insertion into different vessel (33951-33956)
Code also extensive arterial repair/replacement, when performed (35266, 35286, 35371, 35665)
Do not report with (34812, 34820, 34834, 35201, 35206, 35211, 35216, 35226)

#● 33985 **removal of central cannula(e) by sternotomy or thoracotomy, birth through 5 years of age**
Code also new cannula insertion into different vessel (33951-33956)
Code also extensive arterial repair/replacement, when performed (35266, 35286, 35371, 35665)
Do not report with (35201, 35206, 35211, 35216, 35226)

#● 33986 **removal of central cannula(e) by sternotomy or thoracotomy, 6 years and older**
Code also new cannula insertion into different vessel (33951-33956)
Code also extensive arterial repair/replacement, when performed (35266, 35286, 35371, 35665)
Do not report with (35201, 35206, 35211, 35216, 35226)

+ #● 33987 **Arterial exposure with creation of graft conduit (eg, chimney graft) to facilitate arterial perfusion for ECMO/ECLS (List separately in addition to code for primary procedure)**
Code first (33953-33956)
Do not report with (34833)

#● 33988 **Insertion of left heart vent by thoracic incision (eg, sternotomy, thoracotomy) for ECMO/ECLS**

#● 33989 **Removal of left heart vent by thoracic incision (eg, sternotomy, thoracotomy) for ECMO/ECLS**

33960-33999 Mechanical Circulatory Support

CMS 100-4,3,90.2.1 Artificial Hearts and Related Devices

33960 ~~Prolonged extracorporeal circulation for cardiopulmonary insufficiency; initial day~~
To report, see 33946-33949

33961 ~~each subsequent day~~
To report, see 33948-33949

33962 ***Resequenced code. See code following 33959.***

33963 ***Resequenced code. See code following 33959.***

33964 ***Resequenced code. See code following 33959.***

33965 ***Resequenced code. See code following 33959.***

33966 ***Resequenced code. See code following 33959.***

33967 **Insertion of intra-aortic balloon assist device, percutaneous**

7.50 7.50 **FUD** 000

33968 **Removal of intra-aortic balloon assist device, percutaneous**

0.98 0.98 **FUD** 000

33969 ***Resequenced code. See code following 33959.***

33970 **Insertion of intra-aortic balloon assist device through the femoral artery, open approach**

EXCLUDES *Percutaneous insertion of intra-aortic balloon assist device (33967)*

10.33 10.33 **FUD** 000

33971 **Removal of intra-aortic balloon assist device including repair of femoral artery, with or without graft**

20.63 20.63 **FUD** 090

33973 **Insertion of intra-aortic balloon assist device through the ascending aorta**

14.98 14.98 **FUD** 000

33974 **Removal of intra-aortic balloon assist device from the ascending aorta, including repair of the ascending aorta, with or without graft**

25.93 25.93 **FUD** 090

33975 **Insertion of ventricular assist device; extracorporeal, single ventricle**

INCLUDES Insertion of the new pump with de-airing, connection, and initiation
Removal of the old pump with replacement of the entire ventricular assist device system, including pump(s) and cannulas
Transthoracic approach

EXCLUDES *Percutaneous approach (33990-33991)*
Replacement percutaneous transseptal approach (33999)

Code also removal of thrombus through a separate heart incision, when performed (33310-33315); append modifier 59 to (33315)

38.74 38.74 **FUD** XXX

33976 **extracorporeal, biventricular**

INCLUDES Insertion of the new pump with de-airing, connection, and initiation
Removal with replacement of the entire ventricular assist device system, including pump(s) and cannulas
Transthoracic approach

EXCLUDES *Percutaneous approach (33990-33991)*
Replacement percutaneous transseptal approach (33999)

Code also removal of thrombus through a separate heart incision, when performed (33310-33315); append modifier 59 to (33315)

47.18 47.18 **FUD** XXX

33977 **Removal of ventricular assist device; extracorporeal, single ventricle**

INCLUDES Removal of the entire device and the cannulas

EXCLUDES *Replacement percutaneous transseptal approach (33999)*

Code also removal of thrombus through a separate heart incision, when performed (33310-33315); append modifier 59 to (33315)

Do not report removal of the ventricular assist device when performed at the time of insertion of a new device

32.94 32.94 **FUD** XXX

33978 **extracorporeal, biventricular**

INCLUDES Removal of the entire device and the cannulas

EXCLUDES *Replacement percutaneous transseptal approach (33999)*

Code also removal of thrombus through a separate heart incision, when performed (33310-33315); append modifier 59 to (33315)

Do not report removal of the ventricular assist device when performed at the time of insertion of a new device

39.30 39.30 **FUD** XXX

Total Internal Biventricular Heart Replacement System

33979 **Insertion of ventricular assist device, implantable intracorporeal, single ventricle**

INCLUDES New pump insertion with connection, de-airing, and initiation
Removal with replacement of the entire ventricular assist device system, including pump(s) and cannulas
Transthoracic approach

EXCLUDES *Percutaneous approach (33990-33991)*
Replacement percutaneous transseptal approach (33999)

Code also removal of thrombus through a separate heart incision, when performed (33310-33315); append modifier 59 to (33315)

57.08 57.08 **FUD** XXX

33980 **Removal of ventricular assist device, implantable intracorporeal, single ventricle**

INCLUDES Removal of the entire device and the cannulas

EXCLUDES *Percutaneous transseptal approach (33999)*

Code also removal of thrombus through a separate heart incision, when performed (33310-33315); append modifier 59 to (33315)

Do not report removal of the ventricular assist device when performed at the time of insertion of a new device

52.16 52.16 **FUD** XXX

33981 **Replacement of extracorporeal ventricular assist device, single or biventricular, pump(s), single or each pump**

INCLUDES Insertion of the new pump with de-airing, connection, and initiation
Removal of the old pump

EXCLUDES *Percutaneous transseptal approach (33999)*

24.53 24.53 **FUD** XXX

33982 **Replacement of ventricular assist device pump(s); implantable intracorporeal, single ventricle, without cardiopulmonary bypass**

INCLUDES New pump insertion with connection, de-airing, and initiation
Removal of the old pump

EXCLUDES *Percutaneous transseptal approach (33999)*

57.29 57.29 **FUD** XXX

33983 **implantable intracorporeal, single ventricle, with cardiopulmonary bypass**

INCLUDES Insertion of the new pump with de-airing, connection, and initiation
Removal of the old pump

EXCLUDES *Percutaneous transseptal approach (33999)*

C 80 67.51 67.51 FUD XXX

33984 Resequenced code. See code following 33959.

33985 Resequenced code. See code following 33959.

33986 Resequenced code. See code following 33959.

33987 Resequenced code. See code following 33959.

33988 Resequenced code. See code following 33959.

33989 Resequenced code. See code following 33959.

⊙ 33990 **Insertion of ventricular assist device, percutaneous including radiological supervision and interpretation; arterial access only**

INCLUDES Initial insertion and replacement of percutaneous ventricular assist device

EXCLUDES *Extensive artery repair/replacement (35226, 35286)*
Open arterial approach to aid insertion of percutaneous ventricular assist device, when used (34812)
Transthoracic approach (33975-33976)

Do not report removal of percutaneous ventricular assist device at time of replacement of the entire system (33992)

C 80 12.67 12.67 FUD XXX

⊙ 33991 **both arterial and venous access, with transseptal puncture**

INCLUDES Initial insertion as well as replacement of percutaneous ventricular assist device

EXCLUDES *Extensive artery repair/replacement (35226, 35286)*
Open arterial approach to aid with insertion of percutaneous ventricular assist device, when performed (34812)
Transthoracic approach (33975-33976)

Do not report removal of percutaneous ventricular assist device at time of replacement of the entire system (33992)

C 80 18.47 18.47 FUD XXX

⊙ 33992 **Removal of percutaneous ventricular assist device at separate and distinct session from insertion**

INCLUDES Removal of device and cannulas

Code also modifier 59 when percutaneous ventricular assist device is removed on the same day as the insertion, but at a different session

C 80 5.99 5.99 FUD XXX

⊙ 33993 **Repositioning of percutaneous ventricular assist device with imaging guidance at separate and distinct session from insertion**

Code also modifier 59 when percutaneous ventricular assist device is repositioned using imaging guidance on the same day as the insertion, but at a different session

Do not report repositioning of a percutaneous ventricular assist device without image guidance

Do not report repositioning of the percutaneous ventricular assist device at the same session as the insertion

C 80 5.26 5.26 FUD XXX

33999 **Unlisted procedure, cardiac surgery**

T 80 PQ 0.00 0.00 FUD YYY

34001-34530 Surgical Revascularization: Veins and Arteries

INCLUDES Repair of blood vessel
Surgeon's component of operative arteriogram

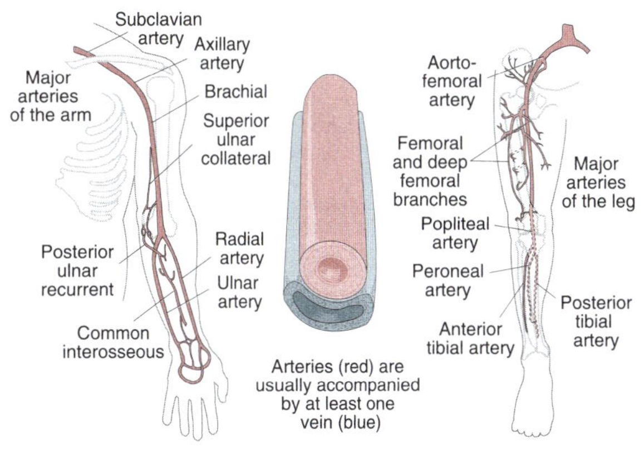

34001 **Embolectomy or thrombectomy, with or without catheter; carotid, subclavian or innominate artery, by neck incision**

C 80 50 28.30 28.30 FUD 090

34051 **innominate, subclavian artery, by thoracic incision**

C 80 50 PQ 29.03 29.03 FUD 090

34101 **axillary, brachial, innominate, subclavian artery, by arm incision**

T 80 50 17.74 17.74 FUD 090

34111 **radial or ulnar artery, by arm incision**

T 80 50 17.73 17.73 FUD 090

34151 **renal, celiac, mesentery, aortoiliac artery, by abdominal incision**

C 80 50 41.43 41.43 FUD 090

34201 **femoropopliteal, aortoiliac artery, by leg incision**

T 80 50 30.52 30.52 FUD 090

34203 **popliteal-tibio-peroneal artery, by leg incision**

T 80 50 28.32 28.32 FUD 090

34401 **Thrombectomy, direct or with catheter; vena cava, iliac vein, by abdominal incision**

C 80 50 42.77 42.77 FUD 090

34421 **vena cava, iliac, femoropopliteal vein, by leg incision**

T 80 50 21.46 21.46 FUD 090

34451 **vena cava, iliac, femoropopliteal vein, by abdominal and leg incision**

C 80 50 42.82 42.82 FUD 090

34471 **subclavian vein, by neck incision**

T 50 31.65 31.65 FUD 090

34490 **axillary and subclavian vein, by arm incision**

T 50 17.85 17.85 FUD 090

34501 **Valvuloplasty, femoral vein**

T 80 50 29.08 29.08 FUD 090

34502 **Reconstruction of vena cava, any method**

C 80 44.53 44.53 FUD 090

34510 **Venous valve transposition, any vein donor**

T 80 50 34.17 34.17 FUD 090

34520 **Cross-over vein graft to venous system**

T 80 50 29.46 29.46 FUD 090

34530 **Saphenopopliteal vein anastomosis**

T 80 50 31.74 31.74 FUD 090

34800-34834 Endovascular Stent Grafting for Abdominal Aneurysms

CMS 100-3,20.23 Fabric Wrapping of Abdominal Aneurysms

INCLUDES Balloon angioplasty/stent deployment within the target treatment zone
Introduction, manipulation, placement, and deployment of the device
Open exposure of femoral or iliac artery/subsequent closure
Thromboendarterectomy at site of aneurysm

EXCLUDES *Additional interventional procedures outside of target treatment zone*
Guidewire and catheter insertion (36140, 36200, 36245-36248)
Study, interpretation, and report of implanted wireless pressure sensor in an aneurysmal sac (93982)
Substantial artery repair/replacement (35226, 35286)
Transcatheter insertion of wireless physiologic sensor in an aneurysmal sac (34806)

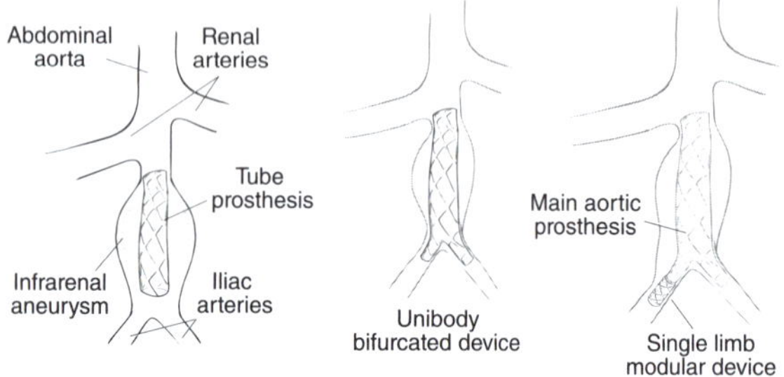

34800 Endovascular repair of infrarenal abdominal aortic aneurysm or dissection; using aorto-aortic tube prosthesis
Code also open arterial exposure as appropriate (34812, 34820, 34833, 34834)
Do not report with (34841-34848)
75952
C 80 PQ 33.20 33.20 FUD 090

34802 using modular bifurcated prosthesis (1 docking limb)
Code also open arterial exposure as appropriate (34812, 34820, 34833, 34834)
Do not report with (34841-34848)
75952
C 80 PQ 36.68 36.68 FUD 090

34803 using modular bifurcated prosthesis (2 docking limbs)
Code also open arterial exposure as appropriate (34812, 34820, 34833, 34834)
Do not report with (34841-34848)
75952
C 80 PQ 37.96 37.96 FUD 090

34804 using unibody bifurcated prosthesis
Code also open arterial exposure as appropriate (34812, 34820, 34833, 34834)
Do not report with (34841-34848)
75952
C 80 PQ 36.64 36.64 FUD 090

34805 using aorto-uniiliac or aorto-unifemoral prosthesis
Code also open arterial exposure as appropriate (34812, 34820, 34833, 34834)
Do not report with (34841-34848)
75952
C 80 PQ 35.21 35.21 FUD 090

\+ **34806 Transcatheter placement of wireless physiologic sensor in aneurysmal sac during endovascular repair, including radiological supervision and interpretation, instrument calibration, and collection of pressure data (List separately in addition to code for primary procedure)**
Code also open arterial exposure as appropriate (34812, 34820, 34833-34834)
Code first (33880-33881, 33886, 34800-34805, 34825, 34900)
Do not report with (93982)
C 80 2.93 2.93 FUD ZZZ

\+ **34808 Endovascular placement of iliac artery occlusion device (List separately in addition to code for primary procedure)**
Code also open arterial exposure as appropriate (34812, 34820, 34833-34834)
Code first (34800, 34805, 34813, 34825-34826)
C 80 6.06 6.06 FUD ZZZ

34812 Open femoral artery exposure for delivery of endovascular prosthesis, by groin incision, unilateral
Code also as appropriate (34800-34808)
Do not report with (33953-33954, 33959, [33962], [33969], [33984])
C 80 50 9.96 9.96 FUD 000

\+ **34813 Placement of femoral-femoral prosthetic graft during endovascular aortic aneurysm repair (List separately in addition to code for primary procedure)**
EXCLUDES *Grafting of femoral artery (35521, 35533, 35539, 35540, 35556, 35558, 35566, 35621, 35646, 35654-35661, 35666, 35700)*
Code first (34812)
C 80 7.01 7.01 FUD ZZZ

34820 Open iliac artery exposure for delivery of endovascular prosthesis or iliac occlusion during endovascular therapy, by abdominal or retroperitoneal incision, unilateral
Code also as appropriate (34800-34808)
Do not report with (33953-33954, 33959, [33962], [33969], [33984])
C 80 50 14.47 14.47 FUD 000

34825 Placement of proximal or distal extension prosthesis for endovascular repair of infrarenal abdominal aortic or iliac aneurysm, false aneurysm, or dissection; initial vessel
Code also as appropriate (34800-34805, 34900)
75953
C 80 PQ 20.53 20.53 FUD 090

\+ **34826 each additional vessel (List separately in addition to code for primary procedure)**
Code also as appropriate (34800-34805, 34900)
Code first (34825)
75953
C 80 PQ 6.04 6.04 FUD ZZZ

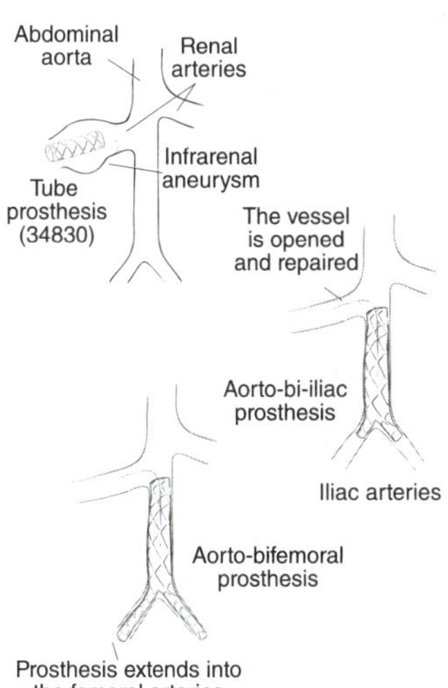

An infrarenal aortic aneurysm or dissection is treated in an open surgical session following an unsuccessful endovascular treatment attempt. A tube prosthesis is placed and any associated arterial trauma is repaired

34830 Open repair of infrarenal aortic aneurysm or dissection, plus repair of associated arterial trauma, following unsuccessful endovascular repair; tube prosthesis
C 80 PQ 52.55 52.55 FUD 090

34831 aorto-bi-iliac prosthesis
C 80 PQ 56.52 56.52 FUD 090

34832 aorto-bifemoral prosthesis
C 80 PQ 56.52 56.52 FUD 090

34833 Open iliac artery exposure with creation of conduit for delivery of aortic or iliac endovascular prosthesis, by abdominal or retroperitoneal incision, unilateral
Code also as appropriate (34800-34805)
Do not report with ([33987], 34820)
C 80 50 18.04 18.04 FUD 000

34834 Open brachial artery exposure to assist in the deployment of aortic or iliac endovascular prosthesis by arm incision, unilateral
Code also as appropriate (34800-34805)
Do not report with (33953-33954, 33959, [33962], [33969], [33984])
C 80 50 8.09 8.09 FUD 000

34839-34848 Repair Visceral Aorta with Fenestrated Endovascular Grafts

INCLUDES Angiography
Balloon angioplasty before and after deployment of graft
Fluoroscopic guidance
Guidewire and catheter insertion of vessels in the target treatment zone
Radiologic supervision and interpretation
Visceral aorta (34841-34844)
Visceral aorta and associated infrarenal abdominal aorta (34845-34848)

EXCLUDES *Catheterization of:*
Arterial families outside treatment zone
Hypogastric arteries
Distal extension prosthesis terminating in the common femoral, external iliac, or internal iliac artery (34825-34826, 75953, 0254T-0255T)
Interventional procedures outside treatment zone
Open exposure of access vessels (34812)
Repair of abdominal aortic aneurysm without a fenestrated graft (34800-34805)
Substantial artery repair (35226, 35286)

Code also associated endovascular repair of descending thoracic aorta (33880-33886, 75956-75959)

Do not report with placement of bare metal or covered intravascular stents in visceral branches in the target treatment zone (37236-37237)

● **34839 Physician planning of a patient-specific fenestrated visceral aortic endograft requiring a minimum of 90 minutes of physician time**
Do not report when total planning time is less than 90 minutes
Do not report on day of or day before endovascular repair procedure
Do not report with (76376-76377)

34841 Endovascular repair of visceral aorta (eg, aneurysm, pseudoaneurysm, dissection, penetrating ulcer, intramural hematoma, or traumatic disruption) by deployment of a fenestrated visceral aortic endograft and all associated radiological supervision and interpretation, including target zone angioplasty, when performed; including one visceral artery endoprosthesis (superior mesenteric, celiac or renal artery)
INCLUDES Repairs extending from the visceral aorta to one or more of the four visceral artery origins to the level of the infrarenal aorta
EXCLUDES *Devices extending into the common iliac arteries (34845-34848)*
Do not report with (34800, 34802-34805, 34839, 34845-34848, 35452, 35472, 75952)
C 80 0.00 0.00 FUD YYY

34842 including two visceral artery endoprostheses (superior mesenteric, celiac and/or renal artery[s])
INCLUDES Repairs extending from the visceral aorta to one or more of the four visceral artery origins to the level of the infrarenal aorta
EXCLUDES *Devices extending into the common iliac arteries (34845-34848)*
Do not report with (34800, 34802-34805, 34839, 34845-34848, 35452, 35472, 75952)
C 80 0.00 0.00 FUD YYY

34843 including three visceral artery endoprostheses (superior mesenteric, celiac and/or renal artery[s])
INCLUDES Repairs extending from the visceral aorta to one or more of the four visceral artery origins to the level of the infrarenal aorta
EXCLUDES *Devices extending into the common iliac arteries (34845-34848)*
Do not report with (34800, 34802-34805, 34839, 34845-34848, 35452, 35472, 75952)
C 80 0.00 0.00 FUD YYY

34844 including four or more visceral artery endoprostheses (superior mesenteric, celiac and/or renal artery[s])
INCLUDES Repairs extending from the visceral aorta to one or more of the four visceral artery origins to the level of the infrarenal aorta
EXCLUDES *Devices extending into the common iliac arteries (34845-34848)*
Do not report with (34800, 34802-34805, 34839, 34845-34848, 35452, 35472, 75952)
C 80 0.00 0.00 FUD YYY

34845 **Endovascular repair of visceral aorta and infrarenal abdominal aorta (eg, aneurysm, pseudoaneurysm, dissection, penetrating ulcer, intramural hematoma, or traumatic disruption) with a fenestrated visceral aortic endograft and concomitant unibody or modular infrarenal aortic endograft and all associated radiological supervision and interpretation, including target zone angioplasty, when performed; including one visceral artery endoprosthesis (superior mesenteric, celiac or renal artery)**

INCLUDES Placement of device and extensions into the common iliac arteries
Repairs extending from the visceral aorta into the common iliac arteries

Code also iliac artery revascularization when performed outside zone of target treatment (37220-37223)
Do not report with (34800, 34802-34805, 34839, 34841-34844, 35081, 35102, 35452, 35472, 75952)

C 80 0.00 0.00 FUD YYY

34846 **including two visceral artery endoprostheses (superior mesenteric, celiac and/or renal artery[s])**

INCLUDES Placement of device and extensions into the common iliac arteries
Repairs extending from the visceral aorta into the common iliac arteries

Code also iliac artery revascularization when performed outside zone of target treatment (37220-37223)
Do not report with (34800, 34802-34805, 34839, 34841-34844, 35081, 35102, 35452, 35472, 75952)

C 80 0.00 0.00 FUD YYY

34847 **including three visceral artery endoprostheses (superior mesenteric, celiac and/or renal artery[s])**

INCLUDES Placement of device and extensions into the common iliac arteries
Repairs extending from the visceral aorta into the common iliac arteries

Code also iliac artery revascularization when performed outside zone of target treatment (37220-37223)
Do not report with (34800, 34802-34805, 34839, 34841-34844, 35081, 35102, 35452, 35472, 75952)

C 80 0.00 0.00 FUD YYY

34848 **including four or more visceral artery endoprostheses (superior mesenteric, celiac and/or renal artery[s])**

INCLUDES Placement of device and extensions into the common iliac arteries
Repairs extending from the visceral aorta into the common iliac arteries

Code also iliac artery revascularization when performed outside zone of target treatment (37220-37223)
Do not report with (34800, 34802-34805, 34839, 34841-34844, 35081, 35102, 35452, 35472, 75952)

C 80 0.00 0.00 FUD YYY

34900 Endovascular Stent Grafting Iliac Artery

INCLUDES Balloon angioplasty/stent deployment within the target treatment zone
Introduction, manipulation, placement, and deployment

EXCLUDES *Endovascular repair of iliac artery bifurcation (e.g., aneurysm, arteriovenous malformation, pseudoaneurysm, trauma) using bifurcated endoprosthesis (0254T)*
Insertion guidewires, catheters (36200, 36245-36248)
Open exposure femoral or iliac artery (34812, 34820)
Other concurrent interventional procedures outside of target zone
Placement extension prosthesis (34825-34826)
Substantial artery repair/replacement (35206-35286)

34900 **Endovascular repair of iliac artery (eg, aneurysm, pseudoaneurysm, arteriovenous malformation, trauma) using ilio-iliac tube endoprosthesis**

75954

C 80 50 PQ 26.26 26.26 FUD 090

35001-35152 Repair Aneurysm, False Aneurysm, Related Arterial Disease

INCLUDES Endarterectomy procedures

EXCLUDES *Endovascular repairs of:*
Abdominal aortic aneurysm (34800-34826)
Aneurysm of iliac artery (34900)
Thoracic aortic aneurysm (33880-33891)
Intracranial aneurysms (61697-61710)
Open repairs thoracic aortic aneurysm (33860-33875)
Repairs related to occlusive disease only (35201-35286)

35001 **Direct repair of aneurysm, pseudoaneurysm, or excision (partial or total) and graft insertion, with or without patch graft; for aneurysm and associated occlusive disease, carotid, subclavian artery, by neck incision**

C 80 50 33.18 33.18 FUD 090

35002 **for ruptured aneurysm, carotid, subclavian artery, by neck incision**

C 80 50 33.33 33.33 FUD 090

An incision is made in the back of the neck to directly approach an aneurysm or false aneurysm of the vertebral artery. The artery is either repaired directly or excised with a graft

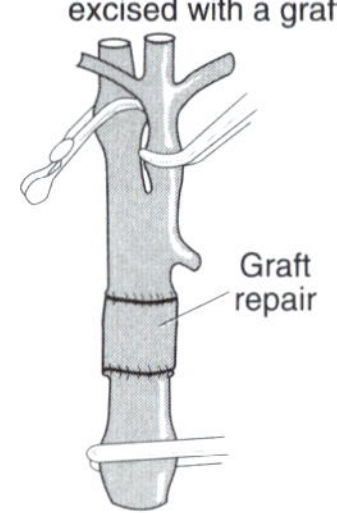

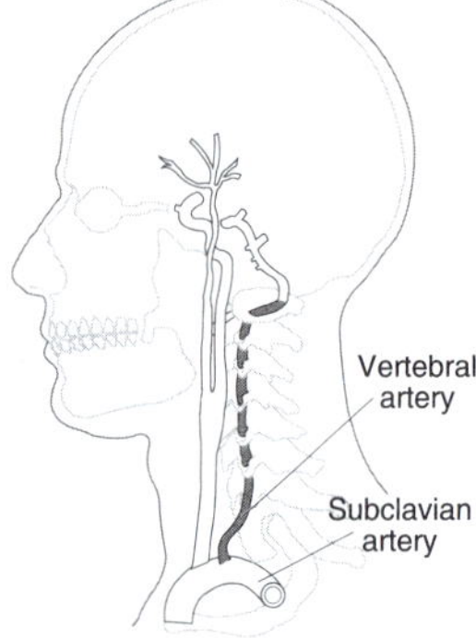

35005 **for aneurysm, pseudoaneurysm, and associated occlusive disease, vertebral artery**

C 80 50 33.76 33.76 FUD 090

35011 **for aneurysm and associated occlusive disease, axillary-brachial artery, by arm incision**

T 80 50 29.48 29.48 FUD 090

35013 **for ruptured aneurysm, axillary-brachial artery, by arm incision**

C 80 50 36.96 36.96 FUD 090

35021 **for aneurysm, pseudoaneurysm, and associated occlusive disease, innominate, subclavian artery, by thoracic incision**

C 80 50 PQ 36.59 36.59 FUD 090

35022 **for ruptured aneurysm, innominate, subclavian artery, by thoracic incision**

C 80 50 42.14 42.14 FUD 090

35045 **for aneurysm, pseudoaneurysm, and associated occlusive disease, radial or ulnar artery**

T 80 50 29.36 29.36 FUD 090

35081 **for aneurysm, pseudoaneurysm, and associated occlusive disease, abdominal aorta**

C 80 PQ 51.82 51.82 FUD 090

35082 **for ruptured aneurysm, abdominal aorta**

C 80 64.84 64.84 FUD 090

35091 **for aneurysm, pseudoaneurysm, and associated occlusive disease, abdominal aorta involving visceral vessels (mesenteric, celiac, renal)**

C 80 50 PQ 53.20 53.20 FUD 090

35092 **for ruptured aneurysm, abdominal aorta involving visceral vessels (mesenteric, celiac, renal)**

C 80 50 77.40 77.40 FUD 090

35102 for aneurysm, pseudoaneurysm, and associated occlusive disease, abdominal aorta involving iliac vessels (common, hypogastric, external)
C 80 50 PQ 56.16 56.16 FUD 090

35103 for ruptured aneurysm, abdominal aorta involving iliac vessels (common, hypogastric, external)
C 80 50 66.65 66.65 FUD 090

35111 for aneurysm, pseudoaneurysm, and associated occlusive disease, splenic artery
C 80 50 44.13 44.13 FUD 090

35112 for ruptured aneurysm, splenic artery
C 80 50 54.12 54.12 FUD 090

35121 for aneurysm, pseudoaneurysm, and associated occlusive disease, hepatic, celiac, renal, or mesenteric artery
C 80 50 48.40 48.40 FUD 090

35122 for ruptured aneurysm, hepatic, celiac, renal, or mesenteric artery
C 80 50 62.45 62.45 FUD 090

35131 for aneurysm, pseudoaneurysm, and associated occlusive disease, iliac artery (common, hypogastric, external)
C 80 50 PQ 41.06 41.06 FUD 090

35132 for ruptured aneurysm, iliac artery (common, hypogastric, external)
C 80 50 48.45 48.45 FUD 090

35141 for aneurysm, pseudoaneurysm, and associated occlusive disease, common femoral artery (profunda femoris, superficial femoral)
C 80 50 PQ 32.75 32.75 FUD 090

35142 for ruptured aneurysm, common femoral artery (profunda femoris, superficial femoral)
C 80 50 39.25 39.25 FUD 090

35151 for aneurysm, pseudoaneurysm, and associated occlusive disease, popliteal artery
C 80 50 PQ 36.84 36.84 FUD 090

35152 for ruptured aneurysm, popliteal artery
C 80 50 41.66 41.66 FUD 090

35180-35190 Surgical Repair Arteriovenous Fistula

35180 Repair, congenital arteriovenous fistula; head and neck
T 80 26.74 26.74 FUD 090

35182 thorax and abdomen
C 80 50.96 50.96 FUD 090

35184 extremities
T 80 30.37 30.37 FUD 090

35188 Repair, acquired or traumatic arteriovenous fistula; head and neck
A2 T 80 34.79 34.79 FUD 090

35189 thorax and abdomen
C 80 45.37 45.37 FUD 090

35190 extremities
T 80 22.27 22.27 FUD 090

35201-35286 Surgical Repair Artery or Vein

EXCLUDES *Arteriovenous fistula repair (35180-35190)*

Do not report with a primary open vascular procedure

35201 Repair blood vessel, direct; neck
Do not report with ([33969, 33984, 33985, 33986])
T 80 50 27.81 27.81 FUD 090

35206 upper extremity
Do not report with ([33969, 33984, 33985, 33986])
T 80 50 22.76 22.76 FUD 090

35207 hand, finger
A2 T 50 21.54 21.54 FUD 090

35211 intrathoracic, with bypass
Do not report with ([33969, 33984, 33985, 33986])
C 80 50 PQ 40.47 40.47 FUD 090

35216 intrathoracic, without bypass
Do not report with ([33969, 33984, 33985, 33986])
C 80 50 PQ 60.07 60.07 FUD 090

35221 intra-abdominal
C 80 50 42.30 42.30 FUD 090

35226 lower extremity
Do not report with ([33969, 33984, 33985, 33986])
T 80 50 24.62 24.62 FUD 090

35231 Repair blood vessel with vein graft; neck
T 80 50 35.51 35.51 FUD 090

35236 upper extremity
T 80 50 28.88 28.88 FUD 090

35241 intrathoracic, with bypass
C 80 50 PQ 41.93 41.93 FUD 090

35246 intrathoracic, without bypass
C 80 50 PQ 45.67 45.67 FUD 090

35251 intra-abdominal
C 80 50 49.38 49.38 FUD 090

35256 lower extremity
T 80 50 30.17 30.17 FUD 090

35261 Repair blood vessel with graft other than vein; neck
Code also (C1768, L8670)
T 80 50 31.25 31.25 FUD 090

35266 upper extremity
Code also (C1768, L8670)
T 80 50 25.64 25.64 FUD 090

35271 intrathoracic, with bypass
C 80 50 PQ 40.42 40.42 FUD 090

35276 intrathoracic, without bypass
C 80 50 PQ 42.37 42.37 FUD 090

35281 intra-abdominal
C 80 50 47.85 47.85 FUD 090

35286 lower extremity
Code also (C1768, L8670)
T 80 50 27.73 27.73 FUD 090

35301-35372 Surgical Thromboendarterectomy Peripheral and Visceral Arteries

CMS 100-3,20.1 Vertebral Artery Surgery
CMS 100-3,160.8 Electroencephalographic Monitoring During Cerebral Vasculature Surgery

INCLUDES Obtaining saphenous or arm vein for graft
Thrombectomy/embolectomy

EXCLUDES *Coronary artery bypass procedures (33510-33536, 33572)*
Thromboendarterectomy for vascular occlusion on a different vessel during the same session

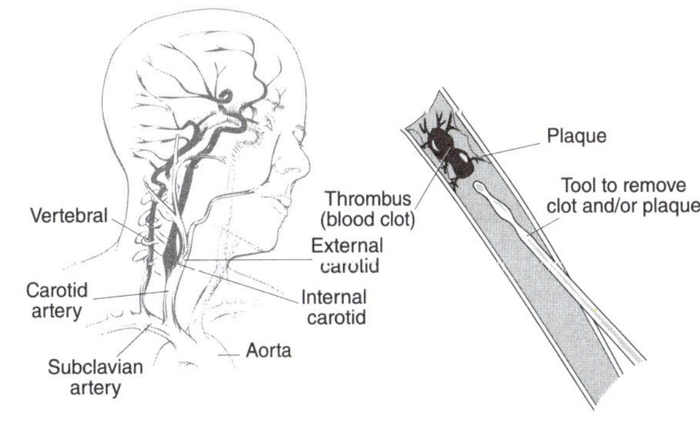

35301 Thromboendarterectomy, including patch graft, if performed; carotid, vertebral, subclavian, by neck incision
C 80 50 PQ 33.51 33.51 FUD 090

35302 **superficial femoral artery**
Do not report with (35500, 37225, 37227)
C 80 50 33.44 33.44 FUD 090

35303 **popliteal artery**
Do not report with (35500, 37225, 37227)
C 80 50 36.92 36.92 FUD 090

35304 **tibioperoneal trunk artery**
Do not report with (35500, 37229, 37231, 37233, 37235)
C 80 50 38.19 38.19 FUD 090

35305 **tibial or peroneal artery, initial vessel**
Do not report with (35500, 37229, 37231, 37233, 37235)
C 80 50 36.67 36.67 FUD 090

\+ **35306** **each additional tibial or peroneal artery (List separately in addition to code for primary procedure)**
Code first (35305)
Do not report with (35500, 37229, 37231, 37233, 37235)
C 80 13.70 13.70 FUD ZZZ

35311 **subclavian, innominate, by thoracic incision**
C 80 50 PQ 42.55 42.55 FUD 090

35321 **axillary-brachial**
T 80 50 26.17 26.17 FUD 090

35331 **abdominal aorta**
C 80 50 42.99 42.99 FUD 090

35341 **mesenteric, celiac, or renal**
C 80 50 40.82 40.82 FUD 090

35351 **iliac**
C 80 50 38.02 38.02 FUD 090

35355 **iliofemoral**
C 80 50 30.80 30.80 FUD 090

35361 **combined aortoiliac**
C 80 50 45.39 45.39 FUD 090

35363 **combined aortoiliofemoral**
C 80 50 51.48 51.48 FUD 090

35371 **common femoral**
C 80 50 24.32 24.32 FUD 090

35372 **deep (profunda) femoral**
C 80 50 29.08 29.08 FUD 090

35390 Surgical Thromboendarterectomy: Carotid Reoperation

\+ **35390** **Reoperation, carotid, thromboendarterectomy, more than 1 month after original operation (List separately in addition to code for primary procedure)**
Code first (35301)
C 80 4.71 4.71 FUD ZZZ

35400 Endoscopic Visualization of Vessels

\+ **35400** **Angioscopy (non-coronary vessels or grafts) during therapeutic intervention (List separately in addition to code for primary procedure)**
Code first the therapeutic intervention
C 80 4.40 4.40 FUD ZZZ

35450-35460 Transluminal Angioplasty: Open

35450 **Transluminal balloon angioplasty, open; renal or other visceral artery**
75962-75968, 75978
C 80 50 15.12 15.12 FUD 000

35452 **aortic**
Do not report with (34841-34848)
75962-75968, 75978
C 80 50 10.10 10.10 FUD 000

35458 **brachiocephalic trunk or branches, each vessel**
Code also (C1725, C1874, C1876, C1885, C2625)
Do not report with transcatheter intravascular stent placement of common carotid or innominate artery on the same side (37217)
75962-75968, 75978
T 80 50 14.48 14.48 FUD 000

35460 **venous**
Code also (C1725, C1874, C1876, C1885, C2625)
75962-75968, 75978
G2 T 50 9.17 9.17 FUD 000

35471-35476 Transluminal Angioplasty: Percutaneous

CMS 100-3,20.7 Percutaneous Transluminal Angioplasty (PTA)

EXCLUDES *Catheter placement*
Radiological supervision and interpretation

A balloon angioplasty is performed on the renal or visceral artery in a percutaneous procedure

⊙ **35471** **Transluminal balloon angioplasty, percutaneous; renal or visceral artery**
Code also (C1725, C1874, C1876, C1885, C2625)
75966, 75968
T 50 15.30 71.63 FUD 000

⊙ **35472** **aortic**
Code also (C1725, C1874, C1876, C1885, C2625)
Do not report with (34841-34848)
75966, 75968
T 80 50 10.45 52.19 FUD 000

⊙ **35475** **brachiocephalic trunk or branches, each vessel**
INCLUDES All work performed for AV shunt to treat lesion(s) from the peri-arterial anastomosis through the axillary vein
EXCLUDES *Removal of arterial plug (36870)*
Code also (C1725, C1874, C1876, C1885, C2625)
75966, 75968
P3 T 50 9.92 44.95 FUD 000

⊙ **35476** **venous**
INCLUDES All services in an AV shunt segment including treatment of multiple distinct lesions
EXCLUDES *Removal of arterial plug (36870)*
Code also (C1725, C1874, C1876, C1885, C2625)
Do not report venous interventional codes for stenosis at the arterial anastomosis (peri-anastomotic or juxta-anastomotic region) (35475)
75978
P3 T 50 7.89 41.01 FUD 000

35500 Obtain Arm Vein for Graft

EXCLUDES *Endoscopic harvest (33508)*
Harvesting of multiple vein segments (35682, 35683)
Code first (33510-33536, 35556, 35566, 35570-35571, 35583-35587)

\+ **35500** **Harvest of upper extremity vein, 1 segment, for lower extremity or coronary artery bypass procedure (List separately in addition to code for primary procedure)**
N 80 PQ 9.47 9.47 FUD ZZZ

35501-35571 Arterial Bypass Using Vein Grafts

CMS 100-3,20.1 Vertebral Artery Surgery
CMS 100-3,20.2 Extracranial-intracranial (EC-IC) Arterial Bypass Surgery
CMS 100-3,160.8 Electroencephalographic Monitoring During Cerebral Vasculature Surgery

INCLUDES Obtaining saphenous vein grafts

EXCLUDES *Obtaining multiple vein segments (35682, 35683)*
Obtaining vein grafts, upper extremity or femoropopliteal (35500, 35572)
Treatment of different sites with different bypass procedures during the same operative session

35501 **Bypass graft, with vein; common carotid-ipsilateral internal carotid**
C 80 50 ▪ 44.34 44.34 **FUD** 090

35506 **carotid-subclavian or subclavian-carotid**
C 80 50 ▪ 38.03 38.03 **FUD** 090

35508 **carotid-vertebral**
INCLUDES Endoscopic procedure
C 80 50 ▪ 39.95 39.95 **FUD** 090

35509 **carotid-contralateral carotid**
C 80 50 ▪ 42.19 42.19 **FUD** 090

35510 **carotid-brachial**
C 80 50 ▪ 36.69 36.69 **FUD** 090

35511 **subclavian-subclavian**
C 80 50 ▪ 37.70 37.70 **FUD** 090

35512 **subclavian-brachial**
C 80 50 ▪ 35.99 35.99 **FUD** 090

35515 **subclavian-vertebral**
C 80 50 ▪ 39.63 39.63 **FUD** 090

35516 **subclavian-axillary**
C 80 50 ▪ 36.40 36.40 **FUD** 090

35518 **axillary-axillary**
C 80 50 ▪ 34.08 34.08 **FUD** 090

35521 **axillary-femoral**
EXCLUDES *Synthetic graft (35621)*
C 80 50 ▪ 36.58 36.58 **FUD** 090

35522 **axillary-brachial**
C 80 50 ▪ 36.00 36.00 **FUD** 090

35523 **brachial-ulnar or -radial**
EXCLUDES *Bypass graft using synthetic conduit (37799)*
Do not report with (35206, 35500, 35525, 36838)
C 80 50 38.03 38.03 **FUD** 090

35525 **brachial-brachial**
C 80 50 ▪ 33.71 33.71 **FUD** 090

35526 **aortosubclavian, aortoinnominate, or aortocarotid**
EXCLUDES *Synthetic graft (35626)*
C 80 50 ▪ PQ 50.95 50.95 **FUD** 090

35531 **aortoceliac or aortomesenteric**
C 80 50 ▪ 59.94 59.94 **FUD** 090

35533 **axillary-femoral-femoral**
EXCLUDES *Synthetic graft (35654)*
C 80 50 ▪ 44.92 44.92 **FUD** 090

35535 **hepatorenal**
Do not report with (35221, 35251, 35281, 35500, 35536, 35560, 35631, 35636)
C 80 50 50.70 50.70 **FUD** 090

35536 **splenorenal**
C 80 50 ▪ 50.41 50.41 **FUD** 090

35537 **aortoiliac**
EXCLUDES *Synthetic graft (35637)*
Do not report with (35538)
C 80 62.20 62.20 **FUD** 090

35538 **aortobi-iliac**
EXCLUDES *Synthetic graft (35638)*
Do not report with (35537)
C 80 69.64 69.64 **FUD** 090

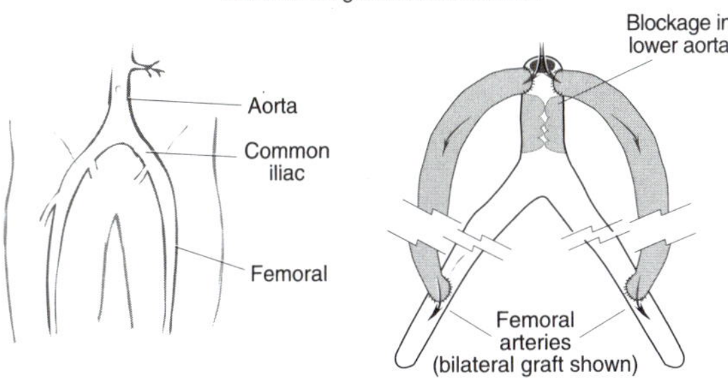

35539 **aortofemoral**
EXCLUDES *Synthetic graft (35647)*
Do not report with (35540)
C 80 50 65.42 65.42 **FUD** 090

35540 **aortobifemoral**
EXCLUDES *Synthetic graft (35646)*
Do not report with (35539)
C 50 72.57 72.57 **FUD** 090

35556 **femoral-popliteal**
C 80 50 ▪ PQ 41.68 41.68 **FUD** 090

35558 **femoral-femoral**
C 80 50 ▪ 36.70 36.70 **FUD** 090

35560 **aortorenal**
C 80 50 ▪ 50.83 50.83 **FUD** 090

35563 **ilioiliac**
C 80 50 ▪ 39.44 39.44 **FUD** 090

35565 **iliofemoral**
C 80 50 ▪ 39.09 39.09 **FUD** 090

35566 **femoral-anterior tibial, posterior tibial, peroneal artery or other distal vessels**
C 80 50 ▪ PQ 49.75 49.75 **FUD** 090

35570 **tibial-tibial, peroneal-tibial, or tibial/peroneal trunk-tibial**
Do not report with (35256, 35286)
C 80 50 40.61 40.61 **FUD** 090

35571 **popliteal-tibial, -peroneal artery or other distal vessels**
C 80 50 ▪ PQ 39.56 39.56 **FUD** 090

35572 Obtain Femoropopliteal Vein for Graft

\+ **35572** **Harvest of femoropopliteal vein, 1 segment, for vascular reconstruction procedure (eg, aortic, vena caval, coronary, peripheral artery) (List separately in addition to code for primary procedure)**
Code first (33510-33523, 33533-33536, 34502, 34520, 35001-35002, 35011-35022, 35102-35103, 35121-35152, 35231-35256, 35501-35587, 35879-35907)
N1 N 80 ▪ 10.21 10.21 **FUD** ZZZ

35583-35587 Lower Extremity Revascularization: In-situ Vein Bypass

INCLUDES Obtaining saphenous vein grafts

EXCLUDES *Obtaining multiple vein segments (35682, 35683)*
Obtaining vein graft, upper extremity or femoropopliteal (35500, 35572)

35583 In-situ vein bypass; femoral-popliteal
Code also aortobifemoral bypass graft other than vein for aortobifemoral bypass using synthetic conduit and femoral-popliteal bypass with vein conduit in situ (35646)
Code also concurrent aortofemoral bypass for aortofemoral bypass graft with synthetic conduit and femoral-popliteal bypass with vein conduit in-situ (35647)
Code also concurrent aortofemoral bypass (vein) for an aortofemoral bypass using a vein conduit or a femoral-popliteal bypass with vein conduit in-situ (35539)
C 80 50 PQ 43.00 43.00 FUD 090

35585 femoral-anterior tibial, posterior tibial, or peroneal artery
C 80 50 PQ 49.87 49.87 FUD 090

35587 popliteal-tibial, peroneal
C 80 50 PQ 40.70 40.70 FUD 090

35600 Obtain Arm Artery for Coronary Bypass

EXCLUDES *Transposition and/or reimplantation of arteries (35691-35695)*

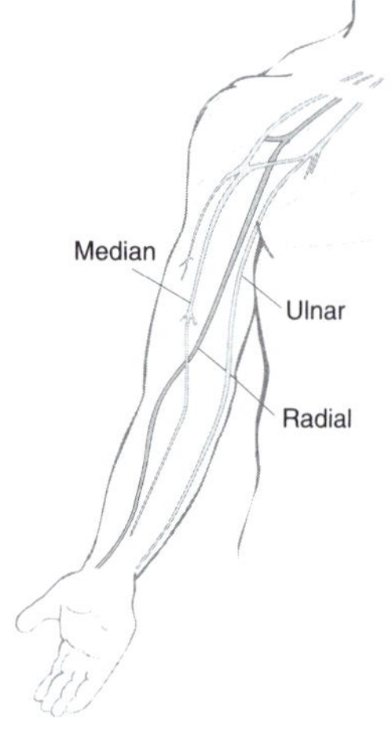

An upper extremity artery or segment is harvested for a coronary artery bypass procedure

+ **35600 Harvest of upper extremity artery, 1 segment, for coronary artery bypass procedure (List separately in addition to code for primary procedure)**
Code first (33533-33536)
C 80 PQ 7.54 7.54 FUD ZZZ

35601-35671 Arterial Bypass: Grafts Other Than Veins

CMS 100-3,20.1 Vertebral Artery Surgery
CMS 100-3,20.2 Extracranial-intracranial (EC-IC) Arterial Bypass Surgery
CMS 100-3,160.8 Electroencephalographic Monitoring During Cerebral Vasculature Surgery

EXCLUDES *Transposition and/or reimplantation of arteries (35691-35695)*

35601 Bypass graft, with other than vein; common carotid-ipsilateral internal carotid
EXCLUDES *Open transcervical common carotid-common carotid bypass with endovascular repair of descending thoracic aorta (33891)*
C 80 50 PQ 41.69 41.69 FUD 090

35606 carotid-subclavian
EXCLUDES *Open subclavian to carotid artery transposition performed with endovascular thoracic aneurysm repair via neck incision (33889)*
C 80 50 PQ 34.91 34.91 FUD 090

35612 subclavian-subclavian
C 80 50 PQ 31.14 31.14 FUD 090

35616 subclavian-axillary
C 80 50 PQ 32.37 32.37 FUD 090

35621 axillary-femoral
C 80 50 PQ 32.67 32.67 FUD 090

35623 axillary-popliteal or -tibial
C 80 50 PQ 39.14 39.14 FUD 090

35626 aortosubclavian, aortoinnominate, or aortocarotid
C 80 50 PQ 46.64 46.64 FUD 090

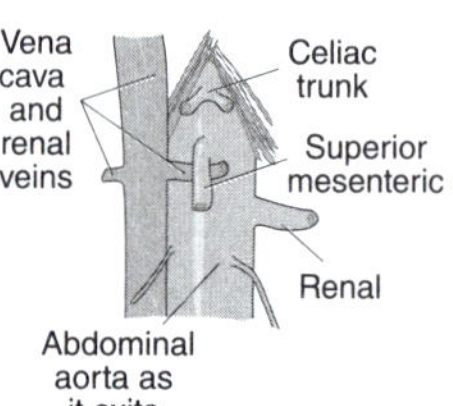

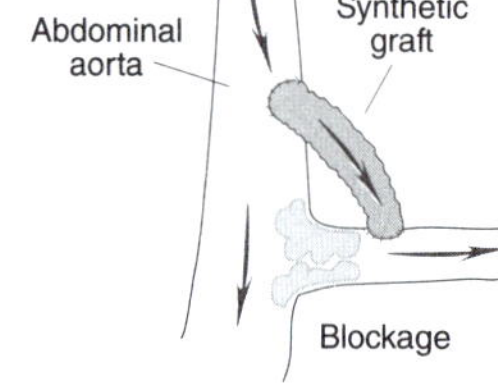

35631 aortoceliac, aortomesenteric, aortorenal
C 80 50 PQ 55.03 55.03 FUD 090

35632 ilio-celiac
Do not report with (35221, 35251, 35281, 35531, 35631)
C 80 50 PQ 48.15 48.15 FUD 090

35633 ilio-mesenteric
Do not report with (35221, 35251, 35281, 35531, 35631)
C 80 50 PQ 53.77 53.77 FUD 090

35634 iliorenal
Do not report with (35221, 35251, 35281, 35536, 35560, 35631)
C 80 50 PQ 47.11 47.11 FUD 090

35636 splenorenal (splenic to renal arterial anastomosis)
C 80 50 PQ 47.55 47.55 FUD 090

35637 aortoiliac
Do not report with (35638, 35646)
C 80 PQ 51.43 51.43 FUD 090

35638 aortobi-iliac
EXCLUDES *Open placement of aorto-bi-iliac prosthesis after a failed endovascular repair (34831)*
Do not report with (35637, 35646)
C 80 PQ 52.45 52.45 FUD 090

35642 carotid-vertebral
C 80 50 PQ 29.40 29.40 FUD 090

35645 subclavian-vertebral
C 80 50 PQ 30.81 30.81 FUD 090

35646 aortobifemoral
EXCLUDES *Bypass graft using vein graft (35540)*
Open placement of aortobifemoral prosthesis after a failed endovascular repair (34832)
C 80 PQ 51.03 51.03 FUD 090

35647 aortofemoral
EXCLUDES *Bypass graft using vein graft (35539)*
C 80 50 PQ 46.29 46.29 FUD 090

35650 **axillary-axillary**
C 80 50 PQ 31.92 31.92 FUD 090

35654 **axillary-femoral-femoral**
C 80 PQ 40.77 40.77 FUD 090

35656 **femoral-popliteal**
C 80 50 PQ 32.23 32.23 FUD 090

35661 **femoral-femoral**
C 80 50 PQ 32.25 32.25 FUD 090

35663 **ilioiliac**
C 80 50 PQ 37.33 37.33 FUD 090

35665 **iliofemoral**
C 80 50 PQ 34.96 34.96 FUD 090

35666 **femoral-anterior tibial, posterior tibial, or peroneal artery**
C 80 50 PQ 37.77 37.77 FUD 090

35671 **popliteal-tibial or -peroneal artery**
C 80 50 PQ 33.35 33.35 FUD 090

35681-35683 Arterial Bypass Using Combination Synthetic and Donor Graft

INCLUDES Acquiring multiple segments of vein from sites other than the extremity for which the arterial bypass is performed
Anastomosis of vein segments to creat bypass graft conduits

\+ 35681 **Bypass graft; composite, prosthetic and vein (List separately in addition to code for primary procedure)**
Code first primary procedure
Do not report with (35682, 35683)
C 80 2.37 2.37 FUD ZZZ

\+ 35682 **autogenous composite, 2 segments of veins from 2 locations (List separately in addition to code for primary procedure)**
Code first (35556, 35566, 35570-35571, 35583-35587)
Do not report with (35681, 35683)
C 80 10.52 10.52 FUD ZZZ

\+ 35683 **autogenous composite, 3 or more segments of vein from 2 or more locations (List separately in addition to code for primary procedure)**
Code first (35556, 35566, 35570-35571, 35583-35587)
Do not report with (35681, 35682)
C 80 12.20 12.20 FUD ZZZ

35685-35686 Supplemental Procedures

INCLUDES Additional procedures that may be needed with a bypass graft to increase the patency of the graft

EXCLUDES *Composite grafts (35681-35683)*

\+ 35685 **Placement of vein patch or cuff at distal anastomosis of bypass graft, synthetic conduit (List separately in addition to code for primary procedure)**
INCLUDES Connection of a segment of vein (cuff or patch) between the distal portion of the synthetic graft and the native artery
Code first (35656, 35666 or 35671)
N 80 5.93 5.93 FUD ZZZ

\+ 35686 **Creation of distal arteriovenous fistula during lower extremity bypass surgery (non-hemodialysis) (List separately in addition to code for primary procedure)**
INCLUDES Creation of a fistula between the peroneal or tibial artery and vein at or past the site of the distal anastomosis
Code first (35556, 35566, 35570-35571, 35583-35587, 35623, 35656, 35666, 35671)
N 80 4.77 4.77 FUD ZZZ

35691-35697 Arterial Translocation

CMS 100-3,20.1 Vertebral Artery Surgery
CMS 100-3,20.2 Extracranial-intracranial (EC-IC) Arterial Bypass Surgery
CMS 100-3,160.8 Electroencephalographic Monitoring During Cerebral Vasculature Surgery

35691 **Transposition and/or reimplantation; vertebral to carotid artery**
C 80 50 28.17 28.17 FUD 090

35693 **vertebral to subclavian artery**
C 80 50 24.87 24.87 FUD 090

35694 **subclavian to carotid artery**
EXCLUDES *Subclavian to carotid artery transposition procedure (open) with concurrent repair of descending thoracic aorta (endovascular) (33889)*
C 80 50 29.41 29.41 FUD 090

35695 **carotid to subclavian artery**
C 80 50 30.54 30.54 FUD 090

\+ 35697 **Reimplantation, visceral artery to infrarenal aortic prosthesis, each artery (List separately in addition to code for primary procedure)**
Code first primary procedure
Do not report with (33877)
C 80 4.39 4.39 FUD ZZZ

35700 Reoperative Bypass Lower Extremities

\+ 35700 **Reoperation, femoral-popliteal or femoral (popliteal)-anterior tibial, posterior tibial, peroneal artery, or other distal vessels, more than 1 month after original operation (List separately in addition to code for primary procedure)**
Code first (35556, 35566, 35570-35571, 35583, 35585, 35587, 35656, 35666, 35671)
C 80 4.54 4.54 FUD ZZZ

35701-35761 Arterial Exploration without Repair

35701 **Exploration (not followed by surgical repair), with or without lysis of artery; carotid artery**
C 80 50 16.65 16.65 FUD 090

35721 **femoral artery**
C 80 50 13.34 13.34 FUD 090

35741 **popliteal artery**
C 80 50 15.12 15.12 FUD 090

35761 **other vessels**
62 T 80 50 11.41 11.41 FUD 090

35800-35860 Arterial Exploration for Postoperative Complication

INCLUDES Return to the operating room for postoperative hemorrhage

35800 **Exploration for postoperative hemorrhage, thrombosis or infection; neck**
C 80 20.97 20.97 FUD 090

35820 **chest**
C 80 58.77 58.77 FUD 090

35840 **abdomen**
C 80 34.41 34.41 FUD 090

35860 **extremity**
T 80 24.87 24.87 FUD 090

35870 Repair Secondary Aortoenteric Fistula

35870 **Repair of graft-enteric fistula**
C 80 37.10 37.10 FUD 090

35875-35876 Removal of Thrombus from Graft

EXCLUDES *Thrombectomy dialysis fistula or graft (36831, 36833)*
Thrombectomy with blood vessel repair, lower extremity, vein graft (35256)
Thrombectomy with blood vessel repair, lower extremity, with/without patch angioplasty (35226)

35875 **Thrombectomy of arterial or venous graft (other than hemodialysis graft or fistula);**
A2 T 17.57 17.57 FUD 090

35876 **with revision of arterial or venous graft**
A2 T 80 28.03 28.03 FUD 090

35879-35884 Revision Lower Extremity Bypass Graft

EXCLUDES *Removal of infected graft (35901-35907)*
Revascularization following removal of infected graft(s)
Thrombectomy dialysis fistula or graft (36831, 36833)
Thrombectomy with blood vessel repair, lower extremity, vein graft (35256)
Thrombectomy with blood vessel repair, lower extremity, with/without patch angioplasty (35226)
Thrombectomy with graft revision (35876)

35879 **Revision, lower extremity arterial bypass, without thrombectomy, open; with vein patch angioplasty**
T 80 50 27.49 27.49 FUD 090

35881 **with segmental vein interposition**
EXCLUDES *Revision of femoral anastomosis of synthetic arterial bypass graft (35883-35884)*
T 80 50 30.33 30.33 FUD 090

35883 **Revision, femoral anastomosis of synthetic arterial bypass graft in groin, open; with nonautogenous patch graft (eg, Dacron, ePTFE, bovine pericardium)**
Do not report with (35700, 35875-35876, 35884)
T 80 50 35.92 35.92 FUD 090

35884 **with autogenous vein patch graft**
Do not report with (35700, 35875-35876, 35883)
T 80 50 36.99 36.99 FUD 090

35901-35907 Removal of Infected Graft

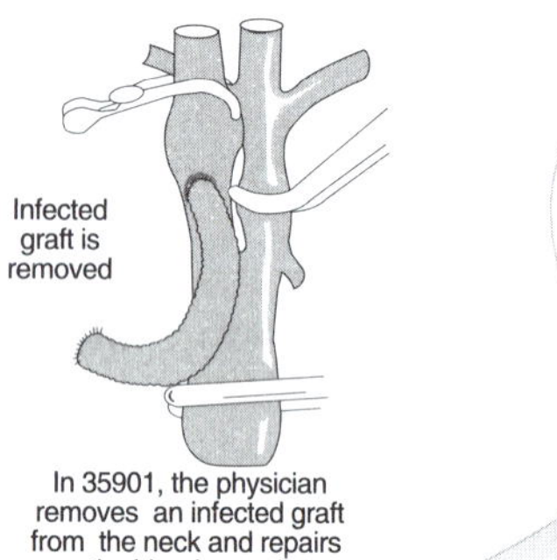

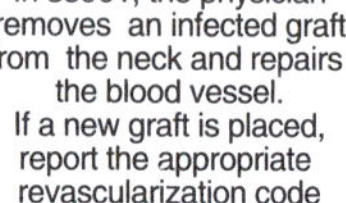
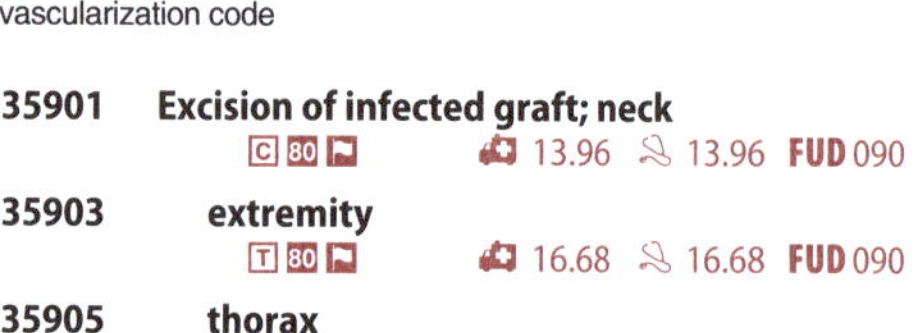

In 35901, the physician removes an infected graft from the neck and repairs the blood vessel. If a new graft is placed, report the appropriate revascularization code

35901 **Excision of infected graft; neck**
C 80 13.96 13.96 FUD 090

35903 **extremity**
T 80 16.68 16.68 FUD 090

35905 **thorax**
C 80 50.09 50.09 FUD 090

35907 **abdomen**
C 80 56.64 56.64 FUD 090

36000 Intravenous Access Established

INCLUDES Venous access for phlebotomy, prophylactic intravenous access, infusion therapy, chemotherapy, hydration, transfusion, drug administration, etc. which is included in the work value of the primary procedure

36000 **Introduction of needle or intracatheter, vein**
N1 N 0.28 0.73 FUD XXX

36002 Injection Treatment of Pseudoaneurysm

INCLUDES Insertion of needle or catheter, local anesthesia, injection of contrast, power injections, and all pre- and postinjection care provided

EXCLUDES *Compression repair pseudoaneurysm, ultrasound guided (76936)*
Medications, contrast material, catheters

Do not report for arteriotomy site sealant

36002 **Injection procedures (eg, thrombin) for percutaneous treatment of extremity pseudoaneurysm**
76942, 77002, 77012, 77021
G2 S 50 3.12 4.64 FUD 000

36005-36015 Insertion Needle or Intracatheter: Venous

INCLUDES Insertion of needle/catheter, local anesthesia, injection of contrast, power injections, all pre- and postinjection care

EXCLUDES *Medications, contrast materials, catheters*

Code also catheterization of second order vessels (or higher) supplied by the same first order branch, same vascular family (36012)
Code also each vascular family (e.g., bilateral procedures are separate vascular families)

36005 **Injection procedure for extremity venography (including introduction of needle or intracatheter)**
75820, 75822
N1 N 80 50 1.40 9.12 FUD 000

⊙ **36010** **Introduction of catheter, superior or inferior vena cava**
N1 N 50 3.52 14.26 FUD XXX

36011 **Selective catheter placement, venous system; first order branch (eg, renal vein, jugular vein)**
N1 N 50 4.56 23.70 FUD XXX

36012 **second order, or more selective, branch (eg, left adrenal vein, petrosal sinus)**
N1 N 50 5.14 24.54 FUD XXX

36013 **Introduction of catheter, right heart or main pulmonary artery**
N1 N 3.79 22.30 FUD XXX

36014 **Selective catheter placement, left or right pulmonary artery**
N1 N 50 4.33 23.04 FUD XXX

36015 **Selective catheter placement, segmental or subsegmental pulmonary artery**
EXCLUDES *Placement of Swan Ganz/other flow directed catheter for monitoring (93503)*
Selective blood sampling, specific organs (36500)
N1 N 50 5.02 24.68 FUD XXX

36100-36218 Insertion Needle or Intracatheter: Arterial

INCLUDES Introduction of the catheter and catheterization of all lesser order vessels used for the approach
Local anesthesia, placement of catheter/needle, injection of contrast, power injections, all pre- and postinjection care

EXCLUDES *Angiography (36222-36228, 75600-75774, 75791)*
Angioplasty (35472, 35475)
Chemotherapy injections (96401-96549)
Injection procedures for cardiac catheterizations (93455, 93457, 93459, 93461, 93530-93533, 93564)
Internal mammary artery angiography without left heart catheterization (36216, 36217)
Medications, contrast, catheters
Transcatheter interventions (37200, [37211], [37213, 37214], 37202, 37236-37239, 37241-37244, 61624, 61626)

Code also additional first order or higher catheterization for vascular families if the vascular family is supplied by a first order vessel that is different from one already coded
Code also catheterization of second and third order vessels supplied by the same first order branch, same vascular family (36218, 36248)

36100 **Introduction of needle or intracatheter, carotid or vertebral artery**
N1 N 50 4.63 14.39 FUD XXX

36120 Introduction of needle or intracatheter; retrograde brachial artery

EXCLUDES *Arteriovenous cannula insertion (36810-36821)*

N1 N 2.91 12.14 FUD XXX

⊙ **36140 extremity artery**

EXCLUDES *Arteriovenous cannula insertion (36810-36821)*

N1 N 2.99 12.44 FUD XXX

⊙ **36147 Introduction of needle and/or catheter, arteriovenous shunt created for dialysis (graft/fistula); initial access with complete radiological evaluation of dialysis access, including fluoroscopy, image documentation and report (includes access of shunt, injection[s] of contrast, and all necessary imaging from the arterial anastomosis and adjacent artery through entire venous outflow including the inferior or superior vena cava)**

INCLUDES Access and imaging of the AV shunt
- Antegrade and/or retrograde punctures for contrast injection through a needle or catheter for imaging
- Catheter manipulation for:
  - Advancement of the tip of the catheter to the vena cava
  - Diagnostic imaging of the AV shunt
  - Visualization of the arterial anastomosis or central veins
- Catheterization of all veins in arteriovenous shunt
- Diagnostic procedures of all upper and lower arteriovenous fistulae and grafts from the arterial anastomosis to the right atrium
- Evaluation of peri-anastomotic portion of the inflow which includes:
  - Portion of the artery bordering the anastomosis
  - Portion of the graft or vessel just distal to the anastomosis
  - Site of the anastomosis

EXCLUDES *Additional catheter work/imaging to evaluate proximal arterial inflow to AV access*
- *Selective catheter advancement from the AV shunt puncture to the inflow artery (most often AV shunt of upper extremity) (36215)*
- *Ultrasound guidance (76937)*

Code also the second shunt catheterization if a need is identified for a therapeutic interventional procedure (36148)

Do not report selective catheterization of inferior/superior vena cava or central veins when performed by direct puncture of the fistula or graft

Do not report with (75791)

P2 T 80 PQ 5.43 23.81 FUD XXX

+ ⊙ **36148 additional access for therapeutic intervention (List separately in addition to code for primary procedure)**

INCLUDES All interventional procedures performed in a single segment no matter how many lesions are taken care of
- Catheterization of all veins in arteriovenous shunt
- Interventional procedures in arteriovenous shunts (arteriovenous fistulae and grafts) considered to be primarily venous
- Two vessel segments:
  - First segment (peripheral) extends from peri-arterial anastomosis through the axillary vein or the complete cephalic vein for cephalic venous outflow
  - Second segment: veins central to the axillary and cephalic veins (eg, subclavian and innominate veins through the vena cava)

EXCLUDES *Arterial intervention with radiological supervision and interpretation in the peri-anastomotic region (35475, 75962)*
- *Catheterization for intervention in an accessory vein (36011-36012)*
- *Embolization of an accessory vein (37241)*
- *Fistula thrombectomy (36870)*
- *Other venous interventional procedures, as appropriate*
- *Radiological supervision and interpretation for venous angioplasty (75978)*
- *Stent placement for central venous stenosis (37239)*
- *Stent placement from the peri-arterial anastomosis through the axillary and cephalic veins (37236 or 37238)*
- *Venous angioplasty, once per vessel only (35476)*

Code first (36147)

Do not report selective catheterization of inferior/superior vena cava or central veins when performed by direct puncture of the fistula or graft

Do not report venous interventional codes for stenosis at the arterial anastomosis (peri-anastomotic or juxta-anastomotic region)

N1 N 80 1.42 7.41 FUD ZZZ

36160 Introduction of needle or intracatheter, aortic, translumbar

N1 N 3.73 14.51 FUD XXX

⊙ **36200 Introduction of catheter, aorta**

EXCLUDES *Nonselective angiography of the extracranial carotid and/or cerebral vessels and cervicocerebral arch (36221)*

N1 N 50 4.44 17.72 FUD 000

36215 Selective catheter placement, arterial system; each first order thoracic or brachiocephalic branch, within a vascular family

INCLUDES Introduction of catheter into the aorta (36200)

EXCLUDES *Placement of catheter for coronary angiography (93454-93461)*

N1 N 7.04 31.28 FUD XXX

36216 initial second order thoracic or brachiocephalic branch, within a vascular family

N1 N 8.04 35.28 FUD XXX

36217 initial third order or more selective thoracic or brachiocephalic branch, within a vascular family

N1 N 9.64 60.64 FUD XXX

+ **36218** **additional second order, third order, and beyond, thoracic or brachiocephalic branch, within a vascular family (List in addition to code for initial second or third order vessel as appropriate)**
Code first (36216-36217, 36225-36226)
N1 N 1.53 5.69 FUD ZZZ

36221-36228 Diagnostic Studies: Aortic Arch/Carotid/Vertebral Arteries

INCLUDES Accessing the vessel
Arterial contrast injection that includes arterial, capillary, and venous phase imaging, when performed
Arteriotomy closure (pressure or closure device)
Catheter placement
Radiologic supervision and interpretation
Reporting of selective catheter placement based on intensity of services in the following hierarchy:
36226>36225
36224>36223>36222

EXCLUDES *3D rendering when performed (76376-76377)*
Interventional procedures
Ultrasound guidance (76937)

Code also diagnostic angiography of upper extremities/other vascular beds during the same session, if performed (75774)
Do not report with angiography of cervicocerebral vessels (75774)

⊙ **36221** **Non-selective catheter placement, thoracic aorta, with angiography of the extracranial carotid, vertebral, and/or intracranial vessels, unilateral or bilateral, and all associated radiological supervision and interpretation, includes angiography of the cervicocerebral arch, when performed**
Do not report with (36222-36226)
Do not report with transcatheter intravascular stent placement of common carotid or innominate artery on the same side (37217)
N1 Q2 6.23 31.61 FUD 000

⊙ **36222** **Selective catheter placement, common carotid or innominate artery, unilateral, any approach, with angiography of the ipsilateral extracranial carotid circulation and all associated radiological supervision and interpretation, includes angiography of the cervicocerebral arch, when performed**
INCLUDES Unilateral catheterization of artery
Code also modifier 59 when different territories on both sides of the body are being studied
Do not report with (37215-37216, 37218)
Do not report with transcatheter intravascular stent placement of common carotid or innominate artery on the same side (37217)
N1 Q2 50 8.47 39.99 FUD 000

⊙ **36223** **Selective catheter placement, common carotid or innominate artery, unilateral, any approach, with angiography of the ipsilateral intracranial carotid circulation and all associated radiological supervision and interpretation, includes angiography of the extracranial carotid and cervicocerebral arch, when performed**
INCLUDES Unilateral catheterization of artery
Code also modifier 59 when different territories on both sides of the body are being studied
Do not report with (37215-37216, 37218)
Do not report with transcatheter intravascular stent placement of common carotid or innominate artery on the same side (37217)
N1 Q2 50 9.14 43.55 FUD 000

⊙ **36224** **Selective catheter placement, internal carotid artery, unilateral, with angiography of the ipsilateral intracranial carotid circulation and all associated radiological supervision and interpretation, includes angiography of the extracranial carotid and cervicocerebral arch, when performed**
INCLUDES Unilateral catheterization of artery
Code also modifier 59 when different territories on both sides of the body are being studied
Do not report with (37215-37216, 37218)
Do not report with transcatheter intravascular stent placement of common carotid or innominate artery on the same side (37217)
N1 Q2 50 10.00 47.87 FUD 000

⊙ **36225** **Selective catheter placement, subclavian or innominate artery, unilateral, with angiography of the ipsilateral vertebral circulation and all associated radiological supervision and interpretation, includes angiography of the cervicocerebral arch, when performed**
Do not report with transcatheter intravascular stent placement of common carotid or innominate artery on the same side (37217)
N1 Q2 50 9.10 43.12 FUD 000

⊙ **36226** **Selective catheter placement, vertebral artery, unilateral, with angiography of the ipsilateral vertebral circulation and all associated radiological supervision and interpretation, includes angiography of the cervicocerebral arch, when performed**
Do not report with transcatheter intravascular stent placement of common carotid or innominate artery on the same side (37217)
N1 Q2 50 10.03 48.83 FUD 000

+ ⊙ **36227** **Selective catheter placement, external carotid artery, unilateral, with angiography of the ipsilateral external carotid circulation and all associated radiological supervision and interpretation (List separately in addition to code for primary procedure)**
INCLUDES Unilateral catheter placement/diagnostic imaging of ipsilateral external carotid circulation
Code first (36222-36224)
Do not report with transcatheter intravascular stent placement of common carotid or innominate artery on the same side (37217)
N1 N 50 3.18 7.05 FUD ZZZ

+ ⊙ **36228** **Selective catheter placement, each intracranial branch of the internal carotid or vertebral arteries, unilateral, with angiography of the selected vessel circulation and all associated radiological supervision and interpretation (eg, middle cerebral artery, posterior inferior cerebellar artery) (List separately in addition to code for primary procedure)**
INCLUDES Unilateral catheter placement/imaging of initial and each additional intracranial branch of internal carotid or vertebral arteries
Code first (36223-36226)
Do not report more than 2 times per side
Do not report with transcatheter intravascular stent placement of common carotid or innominate artery on the same side (37217)
N1 N 50 6.46 33.21 FUD ZZZ

36245-36254 Catheter Placement: Arteries of the Lower Body

INCLUDES Introduction of the catheter and catheterization of all lesser order vessels used for the approach
Local anesthesia, placement of catheter/needle, injection of contrast, power injections

EXCLUDES *Angiography (36147, 36222-36228, 75600-75774, 75791)*
Angioplasty (35471-35472, 35475)
Chemotherapy injections (96401-96549)
Injection procedures for cardiac catheterizations (93455, 93457, 93459, 93461, 93530-93533, 93564)
Internal mammary artery angiography without left heart catheterization (36216-36217)
Medications, contrast, catheters
Transcatheter procedures (37200, [37211], [37213, 37214], 37202, 37236-37239, 37241-37244, 61624, 61626)

Code also additional first order or higher catheterization for vascular families if the vascular family is supplied by a first order vessel that is different from one already coded

Code also catheterization of second and third order vessels supplied by the same first order branch, same vascular family (36218, 36248)

75600-75791

⊙ **36245** **Selective catheter placement, arterial system; each first order abdominal, pelvic, or lower extremity artery branch, within a vascular family**
N1 N 50 — 7.44 — 38.65 FUD XXX

⊙ **36246** **initial second order abdominal, pelvic, or lower extremity artery branch, within a vascular family**
N1 N 50 — 7.82 — 25.31 FUD 000

⊙ **36247** **initial third order or more selective abdominal, pelvic, or lower extremity artery branch, within a vascular family**
N1 N 50 — 9.35 — 44.87 FUD 000

+ ⊙ **36248** **additional second order, third order, and beyond, abdominal, pelvic, or lower extremity artery branch, within a vascular family (List in addition to code for initial second or third order vessel as appropriate)**
Code first (36246, 36247)
N1 N — 1.49 — 4.37 FUD ZZZ

⊙ **36251** **Selective catheter placement (first-order), main renal artery and any accessory renal artery(s) for renal angiography, including arterial puncture and catheter placement(s), fluoroscopy, contrast injection(s), image postprocessing, permanent recording of images, and radiological supervision and interpretation, including pressure gradient measurements when performed, and flush aortogram when performed; unilateral**
INCLUDES Closure device placement at vascular access site
Do not report with (0338T-0339T)
N1 Q2 — 8.15 — 40.08 FUD 000

⊙ **36252** **bilateral**
INCLUDES Closure device placement at vascular access site
Do not report with (0338T-0339T)
N1 Q2 — 10.67 — 43.58 FUD 000

⊙ **36253** **Superselective catheter placement (one or more second order or higher renal artery branches) renal artery and any accessory renal artery(s) for renal angiography, including arterial puncture, catheterization, fluoroscopy, contrast injection(s), image postprocessing, permanent recording of images, and radiological supervision and interpretation, including pressure gradient measurements when performed, and flush aortogram when performed; unilateral**
INCLUDES Closure device placement at vascular access site
Do not report for same kidney with (36251)
Do not report with (0338T-0339T)
N1 Q2 — 11.43 — 64.40 FUD 000

⊙ **36254** **bilateral**
INCLUDES Closure device placement at vascular access site
Do not report with (36252, 0338T-0339T)
N1 Q2 — 12.40 — 61.73 FUD 000

36260-36299 Implanted Infusion Pumps: Intra-arterial

CMS 100-3,280.14 Infusion Pumps

36260 **Insertion of implantable intra-arterial infusion pump (eg, for chemotherapy of liver)**
Code also (C1772, C1891, C2626)
A2 T — 17.82 — 17.82 FUD 090

36261 **Revision of implanted intra-arterial infusion pump**
A2 T 80 — 10.37 — 10.37 FUD 090

36262 **Removal of implanted intra-arterial infusion pump**
A2 Q2 — 8.70 — 8.70 FUD 090

36299 **Unlisted procedure, vascular injection**
N 80 — 0.00 — 0.00 FUD YYY

36400-36425 Specimen Collection: Phlebotomy

EXCLUDES *Collection of specimen from:*
A completely implantable device (36591)
An established catheter (36592)

36400 **Venipuncture, younger than age 3 years, necessitating the skill of a physician or other qualified health care professional, not to be used for routine venipuncture; femoral or jugular vein** A
N1 N — 0.59 — 0.86 FUD XXX

36405 **scalp vein** A
N1 N — 0.49 — 0.76 FUD XXX

36406 **other vein** A
N1 N — 0.27 — 0.54 FUD XXX

36410 **Venipuncture, age 3 years or older, necessitating the skill of a physician or other qualified health care professional (separate procedure), for diagnostic or therapeutic purposes (not to be used for routine venipuncture)** A
N1 N — 0.28 — 0.48 FUD XXX

36415 **Collection of venous blood by venipuncture**
N 63 — 0.00 — 0.00 FUD XXX

36416 **Collection of capillary blood specimen (eg, finger, heel, ear stick)**
N1 N — 0.00 — 0.00 FUD XXX

36420 **Venipuncture, cutdown; younger than age 1 year** A
R2 X 80 63 — 1.40 — 1.40 FUD XXX

36425 **age 1 or over** A
Do not report with (36475-36476, 36478-36479)
R2 X — 1.16 — 1.16 FUD XXX

Cardiovascular System
36245 — 36425

36430-36460 Transfusions

CMS 100-1,3,20.5 Blood Deductibles
CMS 100-1,3,20.5.2 Part B Blood Deductible
CMS 100-2,1,10 Inpatient Hospital Services Covered Under Part A
CMS 100-3,110.5 Granulocyte Transfusions
CMS 100-3,110.7 Blood Transfusions
CMS 100-3,110.8 Blood Platelet Transfusions
CMS 100-3,110.16 Nonselective (Random) Transfusions and Living-Related Donor Specific Transfusions (DST) in Kidney Transplantation
CMS 100-4,3,40.2.2 Beneficiary Charges for Part A Services

36430 **Transfusion, blood or blood components**
P3 S 0.95 0.95 FUD XXX

36440 **Push transfusion, blood, 2 years or younger** A
R2 S 80 1.66 1.66 FUD XXX

36450 **Exchange transfusion, blood; newborn** A
R2 S 80 63 3.10 3.10 FUD XXX

36455 **other than newborn** A
G2 S 3.25 3.25 FUD XXX

36460 **Transfusion, intrauterine, fetal** A ♀
76941
S 80 63 10.53 10.53 FUD XXX

36468-36479 Destruction of Veins

CMS 100-2,16,10 Exclusions from Coverage
CMS 100-2,16,120 Cosmetic Procedures
CMS 100-2,16,180 Services Related to Noncovered Procedures

36468 **Single or multiple injections of sclerosing solutions, spider veins (telangiectasia), limb or trunk**
Do not report in the same operative field with (37241)
R2 T 80 0.00 0.00 FUD 000

36469 **face**

36470 **Injection of sclerosing solution; single vein**
EXCLUDES *Vascular occlusion and embolization services (37241-37244)*
Do not report in same operative field with (37241)
P2 T 50 2.45 4.31 FUD 010

36471 **multiple veins, same leg**
EXCLUDES *Vascular occlusion and embolization services (37241-37244)*
Do not report in same operative field with (37241)
P2 T 50 2.93 4.97 FUD 010

36475 **Endovenous ablation therapy of incompetent vein, extremity, inclusive of all imaging guidance and monitoring, percutaneous, radiofrequency; first vein treated**
Do not report in same operative field with (29581-29582, 36000-36005, 36410, 36425, 36478-36479, 37241-37244, 75894, 76000-76001, 76937, 76942, 76998, 77022, 93970-93971)
A2 T 50 10.35 47.43 FUD 000

+ **36476** **second and subsequent veins treated in a single extremity, each through separate access sites (List separately in addition to code for primary procedure)**
Code first (36475)
Do not report in same operative field with (29581-29582, 36000-36005, 36410, 36425, 36478-36479, 37241-37244, 75894, 76000-76001, 76937, 76942, 76998, 77022, 93970-93971)
N1 N 50 5.08 10.80 FUD ZZZ

36478 **Endovenous ablation therapy of incompetent vein, extremity, inclusive of all imaging guidance and monitoring, percutaneous, laser; first vein treated**
Do not report in same operative field with (29581-29582, 36000-36005, 36410, 36425, 36475-36476, 37241, 75894, 76000-76001, 76937, 76942, 76998, 77022, 93970-93971)
A2 T 50 10.25 37.81 FUD 000

+ **36479** **second and subsequent veins treated in a single extremity, each through separate access sites (List separately in addition to code for primary procedure)**
Code first (36478)
Do not report in same operative field with (29581-29582, 36000-36005, 36410, 36425, 36475-36476, 37241, 75894, 76000-76001, 76937, 76942, 76998, 77022, 93970-93971)
N1 N 50 5.05 11.05 FUD ZZZ

36481-36510 Other Venous Catheterization Procedures

EXCLUDES *Collection of a specimen from:*
A completely implantable device (36591)
An established catheter (36592)

⊙ **36481** **Percutaneous portal vein catheterization by any method**
75885, 75887
N1 N 10.32 57.87 FUD 000

36500 **Venous catheterization for selective organ blood sampling**
EXCLUDES *Inferior or superior vena cava catheterization (36010)*
75893
N1 N 5.23 5.23 FUD 000

36510 **Catheterization of umbilical vein for diagnosis or therapy, newborn** A
EXCLUDES *Collection of a specimen from:*
Capillary blood (36416)
Venipuncture (36415)
N1 N 80 63 1.79 2.82 FUD 000

36511-36516 Apheresis

CMS 100-1,3,20.5.2 Part B Blood Deductible
CMS 100-3,110.14 Apheresis (Therapeutic Pheresis)

EXCLUDES *Collection of a specimen from:*
A completely implantable device (36591)
An established catheter (36592)
Code also modifier 26 for a professional evaluation

36511 **Therapeutic apheresis; for white blood cells**
G2 S 2.74 2.74 FUD 000

36512 **for red blood cells**
G2 S 2.70 2.70 FUD 000

36513 **for platelets**
G2 S 2.86 2.86 FUD 000

36514 **for plasma pheresis**
G2 S 2.72 14.67 FUD 000

36515 **with extracorporeal immunoadsorption and plasma reinfusion**
P2 S 2.52 58.27 FUD 000

36516 **with extracorporeal selective adsorption or selective filtration and plasma reinfusion**
P2 S 2.04 57.02 FUD 000

36522 Extracorporeal Photopheresis

CMS 100-3,110.4 Extracorporeal Photopheresis

36522 **Photopheresis, extracorporeal**
G2 S 2.92 37.92 FUD 000

36555-36571 Placement of Implantable Venous Access Device

INCLUDES Devices accessed by an exposed catheter, or a subcutaneous port or pump
Devices inserted via cutdown or percutaneous access:
Centrally (eg, femoral, jugular, subclavian veins, or inferior vena cava)
Peripherally (eg, basilic or cephalic)
Devices terminating in the brachiocephalic (innominate), iliac, or subclavian veins, vena cava, or right atrium
Venous access obtained by cutdown or percutaneously with any size catheter

EXCLUDES *Maintenance/refilling of implantable pump/reservoir (96522)*

Code also removal of central venous access device (if code available) when a new device is placed through a separate venous access

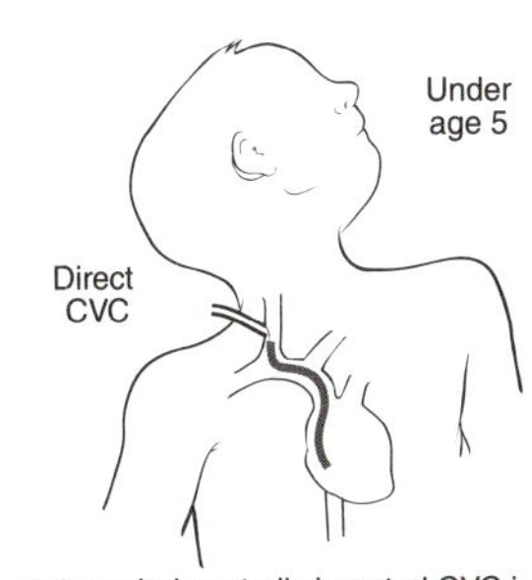

A non-tunneled centrally inserted CVC is inserted. Report 36555 for a patient under age 5 and 36556 for patients older than age 5

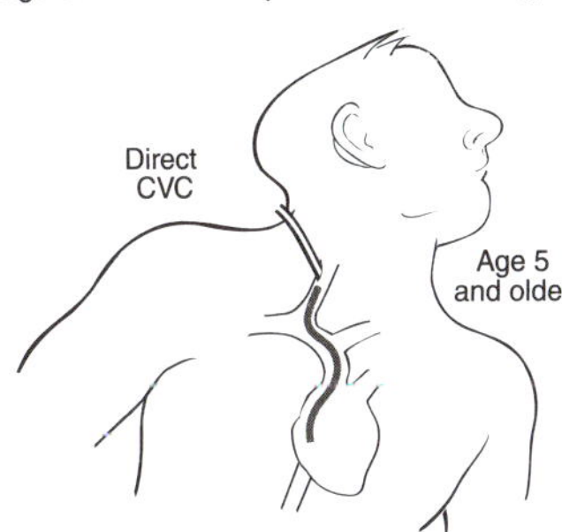

⊙ **36555** **Insertion of non-tunneled centrally inserted central venous catheter; younger than 5 years of age** A

EXCLUDES *Peripheral insertion (36568)*

A2 T PQ 3.40 7.26 FUD 000

36556 **age 5 years or older** A

EXCLUDES *Peripheral insertion (36569)*

A2 T PQ 3.51 6.63 FUD 000

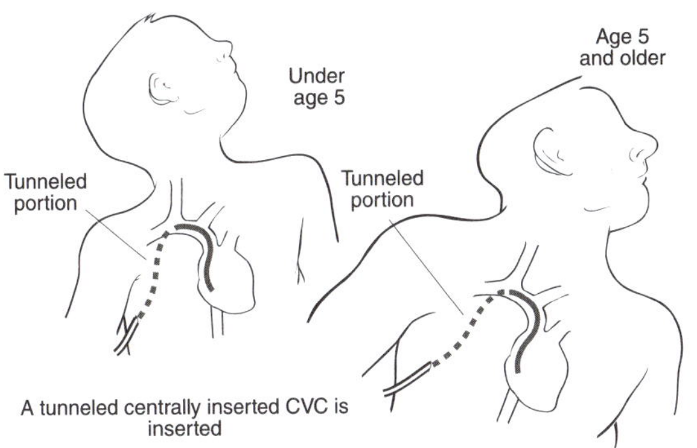

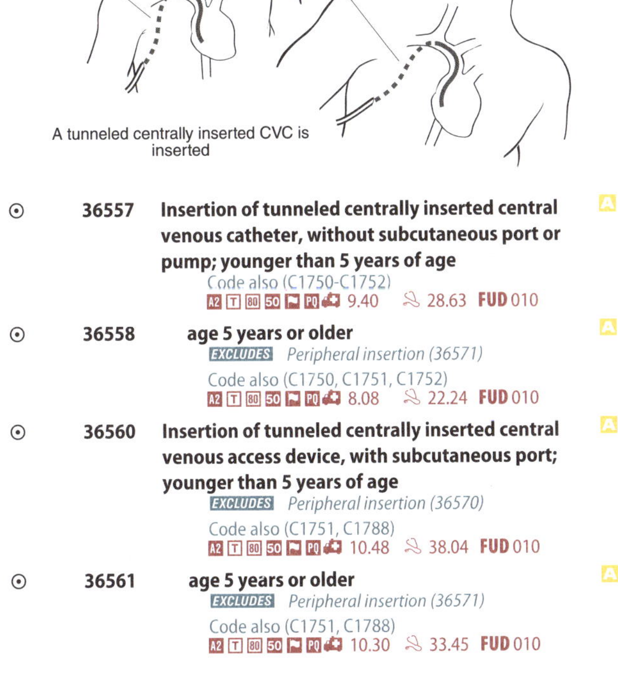

A tunneled centrally inserted CVC is inserted

⊙ **36557** **Insertion of tunneled centrally inserted central venous catheter, without subcutaneous port or pump; younger than 5 years of age** A

Code also (C1750-C1752)

A2 T 80 50 PQ 9.40 28.63 FUD 010

⊙ **36558** **age 5 years or older** A

EXCLUDES *Peripheral insertion (36571)*

Code also (C1750, C1751, C1752)

A2 T 80 50 PQ 8.08 22.24 FUD 010

⊙ **36560** **Insertion of tunneled centrally inserted central venous access device, with subcutaneous port; younger than 5 years of age** A

EXCLUDES *Peripheral insertion (36570)*

Code also (C1751, C1788)

A2 T 80 50 PQ 10.48 38.04 FUD 010

⊙ **36561** **age 5 years or older** A

EXCLUDES *Peripheral insertion (36571)*

Code also (C1751, C1788)

A2 T 80 50 PQ 10.30 33.45 FUD 010

⊙ **36563** **Insertion of tunneled centrally inserted central venous access device with subcutaneous pump**

Code also (C1772, C1891, C2626)

A2 T 80 PQ 10.92 37.39 FUD 010

⊙ **36565** **Insertion of tunneled centrally inserted central venous access device, requiring 2 catheters via 2 separate venous access sites; without subcutaneous port or pump (eg, Tesio type catheter)**

Code also (C1750, C1751, C1752)

A2 T 80 50 PQ 10.14 27.95 FUD 010

⊙ **36566** **with subcutaneous port(s)**

Code also (C1881)

A2 T 80 50 PQ 11.12 151.51 FUD 010

⊙ **36568** **Insertion of peripherally inserted central venous catheter (PICC), without subcutaneous port or pump; younger than 5 years of age** A

EXCLUDES *Centrally inserted placement (36555)*

Do not report removal of PICC lines with codes for removal of tunneled central venous catheters; report appropriate E/M code

A2 T PQ 2.84 8.45 FUD 000

36569 **age 5 years or older** A

EXCLUDES *Centrally inserted placement (36556)*

Do not report removal of PICC lines with codes for removal of tunneled central venous catheters; report appropriate E/M code

A2 T PQ 2.66 7.05 FUD 000

⊙ **36570** **Insertion of peripherally inserted central venous access device, with subcutaneous port; younger than 5 years of age** A

EXCLUDES *Centrally inserted placement (36560)*

Code also (C1751, C1788)

A2 T 80 50 PQ 8.94 33.57 FUD 010

⊙ **36571** **age 5 years or older** A

EXCLUDES *Centrally inserted placement (36561)*

Code also (C1751, C1788)

A2 T 80 50 PQ 9.34 36.96 FUD 010

36575-36590 Repair, Removal, and Replacement Implantable Venous Access Device

EXCLUDES *Mechanical removal obstructive material, pericatheter/intraluminal (36595, 36596)*

Code also a frequency of two for procedures involving both catheters from a multicatheter device

36575 **Repair of tunneled or non-tunneled central venous access catheter, without subcutaneous port or pump, central or peripheral insertion site**

INCLUDES Repair of the device without replacing any parts

A2 T 80 1.03 4.72 FUD 000

⊙ **36576** **Repair of central venous access device, with subcutaneous port or pump, central or peripheral insertion site**

INCLUDES Repair of the device without replacing any parts

A2 T 80 5.68 11.06 FUD 010

⊙ **36578** **Replacement, catheter only, of central venous access device, with subcutaneous port or pump, central or peripheral insertion site**

INCLUDES Partial replacement (catheter only)

EXCLUDES *Total replacement of the entire device using the same venous access sites (36582-36583)*

Code also (C1750, C1751, C1752)

A2 T 80 PQ 6.26 14.87 FUD 010

36580 **Replacement, complete, of a non-tunneled centrally inserted central venous catheter, without subcutaneous port or pump, through same venous access**

INCLUDES Complete replacement (replace all components/same access site)

A2 T PQ 1.95 6.08 FUD 000

⊙ **36581 Replacement, complete, of a tunneled centrally inserted central venous catheter, without subcutaneous port or pump, through same venous access**

INCLUDES Complete replacement (replace all components/same access site)

EXCLUDES *Removal of old device and insertion of new device using a separate venous access site*

Code also (C1750, C1751, C1752)

A2 T 80 PQ 5.71 21.79 FUD 010

⊙ **36582 Replacement, complete, of a tunneled centrally inserted central venous access device, with subcutaneous port, through same venous access**

INCLUDES Complete replacement (replace all components/same access site)

EXCLUDES *Removal of old device and insertion of new device using a separate venous access site*

Code also (C1751, C1788, C1881)

A2 T 80 PQ 8.87 31.52 FUD 010

⊙ **36583 Replacement, complete, of a tunneled centrally inserted central venous access device, with subcutaneous pump, through same venous access**

INCLUDES Complete replacement (replace all components/same access site)

EXCLUDES *Removal of old device and insertion of new device using a separate venous access site*

Code also (C1772, C1891, C2626)

A2 T 80 PQ 9.66 38.45 FUD 010

36584 Replacement, complete, of a peripherally inserted central venous catheter (PICC), without subcutaneous port or pump, through same venous access

INCLUDES Complete replacement (replace all components/same access site)

A2 T PQ 1.93 5.78 FUD 000

⊙ **36585 Replacement, complete, of a peripherally inserted central venous access device, with subcutaneous port, through same venous access**

INCLUDES Complete replacement (replace all components/same access site)

Code also (C1751, C1788)

A2 T 80 PQ 8.15 32.77 FUD 010

36589 Removal of tunneled central venous catheter, without subcutaneous port or pump

INCLUDES Complete removal/all components

EXCLUDES *Non-tunneled central venous catheter removal; report appropriate E/M code*

A2 Q2 80 4.01 4.73 FUD 010

⊙ **36590 Removal of tunneled central venous access device, with subcutaneous port or pump, central or peripheral insertion**

INCLUDES Complete removal/all components

EXCLUDES *Non-tunneled central venous catheter removal; report appropriate E/M code*

A2 Q2 80 5.94 8.39 FUD 010

36591-36592 Obtain Blood Specimen from Implanted Device or Catheter

Do not report with any other service except laboratory services

36591 Collection of blood specimen from a completely implantable venous access device

EXCLUDES *Collection of:*

Capillary blood specimen (36416)

Venous blood specimen by venipuncture (36415)

N1 Q1 TC 80 0.65 0.65 FUD XXX

36592 Collection of blood specimen using established central or peripheral catheter, venous, not otherwise specified

EXCLUDES *Collection of blood from an established arterial catheter (37799)*

N1 Q1 TC 80 0.73 0.73 FUD XXX

36593-36596 Restore Patency of Occluded Catheter or Device

EXCLUDES *Venous catheterization (36010-36012)*

36593 Declotting by thrombolytic agent of implanted vascular access device or catheter

P3 T TC 80 0.86 0.86 FUD XXX

36595 Mechanical removal of pericatheter obstructive material (eg, fibrin sheath) from central venous device via separate venous access

Do not report with (36593)

75901

P3 T 5.36 16.51 FUD 000

36596 Mechanical removal of intraluminal (intracatheter) obstructive material from central venous device through device lumen

Do not report with (36593)

75902

G2 T 1.31 3.81 FUD 000

36597-36598 Repositioning or Assessment of In Situ Venous Access Device

36597 Repositioning of previously placed central venous catheter under fluoroscopic guidance

76000

G2 T 1.77 3.59 FUD 000

36598 Contrast injection(s) for radiologic evaluation of existing central venous access device, including fluoroscopy, image documentation and report

EXCLUDES *Complete venography studies (75820, 75825, 75827)*

Do not report with (36595-36596, 76000)

P3 T 80 50 PQ 1.07 3.13 FUD 000

36600-36660 Insertion Needle or Catheter: Artery

36600 Arterial puncture, withdrawal of blood for diagnosis

Do not report with critical care services

N1 Q3 0.45 0.88 FUD XXX

⊘ **36620 Arterial catheterization or cannulation for sampling, monitoring or transfusion (separate procedure); percutaneous**

N1 N 1.47 1.47 FUD 000

36625 cutdown

N1 N 3.07 3.07 FUD 000

36640 Arterial catheterization for prolonged infusion therapy (chemotherapy), cutdown

EXCLUDES *Intraarterial chemotherapy (96420-96425)*
Transcatheter embolization (75894)

Code also (C1751)

A2 T 3.75 3.75 FUD 000

36660 Catheterization, umbilical artery, newborn, for diagnosis or therapy A

C 80 63 1.97 1.97 FUD 000

36680 Percutaneous Placement of Catheter/Needle into Bone Marrow Cavity

36680 Placement of needle for intraosseous infusion

G2 X 80 1.73 1.73 FUD 000

36800-36821 Vascular Access for Hemodialysis

36800 **Insertion of cannula for hemodialysis, other purpose (separate procedure); vein to vein**
Code also (C1750, C1752)
A2 T CCI 3.63 3.63 FUD 000

36810 **arteriovenous, external (Scribner type)**
Code also (C1750, C1752)
A2 T CCI 6.31 6.31 FUD 000

36815 **arteriovenous, external revision, or closure**
A2 T CCI 4.26 4.26 FUD 000

36818 **Arteriovenous anastomosis, open; by upper arm cephalic vein transposition**
INCLUDES Two incisions in the upper arm; a medial incision over the brachial artery and a lateral incision for exposure of a portion of the cephalic vein
Code also modifier 50 or 59, as appropriate, for a bilateral procedure
Do not report with (for unilateral procedure) (36819-36821, 36830)
A2 T 80 CCI PQ 19.64 19.64 FUD 090

36819 **by upper arm basilic vein transposition**
Code also modifier 50 or 59, as appropriate, for bilateral procedure
Do not report with (for unilateral procedure) (36818, 36820-36821, 36830)
A2 T 80 CCI PQ 21.57 21.57 FUD 090

36820 **by forearm vein transposition**
A2 T 80 50 CCI PQ 23.58 23.58 FUD 090

36821 **direct, any site (eg, Cimino type) (separate procedure)**
A2 T 80 CCI PQ 20.30 20.30 FUD 090

36822-36823 Vascular Access for Extracorporeal Circulation

EXCLUDES *Maintenance for extracorporeal circulation (33946-33949)*

~~**36822** **Insertion of cannula(s) for prolonged extracorporeal circulation for cardiopulmonary insufficiency (ECMO) (separate procedure)**~~
To report, see 33951-33956

36823 **Insertion of arterial and venous cannula(s) for isolated extracorporeal circulation including regional chemotherapy perfusion to an extremity, with or without hyperthermia, with removal of cannula(s) and repair of arteriotomy and venotomy sites**
INCLUDES Chemotherapy perfusion
Do not report with (96409-96425)
C CCI 38.75 38.75 FUD 090

36825-36835 Permanent Vascular Access Procedures

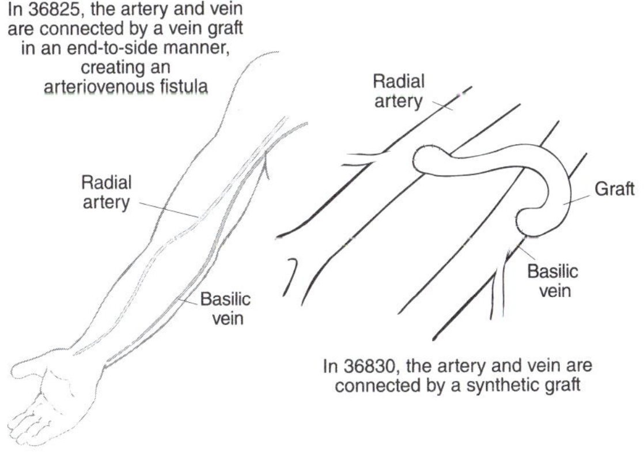

36825 **Creation of arteriovenous fistula by other than direct arteriovenous anastomosis (separate procedure); autogenous graft**
EXCLUDES *Direct arteriovenous (AV) anastomosis (36821)*
A2 T 80 CCI PQ 23.32 23.32 FUD 090

36830 **nonautogenous graft (eg, biological collagen, thermoplastic graft)**
EXCLUDES *Direct arteriovenous (AV) anastomosis (36821)*
A2 T 80 CCI PQ 19.25 19.25 FUD 090

36831 **Thrombectomy, open, arteriovenous fistula without revision, autogenous or nonautogenous dialysis graft (separate procedure)**
A2 T 80 CCI 13.30 13.30 FUD 090

36832 **Revision, open, arteriovenous fistula; without thrombectomy, autogenous or nonautogenous dialysis graft (separate procedure)**
INCLUDES Revision of an arteriovenous access fistula or graft
A2 T 80 CCI 16.97 16.97 FUD 090

36833 **with thrombectomy, autogenous or nonautogenous dialysis graft (separate procedure)**
A2 T 80 CCI 19.24 19.24 FUD 090

36835 **Insertion of Thomas shunt (separate procedure)**
Code also (C1750, C1752)
A2 T CCI 14.58 14.58 FUD 090

36838 DRIL Procedure for Ischemic Steal Syndrome

Do not report with (35512, 35522-35523, 36832, 37607, 37618)

36838 **Distal revascularization and interval ligation (DRIL), upper extremity hemodialysis access (steal syndrome)**
T 80 50 CCI 33.83 33.83 FUD 090

36860-36870 Restore Patency of Occluded Cannula or Arteriovenous Fistula

36860 **External cannula declotting (separate procedure); without balloon catheter**
76000
A2 T CCI 3.29 6.01 FUD 000

36861 **with balloon catheter**
Code also (C1757)
76000
A2 T CCI 3.80 3.80 FUD 000

⊙ **36870** **Thrombectomy, percutaneous, arteriovenous fistula, autogenous or nonautogenous graft (includes mechanical thrombus extraction and intra-graft thrombolysis)**
INCLUDES Declotting using thrombolytics
Moving thrombus using a mechanical methodology including using a balloon catheter
EXCLUDES *Catheterization for arteriovenous (AV) shunt (36147-36148)*
Do not report for removal arterial plug with arterial or venous angioplasty (35475-35476)
Do not report with (36593)
75791
A2 T 50 CCI 8.74 52.10 FUD 090

37140-37181 Open Decompression of Portal Circulation

EXCLUDES *Peritoneal-venous shunt (49425)*

37140 **Venous anastomosis, open; portocaval**
C CCI 65.93 65.93 FUD 090

37145 **renoportal**
C 80 CCI 61.31 61.31 FUD 090

37160 **caval-mesenteric**
C 80 CCI 62.82 62.82 FUD 090

37180 **splenorenal, proximal**

C 80 ⚑ Facility RVU 60.43 Non-Facility RVU 60.43 FUD 090

37181 **splenorenal, distal (selective decompression of esophagogastric varices, any technique)**

EXCLUDES *Percutaneous procedure (37182)*

C 80 ⚑ Facility RVU 65.92 Non-Facility RVU 65.92 FUD 090

37182-37183 Transvenous Decompression of Portal Circulation

Do not report with (75885, 75887)

37182 **Insertion of transvenous intrahepatic portosystemic shunt(s) (TIPS) (includes venous access, hepatic and portal vein catheterization, portography with hemodynamic evaluation, intrahepatic tract formation/dilatation, stent placement and all associated imaging guidance and documentation)**

EXCLUDES *Open procedure (37140)*

C 80 ⚑ PQ Facility RVU 24.43 Non-Facility RVU 24.43 FUD 000

⊙ **37183** **Revision of transvenous intrahepatic portosystemic shunt(s) (TIPS) (includes venous access, hepatic and portal vein catheterization, portography with hemodynamic evaluation, intrahepatic tract recanulization/dilatation, stent placement and all associated imaging guidance and documentation)**

EXCLUDES *Arteriovenous (AV) aneurysm repair (36832)*

T 80 ⚑ PQ Facility RVU 11.49 Non-Facility RVU 166.26 FUD 000

37184-37188 Removal of Thrombus from Vessel: Percutaneous

INCLUDES Fluoroscopic guidance
Injection(s) of thrombolytics during the procedure
Postprocedure evaluation
Pretreatment planning

EXCLUDES *Continuous infusion of thrombolytics prior to and after the procedure ([37211, 37212, 37213, 37214])*
Diagnostic studies
Mechanical thrombectomy, coronary (92973)
Other interventions performed percutaneously (e.g., balloon angioplasty)
Percutaneous thrombectomy of an arteriovenous fistula (36870)
Placement of catheters
Radiological supervision/interpretation

⊙ **37184** **Primary percutaneous transluminal mechanical thrombectomy, noncoronary, arterial or arterial bypass graft, including fluoroscopic guidance and intraprocedural pharmacological thrombolytic injection(s); initial vessel**

EXCLUDES *Mechanical thrombectomy for embolus/thrombus complicating another percutaneous interventional procedure (37186)*
Mechanical thrombectomy of another vascular family/separate access site, append modifier 51 to code, as appropriate

Code also (C1757)
Do not report with (76000-76001, 96374, 99143-99150)

G2 T 50 PQ Facility RVU 13.21 Non-Facility RVU 64.07 FUD 000

+ ⊙ **37185** **second and all subsequent vessel(s) within the same vascular family (List separately in addition to code for primary mechanical thrombectomy procedure)**

INCLUDES Treatment of second and all succeeding vessel(s) in same vascular family

EXCLUDES *Intravenous drug injections administered subsequent to an initial service*
Mechanical thrombectomy for treating of embolus/thrombus complicating another percutaneous interventional procedure (37186)
Mechanical thrombectomy of another vascular family/separate access site, append modifier 51 to code as appropriate

Code first (37184)
Do not report with (76000-76001, 96375)

N1 N Facility RVU 4.86 Non-Facility RVU 20.56 FUD ZZZ

+ ⊙ **37186** **Secondary percutaneous transluminal thrombectomy (eg, nonprimary mechanical, snare basket, suction technique), noncoronary, arterial or arterial bypass graft, including fluoroscopic guidance and intraprocedural pharmacological thrombolytic injections, provided in conjunction with another percutaneous intervention other than primary mechanical thrombectomy (List separately in addition to code for primary procedure)**

INCLUDES Removal of small emboli/thrombi prior to or after another percutaneous procedure

Code first primary procedure
Do not report with (37184-37185, 76000-76001, 96375)

N1 N Facility RVU 7.35 Non-Facility RVU 39.43 FUD ZZZ

⊙ **37187** **Percutaneous transluminal mechanical thrombectomy, vein(s), including intraprocedural pharmacological thrombolytic injections and fluoroscopic guidance**

INCLUDES Secondary or subsequent intravenous injection after another initial service

Code also (C1757)
Do not report with (76000-76001, 96375)

G2 T 50 PQ Facility RVU 11.79 Non-Facility RVU 58.69 FUD 000

⊙ **37188** **Percutaneous transluminal mechanical thrombectomy, vein(s), including intraprocedural pharmacological thrombolytic injections and fluoroscopic guidance, repeat treatment on subsequent day during course of thrombolytic therapy**

Code also (C1757)
Do not report with (76000-76001, 96375)

G2 T 50 PQ Facility RVU 8.46 Non-Facility RVU 50.55 FUD 000

37191-37193 Vena Cava Filters

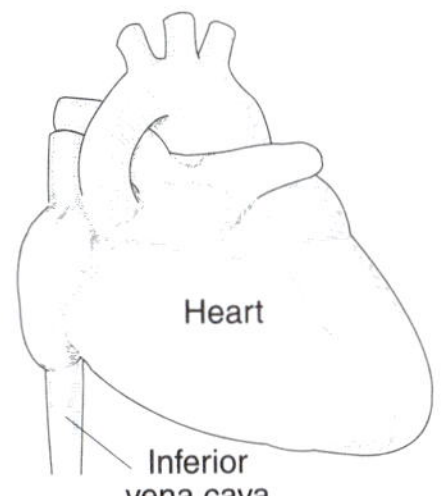

The inverior vena cava (or IVC) is the major return vessel of the lower body. It extends from the right atrium of the heart down to the bifurcation of the iliac veins

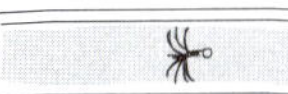

An intravascular "umbrella" device in the IVC. Such devices are intended to entrap clots and prevent clot passage into the pulmonary arteries

⊙ **37191** **Insertion of intravascular vena cava filter, endovascular approach including vascular access, vessel selection, and radiological supervision and interpretation, intraprocedural roadmapping, and imaging guidance (ultrasound and fluoroscopy), when performed**

EXCLUDES *Open ligation of inferior vena cava via laparotomy or retroperitoneal approach (37619)*

T 6.97 74.90 FUD 000

⊙ **37192** **Repositioning of intravascular vena cava filter, endovascular approach including vascular access, vessel selection, and radiological supervision and interpretation, intraprocedural roadmapping, and imaging guidance (ultrasound and fluoroscopy), when performed**

Do not report with (37191)

T 10.51 43.40 FUD 000

⊙ **37193** **Retrieval (removal) of intravascular vena cava filter, endovascular approach including vascular access, vessel selection, and radiological supervision and interpretation, intraprocedural roadmapping, and imaging guidance (ultrasound and fluoroscopy), when performed**

Do not report with (37197)

Q2 10.74 45.73 FUD 000

37195 Intravenous Cerebral Thrombolysis

37195 **Thrombolysis, cerebral, by intravenous infusion**

T 80 0.00 0.00 FUD XXX

37197-37214 [37211, 37212, 37213, 37214] Transcatheter Procedures: Infusions, Biopsy, Foreign Body Removal

⊙ **37197** **Transcatheter retrieval, percutaneous, of intravascular foreign body (eg, fractured venous or arterial catheter), includes radiological supervision and interpretation, and imaging guidance (ultrasound or fluoroscopy), when performed**

EXCLUDES *Percutaneous vena cava filter retrieval (37193)*

62 T 8.84 43.02 FUD 000

37200 **Transcatheter biopsy**

75970

62 T PQ 6.45 6.45 FUD 000

⊙ # **37211** **Transcatheter therapy, arterial infusion for thrombolysis other than coronary, any method, including radiological supervision and interpretation, initial treatment day**

INCLUDES Catheter exchange or position change
Evaluation and management services on the day of and related to thrombolysis
First day of transcatheter thrombolytic infusion
Fluoroscopic guidance
Follow-up arteriography or venography
Radiologic supervision and interpretation

EXCLUDES *Catheter placement*
Declotting of implanted catheter or vascular access device by thrombolytic agent (36593)
Diagnostic studies
Percutaneous interventions
Ultrasound guidance (76937)

Code also significant, separately identifiable evaluation and management services on the day of thrombolysis using modifier 25

Do not report more than one time per date of service

Do not report with (75898)

62 T 50 11.70 11.70 FUD 000

⊙ # **37212** **Transcatheter therapy, venous infusion for thrombolysis, any method, including radiological supervision and interpretation, initial treatment day**

INCLUDES Catheter position change or exchange
Evaluation and management services on the day of and related to thrombolysis
First day of transcatheter thrombolytic infusion
Fluoroscopic guidance
Follow-up arteriography or venography
Initiation and completion of thrombolysis on same date of service
Radiologic supervision and interpretation

EXCLUDES *Catheter placement*
Declotting of implanted catheter or vascular access device by thrombolytic agent (36593)
Diagnostic studies
Percutaneous interventions
Ultrasound guidance (76937)

Code also significant, separately identifiable evaluation and management service on the same day as thrombolysis using modifier 25

Do not report more than one time per date of service

Do not report with (75898)

62 T 50 10.33 10.33 FUD 000

⊙ # **37213 Transcatheter therapy, arterial or venous infusion for thrombolysis other than coronary, any method, including radiological supervision and interpretation, continued treatment on subsequent day during course of thrombolytic therapy, including follow-up catheter contrast injection, position change, or exchange, when performed;**

INCLUDES Continued thrombolytic infusions on subsequent days besides the initial and last days of treatment
Evaluation and management services on the day of and related to the thrombolysis
Fluoroscopic guidance
Radiologic supervision and interpretation

EXCLUDES *Catheter placement*
Declotting of implanted catheter or vascular access device by thrombolytic agent (36593)
Diagnostic studies
Percutaneous interventions
Ultrasound guidance (76937)

Code also significant, separately identifiable evaluation and management services not related to the thrombolysis using modifier 25
Do not report more than one time per date of service
Do not report with (75898)
T 7.20 7.20 FUD 000

⊙ # **37214 cessation of thrombolysis including removal of catheter and vessel closure by any method**

INCLUDES Evaluation and management services on the day of and related to the thrombolysis
Fluoroscopic guidance
Last day of transcatheter thrombolytic infusions
Radiologic supervision and interpretation

EXCLUDES *Catheter placement*
Declotting of implanted catheter or vascular access device by thrombolytic agent (36593)
Diagnostic studies
Percutaneous interventions
Ultrasound guidance (76937)

Code also significant, separately identifiable evaluation and management service not related to thrombolysis using modifier 25
Do not report more than one time per date of service
Do not report with (75898)
T 4.25 4.25 FUD 000

37202 Transcatheter therapy, infusion other than for thrombolysis, any type (eg, spasmolytic, vasoconstrictive)

EXCLUDES *Thrombolysis of coronary vessels (92975-92977)*
Vena cava filter removal (37193)

Code also for nitroglycerin infusion done with a cardiac catheterization
75896
G2 T 8.77 8.77 FUD 000

37211 Resequenced code. See code following 37200.

37212 Resequenced code. See code following 37200.

37213 Resequenced code. See code following 37200.

37214 Resequenced code. See code following 37200.

37215-37216 Stenting of Cervical Carotid Artery with/without Insertion Distal Embolic Protection Device

INCLUDES Carotid stenting, if required
Ipsilateral cerebral and cervical carotid diagnostic imaging/supervision and interpretation
Ipsilateral selective carotid catheterization

EXCLUDES *Carotid catheterization and imaging, if carotid stenting not required*
Transcatheter placement extracranial vertebral artery stents, open or percutaneous (0075T, 0076T)

Do not report with (36222-36224)

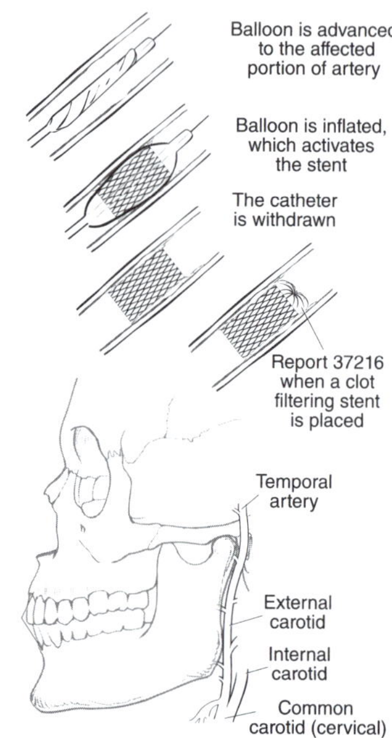

⊙ ▲ **37215 Transcatheter placement of intravascular stent(s), cervical carotid artery, open or percutaneous, including angioplasty, when performed, and radiological supervision and interpretation; with distal embolic protection**
C 80 50 31.47 31.47 FUD 090

⊙ ▲ **37216 without distal embolic protection**
E 29.30 29.30 FUD 090

37217-37218 Stenting of Intrathoracic Carotid Artery/Innominate Artery

INCLUDES Access to vessel (open)
Arteriotomy closure by suture
Catheterization of the vessel (selective)
Imaging during and after the procedure
Radiological supervision and interpretation

EXCLUDES *Transcatheter insertion extracranial vertebral artery stents, open or percutaneous (0075T-0076T)*
Transcatheter insertion intracranial stents (61635)
Transcatheter insertion intravascular cervical carotid artery stents, open or percutaneous (37215-37216)

▲ **37217 Transcatheter placement of intravascular stent(s), intrathoracic common carotid artery or innominate artery by retrograde treatment, open ipsilateral cervical carotid artery exposure, including angioplasty, when performed, and radiological supervision and interpretation**

Code also revascularization of carotid artery, when performed (33891, 35301, 35509-35510, 35601, 35606)
Do not report with the following services performed on the same side (35201, 35458, 36221-36227, 75962)
C 80 50 32.50 32.50 FUD 090

⊙ ● **37218 Transcatheter placement of intravascular stent(s), intrathoracic common carotid artery or innominate artery, open or percutaneous antegrade approach, including angioplasty, when performed, and radiological supervision and interpretation**

Do not report with (36222-36224)

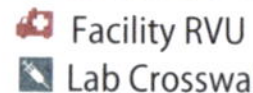

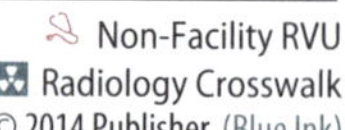

37220-37235 Endovascular Revascularization Lower Extremities

INCLUDES Percutaneous and open interventional and associated procedures for lower extremity occlusive disease; unilateral
- Accessing the vessel
- Arteriotomy closure by suturing of puncture or pressure with application of arterial closure device
- Atherectomy (e.g., directional, laser, rotational)
- Balloon angioplasty (e.g., cryoplasty, cutting balloon, low-profile)
- Catheterization of the vessel (selective)
- Embolic protection
- Imaging once procedure is complete
- Radiological supervision and interpretation of intervention(s)
- Stenting (e.g., bare metal, balloon-expandable, covered, drug-eluting, self-expanding)
- Transversing of the lesion

Reporting the most comprehensive treatment in a given vessel according to the following hierarchy:
1. Stent and atherectomy
2. Atherectomy
3. Stent
4. PTA

Revascularization procedures for three arterial vascular territories:
- Femoral/popliteal vascular territory including the common, deep, and superficial femoral arteries, and the popliteal artery (one extremity = a single vessel) (37224-37227)
- Iliac vascular territory: common iliac, external iliac, internal iliac (37220-37223)
- Tibial/peroneal territory: includes anterior tibial, peroneal artery, posterior tibial (37228-37235)

EXCLUDES *Extensive repair or replacement of artery (35226, 35286)*
Mechanical thrombectomy and/or thrombolysis

Code also add-on codes for different vessels, but not different lesions in the same vessel; and for multiple territories in the same leg
Code also modifier 59 for a bilateral procedure
Code first one primary code for the initial service in each leg
Do not report more than one code from this family for each lower extremity vessel treated
Do not report more than one code when multiple vessels are treated in the femoral/popliteal territory (report the most complex service for more than one lesion in the territory); when a contiguous lesion that spans from one territory to another can be opened with a single procedure; or when more than one stent is deployed in the same vessel

⊙ **37220 Revascularization, endovascular, open or percutaneous, iliac artery, unilateral, initial vessel; with transluminal angioplasty**
Code also (C1725, C1885)
Code also only when transluminal angioplasty is performed outside the treatment target zone of (34802-34805, 34825-34826, 34845-34848, 34900, 0254T)
G2 T 50 PQ 12.15 90.32 FUD 000

⊙ **37221 with transluminal stent placement(s), includes angioplasty within the same vessel, when performed**
Code also (C1874-C1877, C2617, C2625)
Code also only when transluminal angioplasty is performed outside the treatment target zone of (34802-34805, 34825-34826, 34845-34848, 34900, 0254T)
G2 T 80 50 PQ 14.81 132.60 FUD 000

+ ⊙ **37222 Revascularization, endovascular, open or percutaneous, iliac artery, each additional ipsilateral iliac vessel; with transluminal angioplasty (List separately in addition to code for primary procedure)**
Code also (C1725, C1885)
Code also only when transluminal angioplasty is performed outside the treatment target zone of (34802-34805, 34825-34826, 34845-34848, 34900, 0254T)
Code first (37220, 37221)
G2 T 80 50 PQ 5.47 25.44 FUD ZZZ

+ ⊙ **37223 with transluminal stent placement(s), includes angioplasty within the same vessel, when performed (List separately in addition to code for primary procedure)**
Code also (C1874-C1877, C2617, C2625)
Code also only when transluminal angioplasty is performed outside the treatment target zone of (34802-34805, 34825-34826, 34845-34848, 34900, 0254T)
Code first (37221)
G2 T 80 50 PQ 6.26 73.65 FUD ZZZ

⊙ **37224 Revascularization, endovascular, open or percutaneous, femoral, popliteal artery(s), unilateral; with transluminal angioplasty**
Code also (C1725, C1885)
G2 T 80 50 PQ 13.44 109.40 FUD 000

⊙ **37225 with atherectomy, includes angioplasty within the same vessel, when performed**
G2 T 80 50 PQ 18.13 312.36 FUD 000

⊙ **37226 with transluminal stent placement(s), includes angioplasty within the same vessel, when performed**
Code also (C1874-C1877, C2617, C2625)
G2 T 80 50 PQ 14.88 256.48 FUD 000

⊙ **37227 with transluminal stent placement(s) and atherectomy, includes angioplasty within the same vessel, when performed**
Code also (C1874-C1877, C2617, C2625)
J8 T 80 50 PQ 21.84 420.53 FUD 000

⊙ **37228 Revascularization, endovascular, open or percutaneous, tibial, peroneal artery, unilateral, initial vessel; with transluminal angioplasty**
Code also (C1725, C1885)
G2 T 80 50 PQ 16.39 155.46 FUD 000

⊙ **37229 with atherectomy, includes angioplasty within the same vessel, when performed**
G2 T 80 50 PQ 21.20 307.65 FUD 000

⊙ **37230 with transluminal stent placement(s), includes angioplasty within the same vessel, when performed**
Code also (C1874-C1877, C2617, C2625)
G2 T 80 50 PQ 20.55 235.43 FUD 000

⊙ **37231 with transluminal stent placement(s) and atherectomy, includes angioplasty within the same vessel, when performed**
Code also (C1874-C1877, C2617, C2625)
J8 T 80 50 PQ 22.51 375.83 FUD 000

+ ⊙ **37232 Revascularization, endovascular, open or percutaneous, tibial/peroneal artery, unilateral, each additional vessel; with transluminal angioplasty (List separately in addition to code for primary procedure)**
Code also (C1725, C1885)
Code first (37228-37231)
G2 T 80 50 PQ 5.94 34.55 FUD ZZZ

+ ⊙ **37233 with atherectomy, includes angioplasty within the same vessel, when performed (List separately in addition to code for primary procedure)**
Code first (37229, 37231)
G2 T 80 50 9.71 41.49 FUD ZZZ

+ ⊙ **37234 with transluminal stent placement(s), includes angioplasty within the same vessel, when performed (List separately in addition to code for primary procedure)**
Code also (C1874-C1877, C2617, C2625)
Code first (37229-37231)
G2 T 80 50 PQ 8.23 109.85 FUD ZZZ

Cardiovascular System
37220 — 37234

+ ⊙ **37235** **with transluminal stent placement(s) and atherectomy, includes angioplasty within the same vessel, when performed (List separately in addition to code for primary procedure)**
Code also (C1874-C1877, C2617, C2625)
Code first (37231)
G2 T 80 50 P0 11.94 112.14 FUD ZZZ

37236-37239 Endovascular Revascularization Excluding Lower Extremities

INCLUDES Arteriotomy closure by suturing of a puncture, pressure or application of arterial closure device
Balloon angioplasty
Post-dilation after stent deployment
Predilation performed as primary or secondary angioplasty
Treatment of lesion inside same vessel but outside of stented portion
Treatment using different-sized balloons to accomplish the procedure
Endovascular revascularization of arteries and veins other than carotid, coronary, extracranial, intracranial, lower extremities
Imaging once procedure is complete
Radiological supervision and interpretation
Stent placement provided as the only treatment

EXCLUDES *Angioplasty in an unrelated vessel*
Extensive repair or replacement of an artery (35226, 35286)
Intravascular ultrasound (37250-37251)
Mechanical thrombectomy (37184-37188)
Selective and nonselective catheterization (36005, 36010-36015, 36200, 36215-36218, 36245-36248)
Stent placement in:
Arteries of the lower extremities for occlusive disease (37221, 37223, 37226-37227, 37230-37231, 37234-37235)
Cervical carotid artery (37215-37216)
Extracranial vertebral (0075T-0076T)
Intracoronary ([92928, 92929], [92933, 92934], [92937, 92938], [92941], [92943, 92944])
Intracranial (61635)
Intrathoracic common carotid or innominate artery, retrograde or antegrade approach (37217 or 37218)
Visceral arteries with fenestrated aortic repair (34841-34848)
Thrombolytic therapy ([37211, 37212, 37213, 37214])
Ultrasound guidance (76937)

Code also add-on codes for different vessels treated during the same operative session
Do not report insertion of multiple stents in a single vessel with more than one code
Do not report stent placement when performed with embolization procedure

⊙ ▲ **37236** **Transcatheter placement of an intravascular stent(s) (except lower extremity artery(s) for occlusive disease, cervical carotid, extracranial vertebral or intrathoracic carotid, intracranial, or coronary), open or percutaneous, including radiological supervision and interpretation and including all angioplasty within the same vessel, when performed; initial artery**
Do not report in the same target treatment zone with (34841-34848)
G2 T 80 50 13.46 79.91 FUD 000

+ ⊙ ▲ **37237** **each additional artery (List separately in addition to code for primary procedure)**
Code first (37236)
Do not report in the same target treatment zone with (34841-34848)
G2 T 80 50 6.29 34.71 FUD ZZZ

⊙ **37238** **Transcatheter placement of an intravascular stent(s), open or percutaneous, including radiological supervision and interpretation and including angioplasty within the same vessel, when performed; initial vein**
G2 T 80 50 9.43 116.85 FUD 000

+ ⊙ **37239** **each additional vein (List separately in addition to code for primary procedure)**
Code first (37238)
G2 T 80 50 4.39 58.08 FUD ZZZ

37241-37244 Therapeutic Vascular Embolization/Occlusion

INCLUDES Embolization or occlusion of arteries, lymphatics, and veins except for head/neck and central nervous system
Imaging once procedure is complete
Intraprocedural guidance
Radiological supervision and interpretation
Roadmapping
Stent placement provided as support for embolization

EXCLUDES *Head, neck, or central nervous system embolization (61624, 61626, 61710)*
Stent deployment as primary management of aneurysm, pseudoaneurysm, or vascular extravasation

Code also additional embolization procedure(s) and the appropriate modifiers (eg, modifier 59) when embolization procedures are performed in multiple operative fields
Code also diagnostic angiography and catheter placement using modifier 59 when appropriate
Do not report in same operative field with (75894, 75898)
Do not report more than one embolization code per operative field
Do not report multiple codes for indications that overlap, code only the indication needing the most immediate attention

⊙ **37241** **Vascular embolization or occlusion, inclusive of all radiological supervision and interpretation, intraprocedural roadmapping, and imaging guidance necessary to complete the intervention; venous, other than hemorrhage (eg, congenital or acquired venous malformations, venous and capillary hemangiomas, varices, varicoceles)**
INCLUDES Embolization of side branch(s) of an outflow vein from a hemodialysis access
EXCLUDES *Vein destruction (36468-36479)*
Do not report in same operative field with (36468, 36470-36471, 36475-36479)
T 12.95 129.36 FUD 000

⊙ **37242** **arterial, other than hemorrhage or tumor (eg, congenital or acquired arterial malformations, arteriovenous malformations, arteriovenous fistulas, aneurysms, pseudoaneurysms)**
EXCLUDES *Percutaneous treatment of pseudoaneurysm of an extremity (36002)*
T 14.46 217.89 FUD 000

⊙ **37243** **for tumors, organ ischemia, or infarction**
INCLUDES Embolization of uterine fibroids
Code also chemotherapy when provided with embolization procedure (96420-96425)
Code also injection of radioisotopes when provided with embolization procedure (79445)
T 17.24 275.06 FUD 000

⊙ **37244** **for arterial or venous hemorrhage or lymphatic extravasation**
INCLUDES Embolization of uterine arteries for hemorrhage
T 20.11 192.59 FUD 000

37250-37251 Intravascular Ultrasound: Noncoronary

CMS 100-3,220.5 Ultrasound Diagnostic Procedures

INCLUDES Manipulation and repositioning of the transducer prior to and after therapeutic interventional procedures

EXCLUDES *Selective catheter placement for access (36215-36248)*
Transcatheter procedures (37200, 37202, 37236-37239, 37241-37244, 61624, 61626)

+ **37250** **Intravascular ultrasound (non-coronary vessel) during diagnostic evaluation and/or therapeutic intervention; initial vessel (List separately in addition to code for primary procedure)**
Code first primary procedure
75945-75946
N1 N 80 3.13 3.13 FUD ZZZ

+ **37251** **each additional vessel (List separately in addition to code for primary procedure)**
Code first (37250)
75945-75946
N1 N 80 2.34 2.34 FUD ZZZ

37500-37501 Vascular Endoscopic Procedures

INCLUDES Diagnostic endoscopy

EXCLUDES *Open procedure (37760)*

37500 **Vascular endoscopy, surgical, with ligation of perforator veins, subfascial (SEPS)**
A2 T 50 22.14 22.14 FUD 090

37501 **Unlisted vascular endoscopy procedure**
T 50 0.00 0.00 FUD YYY

37565-37606 Ligation Procedures: Jugular Vein, Carotid Arteries

CMS 100-3,160.8 Electroencephalographic Monitoring During Cerebral Vasculature Surgery

EXCLUDES *Arterial balloon occlusion, endovascular, temporary (61623)*
Suture of arteries and veins (35201-35286)
Transcatheter arterial embolization/occlusion, permanent (61624-61626)
Treatment of intracranial aneurysm (61703)

37565 **Ligation, internal jugular vein**
T 80 50 21.25 21.25 FUD 090

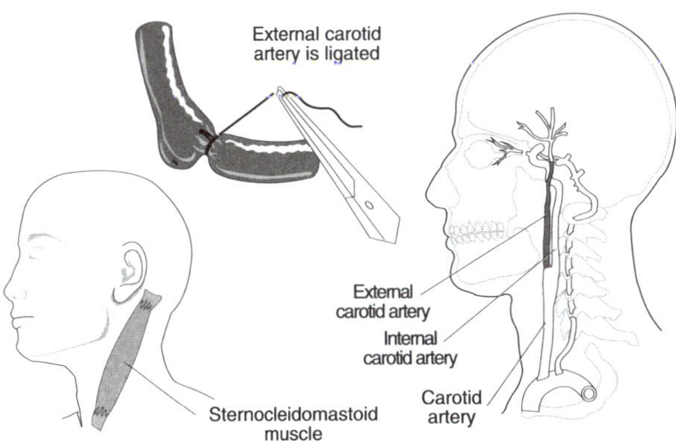

37600 **Ligation; external carotid artery**
T 80 20.74 20.74 FUD 090

37605 **internal or common carotid artery**
T 80 23.42 23.42 FUD 090

37606 **internal or common carotid artery, with gradual occlusion, as with Selverstone or Crutchfield clamp**
T 80 16.55 16.55 FUD 090

37607-37609 Ligation Hemodialysis Angioaccess or Temporal Artery

EXCLUDES *Suture of arteries and veins (35201-35286)*

37607 **Ligation or banding of angioaccess arteriovenous fistula**
A2 T 11.03 11.03 FUD 090

37609 **Ligation or biopsy, temporal artery**
A2 T 50 PQ 6.01 8.88 FUD 010

37615-37618 Arterial Ligation, Major Vessel, for Injury/Rupture

EXCLUDES *Suture of arteries and veins (35201-35286)*

37615 **Ligation, major artery (eg, post-traumatic, rupture); neck**
INCLUDES Touroff ligation
T 80 15.34 15.34 FUD 090

37616 **chest**
INCLUDES Bardenheurer operation
C 80 PQ 31.62 31.62 FUD 090

37617 **abdomen**
C 80 38.68 38.68 FUD 090

37618 **extremity**
C 80 11.27 11.27 FUD 090

37619 Ligation Inferior Vena Cava

EXCLUDES *Suture of arteries and veins (35201-35286)*

37619 **Ligation of inferior vena cava**
EXCLUDES *Endovascular delivery of inferior vena cava filter (37191)*
T 80 47.79 47.79 FUD 090

37650-37660 Venous Ligation, Femoral and Common Iliac

EXCLUDES *Suture of arteries and veins (35201-35286)*

37650 **Ligation of femoral vein**
A2 T 50 14.88 14.88 FUD 090

37660 **Ligation of common iliac vein**
C 80 50 33.02 33.02 FUD 090

37700-37785 Treatment of Varicose Veins of Legs

EXCLUDES *Suture of arteries and veins (35201-35286)*

37700 **Ligation and division of long saphenous vein at saphenofemoral junction, or distal interruptions**
INCLUDES Babcock operation
Do not report with (37718, 37722)
A2 T 50 7.33 7.33 FUD 090

37718 **Ligation, division, and stripping, short saphenous vein**
Do not report with (37700, 37735, 37780)
A2 T 50 12.73 12.73 FUD 090

37722 **Ligation, division, and stripping, long (greater) saphenous veins from saphenofemoral junction to knee or below**
EXCLUDES *Ligation/division/stripping short saphenous vein (37718)*
Do not report with (37700, 37735)
A2 T 50 14.09 14.09 FUD 090

37735 **Ligation and division and complete stripping of long or short saphenous veins with radical excision of ulcer and skin graft and/or interruption of communicating veins of lower leg, with excision of deep fascia**
Do not report with (37700, 37718, 37722, 37780)
A2 T 50 19.90 19.90 FUD 090

37760 **Ligation of perforator veins, subfascial, radical (Linton type), including skin graft, when performed, open,1 leg**
EXCLUDES *Ligation of subfascial perforator veins, endoscopic (37500)*
Do not report with (76937, 76942, 76998, 93971)
A2 T 50 17.98 17.98 FUD 090

37761 **Ligation of perforator vein(s), subfascial, open, including ultrasound guidance, when performed, 1 leg**
EXCLUDES *Ligation of subfascial perforator veins, endoscopic (37500)*
Do not report with (76937, 76942, 76998, 93971)
A2 T 80 50 16.10 16.10 FUD 090

37765 **Stab phlebectomy of varicose veins, 1 extremity; 10-20 stab incisions**
EXCLUDES *Fewer than 10 incisions (37799)*
More than 20 incisions (37766)
P3 T 50 13.16 18.87 FUD 090

37766 **more than 20 incisions**
EXCLUDES *Fewer than 10 incisions (37799)*
10-20 incisions (37765)
P3 T 50 16.19 22.62 FUD 090

37780 **Ligation and division of short saphenous vein at saphenopopliteal junction (separate procedure)**
A2 T 50 7.47 7.47 FUD 090

37785 Ligation, division, and/or excision of varicose vein cluster(s), 1 leg
A2 T 50 ⚑ Facility RVU 7.63 Non-Facility RVU 10.21 FUD 090

37788-37790 Treatment of Vascular Disease of the Penis

37788 Penile revascularization, artery, with or without vein graft ♂
C 80 ⚑ Facility RVU 38.44 Non-Facility RVU 38.44 FUD 090

37790 Penile venous occlusive procedure ♂
A2 T 80 ⚑ Facility RVU 13.81 Non-Facility RVU 13.81 FUD 090

37799 Unlisted Vascular Surgery Procedures

37799 Unlisted procedure, vascular surgery
X 80 Facility RVU 0.00 Non-Facility RVU 0.00 FUD YYY

38100-38200 Splenic Procedures

38100 Splenectomy; total (separate procedure)
C 80 ⚑ PQ Facility RVU 32.86 Non-Facility RVU 32.86 FUD 090

38101 partial (separate procedure)
C 80 ⚑ PQ Facility RVU 33.11 Non-Facility RVU 33.11 FUD 090

\+ **38102** total, en bloc for extensive disease, in conjunction with other procedure (List in addition to code for primary procedure)
Code first primary procedure
C 80 ⚑ Facility RVU 7.49 Non-Facility RVU 7.49 FUD ZZZ

38115 Repair of ruptured spleen (splenorrhaphy) with or without partial splenectomy
C 80 ⚑ PQ Facility RVU 36.18 Non-Facility RVU 36.18 FUD 090

38120 Laparoscopy, surgical, splenectomy
INCLUDES Diagnostic laparoscopy (49320)
T 80 ⚑ PQ Facility RVU 29.98 Non-Facility RVU 29.98 FUD 090

38129 Unlisted laparoscopy procedure, spleen
T 80 Facility RVU 0.00 Non-Facility RVU 0.00 FUD YYY

38200 Injection procedure for splenoportography
Radiology Crosswalk 75810
N1 N 80 ⚑ Facility RVU 3.81 Non-Facility RVU 3.81 FUD 000

38204-38215 Hematopoietic Stem Cell Preparation

CMS 100-3,110.8.1 Stem Cell Transplantation

INCLUDES Preservation, preparation, purification of stem cells before transplant or reinfusion

Do not report each code more than one time per day

38204 Management of recipient hematopoietic progenitor cell donor search and cell acquisition
N1 N Facility RVU 2.90 Non-Facility RVU 2.90 FUD XXX

38205 Blood-derived hematopoietic progenitor cell harvesting for transplantation, per collection; allogeneic
B 80 ⚑ Facility RVU 2.32 Non-Facility RVU 2.32 FUD 000

38206 autologous
62 S 80 ⚑ Facility RVU 2.36 Non-Facility RVU 2.36 FUD 000

38207 Transplant preparation of hematopoietic progenitor cells; cryopreservation and storage
Lab Crosswalk 88240
S Facility RVU 1.28 Non-Facility RVU 1.28 FUD XXX

38208 thawing of previously frozen harvest, without washing, per donor
Lab Crosswalk 88241
S Facility RVU 0.82 Non-Facility RVU 0.82 FUD XXX

38209 thawing of previously frozen harvest, with washing, per donor
S Facility RVU 0.34 Non-Facility RVU 0.34 FUD XXX

38210 specific cell depletion within harvest, T-cell depletion
S Facility RVU 2.27 Non-Facility RVU 2.27 FUD XXX

38211 tumor cell depletion
S Facility RVU 2.07 Non-Facility RVU 2.07 FUD XXX

38212 red blood cell removal
S Facility RVU 1.35 Non-Facility RVU 1.35 FUD XXX

38213 platelet depletion
S Facility RVU 0.34 Non-Facility RVU 0.34 FUD XXX

38214 plasma (volume) depletion
S Facility RVU 1.17 Non-Facility RVU 1.17 FUD XXX

38215 cell concentration in plasma, mononuclear, or buffy coat layer
Do not report with (88182, 88184-88189)
S Facility RVU 1.35 Non-Facility RVU 1.35 FUD XXX

38220-38232 Bone Marrow Procedures

CMS 100-1,5,90.2 Laboratory Defined
CMS 100-2,15,80 Diagnostic Test Requirements
CMS 100-2,15,80.1 Payment for Clinical Laboratory Services
CMS 100-3,110.8.1 Stem Cell Transplantation
CMS 100-4,3,90.3 Stem Cell Transplantation
CMS 100-4,3,90.3.1 Allogeneic Stem Cell Transplantation
CMS 100-4,3,90.3.3 Billing for Stem Cell Transplantation
CMS 100-4,32,90 Billing for Stem Cell Transplantation

38220 Bone marrow; aspiration only
INCLUDES Bone marrow aspiration for bone graft
EXCLUDES *Bone marrow aspiration for platelet rich stem cell injection (0232T)*
P3 T 80 50 ⚑ Facility RVU 1.74 Non-Facility RVU 4.52 FUD XXX

38221 biopsy, needle or trocar
EXCLUDES *Bone marrow aspiration for platelet rich stem cell injection (0232T)*
Lab Crosswalk 88305
P3 T 80 50 ⚑ PQ Facility RVU 2.15 Non-Facility RVU 4.68 FUD XXX

38230 Bone marrow harvesting for transplantation; allogeneic
EXCLUDES *Bone marrow aspiration for platelet rich stem cell injection (0232T)*
Harvesting of blood-derived hematopoietic progenitor cells for transplant (allogeneic) (38205)
62 S 80 ⚑ Facility RVU 6.03 Non-Facility RVU 6.03 FUD 000

38232 autologous
EXCLUDES *Aspiration of bone marrow (38220)*
Harvesting of blood-derived peripheral stem cells for transplant (autologous) (38206)
62 S 80 Facility RVU 5.98 Non-Facility RVU 5.98 FUD 000

38240-38243 [38243] Hematopoietic Progenitor Cell Transplantation

INCLUDES Evaluation of patient prior to, during, and after the infusion
Management of uncomplicated adverse reactions such as hives or nausea
Monitoring of physiological parameters
Physician presence during the infusion
Supervision of clinical staff

EXCLUDES *Cryopreservation, freezing, and storage of hematopoietic progenitor cells for transplant (38207)*
Modification, treatment, processing of hematopoietic progenitor cell specimens for transplant (38210-38215)
Thawing and expansion of hematopoietic progenitor cells for transplant (38208-38209)

Code also administration of medications and/or fluids not related to the transplant with modifier 59
Code also evaluation and management service for the treatment of more complicated adverse reactions after the infusion, as appropriate
Code also separately identifiable evaluation and management service on the same date, using modifier 25 as appropriate
Do not report administration of fluids for the transplant or for incidental hydration separately
Do not report concurrent administration of medications with the infusion for the transplant

38240 **Hematopoietic progenitor cell (HPC); allogeneic transplantation per donor**
Do not report on same date of service with ([38243], 38242)
S 80 6.44 6.44 FUD XXX

38241 **autologous transplantation**
G2 S 80 4.81 4.81 FUD XXX

\# **38243** **Hematopoietic progenitor cell (HPC); HPC boost**
Do not report on same date of service with (38240, 38242)
R2 S 80 3.39 3.39 FUD 000

38242 **Allogeneic lymphocyte infusions**
EXCLUDES *Aspiration of bone marrow (38220)*
Do not report on same date of service with (38240, [38243])
81379-81383, 86812-86822
R2 S 80 3.36 3.36 FUD 000

38243 ***Resequenced code. See code following 38241.***

38300-38382 Incision Lymphatic Vessels

38300 **Drainage of lymph node abscess or lymphadenitis; simple**
A2 T 5.22 7.77 FUD 010

38305 **extensive**
A2 T 13.58 13.58 FUD 090

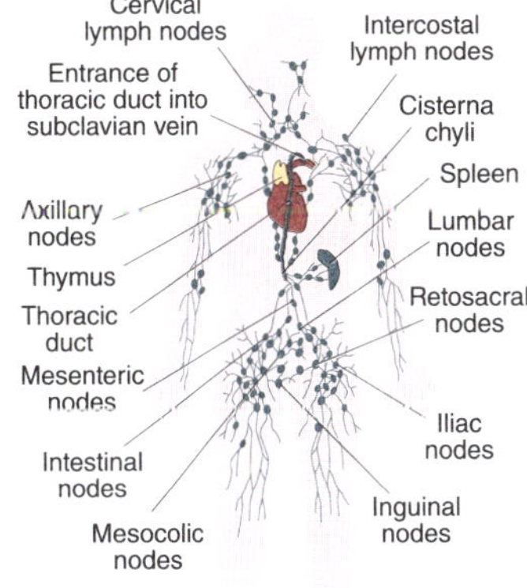

38308 **Lymphangiotomy or other operations on lymphatic channels**
A2 T 80 12.77 12.77 FUD 090

38380 **Suture and/or ligation of thoracic duct; cervical approach**
C 80 16.45 16.45 FUD 090

38381 **thoracic approach**
C 80 PQ 23.12 23.12 FUD 090

38382 **abdominal approach**
C 80 17.21 17.21 FUD 090

38500-38555 Biopsy/Excision Lymphatic Vessels

CMS 100-4,12,30 Correct Coding Policy

EXCLUDES *Injection for sentinel node identification (38792)*
Percutaneous needle biopsy retroperitoneal mass (49180)

38500 **Biopsy or excision of lymph node(s); open, superficial**
Do not report with (38700-38780)
A2 T 50 PQ 7.22 9.37 FUD 010

38505 **by needle, superficial (eg, cervical, inguinal, axillary)**
EXCLUDES *Fine needle aspiration (10021-10022)*
76942, 77012, 77021
88172, 88173
A2 T 50 PQ 2.06 3.59 FUD 000

38510 **open, deep cervical node(s)**
A2 T 50 PQ 12.06 14.83 FUD 010

38520 **open, deep cervical node(s) with excision scalene fat pad**
A2 T 50 PQ 13.32 13.32 FUD 090

38525 **open, deep axillary node(s)**
A2 T 50 PQ 12.38 12.38 FUD 090

38530 **open, internal mammary node(s)**
EXCLUDES *Fine needle aspiration (10022)*
Do not report with (38720-38746)
A2 T 80 50 PQ 15.75 15.75 FUD 090

38542 **Dissection, deep jugular node(s)**
EXCLUDES *Complete cervical lymphadenectomy (38720)*
A2 T 80 50 PQ 14.94 14.94 FUD 090

38550 **Excision of cystic hygroma, axillary or cervical; without deep neurovascular dissection**
A2 T 80 14.40 14.40 FUD 090

38555 **with deep neurovascular dissection**
A2 T 80 28.57 28.57 FUD 090

38562-38564 Limited Lymphadenectomy: Staging

38562 **Limited lymphadenectomy for staging (separate procedure); pelvic and para-aortic**
EXCLUDES *Prostatectomy (55812, 55842)*
Radioactive substance inserted into prostate (55862)
C 80 19.96 19.96 FUD 090

38564 **retroperitoneal (aortic and/or splenic)**
C 80 19.98 19.98 FUD 090

38570-38589 Laparoscopic Lymph Node Procedures

INCLUDES Diagnostic laparoscopy (49320)

EXCLUDES *Laparoscopy with draining of lymphocele to peritoneal cavity (49323)*
Limited lymphadenectomy:
Pelvic (38562)
Retroperitoneal (38564)

38570 **Laparoscopy, surgical; with retroperitoneal lymph node sampling (biopsy), single or multiple**
A2 T 80 PQ 15.22 15.22 FUD 010

38571 **with bilateral total pelvic lymphadenectomy**
A2 T 80 PQ 22.50 22.50 FUD 010

38572 **with bilateral total pelvic lymphadenectomy and peri-aortic lymph node sampling (biopsy), single or multiple**
A2 T 80 PQ 27.40 27.40 FUD 010

38589 **Unlisted laparoscopy procedure, lymphatic system**
T 80 50 Facility RVU 0.00 Non-Facility RVU 0.00 FUD YYY

38700-38780 Lymphadenectomy Procedures

INCLUDES Lymph node biopsy/excision

EXCLUDES *Excision of lymphedematous skin and subcutaneous tissue (15004-15005)*
Limited lymphadenectomy
Pelvic (38562)
Retroperitoneal (38564)
Repair of lymphadematous skin and tissue (15570-15650)

Do not report with (38500)

38700 **Suprahyoid lymphadenectomy**
G2 T 80 50 PQ 23.26 23.26 FUD 090

38720 **Cervical lymphadenectomy (complete)**
T 80 50 PQ 38.86 38.86 FUD 090

38724 **Cervical lymphadenectomy (modified radical neck dissection)**
C 80 50 PQ 42.00 42.00 FUD 090

38740 **Axillary lymphadenectomy; superficial**
A2 T 80 50 PQ 19.71 19.71 FUD 090

38745 **complete**
A2 T 80 50 PQ 24.91 24.91 FUD 090

Parasternal nodes
Central nodes

\+ **38746** **Thoracic lymphadenectomy by thoracotomy, mediastinal and regional lymphadenectomy (List separately in addition to code for primary procedure)**

INCLUDES Left side
Aortopulmonary window
Inferior pulmonary ligament
Paraesophageal
Subcarinal
Right side
Inferior pulmonary ligament
Paraesophageal
Paratracheal
Subcarinal

EXCLUDES *Thoracoscopic mediastinal and regional lymphadenectomy (32674)*

Code first primary procedure (19260, 31760, 31766, 31786, 32096-32200, 32220-32320, 32440-32491, 32503-32505, 33025, 33030, 33050-33130, 39200-39220, 39560-39561, 43101, 43112, 43117-43118, 43122-43123, 43351, 60270, 60505)
C 80 PQ 6.26 6.26 FUD ZZZ

\+ **38747** **Abdominal lymphadenectomy, regional, including celiac, gastric, portal, peripancreatic, with or without para-aortic and vena caval nodes (List separately in addition to code for primary procedure)**
Code first primary procedure
C 80 PQ 7.61 7.61 FUD ZZZ

38760 **Inguinofemoral lymphadenectomy, superficial, including Cloquets node (separate procedure)**
A2 T 80 50 PQ 24.01 24.01 FUD 090

38765 **Inguinofemoral lymphadenectomy, superficial, in continuity with pelvic lymphadenectomy, including external iliac, hypogastric, and obturator nodes (separate procedure)**
C 80 50 PQ 36.77 36.77 FUD 090

38770 **Pelvic lymphadenectomy, including external iliac, hypogastric, and obturator nodes (separate procedure)**
C 80 50 PQ 22.84 22.84 FUD 090

38780 **Retroperitoneal transabdominal lymphadenectomy, extensive, including pelvic, aortic, and renal nodes (separate procedure)**
C 80 PQ 29.29 29.29 FUD 090

38790-38999 Cannulation/Injection/Other Procedures

38790 **Injection procedure; lymphangiography**
75801-75807
N1 N 50 2.41 2.41 FUD 000

38792 **radioactive tracer for identification of sentinel node**
EXCLUDES *Sentinel node excision (38500-38542)*
Sentinel node(s) identification (mapping) intraoperative with nonradioactive dye injection (38900)
78195
N1 Q1 50 1.16 1.16 FUD 000

38794 **Cannulation, thoracic duct**
N1 N 80 8.57 8.57 FUD 090

\+ **38900** **Intraoperative identification (eg, mapping) of sentinel lymph node(s) includes injection of non-radioactive dye, when performed (List separately in addition to code for primary procedure)**
EXCLUDES *Injection of tracer for sentinel node identification (38792)*
Code first (19302, 19307, 38500, 38510, 38520, 38525, 38530, 38542, 38740, 38745)
N1 N 80 50 PQ 3.93 3.93 FUD ZZZ

38999 **Unlisted procedure, hemic or lymphatic system**
S 80 0.00 0.00 FUD YYY

39000-39499 Surgical Procedures: Mediastinum

39000 **Mediastinotomy with exploration, drainage, removal of foreign body, or biopsy; cervical approach**
C 80 PQ 14.35 14.35 FUD 090

39010 **transthoracic approach, including either transthoracic or median sternotomy**
EXCLUDES *Video-assisted thoracic surgery (VATS) pericardial biopsy (32604)*
Do not report with (33955-33956, [33963, 33964])
C 80 PQ 22.84 22.84 FUD 090

39200 **Resection of mediastinal cyst**
C 80 PQ 25.33 25.33 FUD 090

39220 **Resection of mediastinal tumor**
EXCLUDES *Thymectomy (60520)*
Thyroidectomy, substernal (60270)
Video-assisted thoracic surgery (VATS) resection cyst, mass, or tumor of mediastinum (32662)
C 80 PQ 33.11 33.11 FUD 090

39400 **Mediastinoscopy, includes biopsy(ies), when performed**
T PQ 14.64 14.64 FUD 010

39499 **Unlisted procedure, mediastinum**
C 80 0.00 0.00 FUD YYY

39501-39599 Surgical Procedures: Diaphragm

EXCLUDES *Repair of diaphragmatic (esophageal) hernias:*
Laparoscopic with fundoplication (43280-43282)
Laparotomy (43332-43333)
Thoracoabdominal (43336-43337)
Thoracotomy (43334-43335)

39501 **Repair, laceration of diaphragm, any approach**
C 80 PQ 24.34 24.34 FUD 090

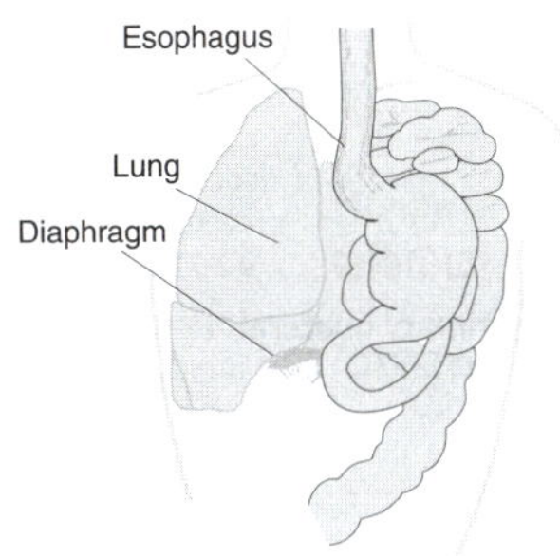

A defect of the diaphragm can allow abdominal contents to herniate into the thoracic cavity

39503 **Repair, neonatal diaphragmatic hernia, with or without chest tube insertion and with or without creation of ventral hernia** A
C 80 CCI PQ 63 175.02 175.02 FUD 090

39540 **Repair, diaphragmatic hernia (other than neonatal), traumatic; acute**
C 80 CCI PQ 24.76 24.76 FUD 090

39541 **chronic**
C 80 CCI PQ 26.97 26.97 FUD 090

39545 **Imbrication of diaphragm for eventration, transthoracic or transabdominal, paralytic or nonparalytic**
C 80 CCI PQ 25.81 25.81 FUD 090

39560 **Resection, diaphragm; with simple repair (eg, primary suture)**
C 80 CCI PQ 22.87 22.87 FUD 090

39561 **with complex repair (eg, prosthetic material, local muscle flap)**
C 80 CCI PQ 35.67 35.67 FUD 090

39599 **Unlisted procedure, diaphragm**
C 80 0.00 0.00 FUD YYY

40490-40799 Resection and Repair Procedures of the Lips

EXCLUDES *Procedures on the skin of lips (10040-17999 [11045, 11046])*

40490 **Biopsy of lip**
P3 T PQ 2.11 3.62 FUD 000

40500 **Vermilionectomy (lip shave), with mucosal advancement**
A2 T 10.49 14.47 FUD 090

40510 **Excision of lip; transverse wedge excision with primary closure**
EXCLUDES *Excision of mucous lesions (40810-40816)*
A2 T 10.32 13.93 FUD 090

40520 **V-excision with primary direct linear closure**
EXCLUDES *Excision of mucous lesions (40810-40816)*
A2 T 10.38 14.06 FUD 090

40525 **full thickness, reconstruction with local flap (eg, Estlander or fan)**
A2 T 16.01 16.01 FUD 090

40527 **full thickness, reconstruction with cross lip flap (Abbe-Estlander)**
INCLUDES Cleft lip repair with cross lip pedicle flap (Abbe-Estlander type), without pedicle sectioning and insertion
EXCLUDES *Cleft lip repair with cross lip pedicle flap (Abbe-Estlander type), with pedicle sectioning and insertion (40761)*
A2 T 80 17.89 17.89 FUD 090

40530 **Resection of lip, more than one-fourth, without reconstruction**
EXCLUDES *Reconstruction (13131-13153)*
A2 T 11.63 15.45 FUD 090

40650 **Repair lip, full thickness; vermilion only**
A2 T 80 8.64 12.58 FUD 090

40652 **up to half vertical height**
A2 T 80 10.11 13.92 FUD 090

40654 **over one-half vertical height, or complex**
A2 T 12.24 16.25 FUD 090

40700 **Plastic repair of cleft lip/nasal deformity; primary, partial or complete, unilateral**
EXCLUDES *Cleft lip repair with cross lip pedicle flap (Abbe-Estlander type):*
With pedicle sectioning and insertion (40761)
Without pedicle sectioning and insertion (40527)
Rhinoplasty for nasal deformity secondary to congenital cleft lip (30460, 30462)
A2 T 80 26.14 26.14 FUD 090

Bilateral cleft lip

Cleft margins on both sides are incised

Margins are closed, correcting cleft

40701 **primary bilateral, 1-stage procedure**
EXCLUDES *Cleft lip repair with cross lip pedicle flap (Abbe-Estlander type):*
With pedicle sectioning and insertion (40761)
Without pedicle sectioning and insertion (40527)
Rhinoplasty for nasal deformity secondary to congenital cleft lip (30460, 30462)
A2 T 80 29.13 29.13 FUD 090

40702 **primary bilateral, 1 of 2 stages**
EXCLUDES *Cleft lip repair with cross lip pedicle flap (Abbe-Estlander type):*
With pedicle sectioning and insertion (40761)
Without pedicle sectioning and insertion (40527)
Rhinoplasty for nasal deformity secondary to congenital cleft lip (30460, 30462)
R2 T 80 25.67 25.67 FUD 090

40720 **secondary, by recreation of defect and reclosure**
EXCLUDES *Cleft lip repair with cross lip pedicle flap (Abbe-Estlander type):*
With pedicle sectioning and insertion (40761)
Without pedicle sectioning and insertion (40527)
Rhinoplasty for nasal deformity secondary to congenital cleft lip (30460, 30462)
A2 T 80 50 29.95 29.95 FUD 090

40761 **with cross lip pedicle flap (Abbe-Estlander type), including sectioning and inserting of pedicle**
EXCLUDES *Cleft lip repair with cross lip pedicle flap (Abbe-Estlander type) without sectioning and insertion of pedicle (40527)*
Cleft palate repair (42200-42225)
Other reconstructive procedures (14060-14061, 15120-15261, 15574, 15576, 15630)
A2 T 31.61 31.61 FUD 090

40799 **Unlisted procedure, lips**
T 80 0.00 0.00 FUD YYY

40800-40819 Incision and Resection of Buccal Cavity

INCLUDES Mucosal/submucosal tissue of lips/cheeks
Oral cavity outside the dentoalveolar structures

40800 **Drainage of abscess, cyst, hematoma, vestibule of mouth; simple**
P2 T 3.83 6.15 FUD 010

40801 **complicated**
A2 T 6.44 9.12 FUD 010

40804 **Removal of embedded foreign body, vestibule of mouth; simple**
P2 X 80 3.88 6.34 FUD 010

40805 **complicated**
P3 T 80 6.84 11.19 FUD 010

40806 **Incision of labial frenum (frenotomy)**
P3 T 80 1.02 3.81 FUD 000

40808 **Biopsy, vestibule of mouth**
P2 T PQ 3.13 5.39 FUD 010

40810 **Excision of lesion of mucosa and submucosa, vestibule of mouth; without repair**
P3 T 3.72 5.99 FUD 010

40812 **with simple repair**
P3 T 5.74 8.34 FUD 010

40814 **with complex repair**
A2 T 8.91 11.16 FUD 090

40816 **complex, with excision of underlying muscle**
A2 T 9.27 11.70 FUD 090

40818 **Excision of mucosa of vestibule of mouth as donor graft**
A2 T 80 7.94 10.36 FUD 090

40819 **Excision of frenum, labial or buccal (frenumectomy, frenulectomy, frenectomy)**
A2 T 80 6.88 9.01 FUD 090

40820 Destruction of Lesion of Buccal Cavity

CMS 100-3,140.5 Laser Procedures

INCLUDES Mucosal/submucosal tissue of lips/cheeks
Oral cavity outside the dentoalveolar structures

40820 **Destruction of lesion or scar of vestibule of mouth by physical methods (eg, laser, thermal, cryo, chemical)**
P3 T 5.00 7.65 FUD 010

40830-40899 Repair Procedures of the Buccal Cavity

INCLUDES Mucosal/submucosal tissue of lips/cheeks
Oral cavity outside the dentoalveolar structures

EXCLUDES *Skin grafts (15002-15630)*

40830 **Closure of laceration, vestibule of mouth; 2.5 cm or less**
G2 T 80 4.85 7.72 FUD 010

40831 **over 2.5 cm or complex**
A2 T 80 6.57 9.82 FUD 010

40840 **Vestibuloplasty; anterior**
A2 T 80 18.07 23.25 FUD 090

40842 **posterior, unilateral**
A2 T 80 17.44 22.57 FUD 090

40843 **posterior, bilateral**
A2 T 80 25.57 32.03 FUD 090

40844 **entire arch**
A2 T 80 31.50 38.38 FUD 090

40845 **complex (including ridge extension, muscle repositioning)**
A2 T 80 35.33 42.05 FUD 090

40899 **Unlisted procedure, vestibule of mouth**
T 80 0.00 0.00 FUD YYY

41000-41018 Surgical Incision of Floor of Mouth or Tongue

EXCLUDES *Frenoplasty (41520)*

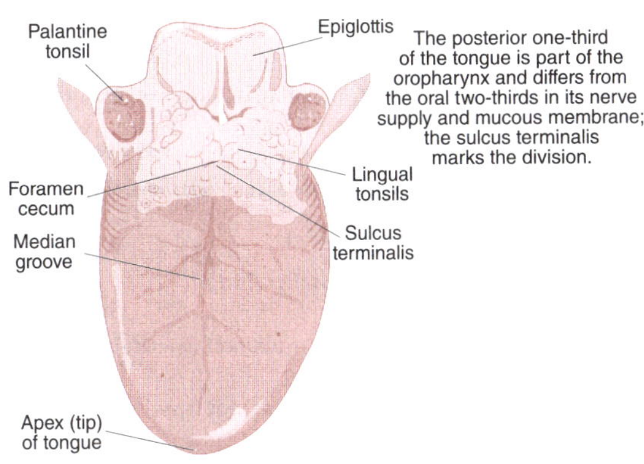

41000 **Intraoral incision and drainage of abscess, cyst, or hematoma of tongue or floor of mouth; lingual**
P3 T 3.26 4.71 FUD 010

41005 **sublingual, superficial**
A2 T 80 3.65 6.62 FUD 010

41006 **sublingual, deep, supramylohyoid**
A2 T 80 7.32 10.36 FUD 090

41007 **submental space**
A2 T 80 7.11 10.19 FUD 090

41008 **submandibular space**
A2 T 80 7.84 10.91 FUD 090

41009 **masticator space**
A2 T 80 8.48 11.60 FUD 090

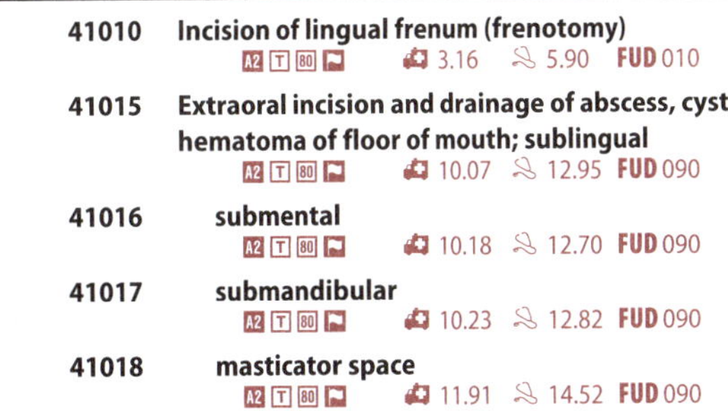

41010 **Incision of lingual frenum (frenotomy)**
A2 T 80 3.16 5.90 FUD 010

41015 **Extraoral incision and drainage of abscess, cyst, or hematoma of floor of mouth; sublingual**
A2 T 80 10.07 12.95 FUD 090

41016 **submental**
A2 T 80 10.18 12.70 FUD 090

41017 **submandibular**
A2 T 80 10.23 12.82 FUD 090

41018 **masticator space**
A2 T 80 11.91 14.52 FUD 090

41019 Placement of Devices for Brachytherapy

EXCLUDES *Application of interstitial radioelements (77776-77787)*
Intracranial brachytherapy radiation sources with stereotactic insertion (61770)

41019 **Placement of needles, catheters, or other device(s) into the head and/or neck region (percutaneous, transoral, or transnasal) for subsequent interstitial radioelement application**
76942, 77002, 77012, 77021
G2 T 80 13.38 13.38 FUD 000

41100-41599 Resection and Repair of the Tongue

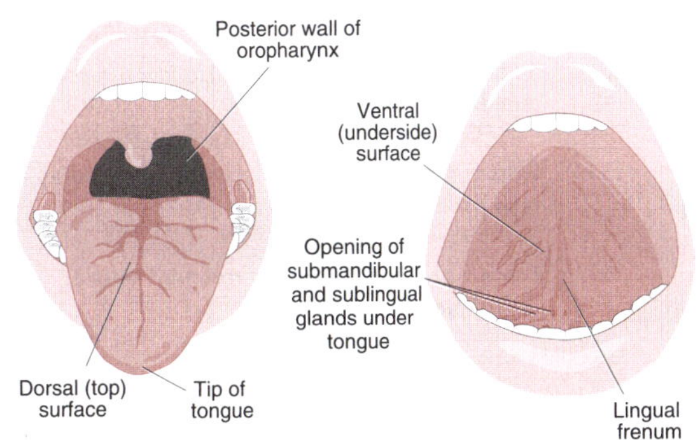

Anterior (front) two-thirds of tongue comprises most of easily visible portions; the base, or root, comprises the remainder of tongue

41100 **Biopsy of tongue; anterior two-thirds**
P3 T PQ 3.15 4.87 FUD 010

41105 **posterior one-third**
P3 T 3.25 4.94 FUD 010

41108 **Biopsy of floor of mouth**
P3 T PQ 2.63 4.28 FUD 010

41110 **Excision of lesion of tongue without closure**
P3 T 3.85 6.19 FUD 010

41112 **Excision of lesion of tongue with closure; anterior two-thirds**
A2 T 7.37 9.69 FUD 090

41113 **posterior one-third**
A2 T 8.14 10.57 FUD 090

41114 **with local tongue flap**
INCLUDES Excision lesion of tongue with closure anterior/posterior two-thirds
Do not report with (41112-41113)
A2 T 80 18.44 18.44 FUD 090

41115 **Excision of lingual frenum (frenectomy)**
P3 T 80 4.44 7.17 FUD 010

41116 **Excision, lesion of floor of mouth**
A2 T 6.44 9.65 FUD 090

41120 **Glossectomy; less than one-half tongue**
A2 T 80 30.22 30.22 FUD 090

41130 **hemiglossectomy**
C 80 PQ 37.46 37.46 FUD 090

41135 **partial, with unilateral radical neck dissection**
C 80 PQ 62.22 62.22 FUD 090

41140 complete or total, with or without tracheostomy, without radical neck dissection
INCLUDES Regnoli's excision
C 80 PQ 62.74 62.74 FUD 090

41145 complete or total, with or without tracheostomy, with unilateral radical neck dissection
C 80 PQ 79.35 79.35 FUD 090

41150 composite procedure with resection floor of mouth and mandibular resection, without radical neck dissection
C 80 PQ 63.06 63.06 FUD 090

41153 composite procedure with resection floor of mouth, with suprahyoid neck dissection
C 80 PQ 68.56 68.56 FUD 090

41155 composite procedure with resection floor of mouth, mandibular resection, and radical neck dissection (Commando type)
C 80 PQ 86.46 86.46 FUD 090

41250 Repair of laceration 2.5 cm or less; floor of mouth and/or anterior two-thirds of tongue
A2 T 80 4.50 7.71 FUD 010

41251 posterior one-third of tongue
A2 T 80 5.23 8.32 FUD 010

41252 Repair of laceration of tongue, floor of mouth, over 2.6 cm or complex
A2 T 80 6.14 9.13 FUD 010

41500 Fixation of tongue, mechanical, other than suture (eg, K-wire)
A2 T 80 10.79 10.79 FUD 090

41510 Suture of tongue to lip for micrognathia (Douglas type procedure)
A2 T 80 12.73 12.73 FUD 090

41512 Tongue base suspension, permanent suture technique
EXCLUDES *Mechanical fixation of tongue, other than suture (41500)*
Suture tongue to lip for micrognathia (41510)
G2 T 80 17.99 17.99 FUD 090

41520 Frenoplasty (surgical revision of frenum, eg, with Z-plasty)
EXCLUDES *Frenotomy (40806, 41010)*
A2 T 80 7.48 10.21 FUD 090

41530 Submucosal ablation of the tongue base, radiofrequency, 1 or more sites, per session
P2 T 80 11.71 92.87 FUD 010

41599 Unlisted procedure, tongue, floor of mouth
T 80 0.00 0.00 FUD YYY

41800-41899 Procedures of the Teeth and Supporting Structures

CMS 100-2,15,150.1 Dental Services

41800 Drainage of abscess, cyst, hematoma from dentoalveolar structures
A2 T 4.28 7.78 FUD 010

41805 Removal of embedded foreign body from dentoalveolar structures; soft tissues
P3 T 80 5.09 7.52 FUD 010

41806 bone
P3 T 80 7.76 10.44 FUD 010

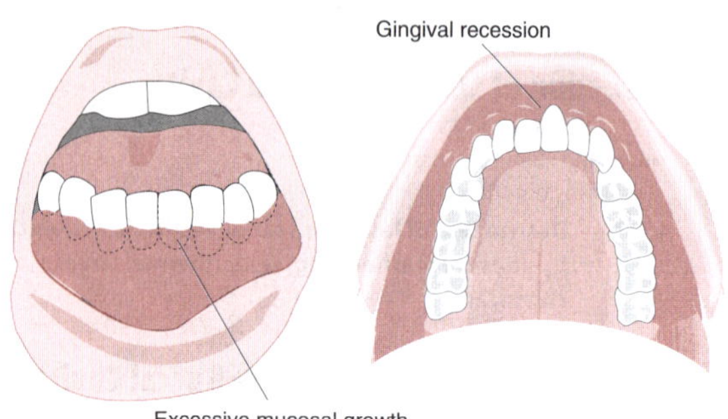

Gingivitis is an inflammatory response to bacteria on the teeth; it is characterized by tender, red, swollen gums and can lead to gingival recession

41820 Gingivectomy, excision gingiva, each quadrant
R2 T 80 0.00 0.00 FUD 000

41821 Operculectomy, excision pericoronal tissues
G2 T 80 0.00 0.00 FUD 000

41822 Excision of fibrous tuberosities, dentoalveolar structures
P3 T 80 5.35 8.44 FUD 010

41823 Excision of osseous tuberosities, dentoalveolar structures
P3 T 80 9.44 12.42 FUD 090

41825 Excision of lesion or tumor (except listed above), dentoalveolar structures; without repair
EXCLUDES *Lesion destruction nonexcisional (41850)*
P3 T 3.57 6.14 FUD 010

41826 with simple repair
EXCLUDES *Lesion destruction nonexcisional (41850)*
P3 T 6.18 9.10 FUD 010

41827 with complex repair
EXCLUDES *Lesion destruction nonexcisional (41850)*
A2 T 8.91 12.74 FUD 090

41828 Excision of hyperplastic alveolar mucosa, each quadrant (specify)
P3 T 80 6.21 8.87 FUD 010

41830 Alveolectomy, including curettage of osteitis or sequestrectomy
P3 T 80 8.28 11.39 FUD 010

41850 Destruction of lesion (except excision), dentoalveolar structures
R2 T 80 0.00 0.00 FUD 000

41870 Periodontal mucosal grafting
G2 T 80 0.00 0.00 FUD 000

41872 Gingivoplasty, each quadrant (specify)
P3 T 80 7.53 10.58 FUD 090

41874 Alveoloplasty, each quadrant (specify)
EXCLUDES *Fracture reduction (21421-21490)*
Laceration closure (40830-40831)
Maxilla osteotomy, segmental (21206)
P3 T 80 7.41 10.84 FUD 090

41899 Unlisted procedure, dentoalveolar structures
T 80 0.00 0.00 FUD YYY

42000-42299 Procedures of the Palate and Uvula

42000 Drainage of abscess of palate, uvula
A2 T 80 3.00 4.56 FUD 010

42100 Biopsy of palate, uvula
P3 T PQ 3.19 4.35 FUD 010

42104 Excision, lesion of palate, uvula; without closure
P3 T 4.06 6.28 FUD 010

42106 with simple primary closure
P3 T 5.20 7.93 FUD 010

42107 with local flap closure
EXCLUDES *Mucosal graft (40818)*
Skin graft (14040-14302)
A2 T 10.07 13.35 FUD 090

42120 Resection of palate or extensive resection of lesion
EXCLUDES *Palate reconstruction using extraoral tissue (14040-14302, 15050, 15120, 15240, 15576)*
A2 T 80 28.70 28.70 FUD 090

42140 Uvulectomy, excision of uvula
A2 T 4.52 7.35 FUD 090

42145 Palatopharyngoplasty (eg, uvulopalatopharyngoplasty, uvulopharyngoplasty)
EXCLUDES *Excision of maxillary torus palatinus (21032)*
Excision of torus mandibularis (21031)
A2 T 20.42 20.42 FUD 090

42160 Destruction of lesion, palate or uvula (thermal, cryo or chemical)
P3 T 80 4.28 6.74 FUD 010

42180 Repair, laceration of palate; up to 2 cm
A2 T 80 5.35 7.09 FUD 010

42182 over 2 cm or complex
A2 T 80 7.43 9.29 FUD 010

42200 Palatoplasty for cleft palate, soft and/or hard palate only
A2 T 80 24.66 24.66 FUD 090

42205 Palatoplasty for cleft palate, with closure of alveolar ridge; soft tissue only
A2 T 80 25.75 25.75 FUD 090

42210 with bone graft to alveolar ridge (includes obtaining graft)
A2 T 80 29.64 29.64 FUD 090

42215 Palatoplasty for cleft palate; major revision
A2 T 80 19.30 19.30 FUD 090

42220 secondary lengthening procedure
A2 T 80 15.01 15.01 FUD 090

42225 attachment pharyngeal flap
G2 T 80 25.34 25.34 FUD 090

42226 Lengthening of palate, and pharyngeal flap
A2 T 80 25.78 25.78 FUD 090

42227 Lengthening of palate, with island flap
G2 T 80 24.19 24.19 FUD 090

42235 Repair of anterior palate, including vomer flap
EXCLUDES *Oronasal fistula repair (30600)*
A2 T 80 21.19 21.19 FUD 090

42260 Repair of nasolabial fistula
EXCLUDES *Cleft lip repair (40700-40761)*
A2 T 80 19.13 23.50 FUD 090

42280 Maxillary impression for palatal prosthesis
P3 T 80 3.30 4.88 FUD 010

42281 Insertion of pin-retained palatal prosthesis
G2 T 80 4.40 5.96 FUD 010

42299 Unlisted procedure, palate, uvula
T 80 0.00 0.00 FUD YYY

42300-42699 Procedures of the Salivary Ducts and Glands

42300 Drainage of abscess; parotid, simple
A2 T 4.44 6.08 FUD 010

42305 parotid, complicated
A2 T 80 12.48 12.48 FUD 090

42310 Drainage of abscess; submaxillary or sublingual, intraoral
A2 T 80 3.62 4.69 FUD 010

42320 submaxillary, external
A2 T 80 5.11 7.26 FUD 010

42330 Sialolithotomy; submandibular (submaxillary), sublingual or parotid, uncomplicated, intraoral
P3 T 4.80 6.74 FUD 010

42335 submandibular (submaxillary), complicated, intraoral
P3 T 7.49 10.87 FUD 090

42340 parotid, extraoral or complicated intraoral
A2 T 80 50 9.76 13.47 FUD 090

42400 Biopsy of salivary gland; needle
EXCLUDES *Fine needle aspiration (10021, 10022)*
76942, 77002, 77012, 77021
88172, 88173
P3 T PQ 1.60 3.06 FUD 000

42405 incisional
76942, 77002, 77012, 77021
A2 T PQ 6.55 8.63 FUD 010

42408 Excision of sublingual salivary cyst (ranula)
A2 T 80 9.47 13.12 FUD 090

42409 Marsupialization of sublingual salivary cyst (ranula)
A2 T 80 6.45 9.67 FUD 090

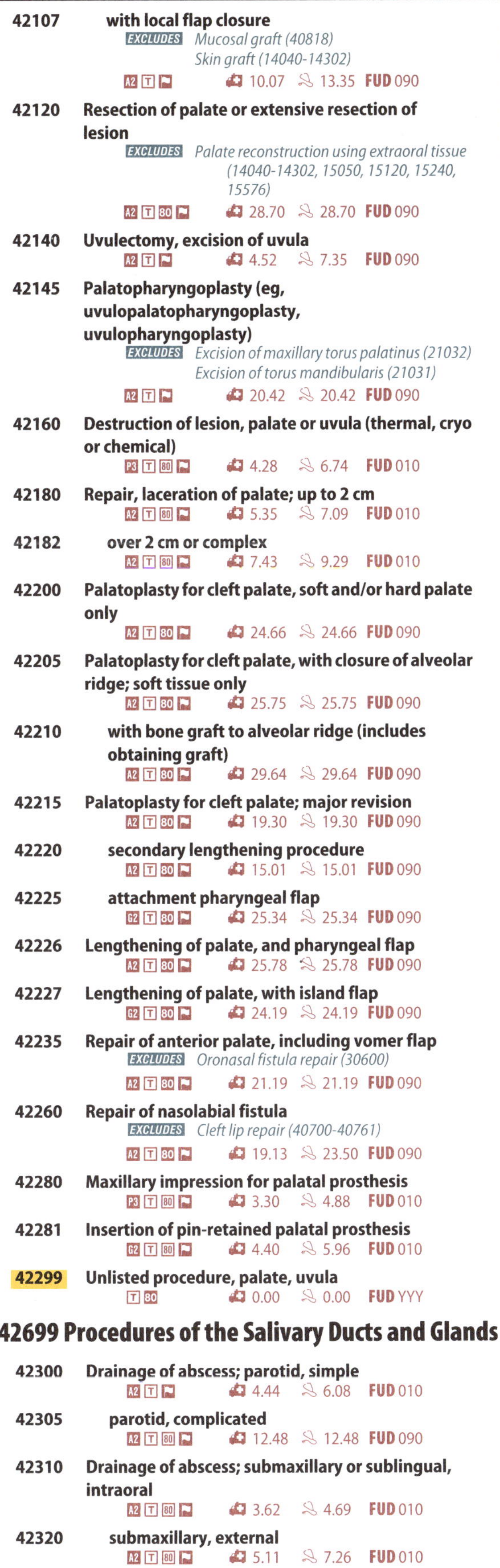

42410 Excision of parotid tumor or parotid gland; lateral lobe, without nerve dissection
EXCLUDES *Facial nerve suture or graft (64864, 64865, 69740, 69745)*
A2 T 80 50 18.03 18.03 FUD 090

42415 lateral lobe, with dissection and preservation of facial nerve
EXCLUDES *Facial nerve suture or graft (64864, 64865, 69740, 69745)*
A2 T 80 50 30.59 30.59 FUD 090

42420 total, with dissection and preservation of facial nerve
EXCLUDES *Facial nerve suture or graft (64864, 64865, 69740, 69745)*
A2 T 80 50 34.34 34.34 FUD 090

42425 total, en bloc removal with sacrifice of facial nerve
EXCLUDES *Facial nerve suture or graft (64864, 64865, 69740, 69745)*
A2 T 80 50 24.23 24.23 FUD 090

42426 total, with unilateral radical neck dissection
EXCLUDES *Facial nerve suture or graft (64864, 64865, 69740, 69745)*
C 80 50 39.12 39.12 FUD 090

42440 Excision of submandibular (submaxillary) gland
A2 T 80 50 11.94 11.94 FUD 090

42450 Excision of sublingual gland
A2 T 80 10.44 13.13 FUD 090

42500 **Plastic repair of salivary duct, sialodochoplasty; primary or simple**
A2 T 80 9.99 12.61 FUD 090

42505 **secondary or complicated**
A2 T 13.21 16.15 FUD 090

42507 **Parotid duct diversion, bilateral (Wilke type procedure);**
A2 T 80 14.90 14.90 FUD 090

~~**42508** **with excision of 1 submandibular gland**~~

42509 **with excision of both submandibular glands**
A2 T 80 25.29 25.29 FUD 090

42510 **with ligation of both submandibular (Wharton's) ducts**
A2 T 80 18.23 18.23 FUD 090

42550 **Injection procedure for sialography**
70390
N1 N 1.82 3.80 FUD 000

42600 **Closure salivary fistula**
A2 T 80 10.11 13.90 FUD 090

42650 **Dilation salivary duct**
P3 T 1.72 2.44 FUD 000

42660 **Dilation and catheterization of salivary duct, with or without injection**
P3 T 80 2.41 3.52 FUD 000

42665 **Ligation salivary duct, intraoral**
A2 T 80 6.02 9.12 FUD 090

42699 **Unlisted procedure, salivary glands or ducts**
T 80 0.00 0.00 FUD YYY

42700-42999 Procedures of the Adenoids/Throat/Tonsils

42700 **Incision and drainage abscess; peritonsillar**
A2 T 3.96 5.51 FUD 010

42720 **retropharyngeal or parapharyngeal, intraoral approach**
A2 T 80 11.37 13.14 FUD 010

42725 **retropharyngeal or parapharyngeal, external approach**
A2 T 80 23.52 23.52 FUD 090

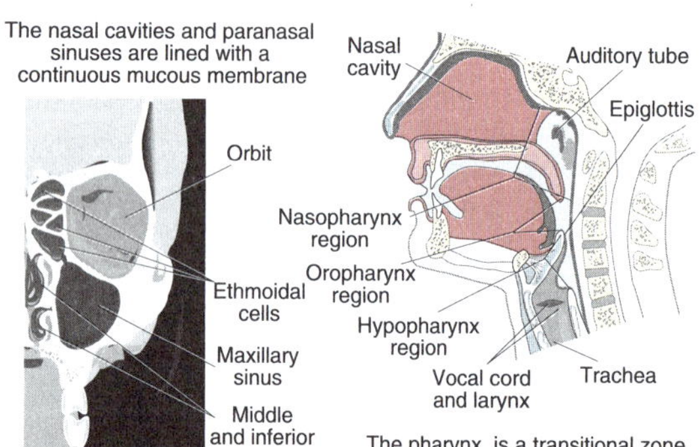

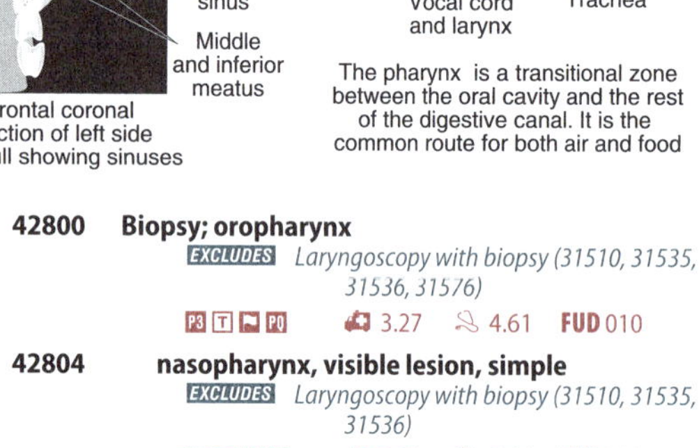

42800 **Biopsy; oropharynx**
EXCLUDES *Laryngoscopy with biopsy (31510, 31535, 31536, 31576)*
P3 T PO 3.27 4.61 FUD 010

42804 **nasopharynx, visible lesion, simple**
EXCLUDES *Laryngoscopy with biopsy (31510, 31535, 31536)*
A2 T PO 3.28 5.66 FUD 010

42806 **nasopharynx, survey for unknown primary lesion**
EXCLUDES *Laryngoscopy with biopsy (31510, 31535, 31536)*
A2 T PO 3.83 6.37 FUD 010

42808 **Excision or destruction of lesion of pharynx, any method**
A2 T 4.70 6.58 FUD 010

42809 **Removal of foreign body from pharynx**
G2 X 3.85 4.99 FUD 010

42810 **Excision branchial cleft cyst or vestige, confined to skin and subcutaneous tissues**
A2 T 80 50 8.41 11.26 FUD 090

42815 **Excision branchial cleft cyst, vestige, or fistula, extending beneath subcutaneous tissues and/or into pharynx**
A2 T 80 50 16.20 16.20 FUD 090

42820 **Tonsillectomy and adenoidectomy; younger than age 12** A
A2 T 80 8.41 8.41 FUD 090

42821 **age 12 or over** A
A2 T 80 8.74 8.74 FUD 090

42825 **Tonsillectomy, primary or secondary; younger than age 12** A
A2 T 80 7.59 7.59 FUD 090

42826 **age 12 or over** A
A2 T 7.29 7.29 FUD 090

42830 **Adenoidectomy, primary; younger than age 12** A
A2 T 80 6.03 6.03 FUD 090

42831 **age 12 or over** A
A2 T 80 6.48 6.48 FUD 090

42835 **Adenoidectomy, secondary; younger than age 12** A
A2 T 80 5.17 5.17 FUD 090

42836 **age 12 or over** A
A2 T 80 6.98 6.98 FUD 090

42842 **Radical resection of tonsil, tonsillar pillars, and/or retromolar trigone; without closure**
T 80 28.74 28.74 FUD 090

42844 **closure with local flap (eg, tongue, buccal)**
T 80 39.45 39.45 FUD 090

42845 **closure with other flap**
Code also closure with other flap(s)
Code also radical neck dissection when combined (38720)
C 80 64.04 64.04 FUD 090

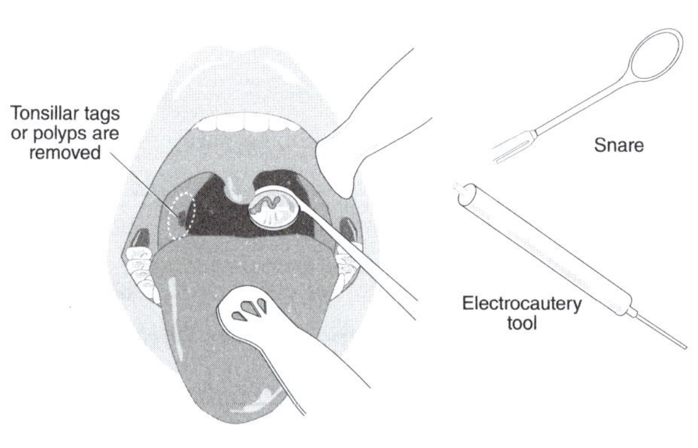

42860 **Excision of tonsil tags**
A2 T 80 5.47 5.47 FUD 090

42870 **Excision or destruction lingual tonsil, any method (separate procedure)**
EXCLUDES *Nasopharynx resection (juvenile angiofibroma) by transzygomatic/bicoronal approach (61586, 61600)*
A2 T 80 16.71 16.71 FUD 090

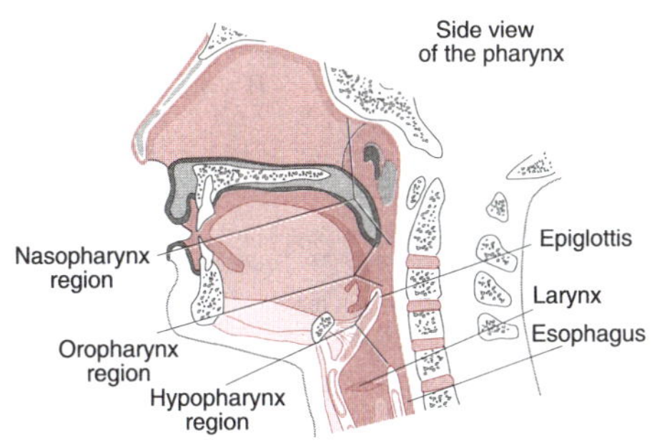

The nasopharynx is the membranous passage above the level of the soft palate; the oropharynx is the region between the soft palate and the upper edge of the epiglottis; the hypopharynx is the region of the epiglottis to the juncture of the larynx and esophagus; the three regions are collectively known as the pharynx

42890 Limited pharyngectomy
Code also radical neck dissection when combined (38720)
A2 T 80 | 40.87 | 40.87 FUD 090

42892 Resection of lateral pharyngeal wall or pyriform sinus, direct closure by advancement of lateral and posterior pharyngeal walls
Code also radical neck dissection when combined (38720)
A2 T 80 | 54.29 | 54.29 FUD 090

42894 Resection of pharyngeal wall requiring closure with myocutaneous or fasciocutaneous flap or free muscle, skin, or fascial flap with microvascular anastomosis
EXCLUDES *Flap used for reconstruction (15732, 15734, 15756-15758)*
Code also radical neck dissection when combined (38720)
C 80 | 68.26 | 68.26 FUD 090

42900 Suture pharynx for wound or injury
A2 T 80 | 9.83 | 9.83 FUD 010

42950 Pharyngoplasty (plastic or reconstructive operation on pharynx)
EXCLUDES *Pharyngeal flap (42225)*
A2 T 80 | 22.92 | 22.92 FUD 090

42953 Pharyngoesophageal repair
Code also closure using myocutaneous or other flap
C 80 | 27.41 | 27.41 FUD 090

42955 Pharyngostomy (fistulization of pharynx, external for feeding)
A2 T 80 | 21.73 | 21.73 FUD 090

42960 Control oropharyngeal hemorrhage, primary or secondary (eg, post-tonsillectomy); simple
A2 T 80 | 4.94 | 4.94 FUD 010

42961 complicated, requiring hospitalization
C 80 | 12.23 | 12.23 FUD 090

42962 with secondary surgical intervention
A2 T | 15.01 | 15.01 FUD 090

42970 Control of nasopharyngeal hemorrhage, primary or secondary (eg, postadenoidectomy); simple, with posterior nasal packs, with or without anterior packs and/or cautery
R2 T | 11.92 | 11.92 FUD 090

42971 complicated, requiring hospitalization
C 80 | 13.26 | 13.26 FUD 090

42972 with secondary surgical intervention
A2 T 80 | 14.85 | 14.85 FUD 090

42999 Unlisted procedure, pharynx, adenoids, or tonsils
T 80 | 0.00 | 0.00 FUD YYY

43020-43135 Incision/Resection of Esophagus

EXCLUDES *Gastrointestinal reconstruction for previous esophagectomy (43360, 43361)*
Gastrotomy with intraluminal tube insertion (43510)

43020 Esophagotomy, cervical approach, with removal of foreign body
EXCLUDES *Laparotomy with esophageal intubation (43510)*
T 80 PQ | 14.30 | 14.30 FUD 090

43030 Cricopharyngeal myotomy
EXCLUDES *Laparotomy with esophageal intubation (43510)*
G2 T 80 PQ | 15.03 | 15.03 FUD 090

43045 Esophagotomy, thoracic approach, with removal of foreign body
EXCLUDES *Laparotomy with esophageal intubation (43510)*
C 80 PQ | 37.65 | 37.65 FUD 090

43100 Excision of lesion, esophagus, with primary repair; cervical approach
EXCLUDES *Wide excision of malignant lesion of cervical esophagus, with total laryngectomy:*
With radical neck dissection (31365, 43107, 43116, 43124)
Without radical neck dissection (31360, 43107, 43116, 43124)
C 80 PQ | 18.17 | 18.17 FUD 090

43101 thoracic or abdominal approach
EXCLUDES *Wide excision of malignant lesion of cervical esophagus with total laryngectomy:*
With radical neck dissection (31365, 43107, 43116, 43124)
Without radical neck dissection (31360, 43107, 43116, 43124)
C 80 PQ | 29.13 | 29.13 FUD 090

43107 Total or near total esophagectomy, without thoracotomy; with pharyngogastrostomy or cervical esophagogastrostomy, with or without pyloroplasty (transhiatal)
C 80 PQ | 73.29 | 73.29 FUD 090

43108 with colon interposition or small intestine reconstruction, including intestine mobilization, preparation and anastomosis(es)
C 80 PQ | 133.81 | 133.81 FUD 090

43112 Total or near total esophagectomy, with thoracotomy; with pharyngogastrostomy or cervical esophagogastrostomy, with or without pyloroplasty
C 80 PQ | 77.54 | 77.54 FUD 090

43113 with colon interposition or small intestine reconstruction, including intestine mobilization, preparation, and anastomosis(es)
C 80 PQ | 130.80 | 130.80 FUD 090

43116 Partial esophagectomy, cervical, with free intestinal graft, including microvascular anastomosis, obtaining the graft and intestinal reconstruction
INCLUDES Operating microscope (69990)
EXCLUDES *Free jejunal graft with microvascular anastomosis done by a different physician (43496)*
Code also modifier 52 if intestinal or free jejunal graft with microvascular anastomosis is done by another physician
C 80 PQ | 151.36 | 151.36 FUD 090

Digestive System

42890 — 43116

43117 **Partial esophagectomy, distal two-thirds, with thoracotomy and separate abdominal incision, with or without proximal gastrectomy; with thoracic esophagogastrostomy, with or without pyloroplasty (Ivor Lewis)**

EXCLUDES *Esophagogastrectomy (lower third) and vagotomy (43122)*
Total esophagectomy with gastropharyngostomy (43107, 43124)

C 80 PQ 71.15 71.15 FUD 090

43118 **with colon interposition or small intestine reconstruction, including intestine mobilization, preparation, and anastomosis(es)**

EXCLUDES *Esophagogastrectomy (lower third) and vagotomy (43122)*
Total esophagectomy with gastropharyngostomy (43107, 43124)

C 80 PQ 104.06 104.06 FUD 090

43121 **Partial esophagectomy, distal two-thirds, with thoracotomy only, with or without proximal gastrectomy, with thoracic esophagogastrostomy, with or without pyloroplasty**

C 80 PQ 82.89 82.89 FUD 090

43122 **Partial esophagectomy, thoracoabdominal or abdominal approach, with or without proximal gastrectomy; with esophagogastrostomy, with or without pyloroplasty**

C 80 PQ 73.64 73.64 FUD 090

43123 **with colon interposition or small intestine reconstruction, including intestine mobilization, preparation, and anastomosis(es)**

C 80 PQ 135.57 135.57 FUD 090

43124 **Total or partial esophagectomy, without reconstruction (any approach), with cervical esophagostomy**

C 80 PQ 110.49 110.49 FUD 090

43130 **Diverticulectomy of hypopharynx or esophagus, with or without myotomy; cervical approach**

EXCLUDES *Diverticulectomy hypopharynx or cervical esophagus, endoscopic (43180)*

G2 T 80 PQ 22.84 22.84 FUD 090

43135 **thoracic approach**

EXCLUDES *Diverticulectomy hypopharynx or cervical esophagus, endoscopic (43180)*

C 80 PQ 43.18 43.18 FUD 090

43180-43233 [43211, 43212, 43213, 43214] Endoscopic Procedures: Esophagus

CMS 100-3,100.2 Endoscopy

INCLUDES Control of bleeding as result of the endoscopic procedure during same operative session
Diagnostic endoscopy with surgical endoscopy
Examination of upper esophageal sphincter (cricopharyngeus muscle) to/including the gastroesophageal junction
Retroflexion examination of proximal region of stomach

● **43180** **Esophagoscopy, rigid, transoral with diverticulectomy of hypopharynx or cervical esophagus (eg, Zenker's diverticulum), with cricopharyngeal myotomy, includes use of telescope or operating microscope and repair, when performed**

INCLUDES Operating microscope (69990)

EXCLUDES *Open diverticulectomy hypopharynx or esophagus (43130-43135)*

43191 **Esophagoscopy, rigid, transoral; diagnostic, including collection of specimen(s) by brushing or washing when performed (separate procedure)**

EXCLUDES *Flexible, transnasal (43197-43198)*
Flexible, transoral (43200)

Do not report with (43192-43198)

G2 T 3.64 3.64 FUD 000

43192 **with directed submucosal injection(s), any substance**

EXCLUDES *Flexible, transoral (43201)*
Injection sclerosis of esophageal varices:
Flexible, transoral (43204)
Rigid, transoral (43499)

Do not report with (43191, 43197-43198)

G2 T 4.34 4.34 FUD 000

43193 **with biopsy, single or multiple**

EXCLUDES *Flexible, transoral (43202)*

Do not report with (43191, 43197-43198)

G2 T 5.17 5.17 FUD 000

▲ **43194** **with removal of foreign body(s)**

EXCLUDES *Flexible, transoral (43215)*

Do not report with (43191, 43197-43198)

76000

G2 T 4.69 4.69 FUD 000

43195 **with balloon dilation (less than 30 mm diameter)**

EXCLUDES *Dilation of esophagus:*
Flexible, with balloon diameter 30 mm or larger ([43214], [43233])
Flexible, with balloon diameter less than 30 mm (43220)
Without endoscopic visualization (43450-43453)

Do not report with (43191, 43197-43198)

74360

G2 T 5.18 5.18 FUD 000

43196 **with insertion of guide wire followed by dilation over guide wire**

EXCLUDES *Flexible, transoral (43226)*

Do not report with (43191, 43197-43198)

74360

G2 T 5.68 5.68 FUD 000

▲ **43197** **Esophagoscopy, flexible, transnasal; diagnostic, including collection of specimen(s) by brushing or washing, when performed (separate procedure)**

EXCLUDES *Flexible, transoral (43200)*
Rigid, transoral (43191)

Do not report with diagnostic nasal endoscopy (31231) unless different type of endoscope used

Do not report with (31575, 43191-43196, 43198, 43200-43232 [43211, 43212, 43213, 43214], 43235-43259 [43233, 43266, 43270], 92511)

G2 T 2.31 5.24 FUD 000

43198 **with biopsy, single or multiple**

EXCLUDES *Flexible, transoral (43202)*
Rigid, transoral (43193)

Do not report with diagnostic nasal endoscopy (31231) unless different type of endoscope used

Do not report with (31575, 43191-43197, 43200-43232 [43211, 43212, 43213, 43214], 43235-43259 [43233, 43266, 43270], 92511)

G2 T 2.75 5.85 FUD 000

⊙ **43200** **Esophagoscopy, flexible, transoral; diagnostic, including collection of specimen(s) by brushing or washing, when performed (separate procedure)**

EXCLUDES *Flexible, transnasal (43197)*
Rigid, transoral (43191)
Upper gastrointestinal endoscopy (43235)

Do not report with (43197-43198, 43201-43232 [43211, 43212, 43213, 43214])

A2 T 2.71 7.67 FUD 000

⊙ 43201 **with directed submucosal injection(s), any substance**

EXCLUDES *Injection sclerosis of esophageal varices:*
Flexible, transoral (43204)
Rigid, transoral (43499)
Rigid, transoral (43192)

Do not report with (43204, [43211], 43227) when on same lesion

Do not report with (43197-43198, 43200)

A2 T CCI 3.18 7.82 FUD 000

⊙ 43202 **with biopsy, single or multiple**

EXCLUDES *Flexible, transnasal (43198)*
Rigid, transoral (43193)

Do not report with ([43211]) when on same lesion

Do not report with (43197-43198, 43200)

A2 T CCI PQ 3.19 10.27 FUD 000

⊙ 43204 **with injection sclerosis of esophageal varices**

EXCLUDES *Rigid, transoral (43499)*

Do not report with (43201, 43227) when on same lesion

Do not report with (43197-43198, 43200)

A2 T CCI 4.20 4.20 FUD 000

⊙ 43205 **with band ligation of esophageal varices**

EXCLUDES *Band ligation non-variceal bleeding (43227)*

Do not report with (43227) when on same lesion

Do not report with (43197-43198, 43200)

A2 T CCI 4.34 4.34 FUD 000

⊙ 43206 **with optical endomicroscopy**

Code also contrast agent

Do not report with (43197-43198, 43200, 88375)

G2 T 4.15 9.41 FUD 000

43211 Resequenced code. See code following 43217.

43212 Resequenced code. See code following 43217.

43213 Resequenced code. See code following 43220.

43214 Resequenced code. See code following 43220.

⊙ ▲ 43215 **with removal of foreign body(s)**

EXCLUDES *Rigid, transoral (43194)*
Upper gastrointestinal endoscopy (43247)

Do not report with (43197-43198, 43200)

76000

A2 T CCI 4.29 11.54 FUD 000

⊙ ▲ 43216 **with removal of tumor(s), polyp(s), or other lesion(s) by hot biopsy forceps**

EXCLUDES *Removal by snare technique (43217)*

Do not report with (43197-43198, 43200)

A2 T CCI 4.17 11.91 FUD 000

⊙ 43217 **with removal of tumor(s), polyp(s), or other lesion(s) by snare technique**

EXCLUDES *Upper gastrointestinal endoscopy with snare technique (43251)*

Do not report with ([43211]) when on same lesion

Do not report with (43197-43198, 43200)

A2 T CCI 4.97 12.73 FUD 000

⊙ # 43211 **with endoscopic mucosal resection**

Do not report with (43201-43202, 43217) when on same lesion

Do not report with (43197-43198, 43200)

G2 T 7.06 7.06 FUD 000

⊙ # 43212 **with placement of endoscopic stent (includes pre- and post-dilation and guide wire passage, when performed)**

Do not report with (43197-43198, 43200, 43220, 43226, 43241)

74360

G2 T 5.57 5.57 FUD 000

⊙ 43220 **with transendoscopic balloon dilation (less than 30 mm diameter)**

EXCLUDES *Dilation of esophagus:*
Rigid, with balloon diameter 30 mm or larger ([43214])
Rigid, with balloon diameter less than 30mm (43195)
Without endoscopic visualization (43450, 43453)

Do not report with (43197-43198, 43200, [43212], 43226, 43229)

74360

A2 T CCI 3.66 28.49 FUD 000

⊙ # 43213 **with dilation of esophagus, by balloon or dilator, retrograde (includes fluoroscopic guidance, when performed)**

Code also each additional stricture treated in same operative session with ([43213]) and append modifier 59

Do not report with (43197-43198, 43200, 74360, 76000-76001)

G2 T 7.85 34.97 FUD 000

⊙ # 43214 **with dilation of esophagus with balloon (30 mm diameter or larger) (includes fluoroscopic guidance, when performed)**

Do not report with (43197-43198, 43200, 74360, 76000 76001)

G2 T 5.68 5.68 FUD 000

⊙ 43226 **with insertion of guide wire followed by passage of dilator(s) over guide wire**

EXCLUDES *Rigid, transoral (43196)*

Do not report with (43229) when on same lesion

Do not report with (43197-43198, 43200, [43212], 43220)

74360

A2 T CCI 4.03 10.84 FUD 000

⊙ 43227 **with control of bleeding, any method**

Do not report with (43201, 43204-43205) when on same lesion

Do not report with (43197-43198, 43200)

A2 T CCI 5.10 11.24 FUD 000

⊙ 43229 **with ablation of tumor(s), polyp(s), or other lesion(s) (includes pre- and post-dilation and guide wire passage, when performed)**

Code also esophagoscopic photodynamic therapy, when performed (96570-96571)

Do not report with (43220, 43226) when on same lesion

Do not report with (43197-43198, 43200)

G2 T 6.00 20.62 FUD 000

⊙ 43231 **with endoscopic ultrasound examination**

Do not report more than one time per operative session

Do not report with (43197-43198, 43200, 43232, 76975)

A2 T CCI 4.97 11.54 FUD 000

⊙ 43232 **with transendoscopic ultrasound-guided intramural or transmural fine needle aspiration/biopsy(s)**

Do not report more than one time per operative session

Do not report with (43197-43198, 43200, 43231, 76942, 76975)

A2 T CCI 5.92 13.60 FUD 000

43233 Resequenced code. See code following 43249.

43235-43259 [43233, 43266, 43270] Endoscopic Procedures: Esophagogastroduodenoscopy (EGD)

INCLUDES Control of bleeding as result of the endoscopic procedure during same operative session
Diagnostic endoscopy with surgical endoscopy

EXCLUDES *Exam of jejunum distal to the anastomosis in surgically altered stomach, including post-gastroenterostomy (Billroth II) and gastric bypass (43235-43259 [43233, 43266, 43270])*
Exam of upper esophageal sphincter (cricopharyngeus muscle) to/including gastroesophageal junction and/or retroflexion exam of proximal region of stomach (43197-43232 [43211, 43212, 43213, 43214])

Code also modifier 52 when duodenum is not examined either deliberately or due to significant issues and repeat procedure will not be performed
Code also modifier 53 when duodenum is not examined either deliberately or due to significant issues and repeat procedure is planned

⊙ **43235 Esophagogastroduodenoscopy, flexible, transoral; diagnostic, including collection of specimen(s) by brushing or washing, when performed (separate procedure)**
Do not report with (43197-43198, 43236-43259 [43233, 43266, 43270], 44360-44379)
A2 T 3.80 8.87 FUD 000

⊙ **43236 with directed submucosal injection(s), any substance**
EXCLUDES *Injection sclerosis of varices, esophageal/gastric (43243)*
Do not report with (43243, 43254-43255) when on same lesion
Do not report with (43197-43198, 43235, 44360-44379)
A2 T 4.27 11.06 FUD 000

⊙ **43237 with endoscopic ultrasound examination limited to the esophagus, stomach or duodenum, and adjacent structures**
Do not report more than one time per operative session
Do not report with (43197-43198, 43235, 43238, 43242, 43253, 43259, 44360-44379, 76975)
A2 T 6.01 6.01 FUD 000

⊙ **43238 with transendoscopic ultrasound-guided intramural or transmural fine needle aspiration/biopsy(s), (includes endoscopic ultrasound examination limited to the esophagus, stomach or duodenum, and adjacent structures)**
Do not report more than one time per operative session
Do not report with (43197-43198, 43235, 43237, 43242, 44360-44379, 76942, 76975)
A2 T 6.86 6.86 FUD 000

⊙ **43239 with biopsy, single or multiple**
Do not report with (43254) when on same lesion
Do not report with (43197-43198, 43235, 44360-44379)
A2 T PQ 4.25 11.32 FUD 000

⊙ **43240 with transmural drainage of pseudocyst (includes placement of transmural drainage catheter[s]/stent[s], when performed, and endoscopic ultrasound, when performed)**
EXCLUDES *Endoscopic pancreatic necrosectomy (48999)*
Do not report more than one time per operative session
Do not report with (43253) when on same lesion
Do not report with (43197-43198, 43235, 43242, [43266], 43259, 44360-44379)
A2 T 11.94 11.94 FUD 000

⊙ **43241 with insertion of intraluminal tube or catheter**
EXCLUDES *Tube placement:*
Enteric, non-endoscopic (44500, 74340)
Naso or oro-gastric requiring professional skill and fluoroscopic guidance (43752)
Do not report with (43197-43198, [43212], 43235, [43266], 44360-44379)
A2 T 4.40 4.40 FUD 000

⊙ **43242 with transendoscopic ultrasound-guided intramural or transmural fine needle aspiration/biopsy(s) (includes endoscopic ultrasound examination of the esophagus, stomach, and either the duodenum or a surgically altered stomach where the jejunum is examined distal to the anastomosis)**
EXCLUDES *Transmural fine needle biopsy/aspiration with ultrasound guidance, transendoscopic, esophagus/stomach/duodenum/neighboring structure (43238)*
Do not report more than one time per operative session
Do not report with (43197-43198, 43235, 43237-43238, 43240, 43259, 44360-44379, 76942, 76975)
88172-88173
A2 T 7.82 7.82 FUD 000

⊙ **43243 with injection sclerosis of esophageal/gastric varices**
Do not report with (43236, 43255) when on same lesion
Do not report with (43197-43198, 43235, 44360-44379)
A2 T 7.25 7.25 FUD 000

⊙ **43244 with band ligation of esophageal/gastric varices**
EXCLUDES *Band ligation, non-variceal bleeding (43255)*
Do not report with (43197-43198, 43235, 43255, 44360-44379)
A2 T 7.51 7.51 FUD 000

⊙ **43245 with dilation of gastric/duodenal stricture(s) (eg, balloon, bougie)**
Do not report with (43197-43198, 43235, [43266], 44360-44379)
74360
A2 T 5.38 17.49 FUD 000

⊙ **43246 with directed placement of percutaneous gastrostomy tube**
EXCLUDES *Gastrostomy tube replacement without endoscopy or imaging (43760)*
Percutaneous insertion of gastrostomy tube, nonendoscopic (49440)
Do not report with (43197-43198, 43235, 44360-44372, 44376-44379)
A2 T 80 6.17 6.17 FUD 000

⊙ ▲ **43247 with removal of foreign body(s)**
Do not report with (43197-43198, 43235, 44360-44379)
76000
A2 T 5.39 11.56 FUD 000

⊙ **43248 with insertion of guide wire followed by passage of dilator(s) through esophagus over guide wire**
Do not report with (43197-43198, 43235, [43266], [43270], 44360-44379)
74360
A2 T 5.13 11.71 FUD 000

⊙ **43249 with transendoscopic balloon dilation of esophagus (less than 30 mm diameter)**
Do not report with (43197-43198, 43235, [43266], [43270], 44360-44379)
74360
A2 T 4.73 29.78 FUD 000

⊙ # **43233** **with dilation of esophagus with balloon (30 mm diameter or larger) (includes fluoroscopic guidance, when performed)**
Do not report with (43197-43198, 43235, 44360-44379, 74360, 76000-76001)
G2 T 6.74 6.74 FUD 000

⊙ ▲ **43250** **with removal of tumor(s), polyp(s), or other lesion(s) by hot biopsy forceps**
Do not report with (43197-43198, 43235, 44360-44379)
A2 T 5.21 13.00 FUD 000

⊙ **43251** **with removal of tumor(s), polyp(s), or other lesion(s) by snare technique**
INCLUDES Do not report with (43254) when on same lesion
EXCLUDES *Endoscopic mucosal resection (43254)*
Do not report with (43197-43198, 43235, 44360-44379)
A2 T 6.03 14.31 FUD 000

⊙ **43252** **with optical endomicroscopy**
Code also contrast agent
Do not report with (43197-43198, 43235, 44360-44379, 88375)
G2 T 5.19 10.50 FUD 000

⊙ **43253** **with transendoscopic ultrasound-guided transmural injection of diagnostic or therapeutic substance(s) (eg, anesthetic, neurolytic agent) or fiducial marker(s) (includes endoscopic ultrasound examination of the esophagus, stomach, and either the duodenum or a surgically altered stomach where the jejunum is examined distal to the anastomosis)**
INCLUDES Do not report with (43240) when on same lesion
EXCLUDES *Transmural fine needle biopsy/aspiration with ultrasound guidance, transendoscopic, esophagus/stomach/duodenum/neighboring structures (43238, 43242)*
Do not report more than one time per operative session
Do not report with (43197-43198, 43235, 43237, 43259, 44360-44379, 76942, 76975)
G2 T 7.82 7.82 FUD 000

⊙ **43254** **with endoscopic mucosal resection**
Do not report with (43236, 43239, 43251) when on same lesion
Do not report with (43197-43198, 43235, 44360-44379)
G2 T 8.12 8.12 FUD 000

⊙ **43255** **with control of bleeding, any method**
Do not report with (43236, 43243-43244) when on same lesion
Do not report with (43197-43198, 43235, 44360-44379)
A2 T 6.18 12.32 FUD 000

⊙ # **43266** **with placement of endoscopic stent (includes pre- and post-dilation and guide wire passage, when performed)**
Do not report with (43197-43198, 43235, 43240-43241, 43245, 43248-43249, 44360-44379)
74360
G2 T 6.72 6.72 FUD 000

⊙ **43257** **with delivery of thermal energy to the muscle of lower esophageal sphincter and/or gastric cardia, for treatment of gastroesophageal reflux disease**
EXCLUDES *Esophageal lesion ablation (43229, [43270])*
Do not report with (43197-43198, 43235, 44360-44379)
A2 T 6.91 6.91 FUD 000

⊙ # **43270** **with ablation of tumor(s), polyp(s), or other lesion(s) (includes pre- and post-dilation and guide wire passage, when performed)**
Code also esophagoscopic photodynamic therapy, when performed (96570-96571)
Do not report with (43248-43249) when on same lesion
Do not report with (43197-43198, 43235, 44360-44379)
G2 T 7.06 20.56 FUD 000

⊙ **43259** **with endoscopic ultrasound examination, including the esophagus, stomach, and either the duodenum or a surgically altered stomach where the jejunum is examined distal to the anastomosis**
Do not report more than one time per operative session
Do not report with (43197-43198, 43235, 43237, 43240, 43242, 43253, 44360-44379, 76975)
A2 T 6.94 6.94 FUD 000

43260-43278 [43274, 43275, 43276, 43277, 43278] Endoscopic Procedures: ERCP

INCLUDES Diagnostic endoscopy with surgical endoscopy
Pancreaticobiliary system:
Biliary tree (right and left hepatic ducts, cystic duct/gallbladder, and common bile ducts)
Pancreas (major and minor ducts)

EXCLUDES *ERCP via Roux-en-Y anatomy (for instance post-gastric or bariatric bypass or post total gastrectomy) or via gastrostomy (open or laparoscopic) (47999, 48999)*
Optical endomicroscopy of biliary tract, report one time per session (47999)
Optical endomicroscopy of pancreas, report one time per session (48999)

Code also appropriate endoscopy of each anatomic site examined
Code also sphincteroplasty or ductal stricture dilation, when performed prior to the debris/stone removal from the duct ([43277])
Code also the appropriate ERCP procedure when performed on altered postoperative anatomy (i.e. Billroth II gastroenterostomy)
74328-74330

⊙ **43260** **Endoscopic retrograde cholangiopancreatography (ERCP); diagnostic, including collection of specimen(s) by brushing or washing, when performed (separate procedure)**
Do not report with (43261-43265 [43274, 43275, 43276, 43277, 43278])
A2 T PQ 9.84 9.84 FUD 000

⊙ **43261** **with biopsy, single or multiple**
Do not report with (43260)
A2 T PQ 10.32 10.32 FUD 000

An endoscope is fed through the stomach and into the duodenum. Usually a smaller sub-scope is fed up the sphincter of Oddi and into the ducts that drain the pancreas and the gallbladder (common bile).

⊙ **43262** **with sphincterotomy/papillotomy**
Code also procedure performed with sphincterotomy (43261, 43263-43265, [43275], [43278])
Do not report with placement or exchange of stent in same location ([43274], [43276])
Do not report with (43260, [43277])
A2 T PQ 10.89 10.89 FUD 000

⊙ **43263** **with pressure measurement of sphincter of Oddi**
Do not report more than one time per session
Do not report with (43260)
A2 T P3 PQ 10.90 10.90 FUD 000

⊙ **43264** **with removal of calculi/debris from biliary/pancreatic duct(s)**
INCLUDES Incidental dilation due to passage of instrument
Code also sphincteroplasty when dilation is necessary in order to access the area of debris/stones ([43277])
Do not report if debris or calculi are not found, even if balloon was used
Do not report with (43260, 43265)
A2 T P3 PQ 11.10 11.10 FUD 000

⊙ **43265** **with destruction of calculi, any method (eg, mechanical, electrohydraulic, lithotripsy)**
INCLUDES Incidental dilation due to passage of instrument
Stone removal when in the same ductal system
Code also sphincteroplasty when dilation is necessary in order to access the area of debris/stones ([43277])
Do not report if debris or calculi are not found, even if balloon was used
Do not report with (43260, 43264)
A2 T P3 PQ 13.18 13.18 FUD 000

⊙ # **43274** **with placement of endoscopic stent into biliary or pancreatic duct, including pre- and post-dilation and guide wire passage, when performed, including sphincterotomy, when performed, each stent**
INCLUDES Balloon dilation when in the same duct
Tube placement for naso-pancreatic or naso-biliary drainage
Code also for each additional stent placement in different ducts or side by side in same duct in same session/day, using modifier 59 with ([43274])
Do not report with the following procedures for stent placement or exchange in the same duct (43262, [43275, 43276, 43277])
G2 T 13.91 13.91 FUD 000

⊙ # **43275** **with removal of foreign body(s) or stent(s) from biliary/pancreatic duct(s)**
EXCLUDES *Pancreatic or biliary duct stent removal without ERCP (43247)*
Do not report more than one time per session
Do not report with (43260, [43274], [43276])
G2 T 11.47 11.47 FUD 000

⊙ # **43276** **with removal and exchange of stent(s), biliary or pancreatic duct, including pre- and post-dilation and guide wire passage, when performed, including sphincterotomy, when performed, each stent exchanged**
INCLUDES Balloon dilation when in the same duct
Stent placement or exchange of one stent
Code also each additional stent exchanged in same session/day, using modifier 59 with ([43276])
Do not report for stent insertion or exchange of stent in same duct (43262, [43274])
Do not report with (43260, [43275])
G2 T 14.47 14.47 FUD 000

43270 Resequenced code. See code following 43257.

⊙ # **43277** **with trans-endoscopic balloon dilation of biliary/pancreatic duct(s) or of ampulla (sphincteroplasty), including sphincterotomy, when performed, each duct**
Code also both right and left hepatic duct (bilateral) balloon dilation, using ([43277]) and append modifier 59 to second procedure
Code also each additional balloon dilation in different ducts or side by side in same duct in same session/day, using modifier 59 with ([43277])
Code also same session sphincterotomy without sphincteroplasty in different duct, using modifier 59 with (43262)
Do not report with ([43274], [43276]) for stent insertion/exchange within the same duct
Do not report with removal of stone/debris (43264-43265) when dilation incidental to instrument passage
Do not report with ([43278]) when on same lesion
Do not report with (43260, 43262)
G2 T 11.54 11.54 FUD 000

⊙ # **43278** **with ablation of tumor(s), polyp(s), or other lesion(s), including pre- and post-dilation and guide wire passage, when performed**
EXCLUDES *Ampullectomy (43254)*
Do not report with ([43277]) when on same lesion
Do not report with (43260)
G2 T 13.12 13.12 FUD 000

+ ⊙ **43273** **Endoscopic cannulation of papilla with direct visualization of pancreatic/common bile duct(s) (List separately in addition to code(s) for primary procedure)**
Code first (43260-43265 [43274, 43275, 43276, 43277, 43278])
Do not report more than one time per session
N1 N 80 3.59 3.59 FUD ZZZ

43274 Resequenced code. See code following 43265.

43275 Resequenced code. See code following 43265.

43276 Resequenced code. See code following 43265.

43277 Resequenced code. See code before 43273.

43278 Resequenced code. See code before 43273.

43279-43289 Laparoscopic Procedures of Esophagus

INCLUDES Diagnostic laparoscopy with surgical laparoscopy

43279 **Laparoscopy, surgical, esophagomyotomy (Heller type), with fundoplasty, when performed**
EXCLUDES *Esophagomyotomy, open method (43330-43331)*
Do not report with (43280)
C 80 PQ 36.83 36.83 FUD 090

43280 **Laparoscopy, surgical, esophagogastric fundoplasty (eg, Nissen, Toupet procedures)**
EXCLUDES *Esophagogastric fundoplasty, open method (43327-43328)*
Do not report with (43279)
T 80 P3 PQ 30.84 30.84 FUD 090

43281 **Laparoscopy, surgical, repair of paraesophageal hernia, includes fundoplasty, when performed; without implantation of mesh**
EXCLUDES *Transabdominal repair of paraesophageal hiatal hernia (43332-43333)*
Transthoracic repair of diaphragmatic hernia (43334-43335)
Do not report with (43280, 43450, 43453, 49568)
T 80 PQ 44.03 44.03 FUD 090

43282 with implantation of mesh
EXCLUDES *Transabdominal paraesophageal hernia repair (43332-43333)*
Transthoracic paraesophageal hernia repair (43334-43335)
Do not report with (43280, 43450, 43453, 49568)
C 80 PQ 49.51 49.51 FUD 090

+ 43283 **Laparoscopy, surgical, esophageal lengthening procedure (eg, Collis gastroplasty or wedge gastroplasty) (List separately in addition to code for primary procedure)**
Code first (43280-43282)
C 80 4.49 4.49 FUD ZZZ

43289 **Unlisted laparoscopy procedure, esophagus**
T 80 50 0.00 0.00 FUD YYY

43300-43425 Open Esophageal Repair Procedures

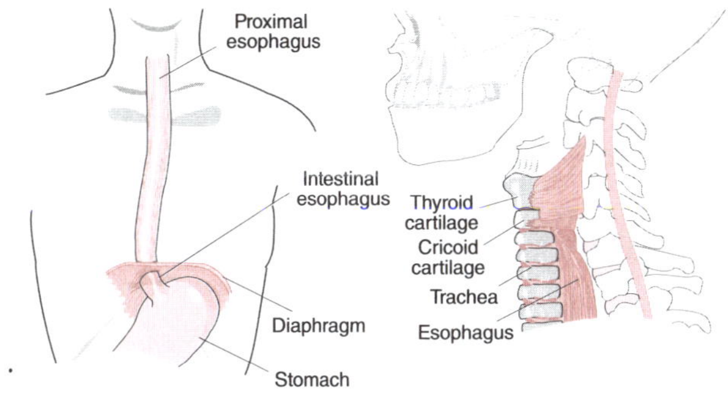

43300 **Esophagoplasty (plastic repair or reconstruction), cervical approach; without repair of tracheoesophageal fistula**
C 80 PQ 17.84 17.84 FUD 090

43305 with repair of tracheoesophageal fistula
C 80 PQ 31.61 31.61 FUD 090

43310 **Esophagoplasty (plastic repair or reconstruction), thoracic approach; without repair of tracheoesophageal fistula**
C 80 PQ 42.98 42.98 FUD 090

43312 with repair of tracheoesophageal fistula
C 80 PQ 46.33 46.33 FUD 090

43313 **Esophagoplasty for congenital defect (plastic repair or reconstruction), thoracic approach; without repair of congenital tracheoesophageal fistula**
C 80 PQ 63 83.16 83.16 FUD 090

43314 with repair of congenital tracheoesophageal fistula
C 80 PQ 63 84.04 84.04 FUD 090

43320 **Esophagogastrostomy (cardioplasty), with or without vagotomy and pyloroplasty, transabdominal or transthoracic approach**
EXCLUDES *Laparoscopic approach (43280)*
C 80 PQ 39.71 39.71 FUD 090

43325 **Esophagogastric fundoplasty; with fundic patch (Thal-Nissen procedure)**
EXCLUDES *Myotomy, cricopharyngeal (43030)*
C 80 PQ 38.32 38.32 FUD 090

43327 **Esophagogastric fundoplasty partial or complete; laparotomy**
C 80 PQ 23.40 23.40 FUD 090

43328 thoracotomy
C 80 PQ 33.30 33.30 FUD 090

43330 **Esophagomyotomy (Heller type); abdominal approach**
EXCLUDES *Esophagomyotomy, laparoscopic method (43279)*
C 80 PQ 38.00 38.00 FUD 090

43331 thoracic approach
EXCLUDES *Thoracoscopy with esophagomyotomy (32665)*
C 80 PQ 38.83 38.83 FUD 090

43332 **Repair, paraesophageal hiatal hernia (including fundoplication), via laparotomy, except neonatal; without implantation of mesh or other prosthesis**
EXCLUDES *Neonatal diaphragmatic hernia repair (39503)*
C 80 PQ 33.15 33.15 FUD 090

43333 with implantation of mesh or other prosthesis
EXCLUDES *Neonatal diaphragmatic hernia repair (39503)*
C 80 PQ 36.07 36.07 FUD 090

43334 **Repair, paraesophageal hiatal hernia (including fundoplication), via thoracotomy, except neonatal; without implantation of mesh or other prosthesis**
EXCLUDES *Neonatal diaphragmatic hernia repair (39503)*
C 80 PQ 35.79 35.79 FUD 090

43335 with implantation of mesh or other prosthesis
EXCLUDES *Neonatal diaphragmatic hernia repair (39503)*
C 80 PQ 38.35 38.35 FUD 090

43336 **Repair, paraesophageal hiatal hernia, (including fundoplication), via thoracoabdominal incision, except neonatal; without implantation of mesh or other prosthesis**
EXCLUDES *Neonatal diaphragmatic hernia repair (39503)*
C 80 PQ 43.47 43.47 FUD 090

43337 with implantation of mesh or other prosthesis
EXCLUDES *Neonatal diaphragmatic hernia repair (39503)*
C 80 PQ 46.93 46.93 FUD 090

+ 43338 **Esophageal lengthening procedure (eg, Collis gastroplasty or wedge gastroplasty) (List separately in addition to code for primary procedure)**
Code first (43280, 43327-43337)
C 80 3.36 3.36 FUD ZZZ

43340 **Esophagojejunostomy (without total gastrectomy); abdominal approach**
C 80 PQ 39.21 39.21 FUD 090

43341 thoracic approach
C 80 PQ 40.39 40.39 FUD 090

43350 ~~Esophagostomy, fistulization of esophagus, external; abdominal approach~~

43351 thoracic approach
C 80 PQ 38.09 38.09 FUD 090

43352 cervical approach
C 80 PQ 30.07 30.07 FUD 090

43360 **Gastrointestinal reconstruction for previous esophagectomy, for obstructing esophageal lesion or fistula, or for previous esophageal exclusion; with stomach, with or without pyloroplasty**
C 80 PQ 68.62 68.62 FUD 090

43361 with colon interposition or small intestine reconstruction, including intestine mobilization, preparation, and anastomosis(es)
C 80 PQ 72.98 72.98 FUD 090

43400 **Ligation, direct, esophageal varices**
C 80 PQ 44.03 44.03 FUD 090

43401 **Transection of esophagus with repair, for esophageal varices**
C 80 PQ 44.54 44.54 FUD 090

43405 **Ligation or stapling at gastroesophageal junction for pre-existing esophageal perforation**
C 80 PQ 41.67 41.67 FUD 090

43410 **Suture of esophageal wound or injury; cervical approach**
C 80 PQ 30.28 30.28 FUD 090

43415 **transthoracic or transabdominal approach**
C 80 PQ 74.41 74.41 FUD 090

43420 **Closure of esophagostomy or fistula; cervical approach**
EXCLUDES *Paraesophageal hiatal hernia repair:*
Transabdominal (43332-43333)
Transthoracic (43334-43335)
T 80 PQ 29.49 29.49 FUD 090

43425 **transthoracic or transabdominal approach**
EXCLUDES *Paraesophageal hiatal hernia repair:*
Transabdominal (43332-43333)
Transthoracic (43334-43335)
C 80 PQ 41.35 41.35 FUD 090

43450-43453 Esophageal Dilation

43450 **Dilation of esophagus, by unguided sound or bougie, single or multiple passes**
74220, 74360
A2 T 2.54 6.05 FUD 000

⊙ **43453** **Dilation of esophagus, over guide wire**
EXCLUDES *Dilation performed with direct visualization (43195, 43226)*
Endoscopic dilation by dilator or balloon:
Balloon diameter 30 mm or larger ([43214], [43233])
Balloon diameter less than 30 mm (43195, 43220, 43249)
74220, 74360
A2 T 2.74 27.67 FUD 000

43460-43499 Other/Unlisted Esophageal Procedures

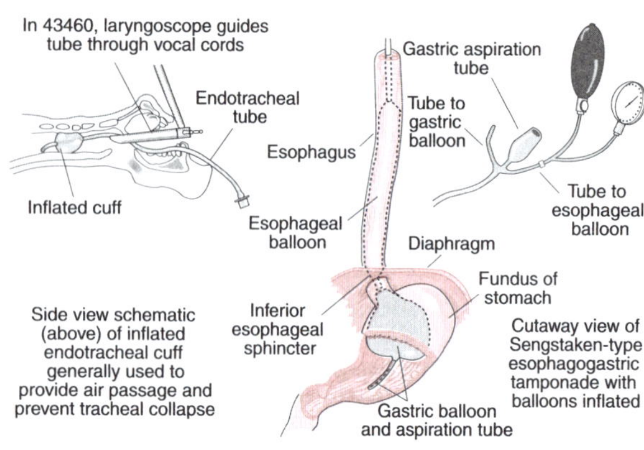

43460 **Esophagogastric tamponade, with balloon (Sengstaken type)**
EXCLUDES *Removal of foreign body of the esophagus with balloon catheter (43499, 74235)*
74220
C 6.37 6.37 FUD 000

43496 **Free jejunum transfer with microvascular anastomosis**
INCLUDES Operating microscope (69990)
C 80 PQ 0.00 0.00 FUD 090

43499 **Unlisted procedure, esophagus**
T 0.00 0.00 FUD YYY

43500-43641 Open Gastric Incisional and Resection Procedures

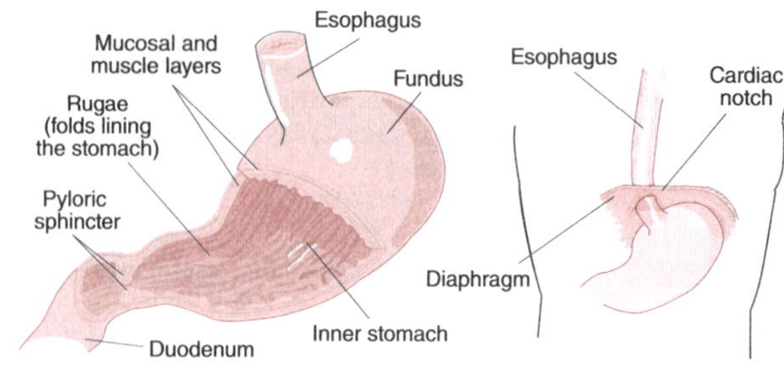

43500 **Gastrotomy; with exploration or foreign body removal**
C 80 PQ 22.44 22.44 FUD 090

43501 **with suture repair of bleeding ulcer**
C 80 PQ 38.38 38.38 FUD 090

43502 **with suture repair of pre-existing esophagogastric laceration (eg, Mallory-Weiss)**
C 80 PQ 43.36 43.36 FUD 090

43510 **with esophageal dilation and insertion of permanent intraluminal tube (eg, Celestin or Mousseaux-Barbin)**
T 80 PQ 25.89 25.89 FUD 090

43520 **Pyloromyotomy, cutting of pyloric muscle (Fredet-Ramstedt type operation)**
C 80 PQ 63 19.61 19.61 FUD 090

43605 **Biopsy of stomach, by laparotomy**
C 80 PQ 23.68 23.68 FUD 090

43610 **Excision, local; ulcer or benign tumor of stomach**
C 80 PQ 27.95 27.95 FUD 090

43611 **malignant tumor of stomach**
C 80 PQ 34.80 34.80 FUD 090

43620 **Gastrectomy, total; with esophagoenterostomy**
C 80 PQ 55.97 55.97 FUD 090

43621 **with Roux-en-Y reconstruction**
C 80 PQ 64.61 64.61 FUD 090

43622 **with formation of intestinal pouch, any type**
C 80 PQ 65.82 65.82 FUD 090

43631 **Gastrectomy, partial, distal; with gastroduodenostomy**
INCLUDES Billroth operation
C 80 PQ 41.31 41.31 FUD 090

43632 **with gastrojejunostomy**
INCLUDES Polya anastomosis
C 80 PQ 57.85 57.85 FUD 090

43633 **with Roux-en-Y reconstruction**
C 80 PQ 54.67 54.67 FUD 090

43634 **with formation of intestinal pouch**
C 80 PQ 60.50 60.50 FUD 090

\+ **43635** **Vagotomy when performed with partial distal gastrectomy (List separately in addition to code[s] for primary procedure)**
Code first as appropriate (43631-43634)
C 80 3.19 3.19 FUD ZZZ

43640 **Vagotomy including pyloroplasty, with or without gastrostomy; truncal or selective**
EXCLUDES *Pyloroplasty (43800)*
Vagotomy (64755, 64760)
C 80 PQ 33.63 33.63 FUD 090

43641 **parietal cell (highly selective)**
EXCLUDES *Upper gastrointestinal endoscopy (43235-43259)*
C 80 PQ 34.17 34.17 FUD 090

43644-43645 Laparoscopic Gastric Bypass with Small Bowel Resection

CMS 100-3,100.1 Bariatric Surgery for Treatment Co-morbid Conditions Due to Morbid Obesity

CMS 100-3,100.8 Intestinal Bypass Surgery

INCLUDES Diagnostic laparoscopy

EXCLUDES *Endoscopy, upper gastrointestinal, (esophagus/stomach/duodenum/jejunum) (43235-43259 [43233, 43266, 43270])*

43644 **Laparoscopy, surgical, gastric restrictive procedure; with gastric bypass and Roux-en-Y gastroenterostomy (roux limb 150 cm or less)**

EXCLUDES *Open method (43846)*
Roux limb greater than 150 cm (43645)

Do not report with (43846, 49320)

C 80 PQ 49.36 49.36 FUD 090

43645 **with gastric bypass and small intestine reconstruction to limit absorption**

Do not report with (43847, 49320)

C 80 PQ 52.77 52.77 FUD 090

43647-43659 Other and Unlisted Laparoscopic Gastric Procedures

INCLUDES Diagnostic laparoscopy

EXCLUDES *Endoscopy, upper gastrointestinal, (esophagus/stomach/duodenum/jejunum) (43235-43259 [43233, 43266, 43270])*

43647 **Laparoscopy, surgical; implantation or replacement of gastric neurostimulator electrodes, antrum**

EXCLUDES *Electronic analysis/programming gastric neurostimulator (95980-95982)*
Insertion gastric neurostimulator pulse generator (64590)
Laparoscopy with implantation, removal, or revision of gastric neurostimulator electrodes on the lesser curvature of the stomach (43659)
Open method (43881)
Vagus nerve blocking pulse generator and/or neurostimulator electrode array implantation, reprogramming, replacement, revision, or removal at the esophagogastric junction performed laparoscopically (0312T-0317T)

Code also (C1778, C1897, L8680)

S 80 0.00 0.00 FUD YYY

43648 **revision or removal of gastric neurostimulator electrodes, antrum**

EXCLUDES *Electronic analysis/programming gastric neurostimulator (95980-95982)*
Laparoscopy with implantation, removal, or revision of gastric neurostimulator electrodes on the lesser curvature of the stomach (43659)
Open method (43882)
Revision/removal gastric neurostimulator pulse generator (64595)
Vagus nerve blocking pulse generator and/or neurostimulator electrode array implantation, reprogramming, replacement, revision, or removal at the esophagogastric junction performed laparoscopically (0312T-0317T)

Q2 80 0.00 0.00 FUD YYY

43651 **Laparoscopy, surgical; transection of vagus nerves, truncal**

T 80 PQ 18.60 18.60 FUD 090

43652 **transection of vagus nerves, selective or highly selective**

T 80 PQ 21.73 21.73 FUD 090

43653 **gastrostomy, without construction of gastric tube (eg, Stamm procedure) (separate procedure)**

A2 T 80 PQ 16.29 16.29 FUD 090

43659 **Unlisted laparoscopy procedure, stomach**

T 80 50 0.00 0.00 FUD YYY

43752-43761 Nonsurgical Gastric Tube Procedures

CMS 100-4,20,50.3 Payment for Replacement of Parenteral and Enteral Pumps

CMS 100-4,20,100.2.2 Medical Necessity for Parenteral and Enteral Nutrition Therapy

43752 **Naso- or oro-gastric tube placement, requiring physician's skill and fluoroscopic guidance (includes fluoroscopy, image documentation and report)**

EXCLUDES *Percutaneous insertion of gastrostomy tube (43246, 49440)*
Placement of enteric tube (44500, 74340)

Do not report with (99291-99292, 99468-99469, 99471-99472, 99478-99479)

G2 Q3 PQ 1.18 1.18 FUD 000

43753 **Gastric intubation and aspiration(s) therapeutic, necessitating physician's skill (eg, for gastrointestinal hemorrhage), including lavage if performed**

G2 X 80 0.60 0.60 FUD 000

43754 **Gastric intubation and aspiration, diagnostic; single specimen (eg, acid analysis)**

EXCLUDES *Naso- or oro-gastric tube placement using fluoroscopic guidance (43752)*

82930

G2 X 80 0.95 2.56 FUD 000

43755 **collection of multiple fractional specimens with gastric stimulation, single or double lumen tube (gastric secretory study) (eg, histamine, insulin, pentagastrin, calcium, secretin), includes drug administration**

EXCLUDES *Naso- or oro-gastric tube placement using fluoroscopic guidance (43752)*

Code also drugs or substances administered

82930

G2 S 80 1.66 3.90 FUD 000

43756 **Duodenal intubation and aspiration, diagnostic, includes image guidance; single specimen (eg, bile study for crystals or afferent loop culture)**

89049-89240

G2 X 80 1.46 5.98 FUD 000

43757 **collection of multiple fractional specimens with pancreatic or gallbladder stimulation, single or double lumen tube, includes drug administration**

Code also drugs or substances administered

89049-89240

G2 X 80 2.21 8.39 FUD 000

43760 **Change of gastrostomy tube, percutaneous, without imaging or endoscopic guidance**

EXCLUDES *Endoscopic placement of gastrostomy tube (43246)*
Gastrostomy tube replacement using fluoroscopy (49450)

A2 T 1.37 13.76 FUD 000

43761 **Repositioning of a naso- or oro-gastric feeding tube, through the duodenum for enteric nutrition**

EXCLUDES *Gastrostomy tube converted endoscopically to jejunostomy tube (44373)*
Introduction of long gastrointestinal tube into the duodenum (44500)

Do not report with (44500, 49446)

76000

A2 T 3.00 3.37 FUD 000

43770-43775 Laparoscopic Bariatric Procedures

CMS 100-3,100.1 Bariatric Surgery for Treatment Co-morbid Conditions Due to Morbid Obesity

INCLUDES Diagnostic laparoscopy
Stomach/duodenum/jejunum/ileum
Subsequent band adjustments (change of the gastric band component diameter by injection/aspiration of fluid through the subcutaneous port component) during the postoperative period

43770 Laparoscopy, surgical, gastric restrictive procedure; placement of adjustable gastric restrictive device (eg, gastric band and subcutaneous port components)
Code also modifier 52 for placement of individual component
T 80 PQ 31.80 31.80 FUD 090

43771 revision of adjustable gastric restrictive device component only
C 80 PQ 36.35 36.35 FUD 090

43772 removal of adjustable gastric restrictive device component only
C 80 PQ 27.17 27.17 FUD 090

43773 removal and replacement of adjustable gastric restrictive device component only
Do not report with (43772)
C 80 PQ 36.17 36.17 FUD 090

43774 removal of adjustable gastric restrictive device and subcutaneous port components
EXCLUDES *Removal/replacement of subcutaneous port components and gastric band (43659)*
C 80 PQ 27.37 27.37 FUD 090

43775 longitudinal gastrectomy (ie, sleeve gastrectomy)
EXCLUDES *Open gastric restrictive procedure for morbid obesity, without gastric bypass, other than vertical-banded gastroplasty (43843)*
Vagus nerve blocking pulse generator and/or neurostimulator electrode array implantation, reprogramming, replacement, revision, or removal at the esophagogastric junction performed laparoscopically (0312T-0317T)
C 80 0.00 0.00 FUD YYY

43800-43840 Open Gastric Incisional/Repair/Resection Procedures

43800 Pyloroplasty
EXCLUDES *Vagotomy with pyloroplasty (43640)*
C 80 PQ 26.52 26.52 FUD 090

43810 Gastroduodenostomy
C 80 PQ 28.93 28.93 FUD 090

43820 Gastrojejunostomy; without vagotomy
C 80 PQ 38.20 38.20 FUD 090

43825 with vagotomy, any type
C 80 PQ 37.23 37.23 FUD 090

43830 Gastrostomy, open; without construction of gastric tube (eg, Stamm procedure) (separate procedure)
T 80 PQ 19.89 19.89 FUD 090

43831 neonatal, for feeding A
EXCLUDES *Change of gastrostomy tube (43760)*
T 80 PQ 63 16.89 16.89 FUD 090

43832 with construction of gastric tube (eg, Janeway procedure)
EXCLUDES *Endoscopic placement of percutaneous gastrostomy tube (43246)*
C 80 PQ 29.70 29.70 FUD 090

43840 Gastrorrhaphy, suture of perforated duodenal or gastric ulcer, wound, or injury
C 80 PQ 38.70 38.70 FUD 090

43842-43848 Open Bariatric Procedures for Morbid Obesity

CMS 100-3,100.1 Bariatric Surgery for Treatment Co-morbid Conditions Due to Morbid Obesity
CMS 100-3,100.8 Intestinal Bypass Surgery

43842 Gastric restrictive procedure, without gastric bypass, for morbid obesity; vertical-banded gastroplasty
E 33.01 33.01 FUD 090

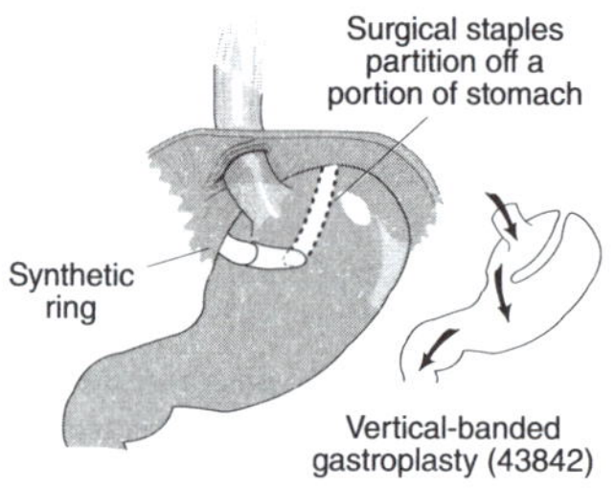

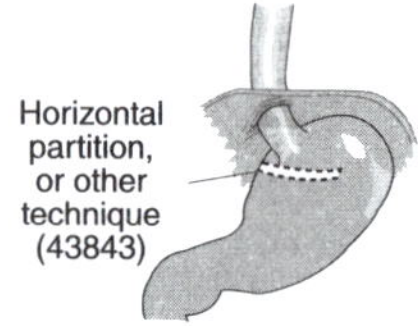

The stomach is surgically restricted to treat morbid obesity. A vertical-banded technique is coded 43842 and any other gastroplasty technique that does not employ gastric bypass is coded 43843. These partitioning techniques give the patient a sensation of fullness, thus decreasing daily caloric intake

43843 other than vertical-banded gastroplasty
EXCLUDES *Laparoscopic longitudinal gastrectomy (e.g., sleeve gastrectomy) (43775)*
C 80 PQ 36.40 36.40 FUD 090

43845 Gastric restrictive procedure with partial gastrectomy, pylorus-preserving duodenoileostomy and ileoileostomy (50 to 100 cm common channel) to limit absorption (biliopancreatic diversion with duodenal switch)
Do not report with (43633, 43847, 44130, 49000)
C 80 PQ 55.80 55.80 FUD 090

43846 Gastric restrictive procedure, with gastric bypass for morbid obesity; with short limb (150 cm or less) Roux-en-Y gastroenterostomy
EXCLUDES *Performed laparoscopically (43644)*
Roux limb more than 150 cm (43847)
C 80 PQ 45.92 45.92 FUD 090

43847 with small intestine reconstruction to limit absorption
EXCLUDES *Performed laparoscopically (43645)*
C 80 PQ 51.26 51.26 FUD 090

43848 Revision, open, of gastric restrictive procedure for morbid obesity, other than adjustable gastric restrictive device (separate procedure)
EXCLUDES *Gastric restrictive port procedures (43886-43888)*
Procedures for adjustable gastric restrictive devices (43770-43774)
C 80 PQ 54.86 54.86 FUD 090

43850-43882 Open Gastric Procedures: Closure/Implantation/Replacement/Revision

43850 Revision of gastroduodenal anastomosis (gastroduodenostomy) with reconstruction; without vagotomy
C 80 PQ 46.32 46.32 FUD 090

43855 **with vagotomy**
C 80 CCI PQ 48.05 48.05 FUD 090

43860 **Revision of gastrojejunal anastomosis (gastrojejunostomy) with reconstruction, with or without partial gastrectomy or intestine resection; without vagotomy**
C 80 CCI PQ 46.62 46.62 FUD 090

43865 **with vagotomy**
C 80 CCI PQ 48.62 48.62 FUD 090

43870 **Closure of gastrostomy, surgical**
A2 T 80 CCI PQ 20.25 20.25 FUD 090

43880 **Closure of gastrocolic fistula**
C 80 CCI PQ 45.55 45.55 FUD 090

43881 **Implantation or replacement of gastric neurostimulator electrodes, antrum, open**
EXCLUDES *Electronic analysis and programming (95980-95982)*
Implantation/removal/revision gastric neurostimulator electrodes, lesser curvature or vagal trunk (EGJ):
Laparoscopically (43659)
Open (43999)
Implantation/replacement performed laparoscopically (43647)
Insertion of gastric neurostimulator pulse generator (64590)
Vagus nerve blocking pulse generator and/or neurostimulator electrode array implantation, reprogramming, replacement, revision, or removal at the esophagogastric junction performed laparoscopically (0312T-0317T)
C 80 0.00 0.00 FUD YYY

43882 **Revision or removal of gastric neurostimulator electrodes, antrum, open**
EXCLUDES *Electronic analysis and programming (95980-95982)*
Implantation/removal/revision gastric neurostimulator electrodes, lesser curvature or vagal trunk (EGJ):
Laparoscopic (43659)
Open (43999)
Revision/removal gastric neurostimulator electrodes, antrum, performed laparoscopically (43648)
Revision/removal gastric neurostimulator pulse generator (64595)
Vagus nerve blocking pulse generator and/or neurostimulator electrode array implantation, reprogramming, replacement, revision, or removal at the esophagogastric junction performed laparoscopically (0312T-0317T)
C 80 0.00 0.00 FUD YYY

43886-43999 Bariatric Procedures: Removal/Replacement/Revision Port Components

CMS 100-3,100.1 Bariatric Surgery for Treatment Co-morbid Conditions Due to Morbid Obesity

43886 **Gastric restrictive procedure, open; revision of subcutaneous port component only**
62 T 80 PQ 10.32 10.32 FUD 090

43887 **removal of subcutaneous port component only**
EXCLUDES *Gastric band and subcutaneous port components:*
Removal and replacement performed laparoscopically (43659)
Removal performed laparoscopically (43774)
62 02 80 PQ 9.27 9.27 FUD 090

43888 **removal and replacement of subcutaneous port component only**
EXCLUDES *Gastric band and subcutaneous port components:*
Removal and replacement performed laparoscopically (43659)
Removal performed laparoscopically (43774)
Do not report with (43774, 43887)
62 T 80 PQ 13.08 13.08 FUD 090

43999 **Unlisted procedure, stomach**
T 80 0.00 0.00 FUD YYY

44005-44130 Incisional and Resection Procedures of Bowel

44005 **Enterolysis (freeing of intestinal adhesion) (separate procedure)**
EXCLUDES *Enterolysis performed laparoscopically (44180)*
Do not report with (45136)
C 80 CCI PQ 31.16 31.16 FUD 090

44010 **Duodenotomy, for exploration, biopsy(s), or foreign body removal**
C 80 CCI PQ 24.86 24.86 FUD 090

+ 44015 **Tube or needle catheter jejunostomy for enteral alimentation, intraoperative, any method (List separately in addition to primary procedure)**
Code first the primary procedure
C 80 CCI 4.08 4.08 FUD ZZZ

44020 **Enterotomy, small intestine, other than duodenum; for exploration, biopsy(s), or foreign body removal**
C 80 CCI PQ 27.68 27.68 FUD 090

44021 **for decompression (eg, Baker tube)**
C 80 CCI PQ 27.97 27.97 FUD 090

44025 **Colotomy, for exploration, biopsy(s), or foreign body removal**
INCLUDES Amussat's operation
EXCLUDES *Intestine exteriorization (Mikulicz resection with crushing of spur) (44602-44605)*
C 80 CCI PQ 28.22 28.22 FUD 090

44050 **Reduction of volvulus, intussusception, internal hernia, by laparotomy**
C 80 CCI PQ 26.65 26.65 FUD 090

44055 **Correction of malrotation by lysis of duodenal bands and/or reduction of midgut volvulus (eg, Ladd procedure)**
C 80 CCI PQ 63 42.64 42.64 FUD 090

44100 **Biopsy of intestine by capsule, tube, peroral (1 or more specimens)**
A2 T CCI PQ 3.23 3.23 FUD 000

44110 **Excision of 1 or more lesions of small or large intestine not requiring anastomosis, exteriorization, or fistulization; single enterotomy**
C 80 CCI PQ 24.30 24.30 FUD 090

44111 **multiple enterotomies**
C 80 CCI PQ 28.12 28.12 FUD 090

44120 **Enterectomy, resection of small intestine; single resection and anastomosis**
Do not report with (45136)
34.88 34.88 FUD 090

+ **44121** **each additional resection and anastomosis (List separately in addition to code for primary procedure)**
Code first single resection of small intestine (44120)
6.91 6.91 FUD ZZZ

44125 **with enterostomy**
33.73 33.73 FUD 090

44126 **Enterectomy, resection of small intestine for congenital atresia, single resection and anastomosis of proximal segment of intestine; without tapering**
70.18 70.18 FUD 090

44127 **with tapering**
81.15 81.15 FUD 090

+ **44128** **each additional resection and anastomosis (List separately in addition to code for primary procedure)**
Code first single resection of small intestine (44126, 44127)
6.94 6.94 FUD ZZZ

44130 **Enteroenterostomy, anastomosis of intestine, with or without cutaneous enterostomy (separate procedure)**
37.48 37.48 FUD 090

44132-44137 Intestine Transplant Procedures

CMS 100-3,260.5 Intestinal and Multi-Visceral Transplantation
CMS 100-4,3,90.6 Intestinal and Multi-Visceral Transplants

44132 **Donor enterectomy (including cold preservation), open; from cadaver donor**
INCLUDES Graft:
Cold preservation
Harvest
0.00 0.00 FUD XXX

44133 **partial, from living donor**
INCLUDES Donor care
Graft:
Cold preservation
Harvest
EXCLUDES *Preparation/reconstruction of backbench intestinal graft (44715, 44720-44721)*
0.00 0.00 FUD XXX

44135 **Intestinal allotransplantation; from cadaver donor**
INCLUDES Allograft transplantation
Recipient care
0.00 0.00 FUD XXX

44136 **from living donor**
INCLUDES Allograft transplantation
Recipient care
0.00 0.00 FUD XXX

44137 **Removal of transplanted intestinal allograft, complete**
EXCLUDES *Partial removal of transplant allograft (44120-44121, 44140)*
0.00 0.00 FUD XXX

44139-44160 Colon Resection Procedures

+ **44139** **Mobilization (take-down) of splenic flexure performed in conjunction with partial colectomy (List separately in addition to primary procedure)**
Code first partial colectomy (44140-44147)
3.46 3.46 FUD ZZZ

44140 **Colectomy, partial; with anastomosis**
EXCLUDES *Laparoscopic method (44204)*
38.26 38.26 FUD 090

44141 **with skin level cecostomy or colostomy**
52.13 52.13 FUD 090

44143 **with end colostomy and closure of distal segment (Hartmann type procedure)**
EXCLUDES *Laparoscopic method (44206)*
47.52 47.52 FUD 090

44144 **with resection, with colostomy or ileostomy and creation of mucofistula**
50.58 50.58 FUD 090

44145 **with coloproctostomy (low pelvic anastomosis)**
EXCLUDES *Laparoscopic method (44207)*
47.47 47.47 FUD 090

44146 **with coloproctostomy (low pelvic anastomosis), with colostomy**
EXCLUDES *Laparoscopic method (44208)*
60.63 60.63 FUD 090

44147 **abdominal and transanal approach**
55.62 55.62 FUD 090

44150 **Colectomy, total, abdominal, without proctectomy; with ileostomy or ileoproctostomy**
INCLUDES Lane's operation
EXCLUDES *Laparoscopic method (44210)*
53.52 53.52 FUD 090

44151 **with continent ileostomy**
61.33 61.33 FUD 090

44155 **Colectomy, total, abdominal, with proctectomy; with ileostomy**
INCLUDES Miles' colectomy
EXCLUDES *Laparoscopic method (44212)*
59.72 59.72 FUD 090

44156 **with continent ileostomy**
65.84 65.84 FUD 090

44157 **with ileoanal anastomosis, includes loop ileostomy, and rectal mucosectomy, when performed**
62.30 62.30 FUD 090

44158 **with ileoanal anastomosis, creation of ileal reservoir (S or J), includes loop ileostomy, and rectal mucosectomy, when performed**
EXCLUDES *Laparoscopic method (44211)*
64.22 64.22 FUD 090

44160 **Colectomy, partial, with removal of terminal ileum with ileocolostomy**
EXCLUDES *Laparoscopic method (44205)*
35.45 35.45 FUD 090

44180 Laparoscopic Enterolysis

INCLUDES Diagnostic laparoscopy
EXCLUDES *Laparoscopic salpingolysis/ovariolysis (58660)*

44180 **Laparoscopy, surgical, enterolysis (freeing of intestinal adhesion) (separate procedure)**
26.20 26.20 FUD 090

44186-44238 Laparoscopic Enterostomy Procedures

INCLUDES Diagnostic laparoscopy with surgical laparoscopy

44186 **Laparoscopy, surgical; jejunostomy (eg, for decompression or feeding)**
18.57 18.57 FUD 090

44187 **ileostomy or jejunostomy, non-tube**
EXCLUDES *Open method (44310)*
31.77 31.77 FUD 090

44188 **Laparoscopy, surgical, colostomy or skin level cecostomy**
EXCLUDES *Open method (44320)*
Do not report with (44970)
35.11 35.11 FUD 090

44202 **Laparoscopy, surgical; enterectomy, resection of small intestine, single resection and anastomosis**
EXCLUDES *Open method (44120)*
C 80 PQ 39.59 39.59 FUD 090

\+ **44203** **each additional small intestine resection and anastomosis (List separately in addition to code for primary procedure)**
EXCLUDES *Open method (44121)*
Code first single resection of small intestine (44202)
C 80 6.92 6.92 FUD ZZZ

44204 **colectomy, partial, with anastomosis**
EXCLUDES *Open method (44140)*
C 80 PQ 44.09 44.09 FUD 090

44205 **colectomy, partial, with removal of terminal ileum with ileocolostomy**
EXCLUDES *Open method (44160)*
C 80 PQ 38.37 38.37 FUD 090

44206 **colectomy, partial, with end colostomy and closure of distal segment (Hartmann type procedure)**
EXCLUDES *Open method (44143)*
C 80 PQ 50.29 50.29 FUD 090

44207 **colectomy, partial, with anastomosis, with coloproctostomy (low pelvic anastomosis)**
EXCLUDES *Open method (44145)*
C 80 PQ 52.44 52.44 FUD 090

44208 **colectomy, partial, with anastomosis, with coloproctostomy (low pelvic anastomosis) with colostomy**
EXCLUDES *Open method (44146)*
C 80 PQ 57.08 57.08 FUD 090

44210 **colectomy, total, abdominal, without proctectomy, with ileostomy or ileoproctostomy**
EXCLUDES *Open method (44150)*
C 80 PQ 51.65 51.65 FUD 090

44211 **colectomy, total, abdominal, with proctectomy, with ileoanal anastomosis, creation of ileal reservoir (S or J), with loop ileostomy, includes rectal mucosectomy, when performed**
EXCLUDES *Open method (44157, 44158)*
C 80 PQ 64.32 64.32 FUD 090

44212 **colectomy, total, abdominal, with proctectomy, with ileostomy**
EXCLUDES *Open method (44155)*
C 80 PQ 59.46 59.46 FUD 090

\+ **44213** **Laparoscopy, surgical, mobilization (take-down) of splenic flexure performed in conjunction with partial colectomy (List separately in addition to primary procedure)**
EXCLUDES *Open method (44139)*
Code first partial colectomy (44204-44208)
C 80 5.42 5.42 FUD ZZZ

44227 **Laparoscopy, surgical, closure of enterostomy, large or small intestine, with resection and anastomosis**
EXCLUDES *Open method (44625-44626)*
C 80 PQ 47.74 47.74 FUD 090

44238 **Unlisted laparoscopy procedure, intestine (except rectum)**
T 80 50 0.00 0.00 FUD YYY

44300-44346 Open Enterostomy Procedures

44300 **Placement, enterostomy or cecostomy, tube open (eg, for feeding or decompression) (separate procedure)**
EXCLUDES *Other gastrointestinal tube(s) placed percutaneously with fluoroscopic imaging guidance (49441-49442)*
C 80 PQ 24.01 24.01 FUD 090

44310 **Ileostomy or jejunostomy, non-tube**
EXCLUDES *Laparoscopic method (44187)*
Do not report with (44144, 44150-44151, 44155-44156, 45113, 45119, 45136)
C 80 PQ 29.88 29.88 FUD 090

44312 **Revision of ileostomy; simple (release of superficial scar) (separate procedure)**
A2 T 80 PQ 16.84 16.84 FUD 090

44314 **complicated (reconstruction in-depth) (separate procedure)**
C 80 PQ 28.84 28.84 FUD 090

44316 **Continent ileostomy (Kock procedure) (separate procedure)**
EXCLUDES *Fiberoptic evaluation (44385)*
C 80 PQ 40.23 40.23 FUD 090

44320 **Colostomy or skin level cecostomy;**
EXCLUDES *Laparoscopic method (44188)*
Do not report with (44141, 44144, 44146, 44605, 45110, 45119, 45126, 45563, 45805, 45825, 50810, 51597, 57307, 58240)
C 80 PQ 34.37 34.37 FUD 090

44322 **with multiple biopsies (eg, for congenital megacolon) (separate procedure)**
C 80 PQ 28.45 28.45 FUD 090

44340 **Revision of colostomy; simple (release of superficial scar) (separate procedure)**
A2 T PQ 17.83 17.83 FUD 090

44345 **complicated (reconstruction in-depth) (separate procedure)**
C 80 PQ 30.12 30.12 FUD 090

Skin
Herniations that have formed around the site of a colostomy are repaired
The colon is mobilized, trimmed if necessary, and a new stoma is often created

44346 **with repair of paracolostomy hernia (separate procedure)**
C 80 PQ 33.85 33.85 FUD 090

44360-44379 Endoscopy of Small Intestine

CMS 100-3,100.2 Endoscopy
INCLUDES Control of bleeding as result of endoscopic procedure during same operative session
EXCLUDES *Retrograde exam through anus/colon stoma (44799)*
Do not report with (43235-43259 [43233, 43266, 43270])

⊙ ▲ **44360** **Small intestinal endoscopy, enteroscopy beyond second portion of duodenum, not including ileum; diagnostic, including collection of specimen(s) by brushing or washing, when performed (separate procedure)**
Do not report with (44376-44379)
A2 T 4.47 4.47 FUD 000

⊙ **44361** **with biopsy, single or multiple**
Do not report with (44376-44379)
A2 T PQ 4.91 4.91 FUD 000

⊙ ▲ **44363** **with removal of foreign body(s)**
Do not report with (44376-44379)
A2 T 80 5.88 5.88 FUD 000

⊙ 44364 **with removal of tumor(s), polyp(s), or other lesion(s) by snare technique**
Do not report with (44376-44379)
A2 T 80 ▶ 6.27 6.27 FUD 000

⊙ 44365 **with removal of tumor(s), polyp(s), or other lesion(s) by hot biopsy forceps or bipolar cautery**
Do not report with (44376-44379)
A2 T 80 ▶ 5.57 5.57 FUD 000

⊙ 44366 **with control of bleeding (eg, injection, bipolar cautery, unipolar cautery, laser, heater probe, stapler, plasma coagulator)**
Do not report with (44376-44379)
A2 T ▶ 7.36 7.36 FUD 000

⊙ 44369 **with ablation of tumor(s), polyp(s), or other lesion(s) not amenable to removal by hot biopsy forceps, bipolar cautery or snare technique**
Do not report with (44376-44379)
A2 T 80 ▶ 7.54 7.54 FUD 000

⊙ 44370 **with transendoscopic stent placement (includes predilation)**
Code also (C1874, C1875, C1876, C1877, C2617, C2625)
Do not report with (44376-44379)
A2 T 80 ▶ 8.13 8.13 FUD 000

⊙ 44372 **with placement of percutaneous jejunostomy tube**
Do not report with (44376-44379)
A2 T ▶ 7.33 7.33 FUD 000

⊙ 44373 **with conversion of percutaneous gastrostomy tube to percutaneous jejunostomy tube**
EXCLUDES *Jejunostomy, fiberoptic, through stoma (43235)*
Do not report with (44376-44379)
A2 T ▶ 5.86 5.86 FUD 000

⊙ 44376 **Small intestinal endoscopy, enteroscopy beyond second portion of duodenum, including ileum; diagnostic, with or without collection of specimen(s) by brushing or washing (separate procedure)**
Do not report with (44360-44373)
A2 T 80 ▶ 8.67 8.67 FUD 000

⊙ 44377 **with biopsy, single or multiple**
Do not report with (44360-44373)
A2 T 80 ▶ PQ 9.13 9.13 FUD 000

⊙ 44378 **with control of bleeding (eg, injection, bipolar cautery, unipolar cautery, laser, heater probe, stapler, plasma coagulator)**
Do not report with (44360-44373)
A2 T 80 ▶ 11.72 11.72 FUD 000

⊙ 44379 **with transendoscopic stent placement (includes predilation)**
Code also (C1874, C1875, C1876, C1877, C2617, C2625)
Do not report with (44360-44373)
A2 T 80 ▶ 12.45 12.45 FUD 000

44380-44384 [44381] Ileoscopy Via Stoma

INCLUDES Control of bleeding as result of endoscopic procedure during same operative session

EXCLUDES *Computed tomographic colonography (74261-74263)*

Code also exam of nonfunctional distal colon/rectum, when performed, with:
Anoscopy (46600, 46604-46606, 46608-46615)
Proctosigmoidoscopy (45300-45327)
Sigmoidoscopy (45330-45347 [45346])

⊙ ▲ 44380 **Ileoscopy, through stoma; diagnostic, including collection of specimen(s) by brushing or washing, when performed (separate procedure)**
Do not report with (44382-44384 [44381])
A2 T ▶ 1.94 1.94 FUD 000

44381 ***Resequenced code. See code following 44382.***

⊙ 44382 **with biopsy, single or multiple**
Do not report with (44380)
A2 T ▶ PQ 2.34 2.34 FUD 000

⊙ #● 44381 **with transendoscopic balloon dilation**
Code also each additional stricture dilated in same session, using modifier 59 with ([44381])
Do not report with (44380, 44384)
74360

~~44383~~ ~~**with transendoscopic stent placement (includes predilation)**~~
To report, see 44384

⊙ ● 44384 **with placement of endoscopic stent (includes pre- and post-dilation and guide wire passage, when performed)**
Do not report with (44380-44381)
74360

44385-44386 Endoscopy of Small Intestinal Pouch

INCLUDES Control of bleeding as result of the endoscopic procedure during same operative session

EXCLUDES *Computed tomographic colonography (74261-74263)*

⊙ ▲ 44385 **Endoscopic evaluation of small intestinal pouch (eg, Kock pouch, ileal reservoir [S or J]); diagnostic, including collection of specimen(s) by brushing or washing, when performed (separate procedure)**
Do not report with (44386)
A2 T ▶ 3.09 7.45 FUD 000

⊙ ▲ 44386 **with biopsy, single or multiple**
Do not report with (44385)
A2 T 80 ▶ 3.67 9.98 FUD 000

44388-44408 [44401] Colonoscopy Via Stoma

CMS 100-3,100.2 Endoscopy

INCLUDES Control of bleeding as result of endoscopic procedure during same operative session

EXCLUDES *Colonoscopy via rectum (45378, 45392-45393 [45390, 45398])*
Computed tomographic colonography (74261-74263)

Code also exam of nonfunctional distal colon/rectum, when performed, with:
Anoscopy (46600, 46604-46606, 46608-46615)
Proctosigmoidoscopy (45300-45327)
Sigmoidoscopy (45330-45347 [45346])

⊙ ▲ 44388 **Colonoscopy through stoma; diagnostic, including collection of specimen(s) by brushing or washing, when performed (separate procedure)**
Code also modifier 53 when planned total colonoscopy cannot be completed
Do not report with (44389-44408 [44401])
A2 T ▶ PQ 4.77 9.97 FUD 000

⊙ 44389 **with biopsy, single or multiple**
Code also modifier 52 when colonoscope fails to reach the junction of the small intestine
Do not report with (44403) when on same lesion
Do not report with (44388)
A2 T ▶ PQ 5.29 11.21 FUD 000

⊙ ▲ 44390 **with removal of foreign body(s)**
Code also modifier 52 when colonoscope fails to reach the junction of the small intestine
Do not report with (44388)
76000
A2 T 80 ▶ 6.44 13.10 FUD 000

⊙ ▲ 44391 **with control of bleeding, any method**
Code also modifier 52 when colonoscope fails to reach the junction of the small intestine
Do not report with (44404) when on same lesion
Do not report with (44388)
A2 T 80 ▶ 7.18 14.08 FUD 000

⊙ ▲ **44392** **with removal of tumor(s), polyp(s), or other lesion(s) by hot biopsy forceps**
Code also modifier 52 when colonoscope fails to reach the junction of the small intestine
Do not report with (44388)
A2 T CCI PQ 6.31 12.46 **FUD** 000

⊙ #● **44401** **with ablation of tumor(s), polyp(s), or other lesion(s) (includes pre-and post-dilation and guide wire passage, when performed)**
Code also modifier 52 when colonoscope fails to reach the junction of the small intestine
Do not report with (44405) when on same lesion
Do not report with (44388)

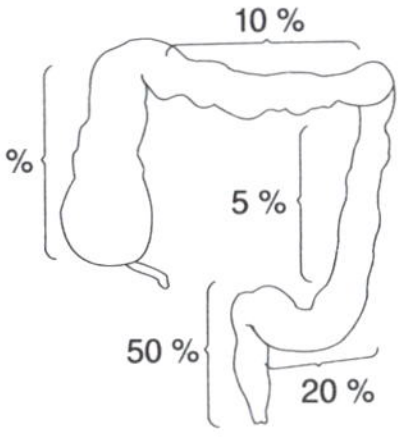

Hepatic flexure
Splenic flexure
Transverse colon
Descending colon
Ascending colon
Sigmoid flexure
Cecum
Ileocecal valve
Rectum
10 %
15 %
5 %
50 %
20 %

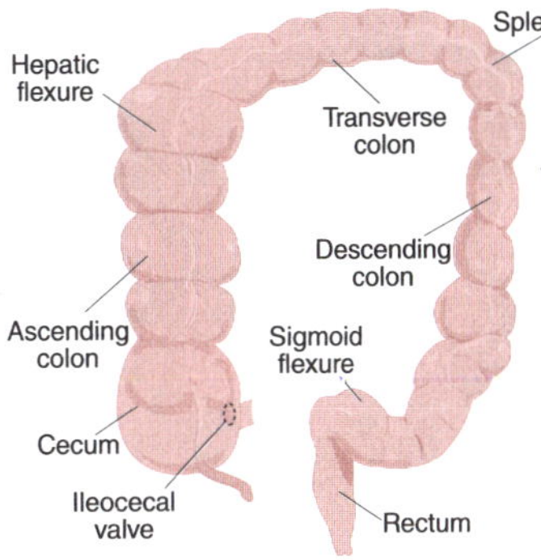

Anatomical distribution of large bowel cancers

~~**44393** **with ablation of tumor(s), polyp(s), or other lesion(s) not amenable to removal by hot biopsy forceps, bipolar cautery or snare technique**~~
To report, see 44401

⊙ **44394** **with removal of tumor(s), polyp(s), or other lesion(s) by snare technique**
INCLUDES Do not report with (44403) when on same lesion
Code also modifier 52 when colonoscope fails to reach the junction of the small intestine
Do not report with (44388)
A2 T CCI PQ 7.34 14.06 **FUD** 000

~~**44397** **with transendoscopic stent placement (includes predilation)**~~
To report, see 44402

44401 Resequenced code. See code following 44392.

⊙ ● **44402** **with endoscopic stent placement (including pre- and post-dilation and guide wire passage, when performed)**
Code also modifier 52 when colonoscope fails to reach the junction of the small intestine
Do not report with (44388, 44405)
74360

⊙ ● **44403** **with endoscopic mucosal resection**
Code also modifier 52 when colonoscope fails to reach the junction of the small intestine
Do not report with (44389, 44394, 44404) when on same lesion
Do not report with (44388)

⊙ ● **44404** **with directed submucosal injection(s), any substance**
Code also modifier 52 when colonoscope fails to reach the junction of the small intestine
Do not report with (44391, 44403) when on same lesion
Do not report with (44388)

⊙ ● **44405** **with transendoscopic balloon dilation**
Code also each additional stricture dilated in same session, using modifier 59 with (44405)
Code also modifier 52 when colonoscope fails to reach the junction of the small intestine
Do not report with (44388, [44401], 44402)
74360

⊙ ● **44406** **with endoscopic ultrasound examination, limited to the sigmoid, descending, transverse, or ascending colon and cecum and adjacent structures**
Code also modifier 52 when colonoscope fails to reach the junction of the small intestine
Do not report more than one time per operative session
Do not report with (44388, 44407, 76975)

⊙ ● **44407** **with transendoscopic ultrasound guided intramural or transmural fine needle aspiration/biopsy(s), includes endoscopic ultrasound examination limited to the sigmoid, descending, transverse, or ascending colon and cecum and adjacent structures**
Code also modifier 52 when colonoscope fails to reach the junction of the small intestine
Do not report more than one time per operative session
Do not report with (44388, 44406, 76942, 76975)

⊙ ● **44408** **with decompression (for pathologic distention) (eg, volvulus, megacolon), including placement of decompression tube, when performed**
Do not report more than one time per operative session
Do not report with (44388)

44500 Gastrointestinal Intubation

⊘ ⊙ **44500** **Introduction of long gastrointestinal tube (eg, Miller-Abbott) (separate procedure)**
EXCLUDES *Placement of oro- or naso-gastric tube (43752)*
74340
02 T 80 CCI PQ 0.71 0.71 **FUD** 000

44602-44680 Open Repair Procedures of Intestines

44602 **Suture of small intestine (enterorrhaphy) for perforated ulcer, diverticulum, wound, injury or rupture; single perforation**
C 80 CCI PQ 40.28 40.28 **FUD** 090

44603 **multiple perforations**
C 80 CCI PQ 46.18 46.18 **FUD** 090

44604 **Suture of large intestine (colorrhaphy) for perforated ulcer, diverticulum, wound, injury or rupture (single or multiple perforations); without colostomy**
C 80 CCI PQ 30.16 30.16 **FUD** 090

44605 **with colostomy**
C 80 CCI PQ 37.30 37.30 **FUD** 090

44615 **Intestinal stricturoplasty (enterotomy and enterorrhaphy) with or without dilation, for intestinal obstruction**
C 80 CCI PQ 30.74 30.74 **FUD** 090

44620 **Closure of enterostomy, large or small intestine;**
C 80 CCI PQ 24.84 24.84 **FUD** 090

44625 **with resection and anastomosis other than colorectal**
EXCLUDES *Laparoscopic method (44227)*
C 80 CCI PQ 29.23 29.23 **FUD** 090

44626 **with resection and colorectal anastomosis (eg, closure of Hartmann type procedure)**
EXCLUDES *Laparoscopic method (44227)*
C 80 CCI PQ 45.89 45.89 **FUD** 090

44640 **Closure of intestinal cutaneous fistula**
C 80 PQ 40.12 40.12 FUD 090

44650 **Closure of enteroenteric or enterocolic fistula**
C 80 PQ 41.48 41.48 FUD 090

44660 **Closure of enterovesical fistula; without intestinal or bladder resection**
EXCLUDES *Closure of fistula:*
Gastrocolic (43880)
Rectovesical (45800, 45805)
Renocolic (50525-50526)
C 80 PQ 38.11 38.11 FUD 090

44661 **with intestine and/or bladder resection**
EXCLUDES *Closure of fistula:*
Gastrocolic (43880)
Rectovesical (45800, 45805)
Renocolic (50525-50526)
C 80 PQ 44.44 44.44 FUD 090

44680 **Intestinal plication (separate procedure)**
INCLUDES Noble intestinal plication
C 80 PQ 30.52 30.52 FUD 090

44700-44705 Other Intestinal Procedures

44700 **Exclusion of small intestine from pelvis by mesh or other prosthesis, or native tissue (eg, bladder or omentum)**
EXCLUDES *Therapeutic radiation clinical treatment (77261-77799 [77295, 77385, 77386, 77387, 77424, 77425])*
C 80 PQ 29.26 29.26 FUD 090

+ **44701** **Intraoperative colonic lavage (List separately in addition to code for primary procedure)**
Code first as appropriate (44140, 44145, 44150, 44604)
Do not report with (44300, 44950-44960)
N1 N 80 4.79 4.79 FUD ZZZ

44705 **Preparation of fecal microbiota for instillation, including assessment of donor specimen**
EXCLUDES *Fecal instillation by enema or oro-nasogastric tube (44799)*
Do not report with (74283)
B 0.00 0.00 FUD XXX

44715-44799 Backbench Transplant Procedures

CMS 100-3,260.5 Intestinal and Multi-Visceral Transplantation
CMS 100-4,3,90.6 Intestinal and Multi-Visceral Transplants

44715 **Backbench standard preparation of cadaver or living donor intestine allograft prior to transplantation, including mobilization and fashioning of the superior mesenteric artery and vein**
INCLUDES Mobilization/fashioning of superior mesenteric vein/artery
C 80 0.00 0.00 FUD XXX

44720 **Backbench reconstruction of cadaver or living donor intestine allograft prior to transplantation; venous anastomosis, each**
C 80 7.24 7.24 FUD XXX

44721 **arterial anastomosis, each**
C 80 11.11 11.11 FUD XXX

▲ **44799** **Unlisted procedure, small intestine**
EXCLUDES *Unlisted colon procedure ([45399])*
Unlisted intestinal procedure performed laparoscopically (44238)
Unlisted rectal procedure (45499, 45999)
T 0.00 0.00 FUD YYY

44800-44899 Meckel's Diverticulum and Mesentery Procedures

44800 **Excision of Meckel's diverticulum (diverticulectomy) or omphalomesenteric duct**
C 80 PQ 21.74 21.74 FUD 090

44820 **Excision of lesion of mesentery (separate procedure)**
EXCLUDES *Resection of intestine (44120-44128, 44140-44160)*
C 80 PQ 23.99 23.99 FUD 090

44850 **Suture of mesentery (separate procedure)**
EXCLUDES *Internal hernia repair/reduction (44050)*
C 80 PQ 21.38 21.38 FUD 090

44899 **Unlisted procedure, Meckel's diverticulum and the mesentery**
C 80 0.00 0.00 FUD YYY

44900-44979 Open and Endoscopic Appendix Procedures

44900 **Incision and drainage of appendiceal abscess, open**
EXCLUDES *Image guided percutaneous catheter drainage (49406)*
C 80 PQ 22.06 22.06 FUD 090

Failure to treat appendicitis can lead to peritonitis
Ascending colon
Ileum
Cecum
Free tenia
Appendix and appendicular artery
Mesoappendix

44950 **Appendectomy;**
INCLUDES Battle's operation
Do not report with other intra-abdominal procedure(s) when appendectomy is incidental
T 80 PQ 18.27 18.27 FUD 090

+ **44955** **when done for indicated purpose at time of other major procedure (not as separate procedure) (List separately in addition to code for primary procedure)**
Code first primary procedure
N 80 2.40 2.40 FUD ZZZ

44960 **for ruptured appendix with abscess or generalized peritonitis**
INCLUDES Battle's operation
C 80 PQ 24.89 24.89 FUD 090

44970 **Laparoscopy, surgical, appendectomy**
INCLUDES Diagnostic laparoscopy
T 80 PQ 17.06 17.06 FUD 090

44979 **Unlisted laparoscopy procedure, appendix**
T 80 50 0.00 0.00 FUD YYY

45000-45190 Open and Transrectal Procedures of Rectum

45000 **Transrectal drainage of pelvic abscess**
EXCLUDES *Image guided transrectal catheter drainage (49407)*
A2 T PQ 12.17 12.17 FUD 090

45005 **Incision and drainage of submucosal abscess, rectum**
A2 T 4.48 7.55 FUD 010

45020 **Incision and drainage of deep supralevator, pelvirectal, or retrorectal abscess**
EXCLUDES *Incision and drainage of perianal, ischiorectal, intramural abscess (46050, 46060)*
A2 T PQ 16.26 16.26 FUD 090

45100 **Biopsy of anorectal wall, anal approach (eg, congenital megacolon)**
EXCLUDES *Biopsy performed endoscopically (45305)*
A2 T CCI PQ 8.57 8.57 FUD 090

45108 **Anorectal myomectomy**
A2 T CCI PQ 10.47 10.47 FUD 090

45110 **Proctectomy; complete, combined abdominoperineal, with colostomy**
EXCLUDES *Laparoscopic method (45395)*
C 80 CCI PQ 53.16 53.16 FUD 090

45111 **partial resection of rectum, transabdominal approach**
INCLUDES Luschka proctectomy
C 80 CCI PQ 31.22 31.22 FUD 090

45112 **Proctectomy, combined abdominoperineal, pull-through procedure (eg, colo-anal anastomosis)**
EXCLUDES *Proctectomy for colo-anal anastomosis with creation of colonic pouch or reservoir (45119)*
C 80 CCI PQ 54.19 54.19 FUD 090

45113 **Proctectomy, partial, with rectal mucosectomy, ileoanal anastomosis, creation of ileal reservoir (S or J), with or without loop ileostomy**
C 80 CCI PQ 57.22 57.22 FUD 090

45114 **Proctectomy, partial, with anastomosis; abdominal and transsacral approach**
C 80 CCI PQ 51.70 51.70 FUD 090

45116 **transsacral approach only (Kraske type)**
C 80 CCI PQ 45.02 45.02 FUD 090

45119 **Proctectomy, combined abdominoperineal pull-through procedure (eg, colo-anal anastomosis), with creation of colonic reservoir (eg, J-pouch), with diverting enterostomy when performed**
EXCLUDES *Laparoscopic method (45397)*
C 80 CCI PQ 56.17 56.17 FUD 090

45120 **Proctectomy, complete (for congenital megacolon), abdominal and perineal approach; with pull-through procedure and anastomosis (eg, Swenson, Duhamel, or Soave type operation)**
C 80 CCI PQ 45.46 45.46 FUD 090

45121 **with subtotal or total colectomy, with multiple biopsies**
C 80 CCI PQ 49.42 49.42 FUD 090

45123 **Proctectomy, partial, without anastomosis, perineal approach**
C 80 CCI PQ 32.20 32.20 FUD 090

45126 **Pelvic exenteration for colorectal malignancy, with proctectomy (with or without colostomy), with removal of bladder and ureteral transplantations, and/or hysterectomy, or cervicectomy, with or without removal of tube(s), with or without removal of ovary(s), or any combination thereof**
C 80 CCI PQ 82.34 82.34 FUD 090

45130 **Excision of rectal procidentia, with anastomosis; perineal approach**
INCLUDES Altemeier procedure
C 80 CCI PQ 31.45 31.45 FUD 090

45135 **abdominal and perineal approach**
INCLUDES Altemeier procedure
C 80 CCI PQ 39.14 39.14 FUD 090

45136 **Excision of ileoanal reservoir with ileostomy**
Do not report with (44005, 44120, 44310)
C 80 CCI PQ 52.53 52.53 FUD 090

45150 **Division of stricture of rectum**
A2 T 80 CCI PQ 11.31 11.31 FUD 090

45160 **Excision of rectal tumor by proctotomy, transsacral or transcoccygeal approach**
A2 T 80 CCI PQ 29.06 29.06 FUD 090

45171 **Excision of rectal tumor, transanal approach; not including muscularis propria (ie, partial thickness)**
EXCLUDES *Transanal destruction of rectal tumor (45190)*
Transanal endoscopic microsurgical tumor excision (TEMS) (0184T)
G2 T 80 PQ 17.17 17.17 FUD 090

45172 **including muscularis propria (ie, full thickness)**
EXCLUDES *Transanal destruction of rectal tumor (45190)*
Transanal endoscopic microsurgical tumor excision (TEMS) (0184T)
G2 T 80 PQ 23.31 23.31 FUD 090

45190 **Destruction of rectal tumor (eg, electrodesiccation, electrosurgery, laser ablation, laser resection, cryosurgery) transanal approach**
EXCLUDES *Transanal endoscopic microsurgical tumor excision (TEMS) (0184T)*
Transanal excision of rectal tumor (45171-45172)
A2 T CCI PQ 19.91 19.91 FUD 090

45300-45327 Rigid Proctosigmoidoscopy Procedures

CMS 100-3,100.2 Endoscopy

INCLUDES Control of bleeding as result of the endoscopic procedure during same operative session
Exam of:
Entire rectum
Portion of sigmoid colon

EXCLUDES *Computed tomographic colonography (74261-74263)*

Code also examination of colon through stoma:
Colonoscopy via stoma (44388-44408 [44401])
Ileoscopy via stoma (44380-44384 [44381])

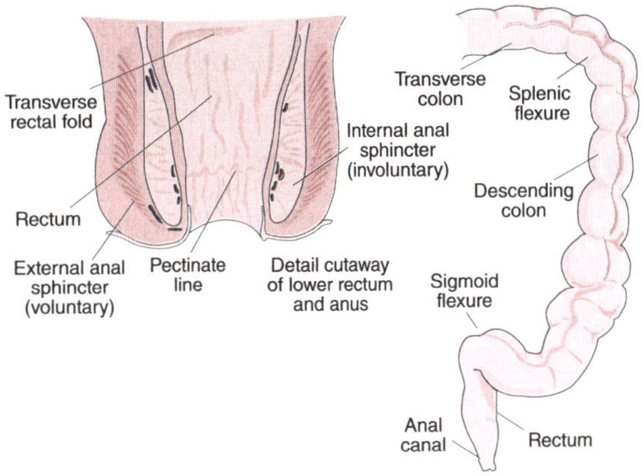

45300 **Proctosigmoidoscopy, rigid; diagnostic, with or without collection of specimen(s) by brushing or washing (separate procedure)**
P3 T CCI 1.55 3.48 FUD 000

⊙ 45303 **with dilation (eg, balloon, guide wire, bougie)**
74360
P2 T CCI 2.65 26.62 FUD 000

⊙ 45305 **with biopsy, single or multiple**
A2 T CCI PQ 2.28 5.56 FUD 000

⊙ 45307 **with removal of foreign body**
A2 T 80 CCI 2.99 6.54 FUD 000

⊙ 45308 **with removal of single tumor, polyp, or other lesion by hot biopsy forceps or bipolar cautery**
A2 T CCI 2.52 6.18 FUD 000

⊙ 45309 **with removal of single tumor, polyp, or other lesion by snare technique**
A2 T CCI 2.66 6.34 FUD 000

⊙ 45315 **with removal of multiple tumors, polyps, or other lesions by hot biopsy forceps, bipolar cautery or snare technique**
A2 T CCI 3.21 6.53 FUD 000

⊙ 45317 **with control of bleeding (eg, injection, bipolar cautery, unipolar cautery, laser, heater probe, stapler, plasma coagulator)**
A2 T ⚑ 3.42 6.95 FUD 000

⊙ 45320 **with ablation of tumor(s), polyp(s), or other lesion(s) not amenable to removal by hot biopsy forceps, bipolar cautery or snare technique (eg, laser)**
A2 T ⚑ 3.08 6.85 FUD 000

⊙ 45321 **with decompression of volvulus**
A2 T ⚑ 3.10 3.10 FUD 000

⊙ 45327 **with transendoscopic stent placement (includes predilation)**
Code also (C1874, C1875, C1876, C1877, C2617, C2625)
A2 T ⚑ 3.48 3.48 FUD 000

45330-45350 [45346] Flexible Sigmoidoscopy Procedures

CMS 100-3,100.2 Endoscopy

INCLUDES Control of bleeding as result of the endoscopic procedure during same operative session
Exam of:
Entire rectum
Entire sigmoid colon
Portion of descending colon (when performed)

EXCLUDES *Computed tomographic colonography (74261-74263)*

Code also examination of colon through stoma when appropriate:
Colonoscopy (44388-44408 [44401])
Ileoscopy (44380-44384 [44381])

▲ 45330 **Sigmoidoscopy, flexible; diagnostic, including collection of specimen(s) by brushing or washing, when performed (separate procedure)**
Do not report with (45331-45349 [45346])
P3 T ⚑ 1.81 3.86 FUD 000

45331 **with biopsy, single or multiple**
Do not report with (45349) when on same lesion
A2 T ⚑ PQ 2.16 4.62 FUD 000

⊙ ▲ 45332 **with removal of foreign body(s)**
76000
Do not report with (45330)
A2 T ⚑ 3.19 8.27 FUD 000

⊙ ▲ 45333 **with removal of tumor(s), polyp(s), or other lesion(s) by hot biopsy forceps**
Do not report with (45330)
A2 T ⚑ 3.16 8.41 FUD 000

⊙ ▲ 45334 **with control of bleeding, any method**
Do not report with (45335, 45350) when on same lesion
Do not report with (45330)
A2 T ⚑ 4.66 4.66 FUD 000

⊙ 45335 **with directed submucosal injection(s), any substance**
Do not report with (45334, 45349) when on same lesion
Do not report with (45330)
A2 T ⚑ 2.64 7.77 FUD 000

⊙ ▲ 45337 **with decompression (for pathologic distention) (eg, volvulus, megacolon), including placement of decompression tube, when performed**
Do not report more than one time per operative session
Do not report with (45330)
A2 T ⚑ 4.08 4.08 FUD 000

⊙ 45338 **with removal of tumor(s), polyp(s), or other lesion(s) by snare technique**
Do not report with (45349) when on same lesion
Do not report with (45330)
A2 T ⚑ 4.04 9.02 FUD 000

⊙ #● 45346 **with ablation of tumor(s), polyp(s), or other lesion(s) (includes pre- and post-dilation and guide wire passage, when performed)**
Do not report with (45340) when on same lesion
Do not report with (45330)

45339 ~~**with ablation of tumor(s), polyp(s), or other lesion(s) not amenable to removal by hot biopsy forceps, bipolar cautery or snare technique**~~
To report, see 45346

⊙ ▲ 45340 **with transendoscopic balloon dilation**
Code also each additional stricture dilated in same session, using modifier 59 with (45340)
Do not report with (45330, [45346], 45347)
74360
A2 T ⚑ 3.32 13.79 FUD 000

⊙ 45341 **with endoscopic ultrasound examination**
Do not report with (45330, 45342, 76872, 76975)
A2 T ⚑ 4.47 4.47 FUD 000

⊙ 45342 **with transendoscopic ultrasound guided intramural or transmural fine needle aspiration/biopsy(s)**
Do not report more than one time per operative session
Do not report with (45330, 45341, 76872, 76942, 76975)
A2 T ⚑ 6.80 6.80 FUD 000

45345 ~~**with transendoscopic stent placement (includes predilation)**~~
To report, see 45347

45346 *Resequenced code. See code following 45338.*

⊙ ● 45347 **with placement of endoscopic stent (includes pre- and post-dilation and guide wire passage, when performed)**
Do not report with (45330, 45340)
74360

⊙ ● 45349 **with endoscopic mucosal resection**
Do not report with (45331, 45335, 45338, 45350) when on same lesion
Do not report with (45330)

⊙ ● 45350 **with band ligation(s) (eg, hemorrhoids)**
EXCLUDES *Bleeding control by band ligation (45334)*
Do not report more than one time per operative session
Do not report with (45334) when on same lesion
Do not report with (45330, 45349, 46221)

45355-45398 [45388, 45390, 45398] Flexible and Rigid Colonoscopy Procedures

CMS 100-3,100.2 Endoscopy

INCLUDES Control of bleeding as result of the endoscopic procedure during same operative session
Exam of:
Entire colon (rectum to cecum)
Terminal ileum (when performed)

EXCLUDES *Computed tomographic colonography (74261-74263)*

Code also modifier 53 (physician), or 73, 74 (facility) for an incomplete colonoscopy

45355 ~~**Colonoscopy, rigid or flexible, transabdominal via colotomy, single or multiple**~~
To report, see 45399

⊙ ▲ 45378 **Colonoscopy, flexible; diagnostic, including collection of specimen(s) by brushing or washing, when performed (separate procedure)**
EXCLUDES *Decompression for pathological distention (45393)*
Code also modifier 53 when planned total colonoscopy cannot be completed
Do not report with (45379-45393 [45388, 45390, 45398])
A2 T CCI PQ 6.19 11.03 FUD 000

⊙ ▲ 45379 **with removal of foreign body(s)**
Code also modifier 52 when colonoscope fails to reach the junction of the small intestine
Do not report with (45378)
76000
A2 T CCI 7.77 14.17 FUD 000

⊙ ▲ 45380 **with biopsy, single or multiple**
Code also modifier 52 when colonoscope fails to reach the junction of the small intestine
Do not report with ([45390]) when on same lesion
Do not report with (45378)
A2 T CCI PQ 7.39 13.13 FUD 000

⊙ ▲ 45381 **with directed submucosal injection(s), any substance**
Code also modifier 52 when colonoscope fails to reach the junction of the small intestine
Do not report with (45382, [45390]) when on same lesion
Do not report with (45378)
A2 T CCI PQ 7.01 13.18 FUD 000

⊙ ▲ 45382 **with control of bleeding, any method**
Code also modifier 52 when colonoscope fails to reach the junction of the small intestine
Do not report with (45381, [45398]) when on same lesion
Do not report with (45378)
A2 T CCI 9.39 17.06 FUD 000

⊙ #● 45388 **with ablation of tumor(s), polyp(s), or other lesion(s) (includes pre- and post-dilation and guide wire passage, when performed)**
Code also modifier 52 when colonoscope fails to reach the junction of the small intestine
Do not report with (45386) when on same lesion
Do not report with (45378)

45383 ~~**with ablation of tumor(s), polyp(s), or other lesion(s) not amenable to removal by hot biopsy forceps, bipolar cautery or snare technique**~~
To report, see 45388

⊙ ▲ 45384 **with removal of tumor(s), polyp(s), or other lesion(s) by hot biopsy forceps**
Code also modifier 52 when colonoscope fails to reach the junction of the small intestine
Do not report with (45378)
A2 T CCI PQ 7.74 13.14 FUD 000

⊙ ▲ 45385 **with removal of tumor(s), polyp(s), or other lesion(s) by snare technique**
Do not report with ([45390]) when on same lesion
Do not report with (45378)
A2 T CCI PQ 8.78 14.82 FUD 000

⊙ ▲ 45386 **with transendoscopic balloon dilation**
Code also each additional stricture dilated in same operative session, using modifier 59 with (45386)
Do not report with (45378, [45388], 45389)
74360
A2 T CCI 7.60 18.87 FUD 000

45387 ~~**with transendoscopic stent placement (includes predilation)**~~
To report, see 45389

45388 Resequenced code. See code following 45382.

⊙ ● 45389 **with endoscopic stent placement (includes pre- and post-dilation and guide wire passage, when performed)**
Do not report with (45378, 45386)
74360

45390 Resequenced code. See code following 45392.

⊙ ▲ 45391 **with endoscopic ultrasound examination limited to the rectum, sigmoid, descending, transverse, or ascending colon and cecum, and adjacent structures**
Do not report with (45378, 45392, 76872, 76975)
A2 T CCI 8.41 8.41 FUD 000

⊙ ▲ 45392 **with transendoscopic ultrasound guided intramural or transmural fine needle aspiration/biopsy(s), includes endoscopic ultrasound examination limited to the rectum, sigmoid, descending, transverse, or ascending colon and cecum, and adjacent structures**
Do not report with (45378, 45391, 76872, 76942, 76975)
A2 T CCI PQ 10.82 10.82 FUD 000

⊙ #● 45390 **with endoscopic mucosal resection**
Do not report with (45380-45381, 45385, [45398]) when on same lesion
Do not report with (45378)

⊙ ● 45393 **with decompression (for pathologic distention) (eg, volvulus, megacolon), including placement of decompression tube, when performed**
Do not report more than one time per operative session
Do not report with (45378)

⊙ #● 45398 **with band ligation(s) (eg, hemorrhoids)**
EXCLUDES *Bleeding control by band ligation (45382)*
Code also modifier 52 when colonoscope fails to reach the junction of the small intestine
Do not report more than one time per operative session
Do not report with (45382) when on same lesion
Do not report with (45378, [45390], 46221)

45395-45499 Laparoscopic Procedures of Rectum

INCLUDES Diagnostic laparoscopy

45395 **Laparoscopy, surgical; proctectomy, complete, combined abdominoperineal, with colostomy**
EXCLUDES *Open method (45110)*
C 80 PQ 57.09 57.09 FUD 090

45397 **proctectomy, combined abdominoperineal pull-through procedure (eg, colo-anal anastomosis), with creation of colonic reservoir (eg, J-pouch), with diverting enterostomy, when performed**
EXCLUDES *Open method (45119)*
C 80 PQ 61.95 61.95 FUD 090

45398 Resequenced code. See code following 45393.

45399 Resequenced code. See code before 45990.

45400 **proctopexy (for prolapse)**
EXCLUDES *Open method (45540-45541)*
C 80 PQ 33.15 33.15 FUD 090

45402 **proctopexy (for prolapse), with sigmoid resection**
EXCLUDES *Open method (45550)*
C 80 PQ 44.08 44.08 FUD 090

45499 **Unlisted laparoscopic procedure, rectum**
EXCLUDES *Unlisted rectal procedure performed via open technique (45999)*
T 80 0.00 0.00 FUD YYY

45500-45825 Open Repairs of Rectum

45500 Proctoplasty; for stenosis
A2 T 80 PQ 15.18 15.18 FUD 090

45505 for prolapse of mucous membrane
A2 T PQ 16.94 16.94 FUD 090

45520 Perirectal injection of sclerosing solution for prolapse
P2 T PQ 1.17 4.46 FUD 000

45540 Proctopexy (eg, for prolapse); abdominal approach
EXCLUDES *Laparoscopic method (45400)*
C 80 PQ 30.43 30.43 FUD 090

45541 perineal approach
G2 T 80 PQ 26.59 26.59 FUD 090

45550 with sigmoid resection, abdominal approach
INCLUDES Frickman proctopexy
EXCLUDES *Laparoscopic method (45402)*
C 80 PQ 42.16 42.16 FUD 090

45560 Repair of rectocele (separate procedure)
EXCLUDES *Posterior colporrhaphy with rectocele repair (57250)*
A2 T 80 PQ 20.03 20.03 FUD 090

45562 Exploration, repair, and presacral drainage for rectal injury;
C 80 PQ 31.95 31.95 FUD 090

45563 with colostomy
INCLUDES Maydl colostomy
C 80 PQ 46.81 46.81 FUD 090

Bladder
Pubic symphysis
Urethra
An anal fistula leading from the rectum to the skin near the anus contains a continual discharge that irritates the skin and causes discomfort or pain
Rectoperineal fistula
Rectum

45800 Closure of rectovesical fistula;
C 80 PQ 34.34 34.34 FUD 090

45805 with colostomy
C 80 PQ 41.52 41.52 FUD 090

45820 Closure of rectourethral fistula;
EXCLUDES *Closure of fistula, rectovaginal (57300-57308)*
C 80 PQ 33.69 33.69 FUD 090

45825 with colostomy
EXCLUDES *Closure of fistula, rectovaginal (57300-57308)*
C 80 PQ 39.57 39.57 FUD 090

45900-45999 [45399] Closed Procedures of Rectum With Anesthesia

45900 Reduction of procidentia (separate procedure) under anesthesia
A2 T 80 5.83 5.83 FUD 010

45905 Dilation of anal sphincter (separate procedure) under anesthesia other than local
A2 T 4.82 4.82 FUD 010

45910 Dilation of rectal stricture (separate procedure) under anesthesia other than local
A2 T 5.59 5.59 FUD 010

45915 Removal of fecal impaction or foreign body (separate procedure) under anesthesia
A2 T 6.47 9.34 FUD 010

⊙ #● **45399 Unlisted procedure, colon**

45990 Anorectal exam, surgical, requiring anesthesia (general, spinal, or epidural), diagnostic
INCLUDES Diagnostic:
- Anoscopy
- Proctoscopy, rigid

Exam:
- Pelvic (when performed)
- Perineal, external
- Rectal, digital

Do not report with (45300-45327, 46600, 57410, 99170)
A2 T 80 3.08 3.08 FUD 000

45999 Unlisted procedure, rectum
EXCLUDES *Unlisted rectal procedure performed laparoscopically (45499)*
T 80 0.00 0.00 FUD YYY

46020-46083 Surgical Incision of Anus

EXCLUDES *Cryosurgical destruction of hemorrhoid(s) (46999)*
Fistulotomy, subcutaneous (46270)
Hemorrhoidopexy ([46947])
Injection of hemorrhoid(s) (46500)
Thermal energy destruction of internal hemorrhoid(s) (46930)

46020 Placement of seton
Do not report with (46060, 46280, 46600, 0249T)
A2 T 6.70 7.85 FUD 010

46030 Removal of anal seton, other marker
A2 T 80 2.60 3.95 FUD 010

46040 Incision and drainage of ischiorectal and/or perirectal abscess (separate procedure)
A2 T 11.74 15.03 FUD 090

46045 Incision and drainage of intramural, intramuscular, or submucosal abscess, transanal, under anesthesia
A2 T 12.31 12.31 FUD 090

46050 Incision and drainage, perianal abscess, superficial
EXCLUDES *Incision and drainage abscess:*
Ischiorectal/intramural (46060)
Supralevator/pelvirectal/retrorectal (45020)
A2 T 2.80 5.70 FUD 010

46060 Incision and drainage of ischiorectal or intramural abscess, with fistulectomy or fistulotomy, submuscular, with or without placement of seton
EXCLUDES *Incision and drainage abscess:*
Supralevator/pelvirectal/retrorectal (45020)
Do not report with (46020)
A2 T 13.55 13.55 FUD 090

46070 Incision, anal septum (infant) A
EXCLUDES *Anoplasty (46700-46705)*
G2 T 80 63 6.84 6.84 FUD 090

46080 Sphincterotomy, anal, division of sphincter (separate procedure)
A2 T 4.57 7.04 FUD 010

46083 Incision of thrombosed hemorrhoid, external
P2 T 3.04 4.97 FUD 010

46200-46262 [46220, 46320, 46945, 46946] Anal Resection and Hemorrhoidectomies

EXCLUDES *Cryosurgical destruction of hemorrhoid(s) (46999)*
Hemorrhoidopexy ([46947])
Injection of hemorrhoid(s) (46500)
Thermal energy destruction of internal hemorrhoid(s) (46930)

46200 Fissurectomy, including sphincterotomy, when performed
A2 T 9.23 12.51 FUD 090

46220 Resequenced code. See code before 46230.

46221 Hemorrhoidectomy, internal, by rubber band ligation(s)
EXCLUDES *Ligation of hemorrhoidal vascular bundles including ultrasound guidance (0249T)*
Do not report with (45350, [45398])
P3 T 5.46 7.60 FUD 010

\# **46945 Hemorrhoidectomy, internal, by ligation other than rubber band; single hemorrhoid column/group**
EXCLUDES *Other hemorrhoid procedures:*
Destruction (46930)
Excision (46250-46262)
Injection sclerosing solution (46500)
Do not report with (0249T)
P3 T 6.36 8.59 FUD 090

\# **46946 2 or more hemorrhoid columns/groups**
Do not report with (0249T)
A2 T 6.38 8.79 FUD 090

\# **46220 Excision of single external papilla or tag, anus**
A2 T 3.41 5.85 FUD 010

46230 Excision of multiple external papillae or tags, anus
A2 T 4.97 7.79 FUD 010

\# **46320 Excision of thrombosed hemorrhoid, external**
P3 T 3.19 5.21 FUD 010

46250 Hemorrhoidectomy, external, 2 or more columns/groups
EXCLUDES *Hemorrhoidectomy, external, single column/group (46999)*
Do not report with (0249T)
A2 T 8.94 13.03 FUD 090

46255 Hemorrhoidectomy, internal and external, single column/group;
Do not report with (0249T)
A2 T 10.06 14.26 FUD 090

46257 with fissurectomy
Do not report with (0249T)
A2 T 11.97 11.97 FUD 090

46258 with fistulectomy, including fissurectomy, when performed
Do not report with (0249T)
A2 T 80 13.20 13.20 FUD 090

46260 Hemorrhoidectomy, internal and external, 2 or more columns/groups;
INCLUDES Whitehead hemorrhoidectomy
Do not report with (0249T)
A2 T 13.51 13.51 FUD 090

46261 with fissurectomy
Do not report with (0249T)
A2 T 14.98 14.98 FUD 090

46262 with fistulectomy, including fissurectomy, when performed
Do not report with (0249T)
A2 T 15.77 15.77 FUD 090

46270-46320 Resection of Anal Fistula

46270 Surgical treatment of anal fistula (fistulectomy/fistulotomy); subcutaneous
A2 T 11.14 14.32 FUD 090

46275 intersphincteric
A2 T 11.82 15.22 FUD 090

46280 transsphincteric, suprasphincteric, extrasphincteric or multiple, including placement of seton, when performed
Do not report with (46020)
A2 T 13.41 13.41 FUD 090

46285 second stage
A2 T 11.80 15.16 FUD 090

46288 Closure of anal fistula with rectal advancement flap
A2 T 15.70 15.70 FUD 090

46320 Resequenced code. See code following 46230.

46500 Other Hemorrhoid Procedures

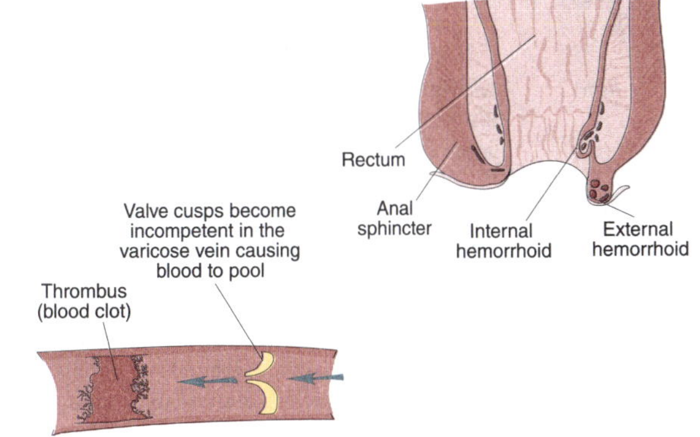

46500 Injection of sclerosing solution, hemorrhoids
EXCLUDES *Anoscopic injection of bulking agent, submucosal, for fecal incontinence (0377T)*
P3 T 3.72 6.76 FUD 010

46505 Chemodenervation Anal Sphincter

EXCLUDES *Chemodenervation of:*
Extremity muscles (64642-64645)
Muscles/facial nerve (64612)
Neck muscles (64616)
Other peripheral nerve/branch (64640)
Pudendal nerve (64630)
Trunk muscles (64646-64647)
Code also drug(s)/substance(s) given

46505 Chemodenervation of internal anal sphincter
G2 T 50 6.88 8.17 FUD 010

46600-46615 Anoscopic Procedures

CMS 100-3,100.2 Endoscopy
INCLUDES Diagnostic endoscopy with surgical endoscopy
EXCLUDES *Delivery of thermal energy via anoscope to the muscle of the anal canal (0288T)*
Injection of bulking agent, submucosal, for fecal incontinence (0377T)

▲ **46600 Anoscopy; diagnostic, including collection of specimen(s) by brushing or washing, when performed (separate procedure)**
EXCLUDES *High-resolution anoscopy (HRA), diagnostic (46601)*
Do not report with (46020, 0249T, 0377T)
P2 X 1.17 2.50 FUD 000

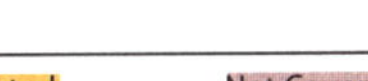

● 46601 diagnostic, with high-resolution magnification (HRA) (eg, colposcope, operating microscope) and chemical agent enhancement, including collection of specimen(s) by brushing or washing, when performed
INCLUDES Operating microscope (69990)

46604 with dilation (eg, balloon, guide wire, bougie)
P2 T 1.91 17.52 FUD 000

46606 with biopsy, single or multiple
EXCLUDES *High resolution anoscopy (HRA) with biopsy (46607)*
P3 T PQ 2.22 6.42 FUD 000

● 46607 with high-resolution magnification (HRA) (eg, colposcope, operating microscope) and chemical agent enhancement, with biopsy, single or multiple
INCLUDES Operating microscope (69990)

46608 with removal of foreign body
A2 T 80 2.31 6.41 FUD 000

46610 with removal of single tumor, polyp, or other lesion by hot biopsy forceps or bipolar cautery
A2 T 2.32 6.41 FUD 000

46611 with removal of single tumor, polyp, or other lesion by snare technique
A2 T 80 2.36 4.98 FUD 000

46612 with removal of multiple tumors, polyps, or other lesions by hot biopsy forceps, bipolar cautery or snare technique
A2 T 80 2.70 7.74 FUD 000

46614 with control of bleeding (eg, injection, bipolar cautery, unipolar cautery, laser, heater probe, stapler, plasma coagulator)
P3 T 1.84 3.63 FUD 000

46615 with ablation of tumor(s), polyp(s), or other lesion(s) not amenable to removal by hot biopsy forceps, bipolar cautery or snare technique
A2 T 80 2.69 4.11 FUD 000

46700-46947 [46947] Anal Repairs and Stapled Hemorrhoidopexy

46700 Anoplasty, plastic operation for stricture; adult
A2 T 18.74 18.74 FUD 090

46705 infant A
EXCLUDES *Anal septum incision (46070)*
C 80 63 13.82 13.82 FUD 090

46706 Repair of anal fistula with fibrin glue
A2 T 4.86 4.86 FUD 010

46707 Repair of anorectal fistula with plug (eg, porcine small intestine submucosa [SIS])
G2 T 80 13.19 13.19 FUD 090

46710 Repair of ileoanal pouch fistula/sinus (eg, perineal or vaginal), pouch advancement; transperineal approach
C 80 31.40 31.40 FUD 090

46712 combined transperineal and transabdominal approach
C 80 58.62 58.62 FUD 090

46715 Repair of low imperforate anus; with anoperineal fistula (cut-back procedure)
C 80 PQ 63 14.23 14.23 FUD 090

46716 with transposition of anoperineal or anovestibular fistula
C 80 PQ 63 30.67 30.67 FUD 090

46730 Repair of high imperforate anus without fistula; perineal or sacroperineal approach
C 80 PQ 63 50.41 50.41 FUD 090

46735 combined transabdominal and sacroperineal approaches
C 80 PQ 63 58.38 58.38 FUD 090

46740 Repair of high imperforate anus with rectourethral or rectovaginal fistula; perineal or sacroperineal approach
C 80 PQ 63 60.96 60.96 FUD 090

46742 combined transabdominal and sacroperineal approaches
C 80 PQ 63 69.65 69.65 FUD 090

46744 Repair of cloacal anomaly by anorectovaginoplasty and urethroplasty, sacroperineal approach ♀
C 80 PQ 63 96.03 96.03 FUD 090

46746 Repair of cloacal anomaly by anorectovaginoplasty and urethroplasty, combined abdominal and sacroperineal approach; ♀
C 80 PQ 101.03 101.03 FUD 090

46748 with vaginal lengthening by intestinal graft or pedicle flaps ♀
C 80 PQ 109.72 109.72 FUD 090

46750 Sphincteroplasty, anal, for incontinence or prolapse; adult
A2 T 80 PQ 21.88 21.88 FUD 090

46751 child A
C 80 PQ 17.34 17.34 FUD 090

46753 Graft (Thiersch operation) for rectal incontinence and/or prolapse
A2 T PQ 16.86 16.86 FUD 090

46754 Removal of Thiersch wire or suture, anal canal
A2 T 80 PQ 6.48 8.25 FUD 010

46760 Sphincteroplasty, anal, for incontinence, adult; muscle transplant
A2 T 80 PQ 31.54 31.54 FUD 090

46761 levator muscle imbrication (Park posterior anal repair)
A2 T 80 PQ 26.73 26.73 FUD 090

46762 implantation artificial sphincter
EXCLUDES *Anoscopic injection of bulking agent, submucosal, for fecal incontinence (0377T)*
A2 T 80 PQ 26.62 26.62 FUD 090

46947 Hemorrhoidopexy (eg, for prolapsing internal hemorrhoids) by stapling
A2 T 10.90 10.90 FUD 090

46900-46999 Destruction Procedures: Anus

46900 Destruction of lesion(s), anus (eg, condyloma, papilloma, molluscum contagiosum, herpetic vesicle), simple; chemical
P2 T 3.95 6.83 FUD 010

46910 electrodesiccation
P3 T 3.87 7.23 FUD 010

46916 cryosurgery
P2 T 4.06 6.42 FUD 010

46917 laser surgery
A2 T 3.84 12.60 FUD 010

46922 surgical excision
A2 T 3.87 7.54 FUD 010

46924 Destruction of lesion(s), anus (eg, condyloma, papilloma, molluscum contagiosum, herpetic vesicle), extensive (eg, laser surgery, electrosurgery, cryosurgery, chemosurgery)
A2 T 5.28 15.14 FUD 010

46930 **Destruction of internal hemorrhoid(s) by thermal energy (eg, infrared coagulation, cautery, radiofrequency)**

EXCLUDES *Other hemorrhoid procedures:*
- *Cryosurgery destruction (46999)*
- *Excision ([46320], 46250-46262)*
- *Hemorrhoidopexy ([46947])*
- *Incision (46083)*
- *Injection sclerosing solution (46500)*
- *Ligation (46221, [46945, 46946])*

P3 T 80 4.20 5.79 FUD 090

46940 **Curettage or cautery of anal fissure, including dilation of anal sphincter (separate procedure); initial**

P3 T 4.21 6.51 FUD 010

46942 **subsequent**

P3 T 80 3.81 6.19 FUD 010

46945 Resequenced code. See code following 46221.

46946 Resequenced code, See code following 46221.

46947 Resequenced code, See code following 46762.

46999 **Unlisted procedure, anus**

T 80 0.00 0.00 FUD YYY

47000-47001 Needle Biopsy of Liver

EXCLUDES *Fine needle aspiration (10021, 10022)*

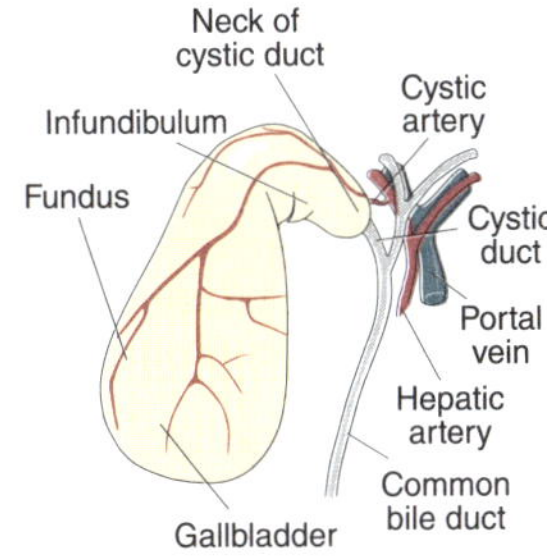

⊙ **47000** **Biopsy of liver, needle; percutaneous**

76942, 77002, 77012, 77021

88172-88173

A2 T PQ 3.00 10.24 FUD 000

\+ **47001** **when done for indicated purpose at time of other major procedure (List separately in addition to code for primary procedure)**

Code first primary procedure

76942, 77002

88172-88173

N1 N PQ 2.94 2.94 FUD ZZZ

47010-47130 Open Incisional and Resection Procedures of Liver

47010 **Hepatotomy, for open drainage of abscess or cyst, 1 or 2 stages**

EXCLUDES *Image guided percutaneous catheter drainage (49505)*

C 80 PQ 34.27 34.27 FUD 090

47015 **Laparotomy, with aspiration and/or injection of hepatic parasitic (eg, amoebic or echinococcal) cyst(s) or abscess(es)**

C 80 32.69 32.69 FUD 090

47100 **Biopsy of liver, wedge**

C 80 PQ 23.98 23.98 FUD 090

47120 **Hepatectomy, resection of liver; partial lobectomy**

C 80 PQ 66.23 66.23 FUD 090

47122 **trisegmentectomy**

C 80 PQ 97.60 97.60 FUD 090

47125 **total left lobectomy**

C 80 PQ 87.43 87.43 FUD 090

47130 **total right lobectomy**

C 80 PQ 93.93 93.93 FUD 090

47133-47147 Liver Transplant Procedures

- CMS 100-3,260.1 Adult Liver Transplantation
- CMS 100-3,260.2 Pediatric Liver Transplantation
- CMS 100-4,3,90.4 Liver Transplants
- CMS 100-4,3,90.4.1 Standard Liver Acquisition Charge
- CMS 100-4,3,90.4.2 Billing for Liver Transplant and Acquisition Services
- CMS 100-4,3,90.6 Intestinal and Multi-Visceral Transplants

47133 **Donor hepatectomy (including cold preservation), from cadaver donor**

INCLUDES Graft:
- Cold preservation
- Harvest

C 0.00 0.00 FUD XXX

47135 **Liver allotransplantation; orthotopic, partial or whole, from cadaver or living donor, any age**

INCLUDES Partial/whole recipient hepatectomy
Partial/whole transplant of allograft
Recipient care

C 80 PQ 139.27 139.27 FUD 090

47136 **heterotopic, partial or whole, from cadaver or living donor, any age**

INCLUDES Partial/whole recipient hepatectomy
Partial/whole transplant of allograft
Recipient care

C 80 PQ 119.31 119.31 FUD 090

47140 **Donor hepatectomy (including cold preservation), from living donor; left lateral segment only (segments II and III)**

INCLUDES Donor care
Graft:
- Cold preservation
- Harvest

C 80 PQ 101.45 101.45 FUD 090

47141 **total left lobectomy (segments II, III and IV)**

INCLUDES Donor care
Graft:
- Cold preservation
- Harvest

C 80 PQ 111.53 111.53 FUD 090

47142 total right lobectomy (segments V, VI, VII and VIII)
INCLUDES Donor care
Graft:
Cold preservation
Harvest
C 80 133.66 133.66 FUD 090

47143 Backbench standard preparation of cadaver donor whole liver graft prior to allotransplantation, including cholecystectomy, if necessary, and dissection and removal of surrounding soft tissues to prepare the vena cava, portal vein, hepatic artery, and common bile duct for implantation; without trisegment or lobe split
Do not report with (47120-47125, 47600, 47610)
C 80 0.00 0.00 FUD XXX

47144 with trisegment split of whole liver graft into 2 partial liver grafts (ie, left lateral segment [segments II and III] and right trisegment [segments I and IV through VIII])
Do not report with (47120-47125, 47600, 47610)
C 80 0.00 0.00 FUD 090

47145 with lobe split of whole liver graft into 2 partial liver grafts (ie, left lobe [segments II, III, and IV] and right lobe [segments I and V through VIII])
Do not report with (47120-47125, 47600, 47610)
C 80 0.00 0.00 FUD XXX

47146 Backbench reconstruction of cadaver or living donor liver graft prior to allotransplantation; venous anastomosis, each
Do not report with (47120-47125, 47600, 47610)
C 80 9.38 9.38 FUD XXX

47147 arterial anastomosis, each
Do not report with (47120-47125, 47600, 47610)
C 80 10.94 10.94 FUD XXX

47300-47362 Open Repair of Liver

47300 Marsupialization of cyst or abscess of liver
C 80 32.08 32.08 FUD 090

47350 Management of liver hemorrhage; simple suture of liver wound or injury
C 80 39.01 39.01 FUD 090

47360 complex suture of liver wound or injury, with or without hepatic artery ligation
C 80 53.07 53.07 FUD 090

47361 exploration of hepatic wound, extensive debridement, coagulation and/or suture, with or without packing of liver
C 80 85.80 85.80 FUD 090

47362 re-exploration of hepatic wound for removal of packing
C 80 41.13 41.13 FUD 090

47370-47379 Laparoscopic Ablation Liver Tumors

INCLUDES Diagnostic laparoscopy

47370 Laparoscopy, surgical, ablation of 1 or more liver tumor(s); radiofrequency
76940
T 80 35.27 35.27 FUD 090

47371 cryosurgical
76940
T 80 34.94 34.94 FUD 090

47379 Unlisted laparoscopic procedure, liver
T 80 0.00 0.00 FUD YYY

47380-47399 Open/Percutaneous Ablation Liver Tumors

47380 Ablation, open, of 1 or more liver tumor(s); radiofrequency
76940
C 80 41.02 41.02 FUD 090

47381 cryosurgical
76940
C 80 41.36 41.36 FUD 090

⊙ **47382** Ablation, 1 or more liver tumor(s), percutaneous, radiofrequency
76940, 77013, 77022
62 T 22.48 141.20 FUD 010

⊙ ● **47383** Ablation, 1 or more liver tumor(s), percutaneous, cryoablation
76940, 77013, 77022

47399 Unlisted procedure, liver
T 0.00 0.00 FUD YYY

47400-47490 Surgical Incision Biliary Tract

47400 Hepaticotomy or hepaticostomy with exploration, drainage, or removal of calculus
C 80 61.26 61.26 FUD 090

47420 Choledochotomy or choledochostomy with exploration, drainage, or removal of calculus, with or without cholecystotomy; without transduodenal sphincterotomy or sphincteroplasty
C 80 38.20 38.20 FUD 090

47425 with transduodenal sphincterotomy or sphincteroplasty
C 80 38.86 38.86 FUD 090

47460 Transduodenal sphincterotomy or sphincteroplasty, with or without transduodenal extraction of calculus (separate procedure)
C 80 36.05 36.05 FUD 090

47480 Cholecystotomy or cholecystostomy, open, with exploration, drainage, or removal of calculus (separate procedure)
EXCLUDES *Percutaneous cholecystostomy (47490)*
C 80 24.88 24.88 FUD 090

47490 Cholecystostomy, percutaneous, complete procedure, including imaging guidance, catheter placement, cholecystogram when performed, and radiological supervision and interpretation
EXCLUDES *Open cholecystostomy (47480)*
Do not report with (47505, 74305, 75989, 76942, 77002, 77012, 77021)
T 9.57 9.57 FUD 010

47500-47530 Injection/Insertion Procedures of Biliary Tract

47500 **Injection procedure for percutaneous transhepatic cholangiography**
74320
NI N PQ 2.81 2.81 FUD 000

47505 **Injection procedure for cholangiography through an existing catheter (eg, percutaneous transhepatic or T-tube)**
Do not report with (47490)
74305
NI N 80 PQ 1.09 1.09 FUD 000

47510 **Introduction of percutaneous transhepatic catheter for biliary drainage**
75980
A2 T 13.60 13.60 FUD 090

47511 **Introduction of percutaneous transhepatic stent for internal and external biliary drainage**
75982
A2 T 50 16.69 16.69 FUD 090

⊙ **47525** **Change of percutaneous biliary drainage catheter**
Code also (C1729)
75984
A2 T 50 2.44 14.56 FUD 000

47530 **Revision and/or reinsertion of transhepatic tube**
75984
A2 T 10.11 38.93 FUD 090

47550-47556 Endoscopic Procedures of the Biliary Tract

CMS 100-3,100.2 Endoscopy
INCLUDES Diagnostic endoscopy with surgical endoscopy

+ **47550** **Biliary endoscopy, intraoperative (choledochoscopy) (List separately in addition to code for primary procedure)**
Code first primary procedure
C 80 4.71 4.71 FUD ZZZ

47552 **Biliary endoscopy, percutaneous via T-tube or other tract; diagnostic, with collection of specimen(s) by brushing and/or washing, when performed (separate procedure)**
A2 T 9.11 9.11 FUD 000

47553 **with biopsy, single or multiple**
A2 T PQ 9.06 9.06 FUD 000

47554 **with removal of calculus/calculi**
A2 T 14.05 14.05 FUD 000

47555 **with dilation of biliary duct stricture(s) without stent**
A2 T 10.75 10.75 FUD 000

47556 **with dilation of biliary duct stricture(s) with stent**
EXCLUDES *Endoscopic retrograde cholangiopancreatography (ERCP) (43260-43273 [43274, 43275, 43276, 43277, 43278], 74328-74330, 74363, 75982)*
74363, 75982
A2 T 12.21 12.21 FUD 000

47560-47579 Laparoscopic Gallbladder Procedures

CMS 100-3,100.13 Laparoscopic Cholecystectomy
INCLUDES Diagnostic laparoscopy

47560 **Laparoscopy, surgical; with guided transhepatic cholangiography, without biopsy**
A2 T 80 PQ 7.63 7.63 FUD 000

47561 **with guided transhepatic cholangiography with biopsy**
A2 T 80 PQ 8.37 8.37 FUD 000

47562 **cholecystectomy**
G2 T 80 PQ 18.69 18.69 FUD 090

47563 **cholecystectomy with cholangiography**
G2 T 80 PQ 20.31 20.31 FUD 090

47564 **cholecystectomy with exploration of common duct**
G2 T 80 PQ 31.67 31.67 FUD 090

47570 **cholecystoenterostomy**
C 80 PQ 22.02 22.02 FUD 090

47579 **Unlisted laparoscopy procedure, biliary tract**
T 80 50 0.00 0.00 FUD YYY

47600-47620 Open Gallbladder Procedures

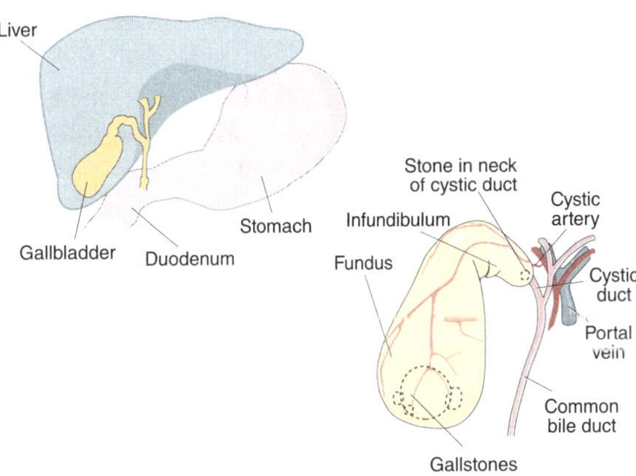

47600 **Cholecystectomy;**
EXCLUDES *Laparoscopic method (47562-47564)*
C 80 PQ 30.40 30.40 FUD 090

47605 **with cholangiography**
EXCLUDES *Laparoscopic method (47563-47564)*
C 80 PQ 31.99 31.99 FUD 090

47610 **Cholecystectomy with exploration of common duct;**
EXCLUDES *Laparoscopic method (47564)*
Code also biliary endoscopy when performed in conjunction with cholecystectomy with exploration of common duct (47550)
C 80 PQ 35.68 35.68 FUD 090

47612 **with choledochoenterostomy**
C 80 PQ 36.12 36.12 FUD 090

47620 **with transduodenal sphincterotomy or sphincteroplasty, with or without cholangiography**
C 80 PQ 39.22 39.22 FUD 090

47630-47999 Open Resection and Repair of Biliary Tract

47630 **Biliary duct stone extraction, percutaneous via T-tube tract, basket, or snare (eg, Burhenne technique)**
74327
A2 T PQ 15.65 15.65 FUD 090

47700 **Exploration for congenital atresia of bile ducts, without repair, with or without liver biopsy, with or without cholangiography**
C 80 PQ 63 29.90 29.90 FUD 090

47701 **Portoenterostomy (eg, Kasai procedure)**
C 80 PQ 63 49.30 49.30 FUD 090

47711 **Excision of bile duct tumor, with or without primary repair of bile duct; extrahepatic**
EXCLUDES *Anastomosis (47760-47800)*
C 80 PQ 44.40 44.40 FUD 090

47712 **intrahepatic**
EXCLUDES *Anastomosis (47760-47800)*
C 80 PQ 56.86 56.86 FUD 090

47715 **Excision of choledochal cyst**
C 80 PQ 37.82 37.82 FUD 090

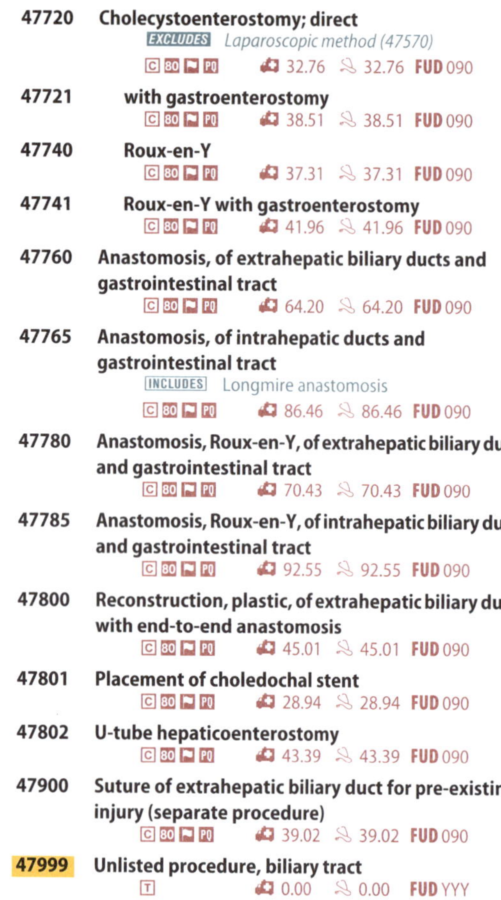

47720 **Cholecystoenterostomy; direct**
EXCLUDES *Laparoscopic method (47570)*
C 80 PQ 32.76 32.76 FUD 090

47721 **with gastroenterostomy**
C 80 PQ 38.51 38.51 FUD 090

47740 **Roux-en-Y**
C 80 PQ 37.31 37.31 FUD 090

47741 **Roux-en-Y with gastroenterostomy**
C 80 PQ 41.96 41.96 FUD 090

47760 **Anastomosis, of extrahepatic biliary ducts and gastrointestinal tract**
C 80 PQ 64.20 64.20 FUD 090

47765 **Anastomosis, of intrahepatic ducts and gastrointestinal tract**
INCLUDES Longmire anastomosis
C 80 PQ 86.46 86.46 FUD 090

47780 **Anastomosis, Roux-en-Y, of extrahepatic biliary ducts and gastrointestinal tract**
C 80 PQ 70.43 70.43 FUD 090

47785 **Anastomosis, Roux-en-Y, of intrahepatic biliary ducts and gastrointestinal tract**
C 80 PQ 92.55 92.55 FUD 090

47800 **Reconstruction, plastic, of extrahepatic biliary ducts with end-to-end anastomosis**
C 80 PQ 45.01 45.01 FUD 090

47801 **Placement of choledochal stent**
C 80 PQ 28.94 28.94 FUD 090

47802 **U-tube hepaticoenterostomy**
C 80 PQ 43.39 43.39 FUD 090

47900 **Suture of extrahepatic biliary duct for pre-existing injury (separate procedure)**
C 80 PQ 39.02 39.02 FUD 090

47999 **Unlisted procedure, biliary tract**
T 0.00 0.00 FUD YYY

48000-48548 Open Procedures of the Pancreas

EXCLUDES *Peroral pancreatic procedures performed endoscopically (43260-43265, [43274, 43275, 43276, 43277, 43278])*

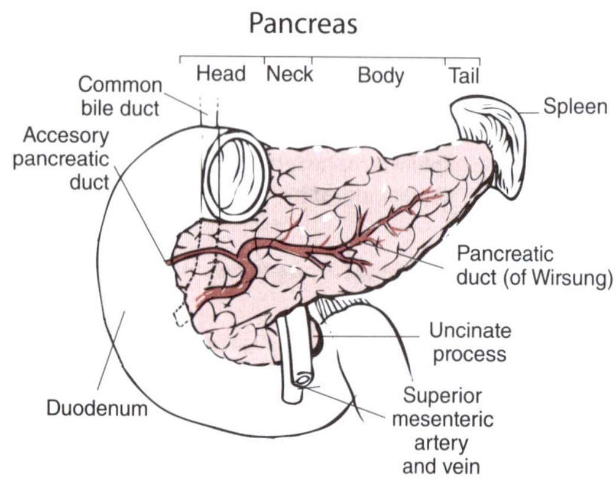

48000 **Placement of drains, peripancreatic, for acute pancreatitis;**
C 80 PQ 52.82 52.82 FUD 090

48001 **with cholecystostomy, gastrostomy, and jejunostomy**
C 80 PQ 65.71 65.71 FUD 090

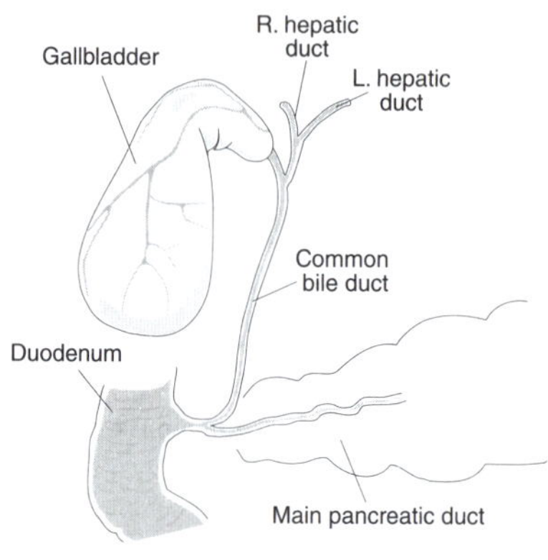

48020 **Removal of pancreatic calculus**
C 80 PQ 33.47 33.47 FUD 090

48100 **Biopsy of pancreas, open (eg, fine needle aspiration, needle core biopsy, wedge biopsy)**
C 80 PQ 25.25 25.25 FUD 090

48102 **Biopsy of pancreas, percutaneous needle**
EXCLUDES *Aspiration, fine needle (10022)*
76942, 77002, 77012, 77021
88172, 88173
A2 T PQ 7.02 15.07 FUD 010

48105 **Resection or debridement of pancreas and peripancreatic tissue for acute necrotizing pancreatitis**
C 80 PQ 81.10 81.10 FUD 090

48120 **Excision of lesion of pancreas (eg, cyst, adenoma)**
C 80 PQ 31.55 31.55 FUD 090

48140 **Pancreatectomy, distal subtotal, with or without splenectomy; without pancreaticojejunostomy**
C 80 PQ 44.48 44.48 FUD 090

48145 **with pancreaticojejunostomy**
C 80 PQ 46.44 46.44 FUD 090

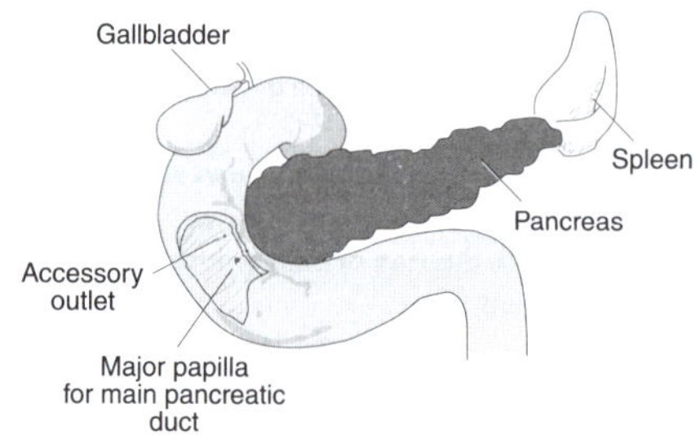

48146 **Pancreatectomy, distal, near-total with preservation of duodenum (Child-type procedure)**
C 80 PQ 53.43 53.43 FUD 090

48148 **Excision of ampulla of Vater**
C 80 PQ 35.49 35.49 FUD 090

48150 **Pancreatectomy, proximal subtotal with total duodenectomy, partial gastrectomy, choledochoenterostomy and gastrojejunostomy (Whipple-type procedure); with pancreatojejunostomy**
C 80 PQ 88.47 88.47 FUD 090

48152 **without pancreatojejunostomy**
C 80 PQ 82.11 82.11 FUD 090

48153 **Pancreatectomy, proximal subtotal with near-total duodenectomy, choledochoenterostomy and duodenojejunostomy (pylorus-sparing, Whipple-type procedure); with pancreatojejunostomy**
C 80 PQ 88.16 88.16 FUD 090

48154 **without pancreatojejunostomy**
C 80 PQ 82.46 82.46 FUD 090

48155 **Pancreatectomy, total**
C 80 PQ 51.69 51.69 FUD 090

48160 **Pancreatectomy, total or subtotal, with autologous transplantation of pancreas or pancreatic islet cells**
E 0.00 0.00 FUD XXX

+ 48400 **Injection procedure for intraoperative pancreatography (List separately in addition to code for primary procedure)**
Code first primary procedure
74300-74305
C 80 3.14 3.14 FUD ZZZ

48500 **Marsupialization of pancreatic cyst**
C 80 PQ 32.71 32.71 FUD 090

48510 **External drainage, pseudocyst of pancreas, open**
EXCLUDES *Image guided percutaneous catheter drainage (49405)*
C 80 PQ 31.01 31.01 FUD 090

48520 **Internal anastomosis of pancreatic cyst to gastrointestinal tract; direct**
C 80 PQ 31.07 31.07 FUD 090

48540 **Roux-en-Y**
C 80 PQ 37.27 37.27 FUD 090

48545 **Pancreatorrhaphy for injury**
C 80 PQ 38.26 38.26 FUD 090

48547 **Duodenal exclusion with gastrojejunostomy for pancreatic injury**
C 80 PQ 50.99 50.99 FUD 090

48548 **Pancreaticojejunostomy, side-to-side anastomosis (Puestow-type operation)**
C 80 PQ 47.37 47.37 FUD 090

48550-48999 Pancreas Transplant Procedures

CMS 100-3,260.3 Pancreas Transplants
CMS 100-4,3,90.5 Pancreas Transplants with Kidney Transplants

48550 **Donor pancreatectomy (including cold preservation), with or without duodenal segment for transplantation**
INCLUDES Graft:
Cold preservation
Harvest (with or without duodenal segment)
E 0.00 0.00 FUD XXX

48551 **Backbench standard preparation of cadaver donor pancreas allograft prior to transplantation, including dissection of allograft from surrounding soft tissues, splenectomy, duodenotomy, ligation of bile duct, ligation of mesenteric vessels, and Y-graft arterial anastomoses from iliac artery to superior mesenteric artery and to splenic artery**
Do not report with (35531, 35563, 35685, 38100-38102, 44010, 44820, 44850, 47460, 47505-47525, 47550-47556, 48100-48120, 48545)
C 80 0.00 0.00 FUD XXX

48552 **Backbench reconstruction of cadaver donor pancreas allograft prior to transplantation, venous anastomosis, each**
Do not report with (35531, 35563, 35685, 38100-38102, 44010, 44820, 44850, 47460, 47505-47525, 47550-47556, 48100-48120, 48545)
C 80 6.71 6.71 FUD XXX

48554 **Transplantation of pancreatic allograft**
INCLUDES Allograft transplant
Recipient care
C 80 PQ 72.89 72.89 FUD 090

48556 **Removal of transplanted pancreatic allograft**
C 80 PQ 36.20 36.20 FUD 090

48999 **Unlisted procedure, pancreas**
T 80 0.00 0.00 FUD YYY

49000-49084 Exploratory and Drainage Procedures: Abdomen/Peritoneum

49000 **Exploratory laparotomy, exploratory celiotomy with or without biopsy(s) (separate procedure)**
EXCLUDES *Exploration of penetrating wound without laparotomy (20102)*
C 80 PQ 21.97 21.97 FUD 090

49002 **Reopening of recent laparotomy**
EXCLUDES *Hepatic wound re-exploration for packing removal (47362)*
C 80 PQ 29.84 29.84 FUD 090

49010 **Exploration, retroperitoneal area with or without biopsy(s) (separate procedure)**
EXCLUDES *Exploration of penetrating wound without laparotomy (20102)*
C 80 PQ 26.69 26.69 FUD 090

49020 **Drainage of peritoneal abscess or localized peritonitis, exclusive of appendiceal abscess, open**
EXCLUDES *Appendiceal abscess (44900)*
Image guided percutaneous catheter drainage (49406)
C 80 PQ 45.31 45.31 FUD 090

49040 **Drainage of subdiaphragmatic or subphrenic abscess, open**
EXCLUDES *Percutaneous drainage (49406)*
C 80 PQ 28.49 28.49 FUD 090

49060 **Drainage of retroperitoneal abscess, open**
EXCLUDES *Drainage performed laparoscopically (49323)*
Percutaneous drainage (49406)
C PQ 31.40 31.40 FUD 090

49062 **Drainage of extraperitoneal lymphocele to peritoneal cavity, open**
C 80 20.92 20.92 FUD 090

49082 **Abdominal paracentesis (diagnostic or therapeutic); without imaging guidance**
G2 T 2.12 5.39 FUD 000

49083 **with imaging guidance**
Do not report with (76942, 77002, 77012, 77021)
G2 T 3.14 8.37 FUD 000

49084 **Peritoneal lavage, including imaging guidance, when performed**
Do not report with (76942, 77002, 77012, 77021)
G2 T 2.90 2.90 FUD 000

49180 Biopsy of Mass: Abdomen/Retroperitoneum

EXCLUDES *Aspiration, fine needle (10021, 10022)*
Lysis of intestinal adhesions (44005)

49180 **Biopsy, abdominal or retroperitoneal mass, percutaneous needle**
76942, 77002, 77012, 77021
88172, 88173
A2 T PQ 2.49 4.62 FUD 000

49203-49205 Open Destruction or Excision: Abdominal Tumors

EXCLUDES *Cryoablation of renal tumor (50250, 50593)*
Lysis of intestinal adhesions (44005)
Primary, recurrent ovarian, uterine, or tubal resection (58957-58958)

Code also colectomy (44140)
Code also small bowel resection (44120)
Code also nephrectomy (50220 or 50240)
Code also vena caval resection with reconstruction (37799)
Do not report with (38770, 38780, 49000, 49010, 49215, 50010, 50205, 50225, 50236, 50250, 50290, 58900-58960)

49203 **Excision or destruction, open, intra-abdominal tumors, cysts or endometriomas, 1 or more peritoneal, mesenteric, or retroperitoneal primary or secondary tumors; largest tumor 5 cm diameter or less**
C 80 PQ 34.14 34.14 FUD 090

49204 **largest tumor 5.1-10.0 cm diameter**
C 80 PQ 43.61 43.61 FUD 090

49205 **largest tumor greater than 10.0 cm diameter**
C 80 PQ 50.12 50.12 FUD 090

49215 Resection Presacral/Sacrococcygeal Tumor

49215 **Excision of presacral or sacrococcygeal tumor**
C 80 PQ 63 63.43 63.43 FUD 090

49220-49255 Other Open Abdominal Procedures

EXCLUDES *Lysis of intestinal adhesions (44005)*

49220 **Staging laparotomy for Hodgkins disease or lymphoma (includes splenectomy, needle or open biopsies of both liver lobes, possibly also removal of abdominal nodes, abdominal node and/or bone marrow biopsies, ovarian repositioning)**
C 80 PQ 27.21 27.21 FUD 090

49250 **Umbilectomy, omphalectomy, excision of umbilicus (separate procedure)**
A2 T PQ 16.60 16.60 FUD 090

49255 **Omentectomy, epiploectomy, resection of omentum (separate procedure)**
C 80 PQ 22.60 22.60 FUD 090

49320-49329 Laparoscopic Procedures of the Abdomen/Peritoneum/Omentum

INCLUDES Diagnostic laparoscopy

EXCLUDES *Fulguration/excision of lesions of ovary/pelvic viscera/peritoneal surface, performed laparoscopically (58662)*

49320 **Laparoscopy, abdomen, peritoneum, and omentum, diagnostic, with or without collection of specimen(s) by brushing or washing (separate procedure)**
A2 T 80 PQ 9.35 9.35 FUD 010

49321 **Laparoscopy, surgical; with biopsy (single or multiple)**
A2 T 80 PQ 9.90 9.90 FUD 010

49322 **with aspiration of cavity or cyst (eg, ovarian cyst) (single or multiple)**
A2 T 80 PQ 10.59 10.59 FUD 010

49323 **with drainage of lymphocele to peritoneal cavity**
EXCLUDES *Retroperitoneal abscess drainage: Open (49062)*
T 80 PQ 18.41 18.41 FUD 090

49324 **with insertion of tunneled intraperitoneal catheter**
EXCLUDES *Open approach (49421)*
Code also insertion of subcutaneous extension to intraperitoneal cannula with remote chest exit site, when appropriate (49435)
G2 T 80 11.16 11.16 FUD 010

49325 **with revision of previously placed intraperitoneal cannula or catheter, with removal of intraluminal obstructive material if performed**
G2 T 80 11.96 11.96 FUD 010

\+ 49326 **with omentopexy (omental tacking procedure) (List separately in addition to code for primary procedure)**
Code first laparoscopy with permanent intraperitoneal cannula or catheter insertion or revision of previously placed catheter/cannula (49324, 49325)
N1 N 80 5.40 5.40 FUD ZZZ

\+ 49327 **with placement of interstitial device(s) for radiation therapy guidance (eg, fiducial markers, dosimeter), intra-abdominal, intrapelvic, and/or retroperitoneum, including imaging guidance, if performed, single or multiple (List separately in addition to code for primary procedure)**
EXCLUDES *Open approach (49412)*
Percutaneous approach (49411)
Code first laparoscopic abdominal, pelvic or retroperitoneal procedures
N1 N 80 3.70 3.70 FUD ZZZ

49329 **Unlisted laparoscopy procedure, abdomen, peritoneum and omentum**
T 80 50 0.00 0.00 FUD YYY

49400-49436 Peritoneal and Visceral Procedures: Drainage/Insertion/Modifications/Removal

49400 **Injection of air or contrast into peritoneal cavity (separate procedure)**
74190
N1 N 2.74 3.88 FUD 000

49402 **Removal of peritoneal foreign body from peritoneal cavity**
EXCLUDES *Enterolysis (44005)*
Percutaneous or open drainage or lavage (49020, 49040, 49082-49084, 49406)
Percutaneous tunneled intraperitoneal catheter insertion without subcutaneous port (49418)
A2 T 24.34 24.34 FUD 090

⊙ 49405 **Image-guided fluid collection drainage by catheter (eg, abscess, hematoma, seroma, lymphocele, cyst); visceral (eg, kidney, liver, spleen, lung/mediastinum), percutaneous**
EXCLUDES *Open drainage (32200, 47010, 48510)*
Percutaneous cholecystostomy (47490)
Pleural drainage (32556-32557)
Pneumonostomy (32200)
Thoracentesis (32554-32555)
Code also each individual collection drained per separate catheter
Do not report with (75989, 76942, 77002-77003, 77012, 77021)
T 6.15 24.74 FUD 000

⊙ 49406 **peritoneal or retroperitoneal, percutaneous**
EXCLUDES *Diagnostic or therapeutic abdominal paracentesis (49082-49083)*
Open drainage (44900, 49020, 49040, 49062, 50020, 58805, 58822)
Percutaneous tunneled intraperitoneal catheter insertion without subcutaneous port (49418)
Peritoneal lavage or paracentesis (49082-49084)
Code also each individual collection drained per separate catheter
Do not report with (75989, 76942, 77002-77003, 77012, 77021)
T 6.16 24.73 FUD 000

⊙ 49407 **peritoneal or retroperitoneal, transvaginal or transrectal**
EXCLUDES *Open drainage (45000, 58800, 58820)*
Percutaneous pleural drainage (32556-32557)
Peritoneal drainage or lavage, open or percutaneous (49020, 49040, 49082)
Image guided percutaneous catheter drainage of soft tissue (ie, abdominal wall, neck, extremity) (10030)
Thoracentesis (32554-32555)
Code also each individual collection drained per separate catheter
Do not report with (75989, 76942, 77002-77003, 77012, 77021)
G2 T 6.56 20.90 FUD 000

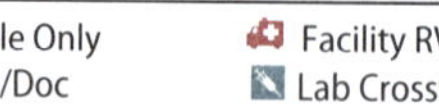

⊙ **49411 Placement of interstitial device(s) for radiation therapy guidance (eg, fiducial markers, dosimeter), percutaneous, intra-abdominal, intra-pelvic (except prostate), and/or retroperitoneum, single or multiple**

EXCLUDES *Placement (percutaneous) of interstitial device(s) for intrathoracic radiation therapy guidance (32553)*

Code also supply of device

76942, 77002, 77012, 77021

P3 X 80 5.71 14.98 FUD 000

\+ **49412 Placement of interstitial device(s) for radiation therapy guidance (eg, fiducial markers, dosimeter), open, intra-abdominal, intrapelvic, and/or retroperitoneum, including image guidance, if performed, single or multiple (List separately in addition to code for primary procedure)**

EXCLUDES *Laparoscopic approach (49327)*
Percutaneous approach (49411)

Code first open abdominal, pelvic or retroperitoneal procedure(s)

C 80 2.33 2.33 FUD ZZZ

⊙ **49418 Insertion of tunneled intraperitoneal catheter (eg, dialysis, intraperitoneal chemotherapy instillation, management of ascites), complete procedure, including imaging guidance, catheter placement, contrast injection when performed, and radiological supervision and interpretation, percutaneous**

G2 T 80 6.52 40.55 FUD 000

49419 Insertion of tunneled intraperitoneal catheter, with subcutaneous port (ie, totally implantable)

EXCLUDES *Removal of catheter/cannula (49422)*

Code also (C1788)

A2 T 12.66 12.66 FUD 090

49421 Insertion of tunneled intraperitoneal catheter for dialysis, open

EXCLUDES *Laparoscopic approach (49324)*

Code also insertion of subcutaneous extension to intraperitoneal cannula with remote chest exit site, when appropriate (49435)

G2 T 6.56 6.56 FUD 000

49422 Removal of tunneled intraperitoneal catheter

EXCLUDES *Removal temporary catheter or cannula (Use appropriate E/M code)*

A2 Q2 10.86 10.86 FUD 010

49423 Exchange of previously placed abscess or cyst drainage catheter under radiological guidance (separate procedure)

Code also drainage catheter (C1729)

75984

G2 T 80 2.09 15.50 FUD 000

49424 Contrast injection for assessment of abscess or cyst via previously placed drainage catheter or tube (separate procedure)

76080

N1 N 80 1.12 4.14 FUD 000

49425 Insertion of peritoneal-venous shunt

C 80 21.42 21.42 FUD 090

49426 Revision of peritoneal-venous shunt

EXCLUDES *Shunt patency test (78291)*

A2 T 17.63 17.63 FUD 090

49427 Injection procedure (eg, contrast media) for evaluation of previously placed peritoneal-venous shunt

75809, 78291

N1 N 80 1.31 1.31 FUD 000

49428 Ligation of peritoneal-venous shunt

C 12.28 12.28 FUD 010

49429 Removal of peritoneal-venous shunt

G2 Q2 13.05 13.05 FUD 010

\+ **49435 Insertion of subcutaneous extension to intraperitoneal cannula or catheter with remote chest exit site (List separately in addition to code for primary procedure)**

Code first permanent insertion of intraperitoneal catheter/cannula (49324, 49421)

G2 T 80 3.42 3.42 FUD ZZZ

49436 Delayed creation of exit site from embedded subcutaneous segment of intraperitoneal cannula or catheter

G2 T 80 5.31 5.31 FUD 010

49440-49442 Insertion of Percutaneous Gastrointestinal Tube

Do not report with (43752)

⊙ **49440 Insertion of gastrostomy tube, percutaneous, under fluoroscopic guidance including contrast injection(s), image documentation and report**

INCLUDES Needle placement with fluoroscopic guidance (77002)

Code also gastrostomy to gastro-jejunostomy tube conversion (49446) with initial gastrostomy tube insertion, when performed

G2 T 80 PQ 6.51 29.67 FUD 010

⊙ **49441 Insertion of duodenostomy or jejunostomy tube, percutaneous, under fluoroscopic guidance including contrast injection(s), image documentation and report**

EXCLUDES *Gastrostomy tube to gastrojejunostomy tube conversion (49446)*

G2 T 80 PQ 7.39 33.45 FUD 010

⊙ **49442 Insertion of cecostomy or other colonic tube, percutaneous, under fluoroscopic guidance including contrast injection(s), image documentation and report**

G2 T 80 PQ 6.39 27.10 FUD 010

49446 Percutaneous Conversion: Gastrostomy to Gastro-jejunostomy Tube

EXCLUDES *Code also initial gastrostomy tube insertion (49440) when conversion is performed at the same time*

⊙ **49446 Conversion of gastrostomy tube to gastro-jejunostomy tube, percutaneous, under fluoroscopic guidance including contrast injection(s), image documentation and report**

G2 T 80 PQ 4.74 28.37 FUD 000

49450-49452 Replacement Gastrointestinal Tube

EXCLUDES *Placement of new tube whether gastrostomy, jejunostomy, duodenostomy, gastro-jejunostomy, or cecostomy at different percutaneous site (49440-49442)*

49450 Replacement of gastrostomy or cecostomy (or other colonic) tube, percutaneous, under fluoroscopic guidance including contrast injection(s), image documentation and report

EXCLUDES *Change of gastrostomy tube, percutaneous, without imaging or endoscopic guidance (43760)*

G2 T 80 PQ 1.94 18.91 FUD 000

49451 Replacement of duodenostomy or jejunostomy tube, percutaneous, under fluoroscopic guidance including contrast injection(s), image documentation and report

G2 T 80 PQ 2.66 20.73 FUD 000

49452 Replacement of gastro-jejunostomy tube, percutaneous, under fluoroscopic guidance including contrast injection(s), image documentation and report

G2 T 80 PQ 4.09 25.57 FUD 000

49460-49465 Removal of Obstruction/Injection for Contrast Through Gastrointestinal Tube

49460 Mechanical removal of obstructive material from gastrostomy, duodenostomy, jejunostomy, gastro-jejunostomy, or cecostomy (or other colonic) tube, any method, under fluoroscopic guidance including contrast injection(s), if performed, image documentation and report

Do not report with (49450-49452, 49465)

G2 T 80 PQ 1.40 20.90 FUD 000

49465 Contrast injection(s) for radiological evaluation of existing gastrostomy, duodenostomy, jejunostomy, gastro-jejunostomy, or cecostomy (or other colonic) tube, from a percutaneous approach including image documentation and report

Do not report with (49450-49460)

N1 Q1 80 PQ 0.89 4.75 FUD 000

49491-49492 Inguinal Hernia Repair on Premature Infant

INCLUDES Hernia repairs done on preterm infants younger than or equal to 50 weeks postconception age but younger than 6 months of age since birth
Initial repair: no previous repair required
Mesh or other prosthesis

EXCLUDES *Abdominal wall debridement (11042, 11043)*
Intra-abdominal hernia repair/reduction (44050)

Code also repair or excision of testicle(s), intestine, ovaries if performed (44120, 54520, 58940)

49491 Repair, initial inguinal hernia, preterm infant (younger than 37 weeks gestation at birth), performed from birth up to 50 weeks postconception age, with or without hydrocelectomy; reducible A

T 80 50 63 22.52 22.52 FUD 090

49492 incarcerated or strangulated A

T 80 50 63 26.83 26.83 FUD 090

49495-49557 Hernia Repair: Femoral/Inguinal/Lumbar

INCLUDES Initial repair: no previous repair required
Mesh or other prosthesis
Recurrent repair: required previous repair(s)

EXCLUDES *Abdominal wall debridement (11042, 11043)*
Intra-abdominal hernia repair/reduction (44050)

Code also repair or excision of testicle(s), intestine, ovaries if performed (44120, 54520, 58940)

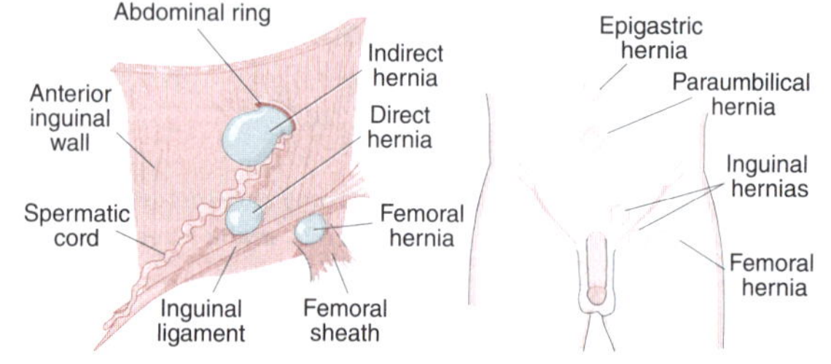

A hernia is a protrusion, usually through an abdominal wall containment

49495 Repair, initial inguinal hernia, full term infant younger than age 6 months, or preterm infant older than 50 weeks postconception age and younger than age 6 months at the time of surgery, with or without hydrocelectomy; reducible A

INCLUDES Hernia repairs done on preterm infants older than 50 weeks postconception age and younger than 6 months

A2 T 80 50 63 11.33 11.33 FUD 090

49496 incarcerated or strangulated A

INCLUDES Hernia repairs done on preterm infants older than 50 weeks postconception age and younger than 6 months

A2 T 80 50 63 17.34 17.34 FUD 090

49500 Repair initial inguinal hernia, age 6 months to younger than 5 years, with or without hydrocelectomy; reducible A

INCLUDES Repairs performed on patients 6 months to younger than 5 years old

A2 T 80 50 10.80 10.80 FUD 090

49501 incarcerated or strangulated A

INCLUDES Repairs performed on patients 6 months to younger than 5 years old

A2 T 80 50 17.16 17.16 FUD 090

49505 Repair initial inguinal hernia, age 5 years or older; reducible A

INCLUDES MacEwen hernia repair

Code also when performed:
Excision of hydrocele (55040)
Excision of spermatocele (54840)
Simple orchiectomy (54520)

A2 T 80 50 14.77 14.77 FUD 090

49507 incarcerated or strangulated A

Code also when performed:
Excision of hydrocele (55040)
Excision of spermatocele (54840)
Simple orchiectomy (54520)

A2 T 80 50 16.63 16.63 FUD 090

49520 Repair recurrent inguinal hernia, any age; reducible

A2 T 80 50 17.93 17.93 FUD 090

49521 incarcerated or strangulated

A2 T 80 50 20.32 20.32 FUD 090

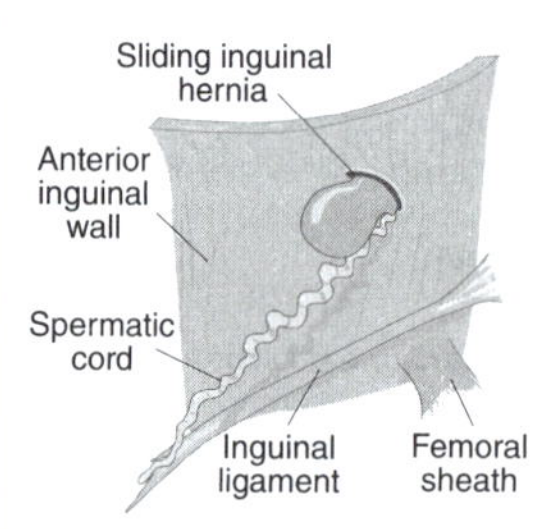

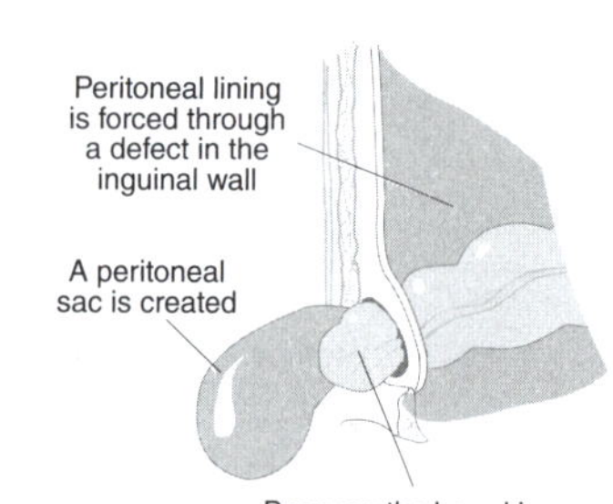

49525 Repair inguinal hernia, sliding, any age

EXCLUDES *Inguinal hernia repair, incarcerated/strangulated (49496, 49501, 49507, 49521)*

A2 T 80 50 16.26 16.26 FUD 090

49540 Repair lumbar hernia

A2 T 80 50 19.11 19.11 FUD 090

49550 Repair initial femoral hernia, any age; reducible

A2 T 80 50 16.32 16.32 FUD 090

49553 incarcerated or strangulated

A2 T 80 50 17.93 17.93 FUD 090

49555 Repair recurrent femoral hernia; reducible

A2 T 80 50 16.90 16.90 FUD 090

49557 incarcerated or strangulated

A2 T 80 50 20.54 20.54 FUD 090

49560-49568 Hernia Repair: Incisional/Ventral

INCLUDES Initial repair: no previous repair required
Recurrent repair: required previous repair(s)

EXCLUDES *Abdominal wall debridement (11042, 11043)*
Intra-abdominal hernia repair/reduction (44050)

Code also repair or excision of testicle(s), intestine, ovaries if performed (44120, 54520, 58940)

49560 Repair initial incisional or ventral hernia; reducible
Code also implantation of mesh or other prosthesis if performed (49568)
A2 T 80 50 PQ 20.95 20.95 FUD 090

49561 incarcerated or strangulated
Code also implantation of mesh or other prosthesis if performed (49568)
A2 T 80 50 PQ 26.45 26.45 FUD 090

49565 Repair recurrent incisional or ventral hernia; reducible
Code also implantation of mesh or other prosthesis if performed (49568)
A2 T 80 50 PQ 21.87 21.87 FUD 090

49566 incarcerated or strangulated
Code also implantation of mesh or other prosthesis if performed (49568)
A2 T 80 50 PQ 26.74 26.74 FUD 090

\+ 49568 Implantation of mesh or other prosthesis for open incisional or ventral hernia repair or mesh for closure of debridement for necrotizing soft tissue infection (List separately in addition to code for the incisional or ventral hernia repair)
Code first (11004-11006, 49560-49566)
N1 N 80 PQ 7.63 7.63 FUD ZZZ

49570-49590 Hernia Repair: Epigastric/Lateral Ventral/Umbilical

INCLUDES Mesh or other prosthesis

EXCLUDES *Abdominal wall debridement (11042, 11043)*
Intra-abdominal hernia repair/reduction (44050)

Code also repair or excision of testicle(s), intestine, ovaries if performed (44120, 54520, 58940)

49570 Repair epigastric hernia (eg, preperitoneal fat); reducible (separate procedure)
A2 T 80 50 PQ 11.83 11.83 FUD 090

49572 incarcerated or strangulated
A2 T 80 50 14.64 14.64 FUD 090

49580 Repair umbilical hernia, younger than age 5 years; reducible A
A2 T 80 9.43 9.43 FUD 090

49582 incarcerated or strangulated A
A2 T 80 13.69 13.69 FUD 090

49585 Repair umbilical hernia, age 5 years or older; reducible A
INCLUDES Mayo hernia repair
A2 T 80 12.61 12.61 FUD 090

49587 incarcerated or strangulated A
A2 T 80 13.50 13.50 FUD 090

49590 Repair spigelian hernia
A2 T 80 50 16.29 16.29 FUD 090

49600-49611 Repair Birth Defect Abdominal Wall: Omphalocele/Gastroschisis

INCLUDES Mesh or other prosthesis

EXCLUDES *Abdominal wall debridement (11042, 11043)*
Intra-abdominal hernia repair/reduction (44050)
Repair of:
Diaphragmatic or hiatal hernia (39503, 43332-43337)
Omentum (49999)

49600 Repair of small omphalocele, with primary closure
A2 T 80 63 20.72 20.72 FUD 090

49605 Repair of large omphalocele or gastroschisis; with or without prosthesis
C 80 63 140.44 140.44 FUD 090

49606 with removal of prosthesis, final reduction and closure, in operating room
C 80 63 32.18 32.18 FUD 090

49610 Repair of omphalocele (Gross type operation); first stage
C 80 63 19.50 19.50 FUD 090

49611 second stage
C 80 63 15.89 15.89 FUD 090

49650-49659 Laparoscopic Hernia Repair

INCLUDES Diagnostic laparoscopy

49650 Laparoscopy, surgical; repair initial inguinal hernia
A2 T 80 50 12.16 12.16 FUD 090

49651 repair recurrent inguinal hernia
A2 T 80 50 15.82 15.82 FUD 090

49652 Laparoscopy, surgical, repair, ventral, umbilical, spigelian or epigastric hernia (includes mesh insertion, when performed); reducible
Do not report with (44180, 49568)
G2 T 80 50 19.54 19.54 FUD 090

49653 incarcerated or strangulated
Do not report with (44180, 49568)
G2 T 80 50 24.41 24.41 FUD 090

49654 Laparoscopy, surgical, repair, incisional hernia (includes mesh insertion, when performed); reducible
Do not report with (44180, 49568)
G2 T 80 50 22.20 22.20 FUD 090

49655 incarcerated or strangulated
Do not report with (44180, 49568)
G2 T 80 50 27.11 27.11 FUD 090

49656 Laparoscopy, surgical, repair, recurrent incisional hernia (includes mesh insertion, when performed); reducible
Do not report with (44180, 49568)
G2 T 80 50 24.11 24.11 FUD 090

49657 incarcerated or strangulated
Do not report with (44180, 49568)
G2 T 80 50 34.61 34.61 FUD 090

49659 Unlisted laparoscopy procedure, hernioplasty, herniorrhaphy, herniotomy
T 80 50 0.00 0.00 FUD YYY

49900 Surgical Repair Abdominal Wall

EXCLUDES *Abdominal wall debridement (11042, 11043)*
Suture of ruptured diaphragm (39540-39541)

49900 Suture, secondary, of abdominal wall for evisceration or dehiscence
C 80 23.20 23.20 FUD 090

49904-49999 Harvesting of Omental Flap

49904 Omental flap, extra-abdominal (eg, for reconstruction of sternal and chest wall defects)
INCLUDES Harvest and transfer
EXCLUDES *Omental flap harvest by second surgeon: both surgeons code 49904 with modifier 62*
C 41.30 41.30 FUD 090

\+ 49905 Omental flap, intra-abdominal (List separately in addition to code for primary procedure)
Code first primary procedure
Do not report with (44700)
C 80 10.09 10.09 FUD ZZZ

49906 Free omental flap with microvascular anastomosis
INCLUDES Operating microscope (69990)
C 0.00 0.00 FUD 090

49999 Unlisted procedure, abdomen, peritoneum and omentum
T 0.00 0.00 FUD YYY

Digestive System

49560 — 49999

50010-50045 Kidney Procedures for Exploration or Drainage

EXCLUDES Retroperitoneal
Abscess drainage (49060)
Exploration (49010)
Tumor/cyst excision (49203-49205)

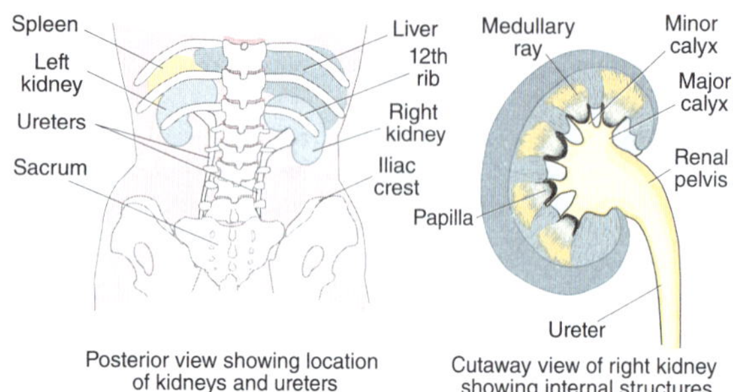

Posterior view showing location of kidneys and ureters

Cutaway view of right kidney showing internal structures

50010 **Renal exploration, not necessitating other specific procedures**
EXCLUDES Laparoscopic ablation of mass lesions of kidney (50542)
C 80 50 21.08 21.08 FUD 090

50020 **Drainage of perirenal or renal abscess, open**
T PQ 29.31 29.31 FUD 090

50040 **Nephrostomy, nephrotomy with drainage**
C 50 26.28 26.28 FUD 090

50045 **Nephrotomy, with exploration**
EXCLUDES Renal endoscopy through nephrotomy (50570-50580)
C 80 50 26.42 26.42 FUD 090

50060-50081 Treatment of Kidney Stones

CMS 100-3,230.1 Treatment of Kidney Stones

EXCLUDES Retroperitoneal:
Abscess drainage (49060)
Exploration (49010)
Tumor/cyst excision (49203-49205)

50060 **Nephrolithotomy; removal of calculus**
C 80 50 32.31 32.31 FUD 090

50065 **secondary surgical operation for calculus**
C 80 50 34.30 34.30 FUD 090

50070 **complicated by congenital kidney abnormality**
C 80 50 33.63 33.63 FUD 090

50075 **removal of large staghorn calculus filling renal pelvis and calyces (including anatrophic pyelolithotomy)**
C 80 50 41.37 41.37 FUD 090

50080 **Percutaneous nephrostolithotomy or pyelostolithotomy, with or without dilation, endoscopy, lithotripsy, stenting, or basket extraction; up to 2 cm**
EXCLUDES Nephrostomy without nephrostolithotomy (50040, 50395, 52334)
76000, 76001
62 T 50 24.68 24.68 FUD 090

50081 **over 2 cm**
EXCLUDES Nephrostomy without nephrostolithotomy (50040, 50395, 52334)
76000, 76001
62 T 80 50 36.23 36.23 FUD 090

50100 Repair of Anomalous Vessels of the Kidney

EXCLUDES Retroperitoneal:
Abscess drainage (49060)
Exploration (49010)
Tumor/cyst excision (49203-49205)

50100 **Transection or repositioning of aberrant renal vessels (separate procedure)**
C 80 50 30.64 30.64 FUD 090

50120-50135 Procedures of Renal Pelvis

EXCLUDES Retroperitoneal:
Abscess drainage (49060)
Exploration (49010)
Tumor/cyst excision (49203-49205)

50120 **Pyelotomy; with exploration**
INCLUDES Gol-Vernet pyelotomy
EXCLUDES Renal endoscopy through pyelotomy (50570-50580)
C 80 50 26.91 26.91 FUD 090

50125 **with drainage, pyelostomy**
C 80 50 27.85 27.85 FUD 090

50130 **with removal of calculus (pyelolithotomy, pelviolithotomy, including coagulum pyelolithotomy)**
C 80 50 29.28 29.28 FUD 090

50135 **complicated (eg, secondary operation, congenital kidney abnormality)**
C 80 50 31.81 31.81 FUD 090

50200-50205 Biopsy of Kidney

CMS 100-3,190.4 Electron Microscope

EXCLUDES Laparoscopic renal mass lesion ablation (50542)
Retroperitoneal tumor/cyst excision (49203-49205)

⊙ **50200** **Renal biopsy; percutaneous, by trocar or needle**
EXCLUDES Fine needle aspiration (10022)
76942, 77002, 77012, 77021
88172, 88173
A2 T 50 PQ 4.15 16.57 FUD 000

50205 **by surgical exposure of kidney**
C 80 50 PQ 21.44 21.44 FUD 090

50220-50240 Nephrectomy Procedures

EXCLUDES Laparoscopic renal mass lesion ablation (50542)
Retroperitoneal tumor/cyst excision (49203-49205)

50220 **Nephrectomy, including partial ureterectomy, any open approach including rib resection;**
C 80 50 PQ 29.66 29.66 FUD 090

50225 **complicated because of previous surgery on same kidney**
C 80 50 PQ 34.03 34.03 FUD 090

50230 **radical, with regional lymphadenectomy and/or vena caval thrombectomy**
EXCLUDES Vena caval resection with reconstruction (37799)
C 80 50 PQ 36.36 36.36 FUD 090

50234 **Nephrectomy with total ureterectomy and bladder cuff; through same incision**
C 80 50 PQ 36.91 36.91 FUD 090

50236 **through separate incision**
C 80 50 PQ 41.58 41.58 FUD 090

50240 **Nephrectomy, partial**
EXCLUDES Laparoscopic partial nephrectomy (50543)
C 80 50 PQ 37.56 37.56 FUD 090

50250-50290 Open Removal Kidney Lesions

50250 Ablation, open, 1 or more renal mass lesion(s), cryosurgical, including intraoperative ultrasound guidance and monitoring, if performed

EXCLUDES *Laparoscopic renal mass lesion ablation (50542)*
Open destruction or excision intra-abdominal tumors (49203-49205)
Percutaneous renal tumor ablation (50592-50593)

C 80 34.51 34.51 FUD 090

50280 Excision or unroofing of cyst(s) of kidney

EXCLUDES *Renal cyst laparoscopic ablation (50541)*

C 80 50 27.09 27.09 FUD 090

50290 Excision of perinephric cyst

EXCLUDES *Open destruction or excision intra-abdominal tumors (49203-49205)*

C 80 25.47 25.47 FUD 090

50300-50380 Kidney Transplant Procedures

CMS 100-3,20.3 Thoracic Duct Drainage (TDD) in Renal Transplants
CMS 100-3,110.16 Nonselective (Random) Transfusions and Living-Related Donor Specific Transfusions (DST) in Kidney Transplantation
CMS 100-3,190.1 Histocompatibility Testing
CMS 100-3,260.7 Lymphocyte Immune Globulin, Anti-Thymocyte Globulin (Equine)
CMS 100-4,3,90.1 Kidney Transplant - General
CMS 100-4,3,90.1.1 Standard Kidney Acquisition Charge
CMS 100-4,3,90.1.2 Billing for Kidney Transplant and Acquisition Services

EXCLUDES *Dialysis procedures (90935-90999)*
Lymphocele drainage to peritoneal cavity performed laparoscopically (49323)

50300 Donor nephrectomy (including cold preservation); from cadaver donor, unilateral or bilateral

INCLUDES Graft:
Cold preservation
Harvesting

C 0.00 0.00 FUD XXX

50320 open, from living donor

INCLUDES Donor care
Graft:
Cold preservation
Harvesting

EXCLUDES *Donor nephrectomy performed laparoscopically (50547)*

C 80 50 PQ 40.52 40.52 FUD 090

50323 Backbench standard preparation of cadaver donor renal allograft prior to transplantation, including dissection and removal of perinephric fat, diaphragmatic and retroperitoneal attachments, excision of adrenal gland, and preparation of ureter(s), renal vein(s), and renal artery(s), ligating branches, as necessary

Do not report with (60540, 60545)

C 80 0.00 0.00 FUD XXX

50325 Backbench standard preparation of living donor renal allograft (open or laparoscopic) prior to transplantation, including dissection and removal of perinephric fat and preparation of ureter(s), renal vein(s), and renal artery(s), ligating branches, as necessary

C 80 0.00 0.00 FUD XXX

50327 Backbench reconstruction of cadaver or living donor renal allograft prior to transplantation; venous anastomosis, each

C 80 6.15 6.15 FUD XXX

50328 arterial anastomosis, each

C 80 5.39 5.39 FUD XXX

50329 ureteral anastomosis, each

C 80 4.98 4.98 FUD XXX

50340 Recipient nephrectomy (separate procedure)

C 80 50 PQ 26.91 26.91 FUD 090

50360 Renal allotransplantation, implantation of graft; without recipient nephrectomy

INCLUDES Allograft transplantation
Recipient care

Code also backbench work (50323, 50325, 50327-50329)
Code also donor nephrectomy (cadaver or living donor) (50300, 50320, 50547)

C 80 PQ 68.65 68.65 FUD 090

50365 with recipient nephrectomy

INCLUDES Allograft transplantation
Recipient care

C 80 50 PQ 80.60 80.60 FUD 090

50370 Removal of transplanted renal allograft

C 80 PQ 34.03 34.03 FUD 090

50380 Renal autotransplantation, reimplantation of kidney

INCLUDES Reimplantation of autograft

EXCLUDES *Secondary backbench procedures:*
Nephrolithotomy (50060-50075)
Partial nephrectomy (50240, 50543)

C 80 PQ 56.80 56.80 FUD 090

50382-50386 Removal With/Without Replacement Internal Ureteral Stent

INCLUDES Radiological supervision and interpretation

⊙ **50382 Removal (via snare/capture) and replacement of internally dwelling ureteral stent via percutaneous approach, including radiological supervision and interpretation**

EXCLUDES *Removal and replacement of an internally dwelling ureteral stent using a transurethral approach (50385)*

Do not report with (50395)

G2 T 50 PQ 7.86 33.62 FUD 000

⊙ **50384 Removal (via snare/capture) of internally dwelling ureteral stent via percutaneous approach, including radiological supervision and interpretation**

EXCLUDES *Removal of an internally dwelling ureteral stent using a transurethral approach (50386)*

Do not report with (50395)

G2 Q2 50 PQ 7.19 26.85 FUD 000

⊙ **50385 Removal (via snare/capture) and replacement of internally dwelling ureteral stent via transurethral approach, without use of cystoscopy, including radiological supervision and interpretation**

G2 T 80 50 PQ 6.63 32.12 FUD 000

⊙ **50386 Removal (via snare/capture) of internally dwelling ureteral stent via transurethral approach, without use of cystoscopy, including radiological supervision and interpretation**

P2 Q2 80 50 PQ 5.03 20.78 FUD 000

50387 Remove/Replace Accessible Ureteral Stent

CMS 100-4,4,61.2 Requirements for Specific Procedures to be Reported With Device Codes

EXCLUDES *Removal and replacement of ureteral stent through ureterostomy tube or ileal conduit (50688)*
Removal without replacement of externally accessible ureteral stent without fluoroscopic guidance, report with appropriate evaluation and management service code

⊙ **50387 Removal and replacement of externally accessible transnephric ureteral stent (eg, external/internal stent) requiring fluoroscopic guidance, including radiological supervision and interpretation**

Code also (C1875, C1877, C2617, C2625)

G2 T 80 50 PQ 2.86 15.55 FUD 000

50389-50398 Percutaneous and Injection Procedures With/Without Indwelling Tube/Catheter Access

50389 **Removal of nephrostomy tube, requiring fluoroscopic guidance (eg, with concurrent indwelling ureteral stent)**

EXCLUDES *Nephrostomy tube removal without fluoroscopic guidance, report with appropriate evaluation and management code*

G2 Q2 50 PQ 1.58 8.51 FUD 000

50390 **Aspiration and/or injection of renal cyst or pelvis by needle, percutaneous**

74425, 74470, 76942, 77002, 77012, 77021

88172-88173

A2 T 50 1.58 2.80 2.80 FUD 000

50391 **Instillation(s) of therapeutic agent into renal pelvis and/or ureter through established nephrostomy, pyelostomy or ureterostomy tube (eg, anticarcinogenic or antifungal agent)**

Code also therapeutic agent

P3 T 50 2.81 3.46 FUD 000

50392 **Introduction of intracatheter or catheter into renal pelvis for drainage and/or injection, percutaneous**

74475, 76942, 77012

A2 T 50 5.17 5.17 FUD 000

50393 **Introduction of ureteral catheter or stent into ureter through renal pelvis for drainage and/or injection, percutaneous**

74480, 76942, 77002, 77012

A2 T 50 6.27 6.27 FUD 000

50394 **Injection procedure for pyelography (as nephrostogram, pyelostogram, antegrade pyeloureterograms) through nephrostomy or pyelostomy tube, or indwelling ureteral catheter**

74425

N1 N 50 1.44 2.88 FUD 000

50395 **Introduction of guide into renal pelvis and/or ureter with dilation to establish nephrostomy tract, percutaneous**

EXCLUDES *Percutaneous nephrostolithotomy (50080, 50081)*
Renal endoscopy (50551-50561)
Retrograde percutaneous nephrostomy (52334)

Do not report with (50382, 50384)

74475, 74480, 74485

A2 T 50 5.18 5.18 FUD 000

50396 **Manometric studies through nephrostomy or pyelostomy tube, or indwelling ureteral catheter**

74425, 74475, 74480

A2 T 80 50 3.40 3.40 FUD 000

50398 **Change of nephrostomy or pyelostomy tube**

Code also (C1729)

75984

A2 T 50 2.10 14.03 FUD 000

50400-50540 Open Surgical Procedures of Kidney

50400 **Pyeloplasty (Foley Y-pyeloplasty), plastic operation on renal pelvis, with or without plastic operation on ureter, nephropexy, nephrostomy, pyelostomy, or ureteral splinting; simple**

EXCLUDES *Laparoscopic pyeloplasty (50544)*

C 80 50 32.83 32.83 FUD 090

50405 **complicated (congenital kidney abnormality, secondary pyeloplasty, solitary kidney, calycoplasty)**

EXCLUDES *Laparoscopic pyeloplasty (50544)*

C 80 50 39.59 39.59 FUD 090

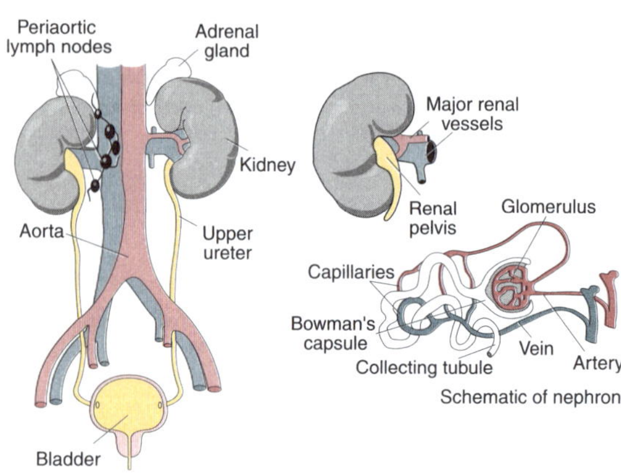

50500 **Nephrorrhaphy, suture of kidney wound or injury**

C 80 36.52 36.52 FUD 090

50520 **Closure of nephrocutaneous or pyelocutaneous fistula**

C 80 30.78 30.78 FUD 090

50525 **Closure of nephrovisceral fistula (eg, renocolic), including visceral repair; abdominal approach**

C 80 41.92 41.92 FUD 090

50526 **thoracic approach**

C 80 40.92 40.92 FUD 090

50540 **Symphysiotomy for horseshoe kidney with or without pyeloplasty and/or other plastic procedure, unilateral or bilateral (1 operation)**

C 80 32.53 32.53 FUD 090

50541-50549 Laparoscopic Surgical Procedures of the Kidney

INCLUDES Diagnostic laparoscopy

EXCLUDES *Diagnostic laparoscopy (peritoneoscopy) performed as a separate procedure (49320)*
Laparoscopic drainage of lymphocele to peritoneal cavity (49323)

50541 **Laparoscopy, surgical; ablation of renal cysts**

T 80 50 26.12 26.12 FUD 090

50542 **ablation of renal mass lesion(s), including intraoperative ultrasound guidance and monitoring, when performed**

EXCLUDES *Open ablation of renal mass lesions (50250)*
Percutaneous ablation of renal tumors (50592-50593)

T 80 50 33.09 33.09 FUD 090

50543 **partial nephrectomy**

EXCLUDES *Partial nephrectomy, open approach (50240)*

T 80 50 PQ 42.25 42.25 FUD 090

50544 **pyeloplasty**

T 80 50 35.37 35.37 FUD 090

50545 **radical nephrectomy (includes removal of Gerota's fascia and surrounding fatty tissue, removal of regional lymph nodes, and adrenalectomy)**

EXCLUDES *Radical nephrectomy, open approach (50230)*

C 80 50 PQ 38.10 38.10 FUD 090

50546 **nephrectomy, including partial ureterectomy**

C 80 50 PQ 34.11 34.11 FUD 090

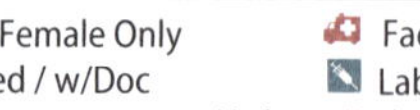

50547 **donor nephrectomy (including cold preservation), from living donor**

INCLUDES Donor care
Graft:
Cold preservation
Harvesting

EXCLUDES *Backbench reconstruction renal allograft prior to transplantation (50327-50329)*
Backbench standard preparation of living donor renal allograft prior to transplantation (50325)
Donor nephrectomy, open approach (50320)

C 80 50 PQ 45.62 45.62 FUD 090

50548 **nephrectomy with total ureterectomy**

EXCLUDES *Nephrectomy, open approach (50234, 50236)*

C 80 50 PQ 38.25 38.25 FUD 090

50549 **Unlisted laparoscopy procedure, renal**

T 80 50 0.00 0.00 FUD YYY

50551-50562 Endoscopic Procedures of Kidney via Established Nephrostomy/Pyelostomy Access

EXCLUDES *Materials and supplies (99070)*

50551 **Renal endoscopy through established nephrostomy or pyelostomy, with or without irrigation, instillation, or ureteropyelography, exclusive of radiologic service;**

A2 T 80 50 8.38 10.11 FUD 000

50553 **with ureteral catheterization, with or without dilation of ureter**

A2 T 50 8.96 10.86 FUD 000

50555 **with biopsy**

A2 T 80 50 PQ 9.71 11.59 FUD 000

50557 **with fulguration and/or incision, with or without biopsy**

A2 T 80 50 PQ 9.83 11.78 FUD 000

50561 **with removal of foreign body or calculus**

A2 T 80 50 11.24 13.40 FUD 000

50562 **with resection of tumor**

G2 T 80 16.52 16.52 FUD 090

50570-50580 Endoscopic Procedures of Kidney via Nephrotomy/Pyelotomy Access

EXCLUDES *Materials and supplies (99070)*
Nephrotomy (50045)
Pyelotomy (50120)

50570 **Renal endoscopy through nephrotomy or pyelotomy, with or without irrigation, instillation, or ureteropyelography, exclusive of radiologic service;**

G2 T 80 50 13.97 13.97 FUD 000

50572 **with ureteral catheterization, with or without dilation of ureter**

G2 T 80 50 15.14 15.14 FUD 000

50574 **with biopsy**

G2 T 80 50 PQ 16.10 16.10 FUD 000

50575 **with endopyelotomy (includes cystoscopy, ureteroscopy, dilation of ureter and ureteral pelvic junction, incision of ureteral pelvic junction and insertion of endopyelotomy stent)**

G2 T 50 PQ 20.34 20.34 FUD 000

50576 **with fulguration and/or incision, with or without biopsy**

G2 T 80 50 PQ 16.04 16.04 FUD 000

50580 **with removal of foreign body or calculus**

G2 T 80 50 17.32 17.32 FUD 000

50590-50593 Noninvasive and Minimally Invasive Procedures of the Kidney

CMS 100-3,230.1 Treatment of Kidney Stones

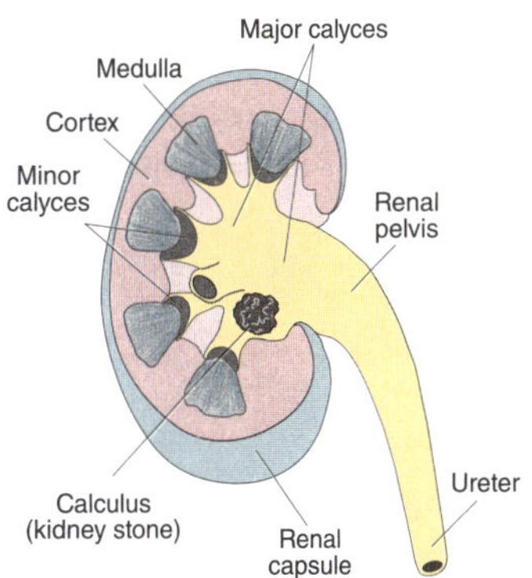

50590 **Lithotripsy, extracorporeal shock wave**

G2 T 50 PQ 16.09 20.23 FUD 090

⊙ **50592** **Ablation, 1 or more renal tumor(s), percutaneous, unilateral, radiofrequency**

76940, 77013, 77022

G2 T 50 10.48 88.10 FUD 010

⊙ **50593** **Ablation, renal tumor(s), unilateral, percutaneous, cryotherapy**

76940, 77013, 77022

G2 T 80 50 13.87 129.27 FUD 010

50600-50940 Open and Injection Procedures of Ureter

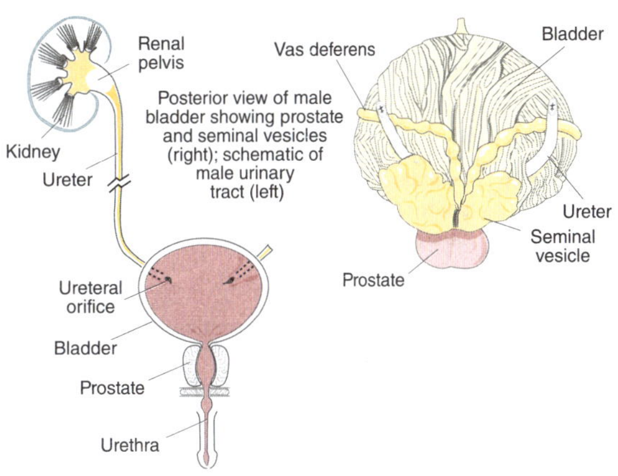

50600 **Ureterotomy with exploration or drainage (separate procedure)**

Code also ureteral endoscopy through ureterotomy when procedures constitute a significant identifiable service (50970-50980)

C 80 50 26.63 26.63 FUD 090

50605 **Ureterotomy for insertion of indwelling stent, all types**

C 80 50 27.72 27.72 FUD 090

50610 **Ureterolithotomy; upper one-third of ureter**

EXCLUDES *Cystotomy with calculus basket extraction of ureteral calculus (51065)*
Transvesical ureterolithotomy (51060)
Ureteral calculus manipulation/extraction performed endoscopically (50080-50081, 50561, 50961, 50980, 52320-52330, 52352-52353, [52356])
Ureterolithotomy performed laparoscopically (50945)

C 80 50 26.81 26.81 FUD 090

50620 **middle one-third of ureter**

EXCLUDES Cystotomy with calculus basket extraction of ureteral calculus (51065)
Transvesical ureterolithotomy (51060)
Ureteral calculus manipulation/extraction performed endoscopically (50080-50081, 50561, 50961, 50980, 52320-52330, 52352-52353, [52356])
Ureterolithotomy performed laparoscopically (50945)

C 80 50 25.64 25.64 FUD 090

50630 **lower one-third of ureter**

EXCLUDES Cystotomy with calculus basket extraction of ureteral calculus (51065)
Transvesical ureterolithotomy (51060)
Ureteral calculus manipulation/extraction performed endoscopically (50080-50081, 50561, 50961, 50980, 52320-52330, 52352-52353, [52356])
Ureterolithotomy performed laparoscopically (50945)

C 80 50 25.32 25.32 FUD 090

50650 **Ureterectomy, with bladder cuff (separate procedure)**

EXCLUDES Ureterocele (51535, 52300)

C 80 50 29.37 29.37 FUD 090

50660 **Ureterectomy, total, ectopic ureter, combination abdominal, vaginal and/or perineal approach**

EXCLUDES Ureterocele (51535, 52300)

C 80 32.43 32.43 FUD 090

50684 **Injection procedure for ureterography or ureteropyelography through ureterostomy or indwelling ureteral catheter**

74425

N1 N 50 1.44 2.97 FUD 000

50686 **Manometric studies through ureterostomy or indwelling ureteral catheter**

P2 T 80 2.68 4.32 FUD 000

50688 **Change of ureterostomy tube or externally accessible ureteral stent via ileal conduit**

Code also (C1729, C1758, C2617, C2625)

75984

A2 T 2.29 2.29 FUD 010

50690 **Injection procedure for visualization of ileal conduit and/or ureteropyelography, exclusive of radiologic service**

74425

N1 N 2.02 2.78 FUD 000

50700 **Ureteroplasty, plastic operation on ureter (eg, stricture)**

C 80 50 26.34 26.34 FUD 090

50715 **Ureterolysis, with or without repositioning of ureter for retroperitoneal fibrosis**

C 80 50 PQ 34.26 34.26 FUD 090

50722 **Ureterolysis for ovarian vein syndrome** ♀

C 80 PQ 30.19 30.19 FUD 090

50725 **Ureterolysis for retrocaval ureter, with reanastomosis of upper urinary tract or vena cava**

C 80 PQ 31.25 31.25 FUD 090

50727 **Revision of urinary-cutaneous anastomosis (any type urostomy);**

G2 T 80 PQ 14.32 14.32 FUD 090

50728 **with repair of fascial defect and hernia**

C 80 PQ 19.79 19.79 FUD 090

50740 **Ureteropyelostomy, anastomosis of ureter and renal pelvis**

C 80 50 34.74 34.74 FUD 090

50750 **Ureterocalycostomy, anastomosis of ureter to renal calyx**

C 80 50 32.71 32.71 FUD 090

50760 **Ureteroureterostomy**

C 80 50 PQ 32.08 32.08 FUD 090

50770 **Transureteroureterostomy, anastomosis of ureter to contralateral ureter**

C 80 PQ 32.71 32.71 FUD 090

50780 **Ureteroneocystostomy; anastomosis of single ureter to bladder**

INCLUDES Minor procedures to prevent vesicoureteral reflux

EXCLUDES Cystourethroplasty with ureteroneocystostomy (51820)

C 80 50 PQ 31.45 31.45 FUD 090

50782 **anastomosis of duplicated ureter to bladder**

INCLUDES Minor procedures to prevent vesicoureteral reflux

C 80 50 PQ 29.79 29.79 FUD 090

50783 **with extensive ureteral tailoring**

INCLUDES Minor procedures to prevent vesicoureteral reflux

C 80 50 PQ 31.97 31.97 FUD 090

50785 **with vesico-psoas hitch or bladder flap**

INCLUDES Minor procedures to prevent vesicoureteral reflux

C 80 50 PQ 34.34 34.34 FUD 090

50800 **Ureteroenterostomy, direct anastomosis of ureter to intestine**

EXCLUDES Cystectomy with ureterosigmoidostomy/ureteroileal conduit (51580-51595)

C 80 50 PQ 26.26 26.26 FUD 090

50810 **Ureterosigmoidostomy, with creation of sigmoid bladder and establishment of abdominal or perineal colostomy, including intestine anastomosis**

EXCLUDES Cystectomy with ureterosigmoidostomy/ureteroileal conduit (51580-51595)

C 80 PQ 37.93 37.93 FUD 090

50815 **Ureterocolon conduit, including intestine anastomosis**

EXCLUDES Cystectomy with ureterosigmoidostomy/ureteroileal conduit (51580-51595)

C 80 50 PQ 34.68 34.68 FUD 090

50820 **Ureteroileal conduit (ileal bladder), including intestine anastomosis (Bricker operation)**

EXCLUDES Cystectomy with ureterosigmoidostomy/ureteroileal conduit (51580-51595)

C 80 50 PQ 37.42 37.42 FUD 090

50825 **Continent diversion, including intestine anastomosis using any segment of small and/or large intestine (Kock pouch or Camey enterocystoplasty)**

C 80 47.03 47.03 FUD 090

50830 **Urinary undiversion (eg, taking down of ureteroileal conduit, ureterosigmoidostomy or ureteroenterostomy with ureteroureterostomy or ureteroneocystostomy)**

C 80 51.17 51.17 FUD 090

50840 **Replacement of all or part of ureter by intestine segment, including intestine anastomosis**

C 80 50 34.86 34.86 FUD 090

50845 **Cutaneous appendico-vesicostomy**

INCLUDES Mitrofanoff operation

C 80 35.41 35.41 FUD 090

50860 **Ureterostomy, transplantation of ureter to skin**

C 80 50 26.80 26.80 FUD 090

50900 **Ureterorrhaphy, suture of ureter (separate procedure)**

C 80 50 24.12 24.12 FUD 090

50920 **Closure of ureterocutaneous fistula**

C 80 24.99 24.99 FUD 090

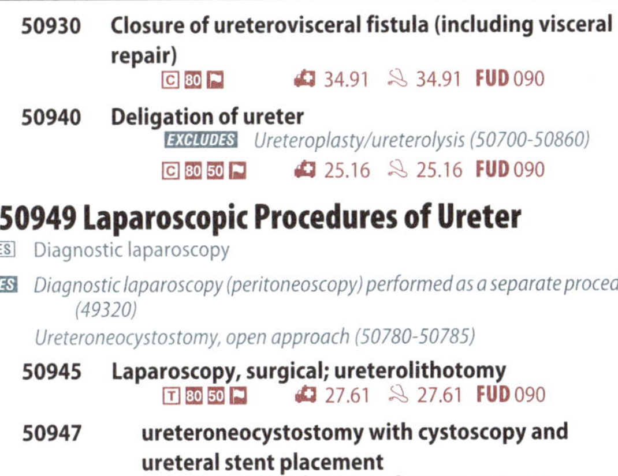

50930 Closure of ureterovisceral fistula (including visceral repair)
C 80 — 34.91 — 34.91 FUD 090

50940 Deligation of ureter
EXCLUDES *Ureteroplasty/ureterolysis (50700-50860)*
C 80 50 — 25.16 — 25.16 FUD 090

50945-50949 Laparoscopic Procedures of Ureter

INCLUDES Diagnostic laparoscopy

EXCLUDES *Diagnostic laparoscopy (peritoneoscopy) performed as a separate procedure (49320)*
Ureteroneocystostomy, open approach (50780-50785)

50945 Laparoscopy, surgical; ureterolithotomy
T 80 50 — 27.61 — 27.61 FUD 090

50947 ureteroneocystostomy with cystoscopy and ureteral stent placement
A2 T 80 50 PQ — 39.36 — 39.36 FUD 090

50948 ureteroneocystostomy without cystoscopy and ureteral stent placement
A2 T 80 50 PQ — 36.18 — 36.18 FUD 090

50949 Unlisted laparoscopy procedure, ureter
T 80 50 — 0.00 — 0.00 FUD YYY

50951-50961 Endoscopic Procedures of Ureter via Established Ureterostomy Access

50951 Ureteral endoscopy through established ureterostomy, with or without irrigation, instillation, or ureteropyelography, exclusive of radiologic service;
A2 T 80 50 — 8.72 — 10.56 FUD 000

50953 with ureteral catheterization, with or without dilation of ureter
A2 T 80 50 — 9.28 — 11.18 FUD 000

50955 with biopsy
A2 T 80 50 PQ — 10.03 — 11.96 FUD 000

50957 with fulguration and/or incision, with or without biopsy
A2 T 80 50 PQ — 10.08 — 12.07 FUD 000

50961 with removal of foreign body or calculus
A2 T 80 50 — 9.02 — 10.86 FUD 000

50970-50980 Endoscopic Procedures of Ureter via Ureterotomy

EXCLUDES *Ureterotomy (50600)*

50970 Ureteral endoscopy through ureterotomy, with or without irrigation, instillation, or ureteropyelography, exclusive of radiologic service;
A2 T 80 50 — 10.54 — 10.54 FUD 000

50972 with ureteral catheterization, with or without dilation of ureter
A2 T 80 50 — 10.19 — 10.19 FUD 000

50974 with biopsy
A2 T 80 50 PQ — 13.45 — 13.45 FUD 000

50976 with fulguration and/or incision, with or without biopsy
A2 T 80 50 PQ — 13.26 — 13.26 FUD 000

50980 with removal of foreign body or calculus
A2 T 80 50 — 10.12 — 10.12 FUD 000

51020-51080 Open Incisional Procedures of Bladder

51020 Cystotomy or cystostomy; with fulguration and/or insertion of radioactive material
A2 T 80 — 13.31 — 13.31 FUD 090

51030 with cryosurgical destruction of intravesical lesion
A2 T 80 — 13.32 — 13.32 FUD 090

51040 Cystostomy, cystotomy with drainage
A2 T 80 — 8.17 — 8.17 FUD 090

51045 Cystotomy, with insertion of ureteral catheter or stent (separate procedure)
A2 T 80 — 13.93 — 13.93 FUD 090

51050 Cystolithotomy, cystotomy with removal of calculus, without vesical neck resection
A2 T 80 — 13.38 — 13.38 FUD 090

51060 Transvesical ureterolithotomy
T 80 — 16.47 — 16.47 FUD 090

51065 Cystotomy, with calculus basket extraction and/or ultrasonic or electrohydraulic fragmentation of ureteral calculus
A2 T 80 — 16.39 — 16.39 FUD 090

51080 Drainage of perivesical or prevesical space abscess
EXCLUDES *Image-guided percutaneous catheter drainage (49406)*
A2 T 80 — 11.56 — 11.56 FUD 090

51100-51102 Bladder Aspiration Procedures

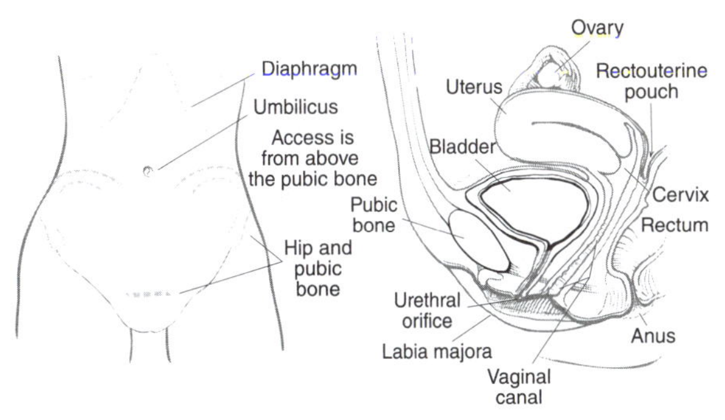

51100 Aspiration of bladder; by needle
76942, 77002, 77012
P3 T — 1.12 — 1.72 FUD 000

51101 by trocar or intracatheter
76942, 77002, 77012
P2 T — 1.50 — 3.48 FUD 000

51102 with insertion of suprapubic catheter
76942, 77002, 77012
A2 T — 4.16 — 6.41 FUD 000

51500-51597 Open Excisional Procedures of Bladder

51500 Excision of urachal cyst or sinus, with or without umbilical hernia repair
A2 T 80 — 18.03 — 18.03 FUD 090

51520 Cystotomy; for simple excision of vesical neck (separate procedure)
A2 T 80 — 16.82 — 16.82 FUD 090

51525 for excision of bladder diverticulum, single or multiple (separate procedure)
EXCLUDES *Transurethral resection (52305)*
C 80 — 24.40 — 24.40 FUD 090

51530 for excision of bladder tumor
EXCLUDES *Transurethral resection (52234-52240)*
C 80 — 22.50 — 22.50 FUD 090

51535 Cystotomy for excision, incision, or repair of ureterocele
EXCLUDES *Transurethral excision (52300)*
G2 T 80 50 — 22.07 — 22.07 FUD 090

51550 Cystectomy, partial; simple
C 80 PQ — 27.47 — 27.47 FUD 090

51555 complicated (eg, postradiation, previous surgery, difficult location)
C 80 PQ — 36.05 — 36.05 FUD 090

51565 Cystectomy, partial, with reimplantation of ureter(s) into bladder (ureteroneocystostomy)
C 80 PQ 36.70 36.70 FUD 090

51570 Cystectomy, complete; (separate procedure)
C 80 PQ 41.98 41.98 FUD 090

51575 with bilateral pelvic lymphadenectomy, including external iliac, hypogastric, and obturator nodes
C 80 PQ 51.66 51.66 FUD 090

51580 Cystectomy, complete, with ureterosigmoidostomy or ureterocutaneous transplantations;
C 80 PQ 53.80 53.80 FUD 090

51585 with bilateral pelvic lymphadenectomy, including external iliac, hypogastric, and obturator nodes
C 80 PQ 59.90 59.90 FUD 090

51590 Cystectomy, complete, with ureteroileal conduit or sigmoid bladder, including intestine anastomosis;
C 80 PQ 54.90 54.90 FUD 090

51595 with bilateral pelvic lymphadenectomy, including external iliac, hypogastric, and obturator nodes
C 80 PQ 62.18 62.18 FUD 090

51596 Cystectomy, complete, with continent diversion, any open technique, using any segment of small and/or large intestine to construct neobladder
C 80 PQ 66.76 66.76 FUD 090

51597 Pelvic exenteration, complete, for vesical, prostatic or urethral malignancy, with removal of bladder and ureteral transplantations, with or without hysterectomy and/or abdominoperineal resection of rectum and colon and colostomy, or any combination thereof
EXCLUDES *Pelvic exenteration for gynecologic malignancy (58240)*
C 80 PQ 65.31 65.31 FUD 090

51600-51720 Injection/Insertion/Instillation Procedures of Bladder

51600 Injection procedure for cystography or voiding urethrocystography
74430, 74455
N1 N 1.27 5.11 FUD 000

51605 Injection procedure and placement of chain for contrast and/or chain urethrocystography
74430
N1 N 1.08 1.08 FUD 000

51610 Injection procedure for retrograde urethrocystography
74450
N1 N 1.84 2.99 FUD 000

51700 Bladder irrigation, simple, lavage and/or instillation
P3 T 1.27 2.32 FUD 000

51701 Insertion of non-indwelling bladder catheter (eg, straight catheterization for residual urine)
EXCLUDES *Catheterization for specimen collection (P9612)*
Do not report with insertion of catheter as an inclusive component of another procedure
P3 X 0.79 1.53 FUD 000

51702 Insertion of temporary indwelling bladder catheter; simple (eg, Foley)
Do not report with (0071T-0072T)
Do not report with insertion of catheter as an inclusive component of another procedure
P3 X 0.86 1.97 FUD 000

51703 complicated (eg, altered anatomy, fractured catheter/balloon)
P3 T 2.31 3.62 FUD 000

51705 Change of cystostomy tube; simple
P3 T 1.48 2.55 FUD 000

51710 complicated
Code also (C2627)
75984
A2 T 2.25 3.58 FUD 000

51715 Endoscopic injection of implant material into the submucosal tissues of the urethra and/or bladder neck
EXCLUDES *Injection of bulking agent (submucosal) for fecal incontinence, via anoscope (0377T)*
Code also (L8603, L8604, L8606)
A2 T 80 5.70 8.12 FUD 000

51720 Bladder instillation of anticarcinogenic agent (including retention time)
Code also bacillus Calmette-Guerin vaccine (BCG) ([90586])
P3 T PQ 2.27 3.05 FUD 000

51725-51798 [51797] Uroflowmetric Evaluations

CMS 100-3,230.2 Uroflowmetric Evaluations

INCLUDES Equipment
Fees for services of technician
Medications
Supplies

Code also modifier 26 if physician/other qualified health care professional provides only interpretation of results and/or operates the equipment

51725 Simple cystometrogram (CMG) (eg, spinal manometer)
P3 T 80 5.22 5.22 FUD 000

51726 Complex cystometrogram (ie, calibrated electronic equipment);
A2 T 7.35 7.35 FUD 000

51727 with urethral pressure profile studies (ie, urethral closure pressure profile), any technique
P3 T 80 8.76 8.76 FUD 000

51728 with voiding pressure studies (ie, bladder voiding pressure), any technique
P3 T 80 8.78 8.78 FUD 000

51729 with voiding pressure studies (ie, bladder voiding pressure) and urethral pressure profile studies (ie, urethral closure pressure profile), any technique
P3 T 80 9.53 9.53 FUD 000

\+ # **51797** **Voiding pressure studies, intra-abdominal (ie, rectal, gastric, intraperitoneal) (List separately in addition to code for primary procedure)**
Code first (51728-51729)
N1 N 80 3.11 3.11 FUD ZZZ

51736 Simple uroflowmetry (UFR) (eg, stop-watch flow rate, mechanical uroflowmeter)
P3 X 80 0.43 0.43 FUD XXX

51741 Complex uroflowmetry (eg, calibrated electronic equipment)
P3 T 0.44 0.44 FUD XXX

51784 Electromyography studies (EMG) of anal or urethral sphincter, other than needle, any technique
Do not report with (51792)
P2 T 5.36 5.36 FUD 000

51785 Needle electromyography studies (EMG) of anal or urethral sphincter, any technique
A2 T 80 7.17 7.17 FUD 000

51792 Stimulus evoked response (eg, measurement of bulbocavernosus reflex latency time)
Do not report with (51784)
P2 T 80 5.88 5.88 FUD 000

51797 ***Resequenced code, See code following 51729.***

51798 **Measurement of post-voiding residual urine and/or bladder capacity by ultrasound, non-imaging**
P3 X TC 80 0.53 0.53 FUD XXX

51800-51980 Open Repairs Urinary System

51800 **Cystoplasty or cystourethroplasty, plastic operation on bladder and/or vesical neck (anterior Y-plasty, vesical fundus resection), any procedure, with or without wedge resection of posterior vesical neck**
C 80 PQ 29.60 29.60 FUD 090

51820 **Cystourethroplasty with unilateral or bilateral ureteroneocystostomy**
C 80 PQ 30.70 30.70 FUD 090

51840 **Anterior vesicourethropexy, or urethropexy (eg, Marshall-Marchetti-Krantz, Burch); simple**
EXCLUDES *Pereyra type urethropexy (57289)*
C 80 18.91 18.91 FUD 090

51841 **complicated (eg, secondary repair)**
EXCLUDES *Pereyra type urethropexy (57289)*
C 80 22.46 22.46 FUD 090

51845 **Abdomino-vaginal vesical neck suspension, with or without endoscopic control (eg, Stamey, Raz, modified Pereyra)** ♀
T 80 16.83 16.83 FUD 090

51860 **Cystorrhaphy, suture of bladder wound, injury or rupture; simple**
T 80 21.33 21.33 FUD 090

51865 **complicated**
C 80 25.48 25.48 FUD 090

51880 **Closure of cystostomy (separate procedure)**
A2 T 80 13.38 13.38 FUD 090

51900 **Closure of vesicovaginal fistula, abdominal approach** ♀
EXCLUDES *Vesicovaginal fistula closure, vaginal approach (57320-57330)*
C 80 PQ 23.55 23.55 FUD 090

51920 **Closure of vesicouterine fistula;** ♀
EXCLUDES *Enterovesical fistula closure (44660-44661)*
Rectovesical fistula closure (45800-45805)
C 80 PQ 22.91 22.91 FUD 090

51925 **with hysterectomy** ♀
EXCLUDES *Enterovesical fistula closure (44660-44661)*
Rectovesical fistula closure (45800-45805)
C 80 PQ 29.99 29.99 FUD 090

51940 **Closure, exstrophy of bladder**
EXCLUDES *Epispadias reconstruction with exstrophy of bladder (54390)*
C 80 46.25 46.25 FUD 090

51960 **Enterocystoplasty, including intestinal anastomosis**
C 80 PQ 39.54 39.54 FUD 090

51980 **Cutaneous vesicostomy**
C 80 20.21 20.21 FUD 090

51990-51999 Laparoscopic Procedures of Urinary System

INCLUDES Diagnostic laparoscopy

EXCLUDES *Diagnostic laparoscopy (peritoneoscopy) performed as a separate procedure (49320)*

51990 **Laparoscopy, surgical; urethral suspension for stress incontinence**
T 80 21.72 21.72 FUD 090

51992 **sling operation for stress incontinence (eg, fascia or synthetic)**
EXCLUDES *Removal/revision of sling for stress incontinence (57287)*
Sling operation for stress incontinence, open approach (57288)
A2 T 80 24.51 24.51 FUD 090

51999 **Unlisted laparoscopy procedure, bladder**
T 80 0.00 0.00 FUD YYY

52000-52318 Endoscopic Procedures via Urethra: Bladder and Urethra

52000 **Cystourethroscopy (separate procedure)**
Do not report with (52001, 52320, 52325, 52327, 52330, 52332, 52334, 52341-52343, [52356])
A2 T 3.59 5.67 FUD 000

52001 **Cystourethroscopy with irrigation and evacuation of multiple obstructing clots**
Do not report with (52000)
A2 T 8.17 10.40 FUD 000

52005 **Cystourethroscopy, with ureteral catheterization, with or without irrigation, instillation, or ureteropyelography, exclusive of radiologic service;**
INCLUDES Howard test
A2 T 3.79 7.36 FUD 000

52007 **with brush biopsy of ureter and/or renal pelvis**
A2 T 50 PQ 4.72 12.30 FUD 000

52010 **Cystourethroscopy, with ejaculatory duct catheterization, with or without irrigation, instillation, or duct radiography, exclusive of radiologic service** ♂
74440
A2 T 4.72 10.18 FUD 000

52204 **Cystourethroscopy, with biopsy(s)**
A2 T PQ 4.03 10.22 FUD 000

52214 **Cystourethroscopy, with fulguration (including cryosurgery or laser surgery) of trigone, bladder neck, prostatic fossa, urethra, or periurethral glands**
Code also modifier 78 when performed by same physician:
During postoperative period (52601, 52630)
During the postoperative period of a related surgical procedure
For postoperative bleeding
A2 T 5.01 18.27 FUD 000

52224 **Cystourethroscopy, with fulguration (including cryosurgery or laser surgery) or treatment of MINOR (less than 0.5 cm) lesion(s) with or without biopsy**
A2 T PQ 5.81 19.14 FUD 000

52234 **Cystourethroscopy, with fulguration (including cryosurgery or laser surgery) and/or resection of; SMALL bladder tumor(s) (0.5 up to 2.0 cm)**
EXCLUDES *Bladder tumor excision through cystotomy (51530)*
A2 T 6.98 6.98 FUD 000

52235 **MEDIUM bladder tumor(s) (2.0 to 5.0 cm)**
EXCLUDES *Bladder tumor excision through cystotomy (51530)*
A2 T 8.20 8.20 FUD 000

52240 **LARGE bladder tumor(s)**
EXCLUDES *Bladder tumor excision through cystotomy (51530)*
A2 T 11.15 11.15 FUD 000

52250 **Cystourethroscopy with insertion of radioactive substance, with or without biopsy or fulguration**
A2 T PQ 6.82 6.82 FUD 000

52260 **Cystourethroscopy, with dilation of bladder for interstitial cystitis; general or conduction (spinal) anesthesia**
A2 T 5.99 5.99 FUD 000

52265 **local anesthesia**
P3 T 4.68 10.20 FUD 000

52270 **Cystourethroscopy, with internal urethrotomy; female** ♀
A2 T 5.18 9.87 FUD 000

52275 **male** ♂
A2 T 7.06 13.33 FUD 000

52276 **Cystourethroscopy with direct vision internal urethrotomy**
A2 T 7.53 7.53 FUD 000

52277 **Cystourethroscopy, with resection of external sphincter (sphincterotomy)**
A2 T 80 7.53 9.19 9.19 FUD 000

52281 **Cystourethroscopy, with calibration and/or dilation of urethral stricture or stenosis, with or without meatotomy, with or without injection procedure for cystography, male or female**
A2 T 4.35 7.57 FUD 000

52282 **Cystourethroscopy, with insertion of permanent urethral stent**
EXCLUDES *Placement of temporary prostatic urethral stent (53855)*
A2 T 9.58 9.58 FUD 000

52283 **Cystourethroscopy, with steroid injection into stricture**
A2 T 5.73 7.72 FUD 000

52285 **Cystourethroscopy for treatment of the female urethral syndrome with any or all of the following: urethral meatotomy, urethral dilation, internal urethrotomy, lysis of urethrovaginal septal fibrosis, lateral incisions of the bladder neck, and fulguration of polyp(s) of urethra, bladder neck, and/or trigone** ♀
A2 T 5.58 7.79 FUD 000

52287 **Cystourethroscopy, with injection(s) for chemodenervation of the bladder**
Code also supply of chemodenervation agent
G2 T 4.82 8.67 FUD 000

52290 **Cystourethroscopy; with ureteral meatotomy, unilateral or bilateral**
A2 T 6.93 6.93 FUD 000

52300 **with resection or fulguration of orthotopic ureterocele(s), unilateral or bilateral**
A2 T 80 8.04 8.04 FUD 000

52301 **with resection or fulguration of ectopic ureterocele(s), unilateral or bilateral**
A2 T 80 8.25 8.25 FUD 000

52305 **with incision or resection of orifice of bladder diverticulum, single or multiple**
A2 T 7.93 7.93 FUD 000

52310 **Cystourethroscopy, with removal of foreign body, calculus, or ureteral stent from urethra or bladder (separate procedure); simple**
Code also modifier 58 for removal of a self-retaining, indwelling ureteral stent
A2 T 4.32 6.77 FUD 000

52315 **complicated**
Code also modifier 58 for removal of a self-retaining, indwelling ureteral stent
A2 T 7.79 11.50 FUD 000

52317 **Litholapaxy: crushing or fragmentation of calculus by any means in bladder and removal of fragments; simple or small (less than 2.5 cm)**
A2 T 9.88 22.33 FUD 000

52318 **complicated or large (over 2.5 cm)**
A2 T 13.46 13.46 FUD 000

52320-52356 [52356] Endoscopic Procedures via Urethra: Renal Pelvis and Ureter

INCLUDES Diagnostic cystourethroscopy when performed with therapeutic cystourethroscopy
Insertion/removal of temporary ureteral catheter

EXCLUDES *Diagnostic cystourethroscopy only (52000)*
Self-retaining/indwelling ureteral stent removal by cystourethroscope, with modifier 58 if appropriate (52310, 52315)

Code also the insertion of an indwelling stent performed in addition to other procedures within this section (52332)
Do not report with (52005)

52320 **Cystourethroscopy (including ureteral catheterization); with removal of ureteral calculus**
Do not report with (52000)
A2 T 50 7.00 7.00 FUD 000

52325 **with fragmentation of ureteral calculus (eg, ultrasonic or electro-hydraulic technique)**
Do not report with (52000)
A2 T 50 9.11 9.11 FUD 000

52327 **with subureteric injection of implant material**
Do not report with (52000)
A2 T 50 7.46 7.46 FUD 000

52330 **with manipulation, without removal of ureteral calculus**
Do not report with (52000)
A2 T 50 7.50 13.73 FUD 000

52332 **Cystourethroscopy, with insertion of indwelling ureteral stent (eg, Gibbons or double-J type)**
Do not report when performed on the same side with (52000, 52353, [52356])
A2 T 50 4.43 13.58 FUD 000

52334 **Cystourethroscopy with insertion of ureteral guide wire through kidney to establish a percutaneous nephrostomy, retrograde**
EXCLUDES *Cystourethroscopy with incision/fulguration/resection of congenital posterior urethral valves/obstructive hypertrophic mucosal folds (52400)*
Cystourethroscopy with pyeloscopy and/or ureteroscopy (52351-52353 [52356])
Nephrostomy tract establishment only (50395)
Percutaneous nephrostolithotomy (50080, 50081)
Do not report with (52000, 52351)
A2 T 50 7.29 7.29 FUD 000

52341 **Cystourethroscopy; with treatment of ureteral stricture (eg, balloon dilation, laser, electrocautery, and incision)**
Do not report with (52000, 52351)
A2 T 50 8.07 8.07 FUD 000

52342 **with treatment of ureteropelvic junction stricture (eg, balloon dilation, laser, electrocautery, and incision)**
Do not report with (52000, 52351)
A2 T 50 8.78 8.78 FUD 000

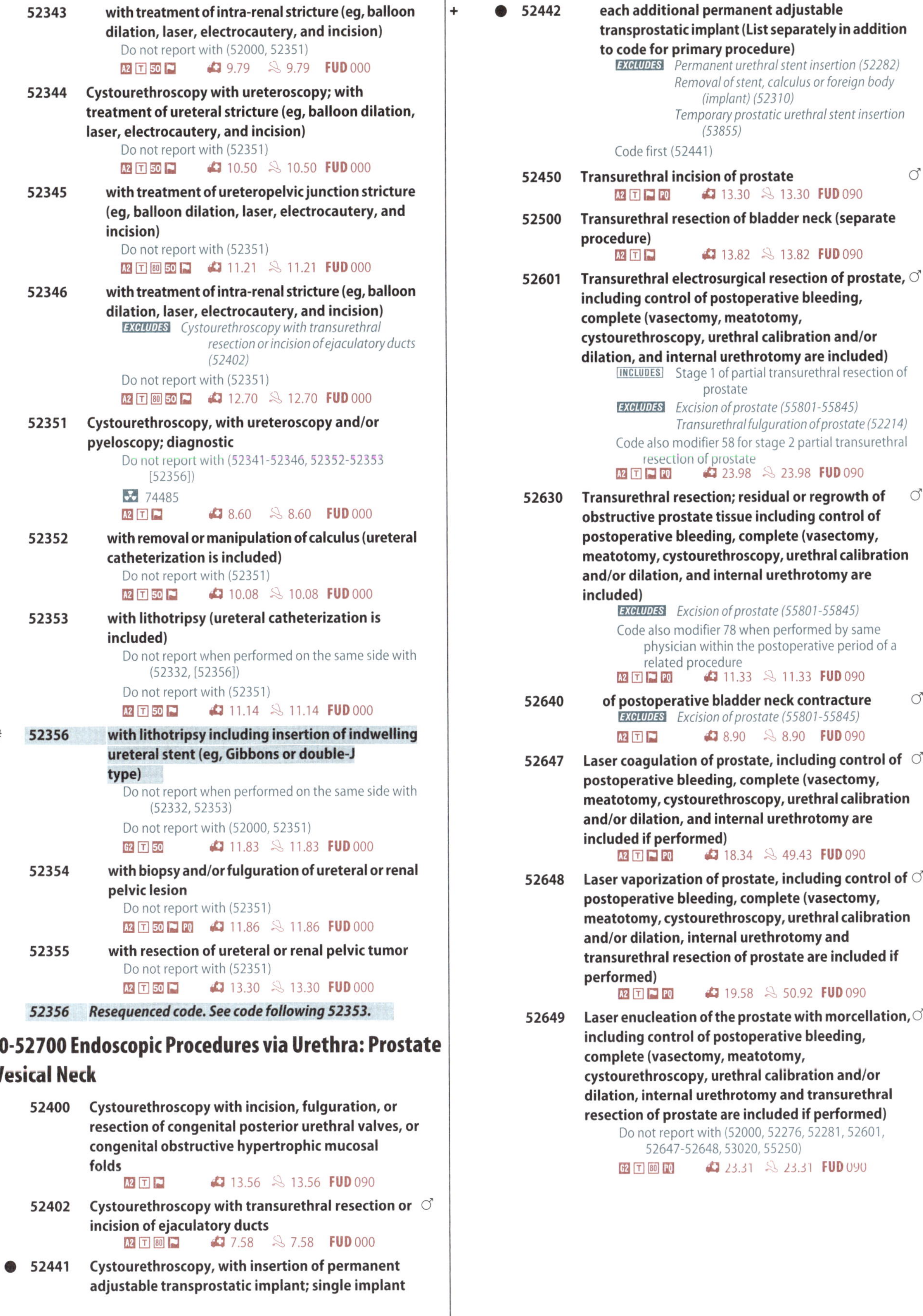

52343 with treatment of intra-renal stricture (eg, balloon dilation, laser, electrocautery, and incision)

Do not report with (52000, 52351)

A2 T 50 9.79 9.79 FUD 000

52344 Cystourethroscopy with ureteroscopy; with treatment of ureteral stricture (eg, balloon dilation, laser, electrocautery, and incision)

Do not report with (52351)

A2 T 50 10.50 10.50 FUD 000

52345 with treatment of ureteropelvic junction stricture (eg, balloon dilation, laser, electrocautery, and incision)

Do not report with (52351)

A2 T 80 50 11.21 11.21 FUD 000

52346 with treatment of intra-renal stricture (eg, balloon dilation, laser, electrocautery, and incision)

EXCLUDES *Cystourethroscopy with transurethral resection or incision of ejaculatory ducts (52402)*

Do not report with (52351)

A2 T 80 50 12.70 12.70 FUD 000

52351 Cystourethroscopy, with ureteroscopy and/or pyeloscopy; diagnostic

Do not report with (52341-52346, 52352-52353 [52356])

74485

A2 T 8.60 8.60 FUD 000

52352 with removal or manipulation of calculus (ureteral catheterization is included)

Do not report with (52351)

A2 T 50 10.08 10.08 FUD 000

52353 with lithotripsy (ureteral catheterization is included)

Do not report when performed on the same side with (52332, [52356])

Do not report with (52351)

A2 T 50 11.14 11.14 FUD 000

\# 52356 with lithotripsy including insertion of indwelling ureteral stent (eg, Gibbons or double-J type)

Do not report when performed on the same side with (52332, 52353)

Do not report with (52000, 52351)

G2 T 50 11.83 11.83 FUD 000

52354 with biopsy and/or fulguration of ureteral or renal pelvic lesion

Do not report with (52351)

A2 T 50 PQ 11.86 11.86 FUD 000

52355 with resection of ureteral or renal pelvic tumor

Do not report with (52351)

A2 T 50 13.30 13.30 FUD 000

52356 Resequenced code. See code following 52353.

52400-52700 Endoscopic Procedures via Urethra: Prostate and Vesical Neck

52400 Cystourethroscopy with incision, fulguration, or resection of congenital posterior urethral valves, or congenital obstructive hypertrophic mucosal folds

A2 T 13.56 13.56 FUD 090

52402 Cystourethroscopy with transurethral resection or incision of ejaculatory ducts ♂

A2 T 80 7.58 7.58 FUD 000

● 52441 Cystourethroscopy, with insertion of permanent adjustable transprostatic implant; single implant

\+ ● 52442 each additional permanent adjustable transprostatic implant (List separately in addition to code for primary procedure)

EXCLUDES *Permanent urethral stent insertion (52282)*

Removal of stent, calculus or foreign body (implant) (52310)

Temporary prostatic urethral stent insertion (53855)

Code first (52441)

52450 Transurethral incision of prostate ♂

A2 T PQ 13.30 13.30 FUD 090

52500 Transurethral resection of bladder neck (separate procedure)

A2 T 13.82 13.82 FUD 090

52601 Transurethral electrosurgical resection of prostate, including control of postoperative bleeding, complete (vasectomy, meatotomy, cystourethroscopy, urethral calibration and/or dilation, and internal urethrotomy are included) ♂

INCLUDES Stage 1 of partial transurethral resection of prostate

EXCLUDES *Excision of prostate (55801-55845)*

Transurethral fulguration of prostate (52214)

Code also modifier 58 for stage 2 partial transurethral resection of prostate

A2 T PQ 23.98 23.98 FUD 090

52630 Transurethral resection; residual or regrowth of obstructive prostate tissue including control of postoperative bleeding, complete (vasectomy, meatotomy, cystourethroscopy, urethral calibration and/or dilation, and internal urethrotomy are included) ♂

EXCLUDES *Excision of prostate (55801-55845)*

Code also modifier 78 when performed by same physician within the postoperative period of a related procedure

A2 T PQ 11.33 11.33 FUD 090

52640 of postoperative bladder neck contracture ♂

EXCLUDES *Excision of prostate (55801-55845)*

A2 T 8.90 8.90 FUD 090

52647 Laser coagulation of prostate, including control of postoperative bleeding, complete (vasectomy, meatotomy, cystourethroscopy, urethral calibration and/or dilation, and internal urethrotomy are included if performed) ♂

A2 T PQ 18.34 49.43 FUD 090

52648 Laser vaporization of prostate, including control of postoperative bleeding, complete (vasectomy, meatotomy, cystourethroscopy, urethral calibration and/or dilation, internal urethrotomy and transurethral resection of prostate are included if performed) ♂

A2 T PQ 19.58 50.92 FUD 090

52649 Laser enucleation of the prostate with morcellation, including control of postoperative bleeding, complete (vasectomy, meatotomy, cystourethroscopy, urethral calibration and/or dilation, internal urethrotomy and transurethral resection of prostate are included if performed) ♂

Do not report with (52000, 52276, 52281, 52601, 52647-52648, 53020, 55250)

G2 T 80 PQ 23.31 23.31 FUD 090

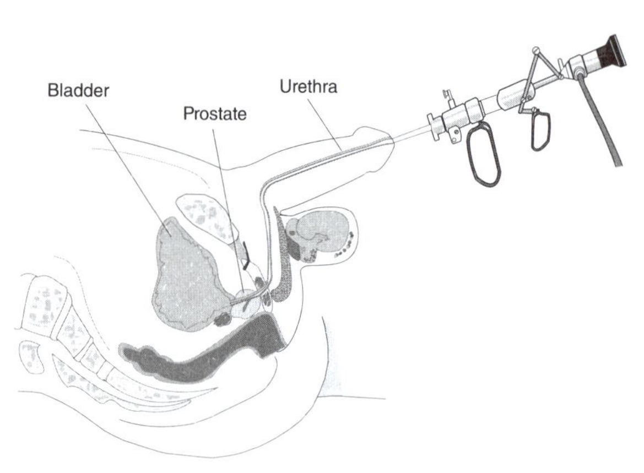

52700 Transurethral drainage of prostatic abscess ♂
EXCLUDES *Lithotomy (52317, 52318)*
A2 T 80 | 12.48 | 12.48 | FUD 090

53000-53520 Open Surgical Procedures of Urethra

EXCLUDES *Endoscopic procedures; cystoscopy, urethroscopy, cystourethroscopy (52000-52700 [52356])*
Urethrocystography injection procedure (51600-51610)

53000 Urethrotomy or urethrostomy, external (separate procedure); pendulous urethra
A2 T | 4.20 | 4.20 | FUD 010

53010 perineal urethra, external
A2 T | 8.31 | 8.31 | FUD 090

53020 Meatotomy, cutting of meatus (separate procedure); except infant
A2 T | 2.76 | 2.76 | FUD 000

53025 infant A
R2 T 80 63 | 1.91 | 1.91 | FUD 000

53040 Drainage of deep periurethral abscess
EXCLUDES *Incision and drainage of subcutaneous abscess (10060, 10061)*
A2 T 80 | 11.12 | 11.12 | FUD 090

53060 Drainage of Skene's gland abscess or cyst ♀
P3 T | 4.83 | 5.33 | FUD 010

53080 Drainage of perineal urinary extravasation; uncomplicated (separate procedure)
A2 T | 11.89 | 11.89 | FUD 090

53085 complicated
G2 T 80 | 18.74 | 18.74 | FUD 090

53200 Biopsy of urethra
A2 T PQ | 4.04 | 4.41 | FUD 000

53210 Urethrectomy, total, including cystostomy; female ♀
A2 T 80 | 21.81 | 21.81 | FUD 090

53215 male ♂
A2 T 80 | 26.32 | 26.32 | FUD 090

53220 Excision or fulguration of carcinoma of urethra
A2 T 80 | 12.83 | 12.83 | FUD 090

53230 Excision of urethral diverticulum (separate procedure); female ♀
● A2 T 80 | 17.28 | 17.28 | FUD 090

53235 male ♂
A2 T 80 | 17.91 | 17.91 | FUD 090

53240 Marsupialization of urethral diverticulum, male or female
A2 T | 12.02 | 12.02 | FUD 090

53250 Excision of bulbourethral gland (Cowper's gland) ♂
A2 T | 11.95 | 11.95 | FUD 090

53260 Excision or fulguration; urethral polyp(s), distal urethra
EXCLUDES *Endoscopic method (52214, 52224)*
A2 T | 5.14 | 5.72 | FUD 010

53265 urethral caruncle
EXCLUDES *Endoscopic method (52214, 52224)*
A2 T | 5.29 | 6.16 | FUD 010

53270 Skene's glands ♀
EXCLUDES *Endoscopic method (52214, 52224)*
A2 T | 5.41 | 6.01 | FUD 010

53275 urethral prolapse
EXCLUDES *Endoscopic method (52214, 52224)*
A2 T | 7.44 | 7.44 | FUD 010

53400 Urethroplasty; first stage, for fistula, diverticulum, or stricture (eg, Johannsen type)
EXCLUDES *Hypospadias repair (54300-54352)*
A2 T 80 | 22.73 | 22.73 | FUD 090

53405 second stage (formation of urethra), including urinary diversion
EXCLUDES *Hypospadias repair (54300-54352)*
A2 T 80 | 24.76 | 24.76 | FUD 090

53410 Urethroplasty, 1-stage reconstruction of male anterior urethra ♂
EXCLUDES *Hypospadias repair (54300-54352)*
A2 T 80 | 27.78 | 27.78 | FUD 090

53415 Urethroplasty, transpubic or perineal, 1-stage, for reconstruction or repair of prostatic or membranous urethra ♂
C 80 | 32.07 | 32.07 | FUD 090

53420 Urethroplasty, 2-stage reconstruction or repair of prostatic or membranous urethra; first stage ♂
A2 T | 23.85 | 23.85 | FUD 090

53425 second stage ♂
A2 T 80 | 26.56 | 26.56 | FUD 090

53430 Urethroplasty, reconstruction of female urethra ♀
A2 T 80 | 27.59 | 27.59 | FUD 090

53431 Urethroplasty with tubularization of posterior urethra and/or lower bladder for incontinence (eg, Tenago, Leadbetter procedure)
A2 T 80 | 32.72 | 32.72 | FUD 090

53440 Sling operation for correction of male urinary incontinence (eg, fascia or synthetic) ♂
Code also (C1762, C1763, C1771, C1781, C2631)
J8 S 80 | 21.34 | 21.34 | FUD 090

53442 Removal or revision of sling for male urinary incontinence (eg, fascia or synthetic) ♂
A2 T 80 | 22.16 | 22.16 | FUD 090

53444 Insertion of tandem cuff (dual cuff)
Code also (C1815)
J8 S 80 | 22.47 | 22.47 | FUD 090

53445 Insertion of inflatable urethral/bladder neck sphincter, including placement of pump, reservoir, and cuff
Code also (C1815)
J8 S 80 | 21.34 | 21.34 | FUD 090

53446 Removal of inflatable urethral/bladder neck sphincter, including pump, reservoir, and cuff
A2 Q2 80 | 18.19 | 18.19 | FUD 090

53447 Removal and replacement of inflatable urethral/bladder neck sphincter including pump, reservoir, and cuff at the same operative session
Code also (C1815)
J8 S 80 | 22.92 | 22.92 | FUD 090

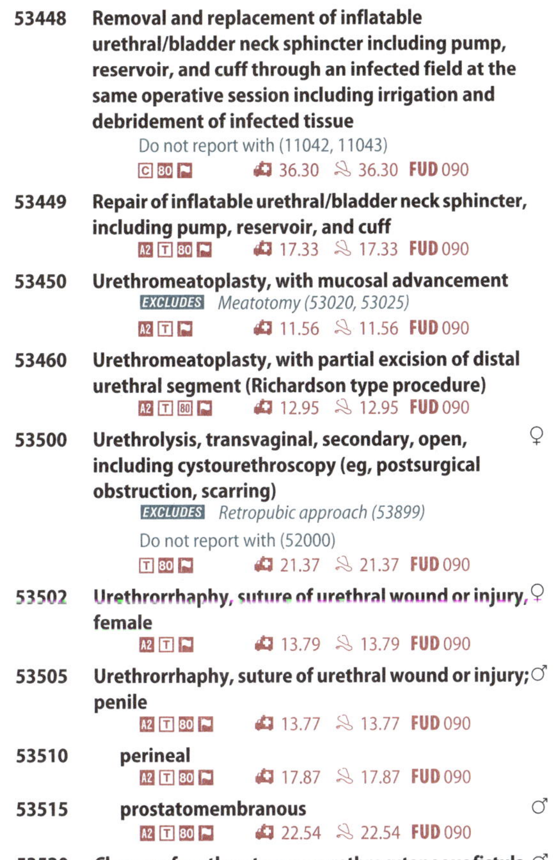

53448 **Removal and replacement of inflatable urethral/bladder neck sphincter including pump, reservoir, and cuff through an infected field at the same operative session including irrigation and debridement of infected tissue**

Do not report with (11042, 11043)

C 80 CCI 36.30 36.30 FUD 090

53449 **Repair of inflatable urethral/bladder neck sphincter, including pump, reservoir, and cuff**

A2 T 80 CCI 17.33 17.33 FUD 090

53450 **Urethromeatoplasty, with mucosal advancement**

EXCLUDES *Meatotomy (53020, 53025)*

A2 T CCI 11.56 11.56 FUD 090

53460 **Urethromeatoplasty, with partial excision of distal urethral segment (Richardson type procedure)**

A2 T 80 CCI 12.95 12.95 FUD 090

53500 **Urethrolysis, transvaginal, secondary, open, including cystourethroscopy (eg, postsurgical obstruction, scarring)** ♀

EXCLUDES *Retropubic approach (53899)*

Do not report with (52000)

T 80 CCI 21.37 21.37 FUD 090

53502 **Urethrorrhaphy, suture of urethral wound or injury, female** ♀

A2 T CCI 13.79 13.79 FUD 090

53505 **Urethrorrhaphy, suture of urethral wound or injury; penile** ♂

A2 T 80 CCI 13.77 13.77 FUD 090

53510 **perineal**

A2 T 80 CCI 17.87 17.87 FUD 090

53515 **prostatomembranous** ♂

A2 T 80 CCI 22.54 22.54 FUD 090

53520 **Closure of urethrostomy or urethrocutaneous fistula, male (separate procedure)** ♂

EXCLUDES *Closure of fistula:*
Urethrorectal (45820, 45825)
Urethrovaginal (57310)

A2 T CCI 15.75 15.75 FUD 090

53600-53665 Urethral Dilation

EXCLUDES *Endoscopic procedures; cystoscopy, urethroscopy, cystourethroscopy (52000-52700 [52356])*
Urethral catheterization (51701-51703)
Urethrocystography injection procedure (51600-51610)

74485

53600 **Dilation of urethral stricture by passage of sound or urethral dilator, male; initial** ♂

P3 T CCI 1.81 2.34 FUD 000

53601 **subsequent** ♂

P3 T CCI 1.51 2.26 FUD 000

53605 **Dilation of urethral stricture or vesical neck by passage of sound or urethral dilator, male, general or conduction (spinal) anesthesia** ♂

EXCLUDES *Procedure performed under local anesthesia (53600-53601, 53620-53621)*

A2 T CCI 1.83 1.83 FUD 000

53620 **Dilation of urethral stricture by passage of filiform and follower, male; initial** ♂

P3 T CCI 2.48 3.26 FUD 000

53621 **subsequent** ♂

P3 T CCI 2.03 3.05 FUD 000

53660 **Dilation of female urethra including suppository and/or instillation; initial** ♀

P3 T CCI 1.18 1.97 FUD 000

53661 **subsequent** ♀

P3 T CCI 1.15 1.94 FUD 000

53665 **Dilation of female urethra, general or conduction (spinal) anesthesia** ♀

EXCLUDES *Procedure performed under local anesthesia (53660-53661)*

A2 T CCI 1.11 1.11 FUD 000

53850-53899 Transurethral Procedures

EXCLUDES *Endoscopic procedures; cystoscopy, urethroscopy, cystourethroscopy (52000-52700 [52356])*
Urethrocystography injection procedure (51600-51610)

53850 **Transurethral destruction of prostate tissue; by microwave thermotherapy** ♂

81020

P3 T CCI 17.19 57.59 FUD 090

53852 **by radiofrequency thermotherapy** ♂

81020

P3 T CCI 17.63 53.02 FUD 090

53855 **Insertion of a temporary prostatic urethral stent, including urethral measurement** ♂

EXCLUDES *Permanent urethral stent insertion (52282)*

P2 T 80 2.35 21.49 FUD 000

53860 **Transurethral radiofrequency micro-remodeling of the female bladder neck and proximal urethra for stress urinary incontinence** ♀

P2 T 80 6.69 43.17 FUD 090

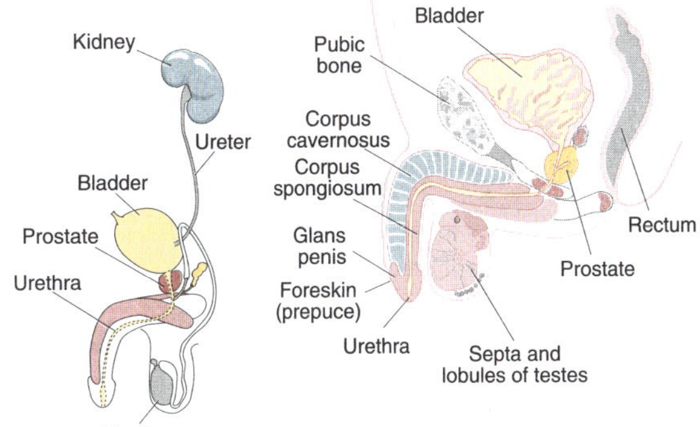

53899 **Unlisted procedure, urinary system**

81020

T 80 0.00 0.00 FUD YYY

54000-54015 Procedures of Penis: Incisional

EXCLUDES *Debridement of abdominal perineal gangrene (11004-11006)*

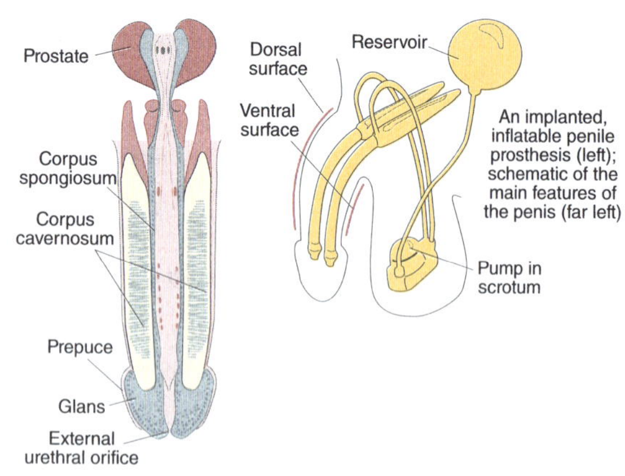

54000 **Slitting of prepuce, dorsal or lateral (separate procedure); newborn** A ♂
A2 T 80 ⚑ 63 — 3.04 — 4.12 — FUD 010

54001 **except newborn** ♂
A2 T ⚑ — 3.94 — 5.18 — FUD 010

54015 **Incision and drainage of penis, deep** ♂
EXCLUDES *Abscess, skin/subcutaneous (10060-10160)*
A2 T 80 ⚑ — 8.77 — 8.77 — FUD 010

54050-54065 Destruction of Penis Lesions: Multiple Methods

CMS 100-3,140.5 Laser Procedures

EXCLUDES *Excision/destruction other lesions (11420-11426, 11620-11626, 17000-17250, 17270-17276)*

54050 **Destruction of lesion(s), penis (eg, condyloma, papilloma, molluscum contagiosum, herpetic vesicle), simple; chemical** ♂
P3 T ⚑ — 2.95 — 3.66 — FUD 010

54055 **electrodesiccation** ♂
P3 T ⚑ — 2.59 — 3.28 — FUD 010

54056 **cryosurgery** ♂
P2 T ⚑ — 3.14 — 3.96 — FUD 010

54057 **laser surgery** ♂
A2 T ⚑ — 2.66 — 3.77 — FUD 010

54060 **surgical excision** ♂
A2 T ⚑ — 3.69 — 5.01 — FUD 010

54065 **Destruction of lesion(s), penis (eg, condyloma, papilloma, molluscum contagiosum, herpetic vesicle), extensive (eg, laser surgery, electrosurgery, cryosurgery, chemosurgery)** ♂
A2 T ⚑ — 4.92 — 6.16 — FUD 010

54100-54115 Procedures of Penis: Excisional

54100 **Biopsy of penis; (separate procedure)** ♂
A2 T ⚑ PQ — 3.55 — 5.50 — FUD 000

54105 **deep structures** ♂
A2 T ⚑ PQ — 6.03 — 7.43 — FUD 010

54110 **Excision of penile plaque (Peyronie disease);** ♂
A2 T 80 ⚑ — 17.68 — 17.68 — FUD 090

54111 **with graft to 5 cm in length** ♂
A2 T 80 ⚑ — 22.70 — 22.70 — FUD 090

54112 **with graft greater than 5 cm in length** ♂
A2 T 80 ⚑ — 26.58 — 26.58 — FUD 090

54115 **Removal foreign body from deep penile tissue (eg, plastic implant)** ♂
A2 T 80 ⚑ — 12.00 — 12.74 — FUD 090

54120-54135 Amputation of Penis

EXCLUDES *Lymphadenectomy (separate procedure) (38760-38770)*

54120 **Amputation of penis; partial** ♂
A2 T 80 ⚑ — 17.91 — 17.91 — FUD 090

54125 **complete** ♂
C 80 ⚑ — 23.05 — 23.05 — FUD 090

54130 **Amputation of penis, radical; with bilateral inguinofemoral lymphadenectomy** ♂
C 80 ⚑ — 33.85 — 33.85 — FUD 090

54135 **in continuity with bilateral pelvic lymphadenectomy, including external iliac, hypogastric and obturator nodes** ♂
C 80 ⚑ — 42.90 — 42.90 — FUD 090

54150-54164 Circumcision Procedures

54150 **Circumcision, using clamp or other device with regional dorsal penile or ring block** A ♂
Code also modifier 52 when performed without dorsal penile or ring block
A2 T 80 ⚑ 63 — 2.81 — 4.36 — FUD 000

54160 **Circumcision, surgical excision other than clamp, device, or dorsal slit; neonate (28 days of age or less)** A ♂
A2 T ⚑ 63 — 4.08 — 6.14 — FUD 010

54161 **older than 28 days of age** A ♂
A2 T ⚑ — 5.58 — 5.58 — FUD 010

54162 **Lysis or excision of penile post-circumcision adhesions** ♂
A2 T ⚑ — 5.64 — 7.23 — FUD 010

54163 **Repair incomplete circumcision** ♂
A2 T ⚑ — 6.18 — 6.18 — FUD 010

54164 **Frenulotomy of penis** ♂
Do not report with (54150-54163)
A2 T ⚑ — 5.48 — 5.48 — FUD 010

54200-54250 Evaluation and Treatment of Erectile Abnormalities

54200 **Injection procedure for Peyronie disease;** ♂
P3 T ⚑ — 2.37 — 2.99 — FUD 010

54205 **with surgical exposure of plaque** ♂
A2 T 80 ⚑ — 15.06 — 15.06 — FUD 090

54220 **Irrigation of corpora cavernosa for priapism** ♂
A2 T ⚑ — 3.81 — 5.71 — FUD 000

54230 **Injection procedure for corpora cavernosography** ♂
74445
N1 N ⚑ — 2.25 — 2.71 — FUD 000

54231 **Dynamic cavernosometry, including intracavernosal injection of vasoactive drugs (eg, papaverine, phentolamine)** ♂
P3 T ⚑ — 3.30 — 3.95 — FUD 000

54235 **Injection of corpora cavernosa with pharmacologic agent(s) (eg, papaverine, phentolamine)** ♂
P3 T ⚑ — 2.09 — 2.54 — FUD 000

54240 **Penile plethysmography** ♂
P3 T 80 ⚑ — 2.80 — 2.80 — FUD 000

54250 **Nocturnal penile tumescence and/or rigidity test** ♂
P3 T 80 ⚑ — 3.40 — 3.40 — FUD 000

54300-54390 Hypospadias Repair and Related Procedures

EXCLUDES *Other urethroplasties (53400-53430)*
Revascularization of penis (37788)

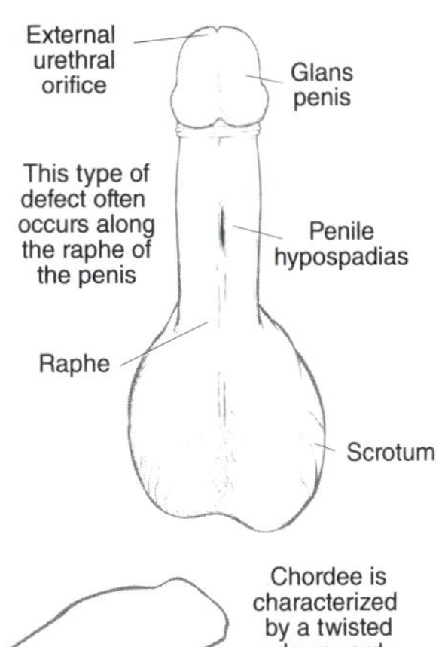

54300 **Plastic operation of penis for straightening of chordee (eg, hypospadias), with or without mobilization of urethra** ♂
A2 T 80 18.16 18.16 FUD 090

54304 **Plastic operation on penis for correction of chordee or for first stage hypospadias repair with or without transplantation of prepuce and/or skin flaps** ♂
A2 T 80 21.24 21.24 FUD 090

54308 **Urethroplasty for second stage hypospadias repair (including urinary diversion); less than 3 cm** ♂
A2 T 80 20.27 20.27 FUD 090

54312 **greater than 3 cm** ♂
A2 T 80 23.19 23.19 FUD 090

54316 **Urethroplasty for second stage hypospadias repair (including urinary diversion) with free skin graft obtained from site other than genitalia** ♂
A2 T 80 28.29 28.29 FUD 090

54318 **Urethroplasty for third stage hypospadias repair to release penis from scrotum (eg, third stage Cecil repair)** ♂
A2 T 80 19.82 19.82 FUD 090

54322 **1-stage distal hypospadias repair (with or without chordee or circumcision); with simple meatal advancement (eg, Magpi, V-flap)** ♂
A2 T 80 22.14 22.14 FUD 090

54324 **with urethroplasty by local skin flaps (eg, flip-flap, prepucial flap)** ♂
INCLUDES Browne's operation
A2 T 80 27.47 27.47 FUD 090

54326 **with urethroplasty by local skin flaps and mobilization of urethra** ♂
A2 T 80 26.82 26.82 FUD 090

54328 **with extensive dissection to correct chordee and urethroplasty with local skin flaps, skin graft patch, and/or island flap** ♂
EXCLUDES *Urethroplasty/straightening of chordee (54308)*
A2 T 80 26.64 26.64 FUD 090

54332 **1-stage proximal penile or penoscrotal hypospadias repair requiring extensive dissection to correct chordee and urethroplasty by use of skin graft tube and/or island flap** ♂
T 80 28.75 28.75 FUD 090

54336 **1-stage perineal hypospadias repair requiring extensive dissection to correct chordee and urethroplasty by use of skin graft tube and/or island flap** ♂
T 80 33.74 33.74 FUD 090

54340 **Repair of hypospadias complications (ie, fistula, stricture, diverticula); by closure, incision, or excision, simple** ♂
A2 T 80 16.13 16.13 FUD 090

54344 **requiring mobilization of skin flaps and urethroplasty with flap or patch graft** ♂
A2 T 80 28.27 28.27 FUD 090

54348 **requiring extensive dissection and urethroplasty with flap, patch or tubed graft (includes urinary diversion)** ♂
A2 T 80 28.28 28.28 FUD 090

54352 **Repair of hypospadias cripple requiring extensive dissection and excision of previously constructed structures including re-release of chordee and reconstruction of urethra and penis by use of local skin as grafts and island flaps and skin brought in as flaps or grafts** ♂
A2 T 80 40.21 40.21 FUD 090

54360 **Plastic operation on penis to correct angulation** ♂
A2 T 80 20.44 20.44 FUD 090

54380 **Plastic operation on penis for epispadias distal to external sphincter;** ♂
INCLUDES Lowsley's operation
A2 T 80 22.65 22.65 FUD 090

54385 **with incontinence** ♂
A2 T 80 28.06 28.06 FUD 090

54390 **with exstrophy of bladder** ♂
C 80 36.45 36.45 FUD 090

54400-54417 Procedures to Treat Impotence

CMS 100-3,230.4 Diagnosis and Treatment of Impotence

EXCLUDES *Other urethroplasties (53400-53430)*
Revascularization of penis (37788)

54400 **Insertion of penile prosthesis; non-inflatable (semi-rigid)** ♂
EXCLUDES *Replacement/removal penile prosthesis (54415, 54416)*
Code also (C2622)
J8 S 14.99 14.99 FUD 090

54401 **inflatable (self-contained)** ♂
EXCLUDES *Replacement/removal penile prosthesis (54415, 54416)*
Code also (C1813)
J8 S PQ 18.56 18.56 FUD 090

54405 **Insertion of multi-component, inflatable penile prosthesis, including placement of pump, cylinders, and reservoir** ♂
Code also (C1813)
Code also modifier 52 for reduced services
J8 S 80 PQ 22.93 22.93 FUD 090

54406 **Removal of all components of a multi-component, inflatable penile prosthesis without replacement of prosthesis** ♂
Code also modifier 52 for reduced services
A2 Q2 80 PQ 20.69 20.69 FUD 090

54408 **Repair of component(s) of a multi-component, inflatable penile prosthesis** ♂
A2 T 80 PQ 22.40 22.40 FUD 090

54410 **Removal and replacement of all component(s) of a multi-component, inflatable penile prosthesis at the same operative session** ♂
Code also (C1813)
J8 S 80 PQ 24.37 24.37 FUD 090

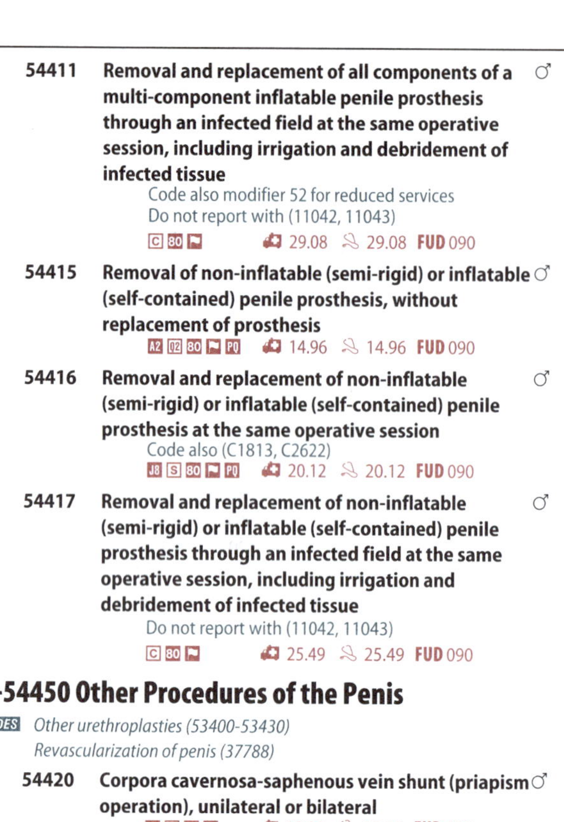

54411 **Removal and replacement of all components of a multi-component inflatable penile prosthesis through an infected field at the same operative session, including irrigation and debridement of infected tissue** ♂
Code also modifier 52 for reduced services
Do not report with (11042, 11043)
C 80 ⚑ Facility RVU 29.08 Non-Facility RVU 29.08 FUD 090

54415 **Removal of non-inflatable (semi-rigid) or inflatable (self-contained) penile prosthesis, without replacement of prosthesis** ♂
A2 Q2 80 ⚑ P0 Facility RVU 14.96 Non-Facility RVU 14.96 FUD 090

54416 **Removal and replacement of non-inflatable (semi-rigid) or inflatable (self-contained) penile prosthesis at the same operative session** ♂
Code also (C1813, C2622)
J8 S 80 ⚑ P0 Facility RVU 20.12 Non-Facility RVU 20.12 FUD 090

54417 **Removal and replacement of non-inflatable (semi-rigid) or inflatable (self-contained) penile prosthesis through an infected field at the same operative session, including irrigation and debridement of infected tissue** ♂
Do not report with (11042, 11043)
C 80 ⚑ Facility RVU 25.49 Non-Facility RVU 25.49 FUD 090

54420-54450 Other Procedures of the Penis

EXCLUDES *Other urethroplasties (53400-53430)*
Revascularization of penis (37788)

54420 **Corpora cavernosa-saphenous vein shunt (priapism operation), unilateral or bilateral** ♂
A2 T 80 ⚑ Facility RVU 19.98 Non-Facility RVU 19.98 FUD 090

54430 **Corpora cavernosa-corpus spongiosum shunt (priapism operation), unilateral or bilateral** ♂
C 80 ⚑ Facility RVU 18.14 Non-Facility RVU 18.14 FUD 090

54435 **Corpora cavernosa-glans penis fistulization (eg, biopsy needle, Winter procedure, rongeur, or punch) for priapism** ♂
A2 T ⚑ Facility RVU 11.79 Non-Facility RVU 11.79 FUD 090

54440 **Plastic operation of penis for injury** ♂
A2 T 80 ⚑ Facility RVU 0.00 Non-Facility RVU 0.00 FUD 090

54450 **Foreskin manipulation including lysis of preputial adhesions and stretching** ♂
A2 T ⚑ Facility RVU 1.63 Non-Facility RVU 1.97 FUD 000

54500-54560 Testicular Procedures: Incisional

EXCLUDES *Debridement of abdominal perineal gangrene (11004-11006)*

54500 **Biopsy of testis, needle (separate procedure)** ♂
EXCLUDES *Fine needle aspiration (10021, 10022)*
Lab Crosswalk 88172, 88173
A2 T 80 50 ⚑ P0 Facility RVU 2.11 Non-Facility RVU 2.11 FUD 000

54505 **Biopsy of testis, incisional (separate procedure)** ♂
Do not report when combined with epididymogram, seminal vesiculogram or vasogram (55300)
A2 T 80 50 ⚑ P0 Facility RVU 5.94 Non-Facility RVU 5.94 FUD 010

54512 **Excision of extraparenchymal lesion of testis** ♂
A2 T 50 ⚑ Facility RVU 15.30 Non-Facility RVU 15.30 FUD 090

54520 **Orchiectomy, simple (including subcapsular), with or without testicular prosthesis, scrotal or inguinal approach** ♂
INCLUDES Huggins' orchiectomy
EXCLUDES *Lymphadenectomy, radical retroperitoneal (38780)*
Code also hernia repair if performed (49505, 49507)
A2 T 50 ⚑ Facility RVU 9.26 Non-Facility RVU 9.26 FUD 090

54522 **Orchiectomy, partial** ♂
EXCLUDES *Lymphadenectomy, radical retroperitoneal (38780)*
A2 T 80 50 ⚑ Facility RVU 17.08 Non-Facility RVU 17.08 FUD 090

54530 **Orchiectomy, radical, for tumor; inguinal approach** ♂
EXCLUDES *Lymphadenectomy, radical retroperitoneal (38780)*
A2 T 80 50 ⚑ Facility RVU 14.34 Non-Facility RVU 14.34 FUD 090

54535 **with abdominal exploration** ♂
EXCLUDES *Lymphadenectomy, radical retroperitoneal (38780)*
T 80 50 ⚑ Facility RVU 21.09 Non-Facility RVU 21.09 FUD 090

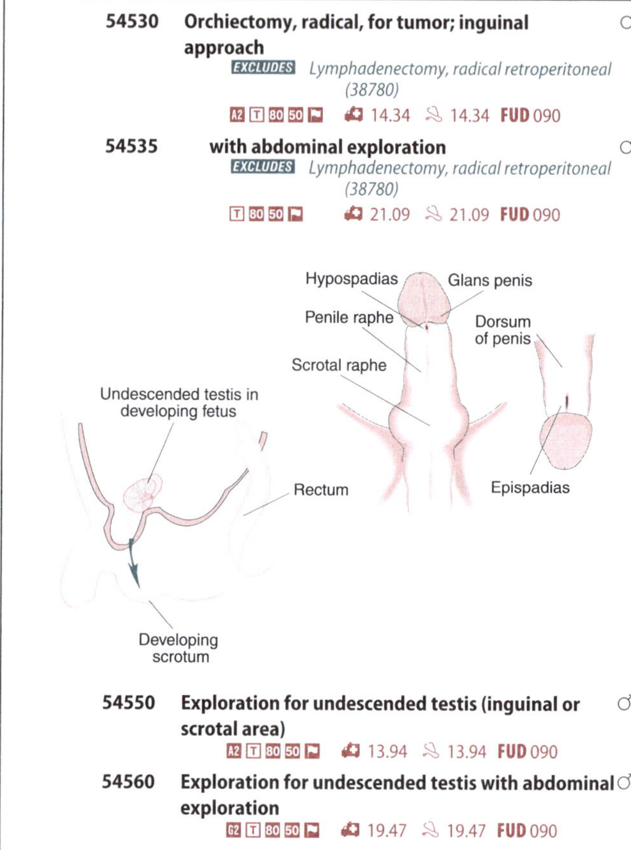

54550 **Exploration for undescended testis (inguinal or scrotal area)** ♂
A2 T 80 50 ⚑ Facility RVU 13.94 Non-Facility RVU 13.94 FUD 090

54560 **Exploration for undescended testis with abdominal exploration** ♂
G2 T 80 50 ⚑ Facility RVU 19.47 Non-Facility RVU 19.47 FUD 090

54600-54699 Open and Laparoscopic Testicular Procedures

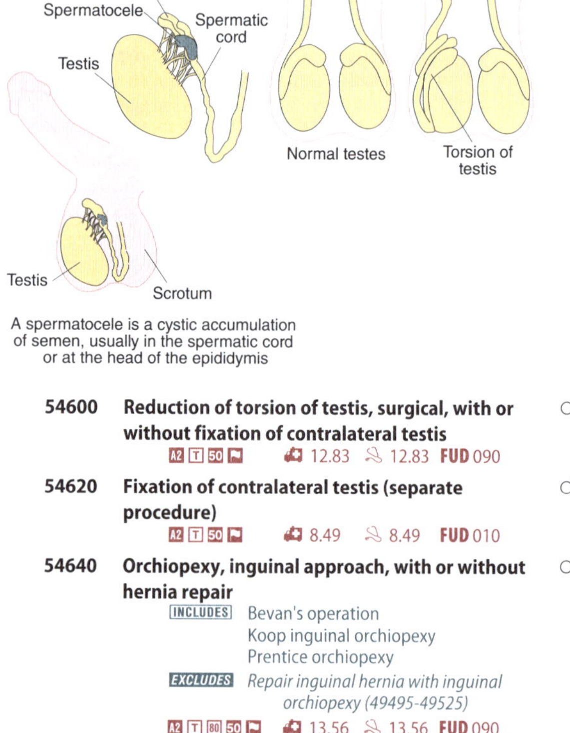

A spermatocele is a cystic accumulation of semen, usually in the spermatic cord or at the head of the epididymis

54600 **Reduction of torsion of testis, surgical, with or without fixation of contralateral testis** ♂
A2 T 50 ⚑ Facility RVU 12.83 Non-Facility RVU 12.83 FUD 090

54620 **Fixation of contralateral testis (separate procedure)** ♂
A2 T 50 ⚑ Facility RVU 8.49 Non-Facility RVU 8.49 FUD 010

54640 **Orchiopexy, inguinal approach, with or without hernia repair** ♂
INCLUDES Bevan's operation
Koop inguinal orchiopexy
Prentice orchiopexy
EXCLUDES *Repair inguinal hernia with inguinal orchiopexy (49495-49525)*
A2 T 80 50 ⚑ Facility RVU 13.56 Non-Facility RVU 13.56 FUD 090

54650 **Orchiopexy, abdominal approach, for intra-abdominal testis (eg, Fowler-Stephens)** ♂
EXCLUDES *Laparoscopic orchiopexy (54692)*
T 80 50 ⚑ Facility RVU 20.17 Non-Facility RVU 20.17 FUD 090

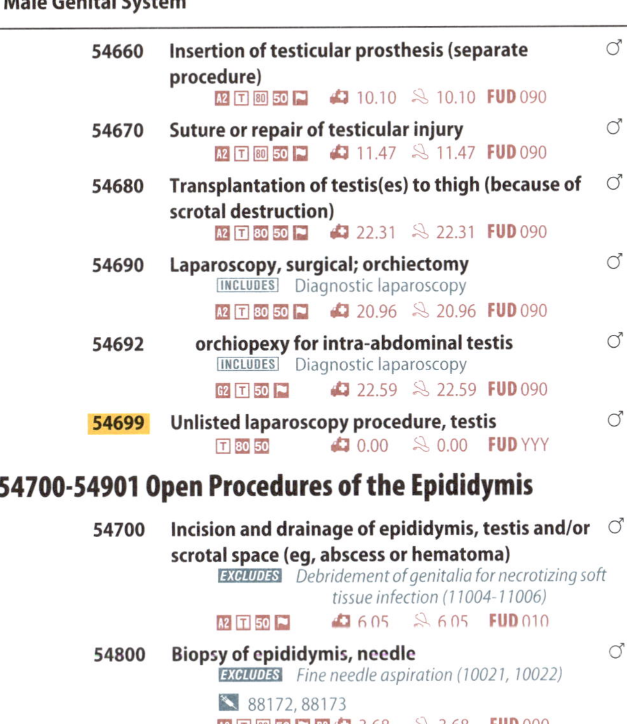

54660 Insertion of testicular prosthesis (separate procedure) ♂
A2 T 80 50 — 10.10 — 10.10 FUD 090

54670 Suture or repair of testicular injury ♂
A2 T 80 50 — 11.47 — 11.47 FUD 090

54680 Transplantation of testis(es) to thigh (because of scrotal destruction) ♂
A2 T 80 50 — 22.31 — 22.31 FUD 090

54690 Laparoscopy, surgical; orchiectomy ♂
INCLUDES Diagnostic laparoscopy
A2 T 80 50 — 20.96 — 20.96 FUD 090

54692 orchiopexy for intra-abdominal testis ♂
INCLUDES Diagnostic laparoscopy
G2 T 50 — 22.59 — 22.59 FUD 090

54699 Unlisted laparoscopy procedure, testis ♂
T 80 50 — 0.00 — 0.00 FUD YYY

54700-54901 Open Procedures of the Epididymis

54700 Incision and drainage of epididymis, testis and/or scrotal space (eg, abscess or hematoma) ♂
EXCLUDES *Debridement of genitalia for necrotizing soft tissue infection (11004-11006)*
A2 T 50 — 6.05 — 6.05 FUD 010

54800 Biopsy of epididymis, needle ♂
EXCLUDES *Fine needle aspiration (10021, 10022)*
88172, 88173
A2 T 80 50 PQ — 3.68 — 3.68 FUD 000

54830 Excision of local lesion of epididymis ♂
A2 T 80 50 — 10.56 — 10.56 FUD 090

54840 Excision of spermatocele, with or without epididymectomy ♂
A2 T 50 — 9.10 — 9.10 FUD 090

54860 Epididymectomy; unilateral ♂
A2 T — 11.86 — 11.86 FUD 090

54861 bilateral ♂
A2 T 80 — 16.02 — 16.02 FUD 090

54865 Exploration of epididymis, with or without biopsy ♂
A2 T 80 PQ — 10.16 — 10.16 FUD 090

54900 Epididymovasostomy, anastomosis of epididymis to vas deferens; unilateral ♂
EXCLUDES *Operating microscope (69990)*
A2 T 80 — 22.35 — 22.35 FUD 090

54901 bilateral ♂
EXCLUDES *Operating microscope (69990)*
A2 T 80 — 30.57 — 30.57 FUD 090

55000-55180 Procedures of the Tunica Vaginalis and Scrotum

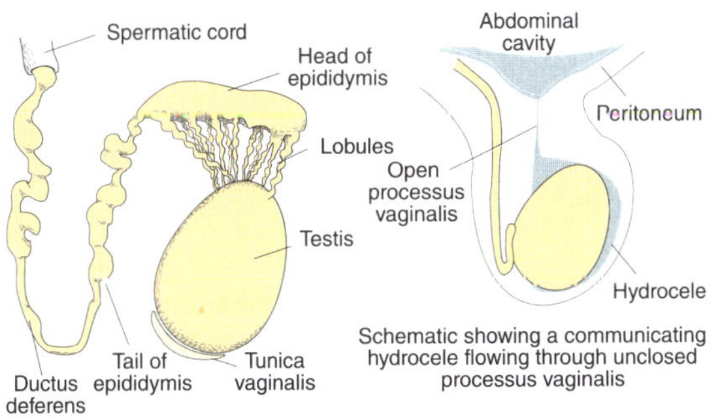

55000 Puncture aspiration of hydrocele, tunica vaginalis, with or without injection of medication ♂
P3 T 50 — 2.40 — 3.28 FUD 000

55040 Excision of hydrocele; unilateral ♂
EXCLUDES *Repair of hernia with hydrocelectomy (49495-49501)*
A2 T — 9.61 — 9.61 FUD 090

55041 bilateral ♂
EXCLUDES *Repair of hernia with hydrocelectomy (49495-49501)*
A2 T — 14.47 — 14.47 FUD 090

55060 Repair of tunica vaginalis hydrocele (Bottle type) ♂
A2 T 80 50 — 10.81 — 10.81 FUD 090

55100 Drainage of scrotal wall abscess ♂
EXCLUDES *Debridement of genitalia for necrotizing soft tissue infection (11004-11006)*
Incision and drainage of scrotal space (54700)
A2 T — 4.74 — 6.10 FUD 010

55110 Scrotal exploration ♂
A2 T — 11.01 — 11.01 FUD 090

55120 Removal of foreign body in scrotum ♂
A2 T 80 — 10.17 — 10.17 FUD 090

55150 Resection of scrotum ♂
EXCLUDES *Lesion excision of skin of scrotum (11420-11426, 11620-11626)*
A2 T 80 — 13.96 — 13.96 FUD 090

55175 Scrotoplasty; simple ♂
A2 T 80 — 10.28 — 10.28 FUD 090

55180 complicated ♂
A2 T 80 — 19.73 — 19.73 FUD 090

55200-55680 Procedures of Other Male Genital Ducts and Glands

55200 Vasotomy, cannulization with or without incision of vas, unilateral or bilateral (separate procedure) ♂
A2 T 80 — 7.93 — 12.30 FUD 090

55250 Vasectomy, unilateral or bilateral (separate procedure), including postoperative semen examination(s) ♂
A2 T — 6.43 — 10.73 FUD 090

55300 Vasotomy for vasograms, seminal vesiculograms, or epididymograms, unilateral or bilateral ♂
Code also biopsy of testis and modifier 51 when combined (54505)
74440
N1 N 80 — 5.33 — 5.33 FUD 000

55400 Vasovasostomy, vasovasorrhaphy ♂
EXCLUDES *Operating microscope (69990)*
A2 T 80 50 — 15.04 — 15.04 FUD 090

55450 Ligation (percutaneous) of vas deferens, unilateral or bilateral (separate procedure) ♂
P3 T 80 — 7.28 — 10.04 FUD 010

55500 Excision of hydrocele of spermatic cord, unilateral (separate procedure) ♂
A2 T 80 50 — 11.29 — 11.29 FUD 090

55520 Excision of lesion of spermatic cord (separate procedure) ♂
A2 T 80 50 — 12.88 — 12.88 FUD 090

55530 Excision of varicocele or ligation of spermatic veins for varicocele; (separate procedure) ♂
A2 T 50 — 10.01 — 10.01 FUD 090

55535 abdominal approach ♂
A2 T 80 50 — 12.18 — 12.18 FUD 090

55540 with hernia repair ♂
A2 T 50 — 15.39 — 15.39 FUD 090

55550 Laparoscopy, surgical, with ligation of spermatic veins for varicocele ♂
INCLUDES Diagnostic laparoscopy
A2 T 80 50 — 12.13 — 12.13 FUD 090

55559 Unlisted laparoscopy procedure, spermatic cord ♂
T 80 50 — 0.00 — 0.00 FUD YYY

55600 **Vesiculotomy;** ♂
A2 T 80 50 ⚑ 11.94 11.94 FUD 090

55605 **complicated** ♂
C 80 50 ⚑ 15.34 15.34 FUD 090

55650 **Vesiculectomy, any approach** ♂
C 80 50 ⚑ 20.34 20.34 FUD 090

55680 **Excision of Mullerian duct cyst** ♂
EXCLUDES *Injection procedure (52010, 55300)*
A2 T 80 50 ⚑ 9.80 9.80 FUD 090

55700-55725 Procedures of Prostate: Incisional

Bladder
Suprapubic approach
Pubic bone
Pubic bone
Ischial tuberosity
Rectum
Vesicle
Prostate
Urethra

Perineal approach (retropubic) to prostate (above) and side view schematic of suprapubic approach

55700 **Biopsy, prostate; needle or punch, single or multiple, any approach** ♂
EXCLUDES *Fine needle aspiration (10021, 10022)*
Needle biopsy of prostate, saturation sampling for prostate mapping (55706)
76942
88172, 88173
A2 T ⚑ PQ 3.97 6.10 FUD 000

55705 **incisional, any approach** ♂
A2 T ⚑ PQ 7.53 7.53 FUD 010

55706 **Biopsies, prostate, needle, transperineal, stereotactic template guided saturation sampling, including imaging guidance** ♂
Do not report with (55700)
G2 T 80 PQ 10.41 10.41 FUD 010

55720 **Prostatotomy, external drainage of prostatic abscess, any approach; simple** ♂
EXCLUDES *Drainage of prostatic abscess, transurethral (52700)*
A2 T 80 ⚑ 12.79 12.79 FUD 090

55725 **complicated** ♂
EXCLUDES *Drainage of prostatic abscess, transurethral (52700)*
A2 T 80 ⚑ 16.81 16.81 FUD 090

55801-55845 Open Prostatectomy

EXCLUDES *Limited pelvic lymphadenectomy for staging (separate procedure) (38562)*
Node dissection, independent (38770-38780)
Transurethral prostate
Destruction (53850-53852)
Resection (52601-52640)

55801 **Prostatectomy, perineal, subtotal (including control of postoperative bleeding, vasectomy, meatotomy, urethral calibration and/or dilation, and internal urethrotomy)** ♂
C 80 ⚑ PQ 31.01 31.01 FUD 090

55810 **Prostatectomy, perineal radical;** ♂
INCLUDES Walsh modified radical prostatectomy
C 80 ⚑ PQ 37.39 37.39 FUD 090

55812 **with lymph node biopsy(s) (limited pelvic lymphadenectomy)** ♂
C 80 ⚑ PQ 45.66 45.66 FUD 090

55815 **with bilateral pelvic lymphadenectomy, including external iliac, hypogastric and obturator nodes** ♂
EXCLUDES *Perineal radical prostatectomy when performed on a separate day from bilateral pelvic lymphadenectomy (38770, 55810)*
C 80 ⚑ PQ 50.04 50.04 FUD 090

55821 **Prostatectomy (including control of postoperative bleeding, vasectomy, meatotomy, urethral calibration and/or dilation, and internal urethrotomy); suprapubic, subtotal, 1 or 2 stages** ♂
C 80 ⚑ PQ 24.79 24.79 FUD 090

55831 **retropubic, subtotal** ♂
C 80 ⚑ PQ 26.81 26.81 FUD 090

55840 **Prostatectomy, retropubic radical, with or without nerve sparing;** ♂
EXCLUDES *Prostatectomy, radical retropubic, performed laparoscopically (55866)*
C 80 ⚑ PQ 37.95 37.95 FUD 090

55842 **with lymph node biopsy(s) (limited pelvic lymphadenectomy)** ♂
EXCLUDES *Prostatectomy, retropubic radical, performed laparoscopically (55866)*
C 80 ⚑ PQ 40.65 40.65 FUD 090

55845 **with bilateral pelvic lymphadenectomy, including external iliac, hypogastric, and obturator nodes** ♂
EXCLUDES *Prostatectomy, retropubic radical, performed laparoscopically (55866)*
Radical retropubic prostatectomy when performed on a separate day from bilateral pelvic lymphadenectomy (38770, 55840)
C 80 ⚑ PQ 46.42 46.42 FUD 090

55860-55865 Prostate Exposure for Radiation Source Application

55860 **Exposure of prostate, any approach, for insertion of radioactive substance;** ♂
77776-77778
G2 T ⚑ 24.80 24.80 FUD 090

55862 **with lymph node biopsy(s) (limited pelvic lymphadenectomy)** ♂
C 80 ⚑ 31.10 31.10 FUD 090

55865 **with bilateral pelvic lymphadenectomy, including external iliac, hypogastric and obturator nodes** ♂
C 80 ⚑ 37.85 37.85 FUD 090

55866 Laparoscopic Prostatectomy

55866 **Laparoscopy, surgical prostatectomy, retropubic radical, including nerve sparing, includes robotic assistance, when performed** ♂
INCLUDES Diagnostic laparoscopy
EXCLUDES *Open method (55840)*
C 80 ⚑ PQ 49.28 49.28 FUD 090

55870-55899 Miscellaneous Prostate Procedures

55870 **Electroejaculation** ♂
EXCLUDES *Artificial insemination (58321-58322)*
P3 T ⚑ 4.05 4.94 FUD 000

55873 **Cryosurgical ablation of the prostate (includes ultrasonic guidance and monitoring)** ♂
Code also (C2618)
J8 T ⚑ PQ 21.71 190.67 FUD 090

55875 Transperineal placement of needles or catheters into prostate for interstitial radioelement application, with or without cystoscopy ♂
EXCLUDES The placement of needles or catheters into the pelvic organs and/or genitalia (except for the prostate) for interstitial radioelement application (55920)
76965, 77776-77787
A2 03 80 PQ 21.63 21.63 FUD 090

55876 Placement of interstitial device(s) for radiation therapy guidance (eg, fiducial markers, dosimeter), prostate (via needle, any approach), single or multiple ♂
Code also supply of device
76942, 77002, 77012, 77021
P3 X PQ 2.85 3.79 FUD 000

55899 Unlisted procedure, male genital system ♂
T 80 0.00 0.00 FUD YYY

55920 Insertion Brachytherapy Catheters/Needles Pelvis/Genitalia, Male/Female

55920 Placement of needles or catheters into pelvic organs and/or genitalia (except prostate) for subsequent interstitial radioelement application
EXCLUDES Insertion of Heyman capsules for purposes of brachytherapy (58346)
Insertion of vaginal ovoids and/or uterine tandems for purposes of brachytherapy (57155)
Placement of catheters or needles, prostate (55875)
G2 T 80 12.74 12.74 FUD 000

55970-55980 Transsexual Surgery

CMS 100-2,16,180 Services Related to Noncovered Procedures
CMS 100-3,140.3 Transexual Surgery

55970 Intersex surgery; male to female ♂
T 0.00 0.00 FUD YYY

55980 female to male ♀
T 0.00 0.00 FUD YYY

56405-56420 Incision and Drainage of Abscess

EXCLUDES Incision and drainage Skene's gland cyst/abscess (53060)
Incision and drainage subcutaneous abscess/cyst/furuncle (10040, 10060, 10061)

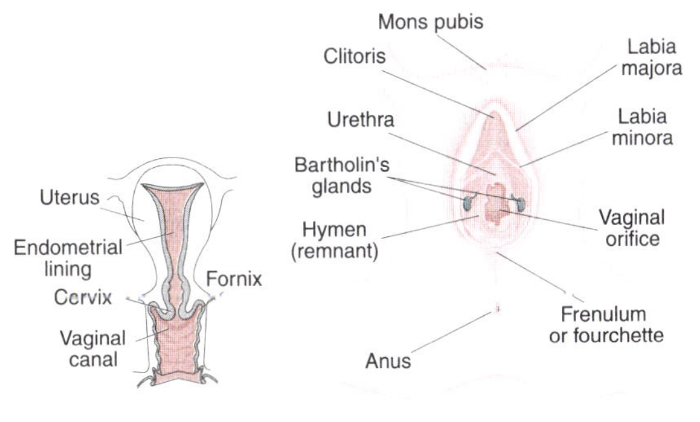

56405 Incision and drainage of vulva or perineal abscess ♀
P3 T 3.13 3.15 FUD 010

56420 Incision and drainage of Bartholin's gland abscess ♀
P3 T 2.64 3.47 FUD 010

56440-56442 Other Female Genital Incisional Procedures

EXCLUDES Incision and drainage subcutaneous abscess/cyst/furuncle (10040, 10060, 10061)

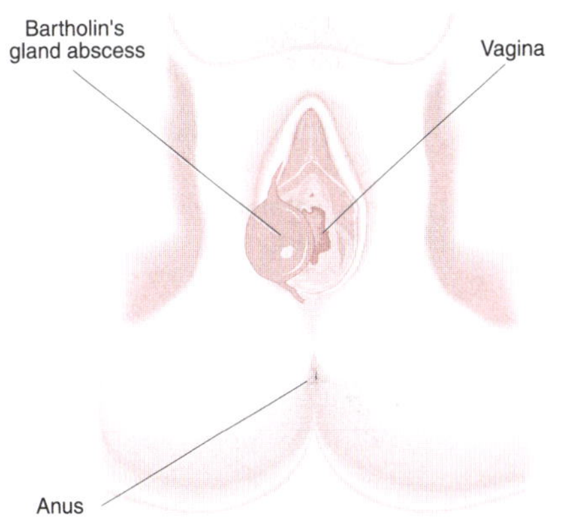

56440 Marsupialization of Bartholin's gland cyst ♀
A2 T 5.28 5.28 FUD 010

56441 Lysis of labial adhesions ♀
A2 T 80 3.97 4.10 FUD 010

56442 Hymenotomy, simple incision ♀
A2 T 80 1.39 1.39 FUD 000

56501-56515 Destruction of Vulvar Lesions, Any Method

CMS 100-3,140.5 Laser Procedures

EXCLUDES Excision/fulguration/destruction
Skene's glands (53270)
Urethral caruncle (53265)

56501 Destruction of lesion(s), vulva; simple (eg, laser surgery, electrosurgery, cryosurgery, chemosurgery) ♀
P3 T 3.31 3.74 FUD 010

56515 extensive (eg, laser surgery, electrosurgery, cryosurgery, chemosurgery) ♀
A2 T 5.76 6.44 FUD 010

56605-56606 Vulvar and Perineal Biopsies

EXCLUDES Excision local lesion (11420-11426, 11620-11626)

56605 Biopsy of vulva or perineum (separate procedure); 1 lesion ♀
P3 T PQ 1.75 2.36 FUD 000

+ 56606 each separate additional lesion (List separately in addition to code for primary procedure) ♀
Code first (56605)
N1 N 0.85 1.07 FUD ZZZ

56620-56640 Vulvectomy Procedures

INCLUDES Removal of:
Greater than 80% of the vulvar area - complete procedure
Less than 80% of the vulvar area - partial procedure
Skin and deep subcutaneous tissue - radical procedure
Skin and superficial subcutaneous tissues - simple procedure

EXCLUDES Skin graft (15004-15005, 15120-15121, 15240-15241)

56620 Vulvectomy simple; partial ♀
A2 T 80 14.70 14.70 FUD 090

56625 complete ♀
A2 T 80 17.66 17.66 FUD 090

56630 Vulvectomy, radical, partial; ♀
C 80 PQ 26.06 26.06 FUD 090

56631 with unilateral inguinofemoral lymphadenectomy ♀
INCLUDES Bassett's operation
C 80 PQ 33.15 33.15 FUD 090

56632 **with bilateral inguinofemoral lymphadenectomy** ♀
INCLUDES Bassett's operation
C 80 ⚑ PQ 38.47 38.47 FUD 090

56633 **Vulvectomy, radical, complete;** ♀
INCLUDES Bassett's operation
C 80 ⚑ PQ 33.97 33.97 FUD 090

56634 **with unilateral inguinofemoral lymphadenectomy** ♀
INCLUDES Bassett's operation
C 80 ⚑ PQ 36.10 36.10 FUD 090

56637 **with bilateral inguinofemoral lymphadenectomy** ♀
INCLUDES Bassett's operation
C 80 ⚑ PQ 42.14 42.14 FUD 090

56640 **Vulvectomy, radical, complete, with inguinofemoral, iliac, and pelvic lymphadenectomy** ♀
INCLUDES Bassett's operation
EXCLUDES *Lymphadenectomy (38760-38780)*
C 80 50 ⚑ PQ 42.21 42.21 FUD 090

56700-56740 Other Excisional Procedures: External Female Genitalia

56700 **Partial hymenectomy or revision of hymenal ring** ♀
A2 T 80 ⚑ 5.41 5.41 FUD 010

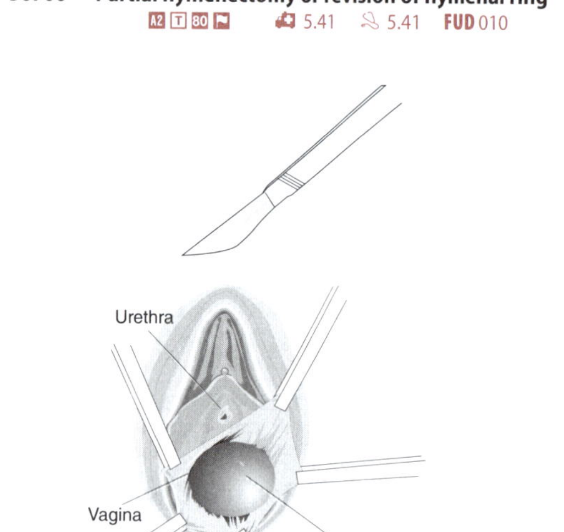

56740 **Excision of Bartholin's gland or cyst** ♀
EXCLUDES *Excision/fulguration/marsupialization:*
Skene's glands (53270)
Urethral carcinoma (53220)
Urethral caruncle (53265)
Urethral diverticulum (53230, 53240)
A2 T 50 ⚑ 8.63 8.63 FUD 010

56800-56810 Repair/Reconstruction External Female Genitalia

EXCLUDES *Repair of urethra for mucosal prolapse (53275)*

56800 **Plastic repair of introitus** ♀
INCLUDES Emmet's operation
A2 T 80 ⚑ 6.93 6.93 FUD 010

56805 **Clitoroplasty for intersex state** ♀
G2 T 80 ⚑ 33.29 33.29 FUD 090

56810 **Perineoplasty, repair of perineum, nonobstetrical (separate procedure)** ♀
INCLUDES Emmet's operation
EXCLUDES *Genitalia wound repair (12001-12007, 12041-12047, 13131-13133)*
Introitus plastic repair (56800)
Sphincteroplasty, anal (46750, 46751)
Vaginal/perineum recent injury repair, nonobstetrical (57210)
Vulva/perineum episiorrhaphy/episioperineorrhaphy for recent injury, nonobstetrical (57210)
A2 T 80 ⚑ 7.50 7.50 FUD 010

56820-56821 Vulvar Colposcopy with/without Biopsy

EXCLUDES *Colposcopic procedures and/or examinations:*
Cervix (57452-57461)
Vagina (57420-57421)

56820 **Colposcopy of the vulva;** ♀
P3 T ⚑ 2.49 3.20 FUD 000

56821 **with biopsy(s)** ♀
P3 T ⚑ PQ 3.34 4.22 FUD 000

57000-57023 Incisional Procedures: Vagina

57000 **Colpotomy; with exploration** ♀
A2 T 80 ⚑ 5.47 5.47 FUD 010

57010 **with drainage of pelvic abscess** ♀
INCLUDES Laroyenne operation
A2 T 80 ⚑ 12.58 12.58 FUD 090

57020 **Colpocentesis (separate procedure)** ♀
A2 T 80 ⚑ 2.38 2.71 FUD 000

57022 **Incision and drainage of vaginal hematoma; obstetrical/postpartum** ♀
A2 T 80 ⚑ 5.00 5.00 FUD 010

57023 **non-obstetrical (eg, post-trauma, spontaneous bleeding)** ♀
A2 T 80 ⚑ 9.00 9.00 FUD 010

57061-57065 Destruction of Vaginal Lesions, Any Method

CMS 100-3,140.5 Laser Procedures

57061 **Destruction of vaginal lesion(s); simple (eg, laser surgery, electrosurgery, cryosurgery, chemosurgery)** ♀
P3 T ⚑ 2.83 3.24 FUD 010

57065 **extensive (eg, laser surgery, electrosurgery, cryosurgery, chemosurgery)** ♀
A2 T ⚑ 4.97 5.53 FUD 010

57100-57135 Excisional Procedures: Vagina

57100 **Biopsy of vaginal mucosa; simple (separate procedure)** ♀
P3 T ⚑ PQ 1.92 2.53 FUD 000

57105 **extensive, requiring suture (including cysts)** ♀
A2 T ⚑ PQ 3.61 3.87 FUD 010

57106 **Vaginectomy, partial removal of vaginal wall;** ♀
T 80 ⚑ 14.00 14.00 FUD 090

57107 **with removal of paravaginal tissue (radical vaginectomy)** ♀
T 80 ⚑ 41.16 41.16 FUD 090

57109 **with removal of paravaginal tissue (radical vaginectomy) with bilateral total pelvic lymphadenectomy and para-aortic lymph node sampling (biopsy)** ♀
T 80 ⚑ 48.28 48.28 FUD 090

57110 **Vaginectomy, complete removal of vaginal wall;** ♀
C 80 ⚑ 26.02 26.02 FUD 090

57111 **with removal of paravaginal tissue (radical vaginectomy)** ♀
C 80 ⚑ 46.65 46.65 FUD 090

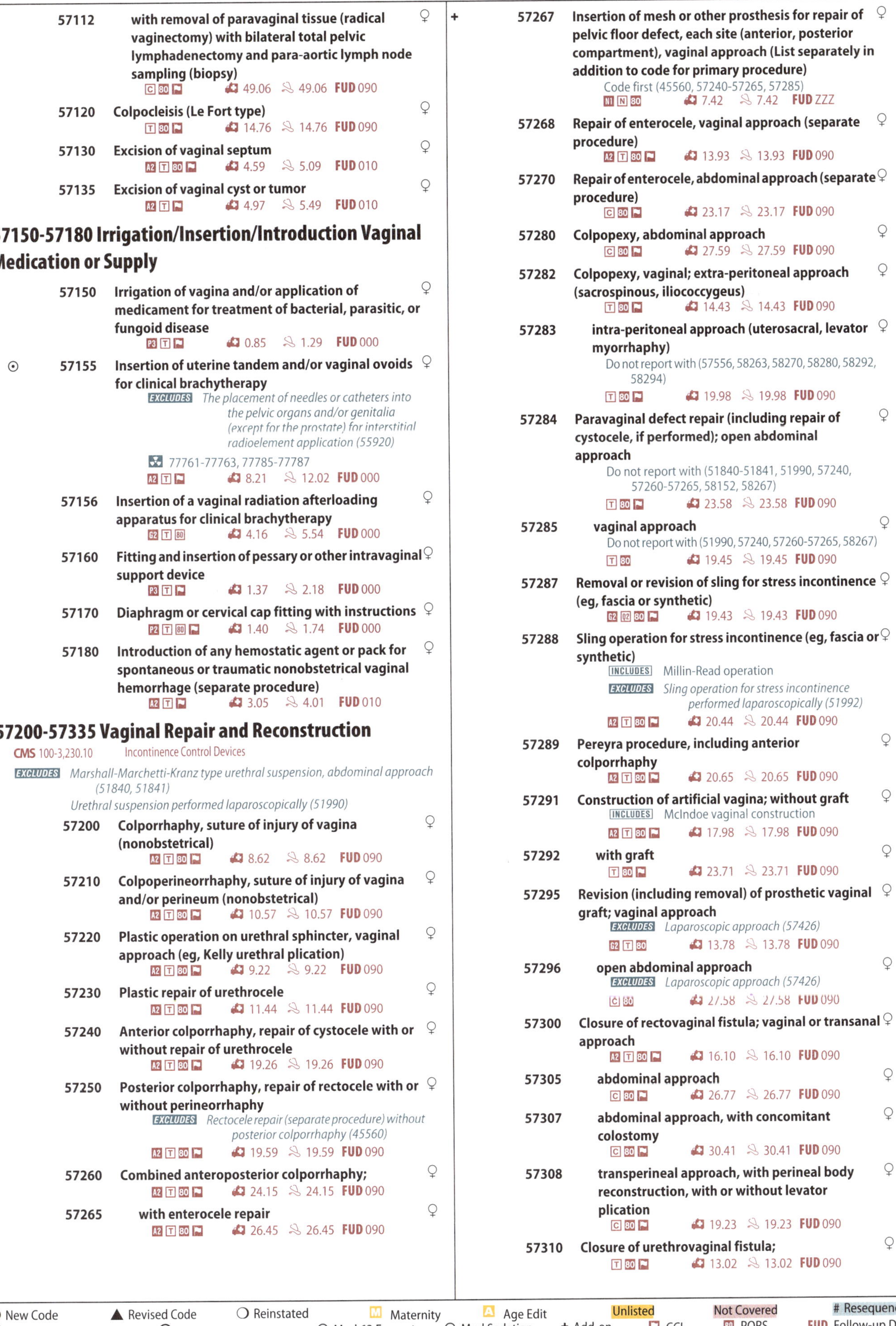

57112 with removal of paravaginal tissue (radical vaginectomy) with bilateral total pelvic lymphadenectomy and para-aortic lymph node sampling (biopsy) ♀
C 80 — 49.06 — 49.06 FUD 090

57120 Colpocleisis (Le Fort type) ♀
T 80 — 14.76 — 14.76 FUD 090

57130 Excision of vaginal septum ♀
A2 T 80 — 4.59 — 5.09 FUD 010

57135 Excision of vaginal cyst or tumor ♀
A2 T — 4.97 — 5.49 FUD 010

57150-57180 Irrigation/Insertion/Introduction Vaginal Medication or Supply

57150 Irrigation of vagina and/or application of medicament for treatment of bacterial, parasitic, or fungoid disease ♀
P3 T — 0.85 — 1.29 FUD 000

⊙ 57155 Insertion of uterine tandem and/or vaginal ovoids for clinical brachytherapy ♀
EXCLUDES *The placement of needles or catheters into the pelvic organs and/or genitalia (except for the prostate) for interstitial radioelement application (55920)*
77761-77763, 77785-77787
A2 T — 8.21 — 12.02 FUD 000

57156 Insertion of a vaginal radiation afterloading apparatus for clinical brachytherapy ♀
G2 T 80 — 4.16 — 5.54 FUD 000

57160 Fitting and insertion of pessary or other intravaginal support device ♀
P3 T — 1.37 — 2.18 FUD 000

57170 Diaphragm or cervical cap fitting with instructions ♀
P2 T 80 — 1.40 — 1.74 FUD 000

57180 Introduction of any hemostatic agent or pack for spontaneous or traumatic nonobstetrical vaginal hemorrhage (separate procedure) ♀
A2 T — 3.05 — 4.01 FUD 010

57200-57335 Vaginal Repair and Reconstruction

CMS 100-3,230.10 Incontinence Control Devices

EXCLUDES *Marshall-Marchetti-Kranz type urethral suspension, abdominal approach (51840, 51841)*
Urethral suspension performed laparoscopically (51990)

57200 Colporrhaphy, suture of injury of vagina (nonobstetrical) ♀
A2 T 80 — 8.62 — 8.62 FUD 090

57210 Colpoperineorrhaphy, suture of injury of vagina and/or perineum (nonobstetrical) ♀
A2 T 80 — 10.57 — 10.57 FUD 090

57220 Plastic operation on urethral sphincter, vaginal approach (eg, Kelly urethral plication) ♀
A2 T 80 — 9.22 — 9.22 FUD 090

57230 Plastic repair of urethrocele ♀
A2 T 80 — 11.44 — 11.44 FUD 090

57240 Anterior colporrhaphy, repair of cystocele with or without repair of urethrocele ♀
A2 T 80 — 19.26 — 19.26 FUD 090

57250 Posterior colporrhaphy, repair of rectocele with or without perineorrhaphy ♀
EXCLUDES *Rectocele repair (separate procedure) without posterior colporrhaphy (45560)*
A2 T 80 — 19.59 — 19.59 FUD 090

57260 Combined anteroposterior colporrhaphy; ♀
A2 T 80 — 24.15 — 24.15 FUD 090

57265 with enterocele repair ♀
A2 T 80 — 26.45 — 26.45 FUD 090

+ 57267 Insertion of mesh or other prosthesis for repair of pelvic floor defect, each site (anterior, posterior compartment), vaginal approach (List separately in addition to code for primary procedure) ♀
Code first (45560, 57240-57265, 57285)
N1 N 80 — 7.42 — 7.42 FUD ZZZ

57268 Repair of enterocele, vaginal approach (separate procedure) ♀
A2 T 80 — 13.93 — 13.93 FUD 090

57270 Repair of enterocele, abdominal approach (separate procedure) ♀
C 80 — 23.17 — 23.17 FUD 090

57280 Colpopexy, abdominal approach ♀
C 80 — 27.59 — 27.59 FUD 090

57282 Colpopexy, vaginal; extra-peritoneal approach (sacrospinous, iliococcygeus) ♀
T 80 — 14.43 — 14.43 FUD 090

57283 intra-peritoneal approach (uterosacral, levator myorrhaphy) ♀
Do not report with (57556, 58263, 58270, 58280, 58292, 58294)
T 80 — 19.98 — 19.98 FUD 090

57284 Paravaginal defect repair (including repair of cystocele, if performed); open abdominal approach ♀
Do not report with (51840-51841, 51990, 57240, 57260-57265, 58152, 58267)
T 80 — 23.58 — 23.58 FUD 090

57285 vaginal approach ♀
Do not report with (51990, 57240, 57260-57265, 58267)
T 80 — 19.45 — 19.45 FUD 090

57287 Removal or revision of sling for stress incontinence (eg, fascia or synthetic) ♀
G2 02 80 — 19.43 — 19.43 FUD 090

57288 Sling operation for stress incontinence (eg, fascia or synthetic) ♀
INCLUDES Millin-Read operation
EXCLUDES *Sling operation for stress incontinence performed laparoscopically (51992)*
A2 T 80 — 20.44 — 20.44 FUD 090

57289 Pereyra procedure, including anterior colporrhaphy ♀
A2 T 80 — 20.65 — 20.65 FUD 090

57291 Construction of artificial vagina; without graft ♀
INCLUDES McIndoe vaginal construction
A2 T 80 — 17.98 — 17.98 FUD 090

57292 with graft ♀
T 80 — 23.71 — 23.71 FUD 090

57295 Revision (including removal) of prosthetic vaginal graft; vaginal approach ♀
EXCLUDES *Laparoscopic approach (57426)*
G2 T 80 — 13.78 — 13.78 FUD 090

57296 open abdominal approach ♀
EXCLUDES *Laparoscopic approach (57426)*
C 80 — 27.58 — 27.58 FUD 090

57300 Closure of rectovaginal fistula; vaginal or transanal approach ♀
A2 T 80 — 16.10 — 16.10 FUD 090

57305 abdominal approach ♀
C 80 — 26.77 — 26.77 FUD 090

57307 abdominal approach, with concomitant colostomy ♀
C 80 — 30.41 — 30.41 FUD 090

57308 transperineal approach, with perineal body reconstruction, with or without levator plication ♀
C 80 — 19.23 — 19.23 FUD 090

57310 Closure of urethrovaginal fistula; ♀
T 80 — 13.02 — 13.02 FUD 090

57311 **with bulbocavernosus transplant** ♀
C 80 ⚑ 14.83 14.83 FUD 090

57320 **Closure of vesicovaginal fistula; vaginal approach** ♀
EXCLUDES *Cystostomy, concomitant (51020-51040, 51101-51102)*
62 T 80 ⚑ 15.16 15.16 FUD 090

57330 **transvesical and vaginal approach** ♀
EXCLUDES *Vesicovaginal fistula closure, abdominal approach (51900)*
T 80 ⚑ 20.94 20.94 FUD 090

57335 **Vaginoplasty for intersex state** ♀
T 80 ⚑ 32.60 32.60 FUD 090

57400-57415 Treatment of Vaginal Disorders Under Anesthesia

57400 **Dilation of vagina under anesthesia (other than local)** ♀
A2 T 80 ⚑ 3.88 3.88 FUD 000

57410 **Pelvic examination under anesthesia (other than local)** ♀
A2 T ⚑ 3.11 3.11 FUD 000

57415 **Removal of impacted vaginal foreign body (separate procedure) under anesthesia (other than local)** ♀
EXCLUDES *Removal of impacted vaginal foreign body without anesthesia, report with appropriate evaluation and management service code*
A2 T 80 ⚑ 4.59 4.59 FUD 010

57420-57426 Endoscopic Vaginal Procedures

57420 **Colposcopy of the entire vagina, with cervix if present;** ♀
EXCLUDES *Colposcopic procedures and/or examinations:*
Cervix (57452-57461)
Vulva (56820-56821)
Endometrial sampling (biopsy) performed at the same time as colposcopy (58110)
Code also modifier 51 for colposcopic procedures of different sites, as appropriate
P3 T ⚑ 2.63 3.34 FUD 000

57421 **with biopsy(s) of vagina/cervix** ♀
EXCLUDES *Colposcopic procedures and/or examinations:*
Cervix (57452-57461)
Vulva (56820-56821)
Endometrial sampling (biopsy) performed at the same time as colposcopy (58110)
Code also modifier 51 for colposcopic procedures of multiple sites, as appropriate
P3 T ⚑ PQ 3.58 4.48 FUD 000

57423 **Paravaginal defect repair (including repair of cystocele, if performed), laparoscopic approach** ♀
Do not report with (49320, 51840-51841, 51990, 57240, 57260, 58152, 58267)
T 80 26.62 26.62 FUD 090

57425 **Laparoscopy, surgical, colpopexy (suspension of vaginal apex)** ♀
T 80 ⚑ 28.07 28.07 FUD 090

57426 **Revision (including removal) of prosthetic vaginal graft, laparoscopic approach** ♀
EXCLUDES *Open abdominal approach (57296)*
Vaginal approach (57295)
62 T 80 24.55 24.55 FUD 090

57452-57461 Endoscopic Cervical Procedures

EXCLUDES *Colposcopic procedures and/or examinations:*
Vagina (57420-57421)
Vulva (56820-56821)
Code also endometrial sampling (biopsy) performed at the same time as colposcopy (58110)

57452 **Colposcopy of the cervix including upper/adjacent vagina;** ♀
Do not report with (57454-57461)
P3 T ⚑ 2.66 3.12 FUD 000

57454 **with biopsy(s) of the cervix and endocervical curettage** ♀
P3 T ⚑ PQ 3.95 4.41 FUD 000

57455 **with biopsy(s) of the cervix** ♀
P3 T ⚑ PQ 3.23 4.10 FUD 000

57456 **with endocervical curettage** ♀
Do not report with (57461)
P3 T ⚑ 3.01 3.88 FUD 000

57460 **with loop electrode biopsy(s) of the cervix** ♀
P3 T ⚑ PQ 4.75 8.06 FUD 000

57461 **with loop electrode conization of the cervix** ♀
Do not report with (57456)
P3 T ⚑ 5.48 9.13 FUD 000

57500-57556 Cervical Procedures: Multiple Techniques

EXCLUDES *Destruction/excision of endometriomas, open method (49203-49205, 58957-58958)*
Radical surgical procedures (58200-58240)

57500 **Biopsy of cervix, single or multiple, or local excision of lesion, with or without fulguration (separate procedure)** ♀
P3 T ⚑ PQ 2.20 3.63 FUD 000

57505 **Endocervical curettage (not done as part of a dilation and curettage)** ♀
P3 T ⚑ 2.64 2.91 FUD 010

57510 **Cautery of cervix; electro or thermal** ♀
P3 T ⚑ 3.36 3.78 FUD 010

57511 **cryocautery, initial or repeat** ♀
P3 T ⚑ 3.83 4.17 FUD 010

57513 **laser ablation** ♀
A2 T ⚑ 3.85 4.15 FUD 010

57520 **Conization of cervix, with or without fulguration, with or without dilation and curettage, with or without repair; cold knife or laser** ♀
EXCLUDES *Dilation and curettage, diagnostic/therapeutic, nonobstetrical (58120)*
A2 T ⚑ PQ 7.88 8.75 FUD 090

57522 **loop electrode excision** ♀
A2 T ⚑ 7.03 7.57 FUD 090

57530 **Trachelectomy (cervicectomy), amputation of cervix (separate procedure)** ♀
A2 T 80 ⚑ 9.95 9.95 FUD 090

57531 **Radical trachelectomy, with bilateral total pelvic lymphadenectomy and para-aortic lymph node sampling biopsy, with or without removal of tube(s), with or without removal of ovary(s)** ♀
C 80 ⚑ 50.98 50.98 FUD 090

57540 **Excision of cervical stump, abdominal approach;** ♀
C 80 ⚑ 22.60 22.60 FUD 090

57545 **with pelvic floor repair** ♀
C 80 ⚑ 23.85 23.85 FUD 090

57550 **Excision of cervical stump, vaginal approach;** ♀
A2 T 80 ⚑ 11.80 11.80 FUD 090

57555 **with anterior and/or posterior repair** ♀
T 80 ⚑ 17.41 17.41 FUD 090

57556 **with repair of enterocele** ♀
EXCLUDES *Insertion of hemostatic agent/pack for spontaneous/traumatic nonobstetrical vaginal hemorrhage (57180)*
Intrauterine device insertion (58300)
A2 T 80 ⚑ 16.38 16.38 FUD 090

57558-57800 Cervical Procedures: Dilation, Suturing, or Instrumentation

EXCLUDES *Destruction/excision of endometriomas, open method (49203-49205, 58957-58958)*

57558 Dilation and curettage of cervical stump ♀
EXCLUDES *Radical surgical procedures (58200-58240)*
A2 T 3.29 3.60 FUD 010

57700 Cerclage of uterine cervix, nonobstetrical ♀
INCLUDES McDonald cerclage
Shirodker operation
A2 T 80 8.95 8.95 FUD 090

57720 Trachelorrhaphy, plastic repair of uterine cervix, vaginal approach ♀
INCLUDES Emmet operation
A2 T 80 8.87 8.87 FUD 090

57800 Dilation of cervical canal, instrumental (separate procedure) ♀
P3 T 1.40 1.72 FUD 000

58100-58120 Procedures Involving the Endometrium

CMS 100-3,230.6 Vabra Aspirator

58100 Endometrial sampling (biopsy) with or without endocervical sampling (biopsy), without cervical dilation, any method (separate procedure) ♀
EXCLUDES *Endocervical curettage only (57505)*
Endometrial sampling (biopsy) performed in conjunction with colposcopy (58110)
P3 T PQ 2.56 3.14 FUD 000

+ **58110 Endometrial sampling (biopsy) performed in conjunction with colposcopy (List separately in addition to code for primary procedure)** ♀
Code first colposcopy (57420-57421, 57452-57461)
N1 N 80 1.19 1.38 FUD ZZZ

58120 Dilation and curettage, diagnostic and/or therapeutic (nonobstetrical) ♀
EXCLUDES *Postpartum hemorrhage (59160)*
A2 T 6.32 7.40 FUD 010

58140-58146 Myomectomy Procedures

58140 Myomectomy, excision of fibroid tumor(s) of uterus, 1 to 4 intramural myoma(s) with total weight of 250 g or less and/or removal of surface myomas; abdominal approach ♀
C 80 26.69 26.69 FUD 090

58145 vaginal approach ♀
A2 T 80 15.77 15.77 FUD 090

58146 Myomectomy, excision of fibroid tumor(s) of uterus, 5 or more intramural myomas and/or intramural myomas with total weight greater than 250 g, abdominal approach ♀
Do not report with (58140-58145, 58150-58240)
C 80 33.53 33.53 FUD 090

58150-58294 Abdominal and Vaginal Hysterectomies

CMS 100-3,230.3 Sterilization

EXCLUDES *Destruction/excision of endometriomas, open method (49203-49205, 58957-58958)*
Paracentesis (49082-49084)
Pelvic laparotomy (49000)
Secondary closure disruption or evisceration of abdominal wall (49900)

58150 Total abdominal hysterectomy (corpus and cervix), with or without removal of tube(s), with or without removal of ovary(s); ♀
C 80 PQ 29.07 29.07 FUD 090

58152 with colpo-urethrocystopexy (eg, Marshall-Marchetti-Krantz, Burch) ♀
EXCLUDES *Urethrocystopexy without hysterectomy (51840-51841)*
C 80 PQ 36.18 36.18 FUD 090

58180 Supracervical abdominal hysterectomy (subtotal hysterectomy), with or without removal of tube(s), with or without removal of ovary(s) ♀
C 80 PQ 27.84 27.84 FUD 090

58200 Total abdominal hysterectomy, including partial vaginectomy, with para-aortic and pelvic lymph node sampling, with or without removal of tube(s), with or without removal of ovary(s) ♀
C 80 PQ 38.56 38.56 FUD 090

58210 Radical abdominal hysterectomy, with bilateral total pelvic lymphadenectomy and para-aortic lymph node sampling (biopsy), with or without removal of tube(s), with or without removal of ovary(s) ♀
INCLUDES Wertheim hysterectomy
EXCLUDES *Chemotherapy (96401-96549)*
Hysterectomy, radical, with transposition of ovary(s) (58825)
C 80 PQ 51.75 51.75 FUD 090

58240 Pelvic exenteration for gynecologic malignancy, with total abdominal hysterectomy or cervicectomy, with or without removal of tube(s), with or without removal of ovary(s), with removal of bladder and ureteral transplantations, and/or abdominoperineal resection of rectum and colon and colostomy, or any combination thereof ♀
EXCLUDES *Chemotherapy (96401-96549)*
Pelvic exenteration for male genital malignancy or lower urinary tract (51597)
C 80 PQ 82.21 82.21 FUD 090

58260 Vaginal hysterectomy, for uterus 250 g or less; ♀
T 80 PQ 24.00 24.00 FUD 090

58262 with removal of tube(s), and/or ovary(s) ♀
T 80 PQ 26.78 26.78 FUD 090

58263 with removal of tube(s), and/or ovary(s), with repair of enterocele ♀
T 80 PQ 28.76 28.76 FUD 090

58267 with colpo-urethrocystopexy (Marshall-Marchetti-Krantz type, Pereyra type) with or without endoscopic control ♀
C 80 PQ 30.64 30.64 FUD 090

58270 with repair of enterocele ♀
EXCLUDES *Vaginal hysterectomy with repair of enterocele and removal of tubes and/or ovaries (58263)*
T 80 PQ 25.60 25.60 FUD 090

58275 Vaginal hysterectomy, with total or partial vaginectomy; ♀
C 80 PQ 28.57 28.57 FUD 090

58280 with repair of enterocele ♀
C 80 PQ 30.54 30.54 FUD 090

58285 Vaginal hysterectomy, radical (Schauta type operation) ♀
C 80 PQ 38.10 38.10 FUD 090

58290 Vaginal hysterectomy, for uterus greater than 250 g; ♀
T 80 PQ 33.44 33.44 FUD 090

58291 with removal of tube(s) and/or ovary(s) ♀
T 80 PQ 36.21 36.21 FUD 090

58292 with removal of tube(s) and/or ovary(s), with repair of enterocele ♀
T 80 PQ 38.20 38.20 FUD 090

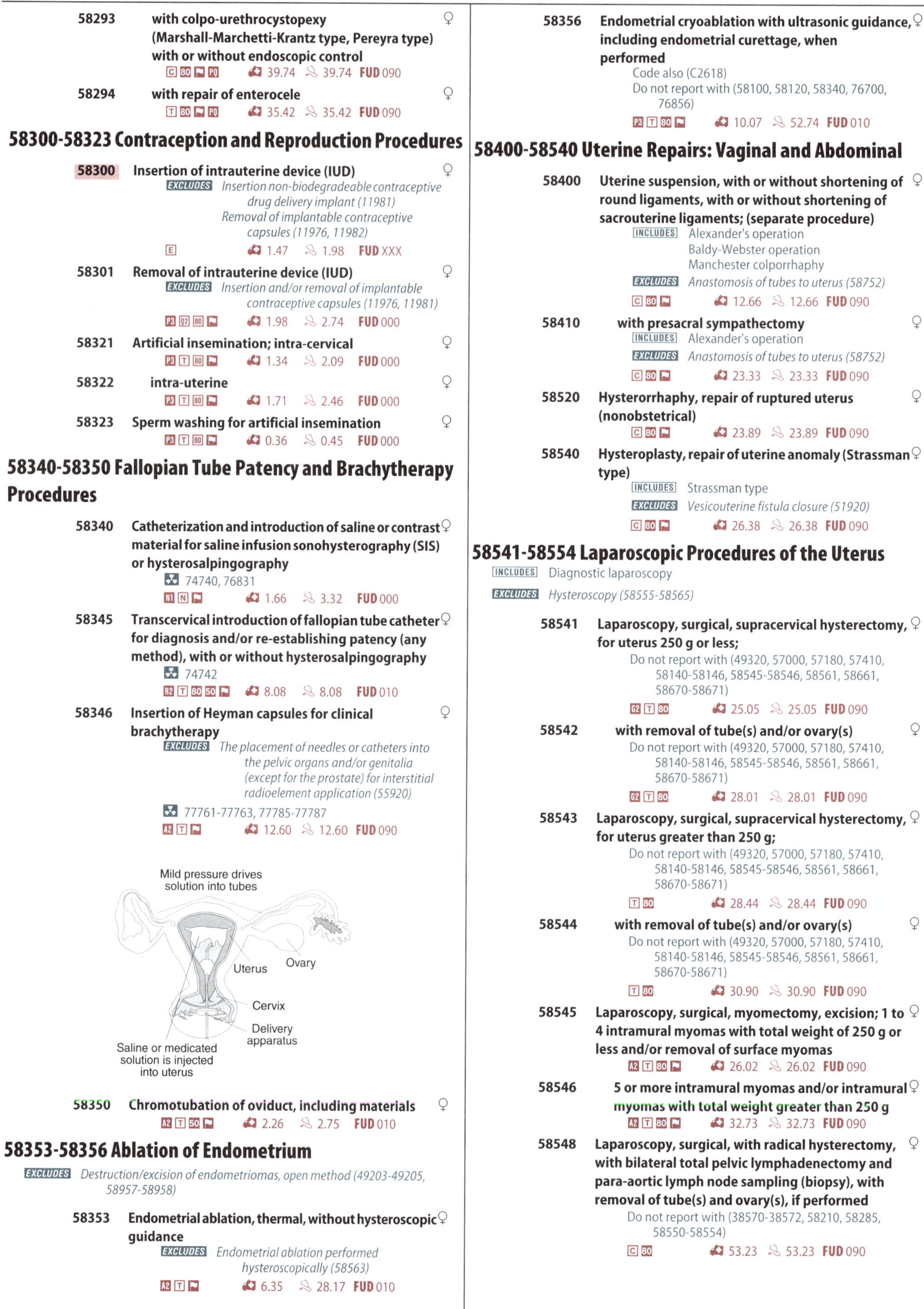

58293 with colpo-urethrocystopexy (Marshall-Marchetti-Krantz type, Pereyra type) with or without endoscopic control ♀
C 80 PQ 39.74 39.74 FUD 090

58294 with repair of enterocele ♀
T 80 PQ 35.42 35.42 FUD 090

58300-58323 Contraception and Reproduction Procedures

58300 Insertion of intrauterine device (IUD) ♀
EXCLUDES *Insertion non-biodegradeable contraceptive drug delivery implant (11981)*
Removal of implantable contraceptive capsules (11976, 11982)
E 1.47 1.98 FUD XXX

58301 Removal of intrauterine device (IUD) ♀
EXCLUDES *Insertion and/or removal of implantable contraceptive capsules (11976, 11981)*
P3 Q2 80 1.98 2.74 FUD 000

58321 Artificial insemination; intra-cervical ♀
P3 T 80 1.34 2.09 FUD 000

58322 intra-uterine ♀
P3 T 80 1.71 2.46 FUD 000

58323 Sperm washing for artificial insemination ♀
P3 T 80 0.36 0.45 FUD 000

58340-58350 Fallopian Tube Patency and Brachytherapy Procedures

58340 Catheterization and introduction of saline or contrast material for saline infusion sonohysterography (SIS) or hysterosalpingography ♀
74740, 76831
N1 N 1.66 3.32 FUD 000

58345 Transcervical introduction of fallopian tube catheter for diagnosis and/or re-establishing patency (any method), with or without hysterosalpingography ♀
74742
R2 T 80 50 8.08 8.08 FUD 010

58346 Insertion of Heyman capsules for clinical brachytherapy ♀
EXCLUDES *The placement of needles or catheters into the pelvic organs and/or genitalia (except for the prostate) for interstitial radioelement application (55920)*
77761-77763, 77785-77787
A2 T 12.60 12.60 FUD 090

58350 Chromotubation of oviduct, including materials ♀
A2 T 50 2.26 2.75 FUD 010

58353-58356 Ablation of Endometrium

EXCLUDES *Destruction/excision of endometriomas, open method (49203-49205, 58957-58958)*

58353 Endometrial ablation, thermal, without hysteroscopic guidance ♀
EXCLUDES *Endometrial ablation performed hysteroscopically (58563)*
A2 T 6.35 28.17 FUD 010

58356 Endometrial cryoablation with ultrasonic guidance, including endometrial curettage, when performed ♀
Code also (C2618)
Do not report with (58100, 58120, 58340, 76700, 76856)
P3 T 80 10.07 52.74 FUD 010

58400-58540 Uterine Repairs: Vaginal and Abdominal

58400 Uterine suspension, with or without shortening of round ligaments, with or without shortening of sacrouterine ligaments; (separate procedure) ♀
INCLUDES Alexander's operation
Baldy-Webster operation
Manchester colporrhaphy
EXCLUDES *Anastomosis of tubes to uterus (58752)*
C 80 12.66 12.66 FUD 090

58410 with presacral sympathectomy ♀
INCLUDES Alexander's operation
EXCLUDES *Anastomosis of tubes to uterus (58752)*
C 80 23.33 23.33 FUD 090

58520 Hysterorrhaphy, repair of ruptured uterus (nonobstetrical) ♀
C 80 23.89 23.89 FUD 090

58540 Hysteroplasty, repair of uterine anomaly (Strassman type) ♀
INCLUDES Strassman type
EXCLUDES *Vesicouterine fistula closure (51920)*
C 80 26.38 26.38 FUD 090

58541-58554 Laparoscopic Procedures of the Uterus

INCLUDES Diagnostic laparoscopy
EXCLUDES *Hysteroscopy (58555-58565)*

58541 Laparoscopy, surgical, supracervical hysterectomy, for uterus 250 g or less; ♀
Do not report with (49320, 57000, 57180, 57410, 58140-58146, 58545-58546, 58561, 58661, 58670-58671)
G2 T 80 25.05 25.05 FUD 090

58542 with removal of tube(s) and/or ovary(s) ♀
Do not report with (49320, 57000, 57180, 57410, 58140-58146, 58545-58546, 58561, 58661, 58670-58671)
G2 T 80 28.01 28.01 FUD 090

58543 Laparoscopy, surgical, supracervical hysterectomy, for uterus greater than 250 g; ♀
Do not report with (49320, 57000, 57180, 57410, 58140-58146, 58545-58546, 58561, 58661, 58670-58671)
T 80 28.44 28.44 FUD 090

58544 with removal of tube(s) and/or ovary(s) ♀
Do not report with (49320, 57000, 57180, 57410, 58140-58146, 58545-58546, 58561, 58661, 58670-58671)
T 80 30.90 30.90 FUD 090

58545 Laparoscopy, surgical, myomectomy, excision; 1 to 4 intramural myomas with total weight of 250 g or less and/or removal of surface myomas ♀
A2 T 80 26.02 26.02 FUD 090

58546 5 or more intramural myomas and/or intramural myomas with total weight greater than 250 g ♀
A2 T 80 32.73 32.73 FUD 090

58548 Laparoscopy, surgical, with radical hysterectomy, with bilateral total pelvic lymphadenectomy and para-aortic lymph node sampling (biopsy), with removal of tube(s) and ovary(s), if performed ♀
Do not report with (38570-38572, 58210, 58285, 58550-58554)
C 80 53.23 53.23 FUD 090

58550 **Laparoscopy, surgical, with vaginal hysterectomy, for uterus 250 g or less;** ♀
Do not report with (49320, 57000, 57180, 57410, 58140-58146, 58545-58546, 58561, 58661, 58670-58671)
A2 T 80 ▣ 25.63 25.63 FUD 090

58552 **with removal of tube(s) and/or ovary(s)** ♀
Do not report with (49320, 57000, 57180, 57410, 58140-58146, 58545-58546, 58561, 58661, 58670-58671)
G2 T 80 ▣ 28.49 28.49 FUD 090

58553 **Laparoscopy, surgical, with vaginal hysterectomy, for uterus greater than 250 g;** ♀
Do not report with (49320, 57000, 57180, 57410, 58140-58146, 58545-58546, 58561, 58661, 58670-58671)
T 80 ▣ 32.99 32.99 FUD 090

58554 **with removal of tube(s) and/or ovary(s)** ♀
Do not report with (49320, 57000, 57180, 57410, 58140-58146, 58545-58546, 58561, 58661, 58670-58671)
T 80 ▣ 38.30 38.30 FUD 090

58555-58565 Hysteroscopy

INCLUDES Diagnostic hysteroscopy

EXCLUDES *Laparoscopy (58541-58554, 58570-58578)*

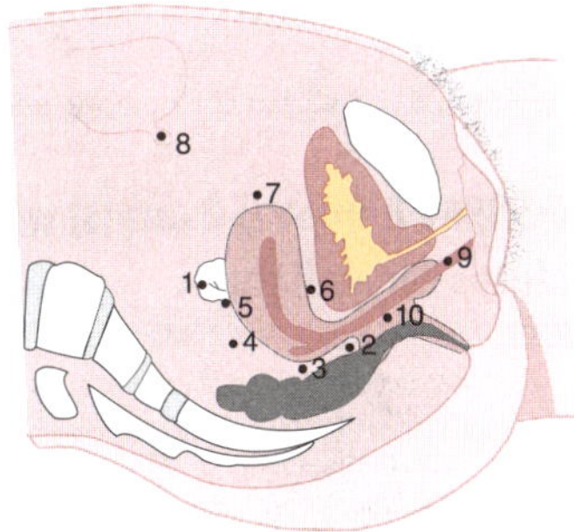

58555 **Hysteroscopy, diagnostic (separate procedure)** ♀
A2 T 80 ▣ 5.53 8.63 FUD 000

58558 **Hysteroscopy, surgical; with sampling (biopsy) of endometrium and/or polypectomy, with or without D & C** ♀
A2 T ▣ PQ 7.75 11.31 FUD 000

58559 **with lysis of intrauterine adhesions (any method)** ♀
A2 T ▣ 9.95 9.95 FUD 000

58560 **with division or resection of intrauterine septum (any method)** ♀
A2 T 80 ▣ 11.25 11.25 FUD 000

58561 **with removal of leiomyomata** ♀
A2 T 80 ▣ 15.92 15.92 FUD 000

58562 **with removal of impacted foreign body** ♀
A2 T ▣ 8.42 11.72 FUD 000

58563 **with endometrial ablation (eg, endometrial resection, electrosurgical ablation, thermoablation)** ♀
A2 T 80 ▣ 9.96 46.51 FUD 000

58565 **with bilateral fallopian tube cannulation to induce occlusion by placement of permanent implants** ♀
Code also modifier 52 when a unilateral procedure is performed
Do not report with (57800, 58555)
A2 T ▣ 12.57 52.33 FUD 090

58570-58579 Other Uterine Endoscopy

INCLUDES Diagnostic laparoscopy

EXCLUDES *Hysteroscopy (58555-58565)*

58570 **Laparoscopy, surgical, with total hysterectomy, for uterus 250 g or less;** ♀
Do not report with (49320, 57000, 57180, 57410, 58140-58146, 58150, 58545-58546, 58561, 58661, 58670-58671)
G2 T 80 26.97 26.97 FUD 090

58571 **with removal of tube(s) and/or ovary(s)** ♀
Do not report with (49320, 57100, 57180, 57410, 58140-58146, 58150, 58545-58546, 58561, 58661, 58670-58671)
G2 T 80 30.20 30.20 FUD 090

58572 **Laparoscopy, surgical, with total hysterectomy, for uterus greater than 250 g;** ♀
Do not report with (49320, 57000, 57180, 57410, 58140-58146, 58150, 58545-58546, 58561, 58661, 58670-58671)
T 80 33.62 33.62 FUD 090

58573 **with removal of tube(s) and/or ovary(s)** ♀
Do not report with (49320, 57000, 57180, 57410, 58140-58146, 58150, 58545-58546, 58561, 58661, 58670-58671)
T 80 38.73 38.73 FUD 090

58578 **Unlisted laparoscopy procedure, uterus** ♀
T 80 50 0.00 0.00 FUD YYY

58579 **Unlisted hysteroscopy procedure, uterus** ♀
T 80 50 0.00 0.00 FUD YYY

58600-58615 Sterilization by Tubal Interruption

CMS 100-3,230.3 Sterilization

EXCLUDES *Destruction/excision of endometriomas, open method (49203-49205, 58957-58958)*

58600 **Ligation or transection of fallopian tube(s), abdominal or vaginal approach, unilateral or bilateral** ♀
INCLUDES Madlener operation
G2 T 80 ▣ 10.57 10.57 FUD 090

58605 **Ligation or transection of fallopian tube(s), abdominal or vaginal approach, postpartum, unilateral or bilateral, during same hospitalization (separate procedure)** ♀
EXCLUDES *Laparoscopic methods (58670, 58671)*
C 80 ▣ 9.53 9.53 FUD 090

\+ 58611 **Ligation or transection of fallopian tube(s) when done at the time of cesarean delivery or intra-abdominal surgery (not a separate procedure) (List separately in addition to code for primary procedure)** ♀
Code first primary procedure
C 80 ▣ 2.26 2.26 FUD ZZZ

58615 **Occlusion of fallopian tube(s) by device (eg, band, clip, Falope ring) vaginal or suprapubic approach** ♀
EXCLUDES *Laparoscopic method (58671)*
Lysis of adnexal adhesions (58740)
G2 T 80 ▣ 7.06 7.06 FUD 010

58660-58679 Endoscopic Procedures Fallopian Tubes and/or Ovaries

CMS 100-3,230.3 Sterilization

INCLUDES Diagnostic laparoscopy

EXCLUDES *Laparoscopy with biopsy of fallopian tube or ovary (49321)*
Laparoscopy with ovarian cyst aspiration (49322)

58660 **Laparoscopy, surgical; with lysis of adhesions (salpingolysis, ovariolysis) (separate procedure)** ♀
A2 T 80 ▣ 19.50 19.50 FUD 090

58661 with removal of adnexal structures (partial or total oophorectomy and/or salpingectomy) ♀
A2 T 80 50 18.71 18.71 FUD 010

58662 with fulguration or excision of lesions of the ovary, pelvic viscera, or peritoneal surface by any method ♀
A2 T 80 20.47 20.47 FUD 090

58670 with fulguration of oviducts (with or without transection) ♀
A2 T 10.58 10.58 FUD 090

58671 with occlusion of oviducts by device (eg, band, clip, or Falope ring) ♀
A2 T 10.59 10.59 FUD 090

58672 with fimbrioplasty ♀
A2 T 80 50 21.36 21.36 FUD 090

58673 with salpingostomy (salpingoneostomy) ♀
A2 T 80 50 23.22 23.22 FUD 090

58679 Unlisted laparoscopy procedure, oviduct, ovary ♀
T 80 50 0.00 0.00 FUD YYY

58700-58770 Open Procedures Fallopian Tubes, with/without Ovaries

EXCLUDES Destruction/excision of endometriomas, open method (49203-49205, 58957-58958)

58700 Salpingectomy, complete or partial, unilateral or bilateral (separate procedure) ♀
C 80 22.45 22.45 FUD 090

58720 Salpingo-oophorectomy, complete or partial, unilateral or bilateral (separate procedure) ♀
C 80 21.04 21.04 FUD 090

58740 Lysis of adhesions (salpingolysis, ovariolysis) ♀
EXCLUDES Excision/fulguration of lesions performed laparoscopically (58662)
Laparoscopic method (58660)
C 80 25.37 25.37 FUD 090

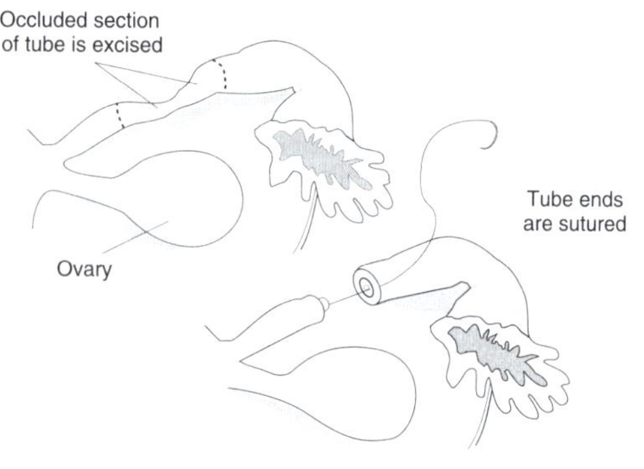

58750 Tubotubal anastomosis ♀
C 80 50 26.53 26.53 FUD 090

58752 Tubouterine implantation ♀
C 80 50 24.71 24.71 FUD 090

58760 Fimbrioplasty ♀
EXCLUDES Laparoscopic method (58672)
C 80 50 23.50 23.50 FUD 090

58770 Salpingostomy (salpingoneostomy) ♀
EXCLUDES Laparoscopic method (58673)
T 80 50 25.09 25.09 FUD 090

58800-58925 Open Procedures: Ovary

CMS 100-3,230.3 Sterilization

EXCLUDES Destruction/excision of endometriomas, open method (49203-49205, 58957-58958)
Paracentesis (49082-49084)
Pelvic laparotomy (49000)
Secondary closure disruption or evisceration (49900)

58800 Drainage of ovarian cyst(s), unilateral or bilateral (separate procedure); vaginal approach ♀
A2 T 8.61 9.15 FUD 090

58805 abdominal approach ♀
G2 T 80 11.71 11.71 FUD 090

58820 Drainage of ovarian abscess; vaginal approach, open ♀
A2 T 80 50 9.02 9.02 FUD 090

58822 abdominal approach ♀
C 80 50 21.36 21.36 FUD 090

58825 Transposition, ovary(s) ♀
C 80 20.14 20.14 FUD 090

58900 Biopsy of ovary, unilateral or bilateral (separate procedure) ♀
EXCLUDES Laparoscopy with biopsy of fallopian tube or ovary (49321)
A2 T 80 PQ 12.88 12.88 FUD 090

58920 Wedge resection or bisection of ovary, unilateral or bilateral ♀
T 80 20.74 20.74 FUD 090

58925 Ovarian cystectomy, unilateral or bilateral ♀
T 80 21.46 21.46 FUD 090

58940-58960 Removal Ovary(s) with/without Multiple Procedures for Malignancy

EXCLUDES Chemotherapy (96401-96549)
Destruction/excision of tumors, cysts, or endometriomas, open method (49203-49205)
Paracentesis (49082-49084)
Pelvic laparotomy (49000)

58940 Oophorectomy, partial or total, unilateral or bilateral; ♀
EXCLUDES Oophorectomy with tumor debulking for ovarian malignancy (58952)
C 80 15.03 15.03 FUD 090

58943 for ovarian, tubal or primary peritoneal malignancy, with para-aortic and pelvic lymph node biopsies, peritoneal washings, peritoneal biopsies, diaphragmatic assessments, with or without salpingectomy(s), with or without omentectomy ♀
C 80 33.23 33.23 FUD 090

58950 Resection (initial) of ovarian, tubal or primary peritoneal malignancy with bilateral salpingo-oophorectomy and omentectomy; ♀
EXCLUDES Resection/tumor debulking of recurrent ovarian/tubal/primary peritoneal/uterine malignancy (58957-58958)
C 80 31.80 31.80 FUD 090

58951 with total abdominal hysterectomy, pelvic and limited para-aortic lymphadenectomy ♀
EXCLUDES Resection/tumor debulking of recurrent ovarian/tubal/primary peritoneal/uterine malignancy (58957-58958)
C 80 PQ 40.83 40.83 FUD 090

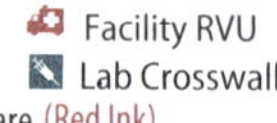

58952 with radical dissection for debulking (ie, radical excision or destruction, intra-abdominal or retroperitoneal tumors) ♀
EXCLUDES *Resection/tumor debulking of recurrent ovarian/tubal/primary peritoneal/uterine malignancy (58957-58958)*
C 80 46.10 46.10 FUD 090

58953 Bilateral salpingo-oophorectomy with omentectomy, total abdominal hysterectomy and radical dissection for debulking; ♀
C 80 PQ 57.02 57.02 FUD 090

58954 with pelvic lymphadenectomy and limited para-aortic lymphadenectomy ♀
C 80 PQ 61.84 61.84 FUD 090

58956 Bilateral salpingo-oophorectomy with total omentectomy, total abdominal hysterectomy for malignancy ♀
Do not report with (49255, 58150, 58180, 58262-58263, 58550, 58661, 58700, 58720, 58900, 58925, 58940, 58957-58958)
C 80 PQ 38.94 38.94 FUD 090

58957 Resection (tumor debulking) of recurrent ovarian, tubal, primary peritoneal, uterine malignancy (intra-abdominal, retroperitoneal tumors), with omentectomy, if performed; ♀
Do not report with (38770, 38780, 44005, 49000, 49203-49215, 49255, 58900-58960)
C 80 44.68 44.68 FUD 090

58958 with pelvic lymphadenectomy and limited para-aortic lymphadenectomy ♀
Do not report with (38770, 38780, 44005, 49000, 49203-49215, 49255, 58900-58960)
C 80 49.02 49.02 FUD 090

58960 Laparotomy, for staging or restaging of ovarian, tubal, or primary peritoneal malignancy (second look), with or without omentectomy, peritoneal washing, biopsy of abdominal and pelvic peritoneum, diaphragmatic assessment with pelvic and limited para-aortic lymphadenectomy ♀
Do not report with (58957-58958)
C 80 27.26 27.26 FUD 090

58970-58999 Procedural Components: In Vitro Fertilization

58970 Follicle puncture for oocyte retrieval, any method M ♀
76948
A2 T 80 5.52 6.11 FUD 000

58974 Embryo transfer, intrauterine M ♀
A2 T 80 0.00 0.00 FUD 000

58976 Gamete, zygote, or embryo intrafallopian transfer, any method M ♀
EXCLUDES *Adnexal procedures performed laparoscopically (58660-58673)*
A2 T 80 5.95 6.90 FUD 000

58999 Unlisted procedure, female genital system (nonobstetrical) ♀
T 0.00 0.00 FUD YYY

59000-59001 Aspiration of Amniotic Fluid

CMS 100-3,220.5 Ultrasound Diagnostic Procedures
EXCLUDES *Intrauterine fetal transfusion (36460)*
Unlisted fetal invasive procedure (59897)

59000 Amniocentesis; diagnostic M ♀
76946
P3 T 2.36 3.60 FUD 000

59001 therapeutic amniotic fluid reduction (includes ultrasound guidance) M ♀
R2 T 5.26 5.26 FUD 000

59012-59076 Fetal Testing and Treatment

EXCLUDES *Intrauterine fetal transfusion (36460)*
Newborn circumcision (54150, 54160)
Unlisted fetal invasive procedures (59897)

59012 Cordocentesis (intrauterine), any method M ♀
76941
G2 T 80 5.95 5.95 FUD 000

59015 Chorionic villus sampling, any method M ♀
76945
P3 T 80 PQ 3.87 4.52 FUD 000

59020 Fetal contraction stress test M ♀
P3 T 80 2.01 2.01 FUD 000

59025 Fetal non-stress test M ♀
P3 T 80 1.36 1.36 FUD 000

59030 Fetal scalp blood sampling M ♀
Code also modifier 76 or 77, as appropriate, for repeat fetal scalp blood sampling
T 80 2.87 2.87 FUD 000

59050 Fetal monitoring during labor by consulting physician (ie, non-attending physician) with written report; supervision and interpretation M ♀
M 80 1.49 1.49 FUD XXX

59051 interpretation only M ♀
B 80 1.24 1.24 FUD XXX

59070 Transabdominal amnioinfusion, including ultrasound guidance M ♀
G2 T 80 9.10 11.86 FUD 000

59072 Fetal umbilical cord occlusion, including ultrasound guidance M ♀
G2 T 15.33 15.33 FUD 000

59074 Fetal fluid drainage (eg, vesicocentesis, thoracocentesis, paracentesis), including ultrasound guidance M ♀
G2 T 80 9.11 11.28 FUD 000

59076 Fetal shunt placement, including ultrasound guidance M ♀
G2 T 80 15.39 15.39 FUD 000

59100-59151 Tubal Pregnancy/Hysterotomy Procedures

CMS 100-3,230.3 Sterilization

59100 Hysterotomy, abdominal (eg, for hydatidiform mole, abortion) M ♀
Code also ligation of fallopian tubes when performed at the same time as hysterotomy (58611)
R2 T 80 24.35 24.35 FUD 090

59120 Surgical treatment of ectopic pregnancy; tubal or ovarian, requiring salpingectomy and/or oophorectomy, abdominal or vaginal approach M ♀
C 80 23.20 23.20 FUD 090

59121 tubal or ovarian, without salpingectomy and/or oophorectomy M ♀
C 80 23.21 23.21 FUD 090

59130 abdominal pregnancy M ♀
C 80 24.00 24.00 FUD 090

59135 interstitial, uterine pregnancy requiring total hysterectomy M ♀
C 80 23.80 23.80 FUD 090

59136 interstitial, uterine pregnancy with partial resection of uterus M ♀
C 80 25.78 25.78 FUD 090

59140 cervical, with evacuation M ♀
C 80 10.83 10.83 FUD 090

59150 Laparoscopic treatment of ectopic pregnancy; without salpingectomy and/or oophorectomy M ♀
G2 T 80 22.47 22.47 FUD 090

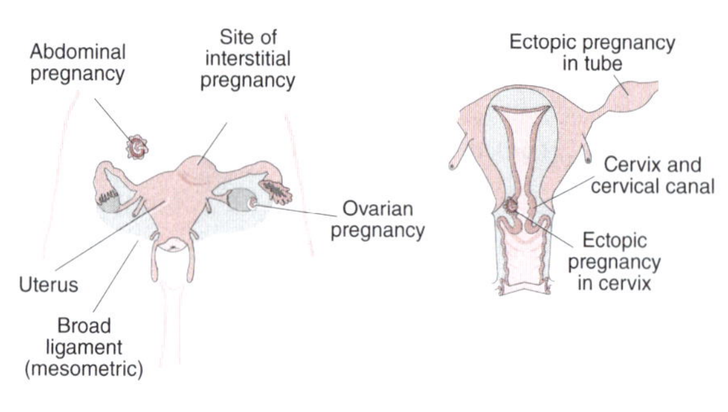

59151 **with salpingectomy and/or oophorectomy** M♀
62 T 80 21.86 21.86 FUD 090

59160-59200 Procedures of Uterus Prior To/After Delivery

59160 **Curettage, postpartum** M♀
A2 T 80 5.05 5.89 FUD 010

59200 **Insertion of cervical dilator (eg, laminaria, prostaglandin) (separate procedure)** M♀
EXCLUDES *Fetal transfusion, intrauterine (36460)*
Hypertonic solution/prostaglandin introduction for labor initiation (59850-59857)
P3 T 1.33 2.08 FUD 000

59300-59350 Postpartum Vaginal/Cervical/Uterine Repairs

EXCLUDES *Nonpregnancy-related cerclage (57700)*

59300 **Episiotomy or vaginal repair, by other than attending** M♀
P3 T 80 4.34 5.56 FUD 000

59320 **Cerclage of cervix, during pregnancy; vaginal** M♀
A2 T 80 4.45 4.45 FUD 000

59325 **abdominal** M♀
C 80 6.27 6.27 FUD 000

59350 **Hysterorrhaphy of ruptured uterus** M♀
C 80 8.21 8.21 FUD 000

59400-59410 Vaginal Delivery: Comprehensive and Component Services

CMS 100-2,15,20.1 Physician Expense for Surgery, Childbirth, and Treatment for Infertility
CMS 100-2,15,180 Nurse-Midwife (CNM) Services

INCLUDES Care provided for an uncomplicated pregnancy including delivery as well as antepartum and postpartum care:
- Admission history
- Admission to hospital
- Artificial rupture of membranes
- Management of uncomplicated labor
- Physical exam
- Vaginal delivery with or without episiotomy or forceps

EXCLUDES *Medical complications of pregnancy, labor, and delivery:*
- *Cardiac problems*
- *Diabetes*
- *Hyperemesis*
- *Hypertension*
- *Neurological problems*
- *Premature rupture of membranes*
- *Pre-term labor*
- *Toxemia*
- *Trauma*

Newborn circumcision (54150, 54160)
Services incidental to or unrelated to the pregnancy

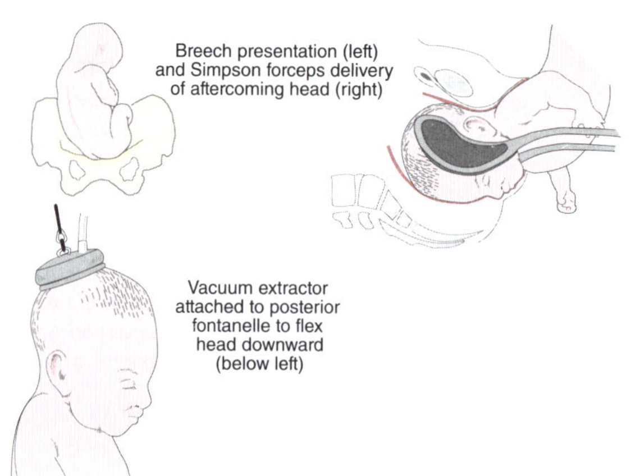

59400 **Routine obstetric care including antepartum care, vaginal delivery (with or without episiotomy, and/or forceps) and postpartum care** M♀
INCLUDES Fetal heart tones
Hospital/office visits following cesarean section or vaginal delivery
Initial/subsequent history
Physical exams
Recording of weight/blood pressures
Routine chemical urinalysis
Routine prenatal visits:
- Each month up to 28 weeks gestation
- Every other week from 29 to 36 weeks gestation
- Weekly from 36 weeks until delivery

B 60.96 60.96 FUD MMM

59409 **Vaginal delivery only (with or without episiotomy and/or forceps);** M♀
EXCLUDES *Inpatient management after delivery/discharge services (99217-99239 [99224, 99225, 99226])*
T 80 23.96 23.96 FUD MMM

59410 **including postpartum care** M♀
INCLUDES Hospital/office visits following cesarean section or vaginal delivery
B 30.51 30.51 FUD MMM

59412-59414 Other Maternity Services

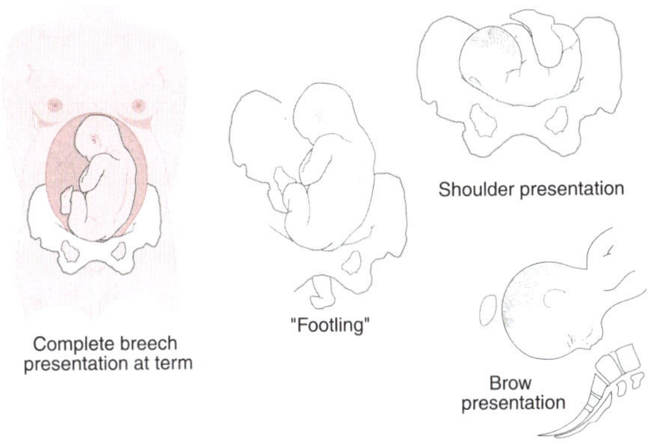

59412 External cephalic version, with or without tocolysis M♀
Code also delivery code(s)
62 T 80 ⚑ 3.03 3.03 FUD MMM

59414 Delivery of placenta (separate procedure) M♀
62 T 80 ⚑ 2.69 2.69 FUD MMM

59425-59430 Prenatal and Postpartum Visits

CMS 100-2,15,20.1 Physician Expense for Surgery, Childbirth, and Treatment for Infertility
CMS 100-2,15,180 Nurse-Midwife (CNM) Services

INCLUDES Physician/other qualified health care professional providing all or a portion of antepartum/postpartum care, but no delivery due to:
- Referral to another physician for delivery
- Termination of pregnancy by abortion

EXCLUDES *Antepartum care, 1-3 visits, report with appropriate evaluation and management service code*
Medical complications of pregnancy, labor, and delivery:
- *Cardiac problems*
- *Diabetes*
- *Hyperemesis*
- *Hypertension*
- *Neurological problems*
- *Premature rupture of membranes*
- *Pre-term labor*
- *Toxemia*
- *Trauma*

Newborn circumcision (54150, 54160)
Services incidental to or unrelated to the pregnancy

59425 Antepartum care only; 4-6 visits M♀
INCLUDES Fetal heart tones
Initial/subsequent history
Physical exams
Recording of weight/blood pressures
Routine chemical urinalysis
Routine prenatal visits:
- Each month up to 28 weeks gestation
- Every other week from 29 to 36 weeks gestation
- Weekly from 36 weeks until delivery

B 80 ⚑ 10.48 13.21 FUD MMM

59426 7 or more visits M♀
INCLUDES Biweekly visits to 36 weeks gestation
Fetal heart tones
Initial/subsequent history
Monthly visits up to 28 weeks gestation
Physical exams
Recording of weight/blood pressures
Routine chemical urinalysis
Weekly visits until delivery

B 80 ⚑ 18.49 23.63 FUD MMM

59430 Postpartum care only (separate procedure) M♀
INCLUDES Office/other outpatient visits following cesarean section or vaginal delivery

B ⚑ 4.09 5.34 FUD MMM

59510-59525 Cesarean Section Delivery: Comprehensive and Components of Care

INCLUDES Classic cesarean section
Low cervical cesarean section

EXCLUDES *Infant standby attendance (99360)*
Medical complications of pregnancy, labor, and delivery:
- *Cardiac problems*
- *Diabetes*
- *Hyperemesis*
- *Hypertension*
- *Neurological problems*
- *Premature rupture of membranes*
- *Pre-term labor*
- *Trauma*
- *Toxemia*

Newborn circumcision (54150, 54160)
Services incidental to or unrelated to the pregnancy
Vaginal delivery after prior cesarean section (59610-59614)

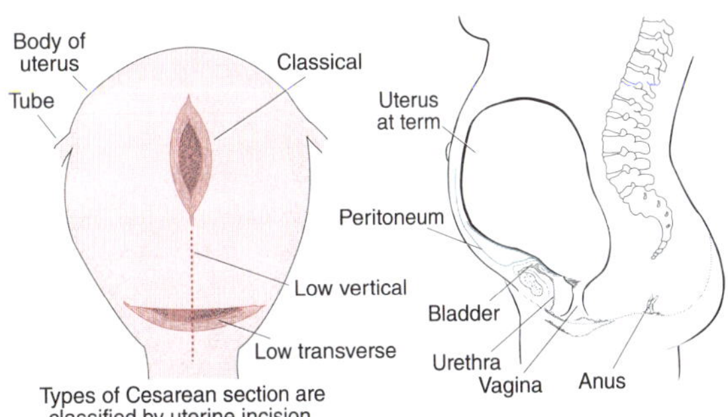

Types of Cesarean section are classified by uterine incision

59510 Routine obstetric care including antepartum care, cesarean delivery, and postpartum care M♀
INCLUDES Admission history
Admission to hospital
Cesarean delivery
Fetal heart tones
Hospital/office visits following cesarean section
Initial/subsequent history
Management of uncomplicated labor
Physical exam
Recording of weight/blood pressures
Routine chemical urinalysis
Routine prenatal visits:
- Each month up to 28 weeks gestation
- Every other week 29 to 36 weeks gestation
- Weekly from 36 weeks until delivery

EXCLUDES *Medical problems complicating labor and delivery*

B ⚑ 67.41 67.41 FUD MMM

59514 Cesarean delivery only; M♀
INCLUDES Admission history
Admission to hospital
Cesarean delivery
Management of uncomplicated labor
Physical exam

EXCLUDES *Inpatient management after delivery/discharge services (99217-99239 [99224, 99225, 99226])*
Medical problems complicating labor and delivery

C 80 ⚑ 26.95 26.95 FUD MMM

59515 **including postpartum care** M ♀
INCLUDES Admission history
Admission to hospital
Cesarean delivery
Hospital/office visits following cesarean section or vaginal delivery
Management of uncomplicated labor
Physical exam
EXCLUDES *Medical problems complicating labor and delivery*
B 36.94 36.94 FUD MMM

\+ **59525** **Subtotal or total hysterectomy after cesarean delivery (List separately in addition to code for primary procedure)** M ♀
Code first cesarean delivery (59510, 59514, 59515, 59618, 59620, 59622)
C 80 14.24 14.24 FUD ZZZ

59610-59614 Vaginal Delivery After Prior Cesarean Section: Comprehensive and Components of Care

CMS 100-2,15,20.1 Physician Expense for Surgery, Childbirth, and Treatment for Infertility
CMS 100-2,15,180 Nurse-Midwife (CNM) Services
INCLUDES Admission history
Admission to hospital
Management of uncomplicated labor
Patients with previous cesarean delivery who present with the expectation of a vaginal delivery
Physical exam
Successful vaginal delivery after previous cesarean delivery (VBAC)
Vaginal delivery with or without episiotomy or forceps
EXCLUDES *Elective cesarean delivery (59510, 59514, 59515)*
Medical complications of pregnancy, labor, and delivery:
Cardiac problems
Diabetes
Hyperemesis
Hypertension
Neurological problems
Premature rupture of membranes
Pre-term labor
Toxemia
Trauma
Newborn circumcision (54150, 54160)
Services incidental to or unrelated to the pregnancy

59610 **Routine obstetric care including antepartum care, vaginal delivery (with or without episiotomy, and/or forceps) and postpartum care, after previous cesarean delivery** M ♀
INCLUDES Fetal heart tones
Hospital/office visits following cesarean section or vaginal delivery
Initial/subsequent history
Physical exams
Recording of weight/blood pressures
Routine chemical urinalysis
Routine prenatal visits:
Each month up to 28 weeks gestation
Every other week 29 to 36 weeks gestation
Weekly from 36 weeks until delivery
B 80 63.92 63.92 FUD MMM

59612 **Vaginal delivery only, after previous cesarean delivery (with or without episiotomy and/or forceps);** M ♀
EXCLUDES *Inpatient management after delivery/discharge services (99217-99239 [99224, 99225, 99226])*
T 80 26.89 26.89 FUD MMM

59614 **including postpartum care** M ♀
INCLUDES Hospital/office visits following cesarean section or vaginal delivery
B 80 33.42 33.42 FUD MMM

59618-59622 Cesarean Section After Attempted Vaginal Birth/Prior C-Section

INCLUDES Admission history
Admission to hospital
Cesarean delivery
Cesarean delivery following an unsuccessful vaginal delivery attempt after previous cesarean delivery
Management of uncomplicated labor
Patients with previous cesarean delivery who present with the expectation of a vaginal delivery
Physical exam
EXCLUDES *Elective cesarean delivery (59510, 59514, 59515)*
Medical complications of pregnancy, labor, and delivery:
Cardiac problems
Diabetes
Hyperemesis
Hypertension
Neurological problems
Premature rupture of membranes
Pre-term labor
Toxemia
Trauma
Newborn circumcision (54150, 54160)
Services incidental to or unrelated to the pregnancy

59618 **Routine obstetric care including antepartum care, cesarean delivery, and postpartum care, following attempted vaginal delivery after previous cesarean delivery** M ♀
INCLUDES Fetal heart tones
Hospital/office visits following cesarean section or vaginal delivery
Initial/subsequent history
Physical exams
Recording of weight/blood pressures
Routine chemical urinalysis
Routine prenatal visits:
Each month up to 28 weeks gestation
Every two weeks 29 to 36 weeks gestation
Weekly from 36 weeks until delivery
B 80 68.33 68.33 FUD MMM

59620 **Cesarean delivery only, following attempted vaginal delivery after previous cesarean delivery;** M ♀
EXCLUDES *Inpatient management after delivery/discharge services (99217-99239 [99224, 99225, 99226])*
C 80 27.84 27.84 FUD MMM

59622 **including postpartum care** M ♀
INCLUDES Hospital/office visits following cesarean section or vaginal delivery
B 80 37.95 37.95 FUD MMM

59812-59830 Treatment of Miscarriage

EXCLUDES *Medical treatment of spontaneous complete abortion, any trimester (99201-99233 [99224, 99225, 99226])*

59812 **Treatment of incomplete abortion, any trimester, completed surgically** M ♀
INCLUDES Surgical treatment of spontaneous abortion
A2 T 8.59 9.21 FUD 090

59820 **Treatment of missed abortion, completed surgically; first trimester** M ♀
A2 T 10.33 10.96 FUD 090

59821 **second trimester** M ♀
A2 T 80 10.38 11.07 FUD 090

59830 **Treatment of septic abortion, completed surgically** M ♀
C 80 12.70 12.70 FUD 090

59840-59866 Elective Abortions

CMS 100-3,140.1 Abortion
CMS 100-4,3,100.1 Billing for Abortion Services

59840 **Induced abortion, by dilation and curettage** M ♀
A2 T 80 ⚑ 5.99 6.23 FUD 010

59841 **Induced abortion, by dilation and evacuation** M ♀
A2 T 80 ⚑ 10.51 11.10 FUD 010

59850 **Induced abortion, by 1 or more intra-amniotic injections (amniocentesis-injections), including hospital admission and visits, delivery of fetus and secundines;** M ♀
EXCLUDES *Cervical dilator insertion (59200)*
C 80 ⚑ 9.84 9.84 FUD 090

59851 **with dilation and curettage and/or evacuation** M ♀
EXCLUDES *Cervical dilator insertion (59200)*
C 80 ⚑ 11.59 11.59 FUD 090

59852 **with hysterotomy (failed intra-amniotic injection)** M ♀
EXCLUDES *Cervical dilator insertion (59200)*
C 80 ⚑ 14.40 14.40 FUD 090

59855 **Induced abortion, by 1 or more vaginal suppositories (eg, prostaglandin) with or without cervical dilation (eg, laminaria), including hospital admission and visits, delivery of fetus and secundines;** M ♀
C 80 ⚑ 12.10 12.10 FUD 090

59856 **with dilation and curettage and/or evacuation** M ♀
C 80 ⚑ 14.22 14.22 FUD 090

59857 **with hysterotomy (failed medical evacuation)** M ♀
C 80 ⚑ 14.76 14.76 FUD 090

59866 **Multifetal pregnancy reduction(s) (MPR)** M ♀
G2 T 80 ⚑ 6.21 6.21 FUD 000

59870-59899 Miscellaneous Obstetrical Procedures

59870 **Uterine evacuation and curettage for hydatidiform mole** M ♀
A2 T 80 ⚑ 13.69 13.69 FUD 090

59871 **Removal of cerclage suture under anesthesia (other than local)** M ♀
A2 02 80 ⚑ 3.91 3.91 FUD 000

59897 **Unlisted fetal invasive procedure, including ultrasound guidance, when performed** ♀
T ⚑ 0.00 0.00 FUD YYY

59898 **Unlisted laparoscopy procedure, maternity care and delivery** M ♀
T 80 50 0.00 0.00 FUD YYY

59899 **Unlisted procedure, maternity care and delivery** M ♀
T 80 0.00 0.00 FUD YYY

60000 I&D of Infected Thyroglossal Cyst

60000 **Incision and drainage of thyroglossal duct cyst, infected**
A2 T 80 🏳 — Facility RVU 4.43 — Non-Facility RVU 4.93 — FUD 010

60100 Core Needle Biopsy: Thyroid

EXCLUDES *Fine needle aspiration (10021-10022)*

60100 **Biopsy thyroid, percutaneous core needle**
Radiology Crosswalk 76942, 77002, 77012, 77021
Lab Crosswalk 88172-88173
P3 T 🏳 — Facility RVU 2.28 — Non-Facility RVU 3.21 — FUD 000

60200 Surgical Removal Thyroid Cyst or Mass; Division of Isthmus

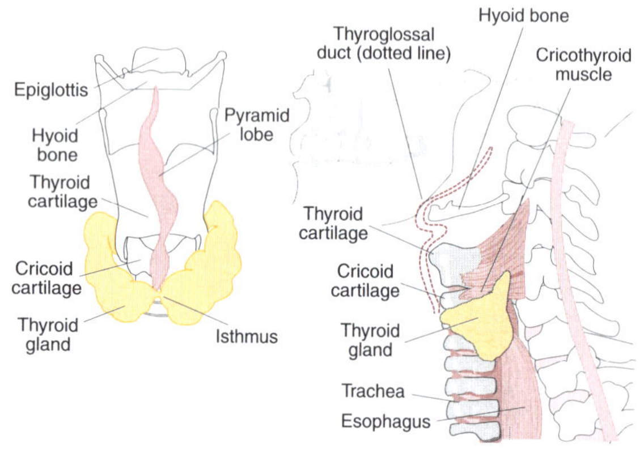

60200 **Excision of cyst or adenoma of thyroid, or transection of isthmus**
A2 T 80 🏳 PQ — Facility RVU 18.91 — Non-Facility RVU 18.91 — FUD 090

60210-60225 Subtotal Thyroidectomy

CMS 100-4,12,40.7 Bilateral Procedures

60210 **Partial thyroid lobectomy, unilateral; with or without isthmusectomy**
G2 T 80 🏳 PQ — Facility RVU 20.23 — Non-Facility RVU 20.23 — FUD 090

60212 **with contralateral subtotal lobectomy, including isthmusectomy**
G2 T 80 🏳 PQ — Facility RVU 28.84 — Non-Facility RVU 28.84 — FUD 090

60220 **Total thyroid lobectomy, unilateral; with or without isthmusectomy**
G2 T 80 🏳 PQ — Facility RVU 20.33 — Non-Facility RVU 20.33 — FUD 090

60225 **with contralateral subtotal lobectomy, including isthmusectomy**
G2 T 80 🏳 PQ — Facility RVU 26.66 — Non-Facility RVU 26.66 — FUD 090

60240-60271 Complete Thyroidectomy Procedures

60240 **Thyroidectomy, total or complete**
EXCLUDES *Subtotal or partial thyroidectomy (60271)*
G2 T 80 🏳 PQ — Facility RVU 26.36 — Non-Facility RVU 26.36 — FUD 090

60252 **Thyroidectomy, total or subtotal for malignancy; with limited neck dissection**
T 80 🏳 PQ — Facility RVU 37.79 — Non-Facility RVU 37.79 — FUD 090

60254 **with radical neck dissection**
C 80 🏳 PQ — Facility RVU 47.81 — Non-Facility RVU 47.81 — FUD 090

60260 **Thyroidectomy, removal of all remaining thyroid tissue following previous removal of a portion of thyroid**
T 80 50 🏳 PQ — Facility RVU 31.38 — Non-Facility RVU 31.38 — FUD 090

60270 **Thyroidectomy, including substernal thyroid; sternal split or transthoracic approach**
C 80 🏳 PQ — Facility RVU 39.19 — Non-Facility RVU 39.19 — FUD 090

60271 **cervical approach**
T 80 🏳 PQ — Facility RVU 30.29 — Non-Facility RVU 30.29 — FUD 090

60280-60300 Treatment of Cyst/Sinus of Thyroid

60280 **Excision of thyroglossal duct cyst or sinus;**
EXCLUDES *Thyroid ultrasound (76536)*
A2 T 80 🏳 PQ — Facility RVU 12.72 — Non-Facility RVU 12.72 — FUD 090

60281 **recurrent**
EXCLUDES *Thyroid ultrasound (76536)*
A2 T 80 🏳 PQ — Facility RVU 16.96 — Non-Facility RVU 16.96 — FUD 090

60300 **Aspiration and/or injection, thyroid cyst**
EXCLUDES *Fine needle aspiration (10021-10022)*
Radiology Crosswalk 76942, 77012
P3 T — Facility RVU 1.44 — Non-Facility RVU 3.33 — FUD 000

60500-60512 Parathyroid Procedures

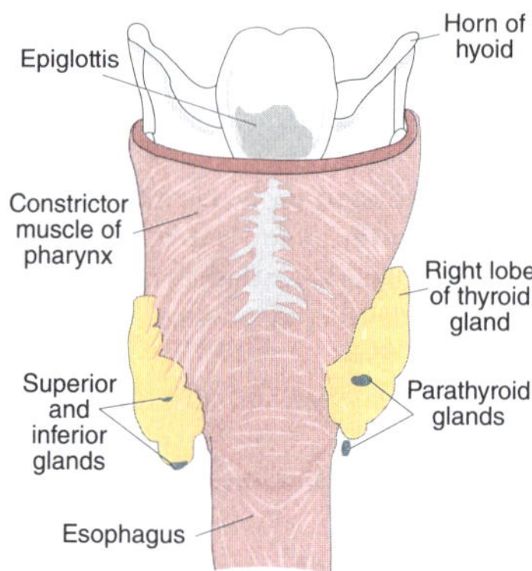

Posterior view of pharynx, thyroid glands, and parathyroid glands

60500 **Parathyroidectomy or exploration of parathyroid(s);**
G2 T 80 🏳 PQ — Facility RVU 27.62 — Non-Facility RVU 27.62 — FUD 090

60502 **re-exploration**
T 80 🏳 PQ — Facility RVU 36.80 — Non-Facility RVU 36.80 — FUD 090

60505 **with mediastinal exploration, sternal split or transthoracic approach**
C 80 🏳 PQ — Facility RVU 39.69 — Non-Facility RVU 39.69 — FUD 090

+ **60512** **Parathyroid autotransplantation (List separately in addition to code for primary procedure)**
Code first (60212, 60225, 60240, 60252, 60254, 60260, 60270-60271, 60500, 60502, 60505)
N 80 — Facility RVU 6.96 — Non-Facility RVU 6.96 — FUD ZZZ

60520-60522 Thymus Procedures

60520 **Thymectomy, partial or total; transcervical approach (separate procedure)**
T 80 🏳 PQ — Facility RVU 29.76 — Non-Facility RVU 29.76 — FUD 090

60521 **sternal split or transthoracic approach, without radical mediastinal dissection (separate procedure)**
C 80 🏳 PQ — Facility RVU 32.49 — Non-Facility RVU 32.49 — FUD 090

60522 **sternal split or transthoracic approach, with radical mediastinal dissection (separate procedure)**
EXCLUDES *Surgical thoracoscopy (video-assisted thoracic surgery (VATS) thymectomy (32673)*
C 80 🏳 PQ — Facility RVU 39.36 — Non-Facility RVU 39.36 — FUD 090

60540-60545 Adrenal Gland Procedures

EXCLUDES *Laparoscopic approach (60650)*
Removal of remote or disseminated pheochromocytoma (49203-49205)

Do not report with (50323)

60540 Adrenalectomy, partial or complete, or exploration of adrenal gland with or without biopsy, transabdominal, lumbar or dorsal (separate procedure);
C 80 50 PQ 30.14 30.14 FUD 090

60545 with excision of adjacent retroperitoneal tumor
C 80 50 PQ 34.68 34.68 FUD 090

60600-60605 Carotid Body Procedures

CMS 100-3,20.18 Carotid Body Resection/Carotid Body Denervation

60600 Excision of carotid body tumor; without excision of carotid artery
C 80 PQ 40.98 40.98 FUD 090

60605 with excision of carotid artery
C 80 PQ 45.50 45.50 FUD 090

60650-60699 Laparoscopic and Unlisted Procedures

INCLUDES Diagnostic laparoscopy

60650 Laparoscopy, surgical, with adrenalectomy, partial or complete, or exploration of adrenal gland with or without biopsy, transabdominal, lumbar or dorsal
C 80 50 PQ 33.96 33.96 FUD 090

60659 Unlisted laparoscopy procedure, endocrine system
T 80 50 0.00 0.00 FUD YYY

60699 Unlisted procedure, endocrine system
T 80 0.00 0.00 FUD YYY

61000-61253 Transcranial Access via Puncture, Burr Hole, Twist Hole, or Trephine

EXCLUDES *Injection for:*
Cerebral angiography (36100-36218)

Overhead view of newborn skull

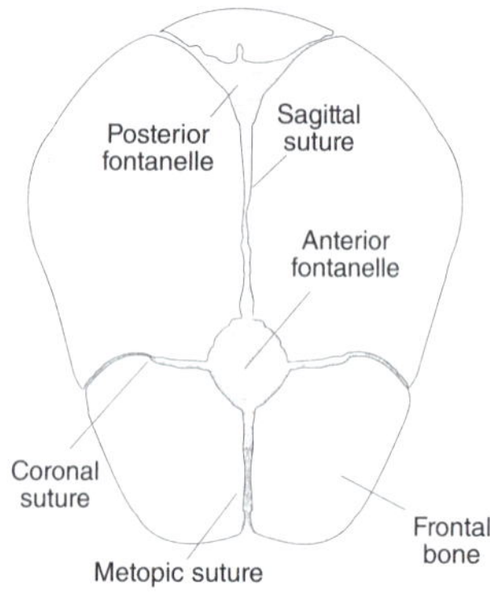

An initial tap through to the subdural level is performed on an infant via a fontanelle or suture, either unilateral or bilateral.

61000 **Subdural tap through fontanelle, or suture, infant, unilateral or bilateral; initial** A
EXCLUDES *Injection for:*
Pneumoencephalography (61055)
Ventriculography (61026, 61120)
A2 T ⚑ 2.54 2.54 FUD 000

61001 **subsequent taps** A
A2 T ⚑ 3.09 3.09 FUD 000

61020 **Ventricular puncture through previous burr hole, fontanelle, suture, or implanted ventricular catheter/reservoir; without injection**
A2 T ⚑ 3.02 3.02 FUD 000

61026 **with injection of medication or other substance for diagnosis or treatment**
A2 T ⚑ 3.07 3.07 FUD 000

61050 **Cisternal or lateral cervical (C1-C2) puncture; without injection (separate procedure)**
A2 T 80 ⚑ 2.46 2.46 FUD 000

▲ **61055** **with injection of medication or other substance for diagnosis or treatment**
INCLUDES Injection for pneumoencephalography
EXCLUDES *Radiology procedures except when furnished by a different provider*
Do not report with (62302-62305)
A2 T ⚑ 3.39 3.39 FUD 000

61070 **Puncture of shunt tubing or reservoir for aspiration or injection procedure**
75809
A2 T ⚑ 1.71 1.71 FUD 000

61105 **Twist drill hole for subdural or ventricular puncture**
C 80 ⚑ 13.20 13.20 FUD 090

⊘ **61107** **Twist drill hole(s) for subdural, intracerebral, or ventricular puncture; for implanting ventricular catheter, pressure recording device, or other intracerebral monitoring device**
Code also intracranial neuroendoscopic ventricular catheter insertion or reinsertion, when performed (62160)
C ⚑ 9.04 9.04 FUD 000

61108 **for evacuation and/or drainage of subdural hematoma**
C ⚑ 25.92 25.92 FUD 090

61120 **Burr hole(s) for ventricular puncture (including injection of gas, contrast media, dye, or radioactive material)**
C 80 ⚑ 21.35 21.35 FUD 090

61140 **Burr hole(s) or trephine; with biopsy of brain or intracranial lesion**
C 80 ⚑ PQ 36.05 36.05 FUD 090

61150 **with drainage of brain abscess or cyst**
C ⚑ 38.69 38.69 FUD 090

61151 **with subsequent tapping (aspiration) of intracranial abscess or cyst**
C ⚑ 28.40 28.40 FUD 090

61154 **Burr hole(s) with evacuation and/or drainage of hematoma, extradural or subdural**
C 80 50 ⚑ PQ 36.33 36.33 FUD 090

61156 **Burr hole(s); with aspiration of hematoma or cyst, intracerebral**
C 80 ⚑ 35.52 35.52 FUD 090

61210 **for implanting ventricular catheter, reservoir, EEG electrode(s), pressure recording device, or other cerebral monitoring device (separate procedure)**
Code also intracranial neuroendoscopic ventricular catheter insertion or reinsertion, when performed (62160)
C ⚑ 10.56 10.56 FUD 000

61215 **Insertion of subcutaneous reservoir, pump or continuous infusion system for connection to ventricular catheter**
EXCLUDES *Chemotherapy (96450)*
Refilling and maintenance of implantable infusion pump (95990)
A2 T ⚑ 14.39 14.39 FUD 090

61250 **Burr hole(s) or trephine, supratentorial, exploratory, not followed by other surgery**
EXCLUDES *Burr hole or trephine followed by craniotomy at same operative session (61304-61321)*
C 80 50 ⚑ 24.76 24.76 FUD 090

61253 **Burr hole(s) or trephine, infratentorial, unilateral or bilateral**
EXCLUDES *Burr hole or trephine followed by craniotomy at same operative session (61304-61321)*
C 80 ⚑ 23.58 23.58 FUD 090

61304-61323 Craniectomy/Craniotomy: By Indication/Specific Area of Brain

EXCLUDES *Injection for:*
Cerebral angiography (36100-36218)
Pneumoencephalography (61055)
Ventriculography (61026, 61120)

61304 **Craniectomy or craniotomy, exploratory; supratentorial**
Do not report with another craniectomy/craniotomy procedure when performed at the same anatomical site and same surgical encounter
C 80 ⚑ 46.88 46.88 FUD 090

61305 **infratentorial (posterior fossa)**
Do not report with another craniectomy/craniotomy procedure when performed at the same anatomical site and same surgical encounter
C 80 57.42 57.42 FUD 090

61312 **Craniectomy or craniotomy for evacuation of hematoma, supratentorial; extradural or subdural**
C 80 PQ 59.52 59.52 FUD 090

61313 **intracerebral**
C 80 PQ 56.73 56.73 FUD 090

61314 **Craniectomy or craniotomy for evacuation of hematoma, infratentorial; extradural or subdural**
C 80 52.34 52.34 FUD 090

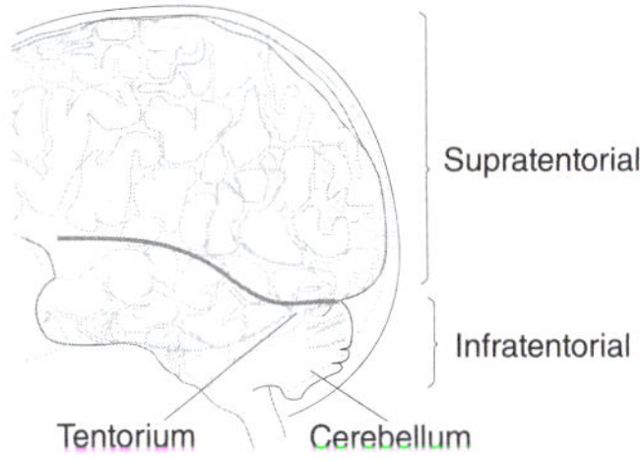

The tentorium is a dural septum that separates the cerebellum from the occipital lobes

61315 **intracerebellar**
C 80 PQ 59.22 59.22 FUD 090

\+ **61316** **Incision and subcutaneous placement of cranial bone graft (List separately in addition to code for primary procedure)**
Code first (61304, 61312-61313, 61322-61323, 61340, 61570-61571, 61680-61705)
C 2.52 2.52 FUD ZZZ

61320 **Craniectomy or craniotomy, drainage of intracranial abscess; supratentorial**
C 80 54.44 54.44 FUD 090

61321 **infratentorial**
C 80 60.86 60.86 FUD 090

61322 **Craniectomy or craniotomy, decompressive, with or without duraplasty, for treatment of intracranial hypertension, without evacuation of associated intraparenchymal hematoma; without lobectomy**
EXCLUDES *Subtemporal decompression (61340)*
Do not report with (61313)
C 80 67.91 67.91 FUD 090

61323 **with lobectomy**
EXCLUDES *Subtemporal decompression (61340)*
Do not report with (61313)
C 68.17 68.17 FUD 090

61330-61530 Craniectomy/Craniotomy/Decompression Brain By Surgical Approach/Specific Area of Brain

EXCLUDES *Injection for:*
Cerebral angiography (36100-36218)
Pneumoencephalography (61055)
Ventriculography (61026, 61120)

61330 **Decompression of orbit only, transcranial approach**
INCLUDES Naffziger operation
62 T 80 50 53.08 53.08 FUD 090

61332 **Exploration of orbit (transcranial approach); with biopsy**
C 80 50 59.26 59.26 FUD 090

61333 **with removal of lesion**
C 80 50 60.60 60.60 FUD 090

~~**61334**~~ ~~**with removal of foreign body**~~

61340 **Subtemporal cranial decompression (pseudotumor cerebri, slit ventricle syndrome)**
EXCLUDES *Decompression craniotomy or craniectomy for intracranial hypertension, without hematoma removal (61322-61323)*
C 80 50 41.31 41.31 FUD 090

61343 **Craniectomy, suboccipital with cervical laminectomy for decompression of medulla and spinal cord, with or without dural graft (eg, Arnold-Chiari malformation)**
C 80 62.90 62.90 FUD 090

61345 **Other cranial decompression, posterior fossa**
EXCLUDES *Kroenlein procedure (67445)*
Orbital decompression using a lateral wall approach (67445)
C 80 58.28 58.28 FUD 090

~~**61440**~~ ~~**Craniotomy for section of tentorium cerebelli (separate procedure)**~~

61450 **Craniectomy, subtemporal, for section, compression, or decompression of sensory root of gasserian ganglion**
INCLUDES Frazier-Spiller procedure
Hartley-Krause
Krause decompression
Taarnhoj procedure
C 80 54.95 54.95 FUD 090

61458 **Craniectomy, suboccipital; for exploration or decompression of cranial nerves**
INCLUDES Jannetta decompression
C 80 57.40 57.40 FUD 090

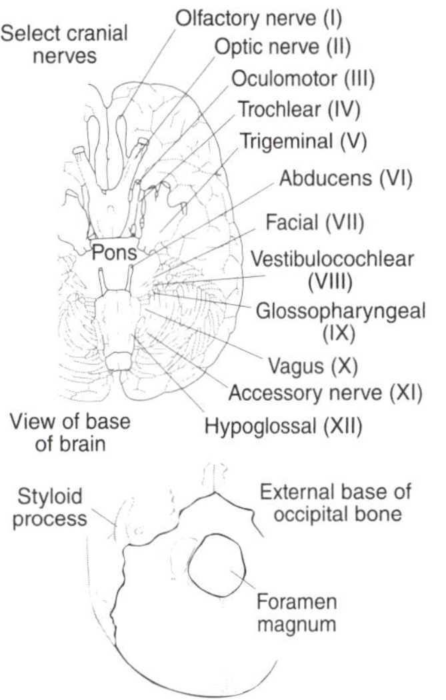

61460 **for section of 1 or more cranial nerves**
C 80 60.12 60.12 FUD 090

~~**61470**~~ ~~**for medullary tractotomy**~~

61480 **for mesencephalic tractotomy or pedunculotomy**
C 80 42.88 42.88 FUD 090

~~**61490**~~ ~~**Craniotomy for lobotomy, including cingulotomy**~~

61500 **Craniectomy; with excision of tumor or other bone lesion of skull**
C 80 38.17 38.17 FUD 090

61501 **for osteomyelitis**
C 80 33.07 33.07 FUD 090

61510 **Craniectomy, trephination, bone flap craniotomy; for excision of brain tumor, supratentorial, except meningioma**
C 80 PQ 62.55 62.55 FUD 090

61512 for excision of meningioma, supratentorial
C 80 PQ 72.96 72.96 FUD 090

61514 for excision of brain abscess, supratentorial
C 80 54.56 54.56 FUD 090

61516 for excision or fenestration of cyst, supratentorial
EXCLUDES *Craniopharyngioma (61545)*
Pituitary tumor removal (61546, 61548)
C 80 53.18 53.18 FUD 090

\+ **61517** Implantation of brain intracavitary chemotherapy agent (List separately in addition to code for primary procedure)
EXCLUDES *Intracavity radioelement source or ribbon implantation (77785-77787)*
Code first (61510, 61518)
C 2.50 2.50 FUD ZZZ

61518 Craniectomy for excision of brain tumor, infratentorial or posterior fossa; except meningioma, cerebellopontine angle tumor, or midline tumor at base of skull
C 80 PQ 78.99 78.99 FUD 090

61519 meningioma
C 80 84.41 84.41 FUD 090

61520 cerebellopontine angle tumor
C 80 PQ 107.18 107.18 FUD 090

61521 midline tumor at base of skull
C 80 91.00 91.00 FUD 090

61522 Craniectomy, infratentorial or posterior fossa; for excision of brain abscess
C 80 62.49 62.49 FUD 090

61524 for excision or fenestration of cyst
C 80 59.50 59.50 FUD 090

61526 Craniectomy, bone flap craniotomy, transtemporal (mastoid) for excision of cerebellopontine angle tumor;
C PQ 104.33 104.33 FUD 090

61530 combined with middle/posterior fossa craniotomy/craniectomy
C PQ 87.96 87.96 FUD 090

61531-61545 Procedures for Seizures/Implanted Electrodes/Choroid Plexus/Craniopharyngioma

CMS 100-3,160.5 Stereotaxic Depth Electrode Implantation

EXCLUDES *Craniotomy for:*
Multiple subpial transections during procedure (61567)
Selective amygdalohippocampectomy (61566)
Injection for:
Cerebral angiography (36100-36218)
Pneumoencephalography (61055)
Ventriculography (61026, 61120)

61531 Subdural implantation of strip electrodes through 1 or more burr or trephine hole(s) for long-term seizure monitoring
EXCLUDES *Craniotomy for intracranial arteriovenous malformation removal (61680-61692)*
Stereotactic insertion of electrodes (61760)
C 80 34.90 34.90 FUD 090

61533 Craniotomy with elevation of bone flap; for subdural implantation of an electrode array, for long-term seizure monitoring
EXCLUDES *Continuous EEG observation (95950-95954)*
C 80 43.51 43.51 FUD 090

61534 for excision of epileptogenic focus without electrocorticography during surgery
C 80 46.99 46.99 FUD 090

61535 for removal of epidural or subdural electrode array, without excision of cerebral tissue (separate procedure)
C 80 28.54 28.54 FUD 090

61536 for excision of cerebral epileptogenic focus, with electrocorticography during surgery (includes removal of electrode array)
C 80 73.71 73.71 FUD 090

61537 for lobectomy, temporal lobe, without electrocorticography during surgery
C 80 70.48 70.48 FUD 090

61538 for lobectomy, temporal lobe, with electrocorticography during surgery
C 80 76.32 76.32 FUD 090

61539 for lobectomy, other than temporal lobe, partial or total, with electrocorticography during surgery
C 80 67.46 67.46 FUD 090

61540 for lobectomy, other than temporal lobe, partial or total, without electrocorticography during surgery
C 80 62.37 62.37 FUD 090

61541 for transection of corpus callosum
C 80 61.39 61.39 FUD 090

~~**61542** for total hemispherectomy~~

61543 for partial or subtotal (functional) hemispherectomy
C 80 62.06 62.06 FUD 090

61544 for excision or coagulation of choroid plexus
C 80 54.36 54.36 FUD 090

61545 for excision of craniopharyngioma
C 80 91.00 91.00 FUD 090

61546-61548 Removal Pituitary Gland/Tumor

EXCLUDES *Injection for:*
Cerebral angiography (36100-36218)
Pneumoencephalography (61055)
Ventriculography (61026, 61120)

61546 Craniotomy for hypophysectomy or excision of pituitary tumor, intracranial approach
C 80 65.93 65.93 FUD 090

61548 **Hypophysectomy or excision of pituitary tumor, transnasal or transseptal approach, nonstereotactic**
INCLUDES Operating microscope (69990)
C 80 PQ 44.54 44.54 FUD 090

61550-61559 Craniosynostosis Procedures

EXCLUDES *Injection for:*
Cerebral angiography (36100-36218)
Pneumoencephalography (61055)
Ventriculography (61026, 61120)
Orbital hypertelorism reconstruction (21260-21263)
Reconstruction (21172-21180)

61550 **Craniectomy for craniosynostosis; single cranial suture**
C 80 25.30 25.30 FUD 090

61552 **multiple cranial sutures**
C 80 32.16 32.16 FUD 090

61556 **Craniotomy for craniosynostosis; frontal or parietal bone flap**
C 80 48.68 48.68 FUD 090

61557 **bifrontal bone flap**
C 80 48.00 48.00 FUD 090

61558 **Extensive craniectomy for multiple cranial suture craniosynostosis (eg, cloverleaf skull); not requiring bone grafts**
C 80 48.44 48.44 FUD 090

61559 **recontouring with multiple osteotomies and bone autografts (eg, barrel-stave procedure) (includes obtaining grafts)**
C 80 50.40 50.40 FUD 090

61563-61564 Removal Cranial Bone Tumor With/Without Optic Nerve Decompression

EXCLUDES *Injection for:*
Cerebral angiography (36100-36218)
Pneumoencephalography (61055)
Ventriculography (61026, 61120)
Reconstruction (21181-21183)

61563 **Excision, intra and extracranial, benign tumor of cranial bone (eg, fibrous dysplasia); without optic nerve decompression**
C 80 56.57 56.57 FUD 090

61564 **with optic nerve decompression**
C 80 50 68.75 68.75 FUD 090

61566-61567 Craniotomy for Seizures

EXCLUDES *Injection for:*
Cerebral angiography (36100-36218)
Pneumoencephalography (61055)
Ventriculography (61026, 61120)

61566 **Craniotomy with elevation of bone flap; for selective amygdalohippocampectomy**
C 80 64.22 64.22 FUD 090

61567 **for multiple subpial transections, with electrocorticography during surgery**
C 80 73.24 73.24 FUD 090

61570-61571 Removal of Foreign Body from Brain

EXCLUDES *Injection for:*
Cerebral angiography (36100-36218)
Pneumoencephalography (61055)
Ventriculography (61026, 61120)
Sequestrectomy for osteomyelitis (61501)

61570 **Craniectomy or craniotomy; with excision of foreign body from brain**
C 80 53.34 53.34 FUD 090

61571 **with treatment of penetrating wound of brain**
C 80 56.81 56.81 FUD 090

61575-61576 Transoral Approach Posterior Cranial Fossa/Upper Cervical Cord

EXCLUDES *Arthrodesis (22548)*
Injection for:
Cerebral angiography (36100-36218)
Pneumoencephalography (61055)
Ventriculography (61026, 61120)

61575 **Transoral approach to skull base, brain stem or upper spinal cord for biopsy, decompression or excision of lesion;**
C 80 PQ 69.02 69.02 FUD 090

61576 **requiring splitting of tongue and/or mandible (including tracheostomy)**
C 80 PQ 98.61 98.61 FUD 090

61580-61598 Surgical Approach: Cranial Fossae

EXCLUDES *Definitive surgery (61600-61616)*
Dural repair and/or reconstruction (61618-61619)
Injection for:
Cerebral angiography (36100-36218)
Pneumoencephalography (61055)
Ventriculography (61026, 61120)
Primary closure (15732, 15756-15758)

61580 **Craniofacial approach to anterior cranial fossa; extradural, including lateral rhinotomy, ethmoidectomy, sphenoidectomy, without maxillectomy or orbital exenteration**
C 50 71.20 71.20 FUD 090

61581 **extradural, including lateral rhinotomy, orbital exenteration, ethmoidectomy, sphenoidectomy and/or maxillectomy**
C 50 77.12 77.12 FUD 090

61582 **extradural, including unilateral or bifrontal craniotomy, elevation of frontal lobe(s), osteotomy of base of anterior cranial fossa**
C 80 84.06 84.06 FUD 090

61583 **intradural, including unilateral or bifrontal craniotomy, elevation or resection of frontal lobe, osteotomy of base of anterior cranial fossa**
C 80 82.99 82.99 FUD 090

61584 **Orbitocranial approach to anterior cranial fossa, extradural, including supraorbital ridge osteotomy and elevation of frontal and/or temporal lobe(s); without orbital exenteration**
C 80 50 81.57 81.57 FUD 090

61585 **with orbital exenteration**
C 80 50 92.44 92.44 FUD 090

61586 **Bicoronal, transzygomatic and/or LeFort I osteotomy approach to anterior cranial fossa with or without internal fixation, without bone graft**
C 80 69.77 69.77 FUD 090

61590 **Infratemporal pre-auricular approach to middle cranial fossa (parapharyngeal space, infratemporal and midline skull base, nasopharynx), with or without disarticulation of the mandible, including parotidectomy, craniotomy, decompression and/or mobilization of the facial nerve and/or petrous carotid artery**
C 80 50 87.66 87.66 FUD 090

61591 **Infratemporal post-auricular approach to middle cranial fossa (internal auditory meatus, petrous apex, tentorium, cavernous sinus, parasellar area, infratemporal fossa) including mastoidectomy, resection of sigmoid sinus, with or without decompression and/or mobilization of contents of auditory canal or petrous carotid artery**
C 80 50 PQ 89.05 89.05 FUD 090

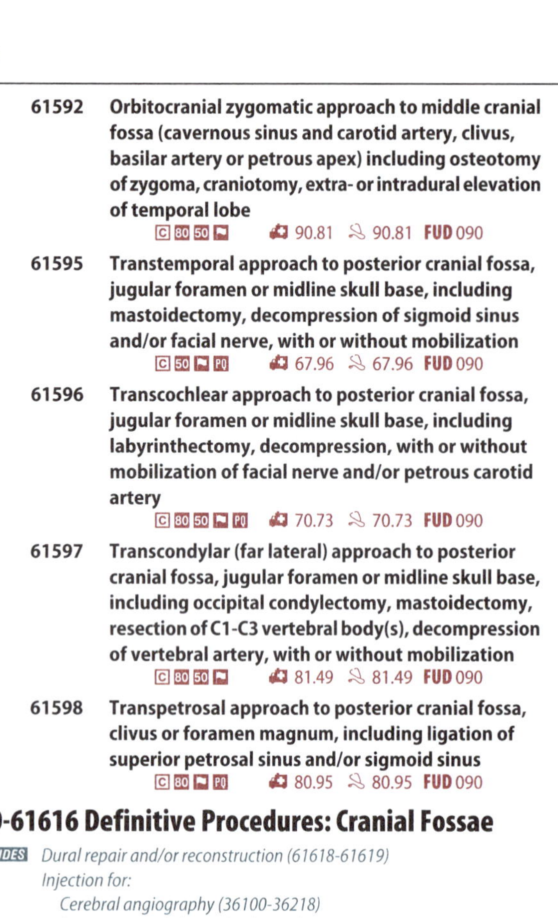

61592 **Orbitocranial zygomatic approach to middle cranial fossa (cavernous sinus and carotid artery, clivus, basilar artery or petrous apex) including osteotomy of zygoma, craniotomy, extra- or intradural elevation of temporal lobe**
C 80 50 ▪ 90.81 90.81 **FUD** 090

61595 **Transtemporal approach to posterior cranial fossa, jugular foramen or midline skull base, including mastoidectomy, decompression of sigmoid sinus and/or facial nerve, with or without mobilization**
C 50 ▪ PQ 67.96 67.96 **FUD** 090

61596 **Transcochlear approach to posterior cranial fossa, jugular foramen or midline skull base, including labyrinthectomy, decompression, with or without mobilization of facial nerve and/or petrous carotid artery**
C 80 50 ▪ PQ 70.73 70.73 **FUD** 090

61597 **Transcondylar (far lateral) approach to posterior cranial fossa, jugular foramen or midline skull base, including occipital condylectomy, mastoidectomy, resection of C1-C3 vertebral body(s), decompression of vertebral artery, with or without mobilization**
C 80 50 ▪ 81.49 81.49 **FUD** 090

61598 **Transpetrosal approach to posterior cranial fossa, clivus or foramen magnum, including ligation of superior petrosal sinus and/or sigmoid sinus**
C 80 ▪ PQ 80.95 80.95 **FUD** 090

61600-61616 Definitive Procedures: Cranial Fossae

EXCLUDES *Dural repair and/or reconstruction (61618-61619)*
Injection for:
Cerebral angiography (36100-36218)
Pneumoencephalography (61055)
Ventriculography (61026, 61120)
Primary closure (15732, 15756-15758)
Surgical approach (61580-61598)

61600 **Resection or excision of neoplastic, vascular or infectious lesion of base of anterior cranial fossa; extradural**
C 80 ▪ 61.46 61.46 **FUD** 090

61601 **intradural, including dural repair, with or without graft**
C 80 ▪ 68.91 68.91 **FUD** 090

61605 **Resection or excision of neoplastic, vascular or infectious lesion of infratemporal fossa, parapharyngeal space, petrous apex; extradural**
C 80 ▪ 62.83 62.83 **FUD** 090

61606 **intradural, including dural repair, with or without graft**
C 80 ▪ PQ 85.88 85.88 **FUD** 090

61607 **Resection or excision of neoplastic, vascular or infectious lesion of parasellar area, cavernous sinus, clivus or midline skull base; extradural**
C 80 ▪ 82.61 82.61 **FUD** 090

61608 **intradural, including dural repair, with or without graft**
C 80 ▪ 92.71 92.71 **FUD** 090

61609 ~~**Transection or ligation, carotid artery in cavernous sinus; without repair (List separately in addition to code for primary procedure)**~~

\+ **61610** **with repair by anastomosis or graft (List separately in addition to code for primary procedure)**
Code first (61605-61608)
C 80 ▪ 50.49 50.49 **FUD** ZZZ

\+ **61611** **Transection or ligation, carotid artery in petrous canal; without repair (List separately in addition to code for primary procedure)**
Code first (61605-61608)
C 80 ▪ 11.36 11.36 **FUD** ZZZ

\+ **61612** **with repair by anastomosis or graft (List separately in addition to code for primary procedure)**
Code first (61605-61608)
C 80 ▪ 40.38 40.38 **FUD** ZZZ

61613 **Obliteration of carotid aneurysm, arteriovenous malformation, or carotid-cavernous fistula by dissection within cavernous sinus**
C 80 50 ▪ 93.76 93.76 **FUD** 090

61615 **Resection or excision of neoplastic, vascular or infectious lesion of base of posterior cranial fossa, jugular foramen, foramen magnum, or C1-C3 vertebral bodies; extradural**
C 80 ▪ 65.08 65.08 **FUD** 090

61616 **intradural, including dural repair, with or without graft**
C 80 ▪ PQ 95.16 95.16 **FUD** 090

61618-61619 Reconstruction Post-Surgical Cranial Fossae Defects

EXCLUDES *Definitive surgery (61600-61616)*
Injection for:
Cerebral angiography (36100-36218)
Pneumoencephalography (61055)
Ventriculography (61026, 61120)
Primary closure (15732, 15756-15758)
Surgical approach (61580-61598)

61618 **Secondary repair of dura for cerebrospinal fluid leak, anterior, middle or posterior cranial fossa following surgery of the skull base; by free tissue graft (eg, pericranium, fascia, tensor fascia lata, adipose tissue, homologous or synthetic grafts)**
C 80 ▪ PQ 37.32 37.32 **FUD** 090

61619 **by local or regionalized vascularized pedicle flap or myocutaneous flap (including galea, temporalis, frontalis or occipitalis muscle)**
C 80 ▪ PQ 42.42 42.42 **FUD** 090

61623-61642 Neurovascular Interventional Procedures

CMS 100-2,16,10 Exclusions from Coverage
CMS 100-2,16,180 Services Related to Noncovered Procedures
CMS 100-3,20.28 Therapeutic Embolization
CMS 100-4,4,61.1 Hospital Requirement for Device Codes on OPPS Claims
CMS 100-4,4,61.2 Requirements for Specific Procedures to be Reported With Device Codes

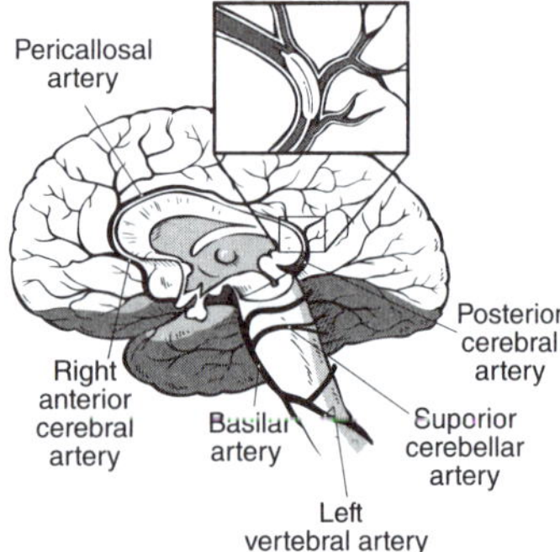

61623 **Endovascular temporary balloon arterial occlusion, head or neck (extracranial/intracranial) including selective catheterization of vessel to be occluded, positioning and inflation of occlusion balloon, concomitant neurological monitoring, and radiologic supervision and interpretation of all angiography required for balloon occlusion and to exclude vascular injury post occlusion**

EXCLUDES *Diagnostic angiography of target artery just before temporary occlusion; report only radiological supervision and interpretation*
Selective catheterization and angiography of artery besides the target artery; report catheterization and radiological supervision and interpretation codes as appropriate

Code also (C2628)

T PQ 15.92 15.92 FUD 000

61624 **Transcatheter permanent occlusion or embolization (eg, for tumor destruction, to achieve hemostasis, to occlude a vascular malformation), percutaneous, any method; central nervous system (intracranial, spinal cord)**

EXCLUDES *Non-central nervous system transcatheter occlusion or embolization other than head or neck (37241-37244)*

75894

C 31.79 31.79 FUD 000

61626 **non-central nervous system, head or neck (extracranial, brachiocephalic branch)**

EXCLUDES *Non-central nervous system transcatheter occlusion or embolization other than head or neck (37241-37244)*

Code also (C1769, C1887, C2628)

75894

T 24.68 24.68 FUD 000

61630 **Balloon angioplasty, intracranial (eg, atherosclerotic stenosis), percutaneous**

INCLUDES Diagnostic arteriogram if stent or angioplasty is necessary
Radiology services for arteriography of target vascular family
Selective catheterization of the target vascular family

EXCLUDES *Diagnostic arteriogram if stent or angioplasty is not necessary (use applicable code for selective catheterization and radiology services)*

C 80 36.57 36.57 FUD XXX

61635 **Transcatheter placement of intravascular stent(s), intracranial (eg, atherosclerotic stenosis), including balloon angioplasty, if performed**

INCLUDES Diagnostic arteriogram if stent or angioplasty is necessary
Radiology services for arteriography of target vascular family
Selective catheterization of the target vascular family

EXCLUDES *Diagnostic arteriogram if stent or angioplasty is not necessary (use applicable code for selective catheterization and radiology services)*

C 80 39.93 39.93 FUD XXX

61640 **Balloon dilatation of intracranial vasospasm, percutaneous; initial vessel**

INCLUDES Angiography after dilation of vessel
Fluoroscopic guidance
Injection of contrast material
Roadmapping
Selective catheterization of target vessel
Vessel analysis

E 17.88 17.88 FUD 000

\+ **61641** **each additional vessel in same vascular family (List separately in addition to code for primary procedure)**

INCLUDES Angiography after dilation of vessel
Fluoroscopic guidance
Injection of contrast material
Roadmapping
Selective catheterization of target vessel
Vessel analysis

Code first (61640)

E 6.29 6.29 FUD ZZZ

\+ **61642** **each additional vessel in different vascular family (List separately in addition to code for primary procedure)**

INCLUDES Angiography after dilation of vessel
Fluoroscopic guidance
Injection of contrast material
Roadmapping
Selective catheterization of target vessel
Vessel analysis

Code first (61640)

E 12.56 12.56 FUD ZZZ

61680-61692 Surgical Treatment of Arteriovenous Malformation of the Brain

CMS 100-4,12,30 Correct Coding Policy

INCLUDES Craniotomy

61680 **Surgery of intracranial arteriovenous malformation; supratentorial, simple**

C 80 64.40 64.40 FUD 090

61682 **supratentorial, complex**

C 80 119.60 119.60 FUD 090

61684 **infratentorial, simple**

C 80 81.30 81.30 FUD 090

61686 **infratentorial, complex**

C 80 128.71 128.71 FUD 090

61690 **dural, simple**

C 80 62.47 62.47 FUD 090

61692 **dural, complex**

C 80 104.69 104.69 FUD 090

61697-61703 Surgical Treatment Brain Aneurysm

INCLUDES Craniotomy

61697 **Surgery of complex intracranial aneurysm, intracranial approach; carotid circulation**

INCLUDES Aneurysms bigger than 15 mm
Calcification of the aneurysm neck
Inclusion of normal vessels in aneurysm neck
Surgery needing temporary vessel occlusion, trapping, or cardiopulmonary bypass to treat aneurysm

C 80 PQ 120.79 120.79 FUD 090

61698 **vertebrobasilar circulation**

INCLUDES Aneurysm bigger than 15 mm
Calcification of aneurysm neck
Inclusion of normal vessels into aneurysm neck
Surgery needing temporary vessel occlusion, trapping, or cardiopulmonary bypass to treat aneurysm

C 80 132.57 132.57 FUD 090

61700 **Surgery of simple intracranial aneurysm, intracranial approach; carotid circulation**

C 80 PQ 97.73 97.73 FUD 090

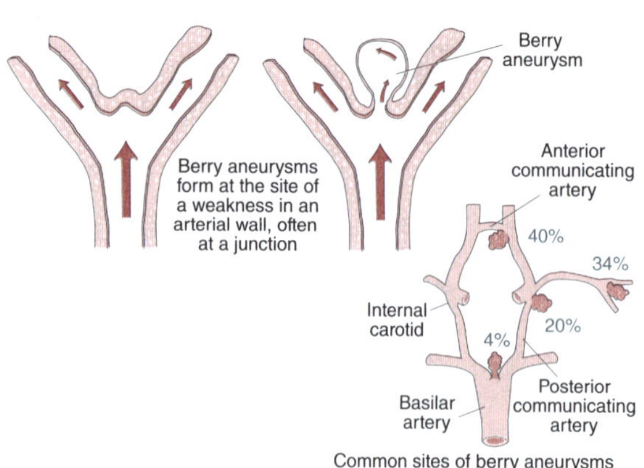

Common sites of berry aneurysms in the circle of Willis arteries

61702 **vertebrobasilar circulation**
C 80 ⚑ Facility RVU 115.15 Non-Facility RVU 115.15 FUD 090

61703 **Surgery of intracranial aneurysm, cervical approach by application of occluding clamp to cervical carotid artery (Selverstone-Crutchfield type)**
EXCLUDES *Cervical approach for direct ligation of carotid artery (37600-37606)*
C 80 ⚑ Facility RVU 38.81 Non-Facility RVU 38.81 FUD 090

61705-61710 Other Procedures for Aneurysm, Arteriovenous Malformation, and Carotid-Cavernous Fistula

INCLUDES Craniotomy

61705 **Surgery of aneurysm, vascular malformation or carotid-cavernous fistula; by intracranial and cervical occlusion of carotid artery**
C 80 ⚑ Facility RVU 74.40 Non-Facility RVU 74.40 FUD 090

61708 **by intracranial electrothrombosis**
EXCLUDES *Ligation or gradual occlusion of internal or common carotid artery (37605-37606)*
C 80 ⚑ Facility RVU 56.17 Non-Facility RVU 56.17 FUD 090

61710 **by intra-arterial embolization, injection procedure, or balloon catheter**
C 80 ⚑ Facility RVU 56.98 Non-Facility RVU 56.98 FUD 090

61711 Extracranial-Intracranial Bypass

INCLUDES Craniotomy

EXCLUDES *Carotid or vertebral thromboendarterectomy (35301)*

Code also operating microscope (69990) when appropriate

61711 **Anastomosis, arterial, extracranial-intracranial (eg, middle cerebral/cortical) arteries**
C 80 ⚑ Facility RVU 74.55 Non-Facility RVU 74.55 FUD 090

61720-61791 Stereotactic Procedures of the Brain

CMS 100-3,160.4 Stereotactic Cingulotomy as a Means of Psychosurgery--Not Covered

CMS 100-3,160.5 Stereotaxic Depth Electrode Implantation

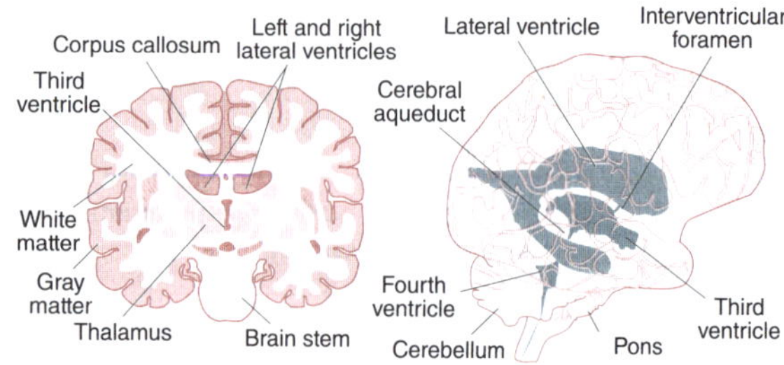

Frontal secion of the brain (left) and lateral view schematic showing the ventricular system in blue (right)

61720 **Creation of lesion by stereotactic method, including burr hole(s) and localizing and recording techniques, single or multiple stages; globus pallidus or thalamus**
T ⚑ Facility RVU 36.27 Non-Facility RVU 36.27 FUD 090

61735 **subcortical structure(s) other than globus pallidus or thalamus**
C ⚑ Facility RVU 45.41 Non-Facility RVU 45.41 FUD 090

61750 **Stereotactic biopsy, aspiration, or excision, including burr hole(s), for intracranial lesion;**
C ⚑ PQ Facility RVU 40.18 Non-Facility RVU 40.18 FUD 090

61751 **with computed tomography and/or magnetic resonance guidance**
Radiology Crosswalk 70450, 70460, 70470, 70551-70553
C ⚑ PQ Facility RVU 39.27 Non-Facility RVU 39.27 FUD 090

61760 **Stereotactic implantation of depth electrodes into the cerebrum for long-term seizure monitoring**
C ⚑ Facility RVU 45.14 Non-Facility RVU 45.14 FUD 090

61770 **Stereotactic localization, including burr hole(s), with insertion of catheter(s) or probe(s) for placement of radiation source**
G2 T ⚑ Facility RVU 46.26 Non-Facility RVU 46.26 FUD 090

+ **61781** **Stereotactic computer-assisted (navigational) procedure; cranial, intradural (List separately in addition to code for primary procedure)**
Code first primary procedure
Do not report for same surgical session by same individual (61782)
Do not report with (61720-61791, 61796-61799, 61863-61868, 62201, 77371-77373, 77432)
N1 N 80 Facility RVU 6.71 Non-Facility RVU 6.71 FUD ZZZ

+ **61782** **cranial, extradural (List separately in addition to code for primary procedure)**
Code first primary procedure
Do not report for same surgical session by same individual (61781)
Do not report with (61796-61799)
N1 N 80 Facility RVU 5.50 Non-Facility RVU 5.50 FUD ZZZ

+ **61783** **spinal (List separately in addition to code for primary procedure)**
Code first primary procedure
Do not report with (61796-61799, 63620-63621)
N1 N 80 Facility RVU 6.73 Non-Facility RVU 6.73 FUD ZZZ

61790 **Creation of lesion by stereotactic method, percutaneous, by neurolytic agent (eg, alcohol, thermal, electrical, radiofrequency); gasserian ganglion**
A2 T 50 ⚑ Facility RVU 24.96 Non-Facility RVU 24.96 FUD 090

61791 **trigeminal medullary tract**
A2 T 80 50 ⚑ Facility RVU 31.79 Non-Facility RVU 31.79 FUD 090

61796-61800 Stereotactic Radiosurgery (SRS): Brain

INCLUDES Planning, dosimetry, targeting, positioning or blocking performed by the neurosurgeon

EXCLUDES *Intensity modulated beam delivery plan and treatment (77301, [77385, 77386])*
Stereotactic body radiation therapy (77373, 77435)
Treatment planning, physics and dosimetry, and treatment delivery performed by the radiation oncologist

Do not report radiation treatment management and radiosurgery by the same provider (77427-77435)

Do not report with (20660)

61796 **Stereotactic radiosurgery (particle beam, gamma ray, or linear accelerator); 1 simple cranial lesion**

INCLUDES Lesions < 3.5 cm

EXCLUDES *Treatment of complex lesions: (61798-61799)*
Arteriovenous malformations (AVM)
Brainstem lesions
Cavernous sinus/parasellar/petroclival tumors, glomus tumors, pituitary tumors, and tumors of pineal region
Lesions located <= 5 mm from the optic nerve, chasm, or tract
Schwannomas

Code also stereotactic headframe application, when performed (61800)

Do not report more than one time per treatment course

Do not report with (61781-61783, 61798)

B 80 28.67 28.67 FUD 090

+ **61797** **each additional cranial lesion, simple (List separately in addition to code for primary procedure)**

INCLUDES Lesions < 3.5 cm

EXCLUDES *Treatment of complex lesions: (61798-61799)*
Arteriovenous malformations (AVM)
Brainstem lesion
Cavernous sinus/parasellar/petroclival tumors, glomus tumors, pituitary tumor, tumors of pineal region
Lesions located <= 5 mm from the optic nerve, chasm, or tract
Schwannomas

Code first (61796 or 61798)

Do not report more than four times in total per treatment course when used alone or in combination with (61799)

Do not report more than one time per lesion per treatment course

Do not report with (61781-61783)

B 80 6.24 6.24 FUD ZZZ

61798 **1 complex cranial lesion**

INCLUDES All therapeutic lesion creation procedures
Treatment of complex lesions:
Arteriovenous malformations (AVM)
Brainstem lesions
Cavernous sinus, parasellar, petroclival, glomus, pineal region, and pituitary tumors
Lesions located <= 5 mm from the optic nerve, chasm, or tract
Lesions >= 3.5 cm
Schwannomas
Treatment of multiple lesions as long as one is complex

Code also stereotactic headframe application, when performed (61800)

Do not report more than one time per treatment course

Do not report with (61781-61783, 61796)

B 80 39.18 39.18 FUD 090

+ **61799** **each additional cranial lesion, complex (List separately in addition to code for primary procedure)**

INCLUDES All therapeutic lesion creation procedures
Treatment of complex lesions:
Arteriovenous malformations (AVM)
Brainstem lesions
Cavernous sinus, parasellar, petroclival, glomus, pineal region, and pituitary tumors
Lesions located <= 5 mm from the optic nerve, chasm, or tract
Lesions >= 3.5 cm
Schwannomas

Code first (61798)

Do not report more than four times in total per treatment course when used alone or in combination with (61799)

Do not report more than once per lesion per treatment course

Do not report with (61781-61783)

B 80 8.60 8.60 FUD ZZZ

+ **61800** **Application of stereotactic headframe for stereotactic radiosurgery (List separately in addition to code for primary procedure)**

Code first (61796, 61798)

B 80 4.36 4.36 FUD ZZZ

61850-61888 Intracranial Neurostimulation

CMS 100-3,160.2 Treatment of Motor Function Disorders with Electric Nerve Stimulation

CMS 100-3,160.7 Electrical Nerve Stimulators

CMS 100-4,32,50 Deep Brain Stimulation for Essential Tremor and Parkinson's Disease

INCLUDES Microelectrode recording by operating surgeon

EXCLUDES *Electronic analysis and reprogramming of neurostimulator pulse generator (95970-95975)*
Neurophysiological mapping by another physician/qualified health care professional (95961-95962)

61850 **Twist drill or burr hole(s) for implantation of neurostimulator electrodes, cortical**

C 80 28.04 28.04 FUD 090

61860 **Craniectomy or craniotomy for implantation of neurostimulator electrodes, cerebral, cortical**

C 80 44.70 44.70 FUD 090

61863 **Twist drill, burr hole, craniotomy, or craniectomy with stereotactic implantation of neurostimulator electrode array in subcortical site (eg, thalamus, globus pallidus, subthalamic nucleus, periventricular, periaqueductal gray), without use of intraoperative microelectrode recording; first array**

C 80 50 42.95 42.95 FUD 090

+ **61864** **each additional array (List separately in addition to primary procedure)**

Code first (61863)

C 80 8.15 8.15 FUD ZZZ

61867 **Twist drill, burr hole, craniotomy, or craniectomy with stereotactic implantation of neurostimulator electrode array in subcortical site (eg, thalamus, globus pallidus, subthalamic nucleus, periventricular, periaqueductal gray), with use of intraoperative microelectrode recording; first array**

C 80 50 PQ 65.21 65.21 FUD 090

+ **61868** **each additional array (List separately in addition to primary procedure)**

Code first (61867)

C 80 14.35 14.35 FUD ZZZ

61870 **Craniectomy for implantation of neurostimulator electrodes, cerebellar, cortical**

C 80 33.80 33.80 FUD 090

~~**61875**~~ ~~**subcortical**~~

61880 **Revision or removal of intracranial neurostimulator electrodes**

62 02 80 50 16.33 16.33 FUD 090

61885 **Insertion or replacement of cranial neurostimulator pulse generator or receiver, direct or inductive coupling; with connection to a single electrode array**

EXCLUDES *Percutaneous procedure to place cranial nerve neurostimulator electrode(s) (64553)*

Revision or replacement cranial nerve neurostimulator electrode array (64569)

Code also (C1767, C1820, L8685, L8686)

J8 S 80 50 — 14.78 — 14.78 FUD 090

61886 **with connection to 2 or more electrode arrays**

EXCLUDES *Percutaneous procedure to place cranial nerve neurostimulator electrode(s) (64553)*

Revision or replacement cranial nerve neurostimulator electrode array (64569)

Code also (C1767, C1820, L8687, L8688)

J8 S 80 — 24.14 — 24.14 FUD 090

61888 **Revision or removal of cranial neurostimulator pulse generator or receiver**

Do not report with (61885-61886)

A2 Q2 50 — 11.18 — 11.18 FUD 010

62000-62148 Repair of Skull and/or Cerebrospinal Fluid Leaks

62000 **Elevation of depressed skull fracture; simple, extradural**

T — 29.43 — 29.43 FUD 090

62005 **compound or comminuted, extradural**

C 80 — 36.29 — 36.29 FUD 090

62010 **with repair of dura and/or debridement of brain**

C 80 — 43.74 — 43.74 FUD 090

62100 **Craniotomy for repair of dural/cerebrospinal fluid leak, including surgery for rhinorrhea/otorrhea**

EXCLUDES *Repair of spinal fluid leak (63707, 63709)*

C 80 — 46.06 — 46.06 FUD 090

62115 **Reduction of craniomegalic skull (eg, treated hydrocephalus); not requiring bone grafts or cranioplasty**

C 80 — 36.24 — 36.24 FUD 090

~~62116~~ ~~with simple cranioplasty~~

62117 **requiring craniotomy and reconstruction with or without bone graft (includes obtaining grafts)**

C 80 — 44.95 — 44.95 FUD 090

62120 **Repair of encephalocele, skull vault, including cranioplasty**

C 80 — 48.05 — 48.05 FUD 090

62121 **Craniotomy for repair of encephalocele, skull base**

C 80 — 48.77 — 48.77 FUD 090

62140 **Cranioplasty for skull defect; up to 5 cm diameter**

C 80 — 29.70 — 29.70 FUD 090

62141 **larger than 5 cm diameter**

C 80 — 32.68 — 32.68 FUD 090

62142 **Removal of bone flap or prosthetic plate of skull**

C 80 — 25.39 — 25.39 FUD 090

62143 **Replacement of bone flap or prosthetic plate of skull**

C 80 — 29.78 — 29.78 FUD 090

62145 **Cranioplasty for skull defect with reparative brain surgery**

C 80 — 40.68 — 40.68 FUD 090

62146 **Cranioplasty with autograft (includes obtaining bone grafts); up to 5 cm diameter**

C 80 — 35.66 — 35.66 FUD 090

62147 **larger than 5 cm diameter**

C 80 — 41.61 — 41.61 FUD 090

\+ **62148** **Incision and retrieval of subcutaneous cranial bone graft for cranioplasty (List separately in addition to code for primary procedure)**

Code first (62140-62147)

C — 3.63 — 3.63 FUD ZZZ

62160-62165 Neuroendoscopic Brain Procedures

INCLUDES Diagnostic endoscopy

\+ **62160** **Neuroendoscopy, intracranial, for placement or replacement of ventricular catheter and attachment to shunt system or external drainage (List separately in addition to code for primary procedure)**

Code first (61107, 61210, 62220-62230, 62258)

N1 N — 5.45 — 5.45 FUD ZZZ

62161 **Neuroendoscopy, intracranial; with dissection of adhesions, fenestration of septum pellucidum or intraventricular cysts (including placement, replacement, or removal of ventricular catheter)**

C 80 — 43.36 — 43.36 FUD 090

62162 **with fenestration or excision of colloid cyst, including placement of external ventricular catheter for drainage**

C 80 — 53.99 — 53.99 FUD 090

62163 **with retrieval of foreign body**

C 80 — 34.94 — 34.94 FUD 090

62164 **with excision of brain tumor, including placement of external ventricular catheter for drainage**

C 80 — 59.69 — 59.69 FUD 090

62165 **with excision of pituitary tumor, transnasal or trans-sphenoidal approach**

C 80 — 44.37 — 44.37 FUD 090

62180-62258 Cerebrospinal Fluid Diversion Procedures

62180 **Ventriculocisternostomy (Torkildsen type operation)**

C 80 — 45.74 — 45.74 FUD 090

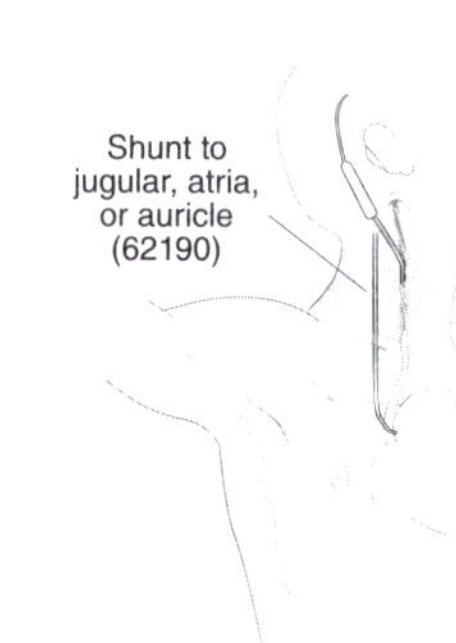

62190 **Creation of shunt; subarachnoid/subdural-atrial, -jugular, -auricular**

C — 26.38 — 26.38 FUD 090

62192 **subarachnoid/subdural-peritoneal, -pleural, other terminus**

C 80 — 27.86 — 27.86 FUD 090

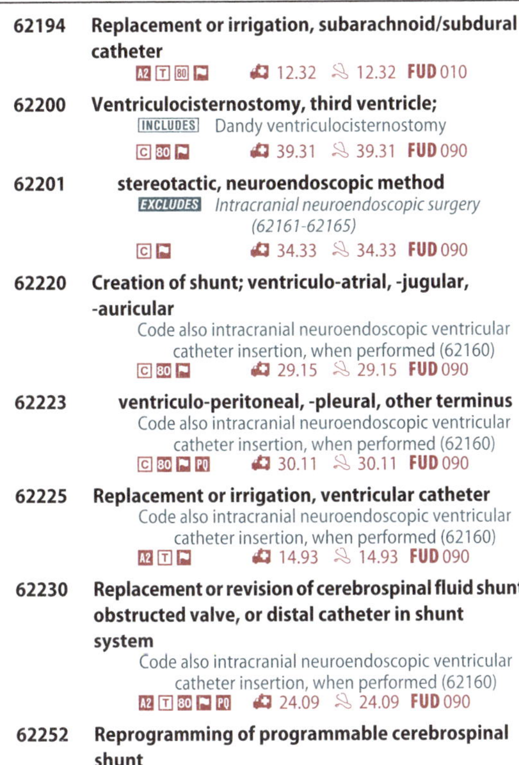

62194 **Replacement or irrigation, subarachnoid/subdural catheter**

A2 T 80 ⚑ 12.32 12.32 FUD 010

62200 **Ventriculocisternostomy, third ventricle;**

INCLUDES Dandy ventriculocisternostomy

C 80 ⚑ 39.31 39.31 FUD 090

62201 **stereotactic, neuroendoscopic method**

EXCLUDES *Intracranial neuroendoscopic surgery (62161-62165)*

C ⚑ 34.33 34.33 FUD 090

62220 **Creation of shunt; ventriculo-atrial, -jugular, -auricular**

Code also intracranial neuroendoscopic ventricular catheter insertion, when performed (62160)

C 80 ⚑ 29.15 29.15 FUD 090

62223 **ventriculo-peritoneal, -pleural, other terminus**

Code also intracranial neuroendoscopic ventricular catheter insertion, when performed (62160)

C 80 ⚑ PQ 30.11 30.11 FUD 090

62225 **Replacement or irrigation, ventricular catheter**

Code also intracranial neuroendoscopic ventricular catheter insertion, when performed (62160)

A2 T ⚑ 14.93 14.93 FUD 090

62230 **Replacement or revision of cerebrospinal fluid shunt, obstructed valve, or distal catheter in shunt system**

Code also intracranial neuroendoscopic ventricular catheter insertion, when performed (62160)

A2 T 80 ⚑ PQ 24.09 24.09 FUD 090

62252 **Reprogramming of programmable cerebrospinal shunt**

P3 S 80 ⚑ 2.41 2.41 FUD XXX

62256 **Removal of complete cerebrospinal fluid shunt system; without replacement**

EXCLUDES *Reprogramming cerebrospinal fluid (CSF) shunt (62252)*

C 80 ⚑ 17.13 17.13 FUD 090

62258 **with replacement by similar or other shunt at same operation**

EXCLUDES *Reprogramming of a cerebrospinal fluid (CSF) shunt (62252)*

Code also intracranial neuroendoscopic ventricular catheter insertion, when performed (62160)

C 80 ⚑ 32.20 32.20 FUD 090

62263-62264 Lysis of Epidural Lesions with Injection of Solution/Mechanical Methods

INCLUDES Contrast injection during fluoroscopic guidance/localization
Fluoroscopic guidance and epidurography (72275, 77003)
Percutaneous mechanical lysis

62263 **Percutaneous lysis of epidural adhesions using solution injection (eg, hypertonic saline, enzyme) or mechanical means (eg, catheter) including radiologic localization (includes contrast when administered), multiple adhesiolysis sessions; 2 or more days**

INCLUDES All adhesiolysis treatments, injections, and infusions during course of treatment
Percutaneous epidural catheter insertion and removal for neurolytic agent injections during a series of treatment sessions

Do not report more than one time for the complete series spanning two or more treatment days

A2 T ⚑ PQ 10.07 19.57 FUD 010

62264 **1 day**

INCLUDES Multiple treatment sessions performed on the same day

Do not report with (62263)

A2 T ⚑ PQ 6.86 11.98 FUD 010

62267-62269 Percutaneous Procedures of Spinal Cord

62267 **Percutaneous aspiration within the nucleus pulposus, intervertebral disc, or paravertebral tissue for diagnostic purposes**

INCLUDES Contrast injection during fluoroscopic guidance/localization

Code also fluoroscopic guidance and localization unless a formal contrast study is performed (77003)

Do not report with (10022, 20225, 62287, 62290-62291)

77003

G2 T 80 4.63 7.07 FUD 000

62268 **Percutaneous aspiration, spinal cord cyst or syrinx**

76942, 77002, 77012

A2 T ⚑ 7.53 7.53 FUD 000

62269 **Biopsy of spinal cord, percutaneous needle**

EXCLUDES *Fine needle aspiration (10021-10022)*

76942, 77002, 77012

88172, 88173

A2 T 80 ⚑ PQ 7.72 7.72 FUD 000

62270-62272 Spinal Puncture, Subarachnoid Space, Diagnostic/Therapeutic

INCLUDES Contrast injection during fluoroscopic guidance/localization

Code also fluoroscopic guidance and localization unless a formal contrast study is performed (77003)

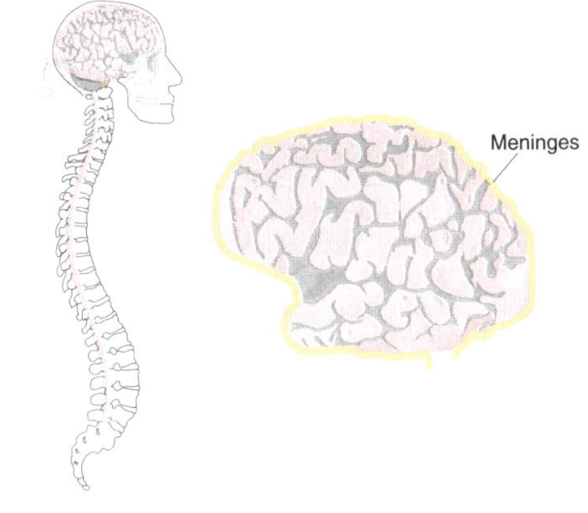

62270 **Spinal puncture, lumbar, diagnostic**

A2 T ⚑ 2.27 4.53 FUD 000

62272 **Spinal puncture, therapeutic, for drainage of cerebrospinal fluid (by needle or catheter)**

A2 T ⚑ 2.45 5.74 FUD 000

62273 Epidural Blood Patch

INCLUDES Contrast injection during fluoroscopic guidance/localization

EXCLUDES *Injection of diagnostic or therapeutic material (62310-62311, 62318-62319)*

Code also fluoroscopic guidance and localization unless a formal contrast study is performed (77003)

62273 **Injection, epidural, of blood or clot patch**

A2 T ⚑ 3.27 4.93 FUD 000

62280-62282 Neurolysis

INCLUDES Contrast injection during fluoroscopic guidance/localization

EXCLUDES *Injection of diagnostic or therapeutic material only (62310-62311, 62318-62319)*

Code also fluoroscopic guidance and localization unless a formal contrast study is performed (77003)

62280 **Injection/infusion of neurolytic substance (eg, alcohol, phenol, iced saline solutions), with or without other therapeutic substance; subarachnoid**

A2 T ⚑ PQ 4.95 9.07 FUD 010

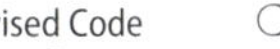
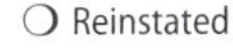
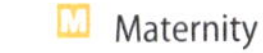
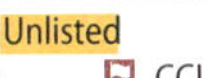

62281 **epidural, cervical or thoracic**
A2 T PQ 4.59 6.91 FUD 010

62282 **epidural, lumbar, sacral (caudal)**
A2 T PQ 4.16 8.15 FUD 010

62284-62294 Injection/Aspiration of Spine, Diagnostic/Therapeutic

▲ 62284 **Injection procedure for myelography and/or computed tomography, lumbar**
EXCLUDES *Injection at C1-C2 (61055)*
Do not report with (62302-62305, 72240, 72255, 72265, 72270)
N1 N 2.49 5.48 FUD 000

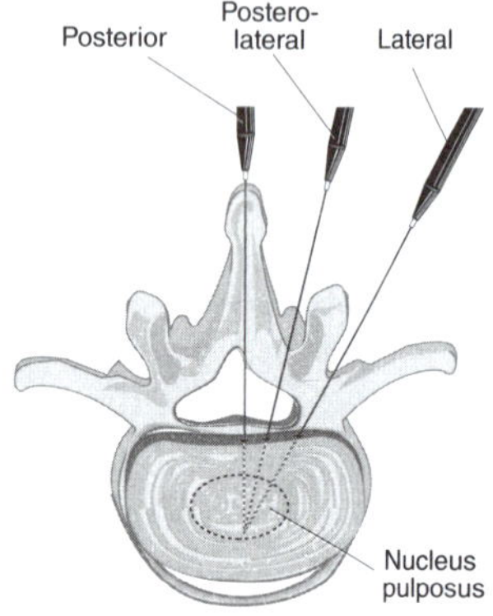

62287 **Decompression procedure, percutaneous, of nucleus pulposus of intervertebral disc, any method utilizing needle based technique to remove disc material under fluoroscopic imaging or other form of indirect visualization, with the use of an endoscope, with discography and/or epidural injection(s) at the treated level(s), when performed, single or multiple levels, lumbar**
INCLUDES Endoscopic approach
EXCLUDES *Percutaneous decompression of nucleus pulposus of an intervertebral disc, non-needle based technique (0274T-0275T)*
Do not report with (62267, 62290, 62311, 72295, 77003, 77012)
A2 T 16.15 16.15 FUD 090

62290 **Injection procedure for discography, each level; lumbar**
72295
N1 N 5.01 9.51 FUD 000

62291 **cervical or thoracic**
72285
N1 N 4.90 9.16 FUD 000

62292 **Injection procedure for chemonucleolysis, including discography, intervertebral disc, single or multiple levels, lumbar**
R2 T 80 16.77 16.77 FUD 090

62294 **Injection procedure, arterial, for occlusion of arteriovenous malformation, spinal**
A2 T 20.60 20.60 FUD 090

62302-62305 Myelography

EXCLUDES *C1-C2 injection (61055)*
Lumbar myelogram furnished by other providers (62284, 72240, 72255, 72265, 72270)

● 62302 **Myelography via lumbar injection, including radiological supervision and interpretation; cervical**
Do not report with (62303-62305)

● 62303 **thoracic**
Do not report with (62302, 62304-62305)

● 62304 **lumbosacral**
Do not report with (62302-62303, 62305)

● 62305 **2 or more regions (eg, lumbar/thoracic, cervical/thoracic, lumbar/cervical, lumbar/thoracic/cervical)**
Do not report with (62302-62305)

62310-62319 Injection/Infusion Diagnostic/Therapeutic Material

INCLUDES Contrast injection during fluoroscopic guidance/localization
EXCLUDES *Daily management of continuous epidural or subarachnoid drug administration (01996)*
Epidurography (72275)
Transforaminal epidural injection (64479-64484)
Code also fluoroscopic guidance and localization unless a formal contrast study is performed (77003)
Do not report more than once, even when catheter tip or substance injected moves into another spinal region

62310 **Injection(s), of diagnostic or therapeutic substance(s) (including anesthetic, antispasmodic, opioid, steroid, other solution), not including neurolytic substances, including needle or catheter placement, includes contrast for localization when performed, epidural or subarachnoid; cervical or thoracic**
INCLUDES Placement and use of a catheter to administer epidural or subarachnoid injection(s), even if more than one injection on a single calendar day
Placement of catheter into the epidural space and then removing the catheter after injecting substance(s) at one or more levels
Do not report with (62318)
A2 T 2.07 3.09 FUD 000

62311 **lumbar or sacral (caudal)**
INCLUDES Placement and use of a catheter to administer epidural or subarachnoid injection(s), even if more than one injection on a single calendar day
Placement of catheter into the epidural space and then removing the catheter after injecting substance(s) at one or more levels
Do not report with (62319)
A2 T 2.03 3.04 FUD 000

62318 **Injection(s), including indwelling catheter placement, continuous infusion or intermittent bolus, of diagnostic or therapeutic substance(s) (including anesthetic, antispasmodic, opioid, steroid, other solution), not including neurolytic substances, includes contrast for localization when performed, epidural or subarachnoid; cervical or thoracic**
INCLUDES Placement of catheter into the epidural space with delivery of substances for more than one calendar day, either continuously or by intermittent bolus
Do not report with (62310)
A2 T 2.22 3.11 FUD 000

62319 **lumbar or sacral (caudal)**
INCLUDES Placement of catheter into the epidural space with delivery of substances for more than one calendar day, either continuously or by intermittent bolus
Do not report with (62311)
A2 T 2.27 3.21 FUD 000

62350-62370 Procedures Related to Epidural and Intrathecal Catheters

CMS 100-3,280.14 Infusion Pumps

EXCLUDES *Infusion pump refilling and maintenance without reprogramming (95990-95991)*
Percutaneous insertion of intrathecal or epidural catheter (62270-62273, 62280-62284, 62310-62319)

62350 **Implantation, revision or repositioning of tunneled intrathecal or epidural catheter, for long-term medication administration via an external pump or implantable reservoir/infusion pump; without laminectomy**
A2 T 11.54 11.54 FUD 010

62351 **with laminectomy**
T 80 25.10 25.10 FUD 090

62355 **Removal of previously implanted intrathecal or epidural catheter**
A2 02 80 7.62 7.62 FUD 010

62360 **Implantation or replacement of device for intrathecal or epidural drug infusion; subcutaneous reservoir**
A2 T 80 8.95 8.95 FUD 010

62361 **nonprogrammable pump**
Code also (C1891, C2626)
J8 T 80 10.01 10.01 FUD 010

62362 **programmable pump, including preparation of pump, with or without programming**
Code also (C1772)
J8 T 80 11.08 11.08 FUD 010

62365 **Removal of subcutaneous reservoir or pump, previously implanted for intrathecal or epidural infusion**
A2 02 80 8.38 8.38 FUD 010

62367 **Electronic analysis of programmable, implanted pump for intrathecal or epidural drug infusion (includes evaluation of reservoir status, alarm status, drug prescription status); without reprogramming or refill**
P3 S 0.73 1.18 FUD XXX

62368 **with reprogramming**
P3 S 0.99 1.59 FUD XXX

62369 **with reprogramming and refill**
P3 S 1.01 3.39 FUD XXX

62370 **with reprogramming and refill (requiring skill of a physician or other qualified health care professional)**
P3 S 1.33 3.57 FUD XXX

63001-63048 Posterior Midline Approach: Laminectomy/Laminotomy/Decompression

INCLUDES Endoscopic assistance through open and direct visualization

EXCLUDES *Arthrodesis (22590-22614)*
Percutaneous laminotomy/hemilaminectomy with imaging guidance and/or endoscope only (0274T, 0275T)

63001 **Laminectomy with exploration and/or decompression of spinal cord and/or cauda equina, without facetectomy, foraminotomy or discectomy (eg, spinal stenosis), 1 or 2 vertebral segments; cervical**
G2 T 80 35.42 35.42 FUD 090

63003 **thoracic**
G2 T 80 35.39 35.39 FUD 090

63005 **lumbar, except for spondylolisthesis**
G2 T 80 33.87 33.87 FUD 090

63011 **sacral**
T 80 31.30 31.30 FUD 090

63012 **Laminectomy with removal of abnormal facets and/or pars inter-articularis with decompression of cauda equina and nerve roots for spondylolisthesis, lumbar (Gill type procedure)**
T 80 34.15 34.15 FUD 090

63015 **Laminectomy with exploration and/or decompression of spinal cord and/or cauda equina, without facetectomy, foraminotomy or discectomy (eg, spinal stenosis), more than 2 vertebral segments; cervical**
T 80 PQ 42.47 42.47 FUD 090

63016 **thoracic**
T 80 43.44 43.44 FUD 090

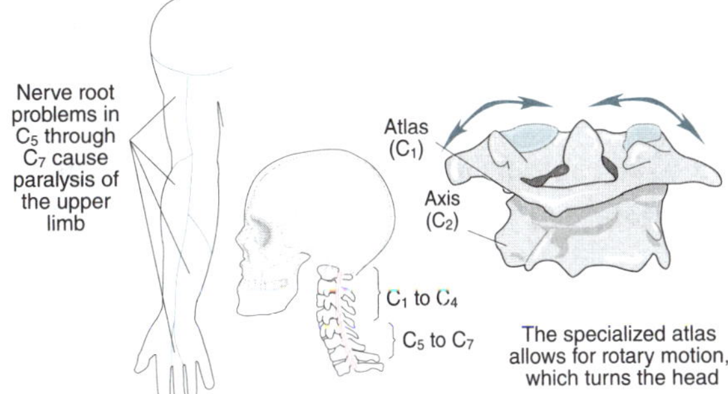

63017 **lumbar**
T 80 35.77 35.77 FUD 090

63020 **Laminotomy (hemilaminectomy), with decompression of nerve root(s), including partial facetectomy, foraminotomy and/or excision of herniated intervertebral disc; 1 interspace, cervical**
T 80 50 PQ 33.52 33.52 FUD 090

63030 **1 interspace, lumbar**
T 80 50 PQ 27.80 27.80 FUD 090

\+ **63035** **each additional interspace, cervical or lumbar (List separately in addition to code for primary procedure)**
Code first (63020-63030)
N 80 50 5.53 5.53 FUD ZZZ

63040 **Laminotomy (hemilaminectomy), with decompression of nerve root(s), including partial facetectomy, foraminotomy and/or excision of herniated intervertebral disc, reexploration, single interspace; cervical**
T 80 50 40.32 40.32 FUD 090

63042 **lumbar**
T 80 50 PQ 37.29 37.29 FUD 090

\+ **63043** **each additional cervical interspace (List separately in addition to code for primary procedure)**
Code first (63040)
C 80 50 0.00 0.00 FUD ZZZ

\+ **63044** **each additional lumbar interspace (List separately in addition to code for primary procedure)**
Code first (63042)
C 80 50 0.00 0.00 FUD ZZZ

63045 **Laminectomy, facetectomy and foraminotomy (unilateral or bilateral with decompression of spinal cord, cauda equina and/or nerve root[s], [eg, spinal or lateral recess stenosis]), single vertebral segment; cervical**
T 80 PQ 36.45 36.45 FUD 090

63046 **thoracic**
T 80 34.71 34.71 FUD 090

63047 **lumbar**
T 80 PQ 31.60 31.60 FUD 090

+ 63048 **each additional segment, cervical, thoracic, or lumbar (List separately in addition to code for primary procedure)**
Code first (63045-63047)
N 80 ⚑ Facility RVU 6.13 Non-Facility RVU 6.13 FUD ZZZ

63050-63051 Cervical Laminoplasty: Posterior Midline Approach

Do not report with procedure performed on the same vertebral segment(s) (22600, 22614, 22840-22842, 63001, 63015, 63045, 63048, 63295)

63050 **Laminoplasty, cervical, with decompression of the spinal cord, 2 or more vertebral segments;**
C 80 ⚑ Facility RVU 44.64 Non-Facility RVU 44.64 FUD 090

63051 **with reconstruction of the posterior bony elements (including the application of bridging bone graft and non-segmental fixation devices [eg, wire, suture, mini-plates], when performed)**
C 80 ⚑ Facility RVU 49.18 Non-Facility RVU 49.18 FUD 090

63055-63066 Spinal Cord/Nerve Root Decompression: Costovertebral or Transpedicular Approach

63055 **Transpedicular approach with decompression of spinal cord, equina and/or nerve root(s) (eg, herniated intervertebral disc), single segment; thoracic**
T 80 ⚑ Facility RVU 46.59 Non-Facility RVU 46.59 FUD 090

63056 **lumbar (including transfacet, or lateral extraforaminal approach) (eg, far lateral herniated intervertebral disc)**
T 80 ⚑ PQ Facility RVU 42.46 Non-Facility RVU 42.46 FUD 090

+ 63057 **each additional segment, thoracic or lumbar (List separately in addition to code for primary procedure)**
Code first (63055-63056)
N 80 ⚑ Facility RVU 9.24 Non-Facility RVU 9.24 FUD ZZZ

63064 **Costovertebral approach with decompression of spinal cord or nerve root(s) (eg, herniated intervertebral disc), thoracic; single segment**
EXCLUDES *Laminectomy with intraspinal thoracic lesion removal (63266, 63271, 63276, 63281, 63286)*
T 80 ⚑ Facility RVU 50.80 Non-Facility RVU 50.80 FUD 090

+ 63066 **each additional segment (List separately in addition to code for primary procedure)**
EXCLUDES *Laminectomy with intraspinal thoracic lesion removal (63266, 63271, 63276, 63281, 63286)*
Code first (63064)
N 80 ⚑ Facility RVU 5.93 Non-Facility RVU 5.93 FUD ZZZ

63075-63078 Discectomy: Anterior or Anterolateral Approach

INCLUDES Operating microscope (69990)

63075 **Discectomy, anterior, with decompression of spinal cord and/or nerve root(s), including osteophytectomy; cervical, single interspace**
EXCLUDES *Anterior cervical discectomy and anterior interbody fusion at same level during same operative session (22551)*
Do not report with anterior interbody arthrodesis (even by another provider) (22554)
T 80 ⚑ PQ Facility RVU 39.19 Non-Facility RVU 39.19 FUD 090

+ 63076 **cervical, each additional interspace (List separately in addition to code for primary procedure)**
EXCLUDES *Anterior cervical discectomy and anterior interbody fusion at same level during same session (22552)*
Code first (63075)
Do not report with anterior interbody arthrodesis (even by another provider) (22554)
N 80 ⚑ Facility RVU 7.16 Non-Facility RVU 7.16 FUD ZZZ

63077 **thoracic, single interspace**
C 80 ⚑ Facility RVU 42.91 Non-Facility RVU 42.91 FUD 090

+ 63078 **thoracic, each additional interspace (List separately in addition to code for primary procedure)**
Code first (63077)
C 80 ⚑ Facility RVU 5.60 Non-Facility RVU 5.60 FUD ZZZ

63081-63091 Vertebral Corpectomy, All Levels, Anterior Approach

INCLUDES Disc removal at the level below and/or above vertebral segment

EXCLUDES *Arthrodesis (22548-22812)*

Code also reconstruction (20930-20938, 22548-22812, 22840-22855)

63081 **Vertebral corpectomy (vertebral body resection), partial or complete, anterior approach with decompression of spinal cord and/or nerve root(s); cervical, single segment**
EXCLUDES *Transoral approach (61575-61576)*
C 80 ⚑ PQ Facility RVU 50.77 Non-Facility RVU 50.77 FUD 090

+ 63082 **cervical, each additional segment (List separately in addition to code for primary procedure)**
EXCLUDES *Transoral approach (61575-61576)*
Code first (63081)
C 80 ⚑ Facility RVU 7.71 Non-Facility RVU 7.71 FUD ZZZ

63085 **Vertebral corpectomy (vertebral body resection), partial or complete, transthoracic approach with decompression of spinal cord and/or nerve root(s); thoracic, single segment**
C 80 ⚑ Facility RVU 54.49 Non-Facility RVU 54.49 FUD 090

+ 63086 **thoracic, each additional segment (List separately in addition to code for primary procedure)**
Code first (63085)
C 80 ⚑ Facility RVU 5.47 Non-Facility RVU 5.47 FUD ZZZ

63087 **Vertebral corpectomy (vertebral body resection), partial or complete, combined thoracolumbar approach with decompression of spinal cord, cauda equina or nerve root(s), lower thoracic or lumbar; single segment**
C 80 ⚑ Facility RVU 68.60 Non-Facility RVU 68.60 FUD 090

+ 63088 **each additional segment (List separately in addition to code for primary procedure)**
Code first (63087)
C 80 ⚑ Facility RVU 7.39 Non-Facility RVU 7.39 FUD ZZZ

63090 **Vertebral corpectomy (vertebral body resection), partial or complete, transperitoneal or retroperitoneal approach with decompression of spinal cord, cauda equina or nerve root(s), lower thoracic, lumbar, or sacral; single segment**
C 80 ⚑ Facility RVU 56.45 Non-Facility RVU 56.45 FUD 090

+ 63091 **each additional segment (List separately in addition to code for primary procedure)**
Code first (63090)
C 80 ⚑ Facility RVU 5.13 Non-Facility RVU 5.13 FUD ZZZ

63101-63103 Corpectomy: Lateral Extracavitary Approach

63101 Vertebral corpectomy (vertebral body resection), partial or complete, lateral extracavitary approach with decompression of spinal cord and/or nerve root(s) (eg, for tumor or retropulsed bone fragments); thoracic, single segment
C 80 66.46 66.46 FUD 090

63102 lumbar, single segment
C 80 64.32 64.32 FUD 090

\+ **63103** thoracic or lumbar, each additional segment (List separately in addition to code for primary procedure)
Code first (63101-63102)
C 80 8.38 8.38 FUD ZZZ

63170-63295 Laminectomies

63170 Laminectomy with myelotomy (eg, Bischof or DREZ type), cervical, thoracic, or thoracolumbar
C 80 45.49 45.49 FUD 090

63172 Laminectomy with drainage of intramedullary cyst/syrinx; to subarachnoid space
C 80 40.31 40.31 FUD 090

63173 to peritoneal or pleural space
C 80 49.33 49.33 FUD 090

63180 Laminectomy and section of dentate ligaments, with or without dural graft, cervical; 1 or 2 segments
C 80 42.44 42.44 FUD 090

63182 more than 2 segments
C 80 41.91 41.91 FUD 090

63185 Laminectomy with rhizotomy; 1 or 2 segments
INCLUDES Dana rhizotomy
Stoffel rhizotomy
C 80 34.28 34.28 FUD 090

63190 more than 2 segments
C 80 36.30 36.30 FUD 090

63191 Laminectomy with section of spinal accessory nerve
EXCLUDES *Division of sternocleidomastoid muscle for torticollis (21720)*
C 80 50 36.45 36.45 FUD 090

63194 Laminectomy with cordotomy, with section of 1 spinothalamic tract, 1 stage; cervical
C 80 35.97 35.97 FUD 090

63195 thoracic
C 80 43.91 43.91 FUD 090

63196 Laminectomy with cordotomy, with section of both spinothalamic tracts, 1 stage; cervical
C 80 39.11 39.11 FUD 090

63197 thoracic
C 80 44.11 44.11 FUD 090

63198 Laminectomy with cordotomy with section of both spinothalamic tracts, 2 stages within 14 days; cervical
INCLUDES Keen laminectomy
C 80 46.06 46.06 FUD 090

63199 thoracic
C 80 48.33 48.33 FUD 090

63200 Laminectomy, with release of tethered spinal cord, lumbar
C 80 44.02 44.02 FUD 090

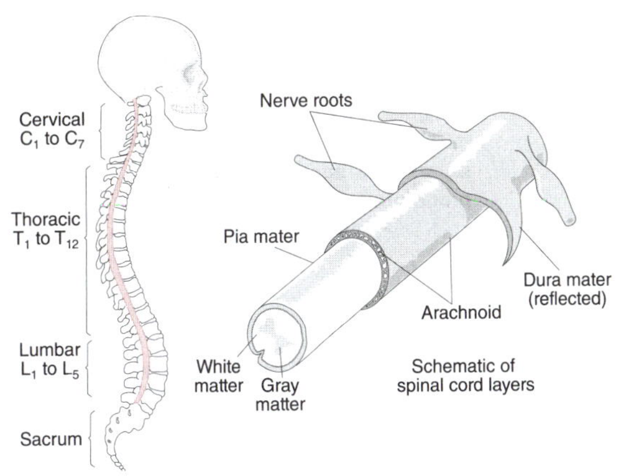

63250 Laminectomy for excision or occlusion of arteriovenous malformation of spinal cord; cervical
C 80 84.86 84.86 FUD 090

63251 thoracic
C 80 86.75 86.75 FUD 090

63252 thoracolumbar
C 80 86.73 86.73 FUD 090

63265 Laminectomy for excision or evacuation of intraspinal lesion other than neoplasm, extradural; cervical
C 80 47.82 47.82 FUD 090

63266 thoracic
C 80 49.36 49.36 FUD 090

63267 lumbar
C 80 PQ 39.44 39.44 FUD 090

63268 sacral
C 80 41.57 41.57 FUD 090

63270 Laminectomy for excision of intraspinal lesion other than neoplasm, intradural; cervical
C 80 59.33 59.33 FUD 090

63271 thoracic
C 80 59.28 59.28 FUD 090

63272 lumbar
C 80 54.54 54.54 FUD 090

63273 sacral
C 80 53.28 53.28 FUD 090

63275 Laminectomy for biopsy/excision of intraspinal neoplasm; extradural, cervical
C 80 PQ 51.60 51.60 FUD 090

63276 extradural, thoracic
C 80 PQ 51.11 51.11 FUD 090

63277 extradural, lumbar
C 80 PQ 44.48 44.48 FUD 090

63278 extradural, sacral
C 80 PQ 45.30 45.30 FUD 090

63280 intradural, extramedullary, cervical
C 80 PQ 60.56 60.56 FUD 090

63281 intradural, extramedullary, thoracic
C 80 PQ 59.81 59.81 FUD 090

63282 intradural, extramedullary, lumbar
C 80 PQ 56.53 56.53 FUD 090

63283 intradural, sacral
C 80 PQ 54.27 54.27 FUD 090

63285 intradural, intramedullary, cervical
C 80 PQ 74.77 74.77 FUD 090

63286 intradural, intramedullary, thoracic
C 80 PQ 73.64 73.64 FUD 090

63287 intradural, intramedullary, thoracolumbar
C 80 PQ 78.48 78.48 FUD 090

63290 combined extradural-intradural lesion, any level

EXCLUDES *Drainage intermedullary cyst or syrinx (63172-63173)*

C 80 PO 79.68 79.68 **FUD** 090

\+ 63295 **Osteoplastic reconstruction of dorsal spinal elements, following primary intraspinal procedure (List separately in addition to code for primary procedure)**

Code first (63172-63173, 63185, 63190, 63200-63290)

Do not report with procedure performed at the same vertebral segment(s) (22590-22614, 22840-22844, 63050-63051)

C 80 9.53 9.53 **FUD** ZZZ

63300-63308 Vertebral Corpectomy for Intraspinal Lesion: Anterior/Anterolateral Approach

EXCLUDES *Arthrodesis (22548-22585)*
Spinal reconstruction (20930-20938)

63300 **Vertebral corpectomy (vertebral body resection), partial or complete, for excision of intraspinal lesion, single segment; extradural, cervical**

C 80 52.64 52.64 **FUD** 090

63301 **extradural, thoracic by transthoracic approach**

C 80 63.01 63.01 **FUD** 090

63302 **extradural, thoracic by thoracolumbar approach**

C 80 62.23 62.23 **FUD** 090

63303 **extradural, lumbar or sacral by transperitoneal or retroperitoneal approach**

C 80 66.12 66.12 **FUD** 090

63304 **intradural, cervical**

C 80 67.14 67.14 **FUD** 090

63305 **intradural, thoracic by transthoracic approach**

C 80 71.49 71.49 **FUD** 090

63306 **intradural, thoracic by thoracolumbar approach**

C 80 62.07 62.07 **FUD** 090

63307 **intradural, lumbar or sacral by transperitoneal or retroperitoneal approach**

C 80 68.79 68.79 **FUD** 090

\+ 63308 **each additional segment (List separately in addition to codes for single segment)**

Code first (63300-63307)

C 80 9.21 9.21 **FUD** ZZZ

63600-63615 Stereotactic Procedures of the Spinal Cord

63600 **Creation of lesion of spinal cord by stereotactic method, percutaneous, any modality (including stimulation and/or recording)**

A2 T 80 26.20 26.20 **FUD** 090

63610 **Stereotactic stimulation of spinal cord, percutaneous, separate procedure not followed by other surgery**

A2 T 80 PQ 11.24 11.24 **FUD** 000

63615 **Stereotactic biopsy, aspiration, or excision of lesion, spinal cord**

A2 T PQ 35.34 35.34 **FUD** 090

63620-63621 Stereotactic Radiosurgery (SRS): Spine

INCLUDES Computer assisted planning
Planning dosimetry, targeting, positioning, or blocking by neurosurgeon

EXCLUDES *Arteriovenous malformations (see Radiation Oncology Section)*
Intensity modulated beam delivery plan and treatment (77301, [77385, 77386])
Stereotactic body radiation therapy (77373, 77435)
Treatment planning, physics, dosimetry, treatment delivery and management provided by the radiation oncologist (77261-77790 [77424, 77425])

Do not report stereotactic radiosurgery services with radiation treatment management by the same provider (77427-77432)

Do not report with (61781-61783)

63620 **Stereotactic radiosurgery (particle beam, gamma ray, or linear accelerator); 1 spinal lesion**

Do not report more than one time per treatment course

B 80 31.62 31.62 **FUD** 090

\+ 63621 **each additional spinal lesion (List separately in addition to code for primary procedure)**

Code first (63620)

Do not report more than one time per lesion

Do not report more than two times per entire treatment course

B 80 7.15 7.15 **FUD** ZZZ

63650-63688 Spinal Neurostimulation

CMS 100-3,160.2 Treatment of Motor Function Disorders with Electric Nerve Stimulation
CMS 100-3,160.7 Electrical Nerve Stimulators

INCLUDES Complex and simple neurostimulators

EXCLUDES *Analysis and programming of neurostimulator pulse generator (95970-95975)*

63650 **Percutaneous implantation of neurostimulator electrode array, epidural**

INCLUDES The following are components of a neurostimulator system:
Collection of contacts of which four or more provide the electrical stimulation in the epidural space
Contacts on a catheter-type lead (array)
Extension
External controller
Implanted neurostimulator

Code also (C1778, C1897, L8680)

J8 S 11.93 37.67 **FUD** 010

63655 **Laminectomy for implantation of neurostimulator electrodes, plate/paddle, epidural**

INCLUDES The following are components of a neurostimulator system:
Collection of contacts of which four or more provide the electrical stimulation in the epidural space
Contacts on a plate or paddle-shaped surface for systems placed by open exposure
Extension
External controller
Implanted neurostimulator

Code also (C1778, C1897, L8680)

J8 S 80 23.65 23.65 **FUD** 090

63661 **Removal of spinal neurostimulator electrode percutaneous array(s), including fluoroscopy, when performed**

INCLUDES The following are components of a neurostimulator system:
Collection of contacts of which four or more provide the electrical stimulation in the epidural space
Contacts on a catheter-type lead (array)
Extension
External controller
Implanted neurostimulator

Do not report when removing or replacing a temporary array placed percutaneously for an external generator

G2 Q2 80 9.20 16.31 **FUD** 010

63662 Removal of spinal neurostimulator electrode plate/paddle(s) placed via laminotomy or laminectomy, including fluoroscopy, when performed

INCLUDES The following are components of a neurostimulator system:
Collection of contacts of which four or more provide the electrical stimulation in the epidural space
Contacts on a plate or paddle-shaped surface for systems placed by open exposure
Extension
External controller
Implanted neurostimulator

G2 Q2 80 22.10 22.10 FUD 090

63663 Revision including replacement, when performed, of spinal neurostimulator electrode percutaneous array(s), including fluoroscopy, when performed

INCLUDES The following are components of a neurostimulator system:
Collection of contacts of which four or more provide the electrical stimulation in the epidural space
Contacts on a catheter-type lead (array)
Extension
External controller
Implanted neurostimulator

Do not report when removing or replacing a temporary array placed percutaneously for an external generator

Do not report with (63661-63662)

J8 S 80 13.24 22.65 FUD 010

63664 Revision including replacement, when performed, of spinal neurostimulator electrode plate/paddle(s) placed via laminotomy or laminectomy, including fluoroscopy, when performed

INCLUDES The following are components of a neurostimulator system:
Collection of contacts of which four or more provide the electrical stimulation in the epidural space
Contacts on a plate or paddle-shaped surface for systems placed by open exposure
Extension
External controller
Implanted neurostimulator

Do not report with (63661-63662)

J8 S 80 22.88 22.88 FUD 090

63685 Insertion or replacement of spinal neurostimulator pulse generator or receiver, direct or inductive coupling

Code also (C1767, C1820, L8685-L8688)

Do not report with 63688 for the same pulse generator or receiver

J8 S 80 10.42 10.42 FUD 010

63688 Revision or removal of implanted spinal neurostimulator pulse generator or receiver

Do not report with 63685 for the same pulse generator or receiver

A2 Q2 10.53 10.53 FUD 010

63700-63706 Repair Congenital Neural Tube Defects

EXCLUDES *Complex skin repair (see appropriate integumentary closure code)*

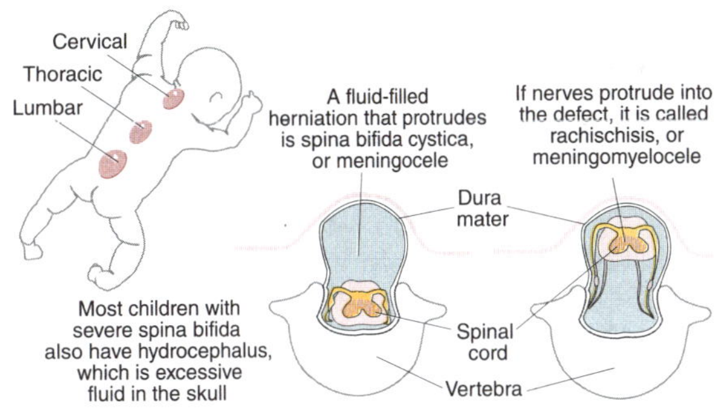

63700 Repair of meningocele; less than 5 cm diameter

C 80 63 36.16 36.16 FUD 090

63702 larger than 5 cm diameter

C 80 63 39.76 39.76 FUD 090

63704 Repair of myelomeningocele; less than 5 cm diameter

C 80 63 47.08 47.08 FUD 090

63706 larger than 5 cm diameter

C 80 63 51.49 51.49 FUD 090

63707-63710 Repair Dural Cerebrospinal Fluid Leak

63707 Repair of dural/cerebrospinal fluid leak, not requiring laminectomy

C 80 26.22 26.22 FUD 090

63709 Repair of dural/cerebrospinal fluid leak or pseudomeningocele, with laminectomy

C 80 31.58 31.58 FUD 090

63710 Dural graft, spinal

EXCLUDES *Laminectomy and section of dentate ligament (63180, 63182)*

C 80 31.65 31.65 FUD 090

63740-63746 Cerebrospinal Fluid (CSF) Shunt: Lumbar

EXCLUDES *Placement of subarachnoid catheter with reservoir and/or pump:*
Not requiring laminectomy (62350, 62360-62362)
With laminectomy (62351, 62360-62362)

63740 Creation of shunt, lumbar, subarachnoid-peritoneal, -pleural, or other; including laminectomy

C 80 27.00 27.00 FUD 090

63741 percutaneous, not requiring laminectomy

T 80 18.65 18.65 FUD 090

63744 Replacement, irrigation or revision of lumbosubarachnoid shunt

A2 T 80 19.54 19.54 FUD 090

63746 Removal of entire lumbosubarachnoid shunt system without replacement

A2 Q2 80 17.12 17.12 FUD 090

64400-64455 Nerve Blocks

EXCLUDES *Epidural or subarachnoid injection (62310-62319)*
Nerve destruction (62280-62282, 64600-64681 [64633, 64634, 64635, 64636])

64400 Injection, anesthetic agent; trigeminal nerve, any division or branch

P3 T 50 1.98 3.52 FUD 000

64402 facial nerve

P2 X 50 2.14 3.48 FUD 000

64405 greater occipital nerve

P3 T 50 1.80 2.85 FUD 000

64408 vagus nerve

P3 T 80 50 2.11 2.82 FUD 000

64410 phrenic nerve
A2 T 80 50 ⚑ 2.18 3.63 FUD 000

64412 spinal accessory nerve
P3 T 50 ⚑ 2.09 3.91 FUD 000

64413 cervical plexus
P3 T 50 ⚑ 2.32 3.52 FUD 000

64415 brachial plexus, single
A2 T 50 ⚑ 1.87 3.35 FUD 000

64416 brachial plexus, continuous infusion by catheter (including catheter placement)
Do not report with (01996)
G2 T 50 ⚑ 2.26 2.26 FUD 000

64417 axillary nerve
A2 T 50 ⚑ 2.02 3.66 FUD 000

64418 suprascapular nerve
P3 T 50 ⚑ 2.16 4.03 FUD 000

64420 intercostal nerve, single
A2 T ⚑ 1.97 3.20 FUD 000

64421 intercostal nerves, multiple, regional block
A2 T 50 ⚑ 2.71 4.34 FUD 000

64425 ilioinguinal, iliohypogastric nerves
P3 T 50 ⚑ 2.72 3.79 FUD 000

64430 pudendal nerve
A2 T 50 ⚑ 2.35 3.90 FUD 000

64435 paracervical (uterine) nerve ♀
P3 T 50 ⚑ 2.44 3.85 FUD 000

64445 sciatic nerve, single
P3 T 50 ⚑ 2.07 3.82 FUD 000

64446 sciatic nerve, continuous infusion by catheter (including catheter placement)
Do not report with (01996)
G2 T 50 ⚑ 2.27 2.27 FUD 000

64447 femoral nerve, single
Do not report with (01996)
P3 T 50 ⚑ 1.89 3.35 FUD 000

64448 femoral nerve, continuous infusion by catheter (including catheter placement)
Do not report with (01996)
G2 T 50 ⚑ 2.03 2.03 FUD 000

64449 lumbar plexus, posterior approach, continuous infusion by catheter (including catheter placement)
Do not report with (01996)
G2 T 50 ⚑ 2.37 2.37 FUD 000

64450 other peripheral nerve or branch
EXCLUDES *Morton's neuroma (64455, 64632)*
P3 T 50 ⚑ 1.31 2.26 FUD 000

64455 Injection(s), anesthetic agent and/or steroid, plantar common digital nerve(s) (eg, Morton's neuroma)
Do not report with (64632)
P3 T 80 50 1.02 1.37 FUD 000

64479-64484 Transforaminal Injection

INCLUDES Imaging guidance (fluoroscopy or CT) and contrast injection

EXCLUDES *Epidural or subarachnoid injection (62310-62319)*
Nerve destruction (62280-62282, 64600-64681 [64633, 64634, 64635, 64636])

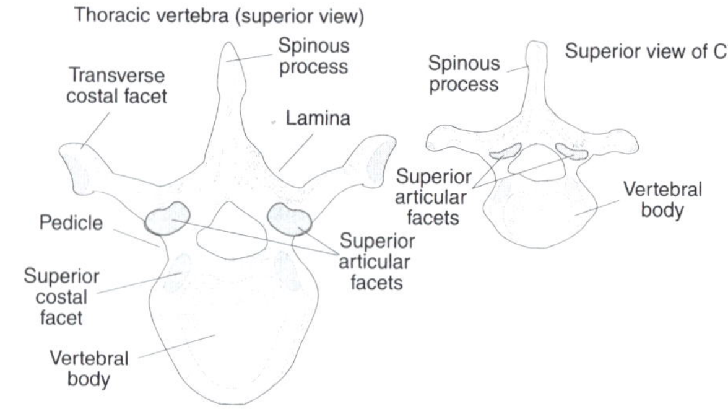

64479 Injection(s), anesthetic agent and/or steroid, transforaminal epidural, with imaging guidance (fluoroscopy or CT); cervical or thoracic, single level
EXCLUDES *Transforaminal epidural injection using ultrasonic guidance (0228T)*
A2 T 50 ⚑ 3.89 6.82 FUD 000

+ 64480 cervical or thoracic, each additional level (List separately in addition to code for primary procedure)
EXCLUDES *Transforaminal epidural injection at T12-L1 level (64479)*
Transforaminal epidural injection using ultrasonic guidance (0229T)
Code first (64479)
N1 N 50 ⚑ 1.89 3.27 FUD ZZZ

64483 lumbar or sacral, single level
EXCLUDES *Transforaminal epidural injection using ultrasonic guidance (0230T)*
A2 T 50 ⚑ 3.25 6.29 FUD 000

+ 64484 lumbar or sacral, each additional level (List separately in addition to code for primary procedure)
EXCLUDES *Transforaminal epidural injection using ultrasonic guidance (0231T)*
Code first (64483)
N1 N 50 ⚑ 1.51 2.50 FUD ZZZ

64486-64489 Transversus Abdominis Plane (TAP) Block

● 64486 Transversus abdominis plane (TAP) block (abdominal plane block, rectus sheath block) unilateral; by injection(s) (includes imaging guidance, when performed)

● 64487 by continuous infusion(s) (includes imaging guidance, when performed)

● 64488 Transversus abdominis plane (TAP) block (abdominal plane block, rectus sheath block) bilateral; by injections (includes imaging guidance, when performed)

● 64489 by continuous infusions (includes imaging guidance, when performed)

64490-64495 Paraspinal Nerve Injections

INCLUDES Image guidance (CT or fluoroscopy) and any contrast injection

EXCLUDES *Injection without imaging (20552-20553)*
Ultrasonic guidance (0213T-0218T)

64490 **Injection(s), diagnostic or therapeutic agent, paravertebral facet (zygapophyseal) joint (or nerves innervating that joint) with image guidance (fluoroscopy or CT), cervical or thoracic; single level**
INCLUDES Injection of T12-L1 joint and nerves that innervate that joint
G2 T 80 50 3.12 5.48 FUD 000

+ **64491** **second level (List separately in addition to code for primary procedure)**
Code first (64490)
N1 N 80 50 1.76 2.69 FUD ZZZ

+ **64492** **third and any additional level(s) (List separately in addition to code for primary procedure)**
Code first (64490-64491)
Do not report more than one time per day
N1 N 80 50 1.78 2.71 FUD ZZZ

64493 **Injection(s), diagnostic or therapeutic agent, paravertebral facet (zygapophyseal) joint (or nerves innervating that joint) with image guidance (fluoroscopy or CT), lumbar or sacral; single level**
G2 T 80 50 2.64 4.95 FUD 000

+ **64494** **second level (List separately in addition to code for primary procedure)**
Code first (64493)
N1 N 80 50 1.50 2.47 FUD ZZZ

+ **64495** **third and any additional level(s) (List separately in addition to code for primary procedure)**
Code first (64493-64494)
Do not report more than one time per day
N1 N 80 50 1.52 2.48 FUD ZZZ

64505-64530 Sympathetic Nerve Blocks

64505 **Injection, anesthetic agent; sphenopalatine ganglion**
P3 T 50 2.46 2.94 FUD 000

64508 **carotid sinus (separate procedure)**
P3 T 80 50 2.24 1.86 FUD 000

64510 **stellate ganglion (cervical sympathetic)**
A2 T 50 2.12 3.60 FUD 000

64517 **superior hypogastric plexus**
A2 T 3.45 4.98 FUD 000

64520 **lumbar or thoracic (paravertebral sympathetic)**
A2 T 50 2.31 5.24 FUD 000

64530 **celiac plexus, with or without radiologic monitoring**
EXCLUDES *Transmural anesthetic injection with transendoscopic ultrasound-guidance (43253)*
A2 T 2.66 5.42 FUD 000

64550 Transcutaneous Electrical Nerve Stimulation

CMS 100-3,160.2 Treatment of Motor Function Disorders with Electric Nerve Stimulation
CMS 100-3,160.7.1 Assessing Patients Suitability for Electrical Nerve Stimulation Therapy
CMS 100-3,160.13 Form-fitting Conductive Garment for TENS or NMES
CMS 100-3,280.13 Transcutaneous Electrical Nerve Stimulators (TENS)

EXCLUDES *Analysis and programming neurostimulator pulse generator (95970-95975)*
Implantation of electrode array(s), either trial or permanent, with pulse generator for peripheral subcutaneous field stimulation (0282T-0284T)

64550 **Application of surface (transcutaneous) neurostimulator**
A 0.26 0.45 FUD 000

64553-64570 Electrical Nerve Stimulation: Insertion/Replacement/Removal/Revision

CMS 100-3,160.2 Treatment of Motor Function Disorders with Electric Nerve Stimulation
CMS 100-3,160.7 Electrical Nerve Stimulators
CMS 100-3,160.7.1 Assessing Patients Suitability for Electrical Nerve Stimulation Therapy
CMS 100-3,160.12 Neuromuscular Electrical Stimulation (NMES)
CMS 100-3,160.13 Form-fitting Conductive Garment for TENS or NMES
CMS 100-4,32,40 Sacral Nerve Stimulation

INCLUDES Simple and complex neurostimulators

EXCLUDES *Analysis and programming of neurostimulator pulse generator (95970-95975)*
Implantation of electrode array(s), either trial or permanent, with pulse generator for peripheral subcutaneous field stimulation (0282T-0284T)

64553 **Percutaneous implantation of neurostimulator electrode array; cranial nerve**
EXCLUDES *Open procedure (61885-61886)*
Code also (C1778, C1897, L8680)
J8 S 80 4.45 5.93 FUD 010

64555 **peripheral nerve (excludes sacral nerve)**
Code also (C1778, C1897, L8680)
Do not report with (64566)
J8 S 4.29 5.74 FUD 010

64561 **sacral nerve (transforaminal placement) including image guidance, if performed**
Code also (C1778, C1897, L8680)
J8 S 50 11.38 22.56 FUD 010

64565 **neuromuscular**
Code also (C1778, C1897, L8680)
J8 S 3.74 5.25 FUD 010

64566 **Posterior tibial neurostimulation, percutaneous needle electrode, single treatment, includes programming**
Do not report with (64555, 95970-95972)
P3 T 80 0.86 3.37 FUD 000

64568 **Incision for implantation of cranial nerve (eg, vagus nerve) neurostimulator electrode array and pulse generator**
Code also (C1767, C1778, C1820, C1897, L8680, L8685-L8688)
Do not report with (61885-61886, 64570)
J8 S 80 50 17.53 17.53 FUD 090

64569 **Revision or replacement of cranial nerve (eg, vagus nerve) neurostimulator electrode array, including connection to existing pulse generator**
EXCLUDES *Replacement of pulse generator (61885)*
Do not report with (61888, 64570)
J8 S 80 50 22.30 22.30 FUD 090

64570 **Removal of cranial nerve (eg, vagus nerve) neurostimulator electrode array and pulse generator**
EXCLUDES *Laparoscopic revision, replacement, removal, or implantation of vagus nerve blocking neurostimulator pulse generator and/or electrode array at the esophagogastric junction (0312T-0317T)*
Do not report with (61888)
G2 02 80 50 19.78 19.78 FUD 090

64575-64595 Implantation/Revision/Removal Neurostimulators: Incisional

INCLUDES Simple and complex neurostimulators

EXCLUDES *Analysis and programming neurostimulator pulse generator (95970-95975)*
Implantation of electrode array(s), either trial or permanent, with pulse generator for peripheral subcutaneous field stimulation (0282T-0284T)

64575 **Incision for implantation of neurostimulator electrode array; peripheral nerve (excludes sacral nerve)**
Code also (C1778, C1897, L8680)
J8 S 8.79 8.79 FUD 090

64580 **neuromuscular**
Code also (C1778, C1897, L8680)
J8 S 80 — 8.49 — 8.49 FUD 090

64581 **sacral nerve (transforaminal placement)**
Code also (C1778, C1897, L8680)
J8 S — 19.10 — 19.10 FUD 090

64585 **Revision or removal of peripheral neurostimulator electrode array**
A2 Q2 — 4.10 — 6.92 FUD 010

64590 **Insertion or replacement of peripheral or gastric neurostimulator pulse generator or receiver, direct or inductive coupling**
Code also (C1767, C1820, L8685-L8688)
Do not report with (64595)
J8 S — 4.56 — 7.43 FUD 010

64595 **Revision or removal of peripheral or gastric neurostimulator pulse generator or receiver**
Do not report with (64590)
A2 Q2 — 3.60 — 6.89 FUD 010

64600-64610 Chemical Denervation Trigeminal Nerve

CMS 100-3,160.1 Induced Lesions of Nerve Tracts

INCLUDES Injection of therapeutic medication

EXCLUDES *The following chemodenervation procedures:*
Bladder (52287)
Internal anal sphincter (46505)
Muscle electrical stimulation or EMG with needle guidance (95873, 95874)
Strabismus that involves the extraocular muscles (67345)
Treatments that do not destroy the target nerve (64999)

Code also chemodenervation agent

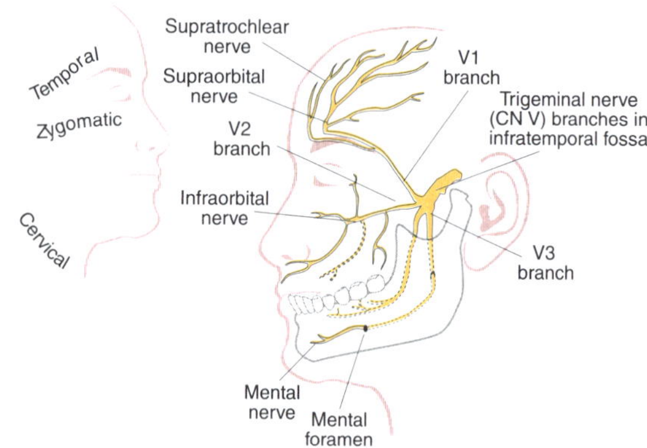

64600 **Destruction by neurolytic agent, trigeminal nerve; supraorbital, infraorbital, mental, or inferior alveolar branch**
A2 T — 6.15 — 10.89 FUD 010

64605 **second and third division branches at foramen ovale**
A2 T 80 50 — 10.45 — 20.92 FUD 010

64610 **second and third division branches at foramen ovale under radiologic monitoring**
A2 T 50 PQ — 13.86 — 20.93 FUD 010

64611-64617 Chemical Denervation Procedures Head and Neck

CMS 100-3,160.1 Induced Lesions of Nerve Tracts

INCLUDES Injection of therapeutic medication

EXCLUDES *Electromyography or muscle electric stimulation guidance (95873-95874)*
Nerve destruction of:
Anal sphincter (46505)
Bladder (52287)
Extraocular muscles to treat strabismus (67345)
Treatments that do not destroy the target nerve (64999)

64611 **Chemodenervation of parotid and submandibular salivary glands, bilateral**
Code also modifier 52 for injection of fewer than four salivary glands
P3 T 80 — 2.80 — 3.19 FUD 010

64612 **Chemodenervation of muscle(s); muscle(s) innervated by facial nerve, unilateral (eg, for blepharospasm, hemifacial spasm)**
P3 T 50 — 3.51 — 3.90 FUD 010

64615 **muscle(s) innervated by facial, trigeminal, cervical spinal and accessory nerves, bilateral (eg, for chronic migraine)**
Code also any guidance performed but report only once (95873-95874)
Do not report more than one time per session
Do not report with (64612, 64616-64617, 64642-64647)
P3 T — 3.62 — 4.07 FUD 010

64616 **neck muscle(s), excluding muscles of the larynx, unilateral (eg, for cervical dystonia, spasmodic torticollis)**
Code also guidance by muscle electrical stimulation or needle electromyography, but report only once (95873-95874)
P3 T 50 — 3.07 — 3.48 FUD 010

64617 **larynx, unilateral, percutaneous (eg, for spasmodic dysphonia), includes guidance by needle electromyography, when performed**
EXCLUDES *Chemodenervation of larynx via direct laryngoscopy (31570-31571)*
Diagnostic needle electromyography of larynx (95865)
Do not report with (95873-95874)
P3 T 50 — 3.26 — 5.40 FUD 010

64620-64640 [64633, 64634, 64635, 64636] Chemical Denervation Intercostal, Facet Joint, Plantar, and Pudendal Nerve(s)

CMS 100-3,160.1 Induced Lesions of Nerve Tracts

INCLUDES Injection of therapeutic medication

EXCLUDES *Treatments that do not destroy the target nerve (64999)*

64620 **Destruction by neurolytic agent, intercostal nerve**
A2 T PQ — 4.97 — 5.86 FUD 010

\# **64633** **Destruction by neurolytic agent, paravertebral facet joint nerve(s), with imaging guidance (fluoroscopy or CT); cervical or thoracic, single facet joint**
INCLUDES Imaging guidance (fluoroscopy or CT) and contrast injection
Paravertebral facet destruction of T12-L1 joint or nerve(s) that innervate that joint
EXCLUDES *Destruction of paravertebral facet joint nerve(s) without imaging guidance (64999)*
Do not report with (77003, 77012)
G2 T 50 — 6.58 — 12.30 FUD 010

\+ # **64634** **cervical or thoracic, each additional facet joint (List separately in addition to code for primary procedure)**

INCLUDES Imaging guidance (fluoroscopy or CT) and contrast injection

EXCLUDES *Destruction of paravertebral facet joint nerve(s) without imaging guidance (64999)*

Code first ([64633])

Do not report with (77003, 77012)

N1 N 50 1.99 5.58 FUD ZZZ

\# **64635** **lumbar or sacral, single facet joint**

INCLUDES Imaging guidance (fluoroscopy or CT) and contrast injection

EXCLUDES *Destruction of paravertebral facet joint nerve(s) without imaging guidance (64999)*

Do not report with (77003, 77012)

G2 T 50 6.48 12.13 FUD 010

\+ # **64636** **lumbar or sacral, each additional facet joint (List separately in addition to code for primary procedure)**

INCLUDES Imaging guidance (fluoroscopy or CT) with contrast injection

EXCLUDES *Destruction of paravertebral facet joint nerve(s) without imaging guidance (64999)*

Code first ([64635])

Do not report with (77003, 77012)

N1 N 50 1.74 5.04 FUD ZZZ

64630 **Destruction by neurolytic agent; pudendal nerve**

A2 T 80 5.41 6.46 FUD 010

64632 **plantar common digital nerve**

Do not report with (64455)

P3 T 80 50 1.99 2.44 FUD 010

64633 ***Resequenced code. See code following 64620.***

64634 ***Resequenced code. See code following 64620.***

64635 ***Resequenced code. See code following 64620.***

64636 ***Resequenced code. See code before 64630.***

64640 **other peripheral nerve or branch**

P3 T 50 2.68 3.78 FUD 010

64642-64645 Chemical Denervation Extremity Muscles

INCLUDES Trunk muscles include erector spine, obliques, paraspinal and rectus abdominus. The rest of the muscles are considered neck, head or extremity muscles.

EXCLUDES *Chemodenervation with needle-guided electromyography or with guidance provided by muscle electrical stimulation (95873-95874)*

Code also other extremities when appropriate, up to a total of 4 units per patient (if all extremities are injected) (64642-64645)

Do not report more than once per extremity

Do not report with modifier 50

64642 **Chemodenervation of one extremity; 1-4 muscle(s)**

Do not report more than one base code per session (64642, 64646)

P3 T 3.06 3.95 FUD 000

\+ **64643** **each additional extremity, 1-4 muscle(s) (List separately in addition to code for primary procedure)**

Code first (64642, 64644)

N1 N 2.05 2.60 FUD ZZZ

64644 **Chemodenervation of one extremity; 5 or more muscles**

P3 T 3.34 4.51 FUD 000

\+ **64645** **each additional extremity, 5 or more muscles (List separately in addition to code for primary procedure)**

Code first (64644)

N1 N 2.35 3.18 FUD ZZZ

64646-64647 Chemical Denervation Trunk Muscles

Do not report more than one time per session

Do not report with modifier 50

64646 **Chemodenervation of trunk muscle(s); 1-5 muscle(s)**

Do not report more than one base code per session (64642, 64646)

P3 T 3.31 4.25 FUD 000

64647 **6 or more muscles**

P3 T 3.82 4.92 FUD 000

64650-64653 Chemical Denervation Eccrine Glands

INCLUDES Injection of therapeutic medication

EXCLUDES *Treatments that do not destroy the target nerve (64999)*

Code also drugs or other substances used

64650 **Chemodenervation of eccrine glands; both axillae**

P3 T 80 1.18 2.15 FUD 000

64653 **other area(s) (eg, scalp, face, neck), per day**

EXCLUDES *Bladder chemodenervation (52287)*

Hands or feet (64999)

P3 T 80 1.55 2.72 FUD 000

64680-64681 Neurolysis: Celiac Plexus, Superior Hypogastric Plexus

INCLUDES Injection of therapeutic medication

Only for lesions that abut the dura matter or that affect the spinal neural tissue

Planning, dosimetry, targeting, positioning, or blocking performed by the surgeon

Radiation treatment management by the same physician (77427-77432)

EXCLUDES *Treatments that do not destroy the target nerve (64999)*

64680 **Destruction by neurolytic agent, with or without radiologic monitoring; celiac plexus**

EXCLUDES *Transmural neurolytic agent injection with transendoscopic ultrasound guidance (43253)*

A2 T 4.83 8.87 FUD 010

64681 **superior hypogastric plexus**

A2 T 5.45 9.62 FUD 010

64702-64727 Decompression and/or Transposition of Nerve

INCLUDES External neurolysis and/or transposition to repair or restore a nerve

Neuroplasty with nerve wrapping

Surgical decompression/freeing of nerve from scar tissue

EXCLUDES *Facial nerve decompression (69720)*

Neuroplasty with operating microscope (64727)

Percutaneous neurolysis (62263-62264, 62280-62282)

64702 **Neuroplasty; digital, 1 or both, same digit**

A2 T 14.13 14.13 FUD 090

64704 **nerve of hand or foot**

A2 T 80 9.10 9.10 FUD 090

64708 **Neuroplasty, major peripheral nerve, arm or leg, open; other than specified**

G2 T 80 14.11 14.11 FUD 090

64712 **sciatic nerve**

G2 T 80 50 16.05 16.05 FUD 090

64713 **brachial plexus**

G2 T 80 50 20.74 20.74 FUD 090

64714 **lumbar plexus**

G2 T 80 50 18.14 18.14 FUD 090

64716 **Neuroplasty and/or transposition; cranial nerve (specify)**

A2 T 80 15.42 15.42 FUD 090

64718 **ulnar nerve at elbow**

A2 T 80 50 16.87 16.87 FUD 090

64719 **ulnar nerve at wrist**

A2 T 50 11.33 11.33 FUD 090

Nervous System

64634 — 64719

64721 median nerve at carpal tunnel
EXCLUDES *Arthroscopic procedure (29848)*
A2 T 50 12.09 12.17 **FUD** 090

64722 **Decompression; unspecified nerve(s) (specify)**
A2 T 80 10.48 10.48 **FUD** 090

64726 plantar digital nerve
A2 T 7.77 7.77 **FUD** 090

\+ 64727 **Internal neurolysis, requiring use of operating microscope (List separately in addition to code for neuroplasty) (Neuroplasty includes external neurolysis)**
INCLUDES Operating microscope (69990)
Code first neuroplasty (64702-64721)
N1 N 5.26 5.26 **FUD** ZZZ

64732-64772 Surgical Avulsion/Transection of Nerve

CMS 100-3,160.1 Induced Lesions of Nerve Tracts

EXCLUDES *Stereotactic lesion of gasserian ganglion (61790)*

64732 **Transection or avulsion of; supraorbital nerve**
A2 T 80 50 11.75 11.75 **FUD** 090

64734 infraorbital nerve
A2 T 80 50 11.10 11.10 **FUD** 090

64736 mental nerve
A2 T 80 50 12.45 12.45 **FUD** 090

64738 inferior alveolar nerve by osteotomy
A2 T 80 50 13.77 13.77 **FUD** 090

64740 lingual nerve
A2 T 80 50 13.14 13.14 **FUD** 090

64742 facial nerve, differential or complete
A2 T 80 50 14.40 14.40 **FUD** 090

64744 greater occipital nerve
A2 T 80 50 14.02 14.02 **FUD** 090

64746 phrenic nerve
EXCLUDES *Section of recurrent unilateral laryngeal nerve (31595)*
A2 T 80 50 PQ 12.40 12.40 **FUD** 090

~~64752 vagus nerve (vagotomy), transthoracic~~

64755 vagus nerves limited to proximal stomach (selective proximal vagotomy, proximal gastric vagotomy, parietal cell vagotomy, supra- or highly selective vagotomy)
EXCLUDES *Laparoscopic procedure (43652)*
C 80 26.10 26.10 **FUD** 090

64760 vagus nerve (vagotomy), abdominal
EXCLUDES *Laparoscopic procedure (43651)*
C 80 14.56 14.56 **FUD** 090

~~64761 pudendal nerve~~

64763 **Transection or avulsion of obturator nerve, extrapelvic, with or without adductor tenotomy**
G2 T 80 50 14.42 14.42 **FUD** 090

64766 **Transection or avulsion of obturator nerve, intrapelvic, with or without adductor tenotomy**
G2 T 80 50 16.05 16.05 **FUD** 090

64771 **Transection or avulsion of other cranial nerve, extradural**
A2 T 80 16.71 16.71 **FUD** 090

64772 **Transection or avulsion of other spinal nerve, extradural**
EXCLUDES *Removal of tender scar and soft tissue including neuroma if necessary (11400-11446, 13100-13153)*
A2 T 80 15.95 15.95 **FUD** 090

64774-64823 Excisional Nerve Procedures

EXCLUDES *Morton neuroma excision (28080)*

64774 **Excision of neuroma; cutaneous nerve, surgically identifiable**
A2 T 11.89 11.89 **FUD** 090

64776 digital nerve, 1 or both, same digit
A2 T 80 11.18 11.18 **FUD** 090

\+ 64778 digital nerve, each additional digit (List separately in addition to code for primary procedure)
Code first (64776)
N1 N 4.45 4.45 **FUD** ZZZ

64782 hand or foot, except digital nerve
A2 T 12.88 12.88 **FUD** 090

\+ 64783 hand or foot, each additional nerve, except same digit (List separately in addition to code for primary procedure)
Code first (64782)
N1 N 6.21 6.21 **FUD** ZZZ

64784 major peripheral nerve, except sciatic
A2 T 80 21.05 21.05 **FUD** 090

64786 sciatic nerve
A2 T 80 50 30.92 30.92 **FUD** 090

\+ 64787 **Implantation of nerve end into bone or muscle (List separately in addition to neuroma excision)**
Code first (64774-64786)
N1 N 80 6.97 6.97 **FUD** ZZZ

64788 **Excision of neurofibroma or neurolemmoma; cutaneous nerve**
A2 T 11.33 11.33 **FUD** 090

64790 major peripheral nerve
A2 T 80 23.58 23.58 **FUD** 090

64792 extensive (including malignant type)
A2 T 80 33.93 33.93 **FUD** 090

64795 **Biopsy of nerve**
A2 T PQ 5.56 5.56 **FUD** 000

64802 **Sympathectomy, cervical**
A2 T 80 50 19.36 19.36 **FUD** 090

64804 **Sympathectomy, cervicothoracic**
T 80 50 29.46 29.46 **FUD** 090

64809 **Sympathectomy, thoracolumbar**
INCLUDES Leriche sympathectomy
C 80 50 20.53 20.53 **FUD** 090

64818 **Sympathectomy, lumbar**
C 80 50 18.48 18.48 **FUD** 090

64820 **Sympathectomy; digital arteries, each digit**
INCLUDES Operating microscope (69990)
G2 T 20.78 20.78 **FUD** 090

64821 radial artery
INCLUDES Operating microscope (69990)
A2 T 50 19.94 19.94 **FUD** 090

64822 ulnar artery
INCLUDES Operating microscope (69990)
G2 T 50 19.94 19.94 **FUD** 090

64823 superficial palmar arch
INCLUDES Operating microscope (69990)
G2 T 50 22.75 22.75 **FUD** 090

64831-64907 Nerve Repair: Suture and Nerve Grafts

64831 **Suture of digital nerve, hand or foot; 1 nerve**
A2 T 50 19.52 19.52 **FUD** 090

\+ 64832 each additional digital nerve (List separately in addition to code for primary procedure)
Code first (64831)
N1 N 80 9.71 9.71 **FUD** ZZZ

64834 **Suture of 1 nerve; hand or foot, common sensory nerve**
A2 T 80 50 21.20 21.20 **FUD** 090

64835 median motor thenar
A2 T 80 50 23.24 23.24 **FUD** 090

64836 ulnar motor
A2 T 80 50 23.24 23.24 **FUD** 090

\+ **64837 Suture of each additional nerve, hand or foot (List separately in addition to code for primary procedure)**
Code first (64834-64836)
N1 N 80 — 10.47 — 10.47 FUD ZZZ

64840 Suture of posterior tibial nerve
A2 T 80 50 — 26.51 — 26.51 FUD 090

64856 Suture of major peripheral nerve, arm or leg, except sciatic; including transposition
A2 T — 28.88 — 28.88 FUD 090

64857 without transposition
A2 T 80 — 30.24 — 30.24 FUD 090

64858 Suture of sciatic nerve
A2 T 80 50 — 30.65 — 30.65 FUD 090

\+ **64859 Suture of each additional major peripheral nerve (List separately in addition to code for primary procedure)**
Code first (64856-64857)
N1 80 — 7.41 — 7.41 FUD ZZZ

64861 Suture of; brachial plexus
A2 T 80 50 — 39.22 — 39.22 FUD 090

64862 lumbar plexus
A2 T 80 50 — 38.92 — 38.92 FUD 090

64864 Suture of facial nerve; extracranial
A2 T 80 — 25.06 — 25.06 FUD 090

64865 infratemporal, with or without grafting
A2 T 80 — 31.98 — 31.98 FUD 090

64866 Anastomosis; facial-spinal accessory
C 80 — 33.18 — 33.18 FUD 090

64868 facial-hypoglossal
INCLUDES Korte-Ballance anastomosis
C 80 — 29.30 — 29.30 FUD 090

~~**64870 facial-phrenic**~~

\+ **64872 Suture of nerve; requiring secondary or delayed suture (List separately in addition to code for primary neurorrhaphy)**
Code first (64831-64865)
N1 N 80 — 3.42 — 3.42 FUD ZZZ

\+ **64874 requiring extensive mobilization, or transposition of nerve (List separately in addition to code for nerve suture)**
Code first (64831-64865)
N1 N 80 — 4.84 — 4.84 FUD ZZZ

\+ **64876 requiring shortening of bone of extremity (List separately in addition to code for nerve suture)**
Code first (64831-64865)
N1 N 80 — 5.29 — 5.29 FUD ZZZ

64885 Nerve graft (includes obtaining graft), head or neck; up to 4 cm in length
A2 T 80 — 32.76 — 32.76 FUD 090

64886 more than 4 cm length
A2 T 80 — 37.32 — 37.32 FUD 090

64890 Nerve graft (includes obtaining graft), single strand, hand or foot; up to 4 cm length
A2 T 80 — 31.79 — 31.79 FUD 090

64891 more than 4 cm length
A2 T 80 — 33.88 — 33.88 FUD 090

64892 Nerve graft (includes obtaining graft), single strand, arm or leg; up to 4 cm length
A2 T 80 — 30.92 — 30.92 FUD 090

64893 more than 4 cm length
A2 T 80 — 33.03 — 33.03 FUD 090

64895 Nerve graft (includes obtaining graft), multiple strands (cable), hand or foot; up to 4 cm length
A2 T 80 — 38.86 — 38.86 FUD 090

64896 more than 4 cm length
A2 T 80 — 45.33 — 45.33 FUD 090

64897 Nerve graft (includes obtaining graft), multiple strands (cable), arm or leg; up to 4 cm length
A2 T 80 — 37.48 — 37.48 FUD 090

64898 more than 4 cm length
A2 T 80 — 39.36 — 39.36 FUD 090

\+ **64901 Nerve graft, each additional nerve; single strand (List separately in addition to code for primary procedure)**
Code first (64885-64893)
N1 N 80 — 16.86 — 16.86 FUD ZZZ

\+ **64902 multiple strands (cable) (List separately in addition to code for primary procedure)**
Code first (64885-64886, 64895-64898)
N1 N 80 — 19.51 — 19.51 FUD ZZZ

64905 Nerve pedicle transfer; first stage
A2 T 80 — 29.79 — 29.79 FUD 090

64907 second stage
A2 T 80 — 34.89 — 34.89 FUD 090

64910-64999 Nerve Repair: Synthetic and Vein Grafts

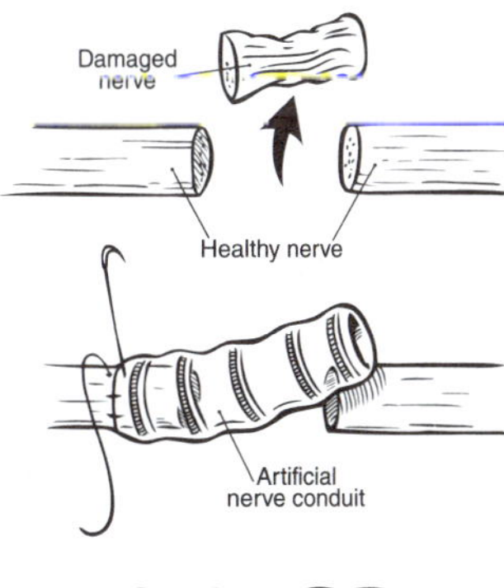

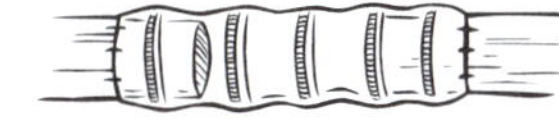

A synthetic "bridge" is affixed to each end of a severed nerve with sutures
This procedure is performed using an operating microscope

64910 Nerve repair; with synthetic conduit or vein allograft (eg, nerve tube), each nerve
INCLUDES Operating microscope (69990)
62 T 80 — 23.54 — 23.54 FUD 090

64911 with autogenous vein graft (includes harvest of vein graft), each nerve
INCLUDES Operating microscope (69990)
T 80 — 29.46 — 29.46 FUD 090

64999 Unlisted procedure, nervous system
T 80 — 0.00 — 0.00 FUD YYY

65091-65093 Surgical Removal of Eyeball Contents

CMS 100-4,12,30 Correct Coding Policy

INCLUDES Operating microscope (69990)

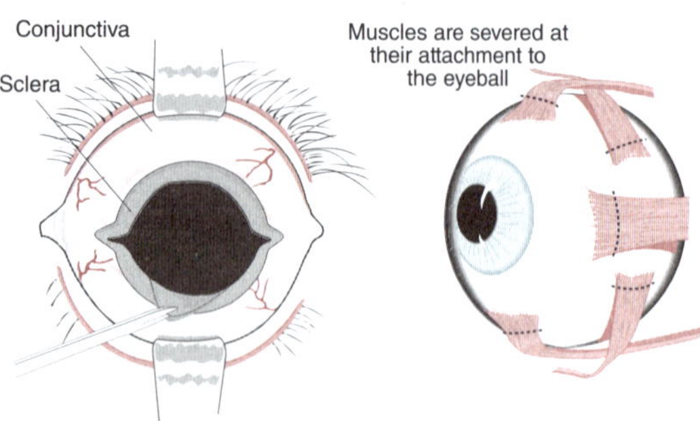

Evisceration involves removal of the contents of the eyeball: the vitreous; retina; choroid; lens; iris; and ciliary muscle. Only the scleral shell remains. A temporary or permanent implant is usually inserted

Enucleation involves severing the extraorbital muscles and optic nerve with removal of the eyeball. An implant is usually inserted and, if permanent, may involve attachment to the severed extraorbital muscles

65091 Evisceration of ocular contents; without implant
A2 T 80 50 ⚑ 18.78 18.78 FUD 090

65093 with implant
A2 T 50 ⚑ 18.53 18.53 FUD 090

65101-65105 Surgical Removal of Eyeball

CMS 100-4,12,30 Correct Coding Policy

INCLUDES Operating microscope (69990)

EXCLUDES *Conjunctivoplasty following enucleation (68320-68328)*

65101 Enucleation of eye; without implant
A2 T 50 ⚑ 21.76 21.76 FUD 090

65103 with implant, muscles not attached to implant
A2 T 50 ⚑ 22.73 22.73 FUD 090

65105 with implant, muscles attached to implant
A2 T 80 50 ⚑ 25.11 25.11 FUD 090

65110-65114 Surgical Removal of Orbital Contents

CMS 100-4,12,30 Correct Coding Policy

INCLUDES Operating microscope (69990)

EXCLUDES *Free full thickness graft (15260-15261)*
Repair more extensive than skin (67930-67975)
Skin graft (15120-15121)

65110 Exenteration of orbit (does not include skin graft), removal of orbital contents; only
A2 T 80 50 ⚑ 35.32 35.32 FUD 090

65112 with therapeutic removal of bone
A2 T 80 50 ⚑ 40.99 40.99 FUD 090

65114 with muscle or myocutaneous flap
A2 T 80 50 ⚑ 43.01 43.01 FUD 090

65125-65175 Implant Procedures: Insertion, Removal, and Revision

CMS 100-4,12,30 Correct Coding Policy

INCLUDES Operating microscope (69990)

EXCLUDES *Orbit implant insertion outside muscle cone (67550)*
Orbital implant removal or revision outside muscle cone (67560)

65125 Modification of ocular implant with placement or replacement of pegs (eg, drilling receptacle for prosthesis appendage) (separate procedure)
G2 T 50 ⚑ 8.64 13.20 FUD 090

65130 Insertion of ocular implant secondary; after evisceration, in scleral shell
A2 T 50 ⚑ 21.63 21.63 FUD 090

65135 after enucleation, muscles not attached to implant
A2 T 50 ⚑ 21.95 21.95 FUD 090

65140 after enucleation, muscles attached to implant
A2 T 50 ⚑ 23.28 23.28 FUD 090

65150 Reinsertion of ocular implant; with or without conjunctival graft
A2 T 80 50 ⚑ 16.26 16.26 FUD 090

65155 with use of foreign material for reinforcement and/or attachment of muscles to implant
A2 T 50 ⚑ 25.04 25.04 FUD 090

65175 Removal of ocular implant
A2 Q2 50 ⚑ 18.92 18.92 FUD 090

65205-65265 Foreign Body Removal By Area of Eye

CMS 100-4,12,30 Correct Coding Policy

INCLUDES Operating microscope (69990)

EXCLUDES *Removal:*
Anterior segment implant (65920)
Ocular implant (65175)
Orbital implant outside muscle cone (67560)
Posterior segment implant (67120)
Removal of foreign body:
Eyelid (67938)
Lacrimal system (68530)
Orbit:
Frontal approach (67413)
Lateral approach (67430)

65205 Removal of foreign body, external eye; conjunctival superficial
70030, 76529
P3 S 50 ⚑ 1.31 1.64 FUD 000

65210 conjunctival embedded (includes concretions), subconjunctival, or scleral nonperforating
70030, 76529
P3 S 50 ⚑ 1.57 1.99 FUD 000

65220 corneal, without slit lamp
EXCLUDES *Repair of corneal wound with foreign body (65275)*
70030, 76529
G2 S 50 ⚑ 1.23 1.66 FUD 000

65222 corneal, with slit lamp
EXCLUDES *Repair of corneal wound with foreign body (65275)*
70030, 76529
P3 S 50 ⚑ 1.56 1.96 FUD 000

65235 Removal of foreign body, intraocular; from anterior chamber of eye or lens
70030, 76529
A2 T 80 50 ⚑ 20.57 20.57 FUD 090

65260 from posterior segment, magnetic extraction, anterior or posterior route
70030, 76529
A2 T 80 50 ⚑ 27.06 27.06 FUD 090

65265 from posterior segment, nonmagnetic extraction
70030, 76529
A2 T 80 50 ⚑ 32.49 32.49 FUD 090

65270-65290 Laceration Repair External Eye

CMS 100-4,12,30 Correct Coding Policy

INCLUDES Conjunctival flap
Operating microscope (69990)
Restoration of anterior chamber with air or saline injection

EXCLUDES *Repair:*
Ciliary body or iris (66680)
Eyelid laceration (12011-12018, 12051-12057, 13151-13160, 67930, 67935)
Lacrimal system injury (68700)
Surgical wound (66250)
Treatment of orbit fracture (21385-21408)

65270 Repair of laceration; conjunctiva, with or without nonperforating laceration sclera, direct closure
A2 T 80 50 ⚑ 4.11 7.60 FUD 010

65272 **conjunctiva, by mobilization and rearrangement, without hospitalization**
A2 T 50 ⚑ 9.94 14.13 FUD 090

65273 **conjunctiva, by mobilization and rearrangement, with hospitalization**
C 50 ⚑ 10.77 10.77 FUD 090

65275 **cornea, nonperforating, with or without removal foreign body**
A2 T 80 50 ⚑ 13.47 16.67 FUD 090

65280 **cornea and/or sclera, perforating, not involving uveal tissue**
Do not report for surgical wound repair
A2 T 80 50 ⚑ 20.10 20.10 FUD 090

65285 **cornea and/or sclera, perforating, with reposition or resection of uveal tissue**
Do not report for surgical wound repair
A2 T 50 ⚑ 32.92 32.92 FUD 090

65286 **application of tissue glue, wounds of cornea and/or sclera**
P2 T 50 ⚑ 14.44 20.22 FUD 090

65290 **Repair of wound, extraocular muscle, tendon and/or Tenon's capsule**
A2 T 50 ⚑ 14.64 14.64 FUD 090

65400-65600 Removal Corneal Lesions

CMS 100-4,12,30 Correct Coding Policy
INCLUDES Operating microscope (69990)

65400 **Excision of lesion, cornea (keratectomy, lamellar, partial), except pterygium**
A2 T 50 ⚑ 17.52 19.64 FUD 090

65410 **Biopsy of cornea**
A2 T 80 50 ⚑ PQ 3.16 4.22 FUD 000

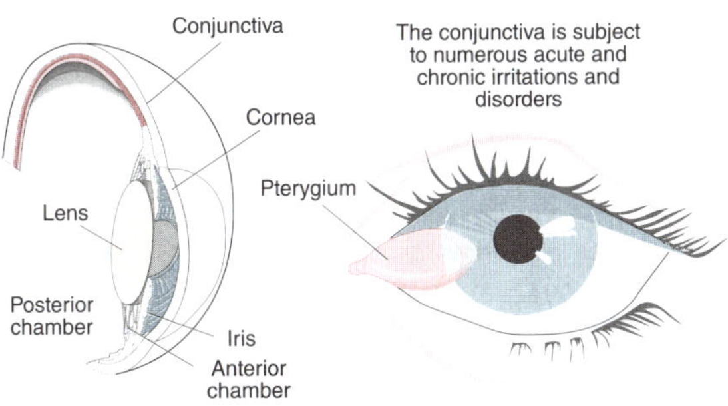

65420 **Excision or transposition of pterygium; without graft**
A2 T 50 ⚑ 10.79 14.58 FUD 090

65426 **with graft**
A2 T 50 ⚑ 13.91 18.72 FUD 090

65430 **Scraping of cornea, diagnostic, for smear and/or culture**
P2 S 50 ⚑ 3.05 3.35 FUD 000

65435 **Removal of corneal epithelium; with or without chemocauterization (abrasion, curettage)**
P3 T 50 ⚑ 2.06 2.34 FUD 000

65436 **with application of chelating agent (eg, EDTA)**
P3 T 50 ⚑ 10.98 11.41 FUD 090

65450 **Destruction of lesion of cornea by cryotherapy, photocoagulation or thermocauterization**
G2 S 50 ⚑ 9.30 9.38 FUD 090

65600 **Multiple punctures of anterior cornea (eg, for corneal erosion, tattoo)**
P3 T 50 ⚑ 10.00 11.39 FUD 090

65710-65757 Corneal Transplants

CMS 100-3,80.7 Refractive Keratoplasty
CMS 100-4,12,30 Correct Coding Policy
INCLUDES Operating microscope (69990)
EXCLUDES *Processing, preserving, and transporting corneal tissue (V2785)*
Do not report with (92025)

65710 **Keratoplasty (corneal transplant); anterior lamellar**
INCLUDES Use and preparation of fresh or preserved graft
EXCLUDES *Refractive keratoplasty surgery (65760-65767)*
A2 T 80 50 ⚑ 32.16 32.16 FUD 090

65730 **penetrating (except in aphakia or pseudophakia)**
INCLUDES Use and preparation of fresh or preserved graft
EXCLUDES *Refractive keratoplasty surgery (65760-65767)*
A2 T 80 50 ⚑ 35.71 35.71 FUD 090

65750 **penetrating (in aphakia)**
INCLUDES Use and preparation of fresh or preserved graft
EXCLUDES *Refractive keratoplasty surgery (65760-65767)*
A2 T 80 50 ⚑ 35.83 35.83 FUD 090

65755 **penetrating (in pseudophakia)**
INCLUDES Use and preparation of fresh or preserved graft
EXCLUDES *Refractive keratoplasty surgery (65760-65767)*
A2 T 80 50 ⚑ 35.76 35.76 FUD 090

65756 **endothelial**
EXCLUDES *Refractive keratoplasty surgery (65760-65767)*
Code also donor material
Code also if appropriate (65757)
G2 T 80 50 33.53 33.53 FUD 090

\+ 65757 **Backbench preparation of corneal endothelial allograft prior to transplantation (List separately in addition to code for primary procedure)**
Code first (65756)
N1 N 80 0.00 0.00 FUD ZZZ

65760-65775 Corneal Refractive Procedures

CMS 100-3,80.7 Refractive Keratoplasty
INCLUDES Operating microscope (69990)
EXCLUDES *Unlisted corneal procedures (66999)*

65760 **Keratomileusis**
Do not report with (92025)
E 0.00 0.00 FUD XXX

65765 **Keratophakia**
Do not report with (92025)
E 0.00 0.00 FUD XXX

65767 **Epikeratoplasty**
Do not report with (92025)
E 0.00 0.00 FUD XXX

65770 **Keratoprosthesis**
Code also (C1818, L8609)
Do not report with (92025)
J8 T 80 50 ⚑ 45.22 45.22 FUD 090

65771 **Radial keratotomy**
Do not report with (92025)
E 0.00 0.00 FUD XXX

65772 **Corneal relaxing incision for correction of surgically induced astigmatism**
A2 T 50 ⚑ 11.76 12.99 FUD 090

65775 **Corneal wedge resection for correction of surgically induced astigmatism**
EXCLUDES *Fitting of contact lens to treat disease (92071-92072)*
A2 T 50 ⚑ Facility RVU 15.58 Non-Facility RVU 15.58 FUD 090

65778-65782 Corneal Surface Reconstruction

CMS 100-4,4,200.4 Billing for Amniotic Membrane
CMS 100-4,12,30 Correct Coding Policy
INCLUDES Operating microscope (69990)

65778 **Placement of amniotic membrane on the ocular surface; without sutures**
EXCLUDES *Placement of amniotic membrane with tissue glue (66999)*
Do not report with (65430, 65435, 65780)
N1 Q2 80 50 Facility RVU 2.11 Non-Facility RVU 38.77 FUD 010

65779 **single layer, sutured**
EXCLUDES *Placement of amniotic membrane with tissue glue (66999)*
Do not report with (65430, 65435, 65780)
N1 Q2 80 50 Facility RVU 8.31 Non-Facility RVU 34.55 FUD 010

65780 **Ocular surface reconstruction; amniotic membrane transplantation, multiple layers**
EXCLUDES *Placement of amniotic membrane without ocular surface reconstruction using:*
No sutures (65778)
Single layer suture technique (65779)
Tissue glue (66999)
A2 T 50 ⚑ Facility RVU 25.72 Non-Facility RVU 25.72 FUD 090

65781 **limbal stem cell allograft (eg, cadaveric or living donor)**
A2 T 80 50 ⚑ Facility RVU 37.71 Non-Facility RVU 37.71 FUD 090

65782 **limbal conjunctival autograft (includes obtaining graft)**
EXCLUDES *Obtaining conjunctival autograft from live donor (68371)*
A2 T 50 ⚑ Facility RVU 34.42 Non-Facility RVU 34.42 FUD 090

65800-66030 Anterior Segment Procedures

INCLUDES Operating microscope (69990)
EXCLUDES *Unlisted procedures of anterior segment (66999)*

65800 **Paracentesis of anterior chamber of eye (separate procedure); with removal of aqueous**
A2 T 50 ⚑ Facility RVU 2.71 Non-Facility RVU 3.47 FUD 000

65810 **with removal of vitreous and/or discission of anterior hyaloid membrane, with or without air injection**
A2 T 50 ⚑ Facility RVU 13.54 Non-Facility RVU 13.54 FUD 090

65815 **with removal of blood, with or without irrigation and/or air injection**
EXCLUDES *Injection only (66020-66030)*
Removal of blood clot only (65930)
A2 T 50 ⚑ Facility RVU 14.10 Non-Facility RVU 18.55 FUD 090

65820 **Goniotomy**
INCLUDES Barkan's operation
Code also ophthalmic endoscope if used (69990)
A2 T 80 50 ⚑ ◎ Facility RVU 21.15 Non-Facility RVU 21.15 FUD 090

65850 **Trabeculotomy ab externo**
A2 T 50 ⚑ Facility RVU 24.89 Non-Facility RVU 24.89 FUD 090

65855 **Trabeculoplasty by laser surgery, 1 or more sessions (defined treatment series)**
EXCLUDES *Trabeculectomy ab externo (66170)*
Code also modifier 22 Increased procedural services, or 52 Reduced services, as appropriate, for re-treatment after several months for advancing disease
P3 T 50 ⚑ Facility RVU 8.75 Non-Facility RVU 9.86 FUD 010

65860 **Severing adhesions of anterior segment, laser technique (separate procedure)**
P3 T 80 50 ⚑ Facility RVU 8.19 Non-Facility RVU 9.73 FUD 090

65865 **Severing adhesions of anterior segment of eye, incisional technique (with or without injection of air or liquid) (separate procedure); goniosynechiae**
EXCLUDES *Laser trabeculectomy (65855)*
A2 T 50 ⚑ Facility RVU 13.33 Non-Facility RVU 13.33 FUD 090

65870 **anterior synechiae, except goniosynechiae**
A2 T 50 ⚑ Facility RVU 17.43 Non-Facility RVU 17.43 FUD 090

65875 **posterior synechiae**
Code also ophthalmic endoscope if used (66990)
A2 T 50 ⚑ Facility RVU 18.29 Non-Facility RVU 18.29 FUD 090

65880 **corneovitreal adhesions**
EXCLUDES *Laser procedure (66821)*
A2 T 50 ⚑ Facility RVU 18.74 Non-Facility RVU 18.74 FUD 090

65900 **Removal of epithelial downgrowth, anterior chamber of eye**
A2 T 80 50 ⚑ Facility RVU 27.22 Non-Facility RVU 27.22 FUD 090

65920 **Removal of implanted material, anterior segment of eye**
Code also ophthalmic endoscope if used (66990)
A2 Q2 50 ⚑ Facility RVU 22.83 Non-Facility RVU 22.83 FUD 090

65930 **Removal of blood clot, anterior segment of eye**
A2 T 50 ⚑ Facility RVU 18.86 Non-Facility RVU 18.86 FUD 090

66020 **Injection, anterior chamber of eye (separate procedure); air or liquid**
A2 T 50 ⚑ Facility RVU 3.71 Non-Facility RVU 5.24 FUD 010

66030 **medication**
A2 T 50 ⚑ Facility RVU 3.20 Non-Facility RVU 4.73 FUD 010

66130 Excision Scleral Lesion

CMS 100-4,12,30 Correct Coding Policy
INCLUDES Operating microscope (69990)
EXCLUDES *Intraocular foreign body removal (65235)*
Surgery on posterior sclera (67250, 67255)

66130 **Excision of lesion, sclera**
A2 T 80 50 ⚑ Facility RVU 17.16 Non-Facility RVU 20.68 FUD 090

66150-66185 Procedures for Glaucoma

INCLUDES Operating microscope (69990)
EXCLUDES *Intraocular foreign body removal (65235)*
Surgery on posterior sclera (67250, 67255)

66150 **Fistulization of sclera for glaucoma; trephination with iridectomy**
A2 T 50 ⚑ Facility RVU 24.73 Non-Facility RVU 24.73 FUD 090

66155 **thermocauterization with iridectomy**
A2 T 50 ⚑ Facility RVU 24.71 Non-Facility RVU 24.71 FUD 090

66160 **sclerectomy with punch or scissors, with iridectomy**
INCLUDES Knapp's operation
A2 T 50 ⚑ Facility RVU 27.90 Non-Facility RVU 27.90 FUD 090

Part of iris cutaway
Iris wick (iris piece) through iris
Iris
Cornea
Lens

In 66165, the wick creates a permanent drainage route for the anterior chamber

66165 ~~**iridencleisis or iridotasis**~~

66170 trabeculectomy ab externo in absence of previous surgery
EXCLUDES *Repair of surgical wound (66250)*
Trabeculectomy ab externo (65850)
A2 T 80 50 ▣ 34.74 ⚲ 34.74 FUD 090

66172 trabeculectomy ab externo with scarring from previous ocular surgery or trauma (includes injection of antifibrotic agents)
A2 T 80 50 ▣ 43.80 ⚲ 43.80 FUD 090

66174 Transluminal dilation of aqueous outflow canal; without retention of device or stent
A2 T 80 50 28.08 ⚲ 28.08 FUD 090

66175 with retention of device or stent
A2 T 80 50 31.81 ⚲ 31.81 FUD 090

● 66179 Aqueous shunt to extraocular equatorial plate reservoir, external approach; without graft

▲ 66180 with graft
Do not report with (67255)
A2 T 80 50 ▣ 33.89 ⚲ 33.89 FUD 090

66183 Insertion of anterior segment aqueous drainage device, without extraocular reservoir, external approach
G2 T 80 50 30.42 ⚲ 30.42 FUD 090

● 66184 Revision of aqueous shunt to extraocular equatorial plate reservoir; without graft

▲ 66185 with graft
EXCLUDES *Implanted shunt removal (67120)*
Do not report with (67255)
A2 T 80 50 ▣ 22.15 ⚲ 22.15 FUD 090

66220-66225 Staphyloma Repair

INCLUDES Operating microscope (69990)

EXCLUDES *Scleral procedures with retinal procedures (67101-67228)*
Scleral reinforcement (67250, 67255)

66220 Repair of scleral staphyloma; without graft
A2 T 80 50 ▣ 21.61 ⚲ 21.61 FUD 090

66225 with graft
A2 T 50 ▣ 27.87 ⚲ 27.87 FUD 090

66250 Anterior Segment Operative Wound Revision or Repair

INCLUDES Operating microscope (69990)

EXCLUDES *Unlisted procedures of anterior sclera (66999)*

66250 Revision or repair of operative wound of anterior segment, any type, early or late, major or minor procedure
A2 T 50 ▣ 16.62 ⚲ 21.93 FUD 090

66500-66505 Iridotomy With/Without Transfixion

CMS 100-4,12,30 Correct Coding Policy

INCLUDES Operating microscope (69990)

EXCLUDES *Photocoagulation iridotomy (66761)*

66500 Iridotomy by stab incision (separate procedure); except transfixion
A2 T 50 ▣ 9.98 ⚲ 9.98 FUD 090

66505 with transfixion as for iris bombe
A2 T 50 ▣ 10.94 ⚲ 10.94 FUD 090

66600-66635 Iridectomy Procedures

CMS 100-4,12,30 Correct Coding Policy

INCLUDES Operating microscope (69990)

EXCLUDES *Photocoagulation coreoplasty (66762)*

Do not report with (0308T)

66600 Iridectomy, with corneoscleral or corneal section; for removal of lesion
A2 T 50 ▣ 23.55 ⚲ 23.55 FUD 090

66605 with cyclectomy
A2 T 50 ▣ 29.88 ⚲ 29.88 FUD 090

66625 peripheral for glaucoma (separate procedure)
A2 T 50 ▣ 12.46 ⚲ 12.46 FUD 090

66630 sector for glaucoma (separate procedure)
A2 T 50 ▣ 16.77 ⚲ 16.77 FUD 090

66635 optical (separate procedure)
A2 T 50 ▣ 16.25 ⚲ 16.25 FUD 090

66680-66770 Other Procedures of the Uveal Tract

CMS 100-4,12,30 Correct Coding Policy

INCLUDES Operating microscope (69990)

EXCLUDES *Unlisted procedures of ciliary body or iris (66999)*

66680 Repair of iris, ciliary body (as for iridodialysis)
EXCLUDES *Resection or repositioning of uveal tissue for perforating laceration of cornea and/or sclera (65285)*
A2 T 50 ▣ 15.48 ⚲ 15.48 FUD 090

66682 Suture of iris, ciliary body (separate procedure) with retrieval of suture through small incision (eg, McCannel suture)
A2 T 50 ▣ 18.89 ⚲ 18.89 FUD 090

66700 Ciliary body destruction; diathermy
INCLUDES Heine's operation
A2 T 80 50 ▣ 11.24 ⚲ 12.81 FUD 090

66710 cyclophotocoagulation, transscleral
A2 T 50 ▣ 11.75 ⚲ 13.04 FUD 090

66711 cyclophotocoagulation, endoscopic
A2 T 50 ▣ 18.15 ⚲ 18.15 FUD 090

⊙ 66720 cryotherapy
A2 T 50 ▣ 12.19 ⚲ 13.58 FUD 090

66740 cyclodialysis
A2 T 50 ▣ 11.10 ⚲ 12.32 FUD 090

66761 Iridotomy/iridectomy by laser surgery (eg, for glaucoma) (per session)
Do not report with (0308T)
P3 T 50 ▣ 6.89 ⚲ 8.57 FUD 010

66762 Iridoplasty by photocoagulation (1 or more sessions) (eg, for improvement of vision, for widening of anterior chamber angle)
P2 T 50 ▣ 12.32 ⚲ 13.66 FUD 090

66770 Destruction of cyst or lesion iris or ciliary body (nonexcisional procedure)
EXCLUDES *Excision:*
Epithelial downgrowth (65900)
Iris, ciliary body lesion (66600-66605)
P2 T 50 ▣ 13.66 ⚲ 14.88 FUD 090

66820-66825 Post-Cataract Surgery Procedures

INCLUDES Operating microscope (69990)

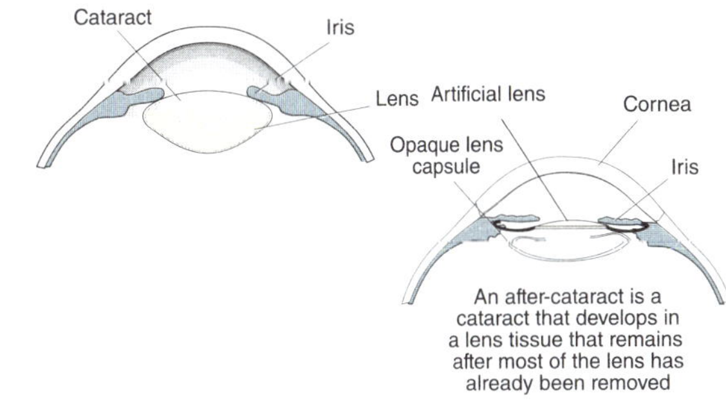

66820 Discission of secondary membranous cataract (opacified posterior lens capsule and/or anterior hyaloid); stab incision technique (Ziegler or Wheeler knife)
G2 T 50 ▣ 11.45 ⚲ 11.45 FUD 090

66821 **laser surgery (eg, YAG laser) (1 or more stages)**
A2 T 50 ▣ 9.06 9.56 FUD 090

66825 **Repositioning of intraocular lens prosthesis, requiring an incision (separate procedure)**
A2 T 80 50 ▣ 21.96 21.96 FUD 090

66830-66940 Cataract Extraction; Without Insertion Intraocular Lens

CMS 100-3,80.10 Phacoemulsification Procedure--Cataract Extraction
CMS 100-3,80.11 Vitrectomy
CMS 100-4,12,30 Correct Coding Policy

INCLUDES Anterior and/or posterior capsulotomy
Enzymatic zonulysis
Iridectomy/iridotomy
Lateral canthotomy
Medications
Operating microscope (69990)
Subconjunctival injection
Subtenon injection
Use of viscoelastic material

EXCLUDES *Removal of intralenticular foreign body without lens excision (65235)*
Repair of surgical laceration (66250)

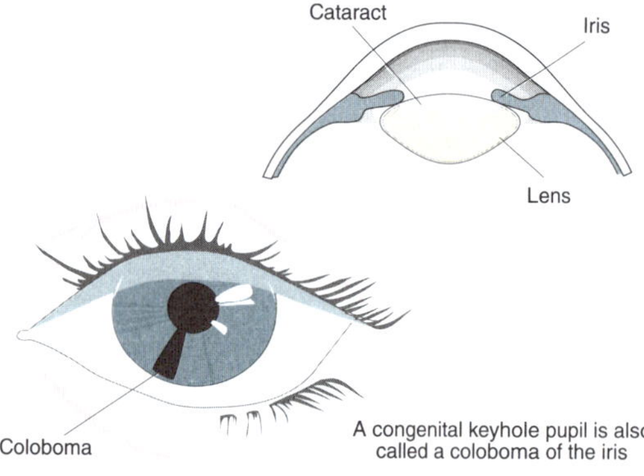

66830 **Removal of secondary membranous cataract (opacified posterior lens capsule and/or anterior hyaloid) with corneo-scleral section, with or without iridectomy (iridocapsulotomy, iridocapsulectomy)**
INCLUDES Graefe's operation
A2 T 50 ▣ 20.15 20.15 FUD 090

66840 **Removal of lens material; aspiration technique, 1 or more stages**
INCLUDES Fukala's operation
A2 T 50 ▣ PQ 20.81 20.81 FUD 090

66850 **phacofragmentation technique (mechanical or ultrasonic) (eg, phacoemulsification), with aspiration**
A2 T 50 ▣ PQ 23.10 23.10 FUD 090

66852 **pars plana approach, with or without vitrectomy**
A2 T 80 50 ▣ PQ 25.03 25.03 FUD 090

66920 **intracapsular**
A2 T 80 50 ▣ PQ 21.32 21.32 FUD 090

66930 **intracapsular, for dislocated lens**
A2 T 80 50 ▣ PQ 24.23 24.23 FUD 090

66940 **extracapsular (other than 66840, 66850, 66852)**
A2 T 80 50 ▣ PQ 23.08 23.08 FUD 090

66982-66984 Cataract Extraction: With Insertion Intraocular Lens

CMS 100-3,80.10 Phacoemulsification Procedure--Cataract Extraction
CMS 100-3,80.12 Intraocular Lenses (IOLs)
CMS 100-4,12,30 Correct Coding Policy

INCLUDES Anterior or posterior capsulotomy
Enzymatic zonulysis
Iridectomy/iridotomy
Lateral canthotomy
Medications
Operating microscope (69990)
Subconjunctival injection
Subtenon injection
Use of viscoelastic material

EXCLUDES *Implanted material removal from the anterior segment (65920)*
Ocular telescope prosthesis insertion with lens removal (0308T)
Secondary fixation (66682)
Supply of intraocular lens

Do not report with (0308T)

66982 **Extracapsular cataract removal with insertion of intraocular lens prosthesis (1-stage procedure), manual or mechanical technique (eg, irrigation and aspiration or phacoemulsification), complex, requiring devices or techniques not generally used in routine cataract surgery (eg, iris expansion device, suture support for intraocular lens, or primary posterior capsulorrhexis) or performed on patients in the amblyogenic developmental stage**
76519
A2 T 50 ▣ PQ 23.39 23.39 FUD 090

66983 **Intracapsular cataract extraction with insertion of intraocular lens prosthesis (1 stage procedure)**
76519
A2 T 50 ▣ PQ 21.20 21.20 FUD 090

66984 **Extracapsular cataract removal with insertion of intraocular lens prosthesis (1 stage procedure), manual or mechanical technique (eg, irrigation and aspiration or phacoemulsification)**
EXCLUDES *Complex extracapsular cataract removal (66982)*
76519
A2 T 50 ▣ PQ 18.79 18.79 FUD 090

66985-66986 Secondary Insertion or Replacement of Intraocular Lens

EXCLUDES *Implanted material removal from the anterior segment (65920)*
Secondary fixation (66682)
Supply of intraocular lens

Code also ophthalmic endoscope if used (66990)
Do not report with (0308T)

66985 **Insertion of intraocular lens prosthesis (secondary implant), not associated with concurrent cataract removal**
EXCLUDES *Insertion of lens at the time of cataract procedure (66982-66984)*
76519
A2 T 50 ▣ 22.34 22.34 FUD 090

66986 **Exchange of intraocular lens**
76519
A2 T 50 ▣ 26.36 26.36 FUD 090

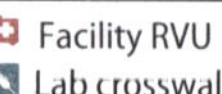

66990-66999 Ophthalmic Endoscopy

CMS 100-3,80.10 Phacoemulsification Procedure--Cataract Extraction
CMS 100-3,80.11 Vitrectomy
CMS 100-4,12,30 Correct Coding Policy
INCLUDES Operating microscope (69990)

+ **66990** **Use of ophthalmic endoscope (List separately in addition to code for primary procedure)**
Code first (65820, 65875, 65920, 66985-66986, 67036, 67039-67043, 67112-67113)
N1 N 2.57 2.57 FUD ZZZ

66999 **Unlisted procedure, anterior segment of eye**
T 80 50 0.00 0.00 FUD YYY

67005-67015 Vitrectomy: Partial and Subtotal

CMS 100-3,80.11 Vitrectomy
CMS 100-4,12,30 Correct Coding Policy
INCLUDES Operating microscope (69990)

67005 **Removal of vitreous, anterior approach (open sky technique or limbal incision); partial removal**
EXCLUDES *Anterior chamber vitrectomy by paracentesis (65810)*
Severing of corneovitreal adhesions (65880)
A2 T 50 14.15 14.15 FUD 090

67010 **subtotal removal with mechanical vitrectomy**
EXCLUDES *Anterior chamber vitrectomy by paracentesis (65810)*
Severing of corneovitreal adhesions (65880)
A2 T 50 15.80 15.80 FUD 090

67015 **Aspiration or release of vitreous, subretinal or choroidal fluid, pars plana approach (posterior sclerotomy)**
A2 T 50 16.85 16.85 FUD 090

67025-67028 Intravitreal Injection/Implantation

CMS 100-3,80.11 Vitrectomy
CMS 100-4,12,30 Correct Coding Policy
INCLUDES Operating microscope (69990)

67025 **Injection of vitreous substitute, pars plana or limbal approach (fluid-gas exchange), with or without aspiration (separate procedure)**
A2 T 50 18.71 21.31 FUD 090

67027 **Implantation of intravitreal drug delivery system (eg, ganciclovir implant), includes concomitant removal of vitreous**
EXCLUDES *Removal of drug delivery system (67121)*
A2 T 80 50 25.26 25.26 FUD 090

67028 **Intravitreal injection of a pharmacologic agent (separate procedure)**
P3 T 50 2.93 2.97 FUD 000

67030-67031 Incision of Vitreous Strands/Membranes

CMS 100-4,12,30 Correct Coding Policy
INCLUDES Operating microscope (69990)

67030 **Discission of vitreous strands (without removal), pars plana approach**
A2 T 50 15.01 15.01 FUD 090

67031 **Severing of vitreous strands, vitreous face adhesions, sheets, membranes or opacities, laser surgery (1 or more stages)**
A2 T 50 10.33 11.21 FUD 090

67036-67043 Pars Plana Mechanical Vitrectomy

CMS Vitrectomy
CMS 100-4,12,30 Correct Coding Policy
INCLUDES Operating microscope (69990)
EXCLUDES *Foreign body removal (65260, 65265)*
Lens removal (66850)
Unlisted vitreal procedures (67299)
Vitrectomy in retinal detachment (67108, 67113)
Code also ophthalmic endoscope if used (66990)

67036 **Vitrectomy, mechanical, pars plana approach;**
Code also placement of intraocular radiation source applicator (0190T)
A2 T 80 50 PQ 27.96 27.96 FUD 090

67039 **with focal endolaser photocoagulation**
A2 T 80 50 PQ 36.59 36.59 FUD 090

67040 **with endolaser panretinal photocoagulation**
A2 T 80 50 PQ 41.38 41.38 FUD 090

67041 **with removal of preretinal cellular membrane (eg, macular pucker)**
G2 T 80 50 PQ 38.71 38.71 FUD 090

67042 **with removal of internal limiting membrane of retina (eg, for repair of macular hole, diabetic macular edema), includes, if performed, intraocular tamponade (ie, air, gas or silicone oil)**
G2 T 80 50 PQ 44.26 44.26 FUD 090

67043 **with removal of subretinal membrane (eg, choroidal neovascularization), includes, if performed, intraocular tamponade (ie, air, gas or silicone oil) and laser photocoagulation**
G2 T 80 50 PQ 47.38 47.38 FUD 090

67101-67115 Detached Retina Repair

CMS 100-4,12,30 Correct Coding Policy
INCLUDES Operating microscope (69990)
Primary technique when cryotherapy and/or diathermy and/or photocoagulation are used in combination

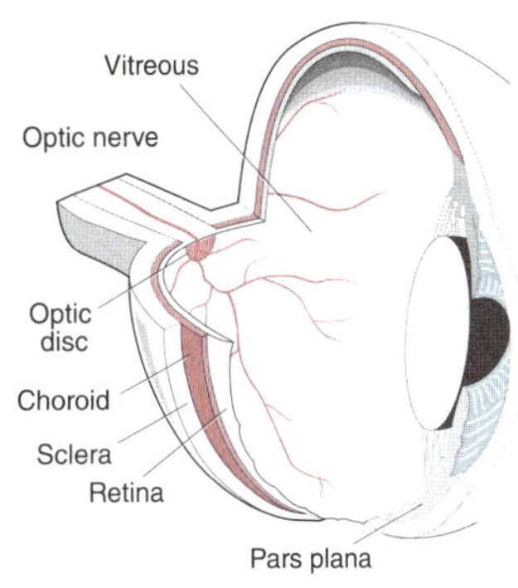

Posterior chamber

67101 **Repair of retinal detachment, 1 or more sessions; cryotherapy or diathermy, with or without drainage of subretinal fluid**
P3 T 50 19.94 22.97 FUD 090

67105 **photocoagulation, with or without drainage of subretinal fluid**
P2 T 50 18.76 20.84 FUD 090

67107 **Repair of retinal detachment; scleral buckling (such as lamellar scleral dissection, imbrication or encircling procedure), with or without implant, with or without cryotherapy, photocoagulation, and drainage of subretinal fluid**
INCLUDES Gonin's operation
A2 T 80 50 36.06 36.06 FUD 090

67108 **with vitrectomy, any method, with or without air or gas tamponade, focal endolaser photocoagulation, cryotherapy, drainage of subretinal fluid, scleral buckling, and/or removal of lens by same technique**
A2 T 80 50 46.86 46.86 FUD 090

67110 **by injection of air or other gas (eg, pneumatic retinopexy)**
P3 T 50 22.47 25.06 FUD 090

Eye and Ocular Adnexa 66990 — 67110

● New Code ▲ Revised Code ○ Reinstated M Maternity A Age Edit Unlisted Not Covered # Resequenced
⊘ AMA Mod 51 Exempt ⑤ Optum Mod 51 Exempt ⑥ Mod 63 Exempt ⊙ Mod Sedation + Add-on CCI PQ PQRS FUD Follow-up Days
 Medicare (Red Ink)

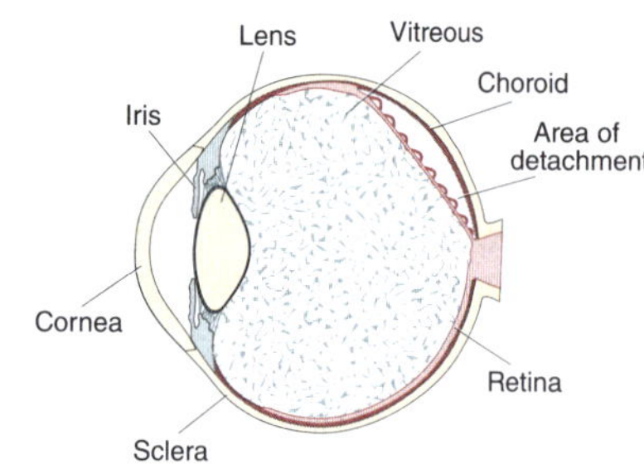

67112 by scleral buckling or vitrectomy, on patient having previous ipsilateral retinal detachment repair(s) using scleral buckling or vitrectomy techniques

EXCLUDES *Aspiration or drainage of subretinal or subchoroidal fluid (67015)*

Code also ophthalmic endoscope if used (66990)

A2 T 80 50 ▶ 38.71 38.71 FUD 090

67113 Repair of complex retinal detachment (eg, proliferative vitreoretinopathy, stage C-1 or greater, diabetic traction retinal detachment, retinopathy of prematurity, retinal tear of greater than 90 degrees), with vitrectomy and membrane peeling, may include air, gas, or silicone oil tamponade, cryotherapy, endolaser photocoagulation, drainage of subretinal fluid, scleral buckling, and/or removal of lens

EXCLUDES *Vitrectomy for other than retinal detachment, pars plana approach (67036-67043)*

Code also ophthalmic endoscope if used (66990)

G2 T 80 50 50.99 50.99 FUD 090

67115 Release of encircling material (posterior segment)

A2 T 50 ▶ 14.44 14.44 FUD 090

67120-67121 Removal of Previously Implanted Prosthetic Device

CMS 100-4,12,30 Correct Coding Policy

INCLUDES Operating microscope (69990)

EXCLUDES *Foreign body removal (65260, 65265)*

Removal of implanted material anterior segment (65920)

67120 Removal of implanted material, posterior segment; extraocular

A2 Q2 50 ▶ 16.65 19.39 FUD 090

67121 intraocular

A2 Q2 80 50 ▶ 26.93 26.93 FUD 090

67141-67145 Retinal Detachment: Preventative Procedures

CMS 100-4,12,30 Correct Coding Policy

INCLUDES Operating microscope (69990)

Treatment at one or more sessions that may occur at different encounters

Do not report more than one time during a defined period of treatment

67141 Prophylaxis of retinal detachment (eg, retinal break, lattice degeneration) without drainage, 1 or more sessions; cryotherapy, diathermy

A2 T 50 ▶ 14.41 15.40 FUD 090

67145 photocoagulation (laser or xenon arc)

P2 T 50 ▶ 14.47 15.26 FUD 090

67208-67218 Destruction of Retinal Lesions

CMS 100-3,140.5 Laser Procedures

CMS 100-4,12,30 Correct Coding Policy

INCLUDES Operating microscope (69990)

Treatment at one or more sessions that may occur at different encounters

EXCLUDES *Unlisted retinal procedures (67299)*

Do not report more than one time during a defined period of treatment

67208 Destruction of localized lesion of retina (eg, macular edema, tumors), 1 or more sessions; cryotherapy, diathermy

P2 T 50 ▶ 16.35 16.92 FUD 090

67210 photocoagulation

P2 T 50 ▶ 14.61 15.10 FUD 090

67218 radiation by implantation of source (includes removal of source)

A2 T 50 ▶ 39.18 39.18 FUD 090

67220-67225 Destruction of Choroidal Lesions

CMS 100-3,80.2 Photodynamic Therapy

CMS 100-3,80.3 Photosensitive Drugs

CMS 100-3,140.5 Laser Procedures

CMS 100-4,12,30 Correct Coding Policy

INCLUDES Operating microscope (69990)

67220 Destruction of localized lesion of choroid (eg, choroidal neovascularization); photocoagulation (eg, laser), 1 or more sessions

INCLUDES Treatment at one or more sessions that may occur at different encounters

Do not report more than one time during a defined period of treatment

P2 T 50 ▶ 14.79 15.73 FUD 090

67221 photodynamic therapy (includes intravenous infusion)

P3 T ▶ 6.29 8.32 FUD 000

\+ 67225 photodynamic therapy, second eye, at single session (List separately in addition to code for primary eye treatment)

Code first (67221)

N1 N ▶ 0.80 0.84 FUD ZZZ

67227-67229 Destruction Retinopathy

CMS 100-4,12,30 Correct Coding Policy

INCLUDES Operating microscope (69990)

Treatment at one or more sessions that may occur at different encounters

EXCLUDES *Unlisted retinal procedures (67299)*

Do not report more than one time during a defined period of treatment

67227 Destruction of extensive or progressive retinopathy (eg, diabetic retinopathy), 1 or more sessions, cryotherapy, diathermy

A2 T 50 ▶ 16.15 17.23 FUD 090

67228 Treatment of extensive or progressive retinopathy, 1 or more sessions; (eg, diabetic retinopathy), photocoagulation

P2 T 50 ▶ 27.90 29.35 FUD 090

67229 preterm infant (less than 37 weeks gestation at birth), performed from birth up to 1 year of age (eg, retinopathy of prematurity), photocoagulation or cryotherapy

R2 T 50 31.41 31.41 FUD 090

67250-67255 Reinforcement of Posterior Sclera

CMS 100-4,12,30 Correct Coding Policy

INCLUDES Operating microscope (69990)

EXCLUDES *Removal of lesion of sclera (66130)*

Repair scleral staphyloma (66220, 66225)

67250 Scleral reinforcement (separate procedure); without graft

A2 T 50 ▶ 22.95 22.95 FUD 090

67255 with graft

Do not report with (66180, 66185)

A2 T 80 50 ▶ 24.97 24.97 FUD 090

67299 Unlisted Posterior Segment Procedure

67299 Unlisted procedure, posterior segment

T 80 50 0.00 0.00 FUD YYY

67311-67334 Strabismus Procedures on Extraocular Muscles

CMS 100-4,12,30 Correct Coding Policy

INCLUDES Operating microscope (69990)

Code also adjustable sutures (67335)

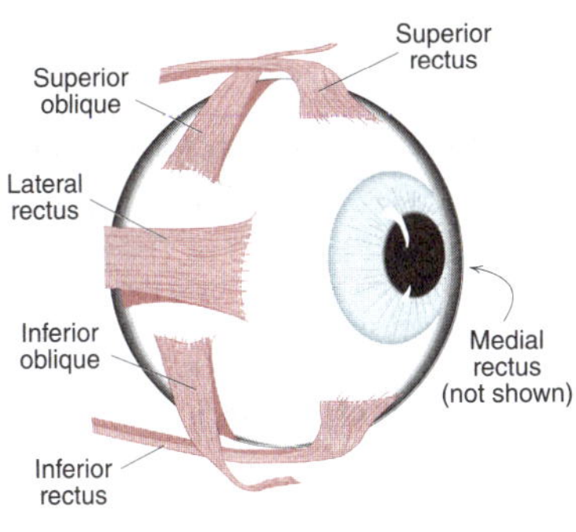

Muscles of the eyeball (right eye shown)

67311 **Strabismus surgery, recession or resection procedure; 1 horizontal muscle**
A2 T 50 ◪ 17.64 17.64 FUD 090

67312 **2 horizontal muscles**
A2 T 50 ◪ 21.32 21.32 FUD 090

67314 **1 vertical muscle (excluding superior oblique)**
A2 T 50 ◪ 19.85 19.85 FUD 090

67316 **2 or more vertical muscles (excluding superior oblique)**
A2 T 80 50 ◪ 23.97 23.97 FUD 090

67318 **Strabismus surgery, any procedure, superior oblique muscle**
A2 T 50 ◪ 19.93 19.93 FUD 090

+ **67320** **Transposition procedure (eg, for paretic extraocular muscle), any extraocular muscle (specify) (List separately in addition to code for primary procedure)**
Code first (67311-67318)
N1 N ◪ 9.15 9.15 FUD ZZZ

+ **67331** **Strabismus surgery on patient with previous eye surgery or injury that did not involve the extraocular muscles (List separately in addition to code for primary procedure)**
Code first (67311-67318)
N1 N 50 ◪ 9.17 9.17 FUD ZZZ

+ **67332** **Strabismus surgery on patient with scarring of extraocular muscles (eg, prior ocular injury, strabismus or retinal detachment surgery) or restrictive myopathy (eg, dysthyroid ophthalmopathy) (List separately in addition to code for primary procedure)**
Code first (67311-67318)
N1 N 50 ◪ 9.96 9.96 FUD ZZZ

+ **67334** **Strabismus surgery by posterior fixation suture technique, with or without muscle recession (List separately in addition to code for primary procedure)**
Code first (67311-67318)
N1 N 50 ◪ 8.57 8.57 FUD ZZZ

67335-67399 Other Procedures of Extraocular Muscles

CMS 100-4,12,30 Correct Coding Policy

INCLUDES Operating microscope (69990)

+ **67335** **Placement of adjustable suture(s) during strabismus surgery, including postoperative adjustment(s) of suture(s) (List separately in addition to code for specific strabismus surgery)**
Code first (67311-67334)
N1 N 50 ◪ 4.46 4.46 FUD ZZZ

+ **67340** **Strabismus surgery involving exploration and/or repair of detached extraocular muscle(s) (List separately in addition to code for primary procedure)**
INCLUDES Hummelsheim operation
Code first (67311-67334)
N1 N 80 ◪ 10.19 10.19 FUD ZZZ

67343 **Release of extensive scar tissue without detaching extraocular muscle (separate procedure)**
Code also 67311-67340 if these procedures are performed on other than the affected muscle
A2 T 50 ◪ 19.48 19.48 FUD 090

67345 **Chemodenervation of extraocular muscle**
EXCLUDES *Nerve destruction for blepharospasm and other neurological disorders (64612, 64616)*
P3 T 50 ◪ 6.56 7.24 FUD 010

67346 **Biopsy of extraocular muscle**
EXCLUDES *Repair laceration extraocular muscle, tendon, or Tenon's capsule (65290)*
A2 T 80 50 PQ 5.89 5.89 FUD 000

▲ **67399** **Unlisted procedure, extraocular muscle**
T 80 50 0.00 0.00 FUD YYY

67400-67415 Frontal Orbitotomy

CMS 100-4,12,30 Correct Coding Policy

INCLUDES Operating microscope (69990)

67400 **Orbitotomy without bone flap (frontal or transconjunctival approach); for exploration, with or without biopsy**
A2 T 50 ◪ PQ 27.44 27.44 FUD 090

67405 **with drainage only**
A2 T 50 ◪ 22.80 22.80 FUD 090

67412 **with removal of lesion**
A2 T 50 ◪ 25.06 25.06 FUD 090

67413 **with removal of foreign body**
A2 T 80 50 ◪ 25.24 25.24 FUD 090

67414 **with removal of bone for decompression**
G2 T 80 50 ◪ 38.39 38.39 FUD 090

67415 **Fine needle aspiration of orbital contents**
EXCLUDES *Decompression optic nerve (67570)*
Exenteration, enucleation, and repair (65101-65175)
A2 T 80 50 ◪ PQ 3.08 3.08 FUD 000

67420-67450 Lateral Orbitotomy

CMS 100-4,12,30 Correct Coding Policy

INCLUDES Operating microscope (69990)

EXCLUDES *Orbital implant (67550, 67560)*
Surgical removal of all or some of the orbital contents or repair after removal (65091-65175)
Transcranial approach orbitotomy (61330-61333)

67420 **Orbitotomy with bone flap or window, lateral approach (eg, Kroenlein); with removal of lesion**
A2 T 80 50 ◪ 48.07 48.07 FUD 090

67430 **with removal of foreign body**
A2 T 80 50 ◪ 35.20 35.20 FUD 090

67440 **with drainage**
A2 T 80 50 ◪ 34.86 34.86 FUD 090

67445 **with removal of bone for decompression**
EXCLUDES *Decompression optic nerve sheath (67570)*
A2 T 80 50 41.81 41.81 FUD 090

67450 **for exploration, with or without biopsy**
A2 T 80 50 36.03 36.03 FUD 090

67500-67515 Eye Injections

CMS 100-4,12,30 Correct Coding Policy
INCLUDES Operating microscope (69990)

67500 **Retrobulbar injection; medication (separate procedure, does not include supply of medication)**
G2 S 50 2.06 2.23 FUD 000

67505 **alcohol**
P3 T 50 2.48 2.69 FUD 000

67515 **Injection of medication or other substance into Tenon's capsule**
EXCLUDES *Subconjunctival injection (68200)*
P3 T 50 2.69 2.90 FUD 000

67550-67560 Orbital Implant

CMS 100-4,12,30 Correct Coding Policy
INCLUDES Operating microscope (69990)
EXCLUDES *Fracture repair malar area, orbit (21355-21408)*
Ocular implant inside muscle cone (65093-65105, 65130-65175)

67550 **Orbital implant (implant outside muscle cone); insertion**
A2 T 50 28.46 28.46 FUD 090

67560 **removal or revision**
A2 T 80 50 28.52 28.52 FUD 090

67570-67599 Other and Unlisted Orbital Procedures

CMS 100-4,12,30 Correct Coding Policy
INCLUDES Operating microscope (69990)

67570 **Optic nerve decompression (eg, incision or fenestration of optic nerve sheath)**
A2 T 80 50 36.11 36.11 FUD 090

67599 **Unlisted procedure, orbit**
T 80 50 0.00 0.00 FUD YYY

67700-67810 [67810] Incisional Procedures of Eyelids

CMS 100-4,12,30 Correct Coding Policy
INCLUDES Operating microscope (69990)

67700 **Blepharotomy, drainage of abscess, eyelid**
P2 T 50 3.40 7.60 FUD 010

67710 **Severing of tarsorrhaphy**
P3 T 50 2.89 6.39 FUD 010

67715 **Canthotomy (separate procedure)**
EXCLUDES *Canthoplasty (67950)*
Symblepharon division (68340)
A2 T 50 3.22 6.78 FUD 010

67810 **Incisional biopsy of eyelid skin including lid margin**
EXCLUDES *Biopsy of eyelid skin (11100-11101, 11310-11313)*
P3 T 50 2.06 4.79 FUD 000

67800-67808 Excision of Chalazion (Meibomian Cyst)

CMS 100-4,12,30 Correct Coding Policy
INCLUDES Lesion removal requiring more than skin:
Lid margin
Palpebral conjunctiva
Tarsus
Operating microscope (69990)
EXCLUDES *Blepharoplasty, graft, or reconstructive procedures (67930-67975)*
Excision skin lesion of eyelid (11310-11313, 11440-11446, 11640-11646, 17000-17004)

67800 **Excision of chalazion; single**
P3 T 3.07 3.71 FUD 010

67801 **multiple, same lid**
P3 T 4.00 4.78 FUD 010

67805 **multiple, different lids**
P3 T 4.92 5.94 FUD 010

67808 **under general anesthesia and/or requiring hospitalization, single or multiple**
A2 T 10.94 10.94 FUD 090

67810-67850 Other Eyelid Procedures

CMS 100-4,12,30 Correct Coding Policy
INCLUDES Operating microscope (69990)

67810 *Resequenced code. See code following 67715.*

67820 **Correction of trichiasis; epilation, by forceps only**
P3 S 50 1.58 1.48 FUD 000

67825 **epilation by other than forceps (eg, by electrosurgery, cryotherapy, laser surgery)**
P3 T 50 3.59 3.78 FUD 010

67830 **incision of lid margin**
A2 T 50 4.10 7.65 FUD 010

67835 **incision of lid margin, with free mucous membrane graft**
A2 T 80 50 13.10 13.10 FUD 090

67840 **Excision of lesion of eyelid (except chalazion) without closure or with simple direct closure**
EXCLUDES *Eyelid resection and reconstruction (67961, 67966)*
P3 T 50 4.65 7.88 FUD 010

67850 **Destruction of lesion of lid margin (up to 1 cm)**
EXCLUDES *Mohs micro procedures (17311-17315)*
Topical chemotherapy (99201-99215)
P3 T 50 3.88 6.04 FUD 010

67875-67882 Suturing of the Eyelids

CMS 100-4,12,30 Correct Coding Policy
INCLUDES Operating microscope (69990)
EXCLUDES *Canthoplasty (67950)*
Canthotomy (67715)
Severing of tarsorrhaphy (67710)

67875 **Temporary closure of eyelids by suture (eg, Frost suture)**
G2 T 50 2.89 4.93 FUD 000

67880 **Construction of intermarginal adhesions, median tarsorrhaphy, or canthorrhaphy;**
A2 T 50 10.86 13.35 FUD 090

67882 **with transposition of tarsal plate**
A2 T 50 14.06 16.58 FUD 090

67900-67912 Repair of Ptosis/Retraction Eyelids, Eyebrows

CMS 100-2,16,120 Cosmetic Procedures
CMS 100-4,12,30 Correct Coding Policy
INCLUDES Operating microscope (69990)

Superior fornix of conjunctiva
Orbital part of superior eyelid
Sulcus of eyelid
Tarsal part of superior eyelid
Lacrimal puncta
Pupil
Opening of tarsal gland
Iris
Cornea
Lens
Lower eyelid
Iris
Inferior fornix of conjunctiva

67900 **Repair of brow ptosis (supraciliary, mid-forehead or coronal approach)**
EXCLUDES *Forehead rhytidectomy (15824)*
A2 T 50 15.03 18.63 FUD 090

67901 **Repair of blepharoptosis; frontalis muscle technique with suture or other material (eg, banked fascia)**
A2 T 50 17.18 22.13 FUD 090

67902 **frontalis muscle technique with autologous fascial sling (includes obtaining fascia)**
A2 T 50 21.59 21.59 FUD 090

67903 **(tarso) levator resection or advancement, internal approach**
A2 T 50 14.42 17.43 FUD 090

67904 **(tarso) levator resection or advancement, external approach**
INCLUDES Everbusch's operation
A2 T 50 17.77 21.47 FUD 090

67906 **superior rectus technique with fascial sling (includes obtaining fascia)**
A2 T 50 14.38 14.38 FUD 090

67908 **conjunctivo-tarso-Muller's muscle-levator resection (eg, Fasanella-Servat type)**
A2 T 50 12.63 14.53 FUD 090

67909 **Reduction of overcorrection of ptosis**
A2 T 50 12.99 15.67 FUD 090

67911 **Correction of lid retraction**
EXCLUDES *Graft harvest (20920, 20922, 20926)*
Mucous membrane graft repair of trichiasis (67835)
A2 T 50 16.71 16.71 FUD 090

67912 **Correction of lagophthalmos, with implantation of upper eyelid lid load (eg, gold weight)**
A2 T 50 14.23 25.11 FUD 090

67914-67924 Repair Ectropion/Entropion

CMS 100-4,12,30 Correct Coding Policy
INCLUDES Operating microscope (69990)
EXCLUDES *Cicatricial ectropion or entropion with scar excision or graft (67961-67966)*

67914 **Repair of ectropion; suture**
A2 T 50 9.62 13.54 FUD 090

67915 **thermocauterization**
P3 T 50 5.71 8.32 FUD 090

67916 **excision tarsal wedge**
A2 T 50 12.69 17.13 FUD 090

67917 **extensive (eg, tarsal strip operations)**
EXCLUDES *Repair of everted punctum (68705)*
A2 T 50 13.59 17.57 FUD 090

67921 **Repair of entropion; suture**
A2 T 50 9.18 13.31 FUD 090

67922 **thermocauterization**
P3 T 50 5.70 8.25 FUD 090

67923 **excision tarsal wedge**
A2 T 50 12.77 17.21 FUD 090

67924 **extensive (eg, tarsal strip or capsulopalpebral fascia repairs operation)**
A2 T 50 13.61 18.37 FUD 090

67930-67935 Repair Eyelid Wound

CMS 100-4,12,30 Correct Coding Policy
INCLUDES Operating microscope (69990)
Repairs involving more than skin:
- Lid margin
- Palpebral conjunctiva
- Tarsus

EXCLUDES *Blepharoplasty for entropion or ectropion (67916-67917, 67923-67924)*
Correction of lid retraction and blepharoptosis (67901-67911)
Free graft (15120-15121, 15260-15261)
Graft preparation (15004)
Plastic repair of lacrimal canaliculi (68700)
Removal of eyelid lesion (67800-67808, 67840-67850)
Repair involving skin of eyelid (12011-12018, 12051-12057, 13151-13153)
Repair of blepharochalasis (15820-15823)
Skin adjacent tissue transfer (14060-14061)
Tarsorrhaphy, canthorrhaphy (67880, 67882)

67930 **Suture of recent wound, eyelid, involving lid margin, tarsus, and/or palpebral conjunctiva direct closure; partial thickness**
P3 T 50 7.18 10.60 FUD 010

67935 **full thickness**
A2 T 50 13.20 17.39 FUD 090

67938-67999 Eyelid Reconstruction/Repair/Removal Deep Foreign Body

CMS 100-4,12,30 Correct Coding Policy
INCLUDES Operating microscope (69990)
EXCLUDES *Blepharoplasty for entropion or ectropion (67916-67917, 67923-67924)*
Correction of lid retraction and blepharoptosis (67901-67911)
Free graft (15120-15121, 15260-15261)
Graft preparation (15004)
Plastic repair of lacrimal canaliculi (68700)
Removal of eyelid lesion (67800-67808, 67840-67850)
Repair involving skin of eyelid (12011-12018, 12051-12053, 13151-13153)
Repair of blepharochalasis (15820-15823)
Skin adjacent tissue transfer (14060-14061)
Tarsorrhaphy, canthorrhaphy (67880, 67882)

67938 **Removal of embedded foreign body, eyelid**
P2 S 50 3.38 6.88 FUD 010

67950 **Canthoplasty (reconstruction of canthus)**
A2 T 50 13.69 16.68 FUD 090

67961 **Excision and repair of eyelid, involving lid margin, tarsus, conjunctiva, canthus, or full thickness, may include preparation for skin graft or pedicle flap with adjacent tissue transfer or rearrangement; up to one-fourth of lid margin**
EXCLUDES *Canthoplasty (67950)*
Delay flap (15630)
Flap attachment (15650)
Free skin grafts (15120-15121, 15260-15261)
Tubed pedicle flap preparation (15576)
A2 T 80 50 13.49 16.79 FUD 090

67966 **over one-fourth of lid margin**
EXCLUDES *Canthoplasty (67950)*
Delay flap (15630)
Flap attachment (15650)
Free skin grafts (15120-15121, 15260-15261)
Tubed pedicle flap preparation (15576)
A2 T 50 19.58 22.62 FUD 090

67971 **Reconstruction of eyelid, full thickness by transfer of tarsoconjunctival flap from opposing eyelid; up to two-thirds of eyelid, 1 stage or first stage**
INCLUDES Dupuy-Dutemp reconstruction
Landboldt's operation
A2 T 50 21.63 21.63 FUD 090

67973 **total eyelid, lower, 1 stage or first stage**
INCLUDES Landboldt's operation
A2 T 80 50 27.88 27.88 FUD 090

67974 **total eyelid, upper, 1 stage or first stage**
INCLUDES Landboldt's operation
A2 T 80 50 27.85 27.85 FUD 090

67975 **second stage**
INCLUDES Landboldt's operation
A2 T 50 20.44 20.44 FUD 090

67999 **Unlisted procedure, eyelids**
T 80 50 0.00 0.00 FUD YYY

68020-68200 Conjunctival Biopsy/Injection/Treatment of Lesions

CMS 100-4,12,30 Correct Coding Policy
INCLUDES Operating microscope (69990)
EXCLUDES *Foreign body removal (65205-65265)*

68020 **Incision of conjunctiva, drainage of cyst**
P3 T 50 3.23 3.46 FUD 010

68040 **Expression of conjunctival follicles (eg, for trachoma)**
EXCLUDES *Automated evacuation meibomian glands with heat/pressure (0207T)*
P3 S 50 1.58 1.91 FUD 000

68100 **Biopsy of conjunctiva**
P3 T 50 PQ 2.85 4.85 FUD 000

68110 **Excision of lesion, conjunctiva; up to 1 cm**
P3 T 50 4.41 6.53 FUD 010

68115 **over 1 cm**
A2 T 50 5.34 8.86 FUD 010

68130 **with adjacent sclera**
A2 T 50 11.63 15.12 FUD 090

68135 **Destruction of lesion, conjunctiva**
P3 T 50 4.39 4.54 FUD 010

68200 **Subconjunctival injection**
EXCLUDES *Retrobulbar or Tenon's capsule injection (67500-67515)*
P3 S 50 1.03 1.21 FUD 000

68320-68340 Conjunctivoplasty Procedures

CMS 100-4,12,30 Correct Coding Policy
INCLUDES Operating microscope (69990)
EXCLUDES *Conjunctival foreign body removal (65205, 65210)*
Laceration repair (65270-65273)

68320 **Conjunctivoplasty; with conjunctival graft or extensive rearrangement**
A2 T 50 16.01 21.11 FUD 090

68325 **with buccal mucous membrane graft (includes obtaining graft)**
A2 T 50 19.63 19.63 FUD 090

68326 **Conjunctivoplasty, reconstruction cul-de-sac; with conjunctival graft or extensive rearrangement**
A2 T 50 19.25 19.25 FUD 090

68328 **with buccal mucous membrane graft (includes obtaining graft)**
A2 T 80 50 21.13 21.13 FUD 090

68330 **Repair of symblepharon; conjunctivoplasty, without graft**
A2 T 80 50 13.72 17.66 FUD 090

68335 **with free graft conjunctiva or buccal mucous membrane (includes obtaining graft)**
A2 T 50 19.33 19.33 FUD 090

68340 **division of symblepharon, with or without insertion of conformer or contact lens**
A2 T 80 50 11.89 15.91 FUD 090

68360-68399 Conjunctival Flaps and Unlisted Procedures

CMS 100-4,12,30 Correct Coding Policy
INCLUDES Operating microscope (69990)

68360 **Conjunctival flap; bridge or partial (separate procedure)**
EXCLUDES *Conjunctival flap for injury (65280, 65285)*
Conjunctival foreign body removal (65205, 65210)
Surgical wound repair (66250)
A2 T 50 12.25 15.56 FUD 090

68362 **total (such as Gunderson thin flap or purse string flap)**
EXCLUDES *Conjunctival flap for injury (65280, 65285)*
Conjunctival foreign body removal (65205, 65210)
Surgical wound repair (66250)
A2 T 50 19.61 19.61 FUD 090

68371 **Harvesting conjunctival allograft, living donor**
A2 T 50 11.65 11.65 FUD 010

68399 **Unlisted procedure, conjunctiva**
T 80 50 0.00 0.00 FUD YYY

68400-68899 Nasolacrimal System Procedures

CMS 100-4,12,30 Correct Coding Policy
INCLUDES Operating microscope (69990)

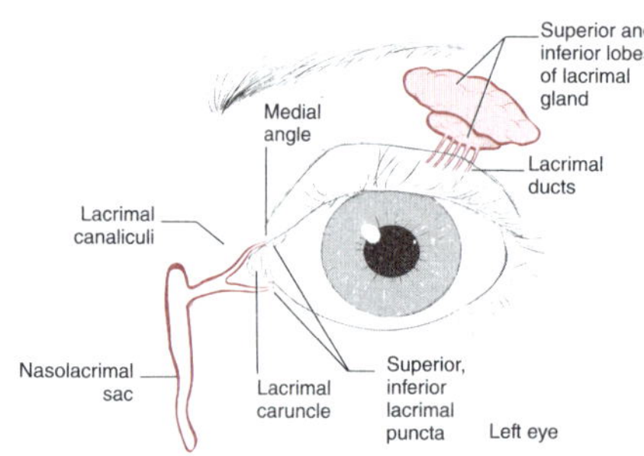

68400 **Incision, drainage of lacrimal gland**
P2 T 50 3.93 8.15 FUD 010

68420 **Incision, drainage of lacrimal sac (dacryocystotomy or dacryocystostomy)**
P3 T 50 4.89 9.11 FUD 010

68440 **Snip incision of lacrimal punctum**
P3 T 50 2.91 2.99 FUD 010

68500 **Excision of lacrimal gland (dacryoadenectomy), except for tumor; total**
A2 T 50 29.57 29.57 FUD 090

68505 **partial**
A2 T 50 28.95 28.95 FUD 090

68510 **Biopsy of lacrimal gland**
A2 T 80 50 PQ 8.88 13.12 FUD 000

68520 **Excision of lacrimal sac (dacryocystectomy)**
A2 T 80 50 19.89 19.89 FUD 090

68525 **Biopsy of lacrimal sac**
A2 T 50 PQ 8.01 8.01 FUD 000

68530 **Removal of foreign body or dacryolith, lacrimal passages**
INCLUDES Meller's excision
P2 T 50 7.73 12.43 FUD 010

68540 **Excision of lacrimal gland tumor; frontal approach**
A2 T 50 26.94 26.94 FUD 090

68550 **involving osteotomy**
A2 T 50 33.02 33.02 FUD 090

68700 **Plastic repair of canaliculi**
A2 T 50 18.00 18.00 FUD 090

68705 **Correction of everted punctum, cautery**
P2 T 50 4.94 6.88 FUD 010

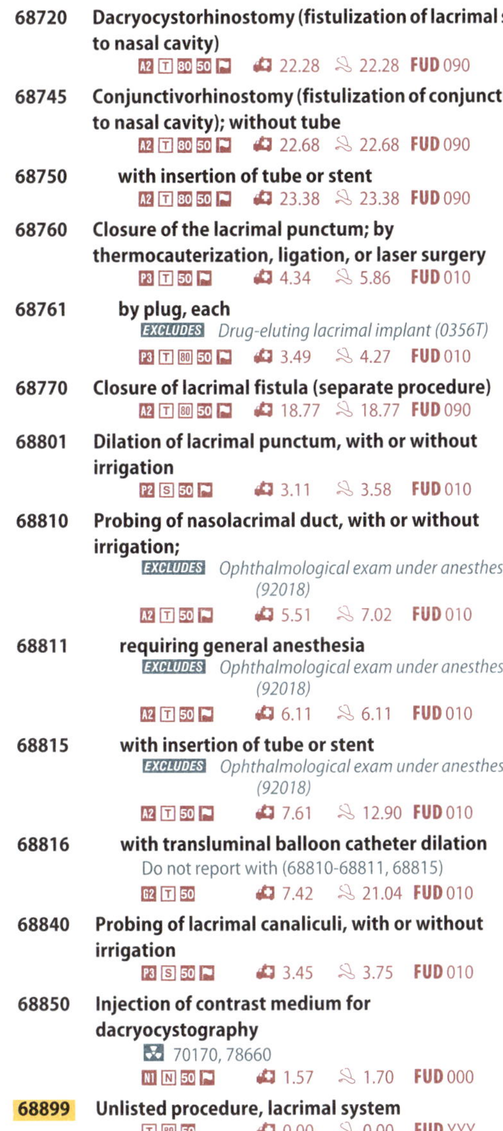

68720 **Dacryocystorhinostomy (fistulization of lacrimal sac to nasal cavity)**
A2 T 80 50 22.28 22.28 FUD 090

68745 **Conjunctivorhinostomy (fistulization of conjunctiva to nasal cavity); without tube**
A2 T 80 50 22.68 22.68 FUD 090

68750 **with insertion of tube or stent**
A2 T 80 50 23.38 23.38 FUD 090

68760 **Closure of the lacrimal punctum; by thermocauterization, ligation, or laser surgery**
P3 T 50 4.34 5.86 FUD 010

68761 **by plug, each**
EXCLUDES *Drug-eluting lacrimal implant (0356T)*
P3 T 80 50 3.49 4.27 FUD 010

68770 **Closure of lacrimal fistula (separate procedure)**
A2 T 80 50 18.77 18.77 FUD 090

68801 **Dilation of lacrimal punctum, with or without irrigation**
P2 S 50 3.11 3.58 FUD 010

68810 **Probing of nasolacrimal duct, with or without irrigation;**
EXCLUDES *Ophthalmological exam under anesthesia (92018)*
A2 T 50 5.51 7.02 FUD 010

68811 **requiring general anesthesia**
EXCLUDES *Ophthalmological exam under anesthesia (92018)*
A2 T 50 6.11 6.11 FUD 010

68815 **with insertion of tube or stent**
EXCLUDES *Ophthalmological exam under anesthesia (92018)*
A2 T 50 7.61 12.90 FUD 010

68816 **with transluminal balloon catheter dilation**
Do not report with (68810-68811, 68815)
G2 T 50 7.42 21.04 FUD 010

68840 **Probing of lacrimal canaliculi, with or without irrigation**
P3 S 50 3.45 3.75 FUD 010

68850 **Injection of contrast medium for dacryocystography**
70170, 78660
N1 N 50 1.57 1.70 FUD 000

68899 **Unlisted procedure, lacrimal system**
T 80 50 0.00 0.00 FUD YYY

69000-69020 Treatment External Abscess/Hematoma

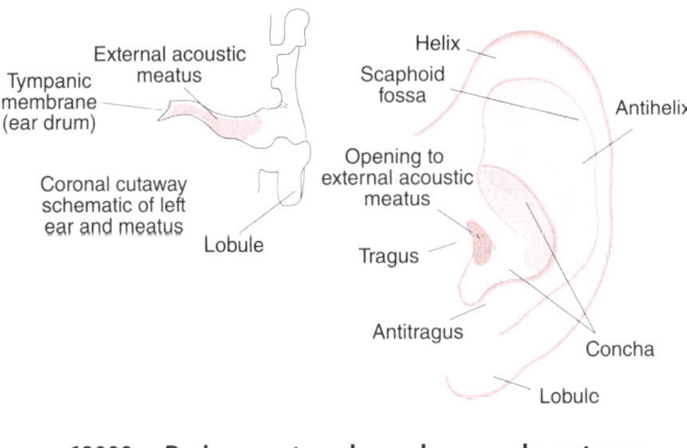

69000 **Drainage external ear, abscess or hematoma; simple**
P2 T 50 3.44 5.36 FUD 010

69005 **complicated**
P3 T 50 4.52 6.15 FUD 010

69020 **Drainage external auditory canal, abscess**
P2 T 50 4.09 6.66 FUD 010

69090 Cosmetic Ear Piercing

CMS 100-2,16,10 Exclusions from Coverage
CMS 100-2,16,120 Cosmetic Procedures

69090 **Ear piercing**
E 0.00 0.00 FUD XXX

69100-69222 Excisional Procedures External Ear/Auditory Canal

CMS 100-4,12,30 Correct Coding Policy
EXCLUDES *Reconstruction of ear (see integumentary section codes)*

69100 **Biopsy external ear**
P3 T PQ 1.40 2.79 FUD 000

69105 **Biopsy external auditory canal**
P3 T 50 PQ 1.83 4.01 FUD 000

69110 **Excision external ear; partial, simple repair**
A2 T 50 9.25 12.99 FUD 090

69120 **complete amputation**
A2 T 11.65 11.65 FUD 090

69140 **Excision exostosis(es), external auditory canal**
A2 T 80 50 25.11 25.11 FUD 090

69145 **Excision soft tissue lesion, external auditory canal**
A2 T 50 7.19 11.39 FUD 090

69150 **Radical excision external auditory canal lesion; without neck dissection**
EXCLUDES *Skin graft (15004-15261)*
Temporal bone resection (69535)
A2 T 30.14 30.14 FUD 090

69155 **with neck dissection**
EXCLUDES *Skin graft (15004-15261)*
Temporal bone resection (69535)
C 80 48.00 48.00 FUD 090

69200 **Removal foreign body from external auditory canal; without general anesthesia**
P2 X 50 1.67 3.50 FUD 000

69205 **with general anesthesia**
A2 T 50 2.92 2.92 FUD 010

69210 **Removal impacted cerumen requiring instrumentation, unilateral**
EXCLUDES *Removal of cerumen by irrigation only (see appropriate E/M code(s))*
P3 X 0.95 1.40 FUD 000

69220 **Debridement, mastoidectomy cavity, simple (eg, routine cleaning)**
P2 T 50 1.79 3.93 FUD 000

69222 **Debridement, mastoidectomy cavity, complex (eg, with anesthesia or more than routine cleaning)**
P3 T 50 3.93 6.30 FUD 010

69300 Plastic Surgery for Prominent Ears

CMS 100-2,16,120 Cosmetic Procedures
CMS 100-2,16,180 Services Related to Noncovered Procedures
EXCLUDES *Suture of laceration of external ear (12011-14302)*

⊙ 69300 **Otoplasty, protruding ear, with or without size reduction**
A2 T 80 50 13.69 20.99 FUD YYY

69310-69399 Reconstruction Auditory Canal: Postaural Approach

CMS 100-4,12,30 Correct Coding Policy
EXCLUDES *Suture of laceration of external ear (12011-14302)*

69310 **Reconstruction of external auditory canal (meatoplasty) (eg, for stenosis due to injury, infection) (separate procedure)**
A2 T 50 31.25 31.25 FUD 090

69320 Reconstruction external auditory canal for congenital atresia, single stage
EXCLUDES *Other reconstruction surgery with graft (13151-15760, 21230-21235)*
Tympanoplasty (69631, 69641)
A2 T 80 50 — 43.78 — 43.78 FUD 090

69399 Unlisted procedure, external ear
EXCLUDES *Otoscopy under general anesthesia (92502)*
T 80 — 0.00 — 0.00 FUD YYY

69400-69405 Treatment of Eustachian Tube Obstruction

CMS 100-4,12,30 — Correct Coding Policy

69400 ~~Eustachian tube inflation, transnasal; with catheterization~~
To report, see 69799

69401 ~~without catheterization~~
To report, see 99201-99205, 99211-99215

69405 ~~Eustachian tube catheterization, transtympanic~~
To report, see 69799

69420-69450 Ear Drum Procedures

CMS 100-4,12,30 — Correct Coding Policy

69420 Myringotomy including aspiration and/or eustachian tube inflation
P3 T 50 — 3.47 — 5.49 FUD 010

69421 Myringotomy including aspiration and/or eustachian tube inflation requiring general anesthesia
A2 T 50 — 4.28 — 4.28 FUD 010

69424 Ventilating tube removal requiring general anesthesia
Do not report with (69205, 69210, 69420-69421, 69433-69676, 69710-69745, 69801-69930)
P3 02 50 — 1.79 — 3.65 FUD 000

69433 Tympanostomy (requiring insertion of ventilating tube), local or topical anesthesia
P3 T 50 — 3.83 — 5.82 FUD 010

69436 Tympanostomy (requiring insertion of ventilating tube), general anesthesia
A2 T 50 — 4.62 — 4.62 FUD 010

69440 Middle ear exploration through postauricular or ear canal incision
EXCLUDES *Atticotomy (69601-69605)*
A2 T 50 — 19.88 — 19.88 FUD 090

69450 Tympanolysis, transcanal
A2 T 80 50 — 15.68 — 15.68 FUD 090

69501-69530 Transmastoid Excision

CMS 100-4,12,30 — Correct Coding Policy

EXCLUDES *Mastoidectomy cavity debridement (69220, 69222)*
Skin graft (15004-15770)

69501 Transmastoid antrotomy (simple mastoidectomy)
A2 T 50 — 21.10 — 21.10 FUD 090

69502 Mastoidectomy; complete
A2 T 80 50 — 28.04 — 28.04 FUD 090

69505 modified radical
A2 T 80 50 — 34.51 — 34.51 FUD 090

69511 radical
A2 T 80 50 — 35.35 — 35.35 FUD 090

69530 Petrous apicectomy including radical mastoidectomy
A2 T 80 50 — 47.42 — 47.42 FUD 090

69535-69554 Polyp and Glomus Tumor Removal

CMS 100-4,12,30 — Correct Coding Policy

69535 Resection temporal bone, external approach
EXCLUDES *Middle fossa approach (69950-69970)*
C 50 — 77.12 — 77.12 FUD 090

69540 Excision aural polyp
P3 T 50 — 3.65 — 5.99 FUD 010

69550 Excision aural glomus tumor; transcanal
A2 T 80 50 — 29.85 — 29.85 FUD 090

69552 transmastoid
A2 T 80 50 — 45.05 — 45.05 FUD 090

69554 extended (extratemporal)
C 80 50 — 72.46 — 72.46 FUD 090

69601-69605 Revised Mastoidectomy

CMS 100-4,12,30 — Correct Coding Policy

EXCLUDES *Skin graft (15120-15121, 15260-15261)*

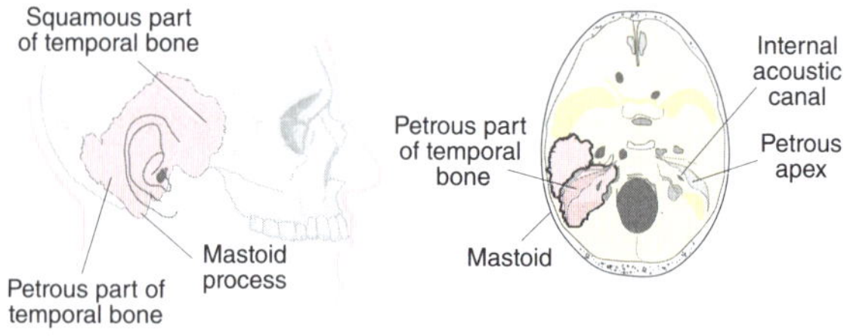

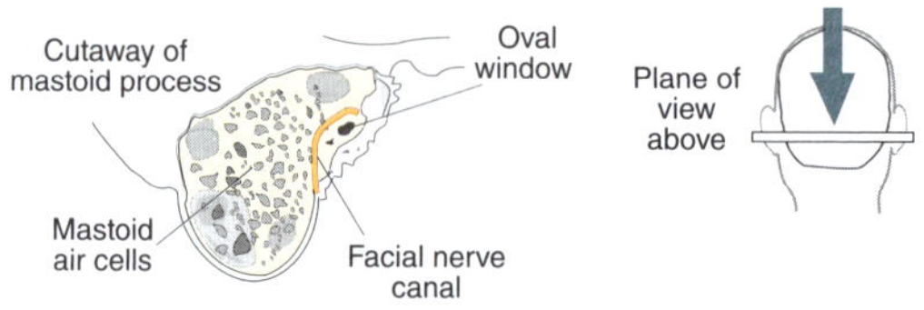

69601 Revision mastoidectomy; resulting in complete mastoidectomy
A2 T 80 50 — 30.17 — 30.17 FUD 090

69602 resulting in modified radical mastoidectomy
A2 T 80 50 — 31.38 — 31.38 FUD 090

69603 resulting in radical mastoidectomy
A2 T 80 50 — 36.13 — 36.13 FUD 090

69604 resulting in tympanoplasty
EXCLUDES *Secondary tympanoplasty following mastoidectomy (69631-69632)*
A2 T 50 — 32.07 — 32.07 FUD 090

69605 with apicectomy
A2 T 80 50 — 44.74 — 44.74 FUD 090

69610-69646 Eardrum Repair with/without Other Procedures

CMS 100-4,12,30 — Correct Coding Policy

69610 Tympanic membrane repair, with or without site preparation of perforation for closure, with or without patch
P3 T 50 — 8.40 — 11.04 FUD 010

69620 Myringoplasty (surgery confined to drumhead and donor area)
A2 T 50 — 14.02 — 19.79 FUD 090

69631 Tympanoplasty without mastoidectomy (including canalplasty, atticotomy and/or middle ear surgery), initial or revision; without ossicular chain reconstruction
A2 T 50 — 25.48 — 25.48 FUD 090

69632 with ossicular chain reconstruction (eg, postfenestration)
A2 T 50 — 31.09 — 31.09 FUD 090

69633 with ossicular chain reconstruction and synthetic prosthesis (eg, partial ossicular replacement prosthesis [PORP], total ossicular replacement prosthesis [TORP])
A2 T 50 — 30.07 — 30.07 FUD 090

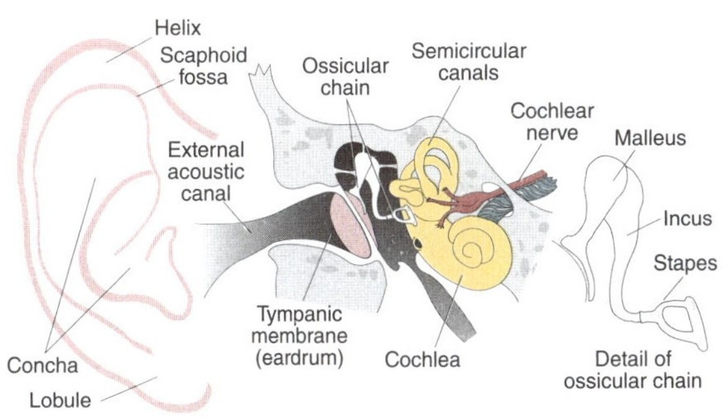

69635 Tympanoplasty with antrotomy or mastoidotomy (including canalplasty, atticotomy, middle ear surgery, and/or tympanic membrane repair); without ossicular chain reconstruction
A2 T 50 35.34 35.34 FUD 090

69636 with ossicular chain reconstruction
A2 T 80 50 39.55 39.55 FUD 090

69637 with ossicular chain reconstruction and synthetic prosthesis (eg, partial ossicular replacement prosthesis [PORP], total ossicular replacement prosthesis [TORP])
A2 T 80 50 39.42 39.42 FUD 090

69641 Tympanoplasty with mastoidectomy (including canalplasty, middle ear surgery, tympanic membrane repair); without ossicular chain reconstruction
A2 T 50 30.03 30.03 FUD 090

69642 with ossicular chain reconstruction
A2 T 50 38.55 38.55 FUD 090

69643 with intact or reconstructed wall, without ossicular chain reconstruction
A2 T 50 35.29 35.29 FUD 090

69644 with intact or reconstructed canal wall, with ossicular chain reconstruction
A2 T 50 42.39 42.39 FUD 090

69645 radical or complete, without ossicular chain reconstruction
A2 T 50 41.69 41.69 FUD 090

69646 radical or complete, with ossicular chain reconstruction
A2 T 80 50 44.24 44.24 FUD 090

69650-69662 Stapes Procedures

CMS 100-4,12,30 Correct Coding Policy

69650 Stapes mobilization
A2 T 50 23.17 23.17 FUD 090

69660 Stapedectomy or stapedotomy with reestablishment of ossicular continuity, with or without use of foreign material;
A2 T 50 26.71 26.71 FUD 090

69661 with footplate drill out
A2 T 80 50 34.79 34.79 FUD 090

69662 Revision of stapedectomy or stapedotomy
A2 T 50 33.31 33.31 FUD 090

69666-69700 Additional Mastoid and Middle Ear Procedures

CMS 100-4,12,30 Correct Coding Policy

69666 Repair oval window fistula
A2 T 80 50 23.31 23.31 FUD 090

69667 Repair round window fistula
A2 T 80 50 23.35 23.35 FUD 090

69670 Mastoid obliteration (separate procedure)
A2 T 80 50 27.21 27.21 FUD 090

69676 Tympanic neurectomy
A2 T 50 23.97 23.97 FUD 090

69700 Closure postauricular fistula, mastoid (separate procedure)
A2 T 50 19.77 19.77 FUD 090

69710-69718 Procedures Related to Hearing Aids/Auditory Implants

CMS 100-2,16,100 Hearing Devices
CMS 100-2,16,180 Services Related to Noncovered Procedures

69710 Implantation or replacement of electromagnetic bone conduction hearing device in temporal bone
INCLUDES Removal of existing device when performing replacement procedure
E 0.00 0.00 FUD XXX

69711 Removal or repair of electromagnetic bone conduction hearing device in temporal bone
A2 02 80 50 24.86 24.86 FUD 090

69714 Implantation, osseointegrated implant, temporal bone, with percutaneous attachment to external speech processor/cochlear stimulator; without mastoidectomy
Code also (L8690)
J8 T 50 31.02 31.02 FUD 090

69715 with mastoidectomy
Code also (L8690)
J8 T 50 38.31 38.31 FUD 090

69717 Replacement (including removal of existing device), osseointegrated implant, temporal bone, with percutaneous attachment to external speech processor/cochlear stimulator; without mastoidectomy
Code also (L8690)
J8 T 50 32.56 32.56 FUD 090

69718 with mastoidectomy
Code also (L8690)
J8 T 50 38.71 38.71 FUD 090

69720-69799 Procedures of the Facial Nerve

CMS 100-4,12,30 Correct Coding Policy

EXCLUDES *Extracranial suture of facial nerve (64864)*

69720 Decompression facial nerve, intratemporal; lateral to geniculate ganglion
A2 T 80 50 PQ 34.41 34.41 FUD 090

69725 including medial to geniculate ganglion
T 80 50 54.24 54.24 FUD 090

69740 Suture facial nerve, intratemporal, with or without graft or decompression; lateral to geniculate ganglion
A2 T 80 50 33.67 33.67 FUD 090

69745 including medial to geniculate ganglion
EXCLUDES *Extracranial suture of facial nerve (64864)*
A2 T 80 50 35.81 35.81 FUD 090

69799 Unlisted procedure, middle ear
T 80 50 0.00 0.00 FUD YYY

69801-69915 Procedures of the Labyrinth

CMS 100-4,12,30 Correct Coding Policy

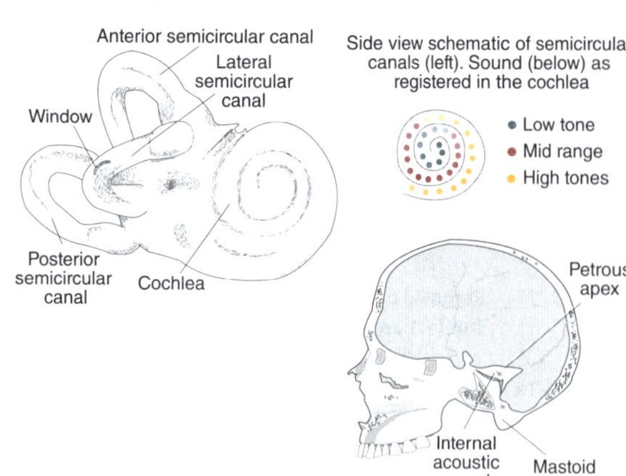

69801 Labyrinthotomy, with perfusion of vestibuloactive drug(s); transcanal
Do not report more than one time per day
Do not report when performed on the same ear (69420-69421, 69433, 69436)
P3 T 80 50 3.64 5.63 FUD 000

69805 Endolymphatic sac operation; without shunt
A2 T 80 50 30.41 30.41 FUD 090

69806 with shunt
A2 T 50 27.31 27.31 FUD 090

69820 Fenestration semicircular canal
INCLUDES Lempert's fenestration
A2 T 80 50 24.72 24.72 FUD 090

69840 Revision fenestration operation
A2 T 80 50 25.53 25.53 FUD 090

69905 Labyrinthectomy; transcanal
A2 T 50 26.48 26.48 FUD 090

69910 with mastoidectomy
A2 T 80 50 29.35 29.35 FUD 090

69915 Vestibular nerve section, translabyrinthine approach
EXCLUDES *Transcranial approach (69950)*
A2 T 80 50 44.43 44.43 FUD 090

69930-69949 Cochlear Implantation

CMS 100-2,16,100 Hearing Devices
CMS 100-3,50.3 Cochlear Implantation
CMS 100-4,32,100 Billing Requirements for Cochlear Implantation

69930 Cochlear device implantation, with or without mastoidectomy
Code also (L8614)
J8 T 80 50 PO 35.32 35.32 FUD 090

69949 Unlisted procedure, inner ear
T 80 50 0.00 0.00 FUD YYY

69950-69979 Inner Ear Procedures via Craniotomy

CMS 100-4,12,30 Correct Coding Policy

EXCLUDES *External approach (69535)*

69950 Vestibular nerve section, transcranial approach
C 80 50 51.42 51.42 FUD 090

69955 Total facial nerve decompression and/or repair (may include graft)
T 80 50 PO 57.08 57.08 FUD 090

69960 Decompression internal auditory canal
T 80 50 PO 55.53 55.53 FUD 090

69970 Removal of tumor, temporal bone
T 80 50 PO 61.82 61.82 FUD 090

69979 Unlisted procedure, temporal bone, middle fossa approach
T 80 50 0.00 0.00 FUD YYY

69990 Operating Microscope

CMS 100-4,12,30 Correct Coding Policy

EXCLUDES *Magnifying loupes*

Do not report with (15756-15758, 15842, 19364, 19368, 20955-20962, 20969-20973, 22551-22552, 22856-22861 [22858], 26551-26554, 26556, 31526, 31531, 31536, 31541, 31545-31546, 31561, 31571, 43116, 43180, 43496, 46601, 46607, 49906, 61548, 63075-63078, 64727, 64820-64823, 65091-68850 [67810], 0184T, 0308T)

+ **69990 Microsurgical techniques, requiring use of operating microscope (List separately in addition to code for primary procedure)**
Code first primary procedure
N1 N 80 6.21 6.21 FUD ZZZ

69801 — 69990

70010-70015 Radiography: Neurodiagnostic

CMS 100-2,6,10 Medical and Other Services Furnished to Inpatients
CMS 100-2,15,80 Diagnostic Test Requirements

70010 **Myelography, posterior fossa, radiological supervision and interpretation**
N1 Q2 80 PQ — 1.84 — 1.84 FUD XXX

70015 **Cisternography, positive contrast, radiological supervision and interpretation**
N1 Q2 80 PQ — 4.32 — 4.32 FUD XXX

70030-70390 Radiography: Head, Neck, Orofacial Structures

CMS 100-2,6,10 Medical and Other Services Furnished to Inpatients
CMS 100-2,15,80 Diagnostic Test Requirements
CMS 100-4,13,10 ICD-9-CM Coding for Diagnostic Tests

INCLUDES Minimum number of views or more views when needed to adequately complete the study
Radiographs that have to be repeated during the encounter due to substandard quality; only one unit of service is reported

EXCLUDES *Obtaining more films after review of initial films, based on the discretion of the radiologist, an order for the test, and a change in the patient's condition*

Do not report with a second interpretation by the requesting physician (included in E/M service)

70030 **Radiologic examination, eye, for detection of foreign body**
Z3 X 80 — 0.84 — 0.84 FUD XXX

70100 **Radiologic examination, mandible; partial, less than 4 views**
Z3 X 80 — 0.99 — 0.99 FUD XXX

70110 **complete, minimum of 4 views**
Z3 X 80 — 1.14 — 1.14 FUD XXX

70120 **Radiologic examination, mastoids; less than 3 views per side**
Z3 X 80 — 1.03 — 1.03 FUD XXX

70130 **complete, minimum of 3 views per side**
Z2 X 80 — 1.65 — 1.65 FUD XXX

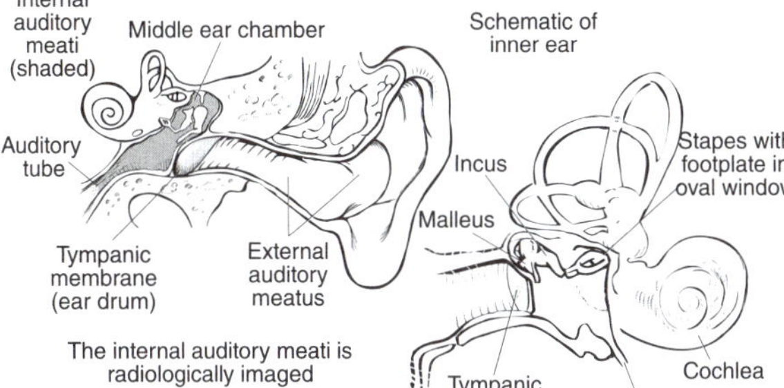

The internal auditory meati is radiologically imaged

70134 **Radiologic examination, internal auditory meati, complete**
Z2 X 80 — 1.58 — 1.58 FUD XXX

An x-ray of the facial bones is performed

70140 **Radiologic examination, facial bones; less than 3 views**
Z3 X 80 — 0.86 — 0.86 FUD XXX

70150 **complete, minimum of 3 views**
Z3 X 80 — 1.22 — 1.22 FUD XXX

70160 **Radiologic examination, nasal bones, complete, minimum of 3 views**
Z3 X 80 — 0.97 — 0.97 FUD XXX

70170 **Dacryocystography, nasolacrimal duct, radiological supervision and interpretation**
EXCLUDES *Injection of contrast (68850)*
N1 Q2 80 PQ — 0.00 — 0.00 FUD XXX

70190 **Radiologic examination; optic foramina**
Z3 X 80 — 1.04 — 1.04 FUD XXX

An x-ray of the orbits is performed

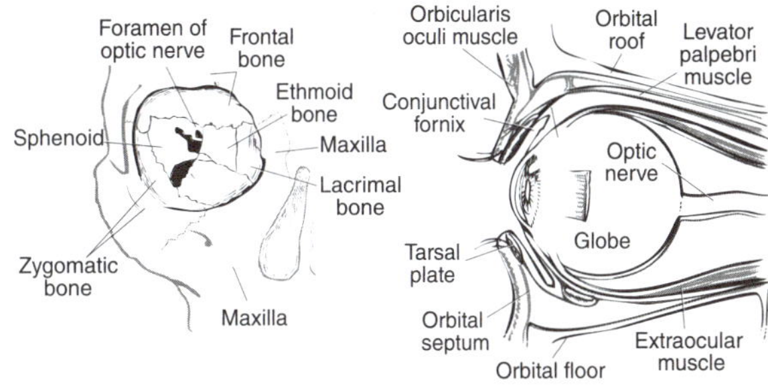

70200 **orbits, complete, minimum of 4 views**
Z3 X 80 — 1.25 — 1.25 FUD XXX

70210 **Radiologic examination, sinuses, paranasal, less than 3 views**
Z3 X 80 — 0.88 — 0.88 FUD XXX

70220 **Radiologic examination, sinuses, paranasal, complete, minimum of 3 views**
Z3 X 80 — 1.11 — 1.11 FUD XXX

70240 **Radiologic examination, sella turcica**
Z3 X 80 — 0.88 — 0.88 FUD XXX

70250 **Radiologic examination, skull; less than 4 views**
Z3 X 80 — 1.07 — 1.07 FUD XXX

70260 **complete, minimum of 4 views**
Z3 X 80 — 1.36 — 1.36 FUD XXX

Radiology
70010 — 70260

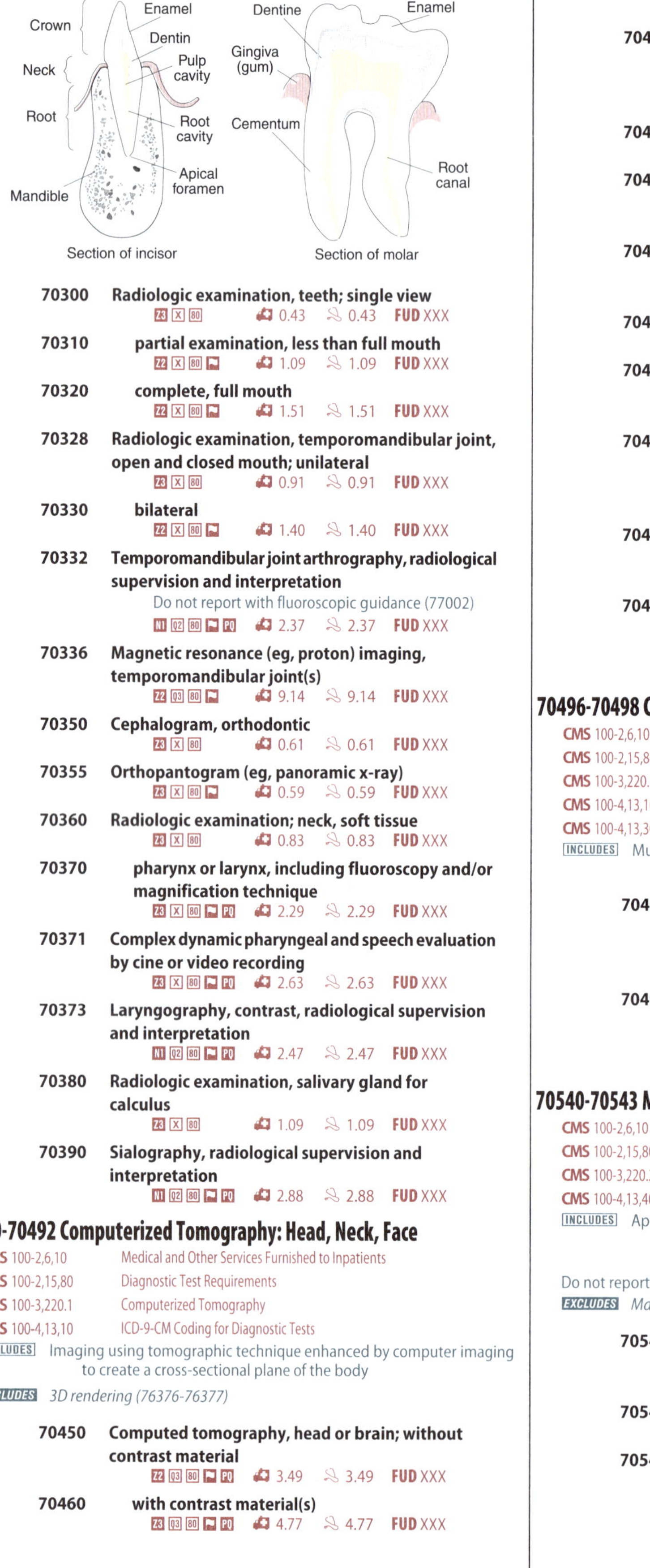

Section of incisor

Section of molar

70300 **Radiologic examination, teeth; single view**
Z3 X 80 — 0.43 — 0.43 — FUD XXX

70310 **partial examination, less than full mouth**
Z2 X 80 — 1.09 — 1.09 — FUD XXX

70320 **complete, full mouth**
Z2 X 80 — 1.51 — 1.51 — FUD XXX

70328 **Radiologic examination, temporomandibular joint, open and closed mouth; unilateral**
Z3 X 80 — 0.91 — 0.91 — FUD XXX

70330 **bilateral**
Z2 X 80 — 1.40 — 1.40 — FUD XXX

70332 **Temporomandibular joint arthrography, radiological supervision and interpretation**
Do not report with fluoroscopic guidance (77002)
N1 Q2 80 PQ — 2.37 — 2.37 — FUD XXX

70336 **Magnetic resonance (eg, proton) imaging, temporomandibular joint(s)**
Z2 Q3 80 — 9.14 — 9.14 — FUD XXX

70350 **Cephalogram, orthodontic**
Z3 X 80 — 0.61 — 0.61 — FUD XXX

70355 **Orthopantogram (eg, panoramic x-ray)**
Z3 X 80 — 0.59 — 0.59 — FUD XXX

70360 **Radiologic examination; neck, soft tissue**
Z3 X 80 — 0.83 — 0.83 — FUD XXX

70370 **pharynx or larynx, including fluoroscopy and/or magnification technique**
Z3 X 80 PQ — 2.29 — 2.29 — FUD XXX

70371 **Complex dynamic pharyngeal and speech evaluation by cine or video recording**
Z3 X 80 PQ — 2.63 — 2.63 — FUD XXX

70373 **Laryngography, contrast, radiological supervision and interpretation**
N1 Q2 80 PQ — 2.47 — 2.47 — FUD XXX

70380 **Radiologic examination, salivary gland for calculus**
Z3 X 80 — 1.09 — 1.09 — FUD XXX

70390 **Sialography, radiological supervision and interpretation**
N1 Q2 80 PQ — 2.88 — 2.88 — FUD XXX

70450-70492 Computerized Tomography: Head, Neck, Face

CMS 100-2,6,10 Medical and Other Services Furnished to Inpatients
CMS 100-2,15,80 Diagnostic Test Requirements
CMS 100-3,220.1 Computerized Tomography
CMS 100-4,13,10 ICD-9-CM Coding for Diagnostic Tests

INCLUDES Imaging using tomographic technique enhanced by computer imaging to create a cross-sectional plane of the body

EXCLUDES *3D rendering (76376-76377)*

70450 **Computed tomography, head or brain; without contrast material**
Z2 Q3 80 PQ — 3.49 — 3.49 — FUD XXX

70460 **with contrast material(s)**
Z3 Q3 80 PQ — 4.77 — 4.77 — FUD XXX

70470 **without contrast material, followed by contrast material(s) and further sections**
Z3 Q3 80 PQ — 5.73 — 5.73 — FUD XXX

70480 **Computed tomography, orbit, sella, or posterior fossa or outer, middle, or inner ear; without contrast material**
Z2 Q3 80 — 7.08 — 7.08 — FUD XXX

70481 **with contrast material(s)**
Z2 Q3 80 — 8.25 — 8.25 — FUD XXX

70482 **without contrast material, followed by contrast material(s) and further sections**
Z2 Q3 80 — 9.12 — 9.12 — FUD XXX

70486 **Computed tomography, maxillofacial area; without contrast material**
Z2 Q3 80 — 5.83 — 5.83 — FUD XXX

70487 **with contrast material(s)**
Z2 Q3 80 — 7.06 — 7.06 — FUD XXX

70488 **without contrast material, followed by contrast material(s) and further sections**
Z2 Q3 80 — 8.45 — 8.45 — FUD XXX

70490 **Computed tomography, soft tissue neck; without contrast material**
EXCLUDES *CT of the cervical spine (72125)*
Z2 Q3 80 — 5.77 — 5.77 — FUD XXX

70491 **with contrast material(s)**
EXCLUDES *CT of the cervical spine (72126)*
Z2 Q3 80 — 6.92 — 6.92 — FUD XXX

70492 **without contrast material followed by contrast material(s) and further sections**
EXCLUDES *CT of the cervical spine (72125-72127)*
Z2 Q3 80 — 8.22 — 8.22 — FUD XXX

70496-70498 Computerized Tomographic Angiography: Head and Neck

CMS 100-2,6,10 Medical and Other Services Furnished to Inpatients
CMS 100-2,15,80 Diagnostic Test Requirements
CMS 100-3,220.1 Computerized Tomography
CMS 100-4,13,10 ICD-9-CM Coding for Diagnostic Tests
CMS 100-4,13,30 Computerized Axial Tomography (CT) Procedures

INCLUDES Multiple rapid thin section CT scans to create cross-sectional images of bones, organs and tissues

70496 **Computed tomographic angiography, head, with contrast material(s), including noncontrast images, if performed, and image postprocessing**
Z2 Q3 80 — 12.59 — 12.59 — FUD XXX

70498 **Computed tomographic angiography, neck, with contrast material(s), including noncontrast images, if performed, and image postprocessing**
Z2 Q3 80 PQ — 13.07 — 13.07 — FUD XXX

70540-70543 Magnetic Resonance Imaging: Face, Neck, Orbits

CMS 100-2,6,10 Medical and Other Services Furnished to Inpatients
CMS 100-2,15,80 Diagnostic Test Requirements
CMS 100-3,220.2 Magnetic Resonance Imaging
CMS 100-4,13,40 Magnetic Resonance Imaging (MRI) Procedures

INCLUDES Application of an external magnetic field that forces alignment of hydrogen atom nuclei in soft tissues which converts to sets of tomographic images that can be displayed as three-dimensional images

Do not report more than one time per session

EXCLUDES *Magnetic resonance angiography head/neck (70544-70549)*

70540 **Magnetic resonance (eg, proton) imaging, orbit, face, and/or neck; without contrast material(s)**
Z2 Q3 80 — 10.19 — 10.19 — FUD XXX

70542 **with contrast material(s)**
Z2 Q3 80 — 11.64 — 11.64 — FUD XXX

70543 **without contrast material(s), followed by contrast material(s) and further sequences**
Z2 Q3 80 — 14.25 — 14.25 — FUD XXX

70544-70549 Magnetic Resonance Angiography: Head and Neck

CMS 100-2,6,10 Medical and Other Services Furnished to Inpatients
CMS 100-2,15,80 Diagnostic Test Requirements
CMS 100-3,220.3 Magnetic Resonance Angiography
CMS 100-4,13,10 ICD-9-CM Coding for Diagnostic Tests
CMS 100-4,13,40.1.1 Magnetic Resonance Angiography

INCLUDES Use of magnetic fields and radio waves to produce detailed cross-sectional images of internal body structures

70544 **Magnetic resonance angiography, head; without contrast material(s)**
Z2 03 80 11.42 11.42 FUD XXX

70545 **with contrast material(s)**
Z2 03 80 11.26 11.26 FUD XXX

70546 **without contrast material(s), followed by contrast material(s) and further sequences**
Z2 03 80 17.17 17.17 FUD XXX

70547 **Magnetic resonance angiography, neck; without contrast material(s)**
Z2 03 80 PQ 11.45 11.45 FUD XXX

70548 **with contrast material(s)**
Z2 03 80 PQ 12.02 12.02 FUD XXX

70549 **without contrast material(s), followed by contrast material(s) and further sequences**
Z2 03 80 PQ 17.28 17.28 FUD XXX

70551-70553 Magnetic Resonance Imaging: Brain and Brain Stem

CMS 100-2,6,10 Medical and Other Services Furnished to Inpatients
CMS 100-2,15,80 Diagnostic Test Requirements
CMS 100-3,220.2 Magnetic Resonance Imaging
CMS 100-4,13,10 ICD-9-CM Coding for Diagnostic Tests
CMS 100-4,13,20.1 Professional Component (PC)
CMS 100-4,13,40 Magnetic Resonance Imaging (MRI) Procedures

INCLUDES Application of an external magnetic field that forces alignment of hydrogen atom nuclei in soft tissues which converts to sets of tomographic images that can be displayed as three-dimensional images

EXCLUDES *Magnetic spectroscopy (76390)*

70551 **Magnetic resonance (eg, proton) imaging, brain (including brain stem); without contrast material**
Z2 03 80 PQ 6.91 6.91 FUD XXX

70552 **with contrast material(s)**
Z2 03 80 PQ 9.40 9.40 FUD XXX

70553 **without contrast material, followed by contrast material(s) and further sequences**
Z2 03 80 PQ 11.09 11.09 FUD XXX

70554-70555 Magnetic Resonance Imaging: Brain Mapping

INCLUDES Neuroimaging technique using MRI to identify and map signals related to brain activity

Do not report with the following codes unless a separate diagnostic MRI is performed (70551-70553)

70554 **Magnetic resonance imaging, brain, functional MRI; including test selection and administration of repetitive body part movement and/or visual stimulation, not requiring physician or psychologist administration**
EXCLUDES *Testing performed by a physician or psychologist (70555)*
Do not report with functional brain mapping (96020)
Z2 03 80 12.76 12.76 FUD XXX

70555 **requiring physician or psychologist administration of entire neurofunctional testing**
EXCLUDES *Testing performed by a technologist, nonphysician, or nonpsychologist (70554)*
Code also (96020)
Z2 S 80 0.00 0.00 FUD XXX

70557-70559 Magnetic Resonance Imaging: Intraoperative

EXCLUDES *Frequency greater than one for each code per operative session*
Intracranial lesion stereotaxic biopsy with magnetic resonance guidance (61751)

Code also only if a separate report is generated (70557-70559)
Do not report with (61751, 77021-77022)

70557 **Magnetic resonance (eg, proton) imaging, brain (including brain stem and skull base), during open intracranial procedure (eg, to assess for residual tumor or residual vascular malformation); without contrast material**
Z2 S 80 0.00 0.00 FUD XXX

70558 **with contrast material(s)**
Z2 S 80 0.00 0.00 FUD XXX

70559 **without contrast material(s), followed by contrast material(s) and further sequences**
Z2 S 80 0.00 0.00 FUD XXX

71010-71130 Radiography: Thorax

CMS 100-2,6,10 Medical and Other Services Furnished to Inpatients
CMS 100-2,15,80 Diagnostic Test Requirements
CMS 100-4,13,10 ICD-9-CM Coding for Diagnostic Tests

EXCLUDES *Needle placement guidance (76942, 77002)*

71010 **Radiologic examination, chest; single view, frontal**
EXCLUDES *Concurrent computer-aided detection (0174T)*
Do not report with (99291-99292)
Do not report with remotely performed CAD (0175T)
Z3 03 80 0.67 0.67 FUD XXX

71015 **stereo, frontal**
Do not report with (99291-99292)
Z3 03 80 0.86 0.86 FUD XXX

71020 **Radiologic examination, chest, 2 views, frontal and lateral;**
EXCLUDES *Concurrent computer-aided detection (0174T)*
Do not report with (99291-99292)
Do not report with remotely performed CAD (0175T)
Z3 03 80 0.87 0.87 FUD XXX

71021 **with apical lordotic procedure**
EXCLUDES *Concurrent computer-aided detection (0174T)*
Do not report with remotely performed CAD (0175T)
Z3 X 80 1.07 1.07 FUD XXX

71022 **with oblique projections**
EXCLUDES *Concurrent computer-aided detection (0174T)*
Do not report with remotely performed CAD (0175T)
Z3 X 80 1.33 1.33 FUD XXX

71023 **with fluoroscopy**
Z3 X 80 PQ 1.88 1.88 FUD XXX

71030 **Radiologic examination, chest, complete, minimum of 4 views;**
EXCLUDES *Concurrent computer-aided detection (0174T)*
Do not report with remotely performed CAD (0175T)
Z3 X 80 1.32 1.32 FUD XXX

71034 **with fluoroscopy**
EXCLUDES *Separate fluoroscopy of chest (76000)*
Z3 X 80 PQ 2.48 2.48 FUD XXX

71035 **Radiologic examination, chest, special views (eg, lateral decubitus, Bucky studies)**
Z3 X 80 1.04 1.04 FUD XXX

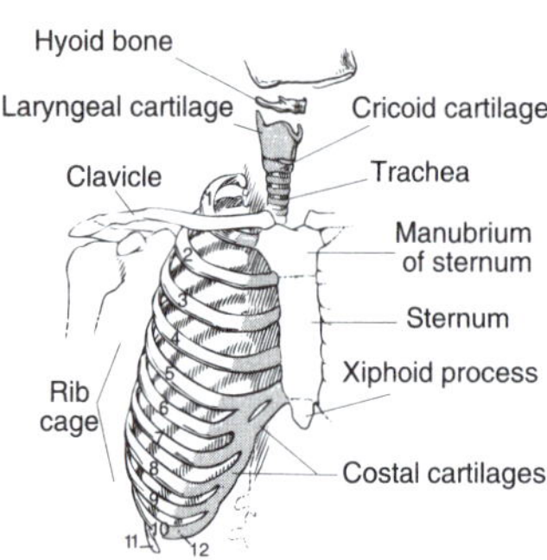

71100 **Radiologic examination, ribs, unilateral; 2 views** Z3 X 80 0.94 0.94 FUD XXX

71101 **including posteroanterior chest, minimum of 3 views** Z3 X 80 1.14 1.14 FUD XXX

71110 **Radiologic examination, ribs, bilateral; 3 views** Z3 X 80 1.17 1.17 FUD XXX

71111 **including posteroanterior chest, minimum of 4 views** Z3 X 80 1.53 1.53 FUD XXX

71120 **Radiologic examination; sternum, minimum of 2 views** Z3 X 80 0.91 0.91 FUD XXX

71130 **sternoclavicular joint or joints, minimum of 3 views** Z3 X 80 1.07 1.07 FUD XXX

71250-71270 Computerized Tomography: Thorax

CMS 100-2,6,10 Medical and Other Services Furnished to Inpatients
CMS 100-2,15,80 Diagnostic Test Requirements
CMS 100-3,220.1 Computerized Tomography
CMS 100-4,13,10 ICD-9-CM Coding for Diagnostic Tests
CMS 100-4,13,30 Computerized Axial Tomography (CT) Procedures

INCLUDES Imaging using tomographic technique enhanced by computer imaging to create a cross-sectional plane of the body

EXCLUDES *3D rendering (76376-76377)*
CT of the heart (75571-75574)

71250 **Computed tomography, thorax; without contrast material** Z2 03 80 5.39 5.39 FUD XXX

71260 **with contrast material(s)** Z2 03 80 6.75 6.75 FUD XXX

71270 **without contrast material, followed by contrast material(s) and further sections** Z2 03 80 8.14 8.14 FUD XXX

71275 Computerized Tomographic Angiography: Thorax

CMS 100-2,6,10 Medical and Other Services Furnished to Inpatients
CMS 100-2,15,80 Diagnostic Test Requirements
CMS 100-3,220.1 Computerized Tomography
CMS 100-4,13,10 ICD-9-CM Coding for Diagnostic Tests
CMS 100-4,13,30 Computerized Axial Tomography (CT) Procedures

INCLUDES Multiple rapid thin section CT scans to create cross-sectional images of bones, organs and tissues

EXCLUDES *CT angiography of coronary arteries that includes calcification score and/or cardiac morphology (75574)*

71275 **Computed tomographic angiography, chest (noncoronary), with contrast material(s), including noncontrast images, if performed, and image postprocessing** Z2 03 80 10.53 10.53 FUD XXX

71550-71552 Magnetic Resonance Imaging: Thorax

CMS 100-2,6,10 Medical and Other Services Furnished to Inpatients
CMS 100-2,15,80 Diagnostic Test Requirements
CMS 100-3,220.2 Magnetic Resonance Imaging
CMS 100-4,13,10 ICD-9-CM Coding for Diagnostic Tests
CMS 100-4,13,40 Magnetic Resonance Imaging (MRI) Procedures

INCLUDES Application of an external magnetic field that forces alignment of hydrogen atom nuclei in soft tissues which converts to sets of tomographic images that can be displayed as three-dimensional images

EXCLUDES *MRI of the breast (77058-77059)*

71550 **Magnetic resonance (eg, proton) imaging, chest (eg, for evaluation of hilar and mediastinal lymphadenopathy); without contrast material(s)** Z2 03 80 11.73 11.73 FUD XXX

71551 **with contrast material(s)** Z2 03 80 13.27 13.27 FUD XXX

71552 **without contrast material(s), followed by contrast material(s) and further sequences** Z2 03 80 16.70 16.70 FUD XXX

71555 Magnetic Resonance Angiography: Thorax

CMS 100-2,6,10 Medical and Other Services Furnished to Inpatients
CMS 100-2,15,80 Diagnostic Test Requirements
CMS 100-3,220.3 Magnetic Resonance Angiography
CMS 100-4,13,10 ICD-9-CM Coding for Diagnostic Tests
CMS 100-4,13,40.1.1 Magnetic Resonance Angiography

71555 **Magnetic resonance angiography, chest (excluding myocardium), with or without contrast material(s)** B 80 11.71 11.71 FUD XXX

72010-72120 Radiography: Spine

CMS 100-2,6,10 Medical and Other Services Furnished to Inpatients
CMS 100-2,15,80 Diagnostic Test Requirements
CMS 100-4,13,10 ICD-9-CM Coding for Diagnostic Tests

INCLUDES Minimum number of views or more views when needed to adequately complete the study
Radiographs that have to be repeated during the encounter due to substandard quality; only one unit of service is reported

EXCLUDES *Obtaining more films after review of initial films, based on the discretion of the radiologist, an order for the test, and a change in the patient's condition*

Do not report with a second interpretation by the requesting physician (included in E/M service)

72010 **Radiologic examination, spine, entire, survey study, anteroposterior and lateral** Z2 X 80 2.26 2.26 FUD XXX

72020 **Radiologic examination, spine, single view, specify level** Z3 X 80 0.66 0.66 FUD XXX

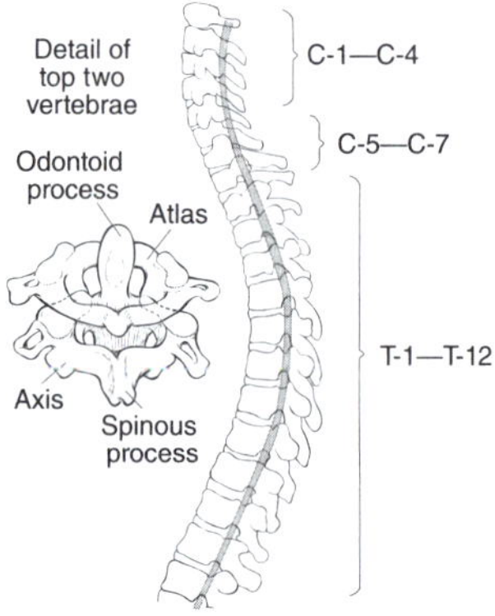

An x-ray of the cervical spine is performed

72040 Radiologic examination, spine, cervical; 2 or 3 views
1.03 1.03 FUD XXX

72050 4 or 5 views
1.39 1.39 FUD XXX

72052 6 or more views
1.78 1.78 FUD XXX

72069 Radiologic examination, spine, thoracolumbar, standing (scoliosis)
1.10 1.10 FUD XXX

72070 Radiologic examination, spine; thoracic, 2 views
0.96 0.96 FUD XXX

72072 thoracic, 3 views
1.07 1.07 FUD XXX

72074 thoracic, minimum of 4 views
1.27 1.27 FUD XXX

72080 thoracolumbar, 2 views
1.04 1.04 FUD XXX

72090 scoliosis study, including supine and erect studies
1.49 1.49 FUD XXX

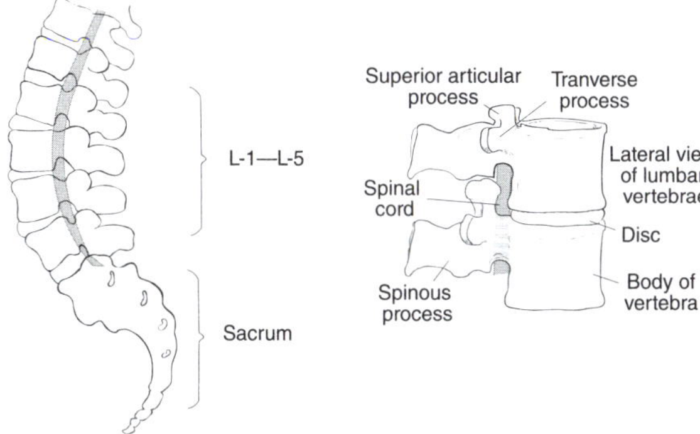

72100 Radiologic examination, spine, lumbosacral; 2 or 3 views
1.03 1.03 FUD XXX

72110 minimum of 4 views
1.41 1.41 FUD XXX

72114 complete, including bending views, minimum of 6 views
1.84 1.84 FUD XXX

72120 bending views only, 2 or 3 views
1.16 1.16 FUD XXX

72125-72133 Computerized Tomography: Spine

CMS 100-2,6,10 Medical and Other Services Furnished to Inpatients
CMS 100-2,15,80 Diagnostic Test Requirements
CMS 100-3,220.1 Computerized Tomography
CMS 100-4,13,10 ICD-9-CM Coding for Diagnostic Tests
CMS 100-4,13,30 Computerized Axial Tomography (CT) Procedures

INCLUDES Imaging using tomographic technique enhanced by computer imaging to create a cross-sectional plane of the body

EXCLUDES *3D rendering (76376-76377)*

Code also intrathecal injection procedure when performed (61055, 62284)

72125 Computed tomography, cervical spine; without contrast material
5.51 5.51 FUD XXX

72126 with contrast material
6.75 6.75 FUD XXX

72127 without contrast material, followed by contrast material(s) and further sections
8.03 8.03 FUD XXX

72128 Computed tomography, thoracic spine; without contrast material
5.40 5.40 FUD XXX

72129 with contrast material
6.75 6.75 FUD XXX

72130 without contrast material, followed by contrast material(s) and further sections
8.12 8.12 FUD XXX

72131 Computed tomography, lumbar spine; without contrast material
5.38 5.38 FUD XXX

72132 with contrast material
6.73 6.73 FUD XXX

72133 without contrast material, followed by contrast material(s) and further sections
8.04 8.04 FUD XXX

72141-72158 Magnetic Resonance Imaging: Spine

CMS 100-2,6,10 Medical and Other Services Furnished to Inpatients
CMS 100-2,15,80 Diagnostic Test Requirements
CMS 100-3,220.2 Magnetic Resonance Imaging
CMS 100-4,13,10 ICD-9-CM Coding for Diagnostic Tests
CMS 100-4,13,40 Magnetic Resonance Imaging (MRI) Procedures

INCLUDES Application of an external magnetic field that forces alignment of hydrogen atom nuclei in soft tissues which converts to sets of tomographic images that can be displayed as three-dimensional images

Code also intrathecal injection procedure when performed (61055, 62284)

72141 Magnetic resonance (eg, proton) imaging, spinal canal and contents, cervical; without contrast material
6.86 6.86 FUD XXX

72142 with contrast material(s)
EXCLUDES *MRI of cervical spinal canal performed without contrast followed by repeating the study with contrast (72156)*
9.43 9.43 FUD XXX

72146 Magnetic resonance (eg, proton) imaging, spinal canal and contents, thoracic; without contrast material
6.86 6.86 FUD XXX

72147 with contrast material(s)
EXCLUDES *MRI of thoracic spinal canal performed without contrast followed by repeating the study with contrast (72157)*
9.34 9.34 FUD XXX

72148 Magnetic resonance (eg, proton) imaging, spinal canal and contents, lumbar; without contrast material
6.87 6.87 FUD XXX

72149 with contrast material(s)
EXCLUDES *MRI of lumbar spinal canal performed without contrast followed by repeating the study with contrast (72158)*
9.31 9.31 FUD XXX

72156 Magnetic resonance (eg, proton) imaging, spinal canal and contents, without contrast material, followed by contrast material(s) and further sequences; cervical
11.10 11.10 FUD XXX

72157 thoracic
11.11 11.11 FUD XXX

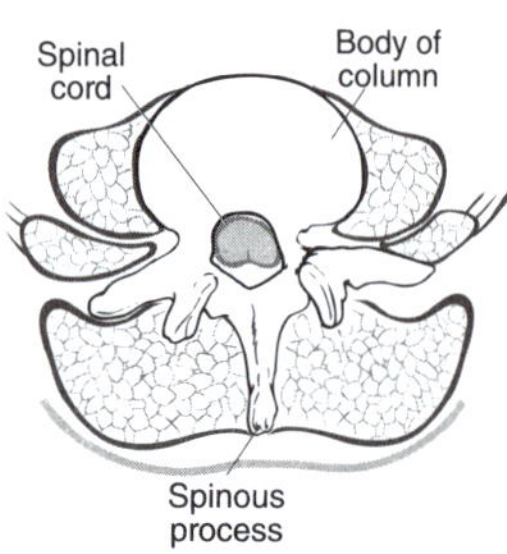

Superior view of thoracic spine and surrounding paraspinal muscles

72158 **lumbar**
Z2 03 80 ▭ 11.07 11.07 FUD XXX

72159 Magnetic Resonance Angiography: Spine

CMS 100-2,6,10 Medical and Other Services Furnished to Inpatients
CMS 100-2,15,80 Diagnostic Test Requirements
CMS 100-3,220.3 Magnetic Resonance Angiography
CMS 100-4,13,10 ICD-9-CM Coding for Diagnostic Tests
CMS 100-4,13,40 Magnetic Resonance Imaging (MRI) Procedures

72159 **Magnetic resonance angiography, spinal canal and contents, with or without contrast material(s)**
B 80 12.20 12.20 FUD XXX

72170-72190 Radiography: Pelvis

CMS 100-2,6,10 Medical and Other Services Furnished to Inpatients
CMS 100-2,15,80 Diagnostic Test Requirements
CMS 100-4,13,10 ICD-9-CM Coding for Diagnostic Tests

INCLUDES Minimum number of views or more views when needed to adequately complete the study
Radiographs that have to be repeated during the encounter due to substandard quality; only one unit of service is reported

EXCLUDES *Combined CT or CT angiography of abdomen and pelvis (74174, 74176-74178)*
Obtaining more films after review of initial films, based on the discretion of the radiologist, an order for the test, and a change in the patient's condition
Pelvimetry (74710)

Do not report with a second interpretation by the requesting physician (included in E/M service)

72170 **Radiologic examination, pelvis; 1 or 2 views**
Z3 X 80 0.83 0.83 FUD XXX

72190 **complete, minimum of 3 views**
Z2 X 80 ▭ 1.23 1.23 FUD XXX

72191 Computerized Tomographic Angiography: Pelvis

CMS 100-2,6,10 Medical and Other Services Furnished to Inpatients
CMS 100-2,15,80 Diagnostic Test Requirements
CMS 100-3,220.1 Computerized Tomography
CMS 100-4,13,10 ICD-9-CM Coding for Diagnostic Tests
CMS 100-4,13,30 Computerized Axial Tomography (CT) Procedures

INCLUDES Multiple rapid thin section CT scans to create cross-sectional images of bones, organs and tissues

Do not report with (73706, 74174-74175, 75635)

72191 **Computed tomographic angiography, pelvis, with contrast material(s), including noncontrast images, if performed, and image postprocessing**
Z2 03 80 ▭ 10.95 10.95 FUD XXX

72192-72194 Computerized Tomography: Pelvis

CMS 100-2,6,10 Medical and Other Services Furnished to Inpatients
CMS 100-2,15,80 Diagnostic Test Requirements
CMS 100-3,220.1 Computerized Tomography
CMS 100-4,13,10 ICD-9-CM Coding for Diagnostic Tests
CMS 100-4,13,30 Computerized Axial Tomography (CT) Procedures

EXCLUDES *3D rendering (76376-76377)*
Combined CT of abdomen and pelvis (74176-74178)
CT colonography, diagnostic (74261-74262)
CT colonography, screening (74263)

Do not report with (74261-74263)

72192 **Computed tomography, pelvis; without contrast material**
Z2 03 80 ▭ 4.26 4.26 FUD XXX

72193 **with contrast material(s)**
Z2 03 80 ▭ 6.64 6.64 FUD XXX

72194 **without contrast material, followed by contrast material(s) and further sections**
Z2 03 80 ▭ 7.77 7.77 FUD XXX

72195-72197 Magnetic Resonance Imaging: Pelvis

CMS 100-2,6,10 Medical and Other Services Furnished to Inpatients
CMS 100-2,15,80 Diagnostic Test Requirements
CMS 100-3,220.2 Magnetic Resonance Imaging
CMS 100-4,13,10 ICD-9-CM Coding for Diagnostic Tests
CMS 100-4,13,40 Magnetic Resonance Imaging (MRI) Procedures

INCLUDES Application of an external magnetic field that forces alignment of hydrogen atom nuclei in soft tissues which converts to sets of tomographic images that can be displayed as three-dimensional images

72195 **Magnetic resonance (eg, proton) imaging, pelvis; without contrast material(s)**
Z2 03 80 ▭ 10.66 10.66 FUD XXX

72196 **with contrast material(s)**
Z2 03 80 ▭ 11.96 11.96 FUD XXX

72197 **without contrast material(s), followed by contrast material(s) and further sequences**
Z2 03 80 ▭ 14.60 14.60 FUD XXX

72198 Magnetic Resonance Angiography: Pelvis

CMS 100-2,6,10 Medical and Other Services Furnished to Inpatients
CMS 100-2,15,80 Diagnostic Test Requirements
CMS 100-3,220.3 Magnetic Resonance Angiography
CMS 100-4,13,10 ICD-9-CM Coding for Diagnostic Tests
CMS 100-4,13,40.1.1 Magnetic Resonance Angiography

INCLUDES Use of magnetic fields and radio waves to produce detailed cross-sectional images of internal body structures

72198 **Magnetic resonance angiography, pelvis, with or without contrast material(s)**
B 80 ▭ 11.85 11.85 FUD XXX

72200-72220 Radiography: Pelvisacral

CMS 100-2,6,10 Medical and Other Services Furnished to Inpatients
CMS 100-2,15,80 Diagnostic Test Requirements
CMS 100-4,13,10 ICD-9-CM Coding for Diagnostic Tests

INCLUDES Minimum number of views or more views when needed to adequately complete the study
Radiographs that have to be repeated during the encounter due to substandard quality; only one unit of service is reported

EXCLUDES *Obtaining more films after review of initial films, based on the discretion of the radiologist, an order for the test, and a change in the patient's condition*

Do not report with second interpretation by the requesting physician (included in E/M service)

72200 **Radiologic examination, sacroiliac joints; less than 3 views**
Z3 X 80 0.85 0.85 FUD XXX

72202 **3 or more views**
Z3 X 80 ▭ 1.00 1.00 FUD XXX

72220 **Radiologic examination, sacrum and coccyx, minimum of 2 views**
Z3 X 80 0.83 0.83 FUD XXX

72240-72270 Myelography with Contrast: Spinal Cord

CMS 100-2,6,10 Medical and Other Services Furnished to Inpatients
CMS 100-2,15,80 Diagnostic Test Requirements
CMS 100-4,13,10 ICD-9-CM Coding for Diagnostic Tests

INCLUDES Fluoroscopic guidance for subarachnoid puncture for diagnostic radiographic myelography (77003)

Code also injection for myelogram at C1-C2 when appropriate (61055)
Do not report with (62284, 62302-62305)

72240 **Myelography, cervical, radiological supervision and interpretation**
N1 02 80 PQ 3.68 3.68 FUD XXX

72255 **Myelography, thoracic, radiological supervision and interpretation**
N1 02 80 PQ 3.50 3.50 FUD XXX

72265 **Myelography, lumbosacral, radiological supervision and interpretation**
N1 02 80 PQ 3.59 3.59 FUD XXX

72270 **Myelography, 2 or more regions (eg, lumbar/thoracic, cervical/thoracic, lumbar/cervical, lumbar/thoracic/cervical), radiological supervision and interpretation**
N1 02 80 PQ 5.58 5.58 FUD XXX

72275 Radiography: Epidural Space

CMS 100-2,15,80 Diagnostic Test Requirements
CMS 100-4,13,10 ICD-9-CM Coding for Diagnostic Tests

INCLUDES Epidurogram, documentation of images, formal written report
Fluoroscopic guidance (77003)

Code also injection procedure as appropriate (62280-62282, 62310-62319, 64479-64484)
Do not report with (22586, 0195T-0196T, 0309T)

72275 **Epidurography, radiological supervision and interpretation**
N1 N PQ 3.30 3.30 FUD XXX

72285 Radiography: Intervertebral Disc (Cervical/Thoracic)

CMS 100-2,6,10 Medical and Other Services Furnished to Inpatients
CMS 100-2,15,80 Diagnostic Test Requirements
CMS 100-4,13,10 ICD-9-CM Coding for Diagnostic Tests

Code also discography injection procedure (62291)

72285 **Discography, cervical or thoracic, radiological supervision and interpretation**
N1 02 80 PQ 3.26 3.26 FUD XXX

72291-72292 Radiography: Percutaneous Vertebral Augmentation

~~72291~~ ~~**Radiological supervision and interpretation, percutaneous vertebroplasty, vertebral augmentation, or sacral augmentation (sacroplasty), including cavity creation, per vertebral body or sacrum; under fluoroscopic guidance**~~
To report, see 0200T-0201T, 22510-22515

~~72292~~ ~~**under CT guidance**~~
To report, see 0200T-0201T, 22510-22515

72295 Radiography: Intervertebral Disc (Lumbar)

CMS 100-2,6,10 Medical and Other Services Furnished to Inpatients
CMS 100-2,15,80 Diagnostic Test Requirements
CMS 100-4,13,10 ICD-9-CM Coding for Diagnostic Tests

Code also discography injection procedure (62290)

72295 **Discography, lumbar, radiological supervision and interpretation**
N1 02 80 PQ 2.82 2.82 FUD XXX

73000-73085 Radiography: Shoulder and Upper Arm

CMS 100-2,15,80 Diagnostic Test Requirements
CMS 100-4,13,10 ICD-9-CM Coding for Diagnostic Tests

INCLUDES Minimum number of views or more views when needed to adequately complete the study
Radiographs that have to be repeated during the encounter due to substandard quality; only one unit of service is reported

EXCLUDES *Obtaining more films after review of initial films, based on the discretion of the radiologist, an order for the test, and a change in the patient's condition*
Stress views of upper body joint(s), when performed (77071)

Do not report with a second interpretation by the requesting physician (included in E/M service)

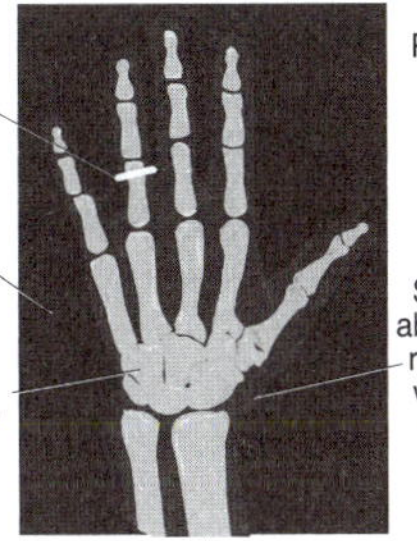

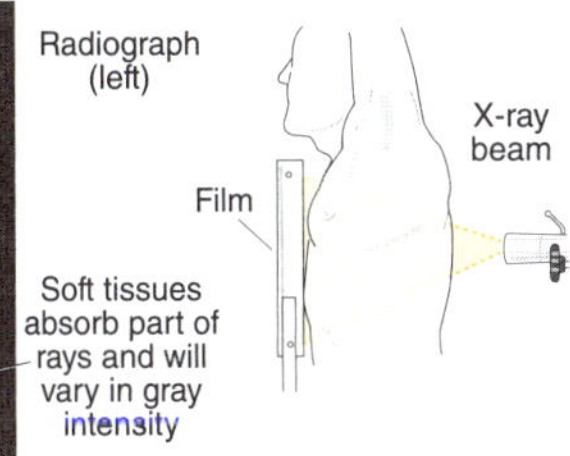

Posterioranterior (PA) chest study, lateral views also common

73000 **Radiologic examination; clavicle, complete**
Z3 X 80 0.83 0.83 FUD XXX

73010 **scapula, complete**
Z3 X 80 0.92 0.92 FUD XXX

73020 **Radiologic examination, shoulder; 1 view**
Z3 X 80 0.68 0.68 FUD XXX

73030 **complete, minimum of 2 views**
Z3 X 80 0.89 0.89 FUD XXX

73040 **Radiologic examination, shoulder, arthrography, radiological supervision and interpretation**
Code also arthrography injection procedure (23350)
Do not report with (77002)
N1 02 80 PQ 3.00 3.00 FUD XXX

73050 **Radiologic examination; acromioclavicular joints, bilateral, with or without weighted distraction**
Z3 X 80 1.14 1.14 FUD XXX

73060 **humerus, minimum of 2 views**
Z3 X 80 0.83 0.83 FUD XXX

73070 **Radiologic examination, elbow; 2 views**
Z3 X 80 0.81 0.81 FUD XXX

73080 **complete, minimum of 3 views**
Z3 X 80 0.96 0.96 FUD XXX

73085 **Radiologic examination, elbow, arthrography, radiological supervision and interpretation**
Do not report with (77002)
Code also arthrography injection procedure (24220)
N1 02 80 PQ 2.90 2.90 FUD XXX

73090-73140 Radiography: Forearm and Hand

CMS 100-2,15,80 Diagnostic Test Requirements
CMS 100-4,13,10 ICD-9-CM Coding for Diagnostic Tests

INCLUDES Minimum number of views or more views when needed to adequately complete the study
Radiographs that have to be repeated during the encounter due to substandard quality; only one unit of service is reported

EXCLUDES *Obtaining more films after review of initial films, based on the discretion of the radiologist, an order for the test, and a change in the patient's condition*
Stress views of upper body joint(s), when performed (77071)

Do not report with a second interpretation by the requesting physician (included in E/M service)

73090 **Radiologic examination; forearm, 2 views**
Z3 X 80 0.80 0.80 FUD XXX

73092 upper extremity, infant, minimum of 2 views
0.81 0.81 FUD XXX

73100 Radiologic examination, wrist; 2 views
0.90 0.90 FUD XXX

73110 complete, minimum of 3 views
1.08 1.08 FUD XXX

73115 Radiologic examination, wrist, arthrography, radiological supervision and interpretation
Code also arthrography injection procedure (25246)
Do not report with (77002)
3.16 3.16 FUD XXX

73120 Radiologic examination, hand; 2 views
0.79 0.79 FUD XXX

73130 minimum of 3 views
0.94 0.94 FUD XXX

73140 Radiologic examination, finger(s), minimum of 2 views
0.95 0.95 FUD XXX

73200-73202 Computerized Tomography: Shoulder, Arm, Hand

CMS 100-2,6,10 Medical and Other Services Furnished to Inpatients
CMS 100-2,15,80 Diagnostic Test Requirements
CMS 100-3,220.1 Computerized Tomography
CMS 100-4,13,10 ICD-9-CM Coding for Diagnostic Tests
CMS 100-4,13,30 Computerized Axial Tomography (CT) Procedures

INCLUDES Imaging using tomographic technique enhanced by computer imaging to create a cross-sectional plane of the body
Intravascular, intrathecal, or intra-articular contrast materials when noted in code descriptor

EXCLUDES *3D rendering (76376-76377)*

73200 Computed tomography, upper extremity; without contrast material
5.39 5.39 FUD XXX

73201 with contrast material(s)
6.59 6.59 FUD XXX

73202 without contrast material, followed by contrast material(s) and further sections
8.40 8.40 FUD XXX

73206 Computerized Tomographic Angiography: Shoulder, Arm, and Hand

CMS 100-2,6,10 Medical and Other Services Furnished to Inpatients
CMS 100-2,15,80 Diagnostic Test Requirements
CMS 100-3,220.1 Computerized Tomography
CMS 100-4,13,10 ICD-9-CM Coding for Diagnostic Tests
CMS 100-4,13,30 Computerized Axial Tomography (CT) Procedures

INCLUDES Intravascular, intrathecal, or intra-articular contrast materials when noted in code descriptor
Multiple rapid thin section CT scans to create cross-sectional images of bones, organs and tissues

73206 Computed tomographic angiography, upper extremity, with contrast material(s), including noncontrast images, if performed, and image postprocessing
9.45 9.45 FUD XXX

73218-73223 Magnetic Resonance Imaging: Shoulder, Arm, Hand

CMS 100-2,6,10 Medical and Other Services Furnished to Inpatients
CMS 100-2,15,80 Diagnostic Test Requirements
CMS 100-3,220.2 Magnetic Resonance Imaging
CMS 100-4,13,10 ICD-9-CM Coding for Diagnostic Tests
CMS 100-4,13,30 Computerized Axial Tomography (CT) Procedures

INCLUDES Application of an external magnetic field that forces alignment of hydrogen atom nuclei in soft tissues which converts to sets of tomographic images that can be displayed as three-dimensional images
Intravascular, intrathecal, or intra-articular contrast materials when noted in code descriptor

73218 Magnetic resonance (eg, proton) imaging, upper extremity, other than joint; without contrast material(s)
10.36 10.36 FUD XXX

73219 with contrast material(s)
11.78 11.78 FUD XXX

73220 without contrast material(s), followed by contrast material(s) and further sequences
14.45 14.45 FUD XXX

73221 Magnetic resonance (eg, proton) imaging, any joint of upper extremity; without contrast material(s)
7.18 7.18 FUD XXX

73222 with contrast material(s)
11.00 11.00 FUD XXX

73223 without contrast material(s), followed by contrast material(s) and further sequences
13.63 13.63 FUD XXX

73225 Magnetic Resonance Angiography: Shoulder, Arm, Hand

CMS 100-2,6,10 Medical and Other Services Furnished to Inpatients
CMS 100-2,15,80 Diagnostic Test Requirements
CMS 100-3,220.3 Magnetic Resonance Angiography
CMS 100-4,13,10 ICD-9-CM Coding for Diagnostic Tests
CMS 100-4,13,40.1.1 Magnetic Resonance Angiography

INCLUDES Intravascular, intrathecal, or intra-articular contrast materials when noted in code descriptor
Use of magnetic fields and radio waves to produce detailed cross-sectional images of internal body structures

73225 Magnetic resonance angiography, upper extremity, with or without contrast material(s)
12.03 12.03 FUD XXX

73500-73550 Radiography: Pelvic Region and Thigh

CMS 100-2,6,10 Medical and Other Services Furnished to Inpatients
CMS 100-2,15,80 Diagnostic Test Requirements
CMS 100-4,13,10 ICD-9-CM Coding for Diagnostic Tests

EXCLUDES *Stress views of lower body joint(s), when performed (77071)*

73500 Radiologic examination, hip, unilateral; 1 view
0.78 0.78 FUD XXX

73510 complete, minimum of 2 views
1.13 1.13 FUD XXX

73520 Radiologic examination, hips, bilateral, minimum of 2 views of each hip, including anteroposterior view of pelvis
1.19 1.19 FUD XXX

73525 Radiologic examination, hip, arthrography, radiological supervision and interpretation
Do not report with (77002)
2.94 2.94 FUD XXX

73530 Radiologic examination, hip, during operative procedure
0.00 0.00 FUD XXX

73540 Radiologic examination, pelvis and hips, infant or child, minimum of 2 views
1.24 1.24 FUD XXX

73550 Radiologic examination, femur, 2 views
0.82 0.82 FUD XXX

73560-73660 Radiography: Lower Leg, Ankle, and Foot

CMS 100-2,15,80 Diagnostic Test Requirements
CMS 100-4,13,10 ICD-9-CM Coding for Diagnostic Tests

EXCLUDES *Stress views of lower body joint(s), when performed (77071)*

73560 Radiologic examination, knee; 1 or 2 views
0.88 0.88 FUD XXX

73562 3 views
1.07 1.07 FUD XXX

73564 complete, 4 or more views
1.24 1.24 FUD XXX

73565 both knees, standing, anteroposterior
1.02 1.02 FUD XXX

73580 **Radiologic examination, knee, arthrography, radiological supervision and interpretation**
Do not report with (77002)
N1 Q2 80 PQ 3.61 3.61 FUD XXX

73590 **Radiologic examination; tibia and fibula, 2 views**
Z3 X 80 0.79 0.79 FUD XXX

73592 **lower extremity, infant, minimum of 2 views** A
Z3 X 80 0.81 0.81 FUD XXX

73600 **Radiologic examination, ankle; 2 views**
Z3 X 80 0.82 0.82 FUD XXX

73610 **complete, minimum of 3 views**
Z3 X 80 0.96 0.96 FUD XXX

73615 **Radiologic examination, ankle, arthrography, radiological supervision and interpretation**
Do not report with (77002)
N1 Q2 80 PQ 2.94 2.94 FUD XXX

73620 **Radiologic examination, foot; 2 views**
Z3 X 80 0.78 0.78 FUD XXX

73630 **complete, minimum of 3 views**
Z3 X 80 0.90 0.90 FUD XXX

73650 **Radiologic examination; calcaneus, minimum of 2 views**
Z3 X 80 0.81 0.81 FUD XXX

73660 **toe(s), minimum of 2 views**
Z3 X 80 0.87 0.87 FUD XXX

73700-73702 Computerized Tomography: Leg, Ankle, and Foot

CMS 100-2,6,10 Medical and Other Services Furnished to Inpatients
CMS 100-2,15,80 Diagnostic Test Requirements
CMS 100-3,220.1 Computerized Tomography
CMS 100-4,13,10 ICD-9-CM Coding for Diagnostic Tests

EXCLUDES *3D rendering (76376-76377)*

73700 **Computed tomography, lower extremity; without contrast material**
Z2 Q3 80 5.39 5.39 FUD XXX

73701 **with contrast material(s)**
Z2 Q3 80 6.67 6.67 FUD XXX

73702 **without contrast material, followed by contrast material(s) and further sections**
Z2 Q3 80 8.33 8.33 FUD XXX

73706 Computerized Tomographic Angiography: Leg, Ankle, and Foot

CMS 100-2,6,10 Medical and Other Services Furnished to Inpatients
CMS 100-2,15,80 Diagnostic Test Requirements
CMS 100-4,13,10 ICD-9-CM Coding for Diagnostic Tests

73706 **Computed tomographic angiography, lower extremity, with contrast material(s), including noncontrast images, if performed, and image postprocessing**
EXCLUDES *CT angiography for aorto-iliofemoral runoff (75635)*
Z2 Q3 80 10.51 10.51 FUD XXX

73718-73723 Magnetic Resonance Imaging: Leg, Ankle, and Foot

CMS 100-2,6,10 Medical and Other Services Furnished to Inpatients
CMS 100-2,15,80 Diagnostic Test Requirements
CMS 100-3,220.2 Magnetic Resonance Imaging
CMS 100-4,13,10 ICD-9-CM Coding for Diagnostic Tests
CMS 100-4,13,40 Magnetic Resonance Imaging (MRI) Procedures

73718 **Magnetic resonance (eg, proton) imaging, lower extremity other than joint; without contrast material(s)**
Z2 Q3 80 10.36 10.36 FUD XXX

73719 **with contrast material(s)**
Z2 Q3 80 11.82 11.82 FUD XXX

73720 **without contrast material(s), followed by contrast material(s) and further sequences**
Z2 Q3 80 14.53 14.53 FUD XXX

73721 **Magnetic resonance (eg, proton) imaging, any joint of lower extremity; without contrast material**
Z2 Q3 80 7.19 7.19 FUD XXX

73722 **with contrast material(s)**
Z2 Q3 80 11.15 11.15 FUD XXX

73723 **without contrast material(s), followed by contrast material(s) and further sequences**
Z2 Q3 80 13.67 13.67 FUD XXX

73725 Magnetic Resonance Angiography: Leg, Ankle, and Foot

CMS 100-2,6,10 Medical and Other Services Furnished to Inpatients
CMS 100-2,15,80 Diagnostic Test Requirements
CMS 100-3,220.3 Magnetic Resonance Angiography
CMS 100-4,13,10 ICD-9-CM Coding for Diagnostic Tests
CMS 100-4,13,40.1.1 Magnetic Resonance Angiography

73725 **Magnetic resonance angiography, lower extremity, with or without contrast material(s)**
B 80 11.88 11.88 FUD XXX

74000-74022 Radiography: Abdomen--General

CMS 100-2,15,80 Diagnostic Test Requirements
CMS 100-4,13,10 ICD-9-CM Coding for Diagnostic Tests

74000 **Radiologic examination, abdomen; single anteroposterior view**
Z3 X 80 0.70 0.70 FUD XXX

74010 **anteroposterior and additional oblique and cone views**
Z3 X 80 1.11 1.11 FUD XXX

74020 **complete, including decubitus and/or erect views**
Z3 X 80 1.16 1.16 FUD XXX

Esophagus
Diaphragm
Liver
Abdomen
Pelvis area

74022 **complete acute abdomen series, including supine, erect, and/or decubitus views, single view chest**
Z3 X 80 1.40 1.40 FUD XXX

74150-74170 Computerized Tomography: Abdomen–General

CMS 100-2,6,10 Medical and Other Services Furnished to Inpatients
CMS 100-2,15,80 Diagnostic Test Requirements
CMS 100-3,220.1 Computerized Tomography
CMS 100-4,13,10 ICD-9-CM Coding for Diagnostic Tests
CMS 100-4,13,30 Computerized Axial Tomography (CT) Procedures

EXCLUDES *3D rendering (76376-76377)*
Combined CT of abdomen and pelvis (74176-74178)
CT colonography, diagnostic (74185-74190)
CT colonography, screening (74263)

Do not report with CT colonography (74185-74210)

74150 **Computed tomography, abdomen; without contrast material**
Z2 Q3 80 4.36 4.36 FUD XXX

74160 **with contrast material(s)**
Z2 Q3 80 6.77 6.77 FUD XXX

74170 without contrast material, followed by contrast material(s) and further sections
Z2 03 80 7.82 7.82 FUD XXX

74174-74175 Computerized Tomographic Angiography: Abdomen and Pelvis

CMS 100-2,6,10 Medical and Other Services Furnished to Inpatients
CMS 100-2,15,80 Diagnostic Test Requirements
CMS 100-3,220.1 Computerized Tomography
CMS 100-4,13,10 ICD-9-CM Coding for Diagnostic Tests
CMS 100-4,13,30 Computerized Axial Tomography (CT) Procedures

EXCLUDES *CT angiography for aorto-iliofemoral runoff (75635)*

74174 Computed tomographic angiography, abdomen and pelvis, with contrast material(s), including noncontrast images, if performed, and image postprocessing
Do not report with (72191, 73706, 74175, 75635, 76376-76377)
Z2 S 80 15.31 15.31 FUD XXX

74175 Computed tomographic angiography, abdomen, with contrast material(s), including noncontrast images, if performed, and image postprocessing
EXCLUDES *Combined CT angiography study of abdomen and pelvis (74174)*
Do not report with (72191, 73706, 75635)
Z2 03 80 10.90 10.90 FUD XXX

74176-74178 Computerized Tomography: Abdomen and Pelvis

Do not report more than one time for each combined examination of the abdomen and pelvis
Do not report with (72192-72194, 74150-74170)

74176 Computed tomography, abdomen and pelvis; without contrast material
Z3 03 6.11 6.11 FUD XXX

74177 with contrast material(s)
Z2 03 9.14 9.14 FUD XXX

74178 without contrast material in one or both body regions, followed by contrast material(s) and further sections in one or both body regions
Z2 03 10.64 10.64 FUD XXX

74181-74183 Magnetic Resonance Imaging: Abdomen–General

CMS 100-2,6,10 Medical and Other Services Furnished to Inpatients
CMS 100-2,15,80 Diagnostic Test Requirements
CMS 100-3,220.2 Magnetic Resonance Imaging
CMS 100-4,13,10 ICD-9-CM Coding for Diagnostic Tests
CMS 100-4,13,40 Magnetic Resonance Imaging (MRI) Procedures

74181 Magnetic resonance (eg, proton) imaging, abdomen; without contrast material(s)
Z2 03 80 9.50 9.50 FUD XXX

74182 with contrast material(s)
Z2 03 80 13.09 13.09 FUD XXX

74183 without contrast material(s), followed by with contrast material(s) and further sequences
Z2 03 80 14.65 14.65 FUD XXX

74185 Magnetic Resonance Angiography: Abdomen–General

CMS 100-2,6,10 Medical and Other Services Furnished to Inpatients
CMS 100-2,15,80 Diagnostic Test Requirements
CMS 100-3,220.3 Magnetic Resonance Angiography
CMS 100-4,13,10 ICD-9-CM Coding for Diagnostic Tests
CMS 100-4,13,40.1.1 Magnetic Resonance Angiography

74185 Magnetic resonance angiography, abdomen, with or without contrast material(s)
B 80 11.88 11.88 FUD XXX

74190 Peritoneography

CMS 100-2,15,80 Diagnostic Test Requirements
CMS 100-4,13,10 ICD-9-CM Coding for Diagnostic Tests

74190 Peritoneogram (eg, after injection of air or contrast), radiological supervision and interpretation
EXCLUDES *Computed tomography, pelvis or abdomen (72192, 74150)*
Code also injection procedure (49400)
N1 Q2 80 PQ 0.00 0.00 FUD XXX

74210-74235 Radiography: Throat and Esophagus

CMS 100-2,15,80 Diagnostic Test Requirements
CMS 100-4,13,10 ICD-9-CM Coding for Diagnostic Tests

EXCLUDES *Percutaneous placement of gastrostomy tube, endoscopic (43246)*
Percutaneous placement of gastrostomy tube, fluoroscopic guidance (49440)

74210 Radiologic examination; pharynx and/or cervical esophagus
Z2 S 80 PQ 2.24 2.24 FUD XXX

74220 esophagus
Z2 S 80 PQ 2.62 2.62 FUD XXX

74230 Swallowing function, with cineradiography/videoradiography
Z2 S 80 PQ 2.62 2.62 FUD XXX

74235 Removal of foreign body(s), esophageal, with use of balloon catheter, radiological supervision and interpretation
Code also procedure (43499)
N1 N 80 PQ 0.00 0.00 FUD XXX

74240-74283 Radiography: Intestines

CMS 100-2,6,10 Medical and Other Services Furnished to Inpatients
CMS 100-2,15,80 Diagnostic Test Requirements
CMS 100-4,13,10 ICD-9-CM Coding for Diagnostic Tests

EXCLUDES *Percutaneous placement of gastrostomy tube, endoscopic (43246)*
Percutaneous placement of gastrostomy tube, fluoroscopic guidance (49440)

74240 Radiologic examination, gastrointestinal tract, upper; with or without delayed films, without KUB
Z3 S 80 PQ 3.28 3.28 FUD XXX

74241 with or without delayed films, with KUB
Z2 S 80 PQ 3.41 3.41 FUD XXX

74245 with small intestine, includes multiple serial films
Z2 S 80 PQ 5.10 5.10 FUD XXX

74246 Radiological examination, gastrointestinal tract, upper, air contrast, with specific high density barium, effervescent agent, with or without glucagon; with or without delayed films, without KUB
INCLUDES Moynihan test
Z2 S 80 PQ 3.69 3.69 FUD XXX

74247 with or without delayed films, with KUB
Z2 S 80 PQ 4.10 4.10 FUD XXX

74249 with small intestine follow-through
Z2 S 80 PQ 5.50 5.50 FUD XXX

74250 Radiologic examination, small intestine, includes multiple serial films;
Z2 S 80 PQ 3.10 3.10 FUD XXX

74251 via enteroclysis tube
Z2 S 80 PQ 11.83 11.83 FUD XXX

74260 Duodenography, hypotonic
Z2 S 80 PQ 9.81 9.81 FUD XXX

74261 Computed tomographic (CT) colonography, diagnostic, including image postprocessing; without contrast material
Do not report with (72192-72194, 74150-74170, 74263, 76376-76377)
Z2 03 80 13.55 13.55 FUD XXX

74262 with contrast material(s) including non-contrast images, if performed
Do not report with (72192-72194, 74150-74170, 74263, 76376-76377)
Z2 03 80 14.88 14.88 FUD XXX

74263 Computed tomographic (CT) colonography, screening, including image postprocessing
Do not report with (72192-72194, 74150-74170, 74261-74262, 76376-76377)
E 21.12 21.12 FUD XXX

74270 Radiologic examination, colon; contrast (eg, barium) enema, with or without KUB
Z2 S 80 PQ 4.51 4.51 FUD XXX

74280 air contrast with specific high density barium, with or without glucagon
Z2 S 80 PQ 6.30 6.30 FUD XXX

74283 Therapeutic enema, contrast or air, for reduction of intussusception or other intraluminal obstruction (eg, meconium ileus)
Z2 S 80 PQ 5.80 5.80 FUD XXX

74290-74330 Radiography: Biliary Tract

CMS 100-2,15,80 Diagnostic Test Requirements
CMS 100-4,13,10 ICD-9-CM Coding for Diagnostic Tests

74290 Cholecystography, oral contrast
Z2 S 80 PQ 2.00 2.00 FUD XXX

~~74291 additional or repeat examination or multiple day examination~~

74300 Cholangiography and/or pancreatography; intraoperative, radiological supervision and interpretation
N1 N 80 PQ 0.00 0.00 FUD XXX

+ 74301 additional set intraoperative, radiological supervision and interpretation (List separately in addition to code for primary procedure)
Code first (74300)
N1 N 80 0.00 0.00 FUD ZZZ

74305 through existing catheter, radiological supervision and interpretation
EXCLUDES *Percutaneous biliary duct stone extraction (47630, 74327)*
Code also procedure performed (47505, 47560-47561, 47563, 48400)
N1 Q2 80 PQ 0.00 0.00 FUD XXX

74320 Cholangiography, percutaneous, transhepatic, radiological supervision and interpretation
INCLUDES Needle placement with fluoroscopic guidance (77002)
N1 Q2 80 PQ 2.77 2.77 FUD XXX

74327 Postoperative biliary duct calculus removal, percutaneous via T-tube tract, basket, or snare (eg, Burhenne technique), radiological supervision and interpretation
Code also percutaneous biliary duct stone extraction (47630)
N1 N 80 PQ 3.98 3.98 FUD XXX

74328 Endoscopic catheterization of the biliary ductal system, radiological supervision and interpretation
Code also ERCP (43260-43272 [43274, 43275, 43276, 43277, 43278])
N1 N 80 PQ 0.00 0.00 FUD XXX

74329 Endoscopic catheterization of the pancreatic ductal system, radiological supervision and interpretation
Code also ERCP (43260-43272 [43274, 43275, 43276, 43277, 43278])
N1 N 80 PQ 0.00 0.00 FUD XXX

74330 Combined endoscopic catheterization of the biliary and pancreatic ductal systems, radiological supervision and interpretation
Code also ERCP (43260-43272 [43274, 43275, 43276, 43277, 43278])
N1 N 80 PQ 0.00 0.00 FUD XXX

74340-74363 Radiography: Bilidigestive Intubation

CMS 100-2,15,80 Diagnostic Test Requirements
CMS 100-4,13,10 ICD-9-CM Coding for Diagnostic Tests
EXCLUDES *Percutaneous insertion of gastrostomy tube, endoscopic (43246)*
Percutaneous placement of gastrotomy tube, fluoroscopic guidance (49440)

74340 Introduction of long gastrointestinal tube (eg, Miller-Abbott), including multiple fluoroscopies and films, radiological supervision and interpretation
Code also placement of tube (44500)
N1 N 80 PQ 0.00 0.00 FUD XXX

74355 Percutaneous placement of enteroclysis tube, radiological supervision and interpretation
INCLUDES Fluoroscopic guidance (77002)
N1 N 80 PQ 0.00 0.00 FUD XXX

74360 Intraluminal dilation of strictures and/or obstructions (eg, esophagus), radiological supervision and interpretation
Do not report with ([43213, 43214], [43233])
N1 N 80 PQ 0.00 0.00 FUD XXX

74363 Percutaneous transhepatic dilation of biliary duct stricture with or without placement of stent, radiological supervision and interpretation
EXCLUDES *Surgical procedure (47510-47511, 47555-47556)*
N1 N 80 PQ 0.00 0.00 FUD XXX

74400-74775 Radiography: Urogenital

CMS 100-2,15,80 Diagnostic Test Requirements
CMS 100-4,13,10 ICD-9-CM Coding for Diagnostic Tests

74400 Urography (pyelography), intravenous, with or without KUB, with or without tomography
Z2 S 80 3.23 3.23 FUD XXX

74410 Urography, infusion, drip technique and/or bolus technique;
Z2 S 80 3.17 3.17 FUD XXX

74415 with nephrotomography
Z2 S 80 3.94 3.94 FUD XXX

74420 Urography, retrograde, with or without KUB
Z2 S 80 0.00 0.00 FUD XXX

74425 Urography, antegrade (pyelostogram, nephrostogram, loopogram), radiological supervision and interpretation
N1 Q2 80 PQ 0.00 0.00 FUD XXX

74430 Cystography, minimum of 3 views, radiological supervision and interpretation
N1 Q2 80 PQ 1.17 1.17 FUD XXX

74440 Vasography, vesiculography, or epididymography, radiological supervision and interpretation ♂
N1 Q2 80 PQ 2.34 2.34 FUD XXX

74445 Corpora cavernosography, radiological supervision and interpretation ♂
INCLUDES Needle placement with fluoroscopic guidance (77002)
N1 Q2 80 PQ 0.00 0.00 FUD XXX

74450 Urethrocystography, retrograde, radiological supervision and interpretation
N1 Q2 80 PQ 0.00 0.00 FUD XXX

74455 Urethrocystography, voiding, radiological supervision and interpretation
N1 Q2 80 PQ 2.38 2.38 FUD XXX

74470 Radiologic examination, renal cyst study, translumbar, contrast visualization, radiological supervision and interpretation
INCLUDES Needle placement with fluoroscopic guidance (77002)
N1 Q2 80 PQ 0.00 0.00 FUD XXX

74475 Introduction of intracatheter or catheter into renal pelvis for drainage and/or injection, percutaneous, radiological supervision and interpretation
INCLUDES Needle placement with fluoroscopic guidance (77002)
N1 Q2 80 PQ 2.75 2.75 FUD XXX

74480 Introduction of ureteral catheter or stent into ureter through renal pelvis for drainage and/or injection, percutaneous, radiological supervision and interpretation
EXCLUDES *Ureter/pelvis transurethral surgery (52320-52353 [52356])*
N1 Q2 80 PQ 2.75 2.75 FUD XXX

74485 Dilation of nephrostomy, ureters, or urethra, radiological supervision and interpretation
EXCLUDES *Change of pyelostomy/nephrostomy tube (50398)*
Ureter dilation without radiologic guidance (52341, 52344)
N1 Q2 80 PQ 2.74 2.74 FUD XXX

74710 Pelvimetry, with or without placental localization ♀
EXCLUDES *Imaging procedures on abdomen and pelvis (72170-72190, 74000-74170)*
Z3 X 80 1.06 1.06 FUD XXX

Tube
Contrast
Ovary
Delivery apparatus
Uterus
Cervix
Vaginal canal

Hysterosalpingography (imaging of the uterus and tubes) is performed. Report for radiological supervision and interpretation

74740 Hysterosalpingography, radiological supervision and interpretation ♀
EXCLUDES *Imaging procedures on abdomen and pelvis (72170-72190, 74000-74170)*
Code also injection of saline/contrast (58340)
N1 Q2 80 PQ 2.20 2.20 FUD XXX

74742 Transcervical catheterization of fallopian tube, radiological supervision and interpretation ♀
EXCLUDES *Imaging procedures on abdomen and pelvis (72170-72190, 74000-74170)*
Code also (58345)
N1 N 80 PQ 0.00 0.00 FUD XXX

74775 Perineogram (eg, vaginogram, for sex determination or extent of anomalies) M ♀
EXCLUDES *Imaging procedures on abdomen and pelvis (72170-72190, 74000-74170)*
Z2 S 80 0.00 0.00 FUD XXX

75557-75565 Magnetic Resonance Imaging: Heart Structure and Physiology

CMS 100-2,15,80 Diagnostic Test Requirements
CMS 100-3,220.2 Magnetic Resonance Imaging
CMS 100-4,13,10 ICD-9-CM Coding for Diagnostic Tests
CMS 100-4,13,40 Magnetic Resonance Imaging (MRI) Procedures
INCLUDES Physiologic evaluation of cardiac function
EXCLUDES *Cardiac catheterization procedures (93451-93572)*
Code also separate vascular injection (36000-36299)
Do not report with (76376-76377)
Do not report with more than one code in this group per session

75557 Cardiac magnetic resonance imaging for morphology and function without contrast material;
Z2 Q3 80 9.26 9.26 FUD XXX

75559 with stress imaging
INCLUDES Pharmacologic wall motion stress evaluation without contrast
Code also stress testing when performed (93015-93018)
Z2 Q3 80 12.52 12.52 FUD XXX

75561 Cardiac magnetic resonance imaging for morphology and function without contrast material(s), followed by contrast material(s) and further sequences;
Z2 Q3 80 12.20 12.20 FUD XXX

75563 with stress imaging
INCLUDES Pharmacologic perfusion stress evaluation with contrast
Code also stress testing when performed (93015-93018)
Z3 Q3 80 14.39 14.39 FUD XXX

\+ **75565 Cardiac magnetic resonance imaging for velocity flow mapping (List separately in addition to code for primary procedure)**
Code first (75557, 75559, 75561, 75563)
Do not report more than one time per session
N1 N 80 1.57 1.57 FUD ZZZ

75571-75574 Computed Tomographic Imaging: Heart

Do not report more than one code in this group per session
Do not report with (76376-76377)

75571 Computed tomography, heart, without contrast material, with quantitative evaluation of coronary calcium
Z2 X 80 2.97 2.97 FUD XXX

75572 Computed tomography, heart, with contrast material, for evaluation of cardiac structure and morphology (including 3D image postprocessing, assessment of cardiac function, and evaluation of venous structures, if performed)
Z2 S 80 8.11 8.11 FUD XXX

75573 Computed tomography, heart, with contrast material, for evaluation of cardiac structure and morphology in the setting of congenital heart disease (including 3D image postprocessing, assessment of LV cardiac function, RV structure and function and evaluation of venous structures, if performed)
Z2 S 80 11.14 11.14 FUD XXX

75574 Computed tomographic angiography, heart, coronary arteries and bypass grafts (when present), with contrast material, including 3D image postprocessing (including evaluation of cardiac structure and morphology, assessment of cardiac function, and evaluation of venous structures, if performed)
Z2 S 80 11.83 11.83 FUD XXX

75600-75791 Radiography: Arterial

CMS 100-2,15,80 Diagnostic Test Requirements

CMS 100-4,13,10 ICD-9-CM Coding for Diagnostic Tests

INCLUDES Diagnostic angiography specifically included in the interventional code description

The following diagnostic procedures with interventional supervision and interpretation:

- Angiography
- Contrast injection
- Fluoroscopic guidance for intervention
- Post-angioplasty/atherectomy/stent angiography
- Roadmapping
- Vessel measurement

EXCLUDES *Catheterization codes for diagnostic angiography of lower extremity when an access site other than the site used for the therapy is required*

Diagnostic angiogram during a separate encounter from the interventional procedure

Diagnostic angiography with interventional procedure if:

1. No previous catheter-based angiogram is accessible and a complete diagnostic procedure is performed and the decision to proceed with an interventional procedure is based on the diagnostic service, OR

2. The previous diagnostic angiogram is accessible but the documentation in the medical record specifies that:

A. the patient's condition has changed

B. there is insufficient imaging of the patient's anatomy and/or disease, OR

C. there is a clinical change during the procedure that necessitates a new examination away from the site of the intervention

3. Modifier 59 is appended to the code(s) for the diagnostic radiological supervision and interpretation service to indicate the guidelines were met

Intra-arterial procedures (36100-36248)

Intravenous procedures (36000, 36005-36015)

75600 Aortography, thoracic, without serialography, radiological supervision and interpretation
EXCLUDES *Supravalvular aortography (93567)*
N1 Q2 80 PQ 5.92 5.92 FUD XXX

75605 Aortography, thoracic, by serialography, radiological supervision and interpretation
EXCLUDES *Supravalvular aortography (93567)*
N1 Q2 80 PQ 4.28 4.28 FUD XXX

75625 Aortography, abdominal, by serialography, radiological supervision and interpretation
EXCLUDES *Supravalvular aortography (93567)*
N1 Q2 80 PQ 4.27 4.27 FUD XXX

75630 Aortography, abdominal plus bilateral iliofemoral lower extremity, catheter, by serialography, radiological supervision and interpretation
EXCLUDES *Supravalvular aortography (93567)*
N1 Q2 80 PQ 5.12 5.12 FUD XXX

75635 Computed tomographic angiography, abdominal aorta and bilateral iliofemoral lower extremity runoff, with contrast material(s), including noncontrast images, if performed, and image postprocessing
Do not report with (72191, 73706, 74174-74175)
N1 Q2 80 11.78 11.78 FUD XXX

75658 Angiography, brachial, retrograde, radiological supervision and interpretation
N1 Q2 80 PQ 4.97 4.97 FUD XXX

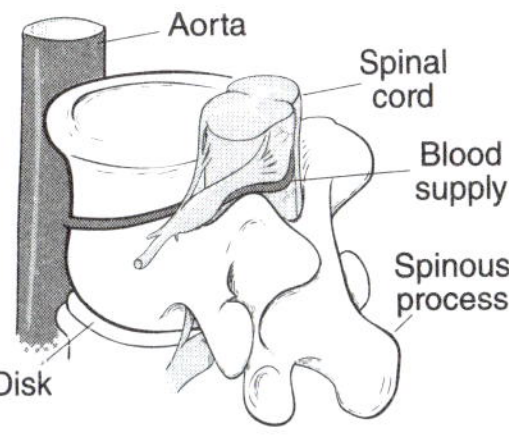

An angiography of a specific area of the spine is performed

75705 Angiography, spinal, selective, radiological supervision and interpretation
N1 Q2 80 PQ 6.97 6.97 FUD XXX

75710 Angiography, extremity, unilateral, radiological supervision and interpretation
N1 Q2 80 PQ 4.93 4.93 FUD XXX

75716 Angiography, extremity, bilateral, radiological supervision and interpretation
N1 Q2 80 PQ 5.90 5.90 FUD XXX

75726 Angiography, visceral, selective or supraselective (with or without flush aortogram), radiological supervision and interpretation
EXCLUDES *Selective angiography, each additional visceral vessel examined after basic examination (75774)*
N1 Q2 80 PQ 4.61 4.61 FUD XXX

75731 Angiography, adrenal, unilateral, selective, radiological supervision and interpretation
N1 Q2 80 PQ 5.11 5.11 FUD XXX

75733 Angiography, adrenal, bilateral, selective, radiological supervision and interpretation
N1 Q2 80 PQ 5.72 5.72 FUD XXX

75736 Angiography, pelvic, selective or supraselective, radiological supervision and interpretation
N1 Q2 80 PQ 4.85 4.85 FUD XXX

75741 Angiography, pulmonary, unilateral, selective, radiological supervision and interpretation
N1 Q2 80 PQ 4.57 4.57 FUD XXX

75743 Angiography, pulmonary, bilateral, selective, radiological supervision and interpretation
EXCLUDES *Injection procedure (93568)*
N1 Q2 80 PQ 5.29 5.29 FUD XXX

75746 Angiography, pulmonary, by nonselective catheter or venous injection, radiological supervision and interpretation
EXCLUDES *Nonselective injection procedure or catheter introduction with cardiac cath (93568)*
N1 Q2 80 PQ 4.74 4.74 FUD XXX

75756 Angiography, internal mammary, radiological supervision and interpretation
EXCLUDES *Internal mammary angiography with cardiac cath (93455, 93457, 93459, 93461, 93564)*
N1 Q2 80 PQ 5.17 5.17 FUD XXX

\+ **75774 Angiography, selective, each additional vessel studied after basic examination, radiological supervision and interpretation (List separately in addition to code for primary procedure)**

EXCLUDES *Angiography (36147, 75600-75756, 75791)*
Cardiac cath procedures (93452-93462, 93531-93533, 93563-93568)
Catheterizations (36215-36248)

Code first diagnostic angiography of upper extremities and other vascular beds (except cervicocerebral vessels)
Code first initial vessel
Do not report with intracranial and extracranial cervicocerebral diagnostic angiography (36221-36228)

N1 N 80 ▭ 2.77 2.77 FUD ZZZ

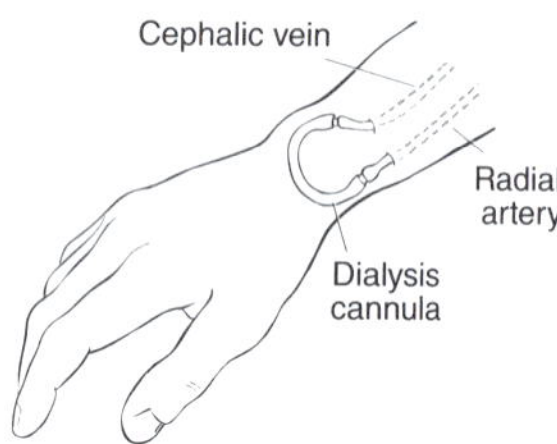

Angiography is performed on an arteriovenous shunt, such as is used in dialysis.

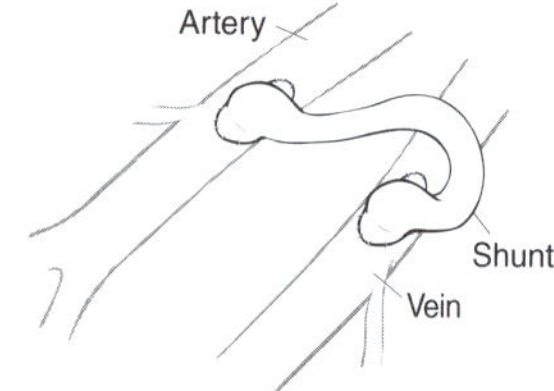

Shunts may be placed for a variety of conditions and are checked radiologically for patency and blood flow

75791 Angiography, arteriovenous shunt (eg, dialysis patient fistula/graft), complete evaluation of dialysis access, including fluoroscopy, image documentation and report (includes injections of contrast and all necessary imaging from the arterial anastomosis and adjacent artery through entire venous outflow including the inferior or superior vena cava), radiological supervision and interpretation

INCLUDES Radiological evaluation performed via existing access into the shunt or from an access that is not a direct puncture of the shunt

EXCLUDES *Catheter introduction, when performed (36140, 36215-36217, 36245-36247)*
Radiological evaluation with introduction of needle/catheter, AV dialysis shunt, complete procedure (36147)

Do not report with (36147-36148)

N1 02 80 PO 9.25 9.25 FUD XXX

75801-75893 Radiography: Lymphatic and Venous

CMS 100-2,15,80 Diagnostic Test Requirements
CMS 100-4,13,10 ICD-9-CM Coding for Diagnostic Tests

INCLUDES Diagnostic venography specifically included in the interventional code description
The following diagnostic procedures with interventional supervision and interpretation:
Contrast injection
Fluoroscopic guidance for intervention
Post-angioplasty/venography
Roadmapping
Venography
Vessel measurement

EXCLUDES *Diagnostic venogram during a separate encounter from the interventional procedure*
Diagnostic venography with interventional procedure if:
1. No previous catheter-based venogram is accessible and a complete diagnostic procedure is performed and the decision to proceed with an interventional procedure is based on the diagnostic service, OR
2. The previous diagnostic venogram is accessible but the documentation in the medical record specifies that:
A. The patient's condition has changed
B. There is insufficient imaging of the patient's anatomy and/or disease, OR
C. There is a clinical change during the procedure that necessitates a new examination away from the site of the intervention
Intravenous procedures (36000-36015, 36400-36510)
Lymphatic injection procedures (38790)

75801 Lymphangiography, extremity only, unilateral, radiological supervision and interpretation
N1 02 80 ▭ PO 0.00 0.00 FUD XXX

75803 Lymphangiography, extremity only, bilateral, radiological supervision and interpretation
N1 02 80 ▭ PO 0.00 0.00 FUD XXX

75805 Lymphangiography, pelvic/abdominal, unilateral, radiological supervision and interpretation
N1 02 80 ▭ PO 0.00 0.00 FUD XXX

75807 Lymphangiography, pelvic/abdominal, bilateral, radiological supervision and interpretation
N1 02 80 ▭ PO 0.00 0.00 FUD XXX

75809 Shuntogram for investigation of previously placed indwelling nonvascular shunt (eg, LeVeen shunt, ventriculoperitoneal shunt, indwelling infusion pump), radiological supervision and interpretation
INCLUDES Needle placement with fluoroscopic guidance (77002)
Code also surgical procedure (49427, 61070)
N1 02 80 ▭ PO 2.92 2.92 FUD XXX

75810 Splenoportography, radiological supervision and interpretation
INCLUDES Needle placement with fluoroscopic guidance (77002)
N1 02 80 ▭ PO 0.00 0.00 FUD XXX

75820 Venography, extremity, unilateral, radiological supervision and interpretation
N1 02 80 ▭ 3.52 3.52 FUD XXX

75822 Venography, extremity, bilateral, radiological supervision and interpretation
N1 02 80 ▭ 4.39 4.39 FUD XXX

75825 Venography, caval, inferior, with serialography, radiological supervision and interpretation
N1 02 80 ▭ PO 4.12 4.12 FUD XXX

75827 Venography, caval, superior, with serialography, radiological supervision and interpretation
N1 02 80 ▭ PO 4.17 4.17 FUD XXX

75831 Venography, renal, unilateral, selective, radiological supervision and interpretation
N1 02 80 ▭ PO 4.45 4.45 FUD XXX

75833 **Venography, renal, bilateral, selective, radiological supervision and interpretation**
N1 Q2 80 CCI PQ 5.06 5.06 FUD XXX

75840 **Venography, adrenal, unilateral, selective, radiological supervision and interpretation**
N1 Q2 80 CCI PQ 4.61 4.61 FUD XXX

75842 **Venography, adrenal, bilateral, selective, radiological supervision and interpretation**
N1 Q2 80 CCI PQ 5.51 5.51 FUD XXX

75860 **Venography, venous sinus (eg, petrosal and inferior sagittal) or jugular, catheter, radiological supervision and interpretation**
N1 Q2 80 CCI PQ 4.33 4.33 FUD XXX

75870 **Venography, superior sagittal sinus, radiological supervision and interpretation**
N1 Q2 80 CCI PQ 4.43 4.43 FUD XXX

75872 **Venography, epidural, radiological supervision and interpretation**
N1 Q2 80 CCI PQ 4.25 4.25 FUD XXX

75880 **Venography, orbital, radiological supervision and interpretation**
N1 Q2 80 CCI PQ 3.83 3.83 FUD XXX

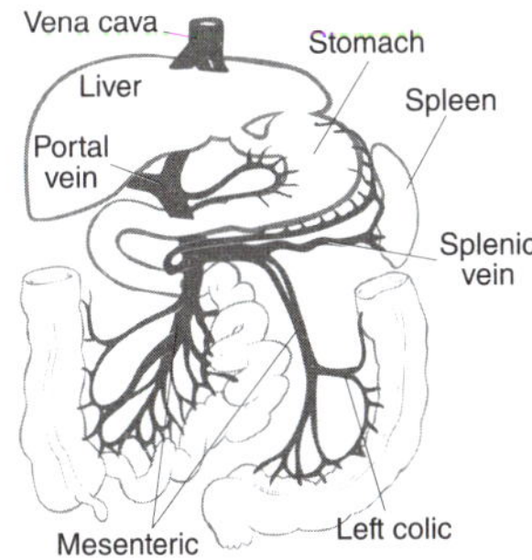

Schematic showing the portal vein

75885 **Percutaneous transhepatic portography with hemodynamic evaluation, radiological supervision and interpretation**
INCLUDES Needle placement with fluoroscopic guidance (77002)
N1 Q2 80 CCI PQ 4.77 4.77 FUD XXX

75887 **Percutaneous transhepatic portography without hemodynamic evaluation, radiological supervision and interpretation**
INCLUDES Needle placement with fluoroscopic guidance (77002)
N1 Q2 80 CCI PQ 4.74 4.74 FUD XXX

75889 **Hepatic venography, wedged or free, with hemodynamic evaluation, radiological supervision and interpretation**
N1 Q2 80 CCI PQ 4.38 4.38 FUD XXX

75891 **Hepatic venography, wedged or free, without hemodynamic evaluation, radiological supervision and interpretation**
N1 Q2 80 CCI PQ 4.41 4.41 FUD XXX

75893 **Venous sampling through catheter, with or without angiography (eg, for parathyroid hormone, renin), radiological supervision and interpretation**
Code also surgical procedure (36500)
N1 Q2 80 CCI PQ 3.57 3.57 FUD XXX

75894-75946 Transcatheter Procedures

CMS 100-2,15,80 Diagnostic Test Requirements
CMS 100-3,20.28 Therapeutic Embolization
CMS 100-4,13,10 ICD-9-CM Coding for Diagnostic Tests

INCLUDES The following diagnostic procedures with interventional supervision and interpretation:
- Angiography/venography
- Completion angiography/venography except for those services allowed by 75898
- Contrast injection
- Fluoroscopic guidance for intervention
- Roadmapping
- Vessel measurement

EXCLUDES *Diagnostic angiography/venography performed at the same session as transcatheter therapy unless it is specifically included in the code descriptor or is excluded in the venography/angiography notes (75600-75893)*

75894 **Transcatheter therapy, embolization, any method, radiological supervision and interpretation**
Do not report with (35475-35476, 36478-36479, 37241-37244)
N1 N 80 CCI PQ 0.00 0.00 FUD XXX

75896 **Transcatheter therapy, infusion, other than for thrombolysis, radiological supervision and interpretation**
EXCLUDES *Coronary disease infusion ([92975], [92977])*
Non-coronary thrombolysis infusion ([37211, 37212, 37213, 37214])
Do not report with ([37211, 37212, 37213, 37214])
N1 N 80 CCI PQ 0.00 0.00 FUD XXX

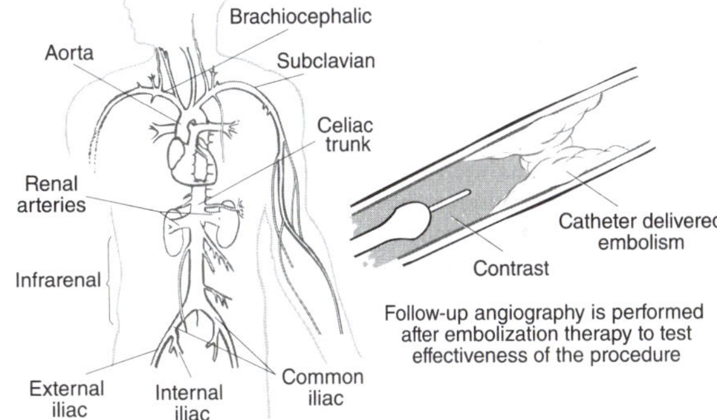

Follow-up angiography is performed after embolization therapy to test effectiveness of the procedure

75898 **Angiography through existing catheter for follow-up study for transcatheter therapy, embolization or infusion, other than for thrombolysis**
EXCLUDES *Noncoronary thrombolysis infusion ([37211, 37212, 37213, 37214])*
Do not report with ([37211, 37212, 37213, 37214], 37241-37244)
N1 Q1 80 CCI PQ 0.00 0.00 FUD XXX

75901 **Mechanical removal of pericatheter obstructive material (eg, fibrin sheath) from central venous device via separate venous access, radiologic supervision and interpretation**
EXCLUDES *Venous catheterization (36010-36012)*
Code also surgical procedure (36595)
N1 N 80 CCI PQ 5.00 5.00 FUD XXX

75902 **Mechanical removal of intraluminal (intracatheter) obstructive material from central venous device through device lumen, radiologic supervision and interpretation**
EXCLUDES *Venous catheterization (36010-36012)*
Code also surgical procedure (36596)
N1 N 80 CCI PQ 2.12 2.12 FUD XXX

75945 **Intravascular ultrasound (non-coronary vessel), radiological supervision and interpretation; initial vessel**
NI Q2 80 ▣ 0.00 0.00 FUD XXX

\+ **75946** **each additional non-coronary vessel (List separately in addition to code for primary procedure)**
EXCLUDES *Selective catheter placement (36215-36248)*
Transcatheter procedures (37200, 37202, 37236-37239, 37241-37244, 61624, 61626)
Code also procedure (37250-37251)
Code first initial vessel (75945)
NI N 80 ▣ 0.00 0.00 FUD ZZZ

75952-75959 Endovascular Aneurysm Repair

INCLUDES The following diagnostic procedures with interventional supervision and interpretation:
- Angiography/venography
- Completion angiography/venography except for those services allowed by 75898
- Contrast injection
- Fluoroscopic guidance for intervention
- Roadmapping
- Vessel measurement

EXCLUDES *Diagnostic angiography/venography performed at the same session as transcatheter therapy unless it is specifically included in the code descriptor (75600-75893)*

75952 **Endovascular repair of infrarenal abdominal aortic aneurysm or dissection, radiological supervision and interpretation**
EXCLUDES *Endovascular repair of visceral aorta with or without infrarenal abdominal aorta repair, radiologic supervision and interpretation (34841-34848)*
Implantation endovascular grafts (34800-34805)
Do not report with (34841-34848)
C 80 ▣ PQ 0.00 0.00 FUD XXX

75953 **Placement of proximal or distal extension prosthesis for endovascular repair of infrarenal aortic or iliac artery aneurysm, pseudoaneurysm, or dissection, radiological supervision and interpretation**
EXCLUDES *Placement of endovascular extension prostheses (34825-34826)*
C 80 ▣ PQ 0.00 0.00 FUD XXX

75954 **Endovascular repair of iliac artery aneurysm, pseudoaneurysm, arteriovenous malformation, or trauma, using ilio-iliac tube endoprosthesis, radiological supervision and interpretation**
EXCLUDES *Endovascular repair of iliac artery aneurysm, arteriovenous malformation, pseudoaneurysm, or trauma with bifurcated endoprosthesis, radiological supervision and interpretation (0255T)*
Placement of endovascular graft (34900)
C 80 ▣ PQ 0.00 0.00 FUD XXX

75956 **Endovascular repair of descending thoracic aorta (eg, aneurysm, pseudoaneurysm, dissection, penetrating ulcer, intramural hematoma, or traumatic disruption); involving coverage of left subclavian artery origin, initial endoprosthesis plus descending thoracic aortic extension(s), if required, to level of celiac artery origin, radiological supervision and interpretation**
INCLUDES All angiography
Fluoroscopy for component delivery
Code also endovascular graft implantation (33880)
C 80 PQ 0.00 0.00 FUD XXX

75957 **not involving coverage of left subclavian artery origin, initial endoprosthesis plus descending thoracic aortic extension(s), if required, to level of celiac artery origin, radiological supervision and interpretation**
INCLUDES All angiography
Fluoroscopy for component delivery
Code also endovascular graft implantation (33881)
C 80 PQ 0.00 0.00 FUD XXX

75958 **Placement of proximal extension prosthesis for endovascular repair of descending thoracic aorta (eg, aneurysm, pseudoaneurysm, dissection, penetrating ulcer, intramural hematoma, or traumatic disruption), radiological supervision and interpretation**
Code also placement of each additional proximal extension(s) (75958)
Code also proximal endovascular extension implantation (33883-33884)
C 80 PQ 0.00 0.00 FUD XXX

75959 **Placement of distal extension prosthesis(s) (delayed) after endovascular repair of descending thoracic aorta, as needed, to level of celiac origin, radiological supervision and interpretation**
INCLUDES Corresponding services for placement of distal thoracic endovascular extension(s) placed during procedure following the principal procedure
Code also placement of distal endovascular extension (33886)
Do not report more than one time no matter how many modules are deployed
Do not report with endovascular repair (75956-75957)
C 80 PQ 0.00 0.00 FUD XXX

75960 Transcatheter Insertion and Removal

CMS 100-2,15,80 Diagnostic Test Requirements
CMS 100-4,13,10 ICD-9-CM Coding for Diagnostic Tests

75962-75978 Percutaneous Transluminal Angioplasty

CMS 100-3,20.7 Percutaneous Transluminal Angioplasty (PTA)

INCLUDES The following diagnostic procedures with interventional supervision and interpretation:
- Angiography/venography
- Completion angiography/venography except for those services allowed by 75898
- Contrast injection
- Fluoroscopic guidance for intervention
- Roadmapping
- Vessel measurement

EXCLUDES *Diagnostic angiography/venography performed at the same session as transcatheter therapy unless it is specifically included in the code descriptor (75600-75893)*
Radiological supervision and interpretation for transluminal balloon angioplasty in:
Femoral/popliteal arteries (37224-37227)
Iliac artery (37220-37223)
Tibial/peroneal artery (37228-37235)

75962 **Transluminal balloon angioplasty, peripheral artery other than renal, or other visceral artery, iliac or lower extremity, radiological supervision and interpretation**
Code also surgical procedure (35458, 35475)
Code also angioplasty catheter (C1725, C1885)
Do not report with (37217)
NI N 80 ▣ PQ 4.11 4.11 FUD XXX

\+ **75964** **Transluminal balloon angioplasty, each additional peripheral artery other than renal or other visceral artery, iliac or lower extremity, radiological supervision and interpretation (List separately in addition to code for primary procedure)**
Code first primary procedure (75962)
NI N 80 ▣ 2.64 2.64 FUD ZZZ

75966 Transluminal balloon angioplasty, renal or other visceral artery, radiological supervision and interpretation

Code also angioplasty catheter (C1725, C1885)

N1 N 80 PQ 4.90 4.90 FUD XXX

+ **75968 Transluminal balloon angioplasty, each additional visceral artery, radiological supervision and interpretation (List separately in addition to code for primary procedure)**

EXCLUDES *Percutaneous transluminal coronary angioplasty ([92920, 92921, 92924, 92925, 92928, 92929, 92933, 92934, 92937, 92938, 92941, 92943, 92944])*

Code first primary procedure (75966)

N1 N 80 2.47 2.47 FUD ZZZ

75970 Transcatheter biopsy, radiological supervision and interpretation

EXCLUDES *Injection procedure only for transcatheter therapy or biopsy (36100-36299)*
Percutaneous needle biopsy
Pancreas (48102)
Retroperitoneal lymph node/mass (49180)
Transcatheter renal/ureteral biopsy (52007)

N1 N 80 PQ 0.00 0.00 FUD XXX

75978 Transluminal balloon angioplasty, venous (eg, subclavian stenosis), radiological supervision and interpretation

Code also angioplasty catheter (C1725, C1885)

N1 Q2 80 PQ 4.06 4.06 FUD XXX

75980-75989 Percutaneous Drainage

CMS 100-3,220.1 Computerized Tomography
CMS 100-3,220.5 Ultrasound Diagnostic Procedures

INCLUDES The following diagnostic procedures with interventional supervision and interpretation:
Angiography/venography
Completion angiography/venography except for those services allowed by 75898
Contrast injection
Fluoroscopic guidance for intervention
Roadmapping
Vessel measurement

EXCLUDES *Diagnostic angiography/venography performed at the same session as transcatheter therapy unless it is specifically included in the code descriptor (75600-75893)*

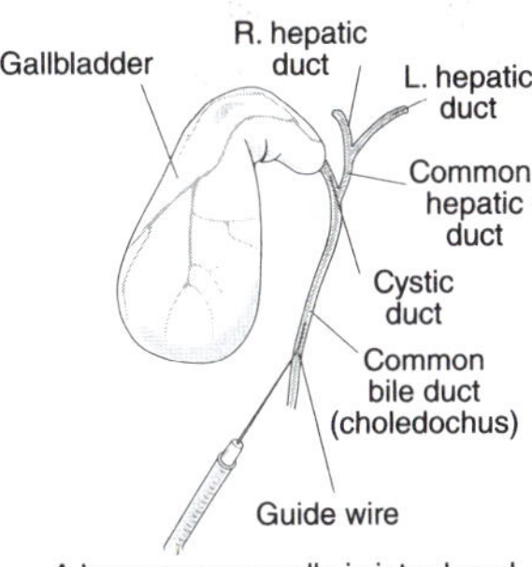

A large gauge needle is introduced into the common bile duct and a guide wire and catheter are introduced Report for radiological supervision and interpretation

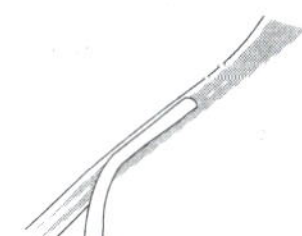

Schematic of a drainage catheter in the bile duct

75980 Percutaneous transhepatic biliary drainage with contrast monitoring, radiological supervision and interpretation

INCLUDES Needle placement with fluoroscopic guidance (77002)

N1 N 80 PQ 0.00 0.00 FUD XXX

75982 Percutaneous placement of drainage catheter for combined internal and external biliary drainage or of a drainage stent for internal biliary drainage in patients with an inoperable mechanical biliary obstruction, radiological supervision and interpretation

INCLUDES Needle placement with fluoroscopic guidance (77002)

N1 N 80 PQ 0.00 0.00 FUD XXX

75984 Change of percutaneous tube or drainage catheter with contrast monitoring (eg, genitourinary system, abscess), radiological supervision and interpretation

EXCLUDES *Change only of nephrostomy/pyelostomy tube (50398)*
Change only of percutaneous biliary drainage catheter (47525)
Cholecystostomy, percutaneous (47490)
Introduction procedure only for percutaneous biliary drainage (47510-47511)
Nephrostolithotomy/pyelostolithotomy, percutaneous (50080-50081)
Percutaneous replacement of gastrointestinal tube using fluoroscopic guidance (49450-49452)
Removal and/or replacement of internal ureteral stent using transurethral approach (50385-50386)

N1 N 80 PQ 3.14 3.14 FUD XXX

75989 Radiological guidance (ie, fluoroscopy, ultrasound, or computed tomography), for percutaneous drainage (eg, abscess, specimen collection), with placement of catheter, radiological supervision and interpretation

INCLUDES Needle placement with fluoroscopic guidance (77002)

Do not report with (10030, 32554-32557, 47490, 49405-49407)

N1 N 80 3.54 3.54 FUD XXX

76000-76140 Miscellaneous Techniques

EXCLUDES *Arthrography:*
Ankle (73615)
Elbow (73085)
Hip (73525)
Knee (73580)
Shoulder (73040)
Wrist (73115)
CT cerebral perfusion test (0042T)

76000 Fluoroscopy (separate procedure), up to 1 hour physician or other qualified health care professional time, other than 71023 or 71034 (eg, cardiac fluoroscopy)

Do not report with (33957-33959, [33962, 33963, 33964])

N1 Q1 80 PQ 1.43 1.43 FUD XXX

76001 Fluoroscopy, physician or other qualified health care professional time more than 1 hour, assisting a nonradiologic physician or other qualified health care professional (eg, nephrostolithotomy, ERCP, bronchoscopy, transbronchial biopsy)

Do not report with (33957-33959, [33962, 33963, 33964])

N1 N 80 PQ 0.00 0.00 FUD XXX

76010 Radiologic examination from nose to rectum for foreign body, single view, child A

Z3 X 80 0.78 0.78 FUD XXX

76080 Radiologic examination, abscess, fistula or sinus tract study, radiological supervision and interpretation
EXCLUDES *Contrast injections, radiology evaluation, and guidance via fluoroscopy of gastrostomy, duodenostomy, jejunostomy, gastro-jejunostomy, or cecostomy tube (49465)*
1.72 1.72 FUD XXX

76098 Radiological examination, surgical specimen
Do not report with (19081-19086)
0.54 0.54 FUD XXX

76100 Radiologic examination, single plane body section (eg, tomography), other than with urography
2.86 2.86 FUD XXX

76101 Radiologic examination, complex motion (ie, hypercycloidal) body section (eg, mastoid polytomography), other than with urography; unilateral
EXCLUDES *Nephrotomography (74415)*
Panoramic x-ray (70355)
Do not report more than one time per day
4.25 4.25 FUD XXX

76102 bilateral
EXCLUDES *Nephrotomography (74415)*
Panoramic x-ray (70355)
Do not report more than one time per day
5.69 5.69 FUD XXX

76120 Cineradiography/videoradiography, except where specifically included
2.63 2.63 FUD XXX

+ **76125 Cineradiography/videoradiography to complement routine examination (List separately in addition to code for primary procedure)**
Code first primary procedure
0.00 0.00 FUD ZZZ

76140 Consultation on X-ray examination made elsewhere, written report
E 0.00 0.00 FUD XXX

76376-76377 Three-dimensional Manipulation

INCLUDES Concurrent physician supervision of image postprocessing
3D manipulation of volumetric data set
Rendering of image

EXCLUDES *Arthrography:*
Ankle (73615)
Elbow (73085)
Hip (73525)
Knee (73580)
Shoulder (73040)
Wrist (73115)
Computer-aided detection of MRI data for lesion, breast MRI (0159T)
CT cerebral perfusion test (0042T)

Code also base imaging procedure(s)

76376 3D rendering with interpretation and reporting of computed tomography, magnetic resonance imaging, ultrasound, or other tomographic modality with image postprocessing under concurrent supervision; not requiring image postprocessing on an independent workstation
Do not report with (31627, 34839, 70496, 70498, 70544-70549, 71275, 71555, 72159, 72191, 72198, 73206, 73225, 73706, 73725, 74174-74175, 74185, 74261-74263, 75557, 75559, 75561, 75563, 75565, 75571-75574, 75635, 76377, 77061-77063, 78012-78999, 93355, 0159T)
N 0.81 0.81 FUD XXX

76377 requiring image postprocessing on an independent workstation
Do not report with (34839, 70496, 70498, 70544-70549, 71275, 71555, 72159, 72191, 72198, 73206, 73225, 73706, 73725, 74174-74175, 74185, 74261-74263, 75557, 75559, 75561, 75563, 75565, 75571-75574, 75635, 76376, 77061-77063, 78012-78999, 93355, 0159T)
N 2.35 2.35 FUD XXX

76380 Computerized Tomography: Delimited

CMS 100-3,220.1 Computerized Tomography

EXCLUDES *Arthrography:*
Ankle (73615)
Elbow (73085)
Hip (73525)
Knee (73580)
Shoulder (73040)
Wrist (73115)
CT cerebral perfusion test (0042T)

76380 Computed tomography, limited or localized follow-up study
4.27 4.27 FUD XXX

76390-76499 Magnetic Resonance Spectroscopy

CMS 100-3,220.2.1 Magnetic Resonance Spectroscopy

EXCLUDES *Arthrography:*
Ankle (73615)
Elbow (73085)
Hip (73525)
Knee (73580)
Shoulder (73040)
Wrist (73115)
CT cerebral perfusion test (0042T)

76390 Magnetic resonance spectroscopy
EXCLUDES *MRI*
E 12.50 12.50 FUD XXX

76496 Unlisted fluoroscopic procedure (eg, diagnostic, interventional)
0.00 0.00 FUD XXX

76497 Unlisted computed tomography procedure (eg, diagnostic, interventional)
0.00 0.00 FUD XXX

76498 Unlisted magnetic resonance procedure (eg, diagnostic, interventional)
0.00 0.00 FUD XXX

76499 Unlisted diagnostic radiographic procedure
0.00 0.00 FUD XXX

76506 Ultrasound: Brain

CMS 100-3,220.5 Ultrasound Diagnostic Procedures

INCLUDES Required permanent documentation of ultrasound images except when diagnostic purpose is biometric measurement
Written documentation

EXCLUDES *Noninvasive vascular studies, diagnostic (93880-93990)*
Ultrasound exam that does not include thorough assessment of organ or site, recorded image, and written report

76506 Echoencephalography, real time with image documentation (gray scale) (for determination of ventricular size, delineation of cerebral contents, and detection of fluid masses or other intracranial abnormalities), including A-mode encephalography as secondary component where indicated
3.49 3.49 FUD XXX

76510-76529 Ultrasound: Eyes

CMS 100-3,220.5 Ultrasound Diagnostic Procedures
CMS 100-3,230.1 NCD for Treatment of Kidney Stones

INCLUDES Required permanent documentation of ultrasound images except when diagnostic purpose is biometric measurement
Written documentation

EXCLUDES *Noninvasive vascular studies, diagnostic (93880-93990)*
Ultrasound exam that does not include thorough assessment of organ or site, recorded image, and written report

76510 **Ophthalmic ultrasound, diagnostic; B-scan and quantitative A-scan performed during the same patient encounter**
Z3 T 80 5.03 5.03 FUD XXX

76511 **quantitative A-scan only**
Z3 S 80 2.89 2.89 FUD XXX

76512 **B-scan (with or without superimposed non-quantitative A-scan)**
Z3 S 80 2.65 2.65 FUD XXX

76513 **anterior segment ultrasound, immersion (water bath) B-scan or high resolution biomicroscopy**
EXCLUDES *Computerized ophthalmic testing other than by ultrasound (92132-92134)*
Z3 Q 80 2.71 2.71 FUD XXX

76514 **corneal pachymetry, unilateral or bilateral (determination of corneal thickness)**
INCLUDES Biometric measurement for which permanent documentation of images is not required
Z3 X 80 0.43 0.43 FUD XXX

76516 **Ophthalmic biometry by ultrasound echography, A-scan;**
INCLUDES Biometric measurement for which permanent documentation of images is not required
Z3 S 80 2.21 2.21 FUD XXX

76519 **with intraocular lens power calculation**
INCLUDES Biometric measurement for which permanent documentation of images is not required
Written prescription that satisfies requirement for written report
EXCLUDES *Partial coherence interferometry (92136)*
Z2 S 80 2.39 2.39 FUD XXX

76529 **Ophthalmic ultrasonic foreign body localization**
Z3 S 80 2.26 2.26 FUD XXX

76536-76800 Ultrasound: Neck, Thorax, Abdomen, and Spine

CMS 100-2,15,80 Diagnostic Test Requirements
CMS 100-3,220.5 Ultrasound Diagnostic Procedures

INCLUDES Required permanent documentation of ultrasound images except when diagnostic purpose is biometric measurement
Written documentation

EXCLUDES *Focused ultrasound ablation of uterine leiomyomata (0071T-0072T)*
Ultrasound exam that does not include thorough assessment of organ or site, recorded image, and written report

76536 **Ultrasound, soft tissues of head and neck (eg, thyroid, parathyroid, parotid), real time with image documentation**
Z2 S 80 3.45 3.45 FUD XXX

76604 **Ultrasound, chest (includes mediastinum), real time with image documentation**
Z3 Q3 80 2.50 2.50 FUD XXX

● **76641** **Ultrasound, breast, unilateral, real time with image documentation, including axilla when performed; complete**
INCLUDES Complete examination of all four quadrants, retroareolar region, and axilla when performed
EXCLUDES *Ultrasound exam that does not include thorough assessment of organ or site, recorded image, and written report*
Do not report more than one time per breast per session

● **76642** **limited**
INCLUDES Examination not including all of the elements in complete examination
EXCLUDES *Ultrasound exam that does not include thorough assessment of organ or site, recorded image, and written report*
Do not report more than one time per breast per session

76645 ~~**Ultrasound, breast(s) (unilateral or bilateral), real time with image documentation**~~
To report, see 76641-76642

76700 **Ultrasound, abdominal, real time with image documentation; complete**
INCLUDES Real time scans of:
Common bile duct
Gall bladder
Inferior vena cava
Kidneys
Liver
Pancreas
Spleen
Upper abdominal aorta
Z2 Q3 80 3.99 3.99 FUD XXX

76705 **limited (eg, single organ, quadrant, follow-up)**
Z2 Q3 80 3.07 3.07 FUD XXX

76770 **Ultrasound, retroperitoneal (eg, renal, aorta, nodes), real time with image documentation; complete**
INCLUDES Complete assessment of kidneys and bladder if history indicates urinary pathology
Real time scans of:
Abdominal aorta
Common iliac artery origins
Inferior vena cava
Kidneys
Z2 Q3 80 3.76 3.76 FUD XXX

76775 **limited**
Z3 Q3 80 1.85 1.85 FUD XXX

76776 **Ultrasound, transplanted kidney, real time and duplex Doppler with image documentation**
EXCLUDES *Transplanted kidney ultrasound without duplex doppler (76775)*
Do not report with abdominal/pelvic/scrotal contents/retroperitoneal duplex scan (93975, 93976)
Z2 Q3 80 4.37 4.37 FUD XXX

76800 **Ultrasound, spinal canal and contents**
Z2 S 80 3.92 3.92 FUD XXX

76801-76802 Ultrasound: Pregnancy Less Than 14 Weeks

CMS 100-2,15,80 Diagnostic Test Requirements
CMS 100-3,220.5 Ultrasound Diagnostic Procedures

INCLUDES Determination of the number of gestational sacs and fetuses
Gestational sac/fetal measurement appropriate for gestational age (younger than 14 weeks 0 days)
Inspection of the maternal uterus and adnexa
Quality analysis of amniotic fluid volume/gestational sac shape
Visualization of fetal and placental anatomic formation
Written documentation of each component of exam

EXCLUDES *Focused ultrasound ablation of uterine leiomyomata (0071T-0072T)*
Ultrasound exam that does not include thorough assessment of organ or site, recorded image, and written report

76801 Ultrasound, pregnant uterus, real time with image documentation, fetal and maternal evaluation, first trimester (< 14 weeks 0 days), transabdominal approach; single or first gestation M ♀
EXCLUDES *Fetal nuchal translucency measurement, first trimester (76813)*
Z2 S 80 3.57 3.57 FUD XXX

+ **76802 each additional gestation (List separately in addition to code for primary procedure)** M ♀
EXCLUDES *Fetal nuchal translucency measurement, first trimester (76814)*
Code first (76801)
N1 N 80 1.90 1.90 FUD ZZZ

76805-76810 Ultrasound: Pregnancy of 14 Weeks or More

CMS 100-2,15,80 Diagnostic Test Requirements
CMS 100-3,220.5 Ultrasound Diagnostic Procedures

INCLUDES Determination of the number of gestational/chorionic sacs and fetuses
Evaluation of:
- Amniotic fluid
- Four chambered heart
- Intracranial, spinal, abdominal anatomy
- Placenta location
- Umbilical cord insertion site

Examination of maternal adnexa if visible
Gestational sac/fetal measurement appropriate for gestational age (older than or equal to 14 weeks 0 days)
Written documentation of each component of exam

EXCLUDES *Focused ultrasound ablation of uterine leiomyomata (0071T-0072T)*
Ultrasound exam that does not include thorough assessment of organ or site, recorded image, and written report

76805 Ultrasound, pregnant uterus, real time with image documentation, fetal and maternal evaluation, after first trimester (> or = 14 weeks 0 days), transabdominal approach; single or first gestation M ♀
Z2 S 80 4.13 4.13 FUD XXX

+ **76810 each additional gestation (List separately in addition to code for primary procedure)** M ♀
Code first (76805)
N1 N 80 2.74 2.74 FUD ZZZ

76811-76812 Ultrasound: Pregnancy, with Additional Studies of Fetus

CMS 100-3,220.5 Ultrasound Diagnostic Procedures

INCLUDES Determination of the number of gestational/chorionic sacs and fetuses
Evaluation of:
- Abdominal organ specific anatomy
- Amniotic fluid
- Chest anatomy
- Face
- Fetal brain/ventricles
- Four chambered heart
- Heart/outflow tracts and chest anatomy
- Intracranial, spinal, abdominal anatomy
- Limbs including number, length, and architecture
- Other fetal anatomy as indicated
- Placenta location
- Umbilical cord insertion site

Examination of maternal adnexa if visible
Gestational sac/fetal measurement appropriate for gestational age (older than or equal to 14 weeks 0 days)
Written documentation of each component of exam, including reason for nonvisualization, when applicable

EXCLUDES *Focused ultrasound ablation of uterine leiomyomata (0071T-0072T)*
Ultrasound exam that does not include thorough assessment organ or site, recorded image, and written report

76811 Ultrasound, pregnant uterus, real time with image documentation, fetal and maternal evaluation plus detailed fetal anatomic examination, transabdominal approach; single or first gestation M ♀
Z3 S 80 5.23 5.23 FUD XXX

+ **76812 each additional gestation (List separately in addition to code for primary procedure)** M ♀
Code first (76811)
N1 N 80 5.93 5.93 FUD ZZZ

76813-76828 Ultrasound: Other Fetal Evaluations

CMS 100-2,15,80 Diagnostic Test Requirements
CMS 100-3,220.5 Ultrasound Diagnostic Procedures

INCLUDES Required permanent documentation of ultrasound images except when diagnostic purpose is biometric measurement
Written documentation

EXCLUDES *Focused ultrasound ablation of uterine leiomyomata (0071T-0072T)*
Ultrasound exam that does not include thorough assessment of organ or site, recorded image, and written report

76813 Ultrasound, pregnant uterus, real time with image documentation, first trimester fetal nuchal translucency measurement, transabdominal or transvaginal approach; single or first gestation M ♀
Z3 S 80 3.42 3.42 FUD XXX

+ **76814 each additional gestation (List separately in addition to code for primary procedure)** M ♀
Code first (76813)
N1 N 80 2.25 2.25 FUD XXX

76815 Ultrasound, pregnant uterus, real time with image documentation, limited (eg, fetal heart beat, placental location, fetal position and/or qualitative amniotic fluid volume), 1 or more fetuses M ♀
INCLUDES Exam concentrating on one or more elements
Reporting only one time per exam, instead of per element
EXCLUDES *Fetal nuchal translucency measurement, first trimester (76813-76814)*
Z3 S 80 2.55 2.55 FUD XXX

76816 Ultrasound, pregnant uterus, real time with image documentation, follow-up (eg, re-evaluation of fetal size by measuring standard growth parameters and amniotic fluid volume, re-evaluation of organ system(s) suspected or confirmed to be abnormal on a previous scan), transabdominal approach, per fetus M ♀

INCLUDES Re-evaluation of fetal size, interval growth, or aberrancies noted on a prior ultrasound

Code also modifier 59 for examination of each additional fetus in a multiple pregnancy

Z2 S 80 ▫ 3.29 3.29 FUD XXX

76817 Ultrasound, pregnant uterus, real time with image documentation, transvaginal M ♀

EXCLUDES Transvaginal ultrasound, non-obstetrical (76830)

Code also transabdominal obstetrical ultrasound, if performed

Z3 S 80 ▫ 2.87 2.87 FUD XXX

76818 Fetal biophysical profile; with non-stress testing M ♀

Code also modifier 59 for each additional fetus

Z3 S 80 ▫ 3.45 3.45 FUD XXX

76819 without non-stress testing M ♀

EXCLUDES Amniotic fluid index without non-stress test (76815)

Code also modifier 59 for each additional fetus

Z3 S 80 ▫ 2.53 2.53 FUD XXX

76820 Doppler velocimetry, fetal; umbilical artery M ♀

Z3 S 80 1.38 1.38 FUD XXX

76821 middle cerebral artery M ♀

Z2 S 80 2.66 2.66 FUD XXX

76825 Echocardiography, fetal, cardiovascular system, real time with image documentation (2D), with or without M-mode recording; M ♀

Z2 S 80 ▫ 7.73 7.73 FUD XXX

76826 follow-up or repeat study M ♀

Z3 S 80 ▫ 4.63 4.63 FUD XXX

76827 Doppler echocardiography, fetal, pulsed wave and/or continuous wave with spectral display; complete M ♀

Z3 S 80 ▫ 2.13 2.13 FUD XXX

76828 follow-up or repeat study M ♀

EXCLUDES Color mapping (93325)

Z3 S 80 ▫ 1.49 1.49 FUD XXX

76830-76873 Ultrasound: Male and Female Genitalia

CMS 100-2,15,80 Diagnostic Test Requirements

CMS 100-3,220.5 Ultrasound Diagnostic Procedures

INCLUDES Required permanent documentation of ultrasound images except when diagnostic purpose is biometric measurement

Written documentation

EXCLUDES Focused ultrasound ablation of uterine leiomyomata (0071T-0072T)

Ultrasound exam that does not include thorough assessment of organ or site, recorded image, and written report

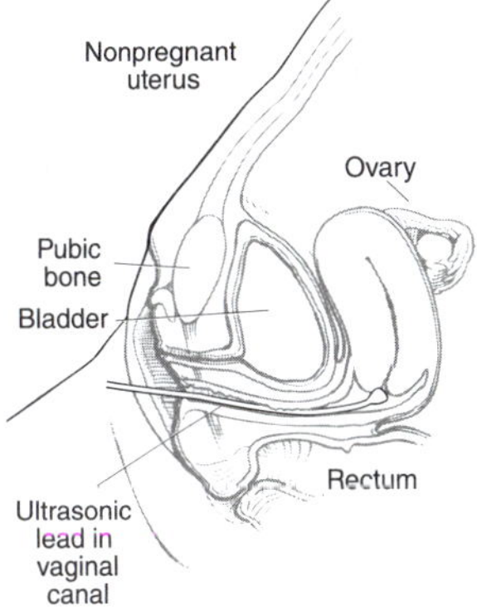

Ultrasound is performed in real time with image documentation by a transvaginal approach

76830 Ultrasound, transvaginal ♀

EXCLUDES Transvaginal ultrasound, obstetric (76817)

Code also transabdominal non-obstetrical ultrasound, if performed

Z2 S 80 ▫ 3.57 3.57 FUD XXX

76831 Saline infusion sonohysterography (SIS), including color flow Doppler, when performed ♀

Code also saline introduction for saline infusion sonohysterography (58340)

Z3 03 80 ▫ 3.50 3.50 FUD XXX

76856 Ultrasound, pelvic (nonobstetric), real time with image documentation; complete

INCLUDES Total examination of the female pelvic anatomy which includes:

- Bladder measurement
- Description and measurement of the uterus and adnexa
- Description of any pelvic pathology
- Measurement of the endometrium

Total examination of the male pelvis which includes:

- Bladder measurement
- Description of any pelvic pathology
- Evaluation of prostate and seminal vesicles

Z2 03 80 ▫ 3.51 3.51 FUD XXX

76857 limited or follow-up (eg, for follicles)

INCLUDES Focused evaluation limited to:

- Evaluation of one or more elements listed in 76856 and/or
- Reevaluation of one or more pelvic aberrancies noted on a prior ultrasound

Urinary bladder alone

EXCLUDES Bladder volume or post-voided residual measurement without imaging the bladder (51798)

Urinary bladder and kidneys (76770)

Z3 03 80 ▫ 1.52 1.52 FUD XXX

76870 Ultrasound, scrotum and contents ♂

Z3 03 80 ▫ 2.09 2.09 FUD XXX

76872 Ultrasound, transrectal;

Do not report with (45341-45342, 45391-45392, 0249T)

Z3 S 80 ▫ 2.62 2.62 FUD XXX

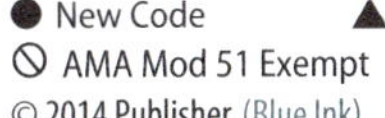

76873 **prostate volume study for brachytherapy treatment planning (separate procedure)** ♂
Z3 S 4.85 4.85 FUD XXX

76881-76886 Ultrasound: Extremities

EXCLUDES *Doppler studies of the extremities (93925-93926, 93930-93931, 93970-93971)*

76881 **Ultrasound, extremity, nonvascular, real-time with image documentation; complete**
INCLUDES Real time scans of a specific joint including assessment of:
Joint
Muscles
Other soft tissue
Tendons
Z2 S 3.35 3.35 FUD XXX

76882 **limited, anatomic specific**
INCLUDES Limited examination of a certain anatomical structure (e.g. muscle or tendon) or for evaluation of a soft-tissue mass
Z3 S 1.01 1.01 FUD XXX

76885 **Ultrasound, infant hips, real time with imaging documentation; dynamic (requiring physician or other qualified health care professional manipulation)** A
Z2 S 80 4.20 4.20 FUD XXX

76886 **limited, static (not requiring physician or other qualified health care professional manipulation)** A
Z2 S 80 3.02 3.02 FUD XXX

76930-76970 Imaging Guidance: Ultrasound

CMS 100-3,220.5 Ultrasound Diagnostic Procedures

INCLUDES Required permanent documentation of ultrasound images except when diagnostic purpose is biometric measurement
Written documentation

EXCLUDES *Focused ultrasound ablation of uterine leiomyomata (0071T-0072T)*
Ultrasound exam that does not include thorough assessment of organ or site, recorded image, and written report

76930 **Ultrasonic guidance for pericardiocentesis, imaging supervision and interpretation**
N1 N 80 2.36 2.36 FUD XXX

76932 **Ultrasonic guidance for endomyocardial biopsy, imaging supervision and interpretation**
N1 N 80 0.00 0.00 FUD XXX

76936 **Ultrasound guided compression repair of arterial pseudoaneurysm or arteriovenous fistulae (includes diagnostic ultrasound evaluation, compression of lesion and imaging)**
Z2 S 80 7.68 7.68 FUD XXX

\+ **76937** **Ultrasound guidance for vascular access requiring ultrasound evaluation of potential access sites, documentation of selected vessel patency, concurrent realtime ultrasound visualization of vascular needle entry, with permanent recording and reporting (List separately in addition to code for primary procedure)**
EXCLUDES *Extremity venous non-invasive vascular diagnostic study performed separately from venous access guidance (93965, 93970-93971)*
Code first primary procedure
Do not report with (37191 37193, 37760 37761, 76942)
N1 N 80 1.02 1.02 FUD ZZZ

76940 **Ultrasound guidance for, and monitoring of, parenchymal tissue ablation**
EXCLUDES *Ablation (32998, 47370-47383, 50592-50593)*
Do not report with (20982-20983, 50250, 50542, 76942, 76998, 0340T)
N1 N 80 0.00 0.00 FUD XXX

76941 **Ultrasonic guidance for intrauterine fetal transfusion or cordocentesis, imaging supervision and interpretation** M ♀
Code also surgical procedure (36460, 59012)
N1 N 80 0.00 0.00 FUD XXX

76942 **Ultrasonic guidance for needle placement (eg, biopsy, aspiration, injection, localization device), imaging supervision and interpretation**
EXCLUDES *Platelet rich plasma injection(s) (0232T)*
Do not report with (10030, 19083, 19285, 20604, 20606, 20611, 27096, 32554-32557, 37760-37761, 43232, 43237, 43242, 45341-45342, 64479-64484, 64490-64495, 76975, 0213T-0218T, 0228T, 0231T-0232T, 0249T, 0301T)
N1 N 80 2.07 2.07 FUD XXX

76945 **Ultrasonic guidance for chorionic villus sampling, imaging supervision and interpretation** M ♀
Code also surgical procedure (59015)
N1 N 80 0.00 0.00 FUD XXX

76946 **Ultrasonic guidance for amniocentesis, imaging supervision and interpretation** M ♀
N1 N 80 0.91 0.91 FUD XXX

76948 **Ultrasonic guidance for aspiration of ova, imaging supervision and interpretation** M ♀
N1 N 80 0.93 0.93 FUD XXX

~~76950~~ ~~**Ultrasonic guidance for placement of radiation therapy fields**~~
To report, see 77387

76965 **Ultrasonic guidance for interstitial radioelement application**
N1 N 80 2.57 2.57 FUD XXX

76970 **Ultrasound study follow-up (specify)**
Z2 S 80 2.67 2.67 FUD XXX

76975 Endoscopic Ultrasound

CMS 100-3,220.5 Ultrasound Diagnostic Procedures
CMS 100-4,12,30.1 Upper Gastrointestinal Endoscopy Including Endoscopic Ultrasound (EUS)

INCLUDES Required permanent documentation of ultrasound images except when diagnostic purpose is biometric measurement
Written documentation

EXCLUDES *Focused ultrasound ablation of uterine leiomyomata (0071T-0072T)*
Ultrasound exam that does not include thorough assessment of organ or site, recorded image, and written report

76975 **Gastrointestinal endoscopic ultrasound, supervision and interpretation**
Do not report with (43231-43232, 43237-43238, 43240, 43242, 43259, 44406-44407, 45341-45342, 45391-45392, 76942)
N1 Q2 80 0.00 0.00 FUD XXX

76977 Bone Density Measurements: Ultrasound

CMS 100-3,220.5 Ultrasound Diagnostic Procedures
CMS 100-4,13,140 Bone Mass Measurements (BMMs)

INCLUDES Required permanent documentation of ultrasound images except when diagnostic purpose is biometric measurement
Written documentation

EXCLUDES *Ultrasound exam that does not include thorough assessment of organ or site, recorded image, and written report*

76977 **Ultrasound bone density measurement and interpretation, peripheral site(s), any method**
Z3 X 80 0.20 0.20 FUD XXX

76998-76999 Imaging Guidance During Surgery: Ultrasound

INCLUDES Required permanent documentation of ultrasound images except when diagnostic purpose is biometric measurement
Written documentation

EXCLUDES *Focused ultrasound ablation of uterine leiomyomata (0071T-0072T)*
Ultrasound exam that does not include thorough assessment of organ or site, recorded image, and written report

76998 Ultrasonic guidance, intraoperative
EXCLUDES *Radiofrequency tissue ablation, open/laparoscopic, ultrasonic guidance (76940)*
Do not report with (36475, 36479, 37760-37761, 47370-47382, 0249T, 0301T)
N1 N 80 0.00 0.00 FUD XXX

76999 Unlisted ultrasound procedure (eg, diagnostic, interventional)
Z2 S 80 0.00 0.00 FUD XXX

77001-77022 Imaging Guidance Techniques

\+ **77001 Fluoroscopic guidance for central venous access device placement, replacement (catheter only or complete), or removal (includes fluoroscopic guidance for vascular access and catheter manipulation, any necessary contrast injections through access site or catheter with related venography radiologic supervision and interpretation, and radiographic documentation of final catheter position) (List separately in addition to code for primary procedure)**
EXCLUDES *Formal extremity venography performed separately from venous access and interpreted separately (36005, 75820, 75822, 75825, 75827)*
Code first primary procedure
Do not report with (33957-33959, [33962, 33963, 33964], 77002)
Do not report with procedure codes that include fluoroscopic guidance in the code descriptor
N1 N PQ 2.23 2.23 FUD ZZZ

77002 Fluoroscopic guidance for needle placement (eg, biopsy, aspiration, injection, localization device)
EXCLUDES *Platelet rich plasma injection(s) (0232T)*
Code also surgical procedure
Do not report with (10030, 19081-19086, 19281-19288, 20982-20983, 32554-32557, 70332, 73040, 73085, 73115, 73525, 73580, 73615, 0232T)
Do not report with arthrography procedure(s)
Do not report with codes that include 77002 in the radiological supervision and interpretation (49440, 74320, 74355, 74445, 74470, 74475, 75809-75810, 75885, 75887, 75980, 75982, 75989)
Do not report with procedure codes that include fluoroscopic guidance in the code descriptor
N1 N PQ 2.88 2.88 FUD XXX

77003 Fluoroscopic guidance and localization of needle or catheter tip for spine or paraspinous diagnostic or therapeutic injection procedures (epidural or subarachnoid)
EXCLUDES *Destruction of paravertebral facet joint nerve by neurolysis ([64633, 64634, 64635, 64636])*
Injection and needle/catheter placement, epidural/subarachnoid (62270-62282, 62310-62319)
Injection, paravertebral facet joint (64490-64495)
Sacroiliac joint arthrography (27096)
Subarachnoid guidance puncture for myelography (72240-72270)
Transforaminal epidural needle placement/injection (64479-64484)
Do not report with (10030, 22586, 27096, 64479-64484, 64490-64495, [64633, 64634, 64635, 64636], 0195T-0196T, 0309T)
Do not report with procedure codes that include fluoroscopic guidance in the code descriptor
N1 N PQ 2.54 2.54 FUD XXX

77011 Computed tomography guidance for stereotactic localization
Do not report with (22586, 0195T-0196T, 0309T)
N1 N 6.31 6.31 FUD XXX

77012 Computed tomography guidance for needle placement (eg, biopsy, aspiration, injection, localization device), radiological supervision and interpretation
EXCLUDES *Platelet rich plasma injection(s) (0232T)*
Do not report with (10030, 22586, 27096, 32554-32557, 64479-64484, 64490-64495, [64633, 64634, 64635, 64636], 0195T-0196T, 0232T, 0309T)
N1 N 3.61 3.61 FUD XXX

77013 Computed tomography guidance for, and monitoring of, parenchymal tissue ablation
EXCLUDES *Percutaneous radiofrequency ablation (32998, 47382-47383, 50592-50593)*
Do not report with (20982-20983, 0340T)
N1 N 80 0.00 0.00 FUD XXX

77014 Computed tomography guidance for placement of radiation therapy fields
Code also placement of interstitial device(s) for radiation therapy guidance (31627, 32553, 49411, 55876)
N1 N 3.46 3.46 FUD XXX

77021 Magnetic resonance guidance for needle placement (eg, for biopsy, needle aspiration, injection, or placement of localization device) radiological supervision and interpretation
EXCLUDES *Platelet rich plasma injection(s) (0232T)*
Surgical procedure
Do not report with (10030, 19085, 19287, 32554-32557, 0232T)
N1 N 11.15 11.15 FUD XXX

77022 Magnetic resonance guidance for, and monitoring of, parenchymal tissue ablation
EXCLUDES *Ablation:*
Percutaneous radiofrequency (32998, 47382-47383, 50592-50593)
Uterine leiomyomata by focused ablation (0071T, 0072T)
Do not report with (20982-20983, 0071T-0072T, 0340T)
N1 N 80 0.00 0.00 FUD XXX

77051-77063 Radiography: Breast

CMS 100-3,220.4 Mammograms
CMS 100-4,18,20 Mammography Services
CMS 100-4,18,20.4 FI/A/B MAC Processing Mammography Services

\+ **77051 Computer-aided detection (computer algorithm analysis of digital image data for lesion detection) with further review for interpretation, with or without digitization of film radiographic images; diagnostic mammography (List separately in addition to code for primary procedure)**
Code first mammography (77055, 77056)
A 0.29 0.29 FUD ZZZ

\+ **77052 screening mammography (List separately in addition to code for primary procedure)**
Code first screening mammography (77057)
A 0.29 0.29 FUD ZZZ

77053 Mammary ductogram or galactogram, single duct, radiological supervision and interpretation
Code also injection procedure (19030)
N1 Q2 1.68 1.68 FUD XXX

77054 Mammary ductogram or galactogram, multiple ducts, radiological supervision and interpretation
N1 Q2 2.27 2.27 FUD XXX

77055 Mammography; unilateral
Do not report with (77063)
Code also computer-aided detection applied to diagnostic mammogram, if performed (77051)
A 2.52 2.52 FUD XXX

77056 bilateral
Code also computer-aided detection applied to diagnostic mammogram, if performed (77051)
Do not report with (77063)
A 3.24 3.24 FUD XXX

77057 Screening mammography, bilateral (2-view film study of each breast) ♀
Code also computer-aided detection applied to screening mammogram, if performed (77052)
Do not report with (77061-77062)
EXCLUDES *Breast electrical impedance scan (76499)*
A PQ 2.31 2.31 FUD XXX

77058 Magnetic resonance imaging, breast, without and/or with contrast material(s); unilateral
B 15.46 15.46 FUD XXX

77059 bilateral
B 15.40 15.40 FUD XXX

● **77061 Digital breast tomosynthesis; unilateral**
Do not report with (76376-76377, 77057)

● **77062 bilateral**
Do not report with (76376-76377, 77057)

\+ ● **77063 Screening digital breast tomosynthesis, bilateral (List separately in addition to code for primary procedure)**
Code first (77057)
Do not report with (76376-76377, 77055-77056)

77071-77086 [77085, 77086] Additional Evaluations of Bones and Joints

77071 Manual application of stress performed by physician or other qualified health care professional for joint radiography, including contralateral joint if indicated
Code also interpretation of stressed images according to anatomical site and number of views
Z2 X 26 80 1.44 1.44 FUD XXX

77072 Bone age studies
Z3 X 80 0.67 0.67 FUD XXX

77073 Bone length studies (orthoroentgenogram, scanogram)
Z3 X 80 1.08 1.08 FUD XXX

77074 Radiologic examination, osseous survey; limited (eg, for metastases)
Z3 X 80 2.02 2.02 FUD XXX

77075 complete (axial and appendicular skeleton)
Z2 X 80 3.02 3.02 FUD XXX

77076 Radiologic examination, osseous survey, infant
Z2 X 80 3.04 3.04 FUD XXX

77077 Joint survey, single view, 2 or more joints (specify)
Z3 X 80 1.14 1.14 FUD XXX

77078 Computed tomography, bone mineral density study, 1 or more sites; axial skeleton (eg, hips, pelvis, spine)
Z2 S 80 3.19 3.19 FUD XXX

77080 Dual-energy X-ray absorptiometry (DXA), bone density study, 1 or more sites; axial skeleton (eg, hips, pelvis, spine)
Do not report with ([77085], [77086])
Z3 S 80 1.38 1.38 FUD XXX

77081 appendicular skeleton (peripheral) (eg, radius, wrist, heel)
Z3 S 80 0.78 0.78 FUD XXX

#● **77085 axial skeleton (eg, hips, pelvis, spine), including vertebral fracture assessment**
Do not report with (77080, [77086])

~~77082 vertebral fracture assessment~~
To report, see 77086

#● **77086 Vertebral fracture assessment via dual-energy X-ray absorptiometry (DXA)**
Do not report with (77080, [77085])

77084 Magnetic resonance (eg, proton) imaging, bone marrow blood supply
Z2 S 80 11.10 11.10 FUD XXX

77085 Resequenced code. See code following 77081.

77086 Resequenced code. See code before 77084.

77261-77263 Therapeutic Radiology: Treatment Planning

CMS 100-2,6,10 Medical and Other Services Furnished to Inpatients

INCLUDES Determination of:
- Appropriate treatment devices
- Number and size of treatment ports
- Treatment method
- Treatment time/dosage
- Treatment volume

Interpretation of special testing
Tumor localization

Do not report with (77401)

77261 Therapeutic radiology treatment planning; simple
INCLUDES Planning for single treatment area included in a single port or simple parallel opposed ports with simple or no blocking
B 26 80 PQ 2.10 2.10 FUD XXX

77262 intermediate
INCLUDES Planning for three or more converging ports, two separate treatment sites, multiple blocks, or special time dose constraints
B 26 80 PQ 3.15 3.15 FUD XXX

77263 complex
INCLUDES Planning for very complex blocking, custom shielding blocks, tangential ports, special wedges or compensators, three or more separate treatment areas, rotational or special beam considerations, combination of treatment modalities
B 26 80 PQ 4.65 4.65 FUD XXX

77280-77299 Radiation Therapy Simulation

CMS 100-2,6,10 Medical and Other Services Furnished to Inpatients
CMS 100-4,4,200.3.2 Additional Billing Instructions for IMRT Planning and Delivery

77280 **Therapeutic radiology simulation-aided field setting; simple**
INCLUDES Simulation of a single treatment site
Z2 X 80 7.58 7.58 FUD XXX

77285 **intermediate**
INCLUDES Two different treatment sites
Z2 X 80 11.81 11.81 FUD XXX

77290 **complex**
INCLUDES Brachytherapy
Complex blocking
Contrast material
Custom shielding blocks
Hyperthermia probe verification
Rotation, arc or particle therapy
Simulation to >= 3 treatment sites
Z2 X 80 14.16 14.16 FUD XXX

\+ **77293** **Respiratory motion management simulation (List separately in addition to code for primary procedure)**
Code first ([77295], 77301)
N 80 12.83 12.83 FUD ZZZ

77295 ***Resequenced code. See code before 77300.***

77299 **Unlisted procedure, therapeutic radiology clinical treatment planning**
Z2 X 80 0.00 0.00 FUD XXX

77295-77370 [77295] Radiation Physics Services

CMS 100-4,4,61.2 Requirements for Specific Procedures to be Reported With Device Codes
CMS 100-4,4,200.3.1 Billing for IMRT Planning and Delivery
CMS 100-4,4,200.3.2 Additional Billing Instructions for IMRT Planning and Delivery
CMS 100-4,4,220.2 Additional Billing Instructions for IMRT Planning

\# **77295** **3-dimensional radiotherapy plan, including dose-volume histograms**
Z3 X 80 PQ 13.54 13.54 FUD XXX

77300 **Basic radiation dosimetry calculation, central axis depth dose calculation, TDF, NSD, gap calculation, off axis factor, tissue inhomogeneity factors, calculation of non-ionizing radiation surface and depth dose, as required during course of treatment, only when prescribed by the treating physician**
Do not report with (77306-77307, 77316-77318, 77321)
Z3 X 80 1.88 1.88 FUD XXX

77301 **Intensity modulated radiotherapy plan, including dose-volume histograms for target and critical structure partial tolerance specifications**
Z2 X 80 54.71 54.71 FUD XXX

~~**77305**~~ ~~**Teletherapy, isodose plan (whether hand or computer calculated); simple (1 or 2 parallel opposed unmodified ports directed to a single area of interest)**~~
To report, see 77306

● **77306** **Teletherapy isodose plan; simple (1 or 2 unmodified ports directed to a single area of interest), includes basic dosimetry calculation(s)**
Do not report more than one time for treatment to a specific area
Do not report with (77300, 77401)

● **77307** **complex (multiple treatment areas, tangential ports, the use of wedges, blocking, rotational beam, or special beam considerations), includes basic dosimetry calculation(s)**
Do not report more than one time for treatment to a specific area
Do not report with (77300, 77401)

~~**77310**~~ ~~**intermediate (3 or more treatment ports directed to a single area of interest)**~~
To report, see 77306-77307

~~**77315**~~ ~~**complex (mantle or inverted Y, tangential ports, the use of wedges, compensators, complex blocking, rotational beam, or special beam considerations)**~~
To report, see 77307

● **77316** **Brachytherapy isodose plan; simple (calculation[s] made from 1 to 4 sources, or remote afterloading brachytherapy, 1 channel), includes basic dosimetry calculation(s)**
Do not report with (77300, 77401)

● **77317** **intermediate (calculation[s] made from 5 to 10 sources, or remote afterloading brachytherapy, 2-12 channels), includes basic dosimetry calculation(s)**
Do not report with (77300, 77401)

● **77318** **complex (calculation[s] made from over 10 sources, or remote afterloading brachytherapy, over 12 channels), includes basic dosimetry calculation(s)**
Do not report with (77300, 77401)

77321 **Special teletherapy port plan, particles, hemibody, total body**
Z3 X 80 2.56 2.56 FUD XXX

~~**77326**~~ ~~**Brachytherapy isodose plan; simple (calculation made from single plane, 1 to 4 sources/ribbon application, remote afterloading brachytherapy, 1 to 8 sources)**~~
To report, see 77316

~~**77327**~~ ~~**intermediate (multiplane dosage calculations, application involving 5 to 10 sources/ribbons, remote afterloading brachytherapy, 9 to 12 sources)**~~
To report, see 77317

~~**77328**~~ ~~**complex (multiplane isodose plan, volume implant calculations, over 10 sources/ribbons used, special spatial reconstruction, remote afterloading brachytherapy, over 12 sources)**~~
To report, see 77318

77331 **Special dosimetry (eg, TLD, microdosimetry) (specify), only when prescribed by the treating physician**
Z3 X 80 1.78 1.78 FUD XXX

77332 **Treatment devices, design and construction; simple (simple block, simple bolus)**
Do not report with (77401)
Z3 X 80 2.25 2.25 FUD XXX

77333 **intermediate (multiple blocks, stents, bite blocks, special bolus)**
Do not report with (77401)
Z3 X 80 1.48 1.48 FUD XXX

77334 **complex (irregular blocks, special shields, compensators, wedges, molds or casts)**
Do not report with (77401)
Z3 X 80 4.20 4.20 FUD XXX

77336 **Continuing medical physics consultation, including assessment of treatment parameters, quality assurance of dose delivery, and review of patient treatment documentation in support of the radiation oncologist, reported per week of therapy**
Do not report with (77401)
Z2 X TC 80 2.09 2.09 FUD XXX

77338 **Multi-leaf collimator (MLC) device(s) for intensity modulated radiation therapy (IMRT), design and construction per IMRT plan**
EXCLUDES *Immobilization in IMRT treatment (77332-77334)*
Do not report with ([77385])
Do not report more than once per IMRT plan
14.01 14.01 FUD XXX

77370 **Special medical radiation physics consultation**
3.20 3.20 FUD XXX

77371-77399 Stereotactic Radiosurgery (SRS) Planning and Delivery

CMS 100-4,4,200.3.3 Billing Multi-Source Photon Stereotactic Radiosurgery Planning and Delivery

77371 **Radiation treatment delivery, stereotactic radiosurgery (SRS), complete course of treatment of cranial lesion(s) consisting of 1 session; multi-source Cobalt 60 based**
0.00 0.00 FUD XXX

77372 **linear accelerator based**
EXCLUDES *Radiation treatment supervision (77432)*
29.18 29.18 FUD XXX

77373 **Stereotactic body radiation therapy, treatment delivery, per fraction to 1 or more lesions, including image guidance, entire course not to exceed 5 fractions**
EXCLUDES *Single fraction cranial lesion(s) (77371-77372)*
Do not report with (77401-77402, 77407, 77412, [77385, 77386])
34.94 34.94 FUD XXX

77385 *Resequenced code. See code following 77417.*

77386 *Resequenced code. See code following 77417.*

77387 *Resequenced code. See code following 77417.*

77399 **Unlisted procedure, medical radiation physics, dosimetry and treatment devices, and special services**
0.00 0.00 FUD XXX

77401-77387 [77385, 77386, 77387] Radiation Treatment

CMS 100-2,6,10 Medical and Other Services Furnished to Inpatients
CMS 100-4,4,220.1 Billing for IMRT Planning and Delivery
CMS 100-4,13,70.3 Radiation Treatment Delivery
INCLUDES Technical component and assorted energy levels
EXCLUDES *Intra-fraction localization and target tracking ([77387])*

▲ **77401** **Radiation treatment delivery, superficial and/or ortho voltage, per day**
Do not report with (77373)
0.56 0.56 FUD XXX

▲ **77402** **Radiation treatment delivery,=>1 MeV; simple**
Do not report with (77373)
3.91 3.91 FUD XXX

~~77403~~ ~~6-10 MeV~~
To report, see 77402

~~77404~~ ~~11-19 MeV~~
To report, see 77402

~~77406~~ ~~20 MeV or greater~~
To report, see 77402

▲ **77407** **intermediate**
Do not report with (77373)
7.10 7.10 FUD XXX

~~77408~~ ~~6-10 MeV~~
To report, see 77407

~~77409~~ ~~11-19 MeV~~
To report, see 77407

~~77411~~ ~~20 MeV or greater~~
To report, see 77407

▲ **77412** **Radiation treatment delivery, =>1 MeV; complex**
Do not report with (77373)
6.74 6.74 FUD XXX

~~77413~~ ~~6-10 MeV~~
To report, see 77412

~~77414~~ ~~11-19 MeV~~
To report, see 77412

~~77416~~ ~~20 MeV or greater~~
To report, see 77412

77417 **Therapeutic radiology port film(s)**
0.39 0.39 FUD XXX

#● **77385** **Intensity modulated radiation treatment delivery (IMRT), includes guidance and tracking, when performed; simple**
Code also modifier 26 for professional component tracking and guidance with ([77387])
Do not report with (77371-77373)

#● **77386** **complex**
Code also modifier 26 for professional component tracking and guidance with ([77387])
Do not report with (77371-77373)

#● **77387** **Guidance for localization of target volume for delivery of radiation treatment delivery, includes intrafraction tracking, when performed**
Do not report technical component with (77371-77373, [77385, 77386])

77418 IMRT Delivery

CMS 100-2,6,10 Medical and Other Services Furnished to Inpatients
CMS 100-4,4,220.1 Billing for IMRT Planning and Delivery

~~77418~~ ~~Intensity modulated treatment delivery, single or multiple fields/arcs, via narrow spatially and temporally modulated beams, binary, dynamic MLC, per treatment session~~

77421 Stereoscopic Imaging Guidance

CMS 100-2,6,10 Medical and Other Services Furnished to Inpatients

~~77421~~ ~~Stereoscopic X-ray guidance for localization of target volume for the delivery of radiation therapy~~
To report, see 77387

77424-77425 [77424, 77425] Intraoperative Radiation Treatment

\# **77424** **Intraoperative radiation treatment delivery, x-ray, single treatment session**
0.00 0.00 FUD XXX

\# **77425** **Intraoperative radiation treatment delivery, electrons, single treatment session**
0.00 0.00 FUD XXX

77422-77425 Neutron Therapy

77422 **High energy neutron radiation treatment delivery; single treatment area using a single port or parallel-opposed ports with no blocks or simple blocking**
1.17 1.17 FUD XXX

77423 **1 or more isocenter(s) with coplanar or non-coplanar geometry with blocking and/or wedge, and/or compensator(s)**
1.39 1.39 FUD XXX

77424 *Resequenced code. See code following 77421.*

77425 *Resequenced code. See code before 77422.*

77427-77499 Radiation Therapy Management

CMS 100-4,13,70.1 Weekly Radiation Therapy Management

INCLUDES Assessment of patient for medical evaluation and management (at least one per treatment management service) that includes:
Coordination of care/treatment
Evaluation of patient's response to treatment
Review of:
Dose delivery
Dosimetry
Lab tests
Patient treatment set-up
Port film
Treatment parameters
X-rays
Units of five fractions or treatment sessions regardless of time. Two or more fractions performed on the same day can be counted separately provided there is a distinct break in service between sessions and the fractions are of the character usually furnished on different days.

Do not report with (77401)

77427 Radiation treatment management, 5 treatments
INCLUDES 3 or 4 fractions beyond a multiple of five at the end of a treatment period
Do not report separately when one or two more fractions are provided beyond a multiple of five at the end of a course of treatment
B 26 PQ 5.20 5.20 FUD XXX

77431 Radiation therapy management with complete course of therapy consisting of 1 or 2 fractions only
Do not report when used to fill in the last week of a long course of therapy
B 26 80 PQ 2.85 2.85 FUD XXX

77432 Stereotactic radiation treatment management of cranial lesion(s) (complete course of treatment consisting of 1 session)
EXCLUDES *Stereotactic body radiation therapy treatment (77435)*
Code also technical component of guidance for localization of target volume by appending modifier TC to ([77387])
Do not report with stereotactic radiosurgery by same physician (61796-61800)
B 26 80 PQ 11.71 11.71 FUD XXX

77435 Stereotactic body radiation therapy, treatment management, per treatment course, to 1 or more lesions, including image guidance, entire course not to exceed 5 fractions
Code also technical component of guidance for localization of target volume by appending modifier TC to ([77387])
Do not report with (77427-77432)
Do not report with stereotactic radiosurgery by same physician (32701, 61796-61800, 63620-63621)
NI N 26 80 PQ 17.69 17.69 FUD XXX

77469 Intraoperative radiation treatment management
EXCLUDES *Medical evaluation and management provided outside of the intraoperative treatment management*
B 80 8.75 8.75 FUD XXX

77470 Special treatment procedure (eg, total body irradiation, hemibody radiation, per oral or endocavitary irradiation)
EXCLUDES *Daily or weekly patient management*
Intraoperative radiation treatment delivery and management ([77424, 77425], 77469)
Do not report more than one time per course of therapy
Z3 S 80 PQ 4.33 4.33 FUD XXX

77499 Unlisted procedure, therapeutic radiology treatment management
B 80 0.00 0.00 FUD XXX

77520-77525 Proton Therapy

CMS 100-2,6,10 Medical and Other Services Furnished to Inpatients

EXCLUDES *High dose rate electronic brachytherapy, per fraction (0182T)*

77520 Proton treatment delivery; simple, without compensation
INCLUDES Single treatment site using:
Single nontangential/oblique port
Z2 S TC 80 0.00 0.00 FUD XXX

77522 simple, with compensation
INCLUDES Single treatment site using:
Custom block with compensation
Single nontangential/oblique port
Z2 S TC 80 0.00 0.00 FUD XXX

77523 intermediate
INCLUDES One or more treatment sites using:
One or more tangential/oblique ports with custom blocks and compensators OR
Two or more ports with custom blocks and compensators
Z2 S TC 80 0.00 0.00 FUD XXX

77525 complex
INCLUDES One or more treatment sites using:
Two or more ports with matching or patching fields and custom blocks and compensators
Z2 S TC 80 0.00 0.00 FUD XXX

77600-77620 Hyperthermia Treatment

CMS 100-3,110.1 Hyperthermia for Treatment of Cancer

INCLUDES Interstitial insertion of temperature sensors
Management during the course of therapy
Normal follow-up care for three months after completion
Physics planning
Use of heat generating devices

EXCLUDES *High dose rate electronic brachytherapy, per fraction (0182T)*
Initial evaluation and management service
Radiation therapy treatment (77371-77373, 77401-77412, 77422-77423)

⊙ **77600 Hyperthermia, externally generated; superficial (ie, heating to a depth of 4 cm or less)**
Z2 S 80 11.11 11.11 FUD XXX

⊙ **77605 deep (ie, heating to depths greater than 4 cm)**
EXCLUDES *Microwave thermotherapy of the breast (0301T)*
Z2 S 80 20.17 20.17 FUD XXX

⊙ **77610 Hyperthermia generated by interstitial probe(s); 5 or fewer interstitial applicators**
Z2 S 80 27.85 27.85 FUD XXX

⊙ **77615 more than 5 interstitial applicators**
Z2 S 80 27.86 27.86 FUD XXX

77620 Hyperthermia generated by intracavitary probe(s)
Z2 S 80 10.20 10.20 FUD XXX

77750-77799 Brachytherapy

CMS 100-4,4,61.4.1 Brachytherapy Sources - General
CMS 100-4,4,61.4.3 Brachytherapy Sources Ordered for a Specific Patient
CMS 100-4,4,61.4.4 Billing for Brachytherapy Source Supervision, Handling, and Loading Costs
CMS 100-4,13,70.4 Clinical Brachytherapy

INCLUDES Hospital admission and daily visits

EXCLUDES *High dose rate electronic brachytherapy, per fraction (0182T)*
Placement of:
Heyman capsules (58346)
Ovoids and tandems (57155)

Code also brachytherapy sources (C1716-C1719, C2616, C2634-C2643, C2698-C2699)

77750 Infusion or instillation of radioelement solution (includes 3-month follow-up care)
EXCLUDES *Monoclonal antibody infusion (79403)*
Nonantibody radiopharmaceutical therapy infusion without follow-up care (79101)
Z2 S 80 10.30 10.30 FUD 090

77761 **Intracavitary radiation source application; simple**
INCLUDES One to four sources/ribbons
Do not report with (0182T)
Z3 S 80 — 10.81 — 10.81 FUD 090

77762 **intermediate**
INCLUDES Five to ten sources/ribbons
Do not report with (0182T)
Z2 S 80 — 14.31 — 14.31 FUD 090

77763 **complex**
INCLUDES More than ten sources/ribbons
Do not report with (0182T)
Z2 S 80 — 20.30 — 20.30 FUD 090

77776 **Interstitial radiation source application; simple**
INCLUDES One to four sources/ribbons
Do not report with (0182T)
Z3 S 80 PQ — 12.14 — 12.14 FUD 090

77777 **intermediate**
INCLUDES Five to ten sources/ribbons
Do not report with (0182T)
Z3 S 80 PQ — 16.38 — 16.38 FUD 090

77778 **complex**
INCLUDES More than ten sources/ribbons
Do not report with (0182T)
Z3 03 80 PQ — 24.33 — 24.33 FUD 090

77785 **Remote afterloading high dose rate radionuclide brachytherapy; 1 channel**
Do not report with (0182T)
Z3 S 80 — 6.63 — 6.63 FUD XXX

77786 **2-12 channels**
Do not report with (0182T)
Z3 S 80 — 13.53 — 13.53 FUD XXX

77787 **over 12 channels**
Do not report with (0182T)
Z2 S 80 PQ — 21.55 — 21.55 FUD XXX

77789 **Surface application of radiation source**
Do not report with (0182T)
Z3 S 80 — 3.30 — 3.30 FUD 000

77790 **Supervision, handling, loading of radiation source**
N1 N 80 — 2.68 — 2.68 FUD XXX

77799 **Unlisted procedure, clinical brachytherapy**
Z2 S 80 — 0.00 — 0.00 FUD XXX

78012-78099 Nuclear Radiology: Thyroid, Parathyroid, Adrenal

CMS 100-3,220.8 Nuclear Radiology Procedure
CMS 100-3,220.12 Single Photon Emission Tomography

EXCLUDES *Diagnostic services (see appropriate sections)*
Follow-up care (see appropriate section)
Radioimmunoassays (82009-84999 [82652])

Code also radiopharmaceutical(s) and/or drug(s) supplied

78012 **Thyroid uptake, single or multiple quantitative measurement(s) (including stimulation, suppression, or discharge, when performed)**
Z2 S 80 — 2.19 — 2.19 FUD XXX

78013 **Thyroid imaging (including vascular flow, when performed);**
Z2 S 80 — 5.52 — 5.52 FUD XXX

78014 **with single or multiple uptake(s) quantitative measurement(s) (including stimulation, suppression, or discharge, when performed)**
Z2 S 80 — 6.69 — 6.69 FUD XXX

78015 **Thyroid carcinoma metastases imaging; limited area (eg, neck and chest only)**
Z2 S 80 — 6.21 — 6.21 FUD XXX

78016 **with additional studies (eg, urinary recovery)**
Z2 S 80 — 8.00 — 8.00 FUD XXX

78018 **whole body**
Z2 S 80 — 8.92 — 8.92 FUD XXX

+ **78020** **Thyroid carcinoma metastases uptake (List separately in addition to code for primary procedure)**
Code first (78018)
N1 N 80 — 2.36 — 2.36 FUD ZZZ

78070 **Parathyroid planar imaging (including subtraction, when performed);**
Z2 S 80 — 8.49 — 8.49 FUD XXX

78071 **with tomographic (SPECT)**
Z2 X 80 — 9.97 — 9.97 FUD XXX

78072 **with tomographic (SPECT), and concurrently acquired computed tomography (CT) for anatomical localization**
Z2 X 80 — 12.46 — 12.46 FUD XXX

78075 **Adrenal imaging, cortex and/or medulla**
Z2 S 80 — 12.12 — 12.12 FUD XXX

78099 **Unlisted endocrine procedure, diagnostic nuclear medicine**
Z2 S 80 — 0.00 — 0.00 FUD XXX

78102-78199 Nuclear Radiology: Blood Forming Organs

EXCLUDES *Diagnostic services (see appropriate sections)*
Follow-up care (see appropriate section)
Radioimmunoassays (82009-84999 [82652])

Code also radiopharmaceutical(s) and/or drug(s) supplied

78102 **Bone marrow imaging; limited area**
Z2 S 80 — 4.82 — 4.82 FUD XXX

78103 **multiple areas**
Z2 S 80 — 6.40 — 6.40 FUD XXX

78104 **whole body**
Z2 S 80 — 6.92 — 6.92 FUD XXX

78110 **Plasma volume, radiopharmaceutical volume-dilution technique (separate procedure); single sampling**
Z2 S 80 — 2.68 — 2.68 FUD XXX

78111 **multiple samplings**
Z2 S 80 — 2.81 — 2.81 FUD XXX

78120 **Red cell volume determination (separate procedure); single sampling**
Z2 S 80 — 2.71 — 2.71 FUD XXX

78121 **multiple samplings**
Z2 S 80 — 2.86 — 2.86 FUD XXX

78122 **Whole blood volume determination, including separate measurement of plasma volume and red cell volume (radiopharmaceutical volume-dilution technique)**
Z2 S 80 — 2.80 — 2.80 FUD XXX

78130 **Red cell survival study;**
Z2 S 80 — 4.85 — 4.85 FUD XXX

78135 **differential organ/tissue kinetics (eg, splenic and/or hepatic sequestration)**
Z2 S 80 — 9.98 — 9.98 FUD XXX

78140 **Labeled red cell sequestration, differential organ/tissue (eg, splenic and/or hepatic)**
Z2 S 80 3.87 3.87 FUD XXX

78185 **Spleen imaging only, with or without vascular flow**
EXCLUDES *Liver imaging (78215-78216)*
Z2 S 80 6.00 6.00 FUD XXX

78190 **Kinetics, study of platelet survival, with or without differential organ/tissue localization**
Z2 S 80 11.30 11.30 FUD XXX

78191 **Platelet survival study**
Z2 S 80 4.85 4.85 FUD XXX

78195 **Lymphatics and lymph nodes imaging**
EXCLUDES *Sentinel node identification without scintigraphy (38792)*
Sentinel node removal (38500-38542)
Z2 S 80 10.17 10.17 FUD XXX

78199 **Unlisted hematopoietic, reticuloendothelial and lymphatic procedure, diagnostic nuclear medicine**
Z2 S 80 0.00 0.00 FUD XXX

78201-78299 Nuclear Radiology: Digestive System

EXCLUDES *Diagnostic services (see appropriate sections)*
Follow-up care (see appropriate section)
Radioimmunoassays (82009-84999 [82652])
Code also radiopharmaceutical(s) and/or drug(s) supplied

78201 **Liver imaging; static only**
EXCLUDES *Spleen imaging only (78185)*
Z2 S 80 5.33 5.33 FUD XXX

78202 **with vascular flow**
EXCLUDES *Spleen imaging only (78185)*
Z2 S 80 5.78 5.78 FUD XXX

78205 **Liver imaging (SPECT);**
Z2 S 80 6.08 6.08 FUD XXX

78206 **with vascular flow**
Z2 S 80 9.67 9.67 FUD XXX

78215 **Liver and spleen imaging; static only**
Z2 S 80 5.55 5.55 FUD XXX

78216 **with vascular flow**
Z2 S 80 3.50 3.50 FUD XXX

78226 **Hepatobiliary system imaging, including gallbladder when present;**
Z2 S 80 9.45 9.45 FUD XXX

78227 **with pharmacologic intervention, including quantitative measurement(s) when performed**
Z2 S 80 12.80 12.80 FUD XXX

78230 **Salivary gland imaging;**
Z2 S 80 3.90 3.90 FUD XXX

78231 **with serial images**
Z2 S 80 3.68 3.68 FUD XXX

78232 **Salivary gland function study**
Z2 S 80 2.83 2.83 FUD XXX

78258 **Esophageal motility**
Z2 S 80 6.30 6.30 FUD XXX

78261 **Gastric mucosa imaging**
Z2 S 80 7.21 7.21 FUD XXX

78262 **Gastroesophageal reflux study**
Z2 S 80 6.95 6.95 FUD XXX

78264 **Gastric emptying study**
Z2 S 80 8.21 8.21 FUD XXX

78267 **Urea breath test, C-14 (isotopic); acquisition for analysis**
EXCLUDES *Breath hydrogen/methane test (91065)*
A 0.00 0.00 FUD XXX

78268 **analysis**
EXCLUDES *Breath hydrogen/methane test (91065)*
A 0.00 0.00 FUD XXX

78270 **Vitamin B-12 absorption study (eg, Schilling test); without intrinsic factor**
Z2 S 80 2.56 2.56 FUD XXX

78271 **with intrinsic factor**
Z2 S 80 2.56 2.56 FUD XXX

78272 **Vitamin B-12 absorption studies combined, with and without intrinsic factor**
Z2 S 80 2.91 2.91 FUD XXX

78278 **Acute gastrointestinal blood loss imaging**
Z2 S 80 9.95 9.95 FUD XXX

78282 **Gastrointestinal protein loss**
Z2 S 80 0.00 0.00 FUD XXX

78290 **Intestine imaging (eg, ectopic gastric mucosa, Meckel's localization, volvulus)**
Z2 S 80 9.53 9.53 FUD XXX

78291 **Peritoneal-venous shunt patency test (eg, for LeVeen, Denver shunt)**
Code also (49427)
Z2 S 80 7.16 7.16 FUD XXX

78299 **Unlisted gastrointestinal procedure, diagnostic nuclear medicine**
Z2 S 80 0.00 0.00 FUD XXX

78300-78399 Nuclear Radiology: Bones and Joints

CMS 100-3,150.3 Bone (Mineral) Density Studies
CMS 100-3,220.8 Nuclear Radiology Procedure

EXCLUDES *Diagnostic services (see appropriate sections)*
Follow-up care (see appropriate section)
Radioimmunoassays (82009-84999 [82652])
Code also radiopharmaceutical(s) and/or drug(s) supplied

78300 **Bone and/or joint imaging; limited area**
Z2 S 80 PQ 5.16 5.16 FUD XXX

78305 **multiple areas**
Z2 S 80 PQ 6.58 6.58 FUD XXX

78306 **whole body**
Z2 S 80 PQ 7.16 7.16 FUD XXX

78315 **3 phase study**
Z2 S 80 PQ 9.93 9.93 FUD XXX

78320 **tomographic (SPECT)**
Z2 S 80 PQ 6.49 6.49 FUD XXX

78350 **Bone density (bone mineral content) study, 1 or more sites; single photon absorptiometry**
E 0.92 0.92 FUD XXX

78351 **dual photon absorptiometry, 1 or more sites**
E 0.43 0.43 FUD XXX

78399 **Unlisted musculoskeletal procedure, diagnostic nuclear medicine**
Z2 S 80 0.00 0.00 FUD XXX

78414-78499 Nuclear Radiology: Heart and Vascular

CMS 100-3,220.6 Positron Emission Tomography (PET) Scans
CMS 100-3,220.6.1 NCD for PET for Perfusion of the Heart (220.6.1)
CMS 100-3,220.6.8 PET (FDG) for Myocardial Viability
CMS 100-3,220.8 Nuclear Radiology Procedure
CMS 100-3,220.12 Single Photon Emission Tomography
CMS 100-4,13,60 Positron Emission Tomography (PET) Scans - General Information
CMS 100-4,13,60.1 Billing for PET Scans
CMS 100-4,13,60.2 Use of Gamma Cameras, Full and Partial Ring PET Scanners
CMS 100-4,13,60.3 PET Scan Qualifying Conditions
CMS 100-4,13,60.4 PET Scans for Imaging of the Perfusion of the Heart Using Rubidium 82
CMS 100-4,13,60.9 Coverage of PET Scans for Myocardial Viability
CMS 100-4,13,60.11 PET Scans for Perfusion of the Heart Using Ammonia N-13

EXCLUDES *Diagnostic services (see appropriate sections)*
Follow-up care (see appropriate section)
Radioimmunoassays (82009-84999 [82652])
Code also radiopharmaceutical(s) and/or drug(s) supplied

78414 **Determination of central c-v hemodynamics (non-imaging) (eg, ejection fraction with probe technique) with or without pharmacologic intervention or exercise, single or multiple determinations**
0.00 0.00 FUD XXX

78428 **Cardiac shunt detection**
5.21 5.21 FUD XXX

78445 **Non-cardiac vascular flow imaging (ie, angiography, venography)**
4.89 4.89 FUD XXX

78451 **Myocardial perfusion imaging, tomographic (SPECT) (including attenuation correction, qualitative or quantitative wall motion, ejection fraction by first pass or gated technique, additional quantification, when performed); single study, at rest or stress (exercise or pharmacologic)**
Code also stress testing when performed (93015-93018)
9.79 9.79 FUD XXX

78452 **multiple studies, at rest and/or stress (exercise or pharmacologic) and/or redistribution and/or rest reinjection**
Code also stress testing when performed (93015-93018)
13.58 13.58 FUD XXX

78453 **Myocardial perfusion imaging, planar (including qualitative or quantitative wall motion, ejection fraction by first pass or gated technique, additional quantification, when performed); single study, at rest or stress (exercise or pharmacologic)**
Code also stress testing when performed (93015-93018)
8.74 8.74 FUD XXX

78454 **multiple studies, at rest and/or stress (exercise or pharmacologic) and/or redistribution and/or rest reinjection**
Code also stress testing when performed (93015-93018)
12.44 12.44 FUD XXX

78456 **Acute venous thrombosis imaging, peptide**
9.13 9.13 FUD XXX

78457 **Venous thrombosis imaging, venogram; unilateral**
5.55 5.55 FUD XXX

78458 **bilateral**
4.63 4.63 FUD XXX

78459 **Myocardial imaging, positron emission tomography (PET), metabolic evaluation**
EXCLUDES *Myocardial perfusion studies (78491-78492)*
0.00 0.00 FUD XXX

78466 **Myocardial imaging, infarct avid, planar; qualitative or quantitative**
5.21 5.21 FUD XXX

78468 **with ejection fraction by first pass technique**
5.61 5.61 FUD XXX

78469 **tomographic SPECT with or without quantification**
EXCLUDES *Myocardial sympathetic innervation imaging (0331T-0332T)*
6.43 6.43 FUD XXX

78472 **Cardiac blood pool imaging, gated equilibrium; planar, single study at rest or stress (exercise and/or pharmacologic), wall motion study plus ejection fraction, with or without additional quantitative processing**
EXCLUDES *Right ventricular ejection fraction by first pass technique (78496)*
Code also stress testing when performed (93015-93018)
Do not report with (78451-78454, 78481, 78483, 78494)
6.55 6.55 FUD XXX

78473 **multiple studies, wall motion study plus ejection fraction, at rest and stress (exercise and/or pharmacologic), with or without additional quantification**
Code also stress testing when performed (93015-93018)
Do not report with (78451-78454, 78481, 78483, 78494)
8.28 8.28 FUD XXX

78481 **Cardiac blood pool imaging (planar), first pass technique; single study, at rest or with stress (exercise and/or pharmacologic), wall motion study plus ejection fraction, with or without quantification**
Code also stress testing when performed (93015-93018)
Do not report with (78451-78454)
5.03 5.03 FUD XXX

78483 **multiple studies, at rest and with stress (exercise and/or pharmacologic), wall motion study plus ejection fraction, with or without quantification**
EXCLUDES *Blood flow studies of the brain (78610)*
Code also stress testing when performed (93015-93018)
Do not report with (78451-78454)
6.86 6.86 FUD XXX

78491 **Myocardial imaging, positron emission tomography (PET), perfusion; single study at rest or stress**
Code also stress testing when performed (93015-93018)
0.00 0.00 FUD XXX

78492 **multiple studies at rest and/or stress**
Code also stress testing when performed (93015-93018)
0.00 0.00 FUD XXX

78494 **Cardiac blood pool imaging, gated equilibrium, SPECT, at rest, wall motion study plus ejection fraction, with or without quantitative processing**
6.47 6.47 FUD XXX

+ 78496 **Cardiac blood pool imaging, gated equilibrium, single study, at rest, with right ventricular ejection fraction by first pass technique (List separately in addition to code for primary procedure)**
Code first (78472)
1.27 1.27 FUD ZZZ

78499 **Unlisted cardiovascular procedure, diagnostic nuclear medicine**
0.00 0.00 FUD XXX

78579-78599 Nuclear Radiology: Lungs

CMS 100-2,15,80 Diagnostic Test Requirements
CMS 100-3,220.7 Xenon Scan
CMS 100-3,220.8 Nuclear Radiology Procedure

EXCLUDES *Diagnostic services (see appropriate sections)*
Follow-up care (see appropriate sections)
Radioimmunoassays (82009-84999 [82652])

Code also radiopharmaceutical(s) and/or drug(s) supplied

78579 **Pulmonary ventilation imaging (eg, aerosol or gas)**
Do not report more than one time per imaging session
5.32 5.32 FUD XXX

78580 **Pulmonary perfusion imaging (eg, particulate)**
Do not report more than one time per imaging session
Do not report with (78451-78454)
6.82 6.82 FUD XXX

78582 **Pulmonary ventilation (eg, aerosol or gas) and perfusion imaging**
Do not report more than one time per imaging session
Do not report with (78451-78454)
9.57 9.57 FUD XXX

78597 **Quantitative differential pulmonary perfusion, including imaging when performed**
Do not report more than one time per imaging session
Do not report with (78451-78454)
5.76 5.76 FUD XXX

78598 **Quantitative differential pulmonary perfusion and ventilation (eg, aerosol or gas), including imaging when performed**
Do not report more than one time per imaging session
Do not report with (78451-78454)
8.76 8.76 FUD XXX

78599 **Unlisted respiratory procedure, diagnostic nuclear medicine**
0.00 0.00 FUD XXX

78600-78650 Nuclear Radiology: Brain/Cerebrospinal Fluid

CMS 100-3,220.6.9 FDG PET for Refractory Seizures
CMS 100-3,220.8 Nuclear Radiology Procedure

EXCLUDES *Diagnostic services (see appropriate sections)*
Follow-up care (see appropriate section)
Radioimmunoassays (82009-84999 [82652])

Code also radiopharmaceutical(s) and/or drug(s) supplied

Diagram of tomography principal (left)

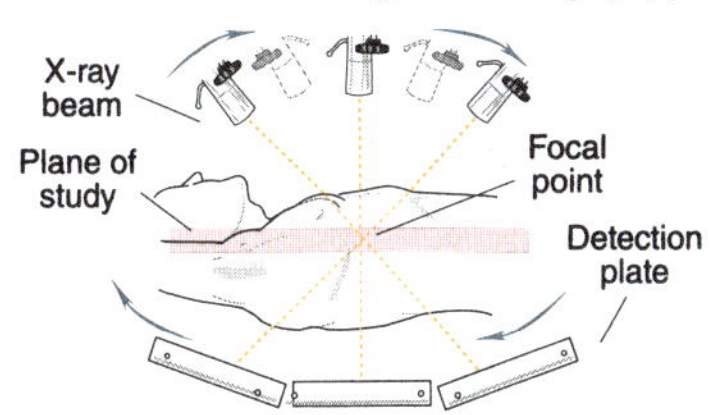

Schematic of frontal coronal CT section of skull

78600 **Brain imaging, less than 4 static views;**
5.22 5.22 FUD XXX

78601 **with vascular flow**
6.17 6.17 FUD XXX

78605 **Brain imaging, minimum 4 static views;**
5.65 5.65 FUD XXX

78606 **with vascular flow**
9.39 9.39 FUD XXX

78607 **Brain imaging, tomographic (SPECT)**
9.94 9.94 FUD XXX

78608 **Brain imaging, positron emission tomography (PET); metabolic evaluation**
0.00 0.00 FUD XXX

78609 **perfusion evaluation**
2.18 2.18 FUD XXX

78610 **Brain imaging, vascular flow only**
4.97 4.97 FUD XXX

78630 **Cerebrospinal fluid flow, imaging (not including introduction of material); cisternography**
Code also injection procedure (61000-61070, 62270-62319)
9.63 9.63 FUD XXX

78635 **ventriculography**
Code also injection procedure (61000-61070, 62270-62294)
9.66 9.66 FUD XXX

78645 **shunt evaluation**
Code also injection procedure (61000-61070, 62270-62294)
9.21 9.21 FUD XXX

78647 **tomographic (SPECT)**
9.99 9.99 FUD XXX

78650 **Cerebrospinal fluid leakage detection and localization**
Code also injection procedure (61000-61070, 62270-62294)
9.58 9.58 FUD XXX

78660-78699 Nuclear Radiology: Lacrimal Duct System

Code also radiopharmaceutical(s) and/or drug(s) supplied

78660 **Radiopharmaceutical dacryocystography**
5.31 5.31 FUD XXX

78699 **Unlisted nervous system procedure, diagnostic nuclear medicine**
0.00 0.00 FUD XXX

78700-78725 Nuclear Radiology: Renal Anatomy and Function

CMS 100-2,15,80 Diagnostic Test Requirements
CMS 100-3,220.8 Nuclear Radiology Procedure
CMS 100-3,220.12 Single Photon Emission Tomography

EXCLUDES *Diagnostic services (see appropriate sections)*
Follow-up care (see appropriate section)
Radioimmunoassays (82009-84999 [82652])
Renal endoscopy with insertion of radioactive substances (77776-77778)

Code also radiopharmaceutical(s) and/or drug(s) supplied

78700 **Kidney imaging morphology;**
4.96 4.96 FUD XXX

78701 **with vascular flow**
6.10 6.10 FUD XXX

78707 **with vascular flow and function, single study without pharmacological intervention**
6.60 6.60 FUD XXX

78708 **with vascular flow and function, single study, with pharmacological intervention (eg, angiotensin converting enzyme inhibitor and/or diuretic)**
4.93 4.93 FUD XXX

78709 **with vascular flow and function, multiple studies, with and without pharmacological intervention (eg, angiotensin converting enzyme inhibitor and/or diuretic)**
10.43 10.43 FUD XXX

78710 **tomographic (SPECT)**
5.67 5.67 FUD XXX

78725 **Kidney function study, non-imaging radioisotopic study**
3.10 3.10 FUD XXX

78730-78799 Nuclear Radiology: Urogenital

CMS 100-2,15,80 Diagnostic Test Requirements
CMS 100-3,220.8 Nuclear Radiology Procedure

EXCLUDES *Diagnostic services (see appropriate sections)*
Follow-up care (see appropriate section)
Radioimmunoassays (82009-84999 [82652])

Code also radiopharmaceutical(s) and/or drug(s) supplied

\+ **78730** **Urinary bladder residual study (List separately in addition to code for primary procedure)**
EXCLUDES *Measurement of postvoid residual urine and/or bladder capacity using ultrasound (51798)*
Ultrasound imaging of the bladder only with measurement of postvoid residual urine (76857)
Code first (78740)
2.16 2.16 FUD ZZZ

78740 **Ureteral reflux study (radiopharmaceutical voiding cystogram)**
EXCLUDES *Catheterization (51701-51703)*
Code also urinary bladder residual study (78730)
Z2 S 80 6.27 6.27 FUD XXX

78761 **Testicular imaging with vascular flow** ♂
Z2 S 80 6.00 6.00 FUD XXX

78799 **Unlisted genitourinary procedure, diagnostic nuclear medicine**
Z2 S 80 0.00 0.00 FUD XXX

78800-78804 Nuclear Radiology: Tumor Localization

CMS 100-2,15,80 Diagnostic Test Requirements
CMS 100-3,220.8 Nuclear Radiology Procedure
CMS 100-3,220.12 Single Photon Emission Tomography
Code also radiopharmaceutical(s) and/or drug(s) supplied

78800 **Radiopharmaceutical localization of tumor or distribution of radiopharmaceutical agent(s); limited area**
INCLUDES Ocular radiophosphorus tumor identification
EXCLUDES *Specific organ (see appropriate site)*
Z2 S 80 5.43 5.43 FUD XXX

78801 **multiple areas**
Z2 S 80 7.14 7.14 FUD XXX

78802 **whole body, single day imaging**
Z2 S 80 9.18 9.18 FUD XXX

78803 **tomographic (SPECT)**
Z2 S 80 9.68 9.68 FUD XXX

78804 **whole body, requiring 2 or more days imaging**
Z2 S 80 16.17 16.17 FUD XXX

78805-78807 Nuclear Radiology: Inflammation and Infection

CMS 100-2,15,80 Diagnostic Test Requirements
CMS 100-3,220.8 Nuclear Radiology Procedure
CMS 100-3,220.12 Single Photon Emission Tomography
EXCLUDES *Imaging bone infectious or inflammatory disease with bone imaging radiopharmaceutical (78300, 78305-78306)*
Code also radiopharmaceutical(s) and/or drug(s) supplied

78805 **Radiopharmaceutical localization of inflammatory process; limited area**
Z2 S 80 5.21 5.21 FUD XXX

78806 **whole body**
Z2 S 80 9.42 9.42 FUD XXX

78807 **tomographic (SPECT)**
Z2 S 80 9.64 9.64 FUD XXX

78808 Intravenous Injection for Radiopharmaceutical Localization

Code also radiopharmaceutical(s) and/or drug(s) supplied

78808 **Injection procedure for radiopharmaceutical localization by non-imaging probe study, intravenous (eg, parathyroid adenoma)**
EXCLUDES *Identification of sentinel node (38792)*
N1 Q1 80 1.32 1.32 FUD XXX

78811-78999 Nuclear Radiology: Diagnosis, Staging, Restaging or Monitoring Cancer

CMS 100-4,13,60.3 PET Scan Qualifying Conditions
CMS 100-4,13,60.3.1 Appropriate Codes for PET Scans
EXCLUDES *CT scan performed for other than attenuation correction and anatomical localization (report with the appropriate site-specific CT code and modifier 59)*
Ocular radiophosphorus tumor identification (78800)
PET brain scan (78608-78609)
PET myocardial imaging (78459, 78491-78492)
Code also radiopharmaceutical(s) and/or drug(s) supplied
Do not report with procedure performed more than one time per session

78811 **Positron emission tomography (PET) imaging; limited area (eg, chest, head/neck)**
Z2 S 80 0.00 0.00 FUD XXX

78812 **skull base to mid-thigh**
Z2 S 80 0.00 0.00 FUD XXX

78813 **whole body**
Z2 S 80 0.00 0.00 FUD XXX

78814 **Positron emission tomography (PET) with concurrently acquired computed tomography (CT) for attenuation correction and anatomical localization imaging; limited area (eg, chest, head/neck)**
Z2 S 80 0.00 0.00 FUD XXX

78815 **skull base to mid-thigh**
Z2 S 80 0.00 0.00 FUD XXX

78816 **whole body**
Z2 S 80 0.00 0.00 FUD XXX

78999 **Unlisted miscellaneous procedure, diagnostic nuclear medicine**
Z2 S 80 0.00 0.00 FUD XXX

79005-79999 Systemic Radiopharmaceutical Therapy

CMS 100-3,220.8 Nuclear Radiology Procedure
EXCLUDES *Imaging guidance*
Injection into artery, body cavity, or joint (see appropriate injection codes)
Radiological supervision and interpretation

79005 **Radiopharmaceutical therapy, by oral administration**
EXCLUDES *Monoclonal antibody treatment (79403)*
Z3 S 80 3.84 3.84 FUD XXX

79101 **Radiopharmaceutical therapy, by intravenous administration**
EXCLUDES *Administration of nonantibody radioelement solution including follow-up care (77750)*
Radiolabeled monoclonal antibody IV infusion (79403)
Do not report with (36400, 36410, 79403, 96360, 96374-96375, 96409)
Z3 S 80 4.06 4.06 FUD XXX

79200 **Radiopharmaceutical therapy, by intracavitary administration**
Z3 S 80 4.46 4.46 FUD XXX

79300 **Radiopharmaceutical therapy, by interstitial radioactive colloid administration**
Z2 S 80 0.00 0.00 FUD XXX

79403 **Radiopharmaceutical therapy, radiolabeled monoclonal antibody by intravenous infusion**
EXCLUDES *Pretreatment imaging (78802, 78804)*
Do not report with (79101)
Z3 S 80 5.46 5.46 FUD XXX

79440 **Radiopharmaceutical therapy, by intra-articular administration**
Z3 S 80 4.11 4.11 FUD XXX

79445 **Radiopharmaceutical therapy, by intra-arterial particulate administration**
EXCLUDES *Procedural and radiological supervision and interpretation for angiographic and interventional procedures before intra-arterial radiopharmaceutical therapy*
Do not report with (96373, 96420)
Z2 S 80 0.00 0.00 FUD XXX

79999 **Radiopharmaceutical therapy, unlisted procedure**
Z2 S 80 0.00 0.00 FUD XXX

80047-80076 Multi-test Laboratory Panels

CMS 100-2,6,10 Medical and Other Services Furnished to Inpatients
CMS 100-2,15,80 Diagnostic Test Requirements

EXCLUDES *Test codes:*
For testing performed at a frequency greater than the number specified by panel definition
Not specified by panel definition

Do not report two or more panel codes comprising the same tests; report the panel with the highest number of tests to meet the definition of the code, and report the remaining tests individually

80047 Basic metabolic panel (Calcium, ionized)
INCLUDES Calcium, ionized (82330)
Carbon dioxide (bicarbonate) (82374)
Chloride (82435)
Creatinine (82565)
Glucose (82947)
Potassium (84132)
Sodium (84295)
Urea nitrogen (BUN) (84520)
N ☒ 0.00 0.00 FUD XXX

80048 Basic metabolic panel (Calcium, total)
INCLUDES Calcium, total (82310)
Carbon dioxide (bicarbonate) (82374)
Chloride (82435)
Creatinine (82565)
Glucose (82947)
Potassium (84132)
Sodium (84295)
Urea nitrogen (BUN) (84520)
N ☒ 0.00 0.00 FUD XXX

80050 General health panel
INCLUDES Complete blood count (CBC), automated, and appropriate manual differential WBC count (85007 or 85009 and 85027)
OR
Complete blood count (CBC), automated, with automated differential WBC count (85004 and 85025 or 85027)
Comprehensive metabolic profile (80053)
Thyroid stimulating hormones (84443)
E 0.00 0.00 FUD XXX

80051 Electrolyte panel
INCLUDES Carbon dioxide (bicarbonate) (82374)
Chloride (82435)
Potassium (84132)
Sodium (84295)
N ☒ 0.00 0.00 FUD XXX

80053 Comprehensive metabolic panel
INCLUDES Albumin (82040)
Bilirubin, total (82247)
Calcium, total (82310)
Carbon dioxide (bicarbonate) (82374)
Chloride (82435)
Creatinine (82565)
Glucose (82947)
Phosphatase, alkaline (84075)
Potassium (84132)
Protein, total (84155)
Sodium (84295)
Transferase, alanine amino (ALT) (SGPT) (84460)
Transferase, aspartate amino (AST) (SGOT) (84450)
Urea nitrogen (BUN) (84520)
N ☒ 0.00 0.00 FUD XXX

80055 Obstetric panel M ♀
INCLUDES Blood typing, ABO and Rh (86900-86901)
Complete blood count (CBC) automated and appropriate manual differential WBC count (85027 and 85007 or 85009)
OR
Complete blood count (CBC) automated and automated differential (85004 and 85025 or 85027)
Hepatitis B surface antigen (HBsAg) (87340)
RBC antibody screen, each serum technique (86850)
Rubella antibody (86762)
Syphilis test, non-treponemal antibody qualitative (86592)

Do not report panel code 80055 when syphilis screening is provided using a treponemal antibody approach (86780); report individual codes for tests performed in the OB panel instead
E 0.00 0.00 FUD XXX

80061 Lipid panel
INCLUDES Cholesterol, serum, total (82465)
Lipoprotein, direct measurement, high density cholesterol (HDL cholesterol) (83718)
Triglycerides (84478)
N ☒ 0.00 0.00 FUD XXX

80069 Renal function panel
INCLUDES Albumin (82040)
Calcium, total (82310)
Carbon dioxide (bicarbonate) (82374)
Chloride (82435)
Creatinine (82565)
Glucose (82947)
Phosphorus inorganic (phosphate) (84100)
Potassium (84132)
Sodium (84295)
Urea nitrogen (BUN) (84520)
N ☒ 0.00 0.00 FUD XXX

80074 Acute hepatitis panel
INCLUDES Hepatitis A antibody (HAAb) IgM (86709)
Hepatitis B core antibody (HBcAb), IgM (86705)
Hepatitis B surface antigen (HBsAg) (87340)
Hepatitis C antibody (86803)
N 0.00 0.00 FUD XXX

80076 Hepatic function panel
INCLUDES Albumin (82040)
Bilirubin, direct (82248)
Bilirubin, total (82247)
Phosphatase, alkaline (84075)
Protein, total (84155)
Transferase, alanine amino (ALT) (SGPT) (84460)
Transferase, aspartate amino (AST) (SGOT) (84450)
N 0.00 0.00 FUD XXX

80100-80104 [80104] Drug Screening Tests

CMS 100-2,6,10 Medical and Other Services Furnished to Inpatients
CMS 100-2,15,80 Diagnostic Test Requirements

~~**80100 Drug screen, qualitative; multiple drug classes chromatographic method, each procedure**~~
To report, see 80300-80304

~~**80101 single drug class method (eg, immunoassay, enzyme assay), each drug class**~~
To report, see 80300-80304

~~**80104 multiple drug classes other than chromatographic method, each procedure**~~
To report, see 80300-80304

~~**80102 Drug confirmation, each procedure**~~
To report, see 80300-80304

~~80103 Tissue preparation for drug analysis~~
To report, see 80300-80304

~~*80104 Resequenced code. See code following 80101.*~~
To report, see 80300-80304

80300-80304 [80300, 80301, 80302, 80303, 80304] Nonspecific Drug Screening

INCLUDES Analytic procedure to identify drugs and drug metabolites in biological specimens based on an antibody-antigen reaction that establishes if a drug metabolite is present

List A drugs
- Alcohol
- Amphetamines
- Barbiturates
- Benzodiazepines
- Buprenorphine
- Cocaine metabolite
- Heroin metabolite
- Marijuana (THC metabolites)
- Methadone and methadone metabolite
- Methamphetamine
- Methaqualone
- Methylenedioxymethamphetamine (MDMA)
- Opiates
- Oxycodone
- Phencyclidine
- Propoxyphene (not available in U.S. after 11/19/2010)
- Tricyclic antidepressants

List B drugs
- Acetaminophen
- Carisoprodol/meprobamate
- Ethyl glucuronide
- Fentanyl
- Ketamine
- Meperidine (Demerol)
- Methylphenidate
- Nicotine and metabolite (Cotinine)
- Salicylate
- Synthetic cannabinoids (K2, spice)
- Tarpentadol
- Tramadol
- Zolpidem
- Other drugs that are not elsewhere classified

#● **80300** **Drug screen, any number of drug classes from Drug Class List A; any number of non-TLC devices or procedures, (eg, immunoassay) capable of being read by direct optical observation, including instrumented-assisted when performed (eg, dipsticks, cups, cards, cartridges), per date of service**
Do not report more than one time per day

#● **80301** **single drug class method, by instrumented test systems (eg, discrete multichannel chemistry analyzers utilizing immunoassay or enzyme assay), per date of service**

#● **80302** **Drug screen, presumptive, single drug class from Drug Class List B, by immunoassay (eg, ELISA) or non-TLC chromatography without mass spectrometry (eg, GC, HPLC), each procedure**

#● **80303** **Drug screen, any number of drug classes, presumptive, single or multiple drug class method; thin layer chromatography procedure(s) (TLC) (eg, acid, neutral, alkaloid plate), per date of service**

#● **80304** **not otherwise specified presumptive procedure (eg, TOF, MALDI, LDTD, DESI, DART), each procedure**

80320-80377 [80320, 80321, 80322, 80323, 80324, 80325, 80326, 80327, 80328, 80329, 80330, 80331, 80332, 80333, 80334, 80335, 80336, 80337, 80338, 80339, 80340, 80341, 80342, 80343, 80344, 80345, 80346, 80347, 80348, 80349, 80350, 80351, 80352, 80353, 80354, 80355, 80356, 80357, 80358, 80359, 80360, 80361, 80362, 80363, 80364, 80365, 80366, 80367, 80368, 80369, 80370, 80371, 80372, 80373, 80374, 80375, 80376, 80377, 83992] Confirmatory Drug Testing

INCLUDES Antihistamine drug tests ([80375, 80376, 80377])
Detection of specific drugs using methods other than immunoassay or enzymatic technique

Do not report metabolites separate from the code for the drug except when a distinct code is available

#● **80320** **Alcohols**

#● **80321** **Alcohol biomarkers; 1 or 2**

#● **80322** **3 or more**

#● **80323** **Alkaloids, not otherwise specified**

#● **80324** **Amphetamines; 1 or 2**

#● **80325** **3 or 4**

#● **80326** **5 or more**

#● **80327** **Anabolic steroids; 1 or 2**

#● **80328** **3 or more**

#● **80329** **Analgesics, non-opioid; 1 or 2**

#● **80330** **3-5**

#● **80331** **6 or more**

#● **80332** **Antidepressants, serotonergic class; 1 or 2**

#● **80333** **3-5**

#● **80334** **6 or more**

#● **80335** **Antidepressants, tricyclic and other cyclicals; 1 or 2**

#● **80336** **3-5**

#● **80337** **6 or more**

#● **80338** **Antidepressants, not otherwise specified**

#● **80339** **Antiepileptics, not otherwise specified; 1-3**

#● **80340** **4-6**

#● **80341** **7 or more**

#● **80342** **Antipsychotics, not otherwise specified; 1-3**

#● **80343** **4-6**

#● **80344** **7 or more**

#● **80345** **Barbiturates**

#● **80346** **Benzodiazepines; 1-12**

#● **80347** **13 or more**

#● **80348** **Buprenorphine**

#● **80349** **Cannabinoids, natural**

#● **80350** **Cannabinoids, synthetic; 1-3**

#● **80351** **4-6**

#● **80352** **7 or more**

#● **80353** **Cocaine**

#● **80354** **Fentanyl**

#● **80355** **Gabapentin, non-blood**

#● **80356** **Heroin metabolite**

#● 80357 Ketamine and norketamine

#● 80358 Methadone

#● 80359 Methylenedioxyamphetamines (MDA, MDEA, MDMA)

#● 80360 Methylphenidate

#● 80361 Opiates, 1 or more

#● 80362 Opioids and opiate analogs; 1 or 2

#● 80363 3 or 4

#● 80364 5 or more

#● 80365 Oxycodone

83992 Phencyclidine (PCP)
N 0.00 0.00 FUD XXX

#● 80366 Pregabalin

#● 80367 Propoxyphene

#● 80368 Sedative hypnotics (non-benzodiazepines)

#● 80369 Skeletal muscle relaxants; 1 or 2

#● 80370 3 or more

#● 80371 Stimulants, synthetic

#● 80372 Tapentadol

#● 80373 Tramadol

#● 80374 Stereoisomer (enantiomer) analysis, single drug class
Code also index drug analysis if appropriate

#● 80375 Drug(s) or substance(s), definitive, qualitative or quantitative, not otherwise specified; 1-3

#● 80376 4-6

#● 80377 7 or more

80150-80377 [80164, 80165, 80171] Therapeutic Drug Levels

CMS 100-2,15,80 Diagnostic Test Requirements
INCLUDES Testing of drug and metabolite(s) in primary code
Tests on specimens from blood and blood components, and spinal fluid

80150 Amikacin
N 0.00 0.00 FUD XXX

~~80152 Amitriptyline~~
To report, see 80335-80337

~~80154 Benzodiazepines~~
To report, see 80346-80347

80155 Caffeine
A 0.00 0.00 FUD XXX

80156 Carbamazepine; total
N 0.00 0.00 FUD XXX

80157 free
N 0.00 0.00 FUD XXX

80158 Cyclosporine
N 0.00 0.00 FUD XXX

80159 Clozapine
A 0.00 0.00 FUD XXX

~~80160 Desipramine~~
To report, see 80335-80337

▲ 80162 Digoxin; total
N 0.00 0.00 FUD XXX

● 80163 free

80164 Resequenced code. See code following 80201.

80165 Resequenced code. See code following 80201.

~~80166 Doxepin~~
To report, see 80335-80337

80168 Ethosuximide
N 0.00 0.00 FUD XXX

80169 Everolimus
A 0.00 0.00 FUD XXX

#▲ 80171 Gabapentin, whole blood, serum, or plasma
A 0.00 0.00 FUD XXX

80170 Gentamicin
N 0.00 0.00 FUD XXX

80171 Resequenced code. See code following 80169.

~~80172 Gold~~
To report, see 80375

80173 Haloperidol
N 0.00 0.00 FUD XXX

~~80174 Imipramine~~
To report, see 80335-80337

80175 Lamotrigine
A 0.00 0.00 FUD XXX

80176 Lidocaine
N 0.00 0.00 FUD XXX

80177 Levetiracetam
A 0.00 0.00 FUD XXX

80178 Lithium
N ☒ 0.00 0.00 FUD XXX

80180 Mycophenolate (mycophenolic acid)
A 0.00 0.00 FUD XXX

~~80182 Nortriptyline~~
To report, see 80335-80337

80183 Oxcarbazepine
A 0.00 0.00 FUD XXX

80184 Phenobarbital
N 0.00 0.00 FUD XXX

80185 Phenytoin; total
N 0.00 0.00 FUD XXX

80186 free
N 0.00 0.00 FUD XXX

80188 Primidone
N 0.00 0.00 FUD XXX

80190 Procainamide;
N 0.00 0.00 FUD XXX

80192 with metabolites (eg, n-acetyl procainamide)
N 0.00 0.00 FUD XXX

80194 Quinidine
N 0.00 0.00 FUD XXX

80195 Sirolimus
N 0.00 0.00 FUD XXX

~~80196 Salicylate~~
To report, see 80329-80331

80197 Tacrolimus
N 0.00 0.00 FUD XXX

80198 Theophylline
N 0.00 0.00 FUD XXX

80199 Tiagabine
A 0.00 0.00 FUD XXX

80200 Tobramycin
N 0.00 0.00 FUD XXX

80201 Topiramate
N 0.00 0.00 FUD XXX

#▲ 80164 Valproic acid (dipropylacetic acid); total
N 0.00 0.00 FUD XXX

#● 80165 free

80202 Vancomycin
N 0.00 0.00 FUD XXX

80203 Zonisamide
A 0.00 0.00 FUD XXX

▲ **80299** **Quantitation of therapeutic drug, not elsewhere specified**
N 0.00 0.00 FUD XXX

80300 Resequenced code. See code before 80150.

80301 Resequenced code. See code before 80150.

80302 Resequenced code. See code before 80150.

80303 Resequenced code. See code before 80150.

80304 Resequenced code. See code before 80150.

80320 Resequenced code. See code before 80150.

80321 Resequenced code. See code before 80150.

80322 Resequenced code. See code before 80150.

80323 Resequenced code. See code before 80150.

80324 Resequenced code. See code before 80150.

80325 Resequenced code. See code before 80150.

80326 Resequenced code. See code before 80150.

80327 Resequenced code. See code before 80150.

80328 Resequenced code. See code before 80150.

80329 Resequenced code. See code before 80150.

80330 Resequenced code. See code before 80150.

80331 Resequenced code. See code before 80150.

80332 Resequenced code. See code before 80150.

80333 Resequenced code. See code before 80150.

80334 Resequenced code. See code before 80150.

80335 Resequenced code. See code before 80150.

80336 Resequenced code. See code before 80150.

80337 Resequenced code. See code before 80150.

80338 Resequenced code. See code before 80150.

80339 Resequenced code. See code before 80150.

80340 Resequenced code. See code before 80150.

80341 Resequenced code. See code before 80150.

80342 Resequenced code. See code before 80150.

80343 Resequenced code. See code before 80150.

80344 Resequenced code. See code before 80150.

80345 Resequenced code. See code before 80150.

80346 Resequenced code. See code before 80150.

80347 Resequenced code. See code before 80150.

80348 Resequenced code. See code before 80150.

80349 Resequenced code. See code before 80150.

80350 Resequenced code. See code before 80150.

80351 Resequenced code. See code before 80150.

80352 Resequenced code. See code before 80150.

80353 Resequenced code. See code before 80150.

80354 Resequenced code. See code before 80150.

80355 Resequenced code. See code before 80150.

80356 Resequenced code. See code before 80150.

80357 Resequenced code. See code before 80150.

80358 Resequenced code. See code before 80150.

80359 Resequenced code. See code before 80150.

80360 Resequenced code. See code before 80150.

80361 Resequenced code. See code before 80150.

80362 Resequenced code. See code before 80150.

80363 Resequenced code. See code before 80150.

80364 Resequenced code. See code before 80150.

80365 Resequenced code. See code following 80364.

80366 Resequenced code. See code following 83992.

80367 Resequenced code. See code following 80366.

80368 Resequenced code. See code following 80367.

80369 Resequenced code. See code following 80368.

80370 Resequenced code. See code following 80369.

80371 Resequenced code. See code following 80370.

80372 Resequenced code. See code following 80371.

80373 Resequenced code. See code following 80372.

80374 Resequenced code. See code following 80373.

80375 Resequenced code. See code following 80374.

80376 Resequenced code. See code following 80375.

80377 Resequenced code. See code following 80376.

80400-80440 Stimulation and Suppression Test Panels

CMS 100-2,15,80 Diagnostic Test Requirements

EXCLUDES *Administration of evocative or suppressive material (96365-96368, 96372, 96374-96376, C8957)*
Evocative or suppression test substances, as applicable
Physician monitoring and attendance during the test (see Evaluation and Management codes)

80400 **ACTH stimulation panel; for adrenal insufficiency**
INCLUDES Cortisol x 2 (82533)
N 0.00 0.00 FUD XXX

80402 **for 21 hydroxylase deficiency**
INCLUDES 17 hydroxyprogesterone X 2 (83498)
Cortisol x 2 (82533)
N 0.00 0.00 FUD XXX

80406 **for 3 beta-hydroxydehydrogenase deficiency**
INCLUDES 17 hydroxypregnenolone x 2 (84143)
Cortisol x 2 (82533)
N 0.00 0.00 FUD XXX

80408 **Aldosterone suppression evaluation panel (eg, saline infusion)**
INCLUDES Aldosterone x 2 (82088)
Renin x 2 (84244)
N 0.00 0.00 FUD XXX

80410 **Calcitonin stimulation panel (eg, calcium, pentagastrin)**
INCLUDES Calcitonin x 3 (82308)
N 0.00 0.00 FUD XXX

80412 **Corticotropic releasing hormone (CRH) stimulation panel**
INCLUDES Adrenocorticotropic hormone (ACTH) x 6 (82024)
Cortisol x 6 (82533)
N 0.00 0.00 FUD XXX

80414 **Chorionic gonadotropin stimulation panel; testosterone response**
INCLUDES Testosterone x 2 on three pooled blood samples (84403)
N 0.00 0.00 FUD XXX

80415 **estradiol response**
INCLUDES Estradiol x 2 on three pooled blood samples (82670)
N 0.00 0.00 FUD XXX

80416 **Renal vein renin stimulation panel (eg, captopril)**
INCLUDES Renin x 6 (84244)
N 0.00 0.00 FUD XXX

80417 **Peripheral vein renin stimulation panel (eg, captopril)**
INCLUDES Renin x 2 (84244)
N 0.00 0.00 FUD XXX

80418 **Combined rapid anterior pituitary evaluation panel**
INCLUDES Adrenocorticotropic hormone (ACTH) x 4 (82024)
Cortisol x 4 (82533)
Follicle stimulating hormone (FSH) x 4 (83001)
Human growth hormone x 4 (83003)
Luteinizing hormone (LH) x 4 (83002)
Prolactin x 4 (84146)
Thyroid stimulating hormone (TSH) x 4 (84443)
N 0.00 0.00 FUD XXX

80420 **Dexamethasone suppression panel, 48 hour**
INCLUDES Cortisol x 2 (82533)
Free cortisol, urine x 2 (82530)
Volume measurement for timed collection x 2 (81050)
EXCLUDES *Single dose dexamethasone (82533)*
N 0.00 0.00 FUD XXX

80422 **Glucagon tolerance panel; for insulinoma**
INCLUDES Glucose x 3 (82947)
Insulin x 3 (83525)
N 0.00 0.00 FUD XXX

80424 **for pheochromocytoma**
INCLUDES Catecholamines, fractionated x 2 (82384)
N 0.00 0.00 FUD XXX

80426 **Gonadotropin releasing hormone stimulation panel**
INCLUDES Follicle stimulating hormone (FSH) x 4 (83001)
Luteinizing hormone (LH) x 4 (83002)
N 0.00 0.00 FUD XXX

80428 **Growth hormone stimulation panel (eg, arginine infusion, l-dopa administration)**
INCLUDES Human growth hormone (HGH) x 4 (83003)
N 0.00 0.00 FUD XXX

80430 **Growth hormone suppression panel (glucose administration)**
INCLUDES Glucose x 3 (82947)
Human growth hormone (HGH) x 4 (83003)
N 0.00 0.00 FUD XXX

80432 **Insulin-induced C-peptide suppression panel**
INCLUDES C-peptide x 5 (84681)
Glucose x 5 (82947)
Insulin (83525)
N 0.00 0.00 FUD XXX

80434 **Insulin tolerance panel; for ACTH insufficiency**
INCLUDES Cortisol x 5 (82533)
Glucose x 5 (82947)
N 0.00 0.00 FUD XXX

80435 **for growth hormone deficiency**
INCLUDES Glucose x 5 (82947)
Human growth hormone (HGH) x 5 (83003)
N 0.00 0.00 FUD XXX

80436 **Metyrapone panel**
INCLUDES 11 deoxycortisol x 2 (82634)
Cortisol x 2 (82533)
N 0.00 0.00 FUD XXX

80438 **Thyrotropin releasing hormone (TRH) stimulation panel; 1 hour**
INCLUDES Thyroid stimulating hormone (TSH) x 3 (84443)
N 0.00 0.00 FUD XXX

80439 **2 hour**
INCLUDES Thyroid stimulating hormone (TSH) x 4 (84443)
N 0.00 0.00 FUD XXX

~~80440~~ **~~for hyperprolactinemia~~**
To report, see 84146

80500-80502 Consultation By Clinical Pathologist

CMS 100-2,15,80 Diagnostic Test Requirements
CMS 100-4,12,60 Payment for Pathology Services
INCLUDES Pharmacokinetic consultations
Written report by pathologist for tests requiring additional medical judgment and requested by a physician or other qualified health care professional
Do not report for consultations that include patient examination
Do not report when a medical interpretive assessment is not provided

80500 **Clinical pathology consultation; limited, without review of patient's history and medical records**
X 80 1.53 0.59 FUD XXX

80502 **comprehensive, for a complex diagnostic problem, with review of patient's history and medical records**
X 80 1.85 1.91 FUD XXX

81000-81099 Urine Tests

CMS 100-2,15,80 Diagnostic Test Requirements

81000 **Urinalysis, by dip stick or tablet reagent for bilirubin, glucose, hemoglobin, ketones, leukocytes, nitrite, pH, protein, specific gravity, urobilinogen, any number of these constituents; non-automated, with microscopy**
N 0.00 0.00 FUD XXX

81001 **automated, with microscopy**
N 0.00 0.00 FUD XXX

81002 **non-automated, without microscopy**
INCLUDES Mosenthal test
N 0.00 0.00 FUD XXX

81003 **automated, without microscopy**
N 0.00 0.00 FUD XXX

81005 **Urinalysis; qualitative or semiquantitative, except immunoassays**
INCLUDES Benedict test for dextrose
EXCLUDES *Immunoassay, qualitative or semiquantitative (83518)*
Microalbumin (82043-82044)
Nonimmunoassay reagent strip analysis (81000, 81002)
N 0.00 0.00 FUD XXX

81007 **bacteriuria screen, except by culture or dipstick**
EXCLUDES *Culture (87086-87088)*
Dipstick (81000, 81002)
N 0.00 0.00 FUD XXX

81015 **microscopic only**
EXCLUDES *Sperm evaluation for retrograde ejaculation (89331)*
N 0.00 0.00 FUD XXX

81020 **2 or 3 glass test**
INCLUDES Valentine's test
N 0.00 0.00 FUD XXX

81025 **Urine pregnancy test, by visual color comparison methods** M ♀
N 0.00 0.00 FUD XXX

81050 **Volume measurement for timed collection, each**
N 0.00 0.00 FUD XXX

81099 **Unlisted urinalysis procedure**
N 0.00 0.00 FUD XXX

81161-81350 [81161, 81287, 81288] Gene Analysis: Tier 1 Procedures

INCLUDES All analytical procedures in the evaluation such as:
- Amplification
- Cell lysis
- Detection
- Digestion
- Extraction
- Nucleic acid stabilization

Code selection based on specific gene being reviewed
Evaluation of constitutional or somatic gene variations
Evaluation of the presence of gene variants using the common gene variant name
Examples of proteins or diseases in the code description that are not all inclusive
Generally all the listed gene variants in the code description would be tested but lists are not all inclusive
Gene specific and genomic testing
Genes described using Human Genome Organization (HUGO) approved names
Qualitative results unless otherwise stated
Tier 1 molecular pathology codes (81200-81355 [81161, 81287])

EXCLUDES *In situ hybridization analyses (88271-88275, 88365-88368)*
Microbial identification (87149-87153, 87470-87801, 87900-87904 [87906])
Tier 1 molecular pathology codes (81370-81383)
Tier 2 codes (81400-81408)
Unlisted molecular pathology procedures (81479)

Code also modifier 26 when only interpretation and report are performed
Code also services required before cell lysis
Do not report full gene sequencing using separately gene variant assessment codes unless it is specifically stated in the code description
Do not report other related gene variants not listed in code

81161 Resequenced code. See code following 81229.

81200 ***ASPA (aspartoacylase)*** **(eg, Canavan disease) gene analysis, common variants (eg, E285A, Y231X)**
A 0.00 0.00 FUD XXX

81201 ***APC (adenomatous polyposis coli)*** **(eg, familial adenomatosis polyposis [FAP], attenuated FAP) gene analysis; full gene sequence**
A 0.00 0.00 FUD XXX

81202 **known familial variants**
A 0.00 0.00 FUD XXX

81203 **duplication/deletion variants**
A 0.00 0.00 FUD XXX

81205 **BCKDHB (branched-chain keto acid dehydrogenase E1, beta polypeptide) (eg, maple syrup urine disease) gene analysis, common variants (eg, R183P, G278S, E422X)**
A 0.00 0.00 FUD XXX

81206 ***BCR/ABL1 (t(9;22))*** **(eg, chronic myelogenous leukemia) translocation analysis; major breakpoint, qualitative or quantitative**
A 0.00 0.00 FUD XXX

81207 **minor breakpoint, qualitative or quantitative**
A 0.00 0.00 FUD XXX

81208 **other breakpoint, qualitative or quantitative**
A 0.00 0.00 FUD XXX

81209 ***BLM (Bloom syndrome, RecQ helicase-like)*** **(eg, Bloom syndrome) gene analysis, 2281del6ins7 variant**
A 0.00 0.00 FUD XXX

81210 ***BRAF (v-raf murine sarcoma viral oncogene homolog B1)*** **(eg, colon cancer), gene analysis, V600E variant**
A 0.00 0.00 FUD XXX

81211 ***BRCA1, BRCA2 (breast cancer 1 and 2)*** **(eg, hereditary breast and ovarian cancer) gene analysis; full sequence analysis and common duplication/deletion variants in BRCA1 (ie, exon 13 del 3.835kb, exon 13 dup 6kb, exon 14-20 del 26kb, exon 22 del 510bp, exon 8-9 del 7.1kb)**
A 0.00 0.00 FUD XXX

81212 **185delAG, 5385insC, 6174delT variants**
A 0.00 0.00 FUD XXX

81213 **uncommon duplication/deletion variants**
A 0.00 0.00 FUD XXX

81214 ***BRCA1 (breast cancer 1)*** **(eg, hereditary breast and ovarian cancer) gene analysis; full sequence analysis and common duplication/deletion variants (ie, exon 13 del 3.835kb, exon 13 dup 6kb, exon 14-20 del 26kb, exon 22 del 510bp, exon 8-9 del 7.1kb)**
EXCLUDES *BRCA1 with BRCA2 full sequence testing (81211)*
A 0.00 0.00 FUD XXX

81215 **known familial variant**
A 0.00 0.00 FUD XXX

81216 ***BRCA2 (breast cancer 2)*** **(eg, hereditary breast and ovarian cancer) gene analysis; full sequence analysis**
EXCLUDES *BRCA1 with BRCA2 full sequence testing (81211)*
A 0.00 0.00 FUD XXX

81217 **known familial variant**
A 0.00 0.00 FUD XXX

81220 ***CFTR (cystic fibrosis transmembrane conductance regulator)*** **(eg, cystic fibrosis) gene analysis; common variants (eg, ACMG/ACOG guidelines)**
Do not report with Intron 8 poly-T analysis performed on a R117H positive patient with (81224)
A 0.00 0.00 FUD XXX

81221 **known familial variants**
A 0.00 0.00 FUD XXX

81222 **duplication/deletion variants**
A 0.00 0.00 FUD XXX

81223 **full gene sequence**
A 0.00 0.00 FUD XXX

81224 **intron 8 poly-T analysis (eg, male infertility)**
A 0.00 0.00 FUD XXX

81225 ***CYP2C19 (cytochrome P450, family 2, subfamily C, polypeptide 19)*** **(eg, drug metabolism), gene analysis, common variants (eg, *2, *3, *4, *8, *17)**
A 0.00 0.00 FUD XXX

81226 ***CYP2D6 (cytochrome P450, family 2, subfamily D, polypeptide 6)*** **(eg, drug metabolism), gene analysis, common variants (eg, *2, *3, *4, *5, *6, *9, *10, *17, *19, *29, *35, *41, *1XN, *2XN, *4XN)**
A 0.00 0.00 FUD XXX

81227 ***CYP2C9 (cytochrome P450, family 2, subfamily C, polypeptide 9)*** **(eg, drug metabolism), gene analysis, common variants (eg, *2, *3, *5, *6)**
A 0.00 0.00 FUD XXX

81228 **Cytogenomic constitutional (genome-wide) microarray analysis; interrogation of genomic regions for copy number variants (eg, bacterial artificial chromosome [BAC] or oligo-based comparative genomic hybridization [CGH] microarray analysis)**
EXCLUDES *Cytogenomic constitutional microarray analysis (not genome-wide), report code for targeted analysis or unlisted molecular pathology (81405, 81479)*
Do not report with analyte-specific procedures when the analytes are included in the microarray analysis
Do not report with (81229, 88271)
A 0.00 0.00 FUD XXX

81229 **interrogation of genomic regions for copy number and single nucleotide polymorphism (SNP) variants for chromosomal abnormalities**

EXCLUDES *Cytogenomic constitutional microarray analysis (not genome-wide), report code for targeted analysis or unlisted molecular pathology (81405, 81479)*

Do not report with analyte-specific procedures when the analytes are included in the microarray analysis

Do not report with (81228, 88271)

A 0.00 0.00 FUD XXX

\# **81161** **DMD (dystrophin) (eg, Duchenne/Becker muscular dystrophy) deletion analysis, and duplication analysis, if performed**

E 0.00 0.00 FUD XXX

81235 ***EGFR (epidermal growth factor receptor)* (eg, non-small cell lung cancer) gene analysis, common variants (eg, exon 19 LREA deletion, L858R, T790M, G719A, G719S, L861Q)**

A 0.00 0.00 FUD XXX

81240 ***F2 (prothrombin, coagulation factor II)* (eg, hereditary hypercoagulability) gene analysis, 20210G>A variant**

A 0.00 0.00 FUD XXX

81241 **F5 (coagulation factor V) (eg, hereditary hypercoagulability) gene analysis, Leiden variant**

A 0.00 0.00 FUD XXX

81242 ***FANCC (Fanconi anemia, complementation group C)* (eg, Fanconi anemia, type C) gene analysis, common variant (eg, IVS4+4A>T)**

A 0.00 0.00 FUD XXX

81243 **FMR1 (fragile X mental retardation 1) (eg, fragile X mental retardation) gene analysis; evaluation to detect abnormal (eg, expanded) alleles**

INCLUDES Testing for detection and characterization of abnormal alleles using a single assay such as PCR

Code also characterization of abnormal alleles, unless performed by a single assay technique (81244)

A 0.00 0.00 FUD XXX

81244 **characterization of alleles (eg, expanded size and methylation status)**

EXCLUDES *Testing for detection and characterization of abnormal alleles using a single assay such as PCR (81243)*

Code also characterization of abnormal alleles, unless performed by a single assay technique (81243)

A 0.00 0.00 FUD XXX

▲ **81245** **FLT3 (fms-related tyrosine kinase 3) (eg, acute myeloid leukemia), gene analysis; internal tandem duplication (ITD) variants (ie, exons 14, 15)**

A 0.00 0.00 FUD XXX

● **81246** **tyrosine kinase domain (TKD) variants (eg, D835, I836)**

81250 **G6PC (glucose-6-phosphatase, catalytic subunit) (eg, Glycogen storage disease, type 1a, von Gierke disease) gene analysis, common variants (eg, R83C, Q347X)**

A 0.00 0.00 FUD XXX

81251 ***GBA (glucosidase, beta, acid)* (eg, Gaucher disease) gene analysis, common variants (eg, N370S, 84GG, L444P, IVS2+1G>A)**

A 0.00 0.00 FUD XXX

81252 ***GJB2 (gap junction protein, beta 2, 26kDa, connexin 26)* (eg, nonsyndromic hearing loss) gene analysis; full gene sequence**

A 0.00 0.00 FUD XXX

81253 **known familial variants**

A 0.00 0.00 FUD XXX

81254 ***GJB6 (gap junction protein, beta 6, 30kDa, connexin 30)* (eg, nonsyndromic hearing loss) gene analysis, common variants (eg, 309kb [del(GJB6-D13S1830)] and 232kb [del(GJB6-D13S1854)])**

A 0.00 0.00 FUD XXX

81255 ***HEXA (hexosaminidase A [alpha polypeptide])* (eg, Tay-Sachs disease) gene analysis, common variants (eg, 1278insTATC, 1421+1G>C, G269S)**

A 0.00 0.00 FUD XXX

81256 ***HFE (hemochromatosis)* (eg, hereditary hemochromatosis) gene analysis, common variants (eg, C282Y, H63D)**

A 0.00 0.00 FUD XXX

81257 ***HBA1/HBA2 (alpha globin 1 and alpha globin 2)* (eg, alpha thalassemia, Hb Bart hydrops fetalis syndrome, HbH disease), gene analysis, for common deletions or variant (eg, Southeast Asian, Thai, Filipino, Mediterranean, alpha3.7, alpha4.2, alpha20.5, and Constant Spring)**

A 0.00 0.00 FUD XXX

81260 ***IKBKAP (inhibitor of kappa light polypeptide gene enhancer in B-cells, kinase complex-associated protein)* (eg, familial dysautonomia) gene analysis, common variants (eg, 2507+6T>C, R696P)**

A 0.00 0.00 FUD XXX

81261 ***IGH@ (Immunoglobulin heavy chain locus)* (eg, leukemias and lymphomas, B-cell), gene rearrangement analysis to detect abnormal clonal population(s); amplified methodology (eg, polymerase chain reaction)**

A 0.00 0.00 FUD XXX

81262 **direct probe methodology (eg, Southern blot)**

A 0.00 0.00 FUD XXX

81263 ***IGH@ (Immunoglobulin heavy chain locus)* (eg, leukemia and lymphoma, B-cell), variable region somatic mutation analysis**

A 0.00 0.00 FUD XXX

81264 ***IGK@ (Immunoglobulin kappa light chain locus)* (eg, leukemia and lymphoma, B-cell), gene rearrangement analysis, evaluation to detect abnormal clonal population(s)**

EXCLUDES *Immunoglobulin kappa deleting element (IGKDEL) analysis (81479)*
Immunoglobulin lambda gene (IGL@) rearrangement (81479)

A 0.00 0.00 FUD XXX

81265 **Comparative analysis using Short Tandem Repeat (STR) markers; patient and comparative specimen (eg, pre-transplant recipient and donor germline testing, post-transplant non-hematopoietic recipient germline [eg, buccal swab or other germline tissue sample] and donor testing, twin zygosity testing, or maternal cell contamination of fetal cells)**

Code also the following codes for chimerism testing if comparative short tandem repeat (STR) analysis of recipient (using buccal swab or other germline tissue sample) and donor are performed after hematopoietic stem cell transplantation (81266-81268)

A 0.00 0.00 FUD XXX

Pathology and Laboratory

81229 — 81265

● New Code ▲ Revised Code 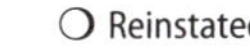 ○ Reinstated 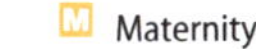 Maternity 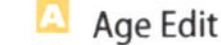 Age Edit 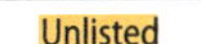 Unlisted Not Covered # Resequenced
⊘ AMA Mod 51 Exempt ⑤ Optum Mod 51 Exempt ⑥ Mod 63 Exempt ⊙ Mod Sedation + Add-on CCI PQRS FUD Follow-up Days

+ 81266 **each additional specimen (eg, additional cord blood donor, additional fetal samples from different cultures, or additional zygosity in multiple birth pregnancies) (List separately in addition to code for primary procedure)**
Code also the following codes for chimerism testing if comparative short tandem repeat (STR) analysis of recipient (using buccal swab or other germline tissue sample) and donor are performed after hematopoietic stem cell transplantation (81267-81268)
Code first (81265)
A 0.00 0.00 FUD XXX

81267 **Chimerism (engraftment) analysis, post transplantation specimen (eg, hematopoietic stem cell), includes comparison to previously performed baseline analyses; without cell selection**
Code also the following codes for chimerism testing if comparative short tandem repeat (STR) analysis of recipient (using buccal swab or other germline tissue sample) and donor are performed after hematopoietic stem cell transplantation (81265-81266, 81268)
A 0.00 0.00 FUD XXX

81268 **with cell selection (eg, CD3, CD33), each cell type**
Code also the following codes for chimerism testing if comparative short tandem repeat (STR) analysis of recipient (using buccal swab or other germline tissue sample) and donor are performed after hematopoietic stem cell transplantation (81265-81267)
A 0.00 0.00 FUD XXX

81270 ***JAK2 (Janus kinase 2)* (eg, myeloproliferative disorder) gene analysis, p.Val617Phe (V617F) variant**
A 0.00 0.00 FUD XXX

81275 ***KRAS (v-Ki-ras2 Kirsten rat sarcoma viral oncogene)* (eg, carcinoma) gene analysis, variants in codons 12 and 13**
A 0.00 0.00 FUD XXX

81280 **Long QT syndrome gene analyses (eg, *KCNQ1, KCNH2, SCN5A, KCNE1, KCNE2, KCNJ2, CACNA1C, CAV3, SCN4B, AKAP, SNTA1, and ANK2*); full sequence analysis**
A 0.00 0.00 FUD XXX

81281 **known familial sequence variant**
A 0.00 0.00 FUD XXX

81282 **duplication/deletion variants**
A 0.00 0.00 FUD XXX

81287 ***Resequenced code. See code following 81290.***

81288 ***Resequenced code. See code following 81292.***

81290 ***MCOLN1 (mucolipin 1)* (eg, Mucolipidosis, type IV) gene analysis, common variants (eg, IVS3-2A>G, del6.4kb)**
A 0.00 0.00 FUD XXX

81287 **MGMT (O-6-methylguanine-DNA methyltransferase) (eg, glioblastoma multiforme), methylation analysis**
A 0.00 0.00 FUD XXX

81291 ***MTHFR (5,10-methylenetetrahydrofolate reductase)* (eg, hereditary hypercoagulability) gene analysis, common variants (eg, 677T, 1298C)**
A 0.00 0.00 FUD XXX

81292 ***MLH1 (mutL homolog 1, colon cancer, nonpolyposis type 2)* (eg, hereditary non-polyposis colorectal cancer, Lynch syndrome) gene analysis; full sequence analysis**
A 0.00 0.00 FUD XXX

#● 81288 **promoter methylation analysis**

81293 **known familial variants**
A 0.00 0.00 FUD XXX

81294 **duplication/deletion variants**
A 0.00 0.00 FUD XXX

81295 ***MSH2 (mutS homolog 2, colon cancer, nonpolyposis type 1)* (eg, hereditary non-polyposis colorectal cancer, Lynch syndrome) gene analysis; full sequence analysis**
A 0.00 0.00 FUD XXX

81296 **known familial variants**
A 0.00 0.00 FUD XXX

81297 **duplication/deletion variants**
A 0.00 0.00 FUD XXX

81298 ***MSH6 (mutS homolog 6 [E. coli])* (eg, hereditary non-polyposis colorectal cancer, Lynch syndrome) gene analysis; full sequence analysis**
A 0.00 0.00 FUD XXX

81299 **known familial variants**
A 0.00 0.00 FUD XXX

81300 **duplication/deletion variants**
A 0.00 0.00 FUD XXX

81301 **Microsatellite instability analysis (eg, hereditary non-polyposis colorectal cancer, Lynch syndrome) of markers for mismatch repair deficiency (eg, BAT25, BAT26), includes comparison of neoplastic and normal tissue, if performed**
A 0.00 0.00 FUD XXX

81302 ***MECP2 (methyl CpG binding protein 2)* (eg, Rett syndrome) gene analysis; full sequence analysis**
A 0.00 0.00 FUD XXX

81303 **known familial variant**
A 0.00 0.00 FUD XXX

81304 **duplication/deletion variants**
A 0.00 0.00 FUD XXX

81310 ***NPM1 (nucleophosmin)* (eg, acute myeloid leukemia) gene analysis, exon 12 variants**
A 0.00 0.00 FUD XXX

● 81313 **PCA3/KLK3 (prostate cancer antigen 3 [non-protein coding]/kallikrein-related peptidase 3 [prostate specific antigen]) ratio (eg, prostate cancer)**

81315 ***PML/RARalpha, (t(15;17)), (promyelocytic leukemia/retinoic acid receptor alpha)* (eg, promyelocytic leukemia) translocation analysis; common breakpoints (eg, intron 3 and intron 6), qualitative or quantitative**
INCLUDES Intron 3 and 6 (and exon 6 if performed) testing
A 0.00 0.00 FUD XXX

81316 **single breakpoint (eg, intron 3, intron 6 or exon 6), qualitative or quantitative**
EXCLUDES *Intron 3 and 6 (and exon 6 if performed) testing (81315)*
Do not report more than one unit of this code for testing intron 6 and exon 6 without intron 3 (81316)
A 0.00 0.00 FUD XXX

81317 ***PMS2 (postmeiotic segregation increased 2 [S. cerevisiae])* (eg, hereditary non-polyposis colorectal cancer, Lynch syndrome) gene analysis; full sequence analysis**
A 0.00 0.00 FUD XXX

81318 **known familial variants**
A 0.00 0.00 FUD XXX

81319 **duplication/deletion variants**
A 0.00 0.00 FUD XXX

81321 ***PTEN (phosphatase and tensin homolog)* (eg, Cowden syndrome, PTEN hamartoma tumor syndrome) gene analysis; full sequence analysis**
A 0.00 0.00 FUD XXX

81322 **known familial variant**
A 0.00 0.00 FUD XXX

81323 **duplication/deletion variant**
A 0.00 0.00 FUD XXX

81324 ***PMP22 (peripheral myelin protein 22)*** **(eg, Charcot-Marie-Tooth, hereditary neuropathy with liability to pressure palsies) gene analysis; duplication/deletion analysis**
A 0.00 0.00 FUD XXX

81325 **full sequence analysis**
A 0.00 0.00 FUD XXX

81326 **known familial variant**
A 0.00 0.00 FUD XXX

81330 ***SMPD1(sphingomyelin phosphodiesterase 1, acid lysosomal)*** **(eg, Niemann-Pick disease, Type A) gene analysis, common variants (eg, R496L, L302P, fsP330)**
A 0.00 0.00 FUD XXX

81331 ***SNRPN/UBE3A (small nuclear ribonucleoprotein polypeptide N and ubiquitin protein ligase E3A)*** **(eg, Prader-Willi syndrome and/or Angelman syndrome), methylation analysis**
A 0.00 0.00 FUD XXX

81332 ***SERPINA1 (serpin peptidase inhibitor, clade A, alpha-1 antiproteinase, antitrypsin, member 1)*** **(eg, alpha-1-antitrypsin deficiency), gene analysis, common variants (eg, *S and *Z)**
A 0.00 0.00 FUD XXX

81340 ***TRB@ (T cell antigen receptor, beta)*** **(eg, leukemia and lymphoma), gene rearrangement analysis to detect abnormal clonal population(s); using amplification methodology (eg, polymerase chain reaction)**
A 0.00 0.00 FUD XXX

81341 **using direct probe methodology (eg, Southern blot)**
A 0.00 0.00 FUD XXX

81342 ***TRG@ (T cell antigen receptor, gamma)*** **(eg, leukemia and lymphoma), gene rearrangement analysis, evaluation to detect abnormal clonal population(s)**

EXCLUDES *T cell antigen alpha [TRA@] gene arrangement testing (81479)*
T cell antigen delta [TRD@] gene arrangement testing (81402)

A 0.00 0.00 FUD XXX

81350 ***UGT1A1 (UDP glucuronosyltransferase 1 family, polypeptide A1)*** **(eg, irinotecan metabolism), gene analysis, common variants (eg, *28, *36, *37)**
A 0.00 0.00 FUD XXX

81355 ***VKORC1 (vitamin K epoxide reductase complex, subunit 1)*** **(eg, warfarin metabolism), gene analysis, common variants (eg, -1639/3673)**
A 0.00 0.00 FUD XXX

81370-81383 Human Leukocyte Antigen (HLA) Testing

INCLUDES Additional testing that must be performed to resolve ambiguous allele combinations for high-resolution typing
All analytical procedures in the evaluation such as:
- Amplification
- Cell lysis
- Detection
- Digestion
- Extraction
- Nucleic acid stabilization

Analysis to identify human leukocyte antigen (HLA) alleles and allele groups connected to specific diseases and individual response to drug therapy in addition to other clinical uses
Code selection based on specific gene being reviewed
Evaluation of the presence of gene variants using the common gene variant name
Examples of proteins or diseases in the code description that are not all inclusive
Generally all the listed gene variants in the code description would be tested but lists are not all inclusive
Genes described using Human Genome Organization (HUGO) approved names
High-resolution typing resolves the common well-defined (CWD) alleles and is usually identified by at least four-digits. There are some instances when high-resolution typing may include some ambiguities for rare alleles, and those may be reported as a string of alleles or an NMDP code
Histocompatibility antigen testing
Intermediate resolution HLA testing is identified by a string of alleles or a National Marrow Donor Program (NMDP) code
Low and intermediate resolution are considered low resolution for code assignment
Low-resolution HLA type reporting is identified by two-digit HLA name
Multiple variant alleles or allele groups that can be identified by typing
One or more HLA genes in specific clinical circumstances
Qualitative results unless otherwise stated
Typing performed to determine the compatibility of recipients and potential donors undergoing solid organ or hematopoietic stem cell pretransplantation testing

EXCLUDES *HLA antigen typing by nonmolecular pathology methods (86812-86822)*
Microbial identification (87149-87153, 87470-87801, 87900-87904 [87906])
Tier 1 molecular pathology codes (81200-81355 [81161, 81287])
Tier 2 codes (81400-81408)
Unlisted molecular pathology procedures (81479)

Code also modifier 26 when only interpretation and report are performed
Code also services required before cell lysis
Do not report full gene sequencing separately using gene variant assessment codes unless it is specifically stated in the code description
Do not report other related gene variants not listed in code

81370 **HLA Class I and II typing, low resolution (eg, antigen equivalents);** ***HLA-A, -B, -C, -DRB1/3/4/5, and -DQB1***
A 0.00 0.00 FUD XXX

81371 **HLA-A, -B, and -DRB1 (eg, verification typing)**
A 0.00 0.00 FUD XXX

81372 **HLA Class I typing, low resolution (eg, antigen equivalents); complete** ***(ie, HLA-A, -B, and -C)***

EXCLUDES *Class I and II low-resolution HLA typing for HLA-A, -B, -C, -DRB1/3/4/5, and -DQB1 (81370)*

A 0.00 0.00 FUD XXX

81373 **one locus** ***(eg, HLA-A, -B, or -C)*****, each**

EXCLUDES *A complete Class 1 (HLA-A, -B, and -C) low-resolution typing (81372)*
Reporting the presence or absence of a single antigen equivalent using low-resolution methodology (81374)

A 0.00 0.00 FUD XXX

81374 **one antigen equivalent** ***(eg, B*27)*****, each**

EXCLUDES *Testing for the presence or absence of more than 2 antigen equivalents at a locus, use the following code for each locus test (81373)*

A 0.00 0.00 FUD XXX

81375 **HLA Class II typing, low resolution (eg, antigen equivalents); *HLA-DRB1/3/4/5 and -DQB1***
EXCLUDES *Class I and II low-resolution HLA typing for HLA-A, -B, -C, -DRB 1/3/4/5, and DQB1 (81370)*
A 0.00 0.00 FUD XXX

81376 **one locus (eg, HLA-DRB1, -DRB3/4/5, -DQB1, -DQA1, -DPB1, or -DPA1), each**
INCLUDES Low-resolution typing, HLA-DRB1/3/4/5 reported as a single locus
EXCLUDES *Low-resolution typing for HLA-DRB1/3/4/5 and -DQB1 (81375)*
A 0.00 0.00 FUD XXX

81377 **one antigen equivalent, each**
EXCLUDES *Testing for presence or absence of more than two antigen equivalents at a locus (81376)*
A 0.00 0.00 FUD XXX

81378 **HLA Class I and II typing, high resolution (ie, alleles or allele groups), *HLA-A, -B, -C, and -DRB1***
A 0.00 0.00 FUD XXX

81379 **HLA Class I typing, high resolution (ie, alleles or allele groups); complete (ie, *HLA-A, -B, and -C*)**
A 0.00 0.00 FUD XXX

81380 **one locus (eg, *HLA-A, -B, or -C*), each**
EXCLUDES *Complete Class I high-resolution typing for HLA-A, -B, and -C (81379)*
Testing for presence or absence of a single allele or allele group using high-resolution methodology (81381)
A 0.00 0.00 FUD XXX

81381 **one allele or allele group (eg, *B*57:01P*), each**
EXCLUDES *Testing for the presence or absence of more than two alleles or allele groups of locus, report the following code for each locus (81380)*
A 0.00 0.00 FUD XXX

81382 **HLA Class II typing, high resolution (ie, alleles or allele groups); one locus (eg, HLA-DRB1, -DRB3/4/5, -DQB1, -DQA1, -DPB1, or -DPA1), each**
INCLUDES Typing of one or all of the DRB3/4/5 genes is regarded as one locus
EXCLUDES *Testing for just the presence or absence of a single allele or allele group using high-resolution methodology (81383)*
A 0.00 0.00 FUD XXX

81383 **1 allele or allele group (eg, *HLA-DQB1*06:02P*), each**
EXCLUDES *For testing for the presence or absence of more than two alleles or allele groups at a locus, report the following code for each locus (81382)*
A 0.00 0.00 FUD XXX

81400-81479 [81479] Molecular Pathology Tier 2 Procedures

INCLUDES All analytical procedures in the evaluation such as:
- Amplification
- Cell lysis
- Detection
- Digestion
- Extraction
- Nucleic acid stabilization

Code selection based on specific gene being reviewed
Codes that are arranged by level of technical resources and work involved
Evaluation of the presence of a gene variant using the common gene variant name
Examples in parentheses at/near the beginning of the code descriptions that are not all-inclusive
Examples of proteins or diseases in the code description that are not all inclusive
Generally all the listed gene variants in the code description would be tested but lists are not all inclusive
Genes described using the Human Genome Organization (HUGO) approved names
Histocompatibility testing
Qualitative results unless otherwise stated
Specific analytes listed after the code description to use for selecting the appropriate molecular pathology procedure
Targeted genomic testing (81410-81471)
Testing for diseases that are more rare

EXCLUDES *Microbial identification (87149-87153, 87470-87801, 87900-87904 [87906])*
Tier 1 molecular pathology (81200-81383 [81161, 81287])
Unlisted molecular pathology procedures (81479)

Code also modifier 26 when only interpretation and report are performed
Code also services required before cell lysis
Do not report full gene sequencing separately using gene variant assessment codes unless it is specifically stated in the code description
Do not report other related gene variants not listed in the code description

81400 **Molecular pathology procedure, Level 1(eg, identification of single germline variant [eg, SNP] by techniques such as restriction enzyme digestion or melt curve analysis)**
INCLUDES *ACADM (acyl-CoA dehydrogenase, C-4 to C-12 straight chain, MCAD)* (eg, medium chain acyl dehydrogenase deficiency), K304E variant
ACE (angiotensin converting enzyme) (eg, hereditary blood pressure regulation), insertion/deletion variant
AGTR1 (angiotensin II receptor, type 1) (eg, essential hypertension), 1166A>C variant
BCKDHA (branched chain keto acid dehydrogenase E1, alpha polypeptide) (eg, maple syrup urine disease, type 1A), Y438N variant
CCR5 (chemokine C-C motif receptor 5) (eg, HIV resistance), 32-bp deletion mutation/794 825del32 deletion
CLRN1 (clarin 1) (eg, Usher syndrome, type 3), N48K variant
DPYD (dihydropyrimidine dehydrogenase) (eg, 5-fluorouracil/5-FU and capecitabine drug metabolism), IVS14+1G>A variant
F2 (coagulation factor 2) (eg, hereditary hypercoagulability), 1199G>A variant
F5 (coagulation factor V) (eg, hereditary hypercoagulability), HR2 variant
F7 (coagulation factor VII [serum prothrombin conversion accelerator]) (eg, hereditary hypercoagulability), R353Q variant

F13B (coagulation factor XIII, B polypeptide) (eg, hereditary hypercoagulability), V34L variant
FGB (fibrinogen beta chain) (eg, hereditary ischemic heart disease), -455G>A variant
FGFR1 (fibroblast growth factor receptor 1) (eg, Pfeiffer syndrome type 1, craniosynostosis), P252R variant
FGFR3 (fibroblast growth factor receptor 3) (eg, Muenke syndrome), P250R variant
FKTN (fukutin) (eg, Fukuyama congenital muscular dystrophy), retrotransposon insertion variant
GNE (glucosamine [UDP-N-acetyl]-2-epimerase/N-acetylmannosamine kinase) (eg, inclusion body myopathy 2 [IBM2], Nonaka myopathy), M712T variant
Human platelet antigen 1 genotyping (HPA-1), ITGB3 (integrin, beta 3 [platelet glycoprotein IIIa], antigen CD61 [GPIIIa]) (eg, neonatal alloimmune thrombocytopenia [NAIT], post-transfusion purpura), HPA-1a/b (L33P)
Human platelet antigen 2 genotyping (HPA-2), GP1BA (glycoprotein Ib [platelet], alpha polypeptide [GPIba]) (eg, neonatal alloimmune thrombocytopenia [NAIT], post-transfusion purpura), HPA-2a/b (T145M)
Human platelet antigen 3 genotyping (HPA-3), ITGA2B (integrin, alpha 2b [platelet glycoprotein IIb of IIb/IIIa complex], antigen CD41 [GPIIb]) (eg, neonatal alloimmune thrombocytopenia [NAIT], post-transfusion purpura), HPA-3a/b (I843S)
Human platelet antigen 4 genotyping (HPA-4), ITGB3 (integrin, beta 3 [platelet glycoprotein IIIa], antigen CD61 [GPIIIa]) (eg, neonatal alloimmune thrombocytopenia [NAIT], post-transfusion purpura), HPA-4a/b (R143Q)
Human platelet antigen 5 genotyping (HPA-5), ITGA2 (integrin, alpha 2 [CD49B, alpha 2 subunit of VLA-2 receptor] [GPIa]) (eg, neonatal alloimmune thrombocytopenia [NAIT], post-transfusion purpura), HPA-5a/b (K505E)
Human platelet antigen 6 genotyping (HPA-6w), ITGB3 (integrin, beta 3 [platelet glycoprotein IIIa, antigen CD61] [GPIIIa]) (eg, neonatal alloimmune thrombocytopenia [NAIT], post-transfusion purpura), HPA-6a/b (R489Q)
Human platelet antigen 9 genotyping (HPA-9w), ITGA2B (integrin, alpha 2b [platelet glycoprotein IIb of IIb/IIIa complex, antigen CD41] [GPIIb]) (eg, neonatal alloimmune thrombocytopenia [NAIT], post-transfusion purpura), HPA-9a/b (V837M)
Human platelet antigen 15 genotyping (HPA-15), CD109 (CD109 molecule) (eg, neonatal alloimmune thrombocytopenia [NAIT], post-transfusion purpura), HPA-15a/b(S682Y)
IL28B (interleukin 28B [interferon, lambda 3]) (eg, drug response), rs12979860 variant
IVD (isovaleryl-CoA dehydrogenase) (eg, isovaleric acidemia), A282V variant
LCT (lactase-phlorizin hydrolase) (eg, lactose intolerance), 13910 C>T variant
NEB (nebulin) (eg, nemaline myopathy 2), exon 55 deletion variant
PCDH15 (protocadherin-related 15) (eg, Usher syndrome type 1F), R245X variant
SERPINE1 (serpine peptidase inhibitor clade E, member 1, plasminogen activator inhibitor -1, PAI-1) (eg, thrombophilia), 4G variant
SHOC2 (soc-2 suppressor of clear homolog) (eg, Noonan-like syndrome with loose anagen hair), S2G variant
SLCO1B1 (solute carrier organic anion transporter family, member 1B1) (eg, adverse drug reaction), V174A variant
SMN1 (survival of motor neuron 1, telomeric) (eg, spinal muscular atrophy), exon 7 deletion
SRY (sex determining region Y) (eg, 46,XX testicular disorder of sex development, gonadal dysgenesis), gene analysis
TOR1A (torsin family 1, member A [torsin A]) (eg, early-onset primary dystonia [DYT1]), 907_909delGAG (904_906delGAG) variant

A 0.00 0.00 FUD XXX

81401 Molecular pathology procedure, Level 2 (eg, 2-10 SNPs, 1 methylated variant, or 1 somatic variant [typically using nonsequencing target variant analysis], or detection of a dynamic mutation disorder/triplet repeat)

INCLUDES *ABCC8 (ATP-binding cassette, sub-family C [CFTR/MRP], member 8)* (eg, familial hyperinsulinism), common variants (eg, c.3898-9G>A [c.3992-9G>A], F1388del)
ABL (c-abl oncogene 1, receptor tyrosine kinase) (eg, acquired imatinib resistance), T315I variant
ACADM (acyl-CoA dehydrogenase, C-4 to C-12 straight chain, MCAD) (eg, medium chain acyl dehydrogenase deficiency), common variants (eg, K304E, Y42H)
ADRB2 (adrenergic beta-2 receptor surface) (eg, drug metabolism), common variants (eg, G16R, Q27E)
AFF2 (AF4/FMR2 family, member 2 [FMR2]) (eg, fragile X mental retardation 2 [FRAXE]), evaluation to detect abnormal (eg, expanded) alleles
APOB (apolipoprotein B) (eg, familial hypercholesterolemia type B), common variants (eg, R3500Q, R3500W)
APOE (apolipoprotein E) (eg, hyperlipoproteinemia type III, cardiovascular disease, Alzheimer disease), common variants (eg, *2, *3, *4)
AR (androgen receptor) (eg, spinal and bulbar muscular atrophy, Kennedy disease, X chromosome inactivation), characterization of alleles (eg, expanded size or methylation status)
ATN1 (atrophin 1) (eg, dentatorubral-pallidoluysian atrophy), evaluation to detect abnormal (eg, expanded) alleles

ATXN1 (ataxin 1) (eg, spinocerebellar ataxia), evaluation to detect abnormal (eg, expanded) alleles
ATXN2 (ataxin 2) (eg, spinocerebellar ataxia), evaluation to detect abnormal (eg, expanded) alleles
ATXN3 (ataxin 3) (eg, spinocerebellar ataxia, Machado-Joseph disease), evaluation to detect abnormal (eg, expanded) alleles
ATXN7 (ataxin 7) (eg, spinocerebellar ataxia), evaluation to detect abnormal (eg, expanded) alleles
ATXN8OS (ATXN8 opposite strand [non-protein coding]) (eg, spinocerebellar ataxia), evaluation to detect abnormal (eg, expanded) alleles
ATXN10 (ataxin 10) (eg, spinocerebellar ataxia), evaluation to detect abnormal (eg, expanded) alleles
CACNA1A (calcium channel, voltage-dependent, P/Q type, alpha 1A subunit) (eg, spinocerebellar ataxia), evaluation to detect abnormal (eg, expanded) alleles
CBFB/MYH11 (inv(16)) (eg, acute myeloid leukemia), qualitative, and quantitative, if performed
CBS (cystathionine-beta-synthase) (eg, homocystinuria, cystathionine beta-synthase deficiency), common variants (eg, I278T, G307S)
CCND1/IGH (BCL1/IgH, t(11;14)) (eg, mantle cell lymphoma) translocation analysis, major breakpoint, qualitative and quantitative, if performed
CFH/ARMS2 (complement factor H/age-related maculopathy susceptibility 2) (eg, macular degeneration), common variants (eg, Y402H [CFH], A69S [ARMS2])
CNBP (CCHC-type zinc finger, nucleic acid binding protein) (eg, myotonic dystrophy type 2), evaluation to detect abnormal (eg, expanded) alleles
CSTB (cystatin B [stefin B]) (eg, Unverricht-Lundborg disease), evaluation to detect abnormal (eg, expanded) alleles
CYP3A4 (cytochrome P450, family 3, subfamily A, polypeptide 4) (eg, drug metabolism), common variants (eg, *2, *3, *4, *5, *6)
CYP3A5 (cytochrome P450, family 3, subfamily A, polypeptide 5) (eg, drug metabolism), common variants (eg, *2, *3, *4, *5, *6)
DMPK (dystrophia myotonica-protein kinase) (eg, myotonic dystrophy, type 1), evaluation to detect abnormal (eg, expanded) alleles
E2A/PBX1 (t(1;19)) (eg, acute lymphocytic leukemia), translocation analysis, qualitative, and quantitative, if performed
EML4/ALK (inv(2)) (eg, non-small cell lung cancer), translocation or inversion analysis
ETV6/NTRK3 (t(12;15)) (eg, congenital/infantile fibrosarcoma), translocation analysis, qualitative, and quantitative, if performed
ETV6/RUNX1 (t(12;21)) (eg, acute lymphocytic leukemia), translocation analysis, qualitative and quantitative, if performed
EWSR1/ATF1 (t(12;22)) (eg, clear cell sarcoma), translocation analysis, qualitative, and quantitative, if performed
EWSR1/ERG (t(21;22)) (eg, Ewing sarcoma/peripheral neuroectodermal tumor), translocation analysis, qualitative and quantitative, if performed
EWSR1/FLI1 (t(11;22)) (eg, Ewing sarcoma/peripheral neuroectodermal tumor), translocation analysis, qualitative and quantitative, if performed
EWSR1/WT1 (t(11;22)) (eg, desmoplastic small round cell tumor), translocation analysis, qualitative and quantitative, if performed
F11 (coagulation factor XI) (eg, coagulation disorder), common variants (eg, E117X [Type II], F283L [Type III], IVS14del14, and IVS14+1G>A [Type I])
FGFR3 (fibroblast growth factor receptor 3) (eg, achondroplasia, hypochondroplasia), common variants (eg, 1138G>A, 1138G>C, 1620C>A, 1620C>G)
FIP1L1/PDGFRA (del[4q12]) (eg, imatinib-sensitive chronic eosinophilic leukemia), qualitative and quantitative, if performed
FLG (filaggrin) (eg, ichthyosis vulgaris), common variants (eg, R501X, 2282del4, R2447X, S3247X, 3702delG)
FOXO1/PAX3 (t(2;13)) (eg, alveolar rhabdomyosarcoma), translocation analysis, qualitative and quantitative, if performed
FOXO1/PAX7 (t(1;13)) (eg, alveolar rhabdomyosarcoma), translocation analysis, qualitative and quantitative, if performed
FUS/DDIT3 (t(12;16)) (eg, myxoid liposarcoma), translocation analysis, qualitative, and quantitative, if performed
FXN (frataxin) (eg, Friedreich ataxia), evaluation to detect abnormal (expanded) alleles
GALC (galactosylceramidase) (eg, Krabbe disease), common variants (eg, c.857G>A, 30-kb deletion)
GALT (galactose-1-phosphate uridylyltransferase) (eg, galactosemia), common variants (eg, Q188R, S135L, K285N, T138M, L195P, Y209C, IVS2-2A>G, P171S, del5kb, N314D, L218L/N314D)
H19 (imprinted maternally expressed transcript [non-protein coding]) (eg, Beckwith-Wiedemann syndrome), methylation analysis
HBB (hemoglobin, beta) (eg, sickle cell anemia, hemoglobin C, hemoglobin E), common variants (eg, HbS, HbC, HbE)
HTT (huntingtin) (eg, Huntington disease), evaluation to detect abnormal (eg, expanded) alleles
KCNQ1OT1 (KCNQ1 overlapping transcript 1 [non-protein coding]) (e.g, Beckwith-Wiedemann syndrome), methylation analysis
LRRK2 (leucine-rich repeat kinase 2) (eg, Parkinson disease), common variants (eg, R1441G, G2019S, I2020T)
MED12 (mediator complex subunit 12) (eg, FG syndrome type 1, Lujan syndrome), common variants (eg, R961W, N1007S)
MEG3/DLK1 (maternally expressed 3 [non-protein coding]/delta-like 1 homolog [Drosophila]) (eg, intrauterine growth retardation), methylation analysis
MLL/AFF1 (t(4;11)) (eg acute lymphoblastic leukemia), translocation analysis, qualitative and quantitative, if performed

MLL/MLLT3 (t(9;11)) (eg, acute myeloid leukemia) translocation analysis, qualitative and quantitative, if performed

MT-RNR1 (mitochondrially encoded 12S RNA) (eg, nonsyndromic hearing loss), common variants (eg, m.1555>G, m1494C>T)

MUTYH (mutY homolog [E.coli]) (eg, MYH-associated polyposis), common variants (eg, Y165C, G382D)

MT-ATP6 (mitochondrially encoded ATP synthase 6) (eg, neuropathy with ataxia and retinitis pigmentosa [NARP], Leigh syndrome), common variants (eg, m.8993T>G, m.8993T>C)

MT-ND4, MT-ND6 (mitochondrially encoded NADH dehydrogenase 4, mitochondrially encoded NADH dehydrogenase 6) (eg, Leber hereditary optic neuropathy [LHON]), common variants (eg m.11778G>A, m3460G>A, m14484T>C)

MT-ND5 (mitochondrially encoded tRNA leucine 1 [UUA/G], mitochondrially encoded NADH dehydrogenase 5) (eg, mitochondrial encephalopathy with lactic acidosis and stroke-like episodes [MELAS]), common variants (eg, m.3243A>G, m.3271T>C, m.3252A>G, m.13513G>A)

MT-TK (mitochondrially encoded tRNA lysine) (eg, myoclonic epilepsy with ragged-red fibers [MERRF]), common variants (eg, m8344A>G, m.8356T>C)

MT-TL1 (mitochondrially encoded tRNA leucine 1[UUA/G]) (eg, diabetes and hearing loss), common variants (eg, m.3243A>G, m.14709 T>C) MT-TL1

MT-TS1, MT-RNR1 (mitochondrially encoded tRNA serine 1 [UCN], mitochondrially encoded 12S RNA) (eg, nonsyndromic sensorineural deafness [including aminoglycoside-induced nonsyndromic deafness]) common variants (eg, m.7445A>G, m.1555A>G)

NOD2 (nucleotide-binding oligomerization domain containing 2) (eg, Crohn's disease, Blau syndrome), common variants (eg, SNP 8, SNP 12, SNP 13)

NPM/ALK (t(2;5)) (eg, anaplastic large cell lymphoma), translocation analysis

PABPN1 (poly[A] binding protein, nuclear 1) (eg, oculopharyngeal muscular dystrophy), evaluation to detect abnormal (eg, expanded) alleles

PAX8/PPARG (t(2;3) (q13;p25)) (eg, follicular thyroid carcinoma), translocation analysis

PPP2R2B (protein phosphatase 2, regulatory subunit B, beta) (eg, spinocerebellar ataxia), evaluation to detect abnormal (eg, expanded) alleles

PRSS1 (protease, serine, 1 [trypsin 1]) (eg, hereditary pancreatitis), common variants (eg, N29I, A16V, R122H)

PYGM (phosphorylase, glycogen, muscle) (eg, glycogen storage disease type V, McArdle disease), common variants (eg, R50X, G205S)

RUNX1/RUNX1T1 (t(8;21)) (eg, acute myeloid leukemia) translocation analysis, qualitative and quantitative, if performed

SEPT9 (septin 9) (eg, colon cancer), methylation analysis

SMN1/SMN2 (survival of motor neuron 1, telomeric/survival of motor neuron 2, centromeric) (eg, spinal muscular atrophy), dosage analysis (eg, carrier testing)

SMN1/SMN2 duplication/deletion analysis

SS18/SSX1 (t(X;18)) (eg, synovial sarcoma), translocation analysis, qualitative and quantitative, if performed

SS18/SSX2 (t(X;18)) (eg, synovial sarcoma), translocation analysis, qualitative and quantitative, if performed

TBP (TATA box binding protein) (eg, spinocerebellar ataxia), evaluation to detect abnormal (eg, expanded) alleles

TPMT (thiopurine S-methyltransferase) (eg, drug metabolism), common variants (eg, *2, *3)

TYMS (thymidylate synthetase) (eg, 5-fluorouracil/5-FU drug metabolism), tandem repeat variant

VWF (von Willebrand factor) (eg, von Willebrand disease type 2N), common variants (eg, T791M, R816W, R854Q)

A 0.00 0.00 FUD XXX

▲ **81402 Molecular pathology procedure, Level 3 (eg, >10 SNPs, 2-10 methylated variants, or 2-10 somatic variants [typically using non-sequencing target variant analysis], immunoglobulin and T-cell receptor gene rearrangements, duplication/deletion variants of 1 exon, loss of heterozygosity [LOH], uniparental disomy [UPD])**

INCLUDES *Chromosome 1p-/19q-* (eg, glial tumors), deletion analysis

Chromosome 18q- (eg, D18S55, D18S58, D18S61, D18S64, and D18S69) (eg, colon cancer), allelic imbalance assessment (ie, loss of heterozygosity)

COL1A1/PDGFB (t(17;22)) (eg, dermatofibrosarcoma protuberans), translocation analysis, multiple breakpoints, qualitative, and quantitative, if performed

CYP21A2 (cytochrome P450, family 21, subfamily A, polypeptide 2) (eg, congenital adrenal hyperplasia, 21-hydroxylase deficiency), common variants (eg, IVS2-13G, P30L, I172N, exon 6 mutation cluster [I235N, V236E, M238K], V281L, L307FfsX6, Q318X, R356W, P453S, G110VfsX21, 30-kb deletion variant)

ESR1/PGR (receptor 1/progesterone receptor) ratio (eg, breast cancer)

IGH@/BCL2 (t(14;18)) (eg, follicular lymphoma), translocation analysis; major breakpoint region (MBR) and minor cluster region (mcr) breakpoints, qualitative or quantitative

KIT (v-kit Hardy-Zuckerman 4 feline sarcoma viral oncogene homolog) (eg, mastocytosis), common variants (eg, D816V, D816Y, D816F)

MEFV (Mediterranean fever) (eg, familial Mediterranean fever), common variants (eg, E148Q, P369S, F479L, M680I, I692del, M694V, M694I, K695R, V726A, A744S, R761H)

MPL (myeloproliferative leukemia virus oncogene, thrombopoietin receptor, TPOR) (eg, myeloproliferative disorder), common variants (eg, W515A, W515K, W515L, W515R)

TRD@ (T cell antigen receptor, delta) (eg, leukemia and lymphoma), gene rearrangement analysis, evaluation to detect abnormal clonal population

Uniparental disomy (UPD) (eg, Russell-Silver syndrome, Prader-Willi/Angelman syndrome), short tandem repeat (STR) analysis

A 0.00 0.00 FUD XXX

▲ 81403 **Molecular pathology procedure, Level 4 (eg, analysis of single exon by DNA sequence analysis, analysis of >10 amplicons using multiplex PCR in 2 or more independent reactions, mutation scanning or duplication/deletion variants of 2-5 exons)**

INCLUDES *ABL1 (c-abl oncogene 1, receptor tyrosine kinase)* (eg, acquired imatinib tyrosine kinase inhibitor resistance), variants in the kinase domain

ANG (angiogenin, ribonuclease, RNase A family, 5) (eg, amyotrophic lateral sclerosis), full gene sequence

ARX (aristaless-related homeobox) (eg, X-linked lissencephaly with ambiguous genitalia, X-linked mental retardation), duplication/deletion analysis

CEBPA (CCAAT/enhancer binding protein [C/EBP], alpha) (eg, acute myeloid leukemia), full gene sequence

CEL (carboxyl ester lipase [bile salt-stimulated lipase]) (eg, maturity-onset diabetes of the young [MODY]), targeted sequence analysis of exon 11 (eg, c.1785delC, c.1686delT)

CTNNB1 (catenin [cadherin-associated protein], beta 1, 88kDa) (eg, desmoid tumors), targeted sequence analysis (eg, exon 3)

DAZ/SRY (deleted in azoospermia and sex determining region Y) (eg, male infertility), common deletions (eg, AZFa, AZFb, AZFc, AZFd)

DNMT3A (DNA [cytosine-5-]-methyltransferase 3 alpha) (eg, acute myeloid leukemia), targeted sequence analysis (eg, exon 23)

EPCAM (epithelial cell adhesion molecule) (eg, Lynch syndrome), duplication/deletion analysis

F8 (coagulation factor VIII) (eg, hemophilia A), inversion analysis, intron 1 and intron 22A

F12 (coagulation factor XII [Hageman factor]) (eg, angioedema, hereditary, type III; factor XII deficiency), targeted sequence analysis of exon 9

FGFR3 (fibroblast growth factor receptor 3) (eg, isolated craniosynostosis), targeted sequence analysis (eg, exon 7)

Excludes targeted sequence analysis of multiple FGFR3 exons (81404)

GJB1 (gap junction protein, beta 1) (eg, Charcot-Marie-Tooth X-linked), full gene sequence

GNAQ (guanine nucleotide-binding protein G[q] subunit alpha) (eg, uveal melanoma), common variants (eg, R183, Q209)

HBB (hemoglobin, beta, beta-globin) (eg, beta thalassemia), duplication/deletion analysis

Human erythrocyte antigen gene analyses (eg, SLC14A1 [Kidd blood group], BCAM [Lutheran blood group], ICAM4 [Landsteiner-Wiener blood group], SLC4A1 [Diego blood group], AQP1 [Colton blood group], ERMAP [Scianna blood group], RHCE [Rh blood group, CcEe antigens], KEL [Kell blood group], DARC [Duffy blood group], GYPA, GYPB, GYPE [MNS blood group], ART4 [Dombrock blood group]) (eg, sickle-cell disease, thalassemia, hemolytic transfusion reactions, hemolytic disease of the fetus or newborn), common variants

HRAS (v-Ha-ras Harvey rat sarcoma viral oncogene homolog) (eg, Costello syndrome), exon 2 sequence

IDH1 (isocitrate dehydrogenase 1 [NADP+], soluble) (eg, glioma), common exon 4 variants (eg, R132H, R132C)

IDH2 (isocitrate dehydrogenase 2 [NADP+], mitochondrial) (eg, glioma), common exon 4 variants (eg, R140W, R172M)

JAK2 (Janus kinase 2) (eg, myeloproliferative disorder), exon 12 sequence and exon 13 sequence, if performed

KCNC3 (potassium voltage-gated channel, Shaw-related subfamily, member 3) (eg, spinocerebellar ataxia), targeted sequence analysis (eg, exon 2)

KCNJ2 (potassium inwardly-rectifying channel, subfamily J, member 2) (eg, Andersen-Tawil syndrome), full gene sequence

KCNJ11 (potassium inwardly-rectifying channel, subfamily J, member 11) (eg, familial hyperinsulinism), full gene sequence

Killer cell immunoglobulin-like receptor (KIR) gene family (eg, hematopoietic stem cell transplantation), genotyping of KIR family genes

Includes known familial variant, not otherwise specified, for gene listed in Tier 1 or Tier 2, DNA sequence analysis, each variant exon

Excludes specific Tier 1 or Tier 2 code for known common variant

KRAS (v-Ki-ras2 Kirsten rat sarcoma viral oncogene) (eg, carcinoma), gene analysis, variant(s) in exon 3 (eg, codon 61)

MC4R (melanocortin 4 receptor) (eg, obesity), full gene sequence

MICA (MHC class I polypeptide-related sequence A) (eg, solid organ transplantation), common variants (eg, *001, *002)

MPL (myeloproliferative leukemia virus oncogene, thrombopoietin receptor, TPOR) (eg, myeloproliferative disorder), exon 10 sequence

MT-RNR1 (mitochondrially encoded 12S RNA) (eg, nonsyndromic hearing loss), full gene sequence

MT-TS1 (mitochondrially encoded tRNA serine 1) (eg, nonsyndromic hearing loss), full gene sequence

NDP (Norrie disease [pseudoglioma]) (eg, Norrie disease), duplication/deletion analysis

NHLRC1 (NHL repeat containing 1) (eg, progressive myoclonus epilepsy), full gene sequence

PHOX2B (paired-like homeobox 2b) (eg, congenital central hypoventilation syndrome), duplication/deletion analysis

PLN (phospholamban) (eg, dilated cardiomyopathy, hypertrophic cardiomyopathy), full gene sequence

RHD (Rh blood group, D antigen) (eg, hemolytic disease of the fetus and newborn, Rh maternal/fetal compatibility), deletion analysis (eg, exons 4, 5, and 7, pseudogene)

RHD (Rh blood group, D antigen) (eg, hemolytic disease of the fetus and newborn, Rh maternal/fetal compatibility), deletion analysis (eg, exons 4, 5, and 7, pseudogene), performed on cell-free fetal DNA in maternal blood

(For human erythrocyte gene analysis of RHD, use a separate unit of 81403)

SH2D1A (SH2 domain containing 1A) (eg, X-linked lymphoproliferative syndrome), duplication/deletion analysis

SMN1 (survival of motor neuron 1, telomeric) (eg, spinal muscular atrophy), known familial sequence variant(s)

TWIST1 (twist homolog 1 [Drosophila]) (eg, Saethre-Chotzen syndrome), duplication/deletion analysis
UBA1 (ubiquitin-like modifier activating enzyme 1) (eg, spinal muscular atrophy, X-linked), targeted sequence analysis (eg, exon 15)
VHL (von Hippel-Lindau tumor suppressor) (eg, von Hippel-Lindau familial cancer syndrome), deletion/duplication analysis
VWF (von Willebrand factor) (eg, von Willebrand disease types 2A, 2B, 2M), targeted sequence analysis (eg, exon 28)

A 0.00 0.00 **FUD** XXX

▲ **81404** **Molecular pathology procedure, Level 5 (eg, analysis of 2-5 exons by DNA sequence analysis, mutation scanning or duplication/deletion variants of 6-10 exons, or characterization of a dynamic mutation disorder/triplet repeat by Southern blot analysis)**

INCLUDES *ACADS (acyl-CoA dehydrogenase, C-2 to C-3 short chain)* (eg, short chain acyl-CoA dehydrogenase deficiency), targeted sequence analysis (eg, exons 5 and 6)
AFF2 (AF4/FMR2 family, member 2 [FMR2]) (eg, fragile X mental retardation 2 [FRAXE]), characterization of alleles (eg, expanded size and methylation status)
AQP2 (aquaporin 2 [collecting duct]) (eg, nephrogenic diabetes insipidus), full gene sequence
ARX (aristaless related homeobox) (eg, X-linked lissencephaly with ambiguous genitalia, X-linked mental retardation), full gene sequence
AVPR2 (arginine vasopressin receptor 2) (eg, nephrogenic diabetes insipidus), full gene sequence
BBS10 (Bardet-Biedl syndrome 10) (eg, Bardet-Biedl syndrome), full gene sequence
BTD (biotinidase) (eg, biotinidase deficiency), full gene sequence
C10orf2 (chromosome 10 open reading frame 2) (eg, mitochondrial DNA depletion syndrome), full gene sequence
CAV3 (caveolin 3) (eg, CAV3-related distal myopathy, limb-girdle muscular dystrophy type 1C), full gene sequence
CD40LG (CD40 ligand) (eg, X-linked hyper IgM syndrome), full gene sequence
CDKN2A (cyclin-dependent kinase inhibitor 2A) (eg, CDKN2A-related cutaneous malignant melanoma, familial atypical mole-malignant melanoma syndrome), full gene sequence
CLRN1 (clarin 1) (eg, Usher syndrome, type 3), full gene sequence
COX6B1 (cytochrome c oxidase subunit VIb polypeptide 1) (eg, mitochondrial respiratory chain complex IV deficiency), full gene sequence
CPT2 (carnitine palmitoyltransferase 2) (eg, carnitine palmitoyltransferase II deficiency), full gene sequence
CRX (cone-rod homeobox) (eg, cone-rod dystrophy 2, Leber congenital amaurosis), full gene sequence
CSTB (cystatin B [stefin B]) (eg, Unverricht-Lundborg disease), full gene sequence
CYP1B1 (cytochrome P450, family 1, subfamily B, polypeptide 1) (eg, primary congenital glaucoma), full gene sequence
DMPK (dystrophia myotonica-protein kinase) (eg, myotonic dystrophy type 1), characterization of abnormal (eg, expanded) alleles
EGR2 (early growth response 2) (eg, Charcot-Marie-Tooth), full gene sequence
EMD (emerin) (eg, Emery-Dreifuss muscular dystrophy), duplication/deletion analysis
EPM2A (epilepsy, progressive myoclonus type 2A, Lafora disease [laforin]) (eg, progressive myoclonus epilepsy), full gene sequence
FGF23 (fibroblast growth factor 23) (eg, hypophosphatemic rickets), full gene sequence
FGFR2 (fibroblast growth factor receptor 2) (eg, craniosynostosis, Apert syndrome, Crouzon syndrome), targeted sequence analysis (eg, exons 8, 10)
FGFR3 (fibroblast growth factor receptor 3) (eg, achondroplasia, hypochondroplasia), targeted sequence analysis (eg, exons 8, 11, 12, 13)
FHL1 (four and a half LIM domains 1) (eg, Emery-Dreifuss muscular dystrophy), full gene sequence
FKRP (Fukutin related protein) (eg, congenital muscular dystrophy type 1C [MDC1C], limb-girdle muscular dystrophy [LGMD] type 2I), full gene sequence
FOXG1 (forkhead box G1) (eg, Rett syndrome), full gene sequence
FSHMD1A (facioscapulohumeral muscular dystrophy 1A) (eg, facioscapulohumeral muscular dystrophy), evaluation to detect abnormal (eg, deleted) alleles
FSHMD1A (facioscapulohumeral muscular dystrophy 1A) (eg, facioscapulohumeral muscular dystrophy), characterization of haplotype(s) (ie, chromosome 4A and 4B haplotypes)
FXN (frataxin) (eg, Friedreich ataxia), full gene sequence
GH1 (growth hormone 1) (eg, growth hormone deficiency), full gene sequence
GP1BB (glycoprotein Ib [platelet], beta polypeptide) (eg, Bernard-Soulier syndrome type B), full gene sequence
HBA1/HBA2 (alpha globin 1 and alpha globin 2) (eg, alpha thalassemia), duplication/deletion analysis
Excludes common deletion variants of alpha globin 1 and 2 genes (81257)
HBB (hemoglobin, beta, beta-globin) (eg, thalassemia), full gene sequence
HNF1B (HNF1 homeobox B) (eg, maturity-onset diabetes of the young [MODY]), duplication/deletion analysis
HRAS (v-Ha-ras Harvey rat sarcoma viral oncogene homolog) (eg, Costello syndrome), full gene sequence
HSD3B2 (hydroxy-delta-5-steroid dehydrogenase, 3 beta- and steroid delta-isomerase 2) (eg, 3-beta-hydroxysteroid dehydrogenase type II deficiency), full gene sequence
HSD11B2 (hydroxysteroid [11-beta] dehydrogenase 2) (eg, mineralocorticoid excess syndrome), full gene sequence
HSPB1 (heat shock 27kDa protein 1) (eg, Charcot-Marie-Tooth disease), full gene sequence
INS (insulin) (eg, diabetes mellitus), full gene sequence
KCNJ1 (potassium inwardly-rectifying channel, subfamily J, member 1) (eg, Bartter syndrome), full gene sequence
KCNJ10 (potassium inwardly-rectifying channel, subfamily J, member 10) (eg, SeSAME syndrome, EAST syndrome, sensorineural hearing loss), full gene sequence

KIT (C-kit) (v-kit Hardy-Zuckerman 4 feline sarcoma viral oncogene homolog) (eg, GIST, acute myeloid leukemia, melanoma), targeted gene analysis (eg, exons 8, 11, 13, 17, 18)

LITAF (lipopolysaccharide-induced TNF factor) (eg, Charcot-Marie-Tooth), full gene sequence

MEFV (Mediterranean fever) (eg, familial Mediterranean fever), full gene sequence

MEN1 (multiple endocrine neoplasia I) (eg, multiple endocrine neoplasia type 1, Wermer syndrome), duplication/deletion analysis

MMACHC (methylmalonic aciduria [cobalamin deficiency] cblC type, with homocystinuria) (eg, methylmalonic acidemia and homocystinuria), full gene sequence

MPV17 (MpV17 mitochondrial inner membrane protein) (eg, mitochondrial DNA depletion syndrome), duplication/deletion analysis

NDP (Norrie disease [pseudoglioma]) (eg, Norrie disease), full gene sequence

NDUFA1 (NADH dehydrogenase [ubiquinone] 1 alpha subcomplex, 1, 7.5kDa) (eg, Leigh syndrome, mitochondrial complex I deficiency), full gene sequence

NDUFAF2 (NADH dehydrogenase [ubiquinone] 1 alpha subcomplex, assembly factor 2) (eg, Leigh syndrome, mitochondrial complex I deficiency), full gene sequence

NDUFS4 (NADH dehydrogenase [ubiquinone] Fe-S protein 4, 18kDa [NADH-coenzyme Q reductase]) (eg, Leigh syndrome, mitochondrial complex I deficiency), full gene sequence

NIPA1 (non-imprinted in Prader-Willi/Angelman syndrome 1) (eg, spastic paraplegia), full gene sequence

NLGN4X (neuroligin 4, X-linked) (eg, autism spectrum disorders), duplication/deletion analysis

NPC2 (Niemann-Pick disease, type C2 [epididymal secretory protein E1]) (eg, Niemann-Pick disease type C2), full gene sequence

NR0B1 (nuclear receptor subfamily 0, group B, member 1) (eg, congenital adrenal hypoplasia), full gene sequence

NRAS (neuroblastoma RAS viral oncogene homolog) (eg, colorectal carcinoma), exon 1 and exon 2 sequences

PDGFRA (platelet-derived growth factor receptor alpha polypeptide) (eg, gastrointestinal stromal tumor), targeted sequence analysis (eg, exons 12, 18)

PDX1 (pancreatic and duodenal homeobox 1) (eg, maturity-onset diabetes of the young [MODY]), full gene sequence

PHOX2B (paired-like homeobox 2b) (eg, congenital central hypoventilation syndrome), full gene sequence

PIK3CA (phosphatidylinositol-4,5-bisphosphate 3-kinase, catalytic subunit alpha) (eg, colorectal cancer), targeted sequence analysis (eg, exons 9 and 20)

PLP1 (proteolipid protein 1) (eg, Pelizaeus-Merzbacher disease, spastic paraplegia), duplication/deletion analysis

PQBP1 (polyglutamine binding protein 1) (eg, Renpenning syndrome), duplication/deletion analysis

PRNP (prion protein) (eg, genetic prion disease), full gene sequence

PROP1 (PROP paired-like homeobox 1) (eg, combined pituitary hormone deficiency), full gene sequence

PRPH2 (peripherin 2 [retinal degeneration, slow]) (eg, retinitis pigmentosa), full gene sequence

PRSS1 (protease, serine, 1 [trypsin 1]) (eg, hereditary pancreatitis), full gene sequence

RAF1 (v-raf-1 murine leukemia viral oncogene homolog 1) (eg, LEOPARD syndrome), targeted sequence analysis (eg, exons 7, 12, 14, 17)

RET (ret proto-oncogene) (eg, multiple endocrine neoplasia, type 2B and familial medullary thyroid carcinoma), common variants (eg, M918T, 2647_2648delinsTT, A883F)

RHO (rhodopsin) (eg, retinitis pigmentosa), full gene sequence

RP1 (retinitis pigmentosa 1) (eg, retinitis pigmentosa), full gene sequence

SCN1B (sodium channel, voltage-gated, type I, beta) (eg, Brugada syndrome), full gene sequence

SCO2 (SCO cytochrome oxidase deficient homolog 2 [SCO1L]) (eg, mitochondrial respiratory chain complex IV deficiency), full gene sequence

SDHC (succinate dehydrogenase complex, subunit C, integral membrane protein, 15kDa) (eg, hereditary paraganglioma-pheochromocytoma syndrome), duplication/deletion analysis

SDHD (succinate dehydrogenase complex, subunit D, integral membrane protein) (eg, hereditary paraganglioma), full gene sequence

SGCG (sarcoglycan, gamma [35kDa dystrophin-associated glycoprotein]) (eg, limb-girdle muscular dystrophy), duplication/deletion analysis

SH2D1A (SH2 domain containing 1A) (eg, X-linked lymphoproliferative syndrome), full gene sequence

SLC16A2 (solute carrier family 16, member 2 [thyroid hormone transporter]) (eg, specific thyroid hormone cell transporter deficiency, Allan-Herndon-Dudley syndrome), duplication/deletion analysis

SLC25A20 (solute carrier family 25 [carnitine/acylcarnitine translocase], member 20) (eg, carnitine-acylcarnitine translocase deficiency), duplication/deletion analysis

SLC25A4 (solute carrier family 25 [mitochondrial carrier; adenine nucleotide translocation], member 4) (eg, progressive external ophthalmoplegia), full gene sequence

SOD1 (superoxide dismutase 1, soluble) (eg, amyotrophic lateral sclerosis), full gene sequence

SPINK1 (serine peptidase inhibitor, Kazal type 1) (eg, hereditary pancreatitis), full gene sequence

STK11 (serine/threonine kinase 11) (eg, Peutz-Jeghers syndrome), duplication/deletion analysis

TACO1 (translational activator of mitochondrial encoded cytochrome c oxidase I) (eg, mitochondrial respiratory chain complex IV deficiency), full gene sequence

THAP1 (THAP domain containing, apoptosis associated protein 1) (eg, torsion dystonia), full gene sequence

TOR1A (torsin family 1, member A [torsin A]) (eg, torsion dystonia), full gene sequence

TP53 (tumor protein 53) (eg, tumor samples), targeted sequence analysis of 2-5 exons

TTPA (tocopherol [alpha] transfer protein) (eg, ataxia), full gene sequence

TTR (transthyretin) (eg, familial transthyretin amyloidosis), full gene sequence
TWIST1 (twist homolog 1 [Drosophila]) (eg, Saethre-Chotzen syndrome), full gene sequence
TYR (tyrosinase [oculocutaneous albinism IA]) (eg, oculocutaneous albinism IA), full gene sequence
USH1G (Usher syndrome 1G [autosomal recessive]) (eg, Usher syndrome, type 1), full gene sequence
VWF (von Willebrand factor) (eg, von Willebrand disease type 1C), targeted sequence analysis (eg, exons 26, 27, 37)
VHL (von Hippel-Lindau tumor suppressor) (eg, von Hippel-Lindau familial cancer syndrome), full gene sequence
ZEB2 (zinc finger E-box binding homeobox 2) (eg, Mowat-Wilson syndrome), duplication/deletion analysis
ZNF41 (zinc finger protein 41) (eg, X-linked mental retardation 89), full gene sequence

A 0.00 0.00 FUD XXX

▲ **81405 Molecular pathology procedure, Level 6 (eg, analysis of 6-10 exons by DNA sequence analysis, mutation scanning or duplication/deletion variants of 11-25 exons, regionally targeted cytogenomic array analysis)**

INCLUDES *ABCD1 (ATP-binding cassette, sub-family D [ALD], member 1)* (eg, adrenoleukodystrophy), full gene sequence
ACADS (acyl-CoA dehydrogenase, C-2 to C-3 short chain) (eg, short chain acyl-CoA dehydrogenase deficiency), full gene sequence
ACTA2 (actin, alpha 2, smooth muscle, aorta) (eg, thoracic aortic aneurysms and aortic dissections), full gene sequence
ACTC1 (actin, alpha, cardiac muscle 1) (eg, familial hypertrophic cardiomyopathy), full gene sequence
ANKRD1 (ankyrin repeat domain 1) (eg, dilated cardiomyopathy), full gene sequence
APTX (aprataxin) (eg, ataxia with oculomotor apraxia 1), full gene sequence
AR (androgen receptor) (eg, androgen insensitivity syndrome), full gene sequence
ARSA (arylsulfatase A) (eg, arylsulfatase A deficiency), full gene sequence
BCKDHA (branched chain keto acid dehydrogenase E1, alpha polypeptide) (eg, maple syrup urine disease, type 1A), full gene sequence
BCS1L (BCS1-like [S. cerevisiae]) (eg, Leigh syndrome, mitochondrial complex III deficiency, GRACILE syndrome), full gene sequence
BMPR2 (bone morphogenetic protein receptor, type II [serine/threonine kinase]) (eg, heritable pulmonary arterial hypertension), duplication/deletion analysis
CASQ2 (calsequestrin 2 [cardiac muscle]) (eg, catecholaminergic polymorphic ventricular tachycardia), full gene sequence
CASR (calcium-sensing receptor) (eg, hypocalcemia), full gene sequence
CDKL5 (cyclin-dependent kinase-like 5) (eg, early infantile epileptic encephalopathy), duplication/deletion analysis
CHRNA4 (cholinergic receptor, nicotinic, alpha 4) (eg, nocturnal frontal lobe epilepsy), full gene sequence
CHRNB2 (cholinergic receptor, nicotinic, beta 2 [neuronal]) (eg, nocturnal frontal lobe epilepsy), full gene sequence
COX10 (COX10 homolog, cytochrome c oxidase assembly protein) (eg, mitochondrial respiratory chain complex IV deficiency), full gene sequence
COX15 (COX15 homolog, cytochrome c oxidase assembly protein) (eg, mitochondrial respiratory chain complex IV deficiency), full gene sequence
CYP11B1 (cytochrome P450, family 11, subfamily B, polypeptide 1) (eg, congenital adrenal hyperplasia), full gene sequence
CYP17A1 (cytochrome P450, family 17, subfamily A, polypeptide 1) (eg, congenital adrenal hyperplasia), full gene sequence
CYP21A2 (cytochrome P450, family 21, subfamily A, polypeptide2) (eg, steroid 21-hydroxylase isoform, congenital adrenal hyperplasia), full gene sequence
Cytogenomic constitutional targeted microarray analysis of chromosome 22q13 by interrogation of genomic regions for copy number and single nucleotide polymorphism (SNP) variants for chromosomal abnormalities
Excludes genome-wide cytogenomic constitutional microarray analysis (81228-81229)
Do not report analyte-specific molecular pathology services separately when the analytes are part of the microarray analysis of chromosome 22q13
Do not report with (88271)
DBT (dihydrolipoamide branched chain transacylase E2) (eg, maple syrup urine disease, type 2), duplication/deletion analysis
DCX (doublecortin) (eg, X-linked lissencephaly), full gene sequence
DES (desmin) (eg, myofibrillar myopathy), full gene sequence
DFNB59 (deafness, autosomal recessive 59) (eg, autosomal recessive nonsyndromic hearing impairment), full gene sequence
DGUOK (deoxyguanosine kinase) (eg, hepatocerebral mitochondrial DNA depletion syndrome), full gene sequence
DHCR7 (7-dehydrocholesterol reductase) (eg, Smith-Lemli-Opitz syndrome), full gene sequence
EIF2B2 (eukaryotic translation initiation factor 2B, subunit 2 beta, 39kDa) (eg, leukoencephalopathy with vanishing white matter), full gene sequence
EMD (emerin) (eg, Emery-Dreifuss muscular dystrophy), full gene sequence
ENG (endoglin) (eg, hereditary hemorrhagic telangiectasia, type 1), duplication/deletion analysis
EYA1 (eyes absent homolog 1 [Drosophila]) (eg, branchio-oto-renal [BOR] spectrum disorders), duplication/deletion analysis
F9 (coagulation factor IX) (eg, hemophilia B), full gene sequence
FGFR1 (fibroblast growth factor receptor 1) (eg, Kallmann syndrome 2), full gene sequence
FH (fumarate hydratase) (eg, fumarate hydratase deficiency, hereditary leiomyomatosis with renal cell cancer), full gene sequence

FKTN (fukutin) (eg, limb-girdle muscular dystrophy [LGMD] type 2M or 2L), full gene sequence

FTSJ1 (FtsJ RNA methyltransferase homolog 1 [E. coli]) (eg, X-linked mental retardation 9), duplication/deletion analysis

GABRG2 (gamma-aminobutyric acid [GABA] A receptor, gamma 2) (eg, generalized epilepsy with febrile seizures), full gene sequence

GCH1 (GTP cyclohydrolase 1) (eg, autosomal dominant dopa-responsive dystonia), full gene sequence

GDAP1 (ganglioside-induced differentiation-associated protein 1) (eg, Charcot-Marie-Tooth disease), full gene sequence

GFAP (glial fibrillary acidic protein) (eg, Alexander disease), full gene sequence

GHR (growth hormone receptor) (eg, Laron syndrome), full gene sequence

GHRHR (growth hormone releasing hormone receptor) (eg, growth hormone deficiency), full gene sequence

GLA (galactosidase, alpha) (eg, Fabry disease), full gene sequence

HBA1/HBA2 (alpha globin 1 and alpha globin 2) (eg, thalassemia), full gene sequence

HNF1A (HNF1 homeobox A) (eg, maturity-onset diabetes of the young [MODY]), full gene sequence

HNF1B (HNF1 homeobox B) (eg, maturity-onset diabetes of the young [MODY]), full gene sequence

HTRA1 (HtrA serine peptidase 1) (eg, macular degeneration), full gene sequence

IDS (iduronate 2-sulfatase) (eg, mucopolysaccharidosis, type II), full gene sequence

IL2RG (interleukin 2 receptor, gamma) (eg, X-linked severe combined immunodeficiency), full gene sequence

ISPD (isoprenoid synthase domain containing) (eg, muscle-eye-brain disease, Walker-Warburg syndrome), full gene sequence

KRAS (v-Ki-ras2 Kirsten rat sarcoma viral oncogene homolog) (eg, Noonan syndrome), full gene sequence

LAMP2 (lysosomal-associated membrane protein 2) (eg, Danon disease), full gene sequence

LDLR (low density lipoprotein receptor) (eg, familial hypercholesterolemia), duplication/deletion analysis

MEN1 (multiple endocrine neoplasia I) (eg, multiple endocrine neoplasia type 1, Wermer syndrome), full gene sequence

MMAA (methylmalonic aciduria [cobalamine deficiency] type A) (eg, MMAA-related methylmalonic acidemia), full gene sequence

MMAB (methylmalonic aciduria [cobalamine deficiency] type B) (eg, MMAA-related methylmalonic acidemia), full gene sequence

MPI (mannose phosphate isomerase) (eg, congenital disorder of glycosylation 1b), full gene sequence

MPV17 (MpV17 mitochondrial inner membrane protein) (eg, mitochondrial DNA depletion syndrome), full gene sequence

MPZ (myelin protein zero) (eg, Charcot-Marie-Tooth), full gene sequence

MTM1 (myotubularin 1) (eg, X-linked centronuclear myopathy), duplication/deletion analysis

MYL2 (myosin, light chain 2, regulatory, cardiac, slow) (eg, familial hypertrophic cardiomyopathy), full gene sequence

MYL3 (myosin, light chain 3, alkali, ventricular, skeletal, slow) (eg, familial hypertrophic cardiomyopathy), full gene sequence

MYOT (myotilin) (eg, limb-girdle muscular dystrophy), full gene sequence

NDUFS7 (NADH dehydrogenase [ubiquinone] Fe-S protein 7, 20kDa [NADH-coenzyme Q reductase]) (eg, Leigh syndrome, mitochondrial complex I deficiency), full gene sequence

NDUFS8 (NADH dehydrogenase [ubiquinone] Fe-S protein 8, 23kDa [NADH-coenzyme Q reductase]) (eg, Leigh syndrome, mitochondrial complex I deficiency), full gene sequence

NDUFV1 (NADH dehydrogenase [ubiquinone] flavoprotein 1, 51kDa) (eg, Leigh syndrome, mitochondrial complex I deficiency), full gene sequence

NEFL (neurofilament, light polypeptide) (eg, Charcot-Marie-Tooth), full gene sequence

NF2 (neurofibromin 2 [merlin]) (eg, neurofibromatosis, type 2), duplication/deletion analysis

NLGN3 (neuroligin 3) (eg, autism spectrum disorders), full gene sequence

NLGN4X (neuroligin 4, X-linked) (eg, autism spectrum disorders), full gene sequence

NPHP1 (nephronophthisis 1 [juvenile]) (eg, Joubert syndrome), deletion analysis, and duplication analysis, if performed

NPHS2 (nephrosis 2, idiopathic, steroid-resistant [podocin]) (eg, steroid-resistant nephrotic syndrome), full gene sequence

NSD1 (nuclear receptor binding SET domain protein 1) (eg, Sotos syndrome), duplication/deletion analysis

OTC (ornithine carbamoyltransferase) (eg, ornithine transcarbamylase deficiency), full gene sequence

PAFAH1B1 (platelet-activating factor acetylhydrolase 1b, regulatory subunit 1 [45kDa]) (eg, lissencephaly, Miller-Dieker syndrome), duplication/deletion analysis

PARK2 (Parkinson protein 2, E3 ubiquitin protein ligase [parkin]) (eg, Parkinson disease), duplication/deletion analysis

PCCA (propionyl CoA carboxylase, alpha polypeptide) (eg, propionic acidemia, type 1), duplication/deletion analysis

PCDH19 (protocadherin 19) (eg, epileptic encephalopathy), full gene sequence

PDHA1 (pyruvate dehydrogenase [lipoamide] alpha 1) (eg, lactic acidosis), duplication/deletion analysis

PDHB (pyruvate dehydrogenase [lipoamide] beta) (eg, lactic acidosis), full gene sequence

PINK1 (PTEN induced putative kinase 1) (eg, Parkinson disease), full gene sequence

PLP1 (proteolipid protein 1) (eg, Pelizaeus-Merzbacher disease, spastic paraplegia), full gene sequence

POU1F1 (POU class 1 homeobox 1) (eg, combined pituitary hormone deficiency), full gene sequence

PQBP1 (polyglutamine binding protein 1) (eg, Renpenning syndrome), full gene sequence

PRX (periaxin) (eg, Charcot-Marie-Tooth disease), full gene sequence

PSEN1 (presenilin 1) (eg, Alzheimer's disease), full gene sequence

RAB7A (RAB7A, member RAS oncogene family) (eg, Charcot-Marie-Tooth disease), full gene sequence

RAI1 (retinoic acid induced 1) (eg, Smith-Magenis syndrome), full gene sequence

REEP1 (receptor accessory protein 1) (eg, spastic paraplegia), full gene sequence

RET (ret proto-oncogene) (eg, multiple endocrine neoplasia, type 2A and familial medullary thyroid carcinoma), targeted sequence analysis (eg, exons 10, 11, 13-16)

RPS19 (ribosomal protein S19) (eg, Diamond-Blackfan anemia), full gene sequence

RRM2B (ribonucleotide reductase M2 B [TP53 inducible]) (eg, mitochondrial DNA depletion), full gene sequence

SCO1 (SCO cytochrome oxidase deficient homolog 1) (eg, mitochondrial respiratory chain complex IV deficiency), full gene sequence

SDHB (succinate dehydrogenase complex, subunit B, iron sulfur) (eg, hereditary paraganglioma), full gene sequence

SDHC (succinate dehydrogenase complex, subunit C, integral membrane protein, 15kDa) (eg, hereditary paraganglioma-pheochromocytoma syndrome), full gene sequence

SGCA (sarcoglycan, alpha [50kDa dystrophin-associated glycoprotein]) (eg, limb-girdle muscular dystrophy), full gene sequence

SGCB (sarcoglycan, beta [43kDa dystrophin-associated glycoprotein]) (eg, limb-girdle muscular dystrophy), full gene sequence

SGCD (sarcoglycan, delta [35kDa dystrophin-associated glycoprotein]) (eg, limb-girdle muscular dystrophy), full gene sequence

SGCE (sarcoglycan, epsilon) (eg, myoclonic dystonia), duplication/deletion analysis

SGCG (sarcoglycan, gamma [35kDa dystrophin-associated glycoprotein]) (eg, limb-girdle muscular dystrophy), full gene sequence

SHOC2 (soc-2 suppressor of clear homolog) (eg, Noonan-like syndrome with loose anagen hair), full gene sequence

SHOX (short stature homeobox) (eg, Langer mesomelic dysplasia), full gene sequence

SIL1 (SIL1 homolog, endoplasmic reticulum chaperone [S. cerevisiae]) (eg, ataxia), full gene sequence

SLC2A1 (solute carrier family 2 [facilitated glucose transporter], member 1) (eg, glucose transporter type 1 [GLUT 1] deficiency syndrome), full gene sequence

SLC16A2 (solute carrier family 16, member 2 [thyroid hormone transporter]) (eg, specific thyroid hormone cell transporter deficiency, Allan-Herndon-Dudley syndrome), full gene sequence

SLC22A5 (solute carrier family 22 [organic cation/carnitine transporter], member 5) (eg, systemic primary carnitine deficiency), full gene sequence

SLC25A20 (solute carrier family 25 [carnitine/acylcarnitine translocase], member 20) (eg, carnitine-acylcarnitine translocase deficiency), full gene sequence

SMAD4 (SMAD family member 4) (eg, hemorrhagic telangiectasia syndrome, juvenile polyposis), duplication/deletion analysis

SMN1 (survival of motor neuron 1, telomeric) (eg, spinal muscular atrophy), full gene sequence

SPAST (spastin) (eg, spastic paraplegia), duplication/deletion analysis

SPG7 (spastic paraplegia 7 [pure and complicated autosomal recessive]) (eg, spastic paraplegia), duplication/deletion analysis

SPRED1 (sprouty-related, EVH1 domain containing 1) (eg, Legius syndrome), full gene sequence

STAT3 (signal transducer and activator of transcription 3 [acute-phase response factor]) (eg, autosomal dominant hyper-IgE syndrome), targeted sequence analysis (eg, exons 12, 13, 14, 16, 17, 20, 21)

STK11 (serine/threonine kinase 11) (eg, Peutz-Jeghers syndrome), full gene sequence

SURF1 (surfeit 1) (eg, mitochondrial respiratory chain complex IV deficiency), full gene sequence

TARDBP (TAR DNA binding protein) (eg, amyotrophic lateral sclerosis), full gene sequence

TBX5 (T-box 5) (eg, Holt-Oram syndrome), full gene sequence

TCF4 (transcription factor 4) (eg, Pitt-Hopkins syndrome), duplication/deletion analysis

TGFBR1 (transforming growth factor, beta receptor 1) (eg, Marfan syndrome), full gene sequence

TGFBR2 (transforming growth factor, beta receptor 2) (eg, Marfan syndrome), full gene sequence

THRB (thyroid hormone receptor, beta) (eg, thyroid hormone resistance, thyroid hormone beta receptor deficiency), full gene sequence or targeted sequence analysis of >5 exons

TK2 (thymidine kinase 2, mitochondrial) (eg, mitochondrial DNA depletion syndrome), full gene sequence

TNNC1 (troponin C type 1 [slow]) (eg, hypertrophic cardiomyopathy or dilated cardiomyopathy), full gene sequence

TNNI3 (troponin I, type 3 [cardiac]) (eg, familial hypertrophic cardiomyopathy), full gene sequence

TP53 (tumor protein 53) (eg, Li-Fraumeni syndrome, tumor samples), full gene sequence or targeted sequence analysis of >5 exons

TPM1 (tropomyosin 1 [alpha]) (eg, familial hypertrophic cardiomyopathy), full gene sequence

TSC1 (tuberous sclerosis 1) (eg, tuberous sclerosis), duplication/deletion analysis

TYMP (thymidine phosphorylase) (eg, mitochondrial DNA depletion syndrome), full gene sequence

VWF (von Willebrand factor) (eg, von Willebrand disease type 2N), targeted sequence analysis (eg, exons 18-20, 23-25)

WT1 (Wilms tumor 1) (eg, Denys-Drash syndrome, familial Wilms tumor), full gene sequence

ZEB2 (zinc finger E-box binding homeobox 2) (eg, Mowat-Wilson syndrome), full gene sequence

A 0.00 0.00 **FUD** XXX

81406 Molecular pathology procedure, Level 7 (eg, analysis of 11-25 exons by DNA sequence analysis, mutation scanning or duplication/deletion variants of 26-50 exons, cytogenomic array analysis for neoplasia)

INCLUDES *ACADVL (acyl-CoA dehydrogenase, very long chain)* (eg, very long chain acyl-coenzyme A dehydrogenase deficiency), full gene sequence

ACTN4 (actinin, alpha 4) (eg, focal segmental glomerulosclerosis), full gene sequence

AFG3L2 (AFG3 ATPase family gene 3-like 2 [S. cerevisiae]) (eg, spinocerebellar ataxia), full gene sequence
AIRE (autoimmune regulator) (eg, autoimmune polyendocrinopathy syndrome type 1), full gene sequence
ALDH7A1 (aldehyde dehydrogenase 7 family, member A1) (eg, pyridoxine-dependent epilepsy), full gene sequence
ANO5 (anoctamin 5) (eg, limb-girdle muscular dystrophy), full gene sequence
APP (amyloid beta [A4] precursor protein) (eg, Alzheimer's disease), full gene sequence
ASS1 (argininosuccinate synthase 1) (eg, citrullinemia type I), full gene sequence
ATL1 (atlastin GTPase 1) (eg, spastic paraplegia), full gene sequence
ATP1A2 (ATPase, Na+/K+ transporting, alpha 2 polypeptide) (eg, familial hemiplegic migraine), full gene sequence
ATP7B (ATPase, Cu++ transporting, beta polypeptide) (eg, Wilson disease), full gene sequence
BBS1 (Bardet-Biedl syndrome 1) (eg, Bardet-Biedl syndrome), full gene sequence
BBS2 (Bardet-Biedl syndrome 2) (eg, Bardet-Biedl syndrome), full gene sequence
BCKDHB (branched-chain keto acid dehydrogenase E1, beta polypeptide) (eg, maple syrup urine disease, type 1B), full gene sequence
BEST1 (bestrophin 1) (eg, vitelliform macular dystrophy), full gene sequence
BMPR2 (bone morphogenetic protein receptor, type II [serine/threonine kinase]) (eg, heritable pulmonary arterial hypertension), full gene sequence
BRAF (v-raf murine sarcoma viral oncogene homolog B1) (eg, Noonan syndrome), full gene sequence
BSCL2 (Berardinelli-Seip congenital lipodystrophy 2 [seipin]) (eg, Berardinelli-Seip congenital lipodystrophy), full gene sequence
BTK (Bruton agammaglobulinemia tyrosine kinase) (eg, X-linked agammaglobulinemia), full gene sequence
CACNB2 (calcium channel, voltage-dependent, beta 2 subunit) (eg, Brugada syndrome), full gene sequence
CAPN3 (calpain 3) (eg, limb-girdle muscular dystrophy [LGMD] type 2A, calpainopathy), full gene sequence
CBS (cystathionine-beta-synthase) (eg, homocystinuria, cystathionine beta-synthase deficiency), full gene sequence
CDH1 (cadherin 1, type 1, E-cadherin [epithelial]) (eg, hereditary diffuse gastric cancer), full gene sequence
CDKL5 (cyclin-dependent kinase-like 5) (eg, early infantile epileptic encephalopathy), full gene sequence
CLCN1 (chloride channel 1, skeletal muscle) (eg, myotonia congenita), full gene sequence
CLCNKB (chloride channel, voltage-sensitive Kb) (eg, Bartter syndrome 3 and 4b), full gene sequence
CNTNAP2 (contactin-associated protein-like 2) (eg, Pitt-Hopkins-like syndrome 1), full gene sequence
COL6A2 (collagen, type VI, alpha 2) (eg, collagen type VI-related disorders), duplication/deletion analysis
CPT1A (carnitine palmitoyltransferase 1A [liver]) (eg, carnitine palmitoyltransferase 1A [CPT1A] deficiency), full gene sequence
CRB1 (crumbs homolog 1 [Drosophila]) (eg, Leber congenital amaurosis), full gene sequence
CREBBP (CREB binding protein) (eg, Rubinstein-Taybi syndrome), duplication/deletion analysis
Cytogenomic microarray analysis, neoplasia (eg, interrogation of copy number, and loss-of-heterozygosity via single nucleotide polymorphism [SNP]-based comparative genomic hybridization [CGH] microarray analysis)
Do not report analyte-specific molecular pathology services separately when the analytes are part of the cytogenomic microarray analysis for neoplasia
Do not report with (88271)
DBT (dihydrolipoamide branched chain transacylase E2) (eg, maple syrup urine disease, type 2), full gene sequence
DLAT (dihydrolipoamide S-acetyltransferase) (eg, pyruvate dehydrogenase E2 deficiency), full gene sequence
DLD (dihydrolipoamide dehydrogenase) (eg, maple syrup urine disease, type III), full gene sequence
DSC2 (desmocollin) (eg, arrhythmogenic right ventricular dysplasia/cardiomyopathy 11), full gene sequence
DSG2 (desmoglein 2) (eg, arrhythmogenic right ventricular dysplasia/cardiomyopathy 10), full gene sequence
DSP (desmoplakin) (eg, arrhythmogenic right ventricular dysplasia/cardiomyopathy 8), full gene sequence
EFHC1 (EF-hand domain [C-terminal] containing 1) (eg, juvenile myoclonic epilepsy), full gene sequence
EIF2B3 (eukaryotic translation initiation factor 2B, subunit 3 gamma, 58kDa) (eg, leukoencephalopathy with vanishing white matter), full gene sequence
EIF2B4 (eukaryotic translation initiation factor 2B, subunit 4 delta, 67kDa) (eg, leukoencephalopathy with vanishing white matter), full gene sequence
EIF2B5 (eukaryotic translation initiation factor 2B, subunit 5 epsilon, 82kDa) (eg, childhood ataxia with central nervous system hypomyelination/vanishing white matter), full gene sequence
ENG (endoglin) (eg, hereditary hemorrhagic telangiectasia, type 1), full gene sequence
EYA1 (eyes absent homolog 1 [Drosophila]) (eg, branchio-oto-renal [BOR] spectrum disorders), full gene sequence
F8 (coagulation factor VIII) (eg, hemophilia A), duplication/deletion analysis
FAH (fumarylacetoacetate hydrolase [fumarylacetoacetase]) (eg, tyrosinemia, type 1), full gene sequence
FASTKD2 (FAST kinase domains 2) (eg, mitochondrial respiratory chain complex IV deficiency), full gene sequence
FIG4 (FIG4 homolog, SAC1 lipid phosphatase domain containing [S. cerevisiae]) (eg, Charcot-Marie-Tooth disease), full gene sequence
FTSJ1 (FtsJ RNA methyltransferase homolog 1 [E. coli]) (eg, X-linked mental retardation 9), full gene sequence
FUS (fused in sarcoma) (eg, amyotrophic lateral sclerosis), full gene sequence

GAA (glucosidase, alpha; acid) (eg, glycogen storage disease type II [Pompe disease]), full gene sequence
GALC (galactosylceramidase) (eg, Krabbe disease), full gene sequence
GALT (galactose-1-phosphate uridylyltransferase) (eg, galactosemia), full gene sequence
GARS (glycyl-tRNA synthetase) (eg, Charcot-Marie-Tooth disease), full gene sequence
GCDH (glutaryl-CoA dehydrogenase) (eg, glutaricacidemia type 1), full gene sequence
GCK (glucokinase [hexokinase 4]) (eg, maturity-onset diabetes of the young [MODY]), full gene sequence
GLUD1 (glutamate dehydrogenase 1) (eg, familial hyperinsulinism), full gene sequence
GNE (glucosamine [UDP-N-acetyl]-2-epimerase/ N-acetylmannosamine kinase) (eg, inclusion body myopathy 2 [IBM2], Nonaka myopathy), full gene sequence
GRN (granulin) (eg, frontotemporal dementia), full gene sequence
HADHA (hydroxyacyl-CoA dehydrogenase/3-ketoacyl-CoA thiolase/enoyl-CoA hydratase [trifunctional protein] alpha subunit) (eg, long chain acyl-coenzyme A dehydrogenase deficiency), full gene sequence
HADHB (hydroxyacyl-CoA dehydrogenase/3-ketoacyl-CoA thiolase/enoyl-CoA hydratase [trifunctional protein], beta subunit) (eg, trifunctional protein deficiency), full gene sequence
HEXA (hexosaminidase A, alpha polypeptide) (eg, Tay-Sachs disease), full gene sequence
HLCS (HLCS holocarboxylase synthetase) (eg, holocarboxylase synthetase deficiency), full gene sequence
HNF4A (hepatocyte nuclear factor 4, alpha) (eg, maturity-onset diabetes of the young [MODY]), full gene sequence
IDUA (iduronidase, alpha-L-) (eg, mucopolysaccharidosis type I), full gene sequence
INF2 (inverted formin, FH2 and WH2 domain containing) (eg, focal segmental glomerulosclerosis), full gene sequence
IVD (isovaleryl-CoA dehydrogenase) (eg, isovaleric acidemia), full gene sequence
JAG1 (jagged 1) (eg, Alagille syndrome), duplication/deletion analysis
JUP (junction plakoglobin) (eg, arrhythmogenic right ventricular dysplasia/cardiomyopathy 11), full gene sequence
KAL1 (Kallmann syndrome 1 sequence) (eg, Kallmann syndrome), full gene sequence
KCNH2 (potassium voltage-gated channel, subfamily H [eag-related], member 2) (eg, short QT syndrome, long QT syndrome), full gene sequence
Do not report with (81280)
KCNQ1 (potassium voltage-gated channel, KQT-like subfamily, member 1) (eg, short QT syndrome, long QT syndrome), full gene sequence
Do not report with (81280)
KCNQ2 (potassium voltage-gated channel, KQT-like subfamily, member 2) (eg, epileptic encephalopathy), full gene sequence
LDB3 (LIM domain binding 3) (eg, familial dilated cardiomyopathy, myofibrillar myopathy), full gene sequence
LDLR (low density lipoprotein receptor) (eg, familial hypercholesterolemia), full gene sequence
LEPR (leptin receptor(eg, obesity with hypogonadism), full gene sequence
LHCGR (luteinizing hormone/choriogonadotropin receptor) (eg, precocious male puberty), full gene sequence
LMNA (lamin A/C) (eg, Emery-Dreifuss muscular dystrophy [EDMD1, 2 and 3] limb-girdle muscular dystrophy [LGMD] type 1B, dilated cardiomyopathy [CMD1A], familial partial lipodystrophy [FPLD2]), full gene sequence
LRP5 (low density lipoprotein receptor-related protein 5) (eg, osteopetrosis), full gene sequence
MAP2K1 (mitogen-activated protein kinase 1) (eg, cardiofaciocutaneous syndrome), full gene sequence
MAP2K2 (mitogen-activated protein kinase 2) (eg, cardiofaciocutaneous syndrome), full gene sequence
MAPT (microtubule-associated protein tau) (eg, frontotemporal dementia), full gene sequence
MCCC1 (methylcrotonoyl-CoA carboxylase 1 [alpha]) (eg, 3-methylcrotonyl-CoA carboxylase deficiency), full gene sequence
MCCC2 (methylcrotonoyl-CoA carboxylase 2 [beta]) (eg, 3-methylcrotonyl carboxylase deficiency), full gene sequence
MFN2 (mitofusin 2) (eg, Charcot-Marie-Tooth disease), full gene sequence
MTM1 (myotubularin 1) (eg, X-linked centronuclear myopathy), full gene sequence
MUT (methylmalonyl CoA mutase) (eg, methylmalonic acidemia), full gene sequence
MUTYH (mutY homolog [E. coli]) (eg, MYH-associated polyposis), full gene sequence
NDUFS1 (NADH dehydrogenase [ubiquinone] Fe-S protein 1, 75kDa [NADH-coenzyme Q reductase]) (eg, Leigh syndrome, mitochondrial complex I deficiency), full gene sequence
NF2 (neurofibromin 2 [merlin]) (eg, neurofibromatosis, type 2), full gene sequence
NOTCH3 (notch 3) (eg, cerebral autosomal dominant arteriopathy with subcortical infarcts and leukoencephalopathy [CADASIL]), targeted sequence analysis (eg, exons 1-23)
NPC1 (Niemann-Pick disease, type C1) (eg, Niemann-Pick disease), full gene sequence
NPHP1 (nephronophthisis 1 [juvenile]) (eg, Joubert syndrome), full gene sequence
NSD1 (nuclear receptor binding SET domain protein 1) (eg, Sotos syndrome), full gene sequence
OPA1 (optic atrophy 1) (eg, optic atrophy), duplication/deletion analysis
OPTN (optineurin) (eg, amyotrophic lateral sclerosis), full gene sequence
PAFAH1B1 (platelet-activating factor acetylhydrolase 1b, regulatory subunit 1 [45kDa]) (eg, lissencephaly, Miller-Dieker syndrome), full gene sequence
PAH (phenylalanine hydroxylase) (eg, phenylketonuria), full gene sequence
PALB2 (partner and localizer of BRCA2) (eg, breast and pancreatic cancer), full gene sequence
PARK2 (Parkinson protein 2, E3 ubiquitin protein ligase [parkin]) (eg, Parkinson disease), full gene sequence

PAX2 (paired box 2) (eg, renal coloboma syndrome), full gene sequence
PC (pyruvate carboxylase) (eg, pyruvate carboxylase deficiency), full gene sequence
PCCA (propionyl CoA carboxylase, alpha polypeptide) (eg, propionic acidemia, type 1), full gene sequence
PCCB (propionyl CoA carboxylase, beta polypeptide) (eg, propionic acidemia), full gene sequence
PCDH15 (protocadherin-related 15) (eg, Usher syndrome type 1F), duplication/deletion analysis
PDHA1 (pyruvate dehydrogenase [lipoamide] alpha 1) (eg, lactic acidosis), full gene sequence
PDHX (pyruvate dehydrogenase complex, component X) (eg, lactic acidosis), full gene sequence
PHEX (phosphate-regulating endopeptidase homolog, X-linked) (eg, hypophosphatemic rickets), full gene sequence
PKD2 (polycystic kidney disease 2 [autosomal dominant]) (eg, polycystic kidney disease), full gene sequence
PKP2 (plakophilin 2) (eg, arrhythmogenic right ventricular dysplasia/cardiomyopathy 9), full gene sequence
PNKD (eg, paroxysmal nonkinesigenic dyskinesia), full gene sequence
POLG (polymerase [DNA directed], gamma) (eg, Alpers-Huttenlocher syndrome, autosomal dominant progressive external ophthalmoplegia), full gene sequence
POMGNT1 (protein O-linked mannose beta1, 2-N acetylglucosaminyltransferase) (eg, muscle-eye-brain disease, Walker-Warburg syndrome), full gene sequence
POMT1 (protein-O-mannosyltransferase 1) (eg, limb-girdle muscular dystrophy [LGMD] type 2K, Walker-Warburg syndrome), full gene sequence
POMT2 (protein-O-mannosyltransferase 2) (eg, limb-girdle muscular dystrophy [LGMD] type 2N, Walker-Warburg syndrome), full gene sequence
PRKAG2 (protein kinase, AMP-activated, gamma 2 non-catalytic subunit) (eg, familial hypertrophic cardiomyopathy with Wolff-Parkinson-White syndrome, lethal congenital glycogen storage disease of heart), full gene sequence
PRKCG (protein kinase C, gamma) (eg, spinocerebellar ataxia), full gene sequence
PSEN2 (presenilin 2[Alzheimer's disease 4]) (eg, Alzheimer's disease), full gene sequence
PTPN11 (protein tyrosine phosphatase, non-receptor type 11) (eg, Noonan syndrome, LEOPARD syndrome), full gene sequence
PYGM (phosphorylase, glycogen, muscle) (eg, glycogen storage disease type V, McArdle disease), full gene sequence
RAF1 (v-raf-1 murine leukemia viral oncogene homolog 1) (eg, LEOPARD syndrome), full gene sequence
RET (ret proto-oncogene) (eg, Hirschsprung disease), full gene sequence
RPE65 (retinal pigment epithelium-specific protein 65kDa) (eg, retinitis pigmentosa, Leber congenital amaurosis), full gene sequence
RYR1 (ryanodine receptor 1, skeletal) (eg, malignant hyperthermia), targeted sequence analysis of exons with functionally-confirmed mutations
SCN4A (sodium channel, voltage-gated, type IV, alpha subunit) (eg, hyperkalemic periodic paralysis), full gene sequence
SCNN1A (sodium channel, nonvoltage-gated 1 alpha) (eg, pseudohypoaldosteronism), full gene sequence
SCNN1B (sodium channel, nonvoltage-gated 1, beta) (eg, Liddle syndrome, pseudohypoaldosteronism), full gene sequence
SCNN1G (sodium channel, nonvoltage-gated 1, gamma) (eg, Liddle syndrome, pseudohypoaldosteronism), full gene sequence
SDHA (succinate dehydrogenase complex, subunit A, flavoprotein [Fp]) (eg, Leigh syndrome, mitochondrial complex II deficiency), full gene sequence
SETX (senataxin) (eg, ataxia), full gene sequence
SGCE (sarcoglycan, epsilon) (eg, myoclonic dystonia), full gene sequence
SH3TC2 (SH3 domain and tetratricopeptide repeats 2) (eg, Charcot-Marie-Tooth disease), full gene sequence
SLC9A6 (solute carrier family 9 [sodium/hydrogen exchanger], member 6) (eg, Christianson syndrome), full gene sequence
SLC26A4 (solute carrier family 26, member 4) (eg, Pendred syndrome), full gene sequence
SLC37A4 (solute carrier family 37 [glucose-6-phosphate transporter], member 4) (eg, glycogen storage disease type Ib), full gene sequence
SMAD4 (SMAD family member 4) (eg, hemorrhagic telangiectasia syndrome, juvenile polyposis), full gene sequence
SOS1 (son of sevenless homolog 1) (eg, Noonan syndrome, gingival fibromatosis), full gene sequence
SPAST (spastin) (eg, spastic paraplegia), full gene sequence
SPG7 (spastic paraplegia 7 [pure and complicated autosomal recessive]) (eg, spastic paraplegia), full gene sequence
STXBP1 (syntaxin-binding protein 1) (eg, epileptic encephalopathy), full gene sequence
TAZ (tafazzin) (eg, methylglutaconic aciduria type 2, Barth syndrome), full gene sequence
TCF4 (transcription factor 4) (eg, Pitt-Hopkins syndrome), full gene sequence
TH (tyrosine hydroxylase) (eg, Segawa syndrome), full gene sequence
TMEM43 (transmembrane protein 43) (eg, arrhythmogenic right ventricular cardiomyopathy), full gene sequence
TNNT2 (troponin T, type 2 [cardiac]) (eg, familial hypertrophic cardiomyopathy), full gene sequence
TRPC6 (transient receptor potential cation channel, subfamily C, member 6) (eg, focal segmental glomerulosclerosis), full gene sequence
TSC1 (tuberous sclerosis 1) (eg, tuberous sclerosis), full gene sequence
TSC2 (tuberous sclerosis 2) (eg, tuberous sclerosis), duplication/deletion analysis
UBE3A (ubiquitin protein ligase E3A) (eg, Angelman syndrome) full gene sequence
UMOD (uromodulin) (eg, glomerulocystic kidney disease with hyperuricemia and isosthenuria), full gene sequence
VWF (von Willebrand factor) (von Willebrand disease type 2A), extended targeted sequence analysis (eg, exons 11-16, 24-26, 51, 52)
WAS (Wiskott-Aldrich syndrome [eczema-thrombocytopenia]) (eg, Wiskott-Aldrich syndrome), full gene sequence

A 0.00 0.00 **FUD** XXX

81407 Molecular pathology procedure, Level 8 (eg, analysis of 26-50 exons by DNA sequence analysis, mutation scanning or duplication/deletion variants of >50 exons, sequence analysis of multiple genes on one platform)

INCLUDES *ABCC8 (ATP-binding cassette, sub-family C [CFTR/MRP], member 8)* (eg, familial hyperinsulinism), full gene sequence

AGL (amylo-alpha-1, 6-glucosidase, 4-alpha-glucanotransferase) (eg, glycogen storage disease type III), full gene sequence

AHI1 (Abelson helper integration site 1) (eg, Joubert syndrome), full gene sequence

ASPM (asp [abnormal spindle] homolog, microcephaly associated [Drosophila]) (eg, primary microcephaly), full gene sequence

CACNA1A (calcium channel, voltage-dependent, P/Q type, alpha 1A subunit) (eg, familial hemiplegic migraine), full gene sequence

CHD7 (chromodomain helicase DNA binding protein 7) (eg, CHARGE syndrome), full gene sequence

COL4A4 (collagen, type IV, alpha 4) (eg, Alport syndrome), full gene sequence

COL6A1 (collagen, type VI, alpha 1) (eg, collagen type VI-related disorders), full gene sequence

COL6A2 (collagen, type VI, alpha 2) (eg, collagen type VI-related disorders), full gene sequence

COL6A3 (collagen, type VI, alpha 3) (eg, collagen type VI-related disorders), full gene sequence

CREBBP (CREB binding protein) (eg, Rubinstein-Taybi syndrome), full gene sequence

F8 (coagulation factor VIII) (eg, hemophilia A), full gene sequence

JAG1 (jagged 1) (eg, Alagille syndrome), full gene sequence

KDM5C (lysine [K]-specific demethylase 5C) (eg, X-linked mental retardation), full gene sequence

KIAA0196 (KIAA0196) (eg, spastic paraplegia), full gene sequence

L1CAM (L1 cell adhesion molecule) (eg, MASA syndrome, X-linked hydrocephaly), full gene sequence

LAMB2 (laminin, beta 2 [laminin S]) (eg, Pierson syndrome), full gene sequence

MYBPC3 (myosin binding protein C, cardiac) (eg, familial hypertrophic cardiomyopathy), full gene sequence

MYH6 (myosin, heavy chain 6, cardiac muscle, alpha) (eg, familial dilated cardiomyopathy), full gene sequence

MYH7 (myosin, heavy chain 7, cardiac muscle, beta) (eg, familial hypertrophic cardiomyopathy, Liang distal myopathy), full gene sequence

MYO7A (myosin VIIA) (eg, Usher syndrome, type 1), full gene sequence

NOTCH1 (notch 1) (eg, aortic valve disease), full gene sequence

NPHS1 (nephrosis 1, congenital, Finnish type [nephrin]) (eg, congenital Finnish nephrosis), full gene sequence

OPA1 (optic atrophy 1) (eg, optic atrophy), full gene sequence

PCDH15 (protocadherin-related 15) (eg, Usher syndrome, type 1), full gene sequence

PKD1 (polycystic kidney disease 1 [autosomal dominant]) (eg, polycystic kidney disease), full gene sequence

PLCE1 (phospholipase C, epsilon 1) (eg, nephrotic syndrome type 3), full gene sequence

SCN1A (sodium channel, voltage-gated, type 1, alpha subunit) (eg, generalized epilepsy with febrile seizures), full gene sequence

SCN5A (sodium channel, voltage-gated, type V, alpha subunit) (eg, familial dilated cardiomyopathy), full gene sequence

SLC12A1 (solute carrier family 12 [sodium/potassium/chloride transporters], member 1) (eg, Bartter syndrome), full gene sequence

SLC12A3 (solute carrier family 12 [sodium/chloride transporters], member 3) (eg, Gitelman syndrome), full gene sequence

SPG11 (spastic paraplegia 11 [autosomal recessive]) (eg, spastic paraplegia), full gene sequence

SPTBN2 (spectrin, beta, non-erythrocytic 2) (eg, spinocerebellar ataxia), full gene sequence

TMEM67 (transmembrane protein 67) (eg, Joubert syndrome), full gene sequence

TSC2 (tuberous sclerosis 2) (eg, tuberous sclerosis), full gene sequence

USH1C (Usher syndrome 1C [autosomal recessive, severe]) (eg, Usher syndrome, type 1), full gene sequence

VPS13B (vacuolar protein sorting 13 homolog B [yeast]) (eg, Cohen syndrome), duplication/deletion analysis

WDR62 (WD repeat domain 62) (eg, primary autosomal recessive microcephaly), full gene sequence

A 0.00 0.00 FUD XXX

Pathology and Laboratory

81407 — 81407

81408 Molecular pathology procedure, Level 9 (eg, analysis of >50 exons in a single gene by DNA sequence analysis)

INCLUDES *ABCA4 (ATP-binding cassette, sub-family A [ABC1], member 4)* (eg, Stargardt disease, age-related macular degeneration), full gene sequence
ATM (ataxia telangiectasia mutated) (eg, ataxia telangiectasia), full gene sequence
CDH23 (cadherin-related 23) (eg, Usher syndrome, type 1), full gene sequence
CEP290 (centrosomal protein 290kDa) (eg, Joubert syndrome), full gene sequence
COL1A1 (collagen, type I, alpha 1) (eg, osteogenesis imperfecta, type I), full gene sequence
COL1A2 (collagen, type I, alpha 2) (eg, osteogenesis imperfecta, type I), full gene sequence
COL4A1 (collagen, type IV, alpha 1) (eg, brain small-vessel disease with hemorrhage), full gene sequence
COL4A3 (collagen, type IV, alpha 3 [Goodpasture antigen]) (eg, Alport syndrome), full gene sequence
COL4A5 (collagen, type IV, alpha 5) (eg, Alport syndrome), full gene sequence
DMD (dystrophin) (eg, Duchenne/Becker muscular dystrophy), full gene sequence
DYSF (dysferlin, limb girdle muscular dystrophy 2B [autosomal recessive]) (eg, limb-girdle muscular dystrophy), full gene sequence
FBN1 (fibrillin 1) (eg, Marfan syndrome), full gene sequence
ITPR1 (inositol 1,4,5-trisphosphate receptor, type 1) (eg, spinocerebellar ataxia), full gene sequence
LAMA2 (laminin, alpha 2) (eg, congenital muscular dystrophy), full gene sequence
LRRK2 (leucine-rich repeat kinase 2) (eg, Parkinson disease), full gene sequence
MYH11 (myosin, heavy chain 11, smooth muscle) (eg, thoracic aortic aneurysms and aortic dissections), full gene sequence
NEB (nebulin) (eg, nemaline myopathy 2), full gene sequence
NF1 (neurofibromin 1) (eg, neurofibromatosis, type 1), full gene sequence
PKHD1 (polycystic kidney and hepatic disease 1) (eg, autosomal recessive polycystic kidney disease), full gene sequence
RYR1 (ryanodine receptor 1, skeletal) (eg, malignant hyperthermia), full gene sequence
RYR2 (ryanodine receptor 2 [cardiac]) (eg, catecholaminergic polymorphic ventricular tachycardia, arrhythmogenic right ventricular dysplasia), full gene sequence or targeted sequence analysis of > 50 exons
USH2A (Usher syndrome 2A [autosomal recessive, mild]) (eg, Usher syndrome, type 2), full gene sequence
VPS13B (vacuolar protein sorting 13 homolog B [yeast]) (eg, Cohen syndrome), full gene sequence
VWF (von Willebrand factor) (eg, von Willebrand disease types 1 and 3), full gene sequence

A 0.00 0.00 FUD XXX

\# **81479 Unlisted molecular pathology procedure**

A 0.00 0.00 FUD XXX

81410-81479 Genomic Sequencing

● **81410 Aortic dysfunction or dilation (eg, Marfan syndrome, Loeys Dietz syndrome, Ehler Danlos syndrome type IV, arterial tortuosity syndrome); genomic sequence analysis panel, must include sequencing of at least 9 genes, including FBN1, TGFBR1, TGFBR2, COL3A1, MYH11, ACTA2, SLC2A10, SMAD3, and MYLK**

● **81411 duplication/deletion analysis panel, must include analyses for TGFBR1, TGFBR2, MYH11, and COL3A1**

● **81415 Exome (eg, unexplained constitutional or heritable disorder or syndrome); sequence analysis**

\+ ● **81416 sequence analysis, each comparator exome (eg, parents, siblings) (List separately in addition to code for primary procedure)**

Code first (81415)

● **81417 re-evaluation of previously obtained exome sequence (eg, updated knowledge or unrelated condition/syndrome)**

Do not report for results that are incidental

● **81420 Fetal chromosomal aneuploidy (eg, trisomy 21, monosomy X) genomic sequence analysis panel, circulating cell-free fetal DNA in maternal blood, must include analysis of chromosomes 13, 18, and 21** M

● **81425 Genome (eg, unexplained constitutional or heritable disorder or syndrome); sequence analysis**

\+ ● **81426 sequence analysis, each comparator genome (eg, parents, siblings) (List separately in addition to code for primary procedure)**

Code first (81425)

● **81427 re-evaluation of previously obtained genome sequence (eg, updated knowledge or unrelated condition/syndrome)**

Do not report for results that are incidental

● **81430 Hearing loss (eg, nonsyndromic hearing loss, Usher syndrome, Pendred syndrome); genomic sequence analysis panel, must include sequencing of at least 60 genes, including CDH23, CLRN1, GJB2, GPR98, MTRNR1, MYO7A, MYO15A, PCDH15, OTOF, SLC26A4, TMC1, TMPRSS3, USH1C, USH1G, USH2A, and WFS1**

● **81431 duplication/deletion analysis panel, must include copy number analyses for STRC and DFNB1 deletions in GJB2 and GJB6 genes**

● **81435 Hereditary colon cancer syndromes (eg, Lynch syndrome, familial adenomatosis polyposis); genomic sequence analysis panel, must include analysis of at least 7 genes, including APC, CHEK2, MLH1, MSH2, MSH6, MUTYH, and PMS2**

● **81436 duplication/deletion gene analysis panel, must include analysis of at least 8 genes, including APC, MLH1, MSH2, MSH6, PMS2, EPCAM, CHEK2, and MUTYH**

● **81440 Nuclear encoded mitochondrial genes (eg, neurologic or myopathic phenotypes), genomic sequence panel, must include analysis of at least 100 genes, including BCS1L, C10orf2, COQ2, COX10, DGUOK, MPV17, OPA1, PDSS2, POLG, POLG2, RRM2B, SCO1, SCO2, SLC25A4, SUCLA2, SUCLG1, TAZ, TK2, and TYMP**

● 81445 **Targeted genomic sequence analysis panel, solid organ neoplasm, DNA analysis, 5-50 genes (eg, ALK, BRAF, CDKN2A, EGFR, ERBB2, KIT, KRAS, NRAS, MET, PDGFRA, PDGFRB, PGR, PIK3CA, PTEN, RET), interrogation for sequence variants and copy number variants or rearrangements, if performed**

● 81450 **Targeted genomic sequence analysis panel, hematolymphoid neoplasm or disorder, DNA and RNA analysis when performed, 5-50 genes (eg, BRAF, CEBPA, DNMT3A, EZH2, FLT3, IDH1, IDH2, JAK2, KRAS, KIT, MLL, NRAS, NPM1, NOTCH1), interrogation for sequence variants, and copy number variants or rearrangements, or isoform expression or mRNA expression levels, if performed**

● 81455 **Targeted genomic sequence analysis panel, solid organ or hematolymphoid neoplasm, DNA and RNA analysis when performed, 51 or greater genes (eg, ALK, BRAF, CDKN2A, CEBPA, DNMT3A, EGFR, ERBB2, EZH2, FLT3, IDH1, IDH2, JAK2, KIT, KRAS, MLL, NPM1, NRAS, MET, NOTCH1, PDGFRA, PDGFRB, PGR, PIK3CA, PTEN, RET), interrogation for sequence variants and copy number variants or rearrangements, if performed**

● 81460 **Whole mitochondrial genome (eg, Leigh syndrome, mitochondrial encephalomyopathy, lactic acidosis, and stroke-like episodes [MELAS], myoclonic epilepsy with ragged-red fibers [MERFF], neuropathy, ataxia, and retinitis pigmentosa [NARP], Leber hereditary optic neuropathy [LHON]), genomic sequence, must include sequence analysis of entire mitochondrial genome with heteroplasmy detection**

● 81465 **Whole mitochondrial genome large deletion analysis panel (eg, Kearns-Sayre syndrome, chronic progressive external ophthalmoplegia), including heteroplasmy detection, if performed**

● 81470 **X-linked intellectual disability (XLID) (eg, syndromic and non-syndromic XLID); genomic sequence analysis panel, must include sequencing of at least 60 genes, including ARX, ATRX, CDKL5, FGD1, FMR1, HUWE1, IL1RAPL, KDM5C, L1CAM, MECP2, MED12, MID1, OCRL, RPS6KA3, and SLC16A2**

● 81471 **duplication/deletion gene analysis, must include analysis of at least 60 genes, including ARX, ATRX, CDKL5, FGD1, FMR1, HUWE1, IL1RAPL, KDM5C, L1CAM, MECP2, MED12, MID1, OCRL, RPS6KA3, and SLC16A2**

81479 Resequenced code. See code following 81408.

81500-81599 Multianalyte Assays

INCLUDES Procedures using results of multiple assay panels (eg, molecular pathology, fluorescent in situ hybridization, non-nucleic acid-based) and other patient information to perform algorithmic analysis

Required analytical services (eg, amplification, cell lysis, detection, digestion, extraction, hybridization, nucleic acid stabilization) and algorithmic analysis

EXCLUDES *Genomic resequencing tests (81410-81471)*

Multianalyte assays with algorithmic analyses without a Category 1 code

Multianalyte assays with algorithmic analyses without a Category 1 or alphanumeric code (81599)

Code also procedures performed prior to cell lysis (eg, microdissection) (88380-88381)

81500 **Oncology (ovarian), biochemical assays of two proteins (CA-125 and HE4), utilizing serum, with menopausal status, algorithm reported as a risk score** ♀

Do not report with (86304-86305)

E 0.00 0.00 FUD XXX

81503 **Oncology (ovarian), biochemical assays of five proteins (CA-125, apolipoprotein A1, beta-2 microglobulin, transferrin, and pre-albumin), utilizing serum, algorithm reported as a risk score** ♀

Do not report with (82172, 82232, 83695, 83700, 84134, 84466, 86304)

E 0.00 0.00 FUD XXX

81504 **Oncology (tissue of origin), microarray gene expression profiling of > 2000 genes, utilizing formalin-fixed paraffin-embedded tissue, algorithm reported as tissue similarity scores**

A 0.00 0.00 FUD XXX

81506 **Endocrinology (type 2 diabetes), biochemical assays of seven analytes (glucose, HbA1c, insulin, hs-CRP, adiponectin, ferritin, interleukin 2-receptor alpha), utilizing serum or plasma, algorithm reporting a risk score**

Do not report with (82728, 82947, 83036, 83520, 83525, 84999, 86141)

E 0.00 0.00 FUD XXX

81507 **Fetal aneuploidy (trisomy 21, 18, and 13) DNA sequence analysis of selected regions using maternal plasma, algorithm reported as a risk score for each trisomy** ♀

A 0.00 0.00 FUD XXX

81508 **Fetal congenital abnormalities, biochemical assays of two proteins (PAPP-A, hCG [any form]), utilizing maternal serum, algorithm reported as a risk score** ♀

Do not report with (84163, 84702)

E 0.00 0.00 FUD XXX

81509 **Fetal congenital abnormalities, biochemical assays of three proteins (PAPP-A, hCG [any form], DIA), utilizing maternal serum, algorithm reported as a risk score** ♀

Do not report with (84163, 84702, 86336)

E 0.00 0.00 FUD XXX

81510 **Fetal congenital abnormalities, biochemical assays of three analytes (AFP, uE3, hCG [any form]), utilizing maternal serum, algorithm reported as a risk score** ♀

Do not report with (82105, 82677, 84702)

E 0.00 0.00 FUD XXX

81511 **Fetal congenital abnormalities, biochemical assays of four analytes (AFP, uE3, hCG [any form], DIA) utilizing maternal serum, algorithm reported as a risk score (may include additional results from previous biochemical testing)** ♀

Do not report with (82105, 82677, 84702, 86336)

E 0.00 0.00 FUD XXX

81512 **Fetal congenital abnormalities, biochemical assays of five analytes (AFP, uE3, total hCG, hyperglycosylated hCG, DIA) utilizing maternal serum, algorithm reported as a risk score** ♀

Do not report with (82105, 82677, 84702, 86336)

E 0.00 0.00 FUD XXX

● 81519 **Oncology (breast), mRNA, gene expression profiling by real-time RT-PCR of 21 genes, utilizing formalin-fixed paraffin embedded tissue, algorithm reported as recurrence score**

81599 **Unlisted multianalyte assay with algorithmic analysis**

Do not report with (0001M-0008M)

E 0.00 0.00 FUD XXX

82000-82030 Chemistry: Acetaldehyde—Adenosine

CMS 100-2,15,80 Diagnostic Test Requirements

INCLUDES Clinical information not requested by the ordering physician
Mathematically calculated results
Quantitative analysis unless otherwise specified
Specimens from any source unless otherwise specified

EXCLUDES *Calculated results that represent a score or probability that was derived by algorithm*
Drug testing ([80300, 80301, 80302, 80303, 80304], [80324, 80325, 80326, 80327, 80328, 80329, 80330, 80331, 80332, 80333, 80334, 80335, 80336, 80337, 80338, 80339, 80340, 80341, 80342, 80343, 80344, 80345, 80346, 80347, 80348, 80349, 80350, 80351, 80352, 80353, 80354, 80355, 80356, 80357, 80358, 80359, 80360, 80361, 80362, 80363, 80364, 80365, 80366, 80367, 80368, 80369, 80370, 80371, 80372, 80373, 80374, 80375, 80376, 80377, 83992])
Organ or disease panels (80048-80076)
Therapeutic drug assays (80150-80299)

Do not report analytes from nonrequested laboratory analysis

~~**82000** **Acetaldehyde, blood**~~

~~**82003** **Acetaminophen**~~
To report, see 80329-80331

82009 **Ketone body(s) (eg, acetone, acetoacetic acid, beta-hydroxybutyrate); qualitative**
N RVU 0.00 Facility RVU 0.00 FUD XXX

82010 **quantitative**
N CLIA RVU 0.00 Facility RVU 0.00 FUD XXX

82013 **Acetylcholinesterase**
EXCLUDES *Acid phosphatase (84060-84066)*
Gastric acid analysis (82930)
N RVU 0.00 Facility RVU 0.00 FUD XXX

82016 **Acylcarnitines; qualitative, each specimen**
N RVU 0.00 Facility RVU 0.00 FUD XXX

82017 **quantitative, each specimen**
EXCLUDES *Carnitine (82379)*
N [icon] RVU 0.00 Facility RVU 0.00 FUD XXX

82024 **Adrenocorticotropic hormone (ACTH)**
N [icon] RVU 0.00 Facility RVU 0.00 FUD XXX

82030 **Adenosine, 5-monophosphate, cyclic (cyclic AMP)**
N RVU 0.00 Facility RVU 0.00 FUD XXX

82040-82045 Chemistry: Albumin

CMS 100-2,15,80 Diagnostic Test Requirements
CMS 100-3,190.10 Laboratory Tests--CRD Patients

INCLUDES Clinical information not requested by the ordering physician
Mathematically calculated results
Quantitative analysis unless otherwise specified
Specimens from any other sources unless otherwise specified

EXCLUDES *Calculated results that represent a score or probability that was derived by algorithm*
Drug testing ([80300, 80301, 80302, 80303, 80304], [80324, 80325, 80326, 80327, 80328, 80329, 80330, 80331, 80332, 80333, 80334, 80335, 80336, 80337, 80338, 80339, 80340, 80341, 80342, 80343, 80344, 80345, 80346, 80347, 80348, 80349, 80350, 80351, 80352, 80353, 80354, 80355, 80356, 80357, 80358, 80359, 80360, 80361, 80362, 80363, 80364, 80365, 80366, 80367, 80368, 80369, 80370, 80371, 80372, 80373, 80374, 80375, 80376, 80377, 83992])
Organ or disease panels (80048-80076)
Therapeutic drug assays (80150-80299)

Do not report analytes from nonrequested laboratory analysis

82040 **Albumin; serum, plasma or whole blood**
N CLIA RVU 0.00 Facility RVU 0.00 FUD XXX

82042 **urine or other source, quantitative, each specimen**
N RVU 0.00 Facility RVU 0.00 FUD XXX

82043 **urine, microalbumin, quantitative**
N [icon] CLIA RVU 0.00 Facility RVU 0.00 FUD XXX

82044 **urine, microalbumin, semiquantitative (eg, reagent strip assay)**
EXCLUDES *Prealbumin (84134)*
N CLIA RVU 0.00 Facility RVU 0.00 FUD XXX

82045 **ischemia modified**
N RVU 0.00 Facility RVU 0.00 FUD XXX

82055-82107 Chemistry: Alcohol—Alpha-fetoprotein (AFP)

CMS 100-2,15,80 Diagnostic Test Requirements

INCLUDES Clinical information not requested by the ordering physician
Mathematically calculated results
Quantitative analysis unless otherwise specified
Specimens from any source unless otherwise specified

EXCLUDES *Calculated results that represent a score or probability that was derived by algorithm*
Drug testing ([80300, 80301, 80302, 80303, 80304], [80324, 80325, 80326, 80327, 80328, 80329, 80330, 80331, 80332, 80333, 80334, 80335, 80336, 80337, 80338, 80339, 80340, 80341, 80342, 80343, 80344, 80345, 80346, 80347, 80348, 80349, 80350, 80351, 80352, 80353, 80354, 80355, 80356, 80357, 80358, 80359, 80360, 80361, 80362, 80363, 80364, 80365, 80366, 80367, 80368, 80369, 80370, 80371, 80372, 80373, 80374, 80375, 80376, 80377, 83992])
Organ or disease panels (80048-80076)
Therapeutic drug assays (80150-80299)

Do not report analytes from nonrequested laboratory analysis

~~**82055** **Alcohol (ethanol); any specimen except breath**~~
To report, see 80320-80322

82075 **Alcohol (ethanol), breath**
N RVU 0.00 Facility RVU 0.00 FUD XXX

82085 **Aldolase**
N RVU 0.00 Facility RVU 0.00 FUD XXX

82088 **Aldosterone**
N [icon] RVU 0.00 Facility RVU 0.00 FUD XXX

~~**82101** **Alkaloids, urine, quantitative**~~
To report, see 80323

82103 **Alpha-1-antitrypsin; total**
N RVU 0.00 Facility RVU 0.00 FUD XXX

82104 **phenotype**
N RVU 0.00 Facility RVU 0.00 FUD XXX

82105 **Alpha-fetoprotein (AFP); serum**
N [icon] RVU 0.00 Facility RVU 0.00 FUD XXX

82106 **amniotic fluid** M ♀
N [icon] RVU 0.00 Facility RVU 0.00 FUD XXX

82107 **AFP-L3 fraction isoform and total AFP (including ratio)**
N RVU 0.00 Facility RVU 0.00 FUD XXX

82108 Chemistry: Aluminum

CMS 100-2,15,80 Diagnostic Test Requirements
CMS 100-3,190.10 Laboratory Tests--CRD Patients

INCLUDES Clinical information not requested by the ordering physician
Mathematically calculated results
Quantitative analysis unless otherwise specified
Specimens from any source unless otherwise specified

EXCLUDES *Calculated results that represent a score or probability that was derived by algorithm*
Drug testing ([80300, 80301, 80302, 80303, 80304], [80324, 80325, 80326, 80327, 80328, 80329, 80330, 80331, 80332, 80333, 80334, 80335, 80336, 80337, 80338, 80339, 80340, 80341, 80342, 80343, 80344, 80345, 80346, 80347, 80348, 80349, 80350, 80351, 80352, 80353, 80354, 80355, 80356, 80357, 80358, 80359, 80360, 80361, 80362, 80363, 80364, 80365, 80366, 80367, 80368, 80369, 80370, 80371, 80372, 80373, 80374, 80375, 80376, 80377, 83992])
Organ or disease panels (80048-80076)
Therapeutic drug assays (80150-80299)

Do not report analytes from nonrequested laboratory analysis

82108 **Aluminum**
N RVU 0.00 Facility RVU 0.00 FUD XXX

82120-82261 Chemistry: Amines—Biotinidase

CMS 100-2,15,80 Diagnostic Test Requirements

INCLUDES Clinical information not requested by the ordering physician
Mathematically calculated results
Quantitative analysis unless otherwise specified
Specimens from any source unless otherwise specified

EXCLUDES *Calculated results that represent a score or probability that was derived by algorithm*
Drug testing ([80300, 80301, 80302, 80303, 80304], [80324, 80325, 80326, 80327, 80328, 80329, 80330, 80331, 80332, 80333, 80334, 80335, 80336, 80337, 80338, 80339, 80340, 80341, 80342, 80343, 80344, 80345, 80346, 80347, 80348, 80349, 80350, 80351, 80352, 80353, 80354, 80355, 80356, 80357, 80358, 80359, 80360, 80361, 80362, 80363, 80364, 80365, 80366, 80367, 80368, 80369, 80370, 80371, 80372, 80373, 80374, 80375, 80376, 80377, 83992])
Organ or disease panels (80048-80076)
Therapeutic drug assays (80150-80299)

Do not report analytes from nonrequested laboratory analysis

82120 **Amines, vaginal fluid, qualitative** ♀
EXCLUDES *Combined pH and amines test for vaginitis (82120, 83986)*
N ☒ 0.00 0.00 FUD XXX

82127 **Amino acids; single, qualitative, each specimen**
N 0.00 0.00 FUD XXX

82128 **multiple, qualitative, each specimen**
N 0.00 0.00 FUD XXX

82131 **single, quantitative, each specimen**
INCLUDES Van Slyke method
N 0.00 0.00 FUD XXX

82135 **Aminolevulinic acid, delta (ALA)**
N 0.00 0.00 FUD XXX

82136 **Amino acids, 2 to 5 amino acids, quantitative, each specimen**
N 0.00 0.00 FUD XXX

82139 **Amino acids, 6 or more amino acids, quantitative, each specimen**
N 0.00 0.00 FUD XXX

82140 **Ammonia**
N 0.00 0.00 FUD XXX

82143 **Amniotic fluid scan (spectrophotometric)** M ♀
EXCLUDES *L/S ratio (83661)*
N 0.00 0.00 FUD XXX

~~**82145** **Amphetamine or methamphetamine**~~
To report, see 80324-80326

82150 **Amylase**
N ☒ 0.00 0.00 FUD XXX

82154 **Androstanediol glucuronide**
N 0.00 0.00 FUD XXX

82157 **Androstenedione**
N 0.00 0.00 FUD XXX

82160 **Androsterone**
N 0.00 0.00 FUD XXX

82163 **Angiotensin II**
N 0.00 0.00 FUD XXX

82164 **Angiotensin I - converting enzyme (ACE)**
N 0.00 0.00 FUD XXX

82172 **Apolipoprotein, each**
N 0.00 0.00 FUD XXX

82175 **Arsenic**
EXCLUDES *Heavy metal screening (83015)*
N 0.00 0.00 FUD XXX

82180 **Ascorbic acid (Vitamin C), blood**
N 0.00 0.00 FUD XXX

82190 **Atomic absorption spectroscopy, each analyte**
N 0.00 0.00 FUD XXX

~~**82205** **Barbiturates, not elsewhere specified**~~
To report, see 80345

82232 **Beta-2 microglobulin**
N 0.00 0.00 FUD XXX

82239 **Bile acids; total**
N 0.00 0.00 FUD XXX

82240 **cholylglycine**
EXCLUDES *Bile pigments, urine (81000-81005)*
N 0.00 0.00 FUD XXX

82247 **Bilirubin; total**
INCLUDES Van Den Bergh test
N ☒ 0.00 0.00 FUD XXX

82248 **direct**
N 0.00 0.00 FUD XXX

82252 **feces, qualitative**
N 0.00 0.00 FUD XXX

82261 **Biotinidase, each specimen**
N 0.00 0.00 FUD XXX

82270-82274 Chemistry: Occult Blood

CMS 100-2,15,80 Diagnostic Test Requirements
CMS 100-3,190.34 Fecal Occult Blood Test (FOBT)
CMS 100-4,18,60 Colorectal Cancer Screening
CMS 100-4,18,60.1 Payment for Colorectal Screening Services
CMS 100-4,18,60.2 Frequency and Age Requirements for Colorectal Screening
CMS 100-4,18,60.2.1 Common Working File Edits: Colorectal Screening
CMS 100-4,18,60.6 Billing for Colorectal Screening Services

INCLUDES Clinical information not requested by the ordering physician
Mathematically calculated results
Quantitative analysis unless otherwise specified
Specimens from any source unless otherwise specified

EXCLUDES *Calculated results that represent a score or probability that was derived by algorithm*
Drug testing ([80300, 80301, 80302, 80303, 80304], [80324, 80325, 80326, 80327, 80328, 80329, 80330, 80331, 80332, 80333, 80334, 80335, 80336, 80337, 80338, 80339, 80340, 80341, 80342, 80343, 80344, 80345, 80346, 80347, 80348, 80349, 80350, 80351, 80352, 80353, 80354, 80355, 80356, 80357, 80358, 80359, 80360, 80361, 80362, 80363, 80364, 80365, 80366, 80367, 80368, 80369, 80370, 80371, 80372, 80373, 80374, 80375, 80376, 80377, 83992])
Organ or disease panels (80048-80076)
Therapeutic drug assays (80150-80299)

Do not report analytes from nonrequested laboratory analysis

82270 **Blood, occult, by peroxidase activity (eg, guaiac), qualitative; feces, consecutive collected specimens with single determination, for colorectal neoplasm screening (ie, patient was provided 3 cards or single triple card for consecutive collection)**
INCLUDES Day test
N ☒ 0.00 0.00 FUD XXX

82271 **other sources**
N ☒ 0.00 0.00 FUD XXX

82272 **Blood, occult, by peroxidase activity (eg, guaiac), qualitative, feces, 1-3 simultaneous determinations, performed for other than colorectal neoplasm screening**
N ☒ 0.00 0.00 FUD XXX

82274 **Blood, occult, by fecal hemoglobin determination by immunoassay, qualitative, feces, 1-3 simultaneous determinations**
N ☒ 0.00 0.00 FUD XXX

82286-82308 [82652] Chemistry: Bradykinin—Calcitonin

CMS 100-2,15,80 Diagnostic Test Requirements

INCLUDES Clinical information not requested by the ordering physician
Mathematically calculated results
Quantitative analysis unless otherwise specified
Specimens from any source unless otherwise specified

EXCLUDES *Calculated results that represent a score or probability that was derived by algorithm*
Drug testing ([80300, 80301, 80302, 80303, 80304], [80324, 80325, 80326, 80327, 80328, 80329, 80330, 80331, 80332, 80333, 80334, 80335, 80336, 80337, 80338, 80339, 80340, 80341, 80342, 80343, 80344, 80345, 80346, 80347, 80348, 80349, 80350, 80351, 80352, 80353, 80354, 80355, 80356, 80357, 80358, 80359, 80360, 80361, 80362, 80363, 80364, 80365, 80366, 80367, 80368, 80369, 80370, 80371, 80372, 80373, 80374, 80375, 80376, 80377, 83992])
Organ or disease panels (80048-80076)
Therapeutic drug assays (80150-80299)

Do not report analytes from nonrequested laboratory analysis

82286 Bradykinin
N 0.00 0.00 FUD XXX

82300 Cadmium
N 0.00 0.00 FUD XXX

82306 Vitamin D; 25 hydroxy, includes fraction(s), if performed
N 0.00 0.00 FUD XXX

82652 1, 25 dihydroxy, includes fraction(s), if performed
N 0.00 0.00 FUD XXX

82308 Calcitonin
N 0.00 0.00 FUD XXX

82310-82373 Chemistry: Calcium, total; Carbohydrate Deficient Transferrin

CMS 100-2,15,80 Diagnostic Test Requirements

INCLUDES Clinical information not requested by the ordering physician
Mathematically calculated results
Quantitative analysis unless otherwise specified
Specimens from any source unless otherwise specified

EXCLUDES *Calculated results that represent a score or probability that was derived by algorithm*
Drug testing ([80300, 80301, 80302, 80303, 80304], [80324, 80325, 80326, 80327, 80328, 80329, 80330, 80331, 80332, 80333, 80334, 80335, 80336, 80337, 80338, 80339, 80340, 80341, 80342, 80343, 80344, 80345, 80346, 80347, 80348, 80349, 80350, 80351, 80352, 80353, 80354, 80355, 80356, 80357, 80358, 80359, 80360, 80361, 80362, 80363, 80364, 80365, 80366, 80367, 80368, 80369, 80370, 80371, 80372, 80373, 80374, 80375, 80376, 80377, 83992])
Organ or disease panels (80048-80076)
Therapeutic drug assays (80150-80299)

82310 Calcium; total
N 0.00 0.00 FUD XXX

82330 ionized
INCLUDES Calcium, ionized (82330)
N 0.00 0.00 FUD XXX

82331 after calcium infusion test
N 0.00 0.00 FUD XXX

82340 urine quantitative, timed specimen
N 0.00 0.00 FUD XXX

82355 Calculus; qualitative analysis
N 0.00 0.00 FUD XXX

82360 quantitative analysis, chemical
N 0.00 0.00 FUD XXX

82365 infrared spectroscopy
N 0.00 0.00 FUD XXX

82370 X-ray diffraction
N 0.00 0.00 FUD XXX

82373 Carbohydrate deficient transferrin
N 0.00 0.00 FUD XXX

82374 Chemistry: Carbon Dioxide

CMS 100-2,15,80 Diagnostic Test Requirements
CMS 100-3,190.10 Laboratory Tests--CRD Patients

INCLUDES Clinical information not requested by the ordering physician
Mathematically calculated results
Quantitative analysis unless otherwise specified
Specimens from any source unless otherwise specified

EXCLUDES *Calculated results that represent a score or probability that was derived by algorithm*
Drug testing ([80300, 80301, 80302, 80303, 80304], [80324, 80325, 80326, 80327, 80328, 80329, 80330, 80331, 80332, 80333, 80334, 80335, 80336, 80337, 80338, 80339, 80340, 80341, 80342, 80343, 80344, 80345, 80346, 80347, 80348, 80349, 80350, 80351, 80352, 80353, 80354, 80355, 80356, 80357, 80358, 80359, 80360, 80361, 80362, 80363, 80364, 80365, 80366, 80367, 80368, 80369, 80370, 80371, 80372, 80373, 80374, 80375, 80376, 80377, 83992])
Organ or disease panels (80048-80076)
Therapeutic drug assays (80150-80299)

Do not report analytes from nonrequested laboratory analysis

82374 Carbon dioxide (bicarbonate)
EXCLUDES *Blood gases (82803)*
N 0.00 0.00 FUD XXX

82375-82376 Chemistry: Carboxyhemoglobin (Carbon Monoxide)

CMS 100-2,15,80 Diagnostic Test Requirements

INCLUDES Clinical information not requested by the ordering physician
Mathematically calculated results
Specimens from any source unless otherwise specified

EXCLUDES *Calculated results that represent a score or probability that was derived by algorithm*
Drug testing ([80300, 80301, 80302, 80303, 80304], [80324, 80325, 80326, 80327, 80328, 80329, 80330, 80331, 80332, 80333, 80334, 80335, 80336, 80337, 80338, 80339, 80340, 80341, 80342, 80343, 80344, 80345, 80346, 80347, 80348, 80349, 80350, 80351, 80352, 80353, 80354, 80355, 80356, 80357, 80358, 80359, 80360, 80361, 80362, 80363, 80364, 80365, 80366, 80367, 80368, 80369, 80370, 80371, 80372, 80373, 80374, 80375, 80376, 80377, 83992])
Organ or disease panels (80048-80076)
Transcutaneous measurement of carboxyhemoglobin (88740)

Do not report analytes from nonrequested laboratory analysis

82375 Carboxyhemoglobin; quantitative
N 0.00 0.00 FUD XXX

82376 qualitative
N 0.00 0.00 FUD XXX

82378 Chemistry: Carcinoembryonic Antigen (CEA)

CMS 100-2,15,80 Diagnostic Test Requirements
CMS 100-3,190.26 Carcinoembryonic Antigen (CEA)

INCLUDES Clinical information not requested by the ordering physician

EXCLUDES *Calculated results that represent a score or probability that was derived by algorithm*

Do not report analytes from nonrequested laboratory analysis

82378 Carcinoembryonic antigen (CEA)
N 0.00 0.00 FUD XXX

82379-82415 Chemistry: Carnitine—Chloramphenicol

CMS 100-2,15,80 Diagnostic Test Requirements

INCLUDES Clinical information not requested by the ordering physician
Mathematically calculated results
Quantitative analysis unless otherwise specified
Specimens from any source unless otherwise specified

EXCLUDES *Calculated results that represent a score or probability that was derived by algorithm*
Drug testing ([80300, 80301, 80302, 80303, 80304], [80324, 80325, 80326, 80327, 80328, 80329, 80330, 80331, 80332, 80333, 80334, 80335, 80336, 80337, 80338, 80339, 80340, 80341, 80342, 80343, 80344, 80345, 80346, 80347, 80348, 80349, 80350, 80351, 80352, 80353, 80354, 80355, 80356, 80357, 80358, 80359, 80360, 80361, 80362, 80363, 80364, 80365, 80366, 80367, 80368, 80369, 80370, 80371, 80372, 80373, 80374, 80375, 80376, 80377, 83992])
Organ or disease panels (80048-80076)
Therapeutic drug assays (80150-80299)

Do not report analytes from nonrequested laboratory analysis

82379 **Carnitine (total and free), quantitative, each specimen**
EXCLUDES *Acylcarnitine (82016-82017)*
N 0.00 0.00 FUD XXX

82380 **Carotene**
N 0.00 0.00 FUD XXX

82382 **Catecholamines; total urine**
N 0.00 0.00 FUD XXX

82383 **blood**
N 0.00 0.00 FUD XXX

82384 **fractionated**
EXCLUDES *Urine metabolites (83835, 84585)*
N 0.00 0.00 FUD XXX

82387 **Cathepsin-D**
N 0.00 0.00 FUD XXX

82390 **Ceruloplasmin**
N 0.00 0.00 FUD XXX

82397 **Chemiluminescent assay**
N 0.00 0.00 FUD XXX

82415 **Chloramphenicol**
N 0.00 0.00 FUD XXX

82435-82438 Chemistry: Chloride

CMS 100-2,15,80 Diagnostic Test Requirements
CMS 100-3,190.10 Laboratory Tests--CRD Patients
INCLUDES Clinical information not requested by the ordering physician
Mathematically calculated results
Quantitative analysis unless otherwise specified
Specimens from any source unless otherwise specified
EXCLUDES *Calculated results that represent a score or probability that was derived by algorithm*
Organ or disease panels (80048-80076)
Therapeutic drug assays (80150-80299)
Do not report analytes from nonrequested laboratory analysis

82435 **Chloride; blood**
N 0.00 0.00 FUD XXX

82436 **urine**
N 0.00 0.00 FUD XXX

82438 **other source**
EXCLUDES *Sweat collections by iontophoresis (89230)*
N 0.00 0.00 FUD XXX

82441 Chemistry: Chlorinated Hydrocarbons

CMS 100-2,15,80 Diagnostic Test Requirements
INCLUDES Clinical information not requested by the ordering physician
Mathematically calculated results
Quantitative analysis unless otherwise specified
Specimens from any source unless otherwise specified
EXCLUDES *Calculated results that represent a score or probability that was derived by algorithm*
Do not report analytes from nonrequested laboratory analysis

82441 **Chlorinated hydrocarbons, screen**
N 0.00 0.00 FUD XXX

82465 Chemistry: Cholesterol, Total

CMS 100-2,15,80 Diagnostic Test Requirements
CMS 100-3,190.23 Lipid Testing
INCLUDES Clinical information not requested by the ordering physician
Mathematically calculated results
Quantitative analysis unless otherwise specified
EXCLUDES *Calculated results that represent a score or probability that was derived by algorithm*
Organ or disease panels (80048-80299 [80104])
Do not report analytes from nonrequested laboratory analysis

82465 **Cholesterol, serum or whole blood, total**
EXCLUDES *High density lipoprotein (HDL) (83718)*
N 0.00 0.00 FUD XXX

82480-82492 Chemistry: Cholinesterase—Chromatography

INCLUDES Clinical information not requested by the ordering physician
Mathematically calculated results
Quantitative analysis unless otherwise specified
Specimens from any source unless otherwise specified
EXCLUDES *Calculated results that represent a score or probability that was derived by algorithm*
Drug testing ([80300, 80301, 80302, 80303, 80304], [80324, 80325, 80326, 80327, 80328, 80329, 80330, 80331, 80332, 80333, 80334, 80335, 80336, 80337, 80338, 80339, 80340, 80341, 80342, 80343, 80344, 80345, 80346, 80347, 80348, 80349, 80350, 80351, 80352, 80353, 80354, 80355, 80356, 80357, 80358, 80359, 80360, 80361, 80362, 80363, 80364, 80365, 80366, 80367, 80368, 80369, 80370, 80371, 80372, 80373, 80374, 80375, 80376, 80377, 83992])
Organ or disease panels (80048-80076)
Therapeutic drug assays (80048-80299 [80104])
Do not report analytes from nonrequested laboratory analysis

82480 **Cholinesterase; serum**
N 0.00 0.00 FUD XXX

82482 **RBC**
N 0.00 0.00 FUD XXX

82485 **Chondroitin B sulfate, quantitative**
N 0.00 0.00 FUD XXX

82486 **Chromatography, qualitative; column (eg, gas liquid or HPLC), analyte not elsewhere specified**
N 0.00 0.00 FUD XXX

82487 **paper, 1-dimensional, analyte not elsewhere specified**
N 0.00 0.00 FUD XXX

82488 **paper, 2-dimensional, analyte not elsewhere specified**
N 0.00 0.00 FUD XXX

82489 **thin layer, analyte not elsewhere specified**
N 0.00 0.00 FUD XXX

82491 **Chromatography, quantitative, column (eg, gas liquid or HPLC); single analyte not elsewhere specified, single stationary and mobile phase**
N 0.00 0.00 FUD XXX

82492 **multiple analytes, single stationary and mobile phase**
N 0.00 0.00 FUD XXX

82495-82520 Chemistry: Chromium—Cocaine

CMS 100-2,15,80 Diagnostic Test Requirements
INCLUDES Clinical information not requested by the ordering physician
Mathematically calculated results
Quantitative analysis unless otherwise specified
Specimens from any source unless otherwise specified
EXCLUDES *Calculated results that represent a score or probability that was derived by algorithm*
Drug testing ([80300, 80301, 80302, 80303, 80304], [80324, 80325, 80326, 80327, 80328, 80329, 80330, 80331, 80332, 80333, 80334, 80335, 80336, 80337, 80338, 80339, 80340, 80341, 80342, 80343, 80344, 80345, 80346, 80347, 80348, 80349, 80350, 80351, 80352, 80353, 80354, 80355, 80356, 80357, 80358, 80359, 80360, 80361, 80362, 80363, 80364, 80365, 80366, 80367, 80368, 80369, 80370, 80371, 80372, 80373, 80374, 80375, 80376, 80377, 83992])
Organ or disease panels (80048-80076)
Therapeutic drug assays (80150-80299)
Do not report analytes from nonrequested laboratory analysis

82495 **Chromium**
N 0.00 0.00 FUD XXX

82507 **Citrate**
N 0.00 0.00 FUD XXX

~~82520~~ ~~**Cocaine or metabolite**~~
To report, see 80353

82523 Chemistry: Collagen Crosslinks, Any Method

CMS 100-2,15,80 Diagnostic Test Requirements

CMS 100-3,190.19 NCD for Collagen Crosslinks, Any Method

INCLUDES Clinical information not requested by the ordering physician
Mathematically calculated results
Quantitative analysis unless otherwise specified
Specimens from any source unless otherwise specified

EXCLUDES *Calculated results that represent a score or probability that was derived by algorithm*
Organ or disease panels (80048-80076)
Therapeutic drug assays (80150-80299)

Do not report analytes from nonrequested laboratory analysis

82523 **Collagen cross links, any method**
N CLIA 0.00 0.00 FUD XXX

82525-82946 Chemistry: Copper—Glucagon Tolerance Test

CMS 100-2,15,80 Diagnostic Test Requirements

INCLUDES Clinical information not requested by the ordering physician
Mathematically calculated results
Quantitative analysis unless otherwise specified
Specimens from any source unless otherwise specified

EXCLUDES *Calculated results that represent a score or probability that was derived by algorithm*
Drug testing ([80300, 80301, 80302, 80303, 80304], [80324, 80325, 80326, 80327, 80328, 80329, 80330, 80331, 80332, 80333, 80334, 80335, 80336, 80337, 80338, 80339, 80340, 80341, 80342, 80343, 80344, 80345, 80346, 80347, 80348, 80349, 80350, 80351, 80352, 80353, 80354, 80355, 80356, 80357, 80358, 80359, 80360, 80361, 80362, 80363, 80364, 80365, 80366, 80367, 80368, 80369, 80370, 80371, 80372, 80373, 80374, 80375, 80376, 80377, 83992])
Organ or disease panels (80048-80076)
Therapeutic drug assays (80150-80299)

Do not report analytes from nonrequested laboratory analysis

82525 **Copper**
N 0.00 0.00 FUD XXX

82528 **Corticosterone**
INCLUDES Porter-Silber test
N 0.00 0.00 FUD XXX

82530 **Cortisol; free**
N 0.00 0.00 FUD XXX

82533 **total**
N 0.00 0.00 FUD XXX

82540 **Creatine**
N 0.00 0.00 FUD XXX

▲ **82541** **Column chromatography/mass spectrometry (eg, GC/MS, or HPLC/MS), non-drug analyte not elsewhere specified; qualitative, single stationary and mobile phase**
N 0.00 0.00 FUD XXX

▲ **82542** **quantitative, single stationary and mobile phase**
N 0.00 0.00 FUD XXX

▲ **82543** **stable isotope dilution, single analyte, quantitative, single stationary and mobile phase**
N 0.00 0.00 FUD XXX

▲ **82544** **stable isotope dilution, multiple analytes, quantitative, single stationary and mobile phase**
N 0.00 0.00 FUD XXX

82550 **Creatine kinase (CK), (CPK); total**
N CLIA 0.00 0.00 FUD XXX

82552 **isoenzymes**
N 0.00 0.00 FUD XXX

82553 **MB fraction only**
N 0.00 0.00 FUD XXX

82554 **isoforms**
N 0.00 0.00 FUD XXX

82565 **Creatinine; blood**
N CLIA 0.00 0.00 FUD XXX

82570 **other source**
N CLIA 0.00 0.00 FUD XXX

82575 **clearance**
INCLUDES Holten test
N 0.00 0.00 FUD XXX

82585 **Cryofibrinogen**
N 0.00 0.00 FUD XXX

82595 **Cryoglobulin, qualitative or semi-quantitative (eg, cryocrit)**
EXCLUDES *Quantitative, cryoglobulin (82784-82785)*
N 0.00 0.00 FUD XXX

82600 **Cyanide**
N 0.00 0.00 FUD XXX

82607 **Cyanocobalamin (Vitamin B-12);**
N 0.00 0.00 FUD XXX

82608 **unsaturated binding capacity**
N 0.00 0.00 FUD XXX

82610 **Cystatin C**
N 0.00 0.00 FUD XXX

82615 **Cystine and homocystine, urine, qualitative**
N 0.00 0.00 FUD XXX

82626 **Dehydroepiandrosterone (DHEA)**
Do not report with ([80327, 80328])
N 0.00 0.00 FUD XXX

82627 **Dehydroepiandrosterone-sulfate (DHEA-S)**
N 0.00 0.00 FUD XXX

82633 **Desoxycorticosterone, 11-**
N 0.00 0.00 FUD XXX

82634 **Deoxycortisol, 11-**
N 0.00 0.00 FUD XXX

82638 **Dibucaine number**
N 0.00 0.00 FUD XXX

~~82646~~ ~~Dihydrocodeinone~~
To report, see 80361

~~82649~~ ~~Dihydromorphinone~~
To report, see 80361

~~82651~~ ~~Dihydrotestosterone (DHT)~~
To report, see 80327-80328

82652 ***Resequenced code, See code following 82306.***

~~82654~~ ~~Dimethadione~~
To report, see 80339-80341

82656 **Elastase, pancreatic (EL-1), fecal, qualitative or semi-quantitative**
N 0.00 0.00 FUD XXX

82657 **Enzyme activity in blood cells, cultured cells, or tissue, not elsewhere specified; nonradioactive substrate, each specimen**
N 0.00 0.00 FUD XXX

82658 **radioactive substrate, each specimen**
N 0.00 0.00 FUD XXX

82664 **Electrophoretic technique, not elsewhere specified**
N 0.00 0.00 FUD XXX

~~82666~~ ~~Epiandrosterone~~
To report, see 80327-80328

82668 **Erythropoietin**
N 0.00 0.00 FUD XXX

82670 **Estradiol**
N 0.00 0.00 FUD XXX

82671 **Estrogens; fractionated**
EXCLUDES *Estrogen receptor assay (84233)*
N 0.00 0.00 FUD XXX

82672 total
EXCLUDES *Estrogen receptor assay (84233)*
N 0.00 0.00 FUD XXX

82677 Estriol
N 0.00 0.00 FUD XXX

82679 Estrone
N 0.00 0.00 FUD XXX

~~82690 Ethchlorvynol~~
To report, see 80320

82693 Ethylene glycol
N 0.00 0.00 FUD XXX

82696 Etiocholanolone
EXCLUDES *Fractionation of ketosteroids (83593)*
N 0.00 0.00 FUD XXX

82705 Fat or lipids, feces; qualitative
N 0.00 0.00 FUD XXX

82710 quantitative
N 0.00 0.00 FUD XXX

82715 Fat differential, feces, quantitative
N 0.00 0.00 FUD XXX

82725 Fatty acids, nonesterified
N 0.00 0.00 FUD XXX

82726 Very long chain fatty acids
EXCLUDES *Long-chain (C20-22) omega-3 fatty acids in red blood cell (RBC) membranes (0111T)*
N 0.00 0.00 FUD XXX

82728 Ferritin
N 0.00 0.00 FUD XXX

82731 Fetal fibronectin, cervicovaginal secretions, semi-quantitative M ♀
N 0.00 0.00 FUD XXX

82735 Fluoride
N 0.00 0.00 FUD XXX

~~82742 Flurazepam~~
To report, see 80346-80347

82746 Folic acid; serum
N 0.00 0.00 FUD XXX

82747 RBC
N 0.00 0.00 FUD XXX

82757 Fructose, semen ♂
EXCLUDES *Fructosamine (82985)*
Fructose, TLC screen (84375)
N 0.00 0.00 FUD XXX

82759 Galactokinase, RBC
N 0.00 0.00 FUD XXX

82760 Galactose
N 0.00 0.00 FUD XXX

82775 Galactose-1-phosphate uridyl transferase; quantitative
N 0.00 0.00 FUD XXX

82776 screen
N 0.00 0.00 FUD XXX

82777 Galectin-3
N 0.00 0.00 FUD XXX

82784 Gammaglobulin (immunoglobulin); IgA, IgD, IgG, IgM, each
INCLUDES Farr test
N 0.00 0.00 FUD XXX

82785 IgE
INCLUDES Farr test
EXCLUDES *Allergen specific, IgE (86003, 86005)*
N 0.00 0.00 FUD XXX

82787 immunoglobulin subclasses (eg, IgG1, 2, 3, or 4), each
EXCLUDES *Gamma-glutamyltransferase (GGT) (82977)*
N 0.00 0.00 FUD XXX

82800 Gases, blood, pH only
N 0.00 0.00 FUD XXX

82803 Gases, blood, any combination of pH, pCO2, pO2, CO2, HCO3 (including calculated O2 saturation);
INCLUDES Two or more of the listed analytes
N 0.00 0.00 FUD XXX

82805 with O2 saturation, by direct measurement, except pulse oximetry
N 0.00 0.00 FUD XXX

82810 Gases, blood, O2 saturation only, by direct measurement, except pulse oximetry
EXCLUDES *Pulse oximetry (94760)*
N 0.00 0.00 FUD XXX

82820 Hemoglobin-oxygen affinity (pO2 for 50% hemoglobin saturation with oxygen)
N 0.00 0.00 FUD XXX

82930 Gastric acid analysis, includes pH if performed, each specimen
N 0.00 0.00 FUD XXX

82938 Gastrin after secretin stimulation
N 0.00 0.00 FUD XXX

82941 Gastrin
N 0.00 0.00 FUD XXX

82943 Glucagon
N 0.00 0.00 FUD XXX

82945 Glucose, body fluid, other than blood
N 0.00 0.00 FUD XXX

82946 Glucagon tolerance test
N 0.00 0.00 FUD XXX

82947-82962 Chemistry: Glucose Testing

CMS 100-2,15,80 Diagnostic Test Requirements
CMS 100-3,190.20 Blood Glucose Testing

INCLUDES Clinical information not requested by the ordering physician
Mathematically calculated results
Quantitative analysis unless otherwise specified
Specimens from any source unless otherwise specified

EXCLUDES *Calculated results that represent a score or probability that was derived by algorithm*
Organ or disease panels (80048-80076)
Therapeutic drug assays (80150-80299)

Code also glucose administration injection (96374)
Do not report analytes from nonrequested laboratory analysis

82947 Glucose; quantitative, blood (except reagent strip)
N 0.00 0.00 FUD XXX

82948 blood, reagent strip
N 0.00 0.00 FUD XXX

82950 post glucose dose (includes glucose)
N 0.00 0.00 FUD XXX

82951 tolerance test (GTT), 3 specimens (includes glucose)
N 0.00 0.00 FUD XXX

+ 82952 tolerance test, each additional beyond 3 specimens (List separately in addition to code for primary procedure)
Code first (82951)
N 0.00 0.00 FUD XXX

~~82953 tolbutamide tolerance test~~

82955 Glucose-6-phosphate dehydrogenase (G6PD); quantitative
N 0.00 0.00 FUD XXX

82960 screen
N 0.00 0.00 FUD XXX

82962 Glucose, blood by glucose monitoring device(s) cleared by the FDA specifically for home use
N 0.00 0.00 FUD XXX

82963-83690 Chemistry: Glucosidase—Lipase

CMS 100-2,15,80 Diagnostic Test Requirements

INCLUDES Clinical information not requested by the ordering physician
Mathematically calculated results
Quantitative analysis unless otherwise specified
Specimens from any source unless otherwise specified

EXCLUDES *Calculated results that represent a score or probability that was derived by algorithm*
Drug testing ([80300, 80301, 80302, 80303, 80304], [80324, 80325, 80326, 80327, 80328, 80329, 80330, 80331, 80332, 80333, 80334, 80335, 80336, 80337, 80338, 80339, 80340, 80341, 80342, 80343, 80344, 80345, 80346, 80347, 80348, 80349, 80350, 80351, 80352, 80353, 80354, 80355, 80356, 80357, 80358, 80359, 80360, 80361, 80362, 80363, 80364, 80365, 80366, 80367, 80368, 80369, 80370, 80371, 80372, 80373, 80374, 80375, 80376, 80377, 83992])
Organ or disease panels (80048-80076)
Therapeutic drug assays (80150-80299)

Do not report analytes from nonrequested laboratory analysis

82963 Glucosidase, beta
N 0.00 0.00 FUD XXX

82965 Glutamate dehydrogenase
N 0.00 0.00 FUD XXX

~~82975 Glutamine (glutamic acid amide)~~
To report, see 82127-82128, 82131

82977 Glutamyltransferase, gamma (GGT)
N ☒ 0.00 0.00 FUD XXX

82978 Glutathione
N 0.00 0.00 FUD XXX

82979 Glutathione reductase, RBC
N 0.00 0.00 FUD XXX

~~82980 Glutethimide~~

82985 Glycated protein
EXCLUDES *Gonadotropin chorionic (hCG) (84702-84703)*
N ☒ 0.00 0.00 FUD XXX

83001 Gonadotropin; follicle stimulating hormone (FSH)
N ☒ 0.00 0.00 FUD XXX

83002 luteinizing hormone (LH)
EXCLUDES *Luteinizing releasing factor (LRH) (83727)*
N ☒ 0.00 0.00 FUD XXX

83003 Growth hormone, human (HGH) (somatotropin)
EXCLUDES *Antibody to human growth hormone (86277)*
N 0.00 0.00 FUD XXX

● **83006 Growth stimulation expressed gene 2 (ST2, Interleukin 1 receptor like-1)**

~~83008 Guanosine monophosphate (GMP), cyclic~~

83009 Helicobacter pylori, blood test analysis for urease activity, non-radioactive isotope (eg, C-13)
EXCLUDES *H. pylori, breath test analysis for urease activity (83013-83014)*
N 0.00 0.00 FUD XXX

83010 Haptoglobin; quantitative
N 0.00 0.00 FUD XXX

83012 phenotypes
N 0.00 0.00 FUD XXX

83013 Helicobacter pylori; breath test analysis for urease activity, non-radioactive isotope (eg, C-13)
N 0.00 0.00 FUD XXX

83014 drug administration
EXCLUDES *H. pylori:*
Blood test analysis for urease activity (83009)
Enzyme immunoassay (87339)
Liquid scintillation counter (78267-78268)
Stool (87338)
N 0.00 0.00 FUD XXX

83015 Heavy metal (eg, arsenic, barium, beryllium, bismuth, antimony, mercury); screen
INCLUDES Reinsch test
N 0.00 0.00 FUD XXX

83018 quantitative, each
N 0.00 0.00 FUD XXX

83020 Hemoglobin fractionation and quantitation; electrophoresis (eg, A2, S, C, and/or F)
N 0.00 0.00 FUD XXX

83021 chromatography (eg, A2, S, C, and/or F)
EXCLUDES *Analysis of glycosylated (A1c) hemoglobin by chromatography or electrophoresis without an identified hemoglobin variant (83036)*
N 0.00 0.00 FUD XXX

83026 Hemoglobin; by copper sulfate method, non-automated
N ☒ 0.00 0.00 FUD XXX

83030 F (fetal), chemical
N 0.00 0.00 FUD XXX

83033 F (fetal), qualitative
N 0.00 0.00 FUD XXX

83036 glycosylated (A1C)
EXCLUDES *Analysis of glycosylated (A1c) hemoglobin by chromatography or electrophoresis without an identified hemoglobin variant (83021)*
Detection of hemoglobin, fecal, by immunoassay (82274)
N ☒ 0.00 0.00 FUD XXX

83037 glycosylated (A1C) by device cleared by FDA for home use
N ☒ 0.00 0.00 FUD XXX

83045 methemoglobin, qualitative
N 0.00 0.00 FUD XXX

83050 methemoglobin, quantitative
EXCLUDES *Transcutaneous methemoglobin test (88741)*
N 0.00 0.00 FUD XXX

83051 plasma
N 0.00 0.00 FUD XXX

~~83055 sulfhemoglobin, qualitative~~

83060 sulfhemoglobin, quantitative
N 0.00 0.00 FUD XXX

83065 thermolabile
N 0.00 0.00 FUD XXX

83068 unstable, screen
N 0.00 0.00 FUD XXX

83069 urine
N 0.00 0.00 FUD XXX

83070 Hemosiderin, qualitative
N 0.00 0.00 FUD XXX

~~83071 quantitative~~

83080 b-Hexosaminidase, each assay
N 0.00 0.00 FUD XXX

83088 Histamine
N 0.00 0.00 FUD XXX

83090 Homocysteine
N 0.00 0.00 FUD XXX

83150 Homovanillic acid (HVA)
N 0.00 0.00 FUD XXX

83491 Hydroxycorticosteroids, 17- (17-OHCS)
EXCLUDES *Cortisol (82530, 82533)*
Deoxycortisol (82634)
N 0.00 0.00 FUD XXX

83497 Hydroxyindolacetic acid, 5-(HIAA)
EXCLUDES *Urine qualitative test (81005)*
N 0.00 0.00 FUD XXX

83498 Hydroxyprogesterone, 17-d
N 0.00 0.00 FUD XXX

83499 **Hydroxyprogesterone, 20-**
N 0.00 0.00 FUD XXX

83500 **Hydroxyproline; free**
N 0.00 0.00 FUD XXX

83505 **total**
N 0.00 0.00 FUD XXX

83516 **Immunoassay for analyte other than infectious agent antibody or infectious agent antigen; qualitative or semiquantitative, multiple step method**
N 0.00 0.00 FUD XXX

83518 **qualitative or semiquantitative, single step method (eg, reagent strip)**
N 0.00 0.00 FUD XXX

83519 **quantitative, by radioimmunoassay (eg, RIA)**
N 0.00 0.00 FUD XXX

83520 **quantitative, not otherwise specified**
N 0.00 0.00 FUD XXX

83525 **Insulin; total**
EXCLUDES *Proinsulin (84206)*
N 0.00 0.00 FUD XXX

83527 **free**
N 0.00 0.00 FUD XXX

83528 **Intrinsic factor**
EXCLUDES *Intrinsic factor antibodies (86340)*
N 0.00 0.00 FUD XXX

83540 **Iron**
N 0.00 0.00 FUD XXX

83550 **Iron binding capacity**
N 0.00 0.00 FUD XXX

83570 **Isocitric dehydrogenase (IDH)**
N 0.00 0.00 FUD XXX

83582 **Ketogenic steroids, fractionation**
N 0.00 0.00 FUD XXX

83586 **Ketosteroids, 17- (17-KS); total**
N 0.00 0.00 FUD XXX

83593 **fractionation**
N 0.00 0.00 FUD XXX

83605 **Lactate (lactic acid)**
N 0.00 0.00 FUD XXX

83615 **Lactate dehydrogenase (LD), (LDH);**
N 0.00 0.00 FUD XXX

83625 **isoenzymes, separation and quantitation**
N 0.00 0.00 FUD XXX

83630 **Lactoferrin, fecal; qualitative**
N 0.00 0.00 FUD XXX

83631 **quantitative**
N 0.00 0.00 FUD XXX

83632 **Lactogen, human placental (HPL) human chorionic somatomammotropin** M ♀
N 0.00 0.00 FUD XXX

83633 **Lactose, urine, qualitative**
N 0.00 0.00 FUD XXX

~~83634 quantitative~~

83655 **Lead**
N 0.00 0.00 FUD XXX

83661 **Fetal lung maturity assessment; lecithin sphingomyelin (L/S) ratio** M ♀
N 0.00 0.00 FUD XXX

83662 **foam stability test** M ♀
N 0.00 0.00 FUD XXX

83663 **fluorescence polarization** M ♀
N 0.00 0.00 FUD XXX

83664 **lamellar body density** M ♀
EXCLUDES *Phosphatidylglycerol (84081)*
N 0.00 0.00 FUD XXX

83670 **Leucine aminopeptidase (LAP)**
N 0.00 0.00 FUD XXX

83690 **Lipase**
N 0.00 0.00 FUD XXX

83695-83727 Chemistry: Lipoprotein—Luteinizing Releasing Factor

CMS 100-2,15,80 Diagnostic Test Requirements
CMS 100-3,190.23 Lipid Testing

INCLUDES Clinical information not requested by the ordering physician
Mathematically calculated results
Quantitative analysis unless otherwise specified
Specimens from any source unless otherwise specified

EXCLUDES *Calculated results that represent a score or probability that was derived by algorithm*
Organ or disease panels (80048-80076)
Therapeutic drug assays (80150-80299)

Do not report analytes from nonrequested laboratory analysis

83695 **Lipoprotein (a)**
N 0.00 0.00 FUD XXX

83698 **Lipoprotein-associated phospholipase A2 (Lp-PLA2)**
N 0.00 0.00 FUD XXX

83700 **Lipoprotein, blood; electrophoretic separation and quantitation**
N 0.00 0.00 FUD XXX

83701 **high resolution fractionation and quantitation of lipoproteins including lipoprotein subclasses when performed (eg, electrophoresis, ultracentrifugation)**
N 0.00 0.00 FUD XXX

83704 **quantitation of lipoprotein particle numbers and lipoprotein particle subclasses (eg, by nuclear magnetic resonance spectroscopy)**
N 0.00 0.00 FUD XXX

83718 **Lipoprotein, direct measurement; high density cholesterol (HDL cholesterol)**
N 0.00 0.00 FUD XXX

83719 **VLDL cholesterol**
N 0.00 0.00 FUD XXX

83721 **LDL cholesterol**
EXCLUDES *Fractionation by high resolution electrophoresis or ultracentrifugation (83701)*
Lipoprotein particle numbers and subclasses analysis by nuclear magnetic resonance spectroscopy (83704)
N 0.00 0.00 FUD XXX

83727 **Luteinizing releasing factor (LRH)**
N 0.00 0.00 FUD XXX

83735-83887 Chemistry: Magnesium—Nicotine

CMS 100-2,15,80 Diagnostic Test Requirements

INCLUDES Clinical information not requested by the ordering physician
Mathematically calculated results
Quantitative analysis unless otherwise specified
Specimens from any source unless otherwise specified

EXCLUDES *Calculated results that represent a score or probability that was derived by algorithm*
Organ or disease panels (80048-80076)
Therapeutic drug assays (80150-80299)

Do not report analytes from nonrequested laboratory analysis

83735 **Magnesium**
N 0.00 0.00 FUD XXX

83775 **Malate dehydrogenase**
N 0.00 0.00 FUD XXX

83785 **Manganese**
N 0.00 0.00 FUD XXX

83788 **Mass spectrometry and tandem mass spectrometry (MS, MS/MS), analyte not elsewhere specified; qualitative, each specimen**
N 0.00 0.00 FUD XXX

83789 **quantitative, each specimen**
N 0.00 0.00 FUD XXX

Pathology and Laboratory

83499 — 83789

● New Code ▲ Revised Code ○ Reinstated M Maternity A Age Edit 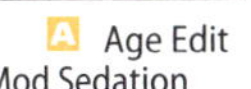 Unlisted 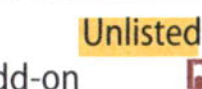 Not Covered # Resequenced
⊘ AMA Mod 51 Exempt ⑤ Optum Mod 51 Exempt ⑥ Mod 63 Exempt ⊙ Mod Sedation + Add-on CCI PQRS FUD Follow-up Days

~~83805 Meprobamate~~
To report, see 80369-80370

83825 Mercury, quantitative
EXCLUDES *Mercury screen (83015)*
N 0.00 0.00 FUD XXX

83835 Metanephrines
EXCLUDES *Catecholamines (82382-82384)*
N 0.00 0.00 FUD XXX

~~83840 Methadone~~
To report, see 80358

83857 Methemalbumin
N 0.00 0.00 FUD XXX

~~83858 Methsuximide~~
To report, see 80339-80341

83861 Microfluidic analysis utilizing an integrated collection and analysis device, tear osmolarity
Code also when performed on both eyes 83861 X 2
N 0.00 0.00 FUD XXX

83864 Mucopolysaccharides, acid, quantitative
N 0.00 0.00 FUD XXX

~~83866 screen~~

83872 Mucin, synovial fluid (Ropes test)
N 0.00 0.00 FUD XXX

83873 Myelin basic protein, cerebrospinal fluid
EXCLUDES *Oligoclonal bands (83916)*
N 0.00 0.00 FUD XXX

83874 Myoglobin
N 0.00 0.00 FUD XXX

83876 Myeloperoxidase (MPO)
N 0.00 0.00 FUD XXX

83880 Natriuretic peptide
N 0.00 0.00 FUD XXX

83883 Nephelometry, each analyte not elsewhere specified
N 0.00 0.00 FUD XXX

83885 Nickel
N 0.00 0.00 FUD XXX

~~83887 Nicotine~~
To report, see 80323

83915-84066 Chemistry: Nucleotidase 5'- —Phosphatase (Acid)

CMS 100-2,15,80 Diagnostic Test Requirements

INCLUDES Clinical information not requested by the ordering physician
Mathematically calculated results
Quantitative analysis unless otherwise specified
Specimens from any source unless otherwise specified

EXCLUDES *Calculated results that represent a score or probability that was derived by algorithm*
Drug testing ([80300, 80301, 80302, 80303, 80304], [80324, 80325, 80326, 80327, 80328, 80329, 80330, 80331, 80332, 80333, 80334, 80335, 80336, 80337, 80338, 80339, 80340, 80341, 80342, 80343, 80344, 80345, 80346, 80347, 80348, 80349, 80350, 80351, 80352, 80353, 80354, 80355, 80356, 80357, 80358, 80359, 80360, 80361, 80362, 80363, 80364, 80365, 80366, 80367, 80368, 80369, 80370, 80371, 80372, 80373, 80374, 80375, 80376, 80377, 83992])
Organ or disease panels (80048-80299 [80104])
Therapeutic drug assays (80150-80299)

Do not report analytes from nonrequested laboratory analysis

83915 Nucleotidase 5'-
N 0.00 0.00 FUD XXX

83916 Oligoclonal immune (oligoclonal bands)
N 0.00 0.00 FUD XXX

83918 Organic acids; total, quantitative, each specimen
N 0.00 0.00 FUD XXX

83919 qualitative, each specimen
N 0.00 0.00 FUD XXX

83921 Organic acid, single, quantitative
N 0.00 0.00 FUD XXX

~~83925 Opiate(s), drug and metabolites, each procedure~~
To report, see specific drug or 80361-80364

83930 Osmolality; blood
EXCLUDES *Tear osmolarity (83861)*
N 0.00 0.00 FUD XXX

83935 urine
EXCLUDES *Tear osmolarity (83861)*
N 0.00 0.00 FUD XXX

83937 Osteocalcin (bone g1a protein)
N 0.00 0.00 FUD XXX

83945 Oxalate
N 0.00 0.00 FUD XXX

83950 Oncoprotein; HER-2/neu
EXCLUDES *Tissue (88342, 88365)*
N 0.00 0.00 FUD XXX

83951 des-gamma-carboxy-prothrombin (DCP)
N 0.00 0.00 FUD XXX

83970 Parathormone (parathyroid hormone)
N 0.00 0.00 FUD XXX

83986 pH; body fluid, not otherwise specified
EXCLUDES *Blood pH (82800, 82803)*
N 0.00 0.00 FUD XXX

83987 exhaled breath condensate
N 0.00 0.00 FUD XXX

83992 Resequenced code. See code following 80365.

83993 Calprotectin, fecal
N 0.00 0.00 FUD XXX

~~84022 Phenothiazine~~
To report, see 80342-80344

84030 Phenylalanine (PKU), blood
INCLUDES Guthrie test
EXCLUDES *Phenylalanine-tyrosine ratio (84030, 84510)*
N 0.00 0.00 FUD XXX

84035 Phenylketones, qualitative
N 0.00 0.00 FUD XXX

84060 Phosphatase, acid; total
N 0.00 0.00 FUD XXX

84061 forensic examination
N 0.00 0.00 FUD XXX

84066 prostatic ♂
N 0.00 0.00 FUD XXX

84075-84080 Chemistry: Phosphatase (Alkaline)

CMS 100-2,15,80 Diagnostic Test Requirements
CMS 100-3,190.10 Laboratory Tests--CRD Patients

INCLUDES Clinical information not requested by the ordering physician
Mathematically calculated results
Quantitative analysis unless otherwise specified
Specimens from any source unless otherwise specified

EXCLUDES *Calculated results that represent a score or probability that was derived by algorithm*
Organ or disease panels (80048-80076)

Do not report analytes from nonrequested laboratory analysis

84075 Phosphatase, alkaline;
N 0.00 0.00 FUD XXX

84078 heat stable (total not included)
N 0.00 0.00 FUD XXX

84080 isoenzymes
N 0.00 0.00 FUD XXX

84081-84150 Chemistry: Phosphatidylglycerol—Prostaglandin

CMS 100-2,15,80 Diagnostic Test Requirements

INCLUDES Clinical information not requested by the ordering physician
Mathematically calculated results
Quantitative analysis unless otherwise specified
Specimens from any source unless otherwise specified

EXCLUDES *Calculated results that represent a score or probability that was derived by algorithm*
Organ or disease panels (80048-80076)
Therapeutic drug assays (80150-80299)

Do not report analytes from nonrequested laboratory analysis

84081 Phosphatidylglycerol
N 0.00 0.00 FUD XXX

84085 Phosphogluconate, 6-, dehydrogenase, RBC
N 0.00 0.00 FUD XXX

84087 Phosphohexose isomerase
N 0.00 0.00 FUD XXX

84100 Phosphorus inorganic (phosphate);
N 0.00 0.00 FUD XXX

84105 urine
N 0.00 0.00 FUD XXX

84106 Porphobilinogen, urine; qualitative
N 0.00 0.00 FUD XXX

84110 quantitative
N 0.00 0.00 FUD XXX

84112 Evaluation of cervicovaginal fluid for specific amniotic fluid protein(s) (eg, placental alpha microglobulin-1 [PAMG-1], placental protein 12 [PP12], alpha-fetoprotein), qualitative, each specimen ♀
N 0.00 0.00 FUD XXX

84119 Porphyrins, urine; qualitative
N 0.00 0.00 FUD XXX

84120 quantitation and fractionation
N 0.00 0.00 FUD XXX

84126 Porphyrins, feces, quantitative
N 0.00 0.00 FUD XXX

~~84127 qualitative~~

84132 Potassium; serum, plasma or whole blood
N 0.00 0.00 FUD XXX

84133 urine
N 0.00 0.00 FUD XXX

84134 Prealbumin
EXCLUDES *Microalbumin (82043-82044)*
N 0.00 0.00 FUD XXX

84135 Pregnanediol ♀
N 0.00 0.00 FUD XXX

84138 Pregnanetriol ♀
N 0.00 0.00 FUD XXX

84140 Pregnenolone
N 0.00 0.00 FUD XXX

84143 17-hydroxypregnenolone
N 0.00 0.00 FUD XXX

84144 Progesterone
EXCLUDES *Progesterone receptor assay (84234)*
N 0.00 0.00 FUD XXX

84145 Procalcitonin (PCT)
N 0.00 0.00 FUD XXX

84146 Prolactin
N 0.00 0.00 FUD XXX

84150 Prostaglandin, each
N 0.00 0.00 FUD XXX

84152-84154 Chemistry: Prostate Specific Antigen

CMS 100-2,15,80 Diagnostic Test Requirements
CMS 100-3,190.31 Prostate Specific Antigen (PSA)
CMS 100-3,210.1 Prostate Cancer Screening Tests

INCLUDES Clinical information not requested by the ordering physician
Mathematically calculated results
Quantitative analysis unless otherwise specified

EXCLUDES *Calculated results that represent a score or probability that was derived by algorithm*

Do not report analytes from nonrequested laboratory analysis

84152 Prostate specific antigen (PSA); complexed (direct measurement) ♂
N 0.00 0.00 FUD XXX

84153 total ♂
N 0.00 0.00 FUD XXX

84154 free ♂
N 0.00 0.00 FUD XXX

84155-84157 Chemistry: Protein, Total (Not by Refractometry)

CMS 100-2,15,80 Diagnostic Test Requirements
CMS 100-3,190.10 Laboratory Tests--CRD Patients

INCLUDES Clinical information not requested by the ordering physician
Mathematically calculated results

EXCLUDES *Calculated results that represent a score or probability that was derived by algorithm*
Organ or disease panels (80048-80076)

Do not report analytes from nonrequested laboratory analysis

84155 Protein, total, except by refractometry; serum, plasma or whole blood
N 0.00 0.00 FUD XXX

84156 urine
N 0.00 0.00 FUD XXX

84157 other source (eg, synovial fluid, cerebrospinal fluid)
N 0.00 0.00 FUD XXX

84160-84432 Chemistry: Protein, Total (Refractometry)—Thyroglobulin

CMS 100-2,15,80 Diagnostic Test Requirements

INCLUDES Clinical information not requested by the ordering physician
Mathematically calculated results
Quantitative analysis unless otherwise specified
Specimens from any source unless otherwise specified

EXCLUDES *Calculated results that represent a score or probability that was derived by algorithm*
Drug testing ([80300, 80301, 80302, 80303, 80304], [80324, 80325, 80326, 80327, 80328, 80329, 80330, 80331, 80332, 80333, 80334, 80335, 80336, 80337, 80338, 80339, 80340, 80341, 80342, 80343, 80344, 80345, 80346, 80347, 80348, 80349, 80350, 80351, 80352, 80353, 80354, 80355, 80356, 80357, 80358, 80359, 80360, 80361, 80362, 80363, 80364, 80365, 80366, 80367, 80368, 80369, 80370, 80371, 80372, 80373, 80374, 80375, 80376, 80377, 83992])
Organ or disease panels (80048-80076)
Therapeutic drug assays (80150-80299)

Do not report analytes from nonrequested laboratory analysis

84160 Protein, total, by refractometry, any source
EXCLUDES *Dipstick urine protein (81000-81003)*
N 0.00 0.00 FUD XXX

84163 Pregnancy-associated plasma protein-A (PAPP-A) ♀
N 0.00 0.00 FUD XXX

84165 Protein; electrophoretic fractionation and quantitation, serum
N 0.00 0.00 FUD XXX

84166 electrophoretic fractionation and quantitation, other fluids with concentration (eg, urine, CSF)
N 0.00 0.00 FUD XXX

84181 Western Blot, with interpretation and report, blood or other body fluid
N 0.00 0.00 FUD XXX

84182 Western Blot, with interpretation and report, blood or other body fluid, immunological probe for band identification, each
EXCLUDES *Western Blot tissue testing (88371)*
0.00 0.00 FUD XXX

84202 Protoporphyrin, RBC; quantitative
0.00 0.00 FUD XXX

84203 screen
0.00 0.00 FUD XXX

84206 Proinsulin
0.00 0.00 FUD XXX

84207 Pyridoxal phosphate (Vitamin B-6)
0.00 0.00 FUD XXX

84210 Pyruvate
0.00 0.00 FUD XXX

84220 Pyruvate kinase
0.00 0.00 FUD XXX

84228 Quinine
0.00 0.00 FUD XXX

84233 Receptor assay; estrogen
0.00 0.00 FUD XXX

84234 progesterone
0.00 0.00 FUD XXX

84235 endocrine, other than estrogen or progesterone (specify hormone)
0.00 0.00 FUD XXX

84238 non-endocrine (specify receptor)
0.00 0.00 FUD XXX

84244 Renin
0.00 0.00 FUD XXX

84252 Riboflavin (Vitamin B-2)
0.00 0.00 FUD XXX

84255 Selenium
0.00 0.00 FUD XXX

84260 Serotonin
EXCLUDES *Urine metabolites (HIAA) (83497)*
0.00 0.00 FUD XXX

84270 Sex hormone binding globulin (SHBG)
0.00 0.00 FUD XXX

84275 Sialic acid
0.00 0.00 FUD XXX

84285 Silica
0.00 0.00 FUD XXX

84295 Sodium; serum, plasma or whole blood
0.00 0.00 FUD XXX

84300 urine
0.00 0.00 FUD XXX

84302 other source
0.00 0.00 FUD XXX

84305 Somatomedin
0.00 0.00 FUD XXX

84307 Somatostatin
0.00 0.00 FUD XXX

84311 Spectrophotometry, analyte not elsewhere specified
0.00 0.00 FUD XXX

84315 Specific gravity (except urine)
EXCLUDES *Urine specific gravity (81000-81003)*
0.00 0.00 FUD XXX

84375 Sugars, chromatographic, TLC or paper chromatography
0.00 0.00 FUD XXX

84376 Sugars (mono-, di-, and oligosaccharides); single qualitative, each specimen
0.00 0.00 FUD XXX

84377 multiple qualitative, each specimen
0.00 0.00 FUD XXX

84378 single quantitative, each specimen
0.00 0.00 FUD XXX

84379 multiple quantitative, each specimen
0.00 0.00 FUD XXX

84392 Sulfate, urine
0.00 0.00 FUD XXX

84402 Testosterone; free
Do not report with ([80327, 80328])
0.00 0.00 FUD XXX

84403 total
Do not report with ([80327, 80328])
0.00 0.00 FUD XXX

84425 Thiamine (Vitamin B-1)
0.00 0.00 FUD XXX

84430 Thiocyanate
0.00 0.00 FUD XXX

84431 Thromboxane metabolite(s), including thromboxane if performed, urine
Code also for determination of concurrent urine creatinine (82570)
0.00 0.00 FUD XXX

84432 Thyroglobulin
EXCLUDES *Thyroglobulin antibody (86800)*
0.00 0.00 FUD XXX

84436-84445 Chemistry: Thyroid Tests

CMS 100-2,15,80 Diagnostic Test Requirements
CMS 100-3,190.22 Thyroid Testing

INCLUDES Clinical information not requested by the ordering physician
Mathematically calculated results
Quantitative analysis unless otherwise specified
Specimens from any source unless otherwise specified

EXCLUDES *Calculated results that represent a score or probability that was derived by algorithm*
Organ or disease panels (80048-80076)
Therapeutic drug assays (80150-80299)

Do not report analytes from nonrequested laboratory analysis

84436 Thyroxine; total
0.00 0.00 FUD XXX

84437 requiring elution (eg, neonatal)
0.00 0.00 FUD XXX

84439 free
0.00 0.00 FUD XXX

84442 Thyroxine binding globulin (TBG)
0.00 0.00 FUD XXX

84443 Thyroid stimulating hormone (TSH)
0.00 0.00 FUD XXX

84445 Thyroid stimulating immune globulins (TSI)
0.00 0.00 FUD XXX

84446-84449 Chemistry: Tocopherol Alpha—Transcortin

CMS 100-2,15,80 Diagnostic Test Requirements

INCLUDES Clinical information not requested by the ordering physician
Mathematically calculated results
Quantitative analysis unless otherwise specified
Specimens from any source unless otherwise specified

EXCLUDES *Calculated results that represent a score or probability that was derived by algorithm*
Organ or disease panels (80048-80076)
Therapeutic drug assays (80150-80299)

Do not report analytes from nonrequested laboratory analysis

84446 Tocopherol alpha (Vitamin E)
0.00 0.00 FUD XXX

84449 Transcortin (cortisol binding globulin)
0.00 0.00 FUD XXX

84450-84460 Chemistry: Transferase

CMS 100-2,15,80 Diagnostic Test Requirements
CMS 100-3,190.10 Laboratory Tests--CRD Patients

INCLUDES Clinical information not requested by the ordering physician
Mathematically calculated results
Quantitative analysis unless otherwise specified

EXCLUDES *Calculated results that represent a score or probability that was derived by algorithm*

Do not report analytes from nonrequested laboratory analysis

84450 Transferase; aspartate amino (AST) (SGOT)
N 0.00 0.00 FUD XXX

84460 alanine amino (ALT) (SGPT)
N 0.00 0.00 FUD XXX

84466 Chemistry: Transferrin

CMS 100-2,15,80 Diagnostic Test Requirements

INCLUDES Clinical information not requested by the ordering physician
Mathematically calculated results
Quantitative analysis unless otherwise specified

EXCLUDES *Calculated results that represent a score or probability that was derived by algorithm*

Do not report analytes from nonrequested laboratory analysis

84466 Transferrin
EXCLUDES *Iron binding capacity (83550)*
N 0.00 0.00 FUD XXX

84478 Chemistry: Triglycerides

CMS 100-2,15,80 Diagnostic Test Requirements
CMS 100-3,190.23 Lipid Testing

INCLUDES Clinical information not requested by the ordering physician
Mathematically calculated results

EXCLUDES *Calculated results that represent a score or probability that was derived by algorithm*
Organ or disease panels (80048-80076)

Do not report analytes from nonrequested laboratory analysis

84478 Triglycerides
N 0.00 0.00 FUD XXX

84479-84482 Chemistry: Thyroid Hormone—Triiodothyronine

CMS 100-2,15,80 Diagnostic Test Requirements
CMS 100-3,190.22 Thyroid Testing

INCLUDES Clinical information not requested by the ordering physician
Mathematically calculated results
Quantitative analysis unless otherwise specified
Specimens from any source unless otherwise specified

EXCLUDES *Calculated results that represent a score or probability that was derived by algorithm*
Organ or disease panels (80048-80076)

Do not report analytes from nonrequested laboratory analysis

84479 Thyroid hormone (T3 or T4) uptake or thyroid hormone binding ratio (THBR)
N 0.00 0.00 FUD XXX

84480 Triiodothyronine T3; total (TT-3)
N 0.00 0.00 FUD XXX

84481 free
N 0.00 0.00 FUD XXX

84482 reverse
N 0.00 0.00 FUD XXX

84484-84512 Chemistry: Troponin (Quantitative)—Troponin (Qualitative)

CMS 100-2,15,80 Diagnostic Test Requirements

INCLUDES Clinical information not requested by the ordering physician
Mathematically calculated results
Specimens from any source unless otherwise specified

EXCLUDES *Calculated results that represent a score or probability that was derived by algorithm*
Organ or disease panels

Do not report analytes from nonrequested laboratory analysis

84484 Troponin, quantitative
EXCLUDES *Qualitative troponin assay (84512)*
N 0.00 0.00 FUD XXX

84485 Trypsin; duodenal fluid
N 0.00 0.00 FUD XXX

84488 feces, qualitative
N 0.00 0.00 FUD XXX

84490 feces, quantitative, 24-hour collection
N 0.00 0.00 FUD XXX

84510 Tyrosine
EXCLUDES *Urate crystal identification (89060)*
N 0.00 0.00 FUD XXX

84512 Troponin, qualitative
EXCLUDES *Quantitative troponin assay (84484)*
N 0.00 0.00 FUD XXX

84520-84525 Chemistry: Urea Nitrogen (Blood)

CMS 100-2,15,80 Diagnostic Test Requirements
CMS 100-3,190.10 Laboratory Tests--CRD Patients

INCLUDES Clinical information not requested by the ordering physician
Mathematically calculated results

EXCLUDES *Calculated results that represent a score or probability that was derived by algorithm*
Organ or disease panels (80048-80076)

Do not report analytes from nonrequested laboratory analysis

84520 Urea nitrogen; quantitative
N 0.00 0.00 FUD XXX

84525 semiquantitative (eg, reagent strip test)
INCLUDES Patterson's test
N 0.00 0.00 FUD XXX

84540-84630 Chemistry: Urea Nitrogen (Urine)—Zinc

CMS 100-2,15,80 Diagnostic Test Requirements

INCLUDES Clinical information not requested by the ordering physician
Mathematically calculated results
Quantitative analysis unless otherwise specified
Specimens from any source unless otherwise specified

EXCLUDES *Calculated results that represent a score or probability that was derived by algorithm*
Organ or disease panels (80048-80076)
Therapeutic drug assays (80150-80299)

Do not report analytes from nonrequested laboratory analysis

84540 Urea nitrogen, urine
N 0.00 0.00 FUD XXX

84545 Urea nitrogen, clearance
N 0.00 0.00 FUD XXX

84550 Uric acid; blood
N 0.00 0.00 FUD XXX

84560 other source
N 0.00 0.00 FUD XXX

84577 Urobilinogen, feces, quantitative
N 0.00 0.00 FUD XXX

84578 Urobilinogen, urine; qualitative
N 0.00 0.00 FUD XXX

84580 quantitative, timed specimen
N 0.00 0.00 FUD XXX

84583 semiquantitative
N 0.00 0.00 FUD XXX

84585 Vanillylmandelic acid (VMA), urine
N 0.00 0.00 FUD XXX

84586 Vasoactive intestinal peptide (VIP)
N 0.00 0.00 FUD XXX

84588 Vasopressin (antidiuretic hormone, ADH)
N 0.00 0.00 FUD XXX

84590 Vitamin A
N 0.00 0.00 FUD XXX

84591 Vitamin, not otherwise specified
N 0.00 0.00 FUD XXX

84597 **Vitamin K**
N 0.00 0.00 FUD XXX

▲ 84600 **Volatiles (eg, acetic anhydride, diethylether)**
EXCLUDES *Carbon tetrachloride, dichloroethane, dichloromethane (82441)*
Isopropyl alcohol and methanol ([80320])
N 0.00 0.00 FUD XXX

84620 **Xylose absorption test, blood and/or urine**
EXCLUDES *Administration (99070)*
N 0.00 0.00 FUD XXX

84630 **Zinc**
N 0.00 0.00 FUD XXX

84681-84999 Other and Unlisted Chemistry Tests

CMS 100-2,15,80 Diagnostic Test Requirements

INCLUDES Clinical information not requested by the ordering physician
Mathematically calculated results
Quantitative analysis unless otherwise specified
Specimens from any source unless otherwise specified

EXCLUDES *Calculated results that represent a score or probability that was derived by algorithm*
Confirmational testing of a not otherwise specified drug ([80375, 80376, 80377], 80299)
Organ or disease panels (80048-80076)

Do not report analytes from nonrequested laboratory analysis

84681 **C-peptide**
N 0.00 0.00 FUD XXX

84702 **Gonadotropin, chorionic (hCG); quantitative**
N 0.00 0.00 FUD XXX

84703 **qualitative**
EXCLUDES *Urine pregnancy test by visual color comparison (81025)*
N 0.00 0.00 FUD XXX

84704 **free beta chain**
N 0.00 0.00 FUD XXX

84830 **Ovulation tests, by visual color comparison methods for human luteinizing hormone** ♀
N 0.00 0.00 FUD XXX

84999 **Unlisted chemistry procedure**
N 0.00 0.00 FUD XXX

85002 Bleeding Time Test

CMS 100-2,15,80 Diagnostic Test Requirements

EXCLUDES *Agglutinins (86000, 86156-86157)*
Antiplasmin (85410)
Antithrombin III (85300-85301)
Blood banking procedures (86850-86999)

85002 **Bleeding time**
N 0.00 0.00 FUD XXX

85004-85049 Blood Counts

CMS 100-2,15,80 Diagnostic Test Requirements
CMS 100-3,190.15 Blood Counts

EXCLUDES *Agglutinins (86000, 86156-86157)*
Antiplasmin (85410)
Antithrombin III (85300-85301)
Blood banking procedures (86850-86999)

85004 **Blood count; automated differential WBC count**
N 0.00 0.00 FUD XXX

85007 **blood smear, microscopic examination with manual differential WBC count**
N 0.00 0.00 FUD XXX

85008 **blood smear, microscopic examination without manual differential WBC count**
EXCLUDES *Cell count other fluids (eg, CSF) (89050-89051)*
N 0.00 0.00 FUD XXX

85009 **manual differential WBC count, buffy coat**
EXCLUDES *Eosinophils, nasal smear (89190)*
N 0.00 0.00 FUD XXX

85013 **spun microhematocrit**
N 0.00 0.00 FUD XXX

85014 **hematocrit (Hct)**
N 0.00 0.00 FUD XXX

85018 **hemoglobin (Hgb)**
EXCLUDES *Immunoassay, hemoglobin, fecal (82274)*
Other hemoglobin determination (83020-83069)
Transcutaneous hemoglobin measurement (88738)
N 0.00 0.00 FUD XXX

85025 **complete (CBC), automated (Hgb, Hct, RBC, WBC and platelet count) and automated differential WBC count**
N 0.00 0.00 FUD XXX

85027 **complete (CBC), automated (Hgb, Hct, RBC, WBC and platelet count)**
N 0.00 0.00 FUD XXX

85032 **manual cell count (erythrocyte, leukocyte, or platelet) each**
N 0.00 0.00 FUD XXX

85041 **red blood cell (RBC), automated**
Do not report with (85025, 85027)
N 0.00 0.00 FUD XXX

85044 **reticulocyte, manual**
N 0.00 0.00 FUD XXX

85045 **reticulocyte, automated**
N 0.00 0.00 FUD XXX

85046 **reticulocytes, automated, including 1 or more cellular parameters (eg, reticulocyte hemoglobin content [CHr], immature reticulocyte fraction [IRF], reticulocyte volume [MRV], RNA content), direct measurement**
N 0.00 0.00 FUD XXX

85048 **leukocyte (WBC), automated**
N 0.00 0.00 FUD XXX

85049 **platelet, automated**
N 0.00 0.00 FUD XXX

85055-85705 Coagulopathy Testing

CMS 100-2,15,80 Diagnostic Test Requirements
CMS 100-4,3,20.7.3 Payment for Blood Clotting Factor for Hemophilia Inpatients

EXCLUDES *Agglutinins (86000, 86156-86157)*
Antiplasmin (85410)
Antithrombin III (85300-85301)
Blood banking procedures (86850-86999)

85055 **Reticulated platelet assay**
N 0.00 0.00 FUD XXX

85060 **Blood smear, peripheral, interpretation by physician with written report**
B 80 0.69 0.69 FUD XXX

85097 **Bone marrow, smear interpretation**
EXCLUDES *Bone biopsy (20220, 20225, 20240, 20245, 20250-20251)*
Special stains (88312-88313)
X 80 1.37 2.41 FUD XXX

85130 **Chromogenic substrate assay**
N 0.00 0.00 FUD XXX

85170 **Clot retraction**
N 0.00 0.00 FUD XXX

85175 **Clot lysis time, whole blood dilution**
N 0.00 0.00 FUD XXX

85210 **Clotting; factor II, prothrombin, specific**
EXCLUDES *Prothrombin time (85610-85611)*
Russell viper venom time (85612-85613)
N 0.00 0.00 FUD XXX

85220 **factor V (AcG or proaccelerin), labile factor**
N 0.00 0.00 FUD XXX

85230 **factor VII (proconvertin, stable factor)**
N 0.00 0.00 FUD XXX

85240 **factor VIII (AHG), 1-stage**
N 0.00 0.00 FUD XXX

85244 factor VIII related antigen
N 0.00 0.00 FUD XXX

85245 factor VIII, VW factor, ristocetin cofactor
N 0.00 0.00 FUD XXX

85246 factor VIII, VW factor antigen
N 0.00 0.00 FUD XXX

85247 factor VIII, von Willebrand factor, multimetric analysis
N 0.00 0.00 FUD XXX

85250 factor IX (PTC or Christmas)
N 0.00 0.00 FUD XXX

85260 factor X (Stuart-Prower)
N 0.00 0.00 FUD XXX

85270 factor XI (PTA)
N 0.00 0.00 FUD XXX

85280 factor XII (Hageman)
N 0.00 0.00 FUD XXX

85290 factor XIII (fibrin stabilizing)
N 0.00 0.00 FUD XXX

85291 factor XIII (fibrin stabilizing), screen solubility
N 0.00 0.00 FUD XXX

85292 prekallikrein assay (Fletcher factor assay)
N 0.00 0.00 FUD XXX

85293 high molecular weight kininogen assay (Fitzgerald factor assay)
N 0.00 0.00 FUD XXX

85300 Clotting inhibitors or anticoagulants; antithrombin III, activity
N 0.00 0.00 FUD XXX

85301 antithrombin III, antigen assay
N 0.00 0.00 FUD XXX

85302 protein C, antigen
N 0.00 0.00 FUD XXX •

85303 protein C, activity
N 0.00 0.00 FUD XXX

85305 protein S, total
N 0.00 0.00 FUD XXX

85306 protein S, free
N 0.00 0.00 FUD XXX

85307 Activated Protein C (APC) resistance assay
N 0.00 0.00 FUD XXX

85335 Factor inhibitor test
N 0.00 0.00 FUD XXX

85337 Thrombomodulin
EXCLUDES *Mixing studies for inhibitors (85732)*
N 0.00 0.00 FUD XXX

85345 Coagulation time; Lee and White
N 0.00 0.00 FUD XXX

85347 activated
N 0.00 0.00 FUD XXX

85348 other methods
N 0.00 0.00 FUD XXX

85360 Euglobulin lysis
N 0.00 0.00 FUD XXX

85362 Fibrin(ogen) degradation (split) products (FDP) (FSP); agglutination slide, semiquantitative
EXCLUDES *Immunoelectrophoresis (86320)*
N 0.00 0.00 FUD XXX

85366 paracoagulation
N 0.00 0.00 FUD XXX

85370 quantitative
N 0.00 0.00 FUD XXX

85378 Fibrin degradation products, D-dimer; qualitative or semiquantitative
N 0.00 0.00 FUD XXX

85379 quantitative
INCLUDES Ultrasensitive and standard sensitivity quantitative D-dimer
N 0.00 0.00 FUD XXX

85380 ultrasensitive (eg, for evaluation for venous thromboembolism), qualitative or semiquantitative
N 0.00 0.00 FUD XXX

85384 Fibrinogen; activity
N 0.00 0.00 FUD XXX

85385 antigen
N 0.00 0.00 FUD XXX

85390 Fibrinolysins or coagulopathy screen, interpretation and report
N 0.00 0.00 FUD XXX

85396 Coagulation/fibrinolysis assay, whole blood (eg, viscoelastic clot assessment), including use of any pharmacologic additive(s), as indicated, including interpretation and written report, per day
N 80 0.57 0.57 FUD XXX

85397 Coagulation and fibrinolysis, functional activity, not otherwise specified (eg, ADAMTS-13), each analyte
N 0.00 0.00 FUD XXX

85400 Fibrinolytic factors and inhibitors; plasmin
N 0.00 0.00 FUD XXX

85410 alpha-2 antiplasmin
N 0.00 0.00 FUD XXX

85415 plasminogen activator
N 0.00 0.00 FUD XXX

85420 plasminogen, except antigenic assay
N 0.00 0.00 FUD XXX

85421 plasminogen, antigenic assay
N 0.00 0.00 FUD XXX

85441 Heinz bodies; direct
N 0.00 0.00 FUD XXX

85445 induced, acetyl phenylhydrazine
N 0.00 0.00 FUD XXX

85460 Hemoglobin or RBCs, fetal, for fetomaternal hemorrhage; differential lysis (Kleihauer-Betke) M ♀
EXCLUDES *Hemoglobin F (83030, 83033)*
Hemolysins (86940-86941)
N 0.00 0.00 FUD XXX

85461 rosette M ♀
N 0.00 0.00 FUD XXX

85475 Hemolysin, acid
INCLUDES Ham test
EXCLUDES *Hemolysins and agglutinins (86940-86941)*
N 0.00 0.00 FUD XXX

85520 Heparin assay
N 0.00 0.00 FUD XXX

85525 Heparin neutralization
N 0.00 0.00 FUD XXX

85530 Heparin-protamine tolerance test
N 0.00 0.00 FUD XXX

85536 Iron stain, peripheral blood
EXCLUDES *Iron stains on bone marrow or other tissues with physician evaluation (88313)*
N 0.00 0.00 FUD XXX

85540 Leukocyte alkaline phosphatase with count
N 0.00 0.00 FUD XXX

85547 Mechanical fragility, RBC
N 0.00 0.00 FUD XXX

85549 Muramidase
N 0.00 0.00 FUD XXX

85555 Osmotic fragility, RBC; unincubated
N 0.00 0.00 FUD XXX

85557 incubated
N 0.00 0.00 FUD XXX

85576 Platelet, aggregation (in vitro), each agent
EXCLUDES *Thromboxane metabolite(s), including thromboxane, when performed, in urine (84431)*
N 0.00 0.00 FUD XXX

85597 Phospholipid neutralization; platelet
N 0.00 0.00 FUD XXX

85598 hexagonal phospholipid
N 0.00 0.00 FUD XXX

85610 Prothrombin time;
N 0.00 0.00 FUD XXX

85611 substitution, plasma fractions, each
N 0.00 0.00 FUD XXX

85612 Russell viper venom time (includes venom); undiluted
N 0.00 0.00 FUD XXX

85613 diluted
N 0.00 0.00 FUD XXX

85635 Reptilase test
N 0.00 0.00 FUD XXX

85651 Sedimentation rate, erythrocyte; non-automated
N 0.00 0.00 FUD XXX

85652 automated
INCLUDES Westergren test
N 0.00 0.00 FUD XXX

85660 Sickling of RBC, reduction
EXCLUDES *Hemoglobin electrophoresis (83020)*
N 0.00 0.00 FUD XXX

85670 Thrombin time; plasma
N 0.00 0.00 FUD XXX

85675 titer
N 0.00 0.00 FUD XXX

85705 Thromboplastin inhibition, tissue
EXCLUDES *Individual clotting factors (85245-85247)*
N 0.00 0.00 FUD XXX

85730-85732 Partial Thromboplastin Time (PTT)

CMS 100-2,15,80 Diagnostic Test Requirements
CMS 100-3,190.16 Partial Thromboplastin Time (PTT)

EXCLUDES *Agglutinins (86000, 86156-86157)*
Antiplasmin (85410)
Antithrombin III (85300-85301)
Blood banking procedures (86850-86999)

85730 Thromboplastin time, partial (PTT); plasma or whole blood
INCLUDES Hicks-Pitney test
N 0.00 0.00 FUD XXX

85732 substitution, plasma fractions, each
N 0.00 0.00 FUD XXX

85810-85999 Blood Viscosity and Unlisted Hematology Procedures

CMS 100-2,15,80 Diagnostic Test Requirements

85810 Viscosity
N 0.00 0.00 FUD XXX

85999 Unlisted hematology and coagulation procedure
N 0.00 0.00 FUD XXX

86000-86063 Antibody Testing

CMS 100-2,15,80 Diagnostic Test Requirements

86000 Agglutinins, febrile (eg, Brucella, Francisella, Murine typhus, Q fever, Rocky Mountain spotted fever, scrub typhus), each antigen
EXCLUDES *Infectious agent antibodies (86602-86804)*
N 0.00 0.00 FUD XXX

86001 Allergen specific IgG quantitative or semiquantitative, each allergen
N 0.00 0.00 FUD XXX

86003 Allergen specific IgE; quantitative or semiquantitative, each allergen
EXCLUDES *Total quantitative IgE (82785)*
N 0.00 0.00 FUD XXX

86005 qualitative, multiallergen screen (dipstick, paddle, or disk)
EXCLUDES *Total qualitative IgE (83518)*
N 0.00 0.00 FUD XXX

86021 Antibody identification; leukocyte antibodies
N 0.00 0.00 FUD XXX

86022 platelet antibodies
N 0.00 0.00 FUD XXX

86023 platelet associated immunoglobulin assay
N 0.00 0.00 FUD XXX

86038 Antinuclear antibodies (ANA);
N 0.00 0.00 FUD XXX

86039 titer
N 0.00 0.00 FUD XXX

86060 Antistreptolysin 0; titer
N 0.00 0.00 FUD XXX

86063 screen
N 0.00 0.00 FUD XXX

86077-86079 Blood Bank Services

CMS 100-2,15,80 Diagnostic Test Requirements
CMS 100-4,12,60 Payment for Pathology Services

86077 Blood bank physician services; difficult cross match and/or evaluation of irregular antibody(s), interpretation and written report
X 80 1.43 1.53 FUD XXX

86078 investigation of transfusion reaction including suspicion of transmissible disease, interpretation and written report
X 80 1.43 1.53 FUD XXX

86079 authorization for deviation from standard blood banking procedures (eg, use of outdated blood, transfusion of Rh incompatible units), with written report
X 80 1.41 1.52 FUD XXX

86140-86344 Diagnostic Immunology Testing

CMS 100-2,15,80 Diagnostic Test Requirements

86140 C-reactive protein;
N 0.00 0.00 FUD XXX

86141 high sensitivity (hsCRP)
N 0.00 0.00 FUD XXX

86146 Beta 2 Glycoprotein I antibody, each
N 0.00 0.00 FUD XXX

86147 Cardiolipin (phospholipid) antibody, each Ig class
N 0.00 0.00 FUD XXX

86152 Cell enumeration using immunologic selection and identification in fluid specimen (eg, circulating tumor cells in blood);
EXCLUDES *Flow cytometric immunophenotyping (88184-88189)*
Flow cytometric quantitation (86355-86357, 86359-86361, 86367)
Code also physician interpretation/report when performed ([86153])
N 0.00 0.00 FUD XXX

86153 physician interpretation and report, when required
EXCLUDES *Flow cytometric immunophenotyping (88184-88189)*
Flow cytometric quantitation (86355-86357, 86359-86361, 86367)
Code first cell enumeration, when performed ([86152])
B

86148 Anti-phosphatidylserine (phospholipid) antibody
EXCLUDES Antiprothrombin (phospholipid cofactor) antibody (86849)
N 0.00 0.00 FUD XXX

86152 *Resequenced code. See code following 86147.*

86153 *Resequenced code. See code before 86148.*

86155 Chemotaxis assay, specify method
N 0.00 0.00 FUD XXX

86156 Cold agglutinin; screen
N 0.00 0.00 FUD XXX

86157 titer
N 0.00 0.00 FUD XXX

86160 Complement; antigen, each component
N 0.00 0.00 FUD XXX

86161 functional activity, each component
N 0.00 0.00 FUD XXX

86162 total hemolytic (CH50)
N 0.00 0.00 FUD XXX

86171 Complement fixation tests, each antigen
N 0.00 0.00 FUD XXX

86185 Counterimmunoelectrophoresis, each antigen
N 0.00 0.00 FUD XXX

86200 Cyclic citrullinated peptide (CCP), antibody
N 0.00 0.00 FUD XXX

86215 Deoxyribonuclease, antibody
N 0.00 0.00 FUD XXX

86225 Deoxyribonucleic acid (DNA) antibody; native or double stranded
EXCLUDES HIV antibody tests (86701-86703)
N 0.00 0.00 FUD XXX

86226 single stranded
EXCLUDES Anti D.S, DNA, IFA, eg, using C. Lucilae (86255-86256)
N 0.00 0.00 FUD XXX

86235 Extractable nuclear antigen, antibody to, any method (eg, nRNP, SS-A, SS-B, Sm, RNP, Sc170, J01), each antibody
N 0.00 0.00 FUD XXX

86243 Fc receptor
N 0.00 0.00 FUD XXX

86255 Fluorescent noninfectious agent antibody; screen, each antibody
N 0.00 0.00 FUD XXX

86256 titer, each antibody
EXCLUDES Fluorescent technique for antigen identification in tissue (88346)
FTA (86780)
Gel (agar) diffusion tests (86331)
Indirect fluorescence (88347)
N 0.00 0.00 FUD XXX

86277 Growth hormone, human (HGH), antibody
N 0.00 0.00 FUD XXX

86280 Hemagglutination inhibition test (HAI)
EXCLUDES Antibodies to infectious agents (86602 86804)
Rubella (86762)
N 0.00 0.00 FUD XXX

86294 Immunoassay for tumor antigen, qualitative or semiquantitative (eg, bladder tumor antigen)
EXCLUDES Qualitative NMP22 protein (86386)
N 0.00 0.00 FUD XXX

86300 Immunoassay for tumor antigen, quantitative; CA 15-3 (27.29)
N 0.00 0.00 FUD XXX

86301 CA 19-9
N 0.00 0.00 FUD XXX

86304 CA 125
EXCLUDES Measurement of serum HER-2/neu oncoprotein (83950)
N 0.00 0.00 FUD XXX

86305 Human epididymis protein 4 (HE4)
N 0.00 0.00 FUD XXX

86308 Heterophile antibodies; screening
EXCLUDES Antibodies to infectious agents (86602-86804)
N 0.00 0.00 FUD XXX

86309 titer
EXCLUDES Antibodies to infectious agents (86602-86804)
N 0.00 0.00 FUD XXX

86310 titers after absorption with beef cells and guinea pig kidney
EXCLUDES Antibodies to infectious agents (86602-86804)
N 0.00 0.00 FUD XXX

86316 Immunoassay for tumor antigen, other antigen, quantitative (eg, CA 50, 72-4, 549), each
N 0.00 0.00 FUD XXX

86317 Immunoassay for infectious agent antibody, quantitative, not otherwise specified
EXCLUDES Immunoassay techniques for antigens (83516, 83518-83520, 87301-87450, 87810-87899)
Particle agglutination test (86403)
N 0.00 0.00 FUD XXX

86318 Immunoassay for infectious agent antibody, qualitative or semiquantitative, single step method (eg, reagent strip)
N 0.00 0.00 FUD XXX

86320 Immunoelectrophoresis; serum
N 0.00 0.00 FUD XXX

86325 other fluids (eg, urine, cerebrospinal fluid) with concentration
N 0.00 0.00 FUD XXX

86327 crossed (2-dimensional assay)
N 0.00 0.00 FUD XXX

86329 Immunodiffusion; not elsewhere specified
N 0.00 0.00 FUD XXX

86331 gel diffusion, qualitative (Ouchterlony), each antigen or antibody
N 0.00 0.00 FUD XXX

86332 Immune complex assay
N 0.00 0.00 FUD XXX

86334 Immunofixation electrophoresis; serum
N 0.00 0.00 FUD XXX

86335 other fluids with concentration (eg, urine, CSF)
N 0.00 0.00 FUD XXX

86336 Inhibin A
N 0.00 0.00 FUD XXX

86337 Insulin antibodies
N 0.00 0.00 FUD XXX

86340 Intrinsic factor antibodies
N 0.00 0.00 FUD XXX

86341 Islet cell antibody
N 0.00 0.00 FUD XXX

86343 Leukocyte histamine release test (LHR)
N 0.00 0.00 FUD XXX

86344 Leukocyte phagocytosis
N 0.00 0.00 FUD XXX

86352 Assay Cellular Function

86352 Cellular function assay involving stimulation (eg, mitogen or antigen) and detection of biomarker (eg, ATP)
N 0.00 0.00 FUD XXX

Pathology and Laboratory

86353 Lymphocyte Mitogen Response Assay

CMS 100-2,15,80 Diagnostic Test Requirements
CMS 100-3,190.8 Lymphocyte Mitogen Response Assays

86353 **Lymphocyte transformation, mitogen (phytomitogen) or antigen induced blastogenesis**
EXCLUDES *Cellular function assay involving stimulation and detection of biomarker (86352)*
N 0.00 0.00 FUD XXX

86355-86593 Additional Diagnostic Immunology Testing

CMS 100-2,15,80 Diagnostic Test Requirements

86355 **B cells, total count**
Do not report with flow cytometry interpretation (88187-88189)
N 0.00 0.00 FUD XXX

86356 **Mononuclear cell antigen, quantitative (eg, flow cytometry), not otherwise specified, each antigen**
Do not report with flow cytometry interpretation (88187-88189)
N 0.00 0.00 FUD XXX

86357 **Natural killer (NK) cells, total count**
Do not report with flow cytometry interpretation (88187-88189)
N 0.00 0.00 FUD XXX

86359 **T cells; total count**
Do not report with flow cytometry interpretation (88187-88189)
N 0.00 0.00 FUD XXX

86360 **absolute CD4 and CD8 count, including ratio**
Do not report with flow cytometry interpretation (88187-88189)
N 0.00 0.00 FUD XXX

86361 **absolute CD4 count**
Do not report with flow cytometry interpretation (88187-88189)
N 0.00 0.00 FUD XXX

86367 **Stem cells (ie, CD34), total count**
Do not report with flow cytometry interpretation (88187-88189)
N 0.00 0.00 FUD XXX

86376 **Microsomal antibodies (eg, thyroid or liver-kidney), each**
N 0.00 0.00 FUD XXX

86378 **Migration inhibitory factor test (MIF)**
N 0.00 0.00 FUD XXX

86382 **Neutralization test, viral**
N 0.00 0.00 FUD XXX

86384 **Nitroblue tetrazolium dye test (NTD)**
N 0.00 0.00 FUD XXX

86386 **Nuclear Matrix Protein 22 (NMP22), qualitative**
N 0.00 0.00 FUD XXX

86403 **Particle agglutination; screen, each antibody**
N 0.00 0.00 FUD XXX

86406 **titer, each antibody**
N 0.00 0.00 FUD XXX

86430 **Rheumatoid factor; qualitative**
N 0.00 0.00 FUD XXX

86431 **quantitative**
N 0.00 0.00 FUD XXX

86480 **Tuberculosis test, cell mediated immunity antigen response measurement; gamma interferon**
N 0.00 0.00 FUD XXX

86481 **enumeration of gamma interferon-producing T-cells in cell suspension**
N 0.00 0.00 FUD XXX

86485 **Skin test; candida**
X TC 80 0.00 0.00 FUD XXX

86486 **unlisted antigen, each**
X TC 80 0.14 0.14 FUD XXX

86490 **coccidioidomycosis**
X TC 80 0.14 0.14 FUD XXX

86510 **histoplasmosis**
X TC 80 0.18 0.18 FUD XXX

86580 **tuberculosis, intradermal**
INCLUDES Heaf test
Intradermal Mantoux test
EXCLUDES *Skin test for allergy (95012-95199)*
Tuberculosis test, cell mediated immunity measurement of gamma interferon antigen response (86480)
X TC 80 0.22 0.22 FUD XXX

86590 **Streptokinase, antibody**
EXCLUDES *Antibodies to infectious agents (86602-86804)*
N 0.00 0.00 FUD XXX

86592 **Syphilis test, non-treponemal antibody; qualitative (eg, VDRL, RPR, ART)**
INCLUDES Wasserman test
EXCLUDES *Antibodies to infectious agents (86602-86804)*
N 0.00 0.00 FUD XXX

86593 **quantitative**
EXCLUDES *Antibodies to infectious agents (86602-86804)*
N 0.00 0.00 FUD XXX

86602-86698 Testing for Antibodies to Infectious Agents: Actinomyces—Histoplasma

CMS 100-2,15,80 Diagnostic Test Requirements

INCLUDES Qualitative or semiquantitative immunoassays performed by multiple-step methods for the detection of antibodies to infectious agents

EXCLUDES *Detection of:*
Antibodies other than those to infectious agents, see specific antibody or method
Infectious agent/antigen (87260-87899)
Immunoassays by single-step method (86318)

86602 **Antibody; actinomyces**
N 0.00 0.00 FUD XXX

86603 **adenovirus**
N 0.00 0.00 FUD XXX

86606 **Aspergillus**
N 0.00 0.00 FUD XXX

86609 **bacterium, not elsewhere specified**
N 0.00 0.00 FUD XXX

86611 **Bartonella**
N 0.00 0.00 FUD XXX

86612 **Blastomyces**
N 0.00 0.00 FUD XXX

86615 **Bordetella**
N 0.00 0.00 FUD XXX

86617 **Borrelia burgdorferi (Lyme disease) confirmatory test (eg, Western Blot or immunoblot)**
N 0.00 0.00 FUD XXX

86618 **Borrelia burgdorferi (Lyme disease)**
N 0.00 0.00 FUD XXX

86619 **Borrelia (relapsing fever)**
N 0.00 0.00 FUD XXX

86622 **Brucella**
N 0.00 0.00 FUD XXX

86625 **Campylobacter**
N 0.00 0.00 FUD XXX

86628 **Candida**
EXCLUDES *Candida skin test (86485)*
N 0.00 0.00 FUD XXX

86631 **Chlamydia**
N 0.00 0.00 FUD XXX

86353 — 86631

86632 **Chlamydia, IgM**
EXCLUDES *Chlamydia antigen (87270, 87320)*
Fluorescent antibody technique (86255-86256)
N 0.00 0.00 FUD XXX

86635 **Coccidioides**
N 0.00 0.00 FUD XXX

86638 **Coxiella burnetii (Q fever)**
N 0.00 0.00 FUD XXX

86641 **Cryptococcus**
N 0.00 0.00 FUD XXX

86644 **cytomegalovirus (CMV)**
N 0.00 0.00 FUD XXX

86645 **cytomegalovirus (CMV), IgM**
N 0.00 0.00 FUD XXX

86648 **Diphtheria**
N 0.00 0.00 FUD XXX

86651 **encephalitis, California (La Crosse)**
N 0.00 0.00 FUD XXX

86652 **encephalitis, Eastern equine**
N 0.00 0.00 FUD XXX

86653 **encephalitis, St. Louis**
N 0.00 0.00 FUD XXX

86654 **encephalitis, Western equine**
N 0.00 0.00 FUD XXX

86658 **enterovirus (eg, coxsackie, echo, polio)**
EXCLUDES *Antibodies to:*
Trichinella (86784)
Trypanosoma—see code for specific methodology
Tuberculosis (86580)
Viral—see code for specific methodology
N 0.00 0.00 FUD XXX

86663 **Epstein-Barr (EB) virus, early antigen (EA)**
N 0.00 0.00 FUD XXX

86664 **Epstein-Barr (EB) virus, nuclear antigen (EBNA)**
N 0.00 0.00 FUD XXX

86665 **Epstein-Barr (EB) virus, viral capsid (VCA)**
N 0.00 0.00 FUD XXX

86666 **Ehrlichia**
N 0.00 0.00 FUD XXX

86668 **Francisella tularensis**
N 0.00 0.00 FUD XXX

86671 **fungus, not elsewhere specified**
N 0.00 0.00 FUD XXX

86674 **Giardia lamblia**
N 0.00 0.00 FUD XXX

86677 **Helicobacter pylori**
N 0.00 0.00 FUD XXX

86682 **helminth, not elsewhere specified**
N 0.00 0.00 FUD XXX

86684 **Haemophilus influenza**
N 0.00 0.00 FUD XXX

86687 **HTLV-I**
N 0.00 0.00 FUD XXX

86688 **HTLV-II**
N 0.00 0.00 FUD XXX

86689 **HTLV or HIV antibody, confirmatory test (eg, Western Blot)**
N 0.00 0.00 FUD XXX

86692 **hepatitis, delta agent**
EXCLUDES *Hepatitis delta agent, antigen (87380)*
N 0.00 0.00 FUD XXX

86694 **herpes simplex, non-specific type test**
N 0.00 0.00 FUD XXX

86695 **herpes simplex, type 1**
N 0.00 0.00 FUD XXX

86696 **herpes simplex, type 2**
N 0.00 0.00 FUD XXX

86698 **histoplasma**
N 0.00 0.00 FUD XXX

86701-86703 Testing for HIV Antibodies

CMS 100-2,15,80 Diagnostic Test Requirements
CMS 100-3,190.9 Serologic Testing for Acquired Immunodeficiency Syndrome (AIDS)
CMS 100-3,190.14 Human Immunodeficiency Virus Testing (Diagnosis)

INCLUDES Qualitative or semiquantitative immunoassays performed by multiple-step methods for the detection of antibodies to infectious agents

EXCLUDES *Confirmatory test for HIV antibody (86689)*
Detection of:
Antibodies other than those to infectious agents, see specific antibody or method
Infectious agent/antigen (87260-87899)
HIV-1 antigen (87390)
HIV-1 antigen(s) with HIV 1 and 2 antibodies, single result (87389)
HIV-2 antigen (87391)
Immunoassays by single-step method (86318)

Code also modifier 92 for test performed using a kit or transportable instrument comprising all or part of a single-use, disposable analytical chamber

86701 **HIV-1**
N 0.00 0.00 FUD XXX

86702 **HIV-2**
N 0.00 0.00 FUD XXX

86703 **HIV-1 and HIV-2, single result**
N 0.00 0.00 FUD XXX

86704-86804 Testing for Infectious Disease Antibodies: Hepatitis—Yersinia

CMS 100-2,15,80 Diagnostic Test Requirements

INCLUDES Qualitative or semiquantitative immunoassays performed by multiple-step methods for the detection of antibodies to infectious agents

EXCLUDES *Detection of:*
Antibodies other than those to infectious agents, see specific antibody or method
Infectious agent/antigen (87260-87899)
Immunoassays by single-step method (86318)

86704 **Hepatitis B core antibody (HBcAb); total**
N 0.00 0.00 FUD XXX

86705 **IgM antibody**
N 0.00 0.00 FUD XXX

86706 **Hepatitis B surface antibody (HBsAb)**
N 0.00 0.00 FUD XXX

86707 **Hepatitis Be antibody (HBeAb)**
N 0.00 0.00 FUD XXX

86708 **Hepatitis A antibody (HAAb); total**
N 0.00 0.00 FUD XXX

86709 **IgM antibody**
N 0.00 0.00 FUD XXX

86710 **Antibody; influenza virus**
N 0.00 0.00 FUD XXX

86711 **JC (John Cunningham) virus**
N 0.00 0.00 FUD XXX

86713 **Legionella**
N 0.00 0.00 FUD XXX

86717 **Leishmania**
N 0.00 0.00 FUD XXX

86720 **Leptospira**
N 0.00 0.00 FUD XXX

86723 **Listeria monocytogenes**
N 0.00 0.00 FUD XXX

86727 **lymphocytic choriomeningitis**
N 0.00 0.00 FUD XXX

86729 **lymphogranuloma venereum**
N 0.00 0.00 FUD XXX

86732 **mucormycosis**
N 0.00 0.00 FUD XXX

86735 mumps
N 0.00 0.00 FUD XXX

86738 mycoplasma
N 0.00 0.00 FUD XXX

86741 Neisseria meningitidis
N 0.00 0.00 FUD XXX

86744 Nocardia
N 0.00 0.00 FUD XXX

86747 parvovirus
N 0.00 0.00 FUD XXX

86750 Plasmodium (malaria)
N 0.00 0.00 FUD XXX

86753 protozoa, not elsewhere specified
N 0.00 0.00 FUD XXX

86756 respiratory syncytial virus
N 0.00 0.00 FUD XXX

86757 Rickettsia
N 0.00 0.00 FUD XXX

86759 rotavirus
N 0.00 0.00 FUD XXX

86762 rubella
N 0.00 0.00 FUD XXX

86765 rubeola
N 0.00 0.00 FUD XXX

86768 Salmonella
N 0.00 0.00 FUD XXX

86771 Shigella
N 0.00 0.00 FUD XXX

86774 tetanus
N 0.00 0.00 FUD XXX

86777 Toxoplasma
N 0.00 0.00 FUD XXX

86778 Toxoplasma, IgM
N 0.00 0.00 FUD XXX

86780 Treponema pallidum
EXCLUDES *Nontreponemal antibody analysis syphilis testing (86592-86593)*
N 0.00 0.00 FUD XXX

86784 Trichinella
N 0.00 0.00 FUD XXX

86787 varicella-zoster
N 0.00 0.00 FUD XXX

86788 West Nile virus, IgM
N 0.00 0.00 FUD XXX

86789 West Nile virus
N 0.00 0.00 FUD XXX

86790 virus, not elsewhere specified
N 0.00 0.00 FUD XXX

86793 Yersinia
N 0.00 0.00 FUD XXX

86800 Thyroglobulin antibody
EXCLUDES *Thyroglobulin (84432)*
N 0.00 0.00 FUD XXX

86803 Hepatitis C antibody;
N 0.00 0.00 FUD XXX

86804 confirmatory test (eg, immunoblot)
N 0.00 0.00 FUD XXX

86805-86808 Pre-Transplant Antibody Cross Matching

CMS 100-2,15,80 Diagnostic Test Requirements

86805 Lymphocytotoxicity assay, visual crossmatch; with titration
N 0.00 0.00 FUD XXX

86806 without titration
N 0.00 0.00 FUD XXX

86807 Serum screening for cytotoxic percent reactive antibody (PRA); standard method
N 0.00 0.00 FUD XXX

86808 quick method
N 0.00 0.00 FUD XXX

86812-86826 Histocompatibility Testing

CMS 100-2,15,80 Diagnostic Test Requirements
CMS 100-3,190.1 Histocompatibility Testing
CMS 100-3,190.8 Lymphocyte Mitogen Response Assays
EXCLUDES *HLA typing by molecular pathology techniques (81370-81383)*

86812 HLA typing; A, B, or C (eg, A10, B7, B27), single antigen
N 0.00 0.00 FUD XXX

86813 A, B, or C, multiple antigens
N 0.00 0.00 FUD XXX

86816 DR/DQ, single antigen
N 0.00 0.00 FUD XXX

86817 DR/DQ, multiple antigens
N 0.00 0.00 FUD XXX

86821 lymphocyte culture, mixed (MLC)
N 0.00 0.00 FUD XXX

86822 lymphocyte culture, primed (PLC)
N 0.00 0.00 FUD XXX

86825 Human leukocyte antigen (HLA) crossmatch, non-cytotoxic (eg, using flow cytometry); first serum sample or dilution
INCLUDES Autologous HLA crossmatch
EXCLUDES *Lymphocytotoxicity visual crossmatch (86805-86806)*
Do not report with (86355, 86359, 88184-88189)
N 0.00 0.00 FUD XXX

+ 86826 each additional serum sample or sample dilution (List separately in addition to primary procedure)
INCLUDES Autologous HLA crossmatch
EXCLUDES *Lymphocytotoxicity visual crossmatch (86805-86806)*
Code first (86825)
Do not report with (86355, 86359, 88184-88189)
N 0.00 0.00 FUD XXX

86828-86849 HLA Antibodies

86828 Antibody to human leukocyte antigens (HLA), solid phase assays (eg, microspheres or beads, ELISA, flow cytometry); qualitative assessment of the presence or absence of antibody(ies) to HLA Class I and Class II HLA antigens
Code also solid phase testing of untreated and treated specimens of either class of HLA after treatment (86828-86833)
N 0.00 0.00 FUD XXX

86829 qualitative assessment of the presence or absence of antibody(ies) to HLA Class I or Class II HLA antigens
Code also solid phase testing of untreated and treated specimens of either class of HLA after treatment (86828-86833)
N 0.00 0.00 FUD XXX

86830 antibody identification by qualitative panel using complete HLA phenotypes, HLA Class I
Code also solid phase testing of untreated and treated specimens of either class of HLA after treatment (86828-86833)
N 0.00 0.00 FUD XXX

86831 antibody identification by qualitative panel using complete HLA phenotypes, HLA Class II
Code also solid phase testing of untreated and treated specimens of either class of HLA after treatment (86828-86833)
N 0.00 0.00 FUD XXX

86832 **high definition qualitative panel for identification of antibody specificities (eg, individual antigen per bead methodology), HLA Class I**
Code also solid phase testing of untreated and treated specimens of either class of HLA after treatment (86828-86833)
N 0.00 0.00 FUD XXX

86833 **high definition qualitative panel for identification of antibody specificities (eg, individual antigen per bead methodology), HLA Class II**
Code also solid phase testing of untreated and treated specimens of either class of HLA after treatment (86828-86833)
N 0.00 0.00 FUD XXX

86834 **semi-quantitative panel (eg, titer), HLA Class I**
N 0.00 0.00 FUD XXX

86835 **semi-quantitative panel (eg, titer), HLA Class II**
N 0.00 0.00 FUD XXX

86849 **Unlisted immunology procedure**
N 0.00 0.00 FUD XXX

86850-86999 Transfusion Services

CMS 100-2,15,80 Diagnostic Test Requirements
CMS 100-3,110.5 Granulocyte Transfusions
CMS 100-3,110.7 Blood Transfusions
CMS 100-3,110.8 Blood Platelet Transfusions

EXCLUDES *Apheresis (36511-36512)*
Therapeutic phlebotomy (99195)

86850 **Antibody screen, RBC, each serum technique**
X 0.00 0.00 FUD XXX

86860 **Antibody elution (RBC), each elution**
X 0.00 0.00 FUD XXX

86870 **Antibody identification, RBC antibodies, each panel for each serum technique**
X 0.00 0.00 FUD XXX

86880 **Antihuman globulin test (Coombs test); direct, each antiserum**
X 0.00 0.00 FUD XXX

86885 **indirect, qualitative, each reagent red cell**
X 0.00 0.00 FUD XXX

86886 **indirect, each antibody titer**
EXCLUDES *Indirect antihuman globulin (Coombs) test for RBC antibody identification using reagent red cell panels (86870)*
Indirect antihuman globulin (Coombs) test for RBC antibody screening (86850)
X 0.00 0.00 FUD XXX

86890 **Autologous blood or component, collection processing and storage; predeposited**
X 0.00 0.00 FUD XXX

86891 **intra- or postoperative salvage**
X 0.00 0.00 FUD XXX

▲ 86900 **Blood typing, serologic; ABO**
X 0.00 0.00 FUD XXX

▲ 86901 **Rh (D)**
X 0.00 0.00 FUD XXX

▲ 86902 **antigen testing of donor blood using reagent serum, each antigen test**
Code also one time for each antigen for each unit when multiple units of blood are tested for the same antigen
X 0.00 0.00 FUD XXX

▲ 86904 **antigen screening for compatible unit using patient serum, per unit screened**
X 0.00 0.00 FUD XXX

▲ 86905 **RBC antigens, other than ABO or Rh (D), each**
X 0.00 0.00 FUD XXX

▲ 86906 **Rh phenotyping, complete**
EXCLUDES *Use of molecular pathology procedures for human erythrocyte antigen typing (81403)*
X 0.00 0.00 FUD XXX

86910 **Blood typing, for paternity testing, per individual; ABO, Rh and MN**
E 0.00 0.00 FUD XXX

86911 **each additional antigen system**
E 0.00 0.00 FUD XXX

86920 **Compatibility test each unit; immediate spin technique**
Code also each antigen for each unit (86902)
Code also same antigen on multiple units (86902)
X 0.00 0.00 FUD XXX

86921 **incubation technique**
X 0.00 0.00 FUD XXX

86922 **antiglobulin technique**
X 0.00 0.00 FUD XXX

86923 **electronic**
Do not report with (86920-86922)
X 0.00 0.00 FUD XXX

86927 **Fresh frozen plasma, thawing, each unit**
S 0.00 0.00 FUD XXX

86930 **Frozen blood, each unit; freezing (includes preparation)**
X 0.00 0.00 FUD XXX

86931 **thawing**
X 0.00 0.00 FUD XXX

86932 **freezing (includes preparation) and thawing**
X 0.00 0.00 FUD XXX

86940 **Hemolysins and agglutinins; auto, screen, each**
N 0.00 0.00 FUD XXX

86941 **incubated**
N 0.00 0.00 FUD XXX

86945 **Irradiation of blood product, each unit**
X 0.00 0.00 FUD XXX

86950 **Leukocyte transfusion**
EXCLUDES *Infusion allogeneic lymphocytes (38242)*
X 0.00 0.00 FUD XXX

86960 **Volume reduction of blood or blood product (eg, red blood cells or platelets), each unit**
X 0.00 0.00 FUD XXX

86965 **Pooling of platelets or other blood products**
EXCLUDES *Injection of platelet rich plasma (0232T)*
X 0.00 0.00 FUD XXX

86970 **Pretreatment of RBCs for use in RBC antibody detection, identification, and/or compatibility testing; incubation with chemical agents or drugs, each**
X 0.00 0.00 FUD XXX

86971 **incubation with enzymes, each**
X 0.00 0.00 FUD XXX

86972 **by density gradient separation**
X 0.00 0.00 FUD XXX

86975 **Pretreatment of serum for use in RBC antibody identification; incubation with drugs, each**
X 0.00 0.00 FUD XXX

86976 **by dilution**
X 0.00 0.00 FUD XXX

86977 **incubation with inhibitors, each**
X 0.00 0.00 FUD XXX

86978 **by differential red cell absorption using patient RBCs or RBCs of known phenotype, each absorption**
X 0.00 0.00 FUD XXX

86985 **Splitting of blood or blood products, each unit**
X 0.00 0.00 FUD XXX

86999 Unlisted transfusion medicine procedure
X 0.00 0.00 FUD XXX

87001-87118 Identification of Microorganisms

CMS 100-2,15,80 Diagnostic Test Requirements
CMS 100-3,190.12 Urine Culture, Bacterial
INCLUDES Bacteriology, mycology, parasitology, and virology
EXCLUDES *Additional tests using molecular probes, chromatography, nucleic acid resequencing, or immunologic techniques (87140-87158)*
Code also modifier 59 for multiple specimens or sites
Code also modifier 91 for repeat procedures performed on the same day

~~87001 Animal inoculation, small animal; with observation~~

87003 Animal inoculation, small animal, with observation and dissection
N 0.00 0.00 FUD XXX

87015 Concentration (any type), for infectious agents
Do not report with (87177)
N 0.00 0.00 FUD XXX

87040 Culture, bacterial; blood, aerobic, with isolation and presumptive identification of isolates (includes anaerobic culture, if appropriate)
N 0.00 0.00 FUD XXX

87045 stool, aerobic, with isolation and preliminary examination (eg, KIA, LIA), Salmonella and Shigella species
N 0.00 0.00 FUD XXX

87046 stool, aerobic, additional pathogens, isolation and presumptive identification of isolates, each plate
N 0.00 0.00 FUD XXX

87070 any other source except urine, blood or stool, aerobic, with isolation and presumptive identification of isolates
EXCLUDES *Urine (87088)*
N 0.00 0.00 FUD XXX

87071 quantitative, aerobic with isolation and presumptive identification of isolates, any source except urine, blood or stool
EXCLUDES *Urine (87088)*
N 0.00 0.00 FUD XXX

87073 quantitative, anaerobic with isolation and presumptive identification of isolates, any source except urine, blood or stool
EXCLUDES *Definitive identification of isolates (87076 or 87077)*
Typing of isolates (87140-87158)
N 0.00 0.00 FUD XXX

87075 any source, except blood, anaerobic with isolation and presumptive identification of isolates
N 0.00 0.00 FUD XXX

87076 anaerobic isolate, additional methods required for definitive identification, each isolate
N 0.00 0.00 FUD XXX

87077 aerobic isolate, additional methods required for definitive identification, each isolate
N 0.00 0.00 FUD XXX

87081 Culture, presumptive, pathogenic organisms, screening only;
N 0.00 0.00 FUD XXX

87084 with colony estimation from density chart
N 0.00 0.00 FUD XXX

87086 Culture, bacterial; quantitative colony count, urine
N 0.00 0.00 FUD XXX

87088 with isolation and presumptive identification of each isolate, urine
N 0.00 0.00 FUD XXX

87101 Culture, fungi (mold or yeast) isolation, with presumptive identification of isolates; skin, hair, or nail
N 0.00 0.00 FUD XXX

87102 other source (except blood)
N 0.00 0.00 FUD XXX

87103 blood
N 0.00 0.00 FUD XXX

87106 Culture, fungi, definitive identification, each organism; yeast
Code also (87101-87103)
N 0.00 0.00 FUD XXX

87107 mold
N 0.00 0.00 FUD XXX

87109 Culture, mycoplasma, any source
N 0.00 0.00 FUD XXX

87110 Culture, chlamydia, any source
EXCLUDES *Immunofluorescence staining of shell vials (87140)*
N 0.00 0.00 FUD XXX

87116 Culture, tubercle or other acid-fast bacilli (eg, TB, AFB, mycobacteria) any source, with isolation and presumptive identification of isolates
EXCLUDES *Concentration (87015)*
N 0.00 0.00 FUD XXX

87118 Culture, mycobacterial, definitive identification, each isolate
EXCLUDES *GLC HPLC identification (87143)*
Nucleic acid probe identification (87149)
N 0.00 0.00 FUD XXX

87140-87158 Additional Culture Typing Techniques

CMS 100-2,15,80 Diagnostic Test Requirements
INCLUDES Bacteriology, mycology, parasitology, and virology
Code also definitive identification
Code also modifier 59 for multiple specimens or sites
Code also modifier 91 for repeat procedures performed on the same day
Do not report molecular procedure codes as a substitute for codes in this range (81200-81408 [81161, 81287, 81288])

87140 Culture, typing; immunofluorescent method, each antiserum
N 0.00 0.00 FUD XXX

87143 gas liquid chromatography (GLC) or high pressure liquid chromatography (HPLC) method
N 0.00 0.00 FUD XXX

87147 immunologic method, other than immunofluoresence (eg, agglutination grouping), per antiserum
N 0.00 0.00 FUD XXX

87149 identification by nucleic acid (DNA or RNA) probe, direct probe technique, per culture or isolate, each organism probed
Do not report with (81200-81408 [81161, 81287, 81288])
N 0.00 0.00 FUD XXX

87150 identification by nucleic acid (DNA or RNA) probe, amplified probe technique, per culture or isolate, each organism probed
Do not report with (81200-81408 [81161, 81287, 81288])
N 0.00 0.00 FUD XXX

87152 identification by pulse field gel typing
Do not report with (81200-81408 [81161, 81287, 81288])
N 0.00 0.00 FUD XXX

87153 identification by nucleic acid sequencing method, each isolate (eg, sequencing of the 16S rRNA gene)
N 0.00 0.00 FUD XXX

87158 other methods
N 0.00 0.00 FUD XXX

87164-87255 Identification of Organism from Primary Source and Sensitivity Studies

CMS 100-2,15,80 Diagnostic Test Requirements

INCLUDES Bacteriology, mycology, parasitology, and virology

EXCLUDES *Additional tests using molecular probes, chromatography, or immunologic techniques (87140-87158)*

Code also modifier 59 for multiple specimens or sites
Code also modifier 91 for repeat procedures performed on the same day

87164 **Dark field examination, any source (eg, penile, vaginal, oral, skin); includes specimen collection**
N 0.00 0.00 FUD XXX

87166 **without collection**
N 0.00 0.00 FUD XXX

87168 **Macroscopic examination; arthropod**
N 0.00 0.00 FUD XXX

87169 **parasite**
N 0.00 0.00 FUD XXX

87172 **Pinworm exam (eg, cellophane tape prep)**
N 0.00 0.00 FUD XXX

87176 **Homogenization, tissue, for culture**
N 0.00 0.00 FUD XXX

87177 **Ova and parasites, direct smears, concentration and identification**
EXCLUDES *Coccidia or microsporidia exam (87207)*
Complex special stain (trichrome, iron hematoxylin) (87209)
Direct smears from primary source (87207)
Nucleic acid probes in cytologic material (88365)
Do not report with (87015)
N 0.00 0.00 FUD XXX

87181 **Susceptibility studies, antimicrobial agent; agar dilution method, per agent (eg, antibiotic gradient strip)**
N 0.00 0.00 FUD XXX

87184 **disk method, per plate (12 or fewer agents)**
N 0.00 0.00 FUD XXX

87185 **enzyme detection (eg, beta lactamase), per enzyme**
N 0.00 0.00 FUD XXX

87186 **microdilution or agar dilution (minimum inhibitory concentration [MIC] or breakpoint), each multi-antimicrobial, per plate**
N 0.00 0.00 FUD XXX

\+ **87187** **microdilution or agar dilution, minimum lethal concentration (MLC), each plate (List separately in addition to code for primary procedure)**
Code first (87186 or 87188)
N 0.00 0.00 FUD XXX

87188 **macrobroth dilution method, each agent**
N 0.00 0.00 FUD XXX

87190 **mycobacteria, proportion method, each agent**
EXCLUDES *Other mycobacterial susceptibility studies (87181, 87184, 87186 or 87188)*
N 0.00 0.00 FUD XXX

87197 **Serum bactericidal titer (Schlicter test)**
N 0.00 0.00 FUD XXX

87205 **Smear, primary source with interpretation; Gram or Giemsa stain for bacteria, fungi, or cell types**
N 0.00 0.00 FUD XXX

87206 **fluorescent and/or acid fast stain for bacteria, fungi, parasites, viruses or cell types**
N 0.00 0.00 FUD XXX

87207 **special stain for inclusion bodies or parasites (eg, malaria, coccidia, microsporidia, trypanosomes, herpes viruses)**
EXCLUDES *Direct smears with concentration and identification (87177)*
Fat, meat, fibers, nasal eosinophils, and starch (see miscellaneous section)
Thick smear preparation (87015)
N 0.00 0.00 FUD XXX

87209 **complex special stain (eg, trichrome, iron hemotoxylin) for ova and parasites**
N 0.00 0.00 FUD XXX

87210 **wet mount for infectious agents (eg, saline, India ink, KOH preps)**
EXCLUDES *KOH evaluation of skin, hair, or nails (87220)*
N 0.00 0.00 FUD XXX

87220 **Tissue examination by KOH slide of samples from skin, hair, or nails for fungi or ectoparasite ova or mites (eg, scabies)**
N 0.00 0.00 FUD XXX

87230 **Toxin or antitoxin assay, tissue culture (eg, Clostridium difficile toxin)**
N 0.00 0.00 FUD XXX

87250 **Virus isolation; inoculation of embryonated eggs, or small animal, includes observation and dissection**
N 0.00 0.00 FUD XXX

87252 **tissue culture inoculation, observation, and presumptive identification by cytopathic effect**
N 0.00 0.00 FUD XXX

87253 **tissue culture, additional studies or definitive identification (eg, hemabsorption, neutralization, immunofluoresence stain), each isolate**
EXCLUDES *Electron microscopy (88348)*
Inclusion bodies in:
Fluids (88106)
Smears (87207-87210)
Tissue sections (88304-88309)
N 0.00 0.00 FUD XXX

87254 **centrifuge enhanced (shell vial) technique, includes identification with immunofluorescence stain, each virus**
Code also (87252)
N 0.00 0.00 FUD XXX

87255 **including identification by non-immunologic method, other than by cytopathic effect (eg, virus specific enzymatic activity)**
N 0.00 0.00 FUD XXX

87260-87300 Fluorescence Microscopy by Organism

CMS 100-2,15,80 Diagnostic Test Requirements

INCLUDES Primary source only

EXCLUDES *Comparable tests on culture material (87140-87158)*
Identification of antibodies (86602-86804)
Nonspecific agent detection (87299, 87449-87450, 87797-87799, 87899)

Code also modifier 59 for different species or strains reported by the same code

87260 **Infectious agent antigen detection by immunofluorescent technique; adenovirus**
N 0.00 0.00 FUD XXX

87265 **Bordetella pertussis/parapertussis**
N 0.00 0.00 FUD XXX

87267 **Enterovirus, direct fluorescent antibody (DFA)**
N 0.00 0.00 FUD XXX

87269 **giardia**
N 0.00 0.00 FUD XXX

87270 **Chlamydia trachomatis**
N 0.00 0.00 FUD XXX

87271 **Cytomegalovirus, direct fluorescent antibody (DFA)**
N 0.00 0.00 FUD XXX

87272 cryptosporidium
N 0.00 0.00 FUD XXX

87273 Herpes simplex virus type 2
N 0.00 0.00 FUD XXX

87274 Herpes simplex virus type 1
N 0.00 0.00 FUD XXX

87275 influenza B virus
N 0.00 0.00 FUD XXX

87276 influenza A virus
N 0.00 0.00 FUD XXX

87277 Legionella micdadei
N 0.00 0.00 FUD XXX

87278 Legionella pneumophila
N 0.00 0.00 FUD XXX

87279 Parainfluenza virus, each type
N 0.00 0.00 FUD XXX

87280 respiratory syncytial virus
N 0.00 0.00 FUD XXX

87281 Pneumocystis carinii
N 0.00 0.00 FUD XXX

87283 Rubeola
N 0.00 0.00 FUD XXX

87285 Treponema pallidum
N 0.00 0.00 FUD XXX

87290 Varicella zoster virus
N 0.00 0.00 FUD XXX

87299 not otherwise specified, each organism
N 0.00 0.00 FUD XXX

87300 **Infectious agent antigen detection by immunofluorescent technique, polyvalent for multiple organisms, each polyvalent antiserum**
EXCLUDES *Physician evaluation of infectious disease agents by immunofluorescence (88346)*
N 0.00 0.00 FUD XXX

87301-87451 Enzyme Immunoassay Technique by Organism

INCLUDES Primary source only

EXCLUDES *Comparable tests on culture material (87140-87158)*
Identification of antibodies (86602-86804)
Nonspecific agent detection (87449-87450, 87797-87799, 87899)

Code also modifier 59 for different species or strains reported by the same code

87301 **Infectious agent antigen detection by enzyme immunoassay technique, qualitative or semiquantitative, multiple-step method; adenovirus enteric types 40/41**
N 0.00 0.00 FUD XXX

87305 Aspergillus
N 0.00 0.00 FUD XXX

87320 Chlamydia trachomatis
N 0.00 0.00 FUD XXX

87324 Clostridium difficile toxin(s)
N 0.00 0.00 FUD XXX

87327 Cryptococcus neoformans
EXCLUDES *Cryptococcus latex agglutination (86403)*
N 0.00 0.00 FUD XXX

87328 cryptosporidium
N 0.00 0.00 FUD XXX

87329 giardia
N 0.00 0.00 FUD XXX

87332 cytomegalovirus
N 0.00 0.00 FUD XXX

87335 Escherichia coli 0157
EXCLUDES *Giardia antigen (87329)*
N 0.00 0.00 FUD XXX

87336 Entamoeba histolytica dispar group
N 0.00 0.00 FUD XXX

87337 Entamoeba histolytica group
N 0.00 0.00 FUD XXX

87338 Helicobacter pylori, stool
N 0.00 0.00 FUD XXX

87339 Helicobacter pylori
EXCLUDES *H. pylori:*
Breath and blood by mass spectrometry (83013-83014)
Liquid scintillation counter (78267-78268)
Stool (87338)
N 0.00 0.00 FUD XXX

87340 hepatitis B surface antigen (HBsAg)
N 0.00 0.00 FUD XXX

87341 hepatitis B surface antigen (HBsAg) neutralization
N 0.00 0.00 FUD XXX

87350 hepatitis Be antigen (HBeAg)
N 0.00 0.00 FUD XXX

87380 hepatitis, delta agent
N 0.00 0.00 FUD XXX

87385 Histoplasma capsulatum
N 0.00 0.00 FUD XXX

87389 HIV-1 antigen(s), with HIV-1 and HIV-2 antibodies, single result
Code also modifier 92 for test performed using a kit or transportable instrument that is all or in part consists of a single-use, disposable analytical chamber
N 0.00 0.00 FUD XXX

87390 HIV-1
N 0.00 0.00 FUD XXX

87391 HIV-2
N 0.00 0.00 FUD XXX

87400 Influenza, A or B, each
N 0.00 0.00 FUD XXX

87420 respiratory syncytial virus
N 0.00 0.00 FUD XXX

87425 rotavirus
N 0.00 0.00 FUD XXX

87427 Shiga-like toxin
N 0.00 0.00 FUD XXX

87430 Streptococcus, group A
N 0.00 0.00 FUD XXX

87449 **Infectious agent antigen detection by enzyme immunoassay technique qualitative or semiquantitative; multiple step method, not otherwise specified, each organism**
N 0.00 0.00 FUD XXX

87450 single step method, not otherwise specified, each organism
N 0.00 0.00 FUD XXX

87451 multiple step method, polyvalent for multiple organisms, each polyvalent antiserum
N 0.00 0.00 FUD XXX

87470-87801 [87623, 87624, 87625] Detection Infectious Agent by Probe Techniques

INCLUDES Primary source only

EXCLUDES *Comparable tests on culture material (87140-87158)*
Identification of antibodies (86602-86804)
Nonspecific agent detection (87299, 87449-87450, 87797-87799, 87899)

Code only modifier 59 for different species or strains reported by the same code
Do not report molecular procedure codes as substitute or with codes in this range (81200-81408 [81161, 81287, 81288])

87470 **Infectious agent detection by nucleic acid (DNA or RNA); Bartonella henselae and Bartonella quintana, direct probe technique**
N 0.00 0.00 FUD XXX

87471 Bartonella henselae and Bartonella quintana, amplified probe technique
N 0.00 0.00 FUD XXX

87472 Bartonella henselae and Bartonella quintana, quantification
N 0.00 0.00 FUD XXX

87475 Borrelia burgdorferi, direct probe technique
N 0.00 0.00 FUD XXX

87476 Borrelia burgdorferi, amplified probe technique
N 0.00 0.00 FUD XXX

87477 Borrelia burgdorferi, quantification
N 0.00 0.00 FUD XXX

87480 Candida species, direct probe technique
N 0.00 0.00 FUD XXX

87481 Candida species, amplified probe technique
N 0.00 0.00 FUD XXX

87482 Candida species, quantification
N 0.00 0.00 FUD XXX

87485 Chlamydia pneumoniae, direct probe technique
N 0.00 0.00 FUD XXX

87486 Chlamydia pneumoniae, amplified probe technique
N 0.00 0.00 FUD XXX

87487 Chlamydia pneumoniae, quantification
N 0.00 0.00 FUD XXX

87490 Chlamydia trachomatis, direct probe technique
N 0.00 0.00 FUD XXX

87491 Chlamydia trachomatis, amplified probe technique
N 0.00 0.00 FUD XXX

87492 Chlamydia trachomatis, quantification
N 0.00 0.00 FUD XXX

87493 Clostridium difficile, toxin gene(s), amplified probe technique
N 0.00 0.00 FUD XXX

87495 cytomegalovirus, direct probe technique
N 0.00 0.00 FUD XXX

87496 cytomegalovirus, amplified probe technique
N 0.00 0.00 FUD XXX

87497 cytomegalovirus, quantification
N 0.00 0.00 FUD XXX

87498 enterovirus, amplified probe technique, includes reverse transcription when performed
N 0.00 0.00 FUD XXX

87500 vancomycin resistance (eg, enterococcus species van A, van B), amplified probe technique
N 0.00 0.00 FUD XXX

▲ 87501 influenza virus, includes reverse transcription, when performed, and amplified probe technique, each type or subtype
N 0.00 0.00 FUD XXX

▲ 87502 influenza virus, for multiple types or sub-types, includes multiplex reverse transcription and multiplex amplified probe technique, first 2 types or sub-types
N 0.00 0.00 FUD XXX

+ ▲ 87503 influenza virus, for multiple types or sub-types, includes multiplex reverse transcription and multiplex amplified probe technique, each additional influenza virus type or sub-type beyond 2 (List separately in addition to code for primary procedure)
Code first (87502)
N 0.00 0.00 FUD XXX

● 87505 gastrointestinal pathogen (eg, Clostridium difficile, E. coli, Salmonella, Shigella, norovirus, Giardia), includes multiplex reverse transcription, when performed, and multiplex amplified probe technique, multiple types or subtypes, 3-5 targets

● 87506 gastrointestinal pathogen (eg, Clostridium difficile, E. coli, Salmonella, Shigella, norovirus, Giardia), includes multiplex reverse transcription, when performed, and multiplex amplified probe technique, multiple types or subtypes, 6-11 targets

● 87507 gastrointestinal pathogen (eg, Clostridium difficile, E. coli, Salmonella, Shigella, norovirus, Giardia), includes multiplex reverse transcription, when performed, and multiplex amplified probe technique, multiple types or subtypes, 12-25 targets

87510 Gardnerella vaginalis, direct probe technique
N 0.00 0.00 FUD XXX

87511 Gardnerella vaginalis, amplified probe technique
N 0.00 0.00 FUD XXX

87512 Gardnerella vaginalis, quantification
N 0.00 0.00 FUD XXX

87515 hepatitis B virus, direct probe technique
N 0.00 0.00 FUD XXX

87516 hepatitis B virus, amplified probe technique
N 0.00 0.00 FUD XXX

87517 hepatitis B virus, quantification
N 0.00 0.00 FUD XXX

87520 hepatitis C, direct probe technique
N 0.00 0.00 FUD XXX

87521 hepatitis C, amplified probe technique, includes reverse transcription when performed
N 0.00 0.00 FUD XXX

87522 hepatitis C, quantification, includes reverse transcription when performed
N 0.00 0.00 FUD XXX

87525 hepatitis G, direct probe technique
N 0.00 0.00 FUD XXX

87526 hepatitis G, amplified probe technique
N 0.00 0.00 FUD XXX

87527 hepatitis G, quantification
N 0.00 0.00 FUD XXX

87528 Herpes simplex virus, direct probe technique
N 0.00 0.00 FUD XXX

87529 Herpes simplex virus, amplified probe technique
N 0.00 0.00 FUD XXX

87530 Herpes simplex virus, quantification
N 0.00 0.00 FUD XXX

87531 Herpes virus-6, direct probe technique
N 0.00 0.00 FUD XXX

87532 Herpes virus-6, amplified probe technique
N 0.00 0.00 FUD XXX

87533 Herpes virus-6, quantification
N 0.00 0.00 FUD XXX

87534 HIV-1, direct probe technique
N 0.00 0.00 FUD XXX

87535 HIV-1, amplified probe technique, includes reverse transcription when performed
N 0.00 0.00 FUD XXX

87536 HIV-1, quantification, includes reverse transcription when performed
N 0.00 0.00 FUD XXX

87537 HIV-2, direct probe technique
N 0.00 0.00 FUD XXX

87538 HIV-2, amplified probe technique, includes reverse transcription when performed
N 0.00 0.00 FUD XXX

87539 HIV-2, quantification, includes reverse transcription when performed
N 0.00 0.00 FUD XXX

#● 87623 Human Papillomavirus (HPV), low-risk types (eg, 6, 11, 42, 43, 44)

#● 87624 Human Papillomavirus (HPV), high-risk types (eg, 16, 18, 31, 33, 35, 39, 45, 51, 52, 56, 58, 59, 68)
INCLUDES Low- and high-risk types in one assay

#● 87625 Human Papillomavirus (HPV), types 16 and 18 only, includes type 45, if performed

87540 Legionella pneumophila, direct probe technique
N 0.00 0.00 FUD XXX

87541 Legionella pneumophila, amplified probe technique
N 0.00 0.00 FUD XXX

87542 Legionella pneumophila, quantification
N 0.00 0.00 FUD XXX

87550 Mycobacteria species, direct probe technique
N 0.00 0.00 FUD XXX

87551 Mycobacteria species, amplified probe technique
N 0.00 0.00 FUD XXX

87552 Mycobacteria species, quantification
N 0.00 0.00 FUD XXX

87555 Mycobacteria tuberculosis, direct probe technique
N 0.00 0.00 FUD XXX

87556 Mycobacteria tuberculosis, amplified probe technique
N 0.00 0.00 FUD XXX

87557 Mycobacteria tuberculosis, quantification
N 0.00 0.00 FUD XXX

87560 Mycobacteria avium-intracellulare, direct probe technique
N 0.00 0.00 FUD XXX

87561 Mycobacteria avium-intracellulare, amplified probe technique
N 0.00 0.00 FUD XXX

87562 Mycobacteria avium-intracellulare, quantification
N 0.00 0.00 FUD XXX

87580 Mycoplasma pneumoniae, direct probe technique
N 0.00 0.00 FUD XXX

87581 Mycoplasma pneumoniae, amplified probe technique
N 0.00 0.00 FUD XXX

87582 Mycoplasma pneumoniae, quantification
N 0.00 0.00 FUD XXX

87590 Neisseria gonorrhoeae, direct probe technique
N 0.00 0.00 FUD XXX

87591 Neisseria gonorrhoeae, amplified probe technique
N 0.00 0.00 FUD XXX

87592 Neisseria gonorrhoeae, quantification
N 0.00 0.00 FUD XXX

~~87620 papillomavirus, human, direct probe technique~~
To report, see 87623-87625

~~87621 papillomavirus, human, amplified probe technique~~
To report, see 87623-87625

~~87622 papillomavirus, human, quantification~~
To report, see 87623-87625

87623 Resequenced code. See code following 87539.

87624 Resequenced code. See code following 87539.

87625 Resequenced code. See code before 87540.

▲ 87631 respiratory virus (eg, adenovirus, influenza virus, coronavirus, metapneumovirus, parainfluenza virus, respiratory syncytial virus, rhinovirus), includes multiplex reverse transcription, when performed, and multiplex amplified probe technique, multiple types or subtypes, 3-5 targets
INCLUDES Detection of multiple respiratory viruses with one test
EXCLUDES *Assays for typing or subtyping influenza viruses only (87501-87503)*
Single test for detection of multiple infectious organisms (87800-87801)
N 0.00 0.00 FUD XXX

▲ 87632 respiratory virus (eg, adenovirus, influenza virus, coronavirus, metapneumovirus, parainfluenza virus, respiratory syncytial virus, rhinovirus), includes multiplex reverse transcription, when performed, and multiplex amplified probe technique, multiple types or subtypes, 6-11 targets
INCLUDES Detection of multiple respiratory viruses with one test
EXCLUDES *Assays for typing or subtyping influenza viruses only (87501-87503)*
Single test to detect multiple infectious organisms (87800-87801)
N 0.00 0.00 FUD XXX

▲ 87633 respiratory virus (eg, adenovirus, influenza virus, coronavirus, metapneumovirus, parainfluenza virus, respiratory syncytial virus, rhinovirus), includes multiplex reverse transcription, when performed, and multiplex amplified probe technique, multiple types or subtypes, 12-25 targets
INCLUDES Detection of multiple respiratory viruses with one test
EXCLUDES *Assays for typing or subtyping influenza viruses only (87501-87503)*
Single test to detect multiple infectious organisms (87800-87801)
N 0.00 0.00 FUD XXX

87640 Staphylococcus aureus, amplified probe technique
N 0.00 0.00 FUD XXX

87641 Staphylococcus aureus, methicillin resistant, amplified probe technique
EXCLUDES *Assays that detect methicillin resistance and identify Staphylococcus aureus using a single nucleic acid sequence (87641)*
N 0.00 0.00 FUD XXX

87650 Streptococcus, group A, direct probe technique
N 0.00 0.00 FUD XXX

87651 Streptococcus, group A, amplified probe technique
N 0.00 0.00 FUD XXX

87652 Streptococcus, group A, quantification
N 0.00 0.00 FUD XXX

87653 Streptococcus, group B, amplified probe technique
N 0.00 0.00 FUD XXX

87660 Trichomonas vaginalis, direct probe technique
N 0.00 0.00 FUD XXX

87661 Trichomonas vaginalis, amplified probe technique
A 0.00 0.00 FUD XXX

87797 Infectious agent detection by nucleic acid (DNA or RNA), not otherwise specified; direct probe technique, each organism
N 0.00 0.00 FUD XXX

87798 amplified probe technique, each organism
N 0.00 0.00 FUD XXX

87799 quantification, each organism
N 0.00 0.00 FUD XXX

87800 Infectious agent detection by nucleic acid (DNA or RNA), multiple organisms; direct probe(s) technique
INCLUDES Single test to detect multiple infectious organisms
EXCLUDES *Detection of specific infectious agents not otherwise specified (87797-87799)*
Each specific organism nucleic acid detection from a primary source (87470-87660)
N 0.00 0.00 FUD XXX

87801 amplified probe(s) technique
INCLUDES Single test to detect multiple infectious organisms
EXCLUDES *Detection of multiple respiratory viruses with one test (87631-87633)*
Detection of specific infectious agents not otherwise specified (87797-87799)
Each specific organism nucleic acid detection from a primary source (87470-87660)
N 0.00 0.00 FUD XXX

87802-87880 [87806] Detection Infectious Agent by Immunoassay with Direct Optical Observation

87802 Infectious agent antigen detection by immunoassay with direct optical observation; Streptococcus, group B
N 0.00 0.00 FUD XXX

87803 Clostridium difficile toxin A
N 0.00 0.00 FUD XXX

#● 87806 Infectious agent antigen detection by immunoassay with direct optical observation; HIV-1 antigen(s), with HIV-1 and HIV-2 antibodies

87804 Influenza
N 0.00 0.00 FUD XXX

87806 Resequenced code. See code following 87803.

87807 respiratory syncytial virus
N 0.00 0.00 FUD XXX

87808 Trichomonas vaginalis
N 0.00 0.00 FUD XXX

87809 adenovirus
N 0.00 0.00 FUD XXX

87810 Chlamydia trachomatis
N 0.00 0.00 FUD XXX

87850 Neisseria gonorrhoeae
N 0.00 0.00 FUD XXX

87880 Streptococcus, group A
N 0.00 0.00 FUD XXX

87899 not otherwise specified
N 0.00 0.00 FUD XXX

87900-87999 [87906, 87910, 87912] Drug Sensitivity Genotype/Phenotype

87900 Infectious agent drug susceptibility phenotype prediction using regularly updated genotypic bioinformatics
N 0.00 0.00 FUD XXX

87910 Infectious agent genotype analysis by nucleic acid (DNA or RNA); cytomegalovirus
N 0.00 0.00 FUD XXX

87901 HIV-1, reverse transcriptase and protease regions
EXCLUDES *Infectious agent drug susceptibility phenotype prediction for HIV-1 (87900)*
N 0.00 0.00 FUD XXX

87906 HIV-1, other region (eg, integrase, fusion)
N 0.00 0.00 FUD XXX

87912 Hepatitis B virus
N 0.00 0.00 FUD XXX

87902 Hepatitis C virus
N 0.00 0.00 FUD XXX

87903 Infectious agent phenotype analysis by nucleic acid (DNA or RNA) with drug resistance tissue culture analysis, HIV 1; first through 10 drugs tested
N 0.00 0.00 FUD XXX

+ 87904 each additional drug tested (List separately in addition to code for primary procedure)
Code first (87903)
N 0.00 0.00 FUD XXX

87905 Infectious agent enzymatic activity other than virus (eg, sialidase activity in vaginal fluid)
EXCLUDES *Isolation of a virus identified by a nonimmunologic method, and by noncytopathic effect (87255)*
N 0.00 0.00 FUD XXX

87906 Resequenced code. See code following 87901.

87910 Resequenced code. See code following 87900.

87912 Resequenced code. See code before 87902.

87999 Unlisted microbiology procedure
N 0.00 0.00 FUD XXX

88000-88099 Autopsy Services

CMS 100-1,5,90.2 Laboratory Defined
CMS 100-2,15,80 Diagnostic Test Requirements
CMS 100-2,15,80.1 Payment for Clinical Laboratory Services
CMS 100-4,16,110.4 Carrier Contacts With Independent Clinical Laboratories
CMS 100-4,16,110.4 Laboratory Definitions
INCLUDES Services for physicians only

88000 Necropsy (autopsy), gross examination only; without CNS
E 0.00 0.00 FUD XXX

88005 with brain
E 0.00 0.00 FUD XXX

88007 with brain and spinal cord
E 0.00 0.00 FUD XXX

88012 infant with brain
E 0.00 0.00 FUD XXX A

88014 stillborn or newborn with brain
E 0.00 0.00 FUD XXX A

88016 macerated stillborn
E 0.00 0.00 FUD XXX A

88020 Necropsy (autopsy), gross and microscopic; without CNS
E 0.00 0.00 FUD XXX

88025 with brain
E 0.00 0.00 FUD XXX

88027 with brain and spinal cord
E 0.00 0.00 FUD XXX

88028 infant with brain
E 0.00 0.00 FUD XXX

88029 stillborn or newborn with brain
E 0.00 0.00 FUD XXX

88036 Necropsy (autopsy), limited, gross and/or microscopic; regional
E 0.00 0.00 FUD XXX

88037 single organ
E 0.00 0.00 FUD XXX

88040 Necropsy (autopsy); forensic examination
E 0.00 0.00 FUD XXX

88045 coroner's call
E 0.00 0.00 FUD XXX

88099 Unlisted necropsy (autopsy) procedure
E 0.00 0.00 FUD XXX

88104-88140 Cytopathology: Other Than Cervical/Vaginal

CMS 100-2,15,80 Diagnostic Test Requirements
CMS 100-4,12,60 Payment for Pathology Services

88104 Cytopathology, fluids, washings or brushings, except cervical or vaginal; smears with interpretation
X 80 2.07 2.07 FUD XXX

88106 simple filter method with interpretation
EXCLUDES *Selective cellular enhancement (nongynecological) including filter transfer techniques (88112)*
Do not report with (88104)
X 80 2.36 2.36 FUD XXX

88108 Cytopathology, concentration technique, smears and interpretation (eg, Saccomanno technique)
EXCLUDES *Cervical or vaginal smears (88150-88155)*
Gastric intubation with lavage (43754-43755)
74340
X 80 2.20 2.20 FUD XXX

88112 Cytopathology, selective cellular enhancement technique with interpretation (eg, liquid based slide preparation method), except cervical or vaginal
Do not report with (88108)
X 80 1.76 1.76 FUD XXX

88120 Cytopathology, in situ hybridization (eg, FISH), urinary tract specimen with morphometric analysis, 3-5 molecular probes, each specimen; manual
EXCLUDES *More than five probes (88399)*
Morphometric in situ hybridization on specimens other than urinary tract (88367-88368)
X 80 17.27 17.27 FUD XXX

88121 using computer-assisted technology
EXCLUDES *More than five probes (88399)*
Morphometric in situ hybridization on specimens other than urinary tract (88367-88368)
X 80 14.94 14.94 FUD XXX

88125 Cytopathology, forensic (eg, sperm)
X 80 0.62 0.62 FUD XXX

88130 Sex chromatin identification; Barr bodies
N 0.00 0.00 FUD XXX

88140 peripheral blood smear, polymorphonuclear drumsticks
EXCLUDES *Guard stain (88313)*
N 0.00 0.00 FUD XXX

88141-88155 Pap Smears

CMS 100-2,15,80 Diagnostic Test Requirements
CMS 100-3,190.2 Diagnostic Pap Smears
CMS 100-3,210.2 Screening Pap Smears/Pelvic Examinations for Early Cancer Detection

88141 Cytopathology, cervical or vaginal (any reporting system), requiring interpretation by physician ♀
Code also (88142-88154, 88164-88167, 88174-88175)
N 26 80 0.89 0.89 FUD XXX

88142 Cytopathology, cervical or vaginal (any reporting system), collected in preservative fluid, automated thin layer preparation; manual screening under physician supervision ♀
INCLUDES Bethesda or non-Bethesda method
N 0.00 0.00 FUD XXX

88143 with manual screening and rescreening under physician supervision ♀
INCLUDES Bethesda or non-Bethesda method
EXCLUDES *Automated screening of automated thin layer preparation (88174-88175)*
N 0.00 0.00 FUD XXX

88147 Cytopathology smears, cervical or vaginal; screening by automated system under physician supervision ♀
N 0.00 0.00 FUD XXX

88148 screening by automated system with manual rescreening under physician supervision ♀
N 0.00 0.00 FUD XXX

88150 Cytopathology, slides, cervical or vaginal; manual screening under physician supervision ♀
EXCLUDES *Bethesda method Pap smears (88164-88167)*
N 0.00 0.00 FUD XXX

88152 with manual screening and computer-assisted rescreening under physician supervision ♀
EXCLUDES *Bethesda method Pap smears (88164-88167)*
N 0.00 0.00 FUD XXX

88153 with manual screening and rescreening under physician supervision ♀
EXCLUDES *Bethesda method Pap smears (88164-88167)*
N 0.00 0.00 FUD XXX

88154 with manual screening and computer-assisted rescreening using cell selection and review under physician supervision ♀
EXCLUDES *Bethesda method Pap smears (88164-88167)*
N 0.00 0.00 FUD XXX

+ 88155 Cytopathology, slides, cervical or vaginal, definitive hormonal evaluation (eg, maturation index, karyopyknotic index, estrogenic index) (List separately in addition to code[s] for other technical and interpretation services) ♀
Code first (88142-88154, 88164-88167, 88174-88175)
N 0.00 0.00 FUD XXX

88160-88162 Cytopathology Smears (Other Than Pap)

CMS 100-2,15,80 Diagnostic Test Requirements
CMS 100-4,12,60 Payment for Pathology Services

88160 Cytopathology, smears, any other source; screening and interpretation
X 80 1.80 1.80 FUD XXX

88161 preparation, screening and interpretation
X 80 1.64 1.64 FUD XXX

88162 extended study involving over 5 slides and/or multiple stains
EXCLUDES *Aerosol collection of sputum (89220)*
Special stains (88312-88314)
X 80 2.69 2.69 FUD XXX

88164-88167 Pap Smears: Bethesda System

CMS 100-2,15,80 Diagnostic Test Requirements
CMS 100-3,190.2 Diagnostic Pap Smears
CMS 100-3,210.2 Screening Pap Smears/Pelvic Examinations for Early Cancer Detection

EXCLUDES *Non-Bethesda method (88150-88154)*

88164 Cytopathology, slides, cervical or vaginal (the Bethesda System); manual screening under physician supervision ♀
N 0.00 0.00 FUD XXX

88165 **with manual screening and rescreening under physician supervision** ♀
N 0.00 0.00 FUD XXX

88166 **with manual screening and computer-assisted rescreening under physician supervision** ♀
N 0.00 0.00 FUD XXX

88167 **with manual screening and computer-assisted rescreening using cell selection and review under physician supervision** ♀
EXCLUDES *Fine needle aspiration (10021-10022)*
N 0.00 0.00 FUD XXX

88172-88177 [88177] Cytopathology of Needle Biopsy

CMS 100-2,15,80 Diagnostic Test Requirements
CMS 100-4,12,60 Payment for Pathology Services

EXCLUDES *Fine needle aspiration (10021-10022)*

88172 **Cytopathology, evaluation of fine needle aspirate; immediate cytohistologic study to determine adequacy for diagnosis, first evaluation episode, each site**
INCLUDES The submission of a complete set of cytologic material for evaluation regardless of the number of needle passes performed or slides prepared from each site
Do not report with same specimen (88333-88334)
X 80 1.52 1.52 FUD XXX

88173 **interpretation and report**
INCLUDES The interpretation and report from each anatomical site no matter how many passes or evaluation episodes are performed during the aspiration
EXCLUDES *Fine needle aspiration (10021-10022)*
Do not report with same specimen (88333-88334)
X 80 4.10 4.10 FUD XXX

+ # 88177 **immediate cytohistologic study to determine adequacy for diagnosis, each separate additional evaluation episode, same site (List separately in addition to code for primary procedure)**
Code also each additional immediate repeat evaluation episode(s) required from the same site (e.g., previous sample is inadequate)
Code first (88172)
N 80 0.83 0.83 FUD ZZZ

88174-88177 Pap Smears: Automated Screening

CMS 100-2,15,80 Diagnostic Test Requirements
CMS 100-3,190.2 Diagnostic Pap Smears
CMS 100-3,210.2 Screening Pap Smears/Pelvic Examinations for Early Cancer Detection

88174 **Cytopathology, cervical or vaginal (any reporting system), collected in preservative fluid, automated thin layer preparation; screening by automated system, under physician supervision** ♀
INCLUDES Bethesda or non-Bethesda method
N 0.00 0.00 FUD XXX

88175 **with screening by automated system and manual rescreening or review, under physician supervision** ♀
INCLUDES Bethesda or non-Bethesda method
EXCLUDES *Manual screening (88142-88143)*
N 0.00 0.00 FUD XXX

88177 Resequenced code, See code following 88173.

88182-88199 Cytopathology Using the Fluorescence-Activated Cell Sorter

CMS 100-2,15,80 Diagnostic Test Requirements
CMS 100-4,12,60 Payment for Pathology Services

88182 **Flow cytometry, cell cycle or DNA analysis**
EXCLUDES *DNA ploidy analysis by morphometric technique (88358)*
X 80 3.07 3.07 FUD XXX

88184 **Flow cytometry, cell surface, cytoplasmic, or nuclear marker, technical component only; first marker**
X TC 80 2.45 2.45 FUD XXX

+ 88185 **each additional marker (List separately in addition to code for first marker)**
Code first (88184)
N TC 80 1.50 1.50 FUD ZZZ

88187 **Flow cytometry, interpretation; 2 to 8 markers**
EXCLUDES *Antibody assessment by flow cytometry (83516-83520, 86000-86849 [86152, 86153])*
Cell enumeration by immunologic selection and identification ([86152, 86153])
Interpretation (86355-86357, 86359-86361, 86367)
X 26 80 2.00 2.00 FUD XXX

88188 **9 to 15 markers**
EXCLUDES *Antibody assessment by flow cytometry (83516-83520, 86000-86849 [86152, 86153])*
Cell enumeration by immunologic selection and identification ([86152, 86153])
Interpretation (86355-86357, 86359-86361, 86367)
X 26 80 2.52 2.52 FUD XXX

88189 **16 or more markers**
EXCLUDES *Antibody assessment by flow cytometry (83516-83520, 86000-86849 [86152, 86153])*
Cell enumeration using immunologic selection and identification in fluid sample ([86152, 86153])
Interpretation (86355-86357, 86359-86361, 86367)
X 26 80 3.09 3.09 FUD XXX

88199 **Unlisted cytopathology procedure**
EXCLUDES *Electron microscopy (88348)*
X 80 0.00 0.00 FUD XXX

88230-88299 Cytogenic Studies

CMS 100-1,5,90.2 Laboratory Defined
CMS 100-2,15,80 Diagnostic Test Requirements
CMS 100-2,15,80.1 Payment for Clinical Laboratory Services
CMS 100-3,190.3 Cytogenic Studies
CMS 100-4,16,110.4 Carrier Contacts With Independent Clinical Laboratories
CMS 100-4,16,110.4 Laboratory Definitions

EXCLUDES *Acetylcholinesterase (82013)*
Alpha-fetoprotein (amniotic fluid or serum) (82105-82106)
Microdissection (88380)
Molecular pathology codes (81200-81383 [81161, 81287, 81288], 81400-81408, [81479], 81410-81471, 81500-81512, 81599)

88230 **Tissue culture for non-neoplastic disorders; lymphocyte**
N 0.00 0.00 FUD XXX

88233 **skin or other solid tissue biopsy**
N 0.00 0.00 FUD XXX

88235 **amniotic fluid or chorionic villus cells** M ♀
N 0.00 0.00 FUD XXX

88237 **Tissue culture for neoplastic disorders; bone marrow, blood cells**
N 0.00 0.00 FUD XXX

88239 **solid tumor**
N 0.00 0.00 FUD XXX

88240 **Cryopreservation, freezing and storage of cells, each cell line**
EXCLUDES *Therapeutic cryopreservation and storage (38207)*
N 0.00 0.00 FUD XXX

88241 **Thawing and expansion of frozen cells, each aliquot**
EXCLUDES *Therapeutic thawing of prior harvest (38208)*
N 0.00 0.00 FUD XXX

Pathology and Laboratory

88165 — 88241

88245 Chromosome analysis for breakage syndromes; baseline Sister Chromatid Exchange (SCE), 20-25 cells
N 0.00 0.00 FUD XXX

88248 baseline breakage, score 50-100 cells, count 20 cells, 2 karyotypes (eg, for ataxia telangiectasia, Fanconi anemia, fragile X)
N 0.00 0.00 FUD XXX

88249 score 100 cells, clastogen stress (eg, diepoxybutane, mitomycin C, ionizing radiation, UV radiation)
N 0.00 0.00 FUD XXX

88261 Chromosome analysis; count 5 cells, 1 karyotype, with banding
N 0.00 0.00 FUD XXX

88262 count 15-20 cells, 2 karyotypes, with banding
N 0.00 0.00 FUD XXX

88263 count 45 cells for mosaicism, 2 karyotypes, with banding
N 0.00 0.00 FUD XXX

88264 analyze 20-25 cells
N 0.00 0.00 FUD XXX

88267 Chromosome analysis, amniotic fluid or chorionic villus, count 15 cells, 1 karyotype, with banding M ♀
N 0.00 0.00 FUD XXX

88269 Chromosome analysis, in situ for amniotic fluid cells, count cells from 6-12 colonies, 1 karyotype, with banding M ♀
N 0.00 0.00 FUD XXX

88271 Molecular cytogenetics; DNA probe, each (eg, FISH)
EXCLUDES *Cytogenomic microarray analysis (81228-81229, 81405-81406, 81479)*
N 0.00 0.00 FUD XXX

88272 chromosomal in situ hybridization, analyze 3-5 cells (eg, for derivatives and markers)
N 0.00 0.00 FUD XXX

88273 chromosomal in situ hybridization, analyze 10-30 cells (eg, for microdeletions)
N 0.00 0.00 FUD XXX

88274 interphase in situ hybridization, analyze 25-99 cells
N 0.00 0.00 FUD XXX

88275 interphase in situ hybridization, analyze 100-300 cells
N 0.00 0.00 FUD XXX

88280 Chromosome analysis; additional karyotypes, each study
N 0.00 0.00 FUD XXX

88283 additional specialized banding technique (eg, NOR, C-banding)
N 0.00 0.00 FUD XXX

88285 additional cells counted, each study
N 0.00 0.00 FUD XXX

88289 additional high resolution study
N 0.00 0.00 FUD XXX

88291 Cytogenetics and molecular cytogenetics, interpretation and report
M 26 80 0.87 0.87 FUD XXX

88299 Unlisted cytogenetic study
X 80 0.00 0.00 FUD XXX

88300 Evaluation of Surgical Specimen: Gross Anatomy

CMS 100-1,5,90.2 Laboratory Defined
CMS 100-4,12,60 Payment for Pathology Services
INCLUDES Attainment, examination, and reporting
Unit of service is the specimen
EXCLUDES *Additional procedures (88311-88365, 88399)*
Microscopic exam (88302-88309)

88300 Level I - Surgical pathology, gross examination only
X 80 0.41 0.41 FUD XXX

88302-88309 Evaluation of Surgical Specimens: Gross and Microscopic Anatomy

CMS 100-1,5,90.2 Laboratory Defined
CMS 100-4,12,60 Payment for Pathology Services
INCLUDES Attainment, examination, and reporting
Unit of service is the specimen
EXCLUDES *Additional procedures (88311-88365, 88399)*
Do not report with Mohs surgery (17311-17315)

88302 Level II - Surgical pathology, gross and microscopic examination
INCLUDES Confirming identification and absence of disease:
- Appendix, incidental
- Fallopian tube, sterilization
- Fingers or toes traumatic amputation
- Foreskin, newborn
- Hernia sac, any site
- Hydrocele sac
- Nerve
- Skin, plastic repair
- Sympathetic ganglion
- Testis, castration
- Vaginal mucosa, incidental
- Vas deferens, sterilization

X 80 0.84 0.84 FUD XXX

88304 **Level III - Surgical pathology, gross and microscopic examination**

INCLUDES Abortion, induced
Abscess
Anal tag
Aneurysm-atrial/ventricular
Appendix, other than incidental
Artery, atheromatous plaque
Bartholin's gland cyst
Bone fragment(s), other than pathologic fracture
Bursa/ synovial cyst
Carpal tunnel tissue
Cartilage, shavings
Cholesteatoma
Colon, colostomy stoma
Conjunctiva-biopsy/pterygium
Cornea
Diverticulum-esophagus/small intestine
Dupuytren's contracture tissue
Femoral head, other than fracture
Fissure/fistula
Foreskin, other than newborn
Gallbladder
Ganglion cyst
Hematoma
Hemorrhoids
Hydatid of Morgagni
Intervertebral disc
Joint, loose body
Meniscus
Mucocele, salivary
Neuroma-Morton's/traumatic
Pilonidal cyst/sinus
Polyps, inflammatory-nasal/sinusoidal
Skin-cyst/tag/debridement
Soft tissue, debridement
Soft tissue, lipoma
Spermatocele
Tendon/tendon sheath
Testicular appendage
Thrombus or embolus
Tonsil and/or adenoids
Varicocele
Vas deferens, other than sterilization
Vein, varicosity

X 80 1.21 1.21 FUD XXX

88305 **Level IV - Surgical pathology, gross and microscopic examination**

INCLUDES Abortion, spontaneous/missed
Artery, biopsy
Bone exostosis
Bone marrow, biopsy
Brain/meninges, other than for tumor resection
Breast biopsy without microscopic assessment of surgical margin
Breast reduction mammoplasty
Bronchus, biopsy
Cell block, any source
Cervix, biopsy
Colon, biopsy
Duodenum, biopsy
Endocervix, curettings/biopsy
Endometrium, curettings/biopsy
Esophagus, biopsy
Extremity, amputation, traumatic
Fallopian tube, biopsy
Fallopian tube, ectopic pregnancy
Femoral head, fracture
Finger/toes, amputation, nontraumatic
Gingiva/oral mucosa, biopsy
Heart valve
Joint resection
Kidney biopsy
Larynx biopsy
Leiomyoma(s), uterine myomectomy-without uterus
Lip, biopsy/wedge resection
Lung, transbronchial biopsy
Lymph node, biopsy
Muscle, biopsy
Nasal mucosa, biopsy
Nasopharynx/oropharynx, biopsy
Nerve biopsy
Odontogenic/dental cyst
Omentum, biopsy
Ovary, biopsy/wedge resection
Ovary with or without tube, nonneoplastic
Parathyroid gland
Peritoneum, biopsy
Pituitary tumor
Placenta, other than third trimester
Pleura/pericardium-biopsy/tissue
Polyp:
- Cervical/endometrial
- Colorectal
- Stomach/small intestine

Prostate:
- Needle biopsy
- TUR

Salivary gland, biopsy
Sinus, paranasal biopsy
Skin, other than cyst/tag/debridement/plastic repair
Small intestine, biopsy
Soft tissue, other than tumor/mas/lipoma/debridement
Spleen
Stomach biopsy
Synovium
Testis, other than tumor/biopsy, castration
Thyroglossal duct/brachial cleft cyst
Tongue, biopsy
Tonsil, biopsy
Trachea biopsy
Ureter, biopsy
Urethra, biopsy
Urinary bladder, biopsy
Uterus, with or without tubes and ovaries, for prolapse
Vagina biopsy
Vulva/labial biopsy

X 80 PQ 1.97 1.97 FUD XXX

88307 Level V - Surgical pathology, gross and microscopic examination

INCLUDES Adrenal resection
Bone, biopsy/curettings
Bone fragment(s), pathologic fractures
Brain, biopsy
Brain meninges, tumor resection
Breast, excision of lesion, requiring microscopic evaluation of surgical margins
Breast, mastectomy-partial/simple
Cervix, conization
Colon, segmental resection, other than for tumor
Extremity, amputation, nontraumatic
Eye, enucleation
Kidney, partial/total nephrectomy
Larynx, partial/total resection
Liver
Biopsy, needle/wedge
Partial resection
Lung, wedge biopsy
Lymph nodes, regional resection
Mediastinum, mass
Myocardium, biopsy
Odontogenic tumor
Ovary with or without tube, neoplastic
Pancreas, biopsy
Placenta, third trimester
Prostate, except radical resection
Salivary gland
Sentinel lymph node
Small intestine, resection, other than for tumor
Soft tissue mass (except lipoma)-biopsy/simple excision
Stomach-subtotal/total resection, other than for tumor
Testis, biopsy
Thymus, tumor
Thyroid, total/lobe
Ureter, resection
Urinary bladder, TUR
Uterus, with or without tubes and ovaries, other than neoplastic/prolapse

X 80 PQ 8.05 8.05 FUD XXX

88309 Level VI - Surgical pathology, gross and microscopic examination

INCLUDES Bone resection
Breast, mastectomy-with regional lymph nodes
Colon:
Segmental resection for tumor
Total resection
Esophagus, partial/total resection
Extremity, disarticulation
Fetus, with dissection
Larynx, partial/total resection-with regional lymph nodes
Lung-total/lobe/segment resection
Pancreas, total/subtotal resection
Prostate, radical resection
Small intestine, resection for tumor
Soft tissue tumor, extensive resection
Stomach, subtotal/total resection for tumor
Testis, tumor
Tongue/tonsil, resection for tumor
Urinary bladder, partial/total resection
Uterus, with or without tubes and ovaries, neoplastic
Vulva, total/subtotal resection

EXCLUDES *Evaluation of fine needle aspirate (88172-88173)*
Fine needle aspiration (10021-10022)

X 80 PQ 12.25 12.25 FUD XXX

88311-88399 [88341, 88364, 88373, 88374, 88377] Additional Surgical Pathology Services

CMS 100-4,12,60 Payment for Pathology Services

\+ **88311 Decalcification procedure (List separately in addition to code for surgical pathology examination)**

Code first surgical pathology exam (88302-88309)
N 80 0.57 0.57 FUD XXX

88312 Special stain including interpretation and report; Group I for microorganisms (eg, acid fast, methenamine silver)

INCLUDES Reporting one unit for each special stain performed on a surgical pathology block, cytologic sample, or hematologic smear
X 80 2.64 2.64 FUD XXX

88313 Group II, all other (eg, iron, trichrome), except stain for microorganisms, stains for enzyme constituents, or immunocytochemistry and immunohistochemistry

INCLUDES Reporting one unit for each special stain performed on a surgical pathology block, cytologic sample, or hematologic smear
EXCLUDES *Immunocytochemistry and immunohistochemistry (88342)*
X 80 1.84 1.84 FUD XXX

\+ **88314 histochemical stain on frozen tissue block (List separately in addition to code for primary procedure)**

INCLUDES Reporting one unit for each special stain on each frozen surgical pathology block
EXCLUDES *Special stain performed on frozen tissue section specimen to identify enzyme constituents (88319)*
Code also modifier 59 for nonroutine histochemical stain on frozen section during Mohs surgery
Code first (17311-17315, 88302-88309, 88331-88332)
Do not report with routine frozen section stain during Mohs surgery (17311-17315)
N 80 2.18 2.18 FUD XXX

88319 Group III, for enzyme constituents

INCLUDES Reporting one unit for each special stain on each frozen surgical pathology block
EXCLUDES *Detection of enzyme constituents by immunohistochemical or immunocytochemical methodology (88342)*
X 80 2.40 2.40 FUD XXX

88321 Consultation and report on referred slides prepared elsewhere

X 80 2.40 2.66 FUD XXX

88323 Consultation and report on referred material requiring preparation of slides

X 80 4.12 4.12 FUD XXX

88325 Consultation, comprehensive, with review of records and specimens, with report on referred material

X 80 3.76 5.94 FUD XXX

88329 Pathology consultation during surgery;

X 80 1.02 1.60 FUD XXX

88331 first tissue block, with frozen section(s), single specimen

Code also cytologic evaluation performed at same time (88334)
X 80 2.76 2.76 FUD XXX

\+ **88332 each additional tissue block with frozen section(s) (List separately in addition to code for primary procedure)**

Code first (88331)
N 80 1.22 1.22 FUD XXX

88333 **cytologic examination (eg, touch prep, squash prep), initial site**
EXCLUDES *Intraprocedural cytologic evaluation of fine needle aspirate (88172)*
Nonintraoperative cytologic examination (88160-88162)
X 80 2.92 2.92 FUD XXX

+ 88334 **cytologic examination (eg, touch prep, squash prep), each additional site (List separately in addition to code for primary procedure)**
EXCLUDES *Intraprocedural cytologic evaluation of fine needle aspirate (88172)*
Nonintraoperative cytologic examination (88160-88162)
Percutaneous needle biopsy requiring intraprocedural cytologic examination (88333)
Code first (88331, 88333)
N 80 1.82 1.82 FUD XXX

*88341 **Resequenced code. See code following 88342.***

▲ 88342 **Immunohistochemistry or immunocytochemistry, per specimen; initial single antibody stain procedure**
Do not report more than one time for each specific antibody
Do not report testing on the same antibody as (88360-88361)
E 80 0.00 0.00 FUD XXX

+ #● 88341 **each additional single antibody stain procedure (List separately in addition to code for primary procedure)**
Code first (88342)
Do not report more than one time for each specific antibody
Do not report testing on the same antibody as (88360-88361)

~~88343 each additional separately identifiable antibody per slide (List separately in addition to code for primary procedure)~~
To report, see 88344

● 88344 **each multiplex antibody stain procedure**
INCLUDES Staining with multiple antibodies on the same slide
Do not report more than one time for each specific antibody
Do not report testing on the same antibody as (88360-88361)

88346 **Immunofluorescent study, each antibody; direct method**
X 80 2.97 2.97 FUD XXX

88347 **indirect method**
X 80 2.48 2.48 FUD XXX

88348 **Electron microscopy, diagnostic**
X 80 19.61 19.61 FUD XXX

~~88349 scanning~~
To report, see 88348

88355 **Morphometric analysis; skeletal muscle**
X 80 4.92 4.92 FUD XXX

88356 **nerve**
X 80 7.81 7.81 FUD XXX

88358 **tumor (eg, DNA ploidy)**
Do not report with 88313 unless each procedure is for a different special stain
X 80 2.33 2.33 FUD XXX

▲ 88360 **Morphometric analysis, tumor immunohistochemistry (eg, Her-2/neu, estrogen receptor/progesterone receptor), quantitative or semiquantitative, per specimen, each single antibody stain procedure; manual**
EXCLUDES *Morphometric analysis using in situ hybridization techniques (88367-88368)*
Do not report additional stain procedures unless each test is for different antibody (88342, [88341], 88344)
X 80 PQ 3.63 3.63 FUD XXX

▲ 88361 **using computer-assisted technology**
EXCLUDES *Morphometric analysis using in situ hybridization techniques (88367-88368)*
Do not report with Do not report additional stain procedures unless each test is for different antibody (88342, [88341], 88344)
X 80 PQ 4.41 4.41 FUD XXX

88362 **Nerve teasing preparations**
X 80 8.60 8.60 FUD XXX

88363 **Examination and selection of retrieved archival (ie, previously diagnosed) tissue(s) for molecular analysis (eg, KRAS mutational analysis)**
INCLUDES Archival retrieval only
X 80 0.54 0.62 FUD XXX

*88364 **Resequenced code. See code following 88365.***

▲ 88365 **In situ hybridization (eg, FISH), per specimen; initial single probe stain procedure**
Do not report for the same probe with (88367, [88374], 88368, [88377])
X 80 4.95 4.95 FUD XXX

+ #● 88364 **each additional single probe stain procedure (List separately in addition to code for primary procedure)**
Code first (88365)

● 88366 **each multiplex probe stain procedure**
Do not report for the same probe with (88367, [88374], 88368, [88377])

▲ 88367 **Morphometric analysis, in situ hybridization (quantitative or semi-quantitative), using computer-assisted technology, per specimen; initial single probe stain procedure**
EXCLUDES *Morphometric in situ hybridization evaluation of urinary tract cytologic specimens (88120-88121)*
Do not report for same probe with (88365, 88366, 88368, [88377])
X 80 7.14 7.14 FUD XXX

+ #● 88373 **each additional single probe stain procedure (List separately in addition to code for primary procedure)**
Code first (88367)

#● 88374 **each multiplex probe stain procedure**
Do not report for same probe with (88365, 88366, 88368, [88377])

▲ 88368 **initial single probe stain procedure**
EXCLUDES *Morphometric in situ hybridization evaluation of urinary tract cytologic specimens (88120-88121)*
Do not report for same probe with (88365, 88366-88367, [88374])
X 80 6.49 6.49 FUD XXX

+ ● 88369 **each additional single probe stain procedure (List separately in addition to code for primary procedure)**
Code first (88368)

#● 88377 **each multiplex probe stain procedure**
Do not report for same probe with (88365, 88366-88367, [88374])

88371 Protein analysis of tissue by Western Blot, with interpretation and report;
N 0.00 0.00 FUD XXX

88372 immunological probe for band identification, each
N 0.00 0.00 FUD XXX

88373 *Resequenced code. See code following 88367.*

88374 *Resequenced code. See code following 88367.*

88375 Optical endomicroscopic image(s), interpretation and report, real-time or referred, each endoscopic session
Do not report with (43206, 43252)
X 80 0.00 0.00 FUD XXX

88377 *Resequenced code. See code following 88369.*

88380 Microdissection (ie, sample preparation of microscopically identified target); laser capture
Do not report with (88381)
N 80 5.32 5.32 FUD XXX

88381 manual
Do not report with (88380)
N 80 4.49 4.49 FUD XXX

88387 Macroscopic examination, dissection, and preparation of tissue for non-microscopic analytical studies (eg, nucleic acid-based molecular studies); each tissue preparation (eg, a single lymph node)
Do not report for tissue preparation for microbiologic cultures or flow cytometric studies
Do not report with (88329-88334, 88388)
N 80 1.00 1.00 FUD XXX

\+ 88388 in conjunction with a touch imprint, intraoperative consultation, or frozen section, each tissue preparation (eg, a single lymph node) (List separately in addition to code for primary procedure)
Code first (88329-88334)
Do not report for tissue preparation for microbiologic cultures or flow cytometric studies
N 80 0.92 0.92 FUD XXX

88399 Unlisted surgical pathology procedure
X 80 0.00 0.00 FUD XXX

88720-88749 Transcutaneous Procedures

EXCLUDES *Transcutaneous oxyhemoglobin measurement in a leg using near infrared spectroscopy (0286T)*
Wavelength fluorescent spectroscopy of advanced glycation end products (skin) (0233T)

88720 Bilirubin, total, transcutaneous
EXCLUDES *Transdermal oxygen saturation testing (94760-94762)*
N 0.00 0.00 FUD XXX

88738 Hemoglobin (Hgb), quantitative, transcutaneous
EXCLUDES *In vitro hemoglobin measurement (85018)*
N 0.00 0.00 FUD XXX

88740 Hemoglobin, quantitative, transcutaneous, per day; carboxyhemoglobin
EXCLUDES *In vitro carboxyhemoglobin measurement (82375)*
N 0.00 0.00 FUD XXX

88741 methemoglobin
EXCLUDES *In vitro quantitative methemoglobin measurement (83050)*
N 0.00 0.00 FUD XXX

88749 Unlisted in vivo (eg, transcutaneous) laboratory service
INCLUDES All in vivo measurements not specifically listed
N 0.00 0.00 FUD XXX

89049-89240 Other Pathology Services

89049 Caffeine halothane contracture test (CHCT) for malignant hyperthermia susceptibility, including interpretation and report
X 80 1.84 7.23 FUD XXX

89050 Cell count, miscellaneous body fluids (eg, cerebrospinal fluid, joint fluid), except blood;
N 0.00 0.00 FUD XXX

89051 with differential count
N 0.00 0.00 FUD XXX

89055 Leukocyte assessment, fecal, qualitative or semiquantitative
N 0.00 0.00 FUD XXX

89060 Crystal identification by light microscopy with or without polarizing lens analysis, tissue or any body fluid (except urine)
Do not report for crystal identification on paraffin embedded tissue
N 0.00 0.00 FUD XXX

89125 Fat stain, feces, urine, or respiratory secretions
N 0.00 0.00 FUD XXX

89160 Meat fibers, feces
N 0.00 0.00 FUD XXX

89190 Nasal smear for eosinophils
EXCLUDES *Occult blood, feces (82270)*
Paternity tests (86910)
N 0.00 0.00 FUD XXX

89220 Sputum, obtaining specimen, aerosol induced technique (separate procedure)
X TC 80 0.48 0.48 FUD XXX

89230 Sweat collection by iontophoresis
X TC 80 0.14 0.14 FUD XXX

89240 Unlisted miscellaneous pathology test
X 80 0.00 0.00 FUD XXX

89250-89398 Infertility Treatment Services

CMS 100-2,1,100 Treatment for Infertility

89250 Culture of oocyte(s)/embryo(s), less than 4 days;
X 0.00 0.00 FUD XXX

89251 with co-culture of oocyte(s)/embryos
EXCLUDES *Extended culture of oocyte(s)/embryo(s) (89272)*
X 0.00 0.00 FUD XXX

89253 Assisted embryo hatching, microtechniques (any method)
X 0.00 0.00 FUD XXX

89254 Oocyte identification from follicular fluid
X 0.00 0.00 FUD XXX

89255 Preparation of embryo for transfer (any method)
X 0.00 0.00 FUD XXX

89257 Sperm identification from aspiration (other than seminal fluid)
EXCLUDES *Semen analysis (89300-89320)*
Sperm identification from testis tissue (89264)
X 0.00 0.00 FUD XXX

89258 Cryopreservation; embryo(s)
X 0.00 0.00 FUD XXX

89259 sperm
EXCLUDES *Cryopreservation of testicular reproductive tissue (89335)*
X 0.00 0.00 FUD XXX

89260 Sperm isolation; simple prep (eg, sperm wash and swim-up) for insemination or diagnosis with semen analysis
X 0.00 0.00 FUD XXX

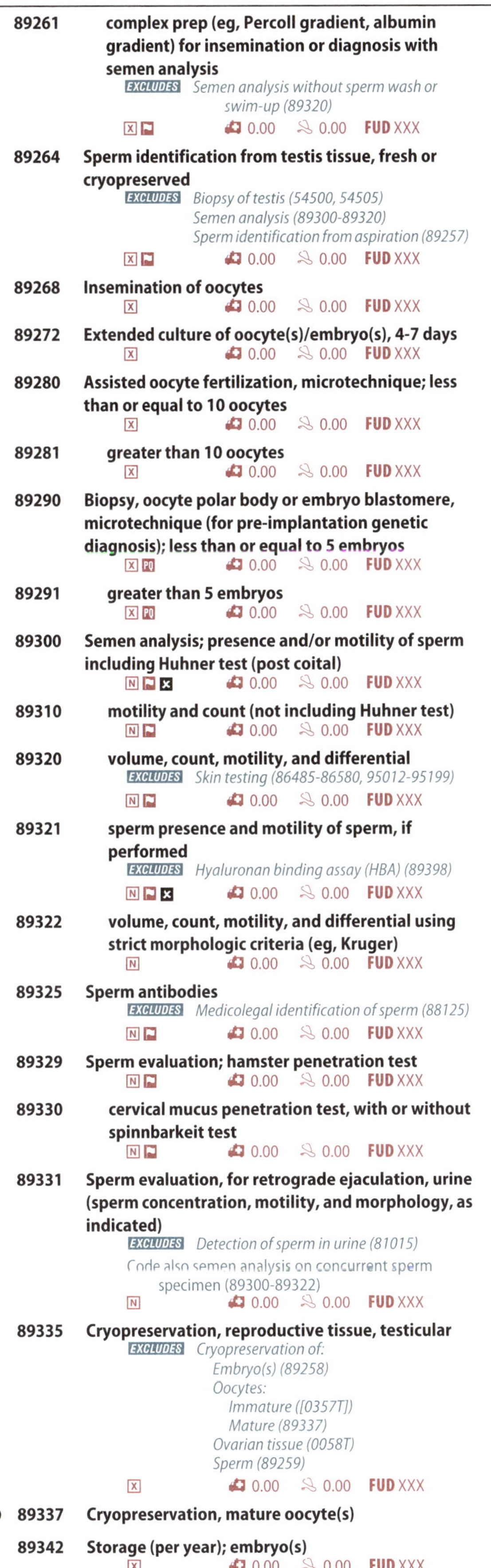

89261 complex prep (eg, Percoll gradient, albumin gradient) for insemination or diagnosis with semen analysis
EXCLUDES *Semen analysis without sperm wash or swim-up (89320)*
0.00 0.00 FUD XXX

89264 Sperm identification from testis tissue, fresh or cryopreserved
EXCLUDES *Biopsy of testis (54500, 54505)*
Semen analysis (89300-89320)
Sperm identification from aspiration (89257)
0.00 0.00 FUD XXX

89268 Insemination of oocytes
0.00 0.00 FUD XXX

89272 Extended culture of oocyte(s)/embryo(s), 4-7 days
0.00 0.00 FUD XXX

89280 Assisted oocyte fertilization, microtechnique; less than or equal to 10 oocytes
0.00 0.00 FUD XXX

89281 greater than 10 oocytes
0.00 0.00 FUD XXX

89290 Biopsy, oocyte polar body or embryo blastomere, microtechnique (for pre-implantation genetic diagnosis); less than or equal to 5 embryos
0.00 0.00 FUD XXX

89291 greater than 5 embryos
0.00 0.00 FUD XXX

89300 Semen analysis; presence and/or motility of sperm including Huhner test (post coital)
N 0.00 0.00 FUD XXX

89310 motility and count (not including Huhner test)
N 0.00 0.00 FUD XXX

89320 volume, count, motility, and differential
EXCLUDES *Skin testing (86485-86580, 95012-95199)*
N 0.00 0.00 FUD XXX

89321 sperm presence and motility of sperm, if performed
EXCLUDES *Hyaluronan binding assay (HBA) (89398)*
N 0.00 0.00 FUD XXX

89322 volume, count, motility, and differential using strict morphologic criteria (eg, Kruger)
N 0.00 0.00 FUD XXX

89325 Sperm antibodies
EXCLUDES *Medicolegal identification of sperm (88125)*
N 0.00 0.00 FUD XXX

89329 Sperm evaluation; hamster penetration test
N 0.00 0.00 FUD XXX

89330 cervical mucus penetration test, with or without spinnbarkeit test
N 0.00 0.00 FUD XXX

89331 Sperm evaluation, for retrograde ejaculation, urine (sperm concentration, motility, and morphology, as indicated)
EXCLUDES *Detection of sperm in urine (81015)*
Code also semen analysis on concurrent sperm specimen (89300-89322)
N 0.00 0.00 FUD XXX

89335 Cryopreservation, reproductive tissue, testicular
EXCLUDES *Cryopreservation of:*
Embryo(s) (89258)
Oocytes:
Immature ([0357T])
Mature (89337)
Ovarian tissue (0058T)
Sperm (89259)
0.00 0.00 FUD XXX

● 89337 Cryopreservation, mature oocyte(s)

89342 Storage (per year); embryo(s)
0.00 0.00 FUD XXX

89343 sperm/semen
0.00 0.00 FUD XXX

89344 reproductive tissue, testicular/ovarian
0.00 0.00 FUD XXX

89346 oocyte(s)
0.00 0.00 FUD XXX

89352 Thawing of cryopreserved; embryo(s)
0.00 0.00 FUD XXX

89353 sperm/semen, each aliquot
0.00 0.00 FUD XXX

89354 reproductive tissue, testicular/ovarian
0.00 0.00 FUD XXX

89356 oocytes, each aliquot
0.00 0.00 FUD XXX

89398 Unlisted reproductive medicine laboratory procedure
INCLUDES Hyaluronan binding assay (HBA)
0.00 0.00 FUD XXX

90281-90399 Immunoglobulin Products

CMS 100-2,15,50 Drugs and Biologicals

INCLUDES Immune globulin product only
Anti-infectives
Antitoxins
Isoantibodies
Monoclonal antibodies

Code also (96365-96368, 96372, 96374-96375)

(51) **90281** **Immune globulin (Ig), human, for intramuscular use**
INCLUDES Gamastan
E 0.00 0.00 FUD XXX

(51) **90283** **Immune globulin (IgIV), human, for intravenous use**
E 0.00 0.00 FUD XXX

(51) **90284** **Immune globulin (SCIg), human, for use in subcutaneous infusions, 100 mg, each**
E 0.00 0.00 FUD XXX

(51) **90287** **Botulinum antitoxin, equine, any route**
E 0.00 0.00 FUD XXX

(51) **90288** **Botulism immune globulin, human, for intravenous use**
E 0.00 0.00 FUD XXX

(51) **90291** **Cytomegalovirus immune globulin (CMV-IgIV), human, for intravenous use**
INCLUDES Cytogram
E 0.00 0.00 FUD XXX

(51) **90296** **Diphtheria antitoxin, equine, any route**
N 0.00 0.00 FUD XXX

(51) **90371** **Hepatitis B immune globulin (HBIg), human, for intramuscular use**
INCLUDES HBIG
K2 K 0.00 0.00 FUD XXX

(51) **90375** **Rabies immune globulin (RIg), human, for intramuscular and/or subcutaneous use**
INCLUDES HyperRAB
K2 K 0.00 0.00 FUD XXX

(51) **90376** **Rabies immune globulin, heat-treated (RIg-HT), human, for intramuscular and/or subcutaneous use**
K2 K 0.00 0.00 FUD XXX

(51) **90378** **Respiratory syncytial virus, monoclonal antibody, recombinant, for intramuscular use, 50 mg, each**
INCLUDES Synagis
K2 K 0.00 0.00 FUD XXX

(51) **90384** **Rho(D) immune globulin (RhIg), human, full-dose, for intramuscular use**
E 0.00 0.00 FUD XXX

(51) **90385** **Rho(D) immune globulin (RhIg), human, mini-dose, for intramuscular use**
N1 N 0.00 0.00 FUD XXX

(51) **90386** **Rho(D) immune globulin (RhIgIV), human, for intravenous use**
E 0.00 0.00 FUD XXX

(51) **90389** **Tetanus immune globulin (TIg), human, for intramuscular use**
E 0.00 0.00 FUD XXX

(51) **90393** **Vaccinia immune globulin, human, for intramuscular use**
E 0.00 0.00 FUD XXX

(51) **90396** **Varicella-zoster immune globulin, human, for intramuscular use**
K2 K 0.00 0.00 FUD XXX

(51) **90399** **Unlisted immune globulin**
E 0.00 0.00 FUD XXX

90460-90461 Injections Provided with Counseling

CMS 100-2,16,90 Routine Services and Appliances

INCLUDES All components of influenza vaccine, report X 1 only
Combination vaccines which comprise multiple vaccine components
Components (all antigens) in vaccines to prevent disease due to specific organisms
Counseling by physician or other qualified health care professional
Multi-valent antigens or multiple antigen serotypes against single organisms are considered one component
Patient/family face-to-face counseling by doctor or qualified health care professional for patients 18 years of age and younger

EXCLUDES *Administration of influenza and pneumococcal vaccine for Medicare patients (G0008-G0009)*
Allergy testing (95004-95028)
Bacterial/viral/fungal skin tests (86485-86580)
Diagnostic or therapeutic injections (96372-96379)
Vaccines provided without face-to-face counseling from a physician or qualified health care professional or to patients over the age of 18 (90471-90474)

Code also significant, separately identifiable evaluation and management or preventive medicine service when appropriate

Code also toxoid/vaccine (90476-90749 [90630, 90672, 90673])

90460 **Immunization administration through 18 years of age via any route of administration, with counseling by physician or other qualified health care professional; first or only component of each vaccine or toxoid administered** A
Code also each additional component in a vaccine (e.g., A 5-year-old receives DtaP-IPV IM administration, and MMR/Varicella vaccines SQ administration. Report 90460 X 2, and 90461 X 6)
B 80 0.70 0.70 FUD XXX

\+ **90461** **each additional vaccine or toxoid component administered (List separately in addition to code for primary procedure)** A
Code also each additional component in a vaccine (e.g., A 5-year-old receives DtaP-IPV IM administration, and MMR/Varicella vaccines SQ administration. Report 90460 X 2, and 90461 X 6)
Code first the initial component in each vaccine provided (90460)
B 80 0.35 0.35 FUD ZZZ

90471-90474 Injections and Other Routes of Administration Without Physician Counseling

CMS 100-2,15,50 Drugs and Biologicals
CMS 100-2,16,90 Routine Services and Appliances
CMS 100-4,18,10.2.1 Vaccines and Administration

EXCLUDES *Administration of influenza and pneumococcal vaccine for Medicare patients (G0008-G0009)*
Administration of vaccine with counseling (90460-90461)
Allergy testing (95004-95028)
Bacterial/viral/fungal skin tests (86485-86580)
Injections, diagnostic/therapeutic (96372-96379)
Patient/family face-to-face counseling

Code also significant separately identifiable evaluation and management or preventive medicine service when appropriate

Code also toxoid/vaccine (90476-90749 [90630, 90672, 90673])

90471 **Immunization administration (includes percutaneous, intradermal, subcutaneous, or intramuscular injections); 1 vaccine (single or combination vaccine/toxoid)**
Do not report with intranasal/oral administration (90473)
S 80 0.70 0.70 FUD XXX

+ **90472** **each additional vaccine (single or combination vaccine/toxoid) (List separately in addition to code for primary procedure)**
EXCLUDES *BCG vaccine, intravesical administration (51720, 90586)*
Immune globulin administration (96365-96368, 96372-96374)
Immune globulin product (90281-90399)
Code first initial vaccine (90460, 90471, 90473)
N 80 0.35 0.35 FUD ZZZ

90473 **Immunization administration by intranasal or oral route; 1 vaccine (single or combination vaccine/toxoid)**
Do not report with (90471)
S 80 0.70 0.70 FUD XXX

+ **90474** **each additional vaccine (single or combination vaccine/toxoid) (List separately in addition to code for primary procedure)**
Code first initial vaccine (90460, 90471, 90473)
N 80 0.35 0.35 FUD ZZZ

90476-90749 [90630, 90672, 90673] Vaccination Products

CMS 100-2,15,50 Drugs and Biologicals
CMS 100-2,16,90 Routine Services and Appliances
INCLUDES Patient's age for coding purposes, not for product license
Vaccine product only
EXCLUDES *Immune globulins and administration (90281-90399, 96365-96368, 96372-96375)*
Code also administration of vaccine (90460-90474)
Code also significant separately identifiable evaluation and management or preventive medicine service when appropriate
Do not report each component of a combination vaccine individually

(51) **90476** **Adenovirus vaccine, type 4, live, for oral use**
INCLUDES Adeno-4
N1 N 0.00 0.00 FUD XXX

(51) **90477** **Adenovirus vaccine, type 7, live, for oral use**
INCLUDES Adeno-7
N1 N 0.00 0.00 FUD XXX

(51) **90581** **Anthrax vaccine, for subcutaneous or intramuscular use**
INCLUDES BioThrax
K2 K 0.00 0.00 FUD XXX

(51) **90585** **Bacillus Calmette-Guerin vaccine (BCG) for tuberculosis, live, for percutaneous use**
INCLUDES Mycobax
K2 K 0.00 0.00 FUD XXX

(51) **90586** **Bacillus Calmette-Guerin vaccine (BCG) for bladder cancer, live, for intravesical use**
INCLUDES TheraCys
TICE BCG
B 0.00 0.00 FUD XXX

(51) ● **90620** **Meningococcal recombinant protein and outer membrane vesicle vaccine, serogroup B, 2 dose schedule, for intramuscular use**
INCLUDES Implementation date 02/01/2015

(51) ● **90621** **Meningococcal recombinant lipoprotein vaccine, serogroup B, 3 dose schedule, for intramuscular use**
INCLUDES Implementation of code prior to 02/01/2015 based on payer discretion

(51) #● **90630** ***Resequenced code. See code following 90654.***

(51) **90632** **Hepatitis A vaccine, adult dosage, for intramuscular use** A
INCLUDES Havrix
Vaqta
N1 N 0.00 0.00 FUD XXX

(51) **90633** **Hepatitis A vaccine, pediatric/adolescent dosage-2 dose schedule, for intramuscular use** A
INCLUDES Havrix
Vaqta
N1 N 0.00 0.00 FUD XXX

(51) **90634** **Hepatitis A vaccine, pediatric/adolescent dosage-3 dose schedule, for intramuscular use** A
INCLUDES Havrix
N1 N 0.00 0.00 FUD XXX

(51) **90636** **Hepatitis A and hepatitis B vaccine (HepA-HepB), adult dosage, for intramuscular use** A
INCLUDES Twinrix
N1 N 0.00 0.00 FUD XXX

(51) **90644** **Meningococcal conjugate vaccine, serogroups C & Y and Hemophilus influenza B vaccine (Hib-MenCY), 4 dose schedule, when administered to children 2-15 months of age, for intramuscular use** A
INCLUDES MenHibrix
E 0.00 0.00 FUD XXX

(51) **90645** **Hemophilus influenza b vaccine (Hib), HbOC conjugate (4 dose schedule), for intramuscular use**
N1 N 0.00 0.00 FUD XXX

(51) **90646** **Hemophilus influenza b vaccine (Hib), PRP-D conjugate, for booster use only, intramuscular use**
N1 N 0.00 0.00 FUD XXX

(51) **90647** **Hemophilus influenza b vaccine (Hib), PRP-OMP conjugate (3 dose schedule), for intramuscular use**
INCLUDES PedvaxHIB
N1 N 0.00 0.00 FUD XXX

(51) **90648** **Hemophilus influenza b vaccine (Hib), PRP-T conjugate (4 dose schedule), for intramuscular use**
INCLUDES ActHIB
Hiberix
N1 N 0.00 0.00 FUD XXX

(51) **90649** **Human Papilloma virus (HPV) vaccine, types 6, 11, 16, 18 (quadrivalent), 3 dose schedule, for intramuscular use**
INCLUDES Gardisil
M 0.00 0.00 FUD XXX

(51) **90650** **Human Papilloma virus (HPV) vaccine, types 16, 18, bivalent, 3 dose schedule, for intramuscular use**
INCLUDES Cervarix
M 0.00 0.00 FUD XXX

(51) ● **90651** **Human Papillomavirus vaccine types 6, 11, 16, 18, 31, 33, 45, 52, 58, nonavalent (HPV), 3 dose schedule, for intramuscular use**

(51) **90653** **Influenza vaccine, inactivated, subunit, adjuvanted, for intramuscular use**
E 0.00 0.00 FUD XXX

(51) ▲ **90654** **Influenza virus vaccine, trivalent (IIV3), split virus, preservative-free, for intradermal use**
INCLUDES Fluzone intradermal
L1 L 0.00 0.00 FUD XXX

(51) #● **90630** **Influenza virus vaccine, quadrivalent (IIV4), split virus, preservative free, for intradermal use**

(51) **90655** **Influenza virus vaccine, trivalent, split virus, preservative free, when administered to children 6-35 months of age, for intramuscular use** A
INCLUDES Afluria
Fluzone, no preservative, pediatric dose
L1 L PQ 0.00 0.00 FUD XXX

(51) **90656** **Influenza virus vaccine, trivalent, split virus, preservative free, when administered to individuals 3 years and older, for intramuscular use** A
INCLUDES Afluria
Fluvarix
Fluvirin
Fluzone, influenza virus vaccine, no preservative
L1 L PQ 0.00 0.00 FUD XXX

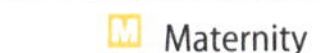
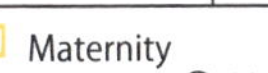
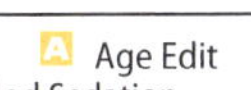
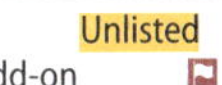

(51) 90657 **Influenza virus vaccine, trivalent, split virus, when administered to children 6-35 months of age, for intramuscular use** A
INCLUDES Afluria
Flulaval
Fluvirin
Fluzone (5 ml vial [0.25ml dose])
L1 L PQ 0.00 0.00 FUD XXX

(51) 90658 **Influenza virus vaccine, trivalent, split virus, when administered to individuals 3 years of age and older, for intramuscular use** A
INCLUDES Afluria
Flulaval
Fluvirin
Fluzone
E 0.00 0.00 FUD XXX

(51) 90660 **Influenza virus vaccine, trivalent, live, for intranasal use**
INCLUDES FluMist
L1 L PQ 0.00 0.00 FUD XXX

(51) # 90672 **Influenza virus vaccine, quadrivalent, live, for intranasal use**
INCLUDES FluMist nasal spray
L1 L 0.00 0.00 FUD XXX

(51) 90661 **Influenza virus vaccine, derived from cell cultures, subunit, preservative and antibiotic free, for intramuscular use**
INCLUDES Flucelvax
L1 L PQ 0.00 0.00 FUD XXX

(51) # 90673 **Influenza virus vaccine, trivalent, derived from recombinant DNA (RIV3), hemagglutinin (HA) protein only, preservative and antibiotic free, for intramuscular use**
INCLUDES Flublok (single dose vial)
L1 L 0.00 0.00 FUD XXX

(51) 90662 **Influenza virus vaccine, split virus, preservative free, enhanced immunogenicity via increased antigen content, for intramuscular use**
INCLUDES Fluzone high-dose
L1 L PQ 0.00 0.00 FUD XXX

(51) 90664 **Influenza virus vaccine, pandemic formulation, live, for intranasal use**
E PQ 0.00 0.00 FUD XXX

(51) ⌿ 90666 **Influenza virus vaccine, pandemic formulation, split virus, preservative free, for intramuscular use**
E PQ 0.00 0.00 FUD XXX

(51) ⌿ 90667 **Influenza virus vaccine, pandemic formulation, split virus, adjuvanted, for intramuscular use**
E PQ 0.00 0.00 FUD XXX

(51) ⌿ 90668 **Influenza virus vaccine, pandemic formulation, split virus, for intramuscular use**
E PQ 0.00 0.00 FUD XXX

(51) 90669 **Pneumococcal conjugate vaccine, 7 valent, for intramuscular use**
INCLUDES Prevnar
L1 L 0.00 0.00 FUD XXX

(51) 90670 **Pneumococcal conjugate vaccine, 13 valent, for intramuscular use**
INCLUDES Prevnar 13
L1 L 0.00 0.00 FUD XXX

90672 Resequenced code. See code following 90660.

90673 Resequenced code. See code following 90661.

(51) 90675 **Rabies vaccine, for intramuscular use**
INCLUDES Imovax
RabAvert
K2 K 0.00 0.00 FUD XXX

(51) 90676 **Rabies vaccine, for intradermal use**
K2 K 0.00 0.00 FUD XXX

(51) 90680 **Rotavirus vaccine, pentavalent, 3 dose schedule, live, for oral use**
INCLUDES RotaTeq
N1 N 0.00 0.00 FUD XXX

(51) 90681 **Rotavirus vaccine, human, attenuated, 2 dose schedule, live, for oral use**
INCLUDES Rotarix
E 0.00 0.00 FUD XXX

(51) 90685 **Influenza virus vaccine, quadrivalent, split virus, preservative free, when administered to children 6-35 months of age, for intramuscular use** A
INCLUDES Fluzone Quadrivalent
L 0.00 0.00 FUD XXX

(51) 90686 **Influenza virus vaccine, quadrivalent, split virus, preservative free, when administered to individuals 3 years of age and older, for intramuscular use** A
INCLUDES Fluarix Quadrivalent
Fluzone Quadrivalent
L 0.00 0.00 FUD XXX

(51) 90687 **Influenza virus vaccine, quadrivalent, split virus, when administered to children 6-35 months of age, for intramuscular use** A
E 0.00 0.00 FUD XXX

(51) 90688 **Influenza virus vaccine, quadrivalent, split virus, when administered to individuals 3 years of age and older, for intramuscular use** A
INCLUDES FluLaval (multidose vial)
L1 L 0.00 0.00 FUD XXX

(51) 90690 **Typhoid vaccine, live, oral**
INCLUDES Vivotif
N1 N 0.00 0.00 FUD XXX

(51) 90691 **Typhoid vaccine, Vi capsular polysaccharide (ViCPs), for intramuscular use**
INCLUDES Typhim Vi
N1 N 0.00 0.00 FUD XXX

(51) 90692 **Typhoid vaccine, heat- and phenol-inactivated (H-P), for subcutaneous or intradermal use**
N1 N 0.00 0.00 FUD XXX

(51) 90693 **Typhoid vaccine, acetone-killed, dried (AKD), for subcutaneous use (U.S. military)**
B 0.00 0.00 FUD XXX

(51) 90696 **Diphtheria, tetanus toxoids, acellular pertussis vaccine and poliovirus vaccine, inactivated (DTaP-IPV), when administered to children 4 through 6 years of age, for intramuscular use** A
INCLUDES KINRIX
N1 N 0.00 0.00 FUD XXX

(51) ⌿● 90697 **Diphtheria, tetanus toxoids, acellular pertussis vaccine, inactivated poliovirus vaccine, Haemophilus influenza type b PRP-OMP conjugate vaccine, and hepatitis B vaccine (DTaP-IPV-Hib-HepB), for intramuscular use**

(51) 90698 **Diphtheria, tetanus toxoids, acellular pertussis vaccine, haemophilus influenza Type B, and poliovirus vaccine, inactivated (DTaP - Hib - IPV), for intramuscular use**
INCLUDES Pentacel
N1 N 0.00 0.00 FUD XXX

(51) 90700 **Diphtheria, tetanus toxoids, and acellular pertussis vaccine (DTaP), when administered to individuals younger than 7 years, for intramuscular use** A
INCLUDES Daptacel
Infanrix
N1 N 0.00 0.00 FUD XXX

⑤ 90702 **Diphtheria and tetanus toxoids (DT) adsorbed when administered to individuals younger than 7 years, for intramuscular use**
INCLUDES Diphtheria and Tetanus Toxoids Adsorbed USP (For Pediatric Use)
N1 N 0.00 0.00 FUD XXX

⑤ 90703 **Tetanus toxoid adsorbed, for intramuscular use**
INCLUDES Tetanus Toxoid Adsorbed
N1 N 0.00 0.00 FUD XXX

⑤ 90704 **Mumps virus vaccine, live, for subcutaneous use**
INCLUDES MumpsVax
K2 K 0.00 0.00 FUD XXX

⑤ 90705 **Measles virus vaccine, live, for subcutaneous use**
INCLUDES AtenuVax
N1 N 0.00 0.00 FUD XXX

⑤ 90706 **Rubella virus vaccine, live, for subcutaneous use**
INCLUDES Meru Vax II
N 0.00 0.00 FUD XXX

⑤ 90707 **Measles, mumps and rubella virus vaccine (MMR), live, for subcutaneous use**
INCLUDES M-M-R II
N1 N 0.00 0.00 FUD XXX

⑤ 90708 **Measles and rubella virus vaccine, live, for subcutaneous use**
N1 N 0.00 0.00 FUD XXX

⑤ 90710 **Measles, mumps, rubella, and varicella vaccine (MMRV), live, for subcutaneous use**
INCLUDES ProQuad
N1 N 0.00 0.00 FUD XXX

⑤ 90712 **Poliovirus vaccine, (any type[s]) (OPV), live, for oral use**
N1 N 0.00 0.00 FUD XXX

⑤ 90713 **Poliovirus vaccine, inactivated (IPV), for subcutaneous or intramuscular use**
INCLUDES IPOL
N1 N 0.00 0.00 FUD XXX

⑤ 90714 **Tetanus and diphtheria toxoids (Td) adsorbed, preservative free, when administered to individuals 7 years or older, for intramuscular use**
INCLUDES DECAVAC/TENIVAC
Tetanus-diphtheria adult
N1 N 0.00 0.00 FUD XXX

⑤ 90715 **Tetanus, diphtheria toxoids and acellular pertussis vaccine (Tdap), when administered to individuals 7 years or older, for intramuscular use**
INCLUDES Adacel
Boostrix
N1 N 0.00 0.00 FUD XXX

⑤ 90716 **Varicella virus vaccine, live, for subcutaneous use**
INCLUDES Varivax
M 0.00 0.00 FUD XXX

⑤ 90717 **Yellow fever vaccine, live, for subcutaneous use**
INCLUDES YF-VAX
N1 N 0.00 0.00 FUD XXX

⑤ 90719 **Diphtheria toxoid, for intramuscular use**
N1 N 0.00 0.00 FUD XXX

⑤ 90720 **Diphtheria, tetanus toxoids, and whole cell pertussis vaccine and Hemophilus influenza B vaccine (DTP-Hib), for intramuscular use**
N1 N 0.00 0.00 FUD XXX

⑤ ▲ 90721 **Diphtheria, tetanus toxoids, and acellular pertussis vaccine and Hemophilus influenza B vaccine (DTaP/Hib), for intramuscular use**
N1 N 0.00 0.00 FUD XXX

⑤ ▲ 90723 **Diphtheria, tetanus toxoids, acellular pertussis vaccine, hepatitis B, and inactivated poliovirus vaccine (DTaP-HepB-IPV), for intramuscular use**
INCLUDES PEDIARIX
E 0.00 0.00 FUD XXX

⑤ 90725 **Cholera vaccine for injectable use**
N 0.00 0.00 FUD XXX

⑤ 90727 **Plague vaccine, for intramuscular use**
E 0.00 0.00 FUD XXX

⑤ 90732 **Pneumococcal polysaccharide vaccine, 23-valent, adult or immunosuppressed patient dosage, when administered to individuals 2 years or older, for subcutaneous or intramuscular use**
INCLUDES Pneumovax 23
L1 L 0.00 0.00 FUD XXX

⑤ 90733 **Meningococcal polysaccharide vaccine (any group(s)), for subcutaneous use**
INCLUDES Menomune-A/C/Y/W-135
K2 K 0.00 0.00 FUD XXX

⑤ ▲ 90734 **Meningococcal conjugate vaccine, serogroups A, C, Y and W-135, quadrivalent, for intramuscular use**
INCLUDES Menactra
Menveo
K2 K 0.00 0.00 FUD XXX

⑤ 90735 **Japanese encephalitis virus vaccine, for subcutaneous use**
K2 K 0.00 0.00 FUD XXX

⑤ 90736 **Zoster (shingles) vaccine, live, for subcutaneous injection**
INCLUDES Zostavax
M 0.00 0.00 FUD XXX

⑤ 90738 **Japanese encephalitis virus vaccine, inactivated, for intramuscular use**
INCLUDES Ixiaro
M 0.00 0.00 FUD XXX

⑤ ✓ 90739 **Hepatitis B vaccine, adult dosage (2 dose schedule), for intramuscular use**
E 0.00 0.00 FUD XXX

⑤ 90740 **Hepatitis B vaccine, dialysis or immunosuppressed patient dosage (3 dose schedule), for intramuscular use**
INCLUDES Recombivax dialysis
F 0.00 0.00 FUD XXX

⑤ 90743 **Hepatitis B vaccine, adolescent (2 dose schedule), for intramuscular use**
INCLUDES Energix-B
Recombivax HB
F 0.00 0.00 FUD XXX

⑤ 90744 **Hepatitis B vaccine, pediatric/adolescent dosage (3 dose schedule), for intramuscular use**
INCLUDES Energix-B
Recombivax HB
F 0.00 0.00 FUD XXX

⑤ 90746 **Hepatitis B vaccine, adult dosage (3 dose schedule), for intramuscular use**
INCLUDES Energix-B
Recombivax HB
F 0.00 0.00 FUD XXX

⑤ 90747 **Hepatitis B vaccine, dialysis or immunosuppressed patient dosage (4 dose schedule), for intramuscular use**
INCLUDES Energix-B
RECOMBIVAX dialysis
F 0.00 0.00 FUD XXX

⑤ 90748 **Hepatitis B and Hemophilus influenza b vaccine (HepB-Hib), for intramuscular use**
INCLUDES COMVAX
E 0.00 0.00 FUD XXX

⑤ 90749 **Unlisted vaccine/toxoid**
N1 N 0.00 0.00 FUD XXX

90785 Complex Interactive Encounter

INCLUDES At least one of the following activities:
- Discussion of a sentinel event demanding third-party involvement (eg, abuse or neglect reported to a state agency)
- Interference by the behavior or emotional state of caregiver to understand and assist in the plan of treatment
- Managing discordant communication complicating care among participating members (eg, arguing, reactivity)
- Use of nonverbal communication methods (eg, toys, other devices, or translator) to eliminate communication barriers

Complicated issues of communication affecting provision of the psychiatric service

Involved communication with:
- Emotionally charged or dissonant family members
- Patients wanting others present during the visit (e.g., family member, translator)
- Patients with impaired or undeveloped verbal skills
- Patients with third parties responsible for their care (eg, parents, guardians)
- Third-party involvement (eg, schools, probation and parole officers, child protective agencies)

Code also evaluation and management codes when reporting with codes for psychotherapy with medical evaluation and management services (99201-99255 [99224, 99225, 99226], 99304-99337, 99341-99350)

Do not report evaluation and management services code when psychotherapy services are not also provided

Do not report with (90839-90840, 0364T-0367T, 0373T-0374T)

+ **90785 Interactive complexity (List separately in addition to the code for primary procedure)**
Code first (99201-99255 [99224, 99225, 99226], 99304-99337, 99341-99350, 90791-90792, 90832-90834, 90836-90838, 90853)
N 0.40 0.40 FUD ZZZ

90791-90792 Psychiatric Evaluations

CMS 100-4,12,110.3 Outpatient Mental Health Limitation
CMS 100-4,12,150 Clinical Social Worker (CSW) Services
CMS 100-4,12,160 Independent Psychologist Services
CMS 100-4,12,160.1 Payment for Independent Psychologists' Services
CMS 100-4,12,170 Clinical Psychologist Services
CMS 100-4,12,170.1 Payment for Clinical Psychologist Services
CMS 100-4,12,210 Outpatient Mental Health Limitation

INCLUDES Diagnostic assessment or reassessment without psychotherapy services

Code also interactive complexity services when applicable (90785)

Do not report on same date of service as (90839-90840, 0364T-0367T, 0373T-0374T)

Do not report with (90839-90840, 0364T-0367T, 0373T-0374T)

Do not report with (99201-99337 [99224, 99225, 99226], 99341-99350, 99366-99368, 99401-99444, 0364T-0367T, 0373T-0374T)

90791 Psychiatric diagnostic evaluation
03 3.62 3.74 FUD XXX

90792 Psychiatric diagnostic evaluation with medical services
03 3.91 4.03 FUD XXX

90832-90838 Psychotherapy Services

CMS 100-3,130.1 Inpatient Stays for Alcoholism Treatment
CMS 100-3,130.2 Outpatient Hospital Services for Alcoholism
CMS 100-3,130.5 Treatment of Alcoholism/Drug Abuse in a Freestanding Clinic
CMS 100-3,130.6 Treatment of Drug Abuse (Chemical Dependency)
CMS 100-3,130.7 Withdrawal Treatments for Narcotic Addictions
CMS 100-4,12,110.3 Outpatient Mental Health Limitation
CMS 100-4,12,150 Clinical Social Worker (CSW) Services
CMS 100-4,12,160 Independent Psychologist Services
CMS 100-4,12,160.1 Payment for Independent Psychologists' Services
CMS 100-4,12,170 Clinical Psychologist Services
CMS 100-4,12,170.1 Payment for Clinical Psychologist Services
CMS 100-4,12,210 Outpatient Mental Health Limitation

INCLUDES Face-to-face time with patient (for part or all of the service) and/or family

Psychotherapy only (90832, 90834, 90837)

Psychotherapy with separately identifiable medical evaluation and management services includes add-on codes (90833, 90836, 90838)

Services provided in all settings

Therapeutic communication to:
- Ameliorate the patient's mental and behavioral symptoms
- Modify behavior
- Support and encourage personality growth and development

Treatment for:
- Behavior disturbances
- Mental illness

EXCLUDES *Family psychotherapy without the patient*

Code also interactive complexity services with the time the provider spends performing the service reflected in the time for the appropriate psychotherapy code (90785)

Do not report time providing pharmacologic management with time allocated to psychotherapy service codes

Do not report with (90839-90840, 0364T-0367T, 0373T-0374T)

90832 Psychotherapy, 30 minutes with patient and/or family member
03 1.79 1.81 FUD XXX

+ **90833 Psychotherapy, 30 minutes with patient and/or family member when performed with an evaluation and management service (List separately in addition to the code for primary procedure)**
Code first (99201-99255 [99224, 99225, 99226], 99304-99337, 99341-99350)
N 1.84 1.85 FUD ZZZ

90834 Psychotherapy, 45 minutes with patient and/or family member
03 2.39 2.40 FUD XXX

+ **90836 Psychotherapy, 45 minutes with patient and/or family member when performed with an evaluation and management service (List separately in addition to the code for primary procedure)**
Code first (99201-99255 [99224, 99225, 99226], 99304-99337, 99341-99350)
N 2.32 2.34 FUD ZZZ

90837 Psychotherapy, 60 minutes with patient and/or family member
Code also prolonged service for psychotherapy performed without evaluation and management service face-to-face with the patient lasting 90 minutes or longer (99354-99357)
03 3.57 3.59 FUD XXX

+ **90838 Psychotherapy, 60 minutes with patient and/or family member when performed with an evaluation and management service (List separately in addition to the code for primary procedure)**
Code first (99201-99255 [99224, 99225, 99226], 99304-99337, 99341-99350)
N 3.07 3.09 FUD ZZZ

90839-90840 Services for Patients in Crisis

INCLUDES 30 minutes or more of face-to-face time with the patient (for all or part of the service) and/or family providing crisis psychotherapy
All time spent exclusively with patient (for all or part of the service) and/or family, even if time is not continuous
Emergent care to a patient in severe distress (eg, life threatening or complex)
Institute interventions to minimize psychological trauma
Measures to ease the crisis and reestablish safety
Psychotherapy

EXCLUDES *Psychotherapy for crisis of less than 30 minutes (90832-90833)*

Do not report with (90785-90899, 0364T-0367T, 0373T-0374T)

90839 Psychotherapy for crisis; first 60 minutes
INCLUDES First 30-74 minutes of crisis psychotherapy per day
Do not report more than one time per day, even when the service is not continuous on that date
03 80 3.72 3.75 FUD XXX

+ **90840 each additional 30 minutes (List separately in addition to code for primary service)**
INCLUDES Up to 30 minutes of time beyond the initial 74 minutes
Code first (90839)
N1 80 1.79 1.00 FUD ZZZ

90845-90863 Additional Psychotherapy Services

CMS 100-2,15,160 Clinical Psychologist Services
CMS 100-3,130.1 Inpatient Stays for Alcoholism Treatment
CMS 100-3,130.2 Outpatient Hospital Services for Alcoholism
CMS 100-3,130.5 Treatment of Alcoholism/Drug Abuse in a Freestanding Clinic
CMS 100-3,130.6 Treatment of Drug Abuse (Chemical Dependency)
CMS 100-3,130.7 Withdrawal Treatments for Narcotic Addictions
CMS 100-4,12,110.3 Outpatient Mental Health Limitation
CMS 100-4,12,150 Clinical Social Worker (CSW) Services
CMS 100-4,12,160 Independent Psychologist Services
CMS 100-4,12,160.1 Payment for Independent Psychologists' Services
CMS 100-4,12,170 Clinical Psychologist Services
CMS 100-4,12,170.1 Payment for Clinical Psychologist Services

EXCLUDES *Analysis/programming of neurostimulators for vagus nerve stimulation therapy (95970, 95974-95975)*

Do not report with (90839-90840, 0364T-0367T, 0373T-0374T)

90845 Psychoanalysis
03 80 PQ 2.57 2.59 FUD XXX

90846 Family psychotherapy (without the patient present)
Do not report with (0368T-0371T)
03 80 2.89 2.91 FUD XXX

90847 Family psychotherapy (conjoint psychotherapy) (with patient present)
Do not report with (0368T-0371T)
03 80 2.98 3.00 FUD XXX

90849 Multiple-family group psychotherapy
03 80 PQ 0.86 0.96 FUD XXX

90853 Group psychotherapy (other than of a multiple-family group)
Do not report with (0372T)
Code also group psychotherapy with interactive complexity (90785)
03 80 PQ 0.72 0.74 FUD XXX

+ **90863 Pharmacologic management, including prescription and review of medication, when performed with psychotherapy services (List separately in addition to the code for primary procedure)**
Code first (90832, 90834, 90837)
Do not report time providing pharmacologic management with time allocated to psychotherapy service codes
E 0.00 0.00 FUD XXX

90865-90870 Other Psychiatric Treatment

CMS 100-4,12,110.3 Outpatient Mental Health Limitation
CMS 100-4,12,150 Clinical Social Worker (CSW) Services
CMS 100-4,12,160 Independent Psychologist Services
CMS 100-4,12,160.1 Payment for Independent Psychologists' Services
CMS 100-4,12,170 Clinical Psychologist Services
CMS 100-4,12,170.1 Payment for Clinical Psychologist Services
CMS 100-4,12,210 Outpatient Mental Health Limitation

EXCLUDES *Analysis/programming of neurostimulators for vagus nerve stimulation therapy (95970, 95974, 95975)*

Do not report with (90839-90840, 0364T-0367T, 0373T-0374T)

90865 Narcosynthesis for psychiatric diagnostic and therapeutic purposes (eg, sodium amobarbital (Amytal) interview)
03 80 3.61 4.73 FUD XXX

90867 Therapeutic repetitive transcranial magnetic stimulation (TMS) treatment; initial, including cortical mapping, motor threshold determination, delivery and management
INCLUDES Evaluation and management services related directly to:
Cortical mapping
Delivery and management of TMS services
Motor threshold determination
EXCLUDES *Medication management*
Significant, separately identifiable evaluation and management service
Significant, separately identifiable psychotherapy service
Transcranial magnetic stimulation (TMS) motor function mapping for treatment planning, upper and lower extremity (0310T)
Do not report more than one time for each course of treatment
Do not report with (90868-90869, 95860, 95870, 95928-95929, [95939])
S 0.00 0.00 FUD 000

90868 subsequent delivery and management, per session
INCLUDES Evaluation and management services related directly to:
Cortical mapping
Delivery and management of TMS services
Motor threshold determination
EXCLUDES *Medication management*
Significant, separately identifiable evaluation and management service
Significant, separately identifiable psychotherapy service
Transcranial magnetic stimulation (TMS) motor function mapping for treatment planning, upper and lower extremity (0310T)
S 0.00 0.00 FUD 000

90869 **subsequent motor threshold re-determination with delivery and management**

INCLUDES Evaluation and management services related directly to:
Cortical mapping
Delivery and management of TMS services
Motor threshold determination

EXCLUDES *Medication management*
Significant, separately identifiable evaluation and management service
Significant, separately identifiable psychotherapy service
Transcranial magnetic stimulation (TMS) motor function mapping for treatment planning, upper and lower extremity (0310T)

Do not report with (90867-90868, 95860-95870, 95928-95929, [95939])

S 0.00 0.00 FUD 000

90870 **Electroconvulsive therapy (includes necessary monitoring)**

S 80 3.14 4.98 FUD 000

90875-90880 Psychiatric Therapy with Biofeedback or Hypnosis

CMS 100-3,30.1 Biofeedback Therapy
CMS 100-4,12,110.3 Outpatient Mental Health Limitation
CMS 100-4,12,150 Clinical Social Worker (CSW) Services
CMS 100-4,12,160 Independent Psychologist Services
CMS 100-4,12,160.1 Payment for Independent Psychologists' Services
CMS 100-4,12,170 Clinical Psychologist Services
CMS 100-4,12,170.1 Payment for Clinical Psychologist Services
CMS 100-4,12,210 Outpatient Mental Health Limitation

EXCLUDES *Analysis/programming of neurostimulators for vagus nerve stimulation therapy (95970, 95974, 95975)*

Do not report with (90839-90840, 0364T-0367T, 0373T-0374T)

90875 **Individual psychophysiological therapy incorporating biofeedback training by any modality (face-to-face with the patient), with psychotherapy (eg, insight oriented, behavior modifying or supportive psychotherapy); 30 minutes**

E 1.74 1.75 FUD XXX

90876 **45 minutes**

E 2.74 3.04 FUD XXX

90880 **Hypnotherapy**

Q3 80 2.65 2.85 FUD XXX

90882-90899 Psychiatric Services without Patient Face-to-Face Contact

CMS 100-1,3,30.3 Mental Health Diagnostic Services
CMS 100-4,12,110.3 Outpatient Mental Health Limitation
CMS 100-4,12,150 Clinical Social Worker (CSW) Services
CMS 100-4,12,160 Independent Psychologist Services
CMS 100-4,12,160.1 Payment for Independent Psychologists' Services
CMS 100-4,12,170 Clinical Psychologist Services
CMS 100-4,12,170.1 Payment for Clinical Psychologist Services
CMS 100-4,12,210 Outpatient Mental Health Limitation

EXCLUDES *Analysis/programming of neurostimulators for vagus nerve stimulation therapy (95970, 95974, 95975)*

Do not report with (90839-90840, 0364T-0367T, 0373T-0374T)

90882 **Environmental intervention for medical management purposes on a psychiatric patient's behalf with agencies, employers, or institutions**

E 0.00 0.00 FUD XXX

90885 **Psychiatric evaluation of hospital records, other psychiatric reports, psychometric and/or projective tests, and other accumulated data for medical diagnostic purposes**

N 1.41 1.41 FUD XXX

90887 **Interpretation or explanation of results of psychiatric, other medical examinations and procedures, or other accumulated data to family or other responsible persons, or advising them how to assist patient**

Do not report with (0368T-0371T)

N 2.15 2.50 FUD XXX

90889 **Preparation of report of patient's psychiatric status, history, treatment, or progress (other than for legal or consultative purposes) for other individuals, agencies, or insurance carriers**

N 0.00 0.00 FUD XXX

90899 **Unlisted psychiatric service or procedure**

Q3 80 0.00 0.00 FUD XXX

90901-90911 Biofeedback Therapy

CMS 100-3,30.1 Biofeedback Therapy
CMS 100-3,30.1.1 Biofeedback for Urinary Incontinence

EXCLUDES *Psychophysiological therapy utilizing biofeedback training (90875-90876)*

90901 **Biofeedback training by any modality**

A 80 0.57 1.12 FUD 000

90911 **Biofeedback training, perineal muscles, anorectal or urethral sphincter, including EMG and/or manometry**

EXCLUDES *Rectal sensation/tone/compliance testing (91120)*
Treatment for incontinence, pulsed magnetic neuromodulation (53899)

T 80 1.28 2.39 FUD 000

90935-90940 Hemodialysis Services: Inpatient ESRD and Outpatient Non-ESRD

CMS 100-2,1,10 Inpatient Hospital Services Covered Under Part A
CMS 100-2,11,20 Coverage of Outpatient Maintenance Dialysis
CMS 100-3,130.8 Hemodialysis for Schizophrenia
CMS 100-3,190.10 Laboratory Tests--CRD Patients
CMS 100-3,230.14 Ultrafiltration Monitor
CMS 100-4,3,100.6 Inpatient Renal Services

EXCLUDES *Attendance by physician or other qualified health care provider for a prolonged period of time (99354-99360)*
Blood specimen collection from partial/complete implantable venous access device (36591)
Declotting of cannula (36831, 36833, 36860-36861)
Hemodialysis home visit by non-physician health care professional (99512)
Thrombolytic agent declotting of implanted vascular access device/catheter (36593)

Code also significant separately identifiable evaluation and management service not related to dialysis procedure or renal failure with modifier 25 (99201-99215, 99217-99223 [99224, 99225, 99226], 99231-99239, 99241-99245, 99281-99285, 99291-99292, 99304-99318, 99324-99337, 99341-99350, 99466-99467, 99468-99476, 99477-99480)

90935 **Hemodialysis procedure with single evaluation by a physician or other qualified health care professional**

INCLUDES All evaluation and management services related to the patient's renal disease rendered on a day dialysis is performed
Inpatient ESRD and non-ESRD procedures
Only one evaluation of the patient related to hemodialysis procedure
Outpatient non-ESRD dialysis

S 80 2.05 2.05 FUD 000

90937 Hemodialysis procedure requiring repeated evaluation(s) with or without substantial revision of dialysis prescription

INCLUDES All evaluation and management services related to the patient's renal disease rendered on a day dialysis is performed
Inpatient ESRD and non-ESRD procedures
Outpatient non-ESRD dialysis
Re-evaluation of the patient during hemodialysis procedure

B 80 2.94 2.94 FUD 000

90940 Hemodialysis access flow study to determine blood flow in grafts and arteriovenous fistulae by an indicator method

EXCLUDES *Hemodialysis access duplex scan (93990)*

N 0.00 0.00 FUD XXX

90945-90947 Dialysis Techniques Other Than Hemodialysis

CMS 100-2,1,10 Inpatient Hospital Services Covered Under Part A
CMS 100-3,110.15 Ultrafiltration, Hemoperfusion, and Hemofiltration
CMS 100-3,190.10 Laboratory Tests--CRD Patients
CMS 100-3,240.6 Transvenous (Catheter) Pulmonary Embolectomy
CMS 100-4,3,100.6 Inpatient Renal Services

INCLUDES All evaluation and management services related to the patient's renal disease rendered on the day dialysis is performed
Procedures other than hemodialysis:
Continuous renal replacement therapies
Hemofiltration
Peritoneal dialysis

EXCLUDES *Attendance by physician or other qualified health care provider for a prolonged period of time (99354-99360)*
Hemodialysis
Tunneled intraperitoneal catheter insertion
Open (49421)
Percutaneous (49418)

Code also significant, separately identifiable evaluation and management service not related to dialysis procedure or renal failure with modifier 25 (99201-99215, 99217-99223 [99224, 99225, 99226], 99231-99239, 99241-99245, 99281-99285, 99291-99292, 99304-99318, 99324-99337, 99341-99350, 99466-99480 [99485, 99486])

90945 Dialysis procedure other than hemodialysis (eg, peritoneal dialysis, hemofiltration, or other continuous renal replacement therapies), with single evaluation by a physician or other qualified health care professional

INCLUDES Only one evaluation of the patient related to the procedure

EXCLUDES *Peritoneal dialysis home infusion (99601, 99602)*

V 80 PQ 2.42 2.42 FUD 000

90947 Dialysis procedure other than hemodialysis (eg, peritoneal dialysis, hemofiltration, or other continuous renal replacement therapies) requiring repeated evaluations by a physician or other qualified health care professional, with or without substantial revision of dialysis prescription

EXCLUDES *Re-evaluation during a procedure*

B 80 PQ 3.51 3.51 FUD 000

90951-90962 End-stage Renal Disease Monthly Outpatient Services

CMS 100-3,190.10 Laboratory Tests--CRD Patients
CMS 100-3,230.14 Ultrafiltration Monitor

INCLUDES Establishing dialyzing cycle
Management of dialysis visits
Outpatient evaluation and management of dialysis visits
Patient management during dialysis for a month
Telephone calls

EXCLUDES *Dialysis services provided during an inpatient hospitalization (90935-90937, 90945-90947)*
ESRD/non-ESRD dialysis services performed in an inpatient setting (90935-90937, 90945-90947)
Non-ESRD dialysis services performed in an outpatient setting (90935-90937, 90945-90947)
Non-ESRD related evaluation and management services that cannot be performed during the dialysis session

Do not report during the time transitional care management services are being provided (99495-99496)
Do not report in the same month with (99487-99489)

90951 End-stage renal disease (ESRD) related services monthly, for patients younger than 2 years of age to include monitoring for the adequacy of nutrition, assessment of growth and development, and counseling of parents; with 4 or more face-to-face visits by a physician or other qualified health care professional per month A

M 80 PQ 26.32 26.32 FUD XXX

90952 with 2-3 face-to-face visits by a physician or other qualified health care professional per month A

M 80 PQ 0.00 0.00 FUD XXX

90953 with 1 face-to-face visit by a physician or other qualified health care professional per month A

M 80 PQ 0.00 0.00 FUD XXX

90954 End-stage renal disease (ESRD) related services monthly, for patients 2-11 years of age to include monitoring for the adequacy of nutrition, assessment of growth and development, and counseling of parents; with 4 or more face-to-face visits by a physician or other qualified health care professional per month A

M 80 PQ 22.84 22.84 FUD XXX

90955 with 2-3 face-to-face visits by a physician or other qualified health care professional per month A

M 80 PQ 12.88 12.88 FUD XXX

90956 with 1 face-to-face visit by a physician or other qualified health care professional per month A

M 80 PQ 8.97 8.97 FUD XXX

90957 End-stage renal disease (ESRD) related services monthly, for patients 12-19 years of age to include monitoring for the adequacy of nutrition, assessment of growth and development, and counseling of parents; with 4 or more face-to-face visits by a physician or other qualified health care professional per month A

M 80 PQ 18.17 18.17 FUD XXX

90958 with 2-3 face-to-face visits by a physician or other qualified health care professional per month A

M 80 PQ 12.29 12.29 FUD XXX

90959 with 1 face-to-face visit by a physician or other qualified health care professional per month A

M 80 PQ 8.32 8.32 FUD XXX

90960 End-stage renal disease (ESRD) related services monthly, for patients 20 years of age and older; with 4 or more face-to-face visits by a physician or other qualified health care professional per month A

M 80 PQ 8.01 8.01 FUD XXX

90961 with 2-3 face-to-face visits by a physician or other qualified health care professional per month A

M 80 PQ 6.74 6.74 FUD XXX

90962 with 1 face-to-face visit by a physician or other qualified health care professional per month A
M 80 PQ 5.20 5.20 FUD XXX

90963-90966 End-stage Renal Disease Monthly Home Dialysis Services

INCLUDES ESRD services for home dialysis patients
Services provided for a full month

Do not report during the time transitional care management services are being provided (99495-99496)
Do not report in the same month with (99487-99489)

90963 End-stage renal disease (ESRD) related services for home dialysis per full month, for patients younger than 2 years of age to include monitoring for the adequacy of nutrition, assessment of growth and development, and counseling of parents A
M 80 PQ 15.40 15.40 FUD XXX

90964 End-stage renal disease (ESRD) related services for home dialysis per full month, for patients 2-11 years of age to include monitoring for the adequacy of nutrition, assessment of growth and development, and counseling of parents A
M 80 PQ 13.42 13.42 FUD XXX

90965 End-stage renal disease (ESRD) related services for home dialysis per full month, for patients 12-19 years of age to include monitoring for the adequacy of nutrition, assessment of growth and development, and counseling of parents A
M 80 PQ 12.73 12.73 FUD XXX

90966 End-stage renal disease (ESRD) related services for home dialysis per full month, for patients 20 years of age and older A
M 80 PQ 6.73 6.73 FUD XXX

90967-90970 End-stage Renal Disease Services: Partial Month

CMS 100-3,190.10 Laboratory Tests--CRD Patients
CMS 100-3,230.14 Ultrafiltration Monitor

INCLUDES ESRD services for less than a full month, such as:
A patient who is transient, dies, recovers, or undergoes kidney transplant
Outpatient ESRD-related services initiated prior to completion of assessment
Patient spending part of the month as a hospital inpatient
Services reported on a daily basis, less the days of hospitalization

Do not report during the time transitional care management services are being provided (99495-99496)
Do not report in the same month with (99487-99489)

90967 End-stage renal disease (ESRD) related services for dialysis less than a full month of service, per day; for patients younger than 2 years of age A
M 80 PQ 0.50 0.50 FUD XXX

90968 for patients 2-11 years of age A
M 80 PQ 0.43 0.43 FUD XXX

90969 for patients 12-19 years of age A
M 80 PQ 0.42 0.42 FUD XXX

90970 for patients 20 years of age and older A
M 80 PQ 0.22 0.22 FUD XXX

90989-90993 Dialysis Training Services

90989 Dialysis training, patient, including helper where applicable, any mode, completed course
B PQ 0.00 0.00 FUD XXX

90993 Dialysis training, patient, including helper where applicable, any mode, course not completed, per training session
B PQ 0.00 0.00 FUD XXX

90997-90999 Hemoperfusion and Unlisted Dialysis Procedures

90997 Hemoperfusion (eg, with activated charcoal or resin)
B 80 PQ 2.61 2.61 FUD 000

90999 Unlisted dialysis procedure, inpatient or outpatient
B 80 PQ 0.00 0.00 FUD XXX

91010-91022 Esophageal Manometry

CMS 100-3,100.4 Esophageal Manometry

91010 Esophageal motility (manometric study of the esophagus and/or gastroesophageal junction) study with interpretation and report;
EXCLUDES *Esophageal motility studies with high-resolution esophageal pressure topography (0240T-0241T)*
Code also for esophageal motility studies with stimulant or perfusion (91013)
X 80 4.97 4.97 FUD 000

\+ **91013** with stimulation or perfusion (eg, stimulant, acid or alkali perfusion) (List separately in addition to code for primary procedure)
EXCLUDES *Esophageal motility studies with high-resolution esophageal pressure topography (0240T-0241T)*
Code first (91010)
Do not report more than one time for each session
N 80 0.67 0.67 FUD ZZZ

91020 Gastric motility (manometric) studies
Do not report with (91112)
X 80 6.60 6.60 FUD 000

91022 Duodenal motility (manometric) study
EXCLUDES *Fluoroscopy (76000)*
Gastric motility study (91020)
Do not report with (91112)
X 80 4.76 4.76 FUD 000

91030-91040 Esophageal Reflux Tests

EXCLUDES *Duodenal intubation/aspiration (43756-43757)*
Esophagoscopy (43180-43232 [43211, 43212, 43213, 43214])
Insertion of:
Esophageal tamponade tube (43460)
Miller-Abbott tube (44500)
Radiologic services, gastrointestinal (74210-74363)
Upper gastrointestinal endoscopy (43235-43259 [43233, 43266, 43270])

91030 Esophagus, acid perfusion (Bernstein) test for esophagitis
X 80 3.88 3.88 FUD 000

91034 Esophagus, gastroesophageal reflux test; with nasal catheter pH electrode(s) placement, recording, analysis and interpretation
X 80 5.34 5.34 FUD 000

91035 with mucosal attached telemetry pH electrode placement, recording, analysis and interpretation
INCLUDES Endoscopy only to place device
X 80 13.58 13.58 FUD 000

91037 **Esophageal function test, gastroesophageal reflux test with nasal catheter intraluminal impedance electrode(s) placement, recording, analysis and interpretation;**
X 80 CCI 4.56 4.56 FUD 000

91038 **prolonged (greater than 1 hour, up to 24 hours)**
X 80 CCI 12.73 12.73 FUD 000

91040 **Esophageal balloon distension provocation study**
X 80 CCI 11.26 11.26 FUD 000

91065 Breath Analysis

CMS 100-3,100.5 Diagnostic Breath Analysis

EXCLUDES *H. pylori breath test analysis, radioactive (C-14) or nonradioactive (C-13) (78268 or 83013)*

Code also each challenge administered

91065 **Breath hydrogen or methane test (eg, for detection of lactase deficiency, fructose intolerance, bacterial overgrowth, or oro-cecal gastrointestinal transit)**
X 80 CCI 2.32 2.32 FUD 000

91110-91299 Additional Gastrointestinal Diagnostic/Therapeutic Procedures

EXCLUDES *Abdominal paracentesis (49082-49084)*
Abdominal paracentesis with medication administration (96440, 96446)
Anoscopy (46600-46615)
Cholangiography (47500, 74320)
Colonoscopy (45378-45393 [45388, 45390, 45398])
Duodenal intubation/aspiration (43756-43757)
Esophagoscopy (43180-43232 [43211, 43212, 43213, 43214])
Proctosigmoidoscopy (45300-45327)
Radiologic services, gastrointestinal (74210-74363)
Sigmoidoscopy (45330-45350 [45346])
Small intestine/stomal endoscopy (44360-44408 [44381, 44401])
Upper gastrointestinal endoscopy (43235-43259 [43233, 43266, 43270])

91110 **Gastrointestinal tract imaging, intraluminal (eg, capsule endoscopy), esophagus through ileum, with interpretation and report**
Code also modifier 52 if ileum is not visualized
Do not report with visualization of the colon separately
Do not report with (91111, 0355T)
T 80 25.12 25.12 FUD XXX

91111 **Gastrointestinal tract imaging, intraluminal (eg, capsule endoscopy), esophagus with interpretation and report**
EXCLUDES *Use of wireless capsule to measure transit times or pressure in gastrointestinal tract (91112)*
Do not report with (91110, 0355T)
T 80 20.55 20.55 FUD XXX

91112 **Gastrointestinal transit and pressure measurement, stomach through colon, wireless capsule, with interpretation and report**
Do not report with (83986, 91020, 91022, 91117)
X 80 30.22 30.22 FUD XXX

91117 **Colon motility (manometric) study, minimum 6 hours continuous recording (including provocation tests, eg, meal, intracolonic balloon distension, pharmacologic agents, if performed), with interpretation and report**
EXCLUDES *Use of wireless capsule to measure transit times or pressure in gastrointestinal tract (91112)*
Do not report more than one time regardless of the number of provocations
Do not report with (91120, 91122)
T 80 4.23 4.23 FUD 000

91120 **Rectal sensation, tone, and compliance test (ie, response to graded balloon distention)**
EXCLUDES *Anorectal manometry (91122)*
Biofeedback training (90911)
Do not report with (91117)
T 80 11.25 11.25 FUD XXX

91122 **Anorectal manometry**
Do not report with (91117)
T 80 CCI 6.25 6.25 FUD 000

91132 **Electrogastrography, diagnostic, transcutaneous;**
X 80 CCI 4.31 4.31 FUD XXX

91133 **with provocative testing**
X 80 CCI 5.04 5.04 FUD XXX

● **91200** **Liver elastography, mechanically induced shear wave (eg, vibration), without imaging, with interpretation and report**

91299 **Unlisted diagnostic gastroenterology procedure**
X 80 0.00 0.00 FUD XXX

92002-92014 Ophthalmic Medical Services

CMS 100-4,4,160 Clinic and Emergency Visits Under OPPS

INCLUDES Routine ophthalmoscopy
Services provided to established patients who have received professional services from the physician or other qualified health care provider or another physician or other qualified health care professional within the same group practice of the exact same specialty and subspecialty within the past three years
Services provided to new patients who have received no professional services from the physician or other qualified health care provider or another physician or other qualified health care professional within the same group practice of the exact same specialty and subspecialty within the past three years

EXCLUDES *Surgical procedures on the eye/ocular adnexa (65091-68899 [67810])*

92002 **Ophthalmological services: medical examination and evaluation with initiation of diagnostic and treatment program; intermediate, new patient**
INCLUDES Evaluation of new/existing condition complicated by new diagnostic or management problem
Integrated services where medical decision making cannot be separated from examination methods
Problems not related to primary diagnosis
The following for intermediate services:
External ocular/adnexal examination
General medical observation
History
Other diagnostic procedures
Biomicroscopy
Mydriasis
Ophthalmoscopy
Tonometry
V 80 CCI PQ 1.40 2.32 FUD XXX

92004 **comprehensive, new patient, 1 or more visits**

INCLUDES General evaluation of complete visual system
Integrated services where medical decision making cannot be separated from examination methods
Single service that need not be performed at one session
The following for comprehensive services:
Basic sensorimotor examination
Biomicroscopy
Dilation (cycloplegia)
External examinations
General medical observation
Gross visual fields
History
Initiation of diagnostic/treatment programs
Mydriasis
Ophthalmoscopic examinations
Other diagnostic procedures
Prescription of medication
Special diagnostic/treatment services
Tonometry

V 80 PQ 2.87 4.22 FUD XXX

92012 **Ophthalmological services: medical examination and evaluation, with initiation or continuation of diagnostic and treatment program; intermediate, established patient**

INCLUDES Evaluation of new/existing condition complicated by new diagnostic or management problem
Integrated services where medical decision making cannot be separated from examination methods
Problems not related to primary diagnosis
The following for intermediate services:
External ocular/adnexal examination
General medical observation
History
Other diagnostic procedures:
Biomicroscopy
Mydriasis
Ophthalmoscopy
Tonometry

V 80 PQ 1.53 2.43 FUD XXX

92014 **comprehensive, established patient, 1 or more visits**

INCLUDES General evaluation of complete visual system
Integrated services where medical decision making cannot be separated from examination methods
Single service that need not be performed at one session
The following for comprehensive services:
Basic sensorimotor examination
Biomicroscopy
Dilation (cycloplegia)
External examinations
General medical observation
Gross visual fields
History
Initiation of diagnostic/treatment programs
Mydriasis
Ophthalmoscopic examinations
Other diagnostic procedures
Prescription of medication
Special diagnostic/treatment services
Tonometry

V 80 PQ 2.31 3.52 FUD XXX

92015-92145 Ophthalmic Special Services

CMS 100-2,16,90 Routine Services and Appliances
CMS 100-3,80.1 Hydrophilic Contact lens for Corneal Bandage
CMS 100-3,80.2 Photodynamic Therapy
CMS 100-3,80.4 Hydrophilic Contact Lens
CMS 100-3,80.6 Intraocular Photography
CMS 100-3,80.8 Endothelial Cell Photography
CMS 100-3,80.9 Computer Enhanced Perimetry

INCLUDES Routine ophthalmoscopy

EXCLUDES *Surgical procedures on the eye/ocular adnexa (65091-68899 [67810])*

Code also evaluation and management services, when performed
Code also general ophthalmological services, when performed (92002-92014)

92015 **Determination of refractive state**

INCLUDES Lens prescription
Absorptive factor
Axis
Impact resistance
Lens power
Prism
Specification of lens type:
Monofocal
Bifocal

EXCLUDES *Bilateral instrument based ocular screening (99174)*

E 0.56 0.57 FUD XXX

92018 **Ophthalmological examination and evaluation, under general anesthesia, with or without manipulation of globe for passive range of motion or other manipulation to facilitate diagnostic examination; complete**

T 80 4.20 4.20 FUD XXX

92019 **limited**

T 80 2.04 2.04 FUD XXX

92020 **Gonioscopy (separate procedure)**

EXCLUDES *Gonioscopy under general anesthesia (92018)*

S 80 0.62 0.78 FUD XXX

92025 **Computerized corneal topography, unilateral or bilateral, with interpretation and report**

EXCLUDES *Manual keratoscopy*

Do not report with (65710-65771)

S 80 1.07 1.07 FUD XXX

92060 **Sensorimotor examination with multiple measurements of ocular deviation (eg, restrictive or paretic muscle with diplopia) with interpretation and report (separate procedure)**

S 80 1.85 1.85 FUD XXX

92065 **Orthoptic and/or pleoptic training, with continuing medical direction and evaluation**

S 80 1.50 1.50 FUD XXX

92071 **Fitting of contact lens for treatment of ocular surface disease**

Code also supply of lens with appropriate supply code or (99070)
Do not report with (92072)

N1 N 80 50 0.97 1.08 FUD XXX

92072 **Fitting of contact lens for management of keratoconus, initial fitting**

EXCLUDES *Subsequent fittings (99211-99215, 92012-92014)*

Code also supply of lens with appropriate supply code or (99070)
Do not report with (92071)

N1 N 80 3.02 3.90 FUD XXX

92081 **Visual field examination, unilateral or bilateral, with interpretation and report; limited examination (eg, tangent screen, Autoplot, arc perimeter, or single stimulus level automated test, such as Octopus 3 or 7 equivalent)**

S 80 0.97 0.97 FUD XXX

92082 **intermediate examination (eg, at least 2 isopters on Goldmann perimeter, or semiquantitative, automated suprathreshold screening program, Humphrey suprathreshold automatic diagnostic test, Octopus program 33)**
S 80 ⊏ 1.39 1.39 FUD XXX

92083 **extended examination (eg, Goldmann visual fields with at least 3 isopters plotted and static determination within the central 30 degrees or quantitative, automated threshold perimetry, Octopus program G-1, 32 or 42, Humphrey visual field analyzer full threshold programs 30-2, 24-2, or 30/60-2)**
EXCLUDES *Assessment of visual field by transmissionof data by patient to a surveillance center (0378T-0379T)*
Do not report gross visual field testing/confrontation testing separately
S 80 ⊏ 1.82 1.82 FUD XXX

92100 **Serial tonometry (separate procedure) with multiple measurements of intraocular pressure over an extended time period with interpretation and report, same day (eg, diurnal curve or medical treatment of acute elevation of intraocular pressure)**
EXCLUDES *Intraocular pressure monitoring for 24 hours or more (0329T)*
Ocular blood flow measurements (0198T)
Single-episode tonometry (99201-99215, 92002-92004)
N 80 ⊏ 0.98 2.26 FUD XXX

92132 **Scanning computerized ophthalmic diagnostic imaging, anterior segment, with interpretation and report, unilateral or bilateral**
EXCLUDES *Imaging of anterior segment with specular microscopy and endothelial cell analysis (92286)*
Scanning computerized ophthalmic diagnostic imaging of optic nerve and retina (92133-92134)
Tear film imaging (0330T)
S 80 1.01 1.01 FUD XXX

92133 **Scanning computerized ophthalmic diagnostic imaging, posterior segment, with interpretation and report, unilateral or bilateral; optic nerve**
Do not report with (92227-92228)
Do not report with scanning computerized ophthalmic imaging of retina at same visit (92134)
S 80 1.26 1.26 FUD XXX

92134 **retina**
Do not report with (92227-92228)
Do not report with scanning computerized ophthalmic imaging of optic nerve at same visit (92133)
S 80 1.29 1.29 FUD XXX

92136 **Ophthalmic biometry by partial coherence interferometry with intraocular lens power calculation**
EXCLUDES *Tear film imaging (0330T)*
S 80 ⊏ 2.53 2.53 FUD XXX

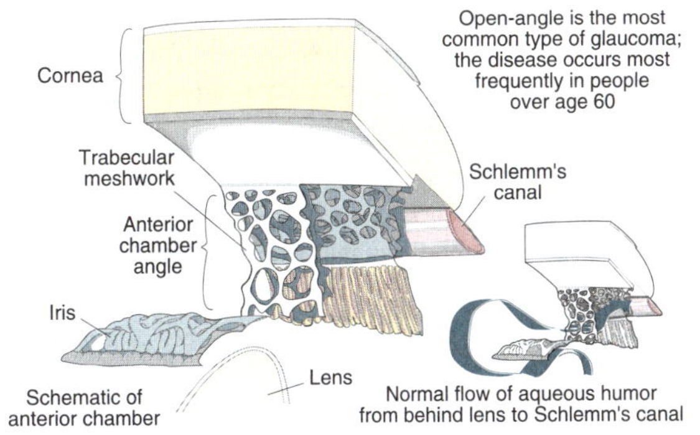

Glaucoma is caused by excessive intraocular pressure and abnormal accumulation of aqueous humor in the anterior chamber of the eye; pressure reduces blood supply to the optic nerve and causes nerve damage

92140 **Provocative tests for glaucoma, with interpretation and report, without tonography**
S 80 ⊏ 0.77 1.78 FUD XXX

● 92145 **Corneal hysteresis determination, by air impulse stimulation, unilateral or bilateral, with interpretation and report**

92225-92287 Other Ophthalmology Services

EXCLUDES *Prescription, fitting, and/or medical supervision of ocular prosthesis adaptation by physician (99201-99215, 99241-99245, 92002-92014)*

92225 **Ophthalmoscopy, extended, with retinal drawing (eg, for retinal detachment, melanoma), with interpretation and report; initial**
EXCLUDES *Ophthalmoscopy under general anesthesia (92018)*
S 80 ⊏ 0.63 0.78 FUD XXX

92226 **subsequent**
S 80 ⊏ 0.54 0.70 FUD XXX

92227 **Remote imaging for detection of retinal disease (eg, retinopathy in a patient with diabetes) with analysis and report under physician supervision, unilateral or bilateral**
Do not report with (99201-99350 [99224, 99225, 99226], 92002-92014, 92133-92134, 92228, 92250)
X TC 80 0.40 0.40 FUD XXX

92228 **Remote imaging for monitoring and management of active retinal disease (eg, diabetic retinopathy) with physician review, interpretation and report, unilateral or bilateral**
Do not report with (99201-99350 [99224, 99225, 99226], 92002-92014, 92133-92134, 92227, 92250)
X 80 0.99 0.99 FUD XXX

92230 **Fluorescein angioscopy with interpretation and report**
S 80 ⊏ 0.98 1.67 FUD XXX

92235 **Fluorescein angiography (includes multiframe imaging) with interpretation and report**
S 80 ⊏ 3.09 3.09 FUD XXX

92240 **Indocyanine-green angiography (includes multiframe imaging) with interpretation and report**
S 80 ⊏ 7.14 7.14 FUD XXX

92250 **Fundus photography with interpretation and report**
S 80 ⊏ 2.21 2.21 FUD XXX

92260 **Ophthalmodynamometry**
EXCLUDES *Ophthalmoscopy under general anesthesia (92018)*
S 80 ⊏ 0.32 0.53 FUD XXX

92265 **Needle oculoelectromyography, 1 or more extraocular muscles, 1 or both eyes, with interpretation and report**
S 80 ⚑ 2.16 2.16 FUD XXX

92270 **Electro-oculography with interpretation and report**
EXCLUDES *Recording of saccadic eye movements (92700)*
Do not report with (92540-92548)
S 80 ⚑ 2.54 2.54 FUD XXX

92275 **Electroretinography with interpretation and report**
EXCLUDES *Vestibular function tests/electronystagmography (92541-92548)*
76511-76529
S 80 ⚑ 4.48 4.48 FUD XXX

92283 **Color vision examination, extended, eg, anomaloscope or equivalent**
EXCLUDES *Color vision testing with pseudoisochromatic plates (e.g., HRR, Ishihara) (92002-92004, 92012-92014, 99172)*
S 80 ⚑ 1.55 1.55 FUD XXX

92284 **Dark adaptation examination with interpretation and report**
S 80 ⚑ 1.70 1.70 FUD XXX

92285 **External ocular photography with interpretation and report for documentation of medical progress (eg, close-up photography, slit lamp photography, goniophotography, stereo-photography)**
EXCLUDES *Tear film imaging (0330T)*
S 80 ⚑ 0.58 0.58 FUD XXX

92286 **Anterior segment imaging with interpretation and report; with specular microscopy and endothelial cell analysis**
S 80 ⚑ 1.08 1.08 FUD XXX

92287 **with fluorescein angiography**
S 80 ⚑ 3.87 3.87 FUD XXX

92310-92326 Services Related to Contact Lenses

CMS 100-2,15,30.4 Optometrist's Services
CMS 100-3,80.1 Hydrophilic Contact lens for Corneal Bandage
CMS 100-3,80.4 Hydrophilic Contact Lens

INCLUDES Incidental revision of lens during training period
Patient training/instruction
Specification of optical/physical characteristics:
- Curvature
- Flexibility
- Gas-permeability
- Power
- Size

EXCLUDES *Extended wear lenses follow up (92012-92014)*
General ophthalmological services
Therapeutic/surgical use of contact lens (68340, 92071-92072)

92310 **Prescription of optical and physical characteristics of and fitting of contact lens, with medical supervision of adaptation; corneal lens, both eyes, except for aphakia**
Code also modifier 52 for one eye
E 1.70 2.70 FUD XXX

92311 **corneal lens for aphakia, 1 eye**
S 80 ⚑ 1.63 2.89 FUD XXX

92312 **corneal lens for aphakia, both eyes**
S 80 ⚑ 1.82 3.26 FUD XXX

92313 **corneoscleral lens**
S 80 ⚑ 1.39 2.77 FUD XXX

92314 **Prescription of optical and physical characteristics of contact lens, with medical supervision of adaptation and direction of fitting by independent technician; corneal lens, both eyes except for aphakia**
Code also modifier 52 for one eye
E 1.00 2.23 FUD XXX

92315 **corneal lens for aphakia, 1 eye**
S 80 ⚑ 0.65 2.07 FUD XXX

92316 **corneal lens for aphakia, both eyes**
S 80 ⚑ 0.96 2.58 FUD XXX

92317 **corneoscleral lens**
S 80 ⚑ 0.62 2.13 FUD XXX

92325 **Modification of contact lens (separate procedure), with medical supervision of adaptation**
S 80 ⚑ 1.16 1.16 FUD XXX

92326 **Replacement of contact lens**
S 80 ⚑ 1.00 1.00 FUD XXX

92340-92499 Services Related to Eyeglasses

CMS 100-2,15,30.4 Optometrist's Services
CMS 100-4,1,30.3.5 Effect of Assignment on Cataract Glasses from Participating Physician/Supplier

INCLUDES Anatomical facial characteristics measurement
Final adjustment of spectacles to visual axes/anatomical topography
Written laboratory specifications

EXCLUDES *Supply of materials*

92340 **Fitting of spectacles, except for aphakia; monofocal**
E 0.54 1.00 FUD XXX

92341 **bifocal**
E 0.68 1.14 FUD XXX

92342 **multifocal, other than bifocal**
E 0.77 1.23 FUD XXX

92352 **Fitting of spectacle prosthesis for aphakia; monofocal**
S 0.54 1.14 FUD XXX

92353 **multifocal**
S 0.72 1.32 FUD XXX

92354 **Fitting of spectacle mounted low vision aid; single element system**
S 0.38 0.38 FUD XXX

92355 **telescopic or other compound lens system**
S 0.58 0.58 FUD XXX

92358 **Prosthesis service for aphakia, temporary (disposable or loan, including materials)**
S 0.32 0.32 FUD XXX

92370 **Repair and refitting spectacles; except for aphakia**
E 0.47 0.87 FUD XXX

92371 **spectacle prosthesis for aphakia**
S 0.32 0.32 FUD XXX

92499 **Unlisted ophthalmological service or procedure**
S 80 0.00 0.00 FUD XXX

92502-92548 Special Procedures of the Ears/Nose/Throat

CMS 100-2,15,80.3 Audiology Services
CMS 100-2,15,230.3 Practice of Speech-Language Pathology

INCLUDES Diagnostic/treatment services not generally included in an evaluation and management service

EXCLUDES *Laryngoscopy with stroboscopy (31579)*

Do not report anterior rhinoscopy, tuning fork testing, otoscopy, or removal of cerumen (non-impacted) separately

92502 **Otolaryngologic examination under general anesthesia**
T 80 ⚑ 2.75 2.75 FUD 000

92504 **Binocular microscopy (separate diagnostic procedure)**
N 80 ⚑ 0.27 0.85 FUD XXX

92507 Treatment of speech, language, voice, communication, and/or auditory processing disorder; individual

EXCLUDES *Auditory rehabilitation:*
Postlingual hearing loss (92633)
Prelingual hearing loss (92630)
Programming of cochlear implant (92601-92604)

Do not report with (0364T-0365T, 0368T-0369T)

A 80 PQ 2.25 2.25 FUD XXX

92508 group, 2 or more individuals

EXCLUDES *Auditory rehabilitation:*
Postlingual hearing loss (92633)
Prelingual hearing loss (92630)
Programming of cochlear implant (92601-92604)

Do not report with (0366T-0367T, 0372T)

A 80 PQ 0.66 0.66 FUD XXX

92511 Nasopharyngoscopy with endoscope (separate procedure)

Do not report with (43197-43198)

T 80 1.38 3.86 FUD 000

92512 Nasal function studies (eg, rhinomanometry)

X 80 0.81 1.72 FUD XXX

92516 Facial nerve function studies (eg, electroneuronography)

X 80 0.66 1.97 FUD XXX

92520 Laryngeal function studies (ie, aerodynamic testing and acoustic testing)

EXCLUDES *Other laryngeal function testing (92700)*
Swallowing/laryngeal sensory testing with flexible fiberoptic endoscope (92611-92617)

Code also modifier 52 for single test

X 80 1.17 2.10 FUD XXX

92521 Evaluation of speech fluency (eg, stuttering, cluttering)

INCLUDES Ability to execute motor movements needed for speech
Comprehension of written and verbal expression
Determination of patient's ability to create and communicate expressive thought
Evaluation of the ability to produce speech sound

A 80 3.19 3.19 FUD XXX

92522 Evaluation of speech sound production (eg, articulation, phonological process, apraxia, dysarthria);

INCLUDES Ability to execute motor movements needed for speech
Comprehension of written and verbal expression
Determination of patient's ability to create and communicate expressive thought
Evaluation of the ability to produce speech sound

A 80 2.59 2.59 FUD XXX

92523 with evaluation of language comprehension and expression (eg, receptive and expressive language)

INCLUDES Ability to execute motor movements needed for speech
Comprehension of written and verbal expression
Determination of patient's ability to create and communicate expressive thought
Evaluation of the ability to produce speech sound

A 80 5.38 5.38 FUD XXX

92524 Behavioral and qualitative analysis of voice and resonance

INCLUDES Ability to execute motor movements needed for speech
Comprehension of written and verbal expression
Determination of patient's ability to create and communicate expressive thought
Evaluation of the ability to produce speech sound

A 80 2.70 2.70 FUD XXX

92526 Treatment of swallowing dysfunction and/or oral function for feeding

A 80 PQ 2.45 2.45 FUD XXX

92531 Spontaneous nystagmus, including gaze

Do not report with evaluation and management services (99201-99215, 99218-99223 [99224, 99225, 99226], 99231-99236, 99241-99245, 99304-99318, 99324-99337)

N 0.00 0.00 FUD XXX

92532 Positional nystagmus test

Do not report with evaluation and management services (99201-99215, 99218-99223 [99224, 99225, 99226], 99231-99236, 99241-99245, 99304-99318, 99324-99337)

N 0.00 0.00 FUD XXX

92533 Caloric vestibular test, each irrigation (binaural, bithermal stimulation constitutes 4 tests)

INCLUDES Barany caloric test

N 0.00 0.00 FUD XXX

92534 Optokinetic nystagmus test

N 0.00 0.00 FUD XXX

92540 Basic vestibular evaluation, includes spontaneous nystagmus test with eccentric gaze fixation nystagmus, with recording, positional nystagmus test, minimum of 4 positions, with recording, optokinetic nystagmus test, bidirectional foveal and peripheral stimulation, with recording, and oscillating tracking test, with recording

Do not report with (92270, 92541-92542, 92544-92545)

X 80 PQ 2.86 2.86 FUD XXX

92541 Spontaneous nystagmus test, including gaze and fixation nystagmus, with recording

Do not report with (92270, 92540, 92542, 92544-92545)

X 80 PQ 0.86 0.86 FUD XXX

92542 Positional nystagmus test, minimum of 4 positions, with recording

Do not report with (92270, 92540-92541, 92544-92545)

X 80 PQ 0.74 0.74 FUD XXX

92543 Caloric vestibular test, each irrigation (binaural, bithermal stimulation constitutes 4 tests), with recording

Do not report with (92270)

X 80 PQ 0.45 0.45 FUD XXX

92544 Optokinetic nystagmus test, bidirectional, foveal or peripheral stimulation, with recording

Do not report with (92270, 92540-92542, 92545)

X 80 PQ 0.67 0.67 FUD XXX

92545 Oscillating tracking test, with recording

Do not report with (92270, 92540-92542, 92544)

X 80 PQ 0.58 0.58 FUD XXX

92546 Sinusoidal vertical axis rotational testing

Do not report with (92270)

X 80 PQ 2.89 2.89 FUD XXX

+ **92547 Use of vertical electrodes (List separately in addition to code for primary procedure)**

EXCLUDES *Unlisted vestibular tests (92700)*

Code first (92540-92546)
Do not report with (92270)

N TC 80 PQ 0.17 0.17 FUD ZZZ

92548 **Computerized dynamic posturography**
Do not report with (92270)
X 80 PQ 2.92 2.92 FUD XXX

92550-92596 [92558] Hearing and Speech Tests

CMS 100-2,15,230.3 Practice of Speech-Language Pathology
CMS 100-4,5,10.2 Financial Limitation for Outpatient Rehabilitation Services
CMS 100-4,12,30.3 Audiological Diagnostic Tests, Speech-Language Evaluations and Treatments

INCLUDES Diagnostic/treatment services not generally included in a comprehensive otorhinolaryngologic evaluation or office visit
Testing of both ears
Use of calibrated electronic equipment, recording of results, and a report with interpretation

EXCLUDES *Evaluation of speech/language/hearing problems using observation/assessment of performance (92521-92524)*

Code also modifier 52 for unilateral testing
Do not report tuning fork or whispered voice hearing tests separately

92550 **Tympanometry and reflex threshold measurements**
Do not report with (92567-92568)
X 80 PQ 0.59 0.59 FUD XXX

92551 **Screening test, pure tone, air only**
E 0.33 0.33 FUD XXX

92552 **Pure tone audiometry (threshold); air only**
EXCLUDES *Automated test (0208T)*
X TC 80 PQ 0.86 0.86 FUD XXX

92553 **air and bone**
EXCLUDES *Automated test (0209T)*
X TC 80 PQ 1.03 1.03 FUD XXX

92555 **Speech audiometry threshold;**
EXCLUDES *Automated test (0210T)*
X TC 80 PQ 0.64 0.64 FUD XXX

92556 **with speech recognition**
EXCLUDES *Automated test (0211T)*
X TC 80 1.02 1.02 FUD XXX

92557 **Comprehensive audiometry threshold evaluation and speech recognition (92553 and 92556 combined)**
EXCLUDES *Automated test (0212T)*
Evaluation/selection of hearing aid (92590-92595)
X 80 PQ 0.92 1.06 FUD XXX

92558 ***Resequenced code. See code following 92586.***

92559 **Audiometric testing of groups**
INCLUDES For group testing, indicate tests performed
E 0.00 0.00 FUD XXX

92560 **Bekesy audiometry; screening**
E 0.00 0.00 FUD XXX

92561 **diagnostic**
X TC 80 PQ 1.05 1.05 FUD XXX

92562 **Loudness balance test, alternate binaural or monaural**
INCLUDES ABLB test
X TC 80 PQ 1.29 1.29 FUD XXX

92563 **Tone decay test**
X TC 80 PQ 0.85 0.85 FUD XXX

92564 **Short increment sensitivity index (SISI)**
X TC 80 PQ 0.79 0.79 FUD XXX

92565 **Stenger test, pure tone**
X TC 80 PQ 0.46 0.46 FUD XXX

92567 **Tympanometry (impedance testing)**
X 80 PQ 0.31 0.41 FUD XXX

92568 **Acoustic reflex testing, threshold**
X 80 PQ 0.44 0.44 FUD XXX

92570 **Acoustic immittance testing, includes tympanometry (impedance testing), acoustic reflex threshold testing, and acoustic reflex decay testing**
Do not report with (92567-92568)
X 80 PQ 0.85 0.91 FUD XXX

92571 **Filtered speech test**
X TC 80 PQ 0.75 0.75 FUD XXX

92572 **Staggered spondaic word test**
X TC 80 PQ 1.43 1.43 FUD XXX

92575 **Sensorineural acuity level test**
X TC 80 PQ 2.09 2.09 FUD XXX

92576 **Synthetic sentence identification test**
X TC 80 PQ 0.97 0.97 FUD XXX

92577 **Stenger test, speech**
X TC 80 PQ 0.54 0.54 FUD XXX

92579 **Visual reinforcement audiometry (VRA)**
X 80 PQ 1.06 1.19 FUD XXX

92582 **Conditioning play audiometry**
X TC 80 PQ 1.91 1.91 FUD XXX

92583 **Select picture audiometry**
X TC 80 1.45 1.45 FUD XXX

92584 **Electrocochleography**
S TC 80 PQ 1.97 1.97 FUD XXX

92585 **Auditory evoked potentials for evoked response audiometry and/or testing of the central nervous system; comprehensive**
S 80 PQ 3.67 3.67 FUD XXX

92586 **limited**
S TC 80 PQ 2.35 2.35 FUD XXX

\# 92558 **Evoked otoacoustic emissions, screening (qualitative measurement of distortion product or transient evoked otoacoustic emissions), automated analysis**
E 0.00 0.00 FUD XXX

92587 **Distortion product evoked otoacoustic emissions; limited evaluation (to confirm the presence or absence of hearing disorder, 3-6 frequencies) or transient evoked otoacoustic emissions, with interpretation and report**
X 80 PQ 0.62 0.62 FUD XXX

92588 **comprehensive diagnostic evaluation (quantitative analysis of outer hair cell function by cochlear mapping, minimum of 12 frequencies), with interpretation and report**
EXCLUDES *Evaluation of central auditory function (92620-92621)*
X 80 PQ 0.94 0.94 FUD XXX

92590 **Hearing aid examination and selection; monaural**
E 0.00 0.00 FUD XXX

92591 **binaural**
E 0.00 0.00 FUD XXX

92592 **Hearing aid check; monaural**
E 0.00 0.00 FUD XXX

92593 **binaural**
E 0.00 0.00 FUD XXX

92594 **Electroacoustic evaluation for hearing aid; monaural**
E 0.00 0.00 FUD XXX

92595 **binaural**
E 0.00 0.00 FUD XXX

92596 **Ear protector attenuation measurements**
X TC 80 1.19 1.19 FUD XXX

92597 Services Related to Voice Prosthesis

INCLUDES Diagnostic/treatment services not generally included in a comprehensive otorhinolaryngologic evaluation or office visit
Use of calibrated electronic equipment

EXCLUDES *Communication device services, augmentative/alternative (92605, 92607-92608)*

92597 **Evaluation for use and/or fitting of voice prosthetic device to supplement oral speech**
A 80 2.05 2.05 FUD XXX

92601-92609 [92618] Services Related to Hearing and Speech Devices

CMS 100-2,15,80.3 Audiology Services
CMS 100-3,50.1 Speech Generating Devices
CMS 100-3,50.2 Electronic Speech Aids
CMS 100-3,50.3 Cochlear Implantation
CMS 100-4,32,100 Billing Requirements for Cochlear Implantation

INCLUDES Diagnostic/treatment services not generally included in a comprehensive otorhinolaryngologic evaluation or office visit

92601 Diagnostic analysis of cochlear implant, patient younger than 7 years of age; with programming
INCLUDES Connection to cochlear implant
Postoperative analysis/fitting of previously placed external devices
Stimulator programming
EXCLUDES *Cochlear implant placement (69930)*
X 80 CCI PQ 3.39 3.93 FUD XXX

92602 subsequent reprogramming
INCLUDES Internal stimulator re-programming
Subsequent sessions for external transmitter measurements/adjustment
EXCLUDES *Aural rehabilitation services after a cochlear implant (92626-92627, 92630-92633)*
Cochlear implant placement (69930)
Do not report with 92601
X 80 CCI PQ 1.87 2.32 FUD XXX

92603 Diagnostic analysis of cochlear implant, age 7 years or older; with programming
INCLUDES Connection to cochlear implant
Post-operative analysis/fitting of previously placed external devices
Stimulator programming
EXCLUDES *Cochlear implant placement (69930)*
X 80 CCI PQ 3.47 4.15 FUD XXX

92604 subsequent reprogramming
INCLUDES Internal stimulator re-programming
Subsequent sessions for external transmitter measurements/adjustment
EXCLUDES *Cochlear implant placement (69930)*
Do not report with 92603
X 80 CCI PQ 1.92 2.50 FUD XXX

92605 Evaluation for prescription of non-speech-generating augmentative and alternative communication device, face-to-face with the patient; first hour
A 2.51 2.63 FUD XXX

\+ # **92618 each additional 30 minutes (List separately in addition to code for primary procedure)**
Code first (92605)
A 0.93 0.95 FUD ZZZ

92606 Therapeutic service(s) for the use of non-speech-generating device, including programming and modification
A 2.01 2.33 FUD XXX

92607 Evaluation for prescription for speech-generating augmentative and alternative communication device, face-to-face with the patient; first hour
EXCLUDES *Evaluation for prescription of non-speech generating device (92605)*
A 80 CCI 3.63 3.63 FUD XXX

\+ **92608 each additional 30 minutes (List separately in addition to code for primary procedure)**
Code first initial hour (92607)
A 80 CCI 1.50 1.50 FUD ZZZ

92609 Therapeutic services for the use of speech-generating device, including programming and modification
EXCLUDES *Therapeutic services for use of non-speech generating device (92606)*
A 80 CCI 3.14 3.14 FUD XXX

92610-92618 Swallowing Evaluations

CMS 100-2,15,230.3 Practice of Speech-Language Pathology
CMS 100-3,170.3 Speech-language Pathology Services for Dysphagia

92610 Evaluation of oral and pharyngeal swallowing function
EXCLUDES *Evaluation with flexible endoscope (92612-92617)*
Motion fluoroscopic evaluation of swallowing function (92611)
A 80 CCI PQ 2.06 2.40 FUD XXX

92611 Motion fluoroscopic evaluation of swallowing function by cine or video recording
EXCLUDES *Evaluation of oral/pharyngeal swallowing function (92610)*
Do not report with diagnostic flexible fiberoptic laryngoscopy (31575)
74230
A 80 CCI PQ 2.57 2.57 FUD XXX

92612 Flexible fiberoptic endoscopic evaluation of swallowing by cine or video recording;
EXCLUDES *Flexible fiberoptic endoscopic examination/testing without cine or video recording (92700)*
Do not report with diagnostic flexible fiberoptic laryngoscopy (31575)
A 80 CCI PQ 1.94 5.00 FUD XXX

92613 interpretation and report only
EXCLUDES *Oral/pharyngeal swallowing function examination (92610)*
Swallowing function motion fluoroscopic examination (92611)
Do not report with diagnostic flexible fiberoptic laryngoscopy (31575)
B 80 CCI 1.07 1.07 FUD XXX

92614 Flexible fiberoptic endoscopic evaluation, laryngeal sensory testing by cine or video recording;
EXCLUDES *Flexible fiberoptic endoscopic examination/testing without cine or video recording (92700)*
Do not report with diagnostic flexible fiberoptic laryngoscopy (31575)
A 80 CCI 1.94 4.23 FUD XXX

92615 interpretation and report only
Do not report with diagnostic flexible fiberoptic laryngoscopy (31575)
E 80 CCI 0.95 0.96 FUD XXX

92616 Flexible fiberoptic endoscopic evaluation of swallowing and laryngeal sensory testing by cine or video recording;
EXCLUDES *Flexible fiberoptic endoscopic examination/testing without cine or video recording (92700)*
Do not report with diagnostic flexible fiberoptic laryngoscopy (31575)
A 80 CCI 2.88 5.96 FUD XXX

92617 interpretation and report only
Do not report with diagnostic flexible fiberoptic laryngoscopy (31575)
E 80 CCI 1.19 1.19 FUD XXX

92618 Resequenced code. See code following 92605.

92620-92700 Diagnostic Hearing Evaluations and Rehabilitation

INCLUDES Diagnostic/treatment services not generally included in a comprehensive otorhinolaryngologic evaluation or office visit

92620 Evaluation of central auditory function, with report; initial 60 minutes
Do not report with (92521-92524)
X 80 CCI PQ 2.37 2.65 FUD XXX

\+ 92621 **each additional 15 minutes (List separately in addition to code for primary procedure)**
Code first (92620)
Do not report with (92521-92524)
N 80 PQ 0.54 0.63 FUD ZZZ

92625 **Assessment of tinnitus (includes pitch, loudness matching, and masking)**
Code also modifier 52 for unilateral procedure
Do not report with (92562)
X 80 PQ 1.77 1.97 FUD XXX

92626 **Evaluation of auditory rehabilitation status; first hour**
INCLUDES Face-to-face time spent with the patient or family
The ability of the patient to use residual hearing in order to identify acoustic characteristics of sounds associated with speech communication
X 80 PQ 2.17 2.54 FUD XXX

\+ 92627 **each additional 15 minutes (List separately in addition to code for primary procedure)**
INCLUDES Face-to-face time spent with the patient or family
The ability of the patient to use residual hearing in order to identify acoustic characteristics of sounds associated with speech communication
Code first initial hour (92626)
N 80 PQ 0.50 0.61 FUD ZZZ

92630 **Auditory rehabilitation; prelingual hearing loss**
E 0.00 0.00 FUD XXX

92633 **postlingual hearing loss**
E 0.00 0.00 FUD XXX

92640 **Diagnostic analysis with programming of auditory brainstem implant, per hour**
EXCLUDES *Nonprogramming services (cardiac monitoring)*
X 80 PQ 3.00 3.49 FUD XXX

92700 **Unlisted otorhinolaryngological service or procedure**
INCLUDES Lombard test
X 80 0.00 0.00 FUD XXX

92920-92953 Emergency Cardiac Procedures

CMS 100-4,12,30.4 Cardiovascular System

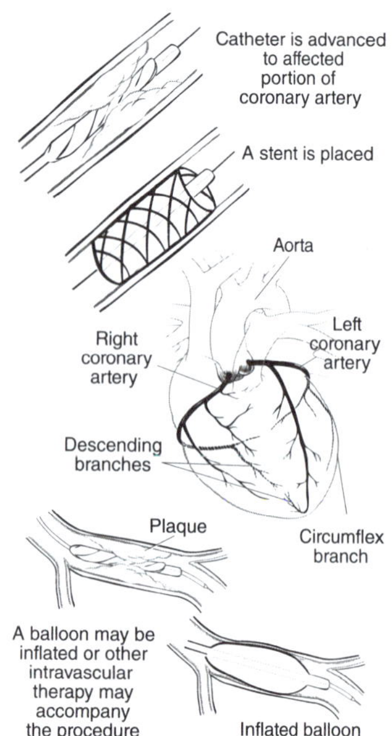

92920 ***Resequenced code. See code following 92998.***

92921 ***Resequenced code. See code following 92998.***

92924 ***Resequenced code. See code following 92998.***

92925 ***Resequenced code. See code following 92998.***

92928 ***Resequenced code. See code following 92998.***

92929 ***Resequenced code. See code following 92998.***

92933 ***Resequenced code. See code following 92998.***

92934 ***Resequenced code. See code following 92998.***

92937 ***Resequenced code. See code following 92998.***

92938 ***Resequenced code. See code following 92998.***

92941 ***Resequenced code. See code following 92998.***

92943 ***Resequenced code. See code following 92998.***

92944 ***Resequenced code. See code following 92998.***

92950 **Cardiopulmonary resuscitation (eg, in cardiac arrest)**
EXCLUDES *Critical care (99291-99292)*
S 80 5.29 8.52 FUD 000

⊙ 92953 **Temporary transcutaneous pacing**
EXCLUDES *Direction of ambulance/rescue personnel by physician or other qualified health care professional outside of the hospital (99288)*
03 80 0.31 0.31 FUD 000

92960-92961 Cardioversion

CMS 100-4,12,30.4 Cardiovascular System

⊙ 92960 **Cardioversion, elective, electrical conversion of arrhythmia; external**
S 80 3.45 5.75 FUD 000

⊙ 92961 **internal (separate procedure)**
Do not report with (93282-93284, 93287, 93289, 93295-93296, 93618-93624, 93631, 93640-93642, 93650, 93653-93657, 93662)
S 6.91 6.91 FUD 000

92970-92979 Circulatory Assist: External/Internal

EXCLUDES *Atrial septostomy, balloon (92992)*
Catheter placement for use in circulatory assist devices (intra-aortic balloon pump) (33970)

92970 **Cardioassist-method of circulatory assist; internal**
C 80 4.99 4.99 FUD 000

92971 **external**
C 80 2.63 2.63 FUD 000

92973 ***Resequenced code. See code following 92998.***

92974 ***Resequenced code. See code following 92998.***

92975 ***Resequenced code. See code following 92998.***

92977 ***Resequenced code. See code following 92998.***

92978 ***Resequenced code. See code following 92998.***

92979 ***Resequenced code. See code following 92998.***

92986-92993 Percutaneous Procedures of Heart Valves and Septum

CMS 100-4,12,30.4 Cardiovascular System

⊙ 92986 **Percutaneous balloon valvuloplasty; aortic valve**
T 80 38.26 38.26 FUD 090

⊙ 92987 **mitral valve**
T 80 39.51 39.51 FUD 090

92990 **pulmonary valve**
T 80 31.07 31.07 FUD 090

92992 **Atrial septectomy or septostomy; transvenous method, balloon (eg, Rashkind type) (includes cardiac catheterization)**
C 80 0.00 0.00 FUD 090

92993 **blade method (Park septostomy) (includes cardiac catheterization)**
C 80 0.00 0.00 FUD 090

92997-92998 Percutaneous Angioplasty: Pulmonary Artery

CMS 100-4,12,30.4 Cardiovascular System

92997 **Percutaneous transluminal pulmonary artery balloon angioplasty; single vessel**
Code also (C1725, C1874, C1876, C1885, C2625)
T 80 18.76 18.76 FUD 000

\+ 92998 **each additional vessel (List separately in addition to code for primary procedure)**
Code also (C1725, C1874, C1876, C1885, C2625)
Code first single vessel (92997)
T 80 9.28 9.28 FUD ZZZ

92920-92944 [92920, 92921, 92924, 92925, 92928, 92929, 92933, 92934, 92937, 92938, 92941, 92943, 92944] Intravascular Coronary Procedures

CMS 100-4,12,30.4 Cardiovascular System

INCLUDES Accessing the vessel
All procedures performed in all segments of branches of coronary arteries
Branches of left anterior descending (diagonals), left circumflex (marginals), and right (posterior descending, posterolaterals)
Distal, proximal, and mid segments
All procedures performed in all segments of major coronary arteries through the native vessels:
Distal, proximal, and mid segments
Left main, left anterior descending, left circumflex, right, and ramus intermedius arteries
All procedures performed in major coronary arteries or recognized coronary artery branches through a coronary artery bypass graft
A sequential bypass graft with more than a single distal anastomosis as one graft
Branching bypass grafts (eg, "Y" grafts) include a coronary vessel for the primary graft, with each branch off the primary graft making up an additional coronary vessel
Each coronary artery bypass graft denotes a single coronary vessel
Embolic protection devices when used
Arteriotomy closure through the access sheath
Atherectomy (eg, directional, laser, rotational)
Balloon angioplasty (eg, cryoplasty, cutting balloon, wired balloons)
Imaging once procedure is complete
Percutaneous coronary interventions (PCI) for disease of coronary vessels, native and bypass grafts
Radiological supervision and interpretation of intervention(s)
Reporting the most comprehensive treatment in a given vessel according to a hierarchy of intensity for the base and add-on codes:
Add-on codes: 92944 = 92938 > 92934 > 92925 > 92929 > 92921
Base codes: 92943 = 92941 = 92933 > 92924 > 92937 = 92928 > 92920
Selective vessel catheterization
Stenting (eg, balloon expandable, bare metal, covered, drug eluting, self-expanding)
Traversing of the lesion

EXCLUDES *Application of intravascular radioelements (77785-77787)*
Insertion of device for coronary intravascular brachytherapy ([92974])
Reduction of septum (eg, alcohol ablation) (93799)

Code also add-on codes for procedures performed during the same session in additional recognized branches of the target vessel
Code also diagnostic angiography at the time of the interventional procedure when:
A previous study is available, but documentation states the patient's condition has changed since the previous study or visualization of the anatomy/pathology is inadequate, or a change occurs during the procedure warranting additional evaluation of an area outside the current target area
No previous catheter-based coronary angiography study is available, and a full diagnostic study is performed, with the decision to perform the intervention based on that study, or
Code also diagnostic angiography performed at a session separate from the interventional procedure
Code also individual base codes for treatment of a segment of a major native coronary artery and another segment of the same artery that requires treatment through a bypass graft when performed at the same time
Code also procedures for both vessels for a bifurcation lesion
Code also procedures performed in second branch of a major coronary artery
Code also treatment of arterial segment requiring access through a bypass graft
Do not report additional procedures performed in a third branch of a major coronary artery
Do not report more than one base code for percutaneous coronary revascularization of recognized branches of a major coronary artery
Do not report more than one code when a single lesion continues from one target vessel (major artery, branch, or bypass graft) to another and revascularization can be achieved with a single procedure
Do not report procedures in branches of the left main and ramus intermedius coronary arteries as they are unrecognized for purposes of reporting
Do not report separately when included in the coronary revascularization service (93454-93461, 93563-93564)

⊙ # 92920 **Percutaneous transluminal coronary angioplasty; single major coronary artery or branch**
Code also (C1725)
T 80 15.67 15.67 FUD 000

\+ ⊙ # 92921 **each additional branch of a major coronary artery (List separately in addition to code for primary procedure)**
Code first ([92920], [92924], [92928], [92933], [92937], [92941], [92943])
T 0.00 0.00 FUD ZZZ

⊙ # 92924 **Percutaneous transluminal coronary atherectomy, with coronary angioplasty when performed; single major coronary artery or branch**
Code also (C1714, C1724, C1885)
T 80 18.64 18.64 FUD 000

\+ ⊙ # 92925 **each additional branch of a major coronary artery (List separately in addition to code for primary procedure)**
Code first ([92924], [92928], [92933], [92937], [92941], [92943])
T 0.00 0.00 FUD ZZZ

⊙ # 92928 **Percutaneous transcatheter placement of intracoronary stent(s), with coronary angioplasty when performed; single major coronary artery or branch**
Code also (C1874, C1875, C1876, C1877)
T 80 17.40 17.40 FUD 000

\+ ⊙ # 92929 **each additional branch of a major coronary artery (List separately in addition to code for primary procedure)**
Code also (C1874-C1877)
Code first ([92928], [92933], [92937], [92941], [92943])
T 0.00 0.00 FUD ZZZ

⊙ # 92933 **Percutaneous transluminal coronary atherectomy, with intracoronary stent, with coronary angioplasty when performed; single major coronary artery or branch**
Code also (C1714, C1724, C1874-C1877, C1885)
T 80 19.47 19.47 FUD 000

\+ ⊙ # 92934 **each additional branch of a major coronary artery (List separately in addition to code for primary procedure)**
Code also (C1714, C1724, C1874-C1877, C1885)
Code first ([92933], [92937], [92941], [92943])
T 0.00 0.00 FUD ZZZ

⊙ # 92937 **Percutaneous transluminal revascularization of or through coronary artery bypass graft (internal mammary, free arterial, venous), any combination of intracoronary stent, atherectomy and angioplasty, including distal protection when performed; single vessel**
Code also (C1714, C1724-C1725, C1874-C1877, C1885)
T 80 17.39 17.39 FUD 000

\+ ⊙ # 92938 **each additional branch subtended by the bypass graft (List separately in addition to code for primary procedure)**
Code first ([92937])
T 0.00 0.00 FUD ZZZ

⊙ # **92941** **Percutaneous transluminal revascularization of acute total/subtotal occlusion during acute myocardial infarction, coronary artery or coronary artery bypass graft, any combination of intracoronary stent, atherectomy and angioplasty, including aspiration thrombectomy when performed, single vessel**

INCLUDES Aspiration thrombectomy, when performed
Embolic protection
Rheolytic thrombectomy

Code also (C1714, C1724-C1725, C1874-C1877, C1885)
Code also treatment of additional vessels, when appropriate ([92920, 92921, 92924, 92925, 92928, 92929, 92933, 92934, 92937, 92938], [92943, 92944])
Code also mechanical thrombectomy, when performed

T 80 19.51 19.51 FUD 000

⊙ # **92943** **Percutaneous transluminal revascularization of chronic total occlusion, coronary artery, coronary artery branch, or coronary artery bypass graft, any combination of intracoronary stent, atherectomy and angioplasty; single vessel**

INCLUDES Lack of antegrade flow with angiography and clinical criteria indicative of chronic total occlusion

EXCLUDES *Presentation with ST elevation or Q wave acute myocardial infarction due to occluded target lesion, subtotal occlusion, and findings indicative of new thrombus*

Code also (C1714, C1724-C1725, C1874-C1877, C1885)

T 80 19.51 19.51 FUD 000

+ ⊙ # **92944** **each additional coronary artery, coronary artery branch, or bypass graft (List separately in addition to code for primary procedure)**

Code first ([92924], [92928], [92933], [92937], [92941, 92943])

T 0.00 0.00 FUD ZZZ

92973-92979 [92973, 92974, 92975, 92977, 92978, 92979] Additional Coronary Artery Procedures

+ ⊙ # **92973** **Percutaneous transluminal coronary thrombectomy mechanical (List separately in addition to code for primary procedure)**

EXCLUDES *Aspiration thrombectomy*

Code first ([92920], [92924], [92928], [92933], [92937], [92941], [92943], [92975], 93454-93461, 93563-93564)

N 80 5.09 5.09 FUD ZZZ

+ ⊙ # **92974** **Transcatheter placement of radiation delivery device for subsequent coronary intravascular brachytherapy (List separately in addition to code for primary procedure)**

EXCLUDES *Application of intravascular radioelements (77785-77787)*

Code first ([92920], [92924], [92928], [92933], [92937], [92941], [92943], 93454-93461)

N 80 4.65 4.65 FUD ZZZ

⊙ # **92975** **Thrombolysis, coronary; by intracoronary infusion, including selective coronary angiography**

EXCLUDES *Thrombolysis, cerebral (37195)*
Thrombolysis other than coronary ([37211, 37212, 37213, 37214])

C 80 11.23 11.23 FUD 000

92977 **by intravenous infusion**

EXCLUDES *Thrombolysis, cerebral (37195)*
Thrombolysis other than coronary ([37211, 37212, 37213, 37214])

T 80 3.54 3.54 FUD XXX

+ ⊙ # **92978** **Intravascular ultrasound (coronary vessel or graft) during diagnostic evaluation and/or therapeutic intervention including imaging supervision, interpretation and report; initial vessel (List separately in addition to code for primary procedure)**

Code also (C1753)
Code first primary procedure ([92920], [92924], [92928], [92933], [92937], [92941], [92943], [92975], 93454-93461, 93563-93564)

N 80 0.00 0.00 FUD ZZZ

+ ⊙ # **92979** **each additional vessel (List separately in addition to code for primary procedure)**

INCLUDES Transducer manipulations/repositioning in the vessel examined, before and after therapeutic intervention

EXCLUDES *Intravascular optic coherence tomography (0291T-0292T)*
Intravascular spectroscopy (0205T)

Code first initial vessel (92978)

N 80 0.00 0.00 FUD ZZZ

93000-93010 Electrocardiographic Services

CMS 100-3,20.15 Electrocardiographic Services
CMS 100-4,12,30.4 Cardiovascular System

INCLUDES Specific order for the service, a separate written and signed report, and documentation of medical necessity

EXCLUDES *Acoustic cardiography (0223T-0225T)*
Echocardiography (93303-93350)
ECG monitoring (99354-99360)
ECG with 64 or more leads, graphic presentation, and analysis (0178T-0180T)
Use of these codes for the review of telemetry monitoring strips

93000 **Electrocardiogram, routine ECG with at least 12 leads; with interpretation and report**

M 80 0.47 0.47 FUD XXX

93005 **tracing only, without interpretation and report**

S TC 80 0.23 0.23 FUD XXX

93010 **interpretation and report only**

B 26 80 0.24 0.24 FUD XXX

Conduction System of the Heart

93015-93018 Stress Test

CMS 100-3,20.10 Cardiac Rehabilitation Programs
CMS 100-3,20.15 Electrocardiographic Services
CMS 100-4,12,30.4 Cardiovascular System

93015 **Cardiovascular stress test using maximal or submaximal treadmill or bicycle exercise, continuous electrocardiographic monitoring, and/or pharmacological stress; with supervision, interpretation and report**

B 80 2.12 2.12 FUD XXX

93016 **supervision only, without interpretation and report**

B 26 80 0.24 0.62 0.62 FUD XXX

93017 **tracing only, without interpretation and report**
01 TC 80 ⊡ 1.09 1.09 FUD XXX

93018 **interpretation and report only**
B 26 80 ⊡ 0.41 0.41 FUD XXX

93024 Provocation Test for Coronary Vasospasm

CMS 100-3,20.15 Electrocardiographic Services
CMS 100-4,12,30.4 Cardiovascular System

93024 **Ergonovine provocation test**
X 80 ⊡ 3.13 3.13 FUD XXX

93025 Microvolt T-Wave Alternans

CMS 100-3,20.30 Microvolt T-Wave Alternans (MTWA)
CMS 100-4,12,30.4 Cardiovascular System

INCLUDES Specific order for the service, a separate written and signed report, and documentation of medical necessity

EXCLUDES *Echocardiography (93303-93350)*
ECG with 64 or more leads, graphic presentation, and analysis (0178T-0180T)
Use of these codes for the review of telemetry monitoring strips

93025 **Microvolt T-wave alternans for assessment of ventricular arrhythmias**
X 80 ⊡ 4.59 4.59 FUD XXX

93040-93042 Rhythm Strips

CMS 100-3,20.15 Electrocardiographic Services
CMS 100-4,12,30.4 Cardiovascular System

INCLUDES Specific order for the service, a separate written and signed report, and documentation of medical necessity

EXCLUDES *Echocardiography (93303-93350)*
ECG with 64 or more leads, graphic presentation, and analysis (0178T-0180T)
Use of these codes for the review of telemetry monitoring strips

Do not report with (93279-93289 [93260], 93285-93289 [93260, 93261], 93291-93296, 93298-93299, 0223T-0225T)

93040 **Rhythm ECG, 1-3 leads; with interpretation and report**
Do not report with ([95943])
B 80 ⊡ 0.36 0.36 FUD XXX

93041 **tracing only without interpretation and report**
X TC 80 0.16 0.16 FUD XXX

93042 **interpretation and report only**
B 26 80 ⊡ 0.20 0.20 FUD XXX

93224-93227 Holter Monitor

CMS 100-3,20.15 Electrocardiographic Services
CMS 100-4,12,30.4 Cardiovascular System

INCLUDES Cardiac monitoring using in-person as well as remote technology for the assessment of electrocardiographic data
Up to 48 hours of recording on a continuous basis

EXCLUDES *Echocardiography (93303-93355)*
ECG with 64 or more leads, graphic presentation, and analysis (0178T-0180T)
Implantable patient activated cardiac event recorders (33282, 93285, 93291, 93298)
More than 48 hours of monitoring (0295T-0298T)

Code also modifier 52 when less than 12 hours of continuous recording is provided

93224 **External electrocardiographic recording up to 48 hours by continuous rhythm recording and storage; includes recording, scanning analysis with report, review and interpretation by a physician or other qualified health care professional**
M 80 ⊡ 2.56 2.56 FUD XXX

93225 **recording (includes connection, recording, and disconnection)**
S TC 80 ⊡ 0.75 0.75 FUD XXX

93226 **scanning analysis with report**
S TC 80 ⊡ 1.06 1.06 FUD XXX

93227 **review and interpretation by a physician or other qualified health care professional**
M 26 80 ⊡ 0.75 0.75 FUD XXX

93228-93229 Remote Cardiovascular Telemetry

INCLUDES Cardiac monitoring using in-person as well as remote technology for the assessment of electrocardiographic data
Mobile telemetry monitors with the capacity to:
Detect arrhythmias
Real-time data analysis for the evaluation quality of the signal
Records ECG rhythm on a continuous basis using external electrodes on the patient
Transmit a tracing at any time
Transmit data to an attended surveillance center where a technician is available to respond to device or rhythm alerts and contact the physician or qualified health care professional if needed

Do not report more than one time in a 30-day period

93228 **External mobile cardiovascular telemetry with electrocardiographic recording, concurrent computerized real time data analysis and greater than 24 hours of accessible ECG data storage (retrievable with query) with ECG triggered and patient selected events transmitted to a remote attended surveillance center for up to 30 days; review and interpretation with report by a physician or other qualified health care professional**
Do not report with (93224, 93227)
M 26 80 0.74 0.74 FUD XXX

93229 **technical support for connection and patient instructions for use, attended surveillance, analysis and transmission of daily and emergent data reports as prescribed by a physician or other qualified health care professional**
EXCLUDES *Cardiovascular monitors that do not perform automatic ECG triggered transmissions to an attended surveillance center (93224-93227, 93268-93272)*
Do not report with (93224, 93226)
S TC 80 18.68 18.68 FUD XXX

93260-93272 Event Monitors

INCLUDES ECG rhythm derived elements, which differ from physiologic data and include rhythm of the heart, rate, ST analysis, heart rate variability, T-wave alternans, among others
Event monitors that:
Record parts of ECGs in response to patient activation or an automatic detection algorithm (or both)
Require attended surveillance
Transmit data upon request (although not immediately when activated)

Do not report with (93279-93289, 93291-93296, 93298-93299)

93260 ***Resequenced code. See code following 93284.***

93261 ***Resequenced code. See code following 93289.***

93268 **External patient and, when performed, auto activated electrocardiographic rhythm derived event recording with symptom-related memory loop with remote download capability up to 30 days, 24-hour attended monitoring; includes transmission, review and interpretation by a physician or other qualified health care professional**
EXCLUDES *Implanted patient activated cardiac event recording (33282, 93285, 93291, 93298)*
M 80 ⊡ 5.73 5.73 FUD XXX

93270 **recording (includes connection, recording, and disconnection)**
S TC 80 ⊡ 0.26 0.26 FUD XXX

93271 **transmission and analysis**
S TC 80 ⊡ 4.76 4.76 FUD XXX

93272 **review and interpretation by a physician or other qualified health care professional**
M 26 80 ⊡ 0.71 0.71 FUD XXX

Medicine

93017 — 93272

93278 Signal-averaged Electrocardiography

CMS 100-3,20.15 Electrocardiographic Services

CMS 100-4,12,30.4 Cardiovascular System

EXCLUDES *Echocardiography (93303-93352)*

Code also modifier 26 for the interpretation and report only

ECG with 64 or more leads, graphic presentation, and analysis (0178T-0180T)

93278 Signal-averaged electrocardiography (SAECG), with or without ECG

X 80 0.85 0.85 FUD XXX

93279-93299 [93260, 93261] Monitoring of Cardiovascular Devices

INCLUDES Implantable defibrillator interrogation:
- Battery
- Capture and sensing functions
- Leads
- Presence or absence of therapy for ventricular tachyarrhythmias
- Programmed parameters
- Underlying heart rhythm

Implantable cardiovascular monitor (ICM) interrogation:
- Analysis of at least one recorded physiologic cardiovascular data element from either internal or external sensors
- Programmed parameters

Implantable loop recorder (ILR) interrogation:
- Heart rate and rhythm during recorded episodes from both patient-initiated and device detected events
- Programmed parameters

Interrogation evaluation of device

Pacemaker interrogation:
- Battery
- Capture and sensing functions
- Heart rhythm
- Leads
- Programmed parameters

Time period established by the initiation of remote monitoring or the 91st day of implantable defibrillator or pacemaker monitoring or the 31st day of ILR monitoring and extending for the succeeding 30- or 90-day period

EXCLUDES *Evaluation of subcutaneous implantable defibrillator device ([93260], [93261])*

Wearable device monitoring (93224-93272)

Do not report in-person and remote interrogation of the same device during the same period

Do not report programming and in-person interrogation on the same day by the same physician

93279 Programming device evaluation (in person) with iterative adjustment of the implantable device to test the function of the device and select optimal permanent programmed values with analysis, review and report by a physician or other qualified health care professional; single lead pacemaker system

Do not report with (93040-93042, 93268-93272, 93286, 93288)

S 80 1.40 1.40 FUD XXX

93280 dual lead pacemaker system

Do not report with (93040-93042, 93268-93272, 93286, 93288)

S 80 1.64 1.64 FUD XXX

93281 multiple lead pacemaker system

Do not report with (93040-93042, 93268-93272, 93286, 93288)

S 80 1.91 1.91 FUD XXX

▲ **93282 single lead transvenous implantable defibrillator system**

Do not report with (93040-93042, 93268-93272, [93260], 93287, 93289, 93745)

S 80 1.76 1.76 FUD XXX

▲ **93283 dual lead transvenous implantable defibrillator system**

Do not report with (93040-93042, 93268-93272, 93287, 93289)

S 80 2.29 2.29 FUD XXX

▲ **93284 multiple lead transvenous implantable defibrillator system**

Do not report with (93040-93042, 93268-93272, 93287, 93289)

S 80 2.52 2.52 FUD XXX

#● **93260 implantable subcutaneous lead defibrillator system**

Do not report with (33240, 33241, [33262], [33270, 33271, 33272, 33273], 93040-93042, 93268-93272, 93282, 93287, [93261])

93285 implantable loop recorder system

Do not report with (33282, 93040-93042, 93268-93272, 93279-93284, 93291)

S 80 1.17 1.17 FUD XXX

93286 Peri-procedural device evaluation (in person) and programming of device system parameters before or after a surgery, procedure, or test with analysis, review and report by a physician or other qualified health care professional; single, dual, or multiple lead pacemaker system

INCLUDES One evaluation and programming (if performed once before and once after, report as two units)

EXCLUDES *Subcutaneous implantable defibrillator peri-procedural device evaluation and programming ([93260], [93261])*

Do not report with (93040-93042, 93268-93272, 93279-93281, 93288)

N 80 0.76 0.76 FUD XXX

▲ **93287 single, dual, or multiple lead implantable defibrillator system**

INCLUDES One evaluation and programming (if performed once before and once after, report as two units)

EXCLUDES *Subcutaneous implantable defibrillator peri-procedural device evaluation and programming ([93260], [93261])*

Do not report with (93040-93042, 93268-93272, 93282-93284, [93260], 93289, [93261])

N 80 1.00 1.00 FUD XXX

93288 Interrogation device evaluation (in person) with analysis, review and report by a physician or other qualified health care professional, includes connection, recording and disconnection per patient encounter; single, dual, or multiple lead pacemaker system

Do not report with (93040-93042, 93268-93272, 93279-93281, 93286, 93294, 93296)

S 80 1.03 1.03 FUD XXX

▲ **93289 single, dual, or multiple lead transvenous implantable defibrillator system, including analysis of heart rhythm derived data elements**

EXCLUDES *Monitoring physiologic cardiovascular data elements derived from an implantable defibrillator (93290)*

Do not report with (93040-93042, 93268-93272, 93282-93284, 93287, [93261], 93295-93296)

S 80 1.83 1.83 FUD XXX

#● **93261 implantable subcutaneous lead defibrillator system**

Do not report with (33240-33241 [33230, 33231], [33262], [33270, 33271, 33272, 33273], 93040-93042, 93268-93272, [93260], 93287, 93289)

93290 implantable cardiovascular monitor system, including analysis of 1 or more recorded physiologic cardiovascular data elements from all internal and external sensors

EXCLUDES *Heart rhythm derived data (93289)*

Do not report with (93297, 93299)

S 80 0.86 0.86 FUD XXX

93291 **implantable loop recorder system, including heart rhythm derived data analysis**
Do not report with (33282, 93040-93042, 93268-93272, 93288-93290, 93298-93299)
S 80 1.01 1.01 FUD XXX

93292 **wearable defibrillator system**
Do not report with (93040-93042, 93268-93272, 93745)
S 80 0.89 0.89 FUD XXX

93293 **Transtelephonic rhythm strip pacemaker evaluation(s) single, dual, or multiple lead pacemaker system, includes recording with and without magnet application with analysis, review and report(s) by a physician or other qualified health care professional, up to 90 days**
EXCLUDES *In-person evaluation (93040-93042)*
Do not report more than one time in a 90 day period
Do not report when monitoring period is less than 30 days
Do not report with (93040-93042, 93268-93272, 93294)
S 80 1.50 1.50 FUD XXX

93294 **Interrogation device evaluation(s) (remote), up to 90 days; single, dual, or multiple lead pacemaker system with interim analysis, review(s) and report(s) by a physician or other qualified health care professional**
Do not report more than one time in a 90 day period
Do not report when monitoring period is less than 30 days
Do not report with (93040-93042, 93268-93272, 93288, 93293)
M 26 80 0.95 0.95 FUD XXX

▲ 93295 **single, dual, or multiple lead implantable defibrillator system with interim analysis, review(s) and report(s) by a physician or other qualified health care professional**
EXCLUDES *Remote monitoring of physiological cardiovascular data (93297)*
Do not report more than one time in a 90 day period
Do not report when monitoring period is less than 30 days
Do not report with (93040-93042, 93268-93272, 93289)
M 26 80 1.89 1.89 FUD XXX

▲ 93296 **single, dual, or multiple lead pacemaker system or implantable defibrillator system, remote data acquisition(s), receipt of transmissions and technician review, technical support and distribution of results**
Do not report more than one time in a 90-day period
Do not report when monitoring period is less than 30 days
Do not report with (93040-93042, 93268-93272, 93288-93289, 93299)
S TC 80 0.72 0.72 FUD XXX

93297 **Interrogation device evaluation(s), (remote) up to 30 days; implantable cardiovascular monitor system, including analysis of 1 or more recorded physiologic cardiovascular data elements from all internal and external sensors, analysis, review(s) and report(s) by a physician or other qualified health care professional**
EXCLUDES *Heart rhythm derived data (93295)*
Do not report more than one time in a 30 day period
Do not report when monitoring period is less than 10 days
Do not report with (93290, 93298)
M 26 80 0.74 0.74 FUD XXX

93298 **implantable loop recorder system, including analysis of recorded heart rhythm data, analysis, review(s) and report(s) by a physician or other qualified health care professional**
Do not report more than one time in a 30 day period
Do not report when monitoring period is less than 10 days
Do not report with (33282, 93040-93042, 93268-93272, 93291, 93297)
M 26 80 0.75 0.75 FUD XXX

93299 **implantable cardiovascular monitor system or implantable loop recorder system, remote data acquisition(s), receipt of transmissions and technician review, technical support and distribution of results**
Do not report more than one time in a 30 day period
Do not report when monitoring period is less than 10 days
Do not report with (93040-93042, 93268-93272, 93290-93291, 93296)
S TC 80 0.00 0.00 FUD XXX

93303-93355 Echocardiography

CMS 100-4,4,200.7.1 Cardiac Echocardiography Without Contrast
CMS 100-4,12,30.4 Cardiovascular System

INCLUDES Interpretation and report
Obtaining ultrasonic signals from heart/great arteries
Report of study which includes:
- Description of recognized abnormalities
- Documentation of all clinically relevant findings which includes obtained quantitative measurements
- Interpretation of all information obtained

Two-dimensional image/doppler ultrasonic signal documentation
Ultrasound exam of:
- Adjacent great vessels
- Cardiac chambers/valves
- Pericardium

EXCLUDES *Contrast agents and/or drugs used for pharmacological stress*
Echocardiography, fetal (76825-76828)
Ultrasound with thorough examination of the organ(s) or anatomic region/documentation of the image/final written report

93303 **Transthoracic echocardiography for congenital cardiac anomalies; complete**
S 80 6.68 6.68 FUD XXX

93304 **follow-up or limited study**
S 80 4.43 4.43 FUD XXX

93306 **Echocardiography, transthoracic, real-time with image documentation (2D), includes M-mode recording, when performed, complete, with spectral Doppler echocardiography, and with color flow Doppler echocardiography**
INCLUDES Doppler and color flow
Two-dimensional and M-mode
EXCLUDES *Transthoracic without spectral and color doppler (93307)*
S 80 6.40 6.40 FUD XXX

93307 **Echocardiography, transthoracic, real-time with image documentation (2D), includes M-mode recording, when performed, complete, without spectral or color Doppler echocardiography**
INCLUDES Additional structures that may be viewed such as pulmonary vein or artery, pulmonic valve, inferior vena cava
Obtaining/recording appropriate measurements
Two-dimensional/selected M-mode exam of:
Adjacent portions of the aorta
Aortic/mitral/tricuspid valves
Left/right atria
Left/right ventricles
Pericardium
Using multiple views as required to obtain a complete functional/anatomic evaluation
Do not report with (93320-93321, 93325)
S 80 3.70 3.70 FUD XXX

93308 **Echocardiography, transthoracic, real-time with image documentation (2D), includes M-mode recording, when performed, follow-up or limited study**
INCLUDES An exam that does not evaluate/document the attempt to evaluate all the structures that comprise the complete echocardiographic exam
S 80 3.45 3.45 FUD XXX

⊙ **93312** **Echocardiography, transesophageal, real-time with image documentation (2D) (with or without M-mode recording); including probe placement, image acquisition, interpretation and report**
Do not report with (93355)
S 80 9.31 9.31 FUD XXX

⊙ **93313** **placement of transesophageal probe only**
Do not report when performed by same person as (93355)
S 80 1.19 1.19 FUD XXX

⊙ **93314** **image acquisition, interpretation and report only**
Do not report with (93355)
N 80 8.63 8.63 FUD XXX

⊙ **93315** **Transesophageal echocardiography for congenital cardiac anomalies; including probe placement, image acquisition, interpretation and report**
Do not report with (93355)
S 80 0.00 0.00 FUD XXX

⊙ **93316** **placement of transesophageal probe only**
Do not report with (93355)
S 80 1.21 1.21 FUD XXX

⊙ **93317** **image acquisition, interpretation and report only**
Do not report with (93355)
N 80 0.00 0.00 FUD XXX

⊙ **93318** **Echocardiography, transesophageal (TEE) for monitoring purposes, including probe placement, real time 2-dimensional image acquisition and interpretation leading to ongoing (continuous) assessment of (dynamically changing) cardiac pumping function and to therapeutic measures on an immediate time basis**
Do not report with (93355)
S 80 0.00 0.00 FUD XXX

\+ **93320** **Doppler echocardiography, pulsed wave and/or continuous wave with spectral display (List separately in addition to codes for echocardiographic imaging); complete**
Code first (93303-93304, 93312, 93314-93315, 93317, 93350-93351, 93355)
Do not report with (93355)
N 80 1.53 1.53 FUD ZZZ

\+ **93321** **follow-up or limited study (List separately in addition to codes for echocardiographic imaging)**
Code first (93303-93304, 93308, 93312, 93314-93315, 93317, 93350-93351)
Do not report with (93355)
N 80 0.87 0.87 FUD ZZZ

\+ **93325** **Doppler echocardiography color flow velocity mapping (List separately in addition to codes for echocardiography)**
Code first (76825-76828, 93303-93304, 93308, 93312, 93314-93315, 93317, 93350-93351)
Do not report with (93355)
N 80 0.73 0.73 FUD ZZZ

93350 **Echocardiography, transthoracic, real-time with image documentation (2D), includes M-mode recording, when performed, during rest and cardiovascular stress test using treadmill, bicycle exercise and/or pharmacologically induced stress, with interpretation and report;**
Code also exercise stress testing (93016-93018)
Do not report with (93015)
S 80 6.76 6.76 FUD XXX

93351 **including performance of continuous electrocardiographic monitoring, with supervision by a physician or other qualified health care professional**
INCLUDES Stress echocardiogram performed with a complete cardiovascular stress test
EXCLUDES *Professional only components of complete stress test and stress echocardiogram performed in a facility by same physician, report with modifier 26*
Code also components of cardiovascular stress test when professional services not performed by same physician performing stress echocardiogram (93016-93018)
Do not report 93351-26 with 93350-26
Do not report 93351-26 with (93016, 93018)
Do not report with (93015-93018, 93350)
S 7.86 7.86 FUD XXX

\+ **93352** **Use of echocardiographic contrast agent during stress echocardiography (List separately in addition to code for primary procedure)**
Code first (93350, 93351)
Do not report more than one time for each stress echocardiogram
M 80 0.94 0.94 FUD ZZZ

● **93355** **Echocardiography, transesophageal (TEE) for guidance of a transcatheter intracardiac or great vessel(s) structural intervention(s) (eg,TAVR, transcathether pulmonary valve replacement, mitral valve repair, paravalvular regurgitation repair, left atrial appendage occlusion/closure, ventricular septal defect closure) (peri-and intra-procedural), real-time image acquisition and documentation, guidance with quantitative measurements, probe manipulation, interpretation, and report, including diagnostic transesophageal echocardiography and, when performed, administration of ultrasound contrast, Doppler, color flow, and 3D**
EXCLUDES *Transesophageal probe positioning by different provider (93313)*
Do not report with (76376-76377, 93312-93318, 93320-93321, 93325)

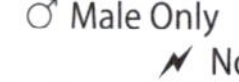
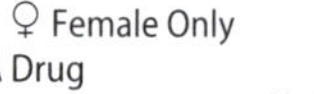

93451-93505 Heart Catheterization

CMS 100-4,12,30.4 Cardiovascular System

INCLUDES Access site imaging and placement of closure device
Catheter insertion and positioning
Contrast injection (except as listed below)
Imaging and insertion of closure device
Radiology supervision and interpretation
Roadmapping angiography

EXCLUDES *Congenital cardiac cath procedures (93530-93533)*

Code also separately identifiable:
Aortography (93567)
Noncardiac angiography (see radiology and vascular codes)
Pulmonary angiography (93568)
Right ventricular or atrial injection (93566)

Arteries of the Heart

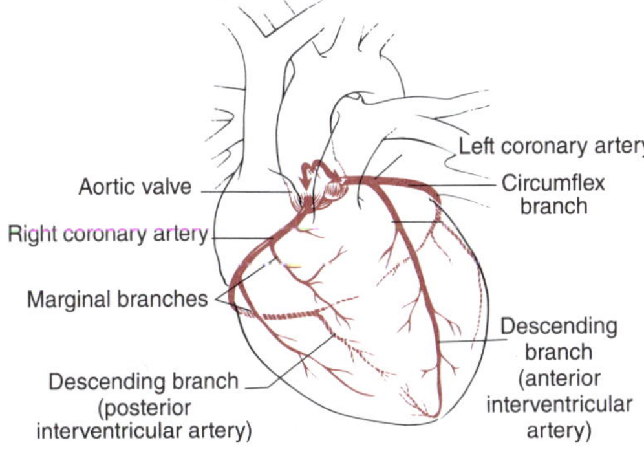

⊘ ⊙ **93451 Right heart catheterization including measurement(s) of oxygen saturation and cardiac output, when performed**

INCLUDES Cardiac output review
Insertion catheter into 1+ right cardiac chambers or areas
Obtaining samples for blood gas

Code also administration of medication or exercise to repeat assessment of hemodynamic measurement (93463-93464)

Do not report with (93453, 93456-93457, 93460-93461, 93503, 93561-93562, 93580, 0345T)

Do not report with insertion of hemodynamic monitor unless done for a reason other than insertion or maintenance of hemodynamic monitoring system (0293T-0294T)

T 80 22.04 22.04 FUD 000

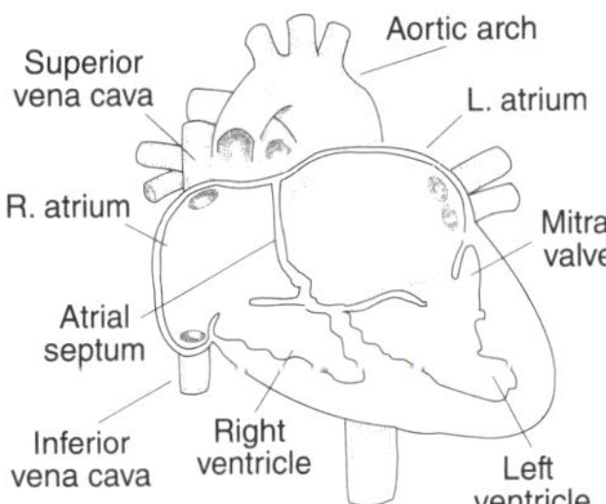

Left heart is catheterized

⊙ **93452 Left heart catheterization including intraprocedural injection(s) for left ventriculography, imaging supervision and interpretation, when performed**

INCLUDES Insertion of catheter into left cardiac chambers

Code also administration of medication or exercise to repeat assessment of hemodynamic measurement (93463-93464)

Code also transapical or transseptal puncture (93462)

Do not report with (93453, 93458-93461, 93503, 93561-93565, 93580)

Do not report with insertion of hemodynamic monitor unless done for a reason other than insertion or maintenance of hemodynamic monitoring system (0293T-0294T)

T 80 24.75 24.75 FUD 000

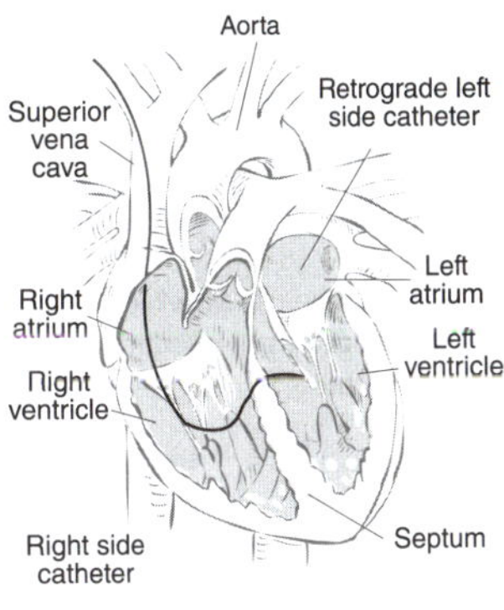

Both sides of the heart are catheterized

⊙ **93453 Combined right and left heart catheterization including intraprocedural injection(s) for left ventriculography, imaging supervision and interpretation, when performed**

INCLUDES Cardiac output review
Insertion catheter into 1+ right cardiac chambers or areas
Insertion of catheter into left cardiac chambers
Obtaining samples for blood gas

Code also administration of medication or exercise to repeat assessment of hemodynamic measurement (93463-93464)

Code also transapical or transseptal puncture (93462)

Do not report with (93451-93452, 93456-93461, 93503, 93561-93565, 93580, 0345T)

Do not report with insertion of hemodynamic monitor unless done for a reason other than insertion or maintenance of hemodynamic monitoring system (0293T-0294T)

T 80 32.07 32.07 FUD 000

⊙ **93454 Catheter placement in coronary artery(s) for coronary angiography, including intraprocedural injection(s) for coronary angiography, imaging supervision and interpretation;**

Do not report with (93503, 93561-93565, 0345T)

T 80 25.22 25.22 FUD 000

⊙ **93455 with catheter placement(s) in bypass graft(s) (internal mammary, free arterial, venous grafts) including intraprocedural injection(s) for bypass graft angiography**

Do not report with (93503, 93561-93565, 93580)

T 80 29.36 29.36 FUD 000

⊘ ⊙ **93456** **with right heart catheterization**

INCLUDES Cardiac output review
Insertion catheter into 1+ right cardiac chambers or areas
Obtaining samples for blood gas

Code also administration of medication or exercise to repeat assessment of hemodynamic measurement (93463-93464)
Do not report with (93503, 93561-93565, 93580, 0345T)

T 80 31.60 31.60 FUD 000

⊙ **93457** **with catheter placement(s) in bypass graft(s) (internal mammary, free arterial, venous grafts) including intraprocedural injection(s) for bypass graft angiography and right heart catheterization**

INCLUDES Cardiac output review
Insertion catheter into 1+ right cardiac chambers or areas
Obtaining samples for blood gas

Code also administration of medication or exercise to repeat assessment of hemodynamic measurement (93463-93464)
Do not report with (93503, 93561-93565, 93580)

T 80 35.72 35.72 FUD 000

⊙ **93458** **with left heart catheterization including intraprocedural injection(s) for left ventriculography, when performed**

INCLUDES Insertion of catheter into left cardiac chambers

Code also administration of medication or exercise to repeat assessment of hemodynamic measurement (93463-93464)
Code also transapical or transseptal puncture (93462)
Do not report with (93503, 93561-93565, 93580)

T 80 30.25 30.25 FUD 000

⊙ **93459** **with left heart catheterization including intraprocedural injection(s) for left ventriculography, when performed, catheter placement(s) in bypass graft(s) (internal mammary, free arterial, venous grafts) with bypass graft angiography**

INCLUDES Insertion of catheter into left cardiac chambers

Code also administration of medication or exercise to repeat assessment of hemodynamic measurement (93463-93464)
Code also transapical or transseptal puncture (93462)
Do not report with (93503, 93561-93565, 93580)

T 80 33.41 33.41 FUD 000

⊙ **93460** **with right and left heart catheterization including intraprocedural injection(s) for left ventriculography, when performed**

INCLUDES Cardiac output review
Insertion catheter into 1+ right cardiac chambers or areas
Insertion of catheter into left cardiac chambers
Obtaining samples for blood gas

Code also administration of medication or exercise to repeat assessment of hemodynamic measurement (93463-93464)
Code also transapical or transseptal puncture (93462)
Do not report with (93503, 93561-93565, 93580)

T 80 35.83 35.83 FUD 000

⊙ **93461** **with right and left heart catheterization including intraprocedural injection(s) for left ventriculography, when performed, catheter placement(s) in bypass graft(s) (internal mammary, free arterial, venous grafts) with bypass graft angiography**

INCLUDES Cardiac output review
Insertion catheter into 1+ right cardiac chambers or areas
Insertion of catheter into left cardiac chambers
Obtaining samples for blood gas

Code also administration of medication or exercise to repeat assessment of hemodynamic measurement (93463-93464)
Code also transapical or transseptal puncture (93462)
Do not report with (93503, 93561-93565, 93580, 0345T)

T 80 40.99 40.99 FUD 000

+ ⊙ **93462** **Left heart catheterization by transseptal puncture through intact septum or by transapical puncture (List separately in addition to code for primary procedure)**

INCLUDES Insertion of catheter into left cardiac chambers

Code first (93452-93453, 93458-93461, 93582, 93653-93654)
Do not report with (93656, 0345T)

N 80 5.99 5.99 FUD ZZZ

+ ⊙ **93463** **Pharmacologic agent administration (eg, inhaled nitric oxide, intravenous infusion of nitroprusside, dobutamine, milrinone, or other agent) including assessing hemodynamic measurements before, during, after and repeat pharmacologic agent administration, when performed (List separately in addition to code for primary procedure)**

Code first (93451-93453, 93456-93461, 93530-93533, 93580-93581)
Do not report more than one time per catheterization
Do not report with coronary interventional procedures ([92920, 92921, 92924, 92925, 92928, 92929, 92933, 92934, 92937, 92938, 92941, 92943, 92944], [92975], [92977])

N 80 3.05 3.05 FUD ZZZ

+ ⊙ **93464** **Physiologic exercise study (eg, bicycle or arm ergometry) including assessing hemodynamic measurements before and after (List separately in addition to code for primary procedure)**

EXCLUDES *Administration of pharmacologic agent (93463)*
Bundle of His recording (93600)

Code first (93451-93453, 93456-93461, 93530-93533)
Do not report more than one time per catheterization

N 80 7.94 7.94 FUD ZZZ

⊘ **93503** **Insertion and placement of flow directed catheter (eg, Swan-Ganz) for monitoring purposes**

EXCLUDES *Subsequent monitoring (99356-99357)*

Do not report with codes for diagnostic cardiac catheterization (93451-93461, 93530-93533)

T 80 3.72 3.72 FUD 000

⊙ 93505 **Endomyocardial biopsy**
EXCLUDES *Intravascular brachytherapy radionuclide insertion (77785-77787)*
Transcatheter insertion of brachytherapy delivery device (92974)
T 80 CCI PQ 21.34 21.34 FUD 000

93530-93533 Congenital Heart Defect Catheterization

INCLUDES Access site imaging and placement of closure device
Cardiac output review
Insertion catheter into 1+ right cardiac chambers or areas
Obtaining samples for blood gas
Radiology supervision and interpretation
Roadmapping angiography

EXCLUDES *Cardiac cath on noncongenital heart (93451-93453, 93456-93461)*

Code also injection procedure (93563-93568)
Do not report with (93503, 93580)

⊙ 93530 **Right heart catheterization, for congenital cardiac anomalies**
T 80 CCI 0.00 0.00 FUD 000

93531 **Combined right heart catheterization and retrograde left heart catheterization, for congenital cardiac anomalies**
T 80 CCI 0.00 0.00 FUD 000

93532 **Combined right heart catheterization and transseptal left heart catheterization through intact septum with or without retrograde left heart catheterization, for congenital cardiac anomalies**
T 80 CCI 0.00 0.00 FUD 000

93533 **Combined right heart catheterization and transseptal left heart catheterization through existing septal opening, with or without retrograde left heart catheterization, for congenital cardiac anomalies**
T 80 CCI 0.00 0.00 FUD 000

93561-93568 Injection Procedures

INCLUDES Catheter repositioning
Radiology supervision and interpretation
Using automatic power injector

⊙ 93561 **Indicator dilution studies such as dye or thermodilution, including arterial and/or venous catheterization; with cardiac output measurement (separate procedure)**
EXCLUDES *Cardiac output, radioisotope method (78472-78473, 78481)*
Do not report with (93451-93462, 93582)
N 80 CCI 0.00 0.00 FUD 000

⊙ 93562 **subsequent measurement of cardiac output**
EXCLUDES *Cardiac output, radioisotope method (78472-78473, 78481)*
Do not report with (93451-93462, 93582)
N 80 CCI 0.00 0.00 FUD 000

+ ⊙ 93563 **Injection procedure during cardiac catheterization including imaging supervision, interpretation, and report; for selective coronary angiography during congenital heart catheterization (List separately in addition to code for primary procedure)**
Code first (93530-93533)
Do not report with (93452-93461, 0345T)
N 80 1.59 1.59 FUD ZZZ

+ ⊙ 93564 **for selective opacification of aortocoronary venous or arterial bypass graft(s) (eg, aortocoronary saphenous vein, free radial artery, or free mammary artery graft) to one or more coronary arteries and in situ arterial conduits (eg, internal mammary), whether native or used for bypass to one or more coronary arteries during congenital heart catheterization, when performed (List separately in addition to code for primary procedure)**
Code first (93530-93533)
Do not report with (93452-93461, 93580, 0345T)
N 80 1.63 1.63 FUD ZZZ

+ ⊙ 93565 **for selective left ventricular or left atrial angiography (List separately in addition to code for primary procedure)**
Code first (93530-93533)
Do not report with (93452-93461, 93580)
N 80 PQ 1.24 1.24 FUD ZZZ

+ ⊙ 93566 **for selective right ventricular or right atrial angiography (List separately in addition to code for primary procedure)**
Code first (93451, 93453, 93456-93457, 93460-93461, 93530-93533)
Do not report with (93580)
N 80 PQ 1.24 4.82 FUD ZZZ

+ ⊙ 93567 **for supravalvular aortography (List separately in addition to code for primary procedure)**
EXCLUDES *Abdominal aortography or non-supravalvular thoracic aortography at same time as cardiac catheterization (36221, 75600-75630)*
Code first (93451-93461, 93530-93533)
N 80 PQ 1.39 3.97 FUD ZZZ

+ ⊙ 93568 **for pulmonary angiography (List separately in addition to code for primary procedure)**
Code first (93451, 93453, 93456-93457, 93460-93461, 93530-93533)
N 80 PQ 1.26 4.31 FUD ZZZ

93571-93572 Coronary Artery Doppler Studies

CMS 100-4,12,30.4 Cardiovascular System

INCLUDES Doppler transducer manipulations/repositioning within the vessel examined, during coronary angiography/therapeutic intervention (angioplasty)

+ ⊙ 93571 **Intravascular Doppler velocity and/or pressure derived coronary flow reserve measurement (coronary vessel or graft) during coronary angiography including pharmacologically induced stress; initial vessel (List separately in addition to code for primary procedure)**
Code first ([92920], [92924], [92928], [92933], [92937], [92941], [92943], [92975], 93454-93461, 93563-93564)
N 80 CCI 0.00 0.00 FUD ZZZ

+ ⊙ 93572 **each additional vessel (List separately in addition to code for primary procedure)**
Code first initial vessel (93571)
N 80 0.00 0.00 FUD ZZZ

93580-93583 Percutaneous Repair of Congenital Heart Defects

CMS 100-4,12,30.4 Cardiovascular System

93580 **Percutaneous transcatheter closure of congenital interatrial communication (ie, Fontan fenestration, atrial septal defect) with implant**
INCLUDES Injection of contrast for atrial/ventricular angiograms
Right heart catheterization
Code also echocardiography, when performed (93303-93317, 93662)
Do not report with (93451-93453, 93455-93461, 93530-93533, 93564-93566)
T 80 CCI 28.24 28.24 FUD 000

93581 Percutaneous transcatheter closure of a congenital ventricular septal defect with implant

INCLUDES Injection of contrast for atrial/ventricular angiograms
Right heart catheterization

Code also echocardiography, when performed (93303-93317, 93662)

Do not report with (93451-93453, 93455-93461, 93530-93533, 93564-93566)

T 80 38.13 38.13 FUD 000

⊙ **93582 Percutaneous transcatheter closure of patent ductus arteriosus**

INCLUDES Right and left heart catheterization, aorta catheter placement, and angiography of the aortic arch when performed

EXCLUDES *Intracardiac echocardiographic services (93662)*
Left heart catheterization performed via transapical puncture or transseptal puncture through intact septum (93462)
Ligation repair (33820, 33822, 33824)
Other cardiac angiographic procedures (93563-93566, 93568)
Other echocardiographic services by different provider (93315-93317)

Do not report with (36013-36014, 36200, 75600, 75605, 93451-93461, 93530-93533, 93567)

T 80 19.47 19.47 FUD 000

⊙ **93583 Percutaneous transcatheter septal reduction therapy (eg, alcohol septal ablation) including temporary pacemaker insertion when performed**

INCLUDES Left anterior descending coronary angiography performed to guide the intervention through roadmapping
Left heart catheterization
Temporary pacemaker insertion

EXCLUDES *Intracardiac echocardiographic services when performed (93662)*
Myectomy (surgical ventriculomyotomy) to treat idiopathic hypertrophic subaortic stenosis (33416)
Other echocardiographic services rendered by different provider (93312-93317)

Code also diagnostic cardiac catheterization procedures if the patient's condition (clinical indication) has changed since the intervention or prior study, there is no available prior catheter-based diagnostic study of the treatment zone, or the prior study is not adequate (93451, 93454-93457, 93530, 93563-93564, 93566-93568)

Do not report alcohol injection (93463)

Do not report for coronary angiography during the procedure in order to roadmap, guide the intervention, measure the vessel, and complete the angiography (93454-93461, 93563)

Do not report with (33210-33211, 93452-93453, 93458-93459, 93460-93461, 93531-93533, 93565)

C 80 21.67 21.67 FUD 000

93600-93603 Recording of Intracardiac Electrograms

CMS 100-3,20.13 HIS Bundle Study
CMS 100-4,12,30.4 Cardiovascular System

INCLUDES Unusual situations where there may be recording/pacing/attempt at arrhythmia induction from only one side of the heart

Do not report with (93619-93620, 93653-93654, 93656)

⊘ **93600 Bundle of His recording**

Code also (C1730, C1731, C1732, C1733, C1766, C1892, C1893, C1894, C2629, C2630)

S 80 0.00 0.00 FUD 000

⊘ **93602 Intra-atrial recording**

Code also (C1730, C1731, C1732, C1733, C1766, C1892, C1893, C1894, C2629, C2630)

S 80 0.00 0.00 FUD 000

⊘ **93603 Right ventricular recording**

Code also (C1730, C1731, C1732, C1733, C1766, C1892, C1893, C1894, C2629, C2630)

S 80 0.00 0.00 FUD 000

93609-93613 Intracardiac Mapping and Pacing

CMS 100-3,20.12 Diagnostic Endocardial Electrical Stimulation (Pacing)
CMS 100-4,12,30.4 Cardiovascular System

+ ⊙ **93609 Intraventricular and/or intra-atrial mapping of tachycardia site(s) with catheter manipulation to record from multiple sites to identify origin of tachycardia (List separately in addition to code for primary procedure)**

Code also (C1730, C1731, C1733, C2629, C2630)
Code first (93620, 93653, 93656)
Do not report with (93613, 93654)

N 80 0.00 0.00 FUD ZZZ

⊘ **93610 Intra-atrial pacing**

INCLUDES Unusual situations where there may be recording/pacing/attempt at arrhythmia induction from only one side of the heart

Code also (C1730, C1731, C1732, C1733, C1766, C1892, C1893, C1894, C2629, C2630)

Do not report with (93619-93620, 93653-93654, 93656)

S 80 0.00 0.00 FUD 000

⊘ **93612 Intraventricular pacing**

INCLUDES Unusual situations where there may be recording/pacing/attempt at arrhythmia induction from only one side of the heart

Code also (C1730, C1731, C1732, C1733, C1766, C1892, C1893, C1894, C2629, C2630)

Do not report with (93619-93622, 93653-93654, 93656)

S 80 0.00 0.00 FUD 000

+ ⊙ **93613 Intracardiac electrophysiologic 3-dimensional mapping (List separately in addition to code for primary procedure)**

Code also (C1730, C1731, C1732, C1733, C2630)
Code first (93620, 93653, 93656)
Do not report with (93609, 93654)

N 80 11.25 11.25 FUD ZZZ

93615-93616 Recording and Pacing via Esophagus

CMS 100-4,12,30.4 Cardiovascular System

⊘ ⊙ **93615 Esophageal recording of atrial electrogram with or without ventricular electrogram(s);**

Code also (C1730, C1731, C1732, C1733, C1766, C1892, C1893, C1894, C2629, C2630)

S 80 0.00 0.00 FUD 000

⊘ ⊙ **93616 with pacing**

Code also (C1730, C1731, C1732, C1733, C1756, C1766, C1892, C1893, C1894, C2629, C2630)

S 80 0.00 0.00 FUD 000

93618 Pacing to Produce an Arrhythmia

CMS 100-4,12,30.4 Cardiovascular System

INCLUDES Unusual situations where there may be recording/pacing/attempt at arrhythmia induction from only one side of the heart

EXCLUDES *Intracardiac phonocardiogram (93799)*

Do not report with (93619-93622, 93653-93654, 93656)

⊘ ⊙ **93618 Induction of arrhythmia by electrical pacing**

Code also (C1730, C1731, C1732, C1733, C1766, C1892, C1893, C1894, C2629, C2630)

S 80 0.00 0.00 FUD 000

93619-93623 Comprehensive Electrophysiological Studies

CMS 100-3,20.12 Diagnostic Endocardial Electrical Stimulation (Pacing)
CMS 100-4,12,30.4 Cardiovascular System

⊙ **93619** **Comprehensive electrophysiologic evaluation with right atrial pacing and recording, right ventricular pacing and recording, His bundle recording, including insertion and repositioning of multiple electrode catheters, without induction or attempted induction of arrhythmia**

INCLUDES Evaluation of sinus node/atrioventricular node/His-Purkinje conduction system without arrhythmia induction

Code also (C1730, C1731, C1732, C1733, C1766, C1892, C1893, C1894, C2629, C2630)

Do not report with (93600, 93602-93603, 93610, 93612, 93618, 93620-93622, 93653-93657)

Q3 80 0.00 0.00 FUD 000

⊙ **93620** **Comprehensive electrophysiologic evaluation including insertion and repositioning of multiple electrode catheters with induction or attempted induction of arrhythmia; with right atrial pacing and recording, right ventricular pacing and recording, His bundle recording**

INCLUDES Recording/pacing/attempted arrhythmia induction from one or more site(s) in the heart

Code also (C1730, C1731, C1732, C1733, C1766, C1892, C1893, C1894, C2629, C2630)

Do not report with (93600, 93602-93603, 93610, 93612, 93618-93619, 93653-93657)

Q3 80 0.00 0.00 FUD 000

+ ⊙ **93621** **with left atrial pacing and recording from coronary sinus or left atrium (List separately in addition to code for primary procedure)**

INCLUDES Recording/pacing/attempted arrhythmia induction from one or more site(s) in the heart

Code also (C1730, C1731, C1732, C1733, C1766, C1892, C1893, C1894, C2629, C2630)

Code first (93620, 93653-93654)

Do not report with (93656)

N 80 0.00 0.00 FUD ZZZ

+ ⊙ **93622** **with left ventricular pacing and recording (List separately in addition to code for primary procedure)**

Code also (C1730, C1731, C1732, C1733, C1766, C1892, C1893, C1894, C2629, C2630)

Code first (93620, 93653, 93656)

Do not report with (93654)

N 80 0.00 0.00 FUD ZZZ

+ **93623** **Programmed stimulation and pacing after intravenous drug infusion (List separately in addition to code for primary procedure)**

INCLUDES Recording/pacing/attempted arrhythmia induction from one or more site(s) in the heart

Code also (C1730, C1731, C1732, C1733, C1766, C1892, C1893, C1894, C2629, C2630)

Code first comprehensive electrophysiologic evaluation (93610, 93612, 93619-93620, 93653-93654, 93656)

N 80 0.00 0.00 FUD ZZZ

93624-93631 Followup and Intraoperative Electrophysiologic Studies

CMS 100-3,20.11 Intraoperative Ventricular Mapping
CMS 100-3,20.12 Diagnostic Endocardial Electrical Stimulation (Pacing)
CMS 100-4,12,30.4 Cardiovascular System

⊙ **93624** **Electrophysiologic follow-up study with pacing and recording to test effectiveness of therapy, including induction or attempted induction of arrhythmia**

INCLUDES Recording/pacing/attempted arrhythmia induction from one or more site(s) in the heart

Code also (C1730, C1731, C1732, C1733, C1766, C1892, C1893, C1894)

T 80 0.00 0.00 FUD 000

⊘ **93631** **Intra-operative epicardial and endocardial pacing and mapping to localize the site of tachycardia or zone of slow conduction for surgical correction**

EXCLUDES *Operative ablation of an arrhythmogenic focus or pathway by a separate provider (33250-33261)*

Code also (C1730, C1731, C1732, C1733, C1766, C1892, C1893, C1894, C2629, C2630)

N 80 0.00 0.00 FUD 000

93640-93644 Electrophysiologic Studies of Cardioverter-Defibrillators

CMS 100-3,20.8.2 Self-contained Pacemaker Monitors
CMS 100-3,20.12 Diagnostic Endocardial Electrical Stimulation (Pacing)
CMS 100-4,12,30.4 Cardiovascular System

INCLUDES Recording/pacing/attempted arrhythmia induction from one or more site(s) in the heart

⊙ **93640** **Electrophysiologic evaluation of single or dual chamber pacing cardioverter-defibrillator leads including defibrillation threshold evaluation (induction of arrhythmia, evaluation of sensing and pacing for arrhythmia termination) at time of initial implantation or replacement;**

N 80 0.00 0.00 FUD 000

⊙ **93641** **with testing of single or dual chamber pacing cardioverter-defibrillator pulse generator**

EXCLUDES *Single/dual chamber pacing cardioverter-defibrillators reprogramming/electronic analysis, subsequent/periodic (93282-93283, 93289, 93292, 93295, 93642)*

N 80 0.00 0.00 FUD 000

⊙ ▲ **93642** **Electrophysiologic evaluation of single or dual chamber transvenous pacing cardioverter-defibrillator (includes defibrillation threshold evaluation, induction of arrhythmia, evaluation of sensing and pacing for arrhythmia termination, and programming or reprogramming of sensing or therapeutic parameters)**

S 80 11.17 11.17 FUD 000

⊙ ● **93644** **Electrophysiologic evaluation of subcutaneous implantable defibrillator (includes defibrillation threshold evaluation, induction of arrhythmia, evaluation of sensing for arrhythmia termination, and programming or reprogramming of sensing or therapeutic parameters)**

EXCLUDES *Subcutaneous cardioverter-defibrillator electrophysiologic evaluation, subsequent/periodic (93285-93289 [93260, 93261])*

Do not report with ([33270])

93650-93657 Intracardiac Ablation

CMS 100-4,12,30.4 Cardiovascular System

INCLUDES Ablation services include selective delivery of cryo-energy or radiofrequency to targeted tissue
Electrophysiologic studies performed in the same session with ablation

⊙ **93650** **Intracardiac catheter ablation of atrioventricular node function, atrioventricular conduction for creation of complete heart block, with or without temporary pacemaker placement**
Code also (C1732, C1733, C1766, C1892, C1893, C1894, C2629, C2630)
Q3 80 17.19 17.19 FUD 000

⊙ **93653** **Comprehensive electrophysiologic evaluation including insertion and repositioning of multiple electrode catheters with induction or attempted induction of an arrhythmia with right atrial pacing and recording, right ventricular pacing and recording (when necessary), and His bundle recording (when necessary) with intracardiac catheter ablation of arrhythmogenic focus; with treatment of supraventricular tachycardia by ablation of fast or slow atrioventricular pathway, accessory atrioventricular connection, cavo-tricuspid isthmus or other single atrial focus or source of atrial re-entry**
Do not report with (93600-93603, 93610, 93612, 93618-93620, 93642, 93654, 93656)
Q3 80 24.15 24.15 FUD 000

⊙ **93654** **with treatment of ventricular tachycardia or focus of ventricular ectopy including intracardiac electrophysiologic 3D mapping, when performed, and left ventricular pacing and recording, when performed**
Do not report with (93279-93284, 93286-93289, 93600-93603, 93609-93610, 93612-93613, 93618-93620, 93622, 93642, 93653, 93656)
Q3 80 32.16 32.16 FUD 000

+ ⊙ **93655** **Intracardiac catheter ablation of a discrete mechanism of arrhythmia which is distinct from the primary ablated mechanism, including repeat diagnostic maneuvers, to treat a spontaneous or induced arrhythmia (List separately in addition to code for primary procedure)**
Code first (93653-93654, 93656)
N 80 12.07 12.07 FUD ZZZ

⊙ **93656** **Comprehensive electrophysiologic evaluation including transseptal catheterizations, insertion and repositioning of multiple electrode catheters with induction or attempted induction of an arrhythmia including left or right atrial pacing/recording when necessary, right ventricular pacing/recording when necessary, and His bundle recording when necessary with intracardiac catheter ablation of atrial fibrillation by pulmonary vein isolation**
INCLUDES His bundle recording when indicated
Left atrial pacing/recording
Right ventricular pacing/recording
Do not report with (93279-93284, 93286-93289, 93600, 93602-93603, 93610, 93612, 93618-93621, 93642, 93653-93654)
Q3 80 32.20 32.20 FUD 000

+ ⊙ **93657** **Additional linear or focal intracardiac catheter ablation of the left or right atrium for treatment of atrial fibrillation remaining after completion of pulmonary vein isolation (List separately in addition to code for primary procedure)**
Code first (93656)
N 80 12.08 12.08 FUD ZZZ

93660-93662 Other Tests for Cardiac Function

CMS 100-4,12,30.4 Cardiovascular System

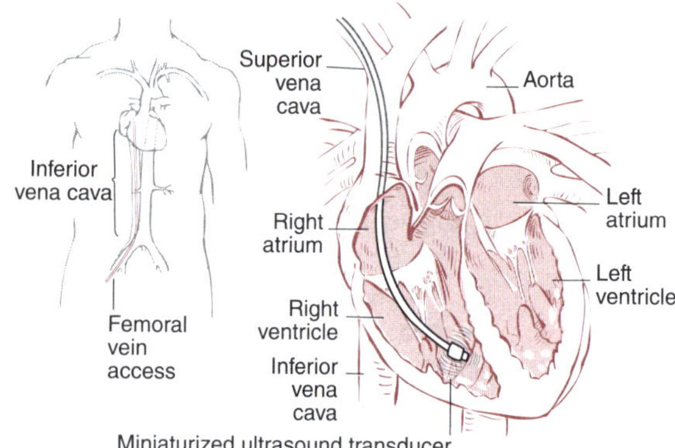

93660 **Evaluation of cardiovascular function with tilt table evaluation, with continuous ECG monitoring and intermittent blood pressure monitoring, with or without pharmacological intervention**
EXCLUDES *Autonomic nervous system function testing (95921, 95924, [95943])*
S 80 4.41 4.41 FUD 000

+ **93662** **Intracardiac echocardiography during therapeutic/diagnostic intervention, including imaging supervision and interpretation (List separately in addition to code for primary procedure)**
Code also (C1759)
Code first (as appropriate) (92987, 93453, 93460-93462, 93532, 93580-93581, 93620-93622, 93653-93654, 93656)
Do not report with internal cardioversion (92961)
N 80 0.00 0.00 FUD ZZZ

93668 Rehabilitation Services: Peripheral Arterial Disease

INCLUDES Monitoring:
Other cardiovascular limitations for adjustment of workload
Patient's claudication threshold
Motorized treadmill or track
Sessions lasting 45-60 minutes
Supervision by exercise physiologist/nurse

Code also appropriate evaluation and management service, when performed

93668 **Peripheral arterial disease (PAD) rehabilitation, per session**
E 0.53 0.53 FUD XXX

93701-93702 Thoracic Electrical Bioimpedance

CMS 100-3,20.16 Cardiac Output Monitoring by Thoracic Electrical Bioimpedance (TEB)
CMS 100-4,12,30.4 Cardiovascular System

EXCLUDES *Indirect measurement of left ventricular filling pressure by computerized calibration of the arterial waveform response to Valsalva (93799)*

93701 **Bioimpedance-derived physiologic cardiovascular analysis**
S TC 80 0.67 0.67 FUD XXX

● **93702** **Bioimpedance spectroscopy (BIS), extracellular fluid analysis for lymphedema assessment(s)**

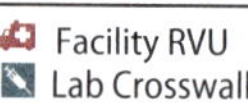

93724 Electronic Analysis of Pacemaker Function

CMS 100-3,20.8 Cardiac Pacemakers
CMS 100-3,20.8.1 Cardiac Pacemaker Evaluation Services
CMS 100-3,20.14 Plethysmography
CMS 100-4,12,30.4 Cardiovascular System

EXCLUDES *Arterial cannulization/recording of direct arterial pressure (36620)*
Radiographic injection services (36000-36299)

93724 Electronic analysis of antitachycardia pacemaker system (includes electrocardiographic recording, programming of device, induction and termination of tachycardia via implanted pacemaker, and interpretation of recordings)
S 80 7.64 7.64 FUD 000

93740 Temperature Gradient Assessment

CMS 100-4,12,30.4 Cardiovascular System

93740 Temperature gradient studies
X 0.25 0.25 FUD XXX

93745 Wearable Cardioverter-Defibrillator System Services

CMS 100-4,12,30.4 Cardiovascular System

EXCLUDES *Arterial cannulization/recording of direct arterial pressure (36620)*
Radiographic injection services (36000-36299)

Do not report with (93282, 93292)

93745 Initial set-up and programming by a physician or other qualified health care professional of wearable cardioverter-defibrillator includes initial programming of system, establishing baseline electronic ECG, transmission of data to data repository, patient instruction in wearing system and patient reporting of problems or events
S 80 0.00 0.00 FUD XXX

93750 Ventricular Assist Device (VAD) Interrogation

Do not report with (33975-33976, 33979, 33981-33983)

93750 Interrogation of ventricular assist device (VAD), in person, with physician or other qualified health care professional analysis of device parameters (eg, drivelines, alarms, power surges), review of device function (eg, flow and volume status, septum status, recovery), with programming, if performed, and report
S 80 1.28 1.53 FUD XXX

93770 Peripheral Venous Blood Pressure Assessment

CMS 100-4,12,30.4 Cardiovascular System

EXCLUDES *Cannulization, central venous (36500, 36555-36556)*

93770 Determination of venous pressure
N 0.25 0.25 FUD XXX

93784-93790 Ambulatory Blood Pressure Monitoring

CMS 100-3,20.19 Ambulatory Blood Pressure Monitoring
CMS 100-4,12,30.4 Cardiovascular System
CMS 100-4,32,10.1 Ambulatory Blood Pressure Monitoring Billing Requirements

93784 Ambulatory blood pressure monitoring, utilizing a system such as magnetic tape and/or computer disk, for 24 hours or longer; including recording, scanning analysis, interpretation and report
B 80 1.51 1.51 FUD XXX

93786 recording only
S TC 80 0.83 0.83 FUD XXX

93788 scanning analysis with report
S TC 80 0.15 0.15 FUD XXX

93790 review with interpretation and report
M 26 80 0.53 0.53 FUD XXX

93797-93799 Cardiac Rehabilitation

CMS 100-3,20.10 Cardiac Rehabilitation Programs
CMS 100-4,4,200.5 Cardiac Rehabilitation Services
CMS 100-4,12,30.4 Cardiovascular System

EXCLUDES *Arterial cannulization/recording of direct arterial pressure (36620)*
Chemotherapy (96409)
Hemodialysis vascular cannulization (36800-36821)
Radiographic injection services (36000-36299)

93797 Physician or other qualified health care professional services for outpatient cardiac rehabilitation; without continuous ECG monitoring (per session)
S 80 0.25 0.46 FUD 000

93798 with continuous ECG monitoring (per session)
S 80 0.39 0.69 FUD 000

93799 Unlisted cardiovascular service or procedure
S 80 0.00 0.00 FUD XXX

93880-93895 Noninvasive Tests Extracranial/Intracranial Arteries

CMS 100-3,20.17 Noninvasive Tests of Carotid Function

INCLUDES Patient care required to perform/supervise studies and interpret results

Do not report for hand-held dopplers that do not provide a hard copy (See E/M codes)
Do not report for hand-held dopplers that do not permit vascular flow bidirectional analysis (see E/M codes)

93880 Duplex scan of extracranial arteries; complete bilateral study
Do not report with (93895, 0126T)
S 80 PQ 5.36 5.36 FUD XXX

93882 unilateral or limited study
Do not report with (93895, 0126T)
S 80 PQ 3.47 3.47 FUD XXX

93886 Transcranial Doppler study of the intracranial arteries; complete study
INCLUDES Complete transcranial doppler (TCD) study
Ultrasound evaluation of right/left anterior circulation territories and posterior circulation territory
S 80 10.09 10.09 FUD XXX

93888 limited study
INCLUDES Limited TCD study
Ultrasound examination of two or fewer of these territories (right/left anterior circulation, posterior circulation)
S 80 5.90 5.90 FUD XXX

93890 vasoreactivity study
Do not report with limited TCD study (93888)
S 80 8.13 8.13 FUD XXX

93892 emboli detection without intravenous microbubble injection
Do not report with limited TCD study (93888)
S 80 9.47 9.47 FUD XXX

93893 emboli detection with intravenous microbubble injection
Do not report with limited TCD study (93888)
S 80 9.78 9.78 FUD XXX

● **93895 Quantitative carotid intima media thickness and carotid atheroma evaluation, bilateral**
Do not report with (93880, 93882, 0126T)

93922-93971 Noninvasive Vascular Studies: Extremities

CMS 100-3,20.14 Plethysmography

INCLUDES Patient care required to perform/supervise studies and interpret results

Do not report for hand-held dopplers that do not permit vascular flow bidirectional analysis (see E/M codes)
Do not report for hand-held dopplers that do not provide a hard copy (See E/M codes)

93922 Limited bilateral noninvasive physiologic studies of upper or lower extremity arteries, (eg, for lower extremity: ankle/brachial indices at distal posterior tibial and anterior tibial/dorsalis pedis arteries plus bidirectional, Doppler waveform recording and analysis at 1-2 levels, or ankle/brachial indices at distal posterior tibial and anterior tibial/dorsalis pedis arteries plus volume plethysmography at 1-2 levels, or ankle/brachial indices at distal posterior tibial and anterior tibial/dorsalis pedis arteries with, transcutaneous oxygen tension measurement at 1-2 levels)

INCLUDES Evaluation of:
- Doppler analysis of bidirectional blood flow
- Nonimaging physiologic recordings of pressure
- Oxygen tension measurements and/or plethysmography

Lower extremity (potential levels include high thigh, low thigh, calf, ankle, metatarsal and toes) limited study includes either:
- Ankle/brachial indices at distal posterior tibial and anterior tibial/dorsalis pedis arteries plus bidirectional Doppler waveform recording and analysis as 1-2 levels; OR
- Ankle/brachial indices at distal posterior tibial and anterior tibial/dorsalis pedis arteries plus volume plethysmography at 1-2 levels; OR
- Ankle/brachial indices at distal posterior tibial and anterior tibial/dorsalis pedis arteries with transcutaneous oxygen tension measurements at 1-2 levels

Unilateral provocative functional measurement

Unilateral study of 3 or move levels

Upper extremity (potential levels include arm, forearm, wrist, and digits) limited study includes:
- Doppler-determined systolic pressures and bidirectional waveform recording with analysis at 1-2 levels; OR
- Doppler-determined systolic pressures and transcutaneous oxygen tension measurements at 1-2 levels; OR
- Doppler-determined systolic pressures and volume plethysmography at 1-2 levels

EXCLUDES *Transcutaneous oxyhemoglobin measurement in wound of lower extremity by near infrared spectroscopy (0286T)*

Code also modifier 52 for unilateral study of 1-2 levels

Code also twice with modifier 59 for upper and lower extremity study

Do not report more than one time for the lower extremity(s)

Do not report more than one time for the upper extremity(s)

Do not report with (0337T)

S 80 ⚑ Facility RVU 2.49 Non-Facility RVU 2.49 FUD XXX

93923 Complete bilateral noninvasive physiologic studies of upper or lower extremity arteries, 3 or more levels (eg, for lower extremity: ankle/brachial indices at distal posterior tibial and anterior tibial/dorsalis pedis arteries plus segmental blood pressure measurements with bidirectional Doppler waveform recording and analysis, at 3 or more levels, or ankle/brachial indices at distal posterior tibial and anterior tibial/dorsalis pedis arteries plus segmental volume plethysmography at 3 or more levels, or ankle/brachial indices at distal posterior tibial and anterior tibial/dorsalis pedis arteries plus segmental transcutaneous oxygen tension measurements at 3 or more levels), or single level study with provocative functional maneuvers (eg, measurements with postural provocative tests, or measurements with reactive hyperemia)

INCLUDES Evaluation of:
- Doppler analysis of bidirectional blood flow
- Nonimaging physiologic recordings of pressures
- Oxygen tension measurements

Lower extremity:
- Ankle/brachial indices at distal posterior tibial and anterior tibial/dorsalis pedis arteries plus bidirectional Doppler waveform recording and analysis at 3 or more levels; OR
- Ankle/brachial indices at distal posterior tibial and anterior tibial/dorsalis pedis arteries with transcutaneous oxygen tension measurements at 3 or more levels; OR
- Ankle/brachial indices at distal posterior tibial and anterior tibial/dorsalis pedis arteries plus volume plethysmography at 3 or more levels; OR

Provocative functional maneuvers and measurement at a single level

Upper extremity complete study:
- Doppler-determined systolic pressures and bidirectional waveform recording with analysis at 3 or more levels; OR
- Doppler-determined systolic pressures and transcutaneous oxygen tension measurements at 3 or more levels; OR
- Doppler-determined systolic pressures and volume plethysmography at 3 or more levels; OR
- Provocative functional maneuvers and measurement at a single level

EXCLUDES *Transcutaneous oxyhemoglobin measurement in wound of lower extremity by near infrared spectroscopy (0286T)*

Unilateral study at 3 or more levels (93922)

Code also twice with modifier 59 for upper and lower extremity study

Do not report more than one time for the lower extremity(s)

Do not report more than one time for the upper extremity(s)

Do not report with (0337T)

S 80 ⚑ Facility RVU 3.91 Non-Facility RVU 3.91 FUD XXX

93924 **Noninvasive physiologic studies of lower extremity arteries, at rest and following treadmill stress testing, (ie, bidirectional Doppler waveform or volume plethysmography recording and analysis at rest with ankle/brachial indices immediately after and at timed intervals following performance of a standardized protocol on a motorized treadmill plus recording of time of onset of claudication or other symptoms, maximal walking time, and time to recovery) complete bilateral study**

INCLUDES Evaluation of:
- Doppler analysis of bidirectional blood flow
- Non-imaging physiologic recordings of pressures
- Oxygen tension measurements
- Plethysmography

Do not report this code for other types of exercise

Do not report with (93922-93923)

S 80 4.91 4.91 FUD XXX

93925 **Duplex scan of lower extremity arteries or arterial bypass grafts; complete bilateral study**

S 80 6.92 6.92 FUD XXX

93926 **unilateral or limited study**

S 80 3.97 3.97 FUD XXX

93930 **Duplex scan of upper extremity arteries or arterial bypass grafts; complete bilateral study**

S 80 6.46 6.46 FUD XXX

93931 **unilateral or limited study**

S 80 4.42 4.42 FUD XXX

93965 **Noninvasive physiologic studies of extremity veins, complete bilateral study (eg, Doppler waveform analysis with responses to compression and other maneuvers, phleborheography, impedance plethysmography)**

INCLUDES Evaluation of:
- Doppler analysis of bidirectional blood flow
- Nonimaging physiologic recordings of pressures
- Oxygen tension measurements
- Plethysmography

S 80 3.40 3.40 FUD XXX

93970 **Duplex scan of extremity veins including responses to compression and other maneuvers; complete bilateral study**

Do not report with (36475-36476, 36478-36479)

S 80 5.27 5.27 FUD XXX

93971 **unilateral or limited study**

Do not report with (36475-36476, 36478-36479)

S 80 3.20 3.20 FUD XXX

93975-93982 Noninvasive Vascular Studies: Abdomen/Chest/Pelvis

93975 **Duplex scan of arterial inflow and venous outflow of abdominal, pelvic, scrotal contents and/or retroperitoneal organs; complete study**

S 80 10.10 10.10 FUD XXX

93976 **limited study**

S 80 5.96 5.96 FUD XXX

93978 **Duplex scan of aorta, inferior vena cava, iliac vasculature, or bypass grafts; complete study**

S 80 6.33 6.33 FUD XXX

93979 **unilateral or limited study**

S 80 4.38 4.38 FUD XXX

93980 **Duplex scan of arterial inflow and venous outflow of penile vessels; complete study** ♂

S 80 3.45 3.45 FUD XXX

93981 **follow-up or limited study** ♂

S 80 2.09 2.09 FUD XXX

93982 **Noninvasive physiologic study of implanted wireless pressure sensor in aneurysmal sac following endovascular repair, complete study including recording, analysis of pressure and waveform tracings, interpretation and report**

Do not report with (34806)

S 80 1.22 1.22 FUD XXX

93990-93998 Noninvasive Vascular Studies: Hemodialysis Access

93990 **Duplex scan of hemodialysis access (including arterial inflow, body of access and venous outflow)**

EXCLUDES *Hemodialysis access flow measurement by indicator method (90940)*

S 80 5.47 5.47 FUD XXX

93998 **Unlisted noninvasive vascular diagnostic study**

X 80 0.00 0.00 FUD XXX

94002-94005 Ventilator Management Services

94002 **Ventilation assist and management, initiation of pressure or volume preset ventilators for assisted or controlled breathing; hospital inpatient/observation, initial day**

Do not report with evaluation and management services

03 80 2.64 2.64 FUD XXX

94003 **hospital inpatient/observation, each subsequent day**

Do not report with evaluation and management services

03 80 1.90 1.90 FUD XXX

94004 **nursing facility, per day**

Do not report with evaluation and management services

B 80 1.40 1.40 FUD XXX

94005 **Home ventilator management care plan oversight of a patient (patient not present) in home, domiciliary or rest home (eg, assisted living) requiring review of status, review of laboratories and other studies and revision of orders and respiratory care plan (as appropriate), within a calendar month, 30 minutes or more**

Code also when a different provider reports care plan oversight in the same 30 days (99339-99340, 99374-99378)

M 2.63 2.63 FUD XXX

94010-94799 Respiratory Services: Diagnostic and Therapeutic

INCLUDES Laboratory procedure(s)
Test results interpretation

EXCLUDES *Separately identifiable evaluation and management service*

94010 **Spirometry, including graphic record, total and timed vital capacity, expiratory flow rate measurement(s), with or without maximal voluntary ventilation**

INCLUDES Measurement of expiratory airflow and volumes

EXCLUDES *Diffusing capacity (94729)*

Do not report with (94150, 94200, 94375, 94728)

X 80 1.01 1.01 FUD XXX

⊙ **94011** **Measurement of spirometric forced expiratory flows in an infant or child through 2 years of age**

X 80 2.90 2.90 FUD XXX

⊙ **94012** **Measurement of spirometric forced expiratory flows, before and after bronchodilator, in an infant or child through 2 years of age**

X 80 4.54 4.54 FUD XXX

⊙ **94013** **Measurement of lung volumes (ie, functional residual capacity [FRC], forced vital capacity [FVC], and expiratory reserve volume [ERV]) in an infant or child through 2 years of age**

X 80 0.90 0.90 FUD XXX

94014 **Patient-initiated spirometric recording per 30-day period of time; includes reinforced education, transmission of spirometric tracing, data capture, analysis of transmitted data, periodic recalibration and review and interpretation by a physician or other qualified health care professional**
X 80 ⚑ 1.46 1.46 FUD XXX

94015 **recording (includes hook-up, reinforced education, data transmission, data capture, trend analysis, and periodic recalibration)**
X TC 80 ⚑ 0.75 0.75 FUD XXX

94016 **review and interpretation only by a physician or other qualified health care professional**
A 26 80 ⚑ 0.71 0.71 FUD XXX

94060 **Bronchodilation responsiveness, spirometry as in 94010, pre- and post-bronchodilator administration**
INCLUDES Spirometry performed prior to and after a bronchodilator has been administered
EXCLUDES *Bronchospasm prolonged exercise test with pre- and post-spirometry (94620)*
Diffusing capacity (94729)
Code also bronchodilator supply with appropriate supply code or 99070
Do not report with (94150, 94200, 94375, 94728)
S 80 ⚑ 1.70 1.70 FUD XXX

94070 **Bronchospasm provocation evaluation, multiple spirometric determinations as in 94010, with administered agents (eg, antigen[s], cold air, methacholine)**
EXCLUDES *Diffusing capacity (94729)*
Code also antigen(s) administration with appropriate supply code or 99070
X 80 ⚑ 1.68 1.68 FUD XXX

94150 **Vital capacity, total (separate procedure)**
EXCLUDES *Thoracic gas volumes (94726-94727)*
Do not report with (94010, 94060, 94728)
X 0.71 0.71 FUD XXX

94200 **Maximum breathing capacity, maximal voluntary ventilation**
Do not report with (94010, 94060)
X 80 0.69 0.69 FUD XXX

94250 **Expired gas collection, quantitative, single procedure (separate procedure)**
X 80 0.74 0.74 FUD XXX

94375 **Respiratory flow volume loop**
INCLUDES Identification of obstruction patterns in central or peripheral airways (inspiratory and/or expiratory)
EXCLUDES *Diffusing capacity (94729)*
Do not report with (94010, 94060, 94728)
X 80 ⚑ 1.10 1.10 FUD XXX

94400 **Breathing response to CO2 (CO2 response curve)**
X 80 ⚑ 1.57 1.57 FUD XXX

94450 **Breathing response to hypoxia (hypoxia response curve)**
EXCLUDES *HAST - high altitude simulation test (94452, 94453)*
X 80 ⚑ 1.91 1.91 FUD XXX

94452 **High altitude simulation test (HAST), with interpretation and report by a physician or other qualified health care professional;**
EXCLUDES *Obtaining arterial blood gases (36600)*
Do not report with (94453, 94760-94761)
X 80 ⚑ 1.62 1.62 FUD XXX

94453 **with supplemental oxygen titration**
EXCLUDES *Obtaining arterial blood gases (36600)*
Do not report with (94452, 94760-94761)
X 80 ⚑ 2.25 2.25 FUD XXX

⊘ **94610** **Intrapulmonary surfactant administration by a physician or other qualified health care professional through endotracheal tube**
INCLUDES Reporting once per dosing episode
EXCLUDES *Intubation, endotracheal (31500)*
Do not report with (99468-99472)
S 80 1.69 1.69 FUD XXX

94620 **Pulmonary stress testing; simple (eg, 6-minute walk test, prolonged exercise test for bronchospasm with pre- and post-spirometry and oximetry)**
X 80 ⚑ 1.57 1.57 FUD XXX

94621 **complex (including measurements of CO2 production, O2 uptake, and electrocardiographic recordings)**
X 80 ⚑ 4.60 4.60 FUD XXX

94640 **Pressurized or nonpressurized inhalation treatment for acute airway obstruction or for sputum induction for diagnostic purposes (eg, with an aerosol generator, nebulizer, metered dose inhaler or intermittent positive pressure breathing [IPPB] device)**
EXCLUDES *1 hour or more of continuous inhalation treatment (94644, 94645)*
Code also modifier 76 when more than 1 inhalation treatment is performed on the same date
S 80 ⚑ 0.51 0.51 FUD XXX

94642 **Aerosol inhalation of pentamidine for pneumocystis carinii pneumonia treatment or prophylaxis**
S 80 ⚑ 0.00 0.00 FUD XXX

94644 **Continuous inhalation treatment with aerosol medication for acute airway obstruction; first hour**
EXCLUDES *Services that are less than 1 hour (94640)*
X 80 1.23 1.23 FUD XXX

\+ **94645** **each additional hour (List separately in addition to code for primary procedure)**
Code first initial hour (94644)
N 80 0.40 0.40 FUD XXX

94660 **Continuous positive airway pressure ventilation (CPAP), initiation and management**
03 80 1.07 1.77 FUD XXX

94662 **Continuous negative pressure ventilation (CNP), initiation and management**
03 80 ⚑ 1.14 1.14 FUD XXX

94664 **Demonstration and/or evaluation of patient utilization of an aerosol generator, nebulizer, metered dose inhaler or IPPB device**
INCLUDES Reporting only one time per day of service
S 80 ⚑ 0.48 0.48 FUD XXX

94667 **Manipulation chest wall, such as cupping, percussing, and vibration to facilitate lung function; initial demonstration and/or evaluation**
S 80 ⚑ 0.71 0.71 FUD XXX

94668 **subsequent**
S 80 ⚑ 0.82 0.82 FUD XXX

94669 **Mechanical chest wall oscillation to facilitate lung function, per session**
INCLUDES Application of an external wrap or vest to provide mechanical oscillation
S 80 0.99 0.99 FUD XXX

94680 **Oxygen uptake, expired gas analysis; rest and exercise, direct, simple**
X 80 ⚑ 1.62 1.62 FUD XXX

94681 **including CO2 output, percentage oxygen extracted**
X 80 ⚑ 1.43 1.43 FUD XXX

94690 **rest, indirect (separate procedure)**
EXCLUDES *Arterial puncture (36600)*
X 80 ⚑ 1.37 1.37 FUD XXX

94726 **Plethysmography for determination of lung volumes and, when performed, airway resistance**
INCLUDES Airway resistance
Determination of:
Functional residual capacity
Residual volume
Total lung capacity
EXCLUDES *Bronchial provocation (94070)*
Diffusing capacity (94729)
Spirometry (94010, 94060)
Do not report with (94727-94728)
X 80 1.49 1.49 FUD XXX

94727 **Gas dilution or washout for determination of lung volumes and, when performed, distribution of ventilation and closing volumes**
EXCLUDES *Bronchial provocation (94070)*
Diffusing capacity (94729)
Spirometry (94010, 94060)
Do not report with (94726)
X 80 1.18 1.18 FUD XXX

94728 **Airway resistance by impulse oscillometry**
EXCLUDES *Diffusing capacity (94729)*
Gas dilution techniques
Do not report with (94010, 94060, 94070, 94375, 94726)
X 80 1.13 1.13 FUD XXX

+ 94729 **Diffusing capacity (eg, carbon monoxide, membrane) (List separately in addition to code for primary procedure)**
Code first (94010, 94060, 94070, 94375, 94726-94728)
N 80 1.52 1.52 FUD ZZZ

94750 **Pulmonary compliance study (eg, plethysmography, volume and pressure measurements)**
X 80 2.28 2.28 FUD XXX

94760 **Noninvasive ear or pulse oximetry for oxygen saturation; single determination**
EXCLUDES *Blood gases (82803-82810)*
N TC 80 0.09 0.09 FUD XXX

94761 **multiple determinations (eg, during exercise)**
N TC 80 0.14 0.14 FUD XXX

94762 **by continuous overnight monitoring (separate procedure)**
03 TC 80 0.69 0.69 FUD XXX

94770 **Carbon dioxide, expired gas determination by infrared analyzer**
EXCLUDES *Arterial catheterization/cannulation (36620)*
Arterial puncture (36600)
Bronchoscopy (31622-31646)
Flow directed catheter placement (93503)
Needle biopsy of the lung (32405)
Orotracheal/nasotracheal intubation (31500)
Placement of central venous catheter (36555-36556)
Therapeutic phlebotomy (99195)
Thoracentesis (32554-32555)
Venipuncture (36410)
X 80 0.23 0.23 FUD XXX

94772 **Circadian respiratory pattern recording (pediatric pneumogram), 12-24 hour continuous recording, infant**
EXCLUDES *Electromyograms/EEG/ECG/respiration recordings*
X 80 0.00 0.00 FUD XXX

94774 **Pediatric home apnea monitoring event recording including respiratory rate, pattern and heart rate per 30-day period of time; includes monitor attachment, download of data, review, interpretation, and preparation of a report by a physician or other qualified health care professional**
INCLUDES Oxygen saturation monitoring
EXCLUDES *Sleep testing (95805-95811 [95800, 95801])*
Do not report with (93224-93272, 94775-94777)
B 80 0.00 0.00 FUD YYY

94775 **monitor attachment only (includes hook-up, initiation of recording and disconnection)**
INCLUDES Oxygen saturation monitoring
EXCLUDES *Sleep testing (95805-95811 [95800, 95801])*
Do not report with 93224-93272
S TC 80 0.00 0.00 FUD YYY

94776 **monitoring, download of information, receipt of transmission(s) and analyses by computer only**
INCLUDES Oxygen saturation monitoring
EXCLUDES *Sleep testing (95805-95811 [95800, 95801])*
Do not report with 93224-93272
S TC 80 0.00 0.00 FUD YYY

94777 **review, interpretation and preparation of report only by a physician or other qualified health care professional**
INCLUDES Oxygen saturation monitoring
EXCLUDES *Sleep testing (95805-95811 [95800, 95801])*
Do not report with (93224-93272)
B 26 80 0.00 0.00 FUD YYY

94780 **Car seat/bed testing for airway integrity, neonate, with continual nursing observation and continuous recording of pulse oximetry, heart rate and respiratory rate, with interpretation and report; 60 minutes**
Do not report for less than 60 minutes
Do not report with (99468-99472, 99477-99480, 93040-93042, 94760-94761)
X 0.65 1.45 FUD XXX

+ 94781 **each additional full 30 minutes (List separately in addition to code for primary procedure)**
Code first (94780)
N 0.24 0.57 FUD ZZZ

94799 **Unlisted pulmonary service or procedure**
X 80 0.00 0.00 FUD XXX

95004-95071 Allergy Tests

CMS 100-2,15,20.2 Physician Expense for Allergy Treatment
CMS 100-3,110.12 Challenge Ingestion Food Testing
CMS 100-3,110.13 Cytotoxic Food Tests
CMS 100-4,12,200 Allergy Testing and Immunotherapy

EXCLUDES *Drugs administered for intractable/severe allergic reaction (eg, antihistamines, epinephrine, steroids) (96372)*
Laboratory tests for allergies (86000-86999 [86152, 86153])

Code also medical conferences regarding use of equipment (eg, air filters, humidifiers, dehumidifiers), climate therapy, physical, occupational, and recreation therapy using appropriate evaluation and management codes

Code also significant, separately identifiable E/M services using modifier 25, when performed (99201-99215, 99217-99223 [99224, 99225, 99226], 99231-99233, 99241-99255, 99281-99285, 99304-99318, 99324-99337, 99341-99350, 99381-99429)

Do not report with codes for evaluation and management services when reporting test interpretation/report

95004 **Percutaneous tests (scratch, puncture, prick) with allergenic extracts, immediate type reaction, including test interpretation and report, specify number of tests**
X 80 0.18 0.18 FUD XXX

95012 **Nitric oxide expired gas determination**
X 80 0.54 0.54 FUD XXX

95017 **Allergy testing, any combination of percutaneous (scratch, puncture, prick) and intracutaneous (intradermal), sequential and incremental, with venoms, immediate type reaction, including test interpretation and report, specify number of tests**
X 80 0.11 0.23 FUD XXX

95018 **Allergy testing, any combination of percutaneous (scratch, puncture, prick) and intracutaneous (intradermal), sequential and incremental, with drugs or biologicals, immediate type reaction, including test interpretation and report, specify number of tests**
X 80 0.20 0.56 FUD XXX

95024 **Intracutaneous (intradermal) tests with allergenic extracts, immediate type reaction, including test interpretation and report, specify number of tests**
X 80 0.03 0.22 FUD XXX

95027 **Intracutaneous (intradermal) tests, sequential and incremental, with allergenic extracts for airborne allergens, immediate type reaction, including test interpretation and report, specify number of tests**
X 80 0.13 0.13 FUD XXX

95028 **Intracutaneous (intradermal) tests with allergenic extracts, delayed type reaction, including reading, specify number of tests**
X TC 80 0.38 0.38 FUD XXX

95044 **Patch or application test(s) (specify number of tests)**
X 80 0.15 0.15 FUD XXX

95052 **Photo patch test(s) (specify number of tests)**
X 80 0.18 0.18 FUD XXX

95056 **Photo tests**
X 80 1.21 1.21 FUD XXX

95060 **Ophthalmic mucous membrane tests**
X TC 80 0.94 0.94 FUD XXX

95065 **Direct nasal mucous membrane test**
X TC 80 0.74 0.74 FUD XXX

95070 **Inhalation bronchial challenge testing (not including necessary pulmonary function tests); with histamine, methacholine, or similar compounds**
EXCLUDES *Pulmonary function tests (94060, 94070)*
X TC 80 0.82 0.82 FUD XXX

95071 **with antigens or gases, specify**
EXCLUDES *Pulmonary function tests (94060, 94070)*
X TC 80 0.98 0.98 FUD XXX

95076-95079 Challenge Ingestion Testing

INCLUDES Assessment and monitoring for allergic reactions (eg, blood pressure, peak flow meter)
Testing time until the test ends or to the point an E&M service is needed

Code also interventions when appropriate (eg, injection of epinephrine or steroid)
Do not report testing time less than 61 minutes, such as a positive challenge resulting in ending the test (use evaluation and management codes as appropriate)

95076 **Ingestion challenge test (sequential and incremental ingestion of test items, eg, food, drug or other substance); initial 120 minutes of testing**
INCLUDES First 120 minutes of testing time (not face-to-face time with physician)
X 80 2.08 3.28 FUD XXX

\+ **95079** **each additional 60 minutes of testing (List separately in addition to code for primary procedure)**
INCLUDES Includes each 60 minutes of additional testing time (not face-to-face time with physician)
Code first (95076)
N 80 1.92 2.35 FUD ZZZ

95115-95199 Allergy Immunotherapy

CMS 100-2,15,20.2 Physician Expense for Allergy Treatment
CMS 100-3,110.9 Antigens Prepared for Sublingual Administration
CMS 100-4,12,200 Allergy Testing and Immunotherapy

INCLUDES Allergen immunotherapy professional services

EXCLUDES *Bacterial/viral/fungal extracts skin testing (86485-86580, 95028)*
Special reports for allergy patients (99080)
The following procedures for testing (see Pathology/Immunology section or 95199):
Leukocyte histamine release (LHR)
Lymphocytic transformation test (LTT)
Mast cell degranulation test (MCDT)
Migration inhibitory factor test (MIF)
Nitroblue tetrazolium dye test (NTD)
Radioallergosorbent testing (RAST)
Rat mast cell technique (RMCT)
Transfer factor test (TFT)

Code also significantly separate identifiable evaluation and management services, when performed

95115 **Professional services for allergen immunotherapy not including provision of allergenic extracts; single injection**
S 80 0.25 0.25 FUD XXX

95117 **2 or more injections**
S 80 0.29 0.29 FUD XXX

95120 **Professional services for allergen immunotherapy in the office or institution of the prescribing physician or other qualified health care professional, including provision of allergenic extract; single injection**
E 0.00 0.00 FUD XXX

95125 **2 or more injections**
E 0.00 0.00 FUD XXX

95130 **single stinging insect venom**
E 0.00 0.00 FUD XXX

95131 **2 stinging insect venoms**
E 0.00 0.00 FUD XXX

95132 **3 stinging insect venoms**
E 0.00 0.00 FUD XXX

95133 **4 stinging insect venoms**
E 0.00 0.00 FUD XXX

95134 **5 stinging insect venoms**
E 0.00 0.00 FUD XXX

95144 **Professional services for the supervision of preparation and provision of antigens for allergen immunotherapy, single dose vial(s) (specify number of vials)**
INCLUDES Single dose vial/single dose of antigen administered in one injection
S 80 0.09 0.35 FUD XXX

95145 **Professional services for the supervision of preparation and provision of antigens for allergen immunotherapy (specify number of doses); single stinging insect venom**
S 80 0.09 0.61 FUD XXX

95146 **2 single stinging insect venoms**
S 80 0.09 1.09 FUD XXX

95147 **3 single stinging insect venoms**
S 80 0.09 0.98 FUD XXX

95148 **4 single stinging insect venoms**
S 80 0.09 1.47 FUD XXX

95149 **5 single stinging insect venoms**
S 80 0.09 1.96 FUD XXX

95165 **Professional services for the supervision of preparation and provision of antigens for allergen immunotherapy; single or multiple antigens (specify number of doses)**
S 80 0.09 0.36 FUD XXX

95170 **whole body extract of biting insect or other arthropod (specify number of doses)**

INCLUDES A dose which is the amount of antigen(s) administered in a single injection from a multiple dose vial

S 80 0.09 0.27 FUD XXX

95180 **Rapid desensitization procedure, each hour (eg, insulin, penicillin, equine serum)**

X 80 2.87 3.78 FUD XXX

95199 **Unlisted allergy/clinical immunologic service or procedure**

X 80 0.00 0.00 FUD XXX

95250-95251 Glucose Monitoring By Subcutaneous Device

Do not report more than one time per month

Do not report with physiologic data collection/interpretation (99091)

95250 **Ambulatory continuous glucose monitoring of interstitial tissue fluid via a subcutaneous sensor for a minimum of 72 hours; sensor placement, hook-up, calibration of monitor, patient training, removal of sensor, and printout of recording**

V TC 80 4.39 4.39 FUD XXX

95251 **interpretation and report**

B 26 80 1.23 1.23 FUD XXX

95782-95783 [95782, 95783, 95800, 95801] Sleep Studies

CMS 100-2,6,50 Sleep Disorder Clinics

INCLUDES Assessment of sleep disorders in adults and children

Continuous and simultaneous monitoring and recording of physiological sleep parameters of 6 hours or more

Evaluation of patient's response to therapies

Physician:

- Interpretation
- Recording
- Report

Recording sessions may be:

- Attended studies that include the presence of a technologist or qualified health care professional to respond to the needs of the patient or technical issues at the bedside
- Remote without the presence of a technologist or a qualified health professional
- Unattended without the presence of a technologist or qualified health care professional

Testing parameters include:

- Actigraphy: Use of a noninvasive portable device to record gross motor movements to approximate periods of sleep and wakefulness
- Electrooculogram (EOG): Records electrical activity associated with eye movements
- Maintenance of wakefulness test (MWT): An attended study used to determine the patient's ability to stay awake
- Multiple sleep latency test (MSLT): Attended study to determine the tendency of the patient to fall asleep
- Peripheral arterial tonometry (PAT): Pulsatile volume changes in a digit are measured to determine activity in the sympathetic nervous system for respiratory analysis
- Polysomnography: An attended continuous, simultaneous recording of physiological parameters of sleep for at least 6 hours in a sleep laboratory setting that also includes four or more of the following:
  1. Airflow-oral and/or nasal
  2. Bilateral anterior tibialis EMG
  3. Electrocardiogram (ECG)
  4. Oxyhemoglobin saturation, SpO_2
  5. Respiratory effort
- Positive airway pressure (PAP): Noninvasive devices used to treat sleep-related disorders
- Respiratory airflow (ventilation): Assessment of air movement during inhalation and exhalation as measured by nasal pressure sensors and thermistor
- Respiratory analysis: Assessment of components of respiration obtained by other methods such as airflow or peripheral arterial tone
- Respiratory effort: Use of the diaphragm and/or intercostal muscle for airflow is measured using transducers to estimate thoracic and abdominal motion
- Respiratory movement: Measures the movement of the chest and abdomen during respiration
- Sleep latency: Pertains to the time it takes to get to sleep
- Sleep staging: Determination of the separate levels of sleep according to physiological measurements
- Total sleep time: Determined by the use of actigraphy and other methods

Use of portable and in-laboratory technology

EXCLUDES *Evaluation and management services*

95782 ***Resequenced code. See code following 95811.***

95783 ***Resequenced code. See code following 95811.***

95800 ***Resequenced code. See code following 95806.***

95801 ***Resequenced code. See code following 95806.***

95803 **Actigraphy testing, recording, analysis, interpretation, and report (minimum of 72 hours to 14 consecutive days of recording)**

Do not report more than one time in a 14 day period

Do not report with (95806-95811 [95800, 95801])

X 80 4.22 4.22 FUD XXX

95805 **Multiple sleep latency or maintenance of wakefulness testing, recording, analysis and interpretation of physiological measurements of sleep during multiple trials to assess sleepiness**

INCLUDES Physiological sleep parameters as measured by:
Frontal, central, and occipital EEG leads (3 leads)
Left and right EOG
Submental EMG lead

EXCLUDES *Polysomnography (95808-95811)*
Sleep study, not attended (95806)

Code also modifier 52 when less than four nap opportunities are recorded

S 80 11.81 11.81 FUD XXX

95806 **Sleep study, unattended, simultaneous recording of, heart rate, oxygen saturation, respiratory airflow, and respiratory effort (eg, thoracoabdominal movement)**

EXCLUDES *Unattended sleep study with measurement of a minimum heart rate, oxygen saturation, and respiratory analysis ([95801])*
Unattended sleep study with measurement of heart rate, oxygen saturation, respiratory analysis, and sleep time ([95800])

Code also modifier 52 for fewer than 6 hours of recording

Do not report with (93041-93229, 93268-93272, [95800, 95801])

S 80 4.83 4.83 FUD XXX

\# **95800** **Sleep study, unattended, simultaneous recording; heart rate, oxygen saturation, respiratory analysis (eg, by airflow or peripheral arterial tone), and sleep time**

EXCLUDES *Unattended sleep study measuring at minimum, heart rate, oxygen saturation, and respiratory analysis ([95801])*

Code also modifier 52 for fewer than 6 hours of recording

Do not report with (93041-93229, 93268-93272, 95803, 95806, [95801])

S 80 5.01 5.01 FUD XXX

\# **95801** **minimum of heart rate, oxygen saturation, and respiratory analysis (eg, by airflow or peripheral arterial tone)**

EXCLUDES *Unattended sleep study measuring heart rate, oxygen saturation, respiratory analysis, and sleep time ([95800])*

Code also modifier 52 for fewer than 6 hours of recording

Do not report with (93041-93229, 93268-93272, 95806, [95800])

S 80 2.66 2.66 FUD XXX

95807 **Sleep study, simultaneous recording of ventilation, respiratory effort, ECG or heart rate, and oxygen saturation, attended by a technologist**

EXCLUDES *Polysomnography (95808-95811)*
Sleep study, not attended (95806)

Code also modifier 52 for fewer than 6 hours of recording

S 80 13.30 13.30 FUD XXX

95808 **Polysomnography; any age, sleep staging with 1-3 additional parameters of sleep, attended by a technologist**

EXCLUDES *Sleep study, not attended (95806)*

S 80 17.83 17.83 FUD XXX

95810 **age 6 years or older, sleep staging with 4 or more additional parameters of sleep, attended by a technologist** A

EXCLUDES *Sleep study, not attended (95806)*

Code also modifier 52 for fewer than 6 hours of recording

S 80 17.34 17.34 FUD XXX

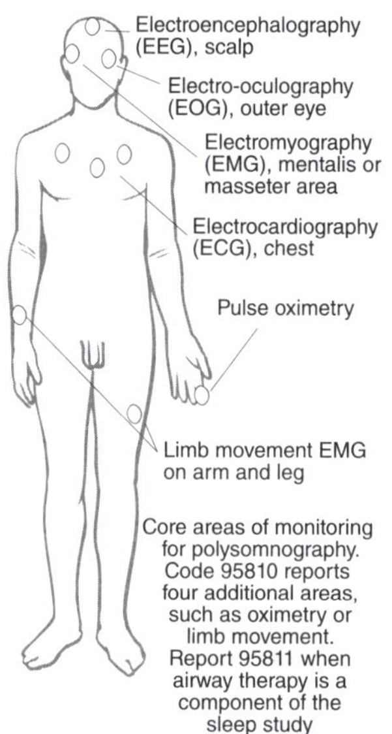

Core areas of monitoring for polysomnography. Code 95810 reports four additional areas, such as oximetry or limb movement. Report 95811 when airway therapy is a component of the sleep study

95811 **age 6 years or older, sleep staging with 4 or more additional parameters of sleep, with initiation of continuous positive airway pressure therapy or bilevel ventilation, attended by a technologist** A

EXCLUDES *Sleep study, not attended (95806)*

Code also modifier 52 for fewer than 6 hours of recording

S 80 18.19 18.19 FUD XXX

\# **95782** **Polysomnography; younger than 6 years, sleep staging with 4 or more additional parameters of sleep, attended by a technologist** A

Code also modifier 52 for fewer than 7 hours of recording

S 80 28.65 28.65 FUD XXX

\# **95783** **younger than 6 years, sleep staging with 4 or more additional parameters of sleep, with initiation of continuous positive airway pressure therapy or bi-level ventilation, attended by a technologist** A

Code also modifier 52 for fewer than 7 hours of recording

S 80 30.54 30.54 FUD XXX

95812-95830 Evaluation of Brain Activity by Electroencephalogram

INCLUDES Only time when time is being recorded and data are being collected and does not include set-up and take-down

EXCLUDES *Evaluation and management services*

95812 **Electroencephalogram (EEG) extended monitoring; 41-60 minutes**

INCLUDES Hyperventilation
Only time when recording is taking place and data are being collected and does not include set-up and take-down
Photic stimulation
Physician interpretation
Recording of 41-60 minutes
Report

EXCLUDES *EEG digital analysis (95957)*
EEG during nonintracranial surgery (95955)
EEG monitoring, 24-hour (95950-95953, 95956)
Wada test (95958)

Code also modifier 26 for physician interpretation only

S 80 12.11 12.11 FUD XXX

95813 **greater than 1 hour**
INCLUDES Hyperventilation
Only time when recording is taking place and data are being collected and does not include set-up and take-down
Photic stimulation
Physician interpretation
Recording of 61 minutes or more
Report
EXCLUDES *EEG digital analysis (95957)*
EEG during nonintracranial surgery (95955)
EEG monitoring, 24-hour (95950-95953, 95956)
Wada test (95958)
Code also modifier 26 for physician interpretation only
S 80 14.17 14.17 FUD XXX

95816 **Electroencephalogram (EEG); including recording awake and drowsy**
INCLUDES Photic stimulation
Physician interpretation
Recording of 20-40 minutes
Report
EXCLUDES *EEG digital analysis (95957)*
EEG during nonintracranial surgery (95955)
EEG monitoring, 24-hour (95950-95953, 95956)
Wada test (95958)
Code also modifier 26 for physician interpretation only
S 80 9.90 9.90 FUD XXX

95819 **including recording awake and asleep**
INCLUDES Hyperventilation
Photic stimulation
Physician interpretation
Recording of 20-40 minutes
Report
EXCLUDES *EEG digital analysis (95957)*
EEG during nonintracranial surgery (95955)
EEG monitoring, 24-hour (95950-95953, 95956)
Wada test (95958)
Code also modifier 26 for interpretation only
S 80 11.30 11.30 FUD XXX

95822 **recording in coma or sleep only**
INCLUDES Hyperventilation
Photic stimulation
Physician interpretation
Recording of 20-40 minutes
Report
EXCLUDES *EEG digital analysis (95957)*
EEG during nonintracranial surgery (95955)
EEG monitoring, 24-hour (95950-95953, 95956)
Wada test (95958)
Code also modifier 26 for interpretation only
S 80 10.07 10.07 FUD XXX

95824 **cerebral death evaluation only**
INCLUDES Physician interpretation
Recording
Report
EXCLUDES *EEG digital analysis (95957)*
EEG during nonintracranial surgery (95955)
EEG monitoring, 24-hour (95950-95953, 95956)
Wada test (95958)
Code also modifier 26 for physician interpretation only
S 80 0.00 0.00 FUD XXX

95827 **all night recording**
INCLUDES Physician interpretation
Recording
Report
EXCLUDES *EEG digital analysis (95957)*
EEG during nonintracranial surgery (95955)
EEG monitoring, 24-hour (95950-95953, 95956)
Wada test (95958)
Code also modifier 26 for interpretation only
S 80 21.76 21.76 FUD XXX

95829 **Electrocorticogram at surgery (separate procedure)**
INCLUDES Physician interpretation
Recording
Report
Code also modifier 26 for interpretation only
N 80 51.86 51.86 FUD XXX

95830 **Insertion by physician or other qualified health care professional of sphenoidal electrodes for electroencephalographic (EEG) recording**
B 80 2.61 7.08 FUD XXX

95831-95857 Evaluation of Muscles and Range of Motion

EXCLUDES *Evaluation and management services*

95831 **Muscle testing, manual (separate procedure) with report; extremity (excluding hand) or trunk**
A 80 0.40 0.77 FUD XXX

95832 **hand, with or without comparison with normal side**
A 80 0.40 0.71 FUD XXX

95833 **total evaluation of body, excluding hands**
A 80 0.61 1.05 FUD XXX

95834 **total evaluation of body, including hands**
A 80 0.89 1.44 FUD XXX

95851 **Range of motion measurements and report (separate procedure); each extremity (excluding hand) or each trunk section (spine)**
A 80 0.22 0.50 FUD XXX

95852 **hand, with or without comparison with normal side**
A 80 0.17 0.47 FUD XXX

95857 **Cholinesterase inhibitor challenge test for myasthenia gravis**
S 80 0.84 1.55 FUD XXX

95860-95887 [95885, 95886, 95887] Evaluation of Nerve and Muscle Function: EMGs with/without Nerve Conduction Studies

CMS 100-2,15,80 Diagnostic Test Requirements
CMS 100-3,160.10 Evoked Response Tests
INCLUDES Physician interpretation
Recording
Report
EXCLUDES *Evaluation and management services*

95860 **Needle electromyography; 1 extremity with or without related paraspinal areas**
INCLUDES Testing of five or more muscles per extremity
EXCLUDES *Dynamic electromyography during motion analysis studies (96002-96003)*
Do not report with (95873-95874, 96002-96003)
S 80 3.40 3.40 FUD XXX

95861 **2 extremities with or without related paraspinal areas**
INCLUDES Testing of five or more muscles per extremity
EXCLUDES *Dynamic electromyography during motion analysis studies (96002-96003)*
Do not report with (95873-95874, 96002-96003)
S 80 4.71 4.71 FUD XXX

95863 **3 extremities with or without related paraspinal areas**
INCLUDES Testing of five or more muscles per extremity
Do not report with (95873-95874, 96002-96003)
S 80 5.73 5.73 FUD XXX

95864 **4 extremities with or without related paraspinal areas**

INCLUDES Testing of five or more muscles per extremity

Do not report with (95873-95874, 96002-96003)

S 80 6.60 6.60 FUD XXX

95865 **larynx**

Code also modifier 52 for unilateral procedure

Do not report with (95873-95874, 96002-96003)

S 80 3.83 3.83 FUD XXX

95866 **hemidiaphragm**

Do not report with (95873-95874, 96002-96003)

S 80 50 3.70 3.70 FUD XXX

95867 **cranial nerve supplied muscle(s), unilateral**

Do not report with (95873-95874)

S 80 2.62 2.62 FUD XXX

95868 **cranial nerve supplied muscles, bilateral**

Do not report with (95873-95874)

S 80 3.65 3.65 FUD XXX

95869 **thoracic paraspinal muscles (excluding T1 or T12)**

Do not report with (95873-95874, 96002-96003)

S 80 2.11 2.11 FUD XXX

95870 **limited study of muscles in 1 extremity or non-limb (axial) muscles (unilateral or bilateral), other than thoracic paraspinal, cranial nerve supplied muscles, or sphincters**

INCLUDES Adson test

Testing of four or less muscles per extremity

EXCLUDES *Anal/urethral sphincter/detrusor/urethra/perineum musculature (51785-51792)*

Complete study of extremities (95860-95864)

Eye muscles (92265)

Do not report with (95873-95874, 96002-96003)

X 80 2.46 2.46 FUD XXX

95872 **Needle electromyography using single fiber electrode, with quantitative measurement of jitter, blocking and/or fiber density, any/all sites of each muscle studied**

Do not report with motion analysis (96002-96003)

S 80 5.73 5.73 FUD XXX

\+ # **95885** **Needle electromyography, each extremity, with related paraspinal areas, when performed, done with nerve conduction, amplitude and latency/velocity study; limited (List separately in addition to code for primary procedure)**

INCLUDES Testing of four or less muscles per extremity

Code also with 95886, when applicable, for a combined maximum total of four units per patient if all four extremities are tested

Code first nerve conduction tests (95907-95913)

Do not report more than one time per extremity

Do not report with (95860-95864, 95870, 95905, 96002-96003)

N 80 1.64 1.64 FUD ZZZ

\+ # **95886** **complete, five or more muscles studied, innervated by three or more nerves or four or more spinal levels (List separately in addition to code for primary procedure)**

INCLUDES Testing of five or more muscles in an extremity

Code also with 95885, when applicable, for a combined maximum total of four units per patient if all four extremities are tested

Code first nerve conduction tests (95907-95913)

Do not report more than one time per extremity

Do not report with (95860-95864, 95870, 95905, 96002-96003)

N 80 2.57 2.57 FUD ZZZ

\+ # **95887** **Needle electromyography, non-extremity (cranial nerve supplied or axial) muscle(s) done with nerve conduction, amplitude and latency/velocity study (List separately in addition to code for primary procedure)**

INCLUDES Testing of cranial nerve innervated muscles on one side, report X2 for a bilateral exam

Code first nerve conduction tests (95907-95913)

Do not report more than one time for each anatomical site

Do not report with (95867-95870, 95905, 96002-96003)

N 80 2.42 2.42 FUD ZZZ

\+ **95873** **Electrical stimulation for guidance in conjunction with chemodenervation (List separately in addition to code for primary procedure)**

Code first chemodenervation (64612, 64615-64616, 64642-64647)

Do not report more than one guidance code for each code for chemodenervation.

Do not report with (64617, 95860-95870, 95874)

N 80 2.09 2.09 FUD ZZZ

\+ **95874** **Needle electromyography for guidance in conjunction with chemodenervation (List separately in addition to code for primary procedure)**

Code first chemodenervation (64612, 64615-64616, 64642-64647)

Do not report more than one guidance code for each code for chemodenervation

Do not report with (64617, 95860-95870, 95873)

N 80 2.02 2.02 FUD ZZZ

95875 **Ischemic limb exercise test with serial specimen(s) acquisition for muscle(s) metabolite(s)**

S 80 3.56 3.56 FUD XXX

95885 ***Resequenced code. See code following 95872.***

95886 ***Resequenced code. See code following 95872.***

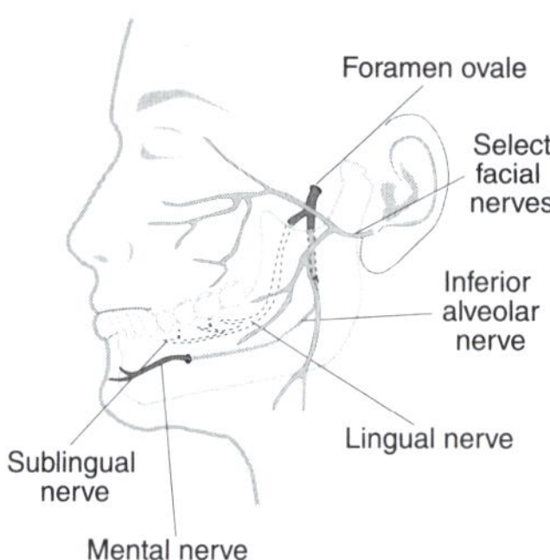

Cranial Nerves: trigeminal branches of lower face and select facial nerves

Needle EMG is performed to determine conduction, amplitude, and latency/velocity

95887 ***Resequenced code. See code before 95873.***

95905-95913 Evaluation of Nerve Function: Nerve Conduction Studies

INCLUDES Conduction studies of motor and sensory nerves

Reports from on-site examiner including the work product of the interpretation of results using established methodologies, calculations, comparisons to normal studies, and interpretation by physician or other qualified health care professional

Single conduction study comprising a sensory and motor conduction test with/without F or H wave testing, and all orthodromic and antidromic impulses

Total number of tests performed indicate which code is appropriate

Code also electromyography performed with nerve conduction studies, as appropriate ([95885, 95886, 95887])

Do not report more than one study when multiple sites on the same nerve are tested

⊘ **95905 Motor and/or sensory nerve conduction, using preconfigured electrode array(s), amplitude and latency/velocity study, each limb, includes F-wave study when performed, with interpretation and report**

INCLUDES Study with preconfigured electrodes that are customized to a specific body location

Do not report this code more than one time for each limb studied

Do not report with ([95885, 95886], 95907-95913)

S 80 1.91 1.91 FUD XXX

95907 Nerve conduction studies; 1-2 studies

S 80 2.66 2.66 FUD XXX

95908 3-4 studies

S 80 3.28 3.28 FUD XXX

95909 5-6 studies

S 80 3.95 3.95 FUD XXX

95910 7-8 studies

S 80 5.19 5.19 FUD XXX

95911 9-10 studies

S 80 6.31 6.31 FUD XXX

95912 11-12 studies

S 80 7.42 7.42 FUD XXX

95913 13 or more studies

S 80 8.59 8.59 FUD XXX

95940-95941 [95940, 95941] Intraoperative Neurophysiological Monitoring

INCLUDES Monitoring, testing, and data evaluation during surgical procedures by a monitoring professional dedicated only to performing the necessary testing and monitoring

EXCLUDES *Baseline neurophysiologic monitoring*
EEG during nonintracranial surgery (95955)
Electrocorticography (95829)
Intraoperative cortical and subcortical mapping (95961-95962)
Neurostimulator programming/analysis (95970-95975)
Time required for set-up, recording, interpretation, and removal of electrodes

Code also baseline studies (eg, EMGs, NCVs), no more than one time per operative session

Code also services provided after midnight using the date when monitoring started and the total monitoring time

Code also standby time prior to procedure (99360)

Code first (92585, 95822, 95860-95870, 95907-95913, 95925-95937 [95938, 95939])

Do not report monitoring services provided by the anesthesiologist or surgeon separately

\+ # **95940 Continuous intraoperative neurophysiology monitoring in the operating room, one on one monitoring requiring personal attendance, each 15 minutes (List separately in addition to code for primary procedure)**

INCLUDES 15 minute increments of monitoring service
A total of all monitoring time for procedures overlapping midnight
Based on time spent monitoring, regardless of number of tests or parameters monitored
Continuous intraoperative neurophysiologic monitoring by a dedicated monitoring professional in the operating room providing one-on-one patient care
Monitoring time may begin prior to the incision
Monitoring time that is distinct from baseline neurophysiologic study/s time or other services (eg, mapping)

EXCLUDES *Time spent in executing or interpreting the baseline neurophysiologic study or studies*

Code also monitoring from outside of the operative room, when applicable ([95941])

NI N 80 0.91 0.91 FUD XXX

\+ # **95941 Continuous intraoperative neurophysiology monitoring, from outside the operating room (remote or nearby) or for monitoring of more than one case while in the operating room, per hour (List separately in addition to code for primary procedure)**

INCLUDES Based on time spent monitoring, regardless of number of tests or parameters monitored
Monitoring time that is distinct from baseline neurophysiologic study/s time or other services (eg, mapping)
One hour increments of monitoring service

NI N 0.00 0.00 FUD XXX

95921-95943 [95943] Evaluation of Autonomic Nervous System

INCLUDES Physician interpretation
Recording
Report
Testing for autonomic dysfunction including site and autonomic subsystems

95921 Testing of autonomic nervous system function; cardiovagal innervation (parasympathetic function), including 2 or more of the following: heart rate response to deep breathing with recorded R-R interval, Valsalva ratio, and 30:15 ratio

INCLUDES Display on a monitor
Minimum of two of the following elements are performed:
Cardiovascular function as indicated by a 30:15 ration (R/R interval at beat 30)/(R-R interval at beat 15)
Heart rate response to deep breathing obtained by visual quantitative analysis of recordings with patient taking 5-6 breaths per minute
Valsalva ratio (at least 2) obtained by dividing the highest heart rate by the lowest
Monitoring of heart rate by electrocardiography of rate obtained from time between two successive R waves (R-R interval)
Storage of data for waveform analysis
Testing most usually in prone position
Tilt table testing, when performed

Do not report with (95922, 95924 [95943])

S 80 2.51 2.51 FUD XXX

95922 vasomotor adrenergic innervation (sympathetic adrenergic function), including beat-to-beat blood pressure and R-R interval changes during Valsalva maneuver and at least 5 minutes of passive tilt

INCLUDES Must include all of the following elements:
Beat-to-beat blood pressure and heart rate recording during at least 2 Valsalva maneuvers
Constant beat-to-beat blood pressure and heart rate recording with EKG equipment that allows for a precise graphical quantitative measurement of R-R interval
Rest period in supine position for at least 20 minutes before test
Tilt table testing with recording of beat-to-beat blood pressure and heart rate recording for at least 5 minutes in the head-up position before tilt-back to supine position

Do not report with (95921, 95924 [95943])

S 80 3.01 3.01 FUD XXX

95923 sudomotor, including 1 or more of the following: quantitative sudomotor axon reflex test (QSART), silastic sweat imprint, thermoregulatory sweat test, and changes in sympathetic skin potential

S 80 5.79 5.79 FUD XXX

95924 **combined parasympathetic and sympathetic adrenergic function testing with at least 5 minutes of passive tilt**
INCLUDES Tilt table testing of adrenergic and parasympathetic function
Do not report with (95921-95922, [95943])
S 80 4.09 4.09 FUD XXX

\# **95943** **Simultaneous, independent, quantitative measures of both parasympathetic function and sympathetic function, based on time-frequency analysis of heart rate variability concurrent with time-frequency analysis of continuous respiratory activity, with mean heart rate and blood pressure measures, during rest, paced (deep) breathing, Valsalva maneuvers, and head-up postural change**
Do not report with (93040, 95921-95922, 95924)
S 80 0.00 0.00 FUD XXX

95925-95943 [95938, 95939] Neurotransmission Studies

95925 **Short-latency somatosensory evoked potential study, stimulation of any/all peripheral nerves or skin sites, recording from the central nervous system; in upper limbs**
EXCLUDES *Auditory evoked potentials (92585)*
Do not report with (95926)
S 80 4.87 4.87 FUD XXX

95926 **in lower limbs**
EXCLUDES *Auditory evoked potentials (92585)*
Do not report with (95925)
S 80 4.07 4.07 FUD XXX

\# **95938** **in upper and lower limbs**
Do not report with (95925-95926)
S 80 9.45 9.45 FUD XXX

95927 **in the trunk or head**
EXCLUDES *Auditory evoked potentials (92585)*
Code also modifier 52 for unilateral test
S 80 4.54 4.54 FUD XXX

95928 **Central motor evoked potential study (transcranial motor stimulation); upper limbs**
Do not report with (95929)
S 80 7.09 7.09 FUD XXX

95929 **lower limbs**
Do not report with (95928)
S 80 6.91 6.91 FUD XXX

\# **95939** **in upper and lower limbs**
Do not report with (95928-95929)
S 80 13.81 13.81 FUD XXX

95930 **Visual evoked potential (VEP) testing central nervous system, checkerboard or flash**
EXCLUDES *Visual acuity screening using automated visual evoked potential devices (0333T)*
S 80 3.74 3.74 FUD XXX

95933 **Orbicularis oculi (blink) reflex, by electrodiagnostic testing**
S 80 2.33 2.33 FUD XXX

A selected neuromuscular junction is repeatedly stimulated. The test is useful to demonstrate reduced muscle action potential from fatique

95937 **Neuromuscular junction testing (repetitive stimulation, paired stimuli), each nerve, any 1 method**
S 80 2.28 2.28 FUD XXX

95938 ***Resequenced code. See code following 95926.***

95939 ***Resequenced code. See code following 95929.***

95940 ***Resequenced code. See code following 95913.***

95941 ***Resequenced code. See code following 95913.***

95943 ***Resequenced code. See code following 95924.***

95950-95962 Electroencephalography For Seizure Monitoring/Intraoperative Use

EXCLUDES *Evaluation and management services*

95950 **Monitoring for identification and lateralization of cerebral seizure focus, electroencephalographic (eg, 8 channel EEG) recording and interpretation, each 24 hours**
INCLUDES Only time when recording is taking place and data are being collected and does not include set-up and take-down
Recording for more than 12 hours up to 24 hours
Code also modifier 52 only when recording is 12 hours or less
Do not report more than one time per 24 hour period
S 80 9.36 9.36 FUD XXX

95951 **Monitoring for localization of cerebral seizure focus by cable or radio, 16 or more channel telemetry, combined electroencephalographic (EEG) and video recording and interpretation (eg, for presurgical localization), each 24 hours**
INCLUDES Interpretations during recording with changes to care of patient
Only time when recording is taking place and data are being collected and does not include set-up and take-down
Recording for more than 12 hours up to 24 hours
Code also modifier 52 only when recording is 12 hours or less
Do not report more than one time per 24 hour period
S 80 0.00 0.00 FUD XXX

95953 **Monitoring for localization of cerebral seizure focus by computerized portable 16 or more channel EEG, electroencephalographic (EEG) recording and interpretation, each 24 hours, unattended**

INCLUDES Only time when recording is taking place and data are being collected and does not include set-up and take-down
Recording for more than 12 hours up to 24 hours

Code also modifier 52 only when recording is 12 hours or less

Do not report more than one time per 24 hour period

S 80 ⚑ 12.12 12.12 FUD XXX

95954 **Pharmacological or physical activation requiring physician or other qualified health care professional attendance during EEG recording of activation phase (eg, thiopental activation test)**

S 80 ⚑ 12.30 12.30 FUD XXX

95955 **Electroencephalogram (EEG) during nonintracranial surgery (eg, carotid surgery)**

N 80 ⚑ 6.41 6.41 FUD XXX

95956 **Monitoring for localization of cerebral seizure focus by cable or radio, 16 or more channel telemetry, electroencephalographic (EEG) recording and interpretation, each 24 hours, attended by a technologist or nurse**

INCLUDES Only time when recording is taking place and data are being collected and does not include set-up and take-down
Recording for more than 12 hours up to 24 hours

Code also modifier 52 only when recording is 12 hours or less

Do not report more than one time per 24 hour period

S 80 ⚑ 46.60 46.60 FUD XXX

95957 **Digital analysis of electroencephalogram (EEG) (eg, for epileptic spike analysis)**

N 80 ⚑ 12.36 12.36 FUD XXX

95958 **Wada activation test for hemispheric function, including electroencephalographic (EEG) monitoring**

S 80 ⚑ 15.85 15.85 FUD XXX

95961 **Functional cortical and subcortical mapping by stimulation and/or recording of electrodes on brain surface, or of depth electrodes, to provoke seizures or identify vital brain structures; initial hour of attendance by a physician or other qualified health care professional**

INCLUDES One hour of attendance by physician or other qualified health care professional

Code also each additional hour of attendance by physician or other qualified health care professional, when appropriate (95962)

Code also modifier 52 for 30 minutes or less of attendance by physician or other qualified health care professional

S 80 ⚑ 8.02 8.02 FUD XXX

+ **95962** **each additional hour of attendance by a physician or other qualified health care professional (List separately in addition to code for primary procedure)**

INCLUDES One hour of attendance by physician or other qualified health care professional

Code first initial hour (95961)

N 80 ⚑ 7.07 7.07 FUD ZZZ

95965-95967 Magnetoencephalography

INCLUDES Physician interpretation
Recording
Report

EXCLUDES *CT provided along with magnetoencephalography (70450-70470, 70496)*
Electroencephalography provided along with magnetoencephalography (95812-95827)
Evaluation and management services
MRI provided along with magnetoencephalography (70551-70553)
Somatosensory evoked potentials/auditory evoked potentials/visual evoked potentials provided along with magnetic evoked field responses (92585, 95925, 95926, 95930)

95965 **Magnetoencephalography (MEG), recording and analysis; for spontaneous brain magnetic activity (eg, epileptic cerebral cortex localization)**

S 80 ⚑ 0.00 0.00 FUD XXX

95966 **for evoked magnetic fields, single modality (eg, sensory, motor, language, or visual cortex localization)**

S 80 ⚑ 0.00 0.00 FUD XXX

+ **95967** **for evoked magnetic fields, each additional modality (eg, sensory, motor, language, or visual cortex localization) (List separately in addition to code for primary procedure)**

Code first single modality (95966)

N 80 0.00 0.00 FUD ZZZ

95970-95982 Evaluation of Implanted Neurostimulator

CMS 100-3,160.12 Neuromuscular Electrical Stimulation (NMES)
CMS 100-3,160.13 Form-fitting Conductive Garment for TENS or NMES
CMS 100-4,32,50 Deep Brain Stimulation for Essential Tremor and Parkinson's Disease

INCLUDES Simple intraoperative or subsequent programming of neurostimulator (three or less of the following); or complex neurostimulator (three or more of the following):
8 or more electrode contacts
Alternating electrode polarities
Cycling
Dose time
More than 1 clinical feature
Number of channels
Number of programs
Pulse amplitude
Pulse duration
Pulse frequency
Rate
Stimulation train duration
Train spacing

EXCLUDES *Electronic analysis and reprogramming of peripheral subcutaneous field stimulation pulse generator (0285T)*
Evaluation and management services
Neurostimulator electrodes:
Implantation (43647, 43881, 61850-61870, 63650-63655, 64553-64580)
Revision/removal (43648, 43882, 61880, 63661-63664, 64585)
Neurostimulator pulse generator/receiver:
Insertion (61885, 63685, 64590)
Revision/removal (61888, 63688, 64595)

95970 **Electronic analysis of implanted neurostimulator pulse generator system (eg, rate, pulse amplitude, pulse duration, configuration of wave form, battery status, electrode selectability, output modulation, cycling, impedance and patient compliance measurements); simple or complex brain, spinal cord, or peripheral (ie, cranial nerve, peripheral nerve, sacral nerve, neuromuscular) neurostimulator pulse generator/transmitter, without reprogramming**

S 80 ⚑ 0.69 1.93 FUD XXX

95971 **simple spinal cord, or peripheral (ie, peripheral nerve, sacral nerve, neuromuscular) neurostimulator pulse generator/transmitter, with intraoperative or subsequent programming**
S 80 ▣ 1.16 1.70 FUD XXX

▲ 95972 **complex spinal cord, or peripheral (ie, peripheral nerve, sacral nerve, neuromuscular) (except cranial nerve) neurostimulator pulse generator/transmitter, with intraoperative or subsequent programming, up to 1 hour**
Code also modifier 52 for service less than 31 minutes
S 80 ▣ 2.22 3.07 FUD XXX

\+ 95973 **complex spinal cord, or peripheral (ie, peripheral nerve, sacral nerve, neuromuscular) (except cranial nerve) neurostimulator pulse generator/transmitter, with intraoperative or subsequent programming, each additional 30 minutes after first hour (List separately in addition to code for primary procedure)**
Code first initial hour (95972)
N 80 1.39 1.78 FUD ZZZ

95974 **complex cranial nerve neurostimulator pulse generator/transmitter, with intraoperative or subsequent programming, with or without nerve interface testing, first hour**
Code also modifier 52 for service less than 31 minutes
S 80 4.63 5.84 FUD XXX

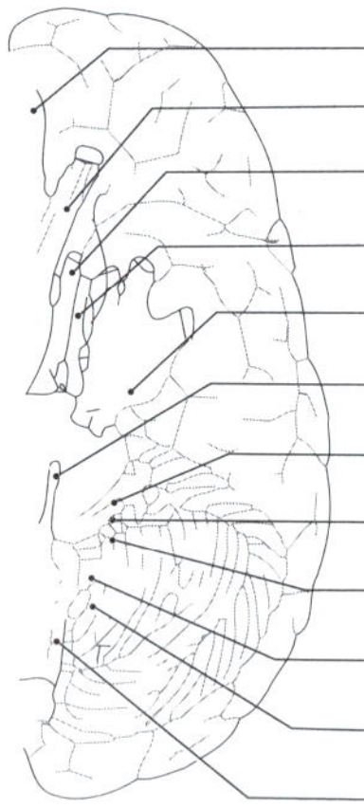

Cranial nerves at base of brain

\+ 95975 **complex cranial nerve neurostimulator pulse generator/transmitter, with intraoperative or subsequent programming, each additional 30 minutes after first hour (List separately in addition to code for primary procedure)**
Code first initial hour (95974)
N 80 2.61 3.12 FUD ZZZ

95978 **Electronic analysis of implanted neurostimulator pulse generator system (eg, rate, pulse amplitude and duration, battery status, electrode selectability and polarity, impedance and patient compliance measurements), complex deep brain neurostimulator pulse generator/transmitter, with initial or subsequent programming; first hour**
Code also modifier 52 for service less than 31 minutes
S 80 ▣ 5.49 7.05 FUD XXX

\+ 95979 **each additional 30 minutes after first hour (List separately in addition to code for primary procedure)**
Code first initial hour (95978)
N 80 2.54 3.05 FUD ZZZ

95980 **Electronic analysis of implanted neurostimulator pulse generator system (eg, rate, pulse amplitude and duration, configuration of wave form, battery status, electrode selectability, output modulation, cycling, impedance and patient measurements) gastric neurostimulator pulse generator/transmitter; intraoperative, with programming**
INCLUDES Gastric neurostimulator of lesser curvature
EXCLUDES *Analysis, with programming when performed, of vagus nerve trunk stimulator for morbid obesity (0312T, 0317T)*
N 80 1.27 1.27 FUD XXX

95981 **subsequent, without reprogramming**
EXCLUDES *Analysis, with programming when performed, of vagus nerve trunk stimulator for morbid obesity (0312T, 0317T)*
S 80 0.50 0.90 FUD XXX

95982 **subsequent, with reprogramming**
EXCLUDES *Analysis, with programming when performed, of vagus nerve trunk stimulator for morbid obesity (0312T, 0317T)*
S 80 1.01 1.45 FUD XXX

95990-95991 Refill/Upkeep of Implanted Drug Delivery Pump to Central Nervous System

CMS 100-3,280.14 Infusion Pumps

EXCLUDES *Analysis/reprogramming of implanted pump for infusion (62367-62370)*
Evaluation and management services

Do not report with (62367-62370)

95990 **Refilling and maintenance of implantable pump or reservoir for drug delivery, spinal (intrathecal, epidural) or brain (intraventricular), includes electronic analysis of pump, when performed;**
S 80 ▣ 2.59 2.59 FUD XXX

95991 **requiring skill of a physician or other qualified health care professional**
S 80 ▣ 1.12 3.41 FUD XXX

95992-95999 Other and Unlisted Neurological Procedures

⊘ 95992 **Canalith repositioning procedure(s) (eg, Epley maneuver, Semont maneuver), per day**
Do not report with (92531-92532)
A 80 1.08 1.23 FUD XXX

95999 **Unlisted neurological or neuromuscular diagnostic procedure**
S 80 0.00 0.00 FUD XXX

96000-96004 Motion Analysis Studies

CMS 100-2,15,80 Diagnostic Test Requirements
CMS 100-2,15,230.4 Services By a Physical/Occupational Therapist in Private Practice

INCLUDES Services provided as part of major therapeutic/diagnostic decision making
Services provided in a dedicated motion analysis department capable of:
3-D kinetics/dynamic electromyography
Computerized 3-D kinematics
Videotaping from the front/back/both sides

EXCLUDES *Evaluation and management services*
Gait training (97116)
Needle electromyography (95860-95872 [95885, 95886, 95887])

96000 **Comprehensive computer-based motion analysis by video-taping and 3D kinematics;**
S 80 ▣ 2.68 2.68 FUD XXX

96001 **with dynamic plantar pressure measurements during walking**
S 80 ▣ 2.79 2.79 FUD XXX

96002 **Dynamic surface electromyography, during walking or other functional activities, 1-12 muscles**
Do not report with (95860-95866, 95869-95872, [95885, 95886, 95887])
S 80 ▣ 0.60 0.60 FUD XXX

96003 Dynamic fine wire electromyography, during walking or other functional activities, 1 muscle

Do not report with (95860-95866, 95869-95872, [95885, 95886, 95887])

S 80 ▭ 0.56 0.56 FUD XXX

96004 Review and interpretation by physician or other qualified health care professional of comprehensive computer-based motion analysis, dynamic plantar pressure measurements, dynamic surface electromyography during walking or other functional activities, and dynamic fine wire electromyography, with written report

B 26 80 ▭ 3.31 3.31 FUD XXX

96020 Neurofunctional Brain Testing

INCLUDES Selection/administration of testing of:
- Cognition
- Determination of validity of neurofunctional testing relative to separately interpreted functional magnetic resonance images
- Functional neuroimaging
- Language
- Memory
- Monitoring performance of testing
- Movement
- Other neurological functions
- Sensation

EXCLUDES *Clinical depression treatment by repetitive transcranial magnetic stimulation (90867-90868)*
Functional MRI of the brain (70555)

Do not report with (70554, 96101-96103, 96116-96120)
Do not report with evaluation and management codes on the same date of service

96020 Neurofunctional testing selection and administration during noninvasive imaging functional brain mapping, with test administered entirely by a physician or other qualified health care professional (ie, psychologist), with review of test results and report

N 80 0.00 0.00 FUD XXX

96040 Genetic Counseling Services

INCLUDES Analysis for genetic risk assessment
- Counseling of patient/family
- Counseling services
- Face-to-face interviews
- Obtaining structured family genetic history
- Pedigree construction
- Review of medical data/family information
- Services provided by trained genetic counselor
- Services provided during one or more sessions
- Thirty minutes of face-to-face time and is reported one time for each 16-30 minutes of the service

EXCLUDES *Education/genetic counseling by a physician or other qualified health care provider to a group (99078)*
Education/genetic counseling by a physician or other qualified health care provider to an individual; use appropriate evaluation and management code
Education regarding genetic risks by a nonphysician to a group (98961, 98962)
Genetic counseling and/or risk factor reduction intervention from a physician or other qualified health care provider provided to patients without symptoms/diagnosis (99401-99412)

Do not report when 15 minutes or less of face-to-face time is provided

96040 Medical genetics and genetic counseling services, each 30 minutes face-to-face with patient/family

B 1.31 1.31 FUD XXX

96101-96127 Cognitive Capability Assessments

CMS 100-1,3,30 Outpatient Mental Health Treatment Limitation
CMS 100-1,3,30.1 Disorders Subject to Mental Health Limitation
CMS 100-1,3,30.1 Application of Mental Health Limitation - Status of Patient
CMS 100-2,15,80.2 Psychological and Neuropsychological Tests
CMS 100-2,15,160 Clinical Psychologist Services
CMS 100-4,12,150 Clinical Social Worker (CSW) Services
CMS 100-4,12,160 Independent Psychologist Services
CMS 100-4,12,170 Clinical Psychologist Services
CMS 100-4,12,170.1 Payment for Clinical Psychologist Services
CMS 100-4,12,210 Outpatient Mental Health Limitation

INCLUDES Cognitive function testing of the central nervous system

EXCLUDES *Cognitive skills development (97532, 97533)*
Physician conducted mini-mental status examination; use appropriate evaluation and management code

96101 Psychological testing (includes psychodiagnostic assessment of emotionality, intellectual abilities, personality and psychopathology, eg, MMPI, Rorschach, WAIS), per hour of the psychologist's or physician's time, both face-to-face time administering tests to the patient and time interpreting these test results and preparing the report

INCLUDES Situations when more time is needed to assimilate other clinical data sources including tests administered by a technician or computer and previously reported
Time spent face to face, interpretation, and preparing report

Do not report less than 31 minutes of time
Do not report with (0364T-0367T, 0373T-0374T)

03 80 2.24 2.26 FUD XXX

96102 Psychological testing (includes psychodiagnostic assessment of emotionality, intellectual abilities, personality and psychopathology, eg, MMPI and WAIS), with qualified health care professional interpretation and report, administered by technician, per hour of technician time, face-to-face

Do not report less than 31 minutes of time
Do not report with (0364T-0367T, 0373T-0374T)

03 80 0.66 1.85 FUD XXX

96103 Psychological testing (includes psychodiagnostic assessment of emotionality, intellectual abilities, personality and psychopathology, eg, MMPI), administered by a computer, with qualified health care professional interpretation and report

Do not report with (0364T-0367T, 0373T-0374T)

03 80 0.75 0.78 FUD XXX

96105 Assessment of aphasia (includes assessment of expressive and receptive speech and language function, language comprehension, speech production ability, reading, spelling, writing, eg, by Boston Diagnostic Aphasia Examination) with interpretation and report, per hour

Do not report with (0364T-0367T, 0373T-0374T)

A 80 ▭ 2.84 2.84 FUD XXX

▲ **96110 Developmental screening (eg, developmental milestone survey, speech and language delay screen), with scoring and documentation, per standardized instrument**

Do not report with (0364T-0367T, 0373T-0374T)

E ▭ 0.23 0.23 FUD XXX

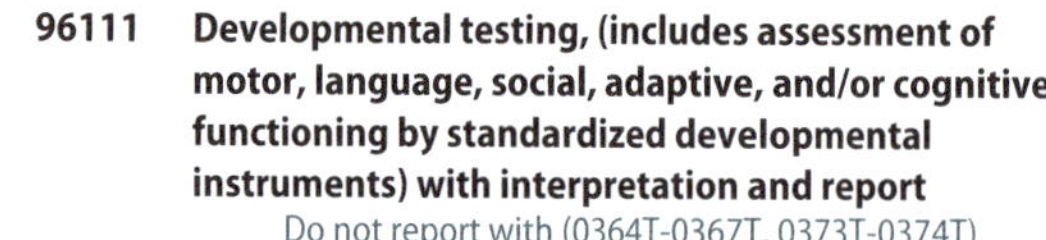

96111 **Developmental testing, (includes assessment of motor, language, social, adaptive, and/or cognitive functioning by standardized developmental instruments) with interpretation and report**
Do not report with (0364T-0367T, 0373T-0374T)
03 80 3.43 3.63 FUD XXX

96116 **Neurobehavioral status exam (clinical assessment of thinking, reasoning and judgment, eg, acquired knowledge, attention, language, memory, planning and problem solving, and visual spatial abilities), per hour of the psychologist's or physician's time, both face-to-face time with the patient and time interpreting test results and preparing the report**
INCLUDES Time spent face to face, interpretation, and preparing report
Do not report less than 31 minutes of time
Do not report with (0364T-0367T, 0373T-0374T)
03 80 PQ 2.48 2.65 FUD XXX

96118 **Neuropsychological testing (eg, Halstead-Reitan Neuropsychological Battery, Wechsler Memory Scales and Wisconsin Card Sorting Test), per hour of the psychologist's or physician's time, both face-to-face time administering tests to the patient and time interpreting these test results and preparing the report**
INCLUDES Situations when more time is needed to assimilate other clinical data sources including tests administered by a technician or computer and previously reported
Time spent face to face, interpretation, and preparing report
Do not report less than 31 minutes of time
Do not report with (0364T-0367T, 0373T-0374T)
03 80 2.23 2.77 FUD XXX

96119 **Neuropsychological testing (eg, Halstead-Reitan Neuropsychological Battery, Wechsler Memory Scales and Wisconsin Card Sorting Test), with qualified health care professional interpretation and report, administered by technician, per hour of technician time, face-to-face**
Do not report less than 31 minutes of time
Do not report with (0364T-0367T, 0373T-0374T)
03 80 0.66 2.27 FUD XXX

96120 **Neuropsychological testing (eg, Wisconsin Card Sorting Test), administered by a computer, with qualified health care professional interpretation and report**
Do not report with (0364T-0367T, 0373T-0374T)
03 80 0.73 1.34 FUD XXX

96125 **Standardized cognitive performance testing (eg, Ross Information Processing Assessment) per hour of a qualified health care professional's time, both face-to-face time administering tests to the patient and time interpreting these test results and preparing the report**
INCLUDES Time spent face to face, interpretation, and preparing report
EXCLUDES *Neuropsychological testing (96118-96120)*
Psychological testing (96101-96103)
Do not report less than 31 minutes of time
Do not report with (0364T-0367T, 0373T-0374T)
A 80 3.20 3.20 FUD XXX

● **96127** **Brief emotional/behavioral assessment (eg, depression inventory, attention-deficit/hyperactivity disorder [ADHD] scale), with scoring and documentation, per standardized instrument**

96150-96155 Biopsychosocial Assessment/Intervention

INCLUDES Services for patients that have primary physical illnesses/diagnoses/symptoms who may benefit from assessments/interventions that focus on the biopsychosocial factors related to the patient's health status
Services used to identify the following factors which are important to the prevention/treatment/management of physical health problems:
Behavioral
Cognitive
Emotional
Psychological
Social

Do not report evaluation and management service codes on the same date of service
Do not report with (0364T-0367T, 0373T-0374T)
Do not report on same date of service with (99401-99412, 90785-90899)

96150 **Health and behavior assessment (eg, health-focused clinical interview, behavioral observations, psychophysiological monitoring, health-oriented questionnaires), each 15 minutes face-to-face with the patient; initial assessment**
03 80 PQ 0.59 0.60 FUD XXX

96151 **re-assessment**
03 80 PQ 0.57 0.58 FUD XXX

96152 **Health and behavior intervention, each 15 minutes, face-to-face; individual**
03 80 PQ 0.54 0.55 FUD XXX

96153 **group (2 or more patients)**
03 80 0.13 0.13 FUD XXX

96154 **family (with the patient present)**
03 80 0.53 0.54 FUD XXX

96155 **family (without the patient present)**
E 0.64 0.64 FUD XXX

96360-96361 Intravenous Fluid Infusion for Hydration (Nonchemotherapy)

CMS 100-4,12,30.5 Payment for Injections and Infusions: Chemotherapy and Nonchemotherapy
INCLUDES Administration of prepackaged fluids and electrolytes
Coding hierarchy rules for facility reporting only:
Chemotherapy services are primary to diagnostic, prophylactic, and therapeutic services
Diagnostic, prophylactic, and therapeutic services are primary to hydration services
Infusions are primary to pushes
Pushes are primary to injections
Constant observance/attendance of person administering the drug or substance
Infusion of 15 minutes or less
Direct supervision by physician or other qualified health care provider:
Direction of personnel
Minimal supervision for:
Consent
Safety oversight
Supervision of personnel
Report the initial code for the primary reason for the visit regardless of the order in which the infusions or injections are given
The following if done to facilitate the injection/infusion:
Flush at the end of infusion
Indwelling IV, subcutaneous catheter/port access
Local anesthesia
Start of IV
Supplies/tubing/syringes
Treatment plan verification
EXCLUDES *Catheter/port declotting (36593)*
Drugs/other substances
Significant separately identifiable evaluation and management service if performed
Code also fluids provided for administration
Do not report a second initial service on the same date for accessing a multi-lumen catheter or restarting an IV, or when two IV lines are needed to meet an infusion rate
Do not report for services provided by physicians or other qualified health care providers in facility settings
Do not report to keep the vein open or during other therapeutic infusions
Do not report with infusion for hydration that is 30 minutes or less

96360 **Intravenous infusion, hydration; initial, 31 minutes to 1 hour**
Do not report hydration infusions of 31 minutes or less
Do not report if performed as a concurrent infusion
S 80 1.59 1.59 FUD XXX

+ 96361 **each additional hour (List separately in addition to code for primary procedure)**
INCLUDES Hydration infusion of more than 30 minutes beyond 1 hour
Hydration provided as a secondary or subsequent service after a different initial service via the same IV access site
Code first (96360)
S 80 0.42 0.42 FUD ZZZ

96365-96371 Infusions: Diagnostic/Preventive/Therapeutic

CMS 100-4,12,30.5 Payment for Injections and Infusions: Chemotherapy and Nonchemotherapy
CMS 100-4,20,160.1 Total Parenteral Nutrition Furnished to Part B Inpatients

INCLUDES Administration of fluid
Administration of substances/drugs
An infusion of 16 minutes or more
Coding hierarchy rules for facility reporting:
- Chemotherapy services are primary to diagnostic, prophylactic, and therapeutic services
- Diagnostic, prophylactic, and therapeutic services are primary to hydration services
- Infusions are primary to pushes
- Pushes are primary to injections

Constant presence of health care professional administering the substance/drug
Direct supervision of physician or other qualified health care provider:
- Consent
- Direction of personnel
- Patient assessment
- Safety oversight
- Supervision of personnel

The following if done to facilitate the injection/infusion:
- Flush at the end of infusion
- Indwelling IV, subcutaneous catheter/port access
- Local anesthesia
- Start of IV
- Supplies/tubing/syringes

Training to assess patient and monitor vital signs
Training to prepare/dose/dispose
Treatment plan verification

EXCLUDES *Catheter/port declotting (36593)*
Significant separately identifiable evaluation and management service, when performed

Code also drugs/materials
Do not report a second initial service on the same date for accessing a multi-lumen catheter or restarting an IV, or when two IV lines are needed to meet an infusion rate
Do not report for services provided by physicians or other qualified health care providers in facility settings
Do not report with codes for which IV push or infusion is an integral part of the procedure

96365 **Intravenous infusion, for therapy, prophylaxis, or diagnosis (specify substance or drug); initial, up to 1 hour**
Code also second initial service with modifier 59 when patient's condition or drug protocol mandates the use of two IV lines
S 80 1.92 1.92 FUD XXX

+ 96366 **each additional hour (List separately in addition to code for primary procedure)**
INCLUDES Additional hours of sequential infusion
Infusion intervals of more than 30 minutes beyond one hour
Second and subsequent infusions of the same drug or substance
Code first (96365)
S 80 0.52 0.52 FUD ZZZ

+ 96367 **additional sequential infusion of a new drug/substance, up to 1 hour (List separately in addition to code for primary procedure)**
INCLUDES A secondary or subsequent service with a new drug or substance after a different initial service via the same IV access
Code first (96365, 96374, 96409, 96413)
Do not report more than one time per sequential infusion of the same mix
S 80 0.84 0.84 FUD ZZZ

+ 96368 **concurrent infusion (List separately in addition to code for primary procedure)**
Code first (96365, 96366, 96413, 96415, 96416)
Do not report more than one time per date of service
N 80 0.57 0.57 FUD ZZZ

96369 **Subcutaneous infusion for therapy or prophylaxis (specify substance or drug); initial, up to 1 hour, including pump set-up and establishment of subcutaneous infusion site(s)**
EXCLUDES *Infusions of 15 minutes or less (96372)*
Do not report more than one time per encounter
S 80 5.44 5.44 FUD XXX

+ 96370 **each additional hour (List separately in addition to code for primary procedure)**
INCLUDES Infusions of more than 30 minutes beyond one hour
Code first (96369)
S 80 0.43 0.43 FUD ZZZ

+ 96371 **additional pump set-up with establishment of new subcutaneous infusion site(s) (List separately in addition to code for primary procedure)**
Code first (96369)
Do not report more than one time per encounter
N 80 2.54 2.54 FUD ZZZ

96372-96379 Injections: Diagnostic/Preventive/Therapeutic

CMS 100-4,12,30.5 Payment for Injections and Infusions: Chemotherapy and Nonchemotherapy

INCLUDES Administration of fluid
Administration of substances/drugs
Coding hierarchy rules for facility reporting:
- Chemotherapy services are primary to diagnostic, prophylactic, and therapeutic services
- Infusions are primary to pushes
- Pushes are primary to injections

Constant presence of health care professional administering the substance/drug
Direct supervision by physician or other qualified health care provider:
- Consent
- Direction of personnel
- Patient assessment
- Safety oversight
- Supervision of personnel

Infusion of 15 minutes or less
The following if done to facilitate the injection/infusion:
- Flush at the end of infusion
- Indwelling IV, subcutaneous catheter/port access
- Local anesthesia
- Start of IV
- Supplies/tubing/syringes

Training to assess patient and monitor vital signs
Training to prepare/dose/dispose
Treatment plan verification

EXCLUDES *Catheter/port declotting (36593)*
Significant separately identifiable evaluation and management service, when performed

Code also drugs/materials
Do not report a second initial service on the same date for accessing a multi-lumen catheter or restarting an IV, or when two IV lines are needed to meet an infusion rate
Do not report services of physicians or other qualified health care providers provided in facility settings
Do not report with codes for which IV push or infusion is an integral part of the procedure

96372 **Therapeutic, prophylactic, or diagnostic injection (specify substance or drug); subcutaneous or intramuscular**

INCLUDES Direct supervision by physician or other qualified health care provider when reported by the physician/other qualified health care provider. When reported by a hospital, physician/other qualified health care provider need not be present.

Hormonal therapy injections (non-antineoplastic) (96372)

EXCLUDES *Administration of vaccines/toxoids (90460-90474)*

Allergen immunotherapy injections (95115-95117)

Antineoplastic hormonal injections (96402)

Antineoplastic nonhormonal injections (96401)

Injections administered without direct supervision by physician or other qualified health care provider (99211)

S 80 Facility RVU 0.70 Non-Facility RVU 0.70 FUD XXX

96373 **intra-arterial**

S 80 Facility RVU 0.54 Non-Facility RVU 0.54 FUD XXX

96374 **intravenous push, single or initial substance/drug**

Code also second initial service with modifier 59 when patient's condition or drug protocol mandates the use of two IV lines

S 80 Facility RVU 1.57 Non-Facility RVU 1.57 FUD XXX

\+ **96375** **each additional sequential intravenous push of a new substance/drug (List separately in addition to code for primary procedure)**

INCLUDES IV push of a new substance/drug provided as a secondary or subsequent service after a different initial service via same IV access site

Code first (96365, 96374, 96409, 96413)

S 80 Facility RVU 0.62 Non-Facility RVU 0.62 FUD ZZZ

\+ **96376** **each additional sequential intravenous push of the same substance/drug provided in a facility (List separately in addition to code for primary procedure)**

INCLUDES Facilities only

EXCLUDES *Services performed by any provider that is not a facility*

Code first (96365, 96374, 96409, 96413)

Do not report a push performed within 30 minutes of a reported push of the same substance or drug

N Facility RVU 0.00 Non-Facility RVU 0.00 FUD ZZZ

96379 **Unlisted therapeutic, prophylactic, or diagnostic intravenous or intra-arterial injection or infusion**

S 80 Facility RVU 0.00 Non-Facility RVU 0.00 FUD XXX

96401-96411 Chemotherapy and Other Complex Drugs, Biologicals: Injection

CMS 100-3,110.2 Certain Drugs Distributed by the National Cancer Institute

CMS 100-3,110.6 Scalp Hypothermia During Chemotherapy, to Prevent Hair Loss

CMS 100-4,4,230.2.2 Chemotherapy Drug Administration

CMS 100-4,12,30.5 Payment for Injections and Infusions: Chemotherapy and Nonchemotherapy

INCLUDES An infusion of 15 minutes or less

Constant presence of the health care professional administering the drug or substance

Highly complex services that require direct supervision for:

- Consent
- Patient assessment
- Safety oversight
- Supervision

Intravenous/intra-arterial push

More intense work and monitoring of clinical staff by physician or other qualified health care provider due to greater risk of severe patient reactions

Parenteral administration of:

- Anti-neoplastic agents for noncancer diagnoses
- Monoclonal antibody agents
- Nonradionuclide antineoplastic drugs
- Other biologic response modifiers

Do not report a second initial service on the same date for accessing a multi-lumen catheter or restarting an IV, or when two IV lines are needed to meet an infusion rate

96401 **Chemotherapy administration, subcutaneous or intramuscular; non-hormonal anti-neoplastic**

Do not report for services of physicians or other qualified health care providers in facility settings

S 80 PQ Facility RVU 2.06 Non-Facility RVU 2.06 FUD XXX

96402 **hormonal anti-neoplastic**

Do not report for services by physician or other qualified health care provider in facility settings

S 80 PQ Facility RVU 0.89 Non-Facility RVU 0.89 FUD XXX

96405 **Chemotherapy administration; intralesional, up to and including 7 lesions**

S PQ Facility RVU 0.85 Non-Facility RVU 2.27 FUD 000

96406 **intralesional, more than 7 lesions**

S PQ Facility RVU 1.30 Non-Facility RVU 3.17 FUD 000

96409 **intravenous, push technique, single or initial substance/drug**

Code also second initial service with modifier 59 when patient's condition or drug protocol mandates the use of two IV lines

Do not report for services by physicians or other qualified health care provider in facility settings

Do not report with 36823

S 80 PQ Facility RVU 3.04 Non-Facility RVU 3.04 FUD XXX

\+ **96411** **intravenous, push technique, each additional substance/drug (List separately in addition to code for primary procedure)**

Code first initial substance/drug (96409, 96413)

Do not report for services of physicians or other qualified health care providers in facility settings

Do not report with 36823

S 80 PQ Facility RVU 1.71 Non-Facility RVU 1.71 FUD ZZZ

96413-96417 Chemotherapy and Complex Drugs, Biologicals: Intravenous Infusion

CMS 100-3,110.2 Certain Drugs Distributed by the National Cancer Institute
CMS 100-3,110.6 Scalp Hypothermia During Chemotherapy, to Prevent Hair Loss
CMS 100-4,4,230.2.2 Chemotherapy Drug Administration
CMS 100-4,4,231 Coding and Payment for Drug Administration
CMS 100-4,12,30.5 Payment for Injections and Infusions: Chemotherapy and Nonchemotherapy

INCLUDES An infusion of 15 minutes or less
Constant presence of the health care professional administering the drug or substance
Highly complex services that require direct supervision for:
- Consent
- Patient assessment
- Safety oversight
- Supervision

Intravenous/intra-arterial push
More intense work and monitoring of clinical staff by physician or other qualified health care provider due to greater risk of severe patient reactions
Parenteral administration of:
- Anti-neoplastic agents for noncancer diagnoses
- Monoclonal antibody agents
- Nonradionuclide antineoplastic drugs
- Other biologic response modifiers

The following in the administration:
- Access to IV/catheter/port
- Drug preparation
- Flushing at the completion of the infusion
- Hydration fluid
- Routine tubing/syringe/supplies
- Starting the IV
- Use of local anesthesia

EXCLUDES *Administration of nonchemotherapy agents such as antibiotics/steroids/analgesics*
Declotting of catheter/port (36593)
Home infusion (99601-99602)

Code also drug or substance
Code also significant separately identifiable evaluation and management service, when performed
Do not report a second initial service on the same date for accessing a multi-lumen catheter or restarting an IV, or when two IV lines are needed to meet an infusion rate
Do not report for services of physicians or other qualified health care providers in facility settings
Do not report with (36823)

96413 Chemotherapy administration, intravenous infusion technique; up to 1 hour, single or initial substance/drug
EXCLUDES *Hydration administered as secondary or subsequent service via same IV access site (96361)*
Therapeutic/prophylactic/diagnostic drug infusion/injection through the same intravenous access (96366, 96367, 96375)
Code also second initial service with modifier 59 when patient's condition or drug protocol mandates the use of two IV lines
S 80 PQ 3.72 3.72 FUD XXX

+ 96415 each additional hour (List separately in addition to code for primary procedure)
INCLUDES Infusion intervals of more than 30 minutes past 1-hour increments
Code first initial hour (96413)
S 80 PQ 0.78 0.78 FUD ZZZ

96416 initiation of prolonged chemotherapy infusion (more than 8 hours), requiring use of a portable or implantable pump
EXCLUDES *Portable or implantable infusion pump/reservoir refilling/maintenance for drug delivery (96521-96523)*
S 80 PQ 3.88 3.88 FUD XXX

+ 96417 each additional sequential infusion (different substance/drug), up to 1 hour (List separately in addition to code for primary procedure)
EXCLUDES *Additional hour(s) of sequential infusion (96415)*
Code first initial substance/drug (96413)
Do not report more than one time per sequential infusion
S 80 PQ 1.73 1.73 FUD ZZZ

96420-96425 Chemotherapy and Complex Drugs, Biologicals: Intra-arterial

CMS 100-3,110.2 Certain Drugs Distributed by the National Cancer Institute
CMS 100-3,110.6 Scalp Hypothermia During Chemotherapy, to Prevent Hair Loss
CMS 100-4,4,230.2.2 Chemotherapy Drug Administration
CMS 100-4,4,231 Coding and Payment for Drug Administration
CMS 100-4,12,30.5 Payment for Injections and Infusions: Chemotherapy and Nonchemotherapy

INCLUDES Highly complex services that require direct supervision for:
- Consent
- Patient assessment
- Safety oversight
- Supervision

More intense work and monitoring of clinical staff by physician or other qualified health care provider due to greater risk of severe patient reactions
Parenteral administration of:
- Anti-neoplastic agents for noncancer diagnoses
- Monoclonal antibody agents
- Non-radionuclide antineoplastic drugs
- Other biologic response modifiers

The following in the administration:
- Access to IV/catheter/port
- Drug preparation
- Flushing at the completion of the infusion
- Hydration fluid
- Routine tubing/syringe/supplies
- Starting the IV
- Use of local anesthesia

EXCLUDES *Administration of non-chemotherapy agents such as antibiotics/steroids/analgesics*
Declotting of catheter/port (36593)
Home infusion (99601-99602)

Code also drug or substance
Code also significant separately identifiable evaluation and management service, when performed
Do not report a second initial service on the same date for accessing a multi-lumen catheter or restarting an IV, or when two IV lines are needed to meet an infusion rate
Do not report for services by physician or other qualified health care provider in facility settings

96420 Chemotherapy administration, intra-arterial; push technique
INCLUDES Regional chemotherapy perfusion
EXCLUDES *Placement of intra-arterial catheter*
Do not report with 36823
S 80 CCI PQ 2.91 2.91 FUD XXX

96422 infusion technique, up to 1 hour
INCLUDES Regional chemotherapy perfusion
EXCLUDES *Placement of intra-arterial catheter*
Do not report with 36823
S 80 CCI PQ 4.68 4.68 FUD XXX

+ 96423 infusion technique, each additional hour (List separately in addition to code for primary procedure)
INCLUDES Infusion intervals of more than 30 minutes past 1-hour increments
Regional chemotherapy perfusion
EXCLUDES *Arterial/venous cannula insertion with regional chemotherapy perfusion to an extremity (36823)*
Placement of intra-arterial catheter
Code first initial hour (96422)
Do not report with 36823
S 80 CCI PQ 2.16 2.16 FUD ZZZ

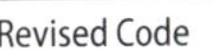
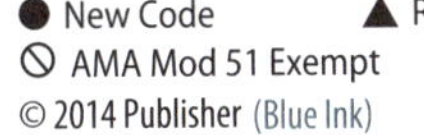

96425 **infusion technique, initiation of prolonged infusion (more than 8 hours), requiring the use of a portable or implantable pump**

INCLUDES Regional chemotherapy perfusion

EXCLUDES *Placement of intra-arterial catheter*
Portable or implantable infusion pump/reservoir refilling/maintenance for drug delivery (96521-96523)

Do not report with (36823)

S 80 PQ 5.04 5.04 FUD XXX

96440-96450 Chemotherapy Administration: Intrathecal/Peritoneal Cavity/Pleural Cavity

96440 **Chemotherapy administration into pleural cavity, requiring and including thoracentesis**

S 80 PQ 3.97 23.86 FUD 000

96446 **Chemotherapy administration into the peritoneal cavity via indwelling port or catheter**

S 80 PQ 0.62 5.40 FUD XXX

96450 **Chemotherapy administration, into CNS (eg, intrathecal), requiring and including spinal puncture**

EXCLUDES *Chemotherapy administration, intravesical/bladder (51720)*
Insertion of catheter/reservoir:
Intraventricular (61210, 61215)
Subarachnoid (62350-62351, 62360-62362)

S 80 PQ 2.29 5.08 FUD 000

96521-96523 Refill/Upkeep of Drug Delivery Device

CMS 100-4,4,231 Coding and Payment for Drug Administration

INCLUDES Highly complex services that require direct supervision for:
- Consent
- Patient assessment
- Safety oversight
- Supervision

Parenteral administration of:
- Anti-neoplastic agents for noncancer diagnoses
- Monoclonal antibody agents
- Non-radionuclide antineoplastic drugs
- Other biologic response modifiers

The following in the administration:
- Access to IV/catheter/port
- Drug preparation
- Flushing at the completion of the infusion
- Hydration fluid
- Routine tubing/syringe/supplies
- Starting the IV
- Use of local anesthesia

Therapeutic drugs other than chemotherapy

EXCLUDES *Administration of non-chemotherapy agents such as antibiotics/steroids/analgesics*
Blood specimen collection from completely implantable venous access device (36591)
Declotting of catheter/port (36593)
Home infusion (99601-99602)

Code also drug or substance
Code also significant separately identifiable evaluation and management service, when performed
Do not report for services by physician or other qualified health care provider in facility settings

96521 **Refilling and maintenance of portable pump**

S 80 PQ 3.77 3.77 FUD XXX

96522 **Refilling and maintenance of implantable pump or reservoir for drug delivery, systemic (eg, intravenous, intra-arterial)**

EXCLUDES *Implantable infusion pump refilling/maintenance for spinal/brain drug delivery (95990-95991)*

S 80 PQ 3.10 3.10 FUD XXX

96523 **Irrigation of implanted venous access device for drug delivery systems**

EXCLUDES *Direct supervision by physician or other qualified health care provider in facility settings*

Do not report with any other services on the same date of service

Q1 80 PQ 0.69 0.69 FUD XXX

96542-96549 Chemotherapy Injection Into Brain

CMS 100-3,110.2 Certain Drugs Distributed by the National Cancer Institute
CMS 100-4,4,230.2.2 Chemotherapy Drug Administration
CMS 100-4,12,30.5 Payment for Injections and Infusions: Chemotherapy and Nonchemotherapy

INCLUDES Highly complex services that require direct supervision for:
- Consent
- Patient assessment
- Safety oversight
- Supervision

Parenteral administration of:
- Anti-neoplastic agents for noncancer diagnoses
- Monoclonal antibody agents
- Non-radionuclide antineoplastic drugs
- Other biologic response modifiers

The following in the administration:
- Access to IV/catheter/port
- Drug preparation
- Flushing at the completion of the infusion
- Hydration fluid
- Routine tubing/syringe/supplies
- Starting the IV
- Use of local anesthesia

EXCLUDES *Administration of non-chemotherapy agents such as antibiotics/steroids/analgesics*
Blood specimen collection from completely implantable venous access device (36591)
Declotting of catheter/port (36593)
Home infusion (99601-99602)

Code also drug or substance
Code also significant separately identifiable evaluation and management service, when performed

96542 **Chemotherapy injection, subarachnoid or intraventricular via subcutaneous reservoir, single or multiple agents**

EXCLUDES *Oral radioactive isotope therapy (79005)*

S 80 PQ 1.19 3.31 FUD XXX

96549 **Unlisted chemotherapy procedure**

S 80 PQ 0.00 0.00 FUD XXX

96567-96571 Destruction of Lesions: Photodynamic Therapy

EXCLUDES *Ocular photodynamic therapy (67221)*

96567 **Photodynamic therapy by external application of light to destroy premalignant and/or malignant lesions of the skin and adjacent mucosa (eg, lip) by activation of photosensitive drug(s), each phototherapy exposure session**

T 80 3.69 3.69 FUD XXX

+ **96570** **Photodynamic therapy by endoscopic application of light to ablate abnormal tissue via activation of photosensitive drug(s); first 30 minutes (List separately in addition to code for endoscopy or bronchoscopy procedures of lung and gastrointestinal tract)**

Code also for 38-52 minutes (96571)
Code also modifier 52 when services with report are less than 23 minutes
Code first (31641, 43229)

N 1.62 1.62 FUD ZZZ

\+ 96571 **each additional 15 minutes (List separately in addition to code for endoscopy or bronchoscopy procedures of lung and gastrointestinal tract)**
EXCLUDES *23-37 minutes of service (96570)*
Code first (96570)
Code first when appropriate (31641, 43229)
N 0.75 0.75 FUD ZZZ

96900-96999 Diagnostic/Therapeutic Skin Procedures

CMS 100-3,190.6 Hair Analysis
CMS 100-3,250.1 Treatment of Psoriasis
CMS 100-3,250.4 Treatment of Actinic Keratosis

EXCLUDES *Evaluation and management services*
Injection, intralesional (11900-11901)

96900 **Actinotherapy (ultraviolet light)**
EXCLUDES *Rhinophototherapy (30999)*
88160-88161
S 80 0.57 0.57 FUD XXX

96902 **Microscopic examination of hairs plucked or clipped by the examiner (excluding hair collected by the patient) to determine telogen and anagen counts, or structural hair shaft abnormality**
88160-88161
N 0.60 0.62 FUD XXX

96904 **Whole body integumentary photography, for monitoring of high risk patients with dysplastic nevus syndrome or a history of dysplastic nevi, or patients with a personal or familial history of melanoma**
88160-88161
N 80 1.87 1.87 FUD XXX

96910 **Photochemotherapy; tar and ultraviolet B (Goeckerman treatment) or petrolatum and ultraviolet B**
88160-88161
S 80 1.94 1.94 FUD XXX

96912 **psoralens and ultraviolet A (PUVA)**
88160-88161
S 80 2.50 2.50 FUD XXX

96913 **Photochemotherapy (Goeckerman and/or PUVA) for severe photoresponsive dermatoses requiring at least 4-8 hours of care under direct supervision of the physician (includes application of medication and dressings)**
88160-88161
S 80 3.52 3.52 FUD XXX

96920 **Laser treatment for inflammatory skin disease (psoriasis); total area less than 250 sq cm**
EXCLUDES *Destruction by laser of:*
Benign lesions (17110-17111)
Cutaneous vascular proliferative lesions (17106-17108)
Malignant lesions (17260-17286)
Premalignant lesions (17000-17004)
88160-88161
T 1.87 4.28 FUD 000

96921 **250 sq cm to 500 sq cm**
EXCLUDES *Destruction by laser of:*
Benign lesions (17110-17111)
Cutaneous vascular proliferative lesions (17106-17108)
Malignant lesions (17260-17286)
Premalignant lesions (17000-17004)
88160-88161
T 2.11 4.72 FUD 000

96922 **over 500 sq cm**
EXCLUDES *Destruction by laser of:*
Benign lesions (17110-17111)
Cutaneous vascular proliferative lesions (17106-17108)
Malignant lesions (17260-17286)
Premalignant lesions (17000-17004)
88160-88161
T 3.43 6.55 FUD 000

96999 **Unlisted special dermatological service or procedure**
T 80 0.00 0.00 FUD XXX

97001-97006 Physical Medicine Assessments

CMS 100-2,15,230.4 Services By a Physical/Occupational Therapist in Private Practice
CMS 100-3,20.10 Cardiac Rehabilitation Programs
CMS 100-4,5,10 Part B Outpatient Rehabilitation and Comprehensive Outpatient Rehabilitation Facility (CORF) Services - General
CMS 100-4,5,10.2 Financial Limitation for Outpatient Rehabilitation Services
CMS 100-4,5,20 HCPCS Coding Requirement

EXCLUDES *Electromyography (95860-95872 [95885, 95886, 95887])*
EMG biofeedback training (90901)
Muscle and range of motion tests (95831-95857)
Nerve conduction studies (95905-95913)
Transcutaneous nerve stimulation (TNS) (64550)

(51) 97001 **Physical therapy evaluation**
A 80 PQ 2.12 2.12 FUD XXX

(51) 97002 **Physical therapy re-evaluation**
A 80 PQ 1.19 1.19 FUD XXX

(51) 97003 **Occupational therapy evaluation**
A 80 PQ 2.38 2.38 FUD XXX

(51) 97004 **Occupational therapy re-evaluation**
A 80 PQ 1.49 1.49 FUD XXX

(51) 97005 **Athletic training evaluation**
E 0.00 0.00 FUD XXX

(51) 97006 **Athletic training re-evaluation**
E 0.00 0.00 FUD XXX

97010-97028 Physical Therapy Treatment Modalities: Supervised

CMS 100-2,15,230 Practice of Physical Therapy, Occupational Therapy, and Speech-Language Pathology
CMS 100-2,15,230.1 Practice of Physical Therapy
CMS 100-2,15,230.4 Services By a Physical/Occupational Therapist in Private Practice
CMS 100-3,20.10 Cardiac Rehabilitation Programs
CMS 100-4,5,10 Part B Outpatient Rehabilitation and Comprehensive Outpatient Rehabilitation Facility (CORF) Services - General
CMS 100-4,5,10.2 Financial Limitation for Outpatient Rehabilitation Services
CMS 100-4,5,20 HCPCS Coding Requirement

EXCLUDES *Direct patient contact by the provider*
Electromyography (95860-95872 [95885, 95886, 95887])
EMG biofeedback training (90901)
Muscle and range of motion tests (95831-95857)
Nerve conduction studies (95905-95913)
Transcutaneous nerve stimulation (TNS) (64550)

(51) 97010 **Application of a modality to 1 or more areas; hot or cold packs**
A 0.17 0.17 FUD XXX

(51) 97012 **traction, mechanical**
A 80 0.45 0.45 FUD XXX

(51) 97014 **electrical stimulation (unattended)**
EXCLUDES *Acupuncture with electrical stimulation (97813, 97814)*
E 0.45 0.45 FUD XXX

(51) 97016 **vasopneumatic devices**
A 80 0.54 0.54 FUD XXX

(51) 97018 **paraffin bath**
A 80 0.31 0.31 FUD XXX

(51) 97022 **whirlpool**
A 80 0.66 0.66 FUD XXX

⑤ **97024** **diathermy (eg, microwave)**

A 80 ▣ 0.18 0.18 FUD XXX

⑤ **97026** **infrared**

A 80 ▣ 0.17 0.17 FUD XXX

⑤ **97028** **ultraviolet**

A 80 ▣ 0.21 0.21 FUD XXX

97032-97039 Physical Therapy Treatment Modalities: Constant Attendance

CMS 100-2,15,230 Practice of Physical Therapy, Occupational Therapy, and Speech-Language Pathology
CMS 100-2,15,230.1 Practice of Physical Therapy
CMS 100-2,15,230.2 Practice of Occupational Therapy
CMS 100-2,15,230.4 Services By a Physical/Occupational Therapist in Private Practice
CMS 100-3,20.10 Cardiac Rehabilitation Programs
CMS 100-4,5,10 Part B Outpatient Rehabilitation and Comprehensive Outpatient Rehabilitation Facility (CORF) Services - General
CMS 100-4,5,10.2 Financial Limitation for Outpatient Rehabilitation Services
CMS 100-4,5,20 HCPCS Coding Requirement

INCLUDES Adding incremental intervals of treatment time for the same visit to calculate the total service time
Direct patient contact by the provider

EXCLUDES *Electromyography (95860-95872 [95885, 95886, 95887])*
EMG biofeedback training (90901)
Muscle and range of motion tests (95831-95857)
Nerve conduction studies (95905-95913)
Transcutaneous nerve stimulation (TNS) (64550)

⑤ **97032** **Application of a modality to 1 or more areas; electrical stimulation (manual), each 15 minutes**

EXCLUDES *Transcutaneous electrical modulation pain reprocessing (TEMPR) (scrambler therapy) (0278T)*

A 80 ▣ 0.54 0.54 FUD XXX

⑤ **97033** **iontophoresis, each 15 minutes**

A 80 ▣ 0.91 0.91 FUD XXX

⑤ **97034** **contrast baths, each 15 minutes**

A 80 ▣ 0.51 0.51 FUD XXX

⑤ **97035** **ultrasound, each 15 minutes**

A 80 ▣ 0.36 0.36 FUD XXX

⑤ **97036** **Hubbard tank, each 15 minutes**

A 80 ▣ 0.92 0.92 FUD XXX

97039 **Unlisted modality (specify type and time if constant attendance)**

A 80 ▣ 0.00 0.00 FUD XXX

97110-97546 Other Therapeutic Techniques With Direct Patient Contact

CMS 100-2,15,230 Practice of Physical Therapy, Occupational Therapy, and Speech-Language Pathology
CMS 100-2,15,230.1 Practice of Physical Therapy
CMS 100-2,15,230.2 Practice of Occupational Therapy
CMS 100-2,15,230.4 Services By a Physical/Occupational Therapist in Private Practice
CMS 100-3,20.10 Cardiac Rehabilitation Programs
CMS 100-4,5,10 Part B Outpatient Rehabilitation and Comprehensive Outpatient Rehabilitation Facility (CORF) Services - General
CMS 100-4,5,10.2 Financial Limitation for Outpatient Rehabilitation Services
CMS 100-4,5,20 HCPCS Coding Requirement

INCLUDES Application of clinical skills/services to improve function
Direct patient contact by the provider
Electromyography (95860-95872 [95885, 95886, 95887])

EXCLUDES *EMG biofeedback training (90901)*
Muscle and range of motion tests (95831-95857)
Nerve conduction studies (95905-95913)
Transcutaneous nerve stimulation (TNS) (64550)

⑤ **97110** **Therapeutic procedure, 1 or more areas, each 15 minutes; therapeutic exercises to develop strength and endurance, range of motion and flexibility**

A 80 ▣ 0.90 0.90 FUD XXX

⑤ **97112** **neuromuscular reeducation of movement, balance, coordination, kinesthetic sense, posture, and/or proprioception for sitting and/or standing activities**

A 80 ▣ 0.94 0.94 FUD XXX

⑤ **97113** **aquatic therapy with therapeutic exercises**

A 80 ▣ 1.21 1.21 FUD XXX

⑤ **97116** **gait training (includes stair climbing)**

EXCLUDES *Comprehensive gait/motion analysis (96000-96003)*

A 80 ▣ 0.80 0.80 FUD XXX

⑤ **97124** **massage, including effleurage, petrissage and/or tapotement (stroking, compression, percussion)**

EXCLUDES *Myofascial release (97140)*

A 80 ▣ 0.74 0.74 FUD XXX

97139 **Unlisted therapeutic procedure (specify)**

A 80 ▣ 0.00 0.00 FUD XXX

⑤ **97140** **Manual therapy techniques (eg, mobilization/ manipulation, manual lymphatic drainage, manual traction), 1 or more regions, each 15 minutes**

A 80 ▣ 0.84 0.84 FUD XXX

⑤ **97150** **Therapeutic procedure(s), group (2 or more individuals)**

INCLUDES Constant attendance by the physician/therapist
Reporting this procedure for each member of group

EXCLUDES *Osteopathic manipulative treatment (98925-98929)*

Do not report with (0364T-0365T, 0368T-0369T)

A 80 ▣ 0.49 0.49 FUD XXX

⑤ **97530** **Therapeutic activities, direct (one-on-one) patient contact (use of dynamic activities to improve functional performance), each 15 minutes**

A 80 ▣ 0.98 0.98 FUD XXX

⑤ **97532** **Development of cognitive skills to improve attention, memory, problem solving (includes compensatory training), direct (one-on-one) patient contact, each 15 minutes**

A 80 ▣ PQ 0.75 0.75 FUD XXX

⑤ **97533** **Sensory integrative techniques to enhance sensory processing and promote adaptive responses to environmental demands, direct (one-on-one) patient contact, each 15 minutes**

A 80 ▣ 0.82 0.82 FUD XXX

⑤ **97535** **Self-care/home management training (eg, activities of daily living (ADL) and compensatory training, meal preparation, safety procedures, and instructions in use of assistive technology devices/adaptive equipment) direct one-on-one contact, each 15 minutes**

A 80 ▣ 0.98 0.98 FUD XXX

⑤ **97537** **Community/work reintegration training (eg, shopping, transportation, money management, avocational activities and/or work environment/modification analysis, work task analysis, use of assistive technology device/adaptive equipment), direct one-on-one contact, each 15 minutes**

EXCLUDES *Wheelchair management/propulsion training (97542)*

A 80 ▣ 0.85 0.85 FUD XXX

⑤ **97542** **Wheelchair management (eg, assessment, fitting, training), each 15 minutes**

A 80 ▣ 0.86 0.86 FUD XXX

⑤ **97545** **Work hardening/conditioning; initial 2 hours**

A 80 ▣ 0.00 0.00 FUD XXX

⑤ + 97546 **each additional hour (List separately in addition to code for primary procedure)**
Code first initial 2 hours (97545)
A 80 0.00 0.00 FUD ZZZ

97597-97610 Treatment of Wounds

CMS 100-2,15,230.4 Services By a Physical/Occupational Therapist in Private Practice
CMS 100-3,270.1 Electrical Stimulation and Electromagnetic Therapy for the Treatment of Wounds
CMS 100-3,270.2 Noncontact Normothermic Wound Therapy
CMS 100-3,270.3 Blood-derived Products for Chronic Nonhealing Wounds
CMS 100-3,270.4 Treatment of Decubitus
CMS 100-4,5,10 Part B Outpatient Rehabilitation and Comprehensive Outpatient Rehabilitation Facility (CORF) Services - General
CMS 100-4,5,20 HCPCS Coding Requirement

INCLUDES Direct patient contact
Removing devitalized/necrotic tissue and promoting healing

EXCLUDES *Burn wound debridement (16020-16030)*

Do not report with other debridement codes for the same wound (11042-11047 [11045, 11046])

Wound may be washed, addressed with scissors, and/or tweezers and scalpel

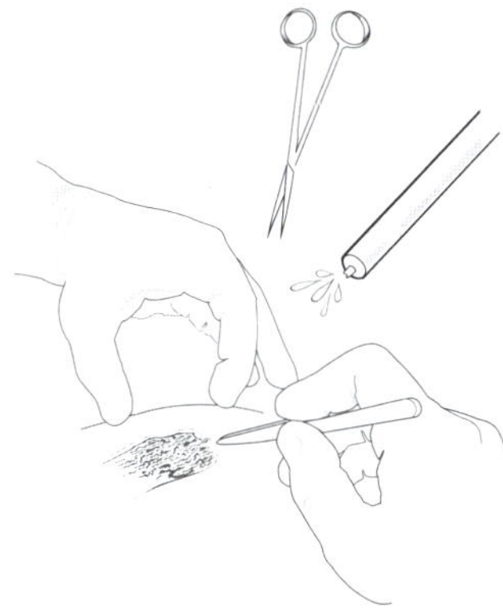

⑤ 97597 **Debridement (eg, high pressure waterjet with/without suction, sharp selective debridement with scissors, scalpel and forceps), open wound, (eg, fibrin, devitalized epidermis and/or dermis, exudate, debris, biofilm), including topical application(s), wound assessment, use of a whirlpool, when performed and instruction(s) for ongoing care, per session, total wound(s) surface area; first 20 sq cm or less**
T 80 CCI PQ 0.69 2.15 FUD 000

⑤ + 97598 **each additional 20 sq cm, or part thereof (List separately in addition to code for primary procedure)**
Code first (97597)
N 80 CCI PQ 0.33 0.71 FUD ZZZ

⑤ 97602 **Removal of devitalized tissue from wound(s), non-selective debridement, without anesthesia (eg, wet-to-moist dressings, enzymatic, abrasion), including topical application(s), wound assessment, and instruction(s) for ongoing care, per session**
T 0.00 0.00 FUD XXX

⑤ ▲ 97605 **Negative pressure wound therapy (eg, vacuum assisted drainage collection), utilizing durable medical equipment (DME), including topical application(s), wound assessment, and instruction(s) for ongoing care, per session; total wound(s) surface area less than or equal to 50 square centimeters**
Do not report with (97607-97608)
T 80 0.77 1.20 FUD XXX

⑤ ▲ 97606 **total wound(s) surface area greater than 50 square centimeters**
Do not report with (97607-97608)
T 80 0.85 1.28 FUD XXX

⑤ ● 97607 **Negative pressure wound therapy, (eg, vacuum assisted drainage collection), utilizing disposable, non-durable medical equipment including provision of exudate management collection system, topical application(s), wound assessment, and instructions for ongoing care, per session; total wound(s) surface area less than or equal to 50 square centimeters**
Do not report with (97605-97606)

⑤ ● 97608 **total wound(s) surface area greater than 50 square centimeters**
Do not report with (97605-97606)

⑤ 97610 **Low frequency, non-contact, non-thermal ultrasound, including topical application(s), when performed, wound assessment, and instruction(s) for ongoing care, per day**
T 80 0.00 0.00 FUD YYY

97750-97799 Assessments and Training

CMS 100-2,15,230 Practice of Physical Therapy, Occupational Therapy, and Speech-Language Pathology
CMS 100-2,15,230.1 Practice of Physical Therapy
CMS 100-2,15,230.2 Practice of Occupational Therapy
CMS 100-2,15,230.4 Services By a Physical/Occupational Therapist in Private Practice
CMS 100-3,20.10 Cardiac Rehabilitation Programs
CMS 100-4,5,10 Part B Outpatient Rehabilitation and Comprehensive Outpatient Rehabilitation Facility (CORF) Services - General
CMS 100-4,5,20 HCPCS Coding Requirement

⑤ 97750 **Physical performance test or measurement (eg, musculoskeletal, functional capacity), with written report, each 15 minutes**
INCLUDES Direct patient contact
EXCLUDES *Muscle/range of motion testing and electromyography/nerve velocity determination (95831-95857, 95860-95872, [95885, 95886, 95887], 95907-95913)*
A 80 CCI PQ 0.94 0.94 FUD XXX

⑤ 97755 **Assistive technology assessment (eg, to restore, augment or compensate for existing function, optimize functional tasks and/or maximize environmental accessibility), direct one-on-one contact, with written report, each 15 minutes**
INCLUDES Direct patient contact
EXCLUDES *Augmentative/alternative communication device (92605, 92607)*
Muscle/range of motion testing and electromyography/nerve velocity determination (95831-95857, 95860-95872, [95885, 95886, 95887], 95907-95913)
A 80 CCI 1.02 1.02 FUD XXX

97760 **Orthotic(s) management and training (including assessment and fitting when not otherwise reported), upper extremity(s), lower extremity(s) and/or trunk, each 15 minutes**
Do not report with gait training, if performed on the same extremity (97116)
A 80 1.08 1.08 FUD XXX

97761 **Prosthetic training, upper and/or lower extremity(s), each 15 minutes**
A 80 0.94 0.94 FUD XXX

97762 **Checkout for orthotic/prosthetic use, established patient, each 15 minutes**
A 80 1.34 1.34 FUD XXX

97799 **Unlisted physical medicine/rehabilitation service or procedure**
A 80 0.00 0.00 FUD XXX

97802-97804 Medical Nutrition Therapy Services

CMS 100-3,40.1 Diabetes Outpatient Self-management Training
CMS 100-3,180.1 Medical Nutrition Therapy
CMS 100-4,4,300 Medical Nutrition Therapy Services

EXCLUDES *Medical nutrition therapy assessment/intervention provided by physician or other qualified health care provider; use appropriate evaluation and management codes*

97802 Medical nutrition therapy; initial assessment and intervention, individual, face-to-face with the patient, each 15 minutes
A 80 PQ 0.93 1.00 FUD XXX

97803 re-assessment and intervention, individual, face-to-face with the patient, each 15 minutes
A 80 PQ 0.80 0.86 FUD XXX

97804 group (2 or more individual(s)), each 30 minutes
A 80 PQ 0.43 0.45 FUD XXX

97810-97814 Acupuncture

CMS 100-3,30.3.1 Acupuncture for Fibromyalgia
CMS 100-3,30.3.2 Acupuncture for Osteoarthritis

INCLUDES 15 minute increments of face-to-face contact with the patient
Reporting only one code for each 15 minute increment

EXCLUDES *Time providing evaluation and management services*

Code also significant separately identifiable evaluation and management code using modifier 25, when performed

97810 Acupuncture, 1 or more needles; without electrical stimulation, initial 15 minutes of personal one-on-one contact with the patient
EXCLUDES *Electrical stimulation (97813-97814)*
Do not report with (97813)
E 0.87 1.02 FUD XXX

\+ **97811 without electrical stimulation, each additional 15 minutes of personal one-on-one contact with the patient, with re-insertion of needle(s) (List separately in addition to code for primary procedure)**
EXCLUDES *Electrical stimulation (97813-97814)*
Code first initial 15 minutes (97810, 97813)
E 0.72 0.77 FUD ZZZ

97813 with electrical stimulation, initial 15 minutes of personal one-on-one contact with the patient
INCLUDES Electrical stimulation
Do not report with (97810)
E 0.94 1.10 FUD XXX

\+ **97814 with electrical stimulation, each additional 15 minutes of personal one-on-one contact with the patient, with re-insertion of needle(s) (List separately in addition to code for primary procedure)**
INCLUDES Electrical stimulation
Code first initial 15 minutes (97810, 97813)
E 0.80 0.88 FUD ZZZ

98925-98929 Osteopathic Manipulation

CMS 100-3,150.1 Manipulation

INCLUDES Physician applied manual treatment done to eliminate/alleviate somatic dysfunction and related disorders using a variety of techniques
The following body regions:
- Abdomen/visceral region
- Cervical region
- Head region
- Lower extremities
- Lumbar region
- Pelvic region
- Rib cage region
- Sacral region
- Thoracic region
- Upper extremities

Code also significant separately identifiable evaluation and management service using modifier 25, when performed

98925 Osteopathic manipulative treatment (OMT); 1-2 body regions involved
S 80 0.67 0.88 FUD 000

98926 3-4 body regions involved
S 80 1.01 1.27 FUD 000

98927 5-6 body regions involved
S 80 1.33 1.66 FUD 000

98928 7-8 body regions involved
S 80 1.70 2.05 FUD 000

98929 9-10 body regions involved
S 80 2.04 2.46 FUD 000

98940-98943 Chiropractic Manipulation

CMS 100-1,5,70.6 Chiropractors
CMS 100-2,15,240 Chiropractic Services - General
CMS 100-3,150.1 Manipulation

INCLUDES Form of manual treatment performed to influence joint/neurophysical function
The following five extraspinal regions:
- Abdomen
- Head, including temporomandibular joint, excluding atlanto-occipital region
- Lower extremities
- Rib cage, not including costotransverse/costovertebral joints
- Upper extremities

The following five spinal regions:
- Cervical region (atlanto-occipital joint)
- Lumbar region
- Pelvic region (sacro-iliac joint)
- Sacral region
- Thoracic region (costovertebral/costotransverse joints)

Code also significant separately identifiable evaluation and management service using modifier 25, when performed

98940 Chiropractic manipulative treatment (CMT); spinal, 1-2 regions
S 80 PQ 0.63 0.79 FUD 000

98941 spinal, 3-4 regions
S 80 PQ 0.99 1.16 FUD 000

98942 spinal, 5 regions
S 80 PQ 1.33 1.50 FUD 000

98943 extraspinal, 1 or more regions
E 0.67 0.77 FUD XXX

98960-98962 Self-Management Training

INCLUDES Education/training services:
- Prescribed by a physician or other qualified health care professional
- Provided by a qualified nonphysician health care provider

Standardized curriculum that may be modified as necessary for:
- Clinical needs
- Cultural norms
- Health literacy

Teaching the patient how to manage the illness/delay the comorbidity(s)

EXCLUDES *Genetic counseling education services (96040, 98961-98962)*
Health/behavior assessment (96150-96155)
Medical nutrition therapy (97802-97804)
The following services:
- *Counseling/education to a group (99078)*
- *Counseling/education to individuals (99201-99215, 99217-99223 [99224, 99225, 99226], 99231-99233, 99241-99255, 99281-99285, 99304-99318, 99324-99337, 99341-99350, 99401-99429)*
- *Counseling/risk factor reduction without symptoms/established disease (99401-99412)*

98960 Education and training for patient self-management by a qualified, nonphysician health care professional using a standardized curriculum, face-to-face with the patient (could include caregiver/family) each 30 minutes; individual patient
E PQ 0.77 0.77 FUD XXX

98961 2-4 patients
INCLUDES Group education regarding genetic risks
E PQ 0.37 0.37 FUD XXX

98962 5-8 patients

INCLUDES Group education regarding genetic risks

E PQ 0.27 0.27 FUD XXX

98966-98968 Nonphysician Telephone Services

CMS 100-1,5,70 Definition of Physician

INCLUDES Assessment and management services provided by telephone by a qualified health care professional

Episode of care initiated by an established patient or his/her guardian

EXCLUDES *Call initiated by the qualified health care professional*

Calls during the postoperative period of a procedure

Decision to see the patient at the next available urgent care appointment

Decision to see the patient within 24 hours of the call

Telephone services provided by a physician (99441-99443)

Telephone services that are considered a part of a previous or subsequent service

Do not report if performed during the service time for (99495-99496)

Do not report if performed in the same month with (99487-99489)

Do not report when performed in the previous seven days as (98966-98969)

98966 Telephone assessment and management service provided by a qualified nonphysician health care professional to an established patient, parent, or guardian not originating from a related assessment and management service provided within the previous 7 days nor leading to an assessment and management service or procedure within the next 24 hours or soonest available appointment; 5-10 minutes of medical discussion

E 0.36 0.39 FUD XXX

98967 11-20 minutes of medical discussion

E 0.72 0.76 FUD XXX

98968 21-30 minutes of medical discussion

E 1.09 1.13 FUD XXX

98969 Nonphysician Online Service

INCLUDES On-line assessment and management service provided by a qualified health care professional

Timely reply to the patient as well as:

Ordering laboratory services

Permanent record of the service; either hard copy or electronic

Providing a prescription

Related telephone calls

EXCLUDES *On-line evaluation service:*

Provided during the postoperative period of a procedure

Provided more than once in a seven day period

Related to a service provided in the previous seven days

Do not report in same month with (99487-99489)

Do not report when performed during the service time for (99495-99496)

Do not report with (99339-99340, 99363-99364, 99374-99380)

98969 Online assessment and management service provided by a qualified nonphysician health care professional to an established patient or guardian, not originating from a related assessment and management service provided within the previous 7 days, using the Internet or similar electronic communications network

F 0.00 0.00 FUD XXX

99000-99091 Supplemental Services and Supplies

INCLUDES Supplemental reporting for services adjunct to the basic service provided

99000 Handling and/or conveyance of specimen for transfer from the office to a laboratory

E 0.00 0.00 FUD XXX

99001 Handling and/or conveyance of specimen for transfer from the patient in other than an office to a laboratory (distance may be indicated)

E 0.00 0.00 FUD XXX

99002 Handling, conveyance, and/or any other service in connection with the implementation of an order involving devices (eg, designing, fitting, packaging, handling, delivery or mailing) when devices such as orthotics, protectives, prosthetics are fabricated by an outside laboratory or shop but which items have been designed, and are to be fitted and adjusted by the attending physician or other qualified health care professional

EXCLUDES *Venous blood routine collection (36415)*

B 0.00 0.00 FUD XXX

99024 Postoperative follow-up visit, normally included in the surgical package, to indicate that an evaluation and management service was performed during a postoperative period for a reason(s) related to the original procedure

B 0.00 0.00 FUD XXX

99026 Hospital mandated on call service; in-hospital, each hour

EXCLUDES *Physician stand-by services with prolonged physician attendance (99360)*

Time spent providing procedures or services that may be separately reported

E 0.00 0.00 FUD XXX

99027 out-of-hospital, each hour

EXCLUDES *Physician stand-by services with prolonged physician attendance (99360)*

Time spent providing procedures or services that may be separately reported

E 0.00 0.00 FUD XXX

⑤ **99050 Services provided in the office at times other than regularly scheduled office hours, or days when the office is normally closed (eg, holidays, Saturday or Sunday), in addition to basic service**

Code first basic service provided

Code also more than one adjunct code per encounter when appropriate

B 0.00 0.00 FUD XXX

⑤ **99051 Service(s) provided in the office during regularly scheduled evening, weekend, or holiday office hours, in addition to basic service**

Code first basic service provided

Code also more than one adjunct code per encounter when appropriate

B 0.00 0.00 FUD XXX

⑤ **99053 Service(s) provided between 10:00 PM and 8:00 AM at 24-hour facility, in addition to basic service**

Code first basic service provided

Code also more than one adjunct code per encounter when appropriate

B 0.00 0.00 FUD XXX

⑤ **99056 Service(s) typically provided in the office, provided out of the office at request of patient, in addition to basic service**

Code first basic service provided

Code also more than one adjunct code per encounter when appropriate

B 0.00 0.00 FUD XXX

⑤ **99058 Service(s) provided on an emergency basis in the office, which disrupts other scheduled office services, in addition to basic service**

Code first basic service provided

Code also more than one adjunct code per encounter when appropriate

B 0.00 0.00 FUD XXX

⑤ **99060 Service(s) provided on an emergency basis, out of the office, which disrupts other scheduled office services, in addition to basic service**

Code first basic service provided

Code also more than one adjunct code per encounter when appropriate

B 0.00 0.00 FUD XXX

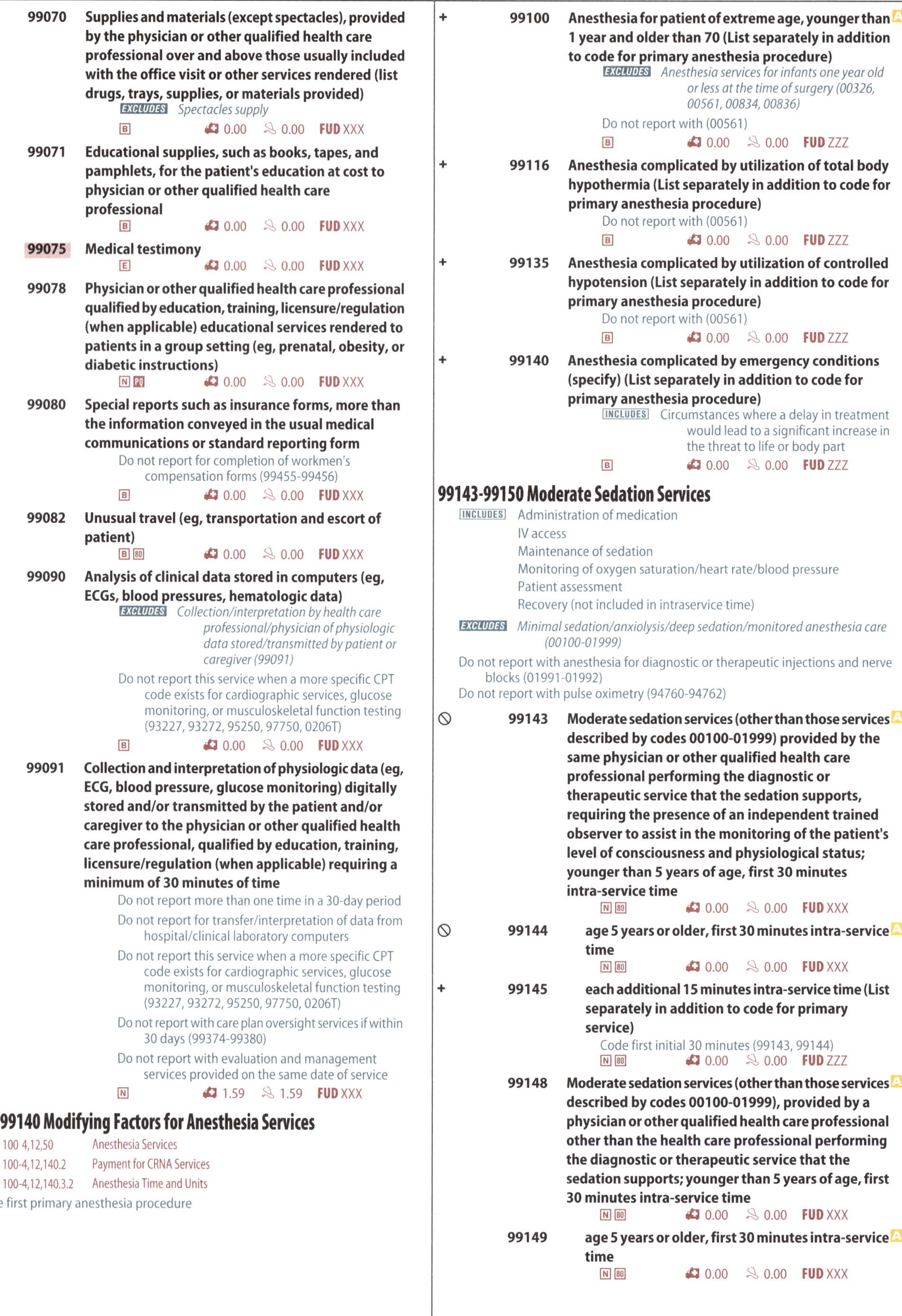

99070 **Supplies and materials (except spectacles), provided by the physician or other qualified health care professional over and above those usually included with the office visit or other services rendered (list drugs, trays, supplies, or materials provided)**
EXCLUDES *Spectacles supply*
B 0.00 0.00 FUD XXX

99071 **Educational supplies, such as books, tapes, and pamphlets, for the patient's education at cost to physician or other qualified health care professional**
B 0.00 0.00 FUD XXX

99075 **Medical testimony**
E 0.00 0.00 FUD XXX

99078 **Physician or other qualified health care professional qualified by education, training, licensure/regulation (when applicable) educational services rendered to patients in a group setting (eg, prenatal, obesity, or diabetic instructions)**
N PQ 0.00 0.00 FUD XXX

99080 **Special reports such as insurance forms, more than the information conveyed in the usual medical communications or standard reporting form**
Do not report for completion of workmen's compensation forms (99455-99456)
B 0.00 0.00 FUD XXX

99082 **Unusual travel (eg, transportation and escort of patient)**
B 80 0.00 0.00 FUD XXX

99090 **Analysis of clinical data stored in computers (eg, ECGs, blood pressures, hematologic data)**
EXCLUDES *Collection/interpretation by health care professional/physician of physiologic data stored/transmitted by patient or caregiver (99091)*
Do not report this service when a more specific CPT code exists for cardiographic services, glucose monitoring, or musculoskeletal function testing (93227, 93272, 95250, 97750, 0206T)
B 0.00 0.00 FUD XXX

99091 **Collection and interpretation of physiologic data (eg, ECG, blood pressure, glucose monitoring) digitally stored and/or transmitted by the patient and/or caregiver to the physician or other qualified health care professional, qualified by education, training, licensure/regulation (when applicable) requiring a minimum of 30 minutes of time**
Do not report more than one time in a 30-day period
Do not report for transfer/interpretation of data from hospital/clinical laboratory computers
Do not report this service when a more specific CPT code exists for cardiographic services, glucose monitoring, or musculoskeletal function testing (93227, 93272, 95250, 97750, 0206T)
Do not report with care plan oversight services if within 30 days (99374-99380)
Do not report with evaluation and management services provided on the same date of service
N 1.59 1.59 FUD XXX

99100-99140 Modifying Factors for Anesthesia Services

CMS 100 4,12,50 Anesthesia Services
CMS 100-4,12,140.2 Payment for CRNA Services
CMS 100-4,12,140.3.2 Anesthesia Time and Units
Code first primary anesthesia procedure

\+ **99100** **Anesthesia for patient of extreme age, younger than 1 year and older than 70 (List separately in addition to code for primary anesthesia procedure)** A
EXCLUDES *Anesthesia services for infants one year old or less at the time of surgery (00326, 00561, 00834, 00836)*
Do not report with (00561)
B 0.00 0.00 FUD ZZZ

\+ **99116** **Anesthesia complicated by utilization of total body hypothermia (List separately in addition to code for primary anesthesia procedure)**
Do not report with (00561)
B 0.00 0.00 FUD ZZZ

\+ **99135** **Anesthesia complicated by utilization of controlled hypotension (List separately in addition to code for primary anesthesia procedure)**
Do not report with (00561)
B 0.00 0.00 FUD ZZZ

\+ **99140** **Anesthesia complicated by emergency conditions (specify) (List separately in addition to code for primary anesthesia procedure)**
INCLUDES Circumstances where a delay in treatment would lead to a significant increase in the threat to life or body part
B 0.00 0.00 FUD ZZZ

99143-99150 Moderate Sedation Services

INCLUDES Administration of medication
IV access
Maintenance of sedation
Monitoring of oxygen saturation/heart rate/blood pressure
Patient assessment
Recovery (not included in intraservice time)

EXCLUDES *Minimal sedation/anxiolysis/deep sedation/monitored anesthesia care (00100-01999)*

Do not report with anesthesia for diagnostic or therapeutic injections and nerve blocks (01991-01992)
Do not report with pulse oximetry (94760-94762)

⊘ **99143** **Moderate sedation services (other than those services described by codes 00100-01999) provided by the same physician or other qualified health care professional performing the diagnostic or therapeutic service that the sedation supports, requiring the presence of an independent trained observer to assist in the monitoring of the patient's level of consciousness and physiological status; younger than 5 years of age, first 30 minutes intra-service time** A
N 80 0.00 0.00 FUD XXX

⊘ **99144** **age 5 years or older, first 30 minutes intra-service time** A
N 80 0.00 0.00 FUD XXX

\+ **99145** **each additional 15 minutes intra-service time (List separately in addition to code for primary service)**
Code first initial 30 minutes (99143, 99144)
N 80 0.00 0.00 FUD ZZZ

99148 **Moderate sedation services (other than those services described by codes 00100-01999), provided by a physician or other qualified health care professional other than the health care professional performing the diagnostic or therapeutic service that the sedation supports; younger than 5 years of age, first 30 minutes intra-service time** A
N 80 0.00 0.00 FUD XXX

99149 **age 5 years or older, first 30 minutes intra-service time** A
N 80 0.00 0.00 FUD XXX

+ 99150 **each additional 15 minutes intra-service time (List separately in addition to code for primary service)**
Code first initial 30 minutes (99148, 99149)
N 80 0.00 0.00 FUD ZZZ

99170 Specialized Examination of Child

EXCLUDES *Moderate sedation (99143-99150)*

99170 **Anogenital examination, magnified, in childhood for suspected trauma, including image recording when performed** A
T 2.53 4.87 FUD 000

99172-99173 Visual Acuity Screening Tests

CMS 100-2,16,90 Routine Services and Appliances

INCLUDES Graduated visual acuity stimuli that allow a quantitative determination/estimation of visual acuity
Ocular photoscreening

99172 **Visual function screening, automated or semi-automated bilateral quantitative determination of visual acuity, ocular alignment, color vision by pseudoisochromatic plates, and field of vision (may include all or some screening of the determination[s] for contrast sensitivity, vision under glare)**
Do not report with (99173)
Do not report with evaluation and management service or general ophthalmological service
E 0.00 0.00 FUD XXX

99173 **Screening test of visual acuity, quantitative, bilateral**
Do not report with (99172)
E 0.08 0.08 FUD XXX

99174 Screening For Amblyogenic Factors

Do not report with (92002-92014, 99172-99173)

99174 **Instrument-based ocular screening (eg, photoscreening, automated-refraction), bilateral**
E 0.21 0.21 FUD XXX

99175 Drug Administration to Induce Vomiting

EXCLUDES *Diagnostic gastric lavage (43754-43755)*
Diagnostic gastric intubation (43754-43755)

99175 **Ipecac or similar administration for individual emesis and continued observation until stomach adequately emptied of poison**
N 80 0.47 0.47 FUD XXX

99183-99184 Hyperbaric Oxygen Therapy

CMS 100-3,20.29 Hyperbaric Oxygen Therapy

EXCLUDES *Evaluation and management services, when performed*
Other procedures such as wound debridement, when performed

99183 **Physician or other qualified health care professional attendance and supervision of hyperbaric oxygen therapy, per session**
B 80 3.45 6.00 FUD XXX

● 99184 **Initiation of selective head or total body hypothermia in the critically ill neonate, includes appropriate patient selection by review of clinical, imaging and laboratory data, confirmation of esophageal temperature probe location, evaluation of amplitude EEG, supervision of controlled hypothermia, and assessment of patient tolerance of cooling** A
Do not report more than one time per hospitalization

99188 Topical Fluoride Application

● 99188 **Application of topical fluoride varnish by a physician or other qualified health care professional**

99190-99192 Assemble and Manage Pump with Oxygenator/Heat Exchange

99190 **Assembly and operation of pump with oxygenator or heat exchanger (with or without ECG and/or pressure monitoring); each hour**
C 0.00 0.00 FUD XXX

99191 **45 minutes**
C 0.00 0.00 FUD XXX

99192 **30 minutes**
C 0.00 0.00 FUD XXX

99195-99199 Therapeutic Phlebotomy and Unlisted Procedures

99195 **Phlebotomy, therapeutic (separate procedure)**
X 80 2.76 2.76 FUD XXX

99199 **Unlisted special service, procedure or report**
B 80 0.00 0.00 FUD XXX

99500-99602 Home Visit By Non-Physician Professionals

INCLUDES Services performed by non-physician providers
Services provided in patient's:
Assisted living apartment
Custodial care facility
Group home
Non-traditional private home
Residence
School

EXCLUDES *Home visits performed by physicians (99341-99350)*
Other services/procedures provided by physicians to patients at home

Code also home visit evaluation and management codes if health care provider is authorized to use (99341-99350)
Code also significant separately identifiable evaluation and management service, when performed

99500 **Home visit for prenatal monitoring and assessment to include fetal heart rate, non-stress test, uterine monitoring, and gestational diabetes monitoring** M ♀
E 0.00 0.00 FUD XXX

99501 **Home visit for postnatal assessment and follow-up care** M ♀
E 0.00 0.00 FUD XXX

99502 **Home visit for newborn care and assessment** A
E 0.00 0.00 FUD XXX

99503 **Home visit for respiratory therapy care (eg, bronchodilator, oxygen therapy, respiratory assessment, apnea evaluation)**
E 0.00 0.00 FUD XXX

99504 **Home visit for mechanical ventilation care**
E 0.00 0.00 FUD XXX

99505 **Home visit for stoma care and maintenance including colostomy and cystostomy**
E 0.00 0.00 FUD XXX

99506 **Home visit for intramuscular injections**
E 0.00 0.00 FUD XXX

99507 **Home visit for care and maintenance of catheter(s) (eg, urinary, drainage, and enteral)**
E 0.00 0.00 FUD XXX

99509 **Home visit for assistance with activities of daily living and personal care**
EXCLUDES *Medical nutrition therapy/assessment home services (97802-97804)*
Self-care/home management training (97535)
Speech therapy home services (92507-92508)
E 0.00 0.00 FUD XXX

99510 **Home visit for individual, family, or marriage counseling**
E 0.00 0.00 FUD XXX

99511 **Home visit for fecal impaction management and enema administration**
E 0.00 0.00 FUD XXX

99512 **Home visit for hemodialysis**
EXCLUDES *Peritoneal dialysis home infusion (99601-99602)*
E 0.00 0.00 FUD XXX

99600 **Unlisted home visit service or procedure**
E 0.00 0.00 FUD XXX

99601 **Home infusion/specialty drug administration, per visit (up to 2 hours);**
E 0.00 0.00 FUD XXX

\+ **99602** **each additional hour (List separately in addition to code for primary procedure)**
Code first (99601)
E 0.00 0.00 FUD XXX

99605-99607 Medication Management By Pharmacist

INCLUDES Direct (face-to-face) assessment and intervention by a pharmacist for the purpose of:
- Managing medication complications and/or interactions
- Maximizing the patient's response to drug therapy

Documenting the following required elements:
- Advice given regarding improvement of treatment compliance and outcomes
- Profile of medications (prescription and nonprescription)
- Review of applicable patient history

EXCLUDES *Routine tasks associated with dispensing and related activities (e.g., providing product information)*

99605 **Medication therapy management service(s) provided by a pharmacist, individual, face-to-face with patient, with assessment and intervention if provided; initial 15 minutes, new patient**
E 0.00 0.00 FUD XXX

99606 **initial 15 minutes, established patient**
E 0.00 0.00 FUD XXX

\+ **99607** **each additional 15 minutes (List separately in addition to code for primary service)**
Code first (99605, 99606)
E 0.00 0.00 FUD XXX

Evaluation and Management (E/M) Services Guidelines

In addition to the information presented in the Introduction, several other items unique to this section are defined or identified here.

CLASSIFICATION OF EVALUATION AND MANAGEMENT (E/M) SERVICES

The E/M section is divided into broad categories such as office visits, hospital visits, and consultations. Most of the categories are further divided into two or more subcategories of E/M services. For example, there are two subcategories of office visits (new patient and established patient) and there are two subcategories of hospital visits (initial and subsequent). The subcategories of E/M services are further classified into levels of E/M services that are identified by specific codes. This classification is important because the nature of work varies by type of service, place of service, and the patient's status.

The basic format of the levels of E/M services is the same for most categories. First, a unique code number is listed. Second, the place and/or type of service is specified, eg, office consultation. Third, the content of the service is defined, eg, comprehensive history and comprehensive examination. (See "Levels of E/M Services," for details on the content of E/M services.) Fourth, the nature of the presenting problem(s) usually associated with a given level is described. Fifth, the time typically required to provide the service is specified. (A detailed discussion of time is provided separately.)

DEFINITIONS OF COMMONLY USED TERMS

Certain key words and phrases are used throughout the E/M section. The following definitions are intended to reduce the potential for differing interpretations and to increase the consistency of reporting by physicians in differing specialties. E/M services may also be reported by other qualified health care professionals who are authorized to perform such services within the scope of their practice.

New and Established Patient

Solely for the purposes of distinguishing between new and established patients, professional services are those face-to-face services rendered by physicians and other qualified health care professionals who may report E/M services with a specific CPT® code or codes. A new patient is one who has not received any professional services from the physician/qualified health care professional or another physician/qualified health care professional of the exact same specialty and subspecialty who belongs to the same group practice, within the past three years.

An established patient is one who has received professional services from the physician/qualified health care professional or another physician/qualified health care professional of the exact same specialty and subspecialty who belongs to the same group practice, within the past three years. See the decision tree at right.

When a physician/qualified health care professional is on call or covering for another physician/qualified health care professional, the patient's encounter is classified as it would have been by the physician/qualified health care professional who is not available. When advanced practice nurses and physician assistants are working with physicians, they are considered as working in the exact same specialty and exact same subspecialties as the physician.

No distinction is made between new and established patients in the emergency department. E/M services in the emergency department category may be reported for any new or established patient who presents for treatment in the emergency department.

The decision tree in the next column is provided to aid in determining whether to report the E/M service provided as a new or an established patient encounter.

Chief Complaint

A chief complaint is a concise statement describing the symptom, problem, condition, diagnosis, or other factor that is the reason for the encounter, usually stated in the patient's words.

Concurrent Care and Transfer of Care

Concurrent care is the provision of similar services (e.g., hospital visits) to the same patient by more than one physician or other qualified health care professional on the same day. When concurrent care is provided, no special reporting is required. Transfer of care is the process whereby a physician or other qualified health care professional who is managing some or all of a patient's problems relinquishes this responsibility to another physician or other qualified health care professional who explicitly agrees to accept this responsibility and who, from the initial encounter, is not providing consultative services. The physician or other qualified health care professional transferring care is then no longer providing care for these problems though he or she may continue providing care for other conditions when appropriate. Consultation codes should not be reported by the physician or other qualified health care professional who has agreed to accept transfer of care before an initial evaluation, but they are appropriate to report if the decision to accept transfer of care cannot be made until after the initial consultation evaluation, regardless of site of service.

Decision Tree for New vs Established Patients

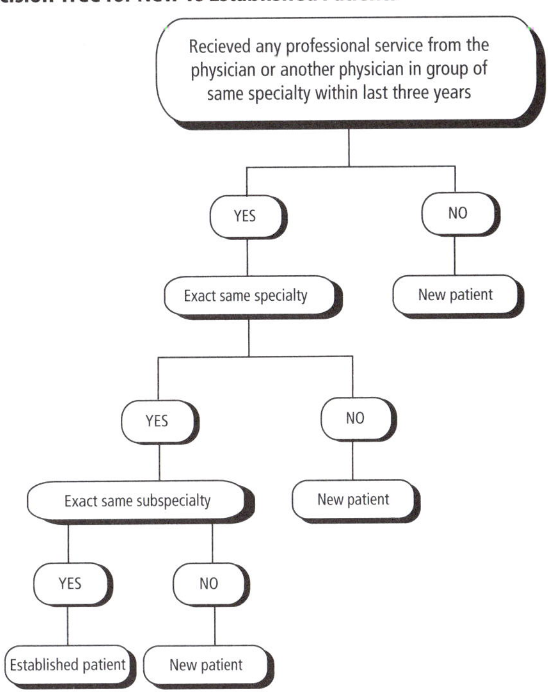

Counseling

Counseling is a discussion with a patient and/or family concerning one or more of the following areas:

- Diagnostic results, impressions, and/or recommended diagnostic studies
- Prognosis
- Risks and benefits of management (treatment) options
- Instructions for management (treatment) and/or follow-up
- Importance of compliance with chosen management (treatment) options
- Risk factor reduction
- Patient and family education
  (For psychotherapy, see 90832–90834, 90836–90840)

Family History

A review of medical events in the patient's family that includes significant information about:

- The health status or cause of death of parents, siblings, and children
- Specific diseases related to problems identified in the Chief Complaint or History of the Present Illness, and/or System Review

- Diseases of family members that may be hereditary or place the patient at risk

History of Present Illness
A chronological description of the development of the patient's present illness from the first sign and/or symptom to the present. This includes a description of location, quality, severity, timing, context, modifying factors, and associated signs and symptoms significantly related to the presenting problem(s).

Levels of E/M Services
Within each category or subcategory of E/M service, there are three to five levels of E/M services available for reporting purposes. Levels of E/M services are not interchangeable among the different categories or subcategories of service. For example, the first level of E/M services in the subcategory of office visit, new patient, does not have the same definition as the first level of E/M services in the subcategory of office visit, established patient.

The levels of E/M services include examinations, evaluations, treatments, conferences with or concerning patients, preventive pediatric and adult health supervision, and similar medical services, such as the determination of the need and/or location for appropriate care. Medical screening includes the history, examination, and medical decision-making required to determine the need and/or location for appropriate care and treatment of the patient (eg, office and other outpatient setting, emergency department, nursing facility). The levels of E/M services encompass the wide variations in skill, effort, time, responsibility, and medical knowledge required for the prevention or diagnosis and treatment of illness or injury and the promotion of optimal health. Each level of E/M services may be used by all physicians or other qualified health care professionals.

The descriptors for the levels of E/M services recognize seven components, six of which are used in defining the levels of E/M services. These components are:

- History
- Examination
- Medical decision making
- Counseling
- Coordination of care
- Nature of presenting problem
- Time

The first three of these components (history, examination, and medical decision making) are considered the key components in selecting a level of E/M services. (See "Determine the Extent of History Obtained.")

The next three components (counseling, coordination of care, and the nature of the presenting problem) are considered contributory factors in the majority of encounters. Although the first two of these contributory factors are important E/M services, it is not required that these services be provided at every patient encounter.

Coordination of care with other physicians, other qualified health care professionals, or agencies without a patient encounter on that day is reported using the case management codes.

The final component, time, is discussed in detail below.

Any specifically identifiable procedure (ie, identified with a specific CPT code) performed on or subsequent to the date of initial or subsequent E/M services should be reported separately.

The actual performance and/or interpretation of diagnostic tests/studies ordered during a patient encounter are not included in the levels of E/M services. Physician performance of diagnostic tests/studies for which specific CPT codes are available may be reported separately, in addition to the appropriate E/M code. The physician's interpretation of the results of diagnostic tests/studies (ie, professional component) with preparation of a separate distinctly identifiable signed written report may also be reported separately, using the appropriate CPT code with modifier 26 appended.

The physician or other health care professional may need to indicate that on the day a procedure or service identified by a CPT code was performed, the patient's condition required a significant separately identifiable E/M service above and beyond other services provided or beyond the usual preservice and postservice care associated with the procedure that was performed. The E/M service may be caused or prompted by the symptoms or condition for which the procedure and/or service was provided. This circumstance may be reported by adding modifier 25 to the appropriate level of E/M service. As such, different diagnoses are not required for reporting of the procedure and the E/M services on the same date.

Nature of Presenting Problem
A presenting problem is a disease, condition, illness, injury, symptom, sign, finding, complaint, or other reason for encounter, with or without a diagnosis being established at the time of the encounter. The E/M codes recognize five types of presenting problems that are defined as follows:

Minimal: A problem that may not require the presence of the physician or other qualified health care professional, but service is provided under the physician's or other qualified health care professional's supervision.

Self-limited or minor: A problem that runs a definite and prescribed course, is transient in nature, and is not likely to permanently alter health status OR has a good prognosis with management/compliance.

Low severity: A problem where the risk of morbidity without treatment is low; there is little to no risk of mortality without treatment; full recovery without functional impairment is expected.

Moderate severity: A problem where the risk of morbidity without treatment is moderate; there is moderate risk of mortality without treatment; uncertain prognosis OR increased probability of prolonged functional impairment.

High severity: A problem where the risk of morbidity without treatment is high to extreme; there is a moderate to high risk of mortality without treatment OR high probability of severe, prolonged functional impairment.

Past History
A review of the patient's past experiences with illnesses, injuries, and treatments that includes significant information about:

- Prior major illnesses and injuries
- Prior operations
- Prior hospitalizations
- Current medications
- Allergies (eg, drug, food)
- Age appropriate immunization status
- Age appropriate feeding/dietary status

Social History
An age appropriate review of past and current activities that includes significant information about:

- Marital status and/or living arrangements
- Current employment
- Occupational history
- Military history
- Use of drugs, alcohol, and tobacco
- Level of education
- Sexual history
- Other relevant social factors

System Review (Review of Systems)
An inventory of body systems obtained through a series of questions seeking to identify signs and/or symptoms that the patient may be experiencing or has experienced. For the purposes of the CPT codebook the following elements of a system review have been identified:

- Constitutional symptoms (fever, weight loss, etc)
- Eyes
- Ears, nose, mouth, throat
- Cardiovascular
- Respiratory
- Gastrointestinal
- Genitourinary
- Musculoskeletal

- Integumentary (skin and/or breast)
- Neurological
- Psychiatric
- Endocrine
- Hematologic/lymphatic
- Allergic/immunologic

The review of systems helps define the problem, clarify the differential diagnosis, identify needed testing, or serves as baseline data on other systems that might be affected by any possible management options.

Time

The inclusion of time in the definitions of levels of E/M services has been implicit in prior editions of the CPT codebook. The inclusion of time as an explicit factor beginning in *CPT 1992* is done to assist in selecting the most appropriate level of E/M services. It should be recognized that the specific times expressed in the visit code descriptors are averages and, therefore, represent a range of times that may be higher or lower depending on actual clinical circumstances.

Time is not a descriptive component for the emergency department levels of E/M services because emergency department services are typically provided on a variable intensity basis, often involving multiple encounters with several patients over an extended period of time. Therefore, it is often difficult to provide accurate estimates of the time spent face-to-face with the patient.

Studies to establish levels of E/M services employed surveys of practicing physicians to obtain data on the amount of time and work associated with typical E/M services. Since "work" is not easily quantifiable, the codes must rely on other objective, verifiable measures that correlate with physicians' estimates of their "work." It has been demonstrated that estimations of intraservice time, both within and across specialties, is a variable that is predictive of the "work" of E/M services. This same research has shown there is a strong relationship between intraservice time and total time for E/M services. Intraservice time, rather than total time, was chosen for inclusion with the codes because of its relative ease of measurement and because of its direct correlation with measurements of the total amount of time and work associated with typical E/M services.

Intraservice times are defined as face-to-face time for office and other outpatient visits and as unit/floor time for hospital and other inpatient visits. This distinction is necessary because most of the work of typical office visits takes place during the face-to-face time with the patient, while most of the work of typical hospital visits takes place during the time spent on the patient's floor or unit. When prolonged time occurs in either the office or the inpatient areas, the appropriate add-on code should be reported.

Face-to-face time (office and other outpatient visits and office consultations): For coding purposes, face-to-face time for these services is defined as only that time spent face-to-face with the patient and/or family. This includes the time spent performing such tasks as obtaining a history, performing an examination, and counseling the patient.

Time is also spent doing work before or after the face-to-face time with the patient, performing such tasks as reviewing records and tests, arranging for further services, and communicating further with other professionals and the patient through written reports and telephone contact.

This non-face-to-face time for office services—also called pre- and postencounter time—is not included in the time component described in the E/M codes. However, the pre- and post-non-face-to-face work associated with an encounter was included in calculating the total work of typical services in physician surveys.

Thus, the face-to-face time associated with the services described by any E/M code is a valid proxy for the total work done before, during, and after the visit.

Unit/floor time (hospital observation services, inpatient hospital care, initial inpatient hospital consultations, nursing facility): For reporting purposes, intraservice time for these services is defined as unit/floor time, which includes the time present on the patient's hospital unit and at the bedside rendering services for that patient. This includes the time to establish and/or review the patient's chart, examine the patient, write notes, and communicate with other professionals and the patient's family.

In the hospital, pre- and post-time includes time spent off the patient's floor performing such tasks as reviewing pathology and radiology findings in another part of the hospital.

This pre- and postvisit time is not included in the time component described in these codes. However, the pre- and postwork performed during the time spent off the floor or unit was included in calculating the total work of typical services in physician surveys.

Thus, the unit/floor time associated with the services described by any code is a valid proxy for the total work done before, during, and after the visit.

UNLISTED SERVICE

An E/M service may be provided that is not listed in this section of the CPT codebook. When reporting such a service, the appropriate unlisted code may be used to indicate the service, identifying it by "Special Report," as discussed in the following paragraph. The "Unlisted Services" and accompanying codes for the E/M section are as follows:

99429 **Unlisted preventive medicine service**

99499 **Unlisted evaluation and management service**

SPECIAL REPORT

An unlisted service or one that is unusual, variable, or new may require a special report demonstrating the medical appropriateness of the service. Pertinent information should include an adequate definition or description of the nature, extent, and need for the procedure and the time, effort, and equipment necessary to provide the service. Additional items that may be included are complexity of symptoms, final diagnosis, pertinent physical findings, diagnostic and therapeutic procedures, concurrent problems, and follow-up care.

INSTRUCTIONS FOR SELECTING A LEVEL OF E/M SERVICE

Review the Reporting Instructions for the Selected Category or Subcategory

Most of the categories and many of the subcategories of service have special guidelines or instructions unique to that category or subcategory. Where these are indicated, eg, "Inpatient Hospital Care," special instructions will be presented preceding the levels of E/M services.

Review the Level of E/M Service Descriptors and Examples in the Selected Category or Subcategory

The descriptors for the levels of E/M services recognize seven components, six of which are used in defining the levels of E/M services. These components are:

- History
- Examination
- Medical decision making
- Counseling
- Coordination of care
- Nature of presenting problem
- Time

The first three of these components (ie, history, examination, and medical decision making) should be considered the key components in selecting the level of E/M services. An exception to this rule is in the case of visits that consist predominantly of counseling or coordination of care.

The nature of the presenting problem and time are provided in some levels to assist the physician in determining the appropriate level of E/M service.

Determine the Extent of History Obtained

The extent of the history is dependent upon clinical judgment and on the nature of the presenting problem(s). The levels of E/M services recognize four types of history that are defined as follows:

Problem focused: Chief complaint; brief history of present illness or problem.

Expanded problem focused: Chief complaint; brief history of present illness; problem pertinent system review.

Detailed: Chief complaint; extended history of present illness; problem pertinent system review extended to include a review of a limited number of additional systems; pertinent past, family, and/or social history directly related to the patient's problems.

Comprehensive: Chief complaint; extended history of present illness; review of systems that is directly related to the problem(s) identified in the history of the present illness plus a review of all additional body systems; complete past, family, and social history.

The comprehensive history obtained as part of the preventive medicine E/M service is not problem-oriented and does not involve a chief complaint or present illness. It does, however, include a comprehensive system review and comprehensive or interval past, family, and social history as well as a comprehensive assessment/history of pertinent risk factors.

Determine the Extent of Examination Performed

The extent of the examination performed is dependent on clinical judgment and on the nature of the presenting problem(s). The levels of E/M services recognize four types of examination that are defined as follows:

Problem focused: A limited examination of the affected body area or organ system.

Expanded problem focused: A limited examination of the affected body area or organ system and other symptomatic or related organ system(s).

Detailed: An extended examination of the affected body area(s) and other symptomatic or related organ system(s).

Comprehensive: A general multisystem examination or a complete examination of a single organ system. Note: The comprehensive examination performed as part of the preventive medicine E/M service is multisystem, but its extent is based on age and risk factors identified.

For the purposes of these CPT definitions, the following body areas are recognized:

- Head, including the face
- Neck
- Chest, including breasts and axilla
- Abdomen
- Genitalia, groin, buttocks
- Back
- Each extremity

For the purposes of these CPT definitions, the following organ systems are recognized:

- Eyes
- Ears, nose, mouth, and throat
- Cardiovascular
- Respiratory
- Gastrointestinal
- Genitourinary
- Musculoskeletal
- Skin
- Neurologic
- Psychiatric
- Hematologic/lymphatic/immunologic

Determine the Complexity of Medical Decision Making

Medical decision making refers to the complexity of establishing a diagnosis and/or selecting a management option as measured by:

- The number of possible diagnoses and/or the number of management options that must be considered
- The amount and/or complexity of medical records, diagnostic tests, and/or other information that must be obtained, reviewed, and analyzed
- The risk of significant complications, morbidity, and/or mortality, as well as comorbidities associated with the patient's presenting problem(s), the diagnostic procedure(s), and/or the possible management options

Four types of medical decision making are recognized: straightforward, low complexity, moderate complexity, and high complexity. To qualify for a given type of decision making, two of the three elements in Table 1 must be met or exceeded.

Comorbidities and underlying diseases, in and of themselves, are not considered in selecting a level of E/M services unless their presence significantly increases the complexity of the medical decision making.

Select the Appropriate Level of E/M Services Based on the Following

For the following categories/subcategories, all of the key components, ie, history, examination, and medical decision making, must meet or exceed the stated requirements to qualify for a particular level of E/M service: office, new patient; hospital observation services; initial hospital care; office consultations; initial inpatient consultations; emergency department services; initial nursing facility care; domiciliary care, new patient; and home, new patient.

For the following categories/subcategories, two of the three key components (ie, history, examination, and medical decision making) must meet or exceed the stated requirements to qualify for a particular level of E/M services: office, established patient; subsequent hospital care; subsequent nursing facility care; domiciliary care, established patient; and home, established patient.

When counseling and/or coordination of care dominates (more than 50 percent) the encounter with the patient and/or family (face-to-face time in the office or other outpatient setting or floor/unit time in the hospital or nursing facility), then time shall be considered the key or controlling factor to qualify for a particular level of E/M services. This includes time spent with parties who have assumed responsibility for the care of the patient or decision making whether or not they are family members (e.g., foster parents, person acting in loco parentis, legal guardian). The extent of counseling and/or coordination of care must be documented in the medical record.

CONSULTATION CODES AND MEDICARE REIMBURSEMENT

The Centers for Medicare and Medicaid Services (CMS) no longer provides benefits for CPT consultation codes. CMS has, however, redistributed the value of the consultation codes across the other E/M codes for services which are covered by Medicare. CMS has retained codes 99241 - 99251 in the Medicare Physician Fee Schedule for those private payers that use this data for reimbursement. Note that private payers may choose to follow CMS or CPT guidelines, and the use of consultation codes should be verified with individual payers.

TABLE 1

Complexity of Medical Decision Making

Number of Diagnoses or Management Options	*Amount and/or Complexity of Data to be Reviewed*	*Risk of Complications and/or Morbidity or Mortality*	*Type of Decision Making*
minimal	minimal or none	minimal	straightforward
limited	limited	low	low complexity
multiple	moderate	moderate	moderate complexity
extensive	extensive	high	high complexity

99201-99215 Outpatient and Other Visits

CMS 100-3,70.3 Physician's Offices Within an Institution--"Incident-to" Provision

CMS 100-4,12,30.6.7 Payment for Office or Other Outpatient E&M Visits

INCLUDES Established patients: received prior professional services from the physician or qualified health care professional or another physician or qualified health care professional in the practice of the exact same specialty and subspecialty in the previous three years (99211-99215)

New patients: have not received professional services from the physician or qualified health care professional or any other physician or qualified health care professional in the same practice in the exact same specialty and subspecialty in the previous three years (99201-99205)

Office visits

Outpatient services (including services prior to a formal admission to a facility)

EXCLUDES *Services provided in:*

Emergency department (99281-99285)

Hospital observation (99217-99223 [99224, 99225, 99226])

Hospital observation or inpatient with same day admission and discharge (99234-99236)

99201 **Office or other outpatient visit for the evaluation and management of a new patient, which requires these 3 key components: A problem focused history; A problem focused examination; Straightforward medical decision making. Counseling and/or coordination of care with other physicians, other qualified health care professionals, or agencies are provided consistent with the nature of the problem(s) and the patient's and/or family's needs. Usually, the presenting problem(s) are self limited or minor. Typically, 10 minutes are spent face-to-face with the patient and/or family.**

B 80 PQ 0.74 1.21 FUD XXX

99202 **Office or other outpatient visit for the evaluation and management of a new patient, which requires these 3 key components: An expanded problem focused history; An expanded problem focused examination; Straightforward medical decision making. Counseling and/or coordination of care with other physicians, other qualified health care professionals, or agencies are provided consistent with the nature of the problem(s) and the patient's and/or family's needs. Usually, the presenting problem(s) are of low to moderate severity. Typically, 20 minutes are spent face-to-face with the patient and/or family.**

B 80 PQ 1.41 2.08 FUD XXX

99203 **Office or other outpatient visit for the evaluation and management of a new patient, which requires these 3 key components: A detailed history; A detailed examination; Medical decision making of low complexity. Counseling and/or coordination of care with other physicians, other qualified health care professionals, or agencies are provided consistent with the nature of the problem(s) and the patient's and/or family's needs. Usually, the presenting problem(s) are of moderate severity. Typically, 30 minutes are spent face-to-face with the patient and/or family.**

B 80 PQ 2.15 3.02 FUD XXX

99204 **Office or other outpatient visit for the evaluation and management of a new patient, which requires these 3 key components: A comprehensive history; A comprehensive examination; Medical decision making of moderate complexity. Counseling and/or coordination of care with other physicians, other qualified health care professionals, or agencies are provided consistent with the nature of the problem(s) and the patient's and/or family's needs. Usually, the presenting problem(s) are of moderate to high severity. Typically, 45 minutes are spent face-to-face with the patient and/or family.**

B 80 PQ 3.68 4.64 FUD XXX

99205 **Office or other outpatient visit for the evaluation and management of a new patient, which requires these 3 key components: A comprehensive history; A comprehensive examination; Medical decision making of high complexity. Counseling and/or coordination of care with other physicians, other qualified health care professionals, or agencies are provided consistent with the nature of the problem(s) and the patient's and/or family's needs. Usually, the presenting problem(s) are of moderate to high severity. Typically, 60 minutes are spent face-to-face with the patient and/or family.**

B 80 PQ 4.75 5.78 FUD XXX

99211 **Office or other outpatient visit for the evaluation and management of an established patient, that may not require the presence of a physician or other qualified health care professional. Usually, the presenting problem(s) are minimal. Typically, 5 minutes are spent performing or supervising these services.**

B 80 PQ 0.26 0.56 FUD XXX

99212 **Office or other outpatient visit for the evaluation and management of an established patient, which requires at least 2 of these 3 key components: A problem focused history; A problem focused examination; Straightforward medical decision making. Counseling and/or coordination of care with other physicians, other qualified health care professionals, or agencies are provided consistent with the nature of the problem(s) and the patient's and/or family's needs. Usually, the presenting problem(s) are self limited or minor. Typically, 10 minutes are spent face-to-face with the patient and/or family.**

B 80 PQ 0.71 1.22 FUD XXX

99213 **Office or other outpatient visit for the evaluation and management of an established patient, which requires at least 2 of these 3 key components: An expanded problem focused history; An expanded problem focused examination; Medical decision making of low complexity. Counseling and coordination of care with other physicians, other qualified health care professionals, or agencies are provided consistent with the nature of the problem(s) and the patient's and/or family's needs. Usually, the presenting problem(s) are of low to moderate severity. Typically, 15 minutes are spent face-to-face with the patient and/or family.**

B 80 PQ 1.44 2.04 FUD XXX

99214 **Office or other outpatient visit for the evaluation and management of an established patient, which requires at least 2 of these 3 key components: A detailed history; A detailed examination; Medical decision making of moderate complexity. Counseling and/or coordination of care with other physicians, other qualified health care professionals, or agencies are provided consistent with the nature of the problem(s) and the patient's and/or family's needs. Usually, the presenting problem(s) are of moderate to high severity. Typically, 25 minutes are spent face-to-face with the patient and/or family.**

B 80 PQ 2.21 3.01 FUD XXX

99215 **Office or other outpatient visit for the evaluation and management of an established patient, which requires at least 2 of these 3 key components: A comprehensive history; A comprehensive examination; Medical decision making of high complexity. Counseling and/or coordination of care with other physicians, other qualified health care professionals, or agencies are provided consistent with the nature of the problem(s) and the patient's and/or family's needs. Usually, the presenting problem(s) are of moderate to high severity. Typically, 40 minutes are spent face-to-face with the patient and/or family.**

B 80 PQ 3.11 4.03 FUD XXX

99217-99220 Facility Observation Visits: Initial and Discharge

CMS 100-1,5,70 Definition of Physician
CMS 100-2,15,30 Physician Services
CMS 100-3,70.1 Consultations with a Beneficiary's Family and Associates
CMS 100-4,12,30.6.8 Payment for Hospital Observation Services

INCLUDES Services provided on the same date in other settings or departments associated with the observation status admission (99201-99215, 99281-99285, 99304-99318, 99324-99337, 99341-99350, 99381-99429)
Services provided to new and established patients admitted to a hospital specifically for observation (not required to be a designated area of the hospital)

EXCLUDES *Services provided by physicians or another qualified health care professional other than the admitting physician ([99224, 99225, 99226], 99241-99245)*
Services provided to a patient admitted to the hospital following observation status (99221-99223)
Services provided to patients who are admitted and discharged from observation status on the same date (99234-99236)

99217 **Observation care discharge day management (This code is to be utilized to report all services provided to a patient on discharge from "observation status" if the discharge is on other than the initial date of "observation status." To report services to a patient designated as "observation status" or "inpatient status" and discharged on the same date, use the codes for Observation or Inpatient Care Services [including Admission and Discharge Services, 99234-99236 as appropriate.])**

INCLUDES Discussing the observation admission with the patient
Final patient evaluation:
Discharge instructions
Sign off on discharge medical records

Do not report with hospital inpatient care
Do not report with hospital discharge day management services (99238-99239)
Do not report with observation/inpatient admission/discharge on the same date (99234-99236)

B 80 PQ 2.03 2.03 FUD XXX

99218 **Initial observation care, per day, for the evaluation and management of a patient which requires these 3 key components: A detailed or comprehensive history; A detailed or comprehensive examination; and Medical decision making that is straightforward or of low complexity. Counseling and/or coordination of care with other physicians, other qualified health care professionals, or agencies are provided consistent with the nature of the problem(s) and the patient's and/or family's needs. Usually, the problem(s) requiring admission to "observation status" are of low severity. Typically, 30 minutes are spent at the bedside and on the patient's hospital floor or unit.**

B 80 PQ 2.78 2.78 FUD XXX

99219 **Initial observation care, per day, for the evaluation and management of a patient, which requires these 3 key components: A comprehensive history; A comprehensive examination; and Medical decision making of moderate complexity. Counseling and/or coordination of care with other physicians, other qualified health care professionals, or agencies are provided consistent with the nature of the problem(s) and the patient's and/or family's needs. Usually, the problem(s) requiring admission to "observation status" are of moderate severity. Typically, 50 minutes are spent at the bedside and on the patient's hospital floor or unit.**

B 80 PQ 3.80 3.80 FUD XXX

99220 **Initial observation care, per day, for the evaluation and management of a patient, which requires these 3 key components: A comprehensive history; A comprehensive examination; and Medical decision making of high complexity. Counseling and/or coordination of care with other physicians, other qualified health care professionals, or agencies are provided consistent with the nature of the problem(s) and the patient's and/or family's needs. Usually, the problem(s) requiring admission to "observation status" are of high severity. Typically, 70 minutes are spent at the bedside and on the patient's hospital floor or unit.**

B 80 PQ 5.20 5.20 FUD XXX

99224-99226 [99224, 99225, 99226] Facility Observation Visits: Subsequent

CMS 100-4,12,30.6.8 Payment for Hospital Observation Services

INCLUDES Changes in patient's status (e.g., physical condition, history; response to medical management)
Medical record review
Review of diagnostic test results

EXCLUDES *Observation admission and discharge on the same day (99234-99236)*

Do not report with (99221-99223, 99231-99233, 99238-99239)

99224 **Subsequent observation care, per day, for the evaluation and management of a patient, which requires at least 2 of these 3 key components: Problem focused interval history; Problem focused examination; Medical decision making that is straightforward or of low complexity. Counseling and/or coordination of care with other physicians, other qualified health care professionals, or agencies are provided consistent with the nature of the problem(s) and the patient's and/or family's needs. Usually, the patient is stable, recovering, or improving. Typically, 15 minutes are spent at the bedside and on the patient's hospital floor or unit.**

B 80 PQ 1.12 1.12 FUD XXX

\# **99225** **Subsequent observation care, per day, for the evaluation and management of a patient, which requires at least 2 of these 3 key components: An expanded problem focused interval history; An expanded problem focused examination; Medical decision making of moderate complexity. Counseling and/or coordination of care with other physicians, other qualified health care professionals, or agencies are provided consistent with the nature of the problem(s) and the patient's and/or family's needs. Usually, the patient is responding inadequately to therapy or has developed a minor complication. Typically, 25 minutes are spent at the bedside and on the patient's hospital floor or unit.**

B 80 PQ 2.03 2.03 FUD XXX

\# **99226** **Subsequent observation care, per day, for the evaluation and management of a patient, which requires at least 2 of these 3 key components: A detailed interval history; A detailed examination; Medical decision making of high complexity. Counseling and/or coordination of care with other physicians, other qualified health care professionals, or agencies are provided consistent with the nature of the problem(s) and the patient's and/or family's needs. Usually, the patient is unstable or has developed a significant complication or a significant new problem. Typically, 35 minutes are spent at the bedside and on the patient's hospital floor or unit.**

B 80 PQ 2.93 2.93 FUD XXX

99221-99233 Inpatient Hospital Visits: Initial and Subsequent

CMS 100-1,5,70 Definition of Physician
CMS 100-2,15,30 Physician Services
CMS 100-3,70.1 Consultations with a Beneficiary's Family and Associates
CMS 100-4,12,30.6.8 Payment for Hospital Observation Services
CMS 100-4,12,30.6.9 Hospital Visit and Critical Care on Same Day
CMS 100-4,12,30.6.9.1 Initial Hospital Care and Observation or Inpatient Care Services

INCLUDES All services provided on the date of admission in other sites of service (e.g., emergency department, office, nursing facility) (99201-99215, 99281-99285, 99304-99318, 99324-99337, 99341-99350, 99381-99397)
Initial physician services provided to the patient in the hospital or "partial" hospital settings (99221-99223)
Physician services provided to the patient in observation status on the same date as inpatient E&M service
Services provided to a new or established patient

EXCLUDES *Inpatient admission and discharge on the same date (99234-99236)*
Inpatient E&M services provided by other than the admitting physician

99221 **Initial hospital care, per day, for the evaluation and management of a patient, which requires these 3 key components: A detailed or comprehensive history; A detailed or comprehensive examination; and Medical decision making that is straightforward or of low complexity. Counseling and/or coordination of care with other physicians, other qualified health care professionals, or agencies are provided consistent with the nature of the problem(s) and the patient's and/or family's needs. Usually, the problem(s) requiring admission are of low severity. Typically, 30 minutes are spent at the bedside and on the patient's hospital floor or unit.**

B 80 CCI PQ 2.85 2.85 FUD XXX

99222 **Initial hospital care, per day, for the evaluation and management of a patient, which requires these 3 key components: A comprehensive history; A comprehensive examination; and Medical decision making of moderate complexity. Counseling and/or coordination of care with other physicians, other qualified health care professionals, or agencies are provided consistent with the nature of the problem(s) and the patient's and/or family's needs. Usually, the problem(s) requiring admission are of moderate severity. Typically, 50 minutes are spent at the bedside and on the patient's hospital floor or unit.**

B 80 CCI PQ 3.87 3.87 FUD XXX

99223 **Initial hospital care, per day, for the evaluation and management of a patient, which requires these 3 key components: A comprehensive history; A comprehensive examination; and Medical decision making of high complexity. Counseling and/or coordination of care with other physicians, other qualified health care professionals, or agencies are provided consistent with the nature of the problem(s) and the patient's and/or family's needs. Usually, the problem(s) requiring admission are of high severity. Typically, 70 minutes are spent at the bedside and on the patient's hospital floor or unit.**

B 80 CCI PQ 5.70 5.70 FUD XXX

99224 *Resequenced code. See code following 99220.*

99225 *Resequenced code. See code following 99220.*

99226 *Resequenced code. See code before 99221.*

99231 **Subsequent hospital care, per day, for the evaluation and management of a patient, which requires at least 2 of these 3 key components: A problem focused interval history; A problem focused examination; Medical decision making that is straightforward or of low complexity. Counseling and/or coordination of care with other physicians, other qualified health care professionals, or agencies are provided consistent with the nature of the problem(s) and the patient's and/or family's needs. Usually, the patient is stable, recovering or improving. Typically, 15 minutes are spent at the bedside and on the patient's hospital floor or unit.**

B 80 CCI PQ 1.10 1.10 FUD XXX

99232 **Subsequent hospital care, per day, for the evaluation and management of a patient, which requires at least 2 of these 3 key components: An expanded problem focused interval history; An expanded problem focused examination; Medical decision making of moderate complexity. Counseling and/or coordination of care with other physicians, other qualified health care professionals, or agencies are provided consistent with the nature of the problem(s) and the patient's and/or family's needs. Usually, the patient is responding inadequately to therapy or has developed a minor complication. Typically, 25 minutes are spent at the bedside and on the patient's hospital floor or unit.**

B 80 CCI PQ 2.02 2.02 FUD XXX

99233 **Subsequent hospital care, per day, for the evaluation and management of a patient, which requires at least 2 of these 3 key components: A detailed interval history; A detailed examination; Medical decision making of high complexity. Counseling and/or coordination of care with other physicians, other qualified health care professionals, or agencies are provided consistent with the nature of the problem(s) and the patient's and/or family's needs. Usually, the patient is unstable or has developed a significant complication or a significant new problem. Typically, 35 minutes are spent at the bedside and on the patient's hospital floor or unit.**

B 80 PQ 2.91 2.91 FUD XXX

99234-99236 Observation/Inpatient Visits: Admitted/Discharged on Same Date

CMS 100-1,5,70 Definition of Physician
CMS 100-2,15,30 Physician Services
CMS 100-3,70.1 Consultations with a Beneficiary's Family and Associates
CMS 100-4,12,30.6.8 Payment for Hospital Observation Services
CMS 100-4,12,30.6.9 Hospital Visit and Critical Care on Same Day
CMS 100-4,12,30.6.9.1 Initial Hospital Care and Observation or Inpatient Care Services
CMS 100-4,12,40.2 Global Surgery Billing Requirements

INCLUDES Admission and discharge services on the same date in an observation or inpatient setting
All services provided by admitting physician or other qualified health care professional on same date of service, even when initiated in another setting (e.g., emergency department, nursing facility, office)

EXCLUDES *Services provided to patients admitted to observation and discharged on a different date (99217-99220, [99224, 99225, 99226])*

99234 **Observation or inpatient hospital care, for the evaluation and management of a patient including admission and discharge on the same date, which requires these 3 key components: A detailed or comprehensive history; A detailed or comprehensive examination; and Medical decision making that is straightforward or of low complexity. Counseling and/or coordination of care with other physicians, other qualified health care professionals, or agencies are provided consistent with the nature of the problem(s) and the patient's and/or family's needs. Usually the presenting problem(s) requiring admission are of low severity. Typically, 40 minutes are spent at the bedside and on the patient's hospital floor or unit.**

B 80 PQ 3.79 3.79 FUD XXX

99235 **Observation or inpatient hospital care, for the evaluation and management of a patient including admission and discharge on the same date, which requires these 3 key components: A comprehensive history; A comprehensive examination; and Medical decision making of moderate complexity. Counseling and/or coordination of care with other physicians, other qualified health care professionals, or agencies are provided consistent with the nature of the problem(s) and the patient's and/or family's needs. Usually the presenting problem(s) requiring admission are of moderate severity. Typically, 50 minutes are spent at the bedside and on the patient's hospital floor or unit.**

B 80 PQ 4.74 4.74 FUD XXX

99236 **Observation or inpatient hospital care, for the evaluation and management of a patient including admission and discharge on the same date, which requires these 3 key components: A comprehensive history; A comprehensive examination; and Medical decision making of high complexity. Counseling and/or coordination of care with other physicians, other qualified health care professionals, or agencies are provided consistent with the nature of the problem(s) and the patient's and/or family's needs. Usually the presenting problem(s) requiring admission are of high severity. Typically, 55 minutes are spent at the bedside and on the patient's hospital floor or unit.**

B 80 PQ 6.12 6.12 FUD XXX

99238-99239 Inpatient Hospital Discharge Services

CMS 100-4,12,30.6.9.2 Hospital Discharge Management

INCLUDES All services on discharge day when discharge and admission are not the same day
Discharge instructions
Final patient evaluation
Final preparation of the patient's medical records
Provision of prescriptions/referrals, as needed
Review of the inpatient admission

EXCLUDES *Admission/discharge on same date (99234-99236)*
Discharge from observation (99217)
Discharge from nursing facility (99315, 99316)
Discharge services for newborns admitted and discharged the same day (99463)
Healthy newborn evaluated and discharged on same date (99463)
Services provided by other than attending physician or other qualified health care professional on date of discharge (99231-99233)

99238 **Hospital discharge day management; 30 minutes or less**

B 80 PQ 2.03 2.03 FUD XXX

99239 **more than 30 minutes**

B 80 PQ 3.00 3.00 FUD XXX

99241-99245 Consultations: Office and Outpatient

CMS 100-1,5,70 Definition of Physician
CMS 100-2,15,30 Physician Services
CMS 100-3,70.1 Consultations with a Beneficiary's Family and Associates
CMS 100-4,12,30.6.10 Consultation Services

INCLUDES A third-party mandated consultation
All outpatient consultations provided in the office, outpatient or other ambulatory facility, domiciliary/rest home, emergency department, patient's home, and hospital observation
Documentation of a request for a consultation from an appropriate source
Documentation of the need for consultation in the patient's medical record
One consultation per consultant
Provision by a physician or qualified nonphysician practitioner whose advice, opinion, recommendation, suggestion, direction, or counsel, etc., is requested for evaluating/treating a patient since that individual's expertise in a specific medical area is beyond the scope of knowledge of the requesting physician
Provision of a written report of findings/recommendations from the consultant to the referring physician

EXCLUDES *Another appropriately requested and documented consultation pertaining to the same/new problem; repeat use of consultation codes*
Any distinctly recognizable procedure/service provided on or following the consultation
Assumption of care (all or partial); report subsequent codes as appropriate for the place of service (99211-99215, 99334-99337, 99347-99350)
Consultation prompted by the patient/family; report codes for office, domiciliary/rest home, or home visits instead (99201-99215, 99324-99337, 99341-99350)

Do not report when services are provided to Medicare and Medicaid patients

99241 **Office consultation for a new or established patient, which requires these 3 key components: A problem focused history; A problem focused examination; and Straightforward medical decision making. Counseling and/or coordination of care with other physicians, other qualified health care professionals, or agencies are provided consistent with the nature of the problem(s) and the patient's and/or family's needs. Usually, the presenting problem(s) are self limited or minor. Typically, 15 minutes are spent face-to-face with the patient and/or family.**

E 0.95 1.37 FUD XXX

99242 **Office consultation for a new or established patient, which requires these 3 key components: An expanded problem focused history; An expanded problem focused examination; and Straightforward medical decision making. Counseling and/or coordination of care with other physicians, other qualified health care professionals, or agencies are provided consistent with the nature of the problem(s) and the patient's and/or family's needs. Usually, the presenting problem(s) are of low severity. Typically, 30 minutes are spent face-to-face with the patient and/or family.**

E 1.98 2.57 FUD XXX

99243 **Office consultation for a new or established patient, which requires these 3 key components: A detailed history; A detailed examination; and Medical decision making of low complexity. Counseling and/or coordination of care with other physicians, other qualified health care professionals, or agencies are provided consistent with the nature of the problem(s) and the patient's and/or family's needs. Usually, the presenting problem(s) are of moderate severity. Typically, 40 minutes are spent face-to-face with the patient and/or family.**

E 2.76 3.51 FUD XXX

99244 **Office consultation for a new or established patient, which requires these 3 key components: A comprehensive history; A comprehensive examination; and Medical decision making of moderate complexity. Counseling and/or coordination of care with other physicians, other qualified health care professionals, or agencies are provided consistent with the nature of the problem(s) and the patient's and/or family's needs. Usually, the presenting problem(s) are of moderate to high severity. Typically, 60 minutes are spent face-to-face with the patient and/or family.**

E 4.37 5.19 FUD XXX

99245 **Office consultation for a new or established patient, which requires these 3 key components: A comprehensive history; A comprehensive examination; and Medical decision making of high complexity. Counseling and/or coordination of care with other physicians, other qualified health care professionals, or agencies are provided consistent with the nature of the problem(s) and the patient's and/or family's needs. Usually, the presenting problem(s) are of moderate to high severity. Typically, 80 minutes are spent face-to-face with the patient and/or family.**

E 5.43 6.35 FUD XXX

99251-99255 Consultations: Inpatient

CMS 100-1,5,70 Definition of Physician
CMS 100-2,15,30 Physician Services
CMS 100-3,70.1 Consultations with a Beneficiary's Family and Associates
CMS 100-4,12,30.6.10 Consultation Services

INCLUDES A third-party mandated consultation
All inpatient consultations include services provided in the hospital inpatient or partial hospital settings and nursing facilities
Documentation of a request for a consultation from an appropriate source
Documentation of the need for consultation in the patient's medical record
One consultation by consultant per admission
Provision by a physician or qualified nonphysician practitioner whose advice, opinion, recommendation, suggestion, direction, or counsel, etc. is requested for evaluating/treating a patient since that individual's expertise in a specific medical area is beyond the scope of knowledge of the requesting physician
Provision of a written report of findings/recommendations from the consultant to the referring physician

EXCLUDES *Another appropriately requested and documented consultation pertaining to the same/new problem: repeat use of consultation codes*
Any distinctly recognizable procedure/service provided on or following the consultation
Assumption of care (all or partial): report subsequent codes as appropriate for the place of service (99231-99233, 99307-99310)
Consultation prompted by the patient/family: report codes for office, domiciliary/rest home, or home visits instead (99201-99215, 99324-99337, 99341-99350)

Do not report an outpatient consultation and an inpatient consultation for the same admission (99241-99245, 99251-99255)
Do not report when services are provided to Medicare and Medicaid patients

99251 **Inpatient consultation for a new or established patient, which requires these 3 key components: A problem focused history; A problem focused examination; and Straightforward medical decision making. Counseling and/or coordination of care with other physicians, other qualified health care professionals, or agencies are provided consistent with the nature of the problem(s) and the patient's and/or family's needs. Usually, the presenting problem(s) are self limited or minor. Typically, 20 minutes are spent at the bedside and on the patient's hospital floor or unit.**

E 1.39 1.39 FUD XXX

99252 **Inpatient consultation for a new or established patient, which requires these 3 key components: An expanded problem focused history; An expanded problem focused examination; and Straightforward medical decision making. Counseling and/or coordination of care with other physicians, other qualified health care professionals, or agencies are provided consistent with the nature of the problem(s) and the patient's and/or family's needs. Usually, the presenting problem(s) are of low severity. Typically, 40 minutes are spent at the bedside and on the patient's hospital floor or unit.**

E 2.13 2.13 FUD XXX

99253 **Inpatient consultation for a new or established patient, which requires these 3 key components: A detailed history; A detailed examination; and Medical decision making of low complexity. Counseling and/or coordination of care with other physicians, other qualified health care professionals, or agencies are provided consistent with the nature of the problem(s) and the patient's and/or family's needs. Usually, the presenting problem(s) are of moderate severity. Typically, 55 minutes are spent at the bedside and on the patient's hospital floor or unit.**

E 3.25 3.25 FUD XXX

99254 Inpatient consultation for a new or established patient, which requires these 3 key components: A comprehensive history; A comprehensive examination; and Medical decision making of moderate complexity. Counseling and/or coordination of care with other physicians, other qualified health care professionals, or agencies are provided consistent with the nature of the problem(s) and the patient's and/or family's needs. Usually, the presenting problem(s) are of moderate to high severity. Typically, 80 minutes are spent at the bedside and on the patient's hospital floor or unit.

E 4.69 4.69 FUD XXX

99255 Inpatient consultation for a new or established patient, which requires these 3 key components: A comprehensive history; A comprehensive examination; and Medical decision making of high complexity. Counseling and/or coordination of care with other physicians, other qualified health care professionals, or agencies are provided consistent with the nature of the problem(s) and the patient's and/or family's needs. Usually, the presenting problem(s) are of moderate to high severity. Typically, 110 minutes are spent at the bedside and on the patient's hospital floor or unit.

E 5.67 5.67 FUD XXX

99281-99288 Emergency Department Visits

CMS 100-1,5,70 Definition of Physician
CMS 100-2,15,30 Physician Services
CMS 100-3,70.1 Consultations with a Beneficiary's Family and Associates
CMS 100-4,12,30.6.11 Emergency Department Visits

INCLUDES Any amount of time spent with the patient, which usually involves a series of encounters while the patient is in the emergency department
Care provided to new and established patients

EXCLUDES *Critical care services (99291-99292)*
Observation services (99217-99220, 99234-99236)

99281 Emergency department visit for the evaluation and management of a patient, which requires these 3 key components: A problem focused history; A problem focused examination; and Straightforward medical decision making. Counseling and/or coordination of care with other physicians, other qualified health care professionals, or agencies are provided consistent with the nature of the problem(s) and the patient's and/or family's needs. Usually, the presenting problem(s) are self limited or minor.

V 80 PQ 0.59 0.59 FUD XXX

99282 Emergency department visit for the evaluation and management of a patient, which requires these 3 key components: An expanded problem focused history; An expanded problem focused examination; and Medical decision making of low complexity. Counseling and/or coordination of care with other physicians, other qualified health care professionals, or agencies are provided consistent with the nature of the problem(s) and the patient's and/or family's needs. Usually, the presenting problem(s) are of low to moderate severity.

V 80 PQ 1.16 1.16 FUD XXX

99283 Emergency department visit for the evaluation and management of a patient, which requires these 3 key components: An expanded problem focused history; An expanded problem focused examination; and Medical decision making of moderate complexity. Counseling and/or coordination of care with other physicians, other qualified health care professionals, or agencies are provided consistent with the nature of the problem(s) and the patient's and/or family's needs. Usually, the presenting problem(s) are of moderate severity.

V 80 PQ 1.73 1.73 FUD XXX

99284 Emergency department visit for the evaluation and management of a patient, which requires these 3 key components: A detailed history; A detailed examination; and Medical decision making of moderate complexity. Counseling and/or coordination of care with other physicians, other qualified health care professionals or agencies are provided consistent with the nature of the problem(s) and the patient's and/or family's needs. Usually, the presenting problem(s) are of high severity, and require urgent evaluation by the physician or other qualified health care professionals but do not pose an immediate significant threat to life or physiologic function.

03 80 PQ 3.30 3.30 FUD XXX

99285 Emergency department visit for the evaluation and management of a patient, which requires these 3 key components within the constraints imposed by the urgency of the patient's clinical condition and/or mental status: A comprehensive history; A comprehensive examination; and Medical decision making of high complexity. Counseling and/or coordination of care with other physicians, other qualified health care professionals, or agencies are provided consistent with the nature of the problem(s) and the patient's and/or family's needs. Usually, the presenting problem(s) are of high severity and pose an immediate significant threat to life or physiologic function.

03 80 PQ 4.85 4.85 FUD XXX

99288 Physician or other qualified health care professional direction of emergency medical systems (EMS) emergency care, advanced life support

INCLUDES Management provided by an emergency/intensive care based physician or other qualified health care professional via voice contact to ambulance/rescue staff for services such as heart monitoring and drug administration

B 0.00 0.00 FUD XXX

99291-99292 Critical Care Visits: Patients 72 Months of Age and Older

CMS 100-1,5,70 Definition of Physician
CMS 100-2,15,30 Physician Services
CMS 100-3,70.1 Consultations with a Beneficiary's Family and Associates
CMS 100-4,12,30.6.9 Hospital Visit and Critical Care on Same Day
CMS 100-4,12,30.6.12 Critical Care Visits

INCLUDES 30 minutes or more of direct care provided by the physician or other qualified health care professional to a critically ill or injured patient, regardless of the location
All time spent exclusively with patient/family/caregivers on the nursing unit or elsewhere
Outpatient critical care provided to neonates and pediatric patients up through 71 months of age
Physician or other qualified health care professional presence during interfacility transfer for critically ill/injured patients over 24 months of age
Professional services for interpretation of:
Blood gases
Chest films (71010, 71015, 71020)
Measurement of cardiac output (93561-93562)
Other computer stored information (99090)
Pulse oximetry (94760-94762)
Professional services for:
Gastric intubation (43752-43753)
Transcutaneous pacing, temporary (92953)
Ventilation assistance and management, includes CPAP, CNP (94002-94004, 94660, 94662)
Venous access, arterial puncture (36000, 36410, 36415, 36591, 36600)

EXCLUDES *All services that are less than 30 minutes; report appropriate E&M code*
Critical care services provided via remote real-time interactive videoconferencing (0188T, 0189T)
Inpatient critical care services provided to child 2 through 5 years of age (99475-99476)
Inpatient critical care services provided to infants 29 days through 24 months of age (99471-99472)
Inpatient critical care services provided to neonates that are age 28 days or less (99468-99469)
Other procedures not listed as included performed by the physician or other qualified health care professional rendering critical care
Patients who are not critically ill but in the critical care department (report appropriate E&M code)
Physician or other qualified health care professional presence during interfacility transfer for critically ill/injured patients under 24 months of age (99466-99467)
Supervisory services of control physician during interfacility transfer for critically ill/injured patients under 24 months of age ([99485, 99486])

Do not report activities performed outside of the unit or off the floor

99291 Critical care, evaluation and management of the critically ill or critically injured patient; first 30-74 minutes
Q3 80 CCI PQ 6.27 7.67 FUD XXX

\+ **99292 each additional 30 minutes (List separately in addition to code for primary service)**
Code first (99291)
N 80 CCI 3.14 3.44 FUD ZZZ

99304-99310 Nursing Facility Visits

CMS 100-1,5,70 Definition of Physician
CMS 100-2,15,30 Physician Services
CMS 100-3,70.1 Consultations with a Beneficiary's Family and Associates
CMS 100-3,70.2 Consultation by a Podiatrist in a Skilled Nursing Facility
CMS 100-3,70.3 Physician's Offices Within an Institution--"Incident-to" Provision
CMS 100-4,12,30.6.9 Swing Bed Visits
CMS 100-4,12,30.6.13 Nursing Facility Visits

INCLUDES All E&M services provided by the admitting physician on the date of nursing facility admission in other locations (e.g., office, emergency department)
Initial care, subsequent care, discharge, and yearly assessments
Initial services include patient assessment and physician participation in developing a plan of care (99304-99306)
Services provided in a psychiatric residential treatment center
Services provided to new and established patients in a nursing facility (skilled, intermediate, and long-term care facilities)
Subsequent services include physician review of medical records, reassessment, and review of test results (99307-99310)

EXCLUDES *Care plan oversight services (99379-99380)*

Code also hospital discharge services on the same date of admission or readmission to the nursing home (99217, 99234-99236, 99238-99239)

99304 Initial nursing facility care, per day, for the evaluation and management of a patient, which requires these 3 key components: A detailed or comprehensive history; A detailed or comprehensive examination; and Medical decision making that is straightforward or of low complexity. Counseling and/or coordination of care with other physicians, other qualified health care professionals, or agencies are provided consistent with the nature of the problem(s) and the patient's and/or family's needs. Usually, the problem(s) requiring admission are of low severity. Typically, 25 minutes are spent at the bedside and on the patient's facility floor or unit.
B 80 PQ 2.61 2.61 FUD XXX

99305 Initial nursing facility care, per day, for the evaluation and management of a patient, which requires these 3 key components: A comprehensive history; A comprehensive examination; and Medical decision making of moderate complexity. Counseling and/or coordination of care with other physicians, other qualified health care professionals, or agencies are provided consistent with the nature of the problem(s) and the patient's and/or family's needs. Usually, the problem(s) requiring admission are of moderate severity. Typically, 35 minutes are spent at the bedside and on the patient's facility floor or unit.
B 80 PQ 3.72 3.72 FUD XXX

99306 Initial nursing facility care, per day, for the evaluation and management of a patient, which requires these 3 key components: A comprehensive history; A comprehensive examination; and Medical decision making of high complexity. Counseling and/or coordination of care with other physicians, other qualified health care professionals, or agencies are provided consistent with the nature of the problem(s) and the patient's and/or family's needs. Usually, the problem(s) requiring admission are of high severity. Typically, 45 minutes are spent at the bedside and on the patient's facility floor or unit.
B 80 PQ 4.71 4.71 FUD XXX

99307 **Subsequent nursing facility care, per day, for the evaluation and management of a patient, which requires at least 2 of these 3 key components: A problem focused interval history; A problem focused examination; Straightforward medical decision making. Counseling and/or coordination of care with other physicians, other qualified health care professionals, or agencies are provided consistent with the nature of the problem(s) and the patient's and/or family's needs. Usually, the patient is stable, recovering, or improving. Typically, 10 minutes are spent at the bedside and on the patient's facility floor or unit.**
B 80 PQ 1.25 1.25 FUD XXX

99308 **Subsequent nursing facility care, per day, for the evaluation and management of a patient, which requires at least 2 of these 3 key components: An expanded problem focused interval history; An expanded problem focused examination; Medical decision making of low complexity. Counseling and/or coordination of care with other physicians, other qualified health care professionals, or agencies are provided consistent with the nature of the problem(s) and the patient's and/or family's needs. Usually, the patient is responding inadequately to therapy or has developed a minor complication. Typically, 15 minutes are spent at the bedside and on the patient's facility floor or unit.**
B 80 PQ 1.93 1.93 FUD XXX

99309 **Subsequent nursing facility care, per day, for the evaluation and management of a patient, which requires at least 2 of these 3 key components: A detailed interval history; A detailed examination; Medical decision making of moderate complexity. Counseling and/or coordination of care with other physicians, other qualified health care professionals, or agencies are provided consistent with the nature of the problem(s) and the patient's and/or family's needs. Usually, the patient has developed a significant complication or a significant new problem. Typically, 25 minutes are spent at the bedside and on the patient's facility floor or unit.**
B 80 PQ 2.54 2.54 FUD XXX

99310 **Subsequent nursing facility care, per day, for the evaluation and management of a patient, which requires at least 2 of these 3 key components: A comprehensive interval history; A comprehensive examination; Medical decision making of high complexity. Counseling and/or coordination of care with other physicians, other qualified health care professionals, or agencies are provided consistent with the nature of the problem(s) and the patient's and/or family's needs. The patient may be unstable or may have developed a significant new problem requiring immediate physician attention. Typically, 35 minutes are spent at the bedside and on the patient's facility floor or unit.**
B 80 PQ 3.78 3.78 FUD XXX

99315-99316 Nursing Home Discharge

INCLUDES Discharge services include all time spent by the physician or other qualified health care professional for:
- Complete discharge records
- Discharge instructions for patient and caregivers
- Discussion regarding the stay in the facility
- Final patient examination
- Provide prescriptions and referrals as appropriate

99315 **Nursing facility discharge day management; 30 minutes or less**
B 80 PQ 2.05 2.05 FUD XXX

99316 **more than 30 minutes**
B 80 PQ 2.94 2.94 FUD XXX

99318 Annual Nursing Home Assessment

Do not report on same date of service as (99304-99316)

99318 **Evaluation and management of a patient involving an annual nursing facility assessment, which requires these 3 key components: A detailed interval history; A comprehensive examination; and Medical decision making that is of low to moderate complexity. Counseling and/or coordination of care with other physicians, other qualified health care professionals, or agencies are provided consistent with the nature of the problem(s) and the patient's and/or family's needs. Usually, the patient is stable, recovering, or improving. Typically, 30 minutes are spent at the bedside and on the patient's facility floor or unit.**
B 80 PQ 2.69 2.69 FUD XXX

99324-99337 Domiciliary Care, Rest Home, Assisted Living Visits

CMS 100-3,70.1 Consultations with a Beneficiary's Family and Associates

CMS 100-4,12,30.6.14 Domiciliary Care, Rest Home, Assisted Living Visits

INCLUDES E&M services for patients residing in assisted living, domiciliary care, and rest homes where medical care is not included

Services provided to new patients or established patients (99324-99328 or 99334-99337)

EXCLUDES *Care plan oversight services provided to a patient in a rest home but under the care of a home health agency (99374-99375)*

Care plan oversight services provided to a patient under the care of a hospice agency (99377-99378)

99324 **Domiciliary or rest home visit for the evaluation and management of a new patient, which requires these 3 key components: A problem focused history; A problem focused examination; and Straightforward medical decision making. Counseling and/or coordination of care with other physicians, other qualified health care professionals, or agencies are provided consistent with the nature of the problem(s) and the patient's and/or family's needs. Usually, the presenting problem(s) are of low severity. Typically, 20 minutes are spent with the patient and/or family or caregiver.**
B 80 PQ 1.56 1.56 FUD XXX

99325 **Domiciliary or rest home visit for the evaluation and management of a new patient, which requires these 3 key components: An expanded problem focused history; An expanded problem focused examination; and Medical decision making of low complexity. Counseling and/or coordination of care with other physicians, other qualified health care professionals, or agencies are provided consistent with the nature of the problem(s) and the patient's and/or family's needs. Usually, the presenting problem(s) are of moderate severity. Typically, 30 minutes are spent with the patient and/or family or caregiver.**
B 80 PQ 2.27 2.27 FUD XXX

99326 **Domiciliary or rest home visit for the evaluation and management of a new patient, which requires these 3 key components: A detailed history; A detailed examination; and Medical decision making of moderate complexity. Counseling and/or coordination of care with other physicians, other qualified health care professionals, or agencies are provided consistent with the nature of the problem(s) and the patient's and/or family's needs. Usually, the presenting problem(s) are of moderate to high severity. Typically, 45 minutes are spent with the patient and/or family or caregiver.**
B 80 PQ 3.91 3.91 FUD XXX

99327 **Domiciliary or rest home visit for the evaluation and management of a new patient, which requires these 3 key components: A comprehensive history; A comprehensive examination; and Medical decision making of moderate complexity. Counseling and/or coordination of care with other physicians, other qualified health care professionals, or agencies are provided consistent with the nature of the problem(s) and the patient's and/or family's needs. Usually, the presenting problem(s) are of high severity. Typically, 60 minutes are spent with the patient and/or family or caregiver.**

B 80 PQ 5.22 5.22 FUD XXX

99328 **Domiciliary or rest home visit for the evaluation and management of a new patient, which requires these 3 key components: A comprehensive history; A comprehensive examination; and Medical decision making of high complexity. Counseling and/or coordination of care with other physicians, other qualified health care professionals, or agencies are provided consistent with the nature of the problem(s) and the patient's and/or family's needs. Usually, the patient is unstable or has developed a significant new problem requiring immediate physician attention. Typically, 75 minutes are spent with the patient and/or family or caregiver.**

B 80 PQ 6.05 6.05 FUD XXX

99334 **Domiciliary or rest home visit for the evaluation and management of an established patient, which requires at least 2 of these 3 key components: A problem focused interval history; A problem focused examination; Straightforward medical decision making. Counseling and/or coordination of care with other physicians, other qualified health care professionals, or agencies are provided consistent with the nature of the problem(s) and the patient's and/or family's needs. Usually, the presenting problem(s) are self-limited or minor. Typically, 15 minutes are spent with the patient and/or family or caregiver.**

B 80 PQ 1.70 1.70 FUD XXX

99335 **Domiciliary or rest home visit for the evaluation and management of an established patient, which requires at least 2 of these 3 key components: An expanded problem focused interval history; An expanded problem focused examination; Medical decision making of low complexity. Counseling and/or coordination of care with other physicians, other qualified health care professionals, or agencies are provided consistent with the nature of the problem(s) and the patient's and/or family's needs. Usually, the presenting problem(s) are of low to moderate severity. Typically, 25 minutes are spent with the patient and/or family or caregiver.**

B 80 PQ 2.66 2.66 FUD XXX

99336 **Domiciliary or rest home visit for the evaluation and management of an established patient, which requires at least 2 of these 3 key components: A detailed interval history; A detailed examination; Medical decision making of moderate complexity. Counseling and/or coordination of care with other physicians, other qualified health care professionals, or agencies are provided consistent with the nature of the problem(s) and the patient's and/or family's needs. Usually, the presenting problem(s) are of moderate to high severity. Typically, 40 minutes are spent with the patient and/or family or caregiver.**

B 80 PQ 3.75 3.75 FUD XXX

99337 **Domiciliary or rest home visit for the evaluation and management of an established patient, which requires at least 2 of these 3 key components: A comprehensive interval history; A comprehensive examination; Medical decision making of moderate to high complexity. Counseling and/or coordination of care with other physicians, other qualified health care professionals, or agencies are provided consistent with the nature of the problem(s) and the patient's and/or family's needs. Usually, the presenting problem(s) are of moderate to high severity. The patient may be unstable or may have developed a significant new problem requiring immediate physician attention. Typically, 60 minutes are spent with the patient and/or family or caregiver.**

B 80 PQ 5.41 5.41 FUD XXX

99339-99340 Care Plan Oversight: Rest Home, Domiciliary Care, Assisted Living, and Home

CMS 100-4,12,30.6.14 Domiciliary Care, Rest Home, Assisted Living Visits

INCLUDES Care plan oversight for patients residing in assisted living, domiciliary care, private residences, and rest homes

EXCLUDES *Care plan oversight services furnished under a home health agency, nursing facility, or hospice (99374 99380)*

Do not report during the same period of time as (99441-99444, 99487, 99489, 99495-99496, 98966-98969)

99339 **Individual physician supervision of a patient (patient not present) in home, domiciliary or rest home (eg, assisted living facility) requiring complex and multidisciplinary care modalities involving regular physician development and/or revision of care plans, review of subsequent reports of patient status, review of related laboratory and other studies, communication (including telephone calls) for purposes of assessment or care decisions with health care professional(s), family member(s), surrogate decision maker(s) (eg, legal guardian) and/or key caregiver(s) involved in patient's care, integration of new information into the medical treatment plan and/or adjustment of medical therapy, within a calendar month; 15-29 minutes**

B 2.19 2.19 FUD XXX

99340 **30 minutes or more**

B PQ 3.06 3.06 FUD XXX

99341-99350 Home Visits

CMS 100-4,12,30.6.14.1 Home Visits

INCLUDES Services for a new patient or an established patient (99341-99345 or 99347-99350)

Services provided to a patient in a private home

EXCLUDES *Services provided to patients under home health agency or hospice care (99374-99378)*

99341 **Home visit for the evaluation and management of a new patient, which requires these 3 key components: A problem focused history; A problem focused examination; and Straightforward medical decision making. Counseling and/or coordination of care with other physicians, other qualified health care professionals, or agencies are provided consistent with the nature of the problem(s) and the patient's and/or family's needs. Usually, the presenting problem(s) are of low severity. Typically, 20 minutes are spent face-to-face with the patient and/or family.**

B 80 CCI PQ 1.55 1.55 FUD XXX

99342 Home visit for the evaluation and management of a new patient, which requires these 3 key components: An expanded problem focused history; An expanded problem focused examination; and Medical decision making of low complexity. Counseling and/or coordination of care with other physicians, other qualified health care professionals, or agencies are provided consistent with the nature of the problem(s) and the patient's and/or family's needs. Usually, the presenting problem(s) are of moderate severity. Typically, 30 minutes are spent face-to-face with the patient and/or family.
B 80 PQ 2.24 2.24 FUD XXX

99343 Home visit for the evaluation and management of a new patient, which requires these 3 key components: A detailed history; A detailed examination; and Medical decision making of moderate complexity. Counseling and/or coordination of care with other physicians, other qualified health care professionals, or agencies are provided consistent with the nature of the problem(s) and the patient's and/or family's needs. Usually, the presenting problem(s) are of moderate to high severity. Typically, 45 minutes are spent face-to-face with the patient and/or family.
B 80 PQ 3.66 3.66 FUD XXX

99344 Home visit for the evaluation and management of a new patient, which requires these 3 key components: A comprehensive history; A comprehensive examination; and Medical decision making of moderate complexity. Counseling and/or coordination of care with other physicians, other qualified health care professionals, or agencies are provided consistent with the nature of the problem(s) and the patient's and/or family's needs. Usually, the presenting problem(s) are of high severity. Typically, 60 minutes are spent face-to-face with the patient and/or family.
B 80 PQ 5.11 5.11 FUD XXX

99345 Home visit for the evaluation and management of a new patient, which requires these 3 key components: A comprehensive history; A comprehensive examination; and Medical decision making of high complexity. Counseling and/or coordination of care with other physicians, other qualified health care professionals, or agencies are provided consistent with the nature of the problem(s) and the patient's and/or family's needs. Usually, the patient is unstable or has developed a significant new problem requiring immediate physician attention. Typically, 75 minutes are spent face-to-face with the patient and/or family.
B 80 PQ 6.16 6.16 FUD XXX

99347 Home visit for the evaluation and management of an established patient, which requires at least 2 of these 3 key components: A problem focused interval history; A problem focused examination; Straightforward medical decision making. Counseling and/or coordination of care with other physicians, other qualified health care professionals, or agencies are provided consistent with the nature of the problem(s) and the patient's and/or family's needs. Usually, the presenting problem(s) are self limited or minor. Typically, 15 minutes are spent face-to-face with the patient and/or family.
B 80 PQ 1.56 1.56 FUD XXX

99348 Home visit for the evaluation and management of an established patient, which requires at least 2 of these 3 key components: An expanded problem focused interval history; An expanded problem focused examination; Medical decision making of low complexity. Counseling and/or coordination of care with other physicians, other qualified health care professionals, or agencies are provided consistent with the nature of the problem(s) and the patient's and/or family's needs. Usually, the presenting problem(s) are of low to moderate severity. Typically, 25 minutes are spent face-to-face with the patient and/or family.
B 80 PQ 2.36 2.36 FUD XXX

99349 Home visit for the evaluation and management of an established patient, which requires at least 2 of these 3 key components: A detailed interval history; A detailed examination; Medical decision making of moderate complexity. Counseling and/or coordination of care with other physicians, other qualified health care professionals, or agencies are provided consistent with the nature of the problem(s) and the patient's and/or family's needs. Usually, the presenting problem(s) are moderate to high severity. Typically, 40 minutes are spent face-to-face with the patient and/or family.
B 80 PQ 3.57 3.57 FUD XXX

99350 Home visit for the evaluation and management of an established patient, which requires at least 2 of these 3 key components: A comprehensive interval history; A comprehensive examination; Medical decision making of moderate to high complexity. Counseling and/or coordination of care with other physicians, other qualified health care professionals, or agencies are provided consistent with the nature of the problem(s) and the patient's and/or family's needs. Usually, the presenting problem(s) are of moderate to high severity. The patient may be unstable or may have developed a significant new problem requiring immediate physician attention. Typically, 60 minutes are spent face-to-face with the patient and/or family.
B 80 PQ 4.98 4.98 FUD XXX

99354-99357 Prolonged Services Direct Contact

CMS 100-1,5,70 Definition of Physician
CMS 100-2,15,30 Physician Services
CMS 100-4,12,30.6.15.1 Prolonged Services With Direct Face-to-Face Patient Contact

INCLUDES Personal contact with the patient by the physician or other qualified health professional (99354-99357)
Services that extend beyond the customary service provided in the inpatient or outpatient setting
Time spent providing additional indirect contact services on the floor or unit of the hospital or nursing facility during the same session as the direct contact
Time spent providing prolonged services on a date of service, even when the time is not continuous

EXCLUDES *Services provided independent of the date of personal contact with the patient (99358-99359)*

Do not report any service of less than 30 minutes, or less than 15 minutes after the first hour or after the final 30 minutes

\+ **99354** Prolonged service in the office or other outpatient setting requiring direct patient contact beyond the usual service; first hour (List separately in addition to code for office or other outpatient Evaluation and Management service)
Code first (99201-99215, 99241-99245, 99324-99337, 99341-99350, 90837)
N 80 2.61 2.80 FUD ZZZ

+ 99355 each additional 30 minutes (List separately in addition to code for prolonged service)

Code first (99354)

N 80 2.55 2.74 FUD ZZZ

+ 99356 Prolonged service in the inpatient or observation setting, requiring unit/floor time beyond the usual service; first hour (List separately in addition to code for inpatient Evaluation and Management service)

Code first (99218-99223 [99224, 99225, 99226], 99231-99236, 99251-99255, 99304-99310, 90837)

C 80 PQ 2.58 2.58 FUD ZZZ

+ 99357 each additional 30 minutes (List separately in addition to code for prolonged service)

Code first (99356)

C 80 PQ 2.56 2.56 FUD ZZZ

99358-99359 Prolonged Services Indirect Contact

CMS 100-1,5,70 Definition of Physician
CMS 100-2,15,30 Physician Services
CMS 100-4,12,30.6.15.2 Prolonged Services Without Face to Face Service

INCLUDES Prolonged services performed in a day that are not continuous
Services provided by the physician or other qualified health care professional in relation to patient management where face-to-face services have or will occur on a different date
Time spent after direct face-to-face contact beyond the usual not necessarily on the same date of service.

EXCLUDES *Anticoagulation services (99363-99364)*
Any additional unit or floor time in the hospital or nursing facility during the same evaluation and management session
Care plan oversight (99339-99340, 99374-99380)
Online medical services (99444)
Other indirect services that have a more specific code and no upper time limit in the code
Time spent in medical team conference (99366-99368)

Code also E&M or other services provided
Code also the code for each additional service for the last 15-30 minutes
Do not report services less than 15 minutes beyond the first hour
Do not report in same month with (99487-99489)
Do not report during time-frame with (99495-99496)
Do not report services less than 30 minutes
Do not report with codes for other face-to-face services without an upper time limit

99358 Prolonged evaluation and management service before and/or after direct patient care; first hour

N 3.08 3.08 FUD XXX

+ 99359 each additional 30 minutes (List separately in addition to code for prolonged service)

Code first (99358)

N 1.49 1.49 FUD ZZZ

99360 Standby Services

CMS 100-4,12,30.6.15.3 Standby Services

INCLUDES Services requested by physician or qualified health care professional that involve no direct patient contact
Total standby time for the day

EXCLUDES *On-call services ordered by the hospital (99026, 99027)*

Do not report less than 30 minutes of standby time

99360 Standby service, requiring prolonged attendance, each 30 minutes (eg, operative standby, standby for frozen section, for cesarean/high risk delivery, for monitoring EEG)

Code also as appropriate (99460, 99465)
Do not report with (99464)

B 1.74 1.74 FUD XXX

99363-99364 Supervision of Warfarin Therapy

INCLUDES Services provided on an outpatient basis only
Supervision of therapy with warfarin: ordering, dosage adjustments, analysis of International Normalized Ration (INR) tests, patient discussion

EXCLUDES *Initial services provided/continued in the hospital or in observation: new period of subsequent therapy starts with discharge (99364)*
Services provided for less than 60 uninterrupted days
Services that fail to meet the required criteria (e.g., at least 8 INR tests/initial 90 days; 3 INR tests/each following 90 days
Warfarin therapy supervision accomplished online or via telephone contact (99441-99444, 98966-98969)

Do not report during the same time frame as (99495-99496)
Do not report in the same month with (99487-99489)
Do not report with (99217-99239 [99224, 99225, 99226], 99291-99292, 99304-99318, 99471-99476, 99477-99480)

99363 Anticoagulant management for an outpatient taking warfarin, physician review and interpretation of International Normalized Ratio (INR) testing, patient instructions, dosage adjustment (as needed), and ordering of additional tests; initial 90 days of therapy (must include a minimum of 8 INR measurements)

B 2.39 3.57 FUD XXX

99364 each subsequent 90 days of therapy (must include a minimum of 3 INR measurements)

B 0.91 1.21 FUD XXX

99366-99368 Interdisciplinary Conferences

CMS 100-1,5,70 Definition of Physician
CMS 100-2,15,30 Physician Services
CMS 100-4,11,40.2 Professional Claims for Hospice

INCLUDES Documentation of participation, contribution, and recommendations of the conference
Face-to-face participation by minimum of three qualified people from different specialties or disciplines
Only participants who have performed face-to-face evaluations or direct treatment to the patient within the previous 60 days
Start of the review of an individual patient and ends at conclusion of review

EXCLUDES *Conferences of less than 30 minutes (not reportable)*
More than one individual from the same specialty at the same encounter
Time spent record keeping or writing a report

Do not report during the same time frame as (99495-99496)
Do not report in the same month with (99487-99489)

99366 Medical team conference with interdisciplinary team of health care professionals, face-to-face with patient and/or family, 30 minutes or more, participation by nonphysician qualified health care professional

INCLUDES Team conferences of 30 minutes or more

EXCLUDES *Team conferences by a physician with patient or family present, see appropriate evaluation and management service code*

N 1.19 1.21 FUD XXX

99367 Medical team conference with interdisciplinary team of health care professionals, patient and/or family not present, 30 minutes or more; participation by physician

INCLUDES Team conferences of 30 minutes or more

N 1.59 1.59 FUD XXX

99368 participation by nonphysician qualified health care professional

INCLUDES Team conferences of 30 minutes or more

N 1.04 1.04 FUD XXX

99374-99380 Care Plan Oversight: Patient Under Care of HHA, Hospice, or Nursing Facility

CMS 100-4,11,40.1.3.1 CPO Services with Hospice Care
CMS 100-4,12,180 Payment of Care Plan Oversight (CPO)
CMS 100-4,12,180.1 Billing for Care Plan Oversight (CPO)

INCLUDES Analysis of reports, diagnostic tests, treatment plans
Discussions with other health care providers, outside of the practice, involved in the patient's care
Establishment of and revisions to care plans within a 30-day period
Payment to one physician per month for covered care plan oversight services (must be the same one who signed the plan of care)

EXCLUDES *Care plan oversight services provided in a hospice agency (99377-99378)*
Care plan oversight services provided in assisted living, domiciliary care, or private residence, not under care of a home health agency or hospice (99339-99340)
Routine postoperative care provided during a global surgery period
Time discussing treatment with patient and/or caregivers

Code also office/outpatient visits, hospital, home, nursing facility, domiciliary, or non-face-to-face services
Do not report during the same time frame as (99495-99496)
Do not report in same month with (99487-99489)
Do not report with (99441-99444, 98966-98969)

99374 **Supervision of a patient under care of home health agency (patient not present) in home, domiciliary or equivalent environment (eg, Alzheimer's facility) requiring complex and multidisciplinary care modalities involving regular development and/or revision of care plans by that individual, review of subsequent reports of patient status, review of related laboratory and other studies, communication (including telephone calls) for purposes of assessment or care decisions with health care professional(s), family member(s), surrogate decision maker(s) (eg, legal guardian) and/or key caregiver(s) involved in patient's care, integration of new information into the medical treatment plan and/or adjustment of medical therapy, within a calendar month; 15-29 minutes**
B 1.59 1.97 FUD XXX

99375 **30 minutes or more**
E 2.51 2.96 FUD XXX

99377 **Supervision of a hospice patient (patient not present) requiring complex and multidisciplinary care modalities involving regular development and/or revision of care plans by that individual, review of subsequent reports of patient status, review of related laboratory and other studies, communication (including telephone calls) for purposes of assessment or care decisions with health care professional(s), family member(s), surrogate decision maker(s) (eg, legal guardian) and/or key caregiver(s) involved in patient's care, integration of new information into the medical treatment plan and/or adjustment of medical therapy, within a calendar month; 15-29 minutes**
B 1.59 1.97 FUD XXX

99378 **30 minutes or more**
E 2.51 2.96 FUD XXX

99379 **Supervision of a nursing facility patient (patient not present) requiring complex and multidisciplinary care modalities involving regular development and/or revision of care plans by that individual, review of subsequent reports of patient status, review of related laboratory and other studies, communication (including telephone calls) for purposes of assessment or care decisions with health care professional(s), family member(s), surrogate decision maker(s) (eg, legal guardian) and/or key caregiver(s) involved in patient's care, integration of new information into the medical treatment plan and/or adjustment of medical therapy, within a calendar month; 15-29 minutes**
B 1.59 1.97 FUD XXX

99380 **30 minutes or more**
B 2.51 2.96 FUD XXX

99381-99397 Preventive Medicine Visits

CMS 100-1,5,70 Definition of Physician
CMS 100-2,15,30 Physician Services
CMS 100-4,12,30.6.2 Medically Necessary and Preventive Medicine Service on Same Date

INCLUDES Care of a small problem or preexisting condition that requires no extra work
New patients or established patients (99381-99387 or 99391-99397)
Regular preventive care (e.g., well-child exams) for all age groups

EXCLUDES *Counseling/risk factor reduction interventions not provided with a preventive medical examination (99401-99412)*
Diagnostic tests and other procedures

Code also immunization administration and product (90460-90461, 90471-90474, 90476-90749 [90630, 90672, 90673])
Code also significant, separately identifiable E&M service on the same date for substantial problems requiring additional work using modifier 25 and (99201-99215)

99381 **Initial comprehensive preventive medicine evaluation and management of an individual including an age and gender appropriate history, examination, counseling/anticipatory guidance/risk factor reduction interventions, and the ordering of laboratory/diagnostic procedures, new patient; infant (age younger than 1 year)** A
E 2.18 3.10 FUD XXX

99382 **early childhood (age 1 through 4 years)** A
E 2.31 3.23 FUD XXX

99383 **late childhood (age 5 through 11 years)** A
E 2.45 3.37 FUD XXX

99384 **adolescent (age 12 through 17 years)** A
E 2.89 3.81 FUD XXX

99385 **18-39 years** A
E 2.78 3.70 FUD XXX

99386 **40-64 years** A
E 3.37 4.27 FUD XXX

99387 **65 years and older** A
E 3.62 4.64 FUD XXX

99391 **Periodic comprehensive preventive medicine reevaluation and management of an individual including an age and gender appropriate history, examination, counseling/anticipatory guidance/risk factor reduction interventions, and the ordering of laboratory/diagnostic procedures, established patient; infant (age younger than 1 year)** A
E 1.99 2.79 FUD XXX

99392 **early childhood (age 1 through 4 years)** A
E 2.18 2.98 FUD XXX

99393 **late childhood (age 5 through 11 years)** A
E 2.18 2.97 FUD XXX

99394 **adolescent (age 12 through 17 years)** A
E 2.45 3.25 FUD XXX

99395 18-39 years A
E 2.52 3.32 FUD XXX

99396 40-64 years A
E 2.74 3.54 FUD XXX

99397 65 years and older A
E 2.89 3.81 FUD XXX

99401-99429 Counseling Services: Risk Factor and Behavioral Change Modification

CMS 100-1,5,70 Definition of Physician
CMS 100-2,15,30 Physician Services
CMS 100-2,16,90 Routine Services and Appliances
CMS 100-3,210.4 Smoking and Tobacco-Use Cessation Counseling
CMS 100-4,4,200.6 Alcohol and/or Substance Abuse Assessment and Intervention Services
CMS 100-4,12,10 General Processing Instructions
CMS 100-4,32,12 Smoking and Tobacco-Use Cessation Counseling Services
CMS 100-4,32,12.1 Smoking And Tobacco- Use Cessation Counseling
CMS 100-4,32,12.2 Carrier Billing: Smoking and Tobacco Use Cessation Counseling
CMS 100-4,32,12.3 FI Billing: Smoking and Tobacco Use Cessation Counseling

INCLUDES Administration and analysis of a health risk assessment (99420)
Face-to-face services for new and established patients based on time increments of 15 to 60 minutes
Issues such as a healthy diet, exercise, alcohol and drug abuse
Services provided by a physician or other qualified healthcare professional for the purpose of promoting health and reducing illness and injury

EXCLUDES *Counseling and risk factor reduction interventions included in preventive medicine services (99381-99397)*
Counseling services provided to patient groups with existing symptoms or illness (99078)

Code also significant, separately identifiable E&M services when performed
Do not report with heath and behavioral services provided on the same day (96150-96155)

99401 **Preventive medicine counseling and/or risk factor reduction intervention(s) provided to an individual (separate procedure); approximately 15 minutes**
E 0.69 1.02 FUD XXX

99402 **approximately 30 minutes**
E 1.43 1.75 FUD XXX

99403 **approximately 45 minutes**
E 2.12 2.44 FUD XXX

99404 **approximately 60 minutes**
E 2.81 3.13 FUD XXX

99406 **Smoking and tobacco use cessation counseling visit; intermediate, greater than 3 minutes up to 10 minutes**
S 80 0.34 0.39 FUD XXX

99407 **intensive, greater than 10 minutes**
Do not report with (99406)
S 80 0.72 0.77 FUD XXX

99408 **Alcohol and/or substance (other than tobacco) abuse structured screening (eg, AUDIT, DAST), and brief intervention (SBI) services; 15 to 30 minutes**
INCLUDES Only initial screening and brief intervention
Services of 15 minutes or more
Do not report with (99420)
E 0.94 0.99 FUD XXX

99409 **greater than 30 minutes**
INCLUDES Only initial screening and brief intervention
Do not report with (99408, 99420)
F 1.88 1.93 FUD XXX

99411 **Preventive medicine counseling and/or risk factor reduction intervention(s) provided to individuals in a group setting (separate procedure); approximately 30 minutes**
E 0.22 0.46 FUD XXX

99412 **approximately 60 minutes**
E 0.36 0.60 FUD XXX

99420 **Administration and interpretation of health risk assessment instrument (eg, health hazard appraisal)**
E 0.30 0.30 FUD XXX

99429 **Unlisted preventive medicine service**
E 0.00 0.00 FUD XXX

99441-99443 Telephone Calls for Patient Management

CMS 100-1,5,70 Definition of Physician
CMS 100-2,15,30 Physician Services
CMS 100-4,11,40.2 Professional Claims for Hospice
CMS 100-4,12,10 General Processing Instructions

INCLUDES Episodes of care initiated by an established patient or the patient or guardian of an established patient
Non-face-to-face E&M services provided by a physician or other health care provider qualified to report E&M services

EXCLUDES *Services provided by a qualified nonphysician health care professional unable to report E&M codes (98966-98968)*

Do not report during the same time frame as (99495-99496)
Do not report in same month with (99487-99489)
Do not report with anticoagulation management reported with codes (99363-99364)
Do not report with a related E&M visit within the next 24 hours or as the next available urgent visit
Do not report with a related E&M service performed and reported within the previous seven days or within the postoperative period of a completed procedure
Do not report with the same call reported with codes (99339-99340, 99374-99380)

99441 **Telephone evaluation and management service by a physician or other qualified health care professional who may report evaluation and management services provided to an established patient, parent, or guardian not originating from a related E/M service provided within the previous 7 days nor leading to an E/M service or procedure within the next 24 hours or soonest available appointment; 5-10 minutes of medical discussion**
E 0.36 0.39 FUD XXX

99442 **11-20 minutes of medical discussion**
E 0.72 0.76 FUD XXX

99443 **21-30 minutes of medical discussion**
E 1.09 1.13 FUD XXX

99444 Online Patient Management Services

INCLUDES All related communications such as related phone calls, prescription and lab orders
Permanent electronic or hardcopy storage
Physician evaluation and management services provided via the internet in response to a patient's on-line inquiry
The physician's personal timely response

EXCLUDES *Online medical evaluation by a qualified nonphysician health care professional (98969)*

Do not report during the same time frame as (99495-99496)
Do not report in same month with (99487-99489)
Do not report more than once per seven-day period for the same episode of care
Do not report when related to an E&M service performed and reported within the previous seven days or within the postoperative period of a completed procedure
Do not report with anticoagulation management reported with codes (99363-99364)
Do not report with (99339-99340, 99374-99380)

99444 **Online evaluation and management service provided by a physician or other qualified health care professional who may report evaluation and management services provided to an established patient or guardian, not originating from a related E/M service provided within the previous 7 days, using the Internet or similar electronic communications network**
E 0.00 0.00 FUD XXX

99446-99449 Online and Telephone Consultative Services

INCLUDES Multiple telephone and/or internet contact needed to complete the consultation (e.g., test result(s) follow-up)
New or established patient with new problem or exacerbation of existing problem and not seen within the last 14 days
Review of pertinent lab, imaging and/or pathology studies, medical records, medications reported only once within a 7 day period

EXCLUDES *Communication with family with or without the patient present (99441-99444, 98966-98969)*
Online services
Physician to patient (99444)
Qualified health care professional to patient (98969)
Requesting physician's time 30 minutes over the typical E/M service and patient is not on-site (99358-99359)
Requesting physician's time 30 minutes over the typical E/M service and patient is on-site (99354-99357)
Telephone services
Physician to patient (99441-99443)
Qualified health care professional to patient (98966-98968)

Do not report if consultation is for transfer of care only
Do not report if consultation is less than 5 minutes

99446 **Interprofessional telephone/Internet assessment and management service provided by a consultative physician including a verbal and written report to the patient's treating/requesting physician or other qualified health care professional; 5-10 minutes of medical consultative discussion and review**
E 0.00 0.00 FUD XXX

99447 **11-20 minutes of medical consultative discussion and review**
E 0.00 0.00 FUD XXX

99448 **21-30 minutes of medical consultative discussion and review**
E 0.00 0.00 FUD XXX

99449 **31 minutes or more of medical consultative discussion and review**
E 0.00 0.00 FUD XXX

99450-99456 Life/Disability Insurance Eligibility Visits

CMS 100-1,5,70 Definition of Physician
CMS 100-2,15,30 Physician Services

INCLUDES Assessment services for insurance eligibility and work-related disability without medical management of the patient's illness/injury
Services provided to new/established patients at any site of service

EXCLUDES *Any additional E&M services or procedures performed on the same date of service: report with appropriate code*

99450 **Basic life and/or disability examination that includes: Measurement of height, weight, and blood pressure; Completion of a medical history following a life insurance pro forma; Collection of blood sample and/or urinalysis complying with "chain of custody" protocols; and Completion of necessary documentation/certificates.**
E 0.00 0.00 FUD XXX

99455 **Work related or medical disability examination by the treating physician that includes: Completion of a medical history commensurate with the patient's condition; Performance of an examination commensurate with the patient's condition; Formulation of a diagnosis, assessment of capabilities and stability, and calculation of impairment; Development of future medical treatment plan; and Completion of necessary documentation/certificates and report.**
Do not report with (99080)
B 80 PQ 0.00 0.00 FUD XXX

99456 **Work related or medical disability examination by other than the treating physician that includes: Completion of a medical history commensurate with the patient's condition; Performance of an examination commensurate with the patient's condition; Formulation of a diagnosis, assessment of capabilities and stability, and calculation of impairment; Development of future medical treatment plan; and Completion of necessary documentation/certificates and report.**
Do not report with (99080)
B 80 PQ 0.00 0.00 FUD XXX

99460-99463 Evaluation and Management Services for Age 28 Days or Less

INCLUDES Family consultation
Healthy newborn history and physical
Medical record documentation
Ordering of diagnostic test and treatments
Services provided to healthy newborns age 28 days or less

EXCLUDES *Neonatal intensive and critical care services (99466-99469, 99477-99480)*
Newborn follow up services in an office or outpatient setting (99201-99215, 99381, 99391)
Newborn hospital discharge services if provided on a date subsequent to the admission date (99238-99239)
Nonroutine neonatal inpatient evaluation and management services (99221-99233)

Code also circumcision (54150)
Code also attendance at delivery (99464)
Code also emergency resuscitation services (99465)

99460 **Initial hospital or birthing center care, per day, for evaluation and management of normal newborn infant** A
V 80 2.65 2.65 FUD XXX

99461 **Initial care, per day, for evaluation and management of normal newborn infant seen in other than hospital or birthing center** A
M 80 1.82 2.75 FUD XXX

99462 **Subsequent hospital care, per day, for evaluation and management of normal newborn** A
C 80 1.18 1.18 FUD XXX

99463 **Initial hospital or birthing center care, per day, for evaluation and management of normal newborn infant admitted and discharged on the same date** A
V 80 3.21 3.21 FUD XXX

99464-99465 Newborn Delivery Attendance/Resuscitation

99464 **Attendance at delivery (when requested by the delivering physician or other qualified health care professional) and initial stabilization of newborn** A
Code also (99460, 99468, 99477)
Do not report with (99465)
N 80 1.99 1.99 FUD XXX

99465 **Delivery/birthing room resuscitation, provision of positive pressure ventilation and/or chest compressions in the presence of acute inadequate ventilation and/or cardiac output** A
Code also any necessary procedures performed as part of the resuscitation
Code also as appropriate (99460, 99468, 99477)
Do not report with (99464)
S 80 4.14 4.14 FUD XXX

99466-99467 Critical Care Transport Age 24 Months or Younger

INCLUDES Face-to-face care starting when the physician assumes responsibility of the patient at the referring facility until the receiving facility accepts the patient
Physician presence during interfacility transfer of critically ill/injured patient 24 months of age or less
Services provided by the physician during transport:
Blood gases
Chest x-rays (71010, 71015, 71020)
Data stored in computers (e.g., ECGs, blood pressures, hematologic data) (99090)
Gastric intubation (43752-43753)
Interpretation of cardiac output measurements (93562)
Pulse oximetry (94760-94762)
Routine monitoring:
Heart rate
Respiratory rate
Temporary transcutaneous pacing (92953)
Vascular access procedures (36000, 36400, 36405-36406, 36415, 36591, 36600)
Ventilatory management (94002-94003, 94660, 94662)

EXCLUDES *Neonatal hypothermia (99184)*
Patient critical care transport services with personal contact with patient of less than 30 minutes
Physician directed emergency care via two-way voice communication with transporting staff (99288)
Services of the physician directing transport (control physician) ([99485, 99486])

Any services not designated as included in the critical care transport service
Do not report for services less than 30 minutes in duration (see E&M codes)
Do not report with non-face-to-face transport when performed by the same physician ([99485, 99486])

99466 **Critical care face-to-face services, during an interfacility transport of critically ill or critically injured pediatric patient, 24 months of age or younger; first 30-74 minutes of hands-on care during transport** A
N 80 7.38 7.38 FUD XXX

+ 99467 **each additional 30 minutes (List separately in addition to code for primary service)** A
Code first (99466)
N 80 3.45 3.45 FUD ZZZ

99485-99486 [99485, 99486] Critical Care Transport Supervision Age 24 Months or Younger

INCLUDES Advice for treatment to the transport team from the control physician
Non face-to-face care starts with first contact by the control physician with the transport team and ends when patient responsibility is assumed by the receiving facility

EXCLUDES *Emergency systems physician direction for pediatric patient older than 24 months (99288)*
Services provided by transport team

Do not report any other services performed by the control physician for the same time period
Do not report if done by same physician (99466-99467)
Do not report services less than 15 minutes

99485 **Supervision by a control physician of interfacility transport care of the critically ill or critically injured pediatric patient, 24 months of age or younger, includes two-way communication with transport team before transport, at the referring facility and during the transport, including data interpretation and report; first 30 minutes** A
B 2.16 2.16 FUD XXX

+ # 99486 **Supervision by a control physician of interfacility transport care of the critically ill or critically injured pediatric patient, 24 months of age or younger, includes two-way communication with transport team before transport, at the referring facility and during the transport, including data interpretation and report; each additional 30 minutes (List separately in addition to code for primary procedure)** A
Code first ([99485])
B 1.88 1.88 FUD XXX

99468-99476 Critical Care Age 5 Years or Younger

INCLUDES All services included in codes 99291-99292 as well as the following which may be reported by facilities only:
Administration of blood/blood components (36430, 36440)
Administration of intravenous fluids (96360-96361)
Administration of surfactant (94610)
Bladder aspiration, suprapubic (51100)
Bladder catheterization (51701, 51702)
Car seat evaluation (94780-94781)
Catheterization umbilical artery (36660)
Catheterization umbilical vein (36510)
Central venous catheter, centrally inserted (36555)
Endotracheal intubation (31500)
Lumbar puncture (62270)
Oral or nasogastric tube placement (43752)
Pulmonary function testing, performed at the bedside (94375)
Pulse or ear oximetry (94760-94762)
Vascular access, arteries (36140, 36620)
Vascular access, venous (36400-36406, 36420, 36600)
Ventilatory management (94002-94004, 94660)
Initial and subsequent care provided to a critically ill infant or child
Other hospital care or intensive care services by same group or individual done on same day that patient was transferred to initial neonatal/pediatric critical care
Readmission to critical unit on same day or during the same stay (subsequent care)

EXCLUDES *Critical care services for patients 6 years of age or older (99291-99292)*
Critical care services provided by a second physician or physician of a different specialty (99291-99292)
Neonatal hypothermia (99184)
Services performed by transferring individual prior to transfer of patient to a different individual in a different group (99221-99233 or 99291-99292 or 99460-99462 or 99477-99480)
Services provided by another individual in another group receiving a patient transferred to a lower level of care (99231-99233, 99478-99480)
Services provided by individual transferring a patient to a lower level of care (99231-99233, 99291-99292)

Code also normal newborn care if done on same day by same group or individual that provides critical care. Report modifier 25 with initial critical care code (99460-99462)
Do not report if performed by same or different individual in same group on same day (99291-99292)
Do not report with remote critical care (0188T-0189T)

99468 **Initial inpatient neonatal critical care, per day, for the evaluation and management of a critically ill neonate, 28 days of age or younger** A
C 80 26.16 26.16 FUD XXX

99469 **Subsequent inpatient neonatal critical care, per day, for the evaluation and management of a critically ill neonate, 28 days of age or younger** A
C 80 11.09 11.09 FUD XXX

99471 **Initial inpatient pediatric critical care, per day, for the evaluation and management of a critically ill infant or young child, 29 days through 24 months of age** A
C 80 23.94 23.94 FUD XXX

99472 **Subsequent inpatient pediatric critical care, per day, for the evaluation and management of a critically ill infant or young child, 29 days through 24 months of age** A
C 80 11.27 11.27 FUD XXX

Evaluation and Management

99475 — 99490

99475 **Initial inpatient pediatric critical care, per day, for the evaluation and management of a critically ill infant or young child, 2 through 5 years of age** A
C 80 16.16 16.16 FUD XXX

99476 **Subsequent inpatient pediatric critical care, per day, for the evaluation and management of a critically ill infant or young child, 2 through 5 years of age** A
C 80 9.77 9.77 FUD XXX

99481-99482 [99481, 99482] Neonatal Hypothermia

~~99481 Total body systemic hypothermia in a critically ill neonate per day (List separately in addition to code for primary procedure)~~
To report, see 99184

~~99482 Selective head hypothermia in a critically ill neonate per day (List separately in addition to code for primary procedure)~~
To report, see 99184

99477-99486 Initial Inpatient Neonatal Intensive Care and Other Services

INCLUDES All services included in codes 99291-99292 as well as the following that may be reported by facilities only:
- Adjustments to enteral and/or parenteral nutrition
- Airway and ventilator management (31500, 94002-94004, 94375, 94610, 94660)
- Bladder catheterization (51701-51702)
- Blood transfusion (36430, 36440)
- Car seat evaluation (94780-94781)
- Constant and/or frequent monitoring of vital signs
- Continuous observation by the healthcare team
- Heat maintenance
- Intensive cardiac or respiratory monitoring
- Oral or nasogastric tube insertion (43752)
- Oxygen saturation (94760-94762)
- Spinal puncture (62270)
- Suprapubic catheterization (51100)
- Vascular access procedures (36000, 36140, 36400, 36405-36406, 36420, 36510, 36555, 36600, 36620, 36660)

EXCLUDES *Initial day intensive care provided by transferring individual same day neonate/infant transferred to a lower level of care (99477)*
Necessary resuscitation services done as part of delivery care prior to admission
Neonatal hypothermia (99184)
Services provided by receiving individual when patient is transferred for critical care (99468-99476)
Services for receiving provider when patient improves after the initial day and is transferred to a lower level of care (99231-99233, 99478-99480)
Subsequent care of a sick neonate, under 28 days of age, more than 5000 grams, not requiring critical or intensive care services (99231-99233)

Code also initial neonatal intensive care service when physician or other qualified health care professional is present for delivery and/or neonate requires resuscitation (99464-99465); append modifier 25 to (99477)
Code also care provided by receiving individual when patient is transferred to another individual in different group (99231-99233 or 99462)
Do not report with critical care services for patient transferred after initial or subsequent intensive care is provided (99291-99292)
Do not report with inpatient neonatal/pediatric critical care services received on same day (99468-99476)

99477 **Initial hospital care, per day, for the evaluation and management of the neonate, 28 days of age or younger, who requires intensive observation, frequent interventions, and other intensive care services** A
EXCLUDES *Initiation of care of a critically ill neonate (99468)*
Initiation of inpatient care of a normal newborn (99460)
C 80 9.73 9.73 FUD XXX

99478 **Subsequent intensive care, per day, for the evaluation and management of the recovering very low birth weight infant (present body weight less than 1500 grams)** A
C 80 3.86 3.86 FUD XXX

99479 **Subsequent intensive care, per day, for the evaluation and management of the recovering low birth weight infant (present body weight of 1500-2500 grams)** A
C 80 3.50 3.50 FUD XXX

99480 **Subsequent intensive care, per day, for the evaluation and management of the recovering infant (present body weight of 2501-5000 grams)** A
C 80 3.37 3.37 FUD XXX

~~99481 Resequenced code. See code following 99476.~~
To report, see 99184

~~99482 Resequenced code. See code following 99476.~~
To report, see 99184

99485 *Resequenced code. See code following 99467.*

99486 *Resequenced code. See code following 99467.*

[99490] Coordination of Services for Chronic Care

INCLUDES Case management services provided to patients that:
- Have two or more conditions anticipated to endure more than 12 months or until the patient's death
- Require at least 20 minutes of staff time monthly
- Risk is high that conditions will result in decompensation, deterioration, or death

Do not report when performed during a postoperative surgical period
Do not report with (99339-99340, 99358-99359, 99363-99364, 99366-99368, 99374-99380, 99441-99444, 99495-99496, 90951-90970, 98960-98962, 98966-98969, 99071, 99078, 99080, 99090-99091, 99605-99607)

#● 99490 **Chronic care management services, at least 20 minutes of clinical staff time directed by a physician or other qualified health care professional, per calendar month, with the following required elements: multiple (two or more) chronic conditions expected to last at least 12 months, or until the death of the patient; chronic conditions place the patient at significant risk of death, acute exacerbation/decompensation, or functional decline; comprehensive care plan established, implemented, revised, or monitored.**

99487-99490 Coordination of Complex Services for Chronic Care

INCLUDES All clinical non-face-to-face time with patient, family, and caregivers
Only services given by physician or other qualified health caregiver who has the role of care coordination for the patient for the month
Services provided to patients in a rest home, domiciliary, assisted living facility, or at home that include:
- Caregiver education to family or patient, addressing independent living and self-management
- Communication with patient and all caregivers and professionals regarding care
- Determining which community and health resources would benefit the patient
- Developing and maintaining a care plan
- Health outcomes data and registry documentation
- Providing communication with home health and other patient utilized services
- Support for treatment and medication adherence
- The facilitation of services and care

Services that address activities of daily living, psychosocial, and medical needs

Do not report in same month with (99339-99340, 99358-99359, 99363-99364, 99366-99368, 99374-99380, 99441-99444, 99495-99496, 90951-90970, 98960-98962, 98966-98969, 99071, 99078, 99080, 99090-99091, 99605-99607)

▲ 99487 **Complex chronic care management services, with the following required elements: multiple (two or more) chronic conditions expected to last at least 12 months, or until the death of the patient, chronic conditions place the patient at significant risk of death, acute exacerbation/decompensation, or functional decline, establishment or substantial revision of a comprehensive care plan, moderate or high complexity medical decision making, 60 minutes of clinical staff time directed by a physician or other qualified health care professional, per calendar month.**

INCLUDES Clinical services, 60 to 74 minutes, during a calendar month

N 1.44 1.44 FUD XXX

99488 ~~**Complex chronic care coordination services; first hour of clinical staff time directed by a physician or other qualified health care professional with one face-to-face visit, per calendar month**~~

To report, see appropriate Evaluation and Management code

+ ▲ 99489 **Complex chronic care management services, with the following required elements: multiple (two or more) chronic conditions expected to last at least 12 months, or until the death of the patient, chronic conditions place the patient at significant risk of death, acute exacerbation/decompensation, or functional decline, establishment or substantial revision of a comprehensive care plan, moderate or high complexity medical decision making, 60 minutes of clinical staff time directed by a physician or other qualified health care professional, per calendar month; each additional 30 minutes of clinical staff time directed by a physician or other qualified health care professional, per calendar month (List separately in addition to code for primary procedure)**

INCLUDES Each 30 additional minutes of clinical services in a calendar month

Code first (99487)

Do not report clinical services less than 30 minutes beyond the initial 60 minutes of care, per calendar month

N 1.36 1.15 FUD ZZZ

99490 Resequenced code. See code before 99487.

99495-99496 Management of Transitional Care Services

INCLUDES First interaction (face-to-face, by telephone, or electronic) with patient or his/her caregiver and must be done within 2 working days of discharge

Initial face-to-face; must be done within code time frame and include medication management

New or established patient with moderate to high complexity medical decision making needs during care transitions

Services from discharge day up to 29 days post discharge

Subsequent discharge within 30 days

Without face-to-face patient care given by physician or other qualified health care professional includes:

- Arrangement of follow-up and referrals with community resources and providers
- Contacting qualified health care professionals for specific problems of patient
- Discharge information review
- Need for follow-up care review based on tests and treatments
- Patient, family, and caregiver education

Without face-to-face patient care given by staff under the guidance of physician or other qualified health care professional includes:

- Caregiver education to family or patient, addressing independent living and self-management
- Communication with patient and all caregivers and professionals regarding care
- Determining which community and health resources would benefit the patient
- Providing communication with home health and other patient utilized services
- Support for treatment and medication adherence
- The facilitation of services and care

EXCLUDES *E&M services after the first face-to-face visit*

Do not report if done during same time frame (99339-99340, 99358-99359, 99363-99364, 99366-99368, 99374-99380, 99441-99444, 99487-99489, 90951-90970, 98960-98962, 98966-98969, 99071, 99078, 99080, 99090-99091, 99605-99607)

99495 **Transitional Care Management Services with the following required elements: Communication (direct contact, telephone, electronic) with the patient and/or caregiver within 2 business days of discharge Medical decision making of at least moderate complexity during the service period Face-to-face visit, within 14 calendar days of discharge**

V 80 3.11 4.58 FUD XXX

99496 **Transitional Care Management Services with the following required elements: Communication (direct contact, telephone, electronic) with the patient and/or caregiver within 2 business days of discharge Medical decision making of high complexity during the service period Face-to-face visit, within 7 calendar days of discharge**

V 80 4.50 6.47 FUD XXX

99497-99498 Advance Directive Guidance

EXCLUDES *Treatment/management for an active problem (see appropriate E&M service)*

Do not report with (99291-99292, 99468-99469, 99471-99472, 99475-99476, 99477-99480)

● 99497 **Advance care planning including the explanation and discussion of advance directives such as standard forms (with completion of such forms, when performed), by the physician or other qualified health care professional; first 30 minutes, face-to-face with the patient, family member(s), and/or surrogate**

+ ● 99498 **each additional 30 minutes (List separately in addition to code for primary procedure)**

Code first (99497)

99499 Unlisted Evaluation and Management Services

99499 **Unlisted evaluation and management service**

B 80 0.00 0.00 FUD XXX

0001F-0015F Quality Measures with Multiple Components

INCLUDES Several measures grouped within a single code descriptor to make possible reporting for clinical conditions when all of the components have been met

0001F Heart failure assessed (includes assessment of all the following components) (CAD): Blood pressure measured (2000F) Level of activity assessed (1003F) Clinical symptoms of volume overload (excess) assessed (1004F) Weight, recorded (2001F) Clinical signs of volume overload (excess) assessed (2002F)

INCLUDES Blood pressure measured (2000F)
Clinical signs of volume overload (excess) assessed (2002F)
Clinical symptoms of volume overload (excess) assessed (1004F)
Level of activity assessed (1003F)
Weight recorded (2001F)

E 0.00 0.00 FUD XXX

0005F Osteoarthritis assessed (OA) Includes assessment of all the following components: Osteoarthritis symptoms and functional status assessed (1006F) Use of anti-inflammatory or over-the-counter (OTC) analgesic medications assessed (1007F) Initial examination of the involved joint(s) (includes visual inspection, palpation, range of motion) (2004F)

INCLUDES Initial examination of the involved joint(s) (includes visual inspection/palpation/range of motion) (2004F)
Osteoarthritis symptoms and functional status assessed (1006F)
Use of anti-inflammatory or over-the-counter (OTC) analgesic medications assessed (1007F)

EXCLUDES *Tobacco use cessation intervention (4001F)*

E 0.00 0.00 FUD XXX

0012F Community-acquired bacterial pneumonia assessment (includes all of the following components) (CAP): Co-morbid conditions assessed (1026F) Vital signs recorded (2010F) Mental status assessed (2014F) Hydration status assessed (2018F)

INCLUDES Co-morbid conditions assessed (1026F)
Hydration status assessed (2018F)
Mental status assessed (2014F)
Vital signs recorded (2010F)

E 0.00 0.00 FUD XXX

0014F Comprehensive preoperative assessment performed for cataract surgery with intraocular lens (IOL) placement (includes assessment of all of the following components) (EC): Dilated fundus evaluation performed within 12 months prior to cataract surgery (2020F) Pre-surgical (cataract) axial length, corneal power measurement and method of intraocular lens power calculation documented (must be performed within 12 months prior to surgery) (3073F) Preoperative assessment of functional or medical indication(s) for surgery prior to the cataract surgery with intraocular lens placement (must be performed within 12 months prior to cataract surgery) (3325F)

INCLUDES Evaluation of dilated fundus done within 12 months prior to surgery (2020F)
Preoperative assessment of functional or medical indications done within 12 months prior to surgery (3325F)
Presurgical measurement of axial length, corneal power, and IOL power calculation performed within 12 months prior to surgery (3073F)

E 0.00 0.00 FUD XXX

0015F Melanoma follow up completed (includes assessment of all of the following components) (ML): History obtained regarding new or changing moles (1050F) Complete physical skin exam performed (2029F) Patient counseled to perform a monthly self skin examination (5005F)

INCLUDES Complete physical skin exam (2029F)
Counseling to perform monthly skin self-examination (5005F)
History obtained of new or changing moles (1050F)

E 0.00 0.00 FUD XXX

0500F-0584F Care Provided According to Prevailing Guidelines

INCLUDES Measures of utilization or patient care provided for certain clinical purposes

0500F Initial prenatal care visit (report at first prenatal encounter with health care professional providing obstetrical care. Report also date of visit and, in a separate field, the date of the last menstrual period [LMP]) (Prenatal) M ♀

E 0.00 0.00 FUD XXX

0501F Prenatal flow sheet documented in medical record by first prenatal visit (documentation includes at minimum blood pressure, weight, urine protein, uterine size, fetal heart tones, and estimated date of delivery). Report also: date of visit and, in a separate field, the date of the last menstrual period [LMP] (Note: If reporting 0501F Prenatal flow sheet, it is not necessary to report 0500F Initial prenatal care visit) (Prenatal) M ♀

E 0.00 0.00 FUD XXX

0502F Subsequent prenatal care visit (Prenatal) [Excludes: patients who are seen for a condition unrelated to pregnancy or prenatal care (eg, an upper respiratory infection; patients seen for consultation only, not for continuing care)] M ♀

EXCLUDES *Patients seen for an unrelated pregnancy/prenatal care condition (e.g., upper respiratory infection; patients seen for consultation only, not for continuing care)*

E 0.00 0.00 FUD XXX

0503F Postpartum care visit (Prenatal) M ♀

E 0.00 0.00 FUD XXX

0505F Hemodialysis plan of care documented (ESRD, P-ESRD)

E 0.00 0.00 FUD XXX

0507F Peritoneal dialysis plan of care documented (ESRD)

E 0.00 0.00 FUD XXX

0509F Urinary incontinence plan of care documented (GER)

M PQ 0.00 0.00 FUD XXX

0513F Elevated blood pressure plan of care documented (CKD)

M PQ 0.00 0.00 FUD XXX

0514F Plan of care for elevated hemoglobin level documented for patient receiving Erythropoiesis-Stimulating Agent therapy (ESA) (CKD)

E 0.00 0.00 FUD XXX

0516F Anemia plan of care documented (ESRD)

E 0.00 0.00 FUD XXX

0517F Glaucoma plan of care documented (EC)

M PQ 0.00 0.00 FUD XXX

0518F Falls plan of care documented (GER)

M PQ 0.00 0.00 FUD XXX

0519F Planned chemotherapy regimen, including at a minimum: drug(s) prescribed, dose, and duration, documented prior to initiation of a new treatment regimen (ONC)
E 0.00 0.00 FUD XXX

0520F Radiation dose limits to normal tissues established prior to the initiation of a course of 3D conformal radiation for a minimum of 2 tissue/organ (ONC)
M PQ 0.00 0.00 FUD XXX

0521F Plan of care to address pain documented (COA) (ONC)
M PQ 0.00 0.00 FUD XXX

0525F Initial visit for episode (BkP)
E 0.00 0.00 FUD XXX

0526F Subsequent visit for episode (BkP)
M PQ 0.00 0.00 FUD XXX

0528F Recommended follow-up interval for repeat colonoscopy of at least 10 years documented in colonoscopy report (End/Polyp)
M 0.00 0.00 FUD XXX

0529F Interval of 3 or more years since patient's last colonoscopy, documented (End/Polyp)
M PQ 0.00 0.00 FUD XXX

0535F Dyspnea management plan of care, documented (Pall Cr)
E 0.00 0.00 FUD XXX

0540F Glucorticoid Management Plan Documented (RA)
M PQ 0.00 0.00 FUD XXX

0545F Plan for follow-up care for major depressive disorder, documented (MDD ADOL)
E 0.00 0.00 FUD XXX

0550F Cytopathology report on routine nongynecologic specimen finalized within two working days of accession date (PATH)
E 0.00 0.00 FUD XXX

0551F Cytopathology report on nongynecologic specimen with documentation that the specimen was non-routine (PATH)
E 0.00 0.00 FUD XXX

0555F Symptom management plan of care documented (HF)
E 0.00 0.00 FUD XXX

0556F Plan of care to achieve lipid control documented (CAD)
M PQ 0.00 0.00 FUD XXX

0557F Plan of care to manage anginal symptoms documented (CAD)
M PQ 0.00 0.00 FUD XXX

0575F HIV RNA control plan of care, documented (HIV)
E PQ 0.00 0.00 FUD XXX

0580F Multidisciplinary care plan developed or updated (ALS)
E 0.00 0.00 FUD XXX

0581F Patient transferred directly from anesthetizing location to critical care unit (Peri2)
E 0.00 0.00 FUD XXX

0582F Patient not transferred directly from anesthetizing location to critical care unit (Peri2)
E 0.00 0.00 FUD XXX

0583F Transfer of care checklist used (Peri2)
E 0.00 0.00 FUD XXX

0584F Transfer of care checklist not used (Peri2)
E 0.00 0.00 FUD XXX

1000F-1505F Elements of History/Review of Systems

INCLUDES Measures for specific aspects of patient history or review of systems

1000F Tobacco use assessed (CAD, CAP, COPD, PV) (DM)
E 0.00 0.00 FUD XXX

1002F Anginal symptoms and level of activity assessed (NMA-No Measure Associated)
E 0.00 0.00 FUD XXX

1003F Level of activity assessed (NMA-No Measure Associated)
E 0.00 0.00 FUD XXX

1004F Clinical symptoms of volume overload (excess) assessed (NMA-No Measure Associated)
E 0.00 0.00 FUD XXX

1005F Asthma symptoms evaluated (includes documentation of numeric frequency of symptoms or patient completion of an asthma assessment tool/survey/questionnaire) (NMA-No Measure Associated)
E 0.00 0.00 FUD XXX

1006F Osteoarthritis symptoms and functional status assessed (may include the use of a standardized scale or the completion of an assessment questionnaire, such as the SF-36, AAOS Hip & Knee Questionnaire) (OA) [Instructions: Report when osteoarthritis is addressed during the patient encounter]
INCLUDES Osteoarthritis when it is addressed during the patient encounter
M PQ 0.00 0.00 FUD XXX

1007F Use of anti-inflammatory or analgesic over-the-counter (OTC) medications for symptom relief assessed (OA)
M PQ 0.00 0.00 FUD XXX

1008F Gastrointestinal and renal risk factors assessed for patients on prescribed or OTC non-steroidal anti-inflammatory drug (NSAID) (OA)
E 0.00 0.00 FUD XXX

1010F Severity of angina assessed by level of activity (CAD)
M PQ 0.00 0.00 FUD XXX

1011F Angina present (CAD)
M PQ 0.00 0.00 FUD XXX

1012F Angina absent (CAD)
M PQ 0.00 0.00 FUD XXX

1015F Chronic obstructive pulmonary disease (COPD) symptoms assessed (Includes assessment of at least 1 of the following: dyspnea, cough/sputum, wheezing), or respiratory symptom assessment tool completed (COPD)
E 0.00 0.00 FUD XXX

1018F Dyspnea assessed, not present (COPD)
E 0.00 0.00 FUD XXX

1019F Dyspnea assessed, present (COPD)
E 0.00 0.00 FUD XXX

1022F Pneumococcus immunization status assessed (CAP, COPD)
E 0.00 0.00 FUD XXX

1026F Co-morbid conditions assessed (eg, includes assessment for presence or absence of: malignancy, liver disease, congestive heart failure, cerebrovascular disease, renal disease, chronic obstructive pulmonary disease, asthma, diabetes, other co-morbid conditions) (CAP)
E 0.00 0.00 FUD XXX

1030F Influenza immunization status assessed (CAP)
E 0.00 0.00 FUD XXX

1031F Smoking status and exposure to second hand smoke in the home assessed (Asthma)
M PQ 0.00 0.00 FUD XXX

1032F Current tobacco smoker or currently exposed to secondhand smoke (Asthma)
M PQ 0.00 0.00 FUD XXX

1033F Current tobacco non-smoker and not currently exposed to secondhand smoke (Asthma)
M PQ 0.00 0.00 FUD XXX

1034F Current tobacco smoker (CAD, CAP, COPD, PV) (DM)
E 0.00 0.00 FUD XXX

1035F Current smokeless tobacco user (eg, chew, snuff) (PV)
E 0.00 0.00 FUD XXX

1036F Current tobacco non-user (CAD, CAP, COPD, PV) (DM) (IBD)
M PQ 0.00 0.00 FUD XXX

1038F Persistent asthma (mild, moderate or severe) (Asthma)
M PQ 0.00 0.00 FUD XXX

1039F Intermittent asthma (Asthma)
M PQ 0.00 0.00 FUD XXX

▲ 1040F DSM-5 criteria for major depressive disorder documented at the initial evaluation (MDD, MDD ADOL)
E PQ 0.00 0.00 FUD XXX

1050F History obtained regarding new or changing moles (ML)
E 0.00 0.00 FUD XXX

1052F Type, anatomic location, and activity all assessed (IBD)
E 0.00 0.00 FUD XXX

1055F Visual functional status assessed (EC)
E 0.00 0.00 FUD XXX

1060F Documentation of permanent or persistent or paroxysmal atrial fibrillation (STR)
E 0.00 0.00 FUD XXX

1061F Documentation of absence of permanent and persistent and paroxysmal atrial fibrillation (STR)
E 0.00 0.00 FUD XXX

1065F Ischemic stroke symptom onset of less than 3 hours prior to arrival (STR)
E 0.00 0.00 FUD XXX

1066F Ischemic stroke symptom onset greater than or equal to 3 hours prior to arrival (STR)
E 0.00 0.00 FUD XXX

1070F Alarm symptoms (involuntary weight loss, dysphagia, or gastrointestinal bleeding) assessed; none present (GERD)
E 0.00 0.00 FUD XXX

1071F 1 or more present (GERD)
E 0.00 0.00 FUD XXX

1090F Presence or absence of urinary incontinence assessed (GER)
M PQ 0.00 0.00 FUD XXX

1091F Urinary incontinence characterized (eg, frequency, volume, timing, type of symptoms, how bothersome) (GER)
M PQ 0.00 0.00 FUD XXX

1100F Patient screened for future fall risk; documentation of 2 or more falls in the past year or any fall with injury in the past year (GER)
M PQ 0.00 0.00 FUD XXX

1101F documentation of no falls in the past year or only 1 fall without injury in the past year (GER)
M PQ 0.00 0.00 FUD XXX

1110F Patient discharged from an inpatient facility (eg, hospital, skilled nursing facility, or rehabilitation facility) within the last 60 days (GER)
E PQ 0.00 0.00 FUD XXX

1111F Discharge medications reconciled with the current medication list in outpatient medical record (COA) (GER)
M PQ 0.00 0.00 FUD XXX

1116F Auricular or periauricular pain assessed (AOE)
E PQ 0.00 0.00 FUD XXX

1118F GERD symptoms assessed after 12 months of therapy (GERD)
E 0.00 0.00 FUD XXX

1119F Initial evaluation for condition (HEP C)(EPI, DSP)
M PQ 0.00 0.00 FUD XXX

1121F Subsequent evaluation for condition (HEP C)(EPI)
E PQ 0.00 0.00 FUD XXX

1123F Advance Care Planning discussed and documented advance care plan or surrogate decision maker documented in the medical record (DEM) (GER, Pall Cr)
M PQ 0.00 0.00 FUD XXX

1124F Advance Care Planning discussed and documented in the medical record, patient did not wish or was not able to name a surrogate decision maker or provide an advance care plan (DEM) (GER, Pall Cr)
M PQ 0.00 0.00 FUD XXX

1125F Pain severity quantified; pain present (COA) (ONC)
M PQ 0.00 0.00 FUD XXX

1126F no pain present (COA) (ONC)
M PQ 0.00 0.00 FUD XXX

1127F New episode for condition (NMA-No Measure Associated)
E 0.00 0.00 FUD XXX

1128F Subsequent episode for condition (NMA-No Measure Associated)
E 0.00 0.00 FUD XXX

1130F Back pain and function assessed, including all of the following: Pain assessment and functional status and patient history, including notation of presence or absence of "red flags" (warning signs) and assessment of prior treatment and response, and employment status (BkP)
M PQ 0.00 0.00 FUD XXX

1134F Episode of back pain lasting 6 weeks or less (BkP)
E 0.00 0.00 FUD XXX

1135F Episode of back pain lasting longer than 6 weeks (BkP)
E 0.00 0.00 FUD XXX

1136F Episode of back pain lasting 12 weeks or less (BkP)
E 0.00 0.00 FUD XXX

1137F Episode of back pain lasting longer than 12 weeks (BkP)
E 0.00 0.00 FUD XXX

1150F Documentation that a patient has a substantial risk of death within 1 year (Pall Cr)
E 0.00 0.00 FUD XXX

1151F Documentation that a patient does not have a substantial risk of death within one year (Pall Cr)
E 0.00 0.00 FUD XXX

1152F Documentation of advanced disease diagnosis, goals of care prioritize comfort (Pall Cr)
E 0.00 0.00 FUD XXX

1153F Documentation of advanced disease diagnosis, goals of care do not prioritize comfort (Pall Cr)
E 0.00 0.00 FUD XXX

1157F Advance care plan or similar legal document present in the medical record (COA)
E 0.00 0.00 FUD XXX

1158F Advance care planning discussion documented in the medical record (COA)
M 0.00 0.00 FUD XXX

1159F Medication list documented in medical record (COA)
E 0.00 0.00 FUD XXX

1160F Review of all medications by a prescribing practitioner or clinical pharmacist (such as, prescriptions, OTCs, herbal therapies and supplements) documented in the medical record (COA)
E 0.00 0.00 FUD XXX

1170F Functional status assessed (COA) (RA)
M PQ 0.00 0.00 FUD XXX

1175F Functional status for dementia assessed and results reviewed (DEM)
M 0.00 0.00 FUD XXX

1180F All specified thromboembolic risk factors assessed (AFIB)
E 0.00 0.00 FUD XXX

1181F Neuropsychiatric symptoms assessed and results reviewed (DEM)
M 0.00 0.00 FUD XXX

1182F Neuropsychiatric symptoms, one or more present (DEM)
E 0.00 0.00 FUD XXX

1183F Neuropsychiatric symptoms, absent (DEM)
E 0.00 0.00 FUD XXX

1200F Seizure type(s) and current seizure frequency(ies) documented (EPI)
M PQ 0.00 0.00 FUD XXX

1205F Etiology of epilepsy or epilepsy syndrome(s) reviewed and documented (EPI)
M PQ 0.00 0.00 FUD XXX

1220F Patient screened for depression (SUD)
M PQ 0.00 0.00 FUD XXX

1400F Parkinson's disease diagnosis reviewed (Prkns)
M 0.00 0.00 FUD XXX

1450F Symptoms improved or remained consistent with treatment goals since last assessment (HF)
E 0.00 0.00 FUD XXX

1451F Symptoms demonstrated clinically important deterioration since last assessment (HF)
E 0.00 0.00 FUD XXX

1460F Qualifying cardiac event/diagnosis in previous 12 months (CAD)
M PQ 0.00 0.00 FUD XXX

1461F No qualifying cardiac event/diagnosis in previous 12 months (CAD)
M PQ 0.00 0.00 FUD XXX

1490F Dementia severity classified, mild (DEM)
M 0.00 0.00 FUD XXX

1491F Dementia severity classified, moderate (DEM)
M 0.00 0.00 FUD XXX

1493F Dementia severity classified, severe (DEM)
M 0.00 0.00 FUD XXX

1494F Cognition assessed and reviewed (DEM)
M 0.00 0.00 FUD XXX

1500F Symptoms and signs of distal symmetric polyneuropathy reviewed and documented (DSP)
E 0.00 0.00 FUD XXX

1501F Not initial evaluation for condition (DSP)
E 0.00 0.00 FUD XXX

1502F Patient queried about pain and pain interference with function using a valid and reliable instrument (DSP)
E 0.00 0.00 FUD XXX

1503F Patient queried about symptoms of respiratory insufficiency (ALS)
E 0.00 0.00 FUD XXX

1504F Patient has respiratory insufficiency (ALS)
E 0.00 0.00 FUD XXX

1505F Patient does not have respiratory insufficiency (ALS)
E 0.00 0.00 FUD XXX

2000F-2060F Elements of Examination

INCLUDES Components of clinical assessment or physical exam

2000F Blood pressure measured (CKD)(DM)
M PQ 0.00 0.00 FUD XXX

2001F Weight recorded (PAG)
E 0.00 0.00 FUD XXX

2002F Clinical signs of volume overload (excess) assessed (NMA-No Measure Associated)
E 0.00 0.00 FUD XXX

2004F Initial examination of the involved joint(s) (includes visual inspection, palpation, range of motion) (OA) [Instructions: Report only for initial osteoarthritis visit or for visits for new joint involvement]
INCLUDES Visits for initial osteoarthritis examination or new joint involvement
E 0.00 0.00 FUD XXX

2010F Vital signs (temperature, pulse, respiratory rate, and blood pressure) documented and reviewed (CAP) (EM)
M PQ 0.00 0.00 FUD XXX

2014F Mental status assessed (CAP) (EM)
E PQ 0.00 0.00 FUD XXX

2015F Asthma impairment assessed (Asthma)
M PQ 0.00 0.00 FUD XXX

2016F Asthma risk assessed (Asthma)
M PQ 0.00 0.00 FUD XXX

2018F Hydration status assessed (normal/mildly dehydrated/severely dehydrated) (CAP)
E 0.00 0.00 FUD XXX

2019F Dilated macular exam performed, including documentation of the presence or absence of macular thickening or hemorrhage and the level of macular degeneration severity (EC)
M PQ 0.00 0.00 FUD XXX

2020F Dilated fundus evaluation performed within 12 months prior to cataract surgery (EC)
E 0.00 0.00 FUD XXX

2021F Dilated macular or fundus exam performed, including documentation of the presence or absence of macular edema and level of severity of retinopathy (EC)
M PQ 0.00 0.00 FUD XXX

2022F Dilated retinal eye exam with interpretation by an ophthalmologist or optometrist documented and reviewed (DM)
M PQ 0.00 0.00 FUD XXX

2024F 7 standard field stereoscopic photos with interpretation by an ophthalmologist or optometrist documented and reviewed (DM)
M PQ 0.00 0.00 FUD XXX

2026F Eye imaging validated to match diagnosis from 7 standard field stereoscopic photos results documented and reviewed (DM)
M PQ 0.00 0.00 FUD XXX

2027F Optic nerve head evaluation performed (EC)
M PQ 0.00 0.00 FUD XXX

2028F Foot examination performed (includes examination through visual inspection, sensory exam with monofilament, and pulse exam - report when any of the 3 components are completed) (DM)
E PQ 0.00 0.00 FUD XXX

2029F Complete physical skin exam performed (ML)
E 0.00 0.00 FUD XXX

2030F Hydration status documented, normally hydrated (PAG)
E 0.00 0.00 FUD XXX

2031F Hydration status documented, dehydrated (PAG)
E 0.00 0.00 FUD XXX

2035F Tympanic membrane mobility assessed with pneumatic otoscopy or tympanometry (OME)
E 0.00 0.00 FUD XXX

2040F Physical examination on the date of the initial visit for low back pain performed, in accordance with specifications (BkP)
M 0.00 0.00 FUD XXX

2044F Documentation of mental health assessment prior to intervention (back surgery or epidural steroid injection) or for back pain episode lasting longer than 6 weeks (BkP)
E 0.00 0.00 FUD XXX

2050F Wound characteristics including size and nature of wound base tissue and amount of drainage prior to debridement documented (CWC)
E 0.00 0.00 FUD XXX

2060F Patient interviewed directly on or before date of diagnosis of major depressive disorder (MDD ADOL)
E 0.00 0.00 FUD XXX

3006F-3776F Findings from Diagnostic or Screening Tests

INCLUDES Results and medical decision making with regards to ordered tests:
Clinical laboratory tests
Other examination procedures
Radiological examinations

3006F Chest X-ray results documented and reviewed (CAP)
E 0.00 0.00 FUD XXX

3008F Body Mass Index (BMI), documented (PV)
E 0.00 0.00 FUD XXX

3011F Lipid panel results documented and reviewed (must include total cholesterol, HDL-C, triglycerides and calculated LDL-C) (CAD)
E 0.00 0.00 FUD XXX

3014F Screening mammography results documented and reviewed (PV)
M PQ 0.00 0.00 FUD XXX

3015F Cervical cancer screening results documented and reviewed (PV) ♀
E 0.00 0.00 FUD XXX

3016F Patient screened for unhealthy alcohol use using a systematic screening method (PV) (DSP)
M PQ 0.00 0.00 FUD XXX

3017F Colorectal cancer screening results documented and reviewed (PV)
M PQ 0.00 0.00 FUD XXX

3018F Pre-procedure risk assessment and depth of insertion and quality of the bowel prep and complete description of polyp(s) found, including location of each polyp, size, number and gross morphology and recommendations for follow-up in final colonoscopy report documented (End/Polyp)
E 0.00 0.00 FUD XXX

3019F Left ventricular ejection fraction (LVEF) assessment planned post discharge (HF)
E 0.00 0.00 FUD XXX

3020F Left ventricular function (LVF) assessment (eg, echocardiography, nuclear test, or ventriculography) documented in the medical record (Includes quantitative or qualitative assessment results) (NMA-No Measure Associated)
E 0.00 0.00 FUD XXX

3021F Left ventricular ejection fraction (LVEF) less than 40% or documentation of moderately or severely depressed left ventricular systolic function (CAD, HF)
M PQ 0.00 0.00 FUD XXX

3022F Left ventricular ejection fraction (LVEF) greater than or equal to 40% or documentation as normal or mildly depressed left ventricular systolic function (CAD, HF)
M PQ 0.00 0.00 FUD XXX

3023F Spirometry results documented and reviewed (COPD)
M PQ 0.00 0.00 FUD XXX

3025F Spirometry test results demonstrate FEV1/FVC less than 70% with COPD symptoms (eg, dyspnea, cough/sputum, wheezing) (CAP, COPD)
E PQ 0.00 0.00 FUD XXX

3027F Spirometry test results demonstrate FEV1/FVC greater than or equal to 70% or patient does not have COPD symptoms (COPD)
E PQ 0.00 0.00 FUD XXX

3028F Oxygen saturation results documented and reviewed (includes assessment through pulse oximetry or arterial blood gas measurement) (CAP, COPD) (EM)
E PQ 0.00 0.00 FUD XXX

3035F Oxygen saturation less than or equal to 88% or a PaO2 less than or equal to 55 mm Hg (COPD)
E 0.00 0.00 FUD XXX

3037F Oxygen saturation greater than 88% or PaO2 greater than 55 mm Hg (COPD)
E 0.00 0.00 FUD XXX

3038F Pulmonary function test performed within 12 months prior to surgery (Lung/Esop Cx)
M PQ 0.00 0.00 FUD XXX

3040F Functional expiratory volume (FEV1) less than 40% of predicted value (COPD)
E 0.00 0.00 FUD XXX

3042F Functional expiratory volume (FEV1) greater than or equal to 40% of predicted value (COPD)
E 0.00 0.00 FUD XXX

3044F Most recent hemoglobin A1c (HbA1c) level less than 7.0% (DM)
M PQ 0.00 0.00 FUD XXX

3045F Most recent hemoglobin A1c (HbA1c) level 7.0-9.0% (DM)
M PQ 0.00 0.00 FUD XXX

3046F Most recent hemoglobin A1c level greater than 9.0% (DM)
EXCLUDES *Levels of hemoglobin A1c less than or equal to 9.0% (3044F-3045F)*
M PQ 0.00 0.00 FUD XXX

3048F Most recent LDL-C less than 100 mg/dL (CAD) (DM)
M PQ 0.00 0.00 FUD XXX

3049F Most recent LDL-C 100-129 mg/dL (CAD) (DM)
M PQ 0.00 0.00 FUD XXX

3050F Most recent LDL-C greater than or equal to 130 mg/dL (CAD) (DM)
M PQ 0.00 0.00 FUD XXX

3055F Left ventricular ejection fraction (LVEF) less than or equal to 35% (HF)
E 0.00 0.00 FUD XXX

3056F Left ventricular ejection fraction (LVEF) greater than 35% or no LVEF result available (HF)
E 0.00 0.00 FUD XXX

3060F Positive microalbuminuria test result documented and reviewed (DM)
M PQ 0.00 0.00 FUD XXX

3061F Negative microalbuminuria test result documented and reviewed (DM)
M PQ 0.00 0.00 FUD XXX

3062F Positive macroalbuminuria test result documented and reviewed (DM)
M PQ 0.00 0.00 FUD XXX

3066F Documentation of treatment for nephropathy (eg, patient receiving dialysis, patient being treated for ESRD, CRF, ARF, or renal insufficiency, any visit to a nephrologist) (DM)
M PQ 0.00 0.00 FUD XXX

3072F Low risk for retinopathy (no evidence of retinopathy in the prior year) (DM)
M PQ 0.00 0.00 FUD XXX

3073F Pre-surgical (cataract) axial length, corneal power measurement and method of intraocular lens power calculation documented within 12 months prior to surgery (EC)
E 0.00 0.00 FUD XXX

3074F Most recent systolic blood pressure less than 130 mm Hg (DM), (HTN, CKD, CAD)
E PQ 0.00 0.00 FUD XXX

3075F Most recent systolic blood pressure 130 - 139 mm Hg (DM),(HTN, CKD, CAD)
E PQ 0.00 0.00 FUD XXX

3077F Most recent systolic blood pressure greater than or equal to 140 mm Hg (HTN, CKD, CAD) (DM)
E PQ 0.00 0.00 FUD XXX

3078F Most recent diastolic blood pressure less than 80 mm Hg (HTN, CKD, CAD) (DM)
E PQ 0.00 0.00 FUD XXX

3079F Most recent diastolic blood pressure 80-89 mm Hg (HTN, CKD, CAD) (DM)
E PQ 0.00 0.00 FUD XXX

3080F Most recent diastolic blood pressure greater than or equal to 90 mm Hg (HTN, CKD, CAD) (DM)
E PQ 0.00 0.00 FUD XXX

3082F Kt/V less than 1.2 (Clearance of urea [Kt]/volume [V]) (ESRD, P-ESRD)
E 0.00 0.00 FUD XXX

3083F Kt/V equal to or greater than 1.2 and less than 1.7 (Clearance of urea [Kt]/volume [V]) (ESRD, P-ESRD)
E 0.00 0.00 FUD XXX

3084F Kt/V greater than or equal to 1.7 (Clearance of urea [Kt]/volume [V]) (ESRD, P-ESRD)
E 0.00 0.00 FUD XXX

3085F Suicide risk assessed (MDD, MDD ADOL)
E PQ 0.00 0.00 FUD XXX

3088F Major depressive disorder, mild (MDD)
E 0.00 0.00 FUD XXX

3089F Major depressive disorder, moderate (MDD)
E 0.00 0.00 FUD XXX

3090F Major depressive disorder, severe without psychotic features (MDD)
E 0.00 0.00 FUD XXX

3091F Major depressive disorder, severe with psychotic features (MDD)
E 0.00 0.00 FUD XXX

3092F Major depressive disorder, in remission (MDD)
E PQ 0.00 0.00 FUD XXX

3093F Documentation of new diagnosis of initial or recurrent episode of major depressive disorder (MDD)
E 0.00 0.00 FUD XXX

3095F Central dual-energy X-ray absorptiometry (DXA) results documented (OP)(IBD)
M PQ 0.00 0.00 FUD XXX

3096F Central dual-energy X-ray absorptiometry (DXA) ordered (OP)(IBD)
M PQ 0.00 0.00 FUD XXX

3100F Carotid imaging study report (includes direct or indirect reference to measurements of distal internal carotid diameter as the denominator for stenosis measurement) (STR, RAD)
M PQ 0.00 0.00 FUD XXX

3110F Documentation in final CT or MRI report of presence or absence of hemorrhage and mass lesion and acute infarction (STR)
E PQ 0.00 0.00 FUD XXX

3111F CT or MRI of the brain performed in the hospital within 24 hours of arrival or performed in an outpatient imaging center, to confirm initial diagnosis of stroke, TIA or intracranial hemorrhage (STR)
E PQ 0.00 0.00 FUD XXX

3112F CT or MRI of the brain performed greater than 24 hours after arrival to the hospital or performed in an outpatient imaging center for purpose other than confirmation of initial diagnosis of stroke, TIA, or intracranial hemorrhage (STR)
E PQ 0.00 0.00 FUD XXX

3115F Quantitative results of an evaluation of current level of activity and clinical symptoms (HF)
E 0.00 0.00 FUD XXX

3117F Heart failure disease specific structured assessment tool completed (HF)
E 0.00 0.00 FUD XXX

3118F New York Heart Association (NYHA) Class documented (HF)
E 0.00 0.00 FUD XXX

3119F No evaluation of level of activity or clinical symptoms (HF)
E 0.00 0.00 FUD XXX

3120F 12-Lead ECG Performed (EM)
M PQ 0.00 0.00 FUD XXX

~~3125F Esophageal biopsy report with a statement about dysplasia (present, absent, or indefinite) (PATH)~~

● 3126F Esophageal biopsy report with a statement about dysplasia (present, absent, or indefinite, and if present, contains appropriate grading) (PATH)

3130F Upper gastrointestinal endoscopy performed (GERD)
E 0.00 0.00 FUD XXX

3132F Documentation of referral for upper gastrointestinal endoscopy (GERD)
E 0.00 0.00 FUD XXX

3140F Upper gastrointestinal endoscopy report indicates suspicion of Barrett's esophagus (GERD)
E 0.00 0.00 FUD XXX

3141F Upper gastrointestinal endoscopy report indicates no suspicion of Barrett's esophagus (GERD)
E 0.00 0.00 FUD XXX

3142F Barium swallow test ordered (GERD)
INCLUDES Documentation of barium swallow test
E 0.00 0.00 FUD XXX

3150F Forceps esophageal biopsy performed (GERD)
E 0.00 0.00 FUD XXX

3155F Cytogenetic testing performed on bone marrow at time of diagnosis or prior to initiating treatment (HEM)
M PQ 0.00 0.00 FUD XXX

3160F Documentation of iron stores prior to initiating erythropoietin therapy (HEM)
M PQ 0.00 0.00 FUD XXX

3170F Flow cytometry studies performed at time of diagnosis or prior to initiating treatment (HEM)
M PQ 0.00 0.00 FUD XXX

3200F Barium swallow test not ordered (GERD)
E 0.00 0.00 FUD XXX

3210F Group A strep test performed (PHAR)
M PQ 0.00 0.00 FUD XXX

3215F Patient has documented immunity to Hepatitis A (HEP-C)
M PQ 0.00 0.00 FUD XXX

3216F Patient has documented immunity to Hepatitis B (HEP-C)(IBD)
E PQ 0.00 0.00 FUD XXX

3218F RNA testing for Hepatitis C documented as performed within 6 months prior to initiation of antiviral treatment for Hepatitis C (HEP-C)
E PQ 0.00 0.00 FUD XXX

3220F Hepatitis C quantitative RNA testing documented as performed at 12 weeks from initiation of antiviral treatment (HEP-C)
E PQ 0.00 0.00 FUD XXX

3230F Documentation that hearing test was performed within 6 months prior to tympanostomy tube insertion (OME)
E 0.00 0.00 FUD XXX

3250F Specimen site other than anatomic location of primary tumor (PATH)
M PQ 0.00 0.00 FUD XXX

3260F pT category (primary tumor), pN category (regional lymph nodes), and histologic grade documented in pathology report (PATH)
M PQ 0.00 0.00 FUD XXX

3265F Ribonucleic acid (RNA) testing for Hepatitis C viremia ordered or results documented (HEP C)
M PQ 0.00 0.00 FUD XXX

3266F Hepatitis C genotype testing documented as performed prior to initiation of antiviral treatment for Hepatitis C (HEP C)
E PQ 0.00 0.00 FUD XXX

3267F Pathology report includes pT category, pN category, Gleason score, and statement about margin status (PATH)
M PQ 0.00 0.00 FUD XXX

3268F Prostate-specific antigen (PSA), and primary tumor (T) stage, and Gleason score documented prior to initiation of treatment (PRCA)
E 0.00 0.00 FUD XXX

3269F Bone scan performed prior to initiation of treatment or at any time since diagnosis of prostate cancer (PRCA)
M PQ 0.00 0.00 FUD XXX

3270F Bone scan not performed prior to initiation of treatment nor at any time since diagnosis of prostate cancer (PRCA)
M PQ 0.00 0.00 FUD XXX

3271F Low risk of recurrence, prostate cancer (PRCA)
M PQ 0.00 0.00 FUD XXX

3272F Intermediate risk of recurrence, prostate cancer (PRCA)
M PQ 0.00 0.00 FUD XXX

3273F High risk of recurrence, prostate cancer (PRCA)
M PQ 0.00 0.00 FUD XXX

3274F Prostate cancer risk of recurrence not determined or neither low, intermediate nor high (PRCA) ♂
M PQ 0.00 0.00 FUD XXX

3278F Serum levels of calcium, phosphorus, intact Parathyroid Hormone (PTH) and lipid profile ordered (CKD)
E 0.00 0.00 FUD XXX

3279F Hemoglobin level greater than or equal to 13 g/dL (CKD, ESRD)
E 0.00 0.00 FUD XXX

3280F Hemoglobin level 11 g/dL to 12.9 g/dL (CKD, ESRD)
E 0.00 0.00 FUD XXX

3281F Hemoglobin level less than 11 g/dL (CKD, ESRD)
E 0.00 0.00 FUD XXX

3284F Intraocular pressure (IOP) reduced by a value of greater than or equal to 15% from the pre-intervention level (EC)
M PQ 0.00 0.00 FUD XXX

3285F Intraocular pressure (IOP) reduced by a value less than 15% from the pre-intervention level (EC)
M PQ 0.00 0.00 FUD XXX

3288F Falls risk assessment documented (GER)
M PQ 0.00 0.00 FUD XXX

3290F Patient is D (Rh) negative and unsensitized (Pre-Cr)
E 0.00 0.00 FUD XXX

3291F Patient is D (Rh) positive or sensitized (Pre-Cr)
E 0.00 0.00 FUD XXX

3292F HIV testing ordered or documented and reviewed during the first or second prenatal visit (Pre-Cr)
E 0.00 0.00 FUD XXX

3293F ABO and Rh blood typing documented as performed (Pre-Cr)
E 0.00 0.00 FUD XXX

3294F Group B Streptococcus (GBS) screening documented as performed during week 35-37 gestation (Pre-Cr)
E 0.00 0.00 FUD XXX

3300F American Joint Committee on Cancer (AJCC) stage documented and reviewed (ONC)
M PQ 0.00 0.00 FUD XXX

3301F Cancer stage documented in medical record as metastatic and reviewed (ONC)
EXCLUDES *Cancer staging measures (3321F-3390F)*
M PQ 0.00 0.00 FUD XXX

3315F Estrogen receptor (ER) or progesterone receptor (PR) positive breast cancer (ONC)
M PQ 0.00 0.00 FUD XXX

3316F Estrogen receptor (ER) and progesterone receptor (PR) negative breast cancer (ONC)
M PQ 0.00 0.00 FUD XXX

3317F Pathology report confirming malignancy documented in the medical record and reviewed prior to the initiation of chemotherapy (ONC)
E 0.00 0.00 FUD XXX

3318F Pathology report confirming malignancy documented in the medical record and reviewed prior to the initiation of radiation therapy (ONC)
E 0.00 0.00 FUD XXX

3319F 1 of the following diagnostic imaging studies ordered: chest x-ray, CT, Ultrasound, MRI, PET, or nuclear medicine scans (ML)
M PQ 0.00 0.00 FUD XXX

3320F None of the following diagnostic imaging studies ordered: chest X-ray, CT, Ultrasound, MRI, PET, or nuclear medicine scans (ML)
M PQ 0.00 0.00 FUD XXX

3321F AJCC cancer Stage 0 or IA melanoma, documented (ML)
M 0.00 0.00 FUD XXX

3322F Melanoma greater than AJCC Stage 0 or IA (ML)
M 0.00 0.00 FUD XXX

3323F Clinical tumor, node and metastases (TNM) staging documented and reviewed prior to surgery (Lung/Esop Cx)
M PQ 0.00 0.00 FUD XXX

3324F MRI or CT scan ordered, reviewed or requested (EPI)
E 0.00 0.00 FUD XXX

3325F Preoperative assessment of functional or medical indication(s) for surgery prior to the cataract surgery with intraocular lens placement (must be performed within 12 months prior to cataract surgery) (EC)
E 0.00 0.00 FUD XXX

3328F Performance status documented and reviewed within 2 weeks prior to surgery (Lung/Esop Cx)
M PQ 0.00 0.00 FUD XXX

3330F Imaging study ordered (BkP)
E 0.00 0.00 FUD XXX

3331F Imaging study not ordered (BkP)
E 0.00 0.00 FUD XXX

3340F Mammogram assessment category of "incomplete: need additional imaging evaluation" documented (RAD)
M PQ 0.00 0.00 FUD XXX

3341F Mammogram assessment category of "negative," documented (RAD)
M PQ 0.00 0.00 FUD XXX

3342F Mammogram assessment category of "benign," documented (RAD)
M PQ 0.00 0.00 FUD XXX

3343F Mammogram assessment category of "probably benign," documented (RAD)
M PQ 0.00 0.00 FUD XXX

3344F Mammogram assessment category of "suspicious," documented (RAD)
M PQ 0.00 0.00 FUD XXX

3345F Mammogram assessment category of "highly suggestive of malignancy," documented (RAD)
M PQ 0.00 0.00 FUD XXX

3350F Mammogram assessment category of "known biopsy proven malignancy," documented (RAD)
M PQ 0.00 0.00 FUD XXX

3351F Negative screen for depressive symptoms as categorized by using a standardized depression screening/assessment tool (MDD)
E 0.00 0.00 FUD XXX

3352F No significant depressive symptoms as categorized by using a standardized depression assessment tool (MDD)
E 0.00 0.00 FUD XXX

3353F Mild to moderate depressive symptoms as categorized by using a standardized depression screening/assessment tool (MDD)
E 0.00 0.00 FUD XXX

3354F Clinically significant depressive symptoms as categorized by using a standardized depression screening/assessment tool (MDD)
E 0.00 0.00 FUD XXX

3370F AJCC breast cancer Stage 0 documented (ONC)
M PQ 0.00 0.00 FUD XXX

3372F AJCC Breast Cancer Stage I: T1mic, T1a or T1b (tumor size </= 1 cm) documented (ONC)
M PQ 0.00 0.00 FUD XXX

3374F AJCC breast cancer Stage I: T1c (tumor size > 1 cm to 2 cm) documented (ONC)
M PQ 0.00 0.00 FUD XXX

3376F AJCC breast cancer Stage II documented (ONC)
M PQ 0.00 0.00 FUD XXX

3378F AJCC breast cancer Stage III documented (ONC)
M PQ 0.00 0.00 FUD XXX

3380F AJCC breast cancer Stage IV documented (ONC)
M PQ 0.00 0.00 FUD XXX

3382F AJCC colon cancer, Stage 0 documented (ONC)
M PQ 0.00 0.00 FUD XXX

3384F AJCC colon cancer, Stage I documented (ONC)
M PQ 0.00 0.00 FUD XXX

3386F AJCC colon cancer, Stage II documented (ONC)
M PQ 0.00 0.00 FUD XXX

3388F AJCC colon cancer, Stage III documented (ONC)
M PQ 0.00 0.00 FUD XXX

3390F AJCC colon cancer, Stage IV documented (ONC)
M PQ 0.00 0.00 FUD XXX

3394F Quantitative HER2 immunohistochemistry (IHC) evaluation of breast cancer consistent with the scoring system defined in the ASCO/CAP guidelines (PATH)
M PQ 0.00 0.00 FUD XXX

3395F Quantitative non-HER2 immunohistochemistry (IHC) evaluation of breast cancer (eg, testing for estrogen or progesterone receptors [ER/PR]) performed (PATH)
M PQ 0.00 0.00 FUD XXX

3450F Dyspnea screened, no dyspnea or mild dyspnea (Pall Cr)
E 0.00 0.00 FUD XXX

3451F Dyspnea screened, moderate or severe dyspnea (Pall Cr)
E 0.00 0.00 FUD XXX

3452F Dyspnea not screened (Pall Cr)
E 0.00 0.00 FUD XXX

3455F TB screening performed and results interpreted within six months prior to initiation of first-time biologic disease modifying anti-rheumatic drug therapy for RA (RA)
M PQ 0.00 0.00 FUD XXX

3470F Rheumatoid arthritis (RA) disease activity, low (RA)
M PQ 0.00 0.00 FUD XXX

3471F Rheumatoid arthritis (RA) disease activity, moderate (RA)
M PQ 0.00 0.00 FUD XXX

3472F Rheumatoid arthritis (RA) disease activity, high (RA)
M PQ 0.00 0.00 FUD XXX

3475F Disease prognosis for rheumatoid arthritis assessed, poor prognosis documented (RA)
M PQ 0.00 0.00 FUD XXX

3476F Disease prognosis for rheumatoid arthritis assessed, good prognosis documented (RA)
M PQ 0.00 0.00 FUD XXX

3490F History of AIDS-defining condition (HIV)
E PQ 0.00 0.00 FUD XXX

3491F HIV indeterminate (infants of undetermined HIV status born of HIV-infected mothers) (HIV)
E 0.00 0.00 FUD XXX

3492F History of nadir CD4+ cell count <350 cells/mm3 (HIV)
E PQ 0.00 0.00 FUD XXX

3493F No history of nadir CD4+ cell count <350 cells/mm3 and no history of AIDS-defining condition (HIV)
E PQ 0.00 0.00 FUD XXX

3494F CD4+ cell count <200 cells/mm3 (HIV)
M PQ 0.00 0.00 FUD XXX

3495F CD4+ cell count 200 - 499 cells/mm3 (HIV)
M PQ 0.00 0.00 FUD XXX

3496F CD4+ cell count >/=500 cells/mm3 (HIV)
M PQ 0.00 0.00 FUD XXX

3497F CD4+ cell percentage <15% (HIV)
E 0.00 0.00 FUD XXX

3498F CD4+ cell percentage >/=15% (HIV)
E 0.00 0.00 FUD XXX

3500F CD4+ cell count or CD4+ cell percentage documented as performed (HIV)
E PQ 0.00 0.00 FUD XXX

3502F HIV RNA viral load below limits of quantification (HIV)
E PQ 0.00 0.00 FUD XXX

3503F HIV RNA viral load not below limits of quantification (HIV)
E PQ 0.00 0.00 FUD XXX

3510F Documentation that tuberculosis (TB) screening test performed and results interpreted (HIV) (IBD)
M 0.00 0.00 FUD XXX

3511F Chlamydia and gonorrhea screenings documented as performed (HIV)
E PQ 0.00 0.00 FUD XXX

3512F Syphilis screening documented as performed (HIV)
E PQ 0.00 0.00 FUD XXX

3513F Hepatitis B screening documented as performed (HIV)
E 0.00 0.00 FUD XXX

3514F Hepatitis C screening documented as performed (HIV)
E 0.00 0.00 FUD XXX

3515F Patient has documented immunity to Hepatitis C (HIV)
E 0.00 0.00 FUD XXX

3517F Hepatitis B Virus (HBV) status assessed and results interpreted within one year prior to receiving a first course of anti-TNF (tumor necrosis factor) therapy (IBD)
M 0.00 0.00 FUD XXX

3520F Clostridium difficile testing performed (IBD)
E 0.00 0.00 FUD XXX

3550F Low risk for thromboembolism (AFIB)
E 0.00 0.00 FUD XXX

3551F Intermediate risk for thromboembolism (AFIB)
E 0.00 0.00 FUD XXX

3552F High risk for thromboembolism (AFIB)
E 0.00 0.00 FUD XXX

3555F Patient had International Normalized Ratio (INR) measurement performed (AFIB)
E 0.00 0.00 FUD XXX

3570F Final report for bone scintigraphy study includes correlation with existing relevant imaging studies (eg, x-ray, MRI, CT) corresponding to the same anatomical region in question (NUC_MED)
M PQ 0.00 0.00 FUD XXX

3572F Patient considered to be potentially at risk for fracture in a weight-bearing site (NUC_MED)
E 0.00 0.00 FUD XXX

3573F Patient not considered to be potentially at risk for fracture in a weight-bearing site (NUC_MED)
E 0.00 0.00 FUD XXX

3650F Electroencephalogram (EEG) ordered, reviewed or requested (EPI)
E 0.00 0.00 FUD XXX

3700F Psychiatric disorders or disturbances assessed (Prkns)
M 0.00 0.00 FUD XXX

3720F Cognitive impairment or dysfunction assessed (Prkns)
M 0.00 0.00 FUD XXX

3725F Screening for depression performed (DEM)
M 0.00 0.00 FUD XXX

3750F Patient not receiving dose of corticosteroids greater than or equal to 10mg/day for 60 or greater consecutive days (IBD)
M 0.00 0.00 FUD XXX

3751F Electrodiagnostic studies for distal symmetric polyneuropathy conducted (or requested), documented, and reviewed within 6 months of initial evaluation for condition (DSP)
E 0.00 0.00 FUD XXX

3752F Electrodiagnostic studies for distal symmetric polyneuropathy not conducted (or requested), documented, or reviewed within 6 months of initial evaluation for condition (DSP)
E 0.00 0.00 FUD XXX

3753F Patient has clear clinical symptoms and signs that are highly suggestive of neuropathy AND cannot be attributed to another condition, AND has an obvious cause for the neuropathy (DSP)
E 0.00 0.00 FUD XXX

3754F Screening tests for diabetes mellitus reviewed, requested, or ordered (DSP)
E 0.00 0.00 FUD XXX

3755F Cognitive and behavioral impairment screening performed (ALS)
E 0.00 0.00 FUD XXX

3756F Patient has pseudobulbar affect, sialorrhea, or ALS-related symptoms (ALS)
E 0.00 0.00 FUD XXX

3757F Patient does not have pseudobulbar affect, sialorrhea, or ALS-related symptoms (ALS)
E 0.00 0.00 FUD XXX

3758F Patient referred for pulmonary function testing or peak cough expiratory flow (ALS)
E 0.00 0.00 FUD XXX

3759F Patient screened for dysphagia, weight loss, and impaired nutrition, and results documented (ALS)
E 0.00 0.00 FUD XXX

3760F Patient exhibits dysphagia, weight loss, or impaired nutrition (ALS)
E 0.00 0.00 FUD XXX

3761F Patient does not exhibit dysphagia, weight loss, or impaired nutrition (ALS)
E 0.00 0.00 FUD XXX

3762F Patient is dysarthric (ALS)
E 0.00 0.00 FUD XXX

3763F Patient is not dysarthric (ALS)
E 0.00 0.00 FUD XXX

● 3775F Adenoma(s) or other neoplasm detected during screening colonoscopy (SCADR)

● 3776F Adenoma(s) or other neoplasm not detected during screening colonoscopy (SCADR)

4000F-4563F Therapies Provided (Includes Preventive Services)

INCLUDES Behavioral/pharmacologic/procedural therapies
Preventive services including patient education/counseling

4000F Tobacco use cessation intervention, counseling (COPD, CAP, CAD, Asthma) (DM) (PV)
M PQ 0.00 0.00 FUD XXX

4001F Tobacco use cessation intervention, pharmacologic therapy (COPD, CAD, CAP, PV, Asthma) (DM) (PV)
M PQ 0.00 0.00 FUD XXX

4003F Patient education, written/oral, appropriate for patients with heart failure, performed (NMA-No Measure Associated)
E 0.00 0.00 FUD XXX

4004F Patient screened for tobacco use and received tobacco cessation intervention (counseling, pharmacotherapy, or both), if identified as a tobacco user (PV, CAD)
M PQ 0.00 0.00 FUD XXX

4005F Pharmacologic therapy (other than minerals/vitamins) for osteoporosis prescribed (OP) (IBD)
M PQ 0.00 0.00 FUD XXX

4008F Beta-blocker therapy prescribed or currently being taken (CAD,HF)
M PQ 0.00 0.00 FUD XXX

4010F Angiotensin converting enzyme (ACE) inhibitor or angiotensin receptor blocker (ARB) therapy prescribed or currently being taken (CAD, CKD, HF) (DM)
M PQ 0.00 0.00 FUD XXX

4011F Oral antiplatelet therapy prescribed (CAD)
E 0.00 0.00 FUD XXX

4012F Warfarin therapy prescribed (NMA-No Measure Associated)
E 0.00 0.00 FUD XXX

4013F Statin therapy prescribed or currently being taken (CAD)
M PQ 0.00 0.00 FUD XXX

4014F Written discharge instructions provided to heart failure patients discharged home (Instructions include all of the following components: activity level, diet, discharge medications, follow-up appointment, weight monitoring, what to do if symptoms worsen) (NMA-No Measure Associated)
EXCLUDES *Patients younger than 18 years of age*
E 0.00 0.00 FUD XXX

4015F Persistent asthma, preferred long term control medication or an acceptable alternative treatment, prescribed (NMA-No Measure Associated)
Code also modifier 2P for patient reasons for not prescribing
Do not report with modifier 1P
E 0.00 0.00 FUD XXX

4016F Anti-inflammatory/analgesic agent prescribed (OA) (Use for prescribed or continued medication[s], including over-the-counter medication[s])
INCLUDES Over-the-counter medication(s)
Prescribed/continued medication(s)
E 0.00 0.00 FUD XXX

4017F Gastrointestinal prophylaxis for NSAID use prescribed (OA)
E 0.00 0.00 FUD XXX

4018F Therapeutic exercise for the involved joint(s) instructed or physical or occupational therapy prescribed (OA)
E 0.00 0.00 FUD XXX

4019F Documentation of receipt of counseling on exercise and either both calcium and vitamin D use or counseling regarding both calcium and vitamin D use (OP)
E 0.00 0.00 FUD XXX

4025F Inhaled bronchodilator prescribed (COPD)
M PQ 0.00 0.00 FUD XXX

4030F Long-term oxygen therapy prescribed (more than 15 hours per day) (COPD)
E 0.00 0.00 FUD XXX

4033F Pulmonary rehabilitation exercise training recommended (COPD)
Code also dyspnea assessed, present (1019F)
E 0.00 0.00 FUD XXX

4035F Influenza immunization recommended (COPD) (IBD)
M 0.00 0.00 FUD XXX

4037F Influenza immunization ordered or administered (COPD, PV, CKD, ESRD)(IBD)
M 0.00 0.00 FUD XXX

4040F Pneumococcal vaccine administered or previously received (COPD) (PV), (IBD)
M PQ 0.00 0.00 FUD XXX

4041F Documentation of order for cefazolin OR cefuroxime for antimicrobial prophylaxis (PERI 2)
E PQ 0.00 0.00 FUD XXX

4042F Documentation that prophylactic antibiotics were neither given within 4 hours prior to surgical incision nor given intraoperatively (PERI 2)
M PQ 0.00 0.00 FUD XXX

4043F Documentation that an order was given to discontinue prophylactic antibiotics within 48 hours of surgical end time, cardiac procedures (PERI 2)
M PQ 0.00 0.00 FUD XXX

4044F Documentation that an order was given for venous thromboembolism (VTE) prophylaxis to be given within 24 hours prior to incision time or 24 hours after surgery end time (PERI 2)
M PQ 0.00 0.00 FUD XXX

4045F Appropriate empiric antibiotic prescribed (CAP), (EM)
M PQ 0.00 0.00 FUD XXX

4046F Documentation that prophylactic antibiotics were given within 4 hours prior to surgical incision or given intraoperatively (PERI 2)
M PQ 0.00 0.00 FUD XXX

4047F Documentation of order for prophylactic parenteral antibiotics to be given within 1 hour (if fluoroquinolone or vancomycin, 2 hours) prior to surgical incision (or start of procedure when no incision is required) (PERI 2)
M PQ 0.00 0.00 FUD XXX

4048F Documentation that administration of prophylactic parenteral antibiotic was initiated within 1 hour (if fluoroquinolone or vancomycin, 2 hours) prior to surgical incision (or start of procedure when no incision is required) as ordered (PERI 2)
M PQ 0.00 0.00 FUD XXX

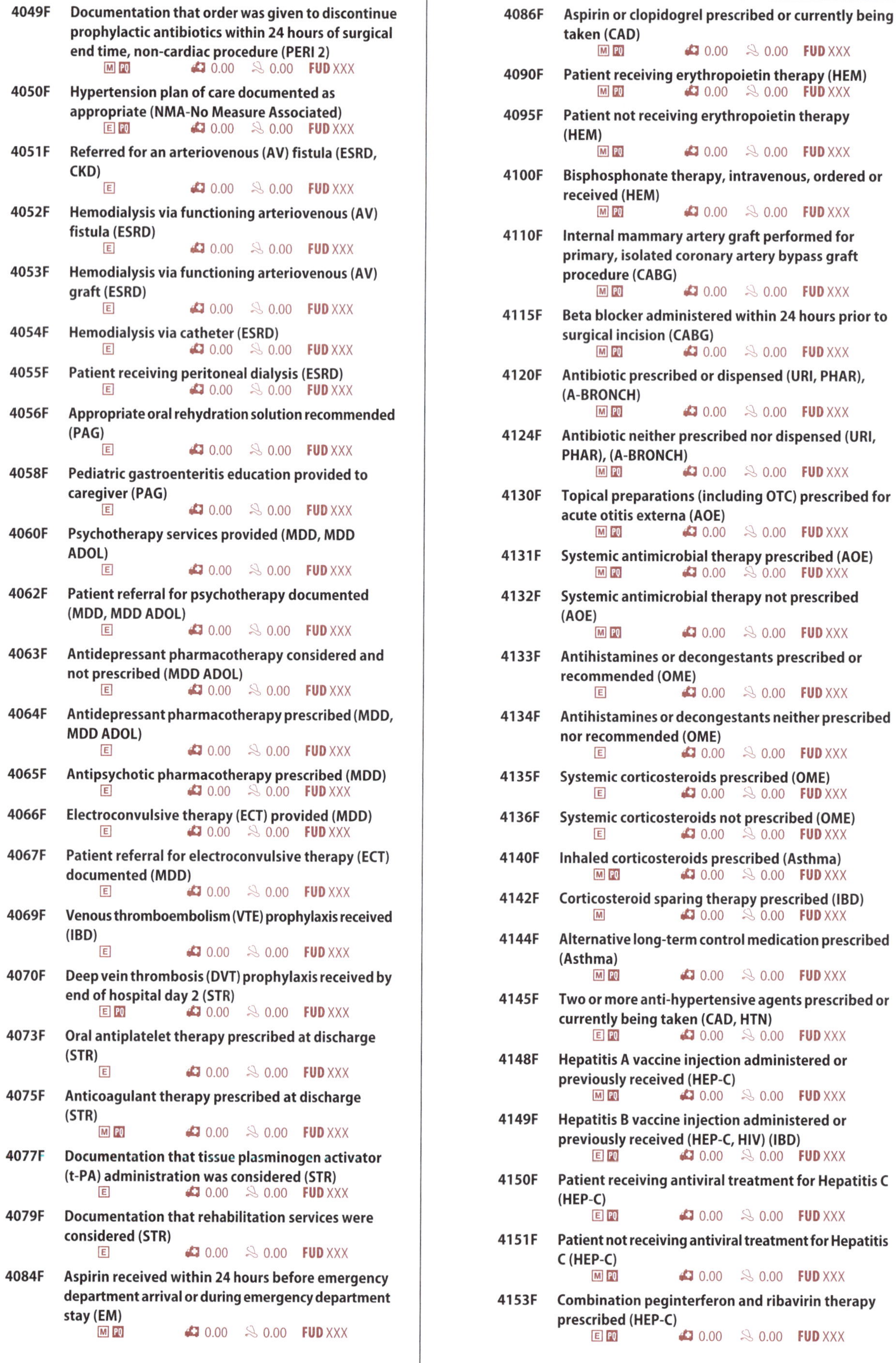

4049F Documentation that order was given to discontinue prophylactic antibiotics within 24 hours of surgical end time, non-cardiac procedure (PERI 2)
M PQ 0.00 0.00 FUD XXX

4050F Hypertension plan of care documented as appropriate (NMA-No Measure Associated)
E PQ 0.00 0.00 FUD XXX

4051F Referred for an arteriovenous (AV) fistula (ESRD, CKD)
E 0.00 0.00 FUD XXX

4052F Hemodialysis via functioning arteriovenous (AV) fistula (ESRD)
E 0.00 0.00 FUD XXX

4053F Hemodialysis via functioning arteriovenous (AV) graft (ESRD)
E 0.00 0.00 FUD XXX

4054F Hemodialysis via catheter (ESRD)
E 0.00 0.00 FUD XXX

4055F Patient receiving peritoneal dialysis (ESRD)
E 0.00 0.00 FUD XXX

4056F Appropriate oral rehydration solution recommended (PAG)
E 0.00 0.00 FUD XXX

4058F Pediatric gastroenteritis education provided to caregiver (PAG)
E 0.00 0.00 FUD XXX

4060F Psychotherapy services provided (MDD, MDD ADOL)
E 0.00 0.00 FUD XXX

4062F Patient referral for psychotherapy documented (MDD, MDD ADOL)
E 0.00 0.00 FUD XXX

4063F Antidepressant pharmacotherapy considered and not prescribed (MDD ADOL)
E 0.00 0.00 FUD XXX

4064F Antidepressant pharmacotherapy prescribed (MDD, MDD ADOL)
E 0.00 0.00 FUD XXX

4065F Antipsychotic pharmacotherapy prescribed (MDD)
E 0.00 0.00 FUD XXX

4066F Electroconvulsive therapy (ECT) provided (MDD)
E 0.00 0.00 FUD XXX

4067F Patient referral for electroconvulsive therapy (ECT) documented (MDD)
E 0.00 0.00 FUD XXX

4069F Venous thromboembolism (VTE) prophylaxis received (IBD)
E 0.00 0.00 FUD XXX

4070F Deep vein thrombosis (DVT) prophylaxis received by end of hospital day 2 (STR)
E PQ 0.00 0.00 FUD XXX

4073F Oral antiplatelet therapy prescribed at discharge (STR)
E 0.00 0.00 FUD XXX

4075F Anticoagulant therapy prescribed at discharge (STR)
M PQ 0.00 0.00 FUD XXX

4077F Documentation that tissue plasminogen activator (t-PA) administration was considered (STR)
E 0.00 0.00 FUD XXX

4079F Documentation that rehabilitation services were considered (STR)
E 0.00 0.00 FUD XXX

4084F Aspirin received within 24 hours before emergency department arrival or during emergency department stay (EM)
M PQ 0.00 0.00 FUD XXX

4086F Aspirin or clopidogrel prescribed or currently being taken (CAD)
M PQ 0.00 0.00 FUD XXX

4090F Patient receiving erythropoietin therapy (HEM)
M PQ 0.00 0.00 FUD XXX

4095F Patient not receiving erythropoietin therapy (HEM)
M PQ 0.00 0.00 FUD XXX

4100F Bisphosphonate therapy, intravenous, ordered or received (HEM)
M PQ 0.00 0.00 FUD XXX

4110F Internal mammary artery graft performed for primary, isolated coronary artery bypass graft procedure (CABG)
M PQ 0.00 0.00 FUD XXX

4115F Beta blocker administered within 24 hours prior to surgical incision (CABG)
M PQ 0.00 0.00 FUD XXX

4120F Antibiotic prescribed or dispensed (URI, PHAR), (A-BRONCH)
M PQ 0.00 0.00 FUD XXX

4124F Antibiotic neither prescribed nor dispensed (URI, PHAR), (A-BRONCH)
M PQ 0.00 0.00 FUD XXX

4130F Topical preparations (including OTC) prescribed for acute otitis externa (AOE)
M PQ 0.00 0.00 FUD XXX

4131F Systemic antimicrobial therapy prescribed (AOE)
M PQ 0.00 0.00 FUD XXX

4132F Systemic antimicrobial therapy not prescribed (AOE)
M PQ 0.00 0.00 FUD XXX

4133F Antihistamines or decongestants prescribed or recommended (OME)
E 0.00 0.00 FUD XXX

4134F Antihistamines or decongestants neither prescribed nor recommended (OME)
E 0.00 0.00 FUD XXX

4135F Systemic corticosteroids prescribed (OME)
E 0.00 0.00 FUD XXX

4136F Systemic corticosteroids not prescribed (OME)
E 0.00 0.00 FUD XXX

4140F Inhaled corticosteroids prescribed (Asthma)
M PQ 0.00 0.00 FUD XXX

4142F Corticosteroid sparing therapy prescribed (IBD)
M 0.00 0.00 FUD XXX

4144F Alternative long-term control medication prescribed (Asthma)
M PQ 0.00 0.00 FUD XXX

4145F Two or more anti-hypertensive agents prescribed or currently being taken (CAD, HTN)
E PQ 0.00 0.00 FUD XXX

4148F Hepatitis A vaccine injection administered or previously received (HEP-C)
M PQ 0.00 0.00 FUD XXX

4149F Hepatitis B vaccine injection administered or previously received (HEP-C, HIV) (IBD)
E PQ 0.00 0.00 FUD XXX

4150F Patient receiving antiviral treatment for Hepatitis C (HEP-C)
E PQ 0.00 0.00 FUD XXX

4151F Patient not receiving antiviral treatment for Hepatitis C (HEP-C)
M PQ 0.00 0.00 FUD XXX

4153F Combination peginterferon and ribavirin therapy prescribed (HEP-C)
E PQ 0.00 0.00 FUD XXX

4155F Hepatitis A vaccine series previously received (HEP-C)
E 0.00 0.00 FUD XXX

4157F Hepatitis B vaccine series previously received (HEP-C)
E 0.00 0.00 FUD XXX

4158F Patient counseled about risks of alcohol use (HEP-C)
E PQ 0.00 0.00 FUD XXX

4159F Counseling regarding contraception received prior to initiation of antiviral treatment (HEP-C)
E PQ 0.00 0.00 FUD XXX

4163F Patient counseling at a minimum on all of the following treatment options for clinically localized prostate cancer: active surveillance, and interstitial prostate brachytherapy, and external beam radiotherapy, and radical prostatectomy, provided prior to initiation of treatment (PRCA)
E 0.00 0.00 FUD XXX

4164F Adjuvant (ie, in combination with external beam radiotherapy to the prostate for prostate cancer) hormonal therapy (gonadotropin-releasing hormone [GnRH] agonist or antagonist) prescribed/administered (PRCA)
M PQ 0.00 0.00 FUD XXX

4165F 3-dimensional conformal radiotherapy (3D-CRT) or intensity modulated radiation therapy (IMRT) received (PRCA)
E PQ 0.00 0.00 FUD XXX

4167F Head of bed elevation (30-45 degrees) on first ventilator day ordered (CRIT)
E 0.00 0.00 FUD XXX

4168F Patient receiving care in the intensive care unit (ICU) and receiving mechanical ventilation, 24 hours or less (CRIT)
E 0.00 0.00 FUD XXX

4169F Patient either not receiving care in the intensive care unit (ICU) OR not receiving mechanical ventilation OR receiving mechanical ventilation greater than 24 hours (CRIT)
E 0.00 0.00 FUD XXX

4171F Patient receiving erythropoiesis-stimulating agents (ESA) therapy (CKD)
M PQ 0.00 0.00 FUD XXX

4172F Patient not receiving erythropoiesis-stimulating agents (ESA) therapy (CKD)
M PQ 0.00 0.00 FUD XXX

4174F Counseling about the potential impact of glaucoma on visual functioning and quality of life, and importance of treatment adherence provided to patient and/or caregiver(s) (EC)
E 0.00 0.00 FUD XXX

4175F Best-corrected visual acuity of 20/40 or better (distance or near) achieved within the 90 days following cataract surgery (EC)
M PQ 0.00 0.00 FUD XXX

4176F Counseling about value of protection from UV light and lack of proven efficacy of nutritional supplements in prevention or progression of cataract development provided to patient and/or caregiver(s) (NMA-No Measure Associated)
E 0.00 0.00 FUD XXX

4177F Counseling about the benefits and/or risks of the age-related eye disease study (AREDS) formulation for preventing progression of age-related macular degeneration (AMD) provided to patient and/or caregiver(s) (EC)
M PQ 0.00 0.00 FUD XXX

4178F Anti-D immune globulin received between 26 and 30 weeks gestation (Pre-Cr) M ♀
E 0.00 0.00 FUD XXX

4179F Tamoxifen or aromatase inhibitor (AI) prescribed (ONC)
M PQ 0.00 0.00 FUD XXX

4180F Adjuvant chemotherapy referred, prescribed, or previously received for Stage III colon cancer (ONC)
E PQ 0.00 0.00 FUD XXX

4181F Conformal radiation therapy received (NMA-No Measure Associated)
E 0.00 0.00 FUD XXX

4182F Conformal radiation therapy not received (NMA-No Measure Associated)
E 0.00 0.00 FUD XXX

4185F Continuous (12-months) therapy with proton pump inhibitor (PPI) or histamine H2 receptor antagonist (H2RA) received (GERD)
E 0.00 0.00 FUD XXX

4186F No continuous (12-months) therapy with either proton pump inhibitor (PPI) or histamine H2 receptor antagonist (H2RA) received (GERD)
E 0.00 0.00 FUD XXX

4187F Disease modifying anti-rheumatic drug therapy prescribed or dispensed (RA)
M PQ 0.00 0.00 FUD XXX

4188F Appropriate angiotensin converting enzyme (ACE)/angiotensin receptor blockers (ARB) therapeutic monitoring test ordered or performed (AM)
E 0.00 0.00 FUD XXX

4189F Appropriate digoxin therapeutic monitoring test ordered or performed (AM)
E 0.00 0.00 FUD XXX

4190F Appropriate diuretic therapeutic monitoring test ordered or performed (AM)
E 0.00 0.00 FUD XXX

4191F Appropriate anticonvulsant therapeutic monitoring test ordered or performed (AM)
E 0.00 0.00 FUD XXX

4192F Patient not receiving glucocorticoid therapy (RA)
M PQ 0.00 0.00 FUD XXX

4193F Patient receiving <10 mg daily prednisone (or equivalent), or RA activity is worsening, or glucocorticoid use is for less than 6 months (RA)
M PQ 0.00 0.00 FUD XXX

4194F Patient receiving >/=10 mg daily prednisone (or equivalent) for longer than 6 months, and improvement or no change in disease activity (RA)
M PQ 0.00 0.00 FUD XXX

4195F Patient receiving first-time biologic disease modifying anti-rheumatic drug therapy for rheumatoid arthritis (RA)
M PQ 0.00 0.00 FUD XXX

4196F Patient not receiving first-time biologic disease modifying anti-rheumatic drug therapy for rheumatoid arthritis (RA)
M PQ 0.00 0.00 FUD XXX

4200F External beam radiotherapy as primary therapy to prostate with or without nodal irradiation (PRCA)
E PQ 0.00 0.00 FUD XXX

4201F External beam radiotherapy with or without nodal irradiation as adjuvant or salvage therapy for prostate cancer patient (PRCA)
E PQ 0.00 0.00 FUD XXX

4210F Angiotensin converting enzyme (ACE) or angiotensin receptor blockers (ARB) medication therapy for 6 months or more (MM)
E 0.00 0.00 FUD XXX

4220F Digoxin medication therapy for 6 months or more (MM)
E 0.00 0.00 FUD XXX

4221F Diuretic medication therapy for 6 months or more (MM)
E 0.00 0.00 FUD XXX

4230F Anticonvulsant medication therapy for 6 months or more (MM)
E 0.00 0.00 FUD XXX

4240F Instruction in therapeutic exercise with follow-up provided to patients during episode of back pain lasting longer than 12 weeks (BkP)
E 0.00 0.00 FUD XXX

4242F Counseling for supervised exercise program provided to patients during episode of back pain lasting longer than 12 weeks (BkP)
E 0.00 0.00 FUD XXX

4245F Patient counseled during the initial visit to maintain or resume normal activities (BkP)
M 0.00 0.00 FUD XXX

4248F Patient counseled during the initial visit for an episode of back pain against bed rest lasting 4 days or longer (BkP)
M 0.00 0.00 FUD XXX

4250F Active warming used intraoperatively for the purpose of maintaining normothermia, or at least 1 body temperature equal to or greater than 36 degrees Centigrade (or 96.8 degrees Fahrenheit) recorded within the 30 minutes immediately before or the 15 minutes immediately after anesthesia end time (CRIT)
M PQ 0.00 0.00 FUD XXX

4255F Duration of general or neuraxial anesthesia 60 minutes or longer, as documented in the anesthesia record (CRIT) (Peri2)
M PQ 0.00 0.00 FUD XXX

4256F Duration of general or neuraxial anesthesia less than 60 minutes, as documented in the anesthesia record (CRIT) (Peri2)
M PQ 0.00 0.00 FUD XXX

4260F Wound surface culture technique used (CWC)
M PQ 0.00 0.00 FUD XXX

4261F Technique other than surface culture of the wound exudate used (eg, Levine/deep swab technique, semi-quantitative or quantitative swab technique) or wound surface culture technique not used (CWC)
M PQ 0.00 0.00 FUD XXX

4265F Use of wet to dry dressings prescribed or recommended (CWC)
M PQ 0.00 0.00 FUD XXX

4266F Use of wet to dry dressings neither prescribed nor recommended (CWC)
M PQ 0.00 0.00 FUD XXX

4267F Compression therapy prescribed (CWC)
E PQ 0.00 0.00 FUD XXX

4268F Patient education regarding the need for long term compression therapy including interval replacement of compression stockings received (CWC)
E 0.00 0.00 FUD XXX

4269F Appropriate method of offloading (pressure relief) prescribed (CWC)
E 0.00 0.00 FUD XXX

4270F Patient receiving potent antiretroviral therapy for 6 months or longer (HIV)
E PQ 0.00 0.00 FUD XXX

4271F Patient receiving potent antiretroviral therapy for less than 6 months or not receiving potent antiretroviral therapy (HIV)
E PQ 0.00 0.00 FUD XXX

4274F Influenza immunization administered or previously received (HIV) (P-ESRD)
E 0.00 0.00 FUD XXX

4276F Potent antiretroviral therapy prescribed (HIV)
E PQ 0.00 0.00 FUD XXX

4279F Pneumocystis jiroveci pneumonia prophylaxis prescribed (HIV)
E 0.00 0.00 FUD XXX

4280F Pneumocystis jiroveci pneumonia prophylaxis prescribed within 3 months of low CD4+ cell count or percentage (HIV)
E PQ 0.00 0.00 FUD XXX

4290F Patient screened for injection drug use (HIV)
E PQ 0.00 0.00 FUD XXX

4293F Patient screened for high-risk sexual behavior (HIV)
E PQ 0.00 0.00 FUD XXX

4300F Patient receiving warfarin therapy for nonvalvular atrial fibrillation or atrial flutter (AFIB)
E 0.00 0.00 FUD XXX

4301F Patient not receiving warfarin therapy for nonvalvular atrial fibrillation or atrial flutter (AFIB)
E 0.00 0.00 FUD XXX

4305F Patient education regarding appropriate foot care and daily inspection of the feet received (CWC)
E 0.00 0.00 FUD XXX

4306F Patient counseled regarding psychosocial and pharmacologic treatment options for opioid addiction (SUD)
E 0.00 0.00 FUD XXX

4320F Patient counseled regarding psychosocial and pharmacologic treatment options for alcohol dependence (SUD)
M PQ 0.00 0.00 FUD XXX

4322F Caregiver provided with education and referred to additional resources for support (DEM)
M 0.00 0.00 FUD XXX

4324F Patient (or caregiver) queried about Parkinson's disease medication related motor complications (Prkns)
E 0.00 0.00 FUD XXX

4325F Medical and surgical treatment options reviewed with patient (or caregiver) (Prkns)
M 0.00 0.00 FUD XXX

4326F Patient (or caregiver) queried about symptoms of autonomic dysfunction (Prkns)
E 0.00 0.00 FUD XXX

4328F Patient (or caregiver) queried about sleep disturbances (Prkns)
M 0.00 0.00 FUD XXX

4330F Counseling about epilepsy specific safety issues provided to patient (or caregiver(s)) (EPI)
E 0.00 0.00 FUD XXX

4340F Counseling for women of childbearing potential with epilepsy (EPI)
M PQ 0.00 0.00 FUD XXX

4350F Counseling provided on symptom management, end of life decisions, and palliation (DEM)
E 0.00 0.00 FUD XXX

4400F Rehabilitative therapy options discussed with patient (or caregiver) (Prkns)
M 0.00 0.00 FUD XXX

4450F Self-care education provided to patient (HF)
E 0.00 0.00 FUD XXX

4470F Implantable cardioverter-defibrillator (ICD) counseling provided (HF)
E 0.00 0.00 FUD XXX

4480F Patient receiving ACE inhibitor/ARB therapy and beta-blocker therapy for 3 months or longer (HF)
E 0.00 0.00 FUD XXX

4481F Patient receiving ACE inhibitor/ARB therapy and beta-blocker therapy for less than 3 months or patient not receiving ACE inhibitor/ARB therapy and beta-blocker therapy (HF)
E 0.00 0.00 FUD XXX

4500F Referred to an outpatient cardiac rehabilitation program (CAD)
M PQ 0.00 0.00 FUD XXX

4510F Previous cardiac rehabilitation for qualifying cardiac event completed (CAD)
M PQ 0.00 0.00 FUD XXX

4525F Neuropsychiatric intervention ordered (DEM)
M 0.00 0.00 FUD XXX

4526F Neuropsychiatric intervention received (DEM)
M 0.00 0.00 FUD XXX

4540F Disease modifying pharmacotherapy discussed (ALS)
E 0.00 0.00 FUD XXX

4541F Patient offered treatment for pseudobulbar affect, sialorrhea, or ALS-related symptoms (ALS)
E 0.00 0.00 FUD XXX

4550F Options for noninvasive respiratory support discussed with patient (ALS)
E 0.00 0.00 FUD XXX

4551F Nutritional support offered (ALS)
E 0.00 0.00 FUD XXX

4552F Patient offered referral to a speech language pathologist (ALS)
E 0.00 0.00 FUD XXX

4553F Patient offered assistance in planning for end of life issues (ALS)
E 0.00 0.00 FUD XXX

4554F Patient received inhalational anesthetic agent (Peri2)
E 0.00 0.00 FUD XXX

4555F Patient did not receive inhalational anesthetic agent (Peri2)
E 0.00 0.00 FUD XXX

4556F Patient exhibits 3 or more risk factors for post-operative nausea and vomiting (Peri2)
E 0.00 0.00 FUD XXX

4557F Patient does not exhibit 3 or more risk factors for post-operative nausea and vomiting (Peri2)
E 0.00 0.00 FUD XXX

4558F Patient received at least 2 prophylactic pharmacologic anti-emetic agents of different classes preoperatively and intraoperatively (Peri2)
E 0.00 0.00 FUD XXX

4559F At least 1 body temperature measurement equal to or greater than 35.5 degrees Celsius (or 95.9 degrees Fahrenheit) recorded within the 30 minutes immediately before or the 15 minutes immediately after anesthesia end time (Peri2)
E 0.00 0.00 FUD XXX

4560F Anesthesia technique did not involve general or neuraxial anesthesia (Peri2)
E 0.00 0.00 FUD XXX

4561F Patient has a coronary artery stent (Peri2)
E 0.00 0.00 FUD XXX

4562F Patient does not have a coronary artery stent (Peri2)
E 0.00 0.00 FUD XXX

4563F Patient received aspirin within 24 hours prior to anesthesia start time (Peri2)
E 0.00 0.00 FUD XXX

5005F-5250F Results Conveyed and Documented

INCLUDES Patient's:
Functional status
Morbidity/mortality
Satisfaction/experience with care
Review/communication of test results to patients

5005F Patient counseled on self-examination for new or changing moles (ML)
E 0.00 0.00 FUD XXX

5010F Findings of dilated macular or fundus exam communicated to the physician or other qualified health care professional managing the diabetes care (EC)
M PQ 0.00 0.00 FUD XXX

5015F Documentation of communication that a fracture occurred and that the patient was or should be tested or treated for osteoporosis (OP)
M PQ 0.00 0.00 FUD XXX

5020F Treatment summary report communicated to physician(s) or other qualified health care professional(s) managing continuing care and to the patient within 1 month of completing treatment (ONC)
E 0.00 0.00 FUD XXX

5050F Treatment plan communicated to provider(s) managing continuing care within 1 month of diagnosis (ML)
M PQ 0.00 0.00 FUD XXX

5060F Findings from diagnostic mammogram communicated to practice managing patient's on-going care within 3 business days of exam interpretation (RAD)
E 0.00 0.00 FUD XXX

5062F Findings from diagnostic mammogram communicated to the patient within 5 days of exam interpretation (RAD)
E 0.00 0.00 FUD XXX

5100F Potential risk for fracture communicated to the referring physician or other qualified health care professional within 24 hours of completion of the imaging study (NUC_MED)
E 0.00 0.00 FUD XXX

5200F Consideration of referral for a neurological evaluation of appropriateness for surgical therapy for intractable epilepsy within the past 3 years (EPI)
E 0.00 0.00 FUD XXX

5250F Asthma discharge plan provided to patient (Asthma)
E 0.00 0.00 FUD XXX

6005F-6150F Elements Related to Patient Safety Processes

INCLUDES Patient safety practices

6005F Rationale (eg, severity of illness and safety) for level of care (eg, home, hospital) documented (CAP)
E 0.00 0.00 FUD XXX

6010F Dysphagia screening conducted prior to order for or receipt of any foods, fluids, or medication by mouth (STR)
M PQ 0.00 0.00 FUD XXX

6015F Patient receiving or eligible to receive foods, fluids, or medication by mouth (STR)
M PQ 0.00 0.00 FUD XXX

6020F NPO (nothing by mouth) ordered (STR)
M PQ 0.00 0.00 FUD XXX

6030F All elements of maximal sterile barrier technique followed including: cap and mask and sterile gown and sterile gloves and a large sterile sheet and hand hygiene and 2% chlorhexidine for cutaneous antisepsis (or acceptable alternative antiseptics, per current guideline) (CRIT)
M PQ 0.00 0.00 FUD XXX

6040F Use of appropriate radiation dose reduction devices OR manual techniques for appropriate moderation of exposure, documented (RAD)
E 0.00 0.00 FUD XXX

6045F Radiation exposure or exposure time in final report for procedure using fluoroscopy, documented (RAD)
M PQ 0.00 0.00 FUD XXX

6070F Patient queried and counseled about anti-epileptic drug (AED) side effects (EPI)
E 0.00 0.00 FUD XXX

6080F Patient (or caregiver) queried about falls (Prkns, DSP)
E 0.00 0.00 FUD XXX

6090F Patient (or caregiver) counseled about safety issues appropriate to patient's stage of disease (Prkns)
E 0.00 0.00 FUD XXX

6100F Timeout to verify correct patient, correct site, and correct procedure, documented (PATH)
E 0.00 0.00 FUD XXX

6101F Safety counseling for dementia provided (DEM)
M 0.00 0.00 FUD XXX

6102F Safety counseling for dementia ordered (DEM)
M 0.00 0.00 FUD XXX

6110F Counseling provided regarding risks of driving and the alternatives to driving (DEM)
M 0.00 0.00 FUD XXX

6150F Patient not receiving a first course of anti-TNF (tumor necrosis factor) therapy (IBD)
M 0.00 0.00 FUD XXX

7010F-7025F Recall/Reminder System in Place

INCLUDES Capabilities of the provider
Measures that address the setting or system of care provided

7010F Patient information entered into a recall system that includes: target date for the next exam specified and a process to follow up with patients regarding missed or unscheduled appointments (ML)
M PQ 0.00 0.00 FUD XXX

7020F Mammogram assessment category (eg, Mammography Quality Standards Act [MQSA], Breast Imaging Reporting and Data System [BI-RADS], or FDA approved equivalent categories) entered into an internal database to allow for analysis of abnormal interpretation (recall) rate (RAD)
E 0.00 0.00 FUD XXX

7025F Patient information entered into a reminder system with a target due date for the next mammogram (RAD)
M PQ 0.00 0.00 FUD XXX

9001F-9007F No Measure Associated

INCLUDES Aspects of care not associated with measures at the current time

9001F Aortic aneurysm less than 5.0 cm maximum diameter on centerline formatted CT or minor diameter on axial formatted CT (NMA-No Measure Associated)
E 0.00 0.00 FUD XXX

9002F Aortic aneurysm 5.0 - 5.4 cm maximum diameter on centerline formatted CT or minor diameter on axial formatted CT (NMA-No Measure Associated)
E 0.00 0.00 FUD XXX

9003F Aortic aneurysm 5.5 - 5.9 cm maximum diameter on centerline formatted CT or minor diameter on axial formatted CT (NMA-No Measure Associated)
M 0.00 0.00 FUD XXX

9004F Aortic aneurysm 6.0 cm or greater maximum diameter on centerline formatted CT or minor diameter on axial formatted CT (NMA-No Measure Associated)
M 0.00 0.00 FUD XXX

9005F Asymptomatic carotid stenosis: No history of any transient ischemic attack or stroke in any carotid or vertebrobasilar territory (NMA-No Measure Associated)
E 0.00 0.00 FUD XXX

9006F Symptomatic carotid stenosis: Ipsilateral carotid territory TIA or stroke less than 120 days prior to procedure (NMA-No Measure Associated)
M 0.00 0.00 FUD XXX

9007F Other carotid stenosis: Ipsilateral TIA or stroke 120 days or greater prior to procedure or any prior contralateral carotid territory or vertebrobasilar TIA or stroke (NMA-No Measure Associated)
M 0.00 0.00 FUD XXX

0019T-0042T

0019T Extracorporeal shock wave involving musculoskeletal system, not otherwise specified, low energy

EXCLUDES *High energy:*
Extracorporeal shock wave (0101T)
Lateral humeral epicondyle extracorporeal shock wave (0102T)

A 80 0.00 0.00 FUD XXX

0042T Cerebral perfusion analysis using computed tomography with contrast administration, including post-processing of parametric maps with determination of cerebral blood flow, cerebral blood volume, and mean transit time

NI N 80 PQ 0.00 0.00 FUD XXX

0051T-0053T

CMS 100-4,3,90.2.1 Artificial Hearts and Related Devices

0051T Implantation of a total replacement heart system (artificial heart) with recipient cardiectomy

EXCLUDES *Ventricular assist device implant (33975-33976)*

C 80 0.00 0.00 FUD XXX

0052T Replacement or repair of thoracic unit of a total replacement heart system (artificial heart)

EXCLUDES *Exchange or repair of other artificial heart components (0053T)*

C 80 0.00 0.00 FUD XXX

0053T Replacement or repair of implantable component or components of total replacement heart system (artificial heart), excluding thoracic unit

EXCLUDES *Exchange or repair of thoracic unit of artificial heart (0052T)*

C 80 0.00 0.00 FUD XXX

0054T-0055T

\+ **0054T Computer-assisted musculoskeletal surgical navigational orthopedic procedure, with image-guidance based on fluoroscopic images (List separately in addition to code for primary procedure)**

Code first primary procedure

N 80 0.00 0.00 FUD XXX

\+ **0055T Computer-assisted musculoskeletal surgical navigational orthopedic procedure, with image-guidance based on CT/MRI images (List separately in addition to code for primary procedure)**

INCLUDES Performance of both CT and MRI in same session (1 unit)

Code first primary procedure

N 80 0.00 0.00 FUD XXX

0058T-0059T [0357T]

EXCLUDES *Cryopreservation of:*
Embryos (89258)
Oocyte(s), mature (89337)
Sperm (89259)
Testicular reproductive tissue (89335)

0058T Cryopreservation; reproductive tissue, ovarian

X 80 0.00 0.00 FUD XXX

#● **0357T Cryopreservation; immature oocyte(s)**

~~0059T~~ ~~oocyte(s)~~

To report, see 89337, 0357T

0071T-0072T

Do not report with (51702, 77022)

0071T Focused ultrasound ablation of uterine leiomyomata, including MR guidance; total leiomyomata volume less than 200 cc of tissue ♀

S 80 0.00 0.00 FUD XXX

0072T total leiomyomata volume greater or equal to 200 cc of tissue ♀

S 80 0.00 0.00 FUD XXX

0073T

CMS 100-4,4,220.1 Billing for IMRT Planning and Delivery

~~**0073T Compensator-based beam modulation treatment delivery of inverse planned treatment using 3 or more high resolution (milled or cast) compensator convergent beam modulated fields, per treatment session**~~

To report, see 77385

0075T-0076T

▲ **0075T Transcatheter placement of extracranial vertebral artery stent(s), including radiologic supervision and interpretation, open or percutaneous; initial vessel**

INCLUDES All diagnostic services for stenting
Ipsilateral extracranial vertebral selective catheterization when confirming the need for stenting

EXCLUDES *Selective catheterization and imaging when stenting is not required (report only selective catheterization codes)*

C 80 PQ 0.00 0.00 FUD XXX

\+ ▲ **0076T each additional vessel (List separately in addition to code for primary procedure)**

Code first (0075T)

C 80 0.00 0.00 FUD XXX

0085T

0085T Breath test for heart transplant rejection

E 0.00 0.00 FUD XXX

0092T-0098T

INCLUDES Fluoroscopy

~~**0092T Total disc arthroplasty (artificial disc), anterior approach, including discectomy with end plate preparation (includes osteophytectomy for nerve root or spinal cord decompression and microdissection), each additional interspace, cervical (List separately in addition to code for primary procedure)**~~

To report cervical arthroplasty on three levels or more, see 0375T

\+ **0095T Removal of total disc arthroplasty (artificial disc), anterior approach, each additional interspace, cervical (List separately in addition to code for primary procedure)**

EXCLUDES *Lumbar disc (0164T)*
Revision of total disc arthroplasty, cervical (22861)
Revision of total disc arthroplasty, lumbar (22862)

Code first (22864)

C 80 0.00 0.00 FUD XXX

\+ **0098T Revision including replacement of total disc arthroplasty (artificial disc), anterior approach, each additional interspace, cervical (List separately in addition to code for primary procedure)**

EXCLUDES *Spinal cord decompression (63001-63048)*

Code first (22861)

Do not report when performed at the same level with (22851)

Do not report with (0095T)

C 80 0.00 0.00 FUD XXX

0099T-0159T

0099T Implantation of intrastromal corneal ring segments

R2 T 80 0.00 0.00 FUD XXX

0100T Placement of a subconjunctival retinal prosthesis receiver and pulse generator, and implantation of intra-ocular retinal electrode array, with vitrectomy

G2 T 80 0.00 0.00 FUD XXX

0101T Extracorporeal shock wave involving musculoskeletal system, not otherwise specified, high energy

EXCLUDES *Extracorporeal shock wave therapy for healing of integumentary system wounds (0299T-0300T)*

Low energy extracorporeal shock wave (0019T)

Do not report for same area with (0299T-0300T)

G2 T 80 0.00 0.00 FUD XXX

0102T Extracorporeal shock wave, high energy, performed by a physician, requiring anesthesia other than local, involving lateral humeral epicondyle

EXCLUDES *Low energy extracorporeal shock wave (0019T)*

G2 T 80 0.00 0.00 FUD XXX

0103T Holotranscobalamin, quantitative

A 80 0.00 0.00 FUD XXX

0106T Quantitative sensory testing (QST), testing and interpretation per extremity; using touch pressure stimuli to assess large diameter sensation

X 80 0.00 0.00 FUD XXX

0107T using vibration stimuli to assess large diameter fiber sensation

X 80 0.00 0.00 FUD XXX

0108T using cooling stimuli to assess small nerve fiber sensation and hyperalgesia

X 80 0.00 0.00 FUD XXX

0109T using heat-pain stimuli to assess small nerve fiber sensation and hyperalgesia

X 80 0.00 0.00 FUD XXX

0110T using other stimuli to assess sensation

X 80 0.00 0.00 FUD XXX

0111T Long-chain (C20-22) omega-3 fatty acids in red blood cell (RBC) membranes

EXCLUDES *Very long chain fatty acids (82726)*

A 80 0.00 0.00 FUD XXX

0123T Fistulization of sclera for glaucoma, through ciliary body

EXCLUDES *Posterior extrascleral placement of pharmacological agent performed with conjunctival incision (68399)*

G2 T 80 0.00 0.00 FUD XXX

0126T Common carotid intima-media thickness (IMT) study for evaluation of atherosclerotic burden or coronary heart disease risk factor assessment

Do not report with (93880, 93882, 93895)

Q1 80 0.00 0.00 FUD XXX

\+ **0159T Computer-aided detection, including computer algorithm analysis of MRI image data for lesion detection/characterization, pharmacokinetic analysis, with further physician review for interpretation, breast MRI (List separately in addition to code for primary procedure)**

Code first (77058-77059)

Do not report with (76376-76377)

N 80 0.00 0.00 FUD ZZZ

0163T-0165T

INCLUDES Fluoroscopy

EXCLUDES *Cervical disc procedures (22856)*

Decompression (63001-63048)

Do not report with these procedures when performed at the same level (22851, 49010)

\+ **0163T Total disc arthroplasty (artificial disc), anterior approach, including discectomy to prepare interspace (other than for decompression), each additional interspace, lumbar (List separately in addition to code for primary procedure)**

Code first (22857)

C 80 0.00 0.00 FUD YYY

\+ **0164T Removal of total disc arthroplasty, (artificial disc), anterior approach, each additional interspace, lumbar (List separately in addition to code for primary procedure)**

Code first (22865)

C 80 0.00 0.00 FUD YYY

\+ **0165T Revision including replacement of total disc arthroplasty (artificial disc), anterior approach, each additional interspace, lumbar (List separately in addition to code for primary procedure)**

Code first (22862)

C 80 0.00 0.00 FUD YYY

0169T-0175T

0169T Stereotactic placement of infusion catheter(s) in the brain for delivery of therapeutic agent(s), including computerized stereotactic planning and burr hole(s)

Do not report with (20660, 61107, 61781-61783)

C 80 0.00 0.00 FUD XXX

0171T Insertion of posterior spinous process distraction device (including necessary removal of bone or ligament for insertion and imaging guidance), lumbar; single level

T 80 0.00 0.00 FUD XXX

\+ **0172T each additional level (List separately in addition to code for primary procedure)**

Code first (0171T)

N 80 0.00 0.00 FUD XXX

\+ **0174T Computer-aided detection (CAD) (computer algorithm analysis of digital image data for lesion detection) with further physician review for interpretation and report, with or without digitization of film radiographic images, chest radiograph(s), performed concurrent with primary interpretation (List separately in addition to code for primary procedure)**

Code first (71010, 71020-71022, 71030)

NI N 80 0.00 0.00 FUD XXX

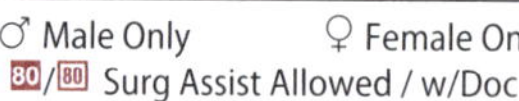
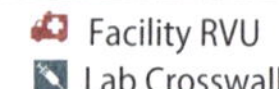

0175T **Computer-aided detection (CAD) (computer algorithm analysis of digital image data for lesion detection) with further physician review for interpretation and report, with or without digitization of film radiographic images, chest radiograph(s), performed remote from primary interpretation**

Do not report with (71010, 71020-71022, 71030)

N1 N 80 0.00 0.00 FUD XXX

0178T-0180T

EXCLUDES *Separately performed 12-lead electrocardiogram (93000-93010)*

0178T **Electrocardiogram, 64 leads or greater, with graphic presentation and analysis; with interpretation and report**

B 80 0.00 0.00 FUD XXX

0179T **tracing and graphics only, without interpretation and report**

X TC 80 0.00 0.00 FUD XXX

0180T **interpretation and report only**

B 26 80 0.00 0.00 FUD XXX

0181T-0184T

~~0181T~~ ~~**Corneal hysteresis determination, by air impulse stimulation, bilateral, with interpretation and report**~~

To report, see 92145

0182T **High dose rate electronic brachytherapy, per fraction**

EXCLUDES *Placement or removal of an applicator into breast for radiation therapy (C9726)*

Do not report with (77761-77763, 77776-77778, 77785-77787, 77789)

Z2 S 80 0.00 0.00 FUD XXX

0184T **Excision of rectal tumor, transanal endoscopic microsurgical approach (ie, TEMS), including muscularis propria (ie, full thickness)**

INCLUDES Operating microscope (66990)

EXCLUDES *Nonendoscopic excision of rectal tumor (45160, 45171-45172)*

Do not report with (45300-45327)

T 80 0.00 0.00 FUD XXX

0188T-0189T

INCLUDES 30 minutes or more of direct medical care by a physician(s) or other qualified health care professional(s) to a critically ill or critically injured patient from an off-site location

Additional on-site critical care services when a critically ill or injured patient requires critical care resources not available on-site

Real time ability to:

- Document the remote care services in the medical record
- Enter orders electronically
- Evaluate patients with high fidelity audio/video capabilities
- Observe patient monitors, infusion pumps, ventilators
- Talk to patients and family members
- Videoconference with the health care team on-site in the patient's room

Real-time access to the patient's:

- Clinical laboratory test results
- Diagnostic test results
- Medical records
- Radiographic images

Review and/or interpretation of all diagnostic information

Time spent with the patient, family, or surrogate decision makers to obtain a medical history, review the patient's condition/prognosis, or discuss treatment options from the remote site

Do not report for same time period with other critical care services rendered by provider or other individual (99291-99292, 99468-99476)

Do not report for time spent away from the remote site without real-time capabilities

Do not report time spent for services that do not directly contribute to patient treatment

0188T **Remote real-time interactive video-conferenced critical care, evaluation and management of the critically ill or critically injured patient; first 30-74 minutes**

INCLUDES First 30 to 74 minutes of remote critical care each day

Do not report remote critical care less than 30 minutes total duration

M 0.00 0.00 FUD XXX

\+ 0189T **each additional 30 minutes (List separately in addition to code for primary service)**

INCLUDES Up to 30 minutes each beyond the first 74 minutes

Code first (0188T)

M 0.00 0.00 FUD XXX

0190T-0253T [0253T, 0376T]

\+ 0190T **Placement of intraocular radiation source applicator (List separately in addition to primary procedure)**

EXCLUDES *Insertion of brachytherapy source by radiation oncologist (see Clinical Brachytherapy Section)*

Code first (67036)

Code also brachytherapy source

N1 N 80 0.00 0.00 FUD XXX

▲ 0191T **Insertion of anterior segment aqueous drainage device, without extraocular reservoir, internal approach, into the trabecular meshwork; initial insertion**

G2 T 80 0.00 0.00 FUD XXX

\+ #● 0376T **Insertion of anterior segment aqueous drainage device, without extraocular reservoir, internal approach, into the trabecular meshwork; each additional device insertion (List separately in addition to code for primary procedure)**

Code first (0191T)

#▲ 0253T **Insertion of anterior segment aqueous drainage device, without extraocular reservoir, internal approach, into the suprachoroidal space**

G2 T 80 0.00 0.00 FUD YYY

0195T-0196T

Do not report with (20930-20938, 22558, 22840, 22845, 22848, 22851, 72275, 76000, 76380, 76496-76497, 77002-77003, 77011-77012)

0195T **Arthrodesis, pre-sacral interbody technique, disc space preparation, discectomy, without instrumentation, with image guidance, includes bone graft when performed; L5-S1 interspace**

C 80 0.00 0.00 FUD XXX

\+ 0196T **L4-L5 interspace (List separately in addition to code for primary procedure)**

Code first (0195T)

C 80 0.00 0.00 FUD XXX

0197T-0199T

~~0197T~~ ~~**Intra-fraction localization and tracking of target or patient motion during delivery of radiation therapy (eg, 3D positional tracking, gating, 3D surface tracking), each fraction of treatment**~~

To report, see 77387

0198T **Measurement of ocular blood flow by repetitive intraocular pressure sampling, with interpretation and report**

S 80 0.00 0.00 FUD XXX

~~0199T~~ ~~**Physiologic recording of tremor using accelerometer(s) and/or gyroscope(s) (including frequency and amplitude), including interpretation and report**~~

To report, see 95999

0200T-0201T

Do not report at same level with (20225)

⊙ ▲ **0200T** **Percutaneous sacral augmentation (sacroplasty), unilateral injection(s), including the use of a balloon or mechanical device, when used, 1 or more needles, includes imaging guidance and bone biopsy, when performed**
G2 T 80 50 0.00 0.00 FUD XXX

⊙ ▲ **0201T** **Percutaneous sacral augmentation (sacroplasty), bilateral injections, including the use of a balloon or mechanical device, when used, 2 or more needles, includes imaging guidance and bone biopsy, when performed**
G2 T 80 0.00 0.00 FUD XXX

0202T-0207T

0202T **Posterior vertebral joint(s) arthroplasty (eg, facet joint[s] replacement), including facetectomy, laminectomy, foraminotomy, and vertebral column fixation, injection of bone cement, when performed, including fluoroscopy, single level, lumbar spine**
Do not report the following codes when performed at the same level: (22511, 22514, 22840, 22851, 22857, 63005, 63012, 63017, 63030, 63042, 63047, 63056)
C 80 0.00 0.00 FUD XXX

+ **0205T** **Intravascular catheter-based coronary vessel or graft spectroscopy (eg, infrared) during diagnostic evaluation and/or therapeutic intervention including imaging supervision, interpretation, and report, each vessel (List separately in addition to code for primary procedure)**
Code first ([92920], [92924], [92928], [92933], [92937], [92941], [92943], [92975], 93454-93461, 93563-93564)
N 80 0.00 0.00 FUD ZZZ

0206T **Computerized database analysis of multiple cycles of digitized cardiac electrical data from two or more ECG leads, including transmission to a remote center, application of multiple nonlinear mathematical transformations, with coronary artery obstruction severity assessment**
Code also 12-lead ECG when performed (93000-93010)
Q1 TC 80 0.00 0.00 FUD XXX

0207T **Evacuation of meibomian glands, automated, using heat and intermittent pressure, unilateral**
S 80 0.00 0.00 FUD XXX

0208T-0212T

EXCLUDES *Manual audiometric testing by a qualified health care professional, using audiometers (92551-92557)*

0208T **Pure tone audiometry (threshold), automated; air only**
X TC 80 0.00 0.00 FUD XXX

0209T **air and bone**
X TC 80 0.00 0.00 FUD XXX

0210T **Speech audiometry threshold, automated;**
X TC 80 0.00 0.00 FUD XXX

0211T **with speech recognition**
X TC 80 0.00 0.00 FUD XXX

0212T **Comprehensive audiometry threshold evaluation and speech recognition (0209T, 0211T combined), automated**
X TC 80 0.00 0.00 FUD XXX

0213T-0215T

0213T **Injection(s), diagnostic or therapeutic agent, paravertebral facet (zygapophyseal) joint (or nerves innervating that joint) with ultrasound guidance, cervical or thoracic; single level**
R2 T 80 50 0.00 0.00 FUD XXX

+ **0214T** **second level (List separately in addition to code for primary procedure)**
Code first (0213T)
N1 N 80 50 0.00 0.00 FUD ZZZ

+ **0215T** **third and any additional level(s) (List separately in addition to code for primary procedure)**
Code first (0213T-0214T)
Do not report more than one time per day
N1 N 80 50 0.00 0.00 FUD ZZZ

0216T-0218T

EXCLUDES *Injection with CT or fluoroscopic guidance (64490-64495)*

0216T **Injection(s), diagnostic or therapeutic agent, paravertebral facet (zygapophyseal) joint (or nerves innervating that joint) with ultrasound guidance, lumbar or sacral; single level**
R2 T 80 50 0.00 0.00 FUD XXX

+ **0217T** **second level (List separately in addition to code for primary procedure)**
Code first (0216T)
N1 N 80 50 0.00 0.00 FUD ZZZ

+ **0218T** **third and any additional level(s) (List separately in addition to code for primary procedure)**
Code first (0216T, 0217T)
Do not report more than one time per day
N1 N 80 50 0.00 0.00 FUD ZZZ

0219T-0222T

Do not report when performed at the same level (20930-20931, 22600-22614, 22840, 22851)
Do not report with any radiology service

0219T **Placement of a posterior intrafacet implant(s), unilateral or bilateral, including imaging and placement of bone graft(s) or synthetic device(s), single level; cervical**
C 80 0.00 0.00 FUD XXX

0220T **thoracic**
C 80 0.00 0.00 FUD XXX

0221T **lumbar**
T 80 0.00 0.00 FUD XXX

+ **0222T** **each additional vertebral segment (List separately in addition to code for primary procedure)**
Code first (0219T-0221T)
N 80 0.00 0.00 FUD ZZZ

0223T-0225T

INCLUDES Assessment of data including heart sounds and limited reprogramming to ensure the best hemodynamics (heart rate parameter and/or automated timing modes, including precise changes of AV/VV intervals)
Evaluation of systolic and diastolic sounds of the heart
Rhythm strip ECG (93040-93042)

EXCLUDES *Complete programming services as separate procedure (93280-93281, 93283-93284)*

0223T **Acoustic cardiography, including automated analysis of combined acoustic and electrical intervals; single, with interpretation and report**
S 80 0.00 0.00 FUD XXX

0224T multiple, including serial trended analysis and limited reprogramming of device parameter, AV or VV delays only, with interpretation and report
Do not report with (93288-93289)
S 80 0.00 0.00 FUD XXX

0225T multiple, including serial trended analysis and limited reprogramming of device parameter, AV and VV delays, with interpretation and report
Do not report with (93288-93299)
S 80 0.00 0.00 FUD XXX

0226T-0233T

~~0226T Anoscopy, high resolution (HRA) (with magnification and chemical agent enhancement); diagnostic, including collection of specimen(s) by brushing or washing when performed~~
To report, see 46601

~~0227T with biopsy(ies)~~
To report, see 46607

0228T Injection(s), anesthetic agent and/or steroid, transforaminal epidural, with ultrasound guidance, cervical or thoracic; single level
62 T 50 0.00 0.00 FUD XXX

+ 0229T each additional level (List separately in addition to code for primary procedure)
Code first (0228T)
N1 N 50 0.00 0.00 FUD XXX

0230T Injection(s), anesthetic agent and/or steroid, transforaminal epidural, with ultrasound guidance, lumbar or sacral; single level
62 T 50 0.00 0.00 FUD XXX

+ 0231T each additional level (List separately in addition to code for primary procedure)
EXCLUDES *Injection performed with CT or fluoroscopic guidance (64479-64484)*
Code first (0230T)
Do not report with (76942, 76998-76999)
N1 N 50 0.00 0.00 FUD XXX

0232T Injection(s), platelet rich plasma, any site, including image guidance, harvesting and preparation when performed
EXCLUDES *Aspiration of bone marrow for grafting, biopsy, harvesting for transplant (38220-38221, 38230)*
Do not report with (20550-20551, 20600-20610, 20926, 76942, 77002, 77012, 77021, 86965)
62 X 0.00 0.00 FUD XXX

0233T Skin advanced glycation endproducts (AGE) measurement by multi-wavelength fluorescent spectroscopy
A 80 0.00 0.00 FUD XXX

0234T-0238T

INCLUDES Atherectomy by any technique in arteries above the inguinal ligaments
Radiology supervision and interpretation

EXCLUDES *Accessing and catheterization of the vessel*
Atherectomy performed below the inguinal ligaments (37225, 37227, 37229, 37231, 37233, 37235)
Closure of the arteriotomy by any technique
Negotiating the lesion
Other interventions to the same or different vessels
Protection from embolism

0234T Transluminal peripheral atherectomy, open or percutaneous, including radiological supervision and interpretation; renal artery
T 80 PQ 0.00 0.00 FUD YYY

0235T visceral artery (except renal), each vessel
C 80 PQ 0.00 0.00 FUD YYY

0236T abdominal aorta
T 80 PQ 0.00 0.00 FUD YYY

0237T brachiocephalic trunk and branches, each vessel
T 80 0.00 0.00 FUD YYY

0238T iliac artery, each vessel
62 T 80 PQ 0.00 0.00 FUD YYY

0239T-0241T

~~0239T Bioimpedance spectroscopy (BIS), measuring 100 frequencies or greater, direct measurement of extracellular fluid differences between the limbs~~
To report, see 93702

0240T Esophageal motility (manometric study of the esophagus and/or gastroesophageal junction) study with interpretation and report; with high resolution esophageal pressure topography
Do not report with (91010, 91013)
X 80 0.00 0.00 FUD YYY

+ 0241T with stimulation or perfusion during high resolution esophageal pressure topography study (eg, stimulant, acid or alkali perfusion) (List separately in addition to code for primary procedure)
Code first (0240T)
Do not report more than one time each session
Do not report with (91010, 91013)
N 80 0.00 0.00 FUD YYY

0243T-0244T

0243T Intermittent measurement of wheeze rate for bronchodilator or bronchial-challenge diagnostic evaluation(s), with interpretation and report
Do not report in the same 24-hour period with (0224T)
Do not report more than one time in a 24 hour period
S 80 0.00 0.00 FUD YYY

0244T Continuous measurement of wheeze rate during treatment assessment or during sleep for documentation of nocturnal wheeze and cough for diagnostic evaluation 3 to 24 hours, with interpretation and report
X 80 0.00 0.00 FUD YYY

0245T-0248T

~~0245T Open treatment of rib fracture requiring internal fixation, unilateral; 1-2 ribs~~
To report, see 21811

~~0246T 3-4 ribs~~
To report, see 21811, 21812

~~0247T 5-6 ribs~~
To report, see 21812

~~0248T 7 or more ribs~~
To report, see 21813

0249T-0255T

0249T Ligation, hemorrhoidal vascular bundle(s), including ultrasound guidance
Do not report with (46020, 46221, [46945, 46946], 46250-46262, 46600, 76872, 76942, 76998)
62 T 80 0.00 0.00 FUD YYY

0253T Resequenced code, See code following 0191T.

0254T **Endovascular repair of iliac artery bifurcation (eg, aneurysm, pseudoaneurysm, arteriovenous malformation, trauma) using bifurcated endoprosthesis from the common iliac artery into both the external and internal iliac artery, unilateral;**
0255T
C 80 0.00 0.00 FUD YYY

0255T **radiological supervision and interpretation**
C 80 0.00 0.00 FUD YYY

0262T

INCLUDES All congenital catheterization(s)
Contrast injections during procedure
Fluoroscopic radiological supervision and interpretation
Imaging guidance for pulmonary valve procedure
Percutaneous balloon angioplasty/valvuloplasty of pulmonary valve/conduit
Stent deployment in pulmonary conduit

Code also cardiovascular stent placement performed at site separate from delivery site of the prosthetic pulmonary valve (37236-37239, [92928, 92929, 92933, 92934, 92937, 92938, 92941, 92943, 92944])
Code also pulmonary artery angioplasty performed at site separate from delivery site of the prosthetic valve (92997-92998)
Do not report with (76000-76001, 92990, 93530, 93563, 93566-93568)

0262T **Implantation of catheter-delivered prosthetic pulmonary valve, endovascular approach**
C 80 0.00 0.00 FUD YYY

0263T-0265T

0263T **Intramuscular autologous bone marrow cell therapy, with preparation of harvested cells, multiple injections, one leg, including ultrasound guidance, if performed; complete procedure including unilateral or bilateral bone marrow harvest**
Do not report with (38204-38242, 76942, 93925-93926)
62 S 80 0.00 0.00 FUD XXX

0264T **complete procedure excluding bone marrow harvest**
Do not report with (38204-38242, 76942, 93925-93926, 0265T)
62 S 80 0.00 0.00 FUD XXX

0265T **unilateral or bilateral bone marrow harvest only for intramuscular autologous bone marrow cell therapy**
EXCLUDES *Complete procedure (0263T)*
Do not report with (38204-38242, 0264T)
62 S 80 0.00 0.00 FUD XXX

0266T-0273T

0266T **Implantation or replacement of carotid sinus baroreflex activation device; total system (includes generator placement, unilateral or bilateral lead placement, intra-operative interrogation, programming, and repositioning, when performed)**
C 80 0.00 0.00 FUD YYY

0267T **lead only, unilateral (includes intra-operative interrogation, programming, and repositioning, when performed)**
Code also (C1778, L8680)
Do not report with (0266T, 0269T-0273T)
T 80 0.00 0.00 FUD YYY

0268T **pulse generator only (includes intra-operative interrogation, programming, and repositioning, when performed)**
Code also (C1767, C1820, L8685-L8688)
Do not report with (0266T, 0269T-0273T)
S 80 0.00 0.00 FUD YYY

0269T **Revision or removal of carotid sinus baroreflex activation device; total system (includes generator placement, unilateral or bilateral lead placement, intra-operative interrogation, programming, and repositioning, when performed)**
Do not report with (0266T-0268T, 0270T-0273T)
62 Q2 80 0.00 0.00 FUD XXX

0270T **lead only, unilateral (includes intra-operative interrogation, programming, and repositioning, when performed)**
EXCLUDES *Removal of total carotid sinus baroreflex activation device (0269T)*
Do not report with (0266T-0269T, 0271T-0273T)
62 Q2 80 0.00 0.00 FUD XXX

0271T **pulse generator only (includes intra-operative interrogation, programming, and repositioning, when performed)**
EXCLUDES *Removal and replacement (0266T-0268T)*
Do not report with (0266T-0270T, 0272T-0273T)
62 Q2 80 0.00 0.00 FUD XXX

0272T **Interrogation device evaluation (in person), carotid sinus baroreflex activation system, including telemetric iterative communication with the implantable device to monitor device diagnostics and programmed therapy values, with interpretation and report (eg, battery status, lead impedance, pulse amplitude, pulse width, therapy frequency, pathway mode, burst mode, therapy start/stop times each day);**
Do not report with (0266T-0271T, 0273T)
S 80 0.00 0.00 FUD XXX

0273T **with programming**
Do not report with (0266T-0272T)
S 80 0.00 0.00 FUD XXX

0274T-0275T

EXCLUDES *Laminotomy/hemilaminectomy by open and endoscopically assisted approach (63020-63035)*
Percutaneous decompression of nucleus pulposus of intervertebral disc by needle-based technique (62287)

0274T **Percutaneous laminotomy/laminectomy (interlaminar approach) for decompression of neural elements, (with or without ligamentous resection, discectomy, facetectomy and/or foraminotomy), any method, under indirect image guidance (eg, fluoroscopic, CT), with or without the use of an endoscope, single or multiple levels, unilateral or bilateral; cervical or thoracic**
62 T 80 0.00 0.00 FUD YYY

0275T **lumbar**
62 T 0.00 0.00 FUD XXX

0278T-0281T

0278T **Transcutaneous electrical modulation pain reprocessing (eg, scrambler therapy), each treatment session (includes placement of electrodes)**
S 80 0.00 0.00 FUD XXX

0281T **Percutaneous transcatheter closure of the left atrial appendage with implant, including fluoroscopy, transseptal puncture, catheter placement(s), left atrial angiography, left atrial appendage angiography, radiological supervision and interpretation**
Code also for right heart catheterization separately for reasons distinct from left atrial appendage closure (93451-93461, 93530-93533)
Code also for separately performed ventriculography with transseptal approach for reasons separate from the left atrial appendage closure. (93565)
Do not report with (93462)
Do not report with the following codes unless the catheterization of the left ventricle is done by a nontransseptal approach for reasons other than the left atrial appendage repair (93452-93453, 93458-93461, 93531-93533)
Do not report with the following codes unless the complete right heart catheterization is done for reasons other than the left atrial appendage repair (93451, 93453, 93456, 93460-93461, 93530-93533)
C 80 0.00 0.00 FUD XXX

0282T-0285T

Do not report with (64550 64595, 77002 77003, 95970 95973)

⊙ **0282T** **Percutaneous or open implantation of neurostimulator electrode array(s), subcutaneous (peripheral subcutaneous field stimulation), including imaging guidance, when performed, cervical, thoracic or lumbar; for trial, including removal at the conclusion of trial period**
Code also (C1778, C1897, L8680)
J8 S 80 50 0.00 0.00 FUD XXX

⊙ **0283T** **permanent, with implantation of a pulse generator**
Code also (C1767, C1778, C1820, C1897, L8680)
J8 S 80 50 0.00 0.00 FUD XXX

⊙ **0284T** **Revision or removal of pulse generator or electrodes, including imaging guidance, when performed, including addition of new electrodes, when performed**
G2 Q2 80 0.00 0.00 FUD XXX

0285T **Electronic analysis of implanted peripheral subcutaneous field stimulation pulse generator, with reprogramming when performed**
S 80 0.00 0.00 FUD XXX

0286T-0287T

0286T **Near-infrared spectroscopy studies of lower extremity wounds (eg, for oxyhemoglobin measurement)**
N1 N 80 0.00 0.00 FUD XXX

0287T **Near-infrared guidance for vascular access requiring real-time digital visualization of subcutaneous vasculature for evaluation of potential access sites and vessel patency**
N1 N 80 0.00 0.00 FUD XXX

0288T

Do not report with (46600-46615)

0288T **Anoscopy, with delivery of thermal energy to the muscle of the anal canal (eg, for fecal incontinence)**
G2 T 80 0.00 0.00 FUD XXX

0289T-0290T

+ **0289T** **Corneal incisions in the donor cornea created using a laser, in preparation for penetrating or lamellar keratoplasty (List separately in addition to code for primary procedure)**
Code first (65710, 65730, 65750, 65755)
N1 N 80 0.00 0.00 FUD ZZZ

+ **0290T** **Corneal incisions in the recipient cornea created using a laser, in preparation for penetrating or lamellar keratoplasty (List separately in addition to code for primary procedure)**
Code first (65710, 65730, 65750, 65755)
N1 N 80 0.00 0.00 FUD ZZZ

0291T-0292T

INCLUDES All manipulations and repositioning inside evaluated vessel including prior to and after the intervention

EXCLUDES *Intravascular spectroscopy (0205T)*

+ ⊙ **0291T** **Intravascular optical coherence tomography (coronary native vessel or graft) during diagnostic evaluation and/or therapeutic intervention, including imaging supervision, interpretation, and report; initial vessel (List separately in addition to primary procedure)**
Code first ([92920], [92924], [92928], [92933], [92937], [92941], [92943], [92975], 93454-93461, 93563-93564)
N1 N 80 0.00 0.00 FUD ZZZ

+ ⊙ **0292T** **each additional vessel (List separately in addition to primary procedure)**
Code first (0291T)
N1 N 80 0.00 0.00 FUD ZZZ

0293T-0294T

Do not report with (93462, 93662)

⊙ **0293T** **Insertion of left atrial hemodynamic monitor; complete system, includes implanted communication module and pressure sensor lead in left atrium including transseptal access, radiological supervision and interpretation, and associated injection procedures, when performed**
Do not report with the following unless performed for separate clinical reason other than calibration or placement of left atrial hemodynamic monitoring system (33202-33249 [33221, 33227, 33228, 33229, 33230, 33231, 33262, 33263, 33264], 93451-93453)
C 80 0.00 0.00 FUD XXX

+ ⊙ **0294T** **pressure sensor lead at time of insertion of pacing cardioverter-defibrillator pulse generator including radiological supervision and interpretation and associated injection procedures, when performed (List separately in addition to code for primary procedure)**
Code first (33240, [33230, 33231], [33262, 33263, 33264], 33249)
Do not report with the following unless performed for separate clinical reason other than calibration or placement of left atrial hemodynamic monitoring system (33202-33249 [33221, 33227, 33228, 33229, 33230, 33231, 33262, 33263, 33264], 93451-93453)
C 80 0.00 0.00 FUD ZZZ

0295T-0298T

Do not report with (93224-93272)

0295T **External electrocardiographic recording for more than 48 hours up to 21 days by continuous rhythm recording and storage; includes recording, scanning analysis with report, review and interpretation**
M 80 0.00 0.00 FUD XXX

0296T recording (includes connection and initial recording)
S 80 0.00 0.00 FUD XXX

0297T scanning analysis with report
S 80 0.00 0.00 FUD XXX

0298T review and interpretation
M 80 0.00 0.00 FUD XXX

0299T-0301T

0299T Extracorporeal shock wave for integumentary wound healing, high energy, including topical application and dressing care; initial wound
R2 T 80 0.00 0.00 FUD XXX

\+ **0300T** each additional wound (List separately in addition to code for primary procedure)
Code first (0299T)
Do not report with (0101T-0102T, 28890) when performed in the same area
N1 N 80 0.00 0.00 FUD ZZZ

⊙ **0301T** Destruction/reduction of malignant breast tumor with externally applied focused microwave, including interstitial placement of disposable catheter with combined temperature monitoring probe and microwave focusing sensocatheter under ultrasound thermotherapy guidance
Do not report with (76641-76642, 76942, 76998, 77600-77615)
G2 S 80 0.00 0.00 FUD XXX

0302T-0304T

Do not report with (93000-93010)

⊙ **0302T** Insertion or removal and replacement of intracardiac ischemia monitoring system including imaging supervision and interpretation when performed and intra-operative interrogation and programming when performed; complete system (includes device and electrode)
J8 T 0.00 0.00 FUD YYY

⊙ **0303T** electrode only
G2 T 0.00 0.00 FUD YYY

⊙ **0304T** device only
J8 T 0.00 0.00 FUD YYY

0305T-0307T

0305T Programming device evaluation (in person) of intracardiac ischemia monitoring system with iterative adjustment of programmed values, with analysis, review, and report
Do not report with (93000-93010, 0302T-0304T, 0306T)
S 80 0.00 0.00 FUD XXX

0306T Interrogation device evaluation (in person) of intracardiac ischemia monitoring system with analysis, review, and report
Do not report with (93000-93010, 0302T-0305T)
S 80 0.00 0.00 FUD XXX

⊙ **0307T** Removal of intracardiac ischemia monitoring device
G2 Q2 0.00 0.00 FUD YYY

0308T-0311T

⊙ **0308T** Insertion of ocular telescope prosthesis including removal of crystalline lens
INCLUDES Operating microscope (69990)
Do not report with (65800-65815, 66020, 66030, 66600-66635, 66761, 66825, 66982-66986)
G2 T 50 0.00 0.00 FUD YYY

\+ **0309T** Arthrodesis, pre-sacral interbody technique, including disc space preparation, discectomy, with posterior instrumentation, with image guidance, includes bone graft, when performed, lumbar, L4-L5 interspace (List separately in addition to code for primary procedure)
Code first (22586)
Do not report with (20930-20938, 22840, 22848, 72275, 77002-77003, 77011-77012)
C 80 0.00 0.00 FUD ZZZ

0310T Motor function mapping using non-invasive navigated transcranial magnetic stimulation (nTMS) for therapeutic treatment planning, upper and lower extremity
Do not report with (95860-95870, 95928-95929, [95939])
S 80 0.00 0.00 FUD XXX

0311T Non-invasive calculation and analysis of central arterial pressure waveforms with interpretation and report
S 80 0.00 0.00 FUD XXX

0312T-0317T

EXCLUDES *Analysis and/or programming (or reprogramming) of vagus nerve stimulator (95970, 95974-95975)*
Implantation, replacement, removal, and/or revision of vagus nerve neurostimulator (electrode array and/or pulse generator) for stimulation of vagus nerve other than at the esophagogastric junction (64568-64570)

0312T Vagus nerve blocking therapy (morbid obesity); laparoscopic implantation of neurostimulator electrode array, anterior and posterior vagal trunks adjacent to esophagogastric junction (EGJ), with implantation of pulse generator, includes programming
C 80 0.00 0.00 FUD XXX

0313T laparoscopic revision or replacement of vagal trunk neurostimulator electrode array, including connection to existing pulse generator
G2 T 80 0.00 0.00 FUD XXX

0314T laparoscopic removal of vagal trunk neurostimulator electrode array and pulse generator
G2 Q2 80 0.00 0.00 FUD XXX

0315T removal of pulse generator
Do not report with (0316T)
G2 Q2 80 0.00 0.00 FUD XXX

0316T replacement of pulse generator
Code also (C1767, C1820, L8685-L8688)
Do not report with (0315T)
J8 S 80 0.00 0.00 FUD XXX

0317T neurostimulator pulse generator electronic analysis, includes reprogramming when performed
S 80 0.00 0.00 FUD XXX

0319T-0325T

~~**0319T** Insertion or replacement of subcutaneous implantable defibrillator system with subcutaneous electrode~~
To report, see 33270

~~**0320T** Insertion of subcutaneous defibrillator electrode~~
To report, see 33271

~~**0321T** Insertion of subcutaneous implantable defibrillator pulse generator only with existing subcutaneous electrode~~
To report, see 33240

~~**0322T** Removal of subcutaneous implantable defibrillator pulse generator only~~
To report, see 33241

~~0323T Removal of subcutaneous implantable defibrillator pulse generator with replacement of subcutaneous implantable defibrillator pulse generator only~~
To report, see 33262-33264

~~0324T Removal of subcutaneous defibrillator electrode~~
To report, see 33272

~~0325T Repositioning of subcutaneous implantable defibrillator electrode and/or pulse generator~~
To report, see 33273

0326T-0328T

~~0326T Electrophysiologic evaluation of subcutaneous implantable defibrillator (includes defibrillation threshold evaluation, induction of arrhythmia, evaluation of sensing for arrhythmia termination, and programming or reprogramming of sensing or therapeutic parameters)~~
To report, see 33270

~~0327T Interrogation device evaluation (in person) with analysis, review and report, includes connection, recording and disconnection per patient encounter; implantable subcutaneous lead defibrillator system~~
To report, see 93261

~~0328T Programming device evaluation (in person) with iterative adjustment of the implantable device to test the function of the device and select optimal permanent programmed values with analysis; implantable subcutaneous lead defibrillator system~~
To report, see 93260

0329T-0330T

0329T Monitoring of intraocular pressure for 24 hours or longer, unilateral or bilateral, with interpretation and report
E 0.00 0.00 FUD YYY

0330T Tear film imaging, unilateral or bilateral, with interpretation and report
S 0.00 0.00 FUD YYY

0331T-0332T

EXCLUDES *Myocardial infarction avid imaging (78466, 78468, 78469)*

0331T Myocardial sympathetic innervation imaging, planar qualitative and quantitative assessment;
Z2 S 0.00 0.00 FUD YYY

0332T with tomographic SPECT
Z2 S 0.00 0.00 FUD YYY

0333T-0337T

0333T Visual evoked potential, screening of visual acuity, automated
E 0.00 0.00 FUD YYY

~~0334T Sacroiliac joint stabilization for arthrodesis, percutaneous or minimally invasive (indirect visualization), includes obtaining and applying autograft or allograft (structural or morselized), when performed, includes image guidance when performed (eg, CT or fluoroscopic)~~
To report, see 27279

⊙ 0335T Extra-osseous subtalar joint implant for talotarsal stabilization
G2 T 0.00 0.00 FUD YYY

0336T Laparoscopy, surgical, ablation of uterine fibroid(s), including intraoperative ultrasound guidance and monitoring, radiofrequency
Do not report with (76998, 0071T)
G2 T 0.00 0.00 FUD YYY

0337T Endothelial function assessment, using peripheral vascular response to reactive hyperemia, non-invasive (eg, brachial artery ultrasound, peripheral artery tonometry), unilateral or bilateral
Do not report with (93922-93923)
S 0.00 0.00 FUD YYY

0338T-0339T

Do not report with (36251-36254)

0338T Transcatheter renal sympathetic denervation, percutaneous approach including arterial puncture, selective catheter placement(s) renal artery(ies), fluoroscopy, contrast injection(s), intraprocedural roadmapping and radiological supervision and interpretation, including pressure gradient measurements, flush aortogram and diagnostic renal angiography when performed; unilateral
G2 E 0.00 0.00 FUD YYY

0339T bilateral
G2 S 0.00 0.00 FUD YYY

0340T-0342T

⊙ 0340T Ablation, pulmonary tumor(s), including pleura or chest wall when involved by tumor extension, percutaneous, cryoablation, unilateral, includes imaging guidance
Do not report with (76940, 77013, 77022)
G2 T 0.00 0.00 FUD YYY

0341T Quantitative pupillometry with interpretation and report, unilateral or bilateral
N1 N 0.00 0.00 FUD YYY

0342T Therapeutic apheresis with selective HDL delipidation and plasma reinfusion
G2 S 0.00 0.00 FUD YYY

0343T-0345T

Do not report with cardiac catheterization procedures inherent to the valve repair (93451-93453, 93456-93461)

~~0343T Transcatheter mitral valve repair percutaneous approach including transseptal puncture when performed; initial prosthesis~~
To report, see 33418

~~0344T additional prosthesis (es) during same session (List separately in addition to code for primary procedure)~~
To report, see 33419

0345T Transcatheter mitral valve repair percutaneous approach via the coronary sinus
Do not report with (93451-93454, 93456-93458, 93460-93461, 93563-93564)
C 0.00 0.00 FUD YYY

0346T

\+ 0346T Ultrasound, elastography (List separately in addition to code for primary procedure)
EXCLUDES *Elastography without other imaging procedures (report with unlisted code)*
Code first (76536, 76604, 76641-76642, 76700, 76705, 76770, 76775, 76830, 76856-76857, 76870, 76872, 76881-76882)
N1 N 0.00 0.00 FUD YYY

0347T

● **0347T** **Placement of interstitial device(s) in bone for radiostereometric analysis (RSA)**
Q2 0.00 0.00 FUD YYY

0348T-0350T

● **0348T** **Radiologic examination, radiostereometric analysis (RSA); spine, (includes, cervical, thoracic and lumbosacral, when performed)**
Z2 X 0.00 0.00 FUD YYY

● **0349T** **upper extremity(ies), (includes shoulder, elbow and wrist, when performed)**
Z2 X 0.00 0.00 FUD YYY

● **0350T** **lower extremity(ies), (includes hip, proximal femur, knee and ankle, when performed)**
Z2 X 0.00 0.00 FUD YYY

0351T-0354T

● **0351T** **Optical coherence tomography of breast or axillary lymph node, excised tissue, each specimen; real time intraoperative**
N 0.00 0.00 FUD YYY

● **0352T** **interpretation and report, real time or referred**
Do not report if provided by same physician (0351T)
B 0.00 0.00 FUD YYY

● **0353T** **Optical coherence tomography of breast, surgical cavity; real time intraoperative**
Do not report more than one time per session
N 0.00 0.00 FUD YYY

● **0354T** **interpretation and report, real time or referred**
Do not report when provided by same physician (0353T)
B 0.00 0.00 FUD YYY

0355T-0358T

● **0355T** **Gastrointestinal tract imaging, intraluminal (eg, capsule endoscopy), colon, with interpretation and report**
INCLUDES Includes distal ileum imaging when performed
Do not report with (91110-91111)
T 0.00 0.00 FUD YYY

● **0356T** **Insertion of drug-eluting implant (including punctal dilation and implant removal when performed) into lacrimal canaliculus, each**
EXCLUDES *Drug-eluting lacrimal implant*
R2 S 0.00 0.00 FUD YYY

0357T ***Resequenced code. See code following 0058T.***

● **0358T** **Bioelectrical impedance analysis whole body composition assessment, supine position, with interpretation and report**
Q1 0.00 0.00 FUD YYY

0359T

INCLUDES Evaluation of adaptive behavior
Provided by physician or other qualified health care professional with assistance of technician(s)

● **0359T** **Behavior identification assessment, by the physician or other qualified health care professional, face-to-face with patient and caregiver(s), includes administration of standardized and non-standardized tests, detailed behavioral history, patient observation and caregiver interview, interpretation of test results, discussion of findings and recommendations with the primary guardian(s)/caregiver(s), and preparation of report**
V 0.00 0.00 FUD YYY

0360T-0363T

INCLUDES Follow-up assessments
Provided to patients with destructive behaviors
Only the time of one technician when more than one is in attendance
Do not report on same date of service with (90785-90899, 96101-96125, 96150-96155)

● **0360T** **Observational behavioral follow-up assessment, includes physician or other qualified health care professional direction with interpretation and report, administered by one technician; first 30 minutes of technician time, face-to-face with the patient**
INCLUDES Time spent by physician or other qualified health care professional involved in technician tasks is considered as technician time
Do not report less than 16 minutes of face-to-face technician time
V 0.00 0.00 FUD YYY

+ ● **0361T** **each additional 30 minutes of technician time, face-to-face with the patient (List separately in addition to code for primary service)**
Code first (0360T)
N 0.00 0.00 FUD ZZZ

● **0362T** **Exposure behavioral follow-up assessment, includes physician or other qualified health care professional direction with interpretation and report, administered by physician or other qualified health care professional with the assistance of one or more technicians; first 30 minutes of technician(s) time, face-to-face with the patient**
INCLUDES Time based on face-to-face time provided by one technician and not the collective time of several technicians
Time spent by physician or other qualified health care professional involved in technician tasks is considered as technician time
V 0.00 0.00 FUD YYY

+ ● **0363T** **each additional 30 minutes of technician(s) time, face-to-face with the patient (List separately in addition to code for primary procedure)**
Code first (0362T)
N 0.00 0.00 FUD ZZZ

0364T-0372T

● **0364T** **Adaptive behavior treatment by protocol, administered by technician, face-to-face with one patient; first 30 minutes of technician time**
Do not report with (90785-90899, 92507, 96101-96155, 97532)
S 0.00 0.00 FUD YYY

+ ● **0365T** **each additional 30 minutes of technician time (List separately in addition to code for primary procedure)**
Code first (0364T)
Do not report with (90785-90899, 92507, 96101-96155, 97532)
N 0.00 0.00 FUD ZZZ

● **0366T** **Group adaptive behavior treatment by protocol, administered by technician, face-to-face with two or more patients; first 30 minutes of technician time**
Do not report when group exceeds eight patients
Do not report with (90785-90899, 92508, 96101-96155, 97150)
S 0.00 0.00 FUD YYY

+ ● 0367T **each additional 30 minutes of technician time (List separately in addition to code for primary procedure)**
Code first (0366T)
Do not report if group exceeds eight patients
Do not report with (90785-90899, 92508, 96101-96155, 97150)
N 0.00 0.00 FUD ZZZ

● 0368T **Adaptive behavior treatment with protocol modification administered by physician or other qualified health care professional with one patient; first 30 minutes of patient face-to-face time**
Do not report with (90791-90792, 90846-90847, 90887, 92507, 97532)
S 0.00 0.00 FUD YYY

+ ● 0369T **each additional 30 minutes of patient face-to-face time (List separately in addition to code for primary procedure)**
Code first (0368T)
Do not report with (90791-90792, 90846-90847, 90887, 92507, 97532)
N 0.00 0.00 FUD ZZZ

● 0370T **Family adaptive behavior treatment guidance, administered by physician or other qualified health care professional (without the patient present)**
Do not report with (90791-90792, 90846-90847, 90887)
S 0.00 0.00 FUD YYY

● 0371T **Multiple-family group adaptive behavior treatment guidance, administered by physician or other qualified health care professional (without the patient present)**
Do not report when group exceeds the families of more than eight patients
Do not report with (90791-90792, 90846-90847, 90887)
S 0.00 0.00 FUD YYY

● 0372T **Adaptive behavior treatment social skills group, administered by physician or other qualified health care professional face-to-face with multiple patients**
Do not report if group exceeds eight patients
Do not report with (90853, 92508, 97150)
S 0.00 0.00 FUD YYY

0373T-0374T

Do not report with (90785-90899, 96101-96155)

● 0373T **Exposure adaptive behavior treatment with protocol modification requiring two or more technicians for severe maladaptive behavior(s); first 60 minutes of technicians' time, face-to-face with patient**
S 0.00 0.00 FUD YYY

+ ● 0374T **each additional 30 minutes of technicians' time face-to-face with patient (List separately in addition to code for primary procedure)**
Code first (0373T)
N 0.00 0.00 FUD ZZZ

0375T

● 0375T **Total disc arthroplasty (artificial disc), anterior approach, including discectomy with end plate preparation (includes osteophytectomy for nerve root or spinal cord decompression and microdissection), cervical, three or more levels**
Do not report at same level with (22851, 22856, [22858])

0376T-0377T

0376T ***Resequenced code. See code following 0191T.***

● 0377T **Anoscopy with directed submucosal injection of bulking agent for fecal incontinence**
Do not report with (46600)

0378T-0380T

● 0378T **Visual field assessment, with concurrent real time data analysis and accessible data storage with patient initiated data transmitted to a remote surveillance center for up to 30 days; review and interpretation with report by a physician or other qualified health care professional**

● 0379T **technical support and patient instructions, surveillance, analysis and transmission of daily and emergent data reports as prescribed by a physician or other qualified health care professional**

● 0380T **Computer-aided animation and analysis of time series retinal images for the monitoring of disease progression, unilateral or bilateral, with interpretation and report**

0381T-0386T

● 0381T **External heart rate and 3-axis accelerometer data recording up to 14 days to assess changes in heart rate and to monitor motion analysis for the purposes of diagnosing nocturnal epilepsy seizure events; includes report, scanning analysis with report, review and interpretation by a physician or other qualified health care professional**

● 0382T **review and interpretation only**

● 0383T **External heart rate and 3-axis accelerometer data recording from 15 to 30 days to assess changes in heart rate to monitor motion analysis for the purposes of diagnosing nocturnal epilepsy seizure events; includes report, scanning analysis with report, review and interpretation by a physician or other qualified health care professional**

● 0384T **review and interpretation only**

● 0385T **External heart rate and 3-axis accelerometer data recording more than 30 days to assess changes in heart rate to monitor motion analysis for the purposes of diagnosing nocturnal epilepsy seizure events; includes report, scanning analysis with report, review and interpretation by a physician or other qualified health care professional**

● 0386T **review and interpretation only**

0387T-0391T

● 0387T **Transcatheter insertion or replacement of permanent leadless pacemaker, ventricular**

● 0388T **Transcatheter removal of permanent leadless pacemaker, ventricular**

● 0389T **Programming device evaluation (in person) with iterative adjustment of the implantable device to test the function of the device and select optimal permanent programmed values with analysis, review and report, leadless pacemaker system**

● 0390T **Peri-procedural device evaluation (in person) and programming of device system parameters before or after a surgery, procedure or test with analysis, review and report, leadless pacemaker system**

● 0391T **Interrogation device evaluation (in person) with analysis, review and report, includes connection, recording and disconnection per patient encounter, leadless pacemaker system**

Appendix A — Modifiers

CPT Modifiers

A modifier is a two-position alpha or numeric code appended to a CPT® code to clarify the services being billed. Modifiers provide a means by which a service can be altered without changing the procedure code. They add more information, such as the anatomical site, to the code. In addition, they help to eliminate the appearance of duplicate billing and unbundling. Modifiers are used to increase accuracy in reimbursement, coding consistency, editing, and to capture payment data.

22 **Increased Procedural Services:** When the work required to provide a service is substantially greater than typically required, it may be identified by adding modifier 22 to the usual procedure code. Documentation must support the substantial additional work and the reason for the additional work (ie, increased intensity, time, technical difficulty of procedure, severity of patient's condition, physical and mental effort required).
Note: This modifier should not be appended to an E/M service.

23 **Unusual Anesthesia:** Occasionally, a procedure, which usually requires either no anesthesia or local anesthesia, because of unusual circumstances must be done under general anesthesia. This circumstance may be reported by adding modifier 23 to the procedure code of the basic service.

24 **Unrelated Evaluation and Management Service by the Same Physician or Other Qualified Health Care Professional During a Postoperative Period:** The physician or other qualified health care professional may need to indicate that an evaluation and management service was performed during a postoperative period for a reason(s) unrelated to the original procedure. This circumstance may be reported by adding modifier 24 to the appropriate level of E/M service.

25 **Significant, Separately Identifiable Evaluation and Management Service by the Same Physician or Other Qualified Health Care Professional on the Same Day of the Procedure or Other Service:** It may be necessary to indicate that on the day a procedure or service identified by a CPT code was performed, the patient's condition required a significant, separately identifiable E/M service above and beyond the other service provided or beyond the usual preoperative and postoperative care associated with the procedure that was performed. A significant, separately identifiable E/M service is defined or substantiated by documentation that satisfies the relevant criteria for the respective E/M service to be reported (see Evaluation and Management Services Guidelines for instructions on determining level of E/M service). The E/M service may be prompted by the symptom or condition for which the procedure and/or service was provided. As such, different diagnoses are not required for reporting of the E/M services on the same date. This circumstance may be reported by adding modifier 25 to the appropriate level of E/M service.
Note: This modifier is not used to report an E/M service that resulted in a decision to perform surgery. See modifier 57. For significant, separately identifiable non-E/M services, see modifier 59.

26 **Professional Component:** Certain procedures are a combination of a physician or other qualified health care professional component and a technical component. When the physician or other qualified health care professional component is reported separately, the service may be identified by adding modifier 26 to the usual procedure number.

32 **Mandated Services:** Services related to mandated consultation and/or related services (eg, third-party payer, governmental, legislative or regulatory requirement) may be identified by adding modifier 32 to the basic procedure.

33 **Preventive Services:** When the primary purpose of the service is the delivery of an evidence-based service in accordance with a U.S. Preventive Services Task Force A or B rating in effect and other preventive services identified in preventive services mandates (legislative or regulatory), the service may be identified by adding 33 to the procedure. For separately reported services specifically identified as preventive, the modifier should not be used.

47 **Anesthesia by Surgeon:** Regional or general anesthesia provided by the surgeon may be reported by adding modifier 47 to the basic service. (This does not include local anesthesia.)
Note: Modifier 47 would not be used as a modifier for the anesthesia procedures 00100-01999.

50 **Bilateral Procedure:** Unless otherwise identified in the listings, bilateral procedures that are performed at the same session should be identified by adding modifier 50 to the appropriate 5-digit code.

51 **Multiple Procedures:** When multiple procedures, other than E/M services, Physical Medicine and Rehabilitation services or provision of supplies (e.g., vaccines), are performed at the same session by the same individual, the primary procedure or service may be reported as listed. The additional procedure(s) or service(s) may be identified by appending modifier 51 to the additional procedure or service code(s).
Note: This modifier should not be appended to designated "add-on" codes.

52 **Reduced Services:** Under certain circumstances a service or procedure is partially reduced or eliminated at the discretion of the physician or other qualified health care professional. Under these circumstances the service provided can be identified by its usual procedure number and the addition of modifier 52, signifying that the service is reduced. This provides a means of reporting reduced services without disturbing the identification of the basic service.
Note: For hospital outpatient reporting of a previously scheduled procedure/service that is partially reduced or cancelled as a result of extenuating circumstances or those that threaten the well-being of the patient prior to or after administration of anesthesia, see modifiers 73 and 74 (see modifiers approved for ASC hospital outpatient use).

53 **Discontinued Procedure:** Under certain circumstances, the physician or other qualified health care professional may elect to terminate a surgical or diagnostic procedure. Due to extenuating circumstances or those that threaten the well being of the patient, it may be necessary to indicate that a surgical or diagnostic procedure was started but discontinued. This circumstance may be reported by adding modifier 53 to the code reported by the physician for the discontinued procedure.
Note: This modifier is not used to report the elective cancellation of a procedure prior to the patient's anesthesia induction and/or surgical preparation in the operating suite. For outpatient hospital/ambulatory surgery center (ASC) reporting of a previously scheduled procedure/service that is partially reduced or cancelled as a result of extenuating circumstances or those that threaten the well being of the patient prior to or after administration of anesthesia, see modifiers 73 and 74 (see modifiers approved for ASC hospital outpatient use).

54 **Surgical Care Only:** When 1 physician or other qualified health care professional performs a surgical procedure and another provides preoperative and/or postoperative management, surgical services may be identified by adding modifier 54 to the usual procedure number.

55 **Postoperative Management Only:** When 1 physician or other qualified health care professional performed the postoperative management and another performed the surgical procedure, the postoperative component may be identified by adding modifier 55 to the usual procedure number.

56 **Preoperative Management Only:** When 1 physician or other qualified health care professional performed the preoperative care and evaluation and another performed the surgical procedure, the preoperative component may be identified by adding modifier 56 to the usual procedure number.

57 **Decision for Surgery:** An evaluation and management service that resulted in the initial decision to perform the surgery may be identified by adding modifier 57 to the appropriate level of E/M service.

58 **Staged or Related Procedure or Service by the Same Physician or Other Qualified Health Care Professional During the Postoperative Period:** It may be necessary to indicate that the performance of a procedure or service during the postoperative period was (a) planned or anticipated (staged); (b) more extensive than the original procedure; or (c) for therapy following a surgical procedure. This circumstance may be reported by adding modifier 58 to the staged or related procedure.
Note: For treatment of a problem that requires a return to the operating or procedure room (eg, unanticipated clinical condition), see modifier 78.

59 **Distinct Procedural Service:** Under certain circumstances, it may be necessary to indicate that a procedure or service was distinct or independent from other non-E/M services performed on the same day. Modifier 59 is used to identify procedures/services, other than E/M services, that are not normally reported together but are appropriate under the circumstances. Documentation must support a different session, different procedure or surgery, different site or organ system, separate incision/excision, separate lesion, or separate injury (or area of injury in extensive injuries) not ordinarily encountered or performed on the same day by the same individual. However, when another already established modifier is appropriate it should be used rather than modifier 59. Only if no more descriptive modifier is available and the use of modifier 59 best explains the circumstances, should modifier 59 be used.
Note: Modifier 59 should not be appended to an E/M service. To report a separate and distinct E/M service with a non-E/M service performed on the same date, see modifier 25. See also "Level II (HCPCS/National) Modifiers."

62 **Two Surgeons:** When 2 surgeons work together as primary surgeons performing distinct part(s) of a procedure, each surgeon should report his/her distinct operative work by adding modifier 62 to the procedure code and any associated add-on code(s) for that procedure as long as both surgeons continue to work together as primary surgeons. Each surgeon should report the cosurgery once using the same procedure code. If additional procedure(s) (including add-on procedure[s]) are performed during the same surgical session, separate code(s) may also be reported with modifier 62 added.
Note: If a cosurgeon acts as an assistant in the performance of additional procedure(s), other than those reported with the modifier 62, during the same surgical session, those services may be reported using separate procedure code(s) with modifier 80 or modifier 82 added, as appropriate.

63 **Procedure Performed on Infants less than 4 kg:** Procedures performed on neonates and infants up to a present body weight of 4 kg may involve significantly increased complexity and physician or other qualified health care professional work commonly associated with these patients. This circumstance may be reported by adding modifier 63 to the procedure number.
Note: Unless otherwise designated, this modifier may only be appended to procedures/services listed in the 20005-69990 code series. Modifier 63 should not be appended to any CPT codes listed in the Evaluation and Management Services, Anesthesia, Radiology, Pathology/Laboratory, or Medicine sections.

66 **Surgical Team:** Under some circumstances, highly complex procedures (requiring the concomitant services of several physicians or other qualified health care professionals, often of different specialties, plus other highly skilled, specially trained personnel, various types of complex equipment) are carried out under the "surgical team" concept. Such circumstances may be identified by each participating individual with the addition of modifier 66 to the basic procedure number used for reporting services.

76 **Repeat Procedure or Service by Same Physician or Other Qualified Health Care Professional:** It may be necessary to indicate that a procedure or service was repeated by the same physician or other qualified health care professional subsequent to the original procedure or service. This circumstance may be reported by adding modifier 76 to the repeated procedure or service.
Note: This modifier should not be appended to an E/M service.

77 **Repeat Procedure by Another Physician or Other Qualified Health Care Professional:** It may be necessary to indicate that a basic procedure or service was repeated by another physician or other qualified health care professional subsequent to the original procedure or service. This circumstance may be reported by adding modifier 77 to the repeated procedure or service.
Note: This modifier should not be appended to an E/M service.

78 **Unplanned Return to the Operating/Procedure Room by the Same Physician or Other Qualified Health Care Professional Following Initial Procedure for a Related Procedure During the Postoperative Period:** It may be necessary to indicate that another procedure was performed during the postoperative period of the initial procedure (unplanned procedure following initial procedure). When this procedure is related to the first, and requires the use of an operating/procedure room, it may be reported by adding modifier 78 to the related procedure. (For repeat procedures, see modifier 76.)

79 **Unrelated Procedure or Service by the Same Physician or Other Qualified Health Care Professional During the Postoperative Period:** The individual may need to indicate that the performance of a procedure or service during the postoperative period was unrelated to the original procedure. This circumstance may be reported by using modifier 79. (For repeat procedures on the same day, see modifier 76.)

80 **Assistant Surgeon:** Surgical assistant services may be identified by adding modifier 80 to the usual procedure number(s).

81 **Minimum Assistant Surgeon:** Minimum surgical assistant services are identified by adding modifier 81 to the usual procedure number.

82 **Assistant Surgeon (when qualified resident surgeon not available):** The unavailability of a qualified resident surgeon is a prerequisite for use of modifier 82 appended to the usual procedure code number(s).

90 **Reference (Outside) Laboratory:** When laboratory procedures are performed by a party other than the treating or reporting physician or other qualified health care professional, the procedure may be identified by adding modifier 90 to the usual procedure number.

91 **Repeat Clinical Diagnostic Laboratory Test:** In the course of treatment of the patient, it may be necessary to repeat the same laboratory test on the same day to obtain subsequent (multiple) test results. Under these circumstances, the laboratory test performed can be identified by its usual procedure number and the addition of modifier 91.
Note: This modifier may not be used when tests are rerun to confirm initial results; due to testing problems with specimens or equipment; or for any other reason when a normal, one-time, reportable result is all that is required. This modifier may not be used when another code(s) describes a series of test results (eg, glucose tolerance tests, evocative/suppression testing). This modifier may only be used for a laboratory test(s) performed more than once on the same day on the same patient.

92 **Alternative Laboratory Platform Testing** When laboratory testing is being performed using a kit or transportable instrument that wholly or in part consists of a single use, disposable analytical chamber, the service may be identified by adding modifier 92 to the usual laboratory procedure code (HIV testing 86701-86703, and 87389). The test does not require permanent dedicated space, hence by its design may be hand carried or transported to the vicinity of the patient for immediate testing at that site, although location of the testing is not in itself determinative of the use of this modifier.

99 **Multiple Modifiers:** Under certain circumstances 2 or more modifiers may be necessary to completely delineate a service. In such situations, modifier 99 should be added to the basic

procedure and other applicable modifiers may be listed as part of the description of the service.

Anesthesia Physical Status Modifiers

All anesthesia services are reported by use of the five-digit anesthesia procedure code with the appropriate physical status modifier appended.

Under certain circumstances, when other modifier(s) are appropriate, they should be reported in addition to the physical status modifier.

P1 A normal healthy patient

P2 A patient with mild systemic disease

P3 A patient with severe systemic disease

P4 A patient with severe systemic disease that is a constant threat to life

P5 A moribund patient who is not expected to survive without the operation

P6 A declared brain-dead patient whose organs are being removed for donor purposes

Modifiers Approved for Ambulatory Surgery Center (ASC) Hospital Outpatient Use

CPT Level I Modifiers

25 **Significant, Separately Identifiable Evaluation and Management Service by the Same Physician or Other Qualified Health Care Professional on the Same Day of the Procedure or Other Service:** It may be necessary to indicate that on the day a procedure or service identified by a CPT code was performed, the patient's condition required a significant, separately identifiable E/M service above and beyond the other service provided or beyond the usual preoperative and postoperative care associated with the procedure that was performed. A significant, separately identifiable E/M service is defined or substantiated by documentation that satisfies the relevant criteria for the respective E/M service to be reported (see Evaluation and Management Services Guidelines for instructions on determining level of E/M service). The E/M service may be prompted by the symptom or condition for which the procedure and/or service was provided. As such, different diagnoses are not required for reporting of the E/M services on the same date. This circumstance may be reported by adding modifier 25 to the appropriate level of E/M service.
Note: This modifier is not used to report an E/M service that resulted in a decision to perform surgery. See modifier 57. For significant, separately identifiable non-E/M services, see modifier 59.

27 **Multiple Outpatient Hospital E/M Encounters on the Same Date:** For hospital outpatient reporting purposes, utilization of hospital resources related to separate and distinct E/M encounters performed in multiple outpatient hospital settings on the same date may be reported by adding modifier 27 to each appropriate level outpatient and/or emergency department E/M code(s). This modifier provides a means of reporting circumstances involving evaluation and management services provided by a physician(s) in more than one (multiple) outpatient hospital setting(s) (eg, hospital emergency department, clinic).
Note: This modifier is not to be used for physician reporting of multiple E/M services performed by the same physician on the same date. For physician reporting of all outpatient evaluation and management services provided by the same physician on the same date and performed in multiple outpatient settings (eg, hospital emergency department, clinic), see Evaluation and Management, Emergency Department, or Preventive Medicine Services codes.

50 **Bilateral Procedure:** Unless otherwise identified in the listings, bilateral procedures that are performed at the same session should be identified by adding modifier 50 to the appropriate 5-digit code.

52 **Reduced Services:** Under certain circumstances a service or procedure is partially reduced or eliminated at the discretion of the physician or other qualified health care professional. Under these circumstances the service provided can be identified by its usual procedure number and the addition of modifier 52, signifying that the service is reduced. This provides a means of reporting reduced services without disturbing the identification of the basic service.
Note: For hospital outpatient reporting of a previously scheduled procedure/service that is partially reduced or cancelled as a result of extenuating circumstances or those that threaten the well-being of the patient prior to or after administration of anesthesia, see modifiers 73 and 74 (see modifiers approved for ASC hospital outpatient use).

58 **Staged or Related Procedure or Service by the Same Physician or Other Qualified Health Care Professional During the Postoperative Period:** It may be necessary to indicate that the performance of a procedure or service during the postoperative period was (a) planned or anticipated (staged); (b) more extensive than the original procedure; or (c) for therapy following a surgical procedure. This circumstance may be reported by adding modifier 58 to the staged or related procedure.
Note: For treatment of a problem that requires a return to the operating or procedure room (eg, unanticipated clinical condition), see modifier 78.

59 **Distinct Procedural Service:** Under certain circumstances, it may be necessary to indicate that a procedure or service was distinct or independent from other non-E/M services performed on the same day. Modifier 59 is used to identify procedures/services, other than E/M services, that are not normally reported together but are appropriate under the circumstances. Documentation must support a different session, different procedure or surgery, different site or organ system, separate incision/excision, separate lesion, or separate injury (or area of injury in extensive injuries) not ordinarily encountered or performed on the same day by the same individual. However, when another already established modifier is appropriate it should be used rather than modifier 59. Only if no more descriptive modifier is available and the use of modifier 59 best explains the circumstances, should modifier 59 be used.
Note: Modifier 59 should not be appended to an E/M service. To report a separate and distinct E/M service with a non-E/M service performed on the same date, see modifier 25. See also "Level II (HCPCS/National) Modifiers."

73 **Discontinued Out-Patient Hospital/Ambulatory Surgery Center (ASC) Procedure Prior to the Administration of Anesthesia:** Due to extenuating circumstances or those that threaten the well being of the patient, the physician may cancel a surgical or diagnostic procedure subsequent to the patient's surgical preparation (including sedation when provided, and being taken to the room where the procedure is to be performed), but prior to the administration of anesthesia (local, regional block(s), or general). Under these circumstances, the intended service that is prepared for but cancelled can be reported by its usual procedure number and the addition of modifier 73.
Note: The elective cancellation of a service prior to the administration of anesthesia and/or surgical preparation of the patient should not be reported. For physician reporting of a discontinued procedure, see modifier 53.

74 **Discontinued Out-Patient Hospital/Ambulatory Surgery Center (ASC) Procedure After Administration of Anesthesia:** Due to extenuating circumstances or those that threaten the well being of the patient, the physician may terminate a surgical or diagnostic procedure after the administration of anesthesia (local, regional block(s), general) or after the procedure was started (incision made, intubation started, scope inserted, etc.). Under these circumstances, the procedure started but terminated can be reported by its usual procedure number and the addition of modifier 74.
Note: The elective cancellation of a service prior to the administration of anesthesia and/or surgical preparation of the patient should not be reported. For physician reporting of a discontinued procedure, see modifier 53.

76 **Repeat Procedure or Service by Same Physician or Other Qualified Health Care Professional:** It may be necessary to indicate that a procedure or service was repeated by the same physician or other qualified health care professional subsequent to the original procedure or service. This circumstance may be reported by adding modifier 76 to the repeated procedure or service.
Note: This modifier should not be appended to an E/M service.

77 **Repeat Procedure by Another Physician or Other Qualified Health Care Professional:** It may be necessary to indicate that a basic procedure or service was repeated by another physician or other qualified health care professional subsequent to the original procedure or service. This circumstance may be reported by adding modifier 77 to the repeated procedure or service.
Note: This modifier should not be appended to an E/M service.

78 **Unplanned Return to the Operating/Procedure Room by the Same Physician or Other Qualified Health Care Professional Following Initial Procedure for a Related Procedure During the Postoperative Period:** It may be necessary to indicate that another procedure was performed during the postoperative period of the initial procedure (unplanned procedure following initial procedure). When this procedure is related to the first, and requires the use of an operating/procedure room, it may be reported by adding modifier 78 to the related procedure. (For repeat procedures, see modifier 76.)

79 **Unrelated Procedure or Service by the Same Physician During the Postoperative Period:** The individual may need to indicate that the performance of a procedure or service during the postoperative period was unrelated to the original procedure. This circumstance may be reported by using modifier 79. (For repeat procedures on the same day, see modifier 76.)

91 **Repeat Clinical Diagnostic Laboratory Test:** In the course of treatment of the patient, it may be necessary to repeat the same laboratory test on the same day to obtain subsequent (multiple) test results. Under these circumstances, the laboratory test performed can be identified by its usual procedure number and the addition of modifier 91.
Note: This modifier may not be used when tests are rerun to confirm initial results; due to testing problems with specimens or equipment; or for any other reason when a normal, one-time, reportable result is all that is required. This modifier may not be used when another code(s) describe a series of test results (eg, glucose tolerance tests, evocative/suppression testing). This modifier may only be used for a laboratory test(s) performed more than once on the same day on the same patient.

Level II (HCPCS/National) Modifiers

Anatomical Modifiers

E1 Upper left, eyelid
E2 Lower left, eyelid
E3 Upper right, eyelid
E4 Lower right, eyelid
F1 Left hand, second digit
F2 Left hand, third digit
F3 Left hand, fourth digit
F4 Left hand, fifth digit
F5 Right hand, thumb
F6 Right hand, second digit
F7 Right hand, third digit
F8 Right hand, fourth digit
F9 Right hand, fifth digit
FA Left hand, thumb
LT Left side (used to identify procedures performed on the left side of the body)
RT Right side (used to identify procedures performed on the right side of the body)
T1 Left foot, second digit
T2 Left foot, third digit
T3 Left foot, fourth digit
T4 Left foot, fifth digit
T5 Right foot, great toe
T6 Right foot, second digit
T7 Right foot, third digit
T8 Right foot, fourth digit
T9 Right foot, fifth digit
TA Left foot, great toe

Anesthesia Modifiers

AA Anesthesia services performed personally by anesthesiologist
AD Medical supervision by a physician: more than four concurrent anesthesia procedures
G8 Monitored anesthesia care (MAC) for deep complex, complicated, or markedly invasive surgical procedure
G9 Monitored anesthesia care for patient who has history of severe cardiopulmonary condition
QK Medical direction of two, three, or four concurrent anesthesia procedures involving qualified individuals
QS Monitored anesthesia care service
QX CRNA service: with medical direction by a physician
QY Medical direction of one certified registered nurse anesthetist (CRNA) by an anesthesiologist
QZ CRNA service: without medical direction by a physician
P1 A normal healthy patient
P2 A patient with mild systemic disease
P3 A patient with severe systemic disease
P4 A patient with severe systemic disease that is a constant threat to life
P5 A moribund patient who is not expected to survive without the operation
P6 A declared brain-dead patient whose organs are being removed for donor purposes

Coronary Artery Modifiers

LC Left circumflex coronary artery
LD Left anterior descending coronary artery
LM Left main coronary artery
RC Right coronary artery
RI Ramus intermedius coronary artery

Ophthalmology Modifiers

AP Determination of refractive state was not performed in the course of diagnostic ophthalmological examination
LS FDA-monitored intraocular lens implant
PL Progressive addition lenses
VP Aphakic patient

Other Modifiers

AE Registered dietician
AF Specialty physician
AG Primary physician
AH Clinical psychologist
AI Principal physician of record
AJ Clinical social worker
AK Nonparticipating physician
AM Physician, team member service

AO Alternate payment method declined by provider of service

AQ Physician providing a service in an unlisted health professional shortage area (HPSA)

AR Physician provider services in a physician scarcity area

AS Physician assistant, nurse practitioner, or clinical nurse specialist services for assistant at surgery

AT Acute treatment (this modifier should be used when reporting service 98940, 98941, 98942)

AY Item or service furnished to an ESRD patient that is not for the treatment of ESRD

CA Procedure payable only in the inpatient setting when performed emergently on an outpatient who expires prior to admission

CB Service ordered by a renal dialysis facility (RDF) physician as part of the ESRD beneficiary's dialysis benefit, is not part of the composite rate, and is separately reimbursable

CC Procedure code change (use 'CC' when the procedure code submitted was changed either for administrative reasons or because an incorrect code was filed)

CG Policy criteria applied

CR Catastrophe/disaster related

CS Item or service related, in whole or in part, to an illness, injury, or condition that was caused by or exacerbated by the effects, direct or indirect, of the 2010 oil spill in the gulf of Mexico, including but not limited to subsequent clean up activities

EA Erythropoetic stimulating agent (ESA) administered to treat anemia due to anticancer chemotherapy

EB Erythropoetic stimulating agent (ESA) administered to treat anemia due to anticancer radiotherapy

EC Erythropoetic stimulating agent (ESA) administered to treat anemia not due to anticancer radiotherapy or anticancer chemotherapy

EP Service provided as part of Medicaid early periodic screening diagnosis and treatment (EPSDT) program

ET Emergency services

EY No physician or other licensed health care provider order for this item or service

FB Item provided without cost to provider, supplier or practitioner, or full credit received for replaced device (examples, but not limited to covered under warranty, replaced due to defect, free samples)

FC Partial credit received for replacement device

FP Service provided as part of family planning program

G7 Pregnancy resulted from rape or incest or pregnancy certified by physician as life threatening

GA Waiver of liability statement issued as required by payer policy, individual case

GB Claim being resubmitted for payment because it is no longer covered under a global payment demonstration

GC This service has been performed in part by a resident under the direction of a teaching physician

GD Units of service exceeds medically unlikely edit value and represents reasonable and necessary services

GE This service has been performed by a resident without the presence of a teaching physician under the primary care exception

GF Non-physician (e.g. nurse practitioner (NP), certified registered nurse anesthetist (CRNA), certified registered nurse (CRN), clinical nurse specialist (CNS), physician assistant (PA)) services in a critical access hospital

GG Performance and payment of a screening mammogram and diagnostic mammogram on the same patient, same day

GH Diagnostic mammogram converted from screening mammogram on same day

GJ Opt out physician or practitioner emergency or urgent service

GK Reasonable and necessary item/service associated with GA or GZ modifier

GN Service delivered under an outpatient speech-language pathology plan of care

GO Service delivered an outpatient occupational therapy plan of care

GP Service delivered under an outpatient physical therapy plan of care

GQ Via asynchronous telecommunications system

GR This service was performed in whole or in part by a resident in a department of veterans affairs medical center or clinic, supervised in accordance with VA policy

GT Via interactive audio and video telecommunication systems

GU Waiver of liability statement issued as required by payer policy, routine notice

GV Attending physician not employed or paid under arrangement by the patient's hospice provider

GW Service not related to the hospice patient's terminal condition

GX Notice of liability issued, voluntary under payer policy

GY Item or service statutorily excluded, does not meet the definition of any Medicare benefit or for non-Medicare insurers, is not a contract benefit

GZ Item or service expected to be denied as not reasonable and necessary

H9 Court-ordered

HA Child/adolescent program

HB Adult program, nongeriatric

HC Adult program, geriatric

HD Pregnant/parenting women's program

HE Mental health program

HF Substance abuse program

HG Opioid addiction treatment program

HH Integrated mental health/substance abuse program

HI Integrated mental health and mental retardation/developmental disabilities program

HJ Employee assistance program

HK Specialized mental health programs for high-risk populations

HL Intern

HM Less than bachelor degree level

HN Bachelors degree level

HO Masters degree level

HP Doctoral level

HQ Group setting

HR Family/couple with client present

HS Family/couple without client present

HT Multi-disciplinary team

HU Funded by child welfare agency

HV Funded state addictions agency

HW Funded by state mental health agency

HX Funded by county/local agency

HY Funded by juvenile justice agency

HZ Funded by criminal justice agency

KB Beneficiary requested upgrade for ABN, more than four modifiers identified on claim

KX Requirements specified in the medical policy have been met

KZ New coverage not implemented by managed care

LR Laboratory round trip

M2 Medicare secondary payer (MSP)

PA Surgical or other invasive procedure on wrong body part

PB Surgical or other invasive procedure on wrong patient

PC Wrong surgery or other invasive procedure on patient

PD Diagnostic or related nondiagnostic item or service provided in a wholly owned or operated entity to a patient who is admitted as an inpatient within 3 days

PI Positron emission tomography (PET) or PET/computed tomography (CT) to inform the initial treatment strategy of tumors that are biopsy proven or strongly suspected of being cancerous based on other diagnostic testing, once per cancer diagnosis

PM Post-mortem visits

PS Positron emission tomography (PET) or PET/computed tomography (CT) to inform the subsequent treatment strategy of cancerous tumor when the beneficiary's treating physician determines that the PET study is needed to inform subsequent anti-tumor strategy

PT Colorectal cancer screening test; converted to diagnostic test or other procedure

Q0 Investigational clinical service provided in a clinical research study that is in an approved clinical research study

Q1 Routine clinical service provided in a clinical research study that is in an approved clinical research study

Q2 HCFA/ORD demonstration project procedure/service

Q3 Live kidney donor surgery and related services

Q4 Service for ordering/referring physician qualifies as a service exemption

Q5 Service furnished by a substitute physician under a reciprocal billing arrangement

Q6 Service furnished by a locum tenens physician

Q7 One Class A finding

Q8 Two Class B findings

Q9 One Class B and two Class C findings

QC Single channel monitoring

QD Recording and storage in solid state memory by a digital recorder

QJ Services/items provided to a prisoner or patient in state or local custody, however the state or local government, as applicable, meets the requirements in 42 CFR 411.4 (B)

QM Ambulance service provided under arrangement by a provider of services

QN Ambulance service furnished directly by a provider of services

QP Documentation is on file showing that the laboratory test(s) was ordered individually or ordered as a CPT-recognized panel other than automated profile codes

QT Recording and storage on tape by an analog tape recorder

QW CLIA waived test

RE Furnished in full compliance with FDA-mandated risk evaluation and mitigation strategy (REMS)

SA Nurse practitioner rendering service in collaboration with a physician

SB Nurse Midwife

SC Medically necessary service or supply

SD Services provided by registered nurse with specialized, highly technical home infusion training

SE State and/or federally funded programs/services

SF Second opinion ordered by a professional review organization (PRO) per section 9401, P.L.99-272 (100% reimbursement - no Medicare deductible or coinsurance)

SG Ambulatory surgical center (ASC) facility service

SH Second concurrently administered infusion therapy

SJ Third or more concurrently administered infusion therapy

SK Member of high risk population (use only with codes for immunization)

SL State supplied vaccine

SM Second surgical opinion

SN Third surgical opinion

SQ Item ordered by home health

SS Home infusion services provided in the infusion suite of the IV therapy provider

ST Related to trauma or injury

SU Procedure performed in physician's office (to denote use of facility and equipment)

SW Services provided by a certified diabetic educator

SY Persons who are in close contact with member of high-risk population (use only with codes for immunization)

TC Technical component. Under certain circumstances, a charge may be made for the technical component alone. Under those circumstances the technical component charge is identified by adding modifier 'TC' to the usual procedure number. Technical component charges are institutional charges and not billed separately by physicians. However, portable x-ray suppliers only bill for technical component and should utilize modifier TC. The charge data from portable x-ray suppliers will then be used to build customary and prevailing profiles.

TD RN

TE LPN/LVN

TF Intermediate level of care

TG Complex/high level of care

TH Obstetrical treatment/services, prenatal or postpartum

TJ Program group, child and/or adolescent

TK Extra patient or passenger, nonambulance

TL Early intervention/individualized family service plan (IFSP)

TM Individualized education program (IEP)

TN Rural/outside providers' customary service area

TR School-based individualized education program (IEP) services provided outside the public school district responsible for the student

TS Follow-up service

TT Individualized service provided to more than one patient in same setting

TU Special payment rate, overtime

TV Special payment rates, holidays/weekends

U1 Medicaid level of care 1, as defined by each state

U2 Medicaid level of care 2, as defined by each state

U3 Medicaid level of care 3, as defined by each state

U4 Medicaid level of care 4, as defined by each state

U5 Medicaid level of care 5, as defined by each state

U6 Medicaid level of care 6, as defined by each state

U7 Medicaid level of care 7, as defined by each state

U8 Medicaid level of care 8, as defined by each state

U9 Medicaid level of care 9, as defined by each state

UA Medicaid level of care 10, as defined by each state

UB Medicaid level of care 11, as defined by each state

UC Medicaid level of care 12, as defined by each state

UD Medicaid level of care 13, as defined by each state

UF Services provided in the morning

UG Services provided in the afternoon

UH Services provided in the evening

UJ Services provided at night

UK Services provided on behalf of the client to someone other than the client (collateral relationship)

UN Two patients served

UP Three patients served

UQ Four patients served

UR Five patients served

US Six or more patients served

V5 Vascular catheter (alone or with any other vascular access)

V6 Arteriovenous graft (or other vascular access not including a vascular catheter)

V7 Arteriovenous fistula only (in use with 2 needles)

XE Separate encounter, a service that Is distinct because it occurred during a separate encounter

XP Separate practitioner, a service that is distinct because it was performed by a different practitioner

XS Separate structure, a service that is distinct because it was performed on a separate organ/structure

XU Unusual non-overlapping service, the use of a service that is distinct because it does not overlap usual components of the main service

Category II Modifiers

1P Performance measure exclusion modifier due to medical reasons

Includes:

- Not indicated (absence of organ/limb, already received/performed, other)
- Contraindicated (patient allergic history, potential adverse drug interaction, other)
- Other medical reasons

2P Performance measure exclusion modifier due to patient reasons

Includes:

- Patient declined
- Economic, social, or religious reasons
- Other patient reasons

3P Performance measure exclusion modifier due to system reasons

Includes:

- Resources to perform the services not available (eg, equipment, supplies)
- Insurance coverage or payer-related limitations
- Other reasons attributable to health care delivery system

8P Performance measure reporting modifier - action not performed, reason not otherwise specified

Dental Modifiers

AZ Physician providing a service in a dental health professional shortage area for the purpose of an electronic health record incentive payment

DA Oral health assessment by a licensed health professional other than a dentist

ET Emergency services (dental procedures performed in emergency situations should show the modifier ET)

ESRD Modifiers

AY Item or service furnished to an ESRD patient that is not for the treatment of ESRD

CD AMCC test has been ordered by an ESRD facility or MCP physician that is a part of the composite rate and is not separately billable

CE AMCC test has been ordered by an ESRD facility or MCP physician that is a composite rate test but is beyond the normal frequency covered under the rate and is separately reimbursable based on medically necessary

CF AMCC test has been ordered by an ESRD facility or MCP physician that is not part of the composite rate and is separately billable

ED Hematocrit level has exceeded 39% (or hemoglobin level has exceeded 13.0 G/dl) for 3 or more consecutive billing cycles immediately prior to and including the current cycle

EE Hematocrit level has not exceeded 39% (or hemoglobin level has not exceeded 13.0 G/dl) for 3 or more consecutive billing cycles immediately prior to and including the current cycle

EJ Subsequent claims for a defined course of therapy, e.g., EPO, sodium hyaluronate, infliximab

EM Emergency reserve supply (for ESRD benefit only)

G1 Most recent URR reading of less than 60

G2 Most recent URR reading of 60 to 64.9

G3 Most recent URR reading of 65 to 69.9

G4 Most recent URR reading of 70 to 74.9

G5 Most recent URR reading of 75 or greater

G6 ESRD patient for whom less than six dialysis sessions have been provided in a month

GS Dosage of EPO or darbepoietin alfa has been reduced and maintained in response to hematocrit or hemoglobin level

JE Administered via dialysate

Q3 Live kidney donor surgery and related services

Appendix B — New, Changed and Deleted Codes

New Codes

0006M Oncology (hepatic), mRNA expression levels of 161 genes, utilizing fresh hepatocellular carcinoma tumor tissue, with alpha-fetoprotein level, algorithm reported as a risk classifier

0007M Oncology (gastrointestinal neuroendocrine tumors), real-time PCR expression analysis of 51 genes, utilizing whole peripheral blood, algorithm reported as a nomogram of tumor disease index

0008M Oncology (breast), mRNA analysis of 58 genes using hybrid capture, on formalin-fixed paraffin-embedded (FFPE) tissue, prognostic algorithm reported as a risk score

3126F Esophageal biopsy report with a statement about dysplasia (present, absent, or indefinite, and if present, contains appropriate grading) (PATH)

3775F Adenoma(s) or other neoplasm detected during screening colonoscopy (SCADR)

3776F Adenoma(s) or other neoplasm not detected during screening colonoscopy (SCADR)

0347T Placement of interstitial device(s) in bone for radiostereometric analysis (RSA)

0348T Radiologic examination, radiostereometric analysis (RSA); spine, (includes, cervical, thoracic and lumbosacral, when performed)

0349T Radiologic examination, radiostereometric analysis (RSA); upper extremity(ies), (includes shoulder, elbow and wrist, when performed)

0350T Radiologic examination, radiostereometric analysis (RSA); lower extremity(ies), (includes hip, proximal femur, knee and ankle, when performed)

0351T Optical coherence tomography of breast or axillary lymph node, excised tissue, each specimen; real time intraoperative

0352T Optical coherence tomography of breast or axillary lymph node, excised tissue, each specimen; interpretation and report, real time or referred

0353T Optical coherence tomography of breast, surgical cavity; real time intraoperative

0354T Optical coherence tomography of breast, surgical cavity; interpretation and report, real time or referred

0355T Gastrointestinal tract imaging, intraluminal (eg, capsule endoscopy), colon, with interpretation and report

0356T Insertion of drug-eluting implant (including punctal dilation and implant removal when performed) into lacrimal canaliculus, each

0357T Cryopreservation; immature oocyte(s)

0358T Bioelectrical impedance analysis whole body composition assessment, supine position, with interpretation and report

0359T Behavior identification assessment, by the physician or other qualified health care professional, face-to-face with patient and caregiver(s), includes administration of standardized and non-standardized tests, detailed behavioral history, patient observation and caregiver interview, interpretation of test results, discussion of findings and recommendations with the primary guardian(s)/caregiver(s), and preparation of report

0360T Observational behavioral follow-up assessment, includes physician or other qualified health care professional direction with interpretation and report, administered by one technician; first 30 minutes of technician time, face-to-face with the patient

0361T Observational behavioral follow-up assessment, includes physician or other qualified health care professional direction with interpretation and report, administered by one technician; each additional 30 minutes of technician time, face-to-face with the patient (List separately in addition to code for primary service)

0362T Exposure behavioral follow-up assessment, includes physician or other qualified health care professional direction with interpretation and report, administered by physician or other qualified health care professional with the assistance of one or more technicians; first 30 minutes of technician(s) time, face-to-face with the patient

0363T Exposure behavioral follow-up assessment, includes physician or other qualified health care professional direction with interpretation and report, administered by physician or other qualified health care professional with the assistance of one or more technicians; each additional 30 minutes of technician(s) time, face-to-face with the patient (List separately in addition to code for primary procedure)

0364T Adaptive behavior treatment by protocol, administered by technician, face-to-face with one patient; first 30 minutes of technician time

0365T Adaptive behavior treatment by protocol, administered by technician, face-to-face with one patient; each additional 30 minutes of technician time (List separately in addition to code for primary procedure)

0366T Group adaptive behavior treatment by protocol, administered by technician, face-to-face with two or more patients; first 30 minutes of technician time

0367T Group adaptive behavior treatment by protocol, administered by technician, face-to-face with two or more patients; each additional 30 minutes of technician time (List separately in addition to code for primary procedure)

0368T Adaptive behavior treatment with protocol modification administered by physician or other qualified health care professional with one patient; first 30 minutes of patient face-to-face time

0369T Adaptive behavior treatment with protocol modification administered by physician or other qualified health care professional with one patient; each additional 30 minutes of patient face-to-face time (List separately in addition to code for primary procedure)

0370T Family adaptive behavior treatment guidance, administered by physician or other qualified health care professional (without the patient present)

0371T Multiple-family group adaptive behavior treatment guidance, administered by physician or other qualified health care professional (without the patient present)

0372T Adaptive behavior treatment social skills group, administered by physician or other qualified health care professional face-to-face with multiple patients

0373T Exposure adaptive behavior treatment with protocol modification requiring two or more technicians for severe maladaptive behavior(s); first 60 minutes of technicians' time, face-to-face with patient

0374T Exposure adaptive behavior treatment with protocol modification requiring two or more technicians for severe maladaptive behavior(s); each additional 30 minutes of technicians' time face-to-face with patient (List separately in addition to code for primary procedure)

0375T Total disc arthroplasty (artificial disc), anterior approach, including discectomy with end plate preparation (includes osteophytectomy for nerve root or spinal cord decompression and microdissection), cervical, three or more levels

0376T Insertion of anterior segment aqueous drainage device, without extraocular reservoir, internal approach, into the trabecular meshwork; each additional device insertion (List separately in addition to code for primary procedure)

0377T Anoscopy with directed submucosal injection of bulking agent for fecal incontinence

0378T Visual field assessment, with concurrent real time data analysis and accessible data storage with patient initiated data transmitted to a remote surveillance center for up to 30 days; review and interpretation with report by a physician or other qualified health care professional

0379T Visual field assessment, with concurrent real time data analysis and accessible data storage with patient initiated data transmitted to a remote surveillance center for up to 30 days; technical support and patient instructions, surveillance, analysis and transmission of daily and emergent data reports as prescribed by a physician or other qualified health care professional

0380T Computer-aided animation and analysis of time series retinal images for the monitoring of disease progression, unilateral or bilateral, with interpretation and report

0381T External heart rate and 3-axis accelerometer data recording up to 14 days to assess changes in heart rate and to monitor motion analysis for the purposes of diagnosing nocturnal epilepsy seizure events; includes report, scanning analysis with report, review and interpretation by a physician or other qualified health care professional

0382T External heart rate and 3-axis accelerometer data recording up to 14 days to assess changes in heart rate and to monitor motion analysis for the purposes of diagnosing nocturnal epilepsy seizure events; review and interpretation only

0383T External heart rate and 3-axis accelerometer data recording from 15 to 30 days to assess changes in heart rate to monitor motion analysis for the purposes of diagnosing nocturnal epilepsy seizure events; includes report, scanning analysis with report, review and interpretation by a physician or other qualified health care professional

0384T External heart rate and 3-axis accelerometer data recording from 15 to 30 days to assess changes in heart rate to monitor motion analysis for the purposes of diagnosing nocturnal epilepsy seizure events; review and interpretation only

0385T External heart rate and 3-axis accelerometer data recording more than 30 days to assess changes in heart rate to monitor motion analysis for the purposes of diagnosing nocturnal epilepsy seizure events; includes report, scanning analysis with report, review and interpretation by a physician or other qualified health care professional

0386T External heart rate and 3-axis accelerometer data recording more than 30 days to assess changes in heart rate to monitor motion analysis for the purposes of diagnosing nocturnal epilepsy seizure events; review and interpretation only

0387T Transcatheter insertion or replacement of permanent leadless pacemaker, ventricular

0388T Transcatheter removal of permanent leadless pacemaker, ventricular

0389T Programming device evaluation (in person) with iterative adjustment of the implantable device to test the function of the device and select optimal permanent programmed values with analysis, review and report, leadless pacemaker system

0390T Peri-procedural device evaluation (in person) and programming of device system parameters before or after a surgery, procedure or test with analysis, review and report, leadless pacemaker system

0391T Interrogation device evaluation (in person) with analysis, review and report, includes connection, recording and disconnection per patient encounter, leadless pacemaker system

20604 Arthrocentesis, aspiration and/or injection, small joint or bursa (eg, fingers, toes); with ultrasound guidance, with permanent recording and reporting

20606 Arthrocentesis, aspiration and/or injection, intermediate joint or bursa (eg, temporomandibular, acromioclavicular, wrist, elbow or ankle, olecranon bursa); with ultrasound guidance, with permanent recording and reporting

20611 Arthrocentesis, aspiration and/or injection, major joint or bursa (eg, shoulder, hip, knee, subacromial bursa); with ultrasound guidance, with permanent recording and reporting

20983 Ablation therapy for reduction or eradication of 1 or more bone tumors (eg, metastasis) including adjacent soft tissue when involved by tumor extension, percutaneous, including imaging guidance when performed; cryoablation

21811 Open treatment of rib fracture(s) with internal fixation, includes thoracoscopic visualization when performed, unilateral; 1-3 ribs

21812 Open treatment of rib fracture(s) with internal fixation, includes thoracoscopic visualization when performed, unilateral; 4-6 ribs

21813 Open treatment of rib fracture(s) with internal fixation, includes thoracoscopic visualization when performed, unilateral; 7 or more ribs

22510 Percutaneous vertebroplasty (bone biopsy included when performed), 1 vertebral body, unilateral or bilateral injection, inclusive of all imaging guidance; cervicothoracic

22511 Percutaneous vertebroplasty (bone biopsy included when performed), 1 vertebral body, unilateral or bilateral injection, inclusive of all imaging guidance; lumbosacral

22512 Percutaneous vertebroplasty (bone biopsy included when performed), 1 vertebral body, unilateral or bilateral injection, inclusive of all imaging guidance; each additional cervicothoracic or lumbosacral vertebral body (List separately in addition to code for primary procedure)

22513 Percutaneous vertebral augmentation, including cavity creation (fracture reduction and bone biopsy included when performed) using mechanical device (eg, kyphoplasty), 1 vertebral body, unilateral or bilateral cannulation, inclusive of all imaging guidance; thoracic

22514 Percutaneous vertebral augmentation, including cavity creation (fracture reduction and bone biopsy included when performed) using mechanical device (eg, kyphoplasty), 1 vertebral body, unilateral or bilateral cannulation, inclusive of all imaging guidance; lumbar

22515 Percutaneous vertebral augmentation, including cavity creation (fracture reduction and bone biopsy included when performed) using mechanical device (eg, kyphoplasty), 1 vertebral body, unilateral or bilateral cannulation, inclusive of all imaging guidance; each additional thoracic or lumbar vertebral body (List separately in addition to code for primary procedure)

22858 Total disc arthroplasty (artificial disc), anterior approach, including discectomy with end plate preparation (includes osteophytectomy for nerve root or spinal cord decompression and microdissection); second level, cervical (List separately in addition to code for primary procedure)

27279 Arthrodesis, sacroiliac joint, percutaneous or minimally invasive (indirect visualization), with image guidance, includes obtaining bone graft when performed, and placement of transfixing device

33270 Insertion or replacement of permanent subcutaneous implantable defibrillator system, with subcutaneous electrode, including defibrillation threshold evaluation, induction of arrhythmia, evaluation of sensing for arrhythmia termination, and programming or reprogramming of sensing or therapeutic parameters, when performed

33271 Insertion of subcutaneous implantable defibrillator electrode

33272 Removal of subcutaneous implantable defibrillator electrode

33273 Repositioning of previously implanted subcutaneous implantable defibrillator electrode

33418 Transcatheter mitral valve repair, percutaneous approach, including transseptal puncture when performed; initial prosthesis

33419 Transcatheter mitral valve repair, percutaneous approach, including transseptal puncture when performed; additional prosthesis(es) during same session (List separately in addition to code for primary procedure)

33946 Extracorporeal membrane oxygenation (ECMO)/extracorporeal life support (ECLS) provided by physician; initiation, veno-venous

33947 Extracorporeal membrane oxygenation (ECMO)/extracorporeal life support (ECLS) provided by physician; initiation, veno-arterial

33948 Extracorporeal membrane oxygenation (ECMO)/extracorporeal life support (ECLS) provided by physician; daily management, each day, veno-venous

33949 Extracorporeal membrane oxygenation (ECMO)/extracorporeal life support (ECLS) provided by physician; daily management, each day, veno-arterial

33951 Extracorporeal membrane oxygenation (ECMO)/extracorporeal life support (ECLS) provided by physician; insertion of peripheral (arterial and/or venous) cannula(e), percutaneous, birth through 5 years of age (includes fluoroscopic guidance, when performed)

33952 Extracorporeal membrane oxygenation (ECMO)/extracorporeal life support (ECLS) provided by physician; insertion of peripheral (arterial and/or venous) cannula(e), percutaneous, 6 years and older (includes fluoroscopic guidance, when performed)

33953 Extracorporeal membrane oxygenation (ECMO)/extracorporeal life support (ECLS) provided by physician; insertion of peripheral (arterial and/or venous) cannula(e), open, birth through 5 years of age

33954 Extracorporeal membrane oxygenation (ECMO)/extracorporeal life support (ECLS) provided by physician; insertion of peripheral (arterial and/or venous) cannula(e), open, 6 years and older

33955 Extracorporeal membrane oxygenation (ECMO)/extracorporeal life support (ECLS) provided by physician; insertion of central cannula(e) by sternotomy or thoracotomy, birth through 5 years of age

33956 Extracorporeal membrane oxygenation (ECMO)/extracorporeal life support (ECLS) provided by physician; insertion of central cannula(e) by sternotomy or thoracotomy, 6 years and older

33957 Extracorporeal membrane oxygenation (ECMO)/extracorporeal life support (ECLS) provided by physician; reposition peripheral (arterial and/or venous) cannula(e), percutaneous, birth through 5 years of age (includes fluoroscopic guidance, when performed)

33958 Extracorporeal membrane oxygenation (ECMO)/extracorporeal life support (ECLS) provided by physician; reposition peripheral (arterial and/or venous) cannula(e), percutaneous, 6 years and older (includes fluoroscopic guidance, when performed)

33959 Extracorporeal membrane oxygenation (ECMO)/extracorporeal life support (ECLS) provided by physician; reposition peripheral (arterial and/or venous) cannula(e), open, birth through 5 years of age (includes fluoroscopic guidance, when performed)

33962 Extracorporeal membrane oxygenation (ECMO)/extracorporeal life support (ECLS) provided by physician; reposition peripheral (arterial and/or venous) cannula(e), open, 6 years and older (includes fluoroscopic guidance, when performed)

33963 Extracorporeal membrane oxygenation (ECMO)/extracorporeal life support (ECLS) provided by physician; reposition of central cannula(e) by sternotomy or thoracotomy, birth through 5 years of age (includes fluoroscopic guidance, when performed)

33964 Extracorporeal membrane oxygenation (ECMO)/extracorporeal life support (ECLS) provided by physician; reposition central cannula(e) by sternotomy or thoracotomy, 6 years and older (includes fluoroscopic guidance, when performed)

33965 Extracorporeal membrane oxygenation (ECMO)/extracorporeal life support (ECLS) provided by physician; removal of peripheral (arterial and/or venous) cannula(e), percutaneous, birth through 5 years of age

33966 Extracorporeal membrane oxygenation (ECMO)/extracorporeal life support (ECLS) provided by physician; removal of peripheral (arterial and/or venous) cannula(e), percutaneous, 6 years and older

33969 Extracorporeal membrane oxygenation (ECMO)/extracorporeal life support (ECLS) provided by physician; removal of peripheral (arterial and/or venous) cannula(e), open, birth through 5 years of age

33984 Extracorporeal membrane oxygenation (ECMO)/extracorporeal life support (ECLS) provided by physician; removal of peripheral (arterial and/or venous) cannula(e), open, 6 years and older

33985 Extracorporeal membrane oxygenation (ECMO)/extracorporeal life support (ECLS) provided by physician; removal of central cannula(e) by sternotomy or thoracotomy, birth through 5 years of age

33986 Extracorporeal membrane oxygenation (ECMO)/extracorporeal life support (ECLS) provided by physician; removal of central cannula(e) by sternotomy or thoracotomy, 6 years and older

33987 Arterial exposure with creation of graft conduit (eg, chimney graft) to facilitate arterial perfusion for ECMO/ECLS (List separately in addition to code for primary procedure)

33988 Insertion of left heart vent by thoracic incision (eg, sternotomy, thoracotomy) for ECMO/ECLS

33989 Removal of left heart vent by thoracic incision (eg, sternotomy, thoracotomy) for ECMO/ECLS

34839 Physician planning of a patient-specific fenestrated visceral aortic endograft requiring a minimum of 90 minutes of physician time

37218 Transcatheter placement of intravascular stent(s), intrathoracic common carotid artery or innominate artery, open or percutaneous antegrade approach, including angioplasty, when performed, and radiological supervision and interpretation

43180 Esophagoscopy, rigid, transoral with diverticulectomy of hypopharynx or cervical esophagus (eg, Zenker's diverticulum), with cricopharyngeal myotomy, includes use of telescope or operating microscope and repair, when performed

44381 Ileoscopy, through stoma; with transendoscopic balloon dilation

44384 Ileoscopy, through stoma; with placement of endoscopic stent (includes pre- and post-dilation and guide wire passage, when performed)

44401 Colonoscopy through stoma; with ablation of tumor(s), polyp(s), or other lesion(s) (includes pre-and post-dilation and guide wire passage, when performed)

44402 Colonoscopy through stoma; with endoscopic stent placement (including pre- and post-dilation and guide wire passage, when performed)

44403 Colonoscopy through stoma; with endoscopic mucosal resection

44404 Colonoscopy through stoma; with directed submucosal injection(s), any substance

44405 Colonoscopy through stoma; with transendoscopic balloon dilation

44406 Colonoscopy through stoma; with endoscopic ultrasound examination, limited to the sigmoid, descending, transverse, or ascending colon and cecum and adjacent structures

44407 Colonoscopy through stoma; with transendoscopic ultrasound guided intramural or transmural fine needle aspiration/biopsy(s), includes endoscopic ultrasound examination limited to the sigmoid, descending, transverse, or ascending colon and cecum and adjacent structures

44408 Colonoscopy through stoma; with decompression (for pathologic distention) (eg, volvulus, megacolon), including placement of decompression tube, when performed

45346 Sigmoidoscopy, flexible; with ablation of tumor(s), polyp(s), or other lesion(s) (includes pre- and post-dilation and guide wire passage, when performed)

45347 Sigmoidoscopy, flexible; with placement of endoscopic stent (includes pre- and post-dilation and guide wire passage, when performed)

45349 Sigmoidoscopy, flexible; with endoscopic mucosal resection

45350 Sigmoidoscopy, flexible; with band ligation(s) (eg, hemorrhoids)

45388 Colonoscopy, flexible; with ablation of tumor(s), polyp(s), or other lesion(s) (includes pre- and post-dilation and guide wire passage, when performed)

45389 Colonoscopy, flexible; with endoscopic stent placement (includes pre- and post-dilation and guide wire passage, when performed)

45390 Colonoscopy, flexible; with endoscopic mucosal resection

45393 Colonoscopy, flexible; with decompression (for pathologic distention) (eg, volvulus, megacolon), including placement of decompression tube, when performed

45398 Colonoscopy, flexible; with band ligation(s) (eg, hemorrhoids)

45399 Unlisted procedure, colon

46601 Anoscopy; diagnostic, with high-resolution magnification (HRA) (eg, colposcope, operating microscope) and chemical agent enhancement, including collection of specimen(s) by brushing or washing, when performed

46607 Anoscopy; with high-resolution magnification (HRA) (eg, colposcope, operating microscope) and chemical agent enhancement, with biopsy, single or multiple

47383 Ablation, 1 or more liver tumor(s), percutaneous, cryoablation

52441 Cystourethroscopy, with insertion of permanent adjustable transprostatic implant; single implant

52442 Cystourethroscopy, with insertion of permanent adjustable transprostatic implant; each additional permanent adjustable transprostatic implant (List separately in addition to code for primary procedure)

62302 Myelography via lumbar injection, including radiological supervision and interpretation; cervical

62303 Myelography via lumbar injection, including radiological supervision and interpretation; thoracic

62304 Myelography via lumbar injection, including radiological supervision and interpretation; lumbosacral

62305 Myelography via lumbar injection, including radiological supervision and interpretation; 2 or more regions (eg, lumbar/thoracic, cervical/thoracic, lumbar/cervical, lumbar/thoracic/cervical)

64486 Transversus abdominis plane (TAP) block (abdominal plane block, rectus sheath block) unilateral; by injection(s) (includes imaging guidance, when performed)

64487 Transversus abdominis plane (TAP) block (abdominal plane block, rectus sheath block) unilateral; by continuous infusion(s) (includes imaging guidance, when performed)

64488 Transversus abdominis plane (TAP) block (abdominal plane block, rectus sheath block) bilateral; by injections (includes imaging guidance, when performed)

64489 Transversus abdominis plane (TAP) block (abdominal plane block, rectus sheath block) bilateral; by continuous infusions (includes imaging guidance, when performed)

66179 Aqueous shunt to extraocular equatorial plate reservoir, external approach; without graft

66184 Revision of aqueous shunt to extraocular equatorial plate reservoir; without graft

76641 Ultrasound, breast, unilateral, real time with image documentation, including axilla when performed; complete

76642 Ultrasound, breast, unilateral, real time with image documentation, including axilla when performed; limited

77061 Digital breast tomosynthesis; unilateral

77062 Digital breast tomosynthesis; bilateral

77063 Screening digital breast tomosynthesis, bilateral (List separately in addition to code for primary procedure)

77085 Dual-energy X-ray absorptiometry (DXA), bone density study, 1 or more sites; axial skeleton (eg, hips, pelvis, spine), including vertebral fracture assessment

77086 Vertebral fracture assessment via dual-energy X-ray absorptiometry (DXA)

77306 Teletherapy isodose plan; simple (1 or 2 unmodified ports directed to a single area of interest), includes basic dosimetry calculation(s)

77307 Teletherapy isodose plan; complex (multiple treatment areas, tangential ports, the use of wedges, blocking, rotational beam, or special beam considerations), includes basic dosimetry calculation(s)

77316 Brachytherapy isodose plan; simple (calculation[s] made from 1 to 4 sources, or remote afterloading brachytherapy, 1 channel), includes basic dosimetry calculation(s)

77317 Brachytherapy isodose plan; intermediate (calculation[s] made from 5 to 10 sources, or remote afterloading brachytherapy, 2-12 channels), includes basic dosimetry calculation(s)

77318 Brachytherapy isodose plan; complex (calculation[s] made from over 10 sources, or remote afterloading brachytherapy, over 12 channels), includes basic dosimetry calculation(s)

77385 Intensity modulated radiation treatment delivery (IMRT), includes guidance and tracking, when performed; simple

77386 Intensity modulated radiation treatment delivery (IMRT), includes guidance and tracking, when performed; complex

77387 Guidance for localization of target volume for delivery of radiation treatment delivery, includes intrafraction tracking, when performed

80163 Digoxin; free

80165 Valproic acid (dipropylacetic acid); free

80300 Drug screen, any number of drug classes from Drug Class List A; any number of non-TLC devices or procedures, (eg, immunoassay) capable of being read by direct optical observation, including instrumented-assisted when performed (eg, dipsticks, cups, cards, cartridges), per date of service

80301 Drug screen, any number of drug classes from Drug Class List A; single drug class method, by instrumented test systems (eg, discrete multichannel chemistry analyzers utilizing immunoassay or enzyme assay), per date of service

80302 Drug screen, presumptive, single drug class from Drug Class List B, by immunoassay (eg, ELISA) or non-TLC chromatography without mass spectrometry (eg, GC, HPLC), each procedure

80303 Drug screen, any number of drug classes, presumptive, single or multiple drug class method; thin layer chromatography procedure(s) (TLC) (eg, acid, neutral, alkaloid plate), per date of service

80304 Drug screen, any number of drug classes, presumptive, single or multiple drug class method; not otherwise specified presumptive procedure (eg, TOF, MALDI, LDTD, DESI, DART), each procedure

80320 Alcohols

80321 Alcohol biomarkers; 1 or 2

80322 Alcohol biomarkers; 3 or more

80323 Alkaloids, not otherwise specified

80324 Amphetamines; 1 or 2

80325 Amphetamines; 3 or 4

80326 Amphetamines; 5 or more

80327 Anabolic steroids; 1 or 2

80328 Anabolic steroids; 3 or more

80329 Analgesics, non-opioid; 1 or 2

80330 Analgesics, non-opioid; 3-5

80331 Analgesics, non-opioid; 6 or more

80332 Antidepressants, serotonergic class; 1 or 2

80333 Antidepressants, serotonergic class; 3-5

80334 Antidepressants, serotonergic class; 6 or more

80335 Antidepressants, tricyclic and other cyclicals; 1 or 2

80336 Antidepressants, tricyclic and other cyclicals; 3-5

80337 Antidepressants, tricyclic and other cyclicals; 6 or more

80338 Antidepressants, not otherwise specified

80339 Antiepileptics, not otherwise specified; 1-3

80340 Antiepileptics, not otherwise specified; 4-6

80341 Antiepileptics, not otherwise specified; 7 or more

80342 Antipsychotics, not otherwise specified; 1-3

80343 Antipsychotics, not otherwise specified; 4-6

80344 Antipsychotics, not otherwise specified; 7 or more

80345 Barbiturates

80346 Benzodiazepines; 1-12

80347 Benzodiazepines; 13 or more

80348 Buprenorphine

80349 Cannabinoids, natural

80350 Cannabinoids, synthetic; 1-3

80351 Cannabinoids, synthetic; 4-6

80352 Cannabinoids, synthetic; 7 or more

80353 Cocaine

80354 Fentanyl

80355 Gabapentin, non-blood

80356 Heroin metabolite

80357 Ketamine and norketamine

80358 Methadone

80359 Methylenedioxyamphetamines (MDA, MDEA, MDMA)

80360 Methylphenidate

80361 Opiates, 1 or more

80362 Opioids and opiate analogs; 1 or 2

80363 Opioids and opiate analogs; 3 or 4

80364 Opioids and opiate analogs; 5 or more

80365 Oxycodone

80366 Pregabalin

80367 Propoxyphene

80368 Sedative hypnotics (non-benzodiazepines)

80369 Skeletal muscle relaxants; 1 or 2

80370 Skeletal muscle relaxants; 3 or more

80371 Stimulants, synthetic

80372 Tapentadol

80373 Tramadol

80374 Stereoisomer (enantiomer) analysis, single drug class

80375 Drug(s) or substance(s), definitive, qualitative or quantitative, not otherwise specified; 1-3

80376 Drug(s) or substance(s), definitive, qualitative or quantitative, not otherwise specified; 4-6

80377 Drug(s) or substance(s), definitive, qualitative or quantitative, not otherwise specified; 7 or more

81246 FLT3 (fms-related tyrosine kinase 3) (eg, acute myeloid leukemia), gene analysis; tyrosine kinase domain (TKD) variants (eg, D835, I836)

81288 MLH1 (mutL homolog 1, colon cancer, nonpolyposis type 2) (eg, hereditary non-polyposis colorectal cancer, Lynch syndrome) gene analysis; promoter methylation analysis

81313 PCA3/KLK3 (prostate cancer antigen 3 [non-protein coding]/kallikrein-related peptidase 3 [prostate specific antigen]) ratio (eg, prostate cancer)

81410 Aortic dysfunction or dilation (eg, Marfan syndrome, Loeys Dietz syndrome, Ehler Danlos syndrome type IV, arterial tortuosity syndrome); genomic sequence analysis panel, must include sequencing of at least 9 genes, including FBN1, TGFBR1, TGFBR2, COL3A1, MYH11, ACTA2, SLC2A10, SMAD3, and MYLK

81411 Aortic dysfunction or dilation (eg, Marfan syndrome, Loeys Dietz syndrome, Ehler Danlos syndrome type IV, arterial tortuosity syndrome); duplication/deletion analysis panel, must include analyses for TGFBR1, TGFBR2, MYH11, and COL3A1

81415 Exome (eg, unexplained constitutional or heritable disorder or syndrome); sequence analysis

81416 Exome (eg, unexplained constitutional or heritable disorder or syndrome); sequence analysis, each comparator exome (eg, parents, siblings) (List separately in addition to code for primary procedure)

81417 Exome (eg, unexplained constitutional or heritable disorder or syndrome); re-evaluation of previously obtained exome sequence (eg, updated knowledge or unrelated condition/syndrome)

81420 Fetal chromosomal aneuploidy (eg, trisomy 21, monosomy X) genomic sequence analysis panel, circulating cell-free fetal DNA in maternal blood, must include analysis of chromosomes 13, 18, and 21

81425 Genome (eg, unexplained constitutional or heritable disorder or syndrome); sequence analysis

81426 Genome (eg, unexplained constitutional or heritable disorder or syndrome); sequence analysis, each comparator genome (eg, parents, siblings) (List separately in addition to code for primary procedure)

81427 Genome (eg, unexplained constitutional or heritable disorder or syndrome); re-evaluation of previously obtained genome sequence (eg, updated knowledge or unrelated condition/syndrome)

81430 Hearing loss (eg, nonsyndromic hearing loss, Usher syndrome, Pendred syndrome); genomic sequence analysis panel, must include sequencing of at least 60 genes, including CDH23, CLRN1, GJB2, GPR98, MTRNR1, MYO7A, MYO15A, PCDH15, OTOF, SLC26A4, TMC1, TMPRSS3, USH1C, USH1G, USH2A, and WFS1

81431 Hearing loss (eg, nonsyndromic hearing loss, Usher syndrome, Pendred syndrome); duplication/deletion analysis panel, must include copy number analyses for STRC and DFNB1 deletions in GJB2 and GJB6 genes

81435 Hereditary colon cancer syndromes (eg, Lynch syndrome, familial adenomatosis polyposis); genomic sequence analysis panel, must include analysis of at least 7 genes, including APC, CHEK2, MLH1, MSH2, MSH6, MUTYH, and PMS2

81436 Hereditary colon cancer syndromes (eg, Lynch syndrome, familial adenomatosis polyposis); duplication/deletion gene analysis panel, must include analysis of at least 8 genes, including APC, MLH1, MSH2, MSH6, PMS2, EPCAM, CHEK2, and MUTYH

81440 Nuclear encoded mitochondrial genes (eg, neurologic or myopathic phenotypes), genomic sequence panel, must include analysis of at least 100 genes, including BCS1L, C10orf2, COQ2, COX10, DGUOK, MPV17, OPA1, PDSS2, POLG, POLG2, RRM2B, SCO1, SCO2, SLC25A4, SUCLA2, SUCLG1, TAZ, TK2, and TYMP

81445 Targeted genomic sequence analysis panel, solid organ neoplasm, DNA analysis, 5-50 genes (eg, ALK, BRAF, CDKN2A, EGFR, ERBB2, KIT, KRAS, NRAS, MET, PDGFRA, PDGFRB, PGR, PIK3CA, PTEN, RET), interrogation for sequence variants and copy number variants or rearrangements, if performed

81450 Targeted genomic sequence analysis panel, hematolymphoid neoplasm or disorder, DNA and RNA analysis when performed, 5-50 genes (eg, BRAF, CEBPA, DNMT3A, EZH2, FLT3, IDH1, IDH2, JAK2, KRAS, KIT, MLL, NRAS, NPM1, NOTCH1), interrogation for sequence variants, and copy number variants or rearrangements, or isoform expression or mRNA expression levels, if performed

81455 Targeted genomic sequence analysis panel, solid organ or hematolymphoid neoplasm, DNA and RNA analysis when performed, 51 or greater genes (eg, ALK, BRAF, CDKN2A, CEBPA, DNMT3A, EGFR, ERBB2, EZH2, FLT3, IDH1, IDH2, JAK2, KIT, KRAS, MLL, NPM1, NRAS, MET, NOTCH1, PDGFRA, PDGFRB, PGR, PIK3CA, PTEN, RET), interrogation for sequence variants and copy number variants or rearrangements, if performed

81460 Whole mitochondrial genome (eg, Leigh syndrome, mitochondrial encephalomyopathy, lactic acidosis, and stroke-like episodes [MELAS], myoclonic epilepsy with ragged-red fibers [MERFF], neuropathy, ataxia, and retinitis pigmentosa [NARP], Leber hereditary optic neuropathy [LHON]), genomic sequence, must include sequence analysis of entire mitochondrial genome with heteroplasmy detection

81465 Whole mitochondrial genome large deletion analysis panel (eg, Kearns-Sayre syndrome, chronic progressive external ophthalmoplegia), including heteroplasmy detection, if performed

81470 X-linked intellectual disability (XLID) (eg, syndromic and non-syndromic XLID); genomic sequence analysis panel, must include sequencing of at least 60 genes, including ARX, ATRX, CDKL5, FGD1, FMR1, HUWE1, IL1RAPL, KDM5C, L1CAM, MECP2, MED12, MID1, OCRL, RPS6KA3, and SLC16A2

81471 X-linked intellectual disability (XLID) (eg, syndromic and non-syndromic XLID); duplication/deletion gene analysis, must include analysis of at least 60 genes, including ARX, ATRX, CDKL5, FGD1, FMR1, HUWE1, IL1RAPL, KDM5C, L1CAM, MECP2, MED12, MID1, OCRL, RPS6KA3, and SLC16A2

81519 Oncology (breast), mRNA, gene expression profiling by real-time RT-PCR of 21 genes, utilizing formalin-fixed paraffin embedded tissue, algorithm reported as recurrence score

83006 Growth stimulation expressed gene 2 (ST2, Interleukin 1 receptor like-1)

87505 Infectious agent detection by nucleic acid (DNA or RNA); gastrointestinal pathogen (eg, Clostridium difficile, E. coli, Salmonella, Shigella, norovirus, Giardia), includes multiplex reverse transcription, when performed, and multiplex amplified probe technique, multiple types or subtypes, 3-5 targets

87506 Infectious agent detection by nucleic acid (DNA or RNA); gastrointestinal pathogen (eg, Clostridium difficile, E. coli, Salmonella, Shigella, norovirus, Giardia), includes multiplex reverse transcription, when performed, and multiplex amplified probe technique, multiple types or subtypes, 6-11 targets

87507 Infectious agent detection by nucleic acid (DNA or RNA); gastrointestinal pathogen (eg, Clostridium difficile, E. coli, Salmonella, Shigella, norovirus, Giardia), includes multiplex reverse transcription, when performed, and multiplex amplified probe technique, multiple types or subtypes, 12-25 targets

87623 Infectious agent detection by nucleic acid (DNA or RNA); Human Papillomavirus (HPV), low-risk types (eg, 6, 11, 42, 43, 44)

87624 Infectious agent detection by nucleic acid (DNA or RNA); Human Papillomavirus (HPV), high-risk types (eg, 16, 18, 31, 33, 35, 39, 45, 51, 52, 56, 58, 59, 68)

87625 Infectious agent detection by nucleic acid (DNA or RNA); Human Papillomavirus (HPV), types 16 and 18 only, includes type 45, if performed

87806 Infectious agent antigen detection by immunoassay with direct optical observation; HIV-1 antigen(s), with HIV-1 and HIV-2 antibodies

88341 Immunohistochemistry or immunocytochemistry, per specimen; each additional single antibody stain procedure (List separately in addition to code for primary procedure)

88344 Immunohistochemistry or immunocytochemistry, per specimen; each multiplex antibody stain procedure

88364 In situ hybridization (eg, FISH), per specimen; each additional single probe stain procedure (List separately in addition to code for primary procedure)

88366 In situ hybridization (eg, FISH), per specimen; each multiplex probe stain procedure

88369 Morphometric analysis, in situ hybridization (quantitative or semi-quantitative), manual, per specimen; each additional single probe stain procedure (List separately in addition to code for primary procedure)

88373 Morphometric analysis, in situ hybridization (quantitative or semi-quantitative), using computer-assisted technology, per specimen; each additional single probe stain procedure (List separately in addition to code for primary procedure)

88374 Morphometric analysis, in situ hybridization (quantitative or semi-quantitative), using computer-assisted technology, per specimen; each multiplex probe stain procedure

88377 Morphometric analysis, in situ hybridization (quantitative or semi-quantitative), manual, per specimen; each multiplex probe stain procedure

89337 Cryopreservation, mature oocyte(s)

90620 Meningococcal recombinant protein and outer membrane vesicle vaccine, serogroup B, 2 dose schedule, for intramuscular

90621 Meningococcal recombinant lipoprotein vaccine, serogroup B, 3 dose schedule, for intramuscular use

90630 Influenza virus vaccine, quadrivalent (IIV4), split virus, preservative free, for intradermal use

90651 Human Papillomavirus vaccine types 6, 11, 16, 18, 31, 33, 45, 52, 58, nonavalent (HPV), 3 dose schedule, for intramuscular use

90697 Diphtheria, tetanus toxoids, acellular pertussis vaccine, inactivated poliovirus vaccine, Haemophilus influenza type b PRP-OMP conjugate vaccine, and hepatitis B vaccine (DTaP-IPV-HibHepB), for intramuscular use

91200 Liver elastography, mechanically induced shear wave (eg, vibration), without imaging, with interpretation and report

92145 Corneal hysteresis determination, by air impulse stimulation, unilateral or bilateral, with interpretation and report

93260 Programming device evaluation (in person) with iterative adjustment of the implantable device to test the function of the device and select optimal permanent programmed values with analysis, review and report by a physician or other qualified health care professional; implantable subcutaneous lead defibrillator system

93261 Interrogation device evaluation (in person) with analysis, review and report by a physician or other qualified health care professional, includes connection, recording and disconnection per patient encounter; implantable subcutaneous lead defibrillator system

93355 Echocardiography, transesophageal (TEE) for guidance of a transcatheter intracardiac or great vessel(s) structural intervention(s) (eg, TAVR, transcatheter pulmonary valve replacement, mitral valve repair, paravalvular regurgitation repair, left atrial appendage occlusion/closure, ventricular septal defect closure) (peri- and intra-procedural), real-time image acquisition and documentation, guidance with quantitative measurements, probe manipulation, interpretation, and report, including diagnostic transesophageal echocardiography and, when performed, administration of ultrasound contrast, Doppler, color flow, and 3D

93644 Electrophysiologic evaluation of subcutaneous implantable defibrillator (includes defibrillation threshold evaluation, induction of arrhythmia, evaluation of sensing for arrhythmia termination, and programming or reprogramming of sensing or therapeutic parameters)

93702 Bioimpedance spectroscopy (BIS), extracellular fluid analysis for lymphedema assessment(s)

93895 Quantitative carotid intima media thickness and carotid atheroma evaluation, bilateral

96127 Brief emotional/behavioral assessment (eg, depression inventory, attention-deficit/hyperactivity disorder [ADHD] scale), with scoring and documentation, per standardized instrument

97607 Negative pressure wound therapy, (eg, vacuum assisted drainage collection), utilizing disposable, non-durable medical equipment including provision of exudate management collection system, topical application(s), wound assessment, and instructions for ongoing care, per session; total wound(s) surface area less than or equal to 50 square centimeters

97608 Negative pressure wound therapy, (eg, vacuum assisted drainage collection), utilizing disposable, non-durable medical equipment including provision of exudate management collection system, topical application(s), wound assessment, and instructions for ongoing care, per session; total wound(s) surface area greater than 50 square centimeters

99184 Initiation of selective head or total body hypothermia in the critically ill neonate, includes appropriate patient selection by review of clinical, imaging and laboratory data, confirmation of esophageal temperature probe location, evaluation of amplitude EEG, supervision of controlled hypothermia, and assessment of patient tolerance of cooling

99188 Application of topical fluoride varnish by a physician or other qualified health care professional

99490 Chronic care management services, at least 20 minutes of clinical staff time directed by a physician or other qualified health care professional, per calendar month, with the following required elements: multiple (two or more) chronic conditions expected to last at least 12 months, or until the death of the patient; chronic conditions place the patient at significant risk of death, acute exacerbation/decompensation, or functional decline; comprehensive care plan established, implemented, revised, or monitored.

99497 Advance care planning including the explanation and discussion of advance directives such as standard forms (with completion of such forms, when performed), by the physician or other qualified health care professional; first 30 minutes, face-to-face with the patient, family member(s), and/or surrogate

99498 Advance care planning including the explanation and discussion of advance directives such as standard forms (with completion of such forms, when performed), by the physician or other qualified health care professional; each additional 30 minutes (List separately in addition to code for primary procedure)

Changed Codes

1040F DSM-5 criteria for major depressive disorder documented at the initial evaluation (MDD, MDD ADOL)

0075T Transcatheter placement of extracranial vertebral artery stent(s), including radiologic supervision and interpretation, open or percutaneous; initial vessel

0076T Transcatheter placement of extracranial vertebral artery stent(s), including radiologic supervision and interpretation, open or percutaneous; each additional vessel (List separately in addition to code for primary procedure)

0191T Insertion of anterior segment aqueous drainage device, without extraocular reservoir, internal approach, into the trabecular meshwork; initial insertion

0200T Percutaneous sacral augmentation (sacroplasty), unilateral injection(s), including the use of a balloon or mechanical device, when used, 1 or more needles, includes imaging guidance and bone biopsy, when performed

0201T Percutaneous sacral augmentation (sacroplasty), bilateral injections, including the use of a balloon or mechanical device, when used, 2 or more needles, includes imaging guidance and bone biopsy, when performed

0253T Insertion of anterior segment aqueous drainage device, without extraocular reservoir, internal approach, into the suprachoroidal space

20600 Arthrocentesis, aspiration and/or injection, small joint or bursa (eg, fingers, toes); without ultrasound guidance

20605 Arthrocentesis, aspiration and/or injection, intermediate joint or bursa (eg, temporomandibular, acromioclavicular, wrist, elbow or ankle, olecranon bursa); without ultrasound guidance

20610 Arthrocentesis, aspiration and/or injection, major joint or bursa (eg, shoulder, hip, knee, subacromial bursa); without ultrasound guidance

20982 Ablation therapy for reduction or eradication of 1 or more bone tumors (eg, metastasis) including adjacent soft tissue when involved by tumor extension, percutaneous, including imaging guidance when performed; radiofrequency

22856 Total disc arthroplasty (artificial disc), anterior approach, including discectomy with end plate preparation (includes osteophytectomy for nerve root or spinal cord decompression and microdissection); single interspace, cervical

27280 Arthrodesis, open, sacroiliac joint, including obtaining bone graft, including instrumentation, when performed

27370 Injection of contrast for knee arthrography

33215 Repositioning of previously implanted transvenous pacemaker or implantable defibrillator (right atrial or right ventricular) electrode

33216 Insertion of a single transvenous electrode, permanent pacemaker or implantable defibrillator

33217 Insertion of 2 transvenous electrodes, permanent pacemaker or implantable defibrillator

33218 Repair of single transvenous electrode, permanent pacemaker or implantable defibrillator

33220 Repair of 2 transvenous electrodes for permanent pacemaker or implantable defibrillator

33223 Relocation of skin pocket for implantable defibrillator

33224 Insertion of pacing electrode, cardiac venous system, for left ventricular pacing, with attachment to previously placed pacemaker or implantable defibrillator pulse generator (including revision of pocket, removal, insertion, and/or replacement of existing generator)

33225 Insertion of pacing electrode, cardiac venous system, for left ventricular pacing, at time of insertion of implantable defibrillator or pacemaker pulse generator (eg, for upgrade to dual chamber system) (List separately in addition to code for primary procedure)

33230 Insertion of implantable defibrillator pulse generator only; with existing dual leads

33231 Insertion of implantable defibrillator pulse generator only; with existing multiple leads

33240 Insertion of implantable defibrillator pulse generator only; with existing single lead

33241 Removal of implantable defibrillator pulse generator only

33243 Removal of single or dual chamber implantable defibrillator electrode(s); by thoracotomy

33244 Removal of single or dual chamber implantable defibrillator electrode(s); by transvenous extraction

33249 Insertion or replacement of permanent implantable defibrillator system, with transvenous lead(s), single or dual chamber

33262 Removal of implantable defibrillator pulse generator with replacement of implantable defibrillator pulse generator; single lead system

33263 Removal of implantable defibrillator pulse generator with replacement of implantable defibrillator pulse generator; dual lead system

33264 Removal of implantable defibrillator pulse generator with replacement of implantable defibrillator pulse generator; multiple lead system

37215 Transcatheter placement of intravascular stent(s), cervical carotid artery, open or percutaneous, including angioplasty, when performed, and radiological supervision and interpretation; with distal embolic protection

37216 Transcatheter placement of intravascular stent(s), cervical carotid artery, open or percutaneous, including angioplasty, when performed, and radiological supervision and interpretation; without distal embolic protection

37217 Transcatheter placement of intravascular stent(s), intrathoracic common carotid artery or innominate artery by retrograde treatment, open ipsilateral cervical carotid artery exposure, including angioplasty, when performed, and radiological supervision and interpretation

37236 Transcatheter placement of an intravascular stent(s) (except lower extremity artery(s) for occlusive disease, cervical carotid, extracranial vertebral or intrathoracic carotid, intracranial, or coronary), open or percutaneous, including radiological supervision and interpretation and including all angioplasty within the same vessel, when performed; initial artery

37237 Transcatheter placement of an intravascular stent(s) (except lower extremity artery(s) for occlusive disease, cervical carotid, extracranial vertebral or intrathoracic carotid, intracranial, or coronary), open or percutaneous, including radiological supervision and interpretation and including all angioplasty within the same vessel, when performed; each additional artery (List separately in addition to code for primary procedure)

43194 Esophagoscopy, rigid, transoral; with removal of foreign body(s)

43197 Esophagoscopy, flexible, transnasal; diagnostic, including collection of specimen(s) by brushing or washing, when performed (separate procedure)

43215 Esophagoscopy, flexible, transoral; with removal of foreign body(s)

43216 Esophagoscopy, flexible, transoral; with removal of tumor(s), polyp(s), or other lesion(s) by hot biopsy forceps

43247 Esophagogastroduodenoscopy, flexible, transoral; with removal of foreign body(s)

43250 Esophagogastroduodenoscopy, flexible, transoral; with removal of tumor(s), polyp(s), or other lesion(s) by hot biopsy forceps

44360 Small intestinal endoscopy, enteroscopy beyond second portion of duodenum, not including ileum; diagnostic, including collection of specimen(s) by brushing or washing, when performed (separate procedure)

44363 Small intestinal endoscopy, enteroscopy beyond second portion of duodenum, not including ileum; with removal of foreign body(s)

44380 Ileoscopy, through stoma; diagnostic, including collection of specimen(s) by brushing or washing, when performed (separate procedure)

44385 Endoscopic evaluation of small intestinal pouch (eg, Kock pouch, ileal reservoir [S or J]); diagnostic, including collection of specimen(s) by brushing or washing, when performed (separate procedure)

44386 Endoscopic evaluation of small intestinal pouch (eg, Kock pouch, ileal reservoir [S or J]); with biopsy, single or multiple

44388 Colonoscopy through stoma; diagnostic, including collection of specimen(s) by brushing or washing, when performed (separate procedure)

44390 Colonoscopy through stoma; with removal of foreign body(s)

44391 Colonoscopy through stoma; with control of bleeding, any method

44392 Colonoscopy through stoma; with removal of tumor(s), polyp(s), or other lesion(s) by hot biopsy forceps

44799 Unlisted procedure, small intestine

45330 Sigmoidoscopy, flexible; diagnostic, including collection of specimen(s) by brushing or washing, when performed (separate procedure)

45332 Sigmoidoscopy, flexible; with removal of foreign body(s)

45333 Sigmoidoscopy, flexible; with removal of tumor(s), polyp(s), or other lesion(s) by hot biopsy forceps

45334 Sigmoidoscopy, flexible; with control of bleeding, any method

45337 Sigmoidoscopy, flexible; with decompression (for pathologic distention) (eg, volvulus, megacolon), including placement of decompression tube, when performed

45340 Sigmoidoscopy, flexible; with transendoscopic balloon dilation

45378 Colonoscopy, flexible; diagnostic, including collection of specimen(s) by brushing or washing, when performed (separate procedure)

45379 Colonoscopy, flexible; with removal of foreign body(s)

45380 Colonoscopy, flexible; with biopsy, single or multiple

45381 Colonoscopy, flexible; with directed submucosal injection(s), any substance

45382 Colonoscopy, flexible; with control of bleeding, any method

45384 Colonoscopy, flexible; with removal of tumor(s), polyp(s), or other lesion(s) by hot biopsy forceps

45385 Colonoscopy, flexible; with removal of tumor(s), polyp(s), or other lesion(s) by snare technique

45386 Colonoscopy, flexible; with transendoscopic balloon dilation

45391 Colonoscopy, flexible; with endoscopic ultrasound examination limited to the rectum, sigmoid, descending, transverse, or ascending colon and cecum, and adjacent structures

45392 Colonoscopy, flexible; with transendoscopic ultrasound guided intramural or transmural fine needle aspiration/biopsy(s), includes endoscopic ultrasound examination limited to the rectum, sigmoid, descending, transverse, or ascending colon and cecum, and adjacent structures

46600 Anoscopy; diagnostic, including collection of specimen(s) by brushing or washing, when performed (separate procedure)

61055 Cisternal or lateral cervical (C1-C2) puncture; with injection of medication or other substance for diagnosis or treatment

62284 Injection procedure for myelography and/or computed tomography, lumbar (other than C1-C2 and posterior fossa)

66180 Aqueous shunt to extraocular equatorial plate reservoir, external approach; with graft

66185 Revision of aqueous shunt to extraocular equatorial plate reservoir; with graft

67399 Unlisted procedure, extraocular muscle

77401 Radiation treatment delivery, superficial and/or ortho voltage, per day

77402 Radiation treatment delivery,=>1 MeV; simple

77407 Radiation treatment delivery, =>1 MeV; intermediate

77412 Radiation treatment delivery, =>1 MeV; complex

80162 Digoxin; total

80164 Valproic acid (dipropylacetic acid); total

80171 Gabapentin, whole blood, serum, or plasma

80299 Quantitation of therapeutic drug, not elsewhere specified

81245 FLT3 (fms-related tyrosine kinase 3) (eg, acute myeloid leukemia), gene analysis; internal tandem duplication (ITD) variants (ie, exons 14, 15)

81402 Molecular pathology procedure, Level 3 (eg, >10 SNPs, 2-10 methylated variants, or 2-10 somatic variants [typically using non-sequencing target variant analysis], immunoglobulin and T-cell receptor gene rearrangements, duplication/deletion variants of 1 exon, loss of heterozygosity [LOH], uniparental disomy [UPD])

81403 Molecular pathology procedure, Level 4 (eg, analysis of single exon by DNA sequence analysis, analysis of >10 amplicons using multiplex PCR in 2 or more independent reactions, mutation scanning or duplication/deletion variants of 2-5 exons)

81404 Molecular pathology procedure, Level 5 (eg, analysis of 2-5 exons by DNA sequence analysis, mutation scanning or duplication/deletion variants of 6-10 exons, or characterization of a dynamic mutation disorder/triplet repeat by Southern blot analysis)

81405 Molecular pathology procedure, Level 6 (eg, analysis of 6-10 exons by DNA sequence analysis, mutation scanning or duplication/deletion variants of 11-25 exons, regionally targeted cytogenomic array analysis)

82541 Column chromatography/mass spectrometry (eg, GC/MS, or HPLC/MS), non-drug analyte not elsewhere specified; qualitative, single stationary and mobile phase

82542 Column chromatography/mass spectrometry (eg, GC/MS, or HPLC/MS), non-drug analyte not elsewhere specified; quantitative, single stationary and mobile phase

82543 Column chromatography/mass spectrometry (eg, GC/MS, or HPLC/MS), non-drug analyte not elsewhere specified; stable isotope dilution, single analyte, quantitative, single stationary and mobile phase

82544 Column chromatography/mass spectrometry (eg, GC/MS, or HPLC/MS), non-drug analyte not elsewhere specified; stable isotope dilution, multiple analytes, quantitative, single stationary and mobile phase

84600 Volatiles (eg, acetic anhydride, diethylether)

86900 Blood typing, serologic; ABO

86901 Blood typing, serologic; Rh (D)

86902 Blood typing, serologic; antigen testing of donor blood using reagent serum, each antigen test

86904 Blood typing, serologic; antigen screening for compatible unit using patient serum, per unit screened

86905 Blood typing, serologic; RBC antigens, other than ABO or Rh (D), each

86906 Blood typing, serologic; Rh phenotyping, complete

87501 Infectious agent detection by nucleic acid (DNA or RNA); influenza virus, includes reverse transcription, when performed, and amplified probe technique, each type or subtype

87502 Infectious agent detection by nucleic acid (DNA or RNA); influenza virus, for multiple types or sub-types, includes multiplex reverse transcription and multiplex amplified probe technique, first 2 types or sub-types

87503 Infectious agent detection by nucleic acid (DNA or RNA); influenza virus, for multiple types or sub-types, includes multiplex reverse transcription and multiplex amplified probe technique, each additional influenza virus type or sub-type beyond 2 (List separately in addition to code for primary procedure)

87631 Infectious agent detection by nucleic acid (DNA or RNA); respiratory virus (eg, adenovirus, influenza virus, coronavirus, metapneumovirus, parainfluenza virus, respiratory syncytial virus, rhinovirus), includes multiplex reverse transcription, when performed, and multiplex amplified probe technique, multiple types or subtypes, 3-5 targets

87632 Infectious agent detection by nucleic acid (DNA or RNA); respiratory virus (eg, adenovirus, influenza virus, coronavirus, metapneumovirus, parainfluenza virus, respiratory syncytial virus, rhinovirus), includes multiplex reverse transcription, when performed, and multiplex amplified probe technique, multiple types or subtypes, 6-11 targets

87633 Infectious agent detection by nucleic acid (DNA or RNA); respiratory virus (eg, adenovirus, influenza virus, coronavirus, metapneumovirus, parainfluenza virus, respiratory syncytial virus, rhinovirus), includes multiplex reverse transcription, when performed, and multiplex amplified probe technique, multiple types or subtypes, 12-25 targets

88342 Immunohistochemistry or immunocytochemistry, per specimen; initial single antibody stain procedure

88360 Morphometric analysis, tumor immunohistochemistry (eg, Her-2/neu, estrogen receptor/progesterone receptor), quantitative or semiquantitative, per specimen, each single antibody stain procedure; manual

88361 Morphometric analysis, tumor immunohistochemistry (eg, Her-2/neu, estrogen receptor/progesterone receptor), quantitative or semiquantitative, per specimen, each single antibody stain procedure; using computer-assisted technology

88365 In situ hybridization (eg, FISH), per specimen; initial single probe stain procedure

88367 Morphometric analysis, in situ hybridization (quantitative or semi-quantitative), using computer-assisted technology, per specimen; initial single probe stain procedure

88368 Morphometric analysis, in situ hybridization (quantitative or semi-quantitative), manual, per specimen; initial single probe stain procedure

90654 Influenza virus vaccine, trivalent (IIV3), split virus, preservative-free, for intradermal use

90721 Diphtheria, tetanus toxoids, and acellular pertussis vaccine and Hemophilus influenza B vaccine (DTaP/Hib), for intramuscular use

90723 Diphtheria, tetanus toxoids, acellular pertussis vaccine, hepatitis B, and inactivated poliovirus vaccine (DTaP-HepB-IPV), for intramuscular use

90734 Meningococcal conjugate vaccine, serogroups A, C, Y and W-135, quadrivalent, for intramuscular use

93282 Programming device evaluation (in person) with iterative adjustment of the implantable device to test the function of the device and select optimal permanent programmed values with analysis, review and report by a physician or other qualified health care professional; single lead transvenous implantable defibrillator system

93283 Programming device evaluation (in person) with iterative adjustment of the implantable device to test the function of the device and select optimal permanent programmed values with analysis, review and report by a physician or other qualified health care professional; dual lead transvenous implantable defibrillator system

93284 Programming device evaluation (in person) with iterative adjustment of the implantable device to test the function of the device and select optimal permanent programmed values with analysis, review and report by a physician or other qualified health care professional; multiple lead transvenous implantable defibrillator system

93287 Peri-procedural device evaluation (in person) and programming of device system parameters before or after a surgery, procedure, or test with analysis, review and report by a physician or other qualified health care professional; single, dual, or multiple lead implantable defibrillator system

93289 Interrogation device evaluation (in person) with analysis, review and report by a physician or other qualified health care professional, includes connection, recording and disconnection per patient encounter; single, dual, or multiple lead transvenous implantable defibrillator system, including analysis of heart rhythm derived data elements

93295 Interrogation device evaluation(s) (remote), up to 90 days; single, dual, or multiple lead implantable defibrillator system with interim analysis, review(s) and report(s) by a physician or other qualified health care professional

93296 Interrogation device evaluation(s) (remote), up to 90 days; single, dual, or multiple lead pacemaker system or implantable defibrillator system, remote data acquisition(s), receipt of transmissions and technician review, technical support and distribution of results

93642 Electrophysiologic evaluation of single or dual chamber transvenous pacing cardioverter-defibrillator (includes defibrillation threshold evaluation, induction of arrhythmia, evaluation of sensing and pacing for arrhythmia termination, and programming or reprogramming of sensing or therapeutic parameters)

95972 Electronic analysis of implanted neurostimulator pulse generator system (eg, rate, pulse amplitude, pulse duration, configuration of wave form, battery status, electrode selectability, output modulation, cycling, impedance and patient compliance measurements); complex spinal cord, or peripheral (ie, peripheral nerve, sacral nerve, neuromuscular) (except cranial nerve) neurostimulator pulse generator/transmitter, with intraoperative or subsequent programming, up to 1 hour

96110 Developmental screening (eg, developmental milestone survey, speech and language delay screen), with scoring and documentation, per standardized instrument

97605 Negative pressure wound therapy (eg, vacuum assisted drainage collection), utilizing durable medical equipment (DME), including topical application(s), wound assessment, and instruction(s) for ongoing care, per session; total wound(s) surface area less than or equal to 50 square centimeters

97606 Negative pressure wound therapy (eg, vacuum assisted drainage collection), utilizing durable medical equipment (DME), including topical application(s), wound assessment, and instruction(s) for ongoing care, per session; total wound(s) surface area greater than 50 square centimeters

99487 Complex chronic care management services, with the following required elements: multiple (two or more) chronic conditions expected to last at least 12 months, or until the death of the patient, chronic conditions place the patient at significant risk of death, acute exacerbation/decompensation, or functional decline, establishment or substantial revision of a comprehensive care plan, moderate or high complexity medical decision making; 60 minutes of clinical staff time directed by a physician or other qualified health care professional, per calendar month

99489 Complex chronic care management services, with the following required elements: multiple (two or more) chronic conditions expected to last at least 12 months, or until the death of the patient, chronic conditions place the patient at significant risk of death, acute exacerbation/decompensation, or functional decline, establishment or substantial revision of a comprehensive care plan, moderate or high complexity medical decision making; each additional 30 minutes of clinical staff time directed by a physician or other qualified health care professional, per calendar month (List separately in addition to code for primary procedure)

Deleted Codes

00452	0059T	00622	00634	0073T	0092T	0181T
0197T	0199T	0226T	0227T	0239T	0245T	0246T
0247T	0248T	0319T	0320T	0321T	0322T	0323T
0324T	0325T	0326T	0327T	0328T	0334T	0343T
0344T	21800	21810	22520	22521	22522	22523
22524	22525	29020	29025	29715	3125F	33332
33472	33960	33961	36469	36822	42508	43350
44383	44393	44397	45339	45345	45355	45383
45387	61334	61440	61470	61490	61542	61609
61875	62116	64752	64761	64870	66165	69400
69401	69405	72291	72292	74291	76645	76950
77082	77305	77310	77315	77326	77327	77328
77403	77404	77406	77408	77409	77411	77413
77414	77416	77418	77421	80100	80101	80102
80103	80104	80152	80154	80160	80166	80172
80174	80182	80196	80440	82000	82003	82055
82101	82145	82205	82520	82646	82649	82651
82654	82666	82690	82742	82953	82975	82980
83008	83055	83071	83634	83805	83840	83858
83866	83887	83925	84022	84127	87001	87620
87621	87622	88343	88349	99481	99482	99488

Appendix C — Crosswalk of Deleted Codes

The deleted code crosswalk is meant to be used as a reference tool to find active codes that could be used in place of the deleted code. This will not always be an exact match. Please review the code descriptions and guidelines before selecting a code.

Code	Cross reference
0059T	To report, see 89337, 0357T
0073T	To report, see 77385
0092T	To report cervical arthroplasty on three levels or more, see 0375T
0181T	To report, see 92145
0197T	To report, see 77387
0199T	To report, see 95999
0226T	To report, see 46601
0227T	To report, see 46607
0239T	To report, see 93702
0245T	To report, see 21811
0246T	To report, see 21811, 21812
0247T	To report, see 21812
0248T	To report, see 21813
0319T	To report, see 33270
0320T	To report, see 33271
0321T	To report, see 33240
0322T	To report, see 33241
0323T	To report, see 33262-33264
0324T	To report, see 33272
0325T	To report, see 33273
0326T	To report, see 33270
0327T	To report, see 93261
0328T	To report, see 93260
0334T	To report, see 27279
0343T	To report, see 33418
0344T	To report, see 33419
21800	To report, see Evaluation and Management Codes
21810	To report, see 21899
22520	To report, see 22510
22521	To report, see 22511
22522	To report, see 22512
22523	To report, see 22513
22524	To report, see 22514
22525	To report, see 22515
33960	To report, see 33946-33949
33961	To report, see 33948-33949
36822	To report, see 33951-33956

Code	Cross reference
44383	To report, see 44384
44393	To report, see 44401
44397	To report, see 44402
45339	To report, see 45346
45345	To report, see 45347
45355	To report, see 45399
45383	To report, see 45388
45387	To report, see 45389
69400	To report, see 69799
69401	To report, see 99201-99205, 99211-99215
69405	To report, see 69799
72291	To report, see 0200T-0201T, 22510-22515
72292	To report, see 0200T-0201T, 22510-22515
76645	To report, see 76641-76642
76950	To report, see 77387
77082	To report, see 77086
77305	To report, see 77306
77310	To report, see 77306-77307
77315	To report, see 77307
77326	To report, see 77316
77327	To report, see 77317
77328	To report, see 77318
77403	To report, see 77402
77404	To report, see 77402
77406	To report, see 77402
77408	To report, see 77407
77409	To report, see 77407
77411	To report, see 77407
77413	To report, see 77412
77414	To report, see 77412
77416	To report, see 77412
77421	To report, see 77387
80100	To report, see 80300-80304
80101	To report, see 80300-80304
80102	To report, see 80300-80304
80103	To report, see 80300-80304
80104	To report, see 80300-80304

Code	Cross reference
80152	To report, see 80335-80337
80154	To report, see 80346-80347
80160	To report, see 80335-80337
80166	To report, see 80335-80337
80172	To report, see 80375
80174	To report, see 80335-80337
80182	To report, see 80335-80337
80196	To report, see 80329-80331
80440	To report, see 84146
82003	To report, see 80329-80331
82055	To report, see 80320-80322
82101	To report, see 80323
82145	To report, see 80324-80326
82205	To report, see 80345
82520	To report, see 80353
82646	To report, see 80361
82649	To report, see 80361
82651	To report, see 80327-80328
82654	To report, see 80339-80341
82666	To report, see 80327-80328
82690	To report, see 80320
82742	To report, see 80346-80347
82975	To report, see 82127-82128, 82131
83805	To report, see 80369-80370
83840	To report, see 80358
83858	To report, see 80339-80341
83887	To report, see 80323
83925	To report, see specific drug or 80361-80364
84022	To report, see 80342-80344
87620	To report, see 87623-87625
87621	To report, see 87623-87625
87622	To report, see 87623-87625
88343	To report, see 88344
88349	To report, see 88348
99481	To report, see 99184
99482	To report, see 99184
99488	To report, see appropriate Evaluation and Management code

Appendix D — Resequenced Codes

Code	Description	Reference
11045	Debridement, subcutaneous tissue (includes epidermis and dermis, if performed); each additional 20 sq cm, or part thereof (List separately in addition to code for primary procedure)	Resequenced code. See code following 11042.
11046	Debridement, muscle and/or fascia (includes epidermis, dermis, and subcutaneous tissue, if performed); each additional 20 sq cm, or part thereof (List separately in addition to code for primary procedure)	Resequenced code. See code following 11043.
21552	Excision, tumor, soft tissue of neck or anterior thorax, subcutaneous; 3 cm or greater	Resequenced code. See code following 21555.
21554	Excision, tumor, soft tissue of neck or anterior thorax, subfascial (eg, intramuscular); 5 cm or greater	Resequenced code. See code following 21556.
22858	Total disc arthroplasty (artificial disc), anterior approach, including discectomy with end plate preparation (includes osteophytectomy for nerve root or spinal cord decompression and microdissection); second level, cervical (List separately in addition to code for primary procedure)	Resequenced code. See code following 22856.
23071	Excision, tumor, soft tissue of shoulder area, subcutaneous; 3 cm or greater	Resequenced code. See code following 23075.
23073	Excision, tumor, soft tissue of shoulder area, subfascial (eg, intramuscular); 5 cm or greater	Resequenced code. See code following 23076.
24071	Excision, tumor, soft tissue of upper arm or elbow area, subcutaneous; 3 cm or greater	Resequenced code. See code following 24075
24073	Excision, tumor, soft tissue of upper arm or elbow area, subfascial (eg, intramuscular); 5 cm or greater	Resequenced code. See code following 24076.
25071	Excision, tumor, soft tissue of forearm and/or wrist area, subcutaneous; 3 cm or greater	Resequenced code. See code following 25075.
25073	Excision, tumor, soft tissue of forearm and/or wrist area, subfascial (eg, intramuscular); 3 cm or greater	Resequenced code. See code following 25076.
26111	Excision, tumor or vascular malformation, soft tissue of hand or finger, subcutaneous; 1.5 cm or greater	Resequenced code. See code following 26115.
26113	Excision, tumor, soft tissue, or vascular malformation, of hand or finger, subfascial (eg, intramuscular); 1.5 cm or greater	Resequenced code. See code following 26116.
27043	Excision, tumor, soft tissue of pelvis and hip area, subcutaneous; 3 cm or greater	Resequenced code. See code following 27047.
27045	Excision, tumor, soft tissue of pelvis and hip area, subfascial (eg, intramuscular); 5 cm or greater	Resequenced code. See code following 27048.
27059	Radical resection of tumor (eg, sarcoma), soft tissue of pelvis and hip area; 5 cm or greater	Resequenced code. See code following 27049.
27329	Radical resection of tumor (eg, sarcoma), soft tissue of thigh or knee area; less than 5 cm	Resequenced code. See code following 27360.
27337	Excision, tumor, soft tissue of thigh or knee area, subcutaneous; 3 cm or greater	Resequenced code. See code following 27327.
27339	Excision, tumor, soft tissue of thigh or knee area, subfascial (eg, intramuscular); 5 cm or greater	Resequenced code. See code following 27328.
27632	Excision, tumor, soft tissue of leg or ankle area, subcutaneous; 3 cm or greater	Resequenced code. See code following 27618.
27634	Excision, tumor, soft tissue of leg or ankle area, subfascial (eg, intramuscular); 5 cm or greater	Resequenced code. See code following 27619.
28039	Excision, tumor, soft tissue of foot or toe, subcutaneous; 1.5 cm or greater	Resequenced code. See code following 28043.
28041	Excision, tumor, soft tissue of foot or toe, subfascial (eg, intramuscular); 1.5 cm or greater	Resequenced code. See code following 28045.
29914	Arthroscopy, hip, surgical; with femoroplasty (ie, treatment of cam lesion)	Resequenced code. See code following 29863.
29915	Arthroscopy, hip, surgical; with acetabuloplasty (ie, treatment of pincer lesion)	Resequenced code. See code following 29863.
29916	Arthroscopy, hip, surgical; with labral repair	Resequenced code. See code before 29866.
31651	Bronchoscopy, rigid or flexible, including fluoroscopic guidance, when performed; with balloon occlusion, when performed, assessment of air leak, airway sizing, and insertion of bronchial valve(s), each additional lobe (List separately in addition to code for primary procedure[s])	Resequenced code. See code following 31647.
33221	Insertion of pacemaker pulse generator only; with existing multiple leads	Resequenced code. See code following 33213.
33227	Removal of permanent pacemaker pulse generator with replacement of pacemaker pulse generator; single lead system	Resequenced code. See code following 33233.
33228	Removal of permanent pacemaker pulse generator with replacement of pacemaker pulse generator; dual lead system	Resequenced code. See code following 33233.
33229	Removal of permanent pacemaker pulse generator with replacement of pacemaker pulse generator; multiple lead system	Resequenced code. See code before 33234.
33230	Insertion of implantable defibrillator pulse generator only; with existing dual leads	Resequenced code. See code following 33240.
33231	Insertion of implantable defibrillator pulse generator only; with existing multiple leads	Resequenced code. See code before 33241.
33262	Removal of implantable defibrillator pulse generator with replacement of implantable defibrillator pulse generator; single lead system	Resequenced code. See code following 33241.
33263	Removal of implantable defibrillator pulse generator with replacement of implantable defibrillator pulse generator; dual lead system	Resequenced code. See code following 33241.
33264	Removal of implantable defibrillator pulse generator with replacement of implantable defibrillator pulse generator; multiple lead system	Resequenced code. See code before 33243.
33270	Insertion or replacement of permanent subcutaneous implantable defibrillator system, with subcutaneous electrode, including defibrillation threshold evaluation, induction of arrhythmia, evaluation of sensing for arrhythmia termination, and programming or reprogramming of sensing or therapeutic parameters, when performed	Resequenced code. See code following 33249.

Code	Description	Reference
33271	Insertion of subcutaneous implantable defibrillator electrode	Resequenced code. See code following 33249.
33272	Removal of subcutaneous implantable defibrillator electrode	Resequenced code. See code following 33249.
33273	Repositioning of previously implanted subcutaneous implantable defibrillator electrode	Resequenced code. See code following 33249.
33962	Extracorporeal membrane oxygenation (ECMO)/extracorporeal life support (ECLS) provided by physician; reposition peripheral (arterial and/or venous) cannula(e), open, 6 years and older (includes fluoroscopic guidance, when performed)	Resequenced code. See code following 33959.
33963	Extracorporeal membrane oxygenation (ECMO)/extracorporeal life support (ECLS) provided by physician; reposition of central cannula(e) by sternotomy or thoracotomy, birth through 5 years of age (includes fluoroscopic guidance, when performed)	Resequenced code. See code following 33959.
33964	Extracorporeal membrane oxygenation (ECMO)/extracorporeal life support (ECLS) provided by physician; reposition central cannula(e) by sternotomy or thoracotomy, 6 years and older (includes fluoroscopic guidance, when performed)	Resequenced code. See code following 33959.
33965	Extracorporeal membrane oxygenation (ECMO)/extracorporeal life support (ECLS) provided by physician; removal of peripheral (arterial and/or venous) cannula(e), percutaneous, birth through 5 years of age	Resequenced code. See code following 33959.
33966	Extracorporeal membrane oxygenation (ECMO)/extracorporeal life support (ECLS) provided by physician; removal of peripheral (arterial and/or venous) cannula(e), percutaneous, 6 years and older	Resequenced code. See code following 33959.
33969	Extracorporeal membrane oxygenation (ECMO)/extracorporeal life support (ECLS) provided by physician; removal of peripheral (arterial and/or venous) cannula(e), open, birth through 5 years of age	Resequenced code. See code following 33959.
33984	Extracorporeal membrane oxygenation (ECMO)/extracorporeal life support (ECLS) provided by physician; removal of peripheral (arterial and/or venous) cannula(e), open, 6 years and older	Resequenced code. See code following 33959.
33985	Extracorporeal membrane oxygenation (ECMO)/extracorporeal life support (ECLS) provided by physician; removal of central cannula(e) by sternotomy or thoracotomy, birth through 5 years of age	Resequenced code. See code following 33959.
33986	Extracorporeal membrane oxygenation (ECMO)/extracorporeal life support (ECLS) provided by physician; removal of central cannula(e) by sternotomy or thoracotomy, 6 years and older	Resequenced code. See code following 33959.
33987	Arterial exposure with creation of graft conduit (eg, chimney graft) to facilitate arterial perfusion for ECMO/ECLS (List separately in addition to code for primary procedure)	Resequenced code. See code following 33959.
33988	Insertion of left heart vent by thoracic incision (eg, sternotomy, thoracotomy) for ECMO/ECLS	Resequenced code. See code following 33959.
33989	Removal of left heart vent by thoracic incision (eg, sternotomy, thoracotomy) for ECMO/ECLS	Resequenced code. See code following 33959.
37211	Transcatheter therapy, arterial infusion for thrombolysis other than coronary, any method, including radiological supervision and interpretation, initial treatment day	Resequenced code. See code following 37200.
37212	Transcatheter therapy, venous infusion for thrombolysis, any method, including radiological supervision and interpretation, initial treatment day	Resequenced code. See code following 37200.
37213	Transcatheter therapy, arterial or venous infusion for thrombolysis other than coronary, any method, including radiological supervision and interpretation, continued treatment on subsequent day during course of thrombolytic therapy, including follow-up catheter contrast injection, position change, or exchange, when performed;	Resequenced code. See code following 37200.
37214	Transcatheter therapy, arterial or venous infusion for thrombolysis other than coronary, any method, including radiological supervision and interpretation, continued treatment on subsequent day during course of thrombolytic therapy, including follow-up catheter contrast injection, position change, or exchange, when performed; cessation of thrombolysis including removal of catheter and vessel closure by any method	Resequenced code. See code following 37200.
38243	Hematopoietic progenitor cell (HPC); HPC boost	Resequenced code. See code following 38241.
43211	Esophagoscopy, flexible, transoral; with endoscopic mucosal resection	Resequenced code. See code following 43217.
43212	Esophagoscopy, flexible, transoral; with placement of endoscopic stent (includes pre- and post-dilation and guide wire passage, when performed)	Resequenced code. See code following 43217.
43213	Esophagoscopy, flexible, transoral; with dilation of esophagus, by balloon or dilator, retrograde (includes fluoroscopic guidance, when performed)	Resequenced code. See code following 43220.
43214	Esophagoscopy, flexible, transoral; with dilation of esophagus with balloon (30 mm diameter or larger) (includes fluoroscopic guidance, when performed)	Resequenced code. See code following 43220.
43233	Esophagogastroduodenoscopy, flexible, transoral; with dilation of esophagus with balloon (30 mm diameter or larger) (includes fluoroscopic guidance, when performed)	Resequenced code. See code following 43249.
43266	Esophagogastroduodenoscopy, flexible, transoral; with placement of endoscopic stent (includes pre- and post-dilation and guide wire passage, when performed)	Resequenced code. See code following 43255.
43270	Esophagogastroduodenoscopy, flexible, transoral; with ablation of tumor(s), polyp(s), or other lesion(s) (includes pre- and post-dilation and guide wire passage, when performed)	Resequenced code. See code following 43257.
43274	Endoscopic retrograde cholangiopancreatography (ERCP); with placement of endoscopic stent into biliary or pancreatic duct, including pre- and post-dilation and guide wire passage, when performed, including sphincterotomy, when performed, each stent	Resequenced code. See code following 43265.
43275	Endoscopic retrograde cholangiopancreatography (ERCP); with removal of foreign body(s) or stent(s) from biliary/pancreatic duct(s)	Resequenced code. See code following 43265.

Code	Description	Reference
43276	Endoscopic retrograde cholangiopancreatography (ERCP); with removal and exchange of stent(s), biliary or pancreatic duct, including pre- and post-dilation and guide wire passage, when performed, including sphincterotomy, when performed, each stent exchanged	Resequenced code. See code following 43265.
43277	Endoscopic retrograde cholangiopancreatography (ERCP); with trans-endoscopic balloon dilation of biliary/pancreatic duct(s) or of ampulla (sphincteroplasty), including sphincterotomy, when performed, each duct	Resequenced code. See code before 43273.
43278	Endoscopic retrograde cholangiopancreatography (ERCP); with ablation of tumor(s), polyp(s), or other lesion(s), including pre- and post-dilation and guide wire passage, when performed	Resequenced code. See code before 43273.
44381	Ileoscopy, through stoma; with transendoscopic balloon dilation	Resequenced code. See code following 44382.
44401	Colonoscopy through stoma; with ablation of tumor(s), polyp(s), or other lesion(s) (includes pre-and post-dilation and guide wire passage, when performed)	Resequenced code. See code following 44392.
45346	Sigmoidoscopy, flexible; with ablation of tumor(s), polyp(s), or other lesion(s) (includes pre- and post-dilation and guide wire passage, when performed)	Resequenced code. See code following 45338.
45388	Colonoscopy, flexible; with ablation of tumor(s), polyp(s), or other lesion(s) (includes pre- and post-dilation and guide wire passage, when performed)	Resequenced code. See code following 45382.
45390	Colonoscopy, flexible; with endoscopic mucosal resection	Resequenced code. See code following 45392.
45398	Colonoscopy, flexible; with band ligation(s) (eg, hemorrhoids)	Resequenced code. See code following 45393.
45399	Unlisted procedure, colon	Resequenced code. See code before 45990.
46220	Excision of single external papilla or tag, anus	Resequenced code. See code before 46230.
46320	Excision of thrombosed hemorrhoid, external	Resequenced code. See code following 46230.
46945	Hemorrhoidectomy, internal, by ligation other than rubber band; single hemorrhoid column/group	Resequenced code. See code following 46221.
46946	Hemorrhoidectomy, internal, by ligation other than rubber band; 2 or more hemorrhoid columns/groups	Resequenced code, See code following 46221.
46947	Hemorrhoidopexy (eg, for prolapsing internal hemorrhoids) by stapling	Resequenced code, See code following 46762.
51797	Voiding pressure studies, intra-abdominal (ie, rectal, gastric, intraperitoneal) (List separately in addition to code for primary procedure)	Resequenced code, See code following 51729.
52356	Cystourethroscopy, with ureteroscopy and/or pyeloscopy; with lithotripsy including insertion of indwelling ureteral stent (eg, Gibbons or double-J type)	Resequenced code. See code following 52353.
64633	Destruction by neurolytic agent, paravertebral facet joint nerve(s), with imaging guidance (fluoroscopy or CT); cervical or thoracic, single facet joint	Resequenced code. See code following 64620.
64634	Destruction by neurolytic agent, paravertebral facet joint nerve(s), with imaging guidance (fluoroscopy or CT); cervical or thoracic, each additional facet joint (List separately in addition to code for primary procedure)	Resequenced code. See code following 64620.
64635	Destruction by neurolytic agent, paravertebral facet joint nerve(s), with imaging guidance (fluoroscopy or CT); lumbar or sacral, single facet joint	Resequenced code. See code following 64620.
64636	Destruction by neurolytic agent, paravertebral facet joint nerve(s), with imaging guidance (fluoroscopy or CT); lumbar or sacral, each additional facet joint (List separately in addition to code for primary procedure)	Resequenced code. See code before 64630.
67810	Incisional biopsy of eyelid skin including lid margin	Resequenced code. See code following 67715.
77085	Dual-energy X-ray absorptiometry (DXA), bone density study, 1 or more sites; axial skeleton (eg, hips, pelvis, spine), including vertebral fracture assessment	Resequenced code. See code following 77081.
77086	Vertebral fracture assessment via dual-energy X-ray absorptiometry (DXA)	Resequenced code. See code before 77084.
77295	3-dimensional radiotherapy plan, including dose-volume histograms	Resequenced code. See code before 77300.
77385	Intensity modulated radiation treatment delivery (IMRT), includes guidance and tracking, when performed; simple	Resequenced code. See code following 77417.
77386	Intensity modulated radiation treatment delivery (IMRT), includes guidance and tracking, when performed; complex	Resequenced code. See code following 77417.
77387	Guidance for localization of target volume for delivery of radiation treatment delivery, includes intrafraction tracking, when performed	Resequenced code. See code following 77417.
77424	Intraoperative radiation treatment delivery, x-ray, single treatment session	Resequenced code. See code following 77421.
77425	Intraoperative radiation treatment delivery, electrons, single treatment session	Resequenced code. See code before 77422.
80164	Valproic acid (dipropylacetic acid); total	Resequenced code. See code following 80201.
80165	Valproic acid (dipropylacetic acid); free	Resequenced code. See code following 80201.
80171	Gabapentin, whole blood, serum, or plasma	Resequenced code. See code following 80169.
80300	Drug screen, any number of drug classes from Drug Class List A; any number of non-TLC devices or procedures, (eg, immunoassay) capable of being read by direct optical observation, including instrumented-assisted when performed (eg, dipsticks, cups, cards, cartridges), per date of service	Resequenced code. See code before 80150.
80301	Drug screen, any number of drug classes from Drug Class List A; single drug class method, by instrumented test systems (eg, discrete multichannel chemistry analyzers utilizing immunoassay or enzyme assay), per date of service	Resequenced code. See code before 80150.
80302	Drug screen, presumptive, single drug class from Drug Class List B, by immunoassay (eg, ELISA) or non-TLC chromatography without mass spectrometry (eg, GC, HPLC), each procedure	Resequenced code. See code before 80150.

Code	Description	Reference
80303	Drug screen, any number of drug classes, presumptive, single or multiple drug class method; thin layer chromatography procedure(s) (TLC) (eg, acid, neutral, alkaloid plate), per date of service	Resequenced code. See code before 80150.
80304	Drug screen, any number of drug classes, presumptive, single or multiple drug class method; not otherwise specified presumptive procedure (eg, TOF, MALDI, LDTD, DESI, DART), each procedure	Resequenced code. See code before 80150.
80320	Alcohols	Resequenced code. See code before 80150.
80321	Alcohol biomarkers; 1 or 2	Resequenced code. See code before 80150.
80322	Alcohol biomarkers; 3 or more	Resequenced code. See code before 80150.
80323	Alkaloids, not otherwise specified	Resequenced code. See code before 80150.
80324	Amphetamines; 1 or 2	Resequenced code. See code before 80150.
80325	Amphetamines; 3 or 4	Resequenced code. See code before 80150.
80326	Amphetamines; 5 or more	Resequenced code. See code before 80150.
80327	Anabolic steroids; 1 or 2	Resequenced code. See code before 80150.
80328	Anabolic steroids; 3 or more	Resequenced code. See code before 80150.
80329	Analgesics, non-opioid; 1 or 2	Resequenced code. See code before 80150.
80330	Analgesics, non-opioid; 3-5	Resequenced code. See code before 80150.
80331	Analgesics, non-opioid; 6 or more	Resequenced code. See code before 80150.
80332	Antidepressants, serotonergic class; 1 or 2	Resequenced code. See code before 80150.
80333	Antidepressants, serotonergic class; 3-5	Resequenced code. See code before 80150.
80334	Antidepressants, serotonergic class; 6 or more	Resequenced code. See code before 80150.
80335	Antidepressants, tricyclic and other cyclicals; 1 or 2	Resequenced code. See code before 80150.
80336	Antidepressants, tricyclic and other cyclicals; 3-5	Resequenced code. See code before 80150.
80337	Antidepressants, tricyclic and other cyclicals; 6 or more	Resequenced code. See code before 80150.
80338	Antidepressants, not otherwise specified	Resequenced code. See code before 80150.
80339	Antiepileptics, not otherwise specified; 1-3	Resequenced code. See code before 80150.
80340	Antiepileptics, not otherwise specified; 4-6	Resequenced code. See code before 80150.
80341	Antiepileptics, not otherwise specified; 7 or more	Resequenced code. See code before 80150.
80342	Antipsychotics, not otherwise specified; 1-3	Resequenced code. See code before 80150.
80343	Antipsychotics, not otherwise specified; 4-6	Resequenced code. See code before 80150.
80344	Antipsychotics, not otherwise specified; 7 or more	Resequenced code. See code before 80150.
80345	Barbiturates	Resequenced code. See code before 80150.
80346	Benzodiazepines; 1-12	Resequenced code. See code before 80150.
80347	Benzodiazepines; 13 or more	Resequenced code. See code before 80150.
80348	Buprenorphine	Resequenced code. See code before 80150.
80349	Cannabinoids, natural	Resequenced code. See code before 80150.
80350	Cannabinoids, synthetic; 1-3	Resequenced code. See code before 80150.
80351	Cannabinoids, synthetic; 4-6	Resequenced code. See code before 80150.
80352	Cannabinoids, synthetic; 7 or more	Resequenced code. See code before 80150.
80353	Cocaine	Resequenced code. See code before 80150.
80354	Fentanyl	Resequenced code. See code before 80150.
80355	Gabapentin, non-blood	Resequenced code. See code before 80150.
80356	Heroin metabolite	Resequenced code. See code before 80150.
80357	Ketamine and norketamine	Resequenced code. See code before 80150.
80358	Methadone	Resequenced code. See code before 80150.
80359	Methylenedioxyamphetamines (MDA, MDEA, MDMA)	Resequenced code. See code before 80150.
80360	Methylphenidate	Resequenced code. See code before 80150.
80361	Opiates, 1 or more	Resequenced code. See code before 80150.
80362	Opioids and opiate analogs; 1 or 2	Resequenced code. See code before 80150.
80363	Opioids and opiate analogs; 3 or 4	Resequenced code. See code before 80150.
80364	Opioids and opiate analogs; 5 or more	Resequenced code. See code before 80150.
80365	Oxycodone	Resequenced code. See code following 80364.
80366	Pregabalin	Resequenced code. See code following 83992.
80367	Propoxyphene	Resequenced code. See code following 80366.
80368	Sedative hypnotics (non-benzodiazepines)	Resequenced code. See code following 80367.
80369	Skeletal muscle relaxants; 1 or 2	Resequenced code. See code following 80368.
80370	Skeletal muscle relaxants; 3 or more	Resequenced code. See code following 80369.
80371	Stimulants, synthetic	Resequenced code. See code following 80370.
80372	Tapentadol	Resequenced code. See code following 80371.
80373	Tramadol	Resequenced code. See code following 80372.

Code	Description	Reference
80374	Stereoisomer (enantiomer) analysis, single drug class	Resequenced code. See code following 80373.
80375	Drug(s) or substance(s), definitive, qualitative or quantitative, not otherwise specified; 1-3	Resequenced code. See code following 80374.
80376	Drug(s) or substance(s), definitive, qualitative or quantitative, not otherwise specified; 4-6	Resequenced code. See code following 80375.
80377	Drug(s) or substance(s), definitive, qualitative or quantitative, not otherwise specified; 7 or more	Resequenced code. See code following 80376.
81161	DMD (dystrophin) (eg, Duchenne/Becker muscular dystrophy) deletion analysis, and duplication analysis, if performed	Resequenced code. See code following 81229.
81287	MGMT (O-6-methylguanine-DNA methyltransferase) (eg, glioblastoma multiforme), methylation analysis	Resequenced code. See code following 81290.
81288	MLH1 (mutL homolog 1, colon cancer, nonpolyposis type 2) (eg, hereditary non-polyposis colorectal cancer, Lynch syndrome) gene analysis; promoter methylation analysis	Resequenced code. See code following 81292.
81479	Unlisted molecular pathology procedure	Resequenced code. See code following 81408.
82652	Vitamin D; 1, 25 dihydroxy, includes fraction(s), if performed	Resequenced code, See code following 82306.
83992	Phencyclidine (PCP)	Resequenced code. See code following 80365.
86152	Cell enumeration using immunologic selection and identification in fluid specimen (eg, circulating tumor cells in blood);	Resequenced code. See code following 86147.
86153	Cell enumeration using immunologic selection and identification in fluid specimen (eg, circulating tumor cells in blood); physician interpretation and report, when required	Resequenced code. See code before 86148.
87623	Infectious agent detection by nucleic acid (DNA or RNA); Human Papillomavirus (HPV), low-risk types (eg, 6, 11, 42, 43, 44)	Resequenced code. See code following 87539.
87624	Infectious agent detection by nucleic acid (DNA or RNA); Human Papillomavirus (HPV), high-risk types (eg, 16, 18, 31, 33, 35, 39, 45, 51, 52, 56, 58, 59, 68)	Resequenced code. See code following 87539.
87625	Infectious agent detection by nucleic acid (DNA or RNA); Human Papillomavirus (HPV), types 16 and 18 only, includes type 45, if performed	Resequenced code. See code before 87540.
87806	Infectious agent antigen detection by immunoassay with direct optical observation; HIV-1 antigen(s), with HIV-1 and HIV-2 antibodies	Resequenced code. See code following 87803.
87906	Infectious agent genotype analysis by nucleic acid (DNA or RNA); HIV-1, other region (eg, integrase, fusion)	Resequenced code. See code following 87901.
87910	Infectious agent genotype analysis by nucleic acid (DNA or RNA); cytomegalovirus	Resequenced code. See code following 87900.
87912	Infectious agent genotype analysis by nucleic acid (DNA or RNA); Hepatitis B virus	Resequenced code. See code before 87902.
88177	Cytopathology, evaluation of fine needle aspirate; immediate cytohistologic study to determine adequacy for diagnosis, each separate additional evaluation episode, same site (List separately in addition to code for primary procedure)	Resequenced code, See code following 88173.
88341	Immunohistochemistry or immunocytochemistry, per specimen; each additional single antibody stain procedure (List separately in addition to code for primary procedure)	Resequenced code. See code following 88342.
88364	In situ hybridization (eg, FISH), per specimen; each additional single probe stain procedure (List separately in addition to code for primary procedure)	Resequenced code. See code following 88365.
88373	Morphometric analysis, in situ hybridization (quantitative or semi-quantitative), using computer-assisted technology, per specimen; each additional single probe stain procedure (List separately in addition to code for primary procedure)	Resequenced code. See code following 88367.
88374	Morphometric analysis, in situ hybridization (quantitative or semi-quantitative), using computer-assisted technology, per specimen; each multiplex probe stain procedure	Resequenced code. See code following 88367.
88377	Morphometric analysis, in situ hybridization (quantitative or semi-quantitative), manual, per specimen; each multiplex probe stain procedure	Resequenced code. See code following 88369.
90630	Influenza virus vaccine, quadrivalent (IIV4), split virus, preservative free, for intradermal use	Resequenced code. See code following 90654.
90672	Influenza virus vaccine, quadrivalent, live, for intranasal use	Resequenced code. See code following 90660.
90673	Influenza virus vaccine, trivalent, derived from recombinant DNA (RIV3), hemagglutinin (HA) protein only, preservative and antibiotic free, for intramuscular use	Resequenced code. See code following 90661.
92558	Evoked otoacoustic emissions, screening (qualitative measurement of distortion product or transient evoked otoacoustic emissions), automated analysis	Resequenced code. See code following 92586.
92618	Evaluation for prescription of non-speech-generating augmentative and alternative communication device, face-to-face with the patient; each additional 30 minutes (List separately in addition to code for primary procedure)	Resequenced code. See code following 92605.
92920	Percutaneous transluminal coronary angioplasty; single major coronary artery or branch	Resequenced code. See code following 92998.
92921	Percutaneous transluminal coronary angioplasty; each additional branch of a major coronary artery (List separately in addition to code for primary procedure)	Resequenced code. See code following 92998.
92924	Percutaneous transluminal coronary atherectomy, with coronary angioplasty when performed; single major coronary artery or branch	Resequenced code. See code following 92998.
92925	Percutaneous transluminal coronary atherectomy, with coronary angioplasty when performed; each additional branch of a major coronary artery (List separately in addition to code for primary procedure)	Resequenced code. See code following 92998.
92928	Percutaneous transcatheter placement of intracoronary stent(s), with coronary angioplasty when performed; single major coronary artery or branch	Resequenced code. See code following 92998.

Code	Description	Reference
92929	Percutaneous transcatheter placement of intracoronary stent(s), with coronary angioplasty when performed; each additional branch of a major coronary artery (List separately in addition to code for primary procedure)	Resequenced code. See code following 92998.
92933	Percutaneous transluminal coronary atherectomy, with intracoronary stent, with coronary angioplasty when performed; single major coronary artery or branch	Resequenced code. See code following 92998.
92934	Percutaneous transluminal coronary atherectomy, with intracoronary stent, with coronary angioplasty when performed; each additional branch of a major coronary artery (List separately in addition to code for primary procedure)	Resequenced code. See code following 92998.
92937	Percutaneous transluminal revascularization of or through coronary artery bypass graft (internal mammary, free arterial, venous), any combination of intracoronary stent, atherectomy and angioplasty, including distal protection when performed; single vessel	Resequenced code. See code following 92998.
92938	Percutaneous transluminal revascularization of or through coronary artery bypass graft (internal mammary, free arterial, venous), any combination of intracoronary stent, atherectomy and angioplasty, including distal protection when performed; each additional branch subtended by the bypass graft (List separately in addition to code for primary procedure)	Resequenced code. See code following 92998.
92941	Percutaneous transluminal revascularization of acute total/subtotal occlusion during acute myocardial infarction, coronary artery or coronary artery bypass graft, any combination of intracoronary stent, atherectomy and angioplasty, including aspiration thrombectomy when performed, single vessel	Resequenced code. See code following 92998.
92943	Percutaneous transluminal revascularization of chronic total occlusion, coronary artery, coronary artery branch, or coronary artery bypass graft, any combination of intracoronary stent, atherectomy and angioplasty; single vessel	Resequenced code. See code following 92998.
92944	Percutaneous transluminal revascularization of chronic total occlusion, coronary artery, coronary artery branch, or coronary artery bypass graft, any combination of intracoronary stent, atherectomy and angioplasty; each additional coronary artery, coronary artery branch, or bypass graft (List separately in addition to code for primary procedure)	Resequenced code. See code following 92998.
92973	Percutaneous transluminal coronary thrombectomy mechanical (List separately in addition to code for primary procedure)	Resequenced code. See code following 92998.
92974	Transcatheter placement of radiation delivery device for subsequent coronary intravascular brachytherapy (List separately in addition to code for primary procedure)	Resequenced code. See code following 92998.
92975	Thrombolysis, coronary; by intracoronary infusion, including selective coronary angiography	Resequenced code. See code following 92998.
92977	Thrombolysis, coronary; by intravenous infusion	Resequenced code. See code following 92998.
92978	Intravascular ultrasound (coronary vessel or graft) during diagnostic evaluation and/or therapeutic intervention including imaging supervision, interpretation and report; initial vessel (List separately in addition to code for primary procedure)	Resequenced code. See code following 92998.
92979	Intravascular ultrasound (coronary vessel or graft) during diagnostic evaluation and/or therapeutic intervention including imaging supervision, interpretation and report; each additional vessel (List separately in addition to code for primary procedure)	Resequenced code. See code following 92998.
93260	Programming device evaluation (in person) with iterative adjustment of the implantable device to test the function of the device and select optimal permanent programmed values with analysis, review and report by a physician or other qualified health care professional; implantable subcutaneous lead defibrillator system	Resequenced code. See code following 93284.
93261	Interrogation device evaluation (in person) with analysis, review and report by a physician or other qualified health care professional, includes connection, recording and disconnection per patient encounter; implantable subcutaneous lead defibrillator system	Resequenced code. See code following 93289.
95782	Polysomnography; younger than 6 years, sleep staging with 4 or more additional parameters of sleep, attended by a technologist	Resequenced code. See code following 95811.
95783	Polysomnography; younger than 6 years, sleep staging with 4 or more additional parameters of sleep, with initiation of continuous positive airway pressure therapy or bi-level ventilation, attended by a technologist	Resequenced code. See code following 95811.
95800	Sleep study, unattended, simultaneous recording; heart rate, oxygen saturation, respiratory analysis (eg, by airflow or peripheral arterial tone), and sleep time	Resequenced code. See code following 95806.
95801	Sleep study, unattended, simultaneous recording; minimum of heart rate, oxygen saturation, and respiratory analysis (eg, by airflow or peripheral arterial tone)	Resequenced code. See code following 95806.
95885	Needle electromyography, each extremity, with related paraspinal areas, when performed, done with nerve conduction, amplitude and latency/velocity study; limited (List separately in addition to code for primary procedure)	Resequenced code. See code following 95872.
95886	Needle electromyography, each extremity, with related paraspinal areas, when performed, done with nerve conduction, amplitude and latency/velocity study; complete, five or more muscles studied, innervated by three or more nerves or four or more spinal levels (List separately in addition to code for primary procedure)	Resequenced code. See code following 95872.
95887	Needle electromyography, non-extremity (cranial nerve supplied or axial) muscle(s) done with nerve conduction, amplitude and latency/velocity study (List separately in addition to code for primary procedure)	Resequenced code. See code before 95873.
95938	Short-latency somatosensory evoked potential study, stimulation of any/all peripheral nerves or skin sites, recording from the central nervous system; in upper and lower limbs	Resequenced code. See code following 95926.

Code	Description	Reference
95939	Central motor evoked potential study (transcranial motor stimulation); in upper and lower limbs	Resequenced code. See code following 95929.
95940	Continuous intraoperative neurophysiology monitoring in the operating room, one on one monitoring requiring personal attendance, each 15 minutes (List separately in addition to code for primary procedure)	Resequenced code. See code following 95913.
95941	Continuous intraoperative neurophysiology monitoring, from outside the operating room (remote or nearby) or for monitoring of more than one case while in the operating room, per hour (List separately in addition to code for primary procedure)	Resequenced code. See code following 95913.
95943	Simultaneous, independent, quantitative measures of both parasympathetic function and sympathetic function, based on time-frequency analysis of heart rate variability concurrent with time-frequency analysis of continuous respiratory activity, with mean heart rate and blood pressure measures, during rest, paced (deep) breathing, Valsalva maneuvers, and head-up postural change	Resequenced code. See code following 95924.
0253T	Insertion of anterior segment aqueous drainage device, without extraocular reservoir, internal approach, into the suprachoroidal space	Resequenced code, See code following 0191T.
0357T	Cryopreservation; immature oocyte(s)	Resequenced code. See code following 0058T.
0376T	Insertion of anterior segment aqueous drainage device, without extraocular reservoir, internal approach, into the trabecular meshwork; each additional device insertion (List separately in addition to code for primary procedure)	Resequenced code. See code following 0191T.
99224	Subsequent observation care, per day, for the evaluation and management of a patient, which requires at least 2 of these 3 key components: Problem focused interval history; Problem focused examination; Medical decision making that is straightforward or of low complexity. Counseling and/or coordination of care with other physicians, other qualified health care professionals, or agencies are provided consistent with the nature of the problem(s) and the patient's and/or family's needs. Usually, the patient is stable, recovering, or improving. Typically, 15 minutes are spent at the bedside and on the patient's hospital floor or unit.	Resequenced code. See code following 99220.
99225	Subsequent observation care, per day, for the evaluation and management of a patient, which requires at least 2 of these 3 key components: An expanded problem focused interval history; An expanded problem focused examination; Medical decision making of moderate complexity. Counseling and/or coordination of care with other physicians, other qualified health care professionals, or agencies are provided consistent with the nature of the problem(s) and the patient's and/or family's needs. Usually, the patient is responding inadequately to therapy or has developed a minor complication. Typically, 25 minutes are spent at the bedside and on the patient's hospital floor or unit.	Resequenced code. See code following 99220.
99226	Subsequent observation care, per day, for the evaluation and management of a patient, which requires at least 2 of these 3 key components: A detailed interval history; A detailed examination; Medical decision making of high complexity. Counseling and/or coordination of care with other physicians, other qualified health care professionals, or agencies are provided consistent with the nature of the problem(s) and the patient's and/or family's needs. Usually, the patient is unstable or has developed a significant complication or a significant new problem. Typically, 35 minutes are spent at the bedside and on the patient's hospital floor or unit.	Resequenced code. See code before 99221.
99485	Supervision by a control physician of interfacility transport care of the critically ill or critically injured pediatric patient, 24 months of age or younger, includes two-way communication with transport team before transport, at the referring facility and during the transport, including data interpretation and report; first 30 minutes	Resequenced code. See code following 99467.
99486	Supervision by a control physician of interfacility transport care of the critically ill or critically injured pediatric patient, 24 months of age or younger, includes two-way communication with transport team before transport, at the referring facility and during the transport, including data interpretation and report; each additional 30 minutes (List separately in addition to code for primary procedure)	Resequenced code. See code following 99467.
99490	Chronic care management services, at least 20 minutes of clinical staff time directed by a physician or other qualified health care professional, per calendar month, with the following required elements: multiple (two or more) chronic conditions expected to last at least 12 months, or until the death of the patient; chronic conditions place the patient at significant risk of death, acute exacerbation/decompensation, or functional decline; comprehensive care plan established, implemented, revised, or monitored.	Resequenced code. See code before 99487.

Appendix E — Add-on Codes, Modifier 51 Exempt, Optum Modifier 51 Exempt, Modifier 63 Exempt, and Moderate Sedation Codes

Codes specified as add-on, exempt from modifier 51 and 63, and that include conscious sedation are listed. The lists are designed to be read left to right rather than vertically.

Add-on Codes

01953	01968	01969	11001	11008	11045	11046
11047	11101	11201	11732	11922	13102	13122
13133	13153	14302	15003	15005	15101	15111
15116	15121	15131	15136	15151	15152	15156
15157	15201	15221	15241	15261	15272	15274
15276	15278	15777	15787	15847	16036	17003
17312	17314	17315	19001	19082	19084	19086
19126	19282	19284	19286	19288	19297	20930
20931	20936	20937	20938	20985	22103	22116
22208	22216	22226	22328	22522	22525	22527
22534	22552	22585	22614	22632	22634	22840
22841	22842	22843	22844	22845	22846	22847
22848	22851	26125	26861	26863	27358	27692
29826	31620	31627	31632	31633	31637	31649
31651	32501	32506	32507	32667	32668	32674
33141	33225	33257	33258	33259	33367	33368
33369	33508	33517	33518	33519	33521	33522
33523	33530	33572	33768	33884	33924	34806
34808	34813	34826	35306	35390	35400	35500
35572	35600	35681	35682	35683	35685	35686
35697	35700	36148	36218	36227	36228	36248
36476	36479	37185	37186	37222	37223	37232
37233	37234	37235	37237	37239	37250	37251
38102	38746	38747	38900	43273	43283	43338
43635	44015	44121	44128	44139	44203	44213
44701	44955	47001	47550	48400	49326	49327
49412	49435	49568	49905	51797	56606	57267
58110	58611	59525	60512	61316	61517	61609
61610	61611	61612	61641	61642	61781	61782
61783	61797	61799	61800	61864	61868	62148
62160	63035	63043	63044	63048	63057	63066
63076	63078	63082	63086	63088	63091	63103
63295	63308	63621	64480	64484	64491	64492
64494	64495	64634	64636	64643	64645	64727
64778	64783	64787	64832	64837	64859	64872
64874	64876	64901	64902	65757	66990	67225
67320	67331	67332	67334	67335	67340	69990
74301	75565	75774	75946	75964	75968	76125
76802	76810	76812	76814	76937	77001	77051
77052	77293	78020	78496	78730	81266	82952
86826	87187	87503	87904	88155	88177	88185
88311	88314	88332	88334	88343	88388	90461
90472	90474	90785	90833	90836	90838	90840
90863	91013	92547	92608	92618	92621	92627
92921	92925	92929	92934	92938	92944	92973
92974	92978	92979	92998	93320	93321	93325
93352	93462	93463	93464	93563	93564	93565
93566	93567	93568	93571	93572	93609	93613
93621	93622	93623	93655	93657	93662	94645
94729	94781	95079	95873	95874	95885	95886
95887	95940	95941	95962	95967	95973	95975
95979	96361	96366	96367	96368	96370	96371
96375	96376	96411	96415	96417	96423	96570
96571	97546	97598	97811	97814	99100	99116
99135	99140	99145	99150	99292	99354	99355
99356	99357	99359	99467	99481	99482	99486
99489	99602	99607	0054T	0055T	0076T	0092T
0095T	0098T	0159T	0163T	0164T	0165T	0172T
0174T	0189T	0190T	0196T	0205T	0214T	0215T
0217T	0218T	0222T	0229T	0231T	0241T	0289T
0290T	0291T	0292T	0294T	0300T	0309T	

AMA Modifer 51 Exempt Codes

17004	20697	20974	20975	31500	33961	36620
44500	61107	93451	93456	93503	93600	93602
93603	93610	93612	93615	93616	93618	93631
94610	95905	95992	99143	99144		

Modifier 63 Exempt Codes

30540	30545	31520	33401	33403	33470	33472
33502	33503	33505	33506	33610	33611	33619
33647	33670	33690	33694	33730	33732	33735
33736	33750	33755	33762	33778	33786	33922
33960	33961	36415	36420	36450	36460	36510
36660	39503	43313	43314	43520	43831	44055
44126	44127	44128	46070	46705	46715	46716
46730	46735	46740	46742	46744	47700	47701
49215	49491	49492	49495	49496	49600	49605
49606	49610	49611	53025	54000	54150	54160
63700	63702	63704	63706	65820		

Moderate Sedation Codes

0200T	0201T	0282T	0283T	0284T	0291T	0292T
0293T	0294T	0301T	0302T	0303T	0304T	0307T
0308T	0335T	10030	19298	20982	22520	22521
22522	22526	22527	31615	31620	31622	31623
31624	31625	31626	31627	31628	31629	31634
31635	31645	31646	31647	31648	31649	31651
31660	31661	31725	32405	32550	32551	32553
33010	33011	33206	33207	33208	33210	33211
33212	33213	33214	33216	33217	33218	33220
33221	33222	33223	33227	33228	33229	33230
33231	33233	33234	33235	33240	33241	33244
33249	33262	33263	33264	33282	33284	33990
33991	33992	33993	35471	35472	35475	35476
36010	36140	36147	36148	36200	36221	36222
36223	36224	36225	36226	36227	36228	36245
36246	36247	36248	36251	36252	36253	36254
36481	36555	36557	36558	36560	36561	36563
36565	36566	36568	36570	36571	36576	36578
36581	36582	36583	36585	36590	36870	37183
37184	37185	37186	37187	37188	37191	37192
37193	37197	37211	37212	37213	37214	37215
37216	37220	37221	37222	37223	37224	37225
37226	37227	37228	37229	37230	37231	37232
37233	37234	37235	37236	37237	37238	37239
37241	37242	37243	37244	43200	43201	43202
43204	43205	43206	43211	43212	43213	43214
43215	43216	43217	43220	43226	43227	43229
43231	43232	43233	43235	43236	43237	43238
43239	43240	43241	43242	43243	43244	43245
43246	43247	43248	43249	43250	43251	43252
43253	43254	43255	43257	43259	43260	43261
43262	43263	43264	43265	43266	43270	43273
43274	43275	43276	43277	43278	43450	43453
44360	44361	44363	44364	44365	44366	44369
44370	44372	44373	44376	44377	44378	44379
44380	44382	44383	44385	44386	44388	44389
44390	44391	44392	44393	44394	44397	44500
45303	45305	45307	45308	45309	45315	45317
45320	45321	45327	45332	45333	45334	45335
45337	45338	45339	45340	45341	45342	45345
45355	45378	45379	45380	45381	45382	45383
45384	45385	45386	45387	45391	45392	47000
47382	47525	49405	49406	49407	49411	49418
49440	49441	49442	49446	50200	50382	50384

50385 50386 50387 50592 50593 57155 66720
69300 77371 77600 77605 77610 77615 92920
92921 92924 92925 92928 92929 92933 92934
92937 92938 92941 92943 92944 92953 92960
92961 92973 92974 92975 92978 92979 92986
92987 93312 93313 93314 93315 93316 93317
93318 93451 93452 93453 93454 93455 93456
93457 93458 93459 93460 93461 93462 93463
93464 93505 93530 93561 93562 93563 93564
93565 93566 93567 93568 93571 93572 93582
93583 93609 93613 93615 93616 93618 93619
93620 93621 93622 93624 93640 93641 93642
93650 93653 93654 93655 93656 93657 94011
94012 94013

Optum Modifier 51 Exempt Codes

90281 90283 90284 90287 90288 90291 90296
90371 90375 90376 90378 90384 90385 90386
90389 90393 90396 90399 90476 90477 90581
90585 90586 90632 90633 90634 90636 90644
90645 90646 90647 90648 90649 90650 90653
90654 90655 90656 90657 90658 90660 90661
90662 90664 90666 90667 90668 90669 90670
90672 90673 90675 90676 90680 90681 90685
90686 90687 90688 90690 90691 90692 90693
90696 90698 90700 90702 90703 90704 90705
90706 90707 90708 90710 90712 90713 90714
90715 90716 90717 90719 90720 90721 90723
90725 90727 90732 90733 90734 90735 90736
90738 90739 90740 90743 90744 90746 90747
90748 90749 97001 97002 97003 97004 97005
97006 97010 97012 97014 97016 97018 97022
97024 97026 97028 97032 97033 97034 97035
97036 97110 97112 97113 97116 97124 97140
97150 97530 97532 97533 97535 97537 97542
97545 97546 97597 97598 97602 97605 97606
97610 97750 97755 99050 99051 99053 99056
99058 99060

Appendix E—Add-on, Modifier 51, Modifier 63, and Moderate Sedation Codes

Appendix F — Place of Service and Type of Service

Place-of-Service Codes for Professional Claims

Listed below are place of service codes and descriptions. These codes should be used on professional claims to specify the entity where service(s) were rendered. Check with individual payers (e.g., Medicare, Medicaid, other private insurance) for reimbursement policies regarding these codes. To comment on a code(s) or description(s), please send your request to posinfo@cms.gov.

01	Pharmacy	A facility or location where drugs and other medically related items and services are sold, dispensed, or otherwise provided directly to patients.
02	Unassigned	N/A
03	School	A facility whose primary purpose is education.
04	Homeless shelter	A facility or location whose primary purpose is to provide temporary housing to homeless individuals (e.g., emergency shelters, individual or family shelters).
05	Indian Health Service freestanding facility	A facility or location, owned and operated by the Indian Health Service, which provides diagnostic, therapeutic (surgical and non-surgical), and rehabilitation services to American Indians and Alaska natives who do not require hospitalization.
06	Indian Health Service provider-based facility	A facility or location, owned and operated by the Indian Health Service, which provides diagnostic, therapeutic (surgical and nonsurgical), and rehabilitation services rendered by, or under the supervision of, physicians to American Indians and Alaska natives admitted as inpatients or outpatients.
07	Tribal 638 freestanding facility	A facility or location owned and operated by a federally recognized American Indian or Alaska native tribe or tribal organization under a 638 agreement, which provides diagnostic, therapeutic (surgical and nonsurgical), and rehabilitation services to tribal members who do not require hospitalization.
08	Tribal 638 Provider-based Facility	A facility or location owned and operated by a federally recognized American Indian or Alaska native tribe or tribal organization under a 638 agreement, which provides diagnostic, therapeutic (surgical and nonsurgical), and rehabilitation services to tribal members admitted as inpatients or outpatients.
09	Prison/correctional facility	A prison, jail, reformatory, work farm, detention center, or any other similar facility maintained by either federal, state or local authorities for the purpose of confinement or rehabilitation of adult or juvenile criminal offenders.
10	Unassigned	N/A
11	Office	Location, other than a hospital, skilled nursing facility (SNF), military treatment facility, community health center, State or local public health clinic, or intermediate care facility (ICF), where the health professional routinely provides health examinations, diagnosis, and treatment of illness or injury on an ambulatory basis.
12	Home	Location, other than a hospital or other facility, where the patient receives care in a private residence.
13	Assisted living facility	Congregate residential facility with self-contained living units providing assessment of each resident's needs and on-site support 24 hours a day, 7 days a week, with the capacity to deliver or arrange for services including some health care and other services.
14	Group home	A residence, with shared living areas, where clients receive supervision and other services such as social and/or behavioral services, custodial service, and minimal services (e.g., medication administration).
15	Mobile unit	A facility/unit that moves from place-to-place equipped to provide preventive, screening, diagnostic, and/or treatment services.
16	Temporary lodging	A short-term accommodation such as a hotel, campground, hostel, cruise ship or resort where the patient receives care, and which is not identified by any other POS code.
17	Walk-in retail health clinic	A walk-in health clinic, other than an office, urgent care facility, pharmacy, or independent clinic and not described by any other place of service code, that is located within a retail operation and provides preventive and primary care services on an ambulatory basis.
18	Place of employment/ worksite	A location, not described by any other POS code, owned or operated by a public or private entity where the patient is employed, and where a health professional provides on-going or episodic occupational medical, therapeutic or rehabilitative services to the individual.
19	Unassigned	N/A
20	Urgent care facility	Location, distinct from a hospital emergency room, an office, or a clinic, whose purpose is to diagnose and treat illness or injury for unscheduled, ambulatory patients seeking immediate medical attention.
21	Inpatient hospital	A facility, other than psychiatric, which primarily provides diagnostic, therapeutic (both surgical and nonsurgical), and rehabilitation services by, or under, the supervision of physicians to patients admitted for a variety of medical conditions.

22	Outpatient hospital	A portion of a hospital which provides diagnostic, therapeutic (both surgical and nonsurgical), and rehabilitation services to sick or injured persons who do not require hospitalization or institutionalization.
23	Emergency room—hospital	A portion of a hospital where emergency diagnosis and treatment of illness or injury is provided.
24	Ambulatory surgical center	A freestanding facility, other than a physician's office, where surgical and diagnostic services are provided on an ambulatory basis.
25	Birthing center	A facility, other than a hospital's maternity facilities or a physician's office, which provides a setting for labor, delivery, and immediate post-partum care as well as immediate care of new born infants.
26	Military treatment facility	A medical facility operated by one or more of the uniformed services. Military treatment facility (MTF) also refers to certain former U.S. Public Health Service (USPHS) facilities now designated as uniformed service treatment facilities (USTF).
27-30	Unassigned	N/A
31	Skilled nursing facility	A facility which primarily provides inpatient skilled nursing care and related services to patients who require medical, nursing, or rehabilitative services but does not provide the level of care or treatment available in a hospital.
32	Nursing facility	A facility which primarily provides to residents skilled nursing care and related services for the rehabilitation of injured, disabled, or sick persons, or, on a regular basis, health-related care services above the level of custodial care to other than mentally retarded individuals.
33	Custodial care facility	A facility which provides room, board, and other personal assistance services, generally on a long-term basis, and which does not include a medical component.
34	Hospice	A facility, other than a patient's home, in which palliative and supportive care for terminally ill patients and their families are provided.
35-40	Unassigned	N/A
41	Ambulance—land	A land vehicle specifically designed, equipped and staffed for lifesaving and transporting the sick or injured.
42	Ambulance—air or water	An air or water vehicle specifically designed, equipped and staffed for lifesaving and transporting the sick or injured.
43-48	Unassigned	N/A
49	Independent clinic	A location, not part of a hospital and not described by any other place-of-service code, that is organized and operated to provide preventive, diagnostic, therapeutic, rehabilitative, or palliative services to outpatients only.
50	Federally qualified health center	A facility located in a medically underserved area that provides Medicare beneficiaries preventive primary medical care under the general direction of a physician.
51	Inpatient psychiatric facility	A facility that provides inpatient psychiatric services for the diagnosis and treatment of mental illness on a 24-hour basis, by or under the supervision of a physician.
52	Psychiatric facility-partial hospitalization	A facility for the diagnosis and treatment of mental illness that provides a planned therapeutic program for patients who do not require full time hospitalization, but who need broader programs than are possible from outpatient visits to a hospital-based or hospital-affiliated facility.
53	Community mental health center	A facility that provides the following services: outpatient services, including specialized outpatient services for children, the elderly, individuals who are chronically ill, and residents of the CMHC's mental health services area who have been discharged from inpatient treatment at a mental health facility; 24 hour a day emergency care services; day treatment, other partial hospitalization services, or psychosocial rehabilitation services; screening for patients being considered for admission to state mental health facilities to determine the appropriateness of such admission; and consultation and education services.
54	Intermediate care facility/mentally retarded	A facility which primarily provides health-related care and services above the level of custodial care to mentally retarded individuals but does not provide the level of care or treatment available in a hospital or SNF.
55	Residential substance abuse treatment facility	A facility which provides treatment for substance (alcohol and drug) abuse to live-in residents who do not require acute medical care. Services include individual and group therapy and counseling, family counseling, laboratory tests, drugs and supplies, psychological testing, and room and board.
56	Psychiatric residential treatment center	A facility or distinct part of a facility for psychiatric care which provides a total 24-hour therapeutically planned and professionally staffed group living and learning environment.
57	Non-residential substance abuse treatment facility	A location which provides treatment for substance (alcohol and drug) abuse on an ambulatory basis. Services include individual and group therapy and counseling, family counseling, laboratory tests, drugs and supplies, and psychological testing.
58-59	Unassigned	N/A
60	Mass immunization center	A location where providers administer pneumococcal pneumonia and influenza virus vaccinations and submit these services as electronic media claims, paper claims, or using the roster billing method. This generally takes place in a mass immunization setting, such as, a public health center, pharmacy, or mall but may include a physician office setting.

61	Comprehensive inpatient rehabilitation facility	A facility that provides comprehensive rehabilitation services under the supervision of a physician to inpatients with physical disabilities. Services include physical therapy, occupational therapy, speech pathology, social or psychological services, and orthotics and prosthetics services.
62	Comprehensive outpatient rehabilitation facility	A facility that provides comprehensive rehabilitation services under the supervision of a physician to outpatients with physical disabilities. Services include physical therapy, occupational therapy, and speech pathology services.
63-64	Unassigned	N/A
65	End-stage renal disease treatment facility	A facility other than a hospital, which provides dialysis treatment, maintenance, and/or training to patients or caregivers on an ambulatory or home-care basis.
66-70	Unassigned	N/A
71	State or local public health clinic	A facility maintained by either state or local health departments that provides ambulatory primary medical care under the general direction of a physician.
72	Rural health clinic	A certified facility which is located in a rural medically underserved area that provides ambulatory primary medical care under the general direction of a physician.
73-80	Unassigned	N/A
81	Independent laboratory	A laboratory certified to perform diagnostic and/or clinical tests independent of an institution or a physician's office.
82-98	Unassigned	N/A
99	Other place of service	Other place of service not identified above.

Type of Service

Common Working File Type of Service (TOS) Indicators

For submitting a claim to the Common Working File (CWF), use the following table to assign the proper TOS. Some procedures may have more than one applicable TOS. CWF will reject alerts on codes with incorrect TOS designations. CWF will produce alerts on codes with incorrect TOS designations.

The only exceptions to this annual update are:

- Surgical services billed for dates of service through December 31, 2007, containing the ASC facility service modifier SG must be reported as TOS F. Effective for services on or after January 1, 2008, the SG modifier is no longer applicable for Medicare services. ASC providers should discontinue applying the SG modifier on ASC facility claims. The indicator F does not appear in the TOS table because its use depends upon claims submitted with POS 24 (ASC facility) from an ASC (specialty 49). This became effective for dates of service January 1, 2008, or after.
- Surgical services billed with an assistant-at-surgery modifier (80-82, AS,) must be reported with TOS 8. The 8 indicator does not appear on the TOS table because its use is dependent upon the use of the appropriate modifier. (See Pub. 100-4 *Medicare Claims Processing Manual,* chapter 12, "Physician/Practitioner Billing," for instructions on when assistant-at-surgery is allowable.)
- Psychiatric treatment services that are subject to the outpatient mental health treatment limitation should be reported with TOS T.
- TOS H appears in the list of descriptors. However, it does not appear in the table. In CWF, "H" is used only as an indicator for hospice. The contractor should not submit TOS H to CWF at this time.
- For outpatient services, when a transfusion medicine code appears on a claim that also contains a blood product, the service is paid under reasonable charge at 80 percent; coinsurance and deductible apply. When transfusion medicine codes are paid under the clinical laboratory fee schedule they are paid at 100 percent; coinsurance and deductible do not apply.

Note: For injection codes with more than one possible TOS designation, use the following guidelines when assigning the TOS:

When the choice is L or 1:

- Use TOS L when the drug is used related to ESRD; or
- Use TOS 1 when the drug is not related to ESRD and is administered in the office.

When the choice is G or 1:

- Use TOS G when the drug is an immunosuppressive drug; or
- Use TOS 1 when the drug is used for other than immunosuppression.

When the choice is P or 1:

- Use TOS P if the drug is administered through durable medical equipment (DME); or
- Use TOS 1 if the drug is administered in the office.

The place of service or diagnosis may be considered when determining the appropriate TOS. The descriptors for each of the TOS codes listed in the annual HCPCS update are:

0	Whole blood
1	Medical care
2	Surgery
3	Consultation
4	Diagnostic radiology
5	Diagnostic laboratory
6	Therapeutic radiology
7	Anesthesia
8	Assistant at surgery
9	Other medical items or services
A	Used DME
B	High risk screening mammography
C	Low risk screening mammography
D	Ambulance
E	Enteral/parenteral nutrients/supplies
F	Ambulatory surgical center (facility usage for surgical services)
G	Immunosuppressive drugs
H	Hospice
J	Diabetic shoes
K	Hearing items and services
L	ESRD supplies
M	Monthly capitation payment for dialysis
N	Kidney donor
P	Lump sum purchase of DME, prosthetics, orthotics
Q	Vision items or services
R	Rental of DME
S	Surgical dressings or other medical supplies
T	Outpatient mental health treatment limitation
U	Occupational therapy
V	Pneumococcal/flu vaccine
W	Physical therapy

Berenson-Eggers Type of Service (BETOS) Codes

The BETOS coding system was developed primarily for analyzing the growth in Medicare expenditures. The coding system covers all HCPCS codes; assigns a HCPCS code to only one BETOS code; consists of readily understood clinical categories (as opposed to statistical or financial categories); consists of categories that permit objective assignment; is stable over time; and is relatively immune to minor changes in technology or practice patterns.

BETOS Codes and Descriptions:

1. **Evaluation and Management**
   1. M1A Office visits—new
   2. M1B Office visits—established
   3. M2A Hospital visit—initial
   4. M2B Hospital visit—subsequent
   5. M2C Hospital visit—critical care
   6. M3 Emergency room visit
   7. M4A Home visit
   8. M4B Nursing home visit
   9. M5A Specialist—pathology
   10. M5B Specialist—psychiatry
   11. M5C Specialist—ophthalmology
   12. M5D Specialist—other
   13. M6 Consultations
2. **Procedures**
   1. P0 Anesthesia
   2. P1A Major procedure—breast
   3. P1B Major procedure—colectomy
   4. P1C Major procedure—cholecystectomy
   5. P1D Major procedure—TURP
   6. P1E Major procedure—hysterectomy
   7. P1F Major procedure—explor/decompr/excis disc
   8. P1G Major procedure—other
   9. P2A Major procedure, cardiovascular—CABG
   10. P2B Major procedure, cardiovascular—aneurysm repair
   11. P2C Major procedure, cardiovascular—thromboendarterectomy
   12. P2D Major procedure, cardiovascular—coronary angioplasty (PTCA)
   13. P2E Major procedure, cardiovascular—pacemaker insertion
   14. P2F Major procedure, cardiovascular—other
   15. P3A Major procedure, orthopedic—hip fracture repair
   16. P3B Major procedure, orthopedic—hip replacement
   17. P3C Major procedure, orthopedic—knee replacement
   18. P3D Major procedure, orthopedic—other
   19. P4A Eye procedure—corneal transplant
   20. P4B Eye procedure—cataract removal/lens insertion
   21. P4C Eye procedure—retinal detachment
   22. P4D Eye procedure—treatment of retinal lesions
   23. P4E Eye procedure—other
   24. P5A Ambulatory procedures—skin
   25. P5B Ambulatory procedures—musculoskeletal
   26. P5C Ambulatory procedures—groin hernia repair
   27. P5D Ambulatory procedures—lithotripsy
   28. P5E Ambulatory procedures—other
   29. P6A Minor procedures—skin
   30. P6B Minor procedures—musculoskeletal
   31. P6C Minor procedures—other (Medicare fee schedule)
   32. P6D Minor procedures—other (non-Medicare fee schedule)
   33. P7A Oncology—radiation therapy
   34. P7B Oncology—other
   35. P8A Endoscopy—arthroscopy
   36. P8B Endoscopy—upper gastrointestinal
   37. P8C Endoscopy—sigmoidoscopy
   38. P8D Endoscopy—colonoscopy
   39. P8E Endoscopy—cystoscopy
   40. P8F Endoscopy—bronchoscopy
   41. P8G Endoscopy—laparoscopic cholecystectomy
   42. P8H Endoscopy—laryngoscopy
   43. P8I Endoscopy—other
   44. P9A Dialysis services (Medicare fee schedule)
   45. P9B Dialysis services (non-Medicare fee schedule)
3. **Imaging**
   1. I1A Standard imaging—chest
   2. I1B Standard imaging—musculoskeletal
   3. I1C Standard imaging—breast
   4. I1D Standard imaging—contrast gastrointestinal
   5. I1E Standard imaging—nuclear medicine
   6. I1F Standard imaging—other
   7. I2A Advanced imaging—CAT/CT/CTA; brain/head/neck
   8. I2B Advanced imaging—CAT/CT/CTA; other
   9. I2C Advanced imaging—MRI/MRA; brain/head/neck
   10. I2D Advanced imaging—MRI/MRA; other
   11. I3A Echography/ultrasoundography—eye
   12. I3B Echography/ultrasoundography—abdomen/pelvis
   13. I3C Echography/ultrasoundography—heart
   14. I3D Echography/ultrasoundography—carotid arteries
   15. I3E Echography/ultrasoundography—prostate, transrectal
   16. I3F Echography/ultrasoundography—other
   17. I4A Imaging/procedure—heart, including cardiac catheterization
   18. I4B Imaging/procedure—other
4. **Tests**
   1. T1A Lab tests—routine venipuncture (non-Medicare fee schedule)
   2. T1B Lab tests—automated general profiles
   3. T1C Lab tests—urinalysis
   4. T1D Lab tests—blood counts
   5. T1E Lab tests—glucose
   6. T1F Lab tests—bacterial cultures
   7. T1G Lab tests—other (Medicare fee schedule)
   8. T1H Lab tests—other (non-Medicare fee schedule)
   9. T2A Other tests—electrocardiograms
   10. T2B Other tests—cardiovascular stress tests
   11. T2C Other tests—EKG monitoring
   12. T2D Other tests—other
5. **Durable Medical Equipment**
   1. D1A Medical/surgical supplies
   2. D1B Hospital beds
   3. D1C Oxygen and supplies
   4. D1D Wheelchairs
   5. D1E Other DME
   6. D1F Prosthetic/orthotic devices
   7. D1G Drugs administered through DME
6. **Other**
   1. O1A Ambulance
   2. O1B Chiropractic
   3. O1C Enteral and parenteral
   4. O1D Chemotherapy
   5. O1E Other drugs
   6. O1F Hearing and speech services
   7. O1G Immunizations/vaccinations
7. **Exceptions/Unclassified**
   1. Y1 Other—Medicare fee schedule
   2. Y2 Other—Non-Medicare fee schedule
   3. Z1 Local codes
   4. Z2 Undefined codes

Appendix G — Pub 100 References

The Centers for Medicare and Medicaid Services restructured its paper-based manual system as a web-based system on October 1, 2003. Called the online CMS manual system, it combines all of the various program instructions into internet-only manuals (IOMs), which are used by all CMS programs and contractors. In many instances, the references from the online manuals in appendix E contain a mention of the old paper manuals from which the current information was obtained when the manuals were converted. This information is shown in the header of the text, in the following format, when applicable, as A3-3101, HO-210, and B3-2049. Complete versions of all of the manuals can be found at http://www.cms.gov/manuals.

Effective with implementation of the IOMs, the former method of publishing program memoranda (PMs) to communicate program instructions was replaced by the following four templates:

- One-time notification
- Manual revisions
- Business requirements
- Confidential requirements

The web-based system has been organized by functional area (e.g., eligibility, entitlement, claims processing, benefit policy, program integrity) in an effort to eliminate redundancy within the manuals, simplify updating, and make CMS program instructions available more quickly. The web-based system contains the functional areas included below:

Pub. 100	Introduction
Pub. 100-1	Medicare General Information, Eligibility, and Entitlement Manual
Pub. 100-2	Medicare Benefit Policy Manual
Pub. 100-3	Medicare National Coverage Determinations (NCD) Manual
Pub. 100-4	Medicare Claims Processing Manual
Pub. 100-5	Medicare Secondary Payer Manual
Pub. 100-6	Medicare Financial Management Manual
Pub. 100-7	State Operations Manual
Pub. 100-8	Medicare Program Integrity Manual
Pub. 100-9	Medicare Contractor Beneficiary and Provider Communications Manual
Pub. 100-10	Quality Improvement Organization Manual
Pub. 100-11	Programs of All-Inclusive Care for the Elderly (PACE) Manual
Pub. 100-12	State Medicaid Manual (under development)
Pub. 100-13	Medicaid State Children's Health Insurance Program (under development)
Pub. 100-14	Medicare ESRD Network Organizations Manual
Pub. 100-15	Medicaid Integrity Program (MIP)
Pub. 100-16	Medicare Managed Care Manual
Pub. 100-17	CMS/Business Partners Systems Security Manual
Pub. 100-18	Medicare Prescription Drug Benefit Manual
Pub. 100-19	Demonstrations
Pub. 100-20	One-Time Notification
Pub. 100-21	Recurring Update Notification
Pub. 100-22	Medicare Quality Reporting Incentive Programs Manual
Pub. 100-24	State Buy-In Manual
Pub. 100-25	Information Security Acceptable Risk Safeguards Manual

A brief description of the Medicare manuals primarily used for *CPC Expert* follows:

The ***National Coverage Determinations Manual*** (NCD), is organized according to categories such as diagnostic services, supplies, and medical procedures. The table of contents lists each category and subject within that category. Revision transmittals identify any new or background material, recap the changes, and provide an effective date for the change.

When complete, the manual will contain two chapters. Chapter 1 currently includes a description of CMS's national coverage determinations. When available, chapter 2 will contain a list of HCPCS codes related to each coverage determination. The manual is organized in accordance with CPT category sequences.

The ***Medicare Benefit Policy Manual*** contains Medicare general coverage instructions that are not national coverage determinations. As a general rule, in the past these instructions have been found in chapter II of the ***Medicare Carriers Manual,*** the ***Medicare Intermediary Manual***, other provider manuals, and program memoranda.

The ***Medicare Claims Processing Manual*** contains instructions for processing claims for contractors and providers.

The ***Medicare Program Integrity Manual*** communicates the priorities and standards for the Medicare integrity programs.

Medicare IOM references

100-1, 3, 20.5

Blood Deductibles (Part A and Part B)

Program payment may not be made for the first 3 pints of whole blood or equivalent units of packed red cells received under Part A and Part B combined in a calendar year. However, blood processing (e.g., administration, storage) is not subject to the deductible.

The blood deductibles are in addition to any other applicable deductible and coinsurance amounts for which the patient is responsible.

The deductible applies only to the first 3 pints of blood furnished in a calendar year, even if more than one provider furnished blood.

100-1, 3, 20.5.2

Part B Blood Deductible

Blood is furnished on an outpatient basis or is subject to the Part B blood deductible and is counted toward the combined limit. It should be noted that payment for blood may be made to the hospital under Part B only for blood furnished in an outpatient setting. Blood is not covered for inpatient Part B services.

100-1, 3, 20.5.3

Items Subject to Blood Deductibles

The blood deductibles apply only to whole blood and packed red cells. The term whole blood means human blood from which none of the liquid or cellular components have been removed. Where packed red cells are furnished, a unit of packed red cells is considered equivalent to a pint of whole blood. Other components of blood such as platelets, fibrinogen, plasma, gamma globulin, and serum albumin are not subject to the blood deductible. However, these components of blood are covered as biologicals.

Refer to Pub. 100-04, Medicare Claims Processing Manual, chapter 4, Sec.231 regarding billing for blood and blood products under the Hospital Outpatient Prospective Payment System (OPPS).

100-1, 3, 30

Outpatient Mental Health Treatment Limitation

Regardless of the actual expenses a beneficiary incurs in connection with the treatment of mental, psychoneurotic, and personality disorders while the beneficiary is not an inpatient of a hospital at the time such expenses are incurred, the amount of those expenses that may be recognized for Part B deductible and payment purposes is limited to 62.5 percent of the Medicare approved amount for those services. The limitation is called the outpatient mental health treatment limitation (the limitation). The 62.5 percent limitation has been in place since the inception of the Medicare Part B program and it will remain effective at this percentage amount until January 1, 2010. However, effective January 1, 2010, through January 1, 2014, the limitation will be phased out as follows:

- January 1, 2010—December 31, 2011, the limitation percentage is 68.75%. (Medicare pays 55% and the patient pays 45%).
- January 1, 2012—December 31, 2012, the limitation percentage is 75%. (Medicare pays 60% and the patient pays 40%).

- January 1, 2013—December 31, 2013, the limitation percentage is 81.25%. (Medicare pays 65% and the patient pays 35%).
- January 1, 2014—onward, the limitation percentage is 100%. (Medicare pays 80% and the patient pays 20%).

For additional details concerning the outpatient mental health treatment limitation, please see the Medicare Claims Processing Manual, Publication 100-04, chapter 9, section 60 and chapter 12, section 210.

100-1, 5, 70

Physician Defined

Physician means doctor of medicine, doctor of osteopathy (including osteopathic practitioner), doctor of dental surgery or dental medicine (within the limitations in subsection Sec.70.2), doctor of podiatric medicine (within the limitations in subsection Sec.70.3), or doctor of optometry (within the limitations of subsection Sec.70.5), and, with respect to certain specified treatment, a doctor of chiropractic legally authorized to practice by a State in which he/she performs this function. The services performed by a physician within these definitions are subject to any limitations imposed by the State on the scope of practice. The issuance by a State of a license to practice medicine constitutes legal authorization. Temporary State licenses also constitute legal authorization to practice medicine. If State law authorizes local political subdivisions to establish higher standards for medical practitioners than those set by the State licensing board, the local standards determine whether a particular physician has legal authorization. If State licensing law limits the scope of practice of a particular type of medical practitioner, only the services within the limitations are covered. The issuance by a State of a license to practice medicine constitutes legal authorization. Temporary State licenses also constitute legal authorization to practice medicine. If State law authorizes local political subdivisions to establish higher standards for medical practitioners than those set by the State licensing board, the local standards determine whether a particular physician has legal authorization. If State licensing law limits the scope of practice of a particular type of medical practitioner, only the services within the limitations are covered. **NOTE:** The term physician does not include such practitioners as a Christian Science practitioner or naturopath.

100-1, 5, 70.6

Chiropractors

A. General

A licensed chiropractor who meets uniform minimum standards (see subsection C) is a physician for specified services. Coverage extends only to treatment by means of manual manipulation of the spine to correct a subluxation demonstrated by X-ray, provided such treatment is legal in the State where performed. All other services furnished or ordered by chiropractors are not covered. An X-ray obtained by a chiropractor for his or her own diagnostic purposes before commencing treatment may suffice for claims documentation purposes. This means that if a chiropractor orders, takes, or interprets an X-ray to demonstrate a subluxation of the spine, the X-ray can be used for claims processing purposes. However, there is no coverage or payment for these services or for any other diagnostic or therapeutic service ordered or furnished by the chiropractor. In addition, in performing manual manipulation of the spine, some chiropractors use manual devices that are hand-held with the thrust of the force of the device being controlled manually. While such manual manipulation may be covered, there is no separate payment permitted for use of this device.

B. Licensure and Authorization to Practice

A chiropractor must be licensed or legally authorized to furnish chiropractic services by the State or jurisdiction in which the services are furnished.

C. Uniform Minimum Standards

1. Prior to July 1, 1974, Chiropractors licensed or authorized to practice prior to July 1, 1974, and those individuals who commenced their studies in a chiropractic college before that date must meet all of the following minimum standards to render payable services under the program:
   a. Preliminary education equal to the requirements for graduation from an accredited high school or other secondary school;
   b. Graduation from a college of chiropractic approved by the State's chiropractic examiners that included the completion of a course of study covering a period of not less than 3 school years of 6 months each year in actual continuous attendance covering adequate course of study in the subjects of anatomy, physiology, symptomatology and diagnosis, hygiene and sanitation, chemistry, histology, pathology, and principles and practice of chiropractic, including clinical instruction in vertebral palpation, nerve tracing and adjusting; and
   c. Passage of an examination prescribed by the State's chiropractic examiners covering the subjects listed in subsection b.
2. After June 30, 1974 - Individuals commencing their studies in a chiropractic college after June 30, 1974, must meet all of the following additional requirements:
   a. Satisfactory completion of 2 years of pre-chiropractic study at the college level;
   b. Satisfactory completion of a 4-year course of 8 months each year (instead of a 3-year course of 6 months each year) at a college or school of chiropractic that includes not less than 4,000 hours in the scientific and chiropractic courses specified in subsection 1.b, plus courses in the use and effect of X-ray and chiropractic analysis; and
   c. The practitioner must be over 21 years of age.

100-1, 5, 90.2

Laboratory Defined

Laboratory means a facility for the biological, microbiological, serological, chemical, immuno-hematological, hematological, biophysical, cytological, pathological, or other examination of materials derived from the human body for the purpose of providing information for the diagnosis, prevention, or treatment of any disease or impairment of, or the assessment of the health of, human beings. These examinations also include procedures to determine, measure, or otherwise describe the presence or absence of various substances or organisms in the body. Facilities only collecting or preparing specimens (or both) or only serving as a mailing service and not performing testing are not considered laboratories.

100-2, 1, 10

Covered Inpatient Hospital Services Covered Under Part A

A3-3101, HO-210

Patients covered under hospital insurance are entitled to have payment made on their behalf for inpatient hospital services. (Inpatient hospital services do not include extended care services provided by hospitals pursuant to swing bed approvals. See Pub. 100-1, Chapter 8, Sec.10.1, "Hospital Providers of Extended Care Services."). However, both inpatient hospital and inpatient SNF benefits are provided under Part A - Hospital Insurance Benefits for the Aged and Disabled, of Title XVIII).

Additional information concerning the following topics can be found in the following manual chapters:

- Benefit periods is found in Chapter 3, "Duration of Covered Inpatient Services";
- Copayment days is found in Chapter 2, "Duration of Covered Inpatient Services";
- Lifetime reserve days is found in Chapter 5, "Lifetime Reserve Days";
- Related payment information is housed in the Provider Reimbursement Manual.

Blood must be furnished on a day which counts as a day of inpatient hospital services to be covered as a Part A service and to count toward the blood deductible. Thus, blood is not covered under Part A and does not count toward the Part A blood deductible when furnished to an inpatient after the inpatient has exhausted all benefit days in a benefit period, or where the individual has elected not to use lifetime reserve days. However, where the patient is discharged on their first day of entitlement or on the hospital's first day of participation, the hospital is permitted to submit a billing form with no accommodation charge, but with ancillary charges including blood.

The records for all Medicare hospital inpatient discharges are maintained in CMS for statistical analysis and use in determining future PPS DRG classifications and rates.

Non-PPS hospitals do not pay for noncovered services generally excluded from coverage in the Medicare Program. This may result in denial of a part of the billed charges or in denial of the entire admission, depending upon circumstance. In PPS hospitals, the following are also possible:

1. In appropriately admitted cases where a noncovered procedure was performed, denied services may result in payment of a different DRG (i.e., one which excludes payment for the noncovered procedure); or
2. In appropriately admitted cases that become cost outlier cases, denied services may lead to denial of some or all of an outlier payment.

The following examples illustrate this principle. If care is noncovered because a patient does not need to be hospitalized, the intermediary denies the admission and makes no Part A (i.e., PPS) payment unless paid under limitation on liability. Under limitation on liability, Medicare payment may be made when the provider and the beneficiary were not aware the services were not necessary and could not reasonably be expected to know that he services were not necessary. For detailed instructions, see the Medicare Claims Processing Manual, Chapter 30,"Limitation on Liability." If a patient is appropriately hospitalized but receives (beyond routine services) only noncovered care, the admission is denied.

NOTE: The intermediary does not deny an admission that includes covered care, even if noncovered care was also rendered. Under PPS, Medicare assumes that it is paying for only the covered care rendered whenever covered services needed to treat and/or diagnose the illness were in fact provided.

If a noncovered procedure is provided along with covered nonroutine care, a DRG change rather than an admission denial might occur. If noncovered procedures are elevating costs into the cost outlier category, outlier payment is denied in whole or in part.

When the hospital is included in PPS, most of the subsequent discussion regarding coverage of inpatient hospital services is relevant only in the context of determining the appropriateness of admissions, which DRG, if any, to pay, and the appropriateness of payment for any outlier cases.

If a patient receives items or services in excess of, or more expensive than, those for which payment can be made, payment is made only for the covered items or services or for only the appropriate prospective payment amount. This provision applies not only to inpatient services, but also to all hospital services under Parts A and B of the program. If the items or services were requested by the patient, the hospital may charge him the difference between the amount customarily charged for the services requested and the amount customarily charged for covered services.

An inpatient is a person who has been admitted to a hospital for bed occupancy for purposes of receiving inpatient hospital services. Generally, a patient is considered an inpatient if formally admitted as inpatient with the expectation that he or she will remain at least overnight and occupy a bed even though it later develops that the patient can be discharged or transferred to another hospital and not actually use a hospital bed overnight.

The physician or other practitioner responsible for a patient's care at the hospital is also responsible for deciding whether the patient should be admitted as an inpatient. Physicians should use a 24-hour period as a benchmark, i.e., they should order admission for patients who are expected to need hospital care for 24 hours or more, and treat other patients on an outpatient basis. However, the decision to admit a patient is a complex medical judgment which can be made only after the physician has considered a number of factors, including the patient's medical history and current medical needs, the types of facilities available to inpatients and to outpatients, the hospital's by-laws and admissions policies, and the relative appropriateness of treatment in each setting. Factors to be considered when making the decision to admit include such things as:

- The severity of the signs and symptoms exhibited by the patient;
- The medical predictability of something adverse happening to the patient;
- The need for diagnostic studies that appropriately are outpatient services (i.e., their performance does not ordinarily require the patient to remain at the hospital for 24 hours or more) to assist in assessing whether the patient should be admitted; and
- The availability of diagnostic procedures at the time when and at the location where the patient presents.

Admissions of particular patients are not covered or noncovered solely on the basis of the length of time the patient actually spends in the hospital. In certain specific situations coverage of services on an inpatient or outpatient basis is determined by the following rules:

Minor Surgery or Other Treatment - When patients with known diagnoses enter a hospital for a specific minor surgical procedure or other treatment that is expected to keep them in the hospital for only a few hours (less than 24), they are considered outpatients for coverage purposes regardless of: the hour they came to the hospital, whether they used a bed, and whether they remained in the hospital past midnight.

Renal Dialysis - Renal dialysis treatments are usually covered only as outpatient services but may under certain circumstances be covered as inpatient services depending on the patient's condition. Patients staying at home, who are ambulatory, whose conditions are stable and who come to the hospital for routine chronic dialysis treatments, and not for a diagnostic workup or a change in therapy, are considered outpatients. On the other hand, patients undergoing short-term dialysis until their kidneys recover from an acute illness (acute dialysis), or persons with borderline renal failure who develop acute renal failure every time they have an illness and require dialysis (episodic dialysis) are usually inpatients. A patient may begin dialysis as an inpatient and then progress to an outpatient status.

Under original Medicare, the Quality Improvement Organization (QIO), for each hospital is responsible for deciding, during review of inpatient admissions on a case-by-case basis, whether the admission was medically necessary. Medicare law authorizes the QIO to make these judgments, and the judgments are binding for purposes of Medicare coverage. In making these judgments, however, QIOs consider only the medical evidence which was available to the physician at the time an admission decision had to be made. They do not take into account other information (e.g., test results) which became available only after admission, except in cases where considering the post-admission information would support a finding that an admission was medically necessary.

Refer to Parts 4 and 7 of the QIO Manual with regard to initial determinations for these services. The QIO will review the swing bed services in these PPS hospitals as well.

NOTE: When patients requiring extended care services are admitted to beds in a hospital, they are considered inpatients of the hospital. In such cases, the services furnished in the hospital will not be considered extended care services, and payment may not be made under the program for such services unless the services are extended care services furnished pursuant to a swing bed agreement granted to the hospital by the Secretary of Health and Human Services.

100-2, 1, 90

Termination of Pregnancy

B3-4276.1,.2

Effective for services furnished on or after October 1, 1998, Medicare will cover abortions procedures in the following situations:

1. If the pregnancy is the result of an act or rape or incest; or
2. In the case where a woman suffers from a physical disorder, physical injury, or physical illness, including a life-endangering physical condition caused by the pregnancy itself that would, as certified by a physician, place the woman in danger of death unless an abortion is performed.

NOTE: The "G7" modifier must be used with the following CPT codes in order for these services to be covered when the pregnancy resulted from rape or incest, or the pregnancy is certified by a physician as life threatening to the mother:

59840, 59841, 59850, 59851, 59852, 59855, 59856, 59857, 59866

100-2, 1, 100

Treatment for Infertility

A3-3101.13

Effective for services rendered on or after January 15, 1980, reasonable and necessary services associated with treatment for infertility are covered under Medicare. Like pregnancy (see Sec. 80 above), infertility is a condition sufficiently at variance with the usual state of health to make it appropriate for a person who normally would be expected to be fertile to seek medical consultation and treatment. Contractors should coordinate with QIOs to see that utilization guidelines are established for this treatment if inappropriate utilization or abuse is suspected.

100-2, 6, 10

Medical and Other Health Services Furnished to Inpatients of Participating Hospitals

Payment may be made under Part B for physician services and for the nonphysician medical and other health services listed below when furnished by a participating hospital (either directly or under arrangements) to an inpatient of the hospital, but only if payment for these services cannot be made under Part A.

In PPS hospitals, this means that Part B payment could be made for these services if:

- No Part A prospective payment is made at all for the hospital stay because of patient exhaustion of benefit days before admission;
- The admission was disapproved as not reasonable and necessary (and waiver of liability payment was not made);
- The day or days of the otherwise covered stay during which the services were provided were not reasonable and necessary (and no payment was made under waiver of liability);
- The patient was not otherwise eligible for or entitled to coverage under Part A (See the Medicare Benefit Policy Manual, Chapter 1, Sec.150, for services received as a result of noncovered services); or
- No Part A day outlier payment is made (for discharges before October 1997) for one or more outlier days due to patient exhaustion of benefit days after admission but before the case's arrival at outlier status, or because outlier days are otherwise not covered and waiver of liability payment is not made.

However, if only day outlier payment is denied under Part A (discharges before October 1997), Part B payment may be made for only the services covered under Part B and furnished on the denied outlier days.

In non-PPS hospitals, Part B payment may be made for services on any day for which Part A payment is denied (i.e., benefit days are exhausted; services are not at the hospital level of care; or patient is not otherwise eligible or entitled to payment under Part A).

Services payable are:

- Diagnostic x-ray tests, diagnostic laboratory tests, and other diagnostic tests;
- X-ray, radium, and radioactive isotope therapy, including materials and services of technicians;
- Surgical dressings, and splints, casts, and other devices used for reduction of fractures and dislocations;
- Prosthetic devices (other than dental) which replace all or part of an internal body organ (including contiguous tissue), or all or part of the function of a permanently inoperative or malfunctioning internal body organ, including replacement or repairs of such devices;
- Leg, arm, back, and neck braces, trusses, and artificial legs, arms, and eyes including adjustments, repairs, and replacements required because of breakage, wear, loss, or a change in the patient's physical condition;
- Outpatient physical therapy, outpatient speech-language pathology services, and outpatient occupational therapy (see the Medicare Benefit Policy Manual, Chapter 15, "Covered Medical and Other Health Services," Sec.Sec.220 and 230);
- Screening mammography services;
- Screening pap smears;
- Influenza, pneumococcal pneumonia, and hepatitis B vaccines;
- Colorectal screening;
- Bone mass measurements;
- Diabetes self-management;
- Prostate screening;
- Ambulance services;
- Hemophilia clotting factors for hemophilia patients competent to use these factors without supervision);
- Immunosuppressive drugs;
- Oral anti-cancer drugs;

- Oral drug prescribed for use as an acute anti-emetic used as part of an anti-cancer chemotherapeutic regimen; and Epoetin Alfa (EPO).

Coverage rules for these services are described in the Medicare Benefit Policy Manual, Chapters: 11, "End Stage Renal Disease (ESRD);" 14, "Medical Devices;" or 15, "Medical and Other Health Services."

For services to be covered under Part A or Part B, a hospital must furnish nonphysician services to its inpatients directly or under arrangements. A nonphysician service is one which does not meet the criteria defining physicians' services specifically provided for in regulation at 42 CFR 415.102. Services "incident to" physicians' services (except for the services of nurse anesthetists employed by anesthesiologists) are nonphysician services for purposes of this provision. This provision is applicable to all hospitals participating in Medicare, including those paid under alternative arrangements such as State cost control systems, and to emergency hospital services furnished by nonparticipating hospitals.

In all hospitals, every service provided to a hospital inpatient other than those listed in the next paragraph must be treated as an inpatient hospital service to be paid for under Part A, if Part A coverage is available and the beneficiary is entitled to Part A. This is because every hospital must provide directly or arrange for any nonphysician service rendered to its inpatients, and a hospital can be paid under Part B for a service provided in this manner only if Part A coverage does not exist.

These services, when provided to a hospital inpatient, may be covered under Part B, even though the patient has Part A coverage for the hospital stay. This is because these services are covered under Part B and not covered under Part A. They are:

- Physicians' services (including the services of residents and interns in unapproved teaching programs);
- Influenza vaccine;
- Pneumoccocal vaccine and its administration;
- Hepatitis B vaccine and its administration;
- Screening mammography services;
- Screening pap smears and pelvic exams;
- Colorectal screening;
- Bone mass measurements;
- Diabetes self management training services; and
- Prostate screening.

However, note that in order to have any Medicare coverage at all (Part A or Part B), any nonphysician service rendered to a hospital inpatient must be provided directly or arranged for by the hospital.

100-2, 6, 50

Sleep Disorder Clinics

A3-3112.5

Sleep disorder clinics are facilities in which certain conditions are diagnosed through the study of sleep. Such clinics are for diagnosis, therapy, and research. Sleep disorder clinics may provide some diagnostic or therapeutic services that are covered under Medicare. These clinics may be affiliated either with a hospital or a freestanding facility. Whether a clinic is hospital-affiliated or freestanding, coverage for diagnostic services under some circumstances is covered under provisions of the law different from those for coverage of therapeutic services.

100-2, 11, 20

Renal Dialysis Items and Services

Medicare provides payment under the ESRD PPS for all renal dialysis services for outpatient maintenance dialysis when they are furnished to Medicare ESRD patients by a Medicare certified ESRD facility or a special purpose dialysis facility. Renal dialysis services are the items and services included under the composite rate and the ESRD-related items and services that were separately paid as of December 31, 2010.

Renal dialysis services are furnished in various settings including hospital outpatient ESRD facilities, independent ESRD facilities, or in the patient? home. Renal dialysis items and services furnished at ESRD facilities differ according to the types of patients being treated, the types of equipment and supplies used, the preferences of the treating physician, and the capability and makeup of the staff. Although not all facilities provide an identical range of services, the most common elements of dialysis treatment include:

- Laboratory Tests;
- Drugs and Biologicals;
- Equipment and supplies - dialysis machine use and maintenance;
- Personnel services;
- Administrative services;
- Overhead costs;
- Monitoring access and related declotting or referring the patient, and
- Direct nursing services include registered nurses, licensed practical nurses, technicians, social workers, and dietitians.

100-2, 12, 40.11

Vaccines

A CORF may provide pneumococcal pneumonia, influenza virus, and hepatitis B vaccines to its patients. While not included as a service under the CORF benefit, Medicare will make payment to the CORF for certain vaccines and their administration provided to CORF patients (CY 2008 PFS Rule 72 FR 66293).

The following three vaccinations are covered in a CORF if a physician who is a doctor of medicine or osteopathy orders it for a CORF patient: Pneumococcal pneumonia vaccine and its administration;

Hepatitis B vaccine and its administration furnished to a beneficiary who is at high or intermediate risk of contracting hepatitis B; and

Influenza virus vaccine and its administration

Payment for covered pneumococcal pneumonia, influenza virus, and hepatitis B vaccines provided in the CORF setting is based on 95 percent of the average wholesale price. The CORF registered nurse provides administration of any of these vaccines using HCPCS codes G0008, G0009 or G0010 with payment based on CPT code 90471.

100-2, 13, 30

Rural Health Clinic and Federally Qualified Health Center Service Defined

Payments for covered RHC/FQHC services furnished to Medicare beneficiaries are made on the basis of an all-inclusive rate per covered visit (except for pneumococcal and influenza vaccines and their administration, which is paid at 100 percent of reasonable cost). The term "visit" is defined as a face-to-face encounter between the patient and a physician, physician assistant, nurse practitioner, certified nurse midwife, visiting nurse, clinical psychologist, or clinical social worker during which an RHC/FQHC service is rendered. As a result of section 5114 of the Deficit Reduction Act of 2005 (DRA), the FQHC definition of a face-to-face encounter is expanded to include encounters with qualified practitioners of Outpatient Diabetes Self-Management Training Services (DSMT) and medical nutrition therapy (MNT) services when the FQHC meets all relevant program requirements for the provision of such services.

Encounters with (1) more than one health professional; and (2) multiple encounters with the same health professional which take place on the same day and at a single location, constitute a single visit. An exception occurs in cases in which the patient, subsequent to the first encounter, suffers an illness or injury requiring additional diagnosis or treatment.

100-2, 15, 20.1

Physician Expense for Surgery, Childbirth, and Treatment for Infertility

B3-2005.I

A. Surgery and Childbirth

Skilled medical management is covered throughout the events of pregnancy, beginning with diagnosis, continuing through delivery and ending after the necessary postnatal care. Similarly, in the event of termination of pregnancy, regardless of whether terminated spontaneously or for therapeutic reasons (i.e., where the life of the mother would be endangered if the fetus were brought to term), the need for skilled medical management and/or medical services is equally important as in those cases carried to full term. After the infant is delivered and is a separate individual, items and services furnished to the infant are not covered on the basis of the mother's eligibility.

Most surgeons and obstetricians bill patients an all-inclusive package charge intended to cover all services associated with the surgical procedure or delivery of the child. All expenses for surgical and obstetrical care, including preoperative/prenatal examinations and tests and post-operative/postnatal services, are considered incurred on the date of surgery or delivery, as appropriate. This policy applies whether the physician bills on a package charge basis, or itemizes the bill separately for these items.

Occasionally, a physician's bill may include charges for additional services not directly related to the surgical procedure or the delivery. Such charges are considered incurred on the date the additional services are furnished.

The above policy applies only where the charges are imposed by one physician or by a clinic on behalf of a group of physicians. Where more than one physician imposes charges for surgical or obstetrical services, all preoperative/prenatal and post-operative/postnatal services performed by the physician who performed the surgery or delivery are considered incurred on the date of the surgery or delivery. Expenses for services rendered by other physicians are considered incurred on the date they were performed.

B. Treatment for Infertility

Reasonable and necessary services associated with treatment for infertility are covered under Medicare. Infertility is a condition sufficiently at variance with the usual state of health to make it appropriate for a person who normally is expected to be fertile to seek medical consultation and treatment.

100-2, 15, 20.2

Physician Expense for Allergy Treatment

B3-2005.2, B3-4145

Allergists commonly bill separately for the initial diagnostic workup and for the treatment (See Sec.60.2). Where it is necessary to provide treatment over an extended period, the allergist may submit a single bill for all of the treatments, or may bill periodically. In either case the Form CMS-1500 claim shows the Healthcare Common Procedure Coding System (HCPCS) codes and from and through dates of service, or the Form CMS-1450 outpatient claim shows the HCPCS code and date of service (except for critical access hospital (CAH) claims).

100-2, 15, 20.3

Artificial Limbs, Braces, and Other Custom Made Items Ordered But Not Furnished

B3-2005.3

A. Date of Incurred Expense

If a custom-made item was ordered but not furnished to a beneficiary because the individual died or because the order was canceled by the beneficiary or because the beneficiary's condition changed and the item was no longer reasonable and necessary or appropriate, payment can be made based on the supplier's expenses. (See subsection B for determination of the allowed amount.) In such cases, the expense is considered incurred on the date the beneficiary died or the date the supplier learned of the cancellation or that the item was no longer reasonable and necessary or appropriate for the beneficiary's condition. If the beneficiary died or the beneficiary's condition changed and the item was no longer reasonable and necessary or appropriate, payment can be made on either an assigned or unassigned claim. If the beneficiary, for any other reason, canceled the order, payment can be made to the supplier only.

B. Determination of Allowed Amount

The allowed amount is based on the services furnished and materials used, up to the date the supplier learned of the beneficiary's death or of the cancellation of the order or that the item was no longer reasonable and necessary or appropriate. The Durable Medical Equipment Regional Carrier (DMERC), carrier or intermediary, as appropriate, determines the services performed and the allowable amount appropriate in the particular situation. It takes into account any salvage value of the device to the supplier. Where a supplier breaches an agreement to make a prosthesis, brace, or other custom-made device for a Medicare beneficiary, e.g., an unexcused failure to provide the article within the time specified in the contract, payment may not be made for any work or material expended on the item. Whether a particular supplier has lived up to its agreement, of course, depends on the facts in the individual case.

100-2, 15, 30

Physician Services

A. General

Physician services are the professional services performed by a physician or physicians for a patient including diagnosis, therapy, surgery, consultation, and care plan oversight.

The physician must render the service for the service to be covered. (See Pub. 100-01, Medicare General Information, Eligibility, and Entitlement Manual, Chapter 5, §70, for definition of physician.) A service may be considered to be a physician's service where the physician either examines the patient in person or is able to visualize some aspect of the patient's condition without the interposition of a third person's judgment. Direct visualization would be possible by means of x-rays, electrocardiogram and electroencephalogram tapes, tissue samples, etc.

For example, the interpretation by a physician of an actual electrocardiogram or electroencephalogram reading that has been transmitted via telephone (i.e., electronically rather than by means of a verbal description) is a covered service.

Professional services of the physician are covered if provided within the United States, and may be performed in a home, office, institution, or at the scene of an accident. A patient's home, for this purpose, is anywhere the patient makes his or her residence, e.g., home for the aged, a nursing home, a relative's home.

B. Telephone Services

Services by means of a telephone call between a physician and a beneficiary, or between a physician and a member of a beneficiary's family, are covered under Medicare, but carriers may not make separate payment for these services under the program. The physician work resulting from telephone calls is considered to be an integral part of the prework and postwork of other physician services, and the fee schedule amount for the latter services already includes payment for the telephone calls. See §270 of this manual for coverage of telehealth services.

C. Consultations

As of January 1, 2010, CMS no longer recognizes consultation codes for Medicare payment, except for inpatient telehealth consultation HCPCS G-codes. Instead, physicians and qualified nonphysician practitioners are instructed to bill a new or established patient office/outpatient visit CPT code or appropriate hospital or nursing facility care code. For further detail regarding reporting services that would otherwise be described by the CPT consultation codes (99241-99245 and 99251-99255), see Pub. 100-04, Medicare Claims Processing Manual, chapter 12, section 30.6. For detailed instructions regarding reporting telehealth consultation services and other telehealth services, see Pub. 100-04, chapter 12, section 190.3.

D. Patient-Initiated Second Opinions

Patient-initiated second opinions that relate to the medical need for surgery or for major nonsurgical diagnostic and therapeutic procedures (e.g., invasive diagnostic techniques such as cardiac catheterization and gastroscopy) are covered under Medicare. In the event that the recommendation of the first and second physician differs regarding the need for surgery (or other major procedure), a third opinion is also covered. Second and third opinions are covered even though the surgery or other procedure, if performed, is determined not covered. Payment may be made for the history and examination of the patient, and for other covered diagnostic services required to properly evaluate the patient's need for a procedure and to render a professional opinion. In some cases, the results of tests done by the first physician may be available to the second physician.

E. Concurrent Care

Concurrent care exists where more than one physician renders services more extensive than consultative services during a period of time. The reasonable and necessary services of each physician rendering concurrent care could be covered where each is required to play an active role in the patient's treatment, for example, because of the existence of more than one medical condition requiring diverse specialized medical services.

In order to determine whether concurrent physicians' services are reasonable and necessary, the carrier must decide the following:

1. Whether the patient's condition warrants the services of more than one physician on an attending (rather than consultative) basis, and
2. Whether the individual services provided by each physician are reasonable and necessary.

In resolving the first question, the carrier should consider the specialties of the physicians as well as the patient's diagnosis, as concurrent care is usually (although not always) initiated because of the existence of more than one medical condition requiring diverse specialized medical or surgical services. The specialties of the physicians are an indication of the necessity for concurrent services, but the patient's condition and the inherent reasonableness and necessity of the services, as determined by the carrier's medical staff in accordance with locality norms, must also be considered. For example, although cardiology is a sub-specialty of internal medicine, the treatment of both diabetes and of a serious heart condition might require the concurrent services of two physicians, each practicing in internal medicine but specializing in different sub-specialties.

While it would not be highly unusual for concurrent care performed by physicians in different specialties (e.g., a surgeon and an internist) or by physicians in different subspecialties of the same specialty (e.g., an allergist and a cardiologist) to be found medically necessary, the need for such care by physicians in the same specialty or subspecialty (e.g., two internists or two cardiologists) would occur infrequently since in most cases both physicians would possess the skills and knowledge necessary to treat the patient. However, circumstances could arise which would necessitate such care. For example, a patient may require the services of two physicians in the same specialty or sub-specialty when one physician has further limited his or her practice to some unusual aspect of that specialty, e.g., tropical medicine. Similarly, concurrent services provided by a family physician and an internist may or may not be found to be reasonable and necessary, depending on the circumstances of the specific case. If it is determined that the services of one of the physicians are not warranted by the patient's condition, payment may be made only for the other physician's (or physicians') services.

Once it is determined that the patient requires the active services of more than one physician, the individual services must be examined for medical necessity, just as where a single physician provides the care. For example, even if it is determined that the patient requires the concurrent services of both a cardiologist and a surgeon, payment may not be made for any services rendered by either physician which, for that condition, exceed normal frequency or duration unless there are special circumstances requiring the additional care.

The carrier must also assure that the services of one physician do not duplicate those provided by another, e.g., where the family physician visits during the post-operative period primarily as a courtesy to the patient.

Hospital admission services performed by two physicians for the same beneficiary on the same day could represent reasonable and necessary services, provided, as stated above, that the patient's condition necessitates treatment by both physicians. The level of difficulty of the service provided may vary between the physicians, depending on the severity of the complaint each one is treating and that physician's prior contact with the patient. For example, the admission services performed by a physician who has been treating a patient over a period of time for a chronic condition would not be as involved as the services performed by a physician who has had no prior contact with the patient and who has been called in to diagnose and treat a major acute condition.

Carriers should have sufficient means for identifying concurrent care situations. A correct coverage determination can be made on a concurrent care case only where the claim is sufficiently documented for the carrier to determine the role each physician played in the patient's care (i.e., the condition or conditions for which the physician treated the patient). If, in any case, the role of each physician involved is not clear, the carrier should request clarification.

F. Completion of Claims Forms

Separate charges for the services of a physician in completing a Form CMS-1500, a statement in lieu of a Form CMS-1500, or an itemized bill are not covered. Payment for completion of the Form CMS-1500 claim form is considered included in the fee schedule amount.

G. Care Plan Oversight Services

Care plan oversight is supervision of patients under care of home health agencies or hospices that require complex and multidisciplinary care modalities involving regular physician development and/or revision of care plans, review of subsequent reports of patient status, review of laboratory and other studies, communication with other health professionals not employed in the same practice who are involved in the patient's care, integration of new information into the care plan, and/or adjustment of medical therapy.

Such services are covered for home health and hospice patients, but are not covered for patients of skilled nursing facilities (SNFs), nursing home facilities, or hospitals.

These services are covered only if all the following requirements are met:

1. The beneficiary must require complex or multi-disciplinary care modalities requiring ongoing physician involvement in the patient's plan of care;
2. The care plan oversight (CPO) services should be furnished during the period in which the beneficiary was receiving Medicare covered HHA or hospice services;
3. The physician who bills CPO must be the same physician who signed the home health or hospice plan of care;
4. The physician furnished at least 30 minutes of care plan oversight within the calendar month for which payment is claimed. Time spent by a physician's nurse or the time spent consulting with one's nurse is not countable toward the 30-minute threshold. Low-intensity services included as part of other evaluation and management services are not included as part of the 30 minutes required for coverage;
5. The work included in hospital discharge day management (codes 99238-99239) and discharge from observation (code 99217) is not countable toward the 30 minutes per month required for work on the same day as discharge but only for those services separately documented as occurring after the patient is actually physically discharged from the hospital;
6. The physician provided a covered physician service that required a face-to-face encounter with the beneficiary within the 6 months immediately preceding the first care plan oversight service. Only evaluation and management services are acceptable prerequisite face-to-face encounters for CPO. EKG, lab, and surgical services are not sufficient face-to-face services for CPO;
7. The care plan oversight billed by the physician was not routine post-operative care provided in the global surgical period of a surgical procedure billed by the physician;
8. If the beneficiary is receiving home health agency services, the physician did not have a significant financial or contractual interest in the home health agency. A physician who is an employee of a hospice, including a volunteer medical director, should not bill CPO services. Payment for the services of a physician employed by the hospice is included in the payment to the hospice;
9. The physician who bills the care plan oversight services is the physician who furnished them;
10. Services provided incident to a physician's service do not qualify as CPO and do not count toward the 30-minute requirement;
11. The physician is not billing for the Medicare end stage renal disease (ESRD) capitation payment for the same beneficiary during the same month; and
12. The physician billing for CPO must document in the patient's record the services furnished and the date and length of time associated with those services

100-2, 15, 30.4

Optometrist's Services

B3-2020.25

Effective April 1, 1987, a doctor of optometry is considered a physician with respect to all services the optometrist is authorized to perform under State law or regulation. To be covered under Medicare, the services must be medically reasonable and necessary for the diagnosis or treatment of illness or injury, and must meet all applicable coverage requirements. See the Medicare Benefit Policy Manual, Chapter 16, "General Exclusions from Coverage," for exclusions from coverage that apply to vision care services, and the Medicare Claims Processing Manual, Chapter 12, "Physician/Practitioner Billing," for information dealing with payment for items and services furnished by optometrists.

A. FDA Monitored Studies of Intraocular Lenses

Special coverage rules apply to situations in which an ophthalmologist is involved in a Food and Drug Administration (FDA) monitored study of the safety and efficacy of an investigational Intraocular Lens (IOL). The investigation process for IOLs is unique in that there is a core period and an adjunct period. The core study is a traditional, well-controlled clinical investigation with full record keeping and reporting requirements. The adjunct study is essentially an extended distribution phase for lenses in which only limited safety data are compiled. Depending on the lens being evaluated, the adjunct study may be an extension of the core study or may be the only type of investigation to which the lens may be subject.

All eye care services related to the investigation of the IOL must be provided by the investigator (i.e., the implanting ophthalmologist) or another practitioner (including a doctor of optometry) who provides services at the direction or under the supervision of the investigator and who has an agreement with the investigator that information on the patient is given to the investigator so that he or she may report on the patient to the IOL manufacturer. Eye care services furnished by anyone other than the investigator (or a practitioner who assists the investigator, as described in the preceding paragraph) are not covered during the period the IOL is being investigated, unless the services are not related to the investigation.

B. Concurrent Care

Where more than one practitioner furnishes concurrent care, services furnished to a beneficiary by both an ophthalmologist and another physician (including an optometrist) may be recognized for payment if it is determined that each practitioner's services were reasonable and necessary. (See Sec.30.E)

100-2, 15, 30.5

Chiropractor's Services

B3-2020.26

A chiropractor must be licensed or legally authorized to furnish chiropractic services by the State or jurisdiction in which the services are furnished. In addition, a licensed chiropractor must meet the following uniform minimum standards to be considered a physician for Medicare coverage. Coverage extends only to treatment by means of manual manipulation of the spine to correct a subluxation provided such treatment is legal in the State where performed. All other services furnished or ordered by chiropractors are not covered. If a chiropractor orders, takes, or interprets an x-ray or other diagnostic procedure to demonstrate a subluxation of the spine, the x-ray can be used for documentation. However, there is no coverage or payment for these services or for any other diagnostic or therapeutic service ordered or furnished by the chiropractor. For detailed information on using x-rays to determine subluxation, see Sec.240.1.2. In addition, in performing manual manipulation of the spine, some chiropractors use manual devices that are hand-held with the thrust of the force of the device being controlled manually. While such manual manipulation may be covered, there is no separate payment permitted for use of this device.

A. Uniform Minimum Standards

Prior to July 1, 1974 Chiropractors licensed or authorized to practice prior to July 1, 1974, and those individuals who commenced their studies in a chiropractic college before that date must meet all of the following three minimum standards to render payable services under the program:

Preliminary education equal to the requirements for graduation from an accredited high school or other secondary school;Graduation from a college of chiropractic approved by the State's chiropractic examiners that included the completion of a course of study covering a period of not less than 3 school years of 6 months each year in actual continuous attendance covering adequate course of study in the subjects of anatomy, physiology, symptomatology and diagnosis, hygiene and sanitation, chemistry, histology, pathology, and principles and practice of chiropractic, including clinical instruction in vertebral palpation, nerve tracing, and adjusting; andPassage of an examination prescribed by the State's chiropractic examiners covering the subjects listed above.

After June 30, 1974 Individuals commencing their studies in a chiropractic college after June 30, 1974, must meet all of the above three standards and all of the following additional requirements:Satisfactory completion of 2 years of pre-chiropractic study at the college level;Satisfactory completion of a 4-year course of 8 months each year (instead of a 3-year course of 6 months each year) at a college or school of chiropractic that includes not less than 4,000 hours in the scientific and chiropractic courses specified in the second bullet under "Prior to July 1, 1974" above, plus courses in the use and effect of x-ray and chiropractic analysis; andThe practitioner must be over 21 years of age.

B. Maintenance Therapy

Under the Medicare program, Chiropractic maintenance therapy is not considered to be medically reasonable or necessary, and is therefore not payable. Maintenance therapy is defined as a treatment plan that seeks to prevent disease, promote health, and prolong and enhance the quality of life; or therapy that is performed to maintain or prevent deterioration of a chronic condition. When further clinical improvement cannot reasonably be expected from continuous ongoing care, and the chiropractic treatment becomes supportive rather than corrective in nature, the treatment is then considered maintenance therapy. For information on how to indicate on a claim a treatment is or is not maintenance, see Sec.240.1.

100-2, 15, 50

Drugs and Biologicals

B3-2049, A3-3112.4.B, HO-230.4.B

The Medicare program provides limited benefits for outpatient drugs. The program covers drugs that are furnished "incident to" a physician's service provided that the drugs are not usually self-administered by the patients who take them. Generally, drugs and biologicals are covered only if all of the following requirements are met:

- They meet the definition of drugs or biologicals (see Sec.50.1);
- They are of the type that are not usually self-administered. (see Sec.50.2);
- They meet all the general requirements for coverage of items as incident to a physician's services (see Secs.50.1 and 50.3);

- They are reasonable and necessary for the diagnosis or treatment of the illness or injury for which they are administered according to accepted standards of medical practice (see Sec.50.4);
- They are not excluded as noncovered immunizations (see Sec.50.4.4.2); and
- They have not been determined by the FDA to be less than effective. (See Sec.50.4.4).

Medicare Part B does generally not cover drugs that can be self-administered, such as those in pill form, or are used for self-injection. However, the statute provides for the coverage of some self-administered drugs. Examples of self-administered drugs that are covered include blood-clotting factors, drugs used in immunosuppressive therapy, erythropoietin for dialysis patients, osteoporosis drugs for certain homebound patients, and certain oral cancer drugs. (See Sec.110.3 for coverage of drugs, which are necessary to the effective use of Durable Medical Equipment (DME) or prosthetic devices.)

100-2, 15, 50.4.4.2

Immunizations

Vaccinations or inoculations are excluded as immunizations unless they are directly related to the treatment of an injury or direct exposure to a disease or condition, such as anti-rabies treatment, tetanus antitoxin or booster vaccine, botulin antitoxin, antivenin sera, or immune globulin. In the absence of injury or direct exposure, preventive immunization (vaccination or inoculation) against such diseases as smallpox, polio, diphtheria, etc., is not covered. However, pneumococcal, hepatitis B, and influenza virus vaccines are exceptions to this rule. (See items A, B, and C below.) In cases where a vaccination or inoculation is excluded from coverage, related charges are also not covered.

A. Pneumococcal Pneumonia Vaccinations

Effective for services furnished on or after May 1, 1981, the Medicare Part B program covers pneumococcal pneumonia vaccine and its administration when furnished in compliance with any applicable State law by any provider of services or any entity or individual with a supplier number. This includes revaccination of patients at highest risk of pneumococcal infection. Typically, these vaccines are administered once in a lifetime except for persons at highest risk. Effective July 1, 2000, Medicare does not require for coverage purposes that a doctor of medicine or osteopathy order the vaccine. Therefore, the beneficiary may receive the vaccine upon request without a physician's order and without physician supervision.

An initial vaccine may be administered only to persons at high risk (see below) of pneumococcal disease. Revaccination may be administered only to persons at highest risk of serious pneumococcal infection and those likely to have a rapid decline in pneumococcal antibody levels, provided that at least 5 years have [passed since the previous dose of pneumococcal vaccine.

Persons at high risk for whom an initial vaccine may be administered include all people age 65 and older; immunocompetent adults who are at increased risk of pneumococcal disease or its complications because of chronic illness (e.g., cardiovascular disease, pulmonary disease, diabetes mellitus, alcoholism, cirrhosis, or cerebrospinal fluid leaks); and individuals with compromised immune systems (e.g., splenic dysfunction or anatomic asplenia, Hodgkin's disease, lymphoma, multiple myeloma, chronic renal failure, HIV infection, nephrotic syndrome, sickle cell disease, or organ transplantation).

Persons at highest risk and those most likely to have rapid declines in antibody levels are those for whom revaccination may be appropriate. This group includes persons with functional or anatomic asplenia (e.g., sickle cell disease, splenectomy), HIV infection, leukemia, lymphoma, Hodgkin's disease, multiple myeloma, generalized malignancy, chronic renal failure, nephrotic syndrome, or other conditions associated with immunosuppression such as organ or bone marrow transplantation, and those receiving immunosuppressive chemotherapy. it is not appropriate for routine revaccination of people age 65 or older that are not at highest risk.

Those administering the vaccine should not require the patient to present an immunization record prior to administering the pneumococcal vaccine, nor should they feel compelled to review the patient's complete medical record if it is not available. Instead, provided that the patient is competent, it is acceptable to rely on the patient's verbal history to determine prior vaccination status. If the patient is uncertain about his or her vaccination history in the past 5 years, the vaccine should be given. However, if the patient is certain he/she was were vaccinated in the last 5 years, the vaccine should not be given. If the patient is certain that the vaccine was given more than 5 years ago, revaccination is covered only if the patient is at high risk.

B. Hepatitis B Vaccine

Effective for services furnished on or after September 1, 1984, P.L. 98-369 provides coverage under Part B for hepatitis B vaccine and its administration, furnished to a Medicare beneficiary who is at high or intermediate risk of contracting hepatitis B. This coverage is effective for services furnished on or after September 1, 1984. High-risk groups currently identified include (see exception below):

- ESRD patients;
- Hemophiliacs who receive Factor VIII or IX concentrates;
- Clients of institutions for the mentally retarded;
- Persons who live in the same household as a Hepatitis B Virus (HBV) carrier;
- Homosexual men; and
- Illicit injectable drug abusers; and
- Persons diagnosed with diabetes mellitus.

Intermediate risk groups currently identified include:

- Staff in institutions for the mentally retarded; and
- Workers in health care professions who have frequent contact with blood or blood-derived body fluids during routine work.

EXCEPTION: Persons in both of the above-listed groups in paragraph B, would not be considered at high or intermediate risk of contracting hepatitis B, however, if there were laboratory evidence positive for antibodies to hepatitis B. (ESRD patients are routinely tested for hepatitis B antibodies as part of their continuing monitoring and therapy.)

For Medicare program purposes, the vaccine may be administered upon the order of a doctor of medicine or osteopathy, by a doctor of medicine or osteopathy, or by home health agencies, skilled nursing facilities, ESRD facilities, hospital outpatient departments, and persons recognized under the incident to physicians' services provision of law.

A charge separate from the ESRD composite rate will be recognized and paid for administration of the vaccine to ESRD patients.

C. Influenza Virus Vaccine

Effective for services furnished on or after May 1, 1993, the Medicare Part B program covers influenza virus vaccine and its administration when furnished in compliance with any applicable State law by any provider of services or any entity or individual with a supplier number. Typically, these vaccines are administered once a flu season. Medicare does not require, for coverage purposes, that a doctor of medicine or osteopathy order the vaccine. Therefore, the beneficiary may receive the vaccine upon request without a physician's order and without physician supervision

100-2, 15, 50.5

Self-Administered Drugs and Biologicals

B3-2049.5

Medicare Part B does not cover drugs that are usually self-administered by the patient unless the statute provides for such coverage. The statute explicitly provides coverage, for blood clotting factors, drugs used in immunosuppressive therapy, erythropoietin for dialysis patients, certain oral anti-cancer drugs and anti-emetics used in certain situations.

100-2, 15, 60.3

Incident to Physician's Service in Clinic

B3-2050.3

Services and supplies incident to a physician's service in a physician directed clinic or group association are generally the same as those described above.

A physician directed clinic is one where:

1. A physician (or a number of physicians) is present to perform medical (rather than administrative) services at all times the clinic is open;
2. Each patient is under the care of a clinic physician; and
3. The nonphysician services are under medical supervision.

In highly organized clinics, particularly those that are departmentalized, direct physician supervision may be the responsibility of several physicians as opposed to an individual attending physician. In this situation, medical management of all services provided in the clinic is assured. The physician ordering a particular service need not be the physician who is supervising the service. Therefore, services performed by auxiliary personnel and other aides are covered even though they are performed in another department of the clinic. Supplies provided by the clinic during the course of treatment are also covered. When the auxiliary personnel perform services outside the clinic premises, the services are covered only if performed under the direct supervision of a clinic physician. If the clinic refers a patient for auxiliary services performed by personnel who are not supervised by clinic physicians, such services are not incident to a physician's service.

100-2, 15, 70

Sleep Disorder Clinics

B3-2055

Sleep disorder clinics are facilities in which certain conditions are diagnosed through the study of sleep. Such clinics are for diagnosis, therapy, and research. Sleep disorder clinics may provide some diagnostic or therapeutic services which are covered under Medicare. These clinics may be affiliated either with a hospital or a freestanding facility. Whether a clinic is hospital-affiliated or freestanding, coverage for diagnostic services under some circumstances is covered under provisions of the law different from those for coverage of therapeutic services.

A. Criteria for Coverage of Diagnostic Tests

- All reasonable and necessary diagnostic tests given for the medical conditions listed in subsection B are covered when the following criteria are met:
- The clinic is either affiliated with a hospital or is under the direction and control of physicians. Diagnostic testing routinely performed in sleep disorder clinics may be covered even in the absence of direct supervision by a physician;

- Patients are referred to the sleep disorder clinic by their attending physicians, and the clinic maintains a record of the attending physician's orders; and
- The need for diagnostic testing is confirmed by medical evidence, e.g., physician examinations and laboratory tests. Diagnostic testing that is duplicative of previous testing done by the attending physician to the extent the results are still pertinent is not covered because it is not reasonable and necessary under §1862(a)(1)(A) of the Act.

B. Medical Conditions for Which Testing is Covered

Diagnostic testing is covered only if the patient has the symptoms or complaints of one of the conditions listed below. Most of the patients who undergo the diagnostic testing are not considered inpatients, although they may come to the facility in the evening for testing and then leave after testing is over. The overnight stay is considered an integral part of these tests.

1. Narcolepsy - This term refers to a syndrome that is characterized by abnormal sleep tendencies, e.g., excessive daytime sleepiness or disturbed nocturnal sleep. Related diagnostic testing is covered if the patient has inappropriate sleep episodes or attacks (e.g., while driving, in the middle of a meal, in the middle of a conversation), amnesiac episodes, or continuous disabling drowsiness. The sleep disorder clinic must submit documentation that this condition is severe enough to interfere with the patient's well being and health before Medicare benefits may be provided for diagnostic testing. Ordinarily, a diagnosis of narcolepsy can be confirmed by three sleep naps. If more than three sleep naps are claimed, the carrier will require persuasive medical evidence justifying the medical necessity for the additional test(s). It will use HCPCS procedure codes 95828 and 95805.
2. Sleep Apnea - This is a potentially lethal condition where the patient stops breathing during sleep. Three types of sleep apnea have been described (central, obstructive, and mixed). The nature of the apnea episodes can be documented by appropriate diagnostic testing. Ordinarily, a single polysomnogram and electroencephalogram (EEG) can diagnose sleep apnea. If more than one such testing session is claimed, the carrier will require persuasive medical evidence justifying the medical necessity for the additional tests. It will use HCPCS procedure codes 95807, 95810, and 95822.
3. Impotence - Diagnostic nocturnal penile tumescence testing may be covered, under limited circumstances, to determine whether erectile impotence in men is organic or psychogenic. Although impotence is not a sleep disorder, the nature of the testing requires that it be performed during sleep. The tests ordinarily are covered only where necessary to confirm the treatment to be given (surgical, medical, or psychotherapeutic). Ordinarily, a diagnosis may be determined by two nights of diagnostic testing. If more than two nights of testing are claimed, the carrier will require persuasive medical evidence justifying the medical necessity for the additional tests. It will have its medical staff review questionable cases to ensure that the tests are reasonable and necessary for the individual. It will use HCPCS procedure code 54250. (See the Medicare National Coverage Determinations Manual, Chapter 1, for policy on coverage of diagnosis and treatment of impotence.)
4. Parasomnia- Parasomnias are a group of conditions that represent undesirable or unpleasant occurrences during sleep. Behavior during these times can often lead to damage to the surroundings and injury to the patient or to others. Parasomnia may include conditions such as sleepwalking, sleep terrors, and rapid eye movement (REM) sleep behavior disorders. In many of these cases, the nature of these conditions may be established by careful clinical evaluation. Suspected seizure disorders as possible cause of the parasomnia are appropriately evaluated by standard or prolonged sleep EEG studies. In cases where seizure disorders have been ruled out and in cases that present a history of repeated violent or injurious episodes during sleep, polysomnography may be useful in providing a diagnostic classification or prognosis. The carrier must use HCPCS procedure codes 95807, 95810, and/or 95822.

C. Polysomnography for Chronic Insomnia Is Not Covered. Evidence at the present time is not convincing that polysomnography in a sleep disorder clinic for chronic insomnia provides definitive diagnostic data or that such information is useful in patient treatment or is associated with improved clinical outcome. The use of polysomnography for diagnosis of patients with chronic insomnia is not covered under Medicare because it is not reasonable and necessary under §1862(a)(1)(A) of the Act.

D. Coverage of Therapeutic Services. Sleep disorder clinics may at times render therapeutic as well as diagnostic services. Therapeutic services may be covered in a hospital outpatient setting or in a freestanding facility provided they meet the pertinent requirements for the particular type of services and are reasonable and necessary for the patient, and are performed under the direct supervision of a physician.

100-2, 15, 80

Requirements for Diagnostic X-Ray, Diagnostic Laboratory, and Other Diagnostic Tests

This section describes the levels of physician supervision required for furnishing the technical component of diagnostic tests for a Medicare beneficiary who is not a hospital inpatient. For hospital outpatient diagnostic services, the supervision levels assigned to each CPT or Level II HCPCS code in the Medicare Physician Fee Schedule Relative Value File that is updated quarterly, apply as described below. For more information, see Chapter 6 (Hospital Services Covered Under Part B), Sec.20.4 (Outpatient Diagnostic Services).

Section 410.32(b) of the Code of Federal Regulations (CFR) requires that diagnostic tests covered under Sec.1861(s)(3) of the Act and payable under the physician fee schedule, with certain exceptions listed in the regulation, have to be performed under the supervision of an individual meeting the definition of a physician (Sec.1861(r) of the Act) to be considered reasonable and necessary and, therefore, covered under Medicare. The regulation defines these levels of physician supervision for diagnostic tests as follows:

General Supervision - means the procedure is furnished under the physician's overall direction and control, but the physician's presence is not required during the performance of the procedure. Under general supervision, the training of the nonphysician personnel who actually performs the diagnostic procedure and the maintenance of the necessary equipment and supplies are the continuing responsibility of the physician.

Direct Supervision - in the office setting means the physician must be present in the office suite and immediately available to furnish assistance and direction throughout the performance of the procedure. It does not mean that the physician must be present in the room when the procedure is performed.

Personal Supervision - means a physician must be in attendance in the room during the performance of the procedure.

One of the following numerical levels is assigned to each CPT or HCPCS code in the Medicare Physician Fee Schedule Database:

0 Procedure is not a diagnostic test or procedure is a diagnostic test which is not subject to the physician supervision policy.

1 Procedure must be performed under the general supervision of a physician.

2 Procedure must be performed under the direct supervision of a physician.

3 Procedure must be performed under the personal supervision of a physician.

4 Physician supervision policy does not apply when procedure is furnished by a qualified, independent psychologist or a clinical psychologist or furnished under the general supervision of a clinical psychologist; otherwise must be performed under the general supervision of a physician.

5 Physician supervision policy does not apply when procedure is furnished by a qualified audiologist; otherwise must be performed under the general supervision of a physician.

6 Procedure must be performed by a physician or by a physical therapist (PT) who is certified by the American Board of Physical Therapy Specialties (ABPTS) as a qualified electrophysiologic clinical specialist and is permitted to provide the procedure under State law.

6a Supervision standards for level 66 apply; in addition, the PT with ABPTS certification may supervise another PT but only the PT with ABPTS certification may bill.

7a Supervision standards for level 77 apply; in addition, the PT with ABPTS certification may supervise another PT but only the PT with ABPTS certification may bill.

9 Concept does not apply.

21 Procedure must be performed by a technician with certification under general supervision of a physician; otherwise must be performed under direct supervision of a physician.

22 Procedure may be performed by a technician with on-line real-time contact with physician.

66 Procedure must be performed by a physician or by a PT with ABPTS certification and certification in this specific procedure.

77 Procedure must be performed by a PT with ABPTS certification or by a PT without certification under direct supervision of a physician, or by a technician with certification under general supervision of a physician.

Nurse practitioners, clinical nurse specialists, and physician assistants are not defined as physicians under Sec.1861(r) of the Act. Therefore, they may not function as supervisory physicians under the diagnostic tests benefit (Sec.1861(s)(3) of the Act). However, when these practitioners personally perform diagnostic tests as provided under Sec.1861(s)(2)(K) of the Act, Sec.1861(s)(3) does not apply and they may perform diagnostic tests pursuant to State scope of practice laws and under the applicable State requirements for physician supervision or collaboration.

Because the diagnostic tests benefit set forth in Sec.1861(s)(3) of the Act is separate and distinct from the incident to benefit set forth in Sec.1861(s)(2) of the Act, diagnostic tests need not meet the incident to requirements. Diagnostic tests may be furnished under situations that meet the incident to requirements but this is not required. However, carriers must not scrutinize claims for diagnostic tests utilizing the incident to requirements.

100-2, 15, 80.1

Clinical Laboratory Services

Section 1833 and 1861 of the Act provides for payment of clinical laboratory services under Medicare Part B. Clinical laboratory services involve the biological, microbiological, serological, chemical, immunohematological, hematological, biophysical, cytological, pathological, or other examination of materials derived from the human body for the diagnosis, prevention, or treatment of a disease or assessment of a medical condition. Laboratory services must meet all applicable requirements of the Clinical Laboratory Improvement Amendments of 1988 (CLIA), as set forth at 42 CFR part 493. Section 1862(a)(1)(A) of the Act provides that Medicare payment may not be made for services that are not reasonable and necessary. Clinical laboratory services must be ordered and used promptly by the physician who is treating the beneficiary as described in 42 CFR 410.32(a), or by a qualified nonphysician practitioner, as described in 42 CFR 410.32(a)(3).

See section 80.6 of this manual for related physician ordering instructions.

See the Medicare Claims Processing Manual Chapter 16 for related claims processing instructions.

100-2, 15, 80.2

Psychological Tests and Neuropsychological Tests

Medicare Part B coverage of psychological tests and neuropsychological tests is authorized under section 1861(s)(3) of the Social Security Act. Payment for psychological and neuropsychological tests is authorized under section 1842(b)(2)(A) of the Social Security Act. The payment amounts for the new psychological and neuropsychological tests (CPT codes 96102, 96103, 96119 and 96120) that are effective January 1, 2006, and are billed for tests administered by a technician or a computer reflect a site of service payment differential for the facility and non-facility settings.

Additionally, there is no authorization for payment for diagnostic tests when performed on an "incident to" basis.

Under the diagnostic tests provision, all diagnostic tests are assigned a certain level of supervision. Generally, regulations governing the diagnostic tests provision require that only physicians can provide the assigned level of supervision for diagnostic tests.

However, there is a regulatory exception to the supervision requirement for diagnostic psychological and neuropsychological tests in terms of who can provide the supervision.

That is, regulations allow a clinical psychologist (CP) or a physician to perform the general supervision assigned to diagnostic psychological and neuropsychological tests.

In addition, nonphysician practitioners such as nurse practitioners (NPs), clinical nurse specialists (CNSs) and physician assistants (PAs) who personally perform diagnostic psychological and neuropsychological tests are excluded from having to perform these tests under the general supervision of a physician or a CP. Rather, NPs and CNSs must perform such tests under the requirements of their respective benefit instead of the requirements for diagnostic psychological and neuropsychological tests. Accordingly, NPs and CNSs must perform tests in collaboration (as defined under Medicare law at section 1861(aa)(6) of the Act) with a physician. PAs perform tests under the general supervision of a physician as required for services furnished under the PA benefit.

Furthermore, physical therapists (PTs), occupational therapists (OTs) and speech language pathologists (SLPs) are authorized to bill three test codes as "sometimes therapy" codes. Specifically, CPT codes 96105, 96110 and 96111 may be performed by these therapists. However, when PTs, OTs and SLPs perform these three tests, they must be performed under the general supervision of a physician or a CP.

(Who May Bill for Diagnostic Psychological and Neuropsychological Tests)

- CPs - see qualifications under chapter 15, section 160 of the Benefits Policy Manual, Pub. 100-02.
- NPs -to the extent authorized under State scope of practice. See qualifications under chapter 15, section 200 of the Benefits Policy Manual, Pub. 100-02.
- CNSs -to the extent authorized under State scope of practice. See qualifications under chapter 15, section 210 of the Benefits Policy Manual, Pub. 100-02.
- PAs - to the extent authorized under State scope of practice. See qualifications under chapter 15, section 190 of the Benefits Policy Manual, Pub. 100-02.
- Independently Practicing Psychologists (IPPs)
- PTs, OTs and SLPs - see qualifications under chapter 15, sections 220-230.6 of the Benefits Policy Manual, Pub. 100-02.

Psychological and neuropsychological tests performed by a psychologist (who is not a CP) practicing independently of an institution, agency, or physician's office are covered when a physician orders such tests. An IPP is any psychologist who is licensed or certified to practice psychology in the State or jurisdiction where furnishing services or, if the jurisdiction does not issue licenses, if provided by any practicing psychologist. (It is CMS' understanding that all States, the District of Columbia, and Puerto Rico license psychologists, but that some trust territories do not. Examples of psychologists, other than CPs, whose psychological and neuropsychological tests are covered under the diagnostic tests provision include, but are not limited to, educational psychologists and counseling psychologists.)

The carrier must secure from the appropriate State agency a current listing of psychologists holding the required credentials to determine whether the tests of a particular IPP are covered under Part B in States that have statutory licensure or certification. In States or territories that lack statutory licensing or certification, the carrier checks individual qualifications before provider numbers are issued. Possible reference sources are the national directory of membership of the American Psychological Association, which provides data about the educational background of individuals and indicates which members are board-certified, the records and directories of the State or territorial psychological association, and the National Register of Health Service Providers. If qualification is dependent on a doctoral degree from a currently accredited program, the carrier verifies the date of accreditation of the school involved, since such accreditation is not retroactive. If the listed reference sources do not provide enough information (e.g., the psychologist is not a member of one of these sources), the carrier contacts the psychologist personally for the required information. Generally, carriers maintain a continuing list of psychologists whose qualifications have been verified.

NOTE: When diagnostic psychological tests are performed by a psychologist who is not practicing independently, but is on the staff of an institution, agency, or clinic, that entity bills for the psychological tests.

The carrier considers psychologists as practicing independently when:

- They render services on their own responsibility, free of the administrative and professional control of an employer such as a physician, institution or agency;
- The persons they treat are their own patients; and
- They have the right to bill directly, collect and retain the fee for their services.

A psychologist practicing in an office located in an institution may be considered an independently practicing psychologist when both of the following conditions exist:

- The office is confined to a separately-identified part of the facility which is used solely as the psychologist's office and cannot be construed as extending throughout the entire institution; and
- The psychologist conducts a private practice, i.e., services are rendered to patients from outside the institution as well as to institutional patients.

(Payment for Diagnostic Psychological and Neuropsychological Tests)

Expenses for diagnostic psychological and neuropsychological tests are not subject to the outpatient mental health treatment limitation, that is, the payment limitation on treatment services for mental, psychoneurotic and personality disorders as authorized under Section 1833(c) of the Act. The payment amount for the new psychological and neuropsychological tests (CPT codes 96102, 96103, 96119 and 96120) that are billed for tests performed by a technician or a computer reflect a site of service payment differential for the facility and non-facility settings. CPs, NPs, CNSs and PAs are required by law to accept assigned payment for psychological and neuropsychological tests. However, while IPPs are not required by law to accept assigned payment for these tests, they must report the name and address of the physician who ordered the test on the claim form when billing for tests.

(CPT Codes for Diagnostic Psychological and Neuropsychological Tests)

The range of CPT codes used to report psychological and neuropsychological tests is 96101-96120. CPT codes 96101, 96102, 96103, 96105, 96110, and 96111 are appropriate for use when billing for psychological tests. CPT codes 96116, 96118, 96119 and 96120 are appropriate for use when billing for neuropsychological tests.

All of the tests under this CPT code range 96101-96120 are indicated as active codes under the physician fee schedule database and are covered if medically necessary.

(Payment and Billing Guidelines for Psychological and Neuropsychological Tests)

The technician and computer CPT codes for psychological and neuropsychological tests include practice expense, malpractice expense and professional work relative value units.

Accordingly, CPT psychological test code 96101 should not be paid when billed for the same tests or services performed under psychological test codes 96102 or 96103. CPT neuropsychological test code 96118 should not be paid when billed for the same tests or services performed under neuropsychological test codes 96119 or 96120. However, CPT codes 96101 and 96118 can be paid separately on the rare occasion when billed on the same date of service for different and separate tests from 96102, 96103, 96119 and 96120.

Under the physician fee schedule, there is no payment for services performed by students or trainees. Accordingly, Medicare does not pay for services represented by CPT codes 96102 and 96119 when performed by a student or a trainee. However, the presence of a student or a trainee while the test is being administered does not prevent a physician, CP, IPP, NP, CNS or PA from performing and being paid for the psychological test under 96102 or the neuropsychological test under 96119.

100-2, 15, 80.3

Audiology Services

References.

1861(ll)(3) of the Social Security Act for the definition of audiology services.

1861(ll)(4)(B) of the Social Security Act for qualifications of audiologists.

42 CFR 410.32(b) for the physician supervision requirements for diagnostic tests.

Pub. 100-04, chapter 12, section 30.3 for coding and billing information related to audiological services and aural rehabilitation.

Pub. 100-02, chapter 15, sections 220 and 230 for the physical therapy and speech-language pathology policies relative to aural rehabilitation and balance, section 60 for services incident to a physician's service, and section 80.6 for policies relevant to ordering for diagnostic tests.

Pub. 100-02, chapter 16, section 100 for hearing aid policies.

A list of audiology service codes is found at: http://www.cms.gov/PhysicianFeeSched/50_Audiology.asp.

A. Benefit.

Hearing and balance assessment services are generally covered as "other diagnostic tests" under section 1861(s)(3) of the Social Security Act. Hearing and balance

Appendix G — Pub 100 References

assessment services furnished to an outpatient of a hospital are covered as "diagnostic services" under section 1861(s)(2)(C).

As defined in the Social Security Act, section 1861(ll)(3), the term "audiology services" specifically means such hearing and balance assessment services furnished by a qualified audiologist as the audiologist is legally authorized to perform under State law (or the State regulatory mechanism provided by State law), as would otherwise be covered if furnished by a physician.

Herein after in this section, hearing and balance assessment services are termed "audiology services," regardless of whether they are furnished by an audiologist, physician, nonphysician practitioner (NPP), or hospital.

Because audiology services are diagnostic tests, when furnished by a physician in an office or hospital outpatient department, they must be furnished under the appropriate level of supervision of a physician as established in 42 CFR 410.32(b)(1) and 410.28(e). However, as specified in 42 CFR 410.32(b)(2)(ii) or (v), respectively, they are excepted from physician supervision when they are personally furnished by a qualified audiologist or performed by a nurse practitioner or clinical nurse specialist authorized to perform the tests under applicable State laws.

Audiological diagnostic testing refers to tests of the audiological and vestibular systems, e.g., hearing, balance, auditory processing, tinnitus and diagnostic programming of certain prosthetic devices, performed by qualified audiologists.

Audiological diagnostic tests are not covered under the benefit for services incident to a physician's service (described in Pub. 100-02, chapter 15, section 60), because they have their own benefit as "other diagnostic tests". See Pub. 100-04, chapter 13 for general diagnostic test policies.

Audiology services, like all other services, should be reported under the most specific HCPCS code that describes the service that was furnished and in accordance with all CPT guidance and Medicare national and local contractor instructions.

B. Orders.

Audiology tests are covered as "other diagnostic tests" under section 1861(s)(3) or 1861(s)(2)(C) of the Act in the physician's office or hospital outpatient settings, respectively, when a physician (or an NPP, as applicable) orders such testing for the purpose of obtaining information necessary for the physician's diagnostic medical evaluation or to determine the appropriate medical or surgical treatment of a hearing deficit or related medical problem. See section 80.6 of this chapter for policies regarding the ordering of diagnostic tests.

If a beneficiary undergoes diagnostic testing performed by an audiologist without a physician order, the tests are not covered even if the audiologist discovers a pathologic condition.

When a qualified physician orders a qualified technician (see definition in subsection D of this section) to furnish an appropriate audiology service, that order must specify which test is to be furnished by the technician under the direct supervision of a physician. Only that test may be provided on that order by the technician.

When the qualified physician or NPP orders diagnostic audiology services furnished by an audiologist without naming specific tests, the audiologist may select the appropriate battery of tests.

C. Coverage and Payment for Audiology Services.

Diagnostic services furnished by a qualified audiologist meeting the requirements in section 80.3.1 of this chapter or physicians and NPPs as described in section 80.6 are covered and payable under the MPFS as "other diagnostic tests."

Services furnished in a hospital outpatient department are covered and payable under the hospital Outpatient Prospective Payment System (OPPS) or other payment methodology applicable to the provider furnishing the services.

Coverage and, therefore, payment for audiological diagnostic tests is determined by the reason the tests were performed, rather than by the diagnosis or the patient's condition.

Under any Medicare payment system, payment for audiological diagnostic tests is not allowed by virtue of their exclusion from coverage in section 1862(a)(7) of the Social Security Act when:

The type and severity of the current hearing, tinnitus or balance status needed to determine the appropriate medical or surgical treatment is known to the physician before the test; or

The test was ordered for the specific purpose of fitting or modifying a hearing aid.

Payment of audiological diagnostic tests is allowed for other reasons and is not limited, for example, by:

- Any information resulting from the test, for example:
- Confirmation of a prior diagnosis;
- Post-evaluation diagnoses; or
- Treatment provided after diagnosis, including hearing aids, or
- The type of evaluation or treatment the physician anticipates before the diagnostic test; or
- Timing of reevaluation. Reevaluation is appropriate at a schedule dictated by the ordering physician when the information provided by the diagnostic test is required, for example, to determine changes in hearing, to evaluate the appropriate medical or surgical treatment or to evaluate the results of treatment. For example, reevaluation may be appropriate, even when the evaluation was recent, in cases where the hearing loss, balance, or tinnitus may be progressive or fluctuating, the patient or caregiver complains of new symptoms, or treatment (such as medication or surgery) may have changed the patient's audiological condition with or without awareness by the patient.

Examples of appropriate reasons for ordering audiological diagnostic tests that could be covered include, but are not limited to:

- Evaluation of suspected change in hearing, tinnitus, or balance; Evaluation of the cause of disorders of hearing, tinnitus, or balance;
- Determination of the effect of medication, surgery, or other treatment; Reevaluation to follow-up changes in hearing, tinnitus, or balance that may be caused by established diagnoses that place the patient at probable risk for a change in status including, but not limited to: otosclerosis, atelectatic tympanic membrane, tympanosclerosis, cholesteatoma, resolving middle ear infection, MeniÐ©re's disease, sudden idiopathic sensorineural hearing loss, autoimmune inner ear disease, acoustic neuroma, demyelinating diseases, ototoxicity secondary to medications, or genetic vascular and viral conditions; Failure of a screening test (although the screening test is not covered);
- Diagnostic analysis of cochlear or brainstem implant and programming; and
- Audiology diagnostic tests before and periodically after implantation of auditory prosthetic devices.

If a physician refers a beneficiary to an audiologist for testing related to signs or symptoms associated with hearing loss, balance disorder, tinnitus, ear disease, or ear injury, the audiologist's diagnostic testing services should be covered even if the only outcome is the prescription of a hearing aid.

D. Individuals Who Furnish Audiology Tests.

1. Qualified Professionals. See section 80.3.1 of this chapter for the qualifications of audiologists. See section 80.6 of this chapter for the qualifications of physicians and NPPs who may furnish diagnostic tests.
2. Qualified Technicians or Other Qualified Staff. References to technicians in this section include other qualified clinical staff. The qualifications for technicians vary locally and may also depend on the type of test, the patient, and the level of participation of the physician who is directly supervising the test. Therefore, an individual must meet qualifications appropriate to the service furnished as determined by the contractor to whom the claim is billed. If it is necessary to determine whether the individual who furnished the labor for appropriate audiology services is qualified, contractors may request verification of any relevant education and training that has been completed by the technician, which shall be available in the records of the clinic or facility.

Depending on the qualifications determined by the contractor, individuals who are also hearing instrument specialists, students of audiology, or other health care professionals may furnish the labor for appropriate audiology services under direct physician supervision when these services are billed by physicians or hospital outpatient departments.

E. Documentation for Audiology Services.

1. Documentation for Orders (Reasons for Tests).

   The reason for the test should be documented either on the order, on the audiological evaluation report, or in the patient's medical record. (See subsection C. of this section concerning reasons for tests.)
2. Documenting skilled services. When the medical record is subject to medical review, it is necessary that the record contains sufficient information so that the contractor may determine that the service qualifies for payment. For example, documentation should indicate that the test was ordered, that the reason for the test results in coverage, and that the test was furnished to the patient by a qualified individual.

   Records that support the appropriate provision of an audiological diagnostic test shall be made available to the contractor on request.

F. Audiological Treatment.

There is no provision in the law for Medicare to pay audiologists for therapeutic services. For example, vestibular treatment, auditory rehabilitation treatment, auditory processing treatment, and canalith repositioning, while they are generally within the scope of practice of audiologists, are not those hearing and balance assessment services that are defined as audiology services in 1861(ll)(3) of the Social Security Act and, therefore, shall not be billed by audiologists to Medicare. Services for the purpose of hearing aid evaluation and fitting are not covered regardless of how they are billed. Services identified as "always" therapy in Pub. 100-04, chapter 5, section 20 may not be billed by hospitals, physicians, NPPs, or audiologists when provided by audiologists. (See also Pub. 100-04, chapter 12, section 30.3.)

Treatment related to hearing may be covered under the speech-language pathology benefit when the services are provided by speech-language pathologists. Treatment related to balance (e.g., services described by "always therapy" codes 97001-97004, 97110, 97112, 97116, and 97750) may be covered under the physical therapy or occupational therapy benefit when the services are provided by therapists or their assistants, where appropriate. Covered therapy services incident to a physician's service must conform to policies in sections 60, 220, and 230 of this chapter. Audiological treatment provided under the benefits for physical therapy and speech-language pathology services may also be personally provided and billed by physicians and NPPs when the services are within their scope of practice and consistent with State and local laws.

For example, aural rehabilitation and signed communication training may be payable according to the benefit for speech-language pathology services or as speech-language pathology services incident to a physician's or NPP's service. Treatment for balance disorders may be payable according to the benefit for physical therapy services or as a physical therapy service incident to the services of a physician or NPP. See the policies in this chapter, sections 220 and 230, for details.

G. Assignment.
Nonhospital entities billing for the audiologist's services may accept assignment under the usual procedure or, if not accepting assignment, may charge the patient and submit a nonassigned claim on their behalf.

H. Opt Out and Mandatory Claims Submissions.
The opt out law does not define "physician" or "practitioner" to include audiologists; therefore, they may not opt out of Medicare and provide services under private contracts. See section 40.4 of this chapter for details.

When a physician or supplier furnishes a service that is covered by Medicare, then it is subject to the mandatory claim submission provisions of section 1848(g)(4) of the Social Security Act. Therefore, if an audiologist charges or attempts to charge a beneficiary any remuneration for a service that is covered by Medicare, then the audiologist must submit a claim to Medicare.

I. Non-Audiology Services Furnished by Audiologists.
Audiologists may be qualified to furnish all or part of some diagnostic tests or treatments that are not defined as audiology services under the MPFS, such as non-auditory evoked potentials or cerumen removal. Audiologists may not bill Medicare for services that are not audiology services according to Medicare's definition (see list at: http://www.cms.gov/PhysicianFeeSched/50_ Audiology.asp). However, the labor for the Technical Component (TC) of certain other diagnostic tests or treatment services may qualify to be billed when furnished by audiologists under physician supervision when all the appropriate policies are followed.

When furnishing services that are not on the Medicare list of audiology services, the audiologist may or may not be working within the scope of practice of an audiologist according to State law. The audiologist furnishing the service must have the qualifications that are ordinarily required of any person providing that service. Consult the following policies for details:

Policies for physical therapy, occupational therapy, and speech-language pathology services are in sections 220 and 230 of this chapter and in Pub. 100-04, chapter 5, sections 10 and 20. Policies for services furnished incident to physicians' services in the physician's office are in section 60 of this chapter.

Policies for therapeutic services furnished incident to physicians' services in the hospital outpatient setting are in chapter 6, section 20.5, of this manual. Policies for diagnostic tests in the physician's office are in section 80 of this chapter. Policies for diagnostic tests furnished in the hospital outpatient setting are in chapter 6, section 20.4, of this manual. Therapeutic or treatment services that are not audiology services and are not "always" therapy (according to the policy in Pub.100-04, chapter 5, section 20) and are furnished by audiologists may be billed incident to the services of a physician when all other appropriate requirements are met.

In addition, the TC or facility services for diagnostic tests that are not audiology services may be billed by physicians or hospital outpatient departments when provided by qualified personnel (who may be audiologists), and physicians and hospital outpatient departments may bill for these diagnostic tests when provided by those qualified personnel under the specified level of physician supervision for the diagnostic test

100-2, 15, 80.5.4

Conditions for Coverage

Medicare covers BMM under the following conditions:

1. Is ordered by the physician or qualified nonphysician practitioner who is treating the beneficiary following an evaluation of the need for a BMM and determination of the appropriate BMM to be used. A physician or qualified nonphysician practitioner treating the beneficiary for purposes of this provision is one who furnishes a consultation or treats a beneficiary for a specific medical problem, and who uses the results in the management of the patient. For the purposes of the BMM benefit, qualified nonphysician practitioners include physician assistants, nurse practitioners, clinical nurse specialists, and certified nurse midwives.
2. Is performed under the appropriate level of physician supervision as defined in 42 CFR 410.32(b).
3. Is reasonable and necessary for diagnosing and treating the condition of a beneficiary who meets the conditions described in Sec.80.5.6.
4. In the case of an individual being monitored to assess the response to or efficacy of an FDA-approved osteoporosis drug therapy, is performed with a dual-energy x-ray absorptiometry system (axial skeleton).
5. In the case of any individual who meets the conditions of 80.5.6 and who has a confirmatory BMM, is performed by a dual-energy x-ray absorptiometry system (axial skeleton) if the initial BMM was not performed by a dual-energy x-ray absorptiometry system (axial skeleton). A confirmatory baseline BMM is not covered if the initial BMM was performed by a dual-energy x-ray absorptiometry system (axial skeleton).

100-2, 15, 80.5.5

Frequency Standards

Medicare pays for a screening BMM once every 2 years (at least 23 months have passed since the month the last covered BMM was performed).

When medically necessary, Medicare may pay for more frequent BMMs. Examples include, but are not limited to, the following medical circumstances:

- Monitoring beneficiaries on long-term glucocorticoid (steroid) therapy of more than 3 months.
- Confirming baseline BMMs to permit monitoring of beneficiaries in the future.

100-2, 15, 80.5.6

Beneficiaries Who May be Covered

To be covered, a beneficiary must meet at least one of the five conditions listed below:

1. A woman who has been determined by the physician or qualified nonphysician practitioner treating her to be estrogen-deficient and at clinical risk for osteoporosis, based on her medical history and other findings.

   NOTE: Since not every woman who has been prescribed estrogen replacement therapy (ERT) may be receiving an "adequate" dose of the therapy, the fact that a woman is receiving ERT should not preclude her treating physician or other qualified treating nonphysician practitioner from ordering a bone mass measurement for her. If a BMM is ordered for a woman following a careful evaluation of her medical need, however, it is expected that the ordering treating physician (or other qualified treating nonphysician practitioner) will document in her medical record why he or she believes that the woman is estrogen-deficient and at clinical risk for osteoporosis.
2. An individual with vertebral abnormalities as demonstrated by an x-ray to be indicative of osteoporosis, osteopenia, or vertebral fracture.
3. An individual receiving (or expecting to receive) glucocorticoid (steroid) therapy equivalent to an average of 5.0 mg of prednisone, or greater, per day, for more than 3 months.
4. An individual with primary hyperparathyroidism.
5. An individual being monitored to assess the response to or efficacy of an FDA-approved osteoporosis drug therapy.

100-2, 15, 100

Surgical Dressings, Splints, Casts, and Other Devices Used for Reductions of Fractures and Dislocations

B3-2079, A3-3110.3, HO-228.3

Surgical dressings are limited to primary and secondary dressings required for the treatment of a wound caused by, or treated by, a surgical procedure that has been performed by a physician or other health care professional to the extent permissible under State law. In addition, surgical dressings required after debridement of a wound are also covered, irrespective of the type of debridement, as long as the debridement was reasonable and necessary and was performed by a health care professional acting within the scope of his/her legal authority when performing this function. Surgical dressings are covered for as long as they are medically necessary.

Primary dressings are therapeutic or protective coverings applied directly to wounds or lesions either on the skin or caused by an opening to the skin. Secondary dressing materials that serve a therapeutic or protective function and that are needed to secure a primary dressing are also covered. Items such as adhesive tape, roll gauze, bandages, and disposable compression material are examples of secondary dressings. Elastic stockings, support hose, foot coverings, leotards, knee supports, surgical leggings, gauntlets, and pressure garments for the arms and hands are examples of items that are not ordinarily covered as surgical dressings. Some items, such as transparent film, may be used as a primary or secondary dressing.

If a physician, certified nurse midwife, physician assistant, nurse practitioner, or clinical nurse specialist applies surgical dressings as part of a professional service that is billed to Medicare, the surgical dressings are considered incident to the professional services of the health care practitioner. (See Sec. 60.1, 180, 190, 200, and 210.) When surgical dressings are not covered incident to the services of a health care practitioner and are obtained by the patient from a supplier (e.g., a drugstore, physician, or other health care practitioner that qualifies as a supplier) on an order from a physician or other health care professional authorized under State law or regulation to make such an order, the surgical dressings are covered separately under Part B.

Splints and casts, and other devices used for reductions of fractures and dislocations are covered under Part B of Medicare. This includes dental splints.

100-2, 15, 120

Prosthetic Devices

B3-2130, A3-3110.4, HO-228.4, A3-3111, HO-229

A. General
Prosthetic devices (other than dental) which replace all or part of an internal body organ (including contiguous tissue), or replace all or part of the function of a permanently inoperative or malfunctioning internal body organ are covered when furnished on a physician's order. This does not require a determination that there is no possibility that the patient's condition may improve sometime in the future. If the medical record, including the judgment of the attending physician, indicates the condition is of long and indefinite duration, the test of permanence is considered

met. (Such a device may also be covered under Sec.60.l as a supply when furnished incident to a physician's service.)

Examples of prosthetic devices include artificial limbs, parenteral and enteral (PEN) nutrition, cardiac pacemakers, prosthetic lenses (see subsection B), breast prostheses (including a surgical brassiere) for postmastectomy patients, maxillofacial devices, and devices which replace all or part of the ear or nose. A urinary collection and retention system with or without a tube is a prosthetic device replacing bladder function in case of permanent urinary incontinence. The foley catheter is also considered a prosthetic device when ordered for a patient with permanent urinary incontinence. However, chucks, diapers, rubber sheets, etc., are supplies that are not covered under this provision. Although hemodialysis equipment is a prosthetic device, payment for the rental or purchase of such equipment in the home is made only for use under the provisions for payment applicable to durable medical equipment.

An exception is that if payment cannot be made on an inpatient's behalf under Part A, hemodialysis equipment, supplies, and services required by such patient could be covered under Part B as a prosthetic device, which replaces the function of a kidney. See the Medicare Benefit Policy Manual, Chapter 11, "End Stage Renal Disease," for payment for hemodialysis equipment used in the home. See the Medicare Benefit Policy Manual, Chapter 1, "Inpatient Hospital Services," Sec.10, for additional instructions on hospitalization for renal dialysis.

NOTE: Medicare does not cover a prosthetic device dispensed to a patient prior to the time at which the patient undergoes the procedure that makes necessary the use of the device. For example, the carrier does not make a separate Part B payment for an intraocular lens (IOL) or pacemaker that a physician, during an office visit prior to the actual surgery, dispenses to the patient for his or her use. Dispensing a prosthetic device in this manner raises health and safety issues. Moreover, the need for the device cannot be clearly established until the procedure that makes its use possible is successfully performed. Therefore, dispensing a prosthetic device in this manner is not considered reasonable and necessary for the treatment of the patient's condition.

Colostomy (and other ostomy) bags and necessary accouterments required for attachment are covered as prosthetic devices. This coverage also includes irrigation and flushing equipment and other items and supplies directly related to ostomy care, whether the attachment of a bag is required. Accessories and/or supplies which are used directly with an enteral or parenteral device to achieve the therapeutic benefit of the prosthesis or to assure the proper functioning of the device may also be covered under the prosthetic device benefit subject to the additional guidelines in the Medicare National Coverage Determinations Manual.

Covered items include catheters, filters, extension tubing, infusion bottles, pumps (either food or infusion), intravenous (I.V.) pole, needles, syringes, dressings, tape, Heparin Sodium (parenteral only), volumetric monitors (parenteral only), and parenteral and enteral nutrient solutions. Baby food and other regular grocery products that can be blenderized and used with the enteral system are not covered. Note that some of these items, e.g., a food pump and an I.V. pole, qualify as DME. Although coverage of the enteral and parenteral nutritional therapy systems is provided on the basis of the prosthetic device benefit, the payment rules relating to lump sum or monthly payment for DME apply to such items.

The coverage of prosthetic devices includes replacement of and repairs to such devices as explained in subsection D.

Finally, the Benefits Improvement and Protection Act of 2000 amended Sec.1834(h)(1) of the Act by adding a provision (1834 (h)(1)(G)(i)) that requires Medicare payment to be made for the replacement of prosthetic devices which are artificial limbs, or for the replacement of any part of such devices, without regard to continuous use or useful lifetime restrictions if an ordering physician determines that the replacement device, or replacement part of such a device, is necessary.

Payment may be made for the replacement of a prosthetic device that is an artificial limb, or replacement part of a device if the ordering physician determines that the replacement device or part is necessary because of any of the following:

1. A change in the physiological condition of the patient;
2. An irreparable change in the condition of the device, or in a part of the device; or
3. The condition of the device, or the part of the device, requires repairs and the cost of such repairs would be more than 60 percent of the cost of a replacement device, or, as the case may be, of the part being replaced.

This provision is effective for items replaced on or after April 1, 2001. It supersedes any rule that that provided a 5-year or other replacement rule with regard to prosthetic devices.

B. Prosthetic Lenses

The term "internal body organ" includes the lens of an eye. Prostheses replacing the lens of an eye include post-surgical lenses customarily used during convalescence from eye surgery in which the lens of the eye was removed. In addition, permanent lenses are also covered when required by an individual lacking the organic lens of the eye because of surgical removal or congenital absence. Prosthetic lenses obtained on or after the beneficiary's date of entitlement to supplementary medical insurance benefits may be covered even though the surgical removal of the crystalline lens occurred before entitlement.

1. Prosthetic Cataract Lenses
   One of the following prosthetic lenses or combinations of prosthetic lenses furnished by a physician (see Sec.30.4 for coverage of prosthetic lenses prescribed by a doctor of optometry) may be covered when determined to be reasonable and necessary to restore essentially the vision provided by the crystalline lens of the eye:
   - Prosthetic bifocal lenses in frames;
   - Prosthetic lenses in frames for far vision, and prosthetic lenses in frames for near vision; or
   - When a prosthetic contact lens(es) for far vision is prescribed (including cases of binocular and monocular aphakia), make payment for the contact lens(es) and prosthetic lenses in frames for near vision to be worn at the same time as the contact lens(es), and prosthetic lenses in frames to be worn when the contacts have been removed.

   Lenses which have ultraviolet absorbing or reflecting properties may be covered, in lieu of payment for regular (untinted) lenses, if it has been determined that such lenses are medically reasonable and necessary for the individual patient.

   Medicare does not cover cataract sunglasses obtained in addition to the regular (untinted) prosthetic lenses since the sunglasses duplicate the restoration of vision function performed by the regular prosthetic lenses.
2. Payment for Intraocular Lenses (IOLs) Furnished in Ambulatory Surgical Centers (ASCs) Effective for services furnished on or after March 12, 1990, payment for intraocular lenses (IOLs) inserted during or subsequent to cataract surgery in a Medicare certified ASC is included with the payment for facility services that are furnished in connection with the covered surgery.

   Refer to the Medicare Claims Processing Manual, Chapter 14, "Ambulatory Surgical Centers," for more information.
3. Limitation on Coverage of Conventional Lenses One pair of conventional eyeglasses or conventional contact lenses furnished after each cataract surgery with insertion of an IOL is covered.

C. Dentures

Dentures are excluded from coverage. However, when a denture or a portion of the denture is an integral part (built-in) of a covered prosthesis (e.g., an obturator to fill an opening in the palate), it is covered as part of that prosthesis.

D. Supplies, Repairs, Adjustments, and Replacement

Supplies are covered that are necessary for the effective use of a prosthetic device (e.g., the batteries needed to operate an artificial larynx). Adjustment of prosthetic devices required by wear or by a change in the patient's condition is covered when ordered by a physician. General provisions relating to the repair and replacement of durable medical equipment in Sec.110.2 for the repair and replacement of prosthetic devices are applicable. (See the Medicare Benefit Policy Manual, Chapter 16, "General Exclusions from Coverage," Sec.40.4, for payment for devices replaced under a warranty.) Replacement of conventional eyeglasses or contact lenses furnished in accordance with Sec.120.B.3 is not covered. Necessary supplies, adjustments, repairs, and replacements are covered even when the device had been in use before the user enrolled in Part B of the program, so long as the device continues to be medically required.

100-2, 15, 150

Dental Services

B3-2136

As indicated under the general exclusions from coverage, items and services in connection with the care, treatment, filling, removal, or replacement of teeth or structures directly supporting the teeth are not covered. "Structures directly supporting the teeth" means the periodontium, which includes the gingivae, dentogingival junction, periodontal membrane, cementum of the teeth, and alveolar process.

In addition to the following, see Pub 100-01, the Medicare General Information, Eligibility, and Entitlement Manual, Chapter 5, Definitions and Pub 3, the Medicare National Coverage Determinations Manual for specific services which may be covered when furnished by a dentist. If an otherwise noncovered procedure or service is performed by a dentist as incident to and as an integral part of a covered procedure or service performed by the dentist, the total service performed by the dentist on such an occasion is covered.

EXAMPLE 1: The reconstruction of a ridge performed primarily to prepare the mouth for dentures is a noncovered procedure. However, when the reconstruction of a ridge is performed as a result of and at the same time as the surgical removal of a tumor (for other than dental purposes), the totality of surgical procedures is a covered service.

EXAMPLE 2: Medicare makes payment for the wiring of teeth when this is done in connection with the reduction of a jaw fracture.

The extraction of teeth to prepare the jaw for radiation treatment of neoplastic disease is also covered. This is an exception to the requirement that to be covered, a noncovered procedure or service performed by a dentist must be an incident to and an integral part of a covered procedure or service performed by the dentist. Ordinarily, the dentist extracts the patient's teeth, but another physician, e.g., a radiologist, administers the radiation treatments.

When an excluded service is the primary procedure involved, it is not covered, regardless of its complexity or difficulty. For example, the extraction of an impacted tooth is not covered. Similarly, an alveoplasty (the surgical improvement of the shape and condition of the alveolar process) and a frenectomy are excluded from coverage when either of these procedures is performed in connection with an excluded service, e.g., the preparation of the mouth for dentures. In a like manner, the removal of a torus palatinus (a bony protuberance of the hard palate) may be a covered service. However, with rare exception, this surgery is performed in connection with an excluded service, i.e., the preparation of the mouth for dentures. Under such circumstances, Medicare does not pay for this procedure.

Dental splints used to treat a dental condition are excluded from coverage under 1862(a)(12) of the Act. On the other hand, if the treatment is determined to be a covered medical condition (i.e., dislocated upper/lower jaw joints), then the splint can be covered.

Whether such services as the administration of anesthesia, diagnostic x-rays, and other related procedures are covered depends upon whether the primary procedure being performed by the dentist is itself covered. Thus, an x-ray taken in connection with the reduction of a fracture of the jaw or facial bone is covered. However, a single x-ray or x-ray survey taken in connection with the care or treatment of teeth or the periodontium is not covered.

Medicare makes payment for a covered dental procedure no matter where the service is performed. The hospitalization or nonhospitalization of a patient has no direct bearing on the coverage or exclusion of a given dental procedure.

Payment may also be made for services and supplies furnished incident to covered dental services. For example, the services of a dental technician or nurse who is under the direct supervision of the dentist or physician are covered if the services are included in the dentist's or physician's bill.

100-2, 15, 160

Clinical Psychologist Services

A. Clinical Psychologist (CP) Defined

To qualify as a clinical psychologist (CP), a practitioner must meet the following requirements:

- Hold a doctoral degree in psychology;
- Be licensed or certified, on the basis of the doctoral degree in psychology, by the State in which he or she practices, at the independent practice level of psychology to furnish diagnostic, assessment, preventive, and therapeutic services directly to individuals.

B. Qualified Clinical Psychologist Services Defined

Effective July 1, 1990, the diagnostic and therapeutic services of CPs and services and supplies furnished incident to such services are covered as the services furnished by a physician or as incident to physician's services are covered. However, the CP must be legally authorized to perform the services under applicable licensure laws of the State in which they are furnished.

C. Types of Clinical Psychologist Services That May Be Covered

Diagnostic and therapeutic services that the CP is legally authorized to perform in accordance with State law and/or regulation. Carriers pay all qualified CPs based on the physician fee schedule for the diagnostic and therapeutic services. (Psychological tests by practitioners who do not meet the requirements for a CP may be covered under the provisions for diagnostic tests as described in Sec.80.2.

Services and supplies furnished incident to a CP's services are covered if the requirements that apply to services incident to a physician's services, as described in Sec.60 are met. These services must be:

- Mental health services that are commonly furnished in CPs' offices;
- An integral, although incidental, part of professional services performed by the CP;
- Performed under the direct personal supervision of the CP; i.e., the CP must be physically present and immediately available;
- Furnished without charge or included in the CP's bill; and
- Performed by an employee of the CP (or an employee of the legal entity that employs the supervising CP) under the common law control test of the Act, as set forth in 20 CFR 404.1007 and Sec.RS 2101.020 of the Retirement and Survivors Insurance part of the Social Security Program Operations Manual System.
- Diagnostic psychological testing services when furnished under the general supervision of a CP.

Carriers are required to familiarize themselves with appropriate State laws and/or regulations governing a CP's scope of practice.

D. Noncovered Services

The services of CPs are not covered if the service is otherwise excluded from Medicare coverage even though a clinical psychologist is authorized by State law to perform them.

For example, Sec.1862(a)(1)(A) of the Act excludes from coverage services that are not "reasonable and necessary for the diagnosis or treatment of an illness or injury or to improve the functioning of a malformed body member." Therefore, even though the services are authorized by State law, the services of a CP that are determined to be not reasonable and necessary are not covered. Additionally, any therapeutic services that are billed by CPs under CPT psychotherapy codes that include medical evaluation and management services are not covered.

E. Requirement for Consultation

When applying for a Medicare provider number, a CP must submit to the carrier a signed Medicare provider/supplier enrollment form that indicates an agreement to the effect that, contingent upon the patient's consent, the CP will attempt to consult with the patient's attending or primary care physician in accordance with accepted professional ethical norms, taking into consideration patient confidentiality.

If the patient assents to the consultation, the CP must attempt to consult with the patient's physician within a reasonable time after receiving the consent. If the CP's attempts to consult directly with the physician are not successful, the CP must notify the physician within a reasonable time that he or she is furnishing services to the patient. Additionally, the CP must document, in the patient's medical record, the date the patient consented or declined consent to consultations, the date of consultation, or, if attempts to consult did not succeed, that date and manner of notification to the physician.

The only exception to the consultation requirement for CPs is in cases where the patient's primary care or attending physician refers the patient to the CP. Also, neither a CP nor a primary care nor attending physician may bill Medicare or the patient for this required consultation.

F. Outpatient Mental Health Services Limitation

All covered therapeutic services furnished by qualified CPs are subject to the outpatient mental health services limitation in Pub 100-01, Medicare General Information, Eligibility, and Entitlement Manual, Chapter 3, "Deductibles, Coinsurance Amounts, and Payment Limitations," Sec.30, (i.e., only 62 1/2 percent of expenses for these services are considered incurred expenses for Medicare purposes). The limitation does not apply to diagnostic services.

G. Assignment Requirement

Assignment Sec. required.

100-2, 15, 170

Clinical Social Worker (CSW) Services

B3-2152

See the Medicare Claims Processing Manual Chapter 12, Physician/Nonphysician Practitioners, Sec.150, "Clinical Social Worker Services," for payment requirements.

A. Clinical Social Worker Defined

Section 1861(hh) of the Act defines a "clinical social worker" as an individual who:

- Possesses a master's or doctor's degree in social work;
- Has performed at least two years of supervised clinical social work; and
- Is licensed or certified as a clinical social worker by the State in which the services are performed; or
- In the case of an individual in a State that does not provide for licensure or certification, has completed at least 2 years or 3,000 hours of post master's degree supervised clinical social work practice under the supervision of a master's level social worker in an appropriate setting such as a hospital, SNF, or clinic.

B. Clinical Social Worker Services Defined

Section 1861(hh)(2) of the Act defines "clinical social worker services" as those services that the CSW is legally authorized to perform under State law (or the State regulatory mechanism provided by State law) of the State in which such services are performed for the diagnosis and treatment of mental illnesses. Services furnished to an inpatient of a hospital or an inpatient of a SNF that the SNF is required to provide as a requirement for participation are not included. The services that are covered are those that are otherwise covered if furnished by a physician or as incident to a physician's professional service.

C. Covered Services

Coverage is limited to the services a CSW is legally authorized to perform in accordance with State law (or State regulatory mechanism established by State law). The services of a CSW may be covered under Part B if they are:

- The type of services that are otherwise covered if furnished by a physician, or as incident to a physician's service. (See Sec.30 for a description of physicians' services and Sec.70 of Pub 100-1, the Medicare General Information, Eligibility, and Entitlement Manual, Chapter 5, for the definition of a physician.);
- Performed by a person who meets the definition of a CSW (See subsection A.); and
- Not otherwise excluded from coverage. Carriers should become familiar with the State law or regulatory mechanism governing a CSW's scope of practice in their service area.

D. Noncovered Services

Services of a CSW are not covered when furnished to inpatients of a hospital or to inpatients of a SNF if the services furnished in the SNF are those that the SNF is required to furnish as a condition of participation in Medicare. In addition, CSW services are not covered if they are otherwise excluded from Medicare coverage even though a CSW is authorized by State law to perform them. For example, the Medicare law excludes from coverage services that are not "reasonable and necessary for the diagnosis or treatment of an illness or injury or to improve the functioning of a malformed body member."

E. Outpatient Mental Health Services Limitation

All covered therapeutic services furnished by qualified CSWs are subject to the outpatient psychiatric services limitation in Pub 100-01, Medicare General Information, Eligibility, and Entitlement Manual, Chapter 3, "Deductibles, Coinsurance Amounts, and Payment Limitations," Sec.30, (i.e., only 62 1/2 percent of expenses for these services are considered incurred expenses for Medicare purposes). The limitation does not apply to diagnostic services.

F. Assignment Requirement

Assignment is required.

100-2, 15, 180

Nurse-Midwife (CNM) Services

B3-2154

A. General

Effective on or after July 1, 1988, the services provided by a certified nurse-midwife or incident to the certified nurse-midwife's services are covered. Payment is made under assignment only. See the Medicare Claims Processing Manual, Chapter 12, "Physician and Nonphysician Practitioners," Sec.130, for payment methodology for nurse midwife services.

B. Certified Nurse-Midwife Defined

A certified nurse-midwife is a registered nurse who has successfully completed a program of study and clinical experience in nurse-midwifery, meeting guidelines prescribed by the Secretary, or who has been certified by an organization recognized by the Secretary. The Secretary has recognized certification by the American College of Nurse-Midwives and State qualifying requirements in those States that specify a program of education and clinical experience for nurse-midwives for these purposes. A nurse-midwife must:

- Be currently licensed to practice in the State as a registered professional nurse; and
- Meet one of the following requirements:
  1. Be legally authorized under State law or regulations to practice as a nurse-midwife and have completed a program of study and clinical experience for nurse-midwives, as specified by the State; or
  2. If the State does not specify a program of study and clinical experience that nurse-midwives must complete to practice in that State, the nurse-midwife must:
     a. Be currently certified as a nurse-midwife by the American College of Nurse-Midwives;
     b. Have satisfactorily completed a formal education program (of at least one academic year) that, upon completion, qualifies the nurse to take the certification examination offered by the American College of Nurse-Midwives; or
     c. Have successfully completed a formal education program for preparing registered nurses to furnish gynecological and obstetrical care to women during pregnancy, delivery, and the postpartum period, and care to normal newborns, and have practiced as a nurse-midwife for a total of 12 months during any 18-month period from August 8, 1976, to July 16, 1982.

C. Covered Services

1. General - Effective January 1, 1988, through December 31, 1993, the coverage of nurse-midwife services was restricted to the maternity cycle. The maternity cycle is a period that includes pregnancy, labor, and the immediate postpartum period.

   Beginning with services furnished on or after January 1, 1994, coverage is no longer limited to the maternity cycle. Coverage is available for services furnished by a nurse-midwife that he or she is legally authorized to perform in the State in which the services are furnished and that would otherwise be covered if furnished by a physician, including obstetrical and gynecological services.
2. Incident To- Services and supplies furnished incident to a nurse midwife's service are covered if they would have been covered when furnished incident to the services of a doctor of medicine or osteopathy, as described in Sec.60.

D. Noncovered Services

The services of nurse-midwives are not covered if they are otherwise excluded from Medicare coverage even though a nurse-midwife is authorized by State law to perform them. For example, the Medicare program excludes from coverage routine physical checkups and services that are not reasonable and necessary for the diagnosis or treatment of an illness or injury or to improve the functioning of a malformed body member. Coverage of service to the newborn continues only to the point that the newborn is or would normally be treated medically as a separate individual. Items and services furnished the newborn from that point are not covered on the basis of the mother's eligibility.

E. Relationship With Physician

Most States have licensure and other requirements applicable to nurse-midwives. For example, some require that the nurse-midwife have an arrangement with a physician for the referral of the patient in the event a problem develops that requires medical attention. Others may require that the nurse-midwife function under the general supervision of a physician. Although these and similar State requirements must be met in order for the nurse-midwife to provide Medicare covered care, they have no effect on the nurse-midwife's right to personally bill for and receive direct Medicare payment. That is, billing does not have to flow through a physician or facility. See Sec.60.2 for coverage of services performed by nurse-midwives incident to the service of physicians.

F. Place of Service

There is no restriction on place of service. Therefore, nurse-midwife services are covered if provided in the nurse-midwife's office, in the patient's home, or in a hospital or other facility, such as a clinic or birthing center owned or operated by a nurse-midwife.

G. Assignment Requirement

Assignment is required.

100-2, 15, 230

Practice of Physical Therapy, Occupational Therapy, and Speech-Language Pathology

A. Group Therapy Services.

Contractors pay for outpatient physical therapy services (which includes outpatient speech-language pathology services) and outpatient occupational therapy services provided simultaneously to two or more individuals by a practitioner as group therapy services (97150). The individuals can be, but need not be performing the same activity. The physician or therapist involved in group therapy services must be in constant attendance, but one-on-one patient contact is not required.

B. Therapy Students

1. General

   Only the services of the therapist can be billed and paid under Medicare Part B. The services performed by a student are not reimbursed even if provided under "line of sight" supervision of the therapist; however, the presence of the student "in the room" does not make the service unbillable. Pay for the direct (one-to-one) patient contact services of the physician or therapist provided to Medicare Part B patients. Group therapy services performed by a therapist or physician may be billed when a student is also present "in the room".

   EXAMPLES:

   Therapists may bill and be paid for the provision of services in the following scenarios:

   - The qualified practitioner is present and in the room for the entire session. The student participates in the delivery of services when the qualified practitioner is directing the service, making the skilled judgment, and is responsible for the assessment and treatment.
   - The qualified practitioner is present in the room guiding the student in service delivery when the therapy student and the therapy assistant student are participating in the provision of services, and the practitioner is not engaged in treating another patient or doing other tasks at the same time
   - The qualified practitioner is responsible for the services and as such, signs all documentation. (A student may, of course, also sign but it is not necessary since the Part B payment is for the clinician's service, not for the student's services).
2. Therapy Assistants as Clinical Instructors

   Physical therapist assistants and occupational therapy assistants are not precluded from serving as clinical instructors for therapy students, while providing services within their scope of work and performed under the direction and supervision of a licensed physical or occupational therapist to a Medicare beneficiary.
3. Services Provided Under Part A and Part B

   The payment methodologies for Part A and B therapy services rendered by a student are different. Under the MPFS (Medicare Part B), Medicare pays for services provided by physicians and practitioners that are specifically authorized by statute. Students do not meet the definition of practitioners under Medicare Part B. Under SNF PPS, payments are based upon the case mix or Resource Utilization Group (RUG) category that describes the patient. In the rehabilitation groups, the number of therapy minutes delivered to the patient determines the RUG category. Payment levels for each category are based upon the costs of caring for patients in each group rather than providing pecific payment for each therapy service as is done in Medicare Part B.

100-2, 15, 230.1

Practice of Physical Therapy

A. General

Physical therapy services are those services provided within the scope of practice of physical therapists and necessary for the diagnosis and treatment of impairments, functional limitations, disabilities or changes in physical function and health status. (See Pub. 100-03, the Medicare National Coverage Determinations Manual, for specific conditions or services.) For descriptions of aquatic therapy in a community center pool see section 220C of this chapter.

B. Qualified Physical Therapist Defined

Reference: 42CFR484.4

The new personnel qualifications for physical therapists were discussed in the 2008 Physician Fee Schedule. See the Federal Register of November 27, 2007, for the full text. See also the correction notice for this rule, published in the Federal Register on January 15, 2008.

The regulation provides that a qualified physical therapist (PT) is a person who is licensed, if applicable, as a PT by the state in which he or she is practicing unless licensure does not apply, has graduated from an accredited PT education program and passed a national examination approved by the state in which PT services are provided. The phrase, "by the state in which practicing" includes any authorization to practice provided by the same state in which the service is provided, including temporary licensure, regardless of the location of the entity billing the services. The curriculum accreditation is provided by the Commission on Accreditation in Physical Therapy Education (CAPTE) or, for those who graduated before CAPTE, curriculum approval was provided by the American Physical Therapy Association (APTA). For internationally educated PTs, curricula are approved by a credentials evaluation organization either approved by the APTA or identified in 8 CFR 212.15(e) as it relates to PTs. For example, in 2007, 8 CFR 212.15(e) approved the credentials evaluation provided by the Federation of State Boards of Physical Therapy (FSBPT) and the Foreign Credentialing Commission on Physical Therapy (FCCPT). The requirements above apply to all PTs effective January 1, 2010, if they have not met any of the following requirements prior to January 1, 2010.

Physical therapists whose current license was obtained on or prior to December 31, 2009, qualify to provide PT services to Medicare beneficiaries if they:

- graduated from a CAPTE approved program in PT on or before December 31, 2009 (examination is not required); or,
- graduated on or before December 31, 2009, from a PT program outside the U.S. that is determined to be substantially equivalent to a U.S. program by a credentials evaluating organization approved by either the APTA or identified in 8 CFR 212.15(e) and also passed an examination for PTs approved by the state in which practicing.

Or, PTs whose current license was obtained before January 1, 2008, may meet the requirements in place on that date (i.e., graduation from a curriculum approved by either the APTA, the Committee on Allied Health Education and Accreditation of the American Medical Association, or both).

Or, PTs meet the requirements who are currently licensed and were licensed or qualified as a PT on or before December 31, 1977, and had 2 years appropriate experience as a PT, and passed a proficiency examination conducted, approved, or sponsored by the U.S. Public Health Service.

Or, PTs meet the requirements if they are currently licensed and before January 1, 1966, they were:

- admitted to membership by the APTA; or
- admitted to registration by the American Registry of Physical Therapists; or
- graduated from a 4-year PT curriculum approved by a State Department of Education; or
- licensed or registered and prior to January 1, 1970, they had 15 years of fulltime experience in PT under the order and direction of attending and referring doctors of medicine or osteopathy.

Or, PTs meet requirements if they are currently licensed and they were trained outside the U.S. before January 1, 2008, and after 1928 graduated from a PT curriculum approved in the country in which the curriculum was located, if that country had an organization that was a member of the World Confederation for Physical Therapy, and that PT qualified as a member of the organization.

For outpatient PT services that are provided incident to the services of physicians/NPPs, the requirement for PT licensure does not apply; all other personnel qualifications do apply. The qualified personnel providing PT services incident to the services of a physician/NPP must be trained in an accredited PT curriculum. For example, a person who, on or before December 31, 2009, graduated from a PT curriculum accredited by CAPTE, but who has not passed the national examination or obtained a license, could provide Medicare outpatient PT therapy services incident to the services of a physician/NPP if the physician assumes responsibility for the services according to the incident to policies. On or after January 1, 2010, although licensure does not apply, both education and examination requirements that are effective January 1, 2010, apply to qualified personnel who provide PT services incident to the services of a physician/NPP.

C. Services of Physical Therapy Support Personnel

Reference: 42CFR 484.4

Personnel Qualifications. The new personnel qualifications for physical therapist assistants (PTA) were discussed in the 2008 Physician Fee Schedule. See the Federal Register of November 27, 2007, for the full text. See also the correction notice for this rule, published in the Federal Register on January 15, 2008.

The regulation provides that a qualified PTA is a person who is licensed as a PTA unless licensure does not apply, is registered or certified, if applicable, as a PTA by the state in which practicing, and graduated from an approved curriculum for PTAs, and passed a national examination for PTAs. The phrase, "by the state in which practicing" includes any authorization to practice provided by the same state in which the service is provided, including temporary licensure, regardless of the location or the entity billing for the services. Approval for the curriculum is provided by CAPTE or, if internationally or military trained PTAs apply, approval will be through a credentialing body for the curriculum for PTAs identified by either the American Physical Therapy Association or identified in 8 CFR 212.15(e). A national examination for PTAs is, for example the one furnished by the Federation of State Boards of Physical Therapy. These requirements above apply to all PTAs effective January 1, 2010, if they have not met any of the following requirements prior to January 1, 2010.

Those PTAs also qualify who, on or before December 31, 2009, are licensed, registered or certified as a PTA and met one of the two following requirements:

1. Is licensed or otherwise regulated in the state in which practicing; or
2. In states that have no licensure or other regulations, or where licensure does not apply, PTAs have:
   - graduated on or before December 31, 2009, from a 2-year college-level program approved by the APTA or CAPTE; and
   - effective January 1, 2010, those PTAs must have both graduated from a CAPTE approved curriculum and passed a national examination for PTAs; or

PTAs may also qualify if they are licensed, registered or certified as a PTA, if applicable and meet requirements in effect before January 1, 2008, that is,

- they have graduated before January 1, 2008, from a 2 year college level program approved by the APTA; or
- on or before December 31, 1977, they were licensed or qualified as a PTA and passed a proficiency examination conducted, approved, or sponsored by the U.S. Public Health Service.

Services. The services of PTAs used when providing covered therapy benefits are included as part of the covered service. These services are billed by the supervising physical therapist. PTAs may not provide evaluation services, make clinical judgments or decisions or take responsibility for the service. They act at the direction and under the supervision of the treating physical therapist and in accordance with state laws.

A physical therapist must supervise PTAs. The level and frequency of supervision differs by setting (and by state or local law). General supervision is required for PTAs in all settings except private practice (which requires direct supervision) unless state practice requirements are more stringent, in which case state or local requirements must be followed. See specific settings for details. For example, in clinics, rehabilitation services, either on or off the organization's premises, those services are supervised by a qualified physical therapist who makes an onsite supervisory visit at least once every 30 days or more frequently if required by state or local laws or regulation.

The services of a PTA shall not be billed as services incident to a physician/NPP's service, because they do not meet the qualifications of a therapist.

The cost of supplies (e.g., theraband, hand putty, electrodes) used in furnishing covered therapy care is included in the payment for the HCPCS codes billed by the physical therapist, and are, therefore, not separately billable. Separate coverage and billing provisions apply to items that meet the definition of brace in Sec.130.

Services provided by aides, even if under the supervision of a therapist, are not therapy services and are not covered by Medicare. Although an aide may help the therapist by providing unskilled services, those services that are unskilled are not covered by Medicare and shall be denied as not reasonable and necessary if they are billed as therapy services.

D. Application of Medicare Guidelines to PT Services

This subsection will be used in the future to illustrate the application of the above guidelines to some of the physical therapy modalities and procedures utilized in the treatment of patient

100-2, 15, 230.2

Practice of Occupational Therapy

(Rev. 88, Issued: 05-07-08, Effective: 01-01-08, Implementation: 06-09-08)

A. General

Occupational therapy services are those services provided within the scope of practice of occupational therapists and necessary for the diagnosis and treatment of impairments, functional disabilities or changes in physical function and health status. (See Pub. 100- 03, the Medicare National Coverage Determinations Manual, for specific conditions or services.)

Occupational therapy is medically prescribed treatment concerned with improving or restoring functions which have been impaired by illness or injury or, where function has been permanently lost or reduced by illness or injury, to improve the individual's ability to perform those tasks required for independent functioning. Such therapy may involve:

The evaluation, and reevaluation as required, of a patient's level of function by administering diagnostic and prognostic tests;

The selection and teaching of task-oriented therapeutic activities designed to restore physical function; e.g., use of woodworking activities on an inclined table to restore shoulder, elbow, and wrist range of motion lost as a result of burns;

The planning, implementing, and supervising of individualized therapeutic activity programs as part of an overall "active treatment" program for a patient with a diagnosed psychiatric illness; e.g., the use of sewing activities which require following a pattern to reduce confusion and restore reality orientation in a schizophrenic patient;

The planning and implementing of therapeutic tasks and activities to restore sensoryintegrative function; e.g., providing motor and tactile activities to increase sensory input and improve response for a stroke patient with functional loss resulting in a distorted body image;

The teaching of compensatory technique to improve the level of independence in the activities of daily living, for example:

- Teaching a patient who has lost the use of an arm how to pare potatoes and chop vegetables with one hand;
- Teaching an upper extremity amputee how to functionally utilize a prosthesis;
- Teaching a stroke patient new techniques to enable the patient to perform feeding, dressing, and other activities as independently as possible; or
- Teaching a patient with a hip fracture/hip replacement techniques of standing tolerance and balance to enable the patient to perform such functional activities as dressing and homemaking tasks.

The designing, fabricating, and fitting of orthotics and self-help devices; e.g., making a hand splint for a patient with rheumatoid arthritis to maintain the hand in a functional position or constructing a device which would enable an individual to hold a utensil and feed independently; or Vocational and prevocational assessment and training, subject to the limitations specified in item B below.

Only a qualified occupational therapist has the knowledge, training, and experience required to evaluate and, as necessary, reevaluate a patient's level of function, determine whether an occupational therapy program could reasonably be expected to improve, restore, or compensate for lost function and, where appropriate, recommend to the physician/NPP a plan of treatment.

B. Qualified Occupational Therapist Defined
Reference: 42CFR484.4 The new personnel qualifications for occupational therapists (OT) were discussed in the 2008 Physician Fee Schedule. See the Federal Register of November 27, 2007, for the full text. See also the correction notice for this rule, published in the Federal Register on January 15, 2008.

The regulation provides that a qualified OT is an individual who is licensed, if licensure applies, or otherwise regulated, if applicable, as an OT by the state in which practicing, and graduated from an accredited education program for OTs, and is eligible to take or has passed the examination for OTs administered by the National Board for Certification in Occupational Therapy, Inc. (NBCOT). The phrase, "by the state in which practicing" includes any authorization to practice provided by the same state in which the service is provided, including temporary licensure, regardless of the location of the entity billing the services. The education program for U.S. trained OTs is accredited by the Accreditation Council for Occupational Therapy Education (ACOTE). The requirements above apply to all OTs effective January 1, 2010, if they have not met any of the following requirements prior to January 1, 2010.

The OTs may also qualify if on or before December 31, 2009:

- they are licensed or otherwise regulated as an OT in the state in which practicing (regardless of the qualifications they met to obtain that licensure or regulation); or
- when licensure or other regulation does not apply, OTs have graduated from an OT education program accredited by ACOTE and are eligible to take, or have successfully completed the NBCOT examination for OTs.

Also, those OTs who met the Medicare requirements for OTs that were in 42CFR484.4 prior to January 1, 2008, qualify to provide OT services for Medicare beneficiaries if:

- on or before January 1, 2008, they graduated an OT program approved jointly by the American Medical Association and the AOTA, or
- they are eligible for the National Registration Examination of AOTA or the National Board for Certification in OT.

Also, they qualify who on or before December 31, 1977, had 2 years of appropriate experience as an occupational therapist, and had achieved a satisfactory grade on a proficiency examination conducted, approved, or sponsored by the U.S. Public Health Service.

Those educated outside the U.S. may meet the same qualifications for domestic trained OTs. For example, they qualify if they were licensed or otherwise regulated by the state in which practicing on or before December 31, 2009. Or they are qualified if they:

- graduated from an OT education program accredited as substantially equivalent to a U.S. OT education program by ACOTE, the World Federation of Occupational Therapists, or a credentialing body approved by AOTA; and
- passed the NBCOT examination for OT; and
- Effective January 1, 2010, are licensed or otherwise regulated, if applicable as an OT by the state in which practicing.

For outpatient OT services that are provided incident to the services of physicians/NPPs, the requirement for OT licensure does not apply; all other personnel qualifications do apply. The qualified personnel providing OT services incident to the services of a physician/NPP must be trained in an accredited OT curriculum. For example, a person who, on or before December 31, 2009, graduated from an OT curriculum accredited by ACOTE and is eligible to take or has successfully completed the entry-level certification examination for OTs developed and administered by NBCOT, could provide Medicare outpatient OT services incident to the services of a physician/NPP if the physician assumes responsibility for the services according to the incident to policies. On or after January 1, 2010, although licensure does not apply, both education and examination requirements that are effective January 1, 2010, apply to qualified personnel who provide OT services incident to the services of a physician/NPP.

C. Services of Occupational Therapy Support Personnel
Reference: 42CFR 484.4

The new personnel qualifications for occupational therapy assistants were discussed in the 2008 Physician Fee Schedule. See the Federal Register of November 27, 2007, for the full text. See also the correction notice for this rule, published in the Federal Register on January 15, 2008.

The regulation provides that an occupational therapy assistant is a person who is licensed, unless licensure does not apply, or otherwise regulated, if applicable, as an OTA by the state in which practicing, and graduated from an OTA education program accredited by ACOTE and is eligible to take or has successfully completed the NBCOT examination for OTAs. The phrase, "by the state in which practicing" includes any authorization to practice provided by the same state in which the service is provided, including temporary licensure, regardless of the location of the entity billing the services.

If the requirements above are not met, an OTA may qualify if, on or before December 31, 2009, the OTA is licensed or otherwise regulated as an OTA, if applicable, by the state in which practicing, or meets any qualifications defined by the state in which practicing.

Or, where licensure or other state regulation does not apply, OTAs may qualify if they have, on or before December 31, 2009:

- completed certification requirements to practice as an OTA established by a credentialing organization approved by AOTA; and
- after January 1, 2010, they have also completed an education program accredited by ACOTE and passed the NBCOT examination for OTAs.

OTAs who qualified under the policies in effect prior to January 1, 2008, continue to qualify to provide OT directed and supervised OTA services to Medicare beneficiaries.

Therefore, OTAs qualify who after December 31, 1977, and on or before December 31, 2007:

- completed certification requirements to practice as an OTA established by a credentialing organization approved by AOTA; or
- completed the requirements to practice as an OTA applicable in the state in which practicing.

Those OTAs who were educated outside the U.S. may meet the same requirements as domestically trained OTAs. Or, if educated outside the U.S. on or after January 1, 2008, they must have graduated from an OTA program accredited as substantially equivalent to OTA entry level education in the U.S. by ACOTE, its successor organization, or the World Federation of Occupational Therapists or a credentialing body approved by AOTA. In addition, they must have passed an exam for OTAs administered by NBCOT.

Services. The services of OTAs used when providing covered therapy benefits are included as part of the covered service. These services are billed by the supervising occupational therapist. OTAs may not provide evaluation services, make clinical judgments or decisions or take responsibility for the service. They act at the direction and under the supervision of the treating occupational therapist and in accordance with state laws.

An occupational therapist must supervise OTAs. The level and frequency of supervision differs by setting (and by state or local law). General supervision is required for OTAs in all settings except private practice (which requires direct supervision) unless state practice requirements are more stringent, in which case state or local requirements must be followed. See specific settings for details. For example, in clinics, rehabilitation agencies, and public health agencies, 42CFR485.713 indicates that when an OTA provides services, either on or off the organization's premises, those services are supervised by a qualified occupational therapist who makes an onsite supervisory visit at least once every 30 days or more frequently if required by state or local laws or regulation.

The services of an OTA shall not be billed as services incident to a physician/NPP's service, because they do not meet the qualifications of a therapist.

The cost of supplies (e.g., looms, ceramic tiles, or leather) used in furnishing covered therapy care is included in the payment for the HCPCS codes billed by the occupational therapist and are, therefore, not separately billable. Separate coverage and billing provisions apply to items that meet the definition of brace in Sec.130 of this manual.

Services provided by aides, even if under the supervision of a therapist, are not therapy services in the outpatient setting and are not covered by Medicare. Although an aide may help the therapist by providing unskilled services, those services that are unskilled are not covered by Medicare and shall be denied as not reasonable and necessary if they are billed as therapy services.

D. Application of Medicare Guidelines to Occupational Therapy Services
Occupational therapy may be required for a patient with a specific diagnosed psychiatric illness. If such services are required, they are covered assuming the coverage criteria are met. However, where an individual's motivational needs are not related to a specific diagnosed psychiatric illness, the meeting of such needs does not usually require an individualized therapeutic program. Such needs can be met through general activity programs or the efforts of other professional personnel involved in the care of the patient. Patient motivation is an appropriate and inherent function of all health disciplines, which is interwoven with other functions performed by such personnel for the patient. Accordingly, since the special skills of an occupational therapist are not required, an occupational therapy program for individuals who do not have a specific diagnosed psychiatric illness is not to be considered reasonable and necessary for the treatment of an illness or injury. Services furnished under such a program are not covered.

Occupational therapy may include vocational and prevocational assessment and training. When services provided by an occupational therapist are related solely to specific employment opportunities, work skills, or work settings, they are not reasonable or necessary for the diagnosis or treatment of an illness or injury and are not covered. However, carriers and intermediaries exercise care in applying this exclusion, because the assessment of level of function and the teaching of compensatory techniques to improve the level of function, especially in activities of daily living, are services which occupational therapists provide for both vocational and nonvocational purposes. For example, an assessment of sitting and standing tolerance might be nonvocational for a mother of young children or a retired individual living alone, but could also be a vocational test for a sales clerk. Training an amputee in the use of prosthesis for telephoning is necessary for everyday activities as well as for employment purposes. Major changes in life style may be mandatory for an individual with a substantial disability. The techniques of adjustment cannot be considered exclusively vocational or nonvocational.

100-2, 15, 230.3

Practice of Speech-Language Pathology

A. General

Speech-language pathology services are those services provided within the scope of practice of speech-language pathologists and necessary for the diagnosis and treatment of speech and language disorders, which result in communication disabilities and for the diagnosis and treatment of swallowing disorders (dysphagia), regardless of the presence of a communication disability. (See Pub. 100-03, chapter 1, Sec.170.3)

B. Qualified Speech-Language Pathologist Defined

A qualified speech-language pathologist for program coverage purposes meets one of the following requirements:

- The education and experience requirements for a Certificate of Clinical Competence in (speech-language pathology) granted by the American Speech-Language Hearing Association; or
- Meets the educational requirements for certification and is in the process of accumulating the supervised experience required for certification.

For outpatient speech-language pathology services that are provided incident to the services of physicians/NPPs, the requirement for speech-language pathology licensure does not apply; all other personnel qualifications do apply. Therefore, qualified personnel providing speech-language pathology services incident to the services of a physician/NPP must meet the above qualifications.

C. Services of Speech-Language Pathology Support Personnel

Services of speech-language pathology assistants are not recognized for Medicare coverage. Services provided by speech-language pathology assistants, even if they are licensed to provide services in their states, will be considered unskilled services and denied as not reasonable and necessary if they are billed as therapy services.

Services provided by aides, even if under the supervision of a therapist, are not therapy services and are not covered by Medicare. Although an aide may help the therapist by providing unskilled services, those services are not covered by Medicare and shall be denied as not reasonable and necessary if they are billed as therapy services.

D. Application of Medicare Guidelines to Speech-Language Pathology Services

1. Evaluation Services
   Speech-language pathology evaluation services are covered if they are reasonable and necessary and not excluded as routine screening by Sec.1862(a)(7) of the Act. The speechlanguage pathologist employs a variety of formal and informal speech, language, and dysphagia assessment tests to ascertain the type, causal factor(s), and severity of the speech and language or swallowing disorders. Reevaluation of patients for whom speech, language and swallowing were previously contraindicated is covered only if the patient exhibits a change in medical condition. However, monthly reevaluations; e.g., a Western Aphasia Battery, for a patient undergoing a rehabilitative speech-language pathology program, are considered a part of the treatment session and shall not be covered as a separate evaluation for billing purposes. Although hearing screening by the speechlanguage pathologist may be part of an evaluation, it is not billable as a separate service.
2. Therapeutic Services
   The following are examples of common medical disorders and resulting communication deficits, which may necessitate active rehabilitative therapy. This list is not all-inclusive:
   - Cerebrovascular disease such as cerebral vascular accidents presenting with dysphagia, aphasia/dysphasia, apraxia, and dysarthria;
   - Neurological disease such as Parkinsonism or
   - Multiple Sclerosis with dysarthria, dysphagia, inadequate respiratory volume/control, or voice disorder; or
   - Laryngeal carcinoma requiring laryngectomy resulting in aphonia.
3. Impairments of the Auditory System
   The terms, aural rehabilitation, auditory rehabilitation, auditory processing, lipreading and speech reading are among the terms used to describe covered services related to perception and comprehension of sound through the auditory system. See Pub. 100-04, chapter 12, section 30.3 for billing instructions. For example:
   - Auditory processing evaluation and treatment may be covered and medically necessary. Examples include but are not limited to services for certain neurological impairments or the absence of natural auditory stimulation that results in impaired ability to process sound. Certain auditory processing disorders require diagnostic audiological tests in addition to speech-language pathology evaluation and treatment.
   - Evaluation and treatment for disorders of the auditory system may be covered and medically necessary, for example, when it has been determined by a speechlanguage pathologist in collaboration with an audiologist that the hearing impaired beneficiary's current amplification options (hearing aid, other amplification device or cochlear implant) will not sufficiently meet the patient's functional communication needs. Audiologists and speech-language pathologists both evaluate beneficiaries for disorders of the auditory system using different skills and techniques, but only speech-language pathologists may provide treatment.

Assessment for the need for rehabilitation of the auditory system (but not the vestibular system) may be done by a speech language pathologist. Examples include but are not limited to: evaluation of comprehension and production of language in oral, signed or written modalities, speech and voice production, listening skills, speech reading, communications strategies, and the impact of the hearing loss on the patient/client and family.

Examples of rehabilitation include but are not limited to treatment that focuses on comprehension, and production of language in oral, signed or written modalities; speech and voice production, auditory training, speech reading, multimodal (e.g., visual, auditory-visual, and tactile) training, communication strategies, education and counseling. In determining the necessity for treatment, the beneficiary's performance in both clinical and natural environment should be considered.

4. Dysphagia
Dysphagia, or difficulty in swallowing, can cause food to enter the airway, resulting in coughing, choking, pulmonary problems, aspiration or inadequate nutrition and hydration with resultant weight loss, failure to thrive, pneumonia and death. It is most often due to complex neurological and/or structural impairments including head and neck trauma, cerebrovascular accident, neuromuscular degenerative diseases, head and neck cancer, dementias, and encephalopathies. For these reasons, it is important that only qualified professionals with specific training and experience in this disorder provide evaluation and treatment.

The speech-language pathologist performs clinical and instrumental assessments and analyzes and integrates the diagnostic information to determine candidacy for intervention as well as appropriate compensations and rehabilitative therapy techniques.

The equipment that is used in the examination may be fixed, mobile or portable.

Professional guidelines recommend that the service be provided in a team setting with a physician/NPP who provides supervision of the radiological examination and interpretation of medical conditions revealed in it.

Swallowing assessment and rehabilitation are highly specialized services. The professional rendering care must have education, experience and demonstrated competencies. Competencies include but are not limited to: identifying abnormal upper aerodigestive tract structure and function; conducting an oral, pharyngeal, laryngeal and respiratory function examination as it relates to the functional assessment of swallowing; recommending methods of oral intake and risk precautions; and developing a treatment plan employing appropriate compensations and therapy techniques.

100-2, 15, 230.4

Services Furnished by a Physical or Occupational Therapist in Private Practice

A. General

See section 220 of this chapter for definitions. Therapist refers only to a qualified physical therapist, occupational therapist or speech-language pathologist. TPP refers to therapists in private practice (qualified physical therapists, occupational therapists and speech-language pathologists).

In order to qualify to bill Medicare directly as a therapist, each individual must be enrolled as a private practitioner and employed in one of the following practice types: an unincorporated solo practice, unincorporated partnership, unincorporated group practice, physician/NPP group or groups that are not professional corporations, if allowed by state and local law. Physician/NPP group practices may employ TPP if state and local law permits this employee relationship.

For purposes of this provision, a physician/NPP group practice is defined as one or more physicians/NPPs enrolled with Medicare who may bill as one entity. For further details on issues concerning enrollment, see the provider enrollment Web site at www.cms.hhs.gov/MedicareProviderSupEnroll and Pub. 100-08, Medicare Program Integrity Manual, chapter10, section 12.4.14.

Private practice also includes therapists who are practicing therapy as employees of another supplier, of a professional corporation or other incorporated therapy practice. Private practice does not include individuals when they are working as employees of an institutional provider.

Services should be furnished in the therapist's or group's office or in the patient's home. The office is defined as the location(s) where the practice is operated, in the state(s) where the therapist (and practice, if applicable) is legally authorized to furnish services, during the hours that the therapist engages in the practice at that location. If services are furnished in a private practice office space, that space shall be owned, leased, or rented by the practice and used for the exclusive purpose of operating the practice. For descriptions of aquatic therapy in a community center pool see section 220C of this chapter.

Therapists in private practice must be approved as meeting certain requirements, but do not execute a formal provider agreement with the Secretary.

If therapists who have their own Medicare National Provider Identifier (NPI) are employed by therapist groups, physician/NPP groups, or groups that are not professional organizations, the requirement that therapy space be owned, leased, or rented may be satisfied by the group that employs the therapist. Each therapist employed by a group should enroll as a TPP.

When therapists with a Medicare NPI provide services in the physician's/NPP's office in which they are employed, and bill using their NPI for each therapy service, then the direct supervision requirement for enrolled staff apply.

When the therapist who has a Medicare NPI is employed in a physician's/NPP's office the services are ordinarily billed as services of the therapist, with the therapist identified on the claim as the supplier of services. However, services of the therapist who has a Medicare NPI may also be billed by the physician/NPP as services incident to the physician's/NPP's service. (See §230.5 for rules related to therapy services incident to a physician.) In that case, the physician/NPP is the supplier of service, the NPI of the supervising physician/NPP is reported on the claim with the service and all the rules for both therapy services and incident to services (§230.5) must be followed.

B. Private Practice Defined

Reference: Federal Register November, 1998, pages 58863-58869; 42CFR 410.38(b), 42CFR410.59, 42CFR410.60, 42CFR410.62

The contractor considers a therapist to be in private practice if the therapist maintains office space at his or her own expense and furnishes services only in that space or the patient's home. Or, a therapist is employed by another supplier and furnishes services in facilities provided at the expense of that supplier.

The therapist need not be in full-time private practice but must be engaged in private practice on a regular basis; i.e., the therapist is recognized as a private practitioner and for that purpose has access to the necessary equipment to provide an adequate program of therapy.

The therapy services must be provided either by or under the direct supervision of the TPP. Each TPP should be enrolled as a Medicare provider. If a therapist is not enrolled, the services of that therapist must be directly supervised by an enrolled therapist. Direct supervision requires that the supervising private practice therapist be present in the office suite at the time the service is performed. These direct supervision requirements apply only in the private practice setting and only for therapists and their assistants. In other outpatient settings, supervision rules differ. The services of support personnel must be included in the therapist's bill. The supporting personnel, including other therapists, must be W-2 or 1099 employees of the TPP or other qualified employer.

Coverage of outpatient therapy under Part B includes the services of a qualified TPP when furnished in the therapist's office or the beneficiary's home. For this purpose, "home" includes an institution that is used as a home, but not a hospital, CAH or SNF, (Federal Register Nov. 2, 1998, pg 58869). Place of Service (POS) includes:

- 03/School, only if residential,
- 04/Homeless Shelter,
- 12/Home, other than a facility that is a private residence,
- 14/Group Home,
- 33/Custodial Care Facility.

C. Assignment

Reference: Nov. 2, 1998 Federal Register, pg. 58863

See also Pub. 100-04 chapter 1, §30.2.

When physicians, NPPs, or TPPs obtain provider numbers, they have the option of accepting assignment (participating) or not accepting assignment (nonparticipating). In contrast, providers, such as outpatient hospitals, SNFs, rehabilitation agencies, and CORFs, do not have the option. For these providers, assignment is mandatory.

If physicians/NPPs, or TPPs accept assignment (are participating), they must accept the Medicare Physician Fee Schedule amount as payment. Medicare pays 80% and the patient is responsible for 20%. In contrast, if they do not accept assignment, Medicare will only pay 95% of the fee schedule amount. However, when these services are not furnished on an assignment-related basis, the limiting charge applies. (See §1848(g)(2)(c) of the Act.)

NOTE: Services furnished by a therapist in the therapist's office under arrangements with hospitals in rural communities and public health agencies (or services provided in the beneficiary's home under arrangements with a provider of outpatient physical or occupational therapy services) are not covered under this provision. See section 230.6.

100-2, 15, 232

Cardiac Rehabilitation (CR) and Intensive Cardiac Rehabilitation (ICR) Services Furnished On or After January 1, 2010

Cardiac rehabilitation (CR) services mean a physician-supervised program that furnishes physician prescribed exercise, cardiac risk factor modification, including education, counseling, and behavioral intervention; psychosocial assessment, outcomes assessment, and other items/services as determined by the Secretary under certain conditions. Intensive cardiac rehabilitation (ICR) services mean a physician-supervised program that furnishes the same items/services under the same conditions as a CR program but must also demonstrate, as shown in peer-reviewed published research, that it improves patients' cardiovascular disease through specific outcome measurements described in 42 CFR 410.49(c). Effective January 1, 2010, Medicare Part B pays for CR/ICR programs and related items/services if specific criteria is met by the Medicare beneficiary, the CR/ICR program itself, the setting in which is it administered, and the physician administering the program, as outlined below:

CR/ICR Program Beneficiary Requirements:

Medicare covers CR/ICR program services for beneficiaries who have experienced one or more of the following:

- Acute myocardial infarction within the preceding 12 months;
- Coronary artery bypass surgery;
- Current stable angina pectoris;
- Heart valve repair or replacement;
- Percutaneous transluminal coronary angioplasty (PTCA) or coronary stenting;
- Heart or heart-lung transplant.

For cardiac rehabilitation only: Stable, chronic heart failure defined as patients with left ventricular ejection fraction of 35% or less and New York Heart Association (NYHA) class II to IV symptoms despite being on optimal heart failure therapy for at least 6 weeks. (Effective February 18, 2014.)

CR/ICR Program Component Requirements:

- Physician-prescribed exercise. This physical activity includes aerobic exercise combined with other types of exercise (i.e., strengthening, stretching) as determined to be appropriate for individual patients by a physician each day CR/ICR items/services are furnished.
- Cardiac risk factor modification. This includes education, counseling, and behavioral intervention, tailored to the patients' individual needs.
- Psychosocial assessment. This assessment means an evaluation of an individual's mental and emotional functioning as it relates to the individual's rehabilitation. It should include: (1) an assessment of those aspects of the individual's family and home situation that affects the individual's rehabilitation treatment, and, (2) a psychosocial evaluation of the individual's response to, and rate of progress under, the treatment plan.
- Outcomes assessment. These should include: (i) minimally, assessments from the commencement and conclusion of CR/ICR, based on patient-centered outcomes which must be measured by the physician immediately at the beginning and end of the program, and, (ii) objective clinical measures of the effectiveness of the CR/ICR program for the individual patient, including exercise performance and self-reported measures of exertion and behavior.
- Individualized treatment plan. This plan should be written and tailored to each individual patient and include (i) a description of the individual's diagnosis; (ii) the type, amount, frequency, and duration of the CR/ICR items/services furnished; and (iii) the goals set for the individual under the plan. The individualized treatment plan must be established, reviewed, and signed by a physician every 30 days.

As specified at 42 CFR 410.49(f)(1), CR sessions are limited to a maximum of 2 1-hour sessions per day for up to 36 sessions over up to 36 weeks with the option for an additional 36 sessions over an extended period of time if approved by the contractor under section 1862(a)(1)(A) of the Act. ICR sessions are limited to 72 1-hour sessions (as defined in section 1848(b)(5) of the Act), up to 6 sessions per day, over a period of up to 18 weeks.

CR/ICR Program Setting Requirements:

CR/ICR services must be furnished in a physician's office or a hospital outpatient setting (for ICR, the hospital outpatient setting must provide ICR using an approved ICR program). All settings must have a physician immediately available and accessible for medical consultations and emergencies at all times when items/services are being furnished under the program. This provision is satisfied if the physician meets the requirements for direct supervision of physician office services as specified at 42 CFR 410.26, and for hospital outpatient services as specified at 42 CFR 410.27.

ICR Program Approval Requirements:

All prospective ICR programs must be approved through the national coverage determination (NCD) process. To be approved as an ICR program, it must demonstrate through peer-reviewed, published research that it has accomplished one or more of the following for its patients: (i) positively affected the progression of coronary heart disease, (ii) reduced the need for coronary bypass surgery, or, (iii) reduced the need for percutaneous coronary interventions.

An ICR program must also demonstrate through peer-reviewed, published research that it accomplished a statistically significant reduction in five or more of the following measures for patients from their levels before CR services to after CR services: (i) low density lipoprotein, (ii) triglycerides, (iii) body mass index, (iv) systolic blood pressure, (v) diastolic blood pressure, and (vi) the need for cholesterol, blood pressure, and diabetes medications.

A list of approved ICR programs, identified through the NCD process, will be posted to the CMS Web site and listed in the Federal Register.

Once an ICR program is approved through the NCD process, all prospective ICR sites wishing to furnish ICR items/services via an approved ICR program may enroll with their local contractor to become an ICR program supplier using the designated forms as specified at 42 CFR 424.510, and report specialty code 31 to be identified as an enrolled ICR supplier. For purposes of appealing an adverse determination concerning site approval, an ICR site is considered a supplier (or prospective supplier) as defined in 42 CFR 498.2.

CR/ICR Program Physician Requirements:

Physicians responsible for CR/ICR programs are identified as medical directors who oversee or supervise the CR/ICR program at a particular site. The medical director, in consultation with staff, is involved in directing the progress of individuals in the program. The medical director, as well as physicians acting as the supervising physician, must possess all of the following: (1) expertise in the management of individuals with cardiac pathophysiology, (2) cardiopulmonary training in basic life support or advanced cardiac life support, and (3) licensed to practice medicine in the state in which the CR/ICR program is offered. Direct physician supervision may be provided by a supervising physician or the medical director.

(See Pub. 100-03, Medicare National Coverage Determinations Manual, Chapter 1, Part 1, section 20.10.1, Pub. 100-04, Medicare Claims Processing Manual, Chapter 32, section 140, Pub. 100-08, Medicare Program Integrity Manual, Chapter 15, section 15.4.2.8, for specific claims processing, coding, and billing requirements for CR/ICR program services.)

100-2, 15, 240

Chiropractic Services - General

B3-2250, B3-4118

The term "physician" under Part B includes a chiropractor who meets the specified qualifying requirements set forth in Sec.30.5 but only for treatment by means of manual manipulation of the spine to correct a subluxation.

Effective for claims with dates of services on or after January 1, 2000, an x-ray is not required to demonstrate the subluxation.

Implementation of the chiropractic benefit requires an appreciation of the differences between chiropractic theory and experience and traditional medicine due to fundamental differences regarding etiology and theories of the pathogenesis of disease. Judgments about the reasonableness of chiropractic treatment must be based on the application of chiropractic principles. So that Medicare beneficiaries receive equitable adjudication of claims based on such principles and are not deprived of the benefits intended by the law, carriers may use chiropractic consultation in carrier review of Medicare chiropractic claims.

Payment is based on the physician fee schedule and made to the beneficiary or, on assignment, to the chiropractor.

A. Verification of Chiropractor's Qualifications
Carriers must establish a reference file of chiropractors eligible for payment as physicians under the criteria in Sec.30.1. They pay only chiropractors on file. Information needed to establish such files is furnished by the CMS RO.

The RO is notified by the appropriate State agency which chiropractors are licensed and whether each meets the national uniform standards.

100-2, 15, 240.1.1

Manual Manipulation

Coverage of chiropractic service is specifically limited to treatment by means of manual manipulation, i.e., by use of the hands. Additionally, manual devices (i.e., those that are hand-held with the thrust of the force of the device being controlled manually) may be used by chiropractors in performing manual manipulation of the spine. However, no additional payment is available for use of the device, nor does Medicare recognize an extra charge for the device itself.

No other diagnostic or therapeutic service furnished by a chiropractor or under the chiropractor's order is covered. This means that if a chiropractor orders, takes, or interprets an x-ray, or any other diagnostic test, the x-ray or other diagnostic test, can be used for claims processing purposes, but Medicare coverage and payment are not available for those services. This prohibition does not affect the coverage of x-rays or other diagnostic tests furnished by other practitioners under the program. For example, an x-ray or any diagnostic test taken for the purpose of determining or demonstrating the existence of a subluxation of the spine is a diagnostic x-ray test covered under §1861(s)(3) of the Act if ordered, taken, and interpreted by a physician who is a doctor of medicine or osteopathy.

Manual devices (i.e., those that are hand-held with the thrust of the force of the device being controlled manually) may be used by chiropractors in performing manual manipulation of the spine. However, no additional payment is available for use of the device, nor does Medicare recognize an extra charge for the device itself.

Effective for claims with dates of service on or after January 1, 2000, an x-ray is not required to demonstrate the subluxation. However, an x-ray may be used for this purpose if the chiropractor so chooses.

The word "correction" may be used in lieu of "treatment." Also, a number of different terms composed of the following words may be used to describe manual manipulation as defined above:

- Spine or spinal adjustment by manual means;
- Spine or spinal manipulation;
- Manual adjustment; and
- Vertebral manipulation or adjustment.

In any case in which the term(s) used to describe the service performed suggests that it may not have been treatment by means of manual manipulation, the carrier analyst refers the claim for professional review and interpretation.

100-2, 15, 240.1.3

Necessity for Treatment

The patient must have a significant health problem in the form of a neuromusculoskeletal condition necessitating treatment, and the manipulative services rendered must have a direct therapeutic relationship to the patient's condition and provide reasonable expectation of recovery or improvement of function. The patient must have a subluxation of the spine as demonstrated by x-ray or physical exam, as described above.

Most spinal joint problems fall into the following categories:

- Acute subluxation-A patient's condition is considered acute when the patient is being treated for a new injury, identified by x-ray or physical exam as specified above. The result of chiropractic manipulation is expected to be an improvement in, or arrest of progression, of the patient's condition.
- Chronic subluxation-A patient's condition is considered chronic when it is not expected to significantly improve or be resolved with further treatment (as is the case with an acute condition), but where the continued therapy can be expected to result in some functional improvement. Once the clinical status has remained stable for a given condition, without expectation of additional objective clinical improvements, further manipulative treatment is considered maintenance therapy and is not covered.

For Medicare purposes, a chiropractor must place an AT modifier on a claim when providing active/corrective treatment to treat acute or chronic subluxation. However the presence of the AT modifier may not in all instances indicate that the service is reasonable and necessary. As always, contractors may deny if appropriate after medical review.

A. Maintenance Therapy
Maintenance therapy includes services that seek to prevent disease, promote health and prolong and enhance the quality of life, or maintain or prevent deterioration of a chronic condition. When further clinical improvement cannot reasonably be expected from continuous ongoing care, and the chiropractic treatment becomes supportive rather than corrective in nature, the treatment is then considered maintenance therapy. The AT modifier must not be placed on the claim when maintenance therapy has been provided. Claims without the AT modifier will be considered as maintenance therapy and denied. Chiropractors who give or receive from beneficiaries an ABN shall follow the instructions in Pub. 100-04, Medicare Claims Processing Manual, chapter 23, section 20.9.1.1 and include a GA (or in rare instances a GZ) modifier on the claim.

B. Contraindications
Dynamic thrust is the therapeutic force or maneuver delivered by the physician during manipulation in the anatomic region of involvement. A relative contraindication is a condition that adds significant risk of injury to the patient from dynamic thrust, but does not rule out the use of dynamic thrust. The doctor should discuss this risk with the patient and record this in the chart. The following are relative contraindications to dynamic thrust:

Articular hyper mobility and circumstances where the stability of the joint is uncertain;

Severe demineralization of bone;

Benign bone tumors (spine);

Bleeding disorders and anticoagulant therapy; and

Radiculopathy with progressive neurological signs.

Dynamic thrust is absolutely contraindicated near the site of demonstrated subluxation and proposed manipulation in the following:

Acute arthropathies characterized by acute inflammation and ligamentous laxity and anatomic subluxation or dislocation; including acute rheumatoid arthritis and ankylosing spondylitis;

Acute fractures and dislocations or healed fractures and dislocations with signs of instability;

An unstable os odontoideum;

Malignancies that involve the vertebral column;

Infection of bones or joints of the vertebral column;

Signs and symptoms of myelopathy or cauda equina syndrome;

For cervical spinal manipulations, vertebrobasilar insufficiency syndrome; and

A significant major artery aneurysm near the proposed manipulation.

100-2, 15, 260

Ambulatory Surgical Center Services

Facility services furnished by ambulatory surgical centers (ASCs) in connection with certain surgical procedures are covered under Part B. To receive coverage of and payment for its services under this provision, a facility must be certified as meeting the requirements for an ASC and enter into a written agreement with CMS. Medicare periodically updates the list of covered procedures and related payment amounts through release of regulations and Program Memoranda. The ASC must accept Medicare's payment for such procedures as payment in full with respect to those services defined as ASC facility services.

Where services are performed in an ASC, the physician and others who perform covered services may also be paid for his/her professional services; however, the "professional" rate is then adjusted since the ASC incurs the facility costs.

100-2, 15, 270

Telehealth Services

Background

Section 223 of the Medicare, Medicaid and SCHIP Benefits Improvement and Protection Act of 2000 (BIPA) - Revision of Medicare Reimbursement for Telehealth Services amended §1834 of the Act to provide for an expansion of Medicare payment for telehealth services.

Effective October 1, 2001, coverage and payment for Medicare telehealth includes consultation, office visits, individual psychotherapy, and pharmacologic management delivered via a telecommunications system. Eligible geographic areas include rural health professional shortage areas (HPSA) and counties not classified as a metropolitan statistical area (MSA). Additionally, Federal telemedicine demonstration projects as of December 31, 2000, may serve as the originating site regardless of geographic location.

An interactive telecommunications system is required as a condition of payment; however, BIPA does allow the use of asynchronous "store and forward" technology in delivering these services when the originating site is a Federal telemedicine demonstration program in Alaska or Hawaii. BIPA does not require that a practitioner present the patient for interactive telehealth services.

With regard to payment amount, BIPA specified that payment for the professional service performed by the distant site practitioner (i.e., where the expert physician or practitioner is physically located at time of telemedicine encounter) is equal to what would have been paid without the use of telemedicine. Distant site practitioners include only a physician as described in §1861(r) of the Act and a medical practitioner as described in §1842(b)(18)(C) of the Act. BIPA also expanded payment under Medicare to include a $20 originating site facility fee (location of beneficiary).

Previously, the Balanced Budget Act of 1997 (BBA) limited the scope of Medicare telehealth coverage to consultation services and the implementing regulation prohibited the use of an asynchronous 'store and forward' telecommunications system. The BBA of 1997 also required the professional fee to be shared between the referring and consulting practitioners, and prohibited Medicare payment for facility fees and line charges associated with the telemedicine encounter.

The BIPA required that Medicare Part B (Supplementary Medical Insurance) pay for this expansion of telehealth services beginning with services furnished on October 1, 2001.

Section 149 of the Medicare Improvements for Patients and Providers Act of 2008 (MIPPA) amended §1834(m) of the Act to add certain entities as originating sites for payment of telehealth services. Effective for services furnished on or after January 1, 2009, eligible originating sites include a hospital-based or critical access hospital-based renal dialysis center (including satellites); a skilled nursing facility (as defined in §1819(a) of the Act); and a community mental health center (as defined in §1861(ff)(3)(B) of the Act). MIPPA also amended§1888(e)(2)(A)(ii) of the Act to exclude telehealth services furnished under §1834(m)(4)(C)(ii)(VII) from the consolidated billing provisions of the skilled nursing facility prospective payment system (SNF PPS).

NOTE: MIPPA did not add independent renal dialysis facilities as originating sites for payment of telehealth services.

The telehealth provisions authorized by §1834(m) of the Act are implemented in 42 CFR 410.78 and 414.65.

100-2, 15, 270.2

List of Medicare Telehealth Services

The use of a telecommunications system may substitute for an in-person encounter for professional consultations, office visits, office psychiatry services, and a limited number of other physician fee schedule (PFS) services. These services are listed below.

Consultations (Effective October 1, 2001- December 31, 2009)

Telehealth consultations, emergency department or initial inpatient (Effective January 1, 2010)

Follow-up inpatient telehealth consultations (Effective January 1, 2009)

Office or other outpatient visits

Subsequent hospital care services (with the limitation of one telehealth visit every 3 days) (Effective January 1, 2011)

Subsequent nursing facility care services (with the limitation of one telehealth visit every 30 days) (Effective January 1, 2011)

Individual psychotherapy

Pharmacologic management (Effective March 1, 2003)

Psychiatric diagnostic interview examination (Effective March 1, 2003)

End stage renal disease related services (Effective January 1, 2005)

Individual and group medical nutrition therapy (Individual effective January 1, 2006; group effective January 1, 2011)

Neurobehavioral status exam (Effective January 1, 2008)

Individual and group health and behavior assessment and intervention (Individual effective January 1, 2010; group effective January 1, 2011)

Individual and group kidney disease education (KDE) services (Effective January 1, 2011)

Individual and group diabetes self-management training (DSMT) services (with a minimum of 1 hour of in-person instruction to be furnished in the initial year training period to ensure effective injection training) (Effective January 1, 2011)

Smoking Cessation Services (Effective January 1, 2012)

Alcohol and/or substance (other than tobacco) abuse structured assessment and intervention services (Effective January 1, 2013)

Annual alcohol misuse screening (Effective January 1, 2013)

Brief face-to-face behavioral counseling for alcohol misuse (Effective January 1, 2013).

Annual Depression Screening (Effective January 1, 2013)

High-intensity behavioral counseling to prevent sexually transmitted infections (Effective January 1, 2013)

Annual, face-to-face Intensive behavioral therapy for cardiovascular disease (Effective January 1, 2013)

Face-to-face behavioral counseling for obesity (Effective January 1, 2013)

NOTE: Beginning January 1, 2010, CMS eliminated the use of all consultation codes, except for inpatient telehealth consultation G-codes. CMS no longer recognizes office/outpatient or inpatient consultation CPT codes for payment of office/outpatient or inpatient visits. Instead, physicians and practitioners are instructed to bill a new or established patient office/outpatient visit CPT code or appropriate hospital or nursing facility care code, as appropriate to the particular patient, for all office/outpatient or inpatient visits. For detailed instructions regarding reporting these and other telehealth services, see Pub. 100-04, Medicare Claims Processing Manual, chapter 12, section 190.3.

The conditions of payment for Medicare telehealth services, including qualifying originating sites and the types of telecommunications systems recognized by Medicare, are subject to the provisions of 42 CFR 410.78. Payment for these services is subject to the provisions of 42 CFR 414.65.

100-2, 15, 270.4

Payment – Physician/Practitioner at a Distant Site

The term "distant site" means the site where the physician or practitioner providing the professional service is located at the time the service is provided via a telecommunications system.

The payment amount for the professional service provided via a telecommunications system by the physician or practitioner at the distant site is equal to the current physician fee schedule amount for the service. Payment for telehealth services (see section 270.2 of this chapter) should be made at the same amount as when these services are furnished without the use of a telecommunications system. For Medicare payment to occur, the service must be within a practitioner's scope of practice under State law. The beneficiary is responsible for any unmet deductible amount and applicable coinsurance.

Medicare Practitioners Who May Receive Payment at the Distant Site (i.e., at a Site Other Than Where the Beneficiary is Located)

As a condition of Medicare Part B payment for telehealth services, the physician or practitioner at the distant site must be licensed to provide the service under State law. When the physician or practitioner at the distant site is licensed under State law to provide a covered telehealth service (see section 270.2 of this chapter) then he or she may bill for and receive payment for this service when delivered via a telecommunications system.

Medicare practitioners who may bill for a covered telehealth service are listed below (subject to State law):

- Physician;
- Nurse practitioner;
- Physician assistant;
- Nurse midwife;
- Clinical nurse specialist;
- Clinical psychologist;
- Clinical social worker; and
- Registered dietitian or nutrition professional.

* Clinical psychologists and clinical social workers cannot bill for psychotherapy services that include medical evaluation and management services under Medicare. These practitioners may not bill or receive payment for the following CPT codes: 90805, 90807, and 90809.

100-2, 15, 270.4.2

Payment for Subsequent Hospital Care Services and Subsequent Nursing Facility Care Services as Telehealth Services

Subsequent hospital care services are limited to one telehealth visit every 3 days. The frequency limit of the benefit is not intended to apply to consulting physicians or practitioners, who should continue to report initial or follow-up inpatient telehealth consultations using the applicable HCPCS G-codes.

Similarly, subsequent nursing facility care services are limited to one telehealth visit every 30 days. Furthermore, subsequent nursing facility care services reported for a Federally-mandated periodic visit under 42 CFR 483.40(c) may not be furnished through telehealth. The frequency limit of the benefit is not intended to apply to consulting physicians or practitioners, who should continue to report initial or follow-up inpatient telehealth consultations using the applicable HCPCS G-codes.

Inpatient telehealth consultations are furnished to beneficiaries in hospitals or skilled nursing facilities via telehealth at the request of the physician of record, the attending physician, or another appropriate source. The physician or practitioner who furnishes the initial inpatient consultation via telehealth cannot be the physician or practitioner of record or the attending physician or practitioner, and the initial inpatient telehealth consultation would be distinct from the care provided by the physician or practitioner of record or the attending physician or practitioner. Counseling and coordination of care with other providers or agencies is included as well, consistent with the nature of the problem(s) and the patient's needs. Initial and follow-up inpatient telehealth consultations are subject to the criteria for inpatient telehealth consultation services, as described in Pub. 100-04, Medicare Claims Processing Manual, chapter 12, section 190.3.

100-2, 15, 290

Foot Care

A. Treatment of Subluxation of Foot

Subluxations of the foot are defined as partial dislocations or displacements of joint surfaces, tendons ligaments, or muscles of the foot. Surgical or nonsurgical treatments undertaken for the sole purpose of correcting a subluxated structure in the foot as an isolated entity are not covered.

However, medical or surgical treatment of subluxation of the ankle joint (talo-crural joint) is covered. In addition, reasonable and necessary medical or surgical services, diagnosis, or treatment for medical conditions that have resulted from or are associated with partial displacement of structures is covered. For example, if a patient has osteoarthritis that has resulted in a partial displacement of joints in the foot, and the primary treatment is for the osteoarthritis, coverage is provided.

B. Exclusions from Coverage

The following foot care services are generally excluded from coverage under both Part A and Part B. (See Sec.290.F and Sec.290.G for instructions on applying foot care exclusions.)

1. Treatment of Flat Foot

   The term "flat foot" is defined as a condition in which one or more arches of the foot have flattened out. Services or devices directed toward the care or correction of such conditions, including the prescription of supportive devices, are not covered.

2. Routine Foot Care

   Except as provided above, routine foot care is excluded from coverage. Services that normally are considered routine and not covered by Medicare include the following:

   - The cutting or removal of corns and calluses;
   - The trimming, cutting, clipping, or debriding of nails; and
   - Other hygienic and preventive maintenance care, such as cleaning and soaking the feet, the use of skin creams to maintain skin tone of either ambulatory or bedfast patients, and any other service performed in the absence of localized illness, injury, or symptoms involving the foot.

3. Supportive Devices for Feet
   Orthopedic shoes and other supportive devices for the feet generally are not covered. However, this exclusion does not apply to such a shoe if it is an integral part of a leg brace, and its expense is included as part of the cost of the brace. Also, this exclusion does not apply to therapeutic shoes furnished to diabetics.

C. Exceptions to Routine Foot Care Exclusion

1. Necessary and Integral Part of Otherwise Covered Services

   In certain circumstances, services ordinarily considered to be routine may be covered if they are performed as a necessary and integral part of otherwise covered services, such as diagnosis and treatment of ulcers, wounds, or infections.

2. Treatment of Warts on Foot

   The treatment of warts (including plantar warts) on the foot is covered to the same extent as services provided for the treatment of warts located elsewhere on the body.

3. Presence of Systemic Condition

   The presence of a systemic condition such as metabolic, neurologic, or peripheral vascular disease may require scrupulous foot care by a professional that in the absence of such condition(s) would be considered routine (and, therefore, excluded from coverage). Accordingly, foot care that would otherwise be considered routine may be covered when systemic condition(s) result in severe circulatory embarrassment or areas of diminished sensation in the individual's legs or feet. (See subsection A.)

   In these instances, certain foot care procedures that otherwise are considered routine (e.g., cutting or removing corns and calluses, or trimming, cutting, clipping, or debriding nails) may pose a hazard when performed by a nonprofessional person on patients with such systemic conditions. (See Sec.290.G for procedural instructions.)

4. Mycotic Nails

   In the absence of a systemic condition, treatment of mycotic nails may be covered.

   The treatment of mycotic nails for an ambulatory patient is covered only when the physician attending the patient's mycotic condition documents that (1) there is clinical evidence of mycosis of the toenail, and (2) the patient has marked limitation of ambulation, pain, or secondary infection resulting from the thickening and dystrophy of the infected toenail plate.

   The treatment of mycotic nails for a nonambulatory patient is covered only when the physician attending the patient's mycotic condition documents that (1) there is clinical evidence of mycosis of the toenail, and (2) the patient suffers from pain or secondary infection resulting from the thickening and dystrophy of the infected toenail plate.

   For the purpose of these requirements, documentation means any written information that is required by the carrier in order for services to be covered. Thus, the information submitted with claims must be substantiated by information found in the patient's medical record. Any information, including that contained in a form letter, used for documentation purposes is subject to carrier verification in order to ensure that the information adequately justifies coverage of the treatment of mycotic nails.

D. Systemic Conditions That Might Justify Coverage

Although not intended as a comprehensive list, the following metabolic, neurologic, and peripheral vascular diseases (with synonyms in parentheses) most commonly represent the underlying conditions that might justify coverage for routine foot care.

- Diabetes mellitus *
- Arteriosclerosis obliterans (A.S.O., arteriosclerosis of the extremities, occlusive peripheral arteriosclerosis)
- Buerger's disease (thromboangiitis obliterans)
- Chronic thrombophlebitis *
- Peripheral neuropathies involving the feet -

  Associated with malnutrition and vitamin deficiency *

  - Malnutrition (general, pellagra)
  - Alcoholism
  - Malabsorption (celiac disease, tropical sprue)
  - Pernicious anemia
    - Associated with carcinoma *
    - Associated with diabetes mellitus *
    - Associated with drugs and toxins *
    - Associated with multiple sclerosis *
    - Associated with uremia (chronic renal disease) *
    - Associated with traumatic injury
    - Associated with leprosy or neurosyphilis
    - Associated with hereditary disorders
  - Hereditary sensory radicular neuropathy
  - Angiokeratoma corporis diffusum (Fabry's)
  - Amyloid neuropathy

When the patient's condition is one of those designated by an asterisk (*), routine procedures are covered only if the patient is under the active care of a doctor of medicine or osteopathy who documents the condition.

E. Supportive Devices for Feet

Orthopedic shoes and other supportive devices for the feet generally are not covered. However, this exclusion does not apply to such a shoe if it is an integral part of a leg brace, and its expense is included as part of the cost of the brace. Also, this exclusion does not apply to therapeutic shoes furnished to diabetics.

F. Presumption of Coverage

In evaluating whether the routine services can be reimbursed, a presumption of coverage may be made where the evidence available discloses certain physical and/or clinical findings consistent with the diagnosis and indicative of severe peripheral involvement. For purposes of applying this presumption the following findings are pertinent:

Class A Findings

- Nontraumatic amputation of foot or integral skeletal portion thereof.

Class B Findings

- Absent posterior tibial pulse;
- Advanced trophic changes as: hair growth (decrease or absence) nail changes (thickening) pigmentary changes (discoloration) skin texture (thin, shiny) skin color (rubor or redness) (Three required); and
- Absent dorsalis pedis pulse.

Class C Findings

- Claudication;
- Temperature changes (e.g., cold feet);
- Edema;
- Paresthesias (abnormal spontaneous sensations in the feet); and
- Burning.

The presumption of coverage may be applied when the physician rendering the routine foot care has identified:

1. A Class A finding;
2. Two of the Class B findings; or
3. One Class B and two Class C findings.

Cases evidencing findings falling short of these alternatives may involve podiatric treatment that may constitute covered care and should be reviewed by the intermediary's medical staff and developed as necessary.

For purposes of applying the coverage presumption where the routine services have been rendered by a podiatrist, the contractor may deem the active care requirement met if the claim or other evidence available discloses that the patient has seen an M.D. or D.O. for treatment and/or evaluation of the complicating disease process during the 6-month period prior to the rendition of the routine-type services. The intermediary may also accept the podiatrist's statement that the diagnosing and treating M.D. or D.O. also concurs with the podiatrist's findings as to the severity of the peripheral involvement indicated.

Services ordinarily considered routine might also be covered if they are performed as a necessary and integral part of otherwise covered services, such as diagnosis and treatment of diabetic ulcers, wounds, and infections.

G. Application of Foot Care Exclusions to Physician's Services
The exclusion of foot care is determined by the nature of the service. Thus, payment for an excluded service should be denied whether performed by a podiatrist, osteopath, or a doctor of medicine, and without regard to the difficulty or complexity of the procedure.

When an itemized bill shows both covered services and noncovered services not integrally related to the covered service, the portion of charges attributable to the noncovered services should be denied. (For example, if an itemized bill shows surgery for an ingrown toenail and also removal of calluses not necessary for the performance of toe surgery, any additional charge attributable to removal of the calluses should be denied.)

In reviewing claims involving foot care, the carrier should be alert to the following exceptional situations:

1. Payment may be made for incidental noncovered services performed as a necessary and integral part of, and secondary to, a covered procedure. For example, if trimming of toenails is required for application of a cast to a fractured foot, the carrier need not allocate and deny a portion of the charge for the trimming of the nails. However, a separately itemized charge for such excluded service should be disallowed. When the primary procedure is covered the administration of anesthesia necessary for the performance of such procedure is also covered.
2. Payment may be made for initial diagnostic services performed in connection with a specific symptom or complaint if it seems likely that its treatment would be covered even though the resulting diagnosis may be one requiring only noncovered care.

The name of the M.D. or D.O. who diagnosed the complicating condition must be submitted with the claim. In those cases, where active care is required, the approximate date the beneficiary was last seen by such physician must also be indicated.

NOTE: Section 939 of P.L. 96-499 removed "warts" from the routine foot care exclusion effective July 1, 1981.

Relatively few claims for routine-type care are anticipated considering the severity of conditions contemplated as the basis for this exception. Claims for this type of foot care should not be paid in the absence of convincing evidence that nonprofessional performance of the service would have been hazardous for the beneficiary because of an underlying systemic disease. The mere statement of a diagnosis such as those mentioned in Sec.D above does not of itself indicate the severity of the condition. Where development is indicated to verify diagnosis and/or severity the carrier should follow existing claims processing practices which may include review of carrier's history and medical consultation as well as physician contacts.

The rules in Sec.290.F concerning presumption of coverage also apply.

Codes and policies for routine foot care and supportive devices for the feet are not exclusively for the use of podiatrists. These codes must be used to report foot care services regardless of the specialty of the physician who furnishes the services. Carriers must instruct physicians to use the most appropriate code available when billing for routine foot care.

100-2, 16, 10

General Exclusions From Coverage

A3-3150, HO-260, HHA-232, B3-2300

No payment can be made under either the hospital insurance or supplementary medical insurance program for certain items and services, when the following conditions exist:

- Not reasonable and necessary (Sec.20);
- No legal obligation to pay for or provide (Sec.40);
- Paid for by a governmental entity (Sec.50);
- Not provided within United States (Sec.60);
- Resulting from war (Sec.70);
- Personal comfort (Sec.80);
- Routine services and appliances (Sec.90);
- Custodial care (Sec.110);
- Cosmetic surgery (Sec.120);
- Charges by immediate relatives or members of household (Sec.130);
- Dental services (Sec.140);
- Paid or expected to be paid under workers' compensation (Sec.150);
- Nonphysician services provided to a hospital inpatient that were not provided directly or arranged for by the hospital (Sec.170);
- Services Related to and Required as a Result of Services Which are not Covered Under Medicare (Sec.180);
- Excluded foot care services and supportive devices for feet (Sec.30); or
- Excluded investigational devices (See Chapter 14, Sec.30).

100-2, 16, 20

Services Not Reasonable and Necessary

A3-3151, HO-260.1, B3-2303, AB-00-52 - 6/00

Items and services which are not reasonable and necessary for the diagnosis or treatment of illness or injury or to improve the functioning of a malformed body member are not covered, e.g., payment cannot be made for the rental of a special hospital bed to be used by the patient in their home unless it was a reasonable and necessary part of the patient's treatment. See also Sec.80.

A health care item or service for the purpose of causing, or assisting to cause, the death of any individual (assisted suicide) is not covered. This prohibition does not apply to the provision of an item or service for the purpose of alleviating pain or discomfort, even if such use may increase the risk of death, so long as the item or service is not furnished for the specific purpose of causing death.

100-2, 16, 90

Routine Services and Appliances

A3-3157, HO-260.7, B3-2320, R-1797A3 - 5/00

Routine physical checkups; eyeglasses, contact lenses, and eye examinations for the purpose of prescribing, fitting, or changing eyeglasses; eye refractions by whatever practitioner and for whatever purpose performed; hearing aids and examinations for hearing aids; and immunizations are not covered.

The routine physical checkup exclusion applies to (a) examinations performed without relationship to treatment or diagnosis for a specific illness, symptom, complaint, or injury; and (b) examinations required by third parties such as insurance companies business establishments, or Government agencies.

If the claim is for a diagnostic test or examination performed solely for the purpose of establishing a claim under title IV of Public Law 91-173, "Black Lung Benefits," the service is not covered under Medicare and the claimant should be advised to contact their Social Security office regarding the filing of a claim for reimbursement under the "Black Lung" program.

The exclusions apply to eyeglasses or contact lenses, and eye examinations for the purpose of prescribing, fitting, or changing eyeglasses or contact lenses for refractive errors. The exclusions do not apply to physicians' services (and services incident to a physicians' service) performed in conjunction with an eye disease, as for example, glaucoma or cataracts, or to post-surgical prosthetic lenses which are customarily used during convalescence from eye surgery in which the lens of the eye was removed, or to permanent prosthetic lenses required by an individual lacking the organic lens of the eye whether by surgical removal or congenital disease. Such prosthetic lens is a replacement for an internal body organ - the lens of the eye. (See the Medicare Benefit Policy Manual, Chapter 15, "Covered Medical and Other Health Services,"Sec.120). Expenses for all refractive procedures, whether performed by an ophthalmologist (or any other physician) or an optometrist and without regard to the reason for performance of the refraction, are excluded from coverage.

A. Immunizations
Vaccinations or inoculations are excluded as immunizations unless they are either

- Directly related to the treatment of an injury or direct exposure to a disease or condition, such as antirabies treatment, tetanus antitoxin or booster vaccine, botulin antitoxin, antivenin sera, or immune globulin. (In the absence of injury or direct exposure, preventive immunization (vaccination or inoculation) against such diseases as smallpox, polio, diphtheria, etc., is not covered.); or

- Specifically covered by statute, as described in the Medicare Benefit Policy Manual, Chapter 15, "Covered Medical and Other Health Services," Sec.50.

B. Antigens

Prior to the Omnibus Reconciliation Act of 1980, a physician who prepared an antigen for a patient could not be reimbursed for that service unless the physician also administered the antigen to the patient. Effective January 1, 1981, payment may be made for a reasonable supply of antigens that have been prepared for a particular patient even though they have not been administered to the patient by the same physician who prepared them if:

- The antigens are prepared by a physician who is a doctor of medicine or osteopathy, and
- The physician who prepared the antigens has examined the patient and has determined a plan of treatment and a dosage regimen.

A reasonable supply of antigens is considered to be not more than a 12-week supply of antigens that has been prepared for a particular patient at any one time. The purpose of the reasonable supply limitation is to assure that the antigens retain their potency and effectiveness over the period in which they are to be administered to the patient. (See the Medicare Benefit Policy Manual, Chapter 15, "Covered Medical and Other Health Services," Sec.50.4.4.2)

100-2, 16, 100

Hearing Aids and Auditory Implants

Section 1862(a)(7) of the Social Security Act states that no payment may be made under part A or part B for any expenses incurred for items or services "where such expenses are for . . . hearing aids or examinations therefore. . . ." This policy is further reiterated at 42 CFR 411.15(d) which specifically states that "hearing aids or examination for the purpose of prescribing, fitting, or changing hearing aids" are excluded from coverage.

Hearing aids are amplifying devices that compensate for impaired hearing. Hearing aids include air conduction devices that provide acoustic energy to the cochlea via stimulation of the tympanic membrane with amplified sound. They also include bone conduction devices that provide mechanical energy to the cochlea via stimulation of the scalp with amplified mechanical vibration or by direct contact with the tympanic membrane or middle ear ossicles.

Certain devices that produce perception of sound by replacing the function of the middle ear, cochlea or auditory nerve are payable by Medicare as prosthetic devices. These devices are indicated only when hearing aids are medically inappropriate or cannot be utilized due to congenital malformations, chronic disease, severe sensorineural hearing loss or surgery. The following are prosthetic devices:

- Cochlear implants and auditory brainstem implants, i.e., devices that replace the function of cochlear structures or auditory nerve and provide electrical energy to auditory nerve fibers and other neural tissue via implanted electrode arrays.
- Osseointegrated implants, i.e., devices implanted in the skull that replace the function of the middle ear and provide mechanical energy to the cochlea via a mechanical transducer.

Medicare contractors deny payment for an item or service that is associated with any hearing aid as defined above. See Sec.180 for policy for the medically necessary treatment of complications of implantable hearing aids, such as medically necessary removals of implantable hearing aids due to infection.

100-2, 16, 120

Cosmetic Surgery

A3-3160, HO-260.11, B3-2329

Cosmetic surgery or expenses incurred in connection with such surgery is not covered. Cosmetic surgery includes any surgical procedure directed at improving appearance, except when required for the prompt (i.e., as soon as medically feasible) repair of accidental injury or for the improvement of the functioning of a malformed body member. For example, this exclusion does not apply to surgery in connection with treatment of severe burns or repair of the face following a serious automobile accident, or to surgery for therapeutic purposes which coincidentally also serves some cosmetic purpose.

100-2, 16, 180

Services Related to and Required as a Result of Services Which Are Not Covered Under Medicare

B3-2300.1, A3-3101.14, HO-210.12

Medical and hospital services are sometimes required to treat a condition that arises as a result of services that are not covered because they are determined to be not reasonable and necessary or because they are excluded from coverage for other reasons. Services "related to" noncovered services (e.g., cosmetic surgery, noncovered organ transplants, noncovered artificial organ implants, etc.), including services related to follow-up care and complications of noncovered services which require treatment during a hospital stay in which the noncovered service was performed, are not covered services under Medicare. Services "not related to" noncovered services are covered under Medicare.

Following are examples of services "related to" and "not related to" noncovered services while the beneficiary is an inpatient:

- A beneficiary was hospitalized for a noncovered service and broke a leg while in the hospital. Services related to care of the broken leg during this stay is a clear example of "not related to" services and are covered under Medicare.
- A beneficiary was admitted to the hospital for covered services, but during the course of hospitalization became a candidate for a noncovered transplant or implant and actually received the transplant or implant during that hospital stay. When the original admission was entirely unrelated to the diagnosis that led to a recommendation for a noncovered transplant or implant, the services related to the admitting condition would be covered.
- A beneficiary was admitted to the hospital for covered services related to a condition which ultimately led to identification of a need for transplant and receipt of a transplant during the same hospital stay. If, on the basis of the nature of the services and a comparison of the date they are received with the date on which the beneficiary is identified as a transplant candidate, the services could reasonably be attributed to preparation for the noncovered transplant, the services would be "related to" noncovered services and would also be noncovered.

Following is an example of services received subsequent to a noncovered inpatient stay:

- After a beneficiary has been discharged from the hospital stay in which the beneficiary received noncovered services, medical and hospital services required to treat a condition or complication that arises as a result of the prior noncovered services may be covered when they are reasonable and necessary in all other respects. Thus, coverage could be provided for subsequent inpatient stays or outpatient treatment ordinarily covered by Medicare, even if the need for treatment arose because of a previous noncovered procedure. Some examples of services that may be found to be covered under this policy are the reversal of intestinal bypass surgery for obesity, repair of complications from transsexual surgery or from cosmetic surgery, removal of a noncovered bladder stimulator, or treatment of any infection at the surgical site of a noncovered transplant that occurred following discharge from the hospital.

However, any subsequent services that could be expected to have been incorporated into a global fee are considered to have been paid in the global fee, and may not be paid again. Thus, where a patient undergoes cosmetic surgery and the treatment regimen calls for a series of postoperative visits to the surgeon for evaluating the patient's progress, these visits are not paid.

100-3, 10.1

Use of Visual Tests Prior to and General Anesthesia during Cataract Surgery

A - Pre-Surgery Evaluations

Cataract surgery with an intraocular lens (IOL) implant is a high volume Medicare procedure. Along with the surgery, a substantial number of preoperative tests are available to the surgeon. In most cases, a comprehensive eye examination (ocular history and ocular examination) and a single scan to determine the appropriate pseudophakic power of the IOL are sufficient. In most cases involving a simple cataract, a diagnostic ultrasound A-scan is used. For patients with a dense cataract, an ultrasound B-scan may be used.

Accordingly, where the only diagnosis is cataract(s), Medicare does not routinely cover testing other than one comprehensive eye examination (or a combination of a brief/intermediate examination not to exceed the charge of a comprehensive examination) and an A-scan or, if medically justified, a B-scan. Claims for additional tests are denied as not reasonable and necessary unless there is an additional diagnosis and the medical need for the additional tests is fully documented.

Because cataract surgery is an elective procedure, the patient may decide not to have the surgery until later, or to have the surgery performed by a physician other than the diagnosing physician. In these situations, it may be medically appropriate for the operating physician to conduct another examination. To the extent the additional tests are considered reasonable and necessary by the carrier's medical staff, they are covered.

B - General Anesthesia

The use of general anesthesia in cataract surgery may be considered reasonable and necessary if, for particular medical indications, it is the accepted procedure among ophthalmologists in the local community to use general anesthesia

100-3, 10.2

Transcutaneous Electrical Nerve Stimulation (TENS) for Acute Post-Operative Pain

The use of transcutaneous electrical nerve stimulation (TENS) for the relief of acute post-operative pain is covered under Medicare. TENS may be covered whether used as an adjunct to the use of drugs, or as an alternative to drugs, in the treatment of acute pain resulting from surgery.

The TENS devices, whether durable or disposable, may be used in furnishing this service. When used for the purpose of treating acute post-operative pain, TENS devices are considered supplies. As such they may be hospital supplies furnished inpatients covered under Part A, or supplies incident to a physician's service when furnished in connection with surgery done on an outpatient basis, and covered under Part B.

It is expected that TENS, when used for acute post-operative pain, will be necessary for relatively short periods of time, usually 30 days or less. In cases when TENS is used for longer periods, contractors should attempt to ascertain whether TENS is no longer being used for acute pain but rather for chronic pain, in which case the TENS device may be covered as durable medical equipment as described in §160.27.

Cross-references:

Medicare Benefit Policy Manual, Chapter 1, "Inpatient Hospital Services," §40;

Medicare Benefit Policy Manual, Chapter 2, "Hospital Services Covered Under Part B," §§20, 20.4, and 80; Medicare Benefit Policy Manual, Chapter 15, "Covered Medical and other Health Services, §110."

100-3, 10.3

Inpatient Hospital Pain Rehabilitation Programs

Since pain rehabilitation programs of a lesser scope than that described above would raise a question as to whether the program could be provided in a less intensive setting than on an inpatient hospital basis, carefully evaluate such programs to determine whether the program does, in fact, necessitate a hospital level of care. Some pain rehabilitation programs may utilize services and devices which are excluded from coverage, e.g., acupuncture (see 35-8), biofeedback (see 35-27), dorsal column stimulator (see 65-8), and family counseling services (see 35-l4). In determining whether the scope of a pain program does necessitate inpatient hospital care, evaluate only those services and devices which are covered. Although diagnostic tests may be an appropriate part of pain rehabilitation programs, such tests would be covered in an individual case only where they can be reasonably related to a patient's illness, complaint, symptom, or injury and where they do not represent an unnecessary duplication of tests previously performed.

An inpatient program of 4 weeks' duration is generally required to modify pain behavior. After this period it would be expected that any additional rehabilitation services which might be required could be effectively provided on an outpatient basis under an outpatient pain rehabilitation program (see 10.4 of the NCD Manual) or other outpatient program. The first 7-l0 days of such an inpatient program constitute, in effect, an evaluation period. If a patient is unable to adjust to the program within this period, it is generally concluded that it is unlikely that the program will be effective and the patient is discharged from the program. On occasions a program longer than 4 weeks may be required in a particular case. In such a case there should be documentation to substantiate that inpatient care beyond a 4-week period was reasonable and necessary. Similarly, where it appears that a patient participating in a program is being granted frequent outside passes, a question would exist as to whether an inpatient program is reasonable and necessary for the treatment of the patient's condition.

An inpatient hospital stay for the purpose of participating in a pain rehabilitation program would be covered as reasonable and necessary to the treatment of a patient's condition where the pain is attributable to a physical cause, the usual methods of treatment have not been successful in alleviating it, and a significant loss of ability to function independently has resulted from the pain. Chronic pain patients often have psychological problems which accompany or stem from the physical pain and it is appropriate to include psychological treatment in the multidisciplinary approach. However, patients whose pain symptoms result from a mental condition, rather than from any physical cause, generally cannot be successfully treated in a pain rehabilitation program.

100-3,10.4

Outpatient Hospital Pain Rehabilitation Programs

Some hospitals also provide pain rehabilitation programs for outpatients. In such programs, services frequently are provided in group settings even though they are being furnished pursuant to each patient's individualized plan of treatment.

Coverage of services furnished under outpatient hospital pain rehabilitation programs, including services furnished in group settings under individualized plans of treatment, is available if the patient's pain is attributable to a physical cause, the usual methods of treatment have not been successful in alleviating it, and a significant loss of ability by the patient to function independently has resulted from the pain. If a patient meets these conditions and the program provides services of the types discussed in 10.3 of the NCD Manual, the services provided under the program may be covered. Noncovered servlces (e.g., vocatlonal counselling, meals for outpatients, or acupuncture) continue to be excluded from coverage, and intermediaries would not be precluded from finding, in the case of particular patients, that the pain rehabilitation program is not reasonable and necessary under 1862(a)(1) of the Act for the treatment of their conditions.

100-3,10.5

Autogenous Epidural Blood Graft

Autogenous epidural blood grafts are considered a safe and effective remedy for severe headaches that may occur after performance of spinal anesthesia, spinal taps or myelograms, and are covered.

100-3, 10.6

Anesthesia in Cardiac Pacemaker Surgery

10.6 - CIM 35-79

The use of general or monitored anesthesia during transvenous cardiac pacemaker surgery may be reasonable and necessary and therefore covered under Medicare only if adequate documentation of medical necessity is provided on a case-by-case basis. The contractor obtains advice from its medical consultants or from appropriate specialty physicians or groups in its locality regarding the adequacy of documentation before deciding whether a particular claim should be covered.

A second type of pacemaker surgery that is sometimes performed involves the use of the thoracic method of implantation which requires open surgery. Where the thoracic method is employed, general anesthesia is always used and should not require special medical documentation.

100-3, 20.1

Vertebral Artery Surgery

- These procedures can be medically reasonable and necessary, but only if each of the following conditions is met:
- Symptoms of vertebral artery obstruction exist;
- Other causes have been considered and ruled out;
- There is radiographic evidence of a valid vertebral artery obstruction; and
- Contraindications to the procedure do not exist, such as coexistent obstructions of multiple cerebral vessels.

Angiograms documenting a valid obstruction should show not only the aortic arch with the vessels off the arch, but also show the vessels in the neck and head (providing biplane views of the carotid and vertebral vascular system). In addition, serial views are needed to diagnose "subclavian steal," the condition in which subclavian artery obstruction causes the symptoms of vertebral artery obstruction. Because the symptoms are not specific for vertebral artery obstruction, other causes must be considered. In addition to vertebral artery obstruction, the differential diagnosis should include various degenerative disorders of the brain, orthostatic hypotension, acoustic neuroma, labyrinthitis, diabetes mellitus and hypoglycemia related disorders.

Obstructions which can cause symptoms of blocked vertebral artery blood flow and which can be documented by an angiogram include:

- Intravascular obstructions - arteriosclerotic lesions within the vertebral artery or in other arteries.
- Extravascular obstructions.
- Bony tissue or osteophytes, located laterally in the C6(C7)-C2 cervical vertebral area course of the vertebral artery, most commonly at C5 -C6.
- Anatomical variations - Anomalous location of the origin of the vertebral artery, a congenital aberration, and tortuosity and kinks of the vertebral artery.
- Fibrous tissue - Tissue changed as a result of manipulation of the neck for neck pain or injury associated with hematoma; external bands, tendinous slings, and fibrous bands.

The most controversial obstructions include vertebral artery tortuosity and kinks and connective tissue along the course of the vertebral artery, and variously called external bands, tendinous slings and fibrous bands. In the absence of symptoms of vertebral artery obstruction, vascular surgeons feel such abnormalities are insignificant. Vascular surgery experts, however, agree that these abnormalities in very rare cases do cause symptoms of vertebral artery obstruction and do necessitate surgical correction.

Vertebral artery construction and vertebral artery surgery are phrases which most physicians interpret to include only surgical cleaning (endarterectomy) and bypass (resection) procedures. However, some physicians who use these terms mean all operative manipulations which remove vertebral artery blood flow obstructions. Also, some physicians use general terms of vascular surgery, such as endarterectomy when vertebral artery related surgery is performed. Use of the above terminology specifies neither the surgical procedure performed nor its relationship to the vertebral artery. Therefore, in developing claims for this type of procedure, require specific identification of the obstruction in question and the surgical procedure performed. Also, in view of the specific coverage criteria given, develop all claims for vertebral artery surgery on a case-by-case basis.

Make payment for a surgical procedure listed above if: (1) it is reasonable and necessary for the individual patient to have the surgery performed to remove or relieve an obstruction to vertebral artery flow, and (2) the four conditions noted are met.

In all other cases, these procedures cannot be considered reasonable and necessary within the meaning of Sec.1862(a)(1) of the Act and are not reimbursable under the program.

100-3, 20.2

Extracranial - Intracranial (EC-IC) Arterial Bypass Surgery

(Rev. 1, 10-03-03) CIM 35-37

Extracranial-Intracranial (EC-IC) arterial bypass surgery is not a covered procedure when it is performed as a treatment for ischemic cerebrovascular disease of the carotid or middle cerebral arteries which includes the treatment or prevention of strokes. The premise that this procedure which bypasses narrowed arterial segments, improves the blood supply to the brain and reduces the risk of having a stroke has not been demonstrated to be any more effective than no surgical intervention. Accordingly, EC-IC arterial bypass surgery is not considered reasonable and necessary within the meaning of §1862(a)(1) of the Act when it is performed as a treatment for ischemic cerebrovascular disease of the carotid or middle cerebral arteries.

100-3, 20.3

Thoracic Duct Drainage (TDD) in Renal Transplants

TDD is performed on an inpatient basis, and the inpatient stay is covered for patients admitted for treatment in advance of a kidney transplant as well as for those receiving it post-transplant. TDD is a covered technique when furnished to a kidney transplant recipient or an individual approved to receive kidney transplantation in a hospital approved to perform kidney transplantation.

100-3, 20.4

Implantable Automatic Defibrillators

A. General

The implantable automatic defibrillator is an electronic device designed to detect and treat life-threatening tachyarrhythmias. The device consists of a pulse generator and electrodes for sensing and defibrillating.

B. Covered Indications

1. Documented episode of cardiac arrest due to ventricular fibrillation (VF), not due to a transient or reversible cause (effective July 1, 1991).
2. Documented sustained ventricular tachyarrhythmia (VT), either spontaneous or induced by an electrophysiology (EP) study, not associated with an acute myocardial infarction (MI) and not due to a transient or reversible cause (effective July 1, 1999).
3. Documented familial or inherited conditions with a high risk of life-threatening VT, such as long QT syndrome or hypertrophic cardiomyopathy (effective July 1, 1999).

   Additional indications effective for services performed on or after October 1, 2003:
4. Coronary artery disease with a documented prior MI, a measured left ventricular ejection fraction (LVEF) <0.35, and inducible, sustained VT or VF at EP study. (The MI must have occurred more than 40 days prior to defibrillator insertion. The EP test must be performed more than 4 weeks after the qualifying MI.)
5. Documented prior MI and a measured LVEF <0.30 and a QRS duration of >120 milliseconds (the QRS restriction does not apply to services performed on or after January 27, 2005) . Patients must not have:
   a. New York Heart Association (NYHC) classification IV;
   b. Cardiogenic shock or symptomatic hypotension while in a stable baseline rhythm;
   c. Had a coronary artery bypass graft (CABG) or percutaneous transluminal coronary angioplasty (PTCA) within past 3 months;
   d. Had an enzyme positive MI within past month (Effective for services on or after January 27, 2005, patients must not have an acute MI in the past 40 days);
   e. Clinical symptoms or findings that would make them a candidate for coronary revascularization; or
   f. Any disease, other than cardiac disease (e.g., cancer, uremia, liver failure), associated with a likelihood of survival less than 1 year.

   Additional indications effective for services performed on or after January 27, 2005:
6. Patients with ischemic dilated cardiomyopathy (IDCM), documented prior MI, NYHA Class II and III heart failure, and measured LVEF <35%;
7. Patients with non-ischemic dilated cardiomyopathy (NIDCM) >9 months, NYHA Class II and III heart failure, and measured LVEF <35%;
8. Patients who meet all current Centers for Medicare & Medicaid Services (CMS) coverage requirements for a cardiac resynchronization therapy (CRT) device and have NYHA Class IV heart failure;

   All indications must meet the following criteria:
   a. Patients must not have irreversible brain damage from preexisting cerebral disease;
   b. MIs must be documented and defined according to the consensus document of the Joint European Society of Cardiology/American College of Cardiology Committee for the Redefinition of Myocardial Infarction[1];

   Either one of the following criteria satisfies the diagnosis for an acute, evolving or recent MI:

1. Alpert and Thygesen et al., 2000. Criteria for acute, evolving or recent MI.

1. Typical rise and gradual fall (troponin) or more rapid rise and fall (CK-MB) of biochemical markers of myocardial necrosis with at least one of the following:
   a. ischemic symptoms;
   b. development of pathologic Q waves on the ECG;
   c. ECG changes indicative of ischemia (ST segment elevation or depression); or
   d. coronary artery intervention (e.g., coronary angioplasty).
2. Pathologic findings of an acute MI.

   Criteria for established MI.

   Any one of the following criteria satisfies the diagnosis for established MI:

   Indications 3-8 (primary prevention of sudden cardiac death) must also meet the following critera:
   a. Patients must be able to give informed consent;
   b. Patients must have:
      - Cardiogenic shock or symptomatic hypotension while in a stable baseline rhythm;
      - Had a CABG or PTCA within the past 3 months;
      - Had an acute MI within the past 40 days;
      - Clinical symptoms or findings that would make them a candidate for coronary revascularization;
      - Any disease, other than cardiac disease (e.g., cancer, uremia, liver failure), associated with a likelihood of survival less than 1 year;
   c. Ejection fractions must be measured by angiography, radionuclide scanning, or echocardiography;
   d. The beneficiary receiving the defibrillator implantation for primary prevention is enrolled in either a Food and Drug Administration (FDA)-approved category B investigational device exemption (IDE) clinical trial (42 CFR Sec.405.201), a trial under the CMS Clinical Trial Policy (National Coverage Determination (NCD) Manual Sec.310.1) or a qualifying data collection system including approved clinical trials and registries. Initially, an implantable cardiac defibrillator (ICD) database will be maintained using a data submission mechanism that is already in use by Medicare participating hospitals to submit data to the Iowa Foundation for Medical Care (IFMC)--a Quality Improvement Organization (QIO) contractor--for determination of reasonable and necessary and quality improvement. Initial hypothesis and data elements are specified in this decision (Appendix VI) and are the minimum necessary to ensure that the device is reasonable and necessary. Data collection will be completed using the ICDA (ICD Abstraction Tool) and transmitted via QNet (Quality Network Exchange) to the IFMC who will collect and maintain the database. Additional stakeholder-developed data collection systems to augment or replace the initial QNet system, addressing at a minimum the hypotheses specified in this decision, must meet the following basic criteria:
      - Written protocol on file;
        1) Development of new pathologic Q waves on serial ECGs. The patient may or may not remember previous symptoms. Biochemical markers of myocardial necrosis may have normalized, depending on the length of time that has passed since the infarct developed.
        2) Pathologic findings of a healed or healing MI.
           - Institutional review board review and approval;
           - Scientific review and approval by two or more qualified individuals who are not part of the research team;
           - Certification that investigators have not been disqualified.
   e. For purposes of this coverage decision, CMS will determine whether specific registries or clinical trials meet these criteria.
   f. Providers must be able to justify the medical necessity of devices other than single lead devices. This justification should be available in the patient's medical record.
9. Patients with NIDCM >3 months, NYHA Class II or III heart failure, and measured LVEF = 35%, only if the following additional criteria are also met:
   a. Patients must be able to give informed consent;
   b. Patients must not have:
      - Cardiogenic shock or symptomatic hypotension while in a stable baseline rhythm;
      - Had a CABG or PTCA within the past 3 months;
      - Had an acute MI within the past 40 days;
      - Clinical symptoms or findings that would make them a candidate for coronary revascularization;
      - Irreversible brain damage from preexisting cerebral disease;
      - Any disease, other than cardiac disease (e.g. cancer, uremia, liver failure), associated with a likelihood of survival less than 1 year;

c. Ejection fractions must be measured by angiography, radionuclide scanning, or echocardiography;

d. MIs must be documented and defined according to the consensus document of the Joint European Society of Cardiology/American College of Cardiology Committee for the Redefinition of Myocardial Infarction;[1]

e. The beneficiary receiving the defibrillator implantation for this indication is enrolled in either an FDA-approved category B IDE clinical trial (42 CFR §405.201), a trial under the CMS Clinical Trial Policy (NCD Manual §310.1), or a prospective data collection system meeting the following basic criteria:

- Written protocol on file;
- Institutional Review Board review and approval;
- Scientific review and approval by two or more qualified individuals who are not part of the research team;
- Certification that investigators have not been disqualified.

For purposes of this coverage decision, CMS will determine whether specific registries or clinical trials meet these criteria.

d. Providers must be able to justify the medical necessity of devices other than single lead devices. This justification should be available in the patient's medical record.

C. Other Indications

All other indications for implantable automatic defibrillators not currently covered in accordance with this decision will continue to be covered under Category B IDE trials (42 CFR §405.201) and the CMS routine clinical trials policy (NCD §310.1).

(This NCD last reviewed February 2005.)

100-3, 20.5

Extracorporeal Immunoadsorption (ECI) Using Protein A Columns

For claims with dates of service on or after January 1, 2001, Medicare covers the use of Protein A columns for the treatment of ITP. In addition, Medicare will cover Protein A columns for the treatment of rheumatoid arthritis (RA) under the following conditions:

- Patient has severe RA. Patient disease is active, having >5 swollen joints, >20 tender joints, and morning stiffness >60 minutes.
- Patient has failed an adequate course of a minimum of 3 Disease Modifying Anti-Rheumatic Drugs (DMARDs). Failure does not include intolerance.

Other uses of these columns are currently considered to be investigational and, therefore, not reasonable and necessary under the Medicare law. (See Sec.1862(a)(1)(A) of the Act.)

100-3, 20.6

Transmyocardial Revascularization (TMR)

CMS therefore covers TMR as a late or last resort for patients with severe (Canadian Cardiovascular Society classification Classes III or IV) angina (stable or unstable), which has been found refractory to standard medical therapy, including drug therapy at the maximum tolerated or maximum safe dosages. In addition, the angina symptoms must be caused by areas of the heart not amenable to surgical therapies such as percutaneous transluminal coronary angioplasty, stenting, coronary atherectomy or coronary bypass. Coverage is further limited to those uses of the laser used in performing the procedure which have been approved by the Food and Drug Administration for the purpose for which they are being used.

Patients would have to meet the following additional selection guidelines:

- An ejection fraction of 25% or greater;
- Have areas of viable ischemic myocardium (as demonstrated by diagnostic study) which are not capable of being revascularized by direct coronary intervention; and
- Have been stabilized, or have had maximal efforts to stabilize acute conditions such as severe ventricular arrhythmias, decompensated congestive heart failure or acute myocardial infarction.

Coverage is limited to physicians who have been properly trained in the procedure. Providers of this service is performed must also document that all ancillary personnel, including physicians, nurses, operating room personnel and technicians, are trained in the procedure and the proper use of the equipment involved. Coverage is further limited to providers which have dedicated cardiac care units, including the diagnostic and support services necessary for care of patients undergoing this therapy. In addition, these providers must conform to the standards for laser safety set by the American National Standards Institute, ANSIZ1363.

100-3, 20.7

Percutaneous Transluminal Angioplasty (PTA)

A. General

This procedure involves inserting a balloon catheter into a narrow or occluded blood vessel to recanalize and dilate the vessel by inflating the balloon. The objective of PTA is to improve the blood flow through the diseased segment of a vessel so that vessel patency is increased and embolization is decreased. With the development and use of balloon angioplasty for treatment of atherosclerotic and other vascular stenoses, PTA (with and without the placement of a stent) is a widely used technique for dilating lesions of peripheral, renal, and coronary arteries.

Indications and Limitations of Coverage

B. Nationally Covered Indications

The PTA is covered when used under the following conditions:

1. Treatment of Atherosclerotic Obstructive Lesions

- In the lower extremities, i.e., the iliac, femoral, and popliteal arteries, or in the upper extremities, i.e., the innominate, subclavian, axillary, and brachial arteries. The upper extremities do not include head or neck vessels.
- Of a single coronary artery for patients for whom the likely alternative treatment is coronary bypass surgery and who exhibit the following characteristics:
  - Angina refractory to optimal medical management;
  - Objective evidence of myocardial ischemia; and
  - Lesions amenable to angioplasty.
- Of the renal arteries for patients in whom there is an inadequate response to a thorough medical management of symptoms and for whom surgery is the likely alternative. PTA for this group of patients is an alternative to surgery, not simply an addition to medical management.
- Of arteriovenous dialysis fistulas and grafts when performed through either a venous or arterial approach.

2. Concurrent with Carotid Stent Placement in Food and Drug Administration (FDA)-Approved Category B Investigational Device Exemption (IDE) Clinical Trials

Effective July 1, 2001, Medicare covers PTA of the carotid artery concurrent with carotid stent placement when furnished in accordance with the FDA-approved protocols governing Category B IDE clinical trials. PTA of the carotid artery, when provided solely for the purpose of carotid artery dilation concurrent with carotid stent placement, is considered to be a reasonable and necessary service when provided in the context of such a clinical trial.

3. Concurrent with Carotid Stent Placement in FDA-Approved Post-Approval Studies

Effective October 12, 2004, Medicare covers PTA of the carotid artery concurrent with the placement of an FDA-approved carotid stent and an FDA-approved or -cleared embolic protection device (effective December 9, 2009) for an FDA-approved indication when furnished in accordance with FDA-approved protocols governing post-approval studies. CMS determines that coverage of PTA of the carotid artery is reasonable and necessary in these circumstances.

4. Concurrent with Carotid Stent Placement in Patients at High Risk for Carotid Endarterectomy (CEA)

Effective March 17, 2005, Medicare covers PTA of the carotid artery concurrent with the placement of an FDA-approved carotid stent with embolic protection for the following:

Patients who are at high risk for CEA and who also have symptomatic carotid artery stenosis >=70%. Coverage is limited to procedures performed using FDA-approved carotid artery stenting systems and FDA-approved or -cleared (effective December 9, 2009) embolic protection devices. If deployment of the embolic protection device is not technically possible, and not performed, then the procedure is not covered by Medicare (effective December 9, 2009);

Patients who are at high risk for CEA and have symptomatic carotid artery stenosis between 50% and 70%, in accordance with the Category B IDE clinical trials regulation (42 CFR 405.201), as a routine cost under the clinical trials policy (Medicare NCD Manual 310.1), or in accordance with the NCD on carotid artery stenting (CAS) post-approval studies (Medicare NCD Manual 20.7);

Patients who are at high risk for CEA and have asymptomatic carotid artery stenosis >=80%, in accordance with the Category B IDE clinical trials regulation (42 CFR 405.201), as a routine cost under the clinical trials policy (Medicare NCD Manual 310.1), or in accordance with the NCD on CAS post-approval studies (Medicare NCD Manual 20.7).

Coverage is limited to procedures performed using FDA-approved carotid artery stents and FDA-approved or -cleared embolic protection devices.

The use of an FDA-approved or cleared embolic protection device is required. If deployment of the embolic protection device is not technically possible, and not performed, then the procedure is not covered by Medicare.

Patients at high risk for CEA are defined as having significant comorbidities and/or anatomic risk factors (i.e., recurrent stenosis and/or previous radical neck dissection), and would be poor candidates for CEA. Significant comorbid conditions include but are not limited to:

- Congestive heart failure (CHF) class III/IV;
- Left ventricular ejection fraction (LVEF) <30%;
- Unstable angina;
- Contralateral carotid occlusion;

1. Ibid.

- Recent myocardial infarction (MI);
- Previous CEA with recurrent stenosis;
- Prior radiation treatment to the neck; and

Other conditions that were used to determine patients at high risk for CEA in the prior carotid artery stenting trials and studies, such as ARCHER, CABERNET, SAPPHIRE, BEACH, and MAVERIC II.

Symptoms of carotid artery stenosis include carotid transient ischemic attack (distinct focal neurological dysfunction persisting less than 24 hours), focal cerebral ischemia producing a non-disabling stroke (modified Rankin scale <3 with symptoms for 24 hours or more), and transient monocular blindness (amaurosis fugax). Patients who have had a disabling stroke (modified Rankin scale >=3) shall be excluded from coverage.

The determination that a patient is at high risk for CEA and the patient's symptoms of carotid artery stenosis shall be available in the patient medical records prior to performing any procedure.

The degree of carotid artery stenosis shall be measured by duplex Doppler ultrasound or carotid artery angiography and recorded in the patient's medical records. If the stenosis is measured by ultrasound prior to the procedure, then the degree of stenosis must be confirmed by angiography at the start of the procedure. If the stenosis is determined to be <70% by angiography, then CAS should not proceed.

In addition, CMS has determined that CAS with embolic protection is reasonable and necessary only if performed in facilities that have been determined to be competent in performing the evaluation, procedure and follow-up necessary to ensure optimal patient outcomes. Standards to determine competency include specific physician training standards, facility support requirements and data collection to evaluate outcomes during a required reevaluation.

The CMS has created a list of minimum standards modeled in part on professional society statements on competency. All facilities must at least meet CMS's standards in order to receive coverage for carotid artery stenting for high-risk patients.

Facilities must have necessary imaging equipment, device inventory, staffing, and infrastructure to support a dedicated carotid stent program. Specifically, high-quality x-ray imaging equipment is a critical component of any carotid interventional suite, such as high-resolution digital imaging systems with the capability of subtraction, magnification, road mapping, and orthogonal angulation.

Advanced physiologic monitoring must be available in the interventional suite. This includes real time and archived physiologic, hemodynamic, and cardiac rhythm monitoring equipment, as well as support staff who are capable of interpreting the findings and responding appropriately.

Emergency management equipment and systems must be readily available in the interventional suite such as resuscitation equipment, a defibrillator, vasoactive and antiarrhythmic drugs, endotracheal intubation capability, and anesthesia support.

Each institution shall have a clearly delineated program for granting carotid stent privileges and for monitoring the quality of the individual interventionalists and the program as a whole. The oversight committee for this program shall be empowered to identify the minimum case volume for an operator to maintain privileges, as well as the (risk-adjusted) threshold for complications that the institution will allow before suspending privileges or instituting measures for remediation. Committees are encouraged to apply published standards from national specialty societies recognized by the American Board of Medical Specialties to determine appropriate physician qualifications. Examples of standards and clinical competence guidelines include those published in the December 2004 edition of the American Journal of Neuroradiology, and those published in the August 18, 2004, Journal of the American College of Cardiology.

To continue to receive Medicare payment for CAS under this decision, the facility or a contractor to the facility must collect data on all CAS procedures done at that particular facility. This data must be analyzed routinely to ensure patient safety. This data must be made available to CMS upon request. The interval for data analysis will be determined by the facility but shall not be less frequent than every 6 months.

Since there currently is no recognized entity that evaluates CAS facilities, CMS has established a mechanism for evaluating facilities. Facilities must provide written documentation to CMS that the facility meets one of the following:

1. The facility was an FDA-approved site that enrolled patients in prior CAS IDE trials, such as SAPPHIRE, and ARCHER;
2. The facility is an FDA-approved site that is participating and enrolling patients in ongoing CAS IDE trials, such as CREST;
3. The facility is an FDA-approved site for one or more FDA post approval studies; or
4. The facility has provided a written affidavit to CMS attesting that the facility has met the minimum facility standards. This should be sent to:

   Director, Coverage and Analysis Group
   7500 Security Boulevard, Mailstop C1-09-06
   Baltimore, MD 21244

   The letter must include the following information:

   Facility's name and complete address;

   Facility's national provider identifier (formerly referred to as the Medicare provider number);

   Point-of-contact for questions with telephone number;

   Discussion of how each standard has been met by the hospital;

   Mechanism of data collection of CAS procedures; and

   Signature of a senior facility administrative official.

   A list of certified facilities will be made available and viewable at: http://www.cms.hhs.gov/coverage/carotid-stent-facilities.asp.

   In addition, CMS will publish a list of approved facilities in the Federal Register.

   Facilities must recertify every two (2) years in order to maintain Medicare coverage of CAS procedures. Recertification will occur when the facility documents that and describes how it continues to meet the CMS standards.

The process for recertification is as follows:

1. At 23 months after initial certification:

   Submission of a letter to CMS stating how the facility continues to meet the minimum facility standards as listed above.

2. At 27 months after initial certification:

   Submission of required data elements for all CAS procedures performed on patients during the previous two (2) years of certification.

   Data elements:

   a. Patients' Medicare identification number if a Medicare beneficiary;

   b. Patients' date of birth;

   c. Date of procedure;

   d. Does the patient meet high surgical risk criteria (defined below)?

   - Age >=80;
   - Recent (<30 days) Myocardial Infarction (MI);
   - Left Ventricle Ejection Fraction (LVEF) <30%;
   - Contralateral carotid occlusion;
   - New York Heart Association (NYHA) Class III or IV congestive heart failure;
   - Unstable angina: Canadian Cardiovascular Society (CCS) Class III/IV;
   - Renal failure: end stage renal disease on dialysis;
   - Common Carotid Artery (CCA) lesion(s) below clavicle;
   - Severe chronic lung disease;
   - Previous neck radiation;
   - High cervical Internal Carotid Artery (ICA) lesion(s);
   - Restenosis of prior carotid endarterectomy (CEA);
   - Tracheostomy;
   - Contralateral laryngeal nerve palsy.

   e. Is the patient symptomatic (defined below)?

   - Carotid Transient Ischemic Attack (TIA) persisting less than 24 hours;
   - Non-disabling stroke: Modified Rankin Scale
   - Transient monocular blindness:amaurosis fugax.

   f. Modified Rankin Scale score if the patient experienced a stroke.

   g. Percent of stenosis of stented lesion(s) by angiography.

   h. Was embolic protection used?

   i. Were there any complications during hospitalization (defined below)?

   - All stroke: an ischemic neurologic deficit that persisted more than 24 hours;
   - MI;
   - All death.

Recertification is effective for two (2) additional years during which facilities will be required to submit the requested data every April 1 and October 1.

The CMS will consider the approval of national CAS registries that provide CMS with a comprehensive overview of the registry and its capabilities, and the manner in which the registry meets CMS data collection and evaluation requirements. Specific standards for CMS approval are listed below. Facilities enrolled in a CMS-approved national CAS registry will automatically meet the data collection standards required for initial and continued facility certification. Hospitals' contracts with an approved registry may include authority for the registry to submit required data to CMS for the hospital. A list of approved registries will be available on the CMS Coverage Web site.

National Registries
As noted above, CMS will approve national registries developed by professional societies and other organizations and allow these entities to collect and submit data to CMS on behalf of participating facilities to meet facility certification and recertification requirements. To be

eligible to perform these functions and become a CMS-approved registry, the national registry, at a minimum, must be able to:

1. Enroll facilities in every U.S. state and territory;
2. Assure data confidentiality and compliance with HIPPA;
3. Collect the required CMS data elements as listed in the above section;
4. Assure data quality and data completeness;
5. Address deficiencies in the facility data collection, quality, and submission;
6. Validate the data submitted by facilities as needed;
7. Track long term outcomes such as stroke and death;
8. Conduct data analyses and produce facility specific data reports and summaries;
9. Submit data to CMS on behalf of the individual facilities; and
10. Provide quarterly reports to CMS on facilities that do not meet or no longer meet the CMS facility certification and recertification requirements pertaining to data collection and analysis.

Registries wishing to receive this designation from CMS must submit evidence that they meet or exceed our standards. Though the registry requirements pertain to CAS, CMS strongly encourages all national registries to establish a similar mechanism to collect comparable data on CEA. Having both CAS and CEA data will help answer questions about carotid revascularization, in general, in the Medicare population.

The CAS for patients who are not at high risk for CEA remains covered only in FDA-approved Category B IDE clinical trials under 42 CFR 405.201.

The CMS has determined that PTA of the carotid artery concurrent with the placement of an FDA-approved carotid stent and an FDA-approved or -cleared embolic protection device is not reasonable and necessary for all other patients.

5. Concurrent with Intracranial Stent Placement in FDA-Approved Category B IDE Clinical Trials

Effective November 6, 2006, Medicare covers PTA and stenting of intracranial arteries for the treatment of cerebral artery stenosis >=50% in patients with intracranial atherosclerotic disease when furnished in accordance with the FDA-approved protocols governing Category B IDE clinical trials. CMS determines that coverage of intracranial PTA and stenting is reasonable and necessary under these circumstances.

C. Nationally Non-Covered Indications
All other indications for PTA with or without stenting to treat obstructive lesions of the vertebral and cerebral arteries remain non-covered. The safety and efficacy of these procedures are not established.

All other indications for PTA without stenting for which CMS has not specifically indicated coverage remain non-covered.

D. Other
Coverage of PTA with stenting not specifically addressed or discussed in this NCD is at local Medicare contractor discretion.

(This NCD last reviewed December 2009.)

100-3, 20.8

Cardiac Pacemakers

Cardiac pacemakers are self-contained, battery-operated units that send electrical stimulation to the heart. They are generally implanted to alleviate symptoms of decreased cardiac output related to abnormal heart rate and/or rhythm. Pacemakers are generally used for persistent, symptomatic second- or third-degree atrioventricular (AV) block and symptomatic sinus bradycardia.

Cardiac pacemakers are covered as prosthetic devices under the Medicare program, subject to the following conditions and limitations. While cardiac pacemakers have been covered under Medicare for many years, there were no specific guidelines for their use other than the general Medicare requirement that covered services be reasonable and necessary for the treatment of the condition. Services rendered for cardiac pacing on or after the effective dates of this instruction are subject to these guidelines, which are based on certain assumptions regarding the clinical goals of cardiac pacing. While some uses of pacemakers are relatively certain or unambiguous, many other uses require considerable expertise and judgment.

Consequently, the medical necessity for permanent cardiac pacing must be viewed in the context of overall patient management. The appropriateness of such pacing may be conditional on other diagnostic or therapeutic modalities having been undertaken. Although significant complications and adverse side effects of pacemaker use are relatively rare, they cannot be ignored when considering the use of pacemakers for dubious medical conditions, or marginal clinical benefit.

These guidelines represent current concepts regarding medical circumstances in which permanent cardiac pacing may be appropriate or necessary. As with other areas of medicine, advances in knowledge and techniques in cardiology are expected. Consequently, judgments about the medical necessity and acceptability of new uses for cardiac pacing in new classes of patients may change as more more conclusive evidence becomes available. This instruction applies only to permanent cardiac pacemakers, and does not address the use of temporary, non-implanted pacemakers.

The two groups of conditions outlined below deal with the necessity for cardiac pacing for patients in general. These are intended as guidelines in assessing the medical necessity for pacing therapies, taking into account the particular circumstances in each case. However, as a general rule, the two groups of current medical concepts may be viewed as representing:

Group I: Single-Chamber Cardiac Pacemakers – a) conditions under which single chamber pacemaker claims may be considered covered without further claims development; and b) conditions under which single-chamber pacemaker claims would be denied unless further claims development shows that they fall into the covered category, or special medical circumstances exist of the sufficiency to convince the contractor that the claim should be paid.

Group II: Dual-Chamber Cardiac Pacemakers - a) conditions under which dual-chamber pacemaker claims may be considered covered without further claims development, and b) conditions under which dual-chamber pacemaker claims would be denied unless further claims development shows that they fall into the covered categories for single- and dual-chamber pacemakers, or special medical circumstances exist sufficient to convince the contractor that the claim should be paid.

The CMS opened the NCD on Cardiac Pacemakers to afford the public an opportunity to comment on the proposal to revise the language contained in the instruction. The revisions transfer the focus of the NCD from the actual pacemaker implantation procedure itself to the reasonable and necessary medical indications that justify cardiac pacing. This is consistent with our findings that pacemaker implantation is no longer considered routinely harmful or an experimental procedure.

Group I: Single-Chamber Cardiac Pacemakers (Effective March 16, 1983)

A. Nationally Covered Indications
Conditions under which cardiac pacing is generally considered acceptable or necessary, provided that the conditions are chronic or recurrent and not due to transient causes such as acute myocardial infarction, drug toxicity, or electrolyte imbalance. (In cases where there is a rhythm disturbance, if the rhythm disturbance is chronic or recurrent, a single episode of a symptom such as syncope or seizure is adequate to establish medical necessity.)

1. Acquired complete (also referred to as third-degree) AV heart block.
2. Congenital complete heart block with severe bradycardia (in relation to age), or significant physiological deficits or significant symptoms due to the bradycardia.
3. Second-degree AV heart block of Type II (i.e., no progressive prolongation of P-R interval prior to each blocked beat. P-R interval indicates the time taken for an impulse to travel from the atria to the ventricles on an electrocardiogram).
4. Second-degree AV heart block of Type I (i.e., progressive prolongation of P-R interval prior to each blocked beat) with significant symptoms due to hemodynamic instability associated with the heart block.
5. Sinus bradycardia associated with major symptoms (e.g., syncope, seizures, congestive heart failure); or substantial sinus bradycardia (heart rate less than 50) associated with dizziness or confusion. The correlation between symptoms and bradycardia must be documented, or the symptoms must be clearly attributable to the bradycardia rather than to some other cause.
6. In selected and few patients, sinus bradycardia of lesser severity (heart rate 50-59) with dizziness or confusion. The correlation between symptoms and bradycardia must be documented, or the symptoms must be clearly attributable to the bradycardia rather than to some other cause.
7. Sinus bradycardia is the consequence of long-term necessary drug treatment for which there is no acceptable alternative when accompanied by significant symptoms (e.g., syncope, seizures, congestive heart failure, dizziness or confusion). The correlation between symptoms and bradycardia must be documented, or the symptoms must be clearly attributable to the bradycardia rather than to some other cause.
8. Sinus node dysfunction with or without tachyarrhythmias or AV conduction block (i.e., the bradycardia-tachycardia syndrome, sino-atrial block, sinus arrest) when accompanied by significant symptoms (e.g., syncope, seizures, congestive heart failure, dizziness or confusion).
9. Sinus node dysfunction with or without symptoms when there are potentially life-threatening ventricular arrhythmias or tachycardia secondary to the bradycardia (e.g., numerous premature ventricular contractions, couplets, runs of premature ventricular contractions, or ventricular tachycardia).
10. Bradycardia associated with supraventricular tachycardia (e.g., atrial fibrillation, atrial flutter, or paroxysmal atrial tachycardia) with high-degree AV block which is unresponsive to appropriate pharmacological management and when the bradycardia is associated with significant symptoms (e.g., syncope, seizures, congestive heart failure, dizziness or confusion).
11. The occasional patient with hypersensitive carotid sinus syndrome with syncope due to bradycardia and unresponsive to prophylactic medical measures.
12. Bifascicular or trifascicular block accompanied by syncope which is attributed to transient complete heart block after other plausible causes of syncope have been reasonably excluded.

13. Prophylactic pacemaker use following recovery from acute myocardial infarction during which there was temporary complete (third-degree) and/or Mobitz Type II second-degree AV block in association with bundle branch block.
14. In patients with recurrent and refractory ventricular tachycardia, "overdrive pacing" (pacing above the basal rate) to prevent ventricular tachycardia.

    (Effective May 9, 1985)
15. Second-degree AV heart block of Type I with the QRS complexes prolonged.

B. Nationally Noncovered Indications
Conditions which, although used by some physicians as a basis for permanent cardiac pacing, are considered unsupported by adequate evidence of benefit and therefore should not generally be considered appropriate uses for single-chamber pacemakers in the absence of the above indications. Contractors should review claims for pacemakers with these indications to determine the need for further claims development prior to denying the claim, since additional claims development may be required. The object of such further development is to establish whether the particular claim actually meets the conditions in a) above. In claims where this is not the case or where such an event appears unlikely, the contractor may deny the claim

1 Syncope of undetermined cause.
2. Sinus bradycardia without significant symptoms.
3. Sino-atrial block or sinus arrest without significant symptoms.
4. Prolonged P-R intervals with atrial fibrillation (without third-degree AV block) or with other causes of transient ventricular pause.
5. Bradycardia during sleep.
6. Right bundle branch block with left axis deviation (and other forms of fascicular or bundle branch block) without syncope or other symptoms of intermittent AV block).
7. Asymptomatic second-degree AV block of Type I unless the QRS complexes are prolonged or electrophysiological studies have demonstrated that the block is at or beyond the level of the His bundle (a component of the electrical conduction system of the heart).

    Effective October 1, 2001
8. Asymptomatic bradycardia in post-mycardial infarction patients about to initiate long-term beta-blocker drug therapy.

C. Other
All other indications for single-chamber cardiac pacing for which CMS has not specifically indicated coverage remain nationally noncovered, except for Category B Investigational Device Exemption (IDE) clinical trials, or as routine costs of single-chamber cardiac pacing associated with clinical trials, in accordance with section 310.1 of the NCD Manual.

Group II: Dual-Chamber Cardiac Pacemakers – (Effective May 9, 1985)

A. Nationally Covered Indications
Conditions under dual-chamber cardiac pacing are considered acceptable or necessary in the general medical community unless conditions 1 and 2 under Group II. B., are present:

1. Patients in who single-chamber (ventricular pacing) at the time of pacemaker insertion elicits a definite drop in blood pressure, retrograde conduction, or discomfort.
2. Patients in whom the pacemaker syndrome (atrial ventricular asynchrony), with significant symptoms, has already been experienced with a pacemaker that is being replaced.
3. Patients in whom even a relatively small increase in cardiac efficiency will importantly improve the quality of life, e.g., patients with congestive heart failure despite adequate other medical measures.
4. Patients in whom the pacemaker syndrome can be anticipated, e.g., in young and active people, etc.

Dual-chamber pacemakers may also be covered for the conditions, as listed in Group I. A., if the medical necessity is sufficiently justified through adequate claims development. Expert physicians differ in their judgments about what constitutes appropriate criteria for dual-chamber pacemaker use. The judgment that such a pacemaker is warranted in the patient meeting accepted criteria must be based upon the individual needs and characteristics of that patient, weighing the magnitude and likelihood of anticipated benefits against the magnitude and likelihood of disadvantages to the patient.

B. Nationally Noncovered Indications
Whenever the following conditions (which represent overriding contraindications) are present, dual-chamber pacemakers are not covered:

1. Ineffective atrial contractions (e.g., chronic atrial fibrillation or flutter, or giant left atrium.
2. Frequent or persistent supraventricular tachycardias, except where the pacemaker is specifically for the control of the tachycardia.
3. A clinical condition in which pacing takes place only intermittently and briefly, and which is not associated with a reasonable likelihood that pacing needs will become prolonged, e.g., the occasional patient with hypersensitive carotid sinus syndrome with syncope due to bradycardia and unresponsive to prophylactic medical measures.
4. Prophylactic pacemaker use following recovery from acute myocardial infarction during which there was temporary complete (third-degree) and/or Type II second-degree AV block in association with bundle branch block.

C. Other
All other indications for dual-chamber cardiac pacing for which CMS has not specifically indicated coverage remain nationally noncovered, except for Category B IDE clinical trials, or as routine costs of dual-chamber cardiac pacing associated with clinical trials, in accordance with section 310.1 of the NCD Manual.

(This NCD last reviewed June 2004.)

100-3, 20.8.1

Cardiac Pacemaker Evaluation Services

Medicare covers a variety of services for the post-implant follow-up and evaluation of implanted cardiac pacemakers. The following guidelines are designed to assist contractors in identifying and processing claims for such services.

NOTE: These new guidelines are limited to lithium battery-powered pacemakers, because mercury-zinc battery-powered pacemakers are no longer being manufactured and virtually all have been replaced by lithium units. Contractors still receiving claims for monitoring such units should continue to apply the guidelines published in 1980 to those units until they are replaced.

One fact of which contractors should be aware is that many dual-chamber units may be programmed to pace only the ventricles; this may be done either at the time the pacemaker is implanted or at some time afterward. In such cases, a dual-chamber unit, when programmed or reprogrammed for ventricular pacing, should be treated as a single-chamber pacemaker in applying screening guidelines.

The decision as to how often any patient's pacemaker should be monitored is the responsibility of the patient's physician who is best able to take into account the condition and circumstances of the individual patient. These may vary over time, requiring modifications of the frequency with which the patient should be monitored. In cases where monitoring is done by some entity other than the patient's physician, such as a commercial monitoring service or hospital outpatient department, the physician's prescription for monitoring is required and should be periodically renewed (at least annually) to assure that the frequency of monitoring is proper for the patient. When a patient is monitered both during clinica visits and transtelephonically, the contractor should be sure to include frequency data on both ypes of monitoring in evaluating the reasonableness of the frequency of monitoring services received by the patient.

Since there are over 200 pacemaker models in service at any given point, and a variety of patient conditions that give rise to the need for pacemakers, the question of the appropriate frequency of monitorings is a complex one. Nevertheless, it is possible to develop guidelines within which the vast majority of pacemaker monitorings will fall and contractors should do this, using their own data and experience, as well as the frequency guidelines which follow, in order to limit extensive claims development to those cases requiring special attention.

100-3, 20.8.1.1

Transtelephonic Monitoring of Cardiac Pacemakers

(Rev. 1, 10-03-03) CIM 50-1

A. General
Transtelephonic monitoring of pacemakers is furnished by commercial suppliers, hospital outpatient departments and physicians offices.

Telephone monitoring of cardiac pacemakers as described below is medically efficacious in identifying early signs of possible pacemaker failure, thus reducing the number of sudden pacemaker failures requiring emergency replacement. All systems that monitor the pacemaker rate (bpm) in both the free-running and/or magnetic mode are effective in detecting subclinical pacemaker failure due to battery depletion. More sophisticated systems are also capable of detecting internal electronic problems within the pulse generator itself and other potential problems. In the case of dual chamber pacemakers in particular, such monitoring may detect failure of synchronization of the atria and ventricles, and the need for adjustment and reprogramming of the device.

NOTE: The transmitting device furnished to the patient is simply one component of the diagnostic system, and is not covered as durable medical equipment. Those engaged in transtelephonic pacemaker monitoring should reflect the costs of the transmitters in setting their charges for monitoring.

B. Definition of Transtelephonic Monitoring
In order for transtelephonic monitoring services to be covered, the services must consist of the following elements:

- A minimum 30-second readable strip of the pacemaker in the free-running mode;
- Unless contraindicated, a minimum 30-second readable strip of the pacemaker in the magnetic mode; and
- A minimum 30 seconds of readable ECG strip.

C. Frequency Guidelines for Transtelephonic Monitoring
The guidelines below constitute a system which contractors should use, in conjunction with their knowledge of local medical practices, to screen claims for transtelephonic monitoring prior to payment. It is important to note that they are not recommendations with respect to a minimum frequency for such monitorings, but rather a maximum frequency (within which payment may be made without further

claims development). As with previous guidelines, more frequent monitorings may be covered in cases where contractors are satisfied that such monitorings are medically necessary; e.g., based on the condition of the patient, or with respect to pacemakers exhibiting unexpected defects or premature failure. Contractors should seek written justification for more frequent monitorings from the patient's physician and/or any monitoring service involved.

These guidelines are divided into two broad categories - Guideline I which will apply to the majority of pacemakers now in use, and Guideline II which will apply only to pacemaker systems (pacemaker and leads) for which sufficient long-term clinical information exists to assure that they meet the standards of the Inter-Society Commission for Heart Disease Resources (ICHD) for longevity and end-of-life decay. (The ICHD standards are: (I) 90 percent cumulative survival at 5 years following implant; and (2) an end-of-life decay of less than a 50 percent drop of output voltage and less than 20 percent deviation of magnet rate, or a drop of 5 beats per minute or less, over a period of 3 months or more.) Contractors should consult with their medical advisers and other appropriate individuals and organizations (such as the North American Society of Pacing and Electrophysiology which publishes product reliability information) should questions arise over whether a pacemaker system meets the ICHD standards.

The two groups of guidelines are then further broken down into two general categories - single chamber and dual-chamber pacemakers. Contractors should be aware that the frequency with which a patient is monitored may be changed from time to time for a number of reasons, such as a change in the patient's overall condition, a reprogramming of the patient's pacemaker, the development of better information on the pacemaker's longevity or failure mode, etc. Consequently, changes in the proper set of guidelines may be required. Contractors should inform physicians and monitoring services to alert contractors to any changes in the patient's monitoring prescription that might necessitate changes in the screening guidelines applied to that patient. (Of particular importance is the reprogramming of a dual-chamber pacemaker to a single-chamber mode of operation.

Such reprogramming would shift the patient from the appropriate dual-chamber guideline to the appropriate single-chamber guideline.)

Guideline I

1 - Single-chamber pacemakers

1st month - every 2 weeks.

2nd through 36th month - every 8 weeks.

37th month to failure - every 4 weeks.

2 - Dual-chamber pacemaker

1st month - every 2 weeks.

2nd through 6th month - every 4 weeks.

7th through 36th month - every 8 weeks.

37th month to failure - every 4 weeks.

Guideline II

1 - Single-chamber pacemakers

1st month - every 2 weeks.

2nd through 48th month - every 12 weeks.

49th through 72nd month - every 8 weeks. Thereafter - every 4 weeks.

2 - Dual-chamber pacemaker

1st month - every 2 weeks.

2nd through 30th month - every 12 weeks.

31st through 48th month - every 8 weeks. Thereafter - every 4 weeks.

D. Pacemaker Clinic Services

1. General
   Pacemaker monitoring is also covered when done by pacemaker clinics. Clinic visits may be done in conjunction with transtelephonic monitoring or as a separate service; however, the services rendered by a pacemaker clinic are more extensive than those currently possible by telephone. They include, for example, physical examination of patients and reprogramming of pacemakers. Thus, the use of one of these types of monitoring does not preclude concurrent use of the other.
2. Frequency Guidelines
   As with transtelephonic pacemaker monitoring, the frequency of clinic visits is the decision of the patient's physician, taking into account, among other things, the medical condition of the patient. However, contractors can develop monitoring guidelines that will prove useful in screening claims. The following are recommendations for monitoring guidelines on lithium-battery pacemakers:
   - For single-chamber pacemakers - twice in the first 6 months following implant, then once every 12 months.
   - For dual-chamber pacemakers - twice in the first 6 months, then once every 6 months.

100-3, 20.8.2

Self-Contained Pacemaker Monitors

Self-contained pacemaker monitors are accepted devices for monitoring cardiac pacemakers. Accordingly, program payment may be made for the rental or purchase of either of the following pacemaker monitors when it is prescribed by a physician for a patient with a cardiac pacemaker:

A. Digital Electronic Pacemaker Monitor.
This device provides the patient with an instantaneous digital readout of his pacemaker pulse rate. Use of this device does not involve professional services until there has been a change of five pulses (or more) per minute above or below the initial rate of the pacemaker; when such change occurs, the patient contacts his physician.

B. Audible/Visible Signal Pacemaker Monitor.
This device produces an audible and visible signal which indicates the pacemaker rate. Use of this device does not involve professional services until a change occurs in these signals; at such time, the patient contacts his physician.

NOTE: The design of the self-contained pacemaker monitor makes it possible for the patient to monitor his pacemaker periodically and minimizes the need for regular visits to the outpatient department of the provider.

Therefore, documentation of the medical necessity for pacemaker evaluation in the outpatient department of the provider should be obtained where such evaluation is employed in addition to the self-contained pacemaker monitor used by the patient in his home.

100-3, 20.10

Cardiac Rehabilitation Programs

A. General
Phase II cardiac rehabilitation, as described by the U.S. Public Health Service, is a comprehensive, long-term program including medical evaluation, prescribed exercise, cardiac risk factor modification, education, and counseling. Phase II refers to outpatient, medically supervised programs that are typically initiated 1-3 weeks after hospital discharge and provide appropriate electrocardiographic monitoring.

B. Nationally Covered Indications
Effective for services performed on or after March 22, 2006, Medicare coverage of cardiac rehabilitation programs is considered reasonable and necessary only for patients who: (1) have a documented diagnosis of acute myocardial infarction within the preceding 12 months; or (2) have had coronary bypass surgery; or (3) have stable angina pectoris; or (4) have had heart valve repair/replacement; or (5) have had percutaneous transluminal coronary angioplasty (PTCA) or coronary stenting; or (6) have had a heart or heart-lung transplant.

1. Program Requirements
   a. Duration

      Services provided in connection with a cardiac rehabilitation exercise program may be considered reasonable and necessary for up to 36 sessions. Patients generally receive 2 to 3 sessions per week for 12 to 18 weeks. Coverage of additional sessions is discussed in section D below.

   b. Components

      Cardiac rehabilitation programs must be comprehensive and to be comprehensive they must include a medical evaluation, a program to modify cardiac risk factors (e.g., nutritional counseling), prescribed exercise, education, and counseling.

   c. Facility

      The facility must have available for immediate use the necessary cardio-pulmonary, emergency, diagnostic, and therapeutic life-saving equipment accepted by the medical community as medically necessary, e.g., oxygen, cardiopulmonary resuscitation equipment, or defibrillator.

   d. Staff

      The program must be staffed by personnel necessary to conduct the program safely and effectively, who are trained in both basic and advanced life support techniques and in exercise therapy for coronary disease. The program must be under the direct supervision of a physician, as defined in 42 CFR Sec.410.26(a)(2) (defined through cross reference to 42 CFR Sec.410.32(b)(3)(ii), or 42 CFR Sec.410.27(f)).

C. Nationally Non-Covered Indications
Except as provided in section D., all other indications are not covered.

D. Other
The contractor has the discretion to cover cardiac rehabilitation services beyond 18 weeks. Coverage must not exceed a total of 72 sessions for 36 weeks.

(This NCD last reviewed March 2006.)

100-3, 20.10.1

A. General
As per sections 1861(s)(2)(CC) and 1861(eee)(1) of the Social Security Act, items and services furnished under a Cardiac Rehabilitation (CR) program may be covered under Medicare Part B. Among other things, Medicare regulations at 42CFR410.49 define key terms, address the components of a CR program, establish the standards for

physician supervision, and limit the maximum number of program sessions that may be furnished. The regulations also describe the cardiac conditions that would enable a beneficiary to obtain CR services.

Effective for dates of service on and after January 1, 2010, coverage is permitted for beneficiaries who have experienced one or more of the following:

- Acute myocardial infarction within the preceding 12 months
- Coronary artery bypasses surgery
- Current stable angina pectoris
- Heart valve repair or replacement
- Percutaneous transluminal coronary angioplasty (PTCA) or coronary stenting
- A heart or heart-lung transplant

The Centers for Medicare & Medicaid Services (CMS) may add "other cardiac conditions as specified through a national coverage determination" (See 42 CFR §410.49(b)(1)(vii).

B. Nationally Covered Indications

Effective for dates of service on and after February 18, 2014, CMS has determined that the evidence is sufficient to expand coverage for cardiac rehabilitation services under 42 CFR § 410.49(b)(1)(vii) to beneficiaries with stable, chronic heart failure, defined as patients with left ventricular ejection fraction of 35% or less and New York Heart Association (NYHA) class II to IV symptoms despite being on optimal heart failure therapy for at least six weeks. Stable patients are defined as patients who have not had recent (=6 weeks) or planned (=6 months) major cardiovascular hospitalizations or procedures. (See section A above for other indications covered under 42 CFR §410.49(b)(1)(vll).

C. Nationally Non-Covered Indications

Any cardiac indication not specifically identified in 42 CFR § 410.49(b)(1)(vii) or identified as covered in this NCD or any other NCD in relation to cardiac rehabilitation services is considered non-covered.

D. Other

NA

(This NCD last reviewed February 2014.)

100-3, 20.11

Intraoperative Ventricular Mapping

Intraoperative ventricular mapping is the technique of recording cardiac electrical activity directly from the heart. The recording sites are usually identified from an anatomical grid and may consist of epicardial, intramural, and endocardial sites. A probe with electrodes is used to explore these surfaces and generate a map that displays the sequence of electrical activation. This information is used by the surgeon to locate precisely the site of an operative intervention.

The intraoperative ventricular mapping procedure is covered under Medicare only for the uses and medical conditions described below:

- Localize accessory pathways associated with the Wolff-Parkinson-White (WPW) and other preexcitation syndromes;
- Map the sequence of atrial and ventricular activation for drug-resistant supraventricular tachycardias;
- Delineate the anatomical course of His bundle and/or bundle branches during corrective cardiac surgery for congenital heart diseases; and
- Direct the surgical treatment of patients with refractory ventricular tachyarrhythmias.

100-3, 20.12

Diagnostic Endocardial Electrical Stimulation (Pacing)

Diagnostic endocardial electrical stimulation (EES), also called programmed electrical stimulation of the heart, is covered under Medicare when used for patients with severe cardiac arrhythmias.

100-3, 20.13

HIS Bundle Study

Medicare coverage of the procedure would be limited to selected patients: those with complex ongoing acute arrhythmias, those with intermittent or permanent heart block in whom pacemaker implantation is being considered, and those patients who have recently developed heart block secondary to a myocardial infarction. When heart catheterization and the HIS Bundle Study are performed at the same time, the program will cover only one catheterization and a small additional charge for the study.

When a HIS bundle cardiogram is obtained as part of a diagnostic endocardial electrical stimulation, no separate charge will be recognized for the His bundle study.

100-3, 20.14

Plethysmography

Medicare coverage is extended to those procedures listed in Category I below when used for the accepted medical indications mentioned above. The procedures in Category II are still considered experimental and are not covered at this time. Denial of claims because a noncovered procedure was used or because there was no medical indication for plethysmographic evaluation of any type should be based on Sec.1862(a)(1) of the Act.

Category I - Covered

Segmental Plethysmography - Included under this procedure are services performed with a regional plethysmograph, differential plethysmograph, recording oscillometer, and a pulse volume recorder.

Electrical Impedance Plethysmography

Ultrasonic Measurement of Blood Flow (Doppler) - While not strictly a plethysmographic method, this is also a useful tool in the evaluation of suspected peripheral vascular disease or preoperative screening of podiatric patients with suspected peripheral vascular compromise. (See Sec.50-7 for the applicable coverage policy on this procedure.)

Oculoplethysmography - See NCD on Noninvasive Tests of Carotid Function, Sec.20.17.

Strain Gauge Plethysmography - This test is based on recording the non-pulsatile aspects of inflowing blood at various points on an extremity by a mercury-in-silastic strain gauge sensor. The instrument consists of a chart recorder, an automatic cuff inflation and deflation system, and a recording manometer.

Category II - Experimental

The following methods have not yet reached a level of development such as to allow their routine use in the evaluation of suspected peripheral vascular disease.

Inductance Plethysmography - This method is considered experimental and does not provide reproducible results.

Capacitance Plethysmography - This method is considered experimental and does not provide reproducible results.

Mechanical Oscillometry - This is a non-standardized method which offers poor sensitivity and is not considered superior to the simple measurement of peripheral blood pressure.

Photoelectric Plethysmography - This method is considered useful only in determining whether or not a pulse is present and does not provide reproducible measurements of blood flow.

Differential plethysmography, on the other hand, is a system which uses an impedance technique to compare pulse pressures at various points along a limb, with a reference pressure at the mid-brachial or wrist level. It is not clear whether this technique, as usually performed in the physician's office, meets the definition of plethysmography because quantitative measurements of blood flow are usually not made. It has been concluded, in any event, that the differential plethysmography system is a blood pulse recorder of undetermined value, which has the potential for significant overutilization. Therefore, reimbursement for studies done by techniques other than venous occlusive pneumoplethysmography should be denied, at least until additional data on these devices, including controlled clinical studies, become available.

100-3, 20.15

Electrocardiographic (EKG) Services

Nationally Covered Indications

1. The following indications are covered nationally unless otherwise indicated:
2. Computer analysis of EKGs when furnished in a setting and under the circumstances required for coverage of other EKG services.
3. EKG services rendered by an independent diagnostic testing facility (IDTF), including physician review and interpretation. Separate physician services are not covered unless he/she is the patient's attending or consulting physician.
4. Emergency EKGs (i.e., when the patient is or may be experiencing a lifethreatening event) performed as a laboratory or diagnostic service by a portable x-ray supplier only when a physician is in attendance at the time the service is performed or immediately thereafter.
5. Home EKG services with documentation of medical necessity.
6. Trans-telephonic EKG transmissions (effective March 1, 1980) as a diagnostic service for the indications described below, when performed with equipment meeting the standards described below, subject to the limitations and conditions specified below. Coverage is further limited to the amounts payable with respect to the physician's service in interpreting the results of such transmissions, including charges for rental of the equipment. The device used by the beneficiary is part of a total diagnostic system and is not considered DME separately. Covered uses are to:
   a. Detect, characterize, and document symptomatic transient arrhythmias;
   b. Initiate, revise, or discontinue arrhythmic drug therapy; or,
   c. Carry out early post-hospital monitoring of patients discharged after myocardial infarction (MI); (only if 24-hour coverage is provided, see C.5. below).

   Certain uses other than those specified above may be covered if, in the judgment of the local contractor, such use is medically necessary.

   Additionally, the transmitting devices must meet at least the following criteria:

   a. They must be capable of transmitting EKG Leads, I, II, or III; and,

b. The tracing must be sufficiently comparable to a conventional EKG.

24-hour attended coverage used as early post-hospital monitoring of patients discharged after MI is only covered if provision is made for such 24-hour attended coverage in the manner described below:

24-hour attended coverage means there must be, at a monitoring site or central data center, an EKG technician or other non-physician, receiving calls and/or EKG data; tape recording devices do not meet this requirement. Further, such technicians should have immediate, 24-hour access to a physician to review transmitted data and make clinical decisions regarding the patient. The technician should also be instructed as to when and how to contact available facilities to assist the patient in case of emergencies.

Nationally Non-covered Indications

The following indications are non-covered nationally unless otherwise specified below:

1. The time-sampling mode of operation of ambulatory EKG cardiac event monitoring/recording.
2. Separate physician services other than those rendered by an IDTF unless rendered by the patient's attending or consulting physician.
3. Home EKG services without documentation of medical necessity.
4. Emergency EKG services by a portable x-ray supplier without a physician in attendance at the time of service or immediately thereafter.
5. 24-hour attended coverage used as early post-hospital monitoring of patients discharged after MI unless provision is made for such 24-hour attended coverage in the manner described in section B.5. above.
6. Any marketed Food and Drug Administration (FDA)-approved ambulatory cardiac monitoring device or service that cannot be categorized according to the framework below.

Other

Ambulatory cardiac monitoring performed with a marketed, FDA-approved device, is eligible for coverage if it can be categorized according to the framework below. Unless there is a specific NCD for that device or service, determination as to whether a device or service that fits into the framework is reasonable and necessary is according to local contractor discretion.

Electrocardiographic Services Framework

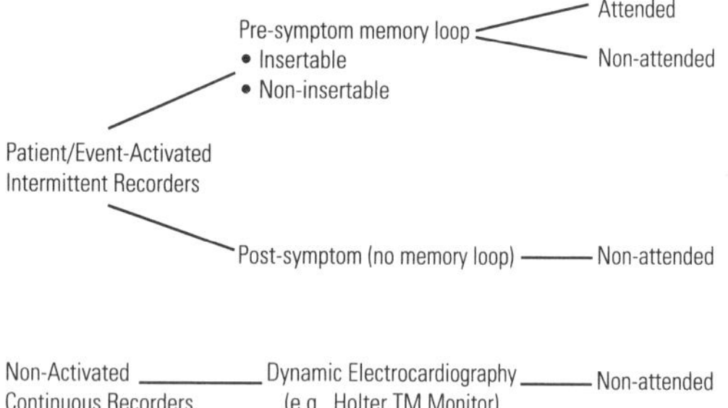

100-3, 20.16

Cardiac Output Monitoring by Thoracic Electrical Bioimpedance (TEB)

Indications and Limitations of Coverage

B. Nationally Covered Indications

Effective for services performed on and after January 23, 2004, TEB is covered for the following uses:

1. Differentiation of cardiogenic from pulmonary causes of acute dyspnea when medical history, physical examination, and standard assessment tools provide insufficient information, and the treating physician has determined that TEB hemodynamic data are necessary for appropriate management of the patient.
2. Optimization of atrioventricular (A/V) interval for patients with A/V sequential cardiac pacemakers when medical history, physical examination, and standard assessment tools provide insufficient information, and the treating physician has determined that TEB hemodynamic data are necessary for appropriate management of the patient.
3. Monitoring of continuous inotropic therapy for patients with terminal congestive heart failure, when those patients have chosen to die with comfort at home, or for patients waiting at home for a heart transplant.
4. Evaluation for rejection in patients with a heart transplant as a predetermined alternative to a myocardial biopsy. Medical necessity must be documented should a biopsy be performed after TEB.
5. Optimization of fluid management in patients with congestive heart failure when medical history, physical examination, and standard assessment tools provide insufficient information, and the treating physician has determined that TEB hemodynamic data are necessary for appropriate management of the patient.

C. Nationally Non-Covered Indications

1. TEB is non-covered when used for patients:
   - With proven or suspected disease involving severe regurgitation of the aorta;
   - With minute ventilation (MV) sensor function pacemakers, since the device may adversely affect the functioning of that type of pacemaker;
   - During cardiac bypass surgery; or,
   - In the management of all forms of hypertension (with the exception of drug-resistant hypertension as outlined below).
2. All other uses of TEB not otherwise specified remain non-covered.

D. Other

Contractors have discretion to determine whether the use of TEB for the management of drug-resistant hypertension is reasonable and necessary. Drug resistant hypertension is defined as failure to achieve goal blood pressure in patients who are adhering to full doses of an appropriate 3-drug regimen that includes a diuretic. Effective November 24, 2006, after reconsideration of Medicare policy, CMS will continue current Medicare policy for TEB.

(This NCD last reviewed November 2006.)

100-3, 20.17

Noninvasive Tests of Carotid Function

It is important to note that the names of these tests are not standardized. Following are some of the acceptable tests, recognizing that this list is not inclusive and that local medical consultants should make determinations:

Direct Tests

- Carotid Phonoangiography
- Direct Bruit Analysis
- Spectral Bruit Analysis
- Doppler Flow Velocity
- Ultrasound Imaging including Real Time
- B-Scan and Doppler Devices

Indirect Tests

- Periorbital Directional Doppler Ultrasonography
- Oculoplethysmography
- Ophthalmodynamometry

100-3, 20.18

Carotid Body Resection/Carotid Body Denervation

Carotid body resection is occasionally used to relieve pulmonary symptoms, including asthma, but has been shown to lack general acceptance of the professional medical community. In addition, controlled clinical studies establishing the safety and effectiveness of this procedure are needed. Therefore, all carotid body resections to relieve pulmonary symptoms must be considered investigational and cannot be considered reasonable and necessary within the meaning of section 1862(a)(l) of the law. No program reimbursement may be made in such cases.

There is, however, one instance where carotid body resection has been accepted by the medical community as effective. That instance is when evidence of a mass in the carotid body,with or without symptoms, indicates the need for surgery to remove the carotid body tumor.

Denervation of a carotid sinus to treat hypersensitive carotid sinus reflex is another procedure performed in the area of the carotid body. In the case of hypersensitive carotid sinus, light pressure on the upper part of the neck (such as might be experienced when turning or raising one's head) results in symptoms such as dizziness or syncope due to hypotension and slowed heart rate. Failure of medical therapy and continued deterioration in the condition of the patient in such cases may indicate need for surgery. Denervation of the carotid sinus is rarely performed, but when elected as the therapy of choice with the above indications, this procedure may be considered reasonable and necessary.

100-3, 20.19

Ambulatory Blood Pressure Monitoring

ABPM must be performed for at least 24 hours to meet coverage criteria.

ABPM is only covered for those patients with suspected white coat hypertension. Suspected white coat hypertension is defined as

1) office blood pressure >140/90 mm Hg on at least three separate clinic/office visits with two separate measurements made at each visit;
2) at least two documented blood pressure measurements taken outside the office which are <140/90 mm Hg; and
3) no evidence of end-organ damage.

The information obtained by ABPM is necessary in order to determine the appropriate management of the patient. ABPM is not covered for any other uses. In the rare circumstance that ABPM needs to be performed more than once in a patient, the qualifying criteria described above must be met for each subsequent ABPM test.

For those patients that undergo ABPM and have an ambulatory blood pressure of <135/85 with no evidence of end-organ damage, it is likely that their cardiovascular risk is similar to that of normotensives. They should be followed over time. Patients for which ABPM demonstrates a blood pressure of >135/85 may be at increased cardiovascular risk, and a physician may wish to consider antihypertensive therapy.

100-3, 20.23

Fabric Wrapping of Abdominal Aneurysms

Fabric wrapping of abdominal aneurysms is not a covered Medicare procedure. This is a treatment for abdominal aneurysms which involves wrapping aneurysms with cellophane or fascia lata. This procedure has not been shown to prevent eventual rupture. In extremely rare instances, external wall reinforcement may be indicated when the current accepted treatment (excision of the aneurysm and reconstruction with synthetic materials) is not a viable alternative, but external wall reinforcement is not fabric wrapping. Accordingly, fabric wrapping of abdominal aneurysms is not considered reasonable and necessary within the meaning of Sec.1862(a)(1) of the Act.

100-3, 20.26

Partial Ventriculectomy

Since the mortality rate is high and there are no published scientific articles or clinical studies regarding partial ventriculectomy, this procedure cannot be considered reasonable and necessary within the meaning of Sec.1862(a)(1) of the Act. Therefore, partial ventriculectomy is not covered by Medicare.

100-3, 20.28

Therapeutic Embolization

Therapeutic embolization is covered when done for hemorrhage, and for other conditions amenable to treatment by the procedure, when reasonable and necessary for the individual patient. Renal embolization for the treatment of renal adenocarcinoma continues to be covered, effective December 15, 1978, as one type of therapeutic embolization, to:

- Reduce tumor vascularity preoperatively;
- Reduce tumor bulk in inoperable cases; or
- Palliate specific symptoms.

100-3, 20.29

Hyperbaric Oxygen Therapy

A. Covered Conditions

Program reimbursement for HBO therapy will be limited to that which is administered in a chamber (including the one man unit) and is limited to the following conditions:

1. Acute carbon monoxide intoxication,
2. Decompression illness,
3. Gas embolism,
4. Gas gangrene,
5. Acute traumatic peripheral ischemia. HBO therapy is a valuable adjunctive treatment to be used in combination with accepted standard therapeutic measures when loss of function, limb, or life is threatened.
6. Crush injuries and suturing of severed limbs. As in the previous conditions, HBO therapy would be an adjunctive treatment when loss of function, limb, or life is threatened.
7. Progressive necrotizing infections (necrotizing fasciitis),
8. Acute peripheral arterial insufficiency,
9. Preparation and preservation of compromised skin grafts (not for primary management of wounds),
10. Chronic refractory osteomyelitis, unresponsive to conventional medical and surgical management,
11. Osteoradionecrosis as an adjunct to conventional treatment,
12. Soft tissue radionecrosis as an adjunct to conventional treatment,
13. Cyanide poisoning,
14. Actinomycosis, only as an adjunct to conventional therapy when the disease process is refractory to antibiotics and surgical treatment,
15. Diabetic wounds of the lower extremities in patients who meet the following three criteria:
    a. Patient has type I or type II diabetes and has a lower extremity wound that is due to diabetes;
    b. Patient has a wound classified as Wagner grade III or higher; and
    c. Patient has failed an adequate course of standard wound therapy.

The use of HBO therapy is covered as adjunctive therapy only after there are no measurable signs of healing for at least 30 -days of treatment with standard wound therapy and must be used in addition to standard wound care. Standard wound care in patients with diabetic wounds includes: assessment of a patient's vascular status and correction of any vascular problems in the affected limb if possible, optimization of nutritional status, optimization of glucose control, debridement by any means to remove devitalized tissue, maintenance of a clean, moist bed of granulation tissue with appropriate moist dressings, appropriate off-loading, and necessary treatment to resolve any infection that might be present. Failure to respond to standard wound care occurs when there are no measurable signs of healing for at least 30 consecutive days. Wounds must be evaluated at least every 30 days during administration of HBO therapy. Continued treatment with HBO therapy is not covered if measurable signs of healing have not been demonstrated within any 30-day period of treatment.

B. Noncovered Conditions

All other indications not specified under Sec.270.4(A) are not covered under the Medicare program. No program payment may be made for any conditions other than those listed in Sec.270.4(A).

No program payment may be made for HBO in the treatment of the following conditions:

1. Cutaneous, decubitus, and stasis ulcers.
2. Chronic peripheral vascular insufficiency.
3. Anaerobic septicemia and infection other than clostridial.
4. Skin burns (thermal).
5. Senility.
6. Myocardial infarction.
7. Cardiogenic shock.
8. Sickle cell anemia.
9. Acute thermal and chemical pulmonary damage, i.e., smoke inhalation with pulmonary insufficiency.
10. Acute or chronic cerebral vascular insufficiency.
11. Hepatic necrosis.
12. Aerobic septicemia.
13. Nonvascular causes of chronic brain syndrome (Pick's disease, Alzheimer's disease, Korsakoff's disease).
14. Tetanus.
15. Systemic aerobic infection.
16. Organ transplantation.
17. Organ storage.
18. Pulmonary emphysema.
19. Exceptional blood loss anemia.
20. Multiple Sclerosis.
21. Arthritic Diseases.
22. Acute cerebral edema.

C. Topical Application of Oxygen

This method of administering oxygen does not meet the definition of HBO therapy as stated above. Also, its clinical efficacy has not been established. Therefore, no Medicare reimbursement may be made for the topical application of oxygen.

100-3, 20.30

Microvolt T-Wave Alternans (MTWA)

B. Nationally Covered Indications

Microvolt T-wave Alternans diagnostic testing is covered for the evaluation of patients at risk for SCD, only when the spectral analysis method is used.

C. Nationally Non-Covered Indications

Microvolt T-wave Alternans diagnostic test is non-covered for the evaluation of patients at risk for SCD if measurement is not performed employing the spectral analysis.

D. Other

N/A

100-3, 20.32

Transcatheter Aortic Valve Replacement (TAVR)

(Rev. 147, Issued: 09-24-12, Effective: 05-01-12, Implementation: 01-07-13)

A. General

Transcatheter aortic valve replacement (TAVR - also known as TAVI or transcatheter aortic valve implantation) is used in the treatment of aortic stenosis. A bioprosthetic valve is inserted percutaneously using a catheter and implanted in the orifice of the aortic valve.

B. Nationally Covered Indications

The Centers for Medicare & Medicaid Services (CMS) covers transcatheter aortic valve replacement (TAVR) under Coverage with Evidence Development (CED) with the following conditions:

A. TAVR is covered for the treatment of symptomatic aortic valve stenosis when furnished according to a Food and Drug Administration (FDA)-approved indication and when all of the following conditions are met:

1. The procedure is furnished with a complete aortic valve and implantation system that has received FDA premarket approval (PMA) for that system's FDA approved indication.
2. Two cardiac surgeons have independently examined the patient face-to-face and evaluated the patient's suitability for open aortic valve replacement (AVR) surgery; and both surgeons have documented the rationale for their clinical judgment and the rationale is available to the heart team.
3. The patient (preoperatively and postoperatively) is under the care of a heart team: a cohesive, multi-disciplinary, team of medical professionals. The heart team concept embodies collaboration and dedication across medical specialties to offer optimal patient-centered care.

   TAVR must be furnished in a hospital with the appropriate infrastructure that includes but is not limited to:

   a. On-site heart valve surgery program,
   b. Cardiac catheterization lab or hybrid operating room/catheterization lab equipped with a fixed radiographic imaging system with flat-panel fluoroscopy, offering quality imaging,
   c. Non-invasive imaging such as echocardiography, vascular ultrasound, computed tomography (CT) and magnetic resonance (MR),
   d. Sufficient space, in a sterile environment, to accommodate necessary equipment for cases with and without complications,
   e. Post-procedure intensive care facility with personnel experienced in managing patients who have undergone open-heart valve procedures,
   f. Appropriate volume requirements per the applicable qualifications below.There are two sets of qualifications; the first set outlined below is for hospital programs and heart teams without previous TAVR experience and the second set is for those with TAVR experience.

   Qualifications to begin a TAVR program for hospitals without TAVR experience:

   The hospital program must have the following:

   a. ≥ 50 total AVRs in the previous year prior to TAVR, including ≥ 10 high-risk patients, and;
   b. ≥ 2 physicians with cardiac surgery privileges, and;
   c. ≥ 1000 catheterizations per year, including ≥ 400 percutaneous coronary interventions (PCIs) per year. Qualifications to begin a TAVR program for heart teams without TAVR experience:

   The heart team must include:

   a. Cardiovascular surgeon with:
      i ≥ 100 career AVRs including 10 high-risk patients; or,
      ii. ≥ 25 AVRs in one year; or,
      iii. ≥ 50 AVRs in 2 years; and which include at least 20 AVRs in the last year prior to TAVR initiation; and,
   b. Interventional cardiologist with:
      i. Professional experience with 100 structural heart disease procedures lifetime; or,
      ii. 30 left-sided structural procedures per year of which 60% should be balloon aortic valvuloplasty (BAV). Atrial septal defect and patent foramen ovale closure are not considered left-sided procedures; and, .
   c. Additional members of the heart team such as echocardiographers, imaging specialists, heart failure specialists, cardiac anesthesiologists, intensivists, nurses, and social workers; and,
   d. Device-specific training as required by the manufacturer.

   Qualifications for hospital programs with TAVR experience:

   The hospital program must maintain the following:

   a ≥ 20 AVRs per year or ≥ 40 AVRs every 2 years; and,
   b. ≥ 2 physicians with cardiac surgery privileges; and,
   c. ≥ 1000 catheterizations per year, including ≥ 400 percutaneous coronary interventions (PCIs) per year.

   Qualifications for heart teams with TAVR experience:

   The heart team must include:

   a. cardiovascular surgeon and an interventional cardiologist whose combined experience maintains the following:
      i. ≥ 20 TAVR procedures in the prior year, or,
      ii. ≥ 40 TAVR procedures in the prior 2 years; and,
   b. Additional members of the heart team such as echocardiographers, imaging specialists, heart failure specialists, cardiac anesthesiologists, intensivists, nurses, and social workers.
4. The heart team's interventional cardiologist(s) and cardiac surgeon(s) must jointly participate in the intra-operative technical aspects of TAVR.
5. The heart team and hospital are participating in a prospective, national, audited registry that: 1) consecutively enrolls TAVR patients; 2) accepts all manufactured devices; 3) follows the patient for at least one year; and, 4) complies with relevant regulations relating to protecting human research subjects, including 45 CFR Part 46 and 21 CFR Parts 50 & 56. The following outcomes must be tracked by the registry; and the registry must be designed to permit identification and analysis of patient, practitioner and facility level variables that predict each of these outcomes:
   i. Stroke;
   ii. All cause mortality;
   iii. Transient Ischemic Attacks (TIAs);
   iv. Major vascular events;
   v. Acute kidney injury;
   vi. Repeat aortic valve procedures;
   vii. Quality of Life (QoL).

   The registry should collect all data necessary and have a written executable analysis plan in place to address the following questions (to appropriately address some questions, Medicare claims or other outside data may be necessary):

   - When performed outside a controlled clinical study, how do outcomes and adverse events compare to the pivotal clinical studies
   - How do outcomes and adverse events in subpopulations compare to patients in the pivotal clinical studies
   - What is the long term (≥ 5 year) durability of the device
   - What are the long term (≥ 5 year) outcomes and adverse events
   - How do the demographics of registry patients compare to the pivotal studies

   Consistent with section 1142 of the Act, the Agency for Healthcare Research and Quality (AHRQ) supports clinical research studies that CMS determines meet the above-listed standards and address the above-listed research questions.

B. TAVR is covered for uses that are not expressly listed as an FDA-approved indication when performed within a clinical study that fulfills all of the following.

1. The heart team's interventional cardiologist(s) and cardiac surgeon(s) must jointly participate in the intra-operative technical aspects of TAVR.
2. As a fully-described, written part of its protocol, the clinical research study must critically evaluate not only each patient's quality of life pre- and post-TAVR (minimum of 1 year), but must also address at least one of the following questions:
   - What is the incidence of stroke
   - What is the rate of all cause mortality
   - What is the incidence of transient ischemic attacks (TIAs)
   - What is the incidence of major vascular events
   - What is the incidence of acute kidney injury
   - What is the incidence of repeat aortic valve procedures
3. The clinical study must adhere to the following standards of scientific integrity and relevance to the Medicare population:
   a. The principal purpose of the research study is to test whether a particular intervention potentially improves the participants's health outcomes.
   b. The research study is well supported by available scientific and medical information or it is intended to clarify or establish the health outcomes of interventions already in common clinical use.
   c. The research study does not unjustifiably duplicate existing studies.
   d. The research study design is appropriate to answer the research question being asked in the study.
   e. The research study is sponsored by an organization or individual capable of executing the proposed study successfully.
   f. The research study is in compliance with all applicable Federal regulations concerning the protection of human subjects found in the Code of Federal Regulations (CFR) at 45 CFR Part 46. If a study is regulated by the Food and Drug Administration (FDA), it also must be in compliance with 21 CFR Parts 50 and 56. In particular, the informed consent includes a straightforward explanation of the reported increased risks of stroke and vascular complications that have been published for TAVR.
   g. All aspects of the research study are conducted according to appropriate standards of scientific integrity (see http://www.icmje.org).
   h. The research study has a written protocol that clearly addresses, or incorporates by reference, the standards listed as Medicare coverage requirements.

i. The clinical research study is not designed to exclusively test toxicity or disease pathophysiology in healthy individuals. Trials of all medical technologies measuring therapeutic outcomes as one of the objectives meet this standard only if the disease or condition being studied is life threatening as defined in 21 CFR section 312.81(a) and the patient has no other viable treatment options.

j. The clinical research study is registered on the www.ClinicalTrials.gov website by the principal sponsor/investigator prior to the enrollment of the first study subject.

k. The research study protocol specifies the method and timing of public release of all pre-specified outcomes to be measured including release of outcomes if outcomes are negative or study is terminated early. The results must be made public within 24 months of the end of data collection. If a report is planned to be published in a peer reviewed journal, then that initial release may be an abstract that meets the requirements of the International Committee of Medical Journal Editors (http://www.icmje.org). However a full report of the outcomes must be made public no later than three (3) years after the end of data collection.

l. The research study protocol must explicitly discuss subpopulations affected by the treatment under investigation, particularly traditionally underrepresented groups in clinical studies, how the inclusion and exclusion criteria affect enrollment of these populations, and a plan for the retention and reporting of said populations on the trial. If the inclusion and exclusion criteria are expected to have a negative effect on the recruitment or retention of underrepresented populations, the protocol must discuss why these criteria are necessary.

m. The research study protocol explicitly discusses how the results are or are not expected to be generalizable to the Medicare population to infer whether Medicare patients may benefit from the intervention. Separate discussions in the protocol may be necessary for populations eligible for Medicare due to age, disability or Medicaid eligibility. Consistent with section 1142 of the Act, AHRQ supports clinical research studies that CMS determines meet the above-listed standards and address the above-listed research questions.

4. The principal investigator must submit the complete study protocol, identify the relevant CMS research question(s) that will be addressed, and cite the location of the detailed analysis plan for those questions in the protocol, plus provide a statement addressing how the study satisfies each of the standards of scientific integrity (a. through m. listed above), as well as the investigator's contact information, to the address below. The information will be reviewed, and approved studies will be identified on the CMS Website.

    Director, Coverage and Analysis Group
    Re: TAVR CED
    Centers for Medicare & Medicaid Services (CMS)
    7500 Security Blvd., Mail Stop S3-02-01
    Baltimore, MD 21244-1850

C. Nationally Non-Covered Indications

TAVR is not covered for patients in whom existing co-morbidities would preclude the expected benefit from correction of the aortic stenosis.

D.

NA

(This NCD last reviewed May 2012.)

100-3, 30.1

Biofeedback Therapy

Biofeedback therapy is covered under Medicare only when it is reasonable and necessary for the individual patient for muscle re-education of specific muscle groups or for treating pathological muscle abnormalities of spasticity, incapacitating muscle spasm, or weakness, and more conventional treatments (heat, cold, massage, exercise, support) have not been successful. This therapy is not covered for treatment of ordinary muscle tension states or for psychosomatic conditions. (See the Medicare Benefit Policy Manual, Chapter 15, for general coverage requirements about physical therapy requirements.)

100-3, 30.1.1

Biofeedback Therapy for the Treatment of Urinary Incontinence

This policy applies to biofeedback therapy rendered by a practitioner in an office or other facility setting.

Biofeedback is covered for the treatment of stress and/or urge incontinence in cognitively intact patients who have failed a documented trial of pelvic muscle exercise (PME)training. Biofeedback is not a treatment, per se, but a tool to help patients learn how to perform PME. Biofeedback-assisted PME incorporates the use of an electronic or mechanical device to relay visual and/or auditory evidence of pelvic floor muscle tone, in order to improve awareness of pelvic floor musculature and to assist patients in the performance of PME.

A failed trial of PME training is defined as no clinically significant improvement in urinary incontinence after completing 4 weeks of an ordered plan of pelvic muscle exercises to increase periurethral muscle strength.

Contractors may decide whether or not to cover biofeedback as an initial treatment modality.

Home use of biofeedback therapy is not covered.

100-3, 30.3

Acupuncture

Although acupuncture has been used for thousands of years in China and for decades in parts of Europe, it is a new agent of unknown use and efficacy in the United States. Even in those areas of the world where it has been widely used, its mechanism is not known. Three units of the National Institutes of Health, the National Institute of General Medical Sciences, National Institute of Neurological Diseases and Stroke, and Fogarty International Center have been designed to assess and identify specific opportunities and needs for research attending the use of acupuncture for surgical anesthesia and relief of chronic pain. Until the pending scientific assessment of the technique has been completed and its efficacy has been established, Medicare reimbursement for acupuncture, as an anesthetic or as an analgesic or for other therapeutic purposes, may not be made. Accordingly, acupuncture is not considered reasonable and necessary within the meaning of §1862(a)(1) of the Act.

100-3, 30.3.1

Acupuncture for Fibromyalgia (Effective April 16, 2004) (30.3.1)

(Rev. 11, 04-16-04)

General

Although acupuncture has been used for thousands of years in China and for decades in parts of Europe, it is still a relatively new agent of unknown use and efficacy in the United States. Even in those areas of the world where it has been widely used, its mechanism is not known. Three units of the National Institutes of Health, the National Institute of General Medical Sciences, National Institute of Neurological Diseases and Stroke, and Fogarty International Center were designated to assess and identify specific opportunities and needs for research attending the use of acupuncture for surgical anesthesia and relief of chronic pain. Following thorough review, and pending completion of the scientific assessment and efficacy of the technique, CMS initially issued a national noncoverage determination for acupuncture in May 1980.

Nationally Covered Indications

Not applicable.

Nationally Noncovered Indications

After careful reconsideration of its initial noncoverage determination for acupuncture, CMS concludes that there is no convincing evidence for the use of acupuncture for pain relief in patients with fibromyalgia. Study design flaws presently prohibit assessing acupuncture's utility for improving health outcomes. Accordingly, CMS determines that acupuncture is not considered reasonable and necessary for the treatment of fibromyalgia within the meaning of §1862(a)(1) of the Social Security Act, and the national noncoverage determination for acupuncture continues.

(This NCD last reviewed April 2004.)

100-3, 30.3.2

30.3.2 – Acupuncture for Osteoarthritis (Effective April 16, 2004) (30.3.2)

(Rev. 11, 04-16-04)

General

Although acupuncture has been used for thousands of years in China and for decades in parts of Europe, it is still a relatively new agent of unknown use and efficacy in the United States. Even in those areas of the world where it has been widely used, its mechanism is not known. Three units of the National Institutes of Health, the National Institute of General Medical Sciences, National Institute of Neurological Diseases and Stroke, and Fogarty International Center were designated to assess and identify specific opportunities and needs for research attending the use of acupuncture for surgical anesthesia and relief of chronic pain. Following thorough review, and pending completion of the scientific assessment and efficacy of the technique, CMS initially issued a national noncoverage determination for acupuncture in May 1980.

Nationally Covered Indications

Not applicable.

Nationally Noncovered Indications

After careful reconsideration of its initial noncoverage determination for acupuncture, CMS concludes that there is no convincing evidence for the use of acupuncture for pain relief in patients with osteoarthritis. Study design flaws presently prohibit assessing acupuncture's utility for improving health outcomes. Accordingly, CMS determines that acupuncture is not considered reasonable and necessary for the treatment of osteoarthritis within the meaning of §1862(a)(1) of the Social Security Act, and the national noncoverage determination for acupuncture continues.

(This NCD last reviewed April 2004.)

100-3, 30.6

Intravenous Histamine Therapy

However, there is no scientifically valid clinical evidence that histamine therapy is effective for any condition regardless of the method of administration, nor is it accepted or widely used by the medical profession. Therefore, histamine therapy cannot be considered reasonable and necessary, and program payment for such therapy is not made.

100-3, 40.1

Diabetes Outpatient Self-Management Training

Please refer to 42 CFR 410.140 - 410.146 for conditions that must be met for Medicare coverage.

100-3, 40.5

Treatment of Obesity

B. Nationally Covered Indications

Certain designated surgical services for the treatment of obesity are covered for Medicare beneficiaries who have a BMI >=35, have at least one co-morbidity related to obesity and have been previously unsuccessful with the medical treatment of obesity. See Sec.100.1.

C. Nationally Noncovered Indications

1. Treatments for obesity alone remain non-covered.
2. Supplemented fasting is not covered under the Medicare program as a general treatment for obesity (see section D. below for discretionary local coverage).

D. Other

Where weight loss is necessary before surgery in order to ameliorate the complications posed by obesity when it coexists with pathological conditions such as cardiac and respiratory diseases, diabetes, or hypertension (and other more conservative techniques to achieve this end are not regarded as appropriate), supplemented fasting with adequate monitoring of the patient is eligible for coverage on a case-by-case basis or pursuant to a local coverage determination. The risks associated with the achievement of rapid weight loss must be carefully balanced against the risk posed by the condition requiring surgical treatment.

(This NCD last reviewed February 2006.)

100-3, 50.1

Speech Generating Devices

Effective January 1, 2001, augmentative and alternative communication devices or communicators, which are hereafter referred to as "speech generating devices" are now considered to fall within the DME benefit category established by Sec.1861(n) of the Act. They may be covered if the contractor's medical staff determines that the patient suffers from a severe speech impairment and that the medical condition warrants the use of a device based on the definitions above.

100-3, 50.2

Electronic Speech Aids

Electronic speech aids are covered under Part B as prosthetic devices when the patient has had a laryngectomy or his larynx is permanently inoperative.

100-3, 50.3

Cochlear Implantation

B. Nationally Covered Indications

1. Effective for services performed on or after April 4, 2005, cochlear implantation may be covered for treatment of bilateral pre- or-post-linguistic, sensorineural, moderate-to-profound hearing loss in individuals who demonstrate limited benefit from amplification. Limited benefit from amplification is defined by test scores of less than or equal to 40% correct in the best-aided listening condition on tape-recorded tests of open-set sentence cognition. Medicare coverage is provided only for those patients who meet all of the following selection guidelines.
   - Diagnosis of bilateral moderate-to-profound sensorineural hearing impairment with limited benefit from appropriate hearing (or vibrotactile) aids;
   - Cognitive ability to use auditory clues and a willingness to undergo an extended program of rehabilitation;
   - Freedom from middle ear infection, an accessible cochlear lumen that is structurally suited to implantation, and freedom from lesions in the auditory nerve and acoustic areas of the central nervous system;
   - No contraindications to surgery; and
   - The device must be used in accordance with Food and Drug Administration (FDA)-approved labeling.
2. Effective for services performed on or after April 4, 2005, cochlear implantation may be covered for individuals meeting the selection guidelines above and with hearing test scores of greater than 40% and less than or equal to 60% only when the provider is participating in, and patients are enrolled in, either an FDA-approved category B investigational device exemption clinical trial as defined at 42 CFR 405.201, a trial under the Centers for Medicare & Medicaid (CMS) Clinical Trial Policy as defined at section 310.1 of the National Coverage Determinations Manual, or a prospective, controlled comparative trial approved by CMS as consistent with the evidentiary requirements for National Coverage Analyses and meeting specific quality standards.

C. Nationally Noncovered Indications

Medicare beneficiaries not meeting all of the coverage criteria for cochlear implantation listed are deemed not eligible for Medicare coverage under section 1862(a)(1)(A) of the Social Security Act.

D. Other

All other indications for cochlear implantation not otherwise indicated as nationally covered or non-covered above remain at local contractor discretion.

(This NCD last reviewed May 2005.)

100-3, 70.1

Consultations with a Beneficiary's Family and Associates

In certain types of medical conditions, including when a patient is withdrawn and uncommunicative due to a mental disorder or comatose, the physician may contact relatives and close associates to secure background information to assist in diagnosis and treatment planning. When a physician contacts his patient's relatives or associates for this purpose, expenses of such interviews are properly chargeable as physician's services to the patient on whose behalf the information was secured. If the beneficiary is not an inpatient of a hospital, Part B reimbursement for such an interview is subject to the special limitation on payments for physicians' services in connection with mental, psychoneurotic, and personality disorders.

A physician may also have contacts with a patient's family and associates for purposes other than securing background information. In some cases, the physician will provide counseling to members of the household. Family counseling services are covered only where the primary purpose of such counseling is the treatment of the patient's condition. For example, two situations where family counseling services would be appropriate are as follows: (1) where there is a need to observe the patient's interaction with family members; and/or (2) where there is a need to assess the capability of and assist the family members in aiding in the management of the patient. Counseling principally concerned with the effects of the patient's condition on the individual being interviewed would not be reimbursable as part of the physician's personal services to the patient. While to a limited degree, the counseling described in the second situation may be used to modify the behavior of the family members, such services nevertheless are covered because they relate primarily to the management of the patient's problems and not to the treatment of the family member's problems.

100-3, 70.2

Consultation Services Rendered by a Podiatrist in a Skilled Nursing Facility

Consultation services rendered by a podiatrist in a skilled nursing facility are covered if the services are reasonable and necessary and do not come within any of the specific statutory exclusions. Section 1862(a)(13) of the Act excludes payment for the treatment of flat foot conditions, the treatment of subluxations of the foot, and routine foot care. To determine whether the consultation comes within the foot care exclusions, apply the same rule as for initial diagnostic examinations, i.e., where services are performed in connection with specific symptoms or complaints which suggest the need for covered services, the services are covered regardless of the resulting diagnosis. The exclusion of routine physician examinations is also pertinent and would generally exclude podiatric consultation performed on all patients in a skilled nursing facility on a routine basis for screening purposes, except in those cases where a specific foot ailment is involved. Section 1862(a)(7) of the Act excludes payment for routine physical checkups.

100-3, 70.2.1

Services Provided for the Diagnosis and Treatment of Diabetic Sensory Neuropathy with Loss of Protective Sensation (AKA Diabetic Peripheral Neuropathy)

Diabetic sensory neuropathy with LOPS is a localized illness of the feet and falls within the regulation's exception to the general exclusionary rule (see 42 CFR Sec.411.15(l)(1)(i)). Foot exams for people with diabetic sensory neuropathy with LOPS are reasonable and necessary to allow for early intervention in serious complications that typically afflict diabetics with the disease.

Effective for services furnished on or after July 1, 2002, Medicare covers, as a physician service, an evaluation (examination and treatment) of the feet no more often than every six months for individuals with a documented diagnosis of diabetic sensory neuropathy and LOPS, as long as the beneficiary has not seen a foot care specialist for some other reason in the interim. LOPS shall be diagnosed through sensory testing with the 5.07 monofilament using established guidelines, such as those developed by the National Institute of Diabetes and Digestive and Kidney Diseases guidelines. Five sites should be tested on the plantar surface of each foot, according to the National Institute of Diabetes and Digestive and Kidney Diseases guidelines. The areas must be tested randomly since the loss of protective sensation may be patchy in distribution, and the patient may get clues if the test is done rhythmically. Heavily callused areas should be avoided. As suggested by the American Podiatric Medicine Association, an absence of sensation at two or more sites out of 5 tested on either foot when tested with the 5.07 Semmes-Weinstein monofilament must be present and documented to diagnose peripheral neuropathy with loss of protective sensation.

The examination includes:

1. A patient history.
2. A physical examination that must consist of at least the following elements:
   - Visual inspection of forefoot and hindfoot (including toe web spaces).
   - Evaluation of protective sensation.
   - Evaluation of foot structure and biomechanics.
   - Evaluation of vascular status and skin integrity.
   - Evaluation of the need for special footwear.
3. Patient education.

A. Treatment includes, but is not limited to:

- Local care of superficial wounds.
- Debridement of corns and calluses.
- Trimming and debridement of nails.

The diagnosis of diabetic sensory neuropathy with LOPS should be established and documented prior to coverage of foot care. Other causes of peripheral neuropathy should be considered and investigated by the primary care physician prior to initiating or referring for foot care for persons with LOPS.

100-3, 80.1

Hydrophilic Contact Lens For Corneal Bandage

Payment may be made under Sec.1861(s)(2) of the Act for a hydrophilic contact les approved by the Food and Drug Administration (FDA) and used as a supply incident to a pphysician's service. Payment for the lens is included in the payment for the physician's service to which the lens is incident. Contractors are authorized to accept an FDA letter of approval or other FDA published material as evidence of FDA approval. (See Sec.80.4 of the NCD Manual for coverage of a hydrophilic contact lens as prosthetic device.)

100-3, 80.2

Photodynamic Therapy

(Rev.155, Issued: 06-14-13, Effective: 04-03-13, Implementation: 07-16-13)

CIM 35-100

Photodynamic therapy is a medical procedure which involves the infusion of a photosensitive (light-activated) drug with a very specific absorption peak. This drug is chemically designed to have a unique affinity for the diseased tissue intended for treatment. Once introduced to the body, the drug accumulates and is retained in diseased tissue to a greater degree than in normal tissue. Infusion is followed by the targeted irradiation of this tissue with a non-thermal laser, calibrated to emit light at a wavelength that corresponds to the drug's absorption peak. The drug then becomes active and locally treats the diseased tissue.

Ocular photodynamic therapy (OPT)

The OPT is used in the treatment of ophthalmologic diseases. OPT is only covered when used in conjunction with verteporfin (see §80.3, "Photosensitive Drugs").

- Classic Subfoveal Choroidal Neovascular (CNV) Lesions - OPT is covered with a diagnosis of neovascular age-related macular degeneration (AMD) with predominately classic subfoveal choroidal neovascular (CNV) lesions (where the area of classic CNV occupies = 50 percent of the area of the entire lesion) at the initial visit as determined by a fluorescein angiogram. Subsequent follow-up visits will require either an optical coherence tomography (OCT) or a fluorescein angiogram (FA) to access treatment response. There are no requirements regarding visual acuity, lesion size, and number of re-treatments.
- Occult Subfoveal Choroidal Neovascular (CNV) Lesions - OPT is noncovered for patients with a diagnosis of age-related macular degeneration (AMD) with occult and no classic CNV lesions.
- Other Conditions - Use of OPT with verteporfin for other types of AMD (e.g., patients with minimally classic CNV lesions, atrophic, or dry AMD) is noncovered. OPT with verteporfin for other ocular indications such as pathologic myopia or presumed ocular histoplasmosis syndrome, is eligible for coverage through individual contractor discretion.

100-3, 80.2.1

Ocular Photodynamic Therapy (OPT)- Effective April 3, 2013

A. General

Ocular Photodynamic Therapy (OPT) is used in the treatment of ophthalmologic diseases; specifically, for age-related macular degeneration (AMD), a common eye disease among the elderly. OPT involves the infusion of an intravenous photosensitizing drug called verteporfin followed by exposure to a laser. OPT is only covered when used in conjunction with verteporfin.

Effective July 1, 2001, OPT with verteporfin was approved for a diagnosis of neovascular AMD with predominately classic subfoveal choroidal neovascularization (CNV) lesions (where the area of classic CNV occupies = 50% of the area of the entire lesion) at the initial visit as determined by a fluorescein angiogram (FA).

On October 17, 2001, the Centers for Medicare & Medicaid Services (CMS) announced its "intent to cover" OPT with verteporfin for AMD patients with occult and no classic subfoveal CNV as determined by an FA. The October 17, 2001, decision was never implemented.

On March 28, 2002, after thorough review and reconsideration of the October 17, 2001, intent to cover policy, CMS determined that the current non-coverage policy for OPT for verteporfin for AMD patients with occult and no classic subfoveal CNV as determined by an FA should remain in effect.

Effective August 20, 2002, CMS issued a non-covered instruction for OPT with verteporfin for AMD patients with occult and no classic subfoveal CNV as determined by an FA.

B. Nationally Covered Indications

Effective April 1, 2004, OPT with verteporfin continues to be approved for a diagnosis of neovascular AMD with predominately classic subfoveal CNV lesions (where the area of classic CNV occupies = 50% of the area of the entire lesion) at the initial visit as determined by an FA. (CNV lesions are comprised of classic and/or occult components.) Subsequent follow-up visits require either an optical coherence tomography (OCT) (effective April 3. 2013) or an FA (effective April 1, 2004) to access treatment response. There are no requirements regarding visual acuity, lesion size, and number of re-treatments when treating predominantly classic lesions.

In addition, after thorough review and reconsideration of the August 20, 2002, non-coverage policy, CMS determines that the evidence is adequate to conclude that OPT with verteporfin is reasonable and necessary for treating:

1. Subfoveal occult with no classic CNV associated with AMD; and,
2. Subfoveal minimally classic CNV (where the area of classic CNV occupies <50% of the area of the entire lesion) associated with AMD.

The above 2 indications are considered reasonable and necessary only when:

1. The lesions are small (4 disk areas or less in size) at the time of initial treatment or within the 3 months prior to initial treatment; and,
2. The lesions have shown evidence of progression within the 3 months prior to initial treatment. Evidence of progression must be documented by deterioration of visual acuity (at least 5 letters on a standard eye examination chart), lesion growth (an increase in at least 1 disk area), or the appearance of blood associated with the lesion.

C. Nationally Non-Covered Indications

Other uses of OPT with verteporfin to treat AMD not already addressed by CMS will continue to be non-covered. These include, but are not limited to, the following AMD indications:

- Juxtafoveal or extrafoveal CNV lesions (lesions outside the fovea),
- Inability to obtain a fluorescein angiogram,
- Atrophic or "dry" AMD.

D. Other

The OPT with verteporfin for other ocular indications, such as pathologic myopia or presumed ocular histoplasmosis syndrome, continue to be eligible for local coverage determinations through individual contractor discretion.

100-3, 80.3

Photosensitive Drugs (80.3)

(Rev. 1, 10-03-03) CIM 45-30

Photosensitive drugs are the light-sensitive agents used in photodynamic therapy. Once introduced into the body, these drugs selectively identify and adhere to diseased tissue. The drugs remain inactive until they are exposed to a specific wavelength of light, by means of a laser, that corresponds to their absorption peak. The activation of a photosensitive drug results in a photochemical reaction which treats the diseased tissue without affecting surrounding normal tissue.

Verteporfin

Verteporfin, a benzoporphyrin derivative, is an intravenous lipophilic photosensitive drug with an absorption peak of 690 nm. This drug was first approved by the Food and Drug Administration (FDA) on April 12, 2000, and subsequently, approved for inclusion in the United States Pharmacopoeia on July 18, 2000, meeting Medicare's definition of a drug when used in conjunction with ocular photodynamic therapy (see §80.2, "Photodynamic Therapy") when furnished intravenously incident to a physician's service. For patients with age-related macular degeneration, Verteporfin is only covered with a diagnosis of neovascular age-related macular degeneration (ICD-9-CM 362.52) with predominately classic subfoveal choroidal neovascular (CNV) lesions (where the area of classic CNV occupies ≥ 50 percent of the area of the entire lesion) at the initial visit as determined by a fluorescein angiogram (CPT code 92235). Subsequent follow-up visits will require a fluorescein angiogram prior to treatment. OPT with verteporfin is covered for the above indication and will remain noncovered for all other indications related to AMD (see §80.2). OPT with Verteporfin for use in non-AMD conditions is eligible for coverage through individual contractor discretion.

100-3, 80.4

Hydrophilic Contact Lenses

Hydrophilic contact lenses are eyeglasses within the meaning of the exclusion in Sec.1862(a)(7) of the Act and are not covered when used in the treatment of nondiseased eyes with spherical ametrophia, refractive astigmatism, and/or corneal astigmatism. Payment may be made under the prosthetic device benefit, however, for hydrophilic contact lenses when prescribed for an aphakic patient.

Contractors are authorized to accept an FDA letter of approval or other FDA published material as evidence of FDA approval. (See Sec.80.1 of the NCD Manual for coverage of a hydrophilic lens as a corneal bandage.)

100-3, 80.6

Intraocular Photography

Intraocular photography is covered when used for the diagnosis of such conditions as macular degeneration, retinal neoplasms, choroid disturbances and diabetic retinopathy, or to identify glaucoma, multiple sclerosis and other central nervous system abnormalities. Make Medicare payment for the use of this procedure by an opthalmologist in these situations when it is reasonable and necessary for the individual patient to receive these services.

100-3, 80.7

Refractive Keratoplasty

The correction of common refractive errors by eyeglasses, contact lenses or other prosthetic devices is specifically excluded from coverage. The use of radial keratotomy and/or keratoplasty for the purpose of refractive error compensation is considered a substitute or alternative to eye glasses or contact lenses, which are specifically excluded by Sec.1862(a)(7) of the Act (except in certain cases in connection with cataract surgery). In addition, many in the medical community consider such procedures cosmetic surgery, which is excluded by section Sec.1862(a)(10) of the Act. Therefore, radial keratotomy and keratoplasty to treat refractive defects are not covered.

Keratoplasty that treats specific lesions of the cornea, such as phototherapeutic keratectomy that removes scar tissue from the visual field, deals with an abnormality of the eye and is not cosmetic surgery. Such cases may be covered under Sec.1862(a)(1)(A) of the Act.

The use of lasers to treat ophthalmic disease constitutes opthalmalogic surgery. Coverage is restricted to practitioners who have completed an approved training program in ophthalmologic surgery.

100-3, 80.8

Endothelial Cell Photography

Endothelial cell photography is a covered procedure under Medicare when reasonable and necessary for patients who meet one or more of the following criteria:

- Have slit lamp evidence of endothelial dystrophy (cornea guttata),
- Have slit lamp evidence of corneal edema (unilateral or bilateral),
- Are about to undergo a secondary intraocular lens implantation,
- Have had previous intraocular surgery and require cataract surgery,
- Are about to undergo a surgical procedure associated with a higher risk to corneal endothelium; i.e., phacoemulsification, or refractive surgery (see Sec.80.7 for excluded refractive procedures),
- With evidence of posterior polymorphous dystrophy of the cornea or irido-corneal-endothelium syndrome, or
- Are about to be fitted with extended wear contact lenses after intraocular surgery.

When a pre-surgical examination for cataract surgery is performed and the conditions of this section are met, if the only visual problem is cataracts, endothelial cell photography is covered as part of the presurgical comprehensive eye examination or combination brief/intermediate examination provided prior to cataract surgery, and not in addition to it. (See Sec.10.1.)

100-3, 80.9

Computer Enhanced Perimetry

It is a covered service when used in assessing visual fields in patients with glaucoma or other neuropathologic defects.

100-3, 80.10

Phaco-Emulsification procedure - cataract extraction

In view of recommendations of authoritative sources in the field of ophthalmology, the subject technique is viewed as an accepted procedure for removal of cataracts. Accordingly, program reimbursement may be made for necessary services furnished in connection with cataract extraction utilizing the phaco-emulsification procedure.

100-3, 80.11

Vitrectomy

Vitrectomy may be considered reasonable and necessary for the following conditions: vitreous loss incident to cataract surgery, vitreous opacities due to vitreous hemorrhage or other causes, retinal detachments secondary to vitreous strands, proliferative retinopathy, and vitreous retraction. See Chapter 23 of the Medicare Claims Manual for how to determine payment for physician vitrectomy services and Chapter 14 Sec.40 for how to determine payment for ASC facility vitrectomy services. Also, see Chapter 23 Sec.20.9 to identify when, for Medicare payment purposes, certain vitrectomy codes are included in other codes or when codes for other services include vitrectomy codes.

100-3, 80.12

Intraocular Lenses (IOLs)

Intraocular lens implantation services, as well as the lens itself, may be covered if reasonable and necessary for the individual. Implantation services may include hospital, surgical, and other medical services, including pre-implantation ultrasound (A-scan) eye measurement of one or both eyes.

100-3, 100.1

Bariatric Surgery for Treatment of Co-Morbid Conditions Related to Morbid Obesity

Please note, sections 40.5, 100.8, 100.11, and 100.14 have been removed from the National Coverage Determination (NCD) Manual and incorporated into NCD 100.1

A. General

Obesity may be caused by medical conditions such as hypothyroidism, Cushing's disease, and hypothalamic lesions, or can aggravate a number of cardiac and respiratory diseases as well as diabetes and hypertension. Non-surgical services in connection with the treatment of obesity are covered when such services are an integral and necessary part of a course of treatment for one of these medical conditions.

In addition, supplemented fasting is a type of very low calorie weight reduction regimen used to achieve rapid weight loss. The reduced calorie intake is supplemented by a mixture of protein, carbohydrates, vitamins, and minerals. Serious questions exist about the safety of prolonged adherence for 2 months or more to a very low calorie weight reduction regimen as a general treatment for obesity, because of instances of cardiopathology and sudden death, as well as possible loss of body protein.

Bariatric surgery procedures are performed to treat comorbid conditions associated with morbid obesity. Two types of surgical procedures are employed. Malabsorptive procedures divert food from the stomach to a lower part of the digestive tract where the normal mixing of digestive fluids and absorption of nutrients cannot occur. Restrictive procedures restrict the size of the stomach and decrease intake. Surgery can combine both types of procedures.

The following are descriptions of bariatric surgery procedures:

1. Roux-en-Y Gastric Bypass (RYGBP)

The RYGBP achieves weight loss by gastric restriction and malabsorption. Reduction of the stomach to a small gastric pouch (30 cc) results in feelings of satiety following even small meals. This small pouch is connected to a segment of the jejunum, bypassing the duodenum and very proximal small intestine, thereby reducing absorption. RYGBP procedures can be open or laparoscopic.

2. Biliopancreatic Diversion with Duodenal Switch (BPD/DS) or Gastric Reduction Duodenal Switch (BPD/GRDS)

The BPD achieves weight loss by gastric restriction and malabsorption. The stomach is partially resected, but the remaining capacity is generous compared to that achieved with RYGBP. As such, patients eat relatively normal-sized meals and do not need to restrict intake radically, since the most proximal areas of the small intestine (i.e., the duodenum and jejunum) are bypassed, and substantial malabsorption occurs. The partial BPD/DS or BPD/GRDS is a variant of the BPD procedure. It involves resection of the greater curvature of the stomach, preservation of the pyloric sphincter, and transection of the duodenum above the ampulla of Vater with a duodeno-ileal anastomosis and a lower ileo-ileal anastomosis. BPD/DS or BPD/GRDS procedures can be open or laparoscopic.

3. Adjustable Gastric Banding (AGB)

The AGB achieves weight loss by gastric restriction only. A band creating a gastric pouch with a capacity of approximately 15 to 30 cc? encircles the uppermost portion of the stomach. The band is an inflatable doughnut-shaped balloon, the diameter of which can be adjusted in the clinic by adding or removing saline via a port that is positioned beneath the skin. The bands are adjustable, allowing the size of the gastric outlet

to be modified as needed, depending on the rate of a patient? weight loss. AGB procedures are laparoscopic only.

4. Sleeve Gastrectomy

Sleeve gastrectomy is a 70%-80% greater curvature gastrectomy (sleeve resection of the stomach) with continuity of the gastric lesser curve being maintained while simultaneously reducing stomach volume. In the past, sleeve gastrectomy was the first step in a two-stage procedure when performing RYGBP, but more recently has been offered as a stand-alone surgery. Sleeve gastrectomy procedures can be open or laparoscopic.

5. Vertical Gastric Banding (VGB)

The VGB achieves weight loss by gastric restriction only. The upper part of the stomach is stapled, creating a narrow gastric inlet or pouch that remains connected with the remainder of the stomach. In addition, a non-adjustable band is placed around this new inlet in an attempt to prevent future enlargement of the stoma (opening). As a result, patients experience a sense of fullness after eating small meals. Weight loss from this procedure results entirely from eating less. VGB procedures are essentially no longer performed.

B. Nationally Covered Indications

Effective for services performed on and after February 21, 2006, Open and laparoscopic Roux-en-Y gastric bypass (RYGBP), open and laparoscopic Biliopancreatic Diversion with Duodenal Switch (BPD/DS) or Gastric Reduction Duodenal Switch (BPD/GRDS), and laparoscopic adjustable gastric banding (LAGB) are covered for Medicare beneficiaries who have a body-mass index = 35, have at least one co-morbidity related to obesity, and have been previously unsuccessful with medical treatment for obesity.

Effective for dates of service on and after February 21, 2006, these procedures are only covered when performed at facilities that are: (1) certified by the American College of Surgeons as a Level 1 Bariatric Surgery Center (program standards and requirements in effect on February 15, 2006); or (2) certified by the American Society for Bariatric Surgery as a Bariatric Surgery Center of Excellence (program standards and requirements in effect on February 15, 2006). Effective for dates of service on and after September 24, 2013, facilities are no longer required to be certified.

Effective for services performed on and after February 12, 2009, the Centers for Medicare & Medicaid Services (CMS) determines that Type 2 diabetes mellitus is a co-morbidity for purposes of this NCD.

A list of approved facilities and their approval dates are listed and maintained on the CMS Coverage Web site at http://www.cms.gov/Medicare/Medicare-General-Information/MedicareApprovedFacilitie/Bariatric-Surgery.html, and published in the Federal Register for services provided up to and including date of service September 23, 2013.

C. Nationally Non-Covered Indications

Treatments for obesity alone remain non-covered.

Supplemented fasting is not covered under the Medicare program as a general treatment for obesity (see section D. below for discretionary local coverage).

The following bariatric surgery procedures are non-covered for all Medicare beneficiaries:

Open adjustable gastric banding;

Open sleeve gastrectomy;

Laparoscopic sleeve gastrectomy (prior to June 27, 2012);

Open and laparoscopic vertical banded gastroplasty;

Intestinal bypass surgery; and,

Gastric balloon for treatment of obesity.

D. Other

Effective for services performed on and after June 27, 2012, Medicare Administrative Contractors (MACs) acting within their respective jurisdictions may determine coverage of stand-alone laparoscopic sleeve gastrectomy (LSG) for the treatment of co-morbid conditions related to obesity in Medicare beneficiaries only when all of the following conditions a.-c. are satisfied.

a. The beneficiary has a body-mass index (BMI) = 35 kg/m2,

b. The beneficiary has at least one co-morbidity related to obesity, and,

c. The beneficiary has been previously unsuccessful with medical treatment for obesity.

The determination of coverage for any bariatric surgery procedures that are not specifically identified in an NCD as covered or non-covered, for Medicare beneficiaries who have a body-mass index = 35, have at least one co-morbidity related to obesity, and have been previously unsuccessful with medical treatment for obesity, is left to the local MACs.

Where weight loss is necessary before surgery in order to ameliorate the complications posed by obesity when it coexists with pathological conditions such as cardiac and respiratory diseases, diabetes, or hypertension (and other more conservative techniques to achieve this end are not regarded as appropriate), supplemented fasting with adequate monitoring of the patient is eligible for coverage on a case-by-case basis or pursuant to a local coverage determination. The risks associated with the achievement of rapid weight loss must be carefully balanced against the risk posed by the condition requiring surgical treatment.

100-3, 100.2

Endoscopy

Endoscopic procedures are covered when reasonable and necessary for the individual patient.

100-3, 100.4

Esophageal Manometry

Esophageal manometry is covered under Medicare where it is determined to be reasonable and necessary for the individual patient.

100-3, 100.5

Diagnostic Breath Analyses

The Following Breath Test is Covered:

- Lactose breath hydrogen to detect lactose malabsorption .

The Following Breath Tests are Excluded from Coverage;

- Lactulose breath hydrogen for diagnosing small bowel bacterial overgrowth and measuring small bowel transit time.
- CO2 for diagnosing bile acid malabsorption.
- CO2 for diagnosing fat malabsorption.

100-3, 100.8

Intestinal By-Pass Surgery

The safety of intestinal bypass surgery for treatment of obesity has not been demonstrated. Severe adverse reactions such as steatorrhea, electrolyte depletion, liver failure, arthralgia, hypoplasia of bone marrow, and avitaminosis have sometimes occurred as a result of this procedure. It does not meet the reasonable and necessary provisions of Sec.1862(a)(1) of the Act and is not a covered Medicare procedure.

100-3, 100.10

Injection Sclerotherapy for Esophageal Variceal Bleeding

Injection sclerotherapy is a technique involving insertion of a flexible fiberoptic endoscope into the esophagus, and the injection of a sclerosing agent or solution into the varicosities to control bleeding. This procedure is covered under Medicare.

100-3, 100.13

Laparoscopic Cholecystectomy

Laparoscopic cholecystectomy is a covered surgical procedure in which a diseased gall bladder is removed through the use of instruments introduced via cannulae, with vision of the operative field maintained by use of a high-resolution television camera-monitor system (video laparoscope). For inpatient claims, use ICD-9-CM code 51.23, Laparoscopic cholecystectomy. For all other claims, use CPT codes 49310 for laparoscopy, surgical; cholecystectomy (any method), and 49311 for laparoscopy, surgical: cholecystectomy with cholangiography.

100-3, 110.1

Hyperthermia for Treatment of Cancer)

Local hyperthermia is covered under Medicare when used in connection with radiation therapy for the treatment of primary or metastatic cutaneous or subcutaneous superficial malignancies. It is not covered when used alone or in connection with chemotherapy.

100-3,110.2

Certain Drugs Distributed by the National Cancer Institute

A physician is eligible to receive Group C drugs from the Division of Cancer Treatment only if the following requirements are met:

A physician must be registered with the NCI as an investigator by having completed an FD-Form 1573;

A written request for the drug, indicating the disease to be treated, must be submitted to the NCI;

The use of the drug must be limited to indications outlined in the NCI's guidelines; and

All adverse reactions must be reported to the Investigational Drug Branch of the Division of Cancer Treatment.

In view of these NCI controls on distribution and use of Group C drugs, intermediaries may assume, in the absence of evidence to the contrary, that a Group C drug and the related hospital stay are covered if all other applicable coverage requirements are satisfied.

If there is reason to question coverage in a particular case, the matter should be resolved with the assistance of the Quality improvemetn organization (QIO), or if there is none, the assistance of your medical consultants.

Information regarding those drugs which are classified as Group C drugs may be obtained from:

Office of the Chief, Investigational Drug Branch
Division of Cancer Treatment, CTEP, Landow Building
Room 4C09, National Cancer Institute
Bethesda, Maryland 20205

100-3, 110.3

Anti-Inhibitor Coagulant Complex (AICC)

Anti-inhibitor coagulant complex, AICC, is a drug used to treat hemophilia in patients with factor VIII inhibitor antibodies. AICC has been shown to be safe and effective and has Medicare coverage when furnished to patients with hemophilia A and inhibitor antibodies to factor VIII who have major bleeding episodes and who fail to respond to other, less expensive therapies.

100-3,110.4

Extracorporeal Photopheresis

A. General

Extracorporeal photopheresis is a medical procedure in which a patient's white blood cells are exposed first to a drug called 8-methoxypsoralen (8-MOP) and then to ultraviolet A (UVA) light. The procedure starts with the removal of the patient's blood, which is centrifuged to isolate the white blood cells. The drug is typically administered directly to the white blood cells after they have been removed from the patient (referred to as ex vivo administration) but the drug can alternatively be administered directly to the patient before the white blood cells are withdrawn. After UVA light exposure, the treated white blood cells are then re-infused into the patient.

B. Nationally Covered Indications

The Centers for Medicare & Medicaid Services (CMS) has determined that extracorporeal photopheresis is reasonable and necessary under section 1862(a)(1)(A) of the Social Security Act (the Act) under the following circumstances:

1. Effective April 8, 1988, Medicare provides coverage for:

   Palliative treatment of skin manifestations of cutaneous T-cell lymphoma that has not responded to other therapy.

2. Effective December 19, 2006, Medicare also provides coverage for:

   Patients with acute cardiac allograft rejection whose disease is refractory to standard immunosuppressive drug treatment; and,

   Patients with chronic graft versus host disease whose disease is refractory to standard immunosuppressive drug treatment.

3. Effective April 30, 2012, Medicare also provides coverage for:

   Extracorporeal photopheresis for the treatment of bronchiolitis obliterans syndrome (BOS) following lung allograft transplantation only when extracorporeal photopheresis is provided under a clinical research study that meets the following conditions:

   The clinical research study meets the requirements specified below to assess the effect of extracorporeal photopheresis for the treatment of BOS following lung allograft transplantation. The clinical study must address one or more aspects of the following question:

   Prospectively, do Medicare beneficiaries who have received lung allografts, developed BOS refractory to standard immunosuppressive therapy, and received extracorporeal photopheresis , experience improved patient-centered health outcomes as indicated by:

   a. improved forced expiratory volume in one second (FEV1);
   b. improved survival after transplant; and/or,
   c. improved quality of life?

   he required clinical study must adhere to the following standards of scientific integrity and relevance to the Medicare population:

   a. The principal purpose of the research study is to test whether extracorporeal photopheresis potentially improves the participants' health outcomes.
   b. The research study is well supported by available scientific and medical information or it is intended to clarify or establish the health outcomes of interventions already in common clinical use.
   c. The research study does not unjustifiably duplicate existing studies.
   d. The research study design is appropriate to answer the research question being asked in the study.
   e. The research study is sponsored by an organization or individual capable of successfully executing the proposed study.
   f. The research study is in compliance with all applicable Federal regulations concerning the protection of human subjects found at 45 CFR Part 46. If a study is regulated by the Food and Drug Administration (FDA), it must also be in compliance with 21 CFR parts 50 and 56.
   g. All aspects of the research study are conducted according to appropriate standards of scientific integrity (see http://www.icmje.org).
   h. The research study has a written protocol that clearly addresses, or incorporates by reference, the standards listed here as Medicare requirements for coverage with evidence development.
   i. The clinical research study is not designed to exclusively test toxicity or disease pathophysiology in healthy individuals. Trials of all medical technologies measuring therapeutic outcomes as one of the objectives meet this standard only if the disease or condition being studied is life threatening as defined in 21 CFR section 312.81(a) and the patient has no other viable treatment options.
   j. The clinical research study is registered on the ClinicalTrials.gov website by the principal sponsor/investigator prior to the enrollment of the first study subject.
   k. The research study protocol specifies the method and timing of public release of all prespecified outcomes to be measured including release of outcomes if outcomes are negative or study is terminated early. The results must be made public within 24 months of the end of data collection. If a report is planned to be published in a peer-reviewed journal, then that initial release may be an abstract that meets the requirements of the International Committee of Medical Journal Editors (http://www.icmje.org).
   l. The research study protocol must explicitly discuss subpopulations affected by the treatment under investigation, particularly traditionally underrepresented groups in clinical studies, how the inclusion and exclusion criteria effect enrollment of these populations, and a plan for the retention and reporting of said populations on the trial. If the inclusion and exclusion criteria are expected to have a negative effect on the recruitment or retention of underrepresented populations, the protocol must discuss why these criteria are necessary.
   m. The research study protocol explicitly discusses how the results are or are not expected to be generalizable to the Medicare population to infer whether Medicare patients may benefit from the intervention. Separate discussions in the protocol may be necessary for populations eligible for Medicare due to age, disability or Medicaid eligibility.

Consistent with section 1142 of the Act, the Agency for Healthcare Research and Quality supports clinical research studies that CMS determines meet the above-listed standards and address the above-listed research questions.

Any clinical study under which there is coverage of extracorporeal photopheresis for this indication pursuant to this national coverage determination (NCD) must be approved by April 30, 2014. If there are no approved clinical studies on this date, this NCD will expire and coverage of extracorporeal photopheresis for BOS will revert to the coverage policy in effect prior to the issuance of the final decision memorandum for this NCD.

C. Nationally Non-Covered Indications

All other indications for extracorporeal photopheresis not otherwise indicated above as covered remain non-covered.

D. Other

Claims processing instructions can be found in chapter 32, section 190 of the Medicare Claims Processing Manual.

(This NCD last reviewed April 2012.)

100-3, 110.5

Granulocyte Transfusions

Granulocyte transfusions to patients suffering from severe infection and granulocytopenia are a covered service under Medicare. Granulocytopenia is usually identified as fewer than 500 granulocytes/mm 3 whole blood. Accepted indications for granulocyte transfusions include:

Granulocytopenia with evidence of gram negative sepsis; and

Granulocytopenia in febrile patients with local progressive infections unresponsive to appropriate antibiotic therapy, thought to be due to gram negative organisms.

100-3, 110.6

Scalp Hypothermia During Chemotherapy, to Prevent Hair Loss

While ice-filled bags or bandages or other devices used for scalp hypothermia during chemotherapy may be covered as supplies of the kind commonly furnished without a separate charge, no separate charge for them would be recognized.

100-3, 110.7

Blood Transfusions

B. Policy Governing Transfusions

For Medicare coverage purposes, it is important to distinguish between a transfusion itself and preoperative blood services; e.g., collection, processing, storage. Medically necessary transfusion of blood, regardless of the type, may generally be a covered service under both Part A and Part B of Medicare. Coverage does not make a distinction between the transfusion of homologous, autologous, or donor-directed blood. With respect to the coverage of the services associated with the preoperative collection, processing, and storage of autologous and donor-directed blood, the following policies apply.

1. Hospital Part A and B Coverage and Payment

   Under Sec.1862(a)(14) of the Act, non-physician services furnished to hospital patients are covered and paid for as hospital services. As provided in Sec.1886 of the Act, under the prospective [payment system (PPS), the diganosis related group (DRG) payment to the hospital includes all covered blood and blood processing expenses, whether or not the blood is eventually used.

Under its provider agreement, a hospital is required to furnish or arrange for all covered services furnished to hospital patients. medicare payment is made to the hospital, under PPS or cost reimbursement, for covered inpatient services, and it is intended to reflect payment for all costs of furnishing those services.

2. Nonhospital Part B Coverage

Under Part B, to be eligible for separate coverage, a service must fit the definition of one of the services authorized by Sec.1832 of the Act. These services are defined in 42 CFR 410.10 and do not include a separate category for a supplier's services associated with blood donation services, either autologous or donor-directed. That is, the collection, processing, and storage of blood for later transfusion into the beneficiary is not recognized as a separate service under Part B. Therefore, there is no avenue through which a blood supplier can receive direct payment under Part B for blood donation services.

C. Perioperative Blood Salvage

When the perioperative blood salvage process is used in surgery on a hospital patient, payment made to the hospital (under PPS or through cost reimbursement) for the procedure in which that process is used is intended to encompass payment for all costs relating to that process.

100-3, 110.8

Blood Platelet Transfusions

Blood platelet transplants are safe and effective for the correction of thrombocytopenia and other blood defects. It is covered under Medicare when treatment is reasonable and necessary for the individual patient.

100-3, 110.8.1

Stem Cell Transplantation

A. General

Stem cell transplantation is a process in which stem cells are harvested from either a patient's (autologous) or donor's (allogeneic) bone marrow or peripheral blood for intravenous infusion. Autologous stem cell transplants (AuSCT) must be used to effect hematopoietic reconstitution following severely myelotoxic doses of chemotherapy (HDCT) and/or radiotherapy used to treat various malignancies. Allogeneic stem cell transplants may be used to restore function in recipients having an inherited or acquired deficiency or defect. Hematopoietic stem cells are multi-potent stem cells that give rise to all the blood cell types; these stem cells form blood and immune cells. A hematopoietic stem cell is a cell isolated from blood or bone marrow that can renew itself, differentiate to a variety of specialized cells, can mobilize out of the bone marrow into circulating blood, and can undergo programmed cell death, called apoptosis - a process by which cells that are unneeded or detrimental self destruct.

The Centers for Medicare & Medicaid Services (CMS) is clarifying that bone marrow and peripheral blood stem cell transplantation is a process which includes mobilization, harvesting, and transplant of bone marrow or peripheral blood stem cells and the administration of high dose chemotherapy or radiotherapy prior to the actual transplant. When bone marrow or peripheral blood stem cell transplantation is covered, all necessary steps are included in coverage. When bone marrow or peripheral blood stem cell transplantation is non-covered, none of the steps are covered.

1. Allogeneic Hematopoietic Stem Cell Transplantation (HSCT)

Allogeneic hematopoietic stem cell transplantation (HSCT) is a procedure in which a portion of a healthy donor's stem cell or bone marrow is obtained and prepared for intravenous infusion.

a. Nationally Covered Indications

The following uses of allogeneic HSCT are covered under Medicare:

i. Effective for services performed on or after August 1, 1978, for the treatment of leukemia, leukemia in remission, or aplastic anemia when it is reasonable and necessary,

ii. Effective for services performed on or after June 3, 1985, for the treatment of severe combined immunodeficiency disease (SCID) and for the treatment of Wiskott-Aldrich syndrome.

iii. Effective for services performed on or after August 4, 2010, for the treatment of Myelodysplastic Syndromes (MDS) pursuant to Coverage with Evidence Development (CED) in the context of a Medicare-approved, prospective clinical study.

The MDS refers to a group of diverse blood disorders in which the bone marrow does not produce enough healthy, functioning blood cells. These disorders are varied with regard to clinical characteristics, cytologic and pathologic features, and cytogenetics. The abnormal production of blood cells in the bone marrow leads to low blood cell counts, referred to as cytopenias, which are a hallmark feature of MDS along with a dysplastic and hypercellular-appearing bone marrow.

Medicare payment for these beneficiaries will be restricted to patients enrolled in an approved clinical study. In accordance with the Stem Cell Therapeutic and Research Act of 2005 (US Public Law 109-129) a standard dataset is collected for all allogeneic transplant patients in the United States by the Center for International Blood and Marrow Transplant Research. The elements in this dataset, comprised of two mandatory forms plus one additional form, encompass the information we require for a study under CED.

A prospective clinical study seeking Medicare payment for treating a beneficiary with allogeneic HSCT for MDS pursuant to CED must meet one or more aspects of the following questions:

- Prospectively, compared to Medicare beneficiaries with MDS who do not receive HSCT, do Medicare beneficiaries with MDS who receive HSCT have improved outcomes as indicated by:
  - Relapse-free mortality,
  - progression free survival,
  - relapse, and
  - overall survival?
- Prospectively, in Medicare beneficiaries with MDS who receive HSCT, how do International Prognostic Scoring System (IPSS) score, patient age, cytopenias and comorbidities predict the following outcomes:
  - Relapse-free mortality,
  - progression free survival,
  - relapse, and
  - overall survival?
- Prospectively, in Medicare beneficiaries with MDS who receive HSCT, what treatment facility characteristics predict meaningful clinical improvement in the following outcomes:
  - Relapse-free mortality,
  - progression free survival,
  - relapse, and
  - overall survival?

In addition, the clinical study must adhere to the following standards of scientific integrity and relevance to the Medicare population:

a. The principal purpose of the research study is to test whether a particular intervention potentially improves the participants' health outcomes.

b. The research study is well supported by available scientific and medical information or it is intended to clarify or establish the health outcomes of interventions already in common clinical use.

c. The research study does not unjustifiably duplicate existing studies.

d. The research study design is appropriate to answer the research question being asked in the study.

e. The research study is sponsored by an organization or individual capable of executing the proposed study successfully.

f. The research study is in compliance with all applicable Federal regulations concerning the protection of human subjects found at 45 CFR Part 46.

g. All aspects of the research study are conducted according to appropriate standards of scientific integrity (see http://www.icmje.org).

h. The research study has a written protocol that clearly addresses, or incorporates by reference, the standards listed here as Medicare requirements for CED coverage.

i. The clinical research study is not designed to exclusively test toxicity or disease pathophysiology in healthy individuals. Trials of all medical technologies measuring therapeutic outcomes as one of the objectives meet this standard only if the disease or condition being studied is life threatening as defined in 21 CFR §312.81(a) and the patient has no other viable treatment options.

j. The clinical research study is registered on the ClinicalTrials.gov Web site by the principal sponsor/investigator prior to the enrollment of the first study subject.

k. The research study protocol specifies the method and timing of public release of all pre-specified outcomes to be measured including release of outcomes if outcomes are negative or study is terminated early. The results must be made public within 24 months of the end of data collection. If a report is planned to be published in a peer-reviewed journal, then that initial release may be an abstract that meets the requirements of the International Committee of Medical Journal Editors (http://www.icmje.org). However a full report of the outcomes must be made public no later than 3 years after the end of data collection.

l. The research study protocol must explicitly discuss subpopulations affected by the treatment under investigation, particularly traditionally underrepresented groups in clinical studies, how the inclusion and exclusion criteria effect enrollment of these populations, and a plan for the retention and reporting of said populations on the trial. If the inclusion and exclusion criteria are expected to have a negative effect on the recruitment or retention of underrepresented populations, the protocol must discuss why these criteria are necessary.

m. The research study protocol explicitly discusses how the results are or are not expected to be generalizable to the Medicare population to infer whether Medicare patients may benefit from the intervention. Separate discussions in the protocol may be necessary for populations eligible for Medicare due to age, disability or Medicaid eligibility. Consistent with section 1142 of the Social Security Act, the Agency for Health Research and Quality (AHRQ) supports clinical research studies that CMS determines meet the above-listed standards and address the above-listed research questions.

The clinical research study should also have the following features:

- It should be a prospective, longitudinal study with clinical information from the period before HSCT and short- and long-term follow-up information.
- Outcomes should be measured and compared among pre-specified subgroups within the cohort.
- The study should be powered to make inferences in subgroup analyses.
- Risk stratification methods should be used to control for selection bias. Data elements to be used in risk stratification models should include:

Patient selection:

- Patient Age at diagnosis of MDS and at transplantation
- Date of onset of MDS
- Disease classification (specific MDS subtype at diagnosis prior to preparative/conditioning regimen using World Health Organization (WHO) classifications). Include presence/absence of refractory cytopenias
- Comorbid conditions
- IPSS score (and WHO-adapted Prognostic Scoring System (WPSS) score, if applicable) at diagnosis and prior to transplantation
- Score immediately prior to transplantation and one year post-transplantation Disease assessment at diagnosis at start of preparative regimen and last assessment prior to preparative regimen Subtype of MDS (refractory anemia with or without blasts, degree of blasts, etc.)

Type of preparative/conditioning regimen administered (myeloabalative, non-myeloablative, reduced–intensity conditioning)

- Donor type
- Cell Source
- IPSS Score at diagnosis Facilities must submit the required transplant essential data to the Stem Cell Therapeutics Outcomes Database.

b. Nationally Non-Covered Indications

Effective for services performed on or after May 24, 1996, allogeneic HSCT is not covered as treatment for multiple myeloma.

2. Autologous Stem Cell Transplantation (AuSCT)

Autologous stem cell transplantation (AuSCT) is a technique for restoring stem cells using the patient's own previously stored cells.

a. Nationally Covered Indications

i. Effective for services performed on or after April 28, 1989, AuSCT is considered reasonable and necessary under §l862(a)(1)(A) of the Social Security Act (the Act) for the following conditions and is covered under Medicare for patients with:
   - Acute leukemia in remission who have a high probability of relapse and who have no human leucocyte antigens (HLA)-matched;
   - Resistant non-Hodgkin's lymphomas or those presenting with poor prognostic features following an initial response;
   - Recurrent or refractory neuroblastoma; or
   - Advanced Hodgkin's disease who have failed conventional therapy and have no HLA-matched donor.

ii. Effective October 1, 2000, single AuSCT is only covered for Durie-Salmon Stage II or III patients that fit the following requirements:
   - Newly diagnosed or responsive multiple myeloma. This includes those patients with previously untreated disease, those with at least a partial response to prior chemotherapy (defined as a 50% decrease either in measurable paraprotein [serum and/or urine] or in bone marrow infiltration, sustained for at least 1 month), and those in responsive relapse; and,
   - Adequate cardiac, renal, pulmonary, and hepatic function.

iii. Effective for services performed on or after March 15, 2005, when recognized clinical risk factors are employed to select patients for transplantation, high dose melphalan (HDM) together with AuSCT is reasonable and necessary for Medicare beneficiaries of any age group with primary amyloid light chain (AL) amyloidosis who meet the following criteria:
   - Amyloid deposition in 2 or fewer organs; and,
   - Cardiac left ventricular ejection fraction (EF) greater than 45%.

b. Nationally Non-Covered Indications

Insufficient data exist to establish definite conclusions regarding the efficacy of AuSCT for the following conditions:

- Acute leukemia not in remission;
- Chronic granulocytic leukemia;
- Solid tumors (other than neuroblastoma);
- Up to October 1, 2000, multiple myeloma;
- Tandem transplantation (multiple rounds of AuSCT) for patients with multiple myeloma;
- Effective October 1, 2000, non primary AL amyloidosis; and,
- Effective October 1, 2000, thru March 14, 2005, primary AL amyloidosis for Medicare beneficiaries age 64 or older.

In these cases, AuSCT is not considered reasonable and necessary within the meaning of §l862(a)(1)(A) of the Act and is not covered under Medicare.

B. Other

All other indications for stem cell transplantation not otherwise noted above as covered or non-covered nationally remain at local contractor discretion.

(This NCD last reviewed August 2010.)

100-3, 110.9

Antigens Prepared for Sublingual Administration

For antigens provided to patients on or after November 17, 1996, Medicare does not cover such antigens if they are to be administered sublingually, i.e., by placing drops under the patient's tongue. This kind of allergy therapy has not been proven to be safe and effective. Antigens are covered only if they are administered by injection.

100-3, 110.10

Intravenous Iron Therapy

Effective December 1, 2000, Medicare covers sodium ferric gluconate complex in sucrose injection as a first line treatment of iron deficiency anemia when furnished intravenously to patients undergoing chronic hemodialysis who are receiving supplemental erythropoeitin therapy.

Effective October 1, 2001, Medicare also covers iron sucrose injection as a first line treatment of iron deficiency anemia when furnished intravenously to patients undergoing chronic hemodialysis who are receiving supplemental erythropoeitin therapy.

100-3, 110.12

Challenge Ingestion Food Testing

This procedure is covered when it is used on an outpatient basis if it is reasonable and necessary for the individual patient.

Challenge ingestion food testing has not been proven to be effective in the diagnosis of rheumatoid arthritis, depression, or respiratory disorders. Accordingly, its use in the diagnosis of these conditions is not reasonable and necessary within the meaning of section 1862(a)(1) of the Medicare law, and no program payment is made for this procedure when it is so used.

100-3, 110.14

Apheresis (Therapeutic Pheresis)

B. Indications

Apheresis is covered for the following indications:

- Plasma exchange for acquired myasthenia gravis;
- Leukapheresis in the treatment of leukemekia
- Plasmapheresis in the treatment of primary macroglobulinemia (Waldenstrom);
- Treatment of hyperglobulinemias, including (but not limited to) multiple myelomas, cryoglobulinemia and hyperviscosity syndromes;
- Plasmapheresis or plasma exchange as a last resort treatment of thromobotic thrombocytopenic purpura (TTP);
- Plasmapheresis or plasma exchange in the last resort treatment of life threatening rheumatoid vasculitis;
- Plasma perfusion of charcoal filters for treatment of pruritis of cholestatic liver disease;
- Plasma exchange in the treatment of Goodpasture's Syndrome;
- Plasma exchange in the treatment of glomerulonephritis associated with antiglomerular basement membrane antibodies and advancing renal failure or pulmonary hemorrhage;
- Treatment of chronic relapsing polyneuropathy for patients with severe or life threatening symptoms who have failed to respond to conventional therapy;
- Treatment of life threatening scleroderma and polymyositis when the patient is unresponsive to conventional therapy;
- Treatment of Guillain-Barre Syndrome; and
- Treatment of last resort for life threatening systemic lupus erythematosus (SLE) when conventional therapy has failed to prevent clinical deterioration.

C. Settings

Apheresis is covered only when performed in a hospital setting (either inpatient or outpatient). or in a nonhospital setting. e.g. physician directed clinic when the following conditions are met:

- A physician (or a number of physicians) is present to perform medical services and to respond to medical emergencies at all times during patient care hours;
- Each patient is under the care of a physician; and
- All nonphysician services are furnished under the direct, personal supervision of a physician.

100-3, 110.15

Ultrafiltration, Hemoperfusion and Hemofiltration

A. Ultrafiltration.

This is a process for removing excess fluid from the blood through the dialysis membrane by means of pressure. It is not a substitute for dialysis. Ultrafiltration is utilized in cases where excess fluid cannot be removed easily during the regular course of hemodialysis. When it is performed, it is commonly done during the first hour or two of each hemodialysis on patients who, e.g., have refractory edema. Ultrafiltration is a covered procedure under the Medicare program (effective for services performed on and after 9/1/79).

Predialysis Ultrafiltration.--While this procedure requires additional staff care, the facility dialysis rate is intended to cover the full range of complicated and uncomplicated nonacute dialysis treatments. Therefore, no additional facility charge is recognized for predialysis ultrafiltration. The physician's role in ultrafiltration varies with the stability of the patient's condition. In unstable patients, the physician may need to be present at the initiation of dialysis, and available either in- house or in close proximity to monitor the patient carefully. In patients who are relatively stable, but who seem to accumulate excessive weight gain, the procedure requires only a modest increase in physician involvement over routine outpatient hemodialysis.

Occasionally, medical complications may occur which require that ultrafiltration be performed separate from the dialysis treatment, and in these cases an additional charge can be recognized. However, the claim must be documented as to why the ultrafiltration could not have been performed at the same time as the dialysis.

B. Hemoperfusion.

This is a process which removes substances from the blood using a charcoal or resin artificial kidney. When used in the treatment of life threatening drug overdose, hemoperfusion is a covered service for patients with or without renal failure (effective for services performed on and after 9/1/79). Hemoperfusion generally requires a physician to be present to initiate treatment and to be present in the hospital or an adjacent medical office during the entire procedure, as changes may be sudden. Special staff training and equipment are required.

Develop charges for hemoperfusion in the same manner as for any new or unusual service. One or two treatments are usually all that is necessary to remove the toxic compound; document additional treatments. Hemoperfusion may be performed concurrently with dialysis, and in those cases payment for the hemoperfusion reflects only the additional care rendered over and above the care given with dialysis.

The effects of using hemoperfusion to improve the results of chronic hemodialysis are not known. Therefore, hemoperfusion is not a covered service when used to improve the results of hemodialysis. In addition, it has not been demonstrated that the use of hemoperfusion in conjunction with deferoxamine (DFO), in treating symptomatic patients with iron overload, is efficacious. There is also a paucity of data regarding its efficacy in treating asymptomatic patients with iron overload. Therefore, hemoperfusion used in conjunction with DFO in treating patients with iron overload is not a covered service; i.e., it is not considered reasonable and necessary within the meaning of Sec.1862(a)(1) of the Act.

However, the use of hemoperfusion in conjunction with DFO for the treatment of patients with aluminum toxicity has been demonstrated to be clinically efficacious and is therefore regarded as a covered service.

C. Hemofiltration.

This is a process which removes fluid, electrolytes and other low molecular weight toxic substances from the blood by filtration through hollow artificial membranes and may be routinely performed in 3 weekly sessions. Hemofiltration (which is also known as diafiltration) is a covered procedure under Medicare and is a safe and effective technique for the treatment of ESRD patients and an alternative to peritoneal dialysis and hemodialysis (effective for services performed on and after August 20, 1987). In contrast to both hemodialysis and peritoneal dialysis treatments, which eliminate dissolved substances via diffusion across semipermeable membranes, hemofiltration mimics the filtration process of the normal kidney. The technique requires an arteriovenous access. Hemofiltration may be performed either in facility or at home.

The procedure is most advantageous when applied to high-risk unstable patients, such as older patients with cardiovascular diseases or diabetes, because there are fewer side effects such as hypotension, hypertension or volume overload.

100-3, 110.16

Nonselective (Random) Transfusions and Living Related Donor Specific Transfusions (DST) in Kidney Transplantation

These pretransplant transfusions are covered under Medicare without a specific limitation on the number of transfusions, subject to the normal Medicare blood deductible provisions. Where blood is given directly to the transplant patient; e.g., in the case of donor specific transfusions, the blood is considered replaced for purposes of the blood deductible provisions.

100-3, 130.1

Inpatient Hospital Stays for the Treatment of Alcoholism

A. Inpatient Hospital Stay for Alcohol Detoxification

Many hospitals provide detoxification services during the more acute stages of alcoholism or alcohol withdrawal. When the high probability or occurrence of medical complications (e.g., delirium, confusion, trauma, or unconsciousness) during detoxification for acute alcoholism or alcohol withdrawal necessitates the constant availability of physicians and/or complex medical equipment found only in the hospital setting, inpatient hospital care during this period is considered reasonable and necessary and is therefore covered under the program. Generally, detoxification can be accomplished within 2-3 days with an occasional need for up to 5 days where the patient's condition dictates. This limit (5 days) may be extended in an individual case where there is a need for a longer period for detoxification for a particular patient. In such cases, however, there should be documentation by a physician which substantiates that a longer period of detoxification was reasonable and necessary. When the detoxification needs of an individual no longer require an inpatient hospital setting, coverage should be denied on the basis that inpatient hospital care is not reasonable and necessary as required by section l862(a)(l) of the Act. Following detoxification a patient may be transferred to an inpatient rehabilitation unit or discharged to a residential treatment program or outpatient treatment setting.

B. Inpatient Hospital Stay for Alcohol Rehabilitation

Hospitals may also provide structured inpatient alcohol rehabilitation programs to the chronic alcoholic. These programs are composed primarily of coordinated educational and psychotherapeutic services provided on a group basis. Depending on the subject matter, a series of lectures, discussions, films, and group therapy sessions are led by either physicians, psychologists, or alcoholism counselors from the hospital or various outside organizations. In addition, individual psychotherapy and family counseling (see Sec.70.1 of the NCD Manual) may be provided in selected cases. These programs are conducted under the supervision and direction of a physician. Patients may directly enter an inpatient hospital rehabilitation program after having undergone detoxification in the same hospital or in another hospital or may enter an inpatient hospital rehabilitation program without prior hospitalization for detoxification.

Alcohol rehabilitation can be provided in a variety of settings other than the hospital setting. In order for an inpatient hospital stay for alcohol rehabilitation to be covered under Medicare it must be medically necessary for the care to be provided in the inpatient hospital setting rather than in a less costly facility or on an outpatient basis. Inpatient hospital care for receipt of an alcohol rehabilitation program would generally be medically necessary where either (l) there is documentation by the physician that recent alcohol rehabilitation services in a less intensive setting or on an outpatient basis have proven unsuccessful and, as a consequence, the patient requires the supervision and intensity of services which can only be found in the controlled environment of the hospital, or (2) only the hospital environment can assure the medical management or control of the patient's concomitant conditions during the course of alcohol rehabilitation. (However, a patient's concomitant condition may make the use of certain alcohol treatment modalities medically inappropriate.) In addition, the "active treatment" criteria (see the Medicare Benefit Policy Manual, Chapter 2, "Inpatient Psychiatric Hospital Services," Sec.20) should be applied to psychiatric care in the general hospital as well as to psychiatric care in a psychiatric hospital. Since alcoholism is classifiable as a psychiatric condition the "active treatment" criteria must also be met in order for alcohol rehabilitation services to be covered under Medicare. (Thus, it is the combined need for "active treatment" and for covered care which can only be provided in the inpatient hospital setting, rather than the fact that rehabilitation immediately follows a period of detoxification, which provides the basis for coverage of inpatient hospital alcohol rehabilitation programs.) Generally 16-19 days of rehabilitation services are sufficient to bring a patient to a point where care could be continued in other than an inpatient hospital setting. An inpatient hospital stay for alcohol rehabilitation may be extended beyond this limit in an individual case where a longer period of alcohol rehabilitation is medically necessary. In such cases, however, there should be documentation by a physician which substantiates the need for such care. Where the rehabilitation needs of an individual no longer require an inpatient hospital setting, coverage should be denied on the basis that inpatient hospital care is not reasonable and necessary as required by section l862(a)(l) of the Act.

Subsequent admissions to the inpatient hospital setting for alcohol rehabilitation followup, reinforcement, or "recap" treatments are considered to be readmissions (rather than an extension of the original stay) and must meet the requirements of this section for coverage under Medicare. Prior admissions to the inpatient hospital setting--either in the same hospital or in a different hospital--may be an indication that the "active treatment" requirements are not met (i.e., there is no reasonable expectation of improvement) and the stay should not be covered. Accordingly, there should be documentation to establish that "readmission" to the hospital setting for alcohol rehabilitation services can reasonably be expected to result in improvement of the patient's condition. For example, the documentation should indicate what changes in the patient's medical condition, social or emotional status, or treatment plan make improvement likely, or why the patient's initial hospital treatment was not sufficient.

C. Combined Alcohol Detoxification/Rehabilitation Programs.

iscal intermediaries should apply the guidelines in A. and B. above to both phases of a combined inpatient hospital alcohol detoxification/rehabilitation program. Not all patients who require the inpatient hospital setting for detoxification also need the inpatient hospital setting for rehabilitation. (See Sec.130.1 of the NCD Manual for coverage of outpatient hospital alcohol rehabilitation services.) Where the inpatient hospital setting is medically necessary for both alcohol detoxification and rehabilitation, generally a 3-week period is reasonable and necessary to bring the patient to the point where care can be continued in other than an inpatient hospital setting.

Decisions regarding reasonableness and necessity of treatment, the need for an inpatient hospital level of care, and length of treatment should be made by intermediaries based on accepted medical practice with the advice of their medical consultant. (In hospitals under PSRO review, PSRO determinations of medical necessity of services and appropriateness of the level of care at which services are provided are binding on the title XVIII fiscal intermediaries for purposes of adjudicating claims for payment.)

100-3, 130.2

Outpatient Hospital Services for Treatment of Alcoholism

Coverage is available for both diagnostic and therapeutic services furnished for the treatment of alcoholism by the hospital to outpatients subject to the same rules applicable to outpatient hospital services in general. While there is no coverage for day hospitalization programs, per se, individual services which meet the requirements in the Medicare Benefit Policy Manual, Chapter 6, Sec.20 may be covered. (Meals, transportation and recreational and social activities do not fall within the scope of covered outpatient hospital services under Medicare.)

All services must be reasonable and necessary for diagnosis or treatment of the patient's condition (see the Medicare Benefit Policy Manual, chapter 16 Sec.20). Thus, educational services and family counseling would only be covered where they are directly related to treatment of the patient's condition. The frequency of treatment and period of time over which it occurs must also be reasonable and necessary.

100-3, 130.3

Chemical Aversion Therapy for Treatment of Alcoholism

Available evidence indicates that chemical aversion therapy may be an effective component of certain alcoholism treatment programs, particularly as part of multimodality treatment programs which include other behavioral techniques and therapies, such as psychotherapy. Based on this evidence, CMS's medical consultants have recommended that chemical aversion therapy be covered under Medicare. However, since chemical aversion therapy is a demanding therapy which may not be appropriate for all Medicare beneficiaries needing treatment for alcoholism, a physician should certify to the appropriateness of chemical aversion therapy in the individual case. Therefore, if chemical aversion therapy for treatment of alcoholism is determined to be reasonable and necessary for an individual patient, it is covered under Medicare.

When it is medically necessary for a patient to receive chemical aversion therapy as a hospital inpatient, coverage for care in that setting is available. (See Sec.130.1 regarding coverage of multimodality treatment programs.) Followup treatments for chemical aversion therapy can generally be provided on an outpatient basis. Thus, where a patient is admitted as an inpatient for receipt of chemical aversion therapy, there must be documentation by the physician of the need in the individual case for the inpatient hospital admission.

Decisions regarding reasonableness and necessity of treatment and the need for an inpatient hospital level of care should be made by intermediaries based on accepted medical practice with the advice of their medical consultant. (In hospitals under QIO review, QIO determinations of medical necessity of services and appropriateness of the level of care at which services are provided are binding on the title XVIII fiscal intermediaries for purposes of adjudicating claims for payment.)

100-3, 130.5

Treatment of Alcoholism and Drug Abuse in a Freestanding Clinic

Coverage is available for alcoholism or drug abuse treatment services (such as drug therapy, psychotherapy, and patient education) that are provided incident to a physician's professional service in a freestanding clinic to patients who, for example, have been discharged from an inpatient hospital stay for the treatment of alcoholism or drug abuse or to individuals who are not in the acute stages of alcoholism or drug abuse but require treatment. The coverage available for these services is subject to the same rules generally applicable to the coverage of clinic services. Of course, the services also must be reasonable and necessary for the diagnosis or treatment of the individual's alcoholism or drug abuse. The Part B psychiatric limitation would apply to alcoholism or drug abuse treatment services furnished by physicians to individuals who are not hospital inpatients.

100-3, 130.6

Treatment of Drug Abuse (Chemical Dependency)

Accordingly, when it is medically necessary for a patient to receive detoxification and/or rehabilitation for drug substance abuse as a hospital inpatient, coverage for care in that setting is available. Coverage is also available for treatment services that are provided in the outpatient department of a hospital to patients who, for example, have been discharged from an inpatient stay for the treatment of drug substance abuse or who require treatment but do not require the availability and intensity of services found only in the inpatient hospital setting. The coverage available for these services is subject to the same rules generally applicable to the coverage of outpatient hospital services. The services must also be reasonable and necessary for treatment of the individual's condition. Decisions regarding reasonableness and necessity of treatment, the need for an inpatient hospital level of care, and length of treatment should be made by intermediaries based on accepted medical practice with the advice of their medical consultant. (In hospitals under QIO review, QIO determinations of medical necessity of services and appropriateness of the level of care at which services are provided are binding on the title XVIII fiscal intermediaries for purposes of adjudicating claims for payment.)

100-3, 130.7

Withdrawal Treatments for Narcotic Addictions

Withdrawal is an accepted treatment for narcotic addiction, and Part B payment can be made for these services if they are provided by the physician directly or under his personal supervision and if they are reasonable and necessary. In reviewing claims, reasonableness and necessity are determined with the aid of the contractor's medical staff.

Drugs that the physician provides in connection with this treatment are also covered if they cannot be self-administered and meet all other statutory requirements.

100-3, 130.8

Hemodialysis for Treatment of Schizophrenia

Scientific evidence supporting use of hemodialysis as a safe and effective means of treatment for schizophrenia is inconclusive at this time. Accordingly, Medicare does not cover hemodialysis for treatment of schizophrenia.

100-3, 140.1

Abortion

Abortions are not covered Medicare procedures except:

1. If the pregnancy is the result of an act of rape or incest; or
2. In the case where a woman suffers from a physical disorder, physical injury, or physical illness, including a life-endangering physical condition caused by or arising from the pregnancy itself, that would, as certified by a physician, place the woman in danger of death unless an abortion is performed.

100-3, 140.2

Breast Reconstruction Following Mastectomy

Reconstruction of the affected and the contralateral unaffected breast following a medically necessary mastectomy is considered a relatively safe and effective noncosmetic procedure. Accordingly, program payment may be made for breast reconstruction surgery following removal of a breast for any medical reason.

Program payment may not be made for breast reconstruction for cosmetic reasons. (Cosmetic surgery is excluded from coverage under Sec.l862(a)(l0) of the Social Security Act.)

100-3, 140.3

Transsexual Surgery

Transsexual surgery for sex reassignment of transsexuals is controversial. Because of the lack of well controlled, long term studies of the safety and effectiveness of the surgical procedures and attendant therapies for transsexualism, the treatment is considered experimental. Moreover, there is a high rate of serious complications for these surgical procedures. For these reasons, transsexual surgery is not covered.

100-3, 140.4

Plastic Surgery to Correct "Moon Face"

The cosmetic surgery exclusion precludes payment for any surgical procedure directed at improving appearance. The condition giving rise to the patient's preoperative appearance is generally not a consideration. The only exception to the exclusion is surgery for the prompt repair of an accidental injury or for the improvement of a malformed body member which coincidentally serves some cosmetic purpose. Since surgery to correct a condition of "moon face" which developed as a side effect of cortisone therapy does not meet the exception to the exclusion, it is not covered under Medicare (Sec.1862(a)(10) of the Act).

100-3, 140.5

Laser Procedures

Medicare recognizes the use of lasers for many medical indications. Procedures performed with lasers are sometimes used in place of more conventional techniques. In the absence of a specific noncoverage instruction, and where a laser has been approved for marketing by the Food and Drug Administration, contractor discretion may be used to determine whether a procedure performed with a laser is reasonable and necessary and, therefore, covered.

The determination of coverage for a procedure performed using a laser is made on the basis that the use of lasers to alter, revise, or destroy tissue is a surgical procedure. Therefore, coverage of laser procedures is restricted to practitioners with training in the surgical management of the disease or condition being treated.

100-3, 150.1

Manipulation

A. Manipulation of the Rib Cage.

Manual manipulation of the rib cage contributes to the treatment of respiratory conditions such as bronchitis, emphysema, and asthma as part of a regimen which includes other elements of therapy, and is covered only under such circumstances.

B. Manipulation of the Head.
Manipulation of the occipitocervical or temporomandibular regions of the head when indicated for conditions affecting those portions of the head and neck is a covered service.

100-3, 150.2

Osteogenic Stimulators

Electrical Osteogenic Stimulators

B. Nationally Covered Indications

1. Noninvasive Stimulator.

   The noninvasive stimulator device is covered only for the following indications:

   - Nonunion of long bone fractures;
   - Failed fusion, where a minimum of nine months has elapsed since the last surgery;
   - Congenital pseudarthroses; and
   - Effective July 1, 1996, as an adjunct to spinal fusion surgery for patients at high risk of pseudarthrosis due to previously failed spinal fusion at the same site or for those undergoing multiple level fusion. A multiple level fusion involves 3 or more vertebrae (e.g., L3-L5, L4-S1, etc).
   - Effective September 15, 1980, nonunion of long bone fractures is considered to exist only after 6 or more months have elapsed without healing of the fracture.
   - Effective April 1, 2000, nonunion of long bone fractures is considered to exist only when serial radiographs have confirmed that fracture healing has ceased for 3 or more months prior to starting treatment with the electrical osteogenic stimulator. Serial radiographs must include a minimum of 2 sets of radiographs, each including multiple views of the fracture site, separated by a minimum of 90 days.

2. Invasive (Implantable) Stimulator.

   The invasive stimulator device is covered only for the following indications:

   - Nonunion of long bone fractures
   - Effective July 1, 1996, as an adjunct to spinal fusion surgery for patients at high risk of pseudarthrosis due to previously failsed spinal fusion at the same site or for those undergoing multiple level fusion. A multiple level fusion involves 3 or more vertebrae (e.g., L3-5, L4-S1, etc.)
   - Effective September 15, 1980, nonunion of long bone fractures is considered to exist only after 6 or more months have elapsed without healing of the fracture.
   - Effective April 1, 2000, non union of long bone fractures is considered to exist only when serial radiographs have confirmed that fracture healing has ceased for 3 or more months prior to starting treatment with the electrical osteogenic stimulator. Serial radiographs must include a minimum of 2 sets of radiographs, each including multiple views of the fracture site, separated by a minimum of 90 days.
   - Effective for services performed on or after January 1, 2001, ultrasonic osteogenic stimulators are covered as medically reasonable and necessary for the treatment of non-union fractures. In demonstrating nonunion of fractures, we would expect:
   - A minimum of two sets of radiographs obtained prior to starting treatment with the osteogenic stimulator, separated by a minimum of 90 days. Each radiograph must include multiple views of the fracture site accompanied with a written interpretation by a physician stating that there has been no clinically significant evidence of fracture healing between the two sets of radiographs.
   - Indications that the patient failed at least one surgical intervention for the treatment of the fracture.
   - Effective April 27, 2005, upon the recommendation of the ultrasound stimulation for nonunion fracture healing, CMS determins that the evidence is adequate to condlude that noninvasive ultrasound stimulation for the treatment of nonunion bone fractures prior to surfical intervention is reasonable and necessary. In demonstrating non-union fracturs, CMS expects:
   - A minimum of 2 sets of radiographs, obtained prior to starting treating with the osteogenic stimulator, separated by a minimum of 90 days. Each radiograph set must include multiple views of the fracture site accompanied with a written interpretation by a physician stating that there has been no clinically significant evidence of fracture healing between the 2 sets of radiographs.

C. Nationally Non-Covered Indications

Nonunion fractures of the skull, vertebrae and those that are tumor-related are excluded from coverage.

Ultrasonic osteogenic stimulators may not be used concurrently with other non-invasive osteogenic devices.

Ultrasonic osteogenic stimulators for fresh fracturs and delayed unions remain non-covered.

(This NCD last reviewed June 2005)

100-3, 150.3

Bone (Mineral) Density Studies

Conditions for coverage of bone mass measurements are now contained in chapter 15, section 80.5 of Pub. 100-02, Medicare Benefit Policy Manual . Claims processing instructions can be found in chapter 13, section 140 of Pub. 100-04, Medicare Claims Processing Manual.

100-3, 150.5

Diathermy Treatment

High energy pulsed wave diathermy machines have been found to produce some degree of therapeutic benefit for essentially the same conditions and to the same extent as standard diathermy. Accordingly, where the contractor's medical staff has determined that the pulsed wave diathermy apparatus used is one which is considered therapeutically effective, the treatments are considered a covered service, but only for those conditions for which standard diathermy is medically indicated and only when rendered by a physician or incident to a physician's professional services.

Cross-reference: §240.3.

100-3, 150.6

Vitamin B12 Injections to Strengthen Tendons, Ligaments, etc., of the Foot

Vitamin B12 injections to strengthen tendons, ligaments, etc., of the foot are not covered under Medicare because (1) there is no evidence that vitamin B12 injections are effective for the purpose of strengthening weakened tendons and ligaments, and (2) this is nonsurgical treatment under the subluxation exclusion. Accordingly, vitamin B12 injections are not considered reasonable and necessary within the meaning of Sec.1862(a)(1) of the Act.

100-3, 150.7

Prolotherapy, Joint Sclerotherapy, and Ligamentous Injections with Sclerosing Agents

The medical effectiveness of the above therapies has not been verified by scientifically controlled studies. Accordingly, reimbursement for these modalities should be denied on the ground that they are not reasonable and necessary as required by Sec.1862(a)(1) of the Act.

100-3, 150.10

Lumbar Artificial Disc Replacement (LADR)

B. Nationally Covered Indications

N/A

C. Nationally Non-Covered Indications

Effective for services performed from May 16, 2006 through August 13, 2007, the Centers for Medicare and Medicaid Services (CMS) has found that LADR with the Charite TM lumbar artificial disc is not reasonable and necessary for the Medicare population over 60 years of age; therefore, LADR with the Charite TM lumbar artificial disc is non-covered for Medicare beneficiaries over 60 years of age.

Effective for services performed on or after August 14, 2007, CMS has found that LADR is not reasonable and necessary for the Medicare population over 60 years of age; therefore, LADR is non-covered for Medicare beneficiaries over 60 years of age.

D. Other

For Medicare beneficiaries 60 years of age and younger, there is no national coverage determination for LADR, leaving such determinations to continue to be made by the local contractors.

For dates of service May 16, 2006 through August 13, 2007, Medicare coverage under the investigational device exemption (IDE) for LADR with a disc other than the Charite TM lumbar disc in eligible clinical trials is not impacted.

(This NCD last reviewed August 2007.)

100-3, 150.11

Thermal Intradiscal Procedures

A. General

Percutaneous thermal intradiscal procedures (TIPs) involve the insertion of a catheter(s)/probe(s) in the spinal disc under fluoroscopic guidance for the purpose of producing or applying heat and/or disruption within the disc to relieve low back pain.

The scope of this national coverage determination on TIPs includes percutaneous intradiscal techniques that employ the use of a radiofrequency energy source or electrothermal energy to apply or create heat and/or disruption within the disc for coagulation and/or decompression of disc material to treat symptomatic patients with annular disruption of a contained herniated disc, to seal annular tears or fissures, or destroy nociceptors for the purpose of relieving pain. This includes techniques that use single or multiple probe(s)/catheter(s), which utilize a resistance coil or other delivery system technology, are flexible or rigid, and are placed within the nucleus, the nuclear-annular junction, or the annulus. Although not intended to be an all inclusive list, TIPs are commonly identified as intradiscal electrothermal therapy

(IDET), intradiscal thermal annuloplasty (IDTA), percutaneous intradiscal radiofrequency thermocoagulation (PIRFT), radiofrequency annuloplasty (RA), intradiscal biacuplasty (IDB), percutaneous (or plasma) disc decompression (PDD) or coblation, or targeted disc decompression (TDD). At times, TIPs are identified or labeled based on the name of the catheter/probe that is used (e.g., SpineCath, discTRODE, SpineWand, Accutherm, or TransDiscal electrodes). Each technique or device has it own protocol for application of the therapy. Percutaneous disc decompression or nucleoplasty procedures that do not utilize a radiofrequency energy source or electrothermal energy (such as the disc decompressor procedure or laser procedure) are not within the scope of this NCD.

B. Nationally Covered Indications

N/A

C. Nationally Non-Covered Indications

Effective for services performed on or after September 29, 2008, the Centers for Medicare and Medicaid Services has determined that TIPs are not reasonable and necessary for the treatment of low back pain. Therefore, TIPs, which include procedures that employ the use of a radiofrequency energy source or electrothermal energy to apply or create heat and/or disruption within the disc for the treatment of low back pain, are noncovered.

D. Other

N/A

(This NCD last reviewed September 2008.)

100-3, 150.12

Collagen Meniscus Implant (Effective May 25, 2010)

A. General

The knee menisci are wedge-shaped, semi-lunar discs of fibrous tissue located in the knee joint between the ends of the femur and the tibia and fibula. There is a lateral and medial meniscus in each knee. It is known now that the menisci provide mechanical support, localized pressure distribution, and lubrication of the knee joint. Initially, meniscal tears were treated with total meniscectomy; however, as knowledge of the function of the menisci and the potential long term effects of total meniscectomy on the knee joint evolved, treatment of symptomatic meniscal tears gravitated to repair of the tear, when possible, or partial meniscectomy.

The collagen meniscus implant (also referred to as collagen scaffold (CS), CMI or MenaflexTM meniscus implant throughout the published literature) is used to fill meniscal defects that result from partial meniscectomy. The collagen meniscus implant is not intended to replace the entire meniscus at it requires a meniscal rim for attachment. The literature describes the placement of the collagen meniscus implant through an arthroscopic procedure with an additional incision for capture of the repair needles and tying of the sutures. After debridement of the damaged meniscus, the implant is trimmed to the size of meniscal defect and sutured into place. The collagen meniscus implant is described as a tissue engineered scaffold to support the generation of new meniscus-like tissue. The collagen meniscus implant is manufactured from bovine collagen and should not be confused with the meniscus transplant which involves the replacement of the meniscus with a transplant meniscus from a cadaver donor. The meniscus transplant is not addressed under this national coverage determination.

B. Nationally Covered Indications

N/A

C. Nationally Non-Covered Indications

Effective for claims with dates of service performed on or after May 25, 2010, the Centers for Medicare & Medicaid Services has determined that the evidence is adequate to conclude that the collagen meniscus implant does not improve health outcomes and, therefore, is not reasonable and necessary for the treatment of meniscal injury/tear under section 1862(a)(1)(A) of the Social Security Act. Thus, the collagen meniscus implant is non-covered by Medicare.

D. Other

N/A

(This NCD last reviewed May 2010.)

100-3, 150.13

Percutaneous Image-guided Lumbar Decompression (PILD) for Lumbar Spinal Stenosis (LSS) (Effective January 09, 2014)

A. General

PILD is a posterior decompression of the lumbar spine performed under indirect image guidance without any direct visualization of the surgical area. This is a procedure proposed as a treatment for symptomatic LSS unresponsive to conservative therapy. This procedure is generally described as a non-invasive procedure using specially designed instruments to percutaneously remove a portion of the lamina and debulk the ligamentum flavum. The procedure is performed under x-ray guidance (e.g., fluoroscopic, CT) with the assistance of contrast media to identify and monitor the compressed area via epiduragram.

B. Nationally Covered Indications

Effective for services performed on or after January 09, 2014, the Centers for Medicare & Medicaid Services (CMS) has determined that PILD will be covered by Medicare when provided in a clinical study under section 1862(a)(1)(E) through Coverage with Evidence Development (CED) for beneficiaries with LSS who are enrolled in an approved clinical study that meets the criteria below.

CMS has a particular interest in improved beneficiary function and quality of life, specific characteristics that identify patients who may benefit from the procedure, and the duration of benefit. A clinical study seeking Medicare payment for PILD for LSS must address one or more aspects of the following questions in a prospective, randomized, controlled design using current validated and reliable measurement instruments and clinically appropriate comparator treatments, including appropriate medical or surgical interventions or a sham controlled arm, for patients randomized to the non-PILD group.

The study protocol must specify a statistical analysis and a minimum length of patient follow up time that evaluates the effect of beneficiary characteristics on patient health outcomes as well as the duration of benefit.

i. Does PILD provide a clinically meaningful improvement of function and/or quality of life in Medicare beneficiaries with LSS compared to other treatments?

ii. Does PILD provide clinically meaningful reduction in pain in Medicare beneficiaries with LSS compared to other treatments?

iii. Does PILD affect the overall clinical management of LSS and decision making, including use of other medical treatments or services, compared to other treatments?

These studies must be designed so that the contribution of treatments in addition to the procedure under study are either controlled for or analyzed in such a way as to determine their impact.

a. The principal purpose of the research study is to test whether a particular intervention potentially improves the participants?health outcomes.

b. The research study is well supported by available scientific and medical information or it is intended to clarify or establish the health outcomes of interventions already in common clinical use.

c. The research study does not unjustifiably duplicate existing studies.

d. The research study design is appropriate to answer the research question being asked in the study.

e. The research study is sponsored by an organization or individual capable of executing the proposed study successfully.

f. The research study is in compliance with all applicable Federal regulations concerning the protection of human subjects found at 45 CFR Part 46. If a study is regulated by the Food and Drug Administration (FDA), it must be in compliance with 21 CFR parts 50 and 56.

g. All aspects of the research study are conducted according to appropriate standards of scientific integrity (see http://www.icmje.org).

h. The research study has a written protocol that clearly addresses, or incorporates by reference, the standards listed here as Medicare requirements for CED coverage.

i. The clinical research study is not designed to exclusively test toxicity or disease pathophysiology in healthy individuals. Trials of all medical technologies measuring therapeutic outcomes as one of the objectives meet this standard only if the disease or condition being studied is life threatening as defined in 21 CFR § 312.81(a) and the patient has no other viable treatment options.

j. The clinical research study is registered on the ClinicalTrials.gov website by the principal sponsor/investigator prior to the enrollment of the first study subject.

k. The research study protocol specifies the method and timing of public release of all prespecified outcomes to be measured including release of outcomes if outcomes are negative or study is terminated early. The results must be made public within 24 months of the end of data collection. If a report is planned to be published in a peer reviewed journal, then that initial release may be an abstract that meets the requirements of the International Committee of Medical Journal Editors (http://www.icmje.org).

l. The research study protocol must explicitly discuss subpopulations affected by the treatment under investigation, particularly traditionally underrepresented groups in clinical studies, how the inclusion and exclusion criteria effect enrollment of these populations, and a plan for the retention and reporting of said populations on the trial. If the inclusion and exclusion criteria are expected to have a negative effect on the recruitment or retention of underrepresented populations, the protocol must discuss why these criteria are necessary.

m. The research study protocol explicitly discusses how the results are or are not expected to be generalizable to the Medicare population to infer whether Medicare patients may benefit from the intervention. Separate discussions in the protocol may be necessary for populations eligible for Medicare due to age, disability or Medicaid eligibility.

Consistent with section 1142 of the Social Security Act, the Agency for Healthcare Research and Quality (AHRQ) supports clinical research studies that CMS determines meet the above-listed standards and address the above-listed research questions.

C. Nationally Non-Covered Indications
Effective for services performed on or after January 09, 2014, CMS has determined that PILD for LSS is not reasonable and necessary under section 1862(a)(1)(A) of the Social Security Act.

D. Other
Endoscopically assisted laminotomy/laminectomy, which requires open and direct visualization, as well as other open lumbar decompression procedures for LSS are not within the scope of this NCD.

100-3, 160.1

Induced Lesions of Nerve Tracts

Accordingly, program payment may be made for these denervation procedures when used in selected cases (concurred in by contractor's medical staff) to treat chronic pain.

100-3, 160.2

Treatment of Motor Function Disorders with Electric Nerve Stimulation

Where electric nerve stimulation is employed to treat motor function disorders, no reimbursement may be made for the stimulator or for the services related to its implantation since this treatment cannot be considered reasonable and necessary.

NOTE: For Medicare coverage of deep brain stimulation for essential tremor and Parkinson's disease, see Sec.160.24 of the NCD Manual.

100-3, 160.4

Stereotactic Cingulotomy as a Means of Psychosurgery

Stereotactic cingulotomy is not covered under Medicare because the procedure is considered to be investigational.

100-3, 160.5

Stereotaxic Depth Electrode Implantation

Stereotaxic depth electrode implantation prior to surgical treatment of focal epilepsy for patients who are unresponsive to anticonvulsant medications has been found both safe and effective for diagnosing resectable seizure foci that may go undetected by conventional scalp electroencephalographs (EEGs).

100-3, 160.6

Carotid Sinus Nerve Stimulator

Implantation of the carotid sinus nerve stimulator is indicated for relief of angina pectoris in carefully selected patients who are refractory to medical therapy and who after undergoing coronary angiography study either are poor candidates for or refuse to have coronary bypass surgery. In such cases, Medicare reimbursement may be made for this device and for the related services required for its implantation.

However, the use of the carotid sinus nerve stimulator in the treatment of paroxysmal supraventricular tachycardia is considered investigational and is not in common use by the medical community. The device and related services in such cases cannot be considered as reasonable and necessary for the treatment of an illness or injury or to improve the functioning of a malformed body member as required by Sec.1862(a)(1) of the Act.

100-3, 160.7

Electrical Nerve Stimulators

Two general classifications of electrical nerve stimulators are employed to treat chronic intractable pain: peripheral nerve stimulators and central nervous system stimulators.

A. Implanted Peripheral Nerve Stimulators
Payment may be made under the prosthetic device benefit for implanted peripheral nerve stimulators. Use of this stimulator involves implantation of electrodes around a selected peripheral nerve. The stimulating electrode is connected by an insulated lead to a receiver unit which is implanted under the skin at a depth not greater than 1/2 inch. Stimulation is induced by a generator connected to an antenna unit which is attached to the skin surface over the receiver unit. Implantation of electrodes requires surgery and usually necessitates an operating room.

NOTE: Peripheral nerve stimulators may also be employed to assess a patient's suitability for continued treatment with an electric nerve stimulator. As explained in Sec.160.7.1, such use of the stimulator is covered as part of the total diagnostic service furnished to the beneficiary rather than as a prosthesis.

B. Central Nervous System Stimulators (Dorsal Column and Depth Brain Stimulators)
The implantation of central nervous system stimulators may be covered as therapies for the relief of chronic intractable pain, subject to the following conditions:

1. Types of Implantations

   There are two types of implantations covered by this instruction:

   Dorsal Column (Spinal Cord) Neurostimulation - The surgical implantation of neurostimulator electrodes within the dura mater (endodural) or the percutaneous insertion of electrodes in the epidural space is covered.

   Depth Brain Neurostimulation - The stereotactic implantation of electrodes in the deep brain (e.g., thalamus and periaqueductal gray matter) is covered.

2. Conditions for Coverage

   No payment may be made for the implantation of dorsal column or depth brain stimulators or services and supplies related to such implantation, unless all of the conditions listed below have been met:

   The implantation of the stimulator is used only as a late resort (if not a last resort) for patients with chronic intractable pain;

   With respect to item a, other treatment modalities (pharmacological, surgical, physical, or psychological therapies) have been tried and did not prove satisfactory, or are judged to be unsuitable or contraindicated for the given patient;

   Patients have undergone careful screening, evaluation and diagnosis by a multidisciplinary team prior to implantation. (Such screening must include psychological, as well as physical evaluation);

   All the facilities, equipment, and professional and support personnel required for the proper diagnosis, treatment training, and followup of the patient (including that required to satisfy item c) must be available; and

   Demonstration of pain relief with a temporarily implanted electrode precedes permanent implantation.

   Contractors may find it helpful to work with QIOs to obtain the information needed to apply these conditions to claims.

100-3, 160.7.1

Assessing Patient's Suitability for Electrical Nerve Stimulation Therapy

Indications and Limitations of Coverage

CIM 35-46

Electrical nerve stimulation is an accepted modality for assessing a patient's suitability for ongoing treatment with a transcutaneous or an implanted nerve stimulator.

Accordingly, program payment may be made for the following techniques when used to determine the potential therapeutic usefulness of an electrical nerve stimulator:

A. Transcutaneous Electrical Nerve Stimulation (TENS)
This technique involves attachment of a transcutaneous nerve stimulator to the surface of the skin over the peripheral nerve to be stimulated. It is used by the patient on a trial basis and its effectiveness in modulating pain is monitored by the physician, or physical therapist. Generally, the physician or physical therapist is able to determine whether the patient is likely to derive a significant therapeutic benefit from continuous use of a transcutaneous stimulator within a trial period of 1 month; in a few cases this determination may take longer to make. Document the medical necessity for such services which are furnished beyond the first month. (See Sec.160.13 for an explanation of coverage of medically necessary supplies for the effective use of TENS.)

If TENS significantly alleviates pain, it may be considered as primary treatment; if it produces no relief or greater discomfort than the original pain electrical nerve stimulation therapy is ruled out. However, where TENS produces incomplete relief, further evaluation with percutaneous electrical nerve stimulation may be considered to determine whether an implanted peripheral nerve stimulator would provide significant relief from pain.

Usually, the physician or physical therapist providing the services will furnish the equipment necessary for assessment. Where the physician or physical therapist advises the patient to rent the TENS from a supplier during the trial period rather than supplying it himself/herself, program payment may be made for rental of the TENS as well as for the services of the physician or physical therapist who is evaluating its use. However, the combined program payment which is made for the physician's or physical therapist's services and the rental of the stimulator from a supplier should not exceed the amount which would be payable for the total service, including the stimulator, furnished by the physician or physical therapist alone.

B. Percutaneous Electrical Nerve Stimulation (PENS)
This diagnostic procedure which involves stimulation of peripheral nerves by a needle electrode inserted through the skin is performed only in a physician's office, clinic, or hospital outpatient department. Therefore, it is covered only when performed by a physician or incident to physician's service. If pain is effectively controlled by percutaneous stimulation, implantation of electrodes is warranted.

As in the case of TENS (described in subsection A), generally the physician should be able to determine whether the patient is likely to derive a significant therapeutic benefit from continuing use of an implanted nerve stimulator within a trial period of 1 month. In a few cases, this determination may take longer to make. The medical necessity for such diagnostic services which are furnished beyond the first month must be documented.

NOTE: Electrical nerve stimulators do not prevent pain but only alleviate pain as it occurs. A patient can be taught how to employ the stimulator, and once this is done, can use it safely and effectively without direct physician supervision. Consequently, it is inappropriate for a patient to visit his/her physician, physical therapist, or an outpatient clinic on a continuing basis for treatment of pain with electrical nerve stimulation. Once it is determined that electrical nerve stimulation should be continued as therapy and the patient has been trained to use the stimulator, it is expected that a stimulator will be implanted or the patient will employ the TENS on a continual basis in his/her home. Electrical nerve stimulation treatments furnished by a physician in his/her office, by a physical therapist or outpatient clinic are excluded from coverage by Sec.1862(a)(1) of the Act. (See Sec.160.7 for an explanation of coverage of the therapeutic use of implanted peripheral nerve stimulators under the prosthetic devices benefit. See Sec.280.13 for an explanation of coverage of the therapeutic use of TENS under the durable medical equipment benefit.)

100-3, 160.8

Electroencephalographic (EEG) Monitoring During Surgical Procedures Involving the Cerebral Vasculature

CIM 35-57

Electroencephalographic (EEG) monitoring is a safe and reliable technique for the assessment of gross cerebral blood flow during general anesthesia and is covered under Medicare. Very characteristic changes in the EEG occur when cerebral perfusion is inadequate for ce rebral function. EEG monitoring as an indirect measure of cerebral perfusion requires the expertise of an electroencephalographer, a neurologist trained in EEG, or an advanced EEG technician for its proper interpretation.

The EEG monitoring may be covered routinely in carotid endarterectomies and in other neurological procedures where cerebral perfusion could be reduced. Such other procedures might include aneurysm surgery where hypotensive anesthesia is used or other cerebral vascular procedures where cerebral blood flow may be interrupted.

100-3, 160.9

Electronecephalographic (EEG) Monitoring during Open-Heart Surgery

The value of EEG monitoring during open heart surgery and in the immediate post-operative period is debatable because there are little published data based on well designed studies regarding its clinical effectiveness. The procedure is not frequently used and does not enjoy widespread acceptance of benefit.

Accordingly, Medicare does not cover EEG monitoring during open heart surgery and during the immediate post-operative period.

100-3, 160.10

Evoked Response Tests

Evoked response tests, including brain stem evoked response and visual evoked response tests, are generally accepted as safe and effective diagnostic tools. Program payment may be made for these procedures.

100-3, 160.12

Neuromuscular Electrical Stimulaton (NMES)

Indications and Limitations of Coverage

Treatment of Muscle Atrophy

Coverage of NMES to treat muscle atrophy is limited to the treatment of disuse atrophy where nerve supply to the muscle is intact, including brain, spinal cord and peripheral nerves, and other non-neurological reasons for disuse atrophy. Some examples would be casting or splinting of a limb, contracture due to scarring of soft tissue as in burn lesions, and hip replacement surgery (until orthotic training begins). (See Sec.160.13 of the NCD Manual for an explanation of coverage of medically necessary supplies for the effective use of NMES.)

Use for Walking in Patients with Spinal Cord Injury (SCI)

The type of NMES that is use to enhance the ability to walk of SCI patients is commonly referred to as functional electrical stimulation (FES). These devices are surface units that use electrical impulses to activate paralyzed or weak muscles in precise sequence. Coverage for the use of NMES/FES is limited to SCI patients for walking, who have completed a training program which consists of at least 32 physical therapy sessions with the device over a period of three months. The trial period of physical therapy will enable the physician treating the patient for his or her spinal cord injury to properly evaluate the person's ability to use these devices frequently and for the long term. Physical therapy necessary to perform this training must be directly performed by the physical therapist as part of a one-on-one training program.

The goal of physical therapy must be to train SCI patients on the use of NMES/FES devices to achieve walking, not to reverse or retard muscle atrophy.

Coverage for NMES/FES for walking will be covered in SCI patients with all of the following characteristics:

- Persons with intact lower motor unite (L1 and below) (both muscle and peripheral nerve);
- Persons with muscle and joint stability for weight bearing at upper and lower extremities that can demonstrate balance and control to maintain an upright support posture independently;
- Persons that demonstrate brisk muscle contraction to NMES and have sensory perception electrical stimulation sufficient for muscle contraction;
- Persons that possess high motivation, commitment and cognitive ability to use such devices for walking;
- Persons that can transfer independently and can demonstrate independent standing tolerance for at least 3 minutes;
- Persons that can demonstrate hand and finger function to manipulate controls;
- Persons with at least 6-month post recovery spinal cord injury and restorative surgery;
- Persons with hip and knee degenerative disease and no history of long bone fracture secondary to osteoporosis; and
- Persons who have demonstrated a willingness to use the device long-term.

NMES/FES for walking will not be covered in SCI patient with any of the following:

- Persons with cardiac pacemakers;
- Severe scoliosis or severe osteoporosis;
- Skin disease or cancer at area of stimulation;
- Irreversible contracture; or
- Autonomic dysflexia.

The only settings where therapists with the sufficient skills to provide these services are employed, are inpatient hospitals; outpatient hospitals; comprehensive outpatient rehabilitation facilities; and outpatient rehabilitation facilities. The physical therapy necessary to perform this training must be part of a one-on-one training program.

Additional therapy after the purchase of the DME would be limited by our general policies in converge of skilled physical therapy.

100-3, 160.13

Supplies Used in the Delivery of Transcutaneous Electrical Nerve Stimulation (TENS) and Neuromuscular Electrical Stimulation (NMES)

A form-fitting conductive garment (and medically necessary related supplies) may be covered under the program only when:

1. It has received permission or approval for marketing by the Food and Drug Administration;
2. It has been prescribed by a physician for use in delivering covered TENS or NMES treatment; and
3. One of the medical indications outlined below is met:
    - The patient cannot manage without the conductive garment because there is such a large area or so many sites to be stimulated and the stimulation would have to be delivered so frequently that it is not feasible to use conventional electrodes, adhesive tapes and lead wires;
    - The patient cannot manage without the conductive garment for the treatment of chronic intractable pain because the areas or sites to be stimulated are inaccessible with the use of conventional electrodes, adhesive tapes and lead wires;
    - The patient has a documented medical condition such as skin problems that preclude the application of conventional electrodes, adhesive tapes and lead wires;
    - The patient requires electrical stimulation beneath a cast either to treat disuse atrophy, where the nerve supply to the muscle is intact, or to treat chronic intractable pain; or
    - The patient has a medical need for rehabilitation strengthening (pursuant to a written plan of rehabilitation) following an injury where the nerve supply to the muscle is intact.

    A conductive garment is not covered for use with a TENS device during the trial period specified in Sec.160.3 unless:

    - The patient has a documented skin problem prior to the start of the trial period; and
    - The carrier's medical consultants are satisfied that use of such an item is medically necessary for the patient.

100-3, 160.15

Electrotherapy for Treatment of Facial Nerve Paralysis (Bell's Palsy)

Electrotherapy for the treatment of facial nerve paralysis, commonly known as Bell's Palsy, is not covered under Medicare because its clinical effectiveness has not been established.

100-3, 160.17

L-DOPA

A. Part A Payment for L-Dopa and Associated Inpatient Hospital Services

A hospital stay and related ancillary services for the administration of L-Dopa are covered if medically required for this purpose. Whether a drug represents an allowable inpatient hospital cost during such stay depends on whether it meets the definition of a drug in Sec.1861(t) of the Act; i.e., on its inclusion in the compendia named in the Act or approval by the hospital's pharmacy and drug therapeutics (P&DT) or equivalent committee. (Levodopa (L-Dopa) has been favorably evaluated for the treatment of Parkinsonism by A.M.A. Drug Evaluations, First Edition 1971, the replacement compendia for "New Drugs.")

Inpatient hospital services are frequently not required in many cases when L-Dopa therapy is initiated. Therefore, determine the medical need for inpatient hospital services on the basis of medical facts in the individual case. It is not necessary to hospitalize the typical, well-functioning, ambulatory Parkinsonian patient who has no concurrent disease at the start of L-Dopa treatment. It is reasonable to provide inpatient hospital services for Parkinsonian patients with concurrent diseases, particularly of the cardiovascular, gastrointestinal, and neuropsychiatric systems. Although many patients require hospitalization for a period of under 2 weeks, a 4-week period of inpatient care is not unreasonable.

Laboratory tests in connection with the administration of L-Dopa - The tests medically warranted in connection with the achievement of optimal dosage and the control of the side effects of L-Dopa include a complete blood count, liver function tests such as SGOT, SGPT, and/or alkaline phosphatase, BUN or creatinine and urinalysis, blood sugar, and electrocardiogram.

Whether or not the patient is hospitalized, laboratory tests in certain cases are reasonable at weekly intervals although some physicians prefer to perform the tests much less frequently.

Physical therapy furnished in connection with administration of L-Dopa - Where, following administration of the drug, the patient experiences a reduction of rigidity which permits the reestablishment of a restorative goal for him/her, physical therapy services required to enable him/her to achieve this goal are payable provided they require the skills of a qualified physical therapist and are furnished by or under the supervision of such a therapist. However, once the individual's restoration potential has been achieved, the services required to maintain him/her at this level do not generally require the skills of a qualified physical therapist. In such situations, the role of the therapist is to evaluate the patient's needs in consultation with his/her physician and design a program of exercise appropriate to the capacity and tolerance of the patient and treatment objectives of the physician, leaving to others the actual carrying out of the program. While the evaluative services rendered by a qualified physical therapist are payable as physical therapy, services furnished by others in connection with the carrying out of the maintenance program established by the therapist are not.

B. Part A Reimbursement for L-Dopa Therapy in SNFs

Initiation of L-Dopa therapy can be appropriately carried out in the SNF setting, applying the same guidelines used for initiation of L-Dopa therapy in the hospital, including the types of patients who should be covered for inpatient services, the role of physical therapy, and the use of laboratory tests. (See subsection A.)

Where inpatient care is required and L-Dopa therapy is initiated in the SNF, limit the stay to a maximum of 4 weeks; but in many cases the need may be no longer than 1 or 2 weeks, depending upon the patient's condition. However, where L-Dopa therapy is begun in the hospital and the patient is transferred to an SNF for continuation of the therapy, a combined length of stay in hospital and SNF of no longer than 4 weeks is reasonable (i.e., 1 week hospital stay followed by 3 weeks SNF stay; or 2 weeks hospital stay followed by 2 weeks SNF stay; etc.). Medical need must be demonstrated in cases where the combined length of stay in hospital and SNF is longer than 4 weeks. The choice of hospital or SNF, and the decision regarding the relative length of time spent in each, should be left to the medical judgment of the treating physician.

C. L-Dopa Coverage Under Part B

Part B reimbursement may not be made for the drug L-Dopa since it is a self-administrable drug. However, physician services rendered in connection with its administration and control of its side effects are covered if determined to be reasonable and necessary. Initiation of L-Dopa therapy on an outpatient basis is possible in most cases. Visit frequency ranging from every week to every 2 or 3 months is acceptable. However, after half a year of therapy, visits more frequent than every month would usually not be reasonable.

100-3, 160.18

Vagus Nerve Stimulation for Treatment of Seizures

B. Nationally Covered Indications

Effective for services performed on or after July 1, 1999, VNS is reasonable and necessary for patients with medically refractory partial onset seizures for whom surgery is not recommended or for whom surgery has failed.

C. Nationally Non-Covered Indications

Effective for services performed on or after July 1, 1999, VNS is not reasonable and necessary for all other types of seizure disorders which are medically refractory and for whom surgery is not recommended or for whom surgery has failed.

Effective for services performed on or after May 4, 2007, VNS is not reasonable and necessary for resistant depression. (Information on the national coverage analysis leading to this determination can be found at: http://www.cms.hhs.gov/mcd/viewnca.asp?where= index&nca_id= 195.)

D. Other

Also see Sec.160, "Electrical Nerve Stimulators."

(This NCD last reviewed May 2007.)

100-3, 160.20

Transfer Factor for Treatment of Multiple Sclerosis

Transfer factor is the dialysate of an extract from sensitized leukocytes which increases cellular immune activity in the recipient. It is not covered as a treatment for multiple sclerosis because its use for the purpose is still experimental.

100-3, 160.21

Telephone Transmission of Electroencephalograms (EEGs)

Telephone transmission of electroencephalograms (EEGs) is covered as a physician's service or as incident to a physician's service when reasonable and necessary for the individual patient, under appropriate circumstances. The service is safe, and may save time and cost in sending EEGs from remote areas without special competence in neurology, neurosurgery, and electroencephalography, by avoiding the need to transport patients to large medical centers for standard EEG testing.

100-3, 160.22

Ambulatory EEG Monitoring

Ambulatory EEG monitoring is a diagnostic procedure for patients in whom a seizure diathesis is suspected but not defined by history, physical or resting EEG. Ambulatory EEG can be utilized in the differential diagnosis of syncope and transient ischemic attacks if not elucidated by conventional studies. Ambulatory EEG should always be preceded by a resting EEG.

Ambulatory EEG monitoring is considered an established technique and covered under Medicare for the above purposes.

100-3, 170.3

Speech Pathology Services for the Treatment of Dysphagia

Speech -language pathology services are covered under Medicare for the treatment of dysphagia, regardless of the presence of a communication disability.

100-3, 180.1

Medical Nutrition Therapy

Effective October 1, 2002, basic coverage of MNT for the first year a beneficiary receives MNT with either a diagnosis of renal disease or diabetes as defined at 42 CFR Sec.410.130 is 3 hours. Also effective October 1, 2002, basic coverage in subsequent years for renal disease or diabetes is 2 hours. The dietitian/nutritionist may choose how many units are performed per day as long as all of the other requirements in this NCD and 42 CFR Secs.410.130-410.134 are met. Pursuant to the exception at 42 CFR Sec.410.132(b)(5), additional hours are considered to be medically necessary and covered if the treating physician determines that there is a change in medical condition, diagnosis, or treatment regimen that requires a change in MNT and orders additional hours during that episode of care.

Effective October 1, 2002, if the treating physician determines that receipt of both MNT and DSMT is medically necessary in the same episode of care, Medicare will cover both DSMT and MNT initial and subsequent years without decreasing either benefit as long as DSMT and MNT are not provided on the same date of service. The dietitian/nutritionist may choose how many units are performed per day as long as all of the other requirements in the NCD and 42 CFR Secs.410.130-410.134 are met. Pursuant to the exception at 42 CFR 410.132(b)(5), additional hours are considered to be medically necessary and covered if the treating physician determines that there is a change in medical condition, diagnosis, or treatment regimen that requires a change in MNT and orders additional hours during that episode of care.

100-3, 190.1

Histocompatibility Testing

This testing is safe and effective when it is performed on patients:

- In preparation for a kidney transplant;
- In preparation for bone marrow transplantation;
- In preparation for blood platelet transfusions (particularly where multiple infusions are involved); or
- Who are suspected of having ankylosing spondylitis.

This testing is covered under Medicare when used for any of the indications listed in A, B, and C and if it is reasonable and necessary for the patient.

It is covered for ankylosing spondylitis in cases where other methods of diagnosis would not be appropriate or have yielded inconclusive results. Request documentation supporting the medical necessity of the test from the physician in all cases where ankylosing spondylitis is indicated as the reason for the test.

100-3, 190.2

Diagnostic Pap Smears

CIM 50-20, CIM 50-20.1

A diagnostic pap smear and related medically necessary services are covered under Medicare Part B when ordered by a physician under one of the following conditions:

- Previous cancer of the cervix, uterus, or vagina that has been or is presently being treated;
- Previous abnormal pap smear;
- Any abnormal findings of the vagina, cervix, uterus, ovaries, or adnexa;
- Any significant complaint by the patient referable to the female reproductive system; or
- Any signs or symptoms that might in the physician's judgment reasonably be related to a gynecologic disorder.

Screening Pap Smears and Pelvic Examinations for Early Detection of Cervical or Vaginal Cancer. (See section 210.2.)

100-3, 190.3

Cytogenetic Studies

Medicare covers these tests when they are reasonable and necessary for the diagnosis or treatment of the following conditions:

Genetic disorders (e.g., mongolism) in a fetus (See Medicare Benefit Policy Manual, Chapter 15, "Covered medical and Other health Services," Sec.20.1)

Failure of sexual development;

Chronic myelogenous leukemia;

Acute leukemias lymphoid (FAB L1-L3), myeloid (FAB M0-M7), and unclassified; or

Mylodysplasia

100-3, 190.4

Electron Microscope

The electron microscope has been used in the examination of biopsies for years; its efficacy, and therefore its Medicare coverage, is not being questioned. However, there are less expensive methods for examining biopsies which are normally adequate. The additional expense for the electron microscope is normally warranted only when distinguishing different types of nephritis from renal needle biopsies or when there is an uncertain diagnosis from the pathologist. When an uncertain diagnosis from the pathologists results from a less expensive method of examination and an electron microscope examination is therefore necessary, both biopsy examinations are covered. Where the additional expense for an electron microscope examination is not warranted, payment is based upon the less costly methods of examining biopsies.

100-3, 190.5

Sweat Test

Indications and Limitations of Coverage

The sweat test is an important diagnostic tool in cystic fibrosis and may be covered when used for that purpose. Usage of the sweat test as a predictor of efficacy of sympathectomy in peripheral vascular disease is unproven and, therefore, is not covered.

100-3, 190.6

Hair Analysis

Indications and Limitations of Coverage

Hair analysis to detect mineral traces as an aid in diagnosing human disease is not a covered service under Medicare.

The correlation of hair analysis to the chemical state of the whole body is not possible at this time, and therefore this diagnostic procedure cannot be considered to be reasonable and necessary under Sec.1862(a)(1) of the Act.

100-3, 190.8

Lymphocyte Mitogen Response Assays

It is a covered test under Medicare when it is medically necessary to assess lymphocytic function in diagnosed immunodeficiency diseases and to monitor immunotherapy.

It is not covered when it is used to monitor the treatment of cancer, because its use for that purpose is experimental.

100-3, 190.9

Serologic Testing for Acquired Immunodeficiency Syndrome (AIDS)

These tests may be covered when performed to help determine a diagnosis for symptomaticpatients. They are not covered when furnished as part of a screening program for asymptomatic persons.

NOTE: Two enzyme-linked immunosorbent assay (ELISA) tests that were conducted on the same specimen must both be positive before Medicare will cover the Western blot test.

100-3, 190.10

Laboratory Tests - CRD Patients

Laboratory tests are essential to monitor the progress of CRD patients. The following list and frequencies of tests constitute the level and types of routine laboratory tests that are covered. Bills for other types of tests are considered nonroutine. Routine tests at greater frequencies must include medical justification. Nonroutine tests generally are justified by the diagnosis.

The routinely covered regimen includes the following tests:

Per Dialysis

- All hematocrit or hemoglobin and clotting time tests furnished incident to dialysis treatments.

Per Week

- Prothrombin time for patients on anticoagulant therapy
- Serum Creatinine

Per Week or Thirteen Per Quarter

- BUN

Monthly

- CBC
- Serum Calcium
- Serum Potassium
- Serum Chloride
- Serum Bicarbonate
- Serum Phosphorous
- Total Protein
- Serum Albumin
- Alkaline Phospatase
- AST, SGOT
- LDH

Guidelines for tests other than those routinely performed include:

- Serum Aluminum - one every 3 months
- Serum Ferritin - one every 3 months

The following tests for hepatitis B are covered when patients first enter a dialysis facility:

- Hepatitis B surface antigen (HBsAg)
- Anti-HBs

Coverage of future testing in these patients depends on their serologic status and on whether they have been successfully immunized against hepatitis B virus. The following table summarizes the frequency of serologic surveillance for hepatitis B. Tests furnished according to this table do not require additional documentation and are paid separately because payment for maintenance dialysis treatments does not take them into account.

Frequency of Screening

	Vaccination and Serologic Status	HbsAg Patients	Anti-HBs Patients
Unvaccinated	Susceptible	Monthly	Semiannually
Unvaccinated	HBsAg Carrier	Annually	None
Unvaccinated	Anti-HBs-Positive (1)	None	Annually
Vaccinated	Anti-HBs-Positive (1)	None	Annually
Vaccinated	Low Level or No Anti-HBs	Monthly	Semiannually

(1) At least 10 sample ration units by radioimmunoassay or positive by enzyme immunoassay.

Patients who are in the process of receiving hepatitis B vaccines, but have not received the complete series, should continue to be routinely screened as susceptible. Between one and six months after the third dose, all vaccines should be tested for anti-HBs to confirm their response to the vaccine. Patients who have a level of anti-HBs of at least 10 sample ratio units (SRUs) by radioimmunoassay (RIA) or who are positive by enzyme immunoassay (EIA) are considered adequate responders to vaccine and need only be tested for anti-HBs annually to verify their immune status. If anti-HBs drops below 10 SRUs by RIA or is negative by EIA, a booster dose of hepatitis B vaccine should be given.

Laboratory tests are subject to the normal coverage requirements. If the laboratory services are performed by a free-standing facility, be sure it meets the conditions of coverage for independent laboratories.

100-3, 190.11

Home Prothrombin Time International Normalized Ratio (INR) Monitoring for Anticoagulation Management

A. General

Use of the International Normalized Ratio (INR) or prothrombin time (PT) - standard measurement for reporting the blood's clotting time) - allows physicians to determine the level of anticoagulation in a patient independent of the laboratory reagents used. The INR is the ratio of the patient's PT (extrinsic or tissue-factor dependent coagulation pathway) compared to the mean PT for a group of normal individuals. Maintaining patients within his/her prescribed therapeutic range minimizes adverse events associated with inadequate or excessive anticoagulation such as serious bleeding or thromboembolic events. Patient self-testing and self-management through the use of a home INR monitor may be used to improve the time in therapeutic rate (TTR) for select groups of patients. Increased TTR leads to improved clinical outcomes and reductions in thromboembolic and hemorrhagic events.

Warfarin (also prescribed under other trade names, e.g., Coumadin(R)) is a self-administered, oral anticoagulant (blood thinner) medication that affects the vitamin K- dependent clotting factors II, VII, IX and X. It is widely used for various medical conditions, and has a narrow therapeutic index, meaning it is a drug with less than a 2-fold difference between median lethal dose and median effective dose. For this reason, since October 4, 2006, it falls under the category of a Food and Drug dministration (FDA) "black-box" drug whose dosage must be closely monitored to avoid serious complications. A PT/INR monitoring system is a portable testing device that includes a finger-stick and an FDA-cleared meter that measures the time it takes for a person's blood plasma to clot.

B. Nationally Covered Indications

For services furnished on or after March 19, 2008, Medicare will cover the use of home PT/INR monitoring for chronic, oral anticoagulation management for patients with mechanical heart valves, chronic atrial fibrillation, or venous thromboembolism (inclusive of deep venous thrombosis and pulmonary embolism) on warfarin. The monitor and the home testing must be prescribed by a treating physician as provided at 42 CFR 410.32(a), and all of the following requirements must be met:

1. The patient must have been anticoagulated for at least 3 months prior to use of the home INR device; and,
2. The patient must undergo a face-to-face educational program on anticoagulation anagement and must have demonstrated the correct use of the device prior to its use in the home; and,
3. The patient continues to correctly use the device in the context of the management of the anticoagulation therapy following the initiation of home monitoring; and,
4. Self-testing with the device should not occur more frequently than once a week.

C. Nationally Non-Covered Indications

N/A

D. Other

1. All other indications for home PT/INR monitoring not indicated as nationally covered above remain at local Medicare contractor discretion.
2. This national coverage determination (NCD) is distinct from, and makes no changes to, the PT clinical laboratory NCD at section 190.17 of Publication 100-03 of the NCD Manual.

100-3, 190.12

Urine Culture, Bacterial

Indications

1. A patient's urinalysis is abnormal suggesting urinary tract infection, for example, abnormal microscopic (hematuria, pyuria, bacteriuria); abnormal biochemical urinalysis (positive leukocyte esterase, nitrite, protein, blood); a Gram's stain positive for microorganisms; positive bacteriuria screen by a non?culture technique; or other significant abnormality of a urinalysis. While it is not essential to evaluate a urine specimen by one of these methods before a urine culture is performed, certain clinical presentations with highly suggestive signs and symptoms may lend themselves to an antecedent urinalysis procedure where follow-up culture depends upon an initial positive or abnormal test result.
2. A patient has clinical signs and symptoms indicative of a possible urinary tract infection (UTI). Acute lower UTI may present with urgency, frequency, nocturia, dysuria, discharge or incontinence. These findings may also be noted in upper UTI with additional systemic symptoms (for example, fever, chills, lethargy); or pain in the costovertebral, abdominal, or pelvic areas. Signs and symptoms may overlap considerably with other inflammatory conditions of the genitourinary tract (for example, prostatitis, urethritis, vaginitis, or cervicitis). Elderly or immunocompromised patients, or patients with neurologic disorders may present atypically (for example, general debility, acute mental status changes, declining functional status).
3. The patient is being evaluated for suspected urosepsis, fever of unknown origin, or other systemic manifestations of infection but without a known source. Signs and symptoms used to define sepsis have been well established.
4. A test-of cure is generally not indicated in an uncomplicated infection. However, it may be indicated if the patient is being evaluated for response to therapy and there is a complicating co-existing urinary abnormality including structural or functional abnormalities, calculi, foreign bodies, or ureteral/renal stents or there is clinical or laboratory evidence of failure to respond as described in Indications 1 and 2.
5. In surgical procedures involving major manipulations of the genitourinary tract, preoperative examination to detect occult infection may be indicated in selected cases (for example, prior to renal transplantation, manipulation or removal of kidney stones, or transurethral surgery of the bladder or prostate).
6. Urine culture may be indicated to detect occult infection in renal transplant recipients on immunosuppressive therapy.

Limitations

1. CPT 87086 may be used one time per encounter.
2. Colony count restrictions on coverage of CPT 87088 do not apply as they may be highly variable according to syndrome or other clinical circumstances (for example, antecedent therapy, collection time, degree of hydration).
3. CPT 87088, 87184, and 87186 may be used multiple times in association with or independent of 87086, as urinary tract infections may be polymicrobial.
4. Testing for asymptomatic bacteriuria as part of a prenatal evaluation may be medically appropriate but is considered screening and, therefore, not covered by Medicare. The US Preventive Services Task Force has concluded that screening for asymptomatic bacteriuria outside of the narrow indication for pregnant women is generally not indicated. There are insufficient data to recommend screening in ambulatory elderly patients including those with diabetes. Testing may be clinically indicated on other grounds including likelihood of recurrence or potential adverse effects of antibiotics, but is considered screening in the absence of clinical or laboratory evidence of infection.

100-3, 190.13

Human Immunodeficiency Virus (HIV) Testing (Prognosis Including Monitoring)

Indications

1. A plasma HIV RNA baseline level may be medically necessary in any patient with confirmed HIV infection.
2. Regular periodic measurement of plasma HIV RNA levels may be medically necessary to determine risk for disease progression in an HIV-infected individual and to determine when to initiate or modify antiretroviral treatment regimens.
3. In clinical situations where the risk of HIV infection is significant and initiation of therapy is anticipated, a baseline HIV quantification may be performed. These situations include:
   a. Persistence of borderline or equivocal serologic reactivity in an at-risk individual.
   b. Signs and symptoms of acute retroviral syndrome characterized by fever, malaise, lymphadenopathy and rash in an at-risk individual.

Limitations

1. Viral quantification may be appropriate for prognostic use including baseline determination, periodic monitoring, and monitoring of response to therapy. Use as a diagnostic test method is not indicated.
2. Measurement of plasma HIV RNA levels should be performed at the time of establishment of an HIV infection diagnosis. For an accurate baseline, 2 specimens in a 2-week period are appropriate.
3. For prognosis including anti-retroviral therapy monitoring, regular, periodic measurements are appropriate. The frequency of viral load testing should be consistent with the most current Centers for Disease Control and Prevention guidelines for use of anti-retroviral agents in adults and adolescents or pediatrics.
4. Because differences in absolute HIV copy number are known to occur using different assays, plasma HIV RNA levels should be measured by the same analytical method. A change in assay method may necessitate re-establishment of a baseline.
5. Nucleic acid quantification techniques are representative of rapidly emerging and evolving new technologies. As such, users are advised to remain current on FDA-approval status.

100-3, 190.14

Human Immunodeficiency Virus (HIV) Testing (Diagnosis)

Indications and Limitations of Coverage

Indications

Diagnostic testing to establish HIV infection may be indicated when there is a strong clinical suspicion supported by one or more of the following clinical findings:

The patient has a documented, otherwise unexplained, AIDS-defining or AIDS-associated opportunistic infection.

The patient has another documented sexually transmitted disease which identifies significant risk of exposure to HIV and the potential for an early or subclinical infection.

The patient has documented acute or chronic hepatitis B or C infection that identifies a significant risk of exposure to HIV and the potential for an early or subclinical infection.

The patient has a documented AIDS-defining or AIDS-associated neoplasm.

The patient has a documented AIDS-associated neurologic disorder or otherwise unexplained dementia.

The patient has another documented AIDS-defining clinical condition, or a history of other severe, recurrent, or persistent conditions which suggest an underlying immune deficiency (for example, cutaneous or mucosal disorders).

The patient has otherwise unexplained generalized signs and symptoms suggestive of a chronic process with an underlying immune deficiency (for example, fever, weight loss, malaise, fatigue, chronic diarrhea, failure to thrive, chronic cough, hemoptysis, shortness of breath, or lymphadenopathy).

The patient has otherwise unexplained laboratory evidence of a chronic disease process with an underlying immune deficiency (for example, anemia, leukopenia, pancytopenia, lymphopenia, or low CD4+ lymphocyte count).

The patient has signs and symptoms of acute retroviral syndrome with fever, malaise, lymphadenopathy, and skin rash.

The patient has documented exposure to blood or body fluids known to be capable of transmitting HIV (for example, needlesticks and other significant blood exposures) and antiviral therapy is initiated or anticipated to be initiated.

The patient is undergoing treatment for rape. (HIV testing is a part of the rape treatment protocol.)

Limitations

HIV antibody testing in the United States is usually performed using HIV-1 or HIV-½ combination tests. HIV-2 testing is indicated if clinical circumstances suggest HIV-2 is likely (that is, compatible clinical findings and HIV-1 test negative). HIV-2 testing may also be indicated in areas of the country where there is greater prevalence of HIV-2 infections.

The Western Blot test should be performed only after documentation that the initial EIA tests are repeatedly positive or equivocal on a single sample.

The HIV antigen tests currently have no defined diagnostic usage.

Direct viral RNA detection may be performed in those situations where serologic

testing does not establish a diagnosis but strong clinical suspicion persists (for example, acute retroviral syndrome, nonspecific serologic evidence of HIV, or perinatal HIV infection).

If initial serologic tests confirm an HIV infection, repeat testing is not indicated.

If initial serologic tests are HIV EIA negative and there is no indication for confirmation of infection by viral RNA detection, the interval prior to retesting is 3-6 months.

Testing for evidence of HIV infection using serologic methods may be medically appropriate in situations where there is a risk of exposure to HIV. However, in the absence of a documented AIDS defining or HIV- associated disease, an HIV associated sign or symptom, or documented exposure to a known HIV-infected source, the testing is considered by Medicare to be screening and thus is not covered by Medicare (for example, history of multiple blood component transfusions, exposure to blood or body fluids not resulting in consideration of therapy, history of transplant, history of illicit drug use, multiple sexual partners, same-sex encounters, prostitution, or contact with prostitutes).

The CPT Editorial Panel has issued a number of codes for infectious agent detection by direct antigen or nucleic acid probe techniques that have not yet been developed or are only being used on an investigational basis. Laboratory providers are advised to remain current on FDA-approval status for these tests.

100-3, 190.15

Blood Counts

Indications

Indications for a CBC or hemogram include red cell, platelet, and white cell disorders. Examples of these indications are enumerated individually below.

1. Indications for a CBC generally include the evaluation of bone marrow dysfunction as a result of neoplasms, therapeutic agents, exposure to toxic substances, or pregnancy. The CBC is also useful in assessing peripheral destruction of blood cells, suspected bone marrow failure or bone marrow infiltrate, suspected myeloproliferative, myelodysplastic, or lymphoproliferative processes, and immune disorders.
2. Indications for hemogram or CBC related to red cell (RBC) parameters of the hemogram include signs, symptoms, test results, illness, or disease that can be associated with anemia or other red blood cell disorder (e.g., pallor, weakness, fatigue, weight loss, bleeding, acute injury associated with blood loss or suspected blood loss, abnormal menstrual bleeding, hematuria, hematemesis, hematochezia, positive fecal occult blood test, malnutrition, vitamin deficiency, malabsorption, neuropathy, known malignancy, presence of acute or chronic disease that may have associated anemia, coagulation or hemostatic disorders, postural dizziness, syncope, abdominal pain, change in bowel habits, chronic marrow hypoplasia or decreased RBC production, tachycardia, systolic heart murmur, congestive heart failure, dyspnea, angina, nailbed deformities, growth retardation, jaundice, hepatomegaly, splenomegaly, lymphadenopathy, ulcers on the lower extremities).
3. Indications for hemogram or CBC related to red cell (RBC) parameters of the hemogram include signs, symptoms, test results, illness, or disease that can be associated with polycythemia (for example, fever, chills, ruddy skin, conjunctival redness, cough, wheezing, cyanosis, clubbing of the fingers, orthopnea, heart murmur, headache, vague cognitive changes including memory changes, sleep apnea, weakness, pruritus, dizziness, excessive sweating, visual symptoms, weight loss, massive obesity, gastrointestinal bleeding, paresthesias, dyspnea, joint symptoms, epigastric distress, pain and erythema of the fingers or toes, venous or arterial thrombosis, thromboembolism, myocardial infarction, stroke, transient ischemic attacks, congenital heart disease, chronic obstructive pulmonary disease, increased erythropoietin production associated with neoplastic, renal or hepatic disorders, androgen or diuretic use, splenomegaly, hepatomegaly, diastolic hypertension.)
4. Specific indications for CBC with differential count related to the WBC include signs, symptoms, test results, illness, or disease associated with leukemia, infections or inflammatory processes, suspected bone marrow failure or bone marrow infiltrate, suspected myeloproliferative, myelodysplastic or lymphoproliferative disorder, use of drugs that may cause leukopenia, and immune disorders (e.g., fever, chills, sweats, shock, fatigue, malaise, tachycardia, tachypnea, heart murmur, seizures, alterations of consciousness, meningismus, pain such as headache, abdominal pain, arthralgia, odynophagia, or dysuria, redness or swelling of skin, soft tissue bone, or joint, ulcers of the skin or mucous membranes, gangrene, mucous membrane discharge, bleeding, thrombosis, respiratory failure, pulmonary infiltrate, jaundice, diarrhea, vomiting, hepatomegaly, splenomegaly, lymphadenopathy, opportunistic infection such as oral candidiasis.)
5. Specific indications for CBC related to the platelet count include signs, symptoms, test results, illness, or disease associated with increased or decreased platelet production and destruction, or platelet dysfunction (e.g., gastrointestinal bleeding, genitourinary tract bleeding, bilateral epistaxis, thrombosis, ecchymosis, purpura, jaundice, petechiae, fever, heparin therapy, suspected DIC, shock, pre-eclampsia, neonate with maternal ITP, massive transfusion, recent platelet transfusion, cardiopulmonary bypass, hemolytic uremic syndrome, renal diseases, lymphadenopathy, hepatomegaly, splenomegaly, hypersplenism, neurologic abnormalities, viral or other infection, myeloproliferative, myelodysplastic, or lymphoproliferative disorder, thrombosis, exposure to toxic agents, excessive alcohol ingestion, autoimmune disorders (SLE, RA and other).
6. Indications for hemogram or CBC related to red cell (RBC) parameters of the hemogram include, in addition to those already listed, thalassemia, suspected hemoglobinopathy, lead poisoning, arsenic poisoning, and spherocytosis.
7. Specific indications for CBC with differential count related to the WBC include, in addition to those already listed, storage diseases; mucopolysaccharidoses, and use of drugs that cause leukocytosis such as G-CSF or GM-CSF
8. Specific indications for CBC related to platelet count include, in addition to those already listed, May-Hegglin syndrome and Wiskott-Aldrich syndrome.

Limitations

1. Testing of patients who are asymptomatic, or who do not have a condition that could be expected to result in a hematological abnormality, is screening and is not a covered service.
2. In some circumstances it may be appropriate to perform only a hemoglobin or hematocrit to assess the oxygen carrying capacity of the blood. When the ordering provider requests only a hemoglobin or hematocrit, the remaining components of the CBC are not covered.
3. When a blood count is performed for an end-stage renal disease (ESRD) patient, and is billed outside the ESRD rate, documentation of the medical necessity for the blood count must be submitted with the claim.
4. In some patients presenting with certain signs, symptoms or diseases, a single CBC may be appropriate. Repeat testing may not be indicated unless abnormal results are found, or unless there is a change in clinical condition. If repeat testing is performed, a more descriptive diagnosis code (e.g., anemia) should be reported to support medical necessity. However, repeat testing may be indicated where results are normal in patients with conditions where there is a continued risk for the development of hematologic abnormality.

100-3, 190.16

Partial Thromboplastin Time (PTT)

Indications and Limitations of Coverage

Indications

1. The PTT is most commonly used to quantitate the effect of therapeutic unfractionated heparin and to regulate its dosing. Except during transitions between heparin and warfarin therapy, in general both the PTT and PT are not

necessary together to assess the effect of anticoagulation therapy. PT and PTT must be justified separately.

2. A PTT may be used to assess patients with signs or symptoms of hemorrhage or thrombosis. For example: abnormal bleeding, hemorrhage or hematoma petechiae or other signs of thrombocytopenia that could be due to disseminated intravascular coagulation; swollen extremity with or without prior trauma.
3. A PTT may be useful in evaluating patients who have a history of a condition known to be associated with the risk of hemorrhage or thrombosis that is related to the intrinsic coagulation pathway. Such abnormalities may be genetic or acquired. For example: dysfibrinogenemia; afibrinogenemia (complete); acute or chronic liver dysfunction or failure, including Wilson's disease; hemophilia; liver disease and failure; infectious processes; bleeding disorders; disseminated intravascular coagulation; lupus erythematosus or other conditions associated with circulating inhibitors, e.g., Factor VIII Inhibitor, lupus-like anticoagulant, etc.; sepsis; von Willebrand's disease; arterial and venous thrombosis, including the evaluation of hypercoagulable states; clinical conditions associated with nephrosis or renal failure; other acquired and congenital coagulopathies as well as thrombotic states.
4. A PTT may be used to assess the risk of thrombosis or hemorrhage in patients who are going to have a medical intervention known to be associated with increased risk of bleeding or thrombosis. An example is as follows: evaluation prior to invasive procedures or operations of patients with personal or family history of bleeding or who are on heparin therapy.

Limitations

1. The PTT is not useful in monitoring the effects of warfarin on a patient's coagulation routinely. However, a PTT may be ordered on a patient being treated with warfarin as heparin therapy is being discontinued. A PTT may also be indicated when the PT is markedly prolonged due to warfarin toxicity.
2. The need to repeat this test is determined by changes in the underlying medical condition and/or the dosing of heparin.
3. Testing prior to any medical intervention associated with a risk of bleeding and thrombosis (other than thrombolytic therapy) will generally be considered medically necessary only where there are signs or symptoms of a bleeding or thrombotic abnormality or a personal history of bleeding, thrombosis or a condition associated with a coagulopathy. Hospital/clinic-specific policies, protocols, etc., in and of themselves, cannot alone justify coverage.

100-3, 190.17

Prothrombin Time (PT)

Basic plasma coagulation function is readily assessed with a few simple laboratory tests: the partial thromboplastin time (PTT), PT, thrombin time, or a quantitative fibrinogen determination. The PT test is one in-vitro laboratory test used to assess coagulation. While the PTT assesses the intrinsic limb of the coagulation system, the PT assesses the extrinsic or tissue factor dependent pathway. Both tests also evaluate the common coagulation pathway involving all the reactions that occur after the activation of factor X.

Extrinsic pathway factors are produced in the liver and their production is dependent on adequate vitamin K activity. Deficiencies of factors may be related to decreased production of increased consumption of coagulation factors. The PR/INR is most commonly used to measure the effect of warfarin and regulate its dosing. Warfarin blocks the effect of vitamin K on hepatic production of extrinsic pathway factors.

A PT is expressed in seconds and/or as an international normalized ration (INR). The INR is the PT ration that would result if the WHO reference thromboplastin had been used in performing the test.

Current medical information does not clarify the role of laboratory PT testing in patients who are self monitoring. Therefore, the indications for testing apply regardless of whether or not the patient is also PT self-testing.

Indications

1. A PT may be used to assess patients taking warfarin. The PT is generally not useful in monitoring patients receiving heparin who are not taking warfarin.
2. A PT may be used to assess patients with signs or symptoms of abnormal bleeding or thrombosis. For example: swollen extremity with or without prior trauma; unexplained bruising; abnormal bleeding, hemorrhage, or hematoma; petechiae or other signs or thrombocytopenia that could be due to disseminated intravascular coagulation.
3. A PT may be useful in evaluating patients who have a history of a condition known to be associated with the risk of bleeding or thrombosis that is related to the extrinsic coagulation pathway. Such abnormalities may be genetic or acquires. For example: dysfibrinogenemia; afibrinogenemia (complete); acute or chronic liver dysfunction or failure, including Wilson? disease and hemochromatosis; disseminated intravascular coagulation (DIC); congenital and acquired deficiencies of factors II, V, VII, X; vitamin K deficiency; lupus erythematosus; hypercoagulable state; paraproteinemia; lymphoma; amyloidosis; acute and chronic leukemias; plasma cell dyscrasia; HIV infection; malignant neoplasms; hemorrhagic fever; salicylate poisoning; obstructive jaundice; intestinal fistula; malabsorption syndrome; colitis; chronic diarrhea; presence of peripheral venous or arterial thrombosis or pulmonary emboli or myocardial infarction; patients with bleeding or clotting tendencies; organ transplantation; presence of circulating coagulation inhibitors.
4. APT may be used to assess the risk of hemorrhage or thrombosis in patients who are going to have a medical intervention known to be associated with increased risk of bleeding or thrombosis. For example: evaluation prior to invasive procedures or operations of patients with personal history of bleeding of a condition associated with coagulopathy; prior to the use of thrombolytic medication.

Limitations

1. When an ESRD patient is tested for PT, testing more frequently than weekly requires documentation of medical necessity, e.g., other than chronic renal failure or renal failure unspecified.
2. The need to repeat this test is determined by changes in the underlying medical condition and/or the dosing of warfarin. In a patient on stable warfarin therapy, it is ordinarily not necessary to repeat testing more than every two to three weeks. When testing is performed to evaluate a patient with signs or symptoms of abnormal bleeding or thrombosis and the initial test result is normal, it is ordinarily not necessary to repeat testing unless there is a change in the patient? medical status.
3. Since the INR is a calculation, it will not be paid in addition to the PT when expressed in seconds, and is considered part of the conventional PT test.
4. Testing prior to any medical intervention associated with a risk of bleeding and thrombosis (other that thrombolytic therapy) will generally be considered medically necessary only where there are signs or symptoms of a bleeding or thrombotic abnormality of a personal history of bleeding, thrombosis or a condition associated with a coagulopathy. Hospital/clinic-specific policies, protocols, etc., in and of themselves, cannot alone justify coverage.

100-3, 190.18

Serum Iron Studies

Serum iron studies are useful in the evaluation of disorders of iron metabolism, particularly iron deficiency and iron excess. Iron studies are best performed when the patients is fasting in the morning and has abstained form medications that may influence iron balance.

Iron deficiency is the most common cause of anemia. In young children on a milk diet, iron deficiency is often secondary to dietary deficiency. In adults, iron deficiency is usually the result of blood loss and is only occasionally secondary to dietary deficiency or malabsorption.

Following major surgery the patient may have iron deficient erythropoiesis for months or years if adequate iron replacement has not been given. High doses of supplemental iron may cause the serum iron to be elevated. Serum iron may also be altered in acute and chronic inflammatory and neoplastic conditions.

Total iron binding capacity (TIBC) is an indirect measure of transferring, a protein that binds and transports iron. TIBC quantifies transferring by the amount of iron that it can bind. TIBC and transferrin are elevated in iron deficiency, and with oral contraceptive use, and during pregnancy. TIBC and transferrin may be decreased in malabsorption syndromes or in those affected with chronic diseases. The percent saturation represents the ratio of iron to the TIBC.

Assays for ferritin are also useful in assessing iron balance. Low concentrations are associated with iron deficiency and are highly specific. High concentrations are found in hemosiderosis (iron overload without associated tissue injury) and hemochromatosis (iron overload with associated tissue injury). In these conditions the iron is elevated, the TIBC and transferring are within the reference range or low, and the percent saturation is elevated. Serum ferritin can be useful for both initiating and monitoring treatment for iron overload.

Transferrin and ferritin belong to a group of serum proteins known as acute phase reactants, and are increased in response to stressful or inflammatory conditions and also can occur with infection and tissue injury due to surgery, trauma or necrosis. Ferritin and iron/TIBC (or transferrin) are affected by acute and chronic inflammatory conditions, and in patients with these disorders, tests of iron status may be difficult to interpret.

Indications

1. Ferritin (82728), iron (83540) and either iron binding capacity (83550) or transferrin (84466) are useful in the differential diagnosis of iron deficiency, anemia, and for iron overload conditions.
   a. The following presentations are examples that may support the use of these studies for evaluating iron deficiency:
      - Certain abnormal blood count values (i.e., decreased mean corpuscular volume (MCV), decreased hemoglobin/hematocrit when the MCV is low or normal, or increased red cell distribution width (RDW) and low or normal MCV);
      - Abnormal appetite (pica);
      - Acute or chronic gastrointestinal blood loss;
      - Hematuria;
      - Menorrhagia;
      - Malabsorption;
      - Status post-gastrectomy;
      - Status post-gastrojejunostomy;

- Malnutrition;
- Preoperative autologous blood collection(s);
- Malignant, chronic inflammatory and infectious conditions associated with anemia which may present in a similar manner to iron deficiency anemia;
- Following a significant surgical procedure where blood loss had occurred and had not been repaired with adequate iron replacement.

b. The following presentations are examples that may support the use of these studies for evaluating iron overload:

- Chronic Hepatitis;
- Diabetes;
- Hyperpigmentation of skin;
- Arthropathy;
- Cirrhosis;
- Hypogonadism;
- Hypopituitarism;
- Impaired porphyrin metabolism;
- Heart failure;
- Multiple transfusions;
- Sideroblastic anemia;
- Thalassemia major;
- Cardiomyopathy, cardiac dysrhythmias and conduction disturbances.

2. Follow-up testing may be appropriate to monitor response to therapy, e.g., oral or parenteral iron, ascorbic acid, and erythropoietin.
3. Iron studies may be appropriate in patients after treatment for other nutritional deficiency anemias, such as folate and vitamin B12, because iron deficiency may not be revealed until such a nutritional deficiency is treated.
4. Serum ferritin may be appropriate for monitoring iron status in patients with chronic renal disease with or without dialysis.
5. Serum iron may also be indicated for evaluation of toxic effects of iron and other metals (e.g., nickel, cadmium, aluminum, lead) whether due to accidental, intentional exposure or metabolic causes.

Limitations

1. Iron studies should be used to diagnose and manage iron deficiency or iron overload states. These tests are not to be used solely to assess acute phase reactants where disease management will be unchanged. For example, infections and malignancies are associated with elevations in acute phase reactants such as ferritin, and decreases in serum iron concentration, but iron studies would only be medically necessary if results of iron studies might alter the management of the primary diagnosis or might warrant direct treatment of an iron disorder or condition.
2. If a normal serum ferritin level is documented, repeat testing would not ordinarily be medically necessary unless there is a change in the patient's condition, and ferritin assessment is needed for the ongoing management of the patient. For example, a patient presents with new onset insulin-dependent diabetes mellitus and has a serum ferritin level performed for the suspicion of hemochromatosis. If the ferritin level is normal, the repeat ferritin for diabetes mellitus would not be medically necessary.
3. When an End Stage Renal Disease (ESRD) patient is tested for ferritin, testing more frequently than every three months (the frequency authorized by 3167.3, Fiscal Intermediary manual) requires documentation of medical necessity [e.g., other than "Chronic Renal Failure" (ICD-9-CM 585) or "Renal Failure, Unspecified" (ICD-9-CM 586)].
4. It is ordinarily not necessary to measure both transferrin and TIBC at the same time because TIBC is an indirect measure of transferrin. When transferrin is ordered as part of the nutritional assessment for evaluating malnutrition, it is not necessary to order other iron studies unless iron deficiency or iron overload is suspected as well.
5. It is not ordinarily necessary to measure both iron/TIBC (or transferrin) and ferritin in initial patient testing. If clinically indicated after evaluation of the initial iron studies, it may be appropriate to perform additional iron studies either on the initial specimen or on a subsequently obtained specimen. After a diagnosis of iron deficiency or iron overload is established, either iron/TIBC (or transferrin) or ferritin may be medically necessary for monitoring, but not both.
6. It would not ordinarily be considered medically necessary to do a ferritin as a preoperative test except in the presence of anemia or recent autologous blood collections prior to the surgery.

100-3, 190.19

Collagen Crosslinks, Any Method

Indications

Generally speaking, collagen crosslink testing is useful mostly in "fast losers" of bone. The age when these bone markers can help direct therapy is often pre-Medicare. By the time a fast loser of bone reaches age 65, she will most likely have been stabilized by appropriate therapy or have lost so much bone mass that further testing is useless. Coverage for bone marker assays may be established, however, for younger Medicare beneficiaries and for those men and women who might become fast losers because of some other therapy such as glucocorticoids. Safeguards should be incorporated to prevent excessive use of tests in patients for whom they have no clinical relevance.

Collagen crosslinks testing is used to:

1. Identify individuals with elevated bone resorption, who have osteoporosis in whom response to treatment is being monitored;
2. Predict response (as assessed by bone mass measurements) to FDA approved antiresorptive therapy in postmenopausal women; and
3. Assess response to treatment of patients with osteoporosis, Paget's disease of the bone, or risk for osteoporosis where treatment may include FDA approved antiresorptive agents, anti-estrogens or selective estrogen receptor moderators.

Limitations

Because of significant specimen to specimen collagen crosslink physiologic variability (15-20%), current recommendations for appropriate utilization include: one or two base-line assays from specified urine collections on separate days; followed by a repeat assay about three months after starting anti-resorptive therapy; followed by a repeat assay in 12 months after the three-month assay; and thereafter not more than annually, unless there is a change in therapy in which circumstance an additional test may be indicated three months after the initiation of new therapy.

Some collagen crosslink assays may not be appropriate for use in some disorders, according to FDA labeling restrictions.

100-3, 190.20

Blood Glucose Testing

Indications

Blood glucose values are often necessary for the management of patients with diabetes mellitus, where hyperglycemia and hypoglycemia are often present. They are also critical in the determination of control of blood glucose levels in the patient with impaired fasting glucose (FPG 110-125 mg/dL), the patient with insulin resistance syndrome and/or carbohydrate intolerance (excessive rise in glucose following ingestion of glucose or glucose sources of food), in the patient with a hypoglycemia disorder such as nesidioblastosis or insulinoma, and in patients with a catabolic or malnutrition state. In addition to those conditions already listed, glucose testing may be medically necessary in patients with tuberculosis, unexplained chronic or recurrent infections, alcoholism, coronary artery disease (especially in women), or unexplained skin conditions (including pruritis, local skin infections, ulceration and gangrene without an established cause).

Many medical conditions may be a consequence of a sustained elevated or depressed glucose level. These include comas, seizures or epilepsy, confusion, abnormal hunger, abnormal weight loss or gain, and loss of sensation. Evaluation of glucose may also be indicated in patients on medications known to affect carbohydrate metabolism.

Effective January 1, 2005, the Medicare law expanded coverage to diabetic screening services. Some forms of blood glucode testing covered under this national coverage determination may be covered for screening purposes subject to specified frequencies. See 42 CFR 410.18 and section 90, chapter 18 of the Claims Processing Manual, for a full description of this screening benefit.

Limitations

Frequent home blood glucose testing by diabetic patients should be encouraged. In stable, non-hospitalized patients who are unable or unwilling to do home monitoring, it may be reasonable and necessary to measure quantitative blood glucose up to four times annually.

Depending upon the age of the patient, type of diabetes, degree of control, complications of diabetes, and other co-morbid conditions, more frequent testing than four times annually may be reasonable and necessary.

In some patients presenting with nonspecific signs, symptoms, or diseases not normally associated with disturbances in glucose metabolism, a single blood glucose test may be medically necessary. Repeat testing may not be indicated unless abnormal results are found or unless there is a change in clinical condition. If repeat testing is performed, a specific diagnosis code (e.g., diabetes) should be reported to support medical necessity. However, repeat testing may be indicated where results are normal in patients with conditions where there is a confirmed continuing risk of glucose metabolism abnormality (e.g., monitoring glucocorticoid therapy).

100-3, 190.21

Glycated Hemoglobin/Glycated Protein

Indications:

Glycated hemoglobin/protein testing is widely accepted as medically necessary for the management and control of diabetes. It is also valuable to assess hyperglycemia, a history of hyperglycemia or dangerous hypoglycemia. Glycated protein testing may be used in place of glycated hemoglobin in the management of diabetic patients, and is particularly useful in patients who have abnormalities of erythrocytes such as hemolytic anemia or hemoglobinopathies.

Limitations:

It is not considered reasonable and necessary to perform glycated hemoglobin tests more often than every three months on a controlled diabetic patient to determine whether the patient's metabolic control has been on average within the target range. It is not considered reasonable and necessary for these tests to be performed more frequently than once a month for diabetic pregnant women. Testing for uncontrolled type one or two diabetes mellitus may require testing more than four times a year. The above Description Section provides the clinical basis for those situations in which testing more frequently than four times per annum is indicated, and medical necessity documentation must support such testing in excess of the above guidelines.

Many methods for the analysis of glycated hemoglobin show significant interference from elevated levels of fetal hemoglobin or by variant hemoglobin molecules. When the glycated hemoglobin assay is initially performed in these patients, the laboratory may inform the ordering physician of a possible analytical interference. Alternative testing, including glycated protein, for example, fructosamine, may be indicated for the monitoring of the degree of glycemic control in this situation. It is therefore conceivable that a patient will have both a glycated hemoglobin and glycated protein ordered on the same day. This should be limited to the initial assay of glycated hemoglobin, with subsequent exclusive use of glycated protein. These tests are not considered to be medically necessary for the diagnosis of diabetes.

100-3, 190.22

Thyroid Testing

Indications

Thyroid function tests are used to define hyper function, euthyroidism, or hypofunction of thyroid disease. Thyroid testing may be reasonable and necessary to:

- Distinguish between primary and secondary hypothyroidism;
- Confirm or rule out primary hypothyroidism;
- Monitor thyroid hormone levels (for example, patients with goiter, thyroid nodules, or thyroid cancer);
- Monitor drug therapy in patients with primary hypothyroidism;
- Confirm or rule out primary hyperthyroidism; and
- Monitor therapy in patients with hyperthyroidism.

Thyroid function testing may be medically necessary in patients with disease or neoplasm of the thyroid and other endocrine glands. Thyroid function testing may also be medically necessary in patients with metabolic disorders; malnutrition; hyperlipidemia; certain types of anemia; psychosis and non-psychotic personality disorders; unexplained depression; ophthalmologic disorders; various cardiac arrhythmias; disorders of menstruation; skin conditions; myalgias; and a wide array of signs and symptoms, including alterations in consciousness; malaise; hypothermia; symptoms of the nervous and musculoskeletal system; skin and integumentary system; nutrition and metabolism; cardiovascular; and gastrointestinal system.

It may be medically necessary to do follow-up thyroid testing in patients with a personal history of malignant neoplasm of the endocrine system and in patients on long-term thyroid drug therapy.

Limitations

Testing may be covered up to two times a year in clinically stable patients; more frequent testing may be reasonable and necessary for patients whose thyroid therapy has been altered or in whom symptoms or signs of hyperthyroidism or hypothyroidism are noted.

100-3, 190.23

Lipid Testing

Indications and Limitations of Coverage

Indications

The medical community recognizes lipid testing as appropriate for evaluating atherosclerotic cardiovascular disease. Conditions in which lipid testing may be indicated include:

- Assessment of patients with atherosclerotic cardiovascular disease.
- Evaluation of primary dyslipidemia.
- Any form of atherosclerotic disease, or any disease leading to the formation of atherosclerotic disease.
- Diagnostic evaluation of diseases associated with altered lipid metabolism, such as: nephrotic syndrome, pancreatitis, hepatic disease, and hypo and hyperthyroidism.
- Secondary dyslipidemia, including diabetes mellitus, disorders of gastrointestinal absorption, chronic renal failure.
- Signs or symptoms of dyslipidemias, such as skin lesions.
- As follow-up to the initial screen for coronary heart disease (total cholesterol + HDL cholesterol) when total cholesterol is determined to be high (>240 mg/dL), or borderline-high (200-240 mg/dL) plus two or more coronary heart disease risk factors, or an HDL cholesterol, <35 mg/dl.

To monitor the progress of patients on anti-lipid dietary management and pharmacologic therapy for the treatment of elevated blood lipid disorders, total cholesterol, HDL cholesterol and LDL cholesterol may be used. Triglycerides may be obtained if this lipid fraction is also elevated or if the patient is put on drugs (for example, thiazide diuretics, beta blockers, estrogens, glucocorticoids, and tamoxifen) which may raise the triglyceride level.

When monitoring long term anti-lipid dietary or pharmacologic therapy and when following patients with borderline high total or LDL cholesterol levels, it may be reasonable to perform the lipid panel annually. A lipid panel at a yearly interval will usually be adequate while measurement of the serum total cholesterol or a measured LDL should suffice for interim visits if the patient does not have hypertriglyceridemia.

Any one component of the panel or a measured LDL may be reasonable and necessary up to six times the first year for monitoring dietary or pharmacologic therapy. More frequent total cholesterol HDL cholesterol, LDL cholesterol and triglyceride testing may be indicated for marked elevations or for changes to anti-lipid therapy due to inadequate initial patient response to dietary or pharmacologic therapy. The LDL cholesterol or total cholesterol may be measured three times yearly after treatment goals have been achieved.

Electrophoretic or other quantitation of lipoproteins may be indicated if the patient has a primary disorder of lipoid metabolism.

Effective January 1, 2005, the Medicare law expanded coverage to cardiovascular screening services. Several of the procedures included in this NCD may be covered for screening purposes subject to specified frequencies. See 42 CFR 410.17 and section 100, chapter 18, of the Claims Processing Manual, for a full description of this benefit.

Limitations

Lipid panel and hepatic panel testing may be used for patients with severe psoriasis which has not responded to conventional therapy and for which the retinoid etretinate has been prescribed and who have developed hyperlipidemia or hepatic toxicity. Specific examples include erythroderma and generalized pustular type and psoriasis associated with arthritis.

Routine screening and prophylactic testing for lipid disorder are not covered by Medicare. While lipid screening may be medically appropriate, Medicare by statute does not pay for it. Lipid testing in asymptomatic individuals is considered to be screening regardless of the presence of other risk factors such as family history, tobacco use, etc.

Once a diagnosis is established, one or several specific tests are usually adequate for monitoring the course of the disease. Less specific diagnoses (for example, other chest pain) alone do not support medical necessity of these tests.

When monitoring long term anti-lipid dietary or pharmacologic therapy and when following patients with borderline high total or LDL cholesterol levels, it is reasonable to perform the lipid panel annually. A lipid panel at a yearly interval will usually be adequate while measurement of the serum total cholesterol or a measured LDL should suffice for interim visits if the patient does not have hypertriglyceridemia.

Any one component of the panel or a measured LDL may be medically necessary up to six times the first year for monitoring dietary or pharmacologic therapy. More frequent total cholesterol HDL cholesterol, LDL cholesterol and triglyceride testing may be indicated for marked elevations or for changes to anti-lipid therapy due to inadequate initial patient response to dietary or pharmacologic therapy. The LDL cholesterol or total cholesterol may be measured three times yearly after treatment goals have been achieved.

If no dietary or pharmacological therapy is advised, monitoring is not necessary.

When evaluating non-specific chronic abnormalities of the liver (for example, elevations of transaminase, alkaline phosphatase, abnormal imaging studies, etc.), a lipid panel would generally not be indicated more than twice per year

100-3, 190.24

Digoxin Therapeutic Drug Assay

Indications and Limitations of Coverage

Indications

Digoxin levels may be performed to monitor drug levels of individuals receiving digoxin therapy because the margin of safety between side effects and toxicity is narrow or because the blood level may not be high enough to achieve the desired clinical effect.

Clinical indications may include individuals on digoxin:

- With symptoms, signs or electrocardiogram (ECG) suggestive of digoxin toxicity.
- Taking medications that influence absorption, bioavailability, distribution, and/or elimination of digoxin.
- With impaired renal, hepatic, gastrointestinal, or thyroid function.
- With pH and/or electrolyte abnormalities.
- With unstable cardiovascular status, including myocarditis.
- Requiring monitoring of patient compliance.

Clinical indications may include individuals:

- Suspected of accidental or intended overdose.
- Who have an acceptable cardiac diagnosis (as listed) and for whom an accurate history of use of digoxin is unobtainable.

The value of obtaining regular serum digoxin levels is uncertain, but it may be reasonable to check levels once yearly after a steady state is achieved. In addition, it may be reasonable to check the level if:

- Heart failure status worsens.

- Renal function deteriorates.
- Additional medications are added that could affect the digoxin level.
- Signs or symptoms of toxicity develop.

Steady state will be reached in approximately 1 week in patients with normal renal function, although 2-3 weeks may be needed in patients with renal impairment. After changes in dosages or the addition of a medication that could affect the digoxin level, it is reasonable to check the digoxin level one week after the change or addition. Based on the clinical situation, in cases of digoxin toxicity, testing may need to be done more than once a week.

Digoxin is indicated for the treatment of patients with heart failure due to systolic dysfunction and for reduction of the ventricular response in patients with atrial fibrillation or flutter. Digoxin may also be indicated for the treatment of other supraventricular arrhythmias, particularly in the presence of heart failure.

Limitations

This test is not appropriate for patients on digitoxin or treated with digoxin FAB (fragment antigen binding) antibody.

100-3, 190.25

Alpha-fetoprotein (AFP)

Indications and Limitations of Coverage

AFP is useful for the diagnosis of hepatocellular carcinoma in high-risk patients (such as alcoholic cirrhosis, cirrhosis of viral etiology, hemochromatosis, and alpha 1-antitrypsin deficiency) and in separating patients with benign hepatocellular neoplasms or metastases from those with hepatocellular carcinoma and, as a non-specific tumor associated antigen, serves in marking germ cell neoplasms of the testis, ovary, retro peritoneum, and mediastinum.

100-3, 190.26

Carcinoembryonic Antigen (CEA)

Indications

CEA may be medically necessary for follow-up of patients with colorectal carcinoma. It would however only be medically necessary at treatment decision?making points. In some clinical situations (e.g. adenocarcinoma of the lung, small cell carcinoma of the lung, and some gastrointestinal carcinomas) when a more specific marker is not expressed by the tumor, CEA may be a medically necessary alternative marker for monitoring. Preoperative CEA may also be helpful in determining the post?operative adequacy of surgical resection and subsequent medical management. In general, a single tumor marker will suffice in following patients with colorectal carcinoma or other malignancies that express such tumor markers.

In following patients who have had treatment for colorectal carcinoma, ASCO guideline suggests that if resection of liver metastasis would be indicated, it is recommended that post-operative CEA testing be performed every two to three months in patients with initial stage II or stage III disease for at least two years after diagnosis.

For patients with metastatic solid tumors which express CEA, CEA may be measured at the start of the treatment and with subsequent treatment cycles to assess the tumor's response to therapy.

Limitations

Serum CEA determinations are generally not indicated more frequently than once per chemotherapy treatment cycle for patients with metastatic solid tumors which express CEA or every two months post-surgical treatment for patients who have had colorectal carcinoma. However, it may be proper to order the test more frequently in certain situations, for example, when there has been a significant change from prior CEA level or a significant change in patient status which could reflect disease progression or recurrence.

Testing with a diagnosis of an in situ carcinoma is not reasonably done more frequently than once, unless the result is abnormal, in which case the test may be repeated once.

100-3, 190.27

Human Chorionic Gonadotropin (hCG)

Indications and Limitations of Coverage

Indications

hCG is useful for monitoring and diagnosis of germ cell neoplasms of the ovary, testis, mediastinum, retroperitoneum, and central nervous system. In addition, hCG is useful for monitoring pregnant patients with vaginal bleeding, hypertension and/or suspected fetal loss.

Limitations

It is not reasonable and necessary to perform hCG testing more than once per month for diagnostic purposes. It may be performed as needed for monitoring of patient progress and treatment. Qualitative hCG assays are not appropriate for medically managing patients with known or suspected germ cell neoplasms.

100-3, 190.28

Tumor Antigen by Immunoassay - CA125

Indications

CA 125 is a high molecular weight serum tumor marker elevated in 80% of patients who present with epithelial ovarian carcinoma. It is also elevated in carcinomas of the fallopian tube, endometrium, and endocervix. An elevated level may also be associated with the presence of a malignant mesothelioma or primary peritoneal carcinoma.

A CA125 level may be obtained as part of the initial pre-operative work-up for women presenting with a suspicious pelvic mass to be used as a baseline for purposes of post-operative monitoring. Initial declines in CA 125 after initial surgery and/or chemotherapy for ovarian carcinoma are also measured by obtaining three serum levels during the first month post treatment to determine the patient's CA 125 half-life, which has significant prognostic implications.

The CA 125 levels are again obtained at the completion of chemotherapy as an index of residual disease. Surveillance CA125 measurements are generally obtained every 3 months for 2 years, every 6 months for the next 3 years, and yearly thereafter. CA 125 levels are also an important indicator of a patient's response to therapy in the presence of advanced or recurrent disease. In this setting, CA 125 levels may be obtained prior to each treatment cycle.

Limitations

These services are not covered for the evaluation of patients with signs or symptoms suggestive of malignancy. The service may be ordered at times necessary to assess either the presence of recurrent disease or the patient's response to treatment with subsequent treatment cycles.

The CA 125 is specifically not covered for aiding in the differential diagnosis of patients with a pelvic mass as the sensitivity and specificity of the test is not sufficient. In general, a single "tumor marker" will suffice in following a patient with one of these malignancies.

100-3, 190.29

Tumor Antigen by Immunoassay CA 15-3/CA 27.29

Indications

Multiple tumor markers are available for monitoring the response of certain malignancies to therapy and assessing whether residual tumor exists post-surgical therapy.

CA 15-3 is often medically necessary to aid in the management of patients with breast cancer. Serial testing must be used in conjunction with other clinical methods for monitoring breast cancer. For monitoring, if medically necessary, use consistently either CA 15-3 or CA 27.29, not both.

CA 27.29 is equivalent to CA 15-3 in its usage in management of patients with breast cancer.

Limitations

These services are not covered for the evaluation of patients with signs or symptoms suggestive of malignancy. The service may be ordered at times necessary to assess either the presence of recurrent disease or the patient's response to treatment with subsequent treatment cycles.

100-3, 190.30

Tumor Antigen by Immunoassay CA 19-9

Indications

Multiple tumor markers are available for monitoring the response of certain malignancies to therapy and assessing whether residual tumor exists post-surgical therapy.

Levels are useful in following the course of patients with established diagnosis of pancreatic and biliary ductal carcinoma. The test is not indicated for diagnosing these two diseases.

Limitations

These services are not covered for the evaluation of patients with signs or symptoms suggestive of malignancy. The service may be ordered at times necessary to assess either the presence of recurrent disease or the patient's response to treatment with subsequent treatment cycles.

100-3, 190.31

Prostate Specific Antigen (PSA)

Indications

PSA is of proven value in differentiating benign from malignant disease in men with lower urinary tract signs and symptoms (e.g., hematuria, slow urine stream, hesitancy, urgency, frequency, nocturia and incontinence) as well as with patients with palpably abnormal prostate glands on physician exam, and in patients with other laboratory or imaging studies that suggest the possibility of a malignant prostate disorder. PSA is also a marker used to follow the progress of prostate cancer once a diagnosis has been established, such as in detecting metastatic or persistent disease in patients who may require additional treatment. PSA testing may also be useful in the differential diagnosis of men presenting with as yet undiagnosed disseminated metastatic disease.

Limitations

Generally, for patients with lower urinary tract signs or symptoms, the test is performed only once per year unless there is a change in the patient's medical condition.

Testing with a diagnosis of in situ carcinoma is not reasonably done more frequently than once, unless the result is abnormal, in which case the test may be repeated once.

100-3, 190.32

Gamma Glutamyl Transferase (GGT)

Indications

1. To provide information about known or suspected hepatobiliary disease, for example:
   a. Following chronic alcohol or drug ingestion.
   b. Following exposure to hepatotoxins.
   c. When using medication known to have a potential for causing liver toxicity (e.g., following the drug manufacturer's recommendations).
   d. Following infection (e.g., viral hepatitis and other specific infections such as amoebiasis, tuberculosis, psittacosis, and similar infections).
2. To assess liver injury/function following diagnosis of primary or secondary malignant neoplasms.
3. To assess liver injury/function in a wide variety of disorders and diseases known to cause liver involvement (e.g., diabetes mellitus, malnutrition, disorders of iron and mineral metabolism, sarcoidosis, amyloidosis, lupus, and hypertension).
4. To assess liver function related to gastrointestinal disease.
5. To assess liver function related to pancreatic disease.
6. To assess liver function in patients subsequent to liver transplantation.
7. To differentiate between the different sources of elevated alkaline phosphatase activity.

Limitations

When used to assess liver dysfunction secondary to existing non-hepatobiliary disease with no change in signs, symptoms, or treatment, it is generally not necessary to repeat a GGT determination after a normal result has been obtained unless new indications are present.

If the GGT is the only "liver" enzyme abnormally high, it is generally not necessary to pursue further evaluation for liver disease for this specific indication.

When used to determine if other abnormal enzyme tests reflect liver abnormality rather than other tissue, it generally is not necessary to repeat a GGT more than one time per week.

Because of the extreme sensitivity of GGT as a marker for cytochrome oxidase induction or cell membrane permeability, it is generally not useful in monitoring patients with known liver disease.

100-3, 190.33

Hepatitis Panel/Acute Hepatitis Panel

Indications

1. To detect viral hepatitis infection when there are abnormal liver function test results, with or without signs or symptoms of hepatitis.
2. Prior to and subsequent to liver transplantation.

Limitations

After a hepatitis diagnosis has been established, only individual tests, rather than the entire panel, are needed.

100-3, 190.34

Fecal Occult Blood Test (FOBT)

NCD for Fecal Occult Blood Test (FOBT) (190.34)

Indications

1. To evaluate known or suspected alimentary tract conditions that might cause bleeding into the intestinal tract.
2. To evaluate unexpected anemia.
3. To evaluate abnormal signs, symptoms, or complaints that might be associated with loss of blood.
4. To evaluate patient complaints of black or red-tinged stools.

Limitations

1. The FOBT is reported once for the testing of up to three separate specimens (comprising either one or two tests per specimen).
2. In patients who are taking non-steroidal anti-inflammatory drugs and have a history of gastrointestinal bleeding but no other signs, symptoms, or complaints associated with gastrointestinal blood loss, testing for occult blood may generally be appropriate no more than once every three months.

When testing is done for the purpose of screening for colorectal cancer in the absence of signs, symptoms, conditions, or complaints associated with gastrointestinal blood loss, report the HCPCS code for colorectal cancer screening; fecal-occult blood test, 1-3 simultaneous determinations should be used.

100-3, 210.1

Prostate Cancer Screening Tests

Indications and Limitations of Coverage

CIM 50-55

Covered

A. General

Section 4103 of the Balanced Budget Act of 1997 provides for coverage of certain prostate cancer screening tests subject to certain coverage, frequency, and payment limitations. Medicare will cover prostate cancer screening tests/procedures for the early detection of prostate cancer. Coverage of prostate cancer screening tests includes the following procedures furnished to an individual for the early detection of prostate cancer:

- Screening digital rectal examination; and
- Screening prostate specific antigen blood test

B. Screening Digital Rectal Examinations

Screening digital rectal examinations are covered at a frequency of once every 12 months for men who have attained age 50 (at least 11 months have passed following the month in which the last Medicare-covered screening digital rectal examination was performed). Screening digital rectal examination means a clinical examination of an individual's prostate for nodules or other abnormalities of the prostate. This screening must be performed by a doctor of medicine or osteopathy (as defined in §1861(r)(1) of the Act), or by a physician assistant, nurse practitioner, clinical nurse specialist, or certified nurse midwife (as defined in §1861(aa) and §1861(gg) of the Act) who is authorized under State law to perform the examination, fully knowledgeable about the beneficiary's medical condition, and would be responsible for using the results of any examination performed in the overall management of the beneficiary's specific medical problem.

C. Screening Prostate Specific Antigen Tests

Screening prostate specific antigen tests are covered at a frequency of once every 12 months for men who have attained age 50 (at least 11 months have passed following the month in which the last Medicare-covered screening prostate specific antigen test was performed). Screening prostate specific antigen tests (PSA) means a test to detect the marker for adenocarcinoma of prostate. PSA is a reliable immunocytochemical marker for primary and metastatic adenocarcinoma of prostate. This screening must be ordered by the beneficiary's physician or by the beneficiary's physician assistant, nurse practitioner, clinical nurse specialist, or certified nurse midwife (the term "attending physician" is defined in §1861(r)(1) of the Act to mean a doctor of medicine or osteopathy and the terms "physician assistant, nurse practitioner, clinical nurse specialist, or certified nurse midwife" are defined in §1861(aa) and §1861(gg) of the Act) who is fully knowledgeable about the beneficiary's medical condition, and who would be responsible for using the results of any examination (test) performed in the overall management of the beneficiary's specific medical problem.

100-3, 210.2

Screening Pap Smears and Pelvic Examinations for Early Detection of Cervical or Vaginal Cancer

Indications and Limitations of Coverage

CIM 50-20.1

Screening Pap Smear

A screening pap smear and related medically necessary services provided to a woman for the early detection of cervical cancer (including collection of the sample of cells and a physician's interpretation of the test results) and pelvic examination (including clinical breast examination) are covered under Medicare Part B when ordered by a physician (or authorized practitioner) under one of the following conditions:

- She has not had such a test during the preceding two years or is a woman of childbearing age (§1861(nn) of the Act).
- There is evidence (on the basis of her medical history or other findings) that she is at high risk of developing cervical cancer and her physician (or authorized practitioner) recommends that she have the test performed more frequently than every two years.

High risk factors for cervical and vaginal cancer are:

- Early onset of sexual activity (under 16 years of age).
- Multiple sexual partners (five or more in a lifetime).
- History of sexually transmitted disease (including HIV infection).
- Fewer than three negative or any pap smears within the previous 7 years.; and
- DES (diethylstilbestrol) - exposed daughters of women who took DES during pregnancy.

NOTE: Claims for pap smears must indicate the beneficiary's low or high risk status by including the appropriate ICD-9-CM on the line item (Item 24E of the Form CMS-1500).

Definitions

- A woman as described in §1861(nn) of the Act is a woman who is of childbearing age and has had a pap smear test during any of the preceding three years that indicated the presence of cervical or vaginal cancer or other abnormality, or is at high risk of developing cervical or vaginal cancer.
- A woman of childbearing age is one who is premenopausal and has been determined by a physician or other qualified practitioner to be of childbearing age, based upon the medical history or other findings.
- Other qualified practitioner, as defined in 42 CFR 410.56(a) includes a certified nurse midwife (as defined in §1861(gg) of the Act), or a physician assistant, nurse practitioner, or clinical nurse specialist (as defined in §1861(aa) of the Act) who is authorized under State law to perform the examination.

Screening Pelvic Examination

Section 4102 of the Balanced Budget Act of 1997 provides for coverage of screening pelvic examinations (including a clinical breast examination) for all female beneficiaries, subject to certain frequency and other limitations. A screening pelvic examination (including a clinical breast examination) should include at least seven of the following eleven elements:

- Inspection and palpation of breasts for masses or lumps, tenderness, symmetry, or nipple discharge.
- Digital rectal examination including sphincter tone, presence of hemorrhoids, and rectal masses. Pelvic examination (with or without specimen collection for smears and cultures) including:
- External genitalia (for example, general appearance, hair distribution, or lesions).
- Urethral maetus (for example, size, location, lesions, or prolapse).
- Urethra (for example, masses, tenderness, or scarring).
- Bladder (for example, fullness, masses, or tenderness).
- Vagina (for example, general appearance, estrogen effect, discharge lesions, pelvic support, cystocele, or rectocele).
- Cervix (for example, general appearance, lesions, or discharge).
- Uterus (for example, size, contour, position, mobility, tenderness, consistency, descent, or support).
- Adnexa/parametria (for example, masses, tenderness, organomegaly, or nodularity).
- Anus and perineum.

This description is from Documentation Guidelines for Evaluation and Management Services, published in May 1997 and was developed by the Centers for Medicare and Medicaid Services and the American Medical Association.

100-3, 210.3

Colorectal Cancer Screening Tests

A. General

Section 4104 of the Balanced Budget Act of 1997 provides for coverage of screening colorectal cancer procedures under Medicare Part B. Medicare currently covers: (1) annual fecal occult blood tests (FOBTs); (2) flexible sigmoidoscopy over 4 years; (3) screening colonoscopy for persons at average risk for colorectal cancer every 10 years, or for persons at high risk for colorectal cancer every 2 years; (4) barium enema every 4 years as an alternative to flexible sigmoidoscopy, or every 2 years as an alternative to colonoscopy for persons at high risk for colorectal cancer; and, (5) other procedures the Secretary finds appropriate based on consultation with appropriate experts and organizations.

Coverage of the above screening examinations was implemented in regulations through a final rule that was published on October 31, 1997 (62 FR 59079), and was effective January 1, 1998. At that time, based on consultation with appropriate experts and organizations, the definition of the term "FOBT" was defined in 42 CFR Sec.410.37(a)(2) of the regulation to mean a "guaiac-based test for peroxidase activity, testing two samples from each of three consecutive stools."

In the 2003 Physician Fee Schedule Final Rule (67 FR 79966) effective March 1, 2003, the Centers for Medicare & Medicaid Services (CMS) amended the FOBT screening test regulation definition to provide that it could include either: (1) a guaiac-based FOBT, or, (2) other tests determined by the Secretary through a national coverage determination.

B. Nationally Covered Indications

Fecal Occult Blood Tests (FOBT) (effective for services performed on or after January 1, 2004)

1. History

   The FOBTs are generally divided into two types: immunoassay and guaiac types. Immunoassay (or immunochemical) fecal occult blood tests (iFOBT) use "antibodies directed against human globin epitopes. While most iFOBTs use spatulas to collect stool samples, some use a brush to collect toilet water surrounding the stool. Most iFOBTs require laboratory processing.

   Guaiac fecal occult blood tests (gFOBT) use a peroxidase reaction to indicate presence of the heme portion of hemoglobin. Guaiac turns blue after oxidation by oxidants or peroxidases in the presence of an oxygen donor such as hydrogen peroxide. Most FOBTs use sticks to collect stool samples and may be developed in a physician's office or a laboratory. In 1998, Medicare began reimbursement for guaiac FOBTs, but not immunoassay type tests for colorectal cancer screening.

   Since the fundamental process is similar for other iFOBTs, CMS evaluated colorectal cancer screening using immunoassay FOBTs in general.

2. Expanded Coverage

   Medicare covers one screening FOBT per annum for the early detection of colorectal cancer. This means that Medicare will cover one guaiac-based (gFOBT) or one immunoassay-based (iFOBT) at a frequency of every 12 months; i.e., at least 11 months have passed following the month in which the last covered screening FOBT was performed, for beneficiaries aged 50 years and older. The beneficiary completes the existing gFOBT by taking samples from two different sites of three consecutive stools; the beneficiary completes the iFOBT by taking the appropriate number of stool samples according to the specific manufacturer's instructions. This screening requires a written order from the beneficiary's attending physician. ("Attending physician means a doctor of medicine or osteopathy (as defined in Sec.1861(r)(1) of the Social Security Act) who is fully knowledgeable about the beneficiary's medical condition, and who would be responsible for using the results of any examination performed in the overall management of the beneficiary's specific medical problem.)

C. Nationally Non-Covered Indications

All other indications for colorectal cancer screening not otherwise specified above remain non-covered. Non-coverage specifically includes:

1. Screening DNA (Deoxyribonucleic acid) stool tests, effective April 28, 2008, and,
2. Screening computed tomographic colonography (CTC), effective May 12, 2009.

D. Other

N/A

(This NCD last reviewed May 2009.)

100-3, 210.4

Smoking and Tobacco-Use Cessation Counseling (Effective March 22, 2005)

(Rev. 36, Issued: 05-20-05; Effective: 03-22-05; Implementation: 07-05-05)

A. General

Tobacco use continues to be the leading cause of preventable death in the United States. In 1964, the Surgeon General of the U.S. Public Health Service (PHS) issued the report of his Advisory Committee on Smoking and Health, officially recognizing that cigarette smoking is a cause of cancer and other serious diseases. Though smoking rates have significantly declined, 9.3% of the population age 65 and older smokes cigarettes. Approximately 440,000 people die annually from smoking related disease, with 68% (300,000) age 65 or older. Many more people of all ages suffer from serious illness caused from smoking, leading to disability and decreased quality of life. Reduction in smoking prevalence is a national objective in Healthy People 2010.

B. Nationally Covered Indications

Effective March 22, 2005, the Centers for Medicare and Medicaid Services (CMS) has determined that the evidence is adequate to conclude that smoking and tobacco use cessation counseling, based on the current PHS Guideline, is reasonable and necessary for a patient with a disease or an adverse health effect that has been found by the U.S. Surgeon General to be linked to tobacco use, or who is taking a therapeutic agent whose metabolism or dosing is affected by tobacco use as based on FDA-approved information.

Patients must be competent and alert at the time that services are provided. Minimal counseling is already covered at each evaluation and management (E&M) visit. Beyond that, Medicare will cover 2 cessation attempts per year. Each attempt may include a maximum of 4 intermediate or intensive sessions, with the total annual benefit covering up to 8 sessions in a 12-month period. The practitioner and patient have flexibility to choose between intermediate or intensive cessation strategies for each attempt.

Intermediate and intensive smoking cessation counseling services will be covered for outpatient and hospitalized beneficiaries who are smokers and who qualify as above, as long as those services are furnished by qualified physicians and other Medicare-recognized practitioners.

C. Nationally Non-Covered Indications

Inpatient hospital stays with the principal diagnosis of Tobacco Use Disorder are not reasonable and necessary for the effective delivery of tobacco cessation counseling services. Therefore, we will not cover tobacco cessation services if tobacco cessation is the primary reason for the patient's hospital stay.

D. Other

N/A

(This NCD last reviewed May 2005.)

100-3, 210.10

Screening for Sexually Transmitted Infections (STIs) and High Intensity Behavioral Counseling (HIBC) to Prevent STIs

A. General

Sexually transmitted infections (STIs) are infections that are passed from one person to another through sexual contact. STIs remain an important cause of morbidity in the United States and have both health and economic consequences. Many of the complications of STIs are borne by women and children. Often, STIs do not present any symptoms so can go untreated for long periods of time The presence of an STI during pregnancy may result in significant health complications for the woman and infant. In fact, any person who has an STI may develop health complications. Screening tests for the STIs in this national coverage determination (NCD) are laboratory tests.

Under Section 1861(ddd) of the Social Security Act (the Act), the Centers for Medicare & Medicaid Services (CMS) has the authority to add coverage of additional preventive services if certain statutory requirements are met. The regulations provide:

Section 410.64 Additional preventive services

(a) Medicare Part B pays for additional preventive services not described in paragraph (1) or (3) of the definition of "preventive services" under section 410.2, that identify medical conditions or risk factors for individuals if the Secretary determines through the national coverage determination process (as defined in section 1869(f)(1)(B) of the Act) that these services are all of the following: (1) reasonable and necessary for the prevention or early detection of illness or disability.(2) recommended with a grade of A or B by the United States Preventive Services Task Force, (3) appropriate for individuals entitled to benefits under Part A or enrolled under Part B.

(b) In making determinations under paragraph (a) of this section regarding the coverage of a new preventive service, the Secretary may conduct an assessment of the relation between predicted outcomes and the expenditures for such services and may take into account the results of such an assessment in making such national coverage determinations.

The scope of the national coverage analysis for this NCD evaluated the evidence for the following STIs and high intensity behavioral counseling (HIBC) to prevent STIs for which the United States Preventive Services Task Force (USPSTF) has issued either an A or B recommendation.

- Screening for chlamydial infection for all sexually active non-pregnant young women aged 24 and younger and for older non-pregnant women who are at increased risk,
- Screening for chlamydial infection for all pregnant women aged 24 and younger and for older pregnant women who are at increased risk,
- Screening for gonorrhea infection in all sexually active women, including those who are pregnant, if they are at increased risk,
- Screening for syphilis infection for all pregnant women and for all persons at increased risk,
- Screening for hepatitis B virus (HBV) infection in pregnant women at their first prenatal visit,
- HIBC for the prevention of STIs for all sexually active adolescents, and for adults at increased risk for STIs.

B. Nationally Covered Indications

CMS has determined that the evidence is adequate to conclude that screening for chlamydia, gonorrhea, syphilis, and hepatitis B, as well as HIBC to prevent STIs, consistent with the grade A and B recommendations by the USPSTF, is reasonable and necessary for the early detection or prevention of an illness or disability and is appropriate for individuals entitled to benefits under Part A or enrolled under Part B.

Therefore, effective for claims with dates of services on or after November 8, 2011, CMS will cover screening for these USPSTF-indicated STIs with the appropriate Food and Drug Administration (FDA)-approved/cleared laboratory tests, used consistent with FDA-approved labeling, and in compliance with the Clinical Laboratory Improvement Act (CLIA) regulations, when ordered by the primary care physician or practitioner, and performed by an eligible Medicare provider for these services.

Screening for chlamydia and gonorrhea:

- Pregnant women who are 24 years old or younger when the diagnosis of pregnancy is known, and then repeat screening during the third trimester if high-risk sexual behavior has occurred since the initial screening test.
- Pregnant women who are at increased risk for STIs when the diagnosis of pregnancy is known, and then repeat screening during the third trimester if high-risk sexual behavior has occurred since the initial screening test.
- Women at increased risk for STIs annually. Screening for syphilis:
- Pregnant women when the diagnosis of pregnancy is known, and then repeat screening during the third trimester and at delivery if high-risk sexual behavior has occurred since the previous screening test.
- Men and women at increased risk for STIs annually.

Screening for hepatitis B:

- Pregnant women at the first prenatal visit when the diagnosis of pregnancy is known, and then rescreening at time of delivery for those with new or continuing risk factors.

In addition, effective for claims with dates of service on or after November 8, 2011, CMS will cover up to two individual 20- to 30-minute, face-to-face counseling sessions annually for Medicare beneficiaries for HIBC to prevent STIs, for all sexually active adolescents, and for adults at increased risk for STIs, if referred for this service by a primary care physician or practitioner, and provided by a Medicare eligible primary care provider in a primary care setting. Coverage of HIBC to prevent STIs is consistent with the USPSTF recommendation.

HIBC is defined as a program intended to promote sexual risk reduction or risk avoidance, which includes each of these broad topics, allowing flexibility for appropriate patient-focused elements:

- education,
- skills training,
- guidance on how to change sexual behavior.

The high/increased risk individual sexual behaviors, based on the USPSTF guidelines, include any of the following:

- Multiple sex partners
- Using barrier protection inconsistently
- Having sex under the influence of alcohol or drugs
- Having sex in exchange for money or drugs
- Age (24 years of age or younger and sexually active for women for chlamydia and gonorrhea)
- Having an STI within the past year
- IV drug use (for hepatitis B only)

In addition for men

- men having sex with men (MSM) and engaged in high risk sexual behavior, but no regard to age

In addition to individual risk factors, in concurrence with the USPSTF recommendations, community social factors such as high prevalence of STIs in the community populations should be considered in determining high/increased risk for chlamydia, gonorrhea, syphilis, and for recommending HIBC.

High/increased risk sexual behavior for STIs is determined by the primary care provider by assessing the patient's sexual history which is part of any complete medical history, typically part of an annual wellness visit or prenatal visit and considered in the development of a comprehensive prevention plan. The medical record should be a reflection of the service provided.

For the purposes of this NCD, a primary care setting is defined as the provision of integrated, accessible health care services by clinicians who are accountable for addressing a large majority of personal health care needs, developing a sustained partnership with patients, and practicing in the context of family and community. Emergency departments, inpatient hospital settings, ambulatory surgical centers, independent diagnostic testing facilities, skilled nursing facilities, inpatient rehabilitation facilities, clinics providing a limited focus of health care services, and hospice are examples of settings not considered primary care settings under this definition.

For the purposes of this NCD, a "primary care physician" and "primary care practitioner" will be defined based on existing sections of the Social Security Act (section 1833(u)(6), section 1833(x)(2)(A)(i)(I) and section 1833(x)(2)(A)(i)(II)).

Section 1833(u)

(6) Physician Defined. For purposes of this paragraph, the term "physician" means a physician described in section 1861(r)(1) and the term "primary care physician" means a physician who is identified in the available data as a general practitioner, family practice practitioner, general internist, or obstetrician or gynecologist.

Section 1833(x)(2)(A)(i)

(I) is a physician (as described in section 1861(r)(1)) who has a primary specialty designation of family medicine, internal medicine, geriatric medicine, or pediatric medicine; or

(II) is a nurse practitioner, clinical nurse specialist, or physician assistant (as those terms are defined in section 1861(aa)(5));

C. Nationally Non-Covered Indications

Unless specifically covered in this NCD, any other NCD, or in statute, preventive services are non-covered by Medicare.

D. Other

Medicare coinsurance and Part B deductible are waived for these preventive services.

HIBC to prevent STIs may be provided on the same date of services as an annual wellness visit, evaluation and management (E&M) service, or during the global billing period for obstetrical car, but only one HIBC may be provided on any one date of service. See the claims processing manual for further instructions on claims processing.

For services provided on an annual basis, this is defined as a 12-month period.

(This NCD last reviewed November 2011.)

100-3, 220.1

Computerized Tomography

A. General

Diagnostic examinations of the head (head scans) and of other parts of the body (body scans) performed by computerized tomography (CT) scanners are covered if you find that the medical and scientific literature and opinion support the effective use of a scan for the condition, and the scan is: (1) reasonable and necessary for the individual patient; and (2) performed on a model of CT equipment that meets the criteria in C below.

CT scans have become the primary diagnostic tool for many conditions and symptoms. CT scanning used as the primary diagnostic tool can be cost effective because it can eliminate the need for a series of other tests, is non-invasive and thus virtually eliminates complications, and does not require hospitalization.

B. Determining Whether a CT Scan Is Reasonable and Necessary
Sufficient information must be provided with claims to differentiate CT scans from other radiology services and to make coverage determinations. Carefully review claims to insure that a scan is reasonable and necessary for the individual patient; i.e., the use must be found to be medically appropriate considering the patient's symptoms and preliminary diagnosis.

There is no general rule that requires other diagnostic tests to be tried before CT scanning is used. However, in an individual case the contractor's medical staff may determine that use of a CT scan as the initial diagnostic test was not reasonable and necessary because it was not supported by the patient's symptoms or complaints stated on the claim form; e.g., "periodic headaches."

Claims for CT scans are reviewed for evidence of abuse which might include the absence of reasonable indications for the scans, an excessive number of scans or unnecessarily expensive types of scans considering the facts in the particular cases.

C-Approved Models of CT Equipment

1. Criteria for Approval

   In the absence of evidence to the contrary, you may assume that a CT scan for which payment is requested has been performed on equipment that meets the following criteria:

   a. The model must be known to the Food and Drug Administration, and

   b. Must be in the full market release phase of development.

   Should it be necessary to confirm that those criteria are met, ask the manufacturer to submit the information in subsection C.2. If manufacturers inquire about obtaining Medicare approval for their equipment, inform them of the foregoing criteria.

2. Evidence of Approval

   a. The letter sent by the Bureau of Radiological Health, Food and Drug Administration (FDA), to the manufacturer acknowledging the FDA's receipt of information on the specific CT scanner system model submitted as required under Public Law 90-602, "The Radiation Control for Health and Safety Act of 1968."

   b. A letter signed by the chief executive officer or other officer acting in a similar capacity for the manufacturer which:

      1) Furnishes the CT scanner system model number, all names that hospitals and physicians' offices may use to refer to the CT scanner system on claims, and the accession number assigned by FDA to the specific model;

      2) Specifies whether the scanner performs head scans only, body scans only (i.e., scans of parts of the body other than the head), or head and body scans;

      3) States that the company or corporation is satisfied with the results of the developmental stages that preceded the full market release phase of the equipment, that the equipment is in the full market release phase, and the date on which it was decided to put the product into the full market release phase.

D-Mobile CT Equipment
CT scans performed on mobile units are subject to the same Medicare coverage requirements applicable to scans performed on stationary units, as well as certain health and safety requirements recommended by PHS. As with scans performed on stationary units, the scans must be determined medically necessary for the individual patient. The scans must be performed on types of CT scanning equipment that have been approved for use as stationary units (see C above), and must be in compliance with applicable State laws and regulations for control of radiation.

1. Hospital Setting

   The hospital must assume responsibility for the quality of the scan furnished to inpatients and outpatients and must assure that a radiologist or other qualified physician is in charge of the procedure. The radiologist or other physician (i.e., one who is with the mobile unit) who is responsible for the procedure must be approved by the hospital for similar privileges.

2. Ambulatory Setting

   If mobile CT scan services are furnished at an ambulatory health care facility other than a hospital-based facility, e.g., a freestanding physician-directed clinic, the diagnostic procedure must be performed by or under the direct personal supervision of a radiologist or other qualified physician. In addition, the facility must maintain a record of the attending physician's order for a scan performed on a mobile unit.

3. Billing for Mobile CT Scans

   Hospitals, hospital-associated radiologists, ambulatory health care facilities, and physician owner/operators of mobile units may bill for mobile scans as they would for scans performed on stationary equipment.

4. Claims Review

   Evidence of compliance with applicable State laws and regulations for control of radiation should be requested from owners of mobile CT scan units upon receipt of the first claims. All mobile scan claims should be reviewed very carefully in accordance with instructions applicable to scans performed on fixed units, with particular emphasis on the medical necessity for scans performed in an ambulatory setting.

E-Multi-Planar Diagnostic Imaging (MPDI)
In usual computerized tomography (CT) scanning procedures, a series of transverse or axial images are reproduced. These transverse images are routinely translated into coronal and/or sagittal views. Multiplanar diagnostic imaging (MPDI) is a process which further translates the data produced by CT scanning by providing reconstructed oblique images which can contribute to diagnostic information. MPDI, also known as planar image reconstruction or reformatted imaging, is covered under Medicare when provided as a service to an entity performing a covered CT scan.

Magnetic Resonance Imaging

A. General

1. Method of Operation

   Magnetic Resonance Imaging (MRI), formerly called nuclear magnetic resonance (NMR), is a non-invasive method of graphically representing the distribution of water and other hydrogen-rich molecules in the human body. In contrast to conventional radiographs or computed tomography (CT) scans, in which the image is produced by x-ray beam attenuation by an object, MRI is capable of producing images by several techniques. In fact, various combinations of MRI image production methods may be employed to emphasize particular characteristics of the tissue or body part being examined. The basic elements by which MRI produces an image are the density of hydrogen nuclei in the object being examined, their motion, and the relaxation times, and the period of time required for the nuclei to return to their original states in the main, static magnetic field after being subjected to a brief additional magnetic field. These relaxation times reflect the physical-chemical properties of tissue and the molecular environment of its hydrogen nuclei. Only hydrogen atoms are present in human tissues in sufficient concentration for current use in clinical MRI.

   Magnetic Resonance Angiography (MRA) is a non-invasive diagnostic test that is an application of MRI. By analyzing the amount of energy released from tissues exposed to a strong magnetic field, MRA provides images of normal and diseased blood vessels, as well as visualization and quantification of blood flow through these vessels.

2. General Clinical Utility

   Overall, MRI is a useful diagnostic imaging modality that is capable of demonstrating a wide variety of soft-tissue lesions with contrast resolution equal or superior to CT scanning in various parts of the body.

   Among the advantages of MRI are the absence of ionizing radiation and the ability to achieve high levels of tissue contrast resolution without injected iodinated radiological contrast agents. Recent advances in technology have resulted in development and Food and Drug Administration (FDA) approval of new paramagnetic contrast agents for MRI which allow even better visualization in some instances. Multislice imaging and the ability to image in multiple planes, especially sagittal and coronal, have provided flexibility not easily available with other modalities. Because cortical (outer layer) bone and metallic prostheses do not cause distortion of MR images, it has been possible to visualize certain lesions and body regions with greater certainty than has been possible with CT. The use of MRI on certain soft tissue structures for the purpose of detecting disruptive, neoplastic, degenerative, or inflammatory lesions has now become established in medical practice.

   Phase contrast (PC) and time-of-flight (TOF) are some of the available MRA techniques at the time these instructions are being issued. PC measures the difference between the phases of proton spins in tissue and blood and measures both the venous and arterial blood flow at any point in the cardiac cycle. TOF measures the difference between the amount of magnetization of tissue and blood and provides information on the structure of blood vessels, thus indirectly indicating blood flow. Two-dimensional (2D) and three-dimensional (3D) images can be obtained using each method.

   Contrast-enhanced MRA (CE-MRA) involves blood flow imaging after the patient receives an intravenous injection of a contrast agent. Gadolinium, a non-ionic element, is the foundation of all contrast agents currently in use. Gadolinium affects the way in which tissues respond to magnetization, resulting in better visualization of structures when compared to un-enhanced studies. Unlike ionic (i.e., iodine-based) contrast agents used in conventional contrast angiography (CA), allergic reactions to gadolinium are extremely rare. Additionally, gadolinium does not cause the kidney failure occasionally seen with ionic contrast agents. Digital subtraction angiography (DSA) is a computer-augmented form of CA that obtains digital blood flow images as contrast agent courses through a blood vessel. The computer "subtracts" bone and other tissue from the image, thereby improving visualization of blood vessels. Physicians elect to use a specific MRA or CA technique based upon clinical information from each patient.

B. Nationally Covered MRI and MRA Indications

1. MRI

   Although several uses of MRI are still considered investigational and some uses are clearly contraindicated (see subsection C), MRI is considered medically efficacious for a number of uses. Use the following descriptions as general guidelines or examples of what may be considered covered rather than as a restrictive list of specific covered indications. Coverage is limited to MRI units that have received FDA premarket approval, and such units must be operated within the parameters specified by the approval. In addition, the services must be reasonable and necessary for the diagnosis or treatment of the specific patient involved.

a. Effective November 22, 1985, MRI is useful in examining the head, central nervous system, and spine. Multiple sclerosis can be diagnosed with MRI and the contents of the posterior fossa are visible. The inherent tissue contrast resolution of MRI makes it an appropriate standard diagnostic modality for general neuroradiology.

b. Effective November 22, 1985, MRI can assist in the differential diagnosis of mediastinal and retroperitoneal masses, including abnormalities of the large vessels such as aneurysms and dissection. When a clinical need exists to visualize the parenchyma of solid organs to detect anatomic disruption or neoplasia, this can be accomplished in the liver, urogenital system, adrenals, and pelvic organs without the use of radiological contrast materials. When MRI is considered reasonable and necessary, the use of paramagnetic contrast materials may be covered as part of the study. MRI may also be used to detect and stage pelvic and retroperitoneal neoplasms and to evaluate disorders of cancellous bone and soft tissues. It may also be used in the detection of pericardial thickening. Primary and secondary bone neoplasm and aseptic necrosis can be detected at an early stage and monitored with MRI. Patients with metallic prostheses, especially of the hip, can be imaged in order to detect the early stages of infection of the bone to which the prosthesis is attached.

c. Effective March 22, 1994, MRI may also be covered to diagnose disc disease without regard to whether radiological imaging has been tried first to diagnose the problem.

d. Effective March 4, 1991, MRI with gating devices and surface coils, and gating devices that eliminate distorted images caused by cardiac and respiratory movement cycles are now considered state of the art techniques and may be covered. Surface and other specialty coils may also be covered, as they are used routinely for high resolution imaging where small limited regions of the body are studied. They produce high signal-to-noise ratios resulting in images of enhanced anatomic detail.

2. MRA (MRI for Blood Flow)

Currently covered indications include using MRA for specific conditions to evaluate flow in internal carotid vessels of the head and neck, peripheral arteries of lower extremities, abdomen and pelvis, and the chest. Coverage is limited to MRA units that have received FDA premarket approval, and such units must be operated within the parameters specified by the approval. In addition, the services must be reasonable and necessary for the diagnosis or treatment of the specific patient involved.

a. Head and Neck

Effective April 15, 2003, studies have proven that MRA is effective for evaluating flow in internal carotid vessels of the head and neck. However, not all potential applications of MRA have been shown to be reasonable and necessary. All of the following criteria must apply in order for Medicare to provide coverage for MRA of the head and neck:

MRA is used to evaluate the carotid arteries, the circle of Willis, the anterior, middle or posterior cerebral arteries, the vertebral or basilar arteries or the venous sinuses;

MRA is performed on patients with conditions of the head and neck for which surgery is anticipated and may be found to be appropriate based on the MRA. These conditions include, but are not limited to, tumor, aneurysms, vascular malformations, vascular occlusion or thrombosis. Within this broad category of disorders, medical necessity is the underlying determinant of the need for an MRA in specific diseases. The medical records should clearly justify and demonstrate the existence of medical necessity; and

MRA and CA are not expected to be performed on the same patient for diagnostic purposes prior to the application of anticipated therapy. Only one of these tests will be covered routinely unless the physician can demonstrate the medical need to perform both tests.

b. Peripheral Arteries of Lower Extremities

Effective April 15, 2003, studies have proven that MRA of peripheral arteries is useful in determining the presence and extent of peripheral vascular disease in lower extremities. This procedure is non-invasive and has been shown to find occult vessels in some patients for which those vessels were not apparent when CA was performed. Medicare will cover either MRA or CA to evaluate peripheral arteries of the lower extremities. However, both MRA and CA may be useful in some cases, such as:

A patient has had CA and this test was unable to identify a viable run-off vessel for bypass. When exploratory surgery is not believed to be a reasonable medical course of action for this patient, MRA may be performed to identify the viable runoff vessel; or

A patient has had MRA, but the results are inconclusive.

c. Abdomen and Pelvis

i. Pre-operative Evaluation of Patients Undergoing Elective Abdominal Aortic Aneurysm (AAA) Repair

Effective July 1, 1999, MRA is covered for pre-operative evaluation of patients undergoing elective AAA repair if the scientific evidence reveals MRA is considered comparable to CA in determining the extent of AAA, as well as in evaluating aortoiliac occlusion disease and renal artery pathology that may be necessary in the surgical planning of AAA repair. These studies also reveal that MRA could provide a net benefit to the patient. If preoperative CA is avoided, then patients are not exposed to the risks associated with invasive procedures, contrast media, end-organ damage, or arterial injury.

ii. Imaging the Renal Arteries and the Aortoiliac Arteries in the Absence of AAA or Aortic Dissection

Effective July 1, 2003, MRA coverage is expanded to include imaging the renal arteries and the aortoiliac arteries in the absence of AAA or aortic dissection. MRA should be obtained in those circumstances in which using MRA is expected to avoid obtaining CA, when physician history, physical examination, and standard assessment tools provide insufficient information for patient management, and obtaining an MRA has a high probability of positively affecting patient management. However, CA may be ordered after obtaining the results of an MRA in those rare instances where medical necessity is demonstrated.

d. Chest

i. Diagnosis of Pulmonary Embolism

Current scientific data has shown that diagnostic pulmonary MRAs are improving due to recent developments such as faster imaging capabilities and gadolinium-enhancement. However, these advances in MRA are not significant enough to warrant replacement of pulmonary angiography in the diagnosis of pulmonary embolism for patients who have no contraindication to receiving intravenous iodinated contrast material. Patients who are allergic to iodinated contrast material face a high risk of developing complications if they undergo pulmonary angiography or computed tomography angiography. Therefore, Medicare will cover MRA of the chest for diagnosing a suspected pulmonary embolism when it is contraindicated for the patient to receive intravascular iodinated contrast material.

ii. Evaluation of Thoracic Aortic Dissection and Aneurysm

Studies have shown that MRA of the chest has a high level of diagnostic accuracy for pre-operative and post-operative evaluation of aortic dissection of aneurysm. Depending on the clinical presentation, MRA may be used as an alternative to other non-invasive imaging technologies, such as transesophageal echocardiography and CT. Generally, Medicare will provide coverage only for MRA or for CA when used as a diagnostic test. However, if both MRA and CA of the chest are used, the physician must demonstrate the medical need for performing these tests.

While the intent of this policy is to provide reimbursement for either MRA or CA, CMS is also allowing flexibility for physicians to make appropriate decisions concerning the use of these tests based on the needs of individual patients. CMS anticipates, however, low utilization of the combined use of MRA and CA. As a result, CMS encourages contractors to monitor the use of these tests and, where indicated, require evidence of the need to perform both MRA and CA.

C. Contraindications and Nationally Non-Covered Indications

1. Contraindications

The MRI is not covered when the following patient-specific contraindications are present:

MRI is not covered for patients with cardiac pacemakers or with metallic clips on vascular aneurysms unless the Medicare beneficiary meets the provisions of the following exceptions:

Effective July 7, 2011, the contraindications will not apply to pacemakers when used according to the FDA-approved labeling in an MRI environment, or

Effective February 24, 2011, CMS believes that the evidence is promising although not yet convincing that MRI will improve patient health outcomes if certain safeguards are in place to ensure that the exposure of the device to an MRI environment adversely affects neither the interpretation of the MRI result nor the proper functioning of the implanted device itself. We believe that specific precautions (as listed below) could maximize benefits of MRI exposure for beneficiaries enrolled in clinical trials designed to assess the utility and safety of MRI exposure. Therefore, CMS determines that MRI will be covered by Medicare when provided in a clinical study under section 1862(a)(1)(E) (consistent with section 1142 of the Act) through the Coverage with Study Participation (CSP) form of Coverage with Evidence Development (CED) if the study meets the criteria in each of the three paragraphs below:

The approved prospective clinical study of MRI must, with appropriate methodology, address one or more aspects of the following questions:

1. Do results of MRI in implanted permanent pacemaker (PM)/implantable cardioverter defibrillator (ICD) beneficiaries with implanted cardiac devices affect physician decision making related to: a. Clinical management strategy (e.g., in oncology, toward palliative or curative care)?

   b. Planning of treatment interventions?; or

   c. Prevention of unneeded diagnostic studies or interventions, or preventable exposures?

2. Do results of MRI in PM/ICD beneficiaries with implanted cardiac devices affect patient outcomes related to:

a. Survival?
b. Quality of life?; or
c. Adverse events during and after MR scanning?

In addition, the prospective clinical study of MRI must include safety criteria for all participants. Such required safety measures for such studies, as further explained in guidance documents from professional societies must include, but are not limited to:

1. MRI should be done on a case-by-case and site-by-site basis.
2. MRI scan sequences, field intensity, and field(s) of exposure should be selected to minimize risk to the patient while gaining needed diagnostic information for diagnosis or for managing therapy.
3. MRI scanning should be done only if the site is staffed with individuals with the appropriate radiology and cardiology knowledge and expertise on hand.
4. Implanted device patients who are candidates for recruitment for an MRI clinical study should be advised that life-threatening arrhythmias might occur during MRI and serious device malfunction might occur, requiring replacement of the device.
5. Radiology and cardiology personnel and a fully stocked crash cart should be readily available throughout the procedure in case a significant arrhythmia develops during the examination that does not terminate with the cessation of the MRI study. The cardiologist should be familiar with the patient's arrhythmia history and the implanted device. A programmer that can be used to adjust the device as necessary should be readily available.
6. All such patients should be actively monitored for cardiac and respiratory function throughout the examination. At a minimum, ECG and pulse oximetry should be used. Visual and verbal contact with the patient must be maintained throughout the MRI scan. The patient should be instructed to alert the MRI staff on hand to any unusual sensations, pains, or to any problems.
7. At the conclusion of the examination, the cardiologist should examine the device to confirm that the function is consistent with its pre-examination state.
8. Follow-up should include a check of the patient's device at a time remote (1,Äì6 weeks) after the scan to confirm appropriate function.
9. If the implanted device manufacturer has indicated additional safety precautions appropriate for safe MRI performance, these must be included in the study protocol.

   The clinical study must adhere to the following standards of scientific integrity and relevance to the Medicare population:

   a. The principal purpose of the research study is to test whether a particular intervention potentially improves the participants' health outcomes.
   b. The research study is well supported by available scientific and medical information or it is intended to clarify or establish the health outcomes of interventions already in common clinical use.
   c. The research study does not unjustifiably duplicate existing studies.
   d. The research study design is appropriate to answer the research question being asked in the study.
   e. The research study is sponsored by an organization or individual capable of executing the proposed study successfully.
   f. The research study is in compliance with all applicable Federal regulations concerning the protection of human subjects found at 45 CFR Part 46. If a study is regulated by the FDA, it must be in compliance with 21 CFR Parts 50 and 56.
   g. All aspects of the research study are conducted according to appropriate standards of scientific integrity (see http://www.icmje.org).
   h. The research study has a written protocol that clearly addresses, or incorporates by reference, the standards listed here as Medicare requirements for CED coverage.
   i. The clinical research study is not designed to exclusively test toxicity or disease pathophysiology in healthy individuals. Trials of all medical technologies measuring therapeutic outcomes as one of the objectives meet this standard only if the disease or condition being studied is life threatening as defined in 21 CFR § 312.81(a) and the patient has no other viable treatment options.
   j. The clinical research study is registered on the ClinicalTrials.gov website by the principal sponsor/investigator prior to the enrollment of the first study subject.
   k. The research study protocol specifies the method and timing of public release of all pre-specified outcomes to be measured, including release of outcomes if outcomes are negative or study is terminated early. The results must be made public within 24 months of the end of data collection. If a report is planned to be published in a peer reviewed journal, then that initial release may be an abstract that meets the requirements of the International Committee of Medical Journal Editors (http://www.icmje.org). However, a full report of the outcomes must be made public no later than three (3) years after the end of data collection.
   l. The research study protocol must explicitly discuss subpopulations affected by the treatment under investigation, particularly traditionally underrepresented groups in clinical studies, how the inclusion and exclusion criteria effect enrollment of these populations, and a plan for the retention and reporting of said populations in the trial. If the inclusion and exclusion criteria are expected to have a negative effect on the recruitment or retention of underrepresented populations, the protocol must discuss why these criteria are necessary.
   m. The research study protocol explicitly discusses how the results are or are not expected to be generalizable to the Medicare population to infer whether Medicare patients may benefit from the intervention. Separate discussions in the protocol may be necessary for populations eligible for Medicare due to age, disability, or Medicaid eligibility.

Consistent with section 1142 of the Act, the Agency for Healthcare Research and Quality (AHRQ) supports clinical research studies that CMS determines meet the above-listed standards and address the above-listed research questions.

- MRI during a viable pregnancy is also contraindicated at this time.
- The danger inherent in bringing ferromagnetic materials within range of MRI units generally constrains the use of MRI on acutely ill patients requiring life support systems and monitoring devices that employ ferromagnetic materials.
- In addition, the long imaging time and the enclosed position of the patient may result in claustrophobia, making patients who have a history of claustrophobia unsuitable candidates for MRI procedures.

2. Nationally Non-Covered Indications

   CMS has determined that MRI of cortical bone and calcifications, and procedures involving spatial resolution of bone and calcifications, are not considered reasonable and necessary indications within the meaning of section 1862(a)(1)(A) of the Act, and are therefore non-covered.

D. Other

Effective June 3, 2010, all other uses of MRI or MRA for which CMS has not specifically indicated coverage or non-coverage continue to be eligible for coverage through individual local contractor discretion.

(This NCD last reviewed July 2011.)

100-3, 220.2

Magnetic Resonance Imaging (MRI) (Various Effective Dates Below)

(Rev. 135, Issued: 09-22-11, Effective: 07-07-11/02-24-11(CR 7296), Implementation: 09-26-11)

A. General

1. Method of Operation

Magnetic Resonance Imaging (MRI), formerly called nuclear magnetic resonance (NMR), is a non-invasive method of graphically representing the distribution of water and other hydrogen-rich molecules in the human body. In contrast to conventional radiographs or computed tomography (CT) scans, in which the image is produced by x- ray beam attenuation by an object, MRI is capable of producing images by several techniques. In fact, various combinations of MRI image production methods may be employed to emphasize particular characteristics of the tissue or body part being examined. The basic elements by which MRI produces an image are the density of hydrogen nuclei in the object being examined, their motion, and the relaxation times, and the period of time required for the nuclei to return to their original states in the main, static magnetic field after being subjected to a brief additional magnetic field. These relaxation times reflect the physical-chemical properties of tissue and the molecular environment of its hydrogen nuclei. Only hydrogen atoms are present in human tissues in sufficient concentration for current use in clinical MRI.

Magnetic Resonance Angiography (MRA) is a non-invasive diagnostic test that is an application of MRI. By analyzing the amount of energy released from tissues exposed to a strong magnetic field, MRA provides images of normal and diseased blood vessels, as well as visualization and quantification of blood flow through these vessels.

2. General Clinical Utility

Overall, MRI is a useful diagnostic imaging modality that is capable of demonstrating a wide variety of soft-tissue lesions with contrast resolution equal or superior to CT scanning in various parts of the body.

Among the advantages of MRI are the absence of ionizing radiation and the ability to achieve high levels of tissue contrast resolution without injected iodinated radiological contrast agents. Recent advances in technology have resulted in development and Food and Drug Administration (FDA) approval of new paramagnetic contrast agents for MRI which allow even better visualization in some instances. Multislice imaging and the ability to image in multiple planes, especially sagittal and coronal, have provided flexibility not easily available with other modalities. Because cortical (outer layer) bone and metallic prostheses do not cause distortion of MR images, it has been possible to visualize certain lesions and body regions with greater certainty than has been possible with CT. The use of MRI on certain soft tissue structures for the purpose of detecting disruptive, neoplastic, degenerative, or inflammatory lesions has now become established in medical practice.

Phase contrast (PC) and time-of-flight (TOF) are some of the available MRA techniques at the time these instructions are being issued. PC measures the difference between the phases of proton spins in tissue and blood and measures both the venous and arterial blood flow at any point in the cardiac cycle. TOF measures the difference between the amount of magnetization of tissue and blood and provides information on the structure of blood vessels, thus indirectly indicating blood flow. Two-dimensional (2D) and three- dimensional (3D) images can be obtained using each method.

Contrast-enhanced MRA (CE-MRA) involves blood flow imaging after the patient receives an intravenous injection of a contrast agent. Gadolinium, a non-ionic element, is the foundation of all contrast agents currently in use. Gadolinium affects the way in which tissues respond to magnetization, resulting in better visualization of structures when compared to un-enhanced studies. Unlike ionic (i.e., iodine-based) contrast agents used in conventional contrast angiography (CA), allergic reactions to gadolinium are extremely rare. Additionally, gadolinium does not cause the kidney failure occasionally seen with ionic contrast agents. Digital subtraction angiography (DSA) is a computer- augmented form of CA that obtains digital blood flow images as contrast agent courses through a blood vessel. The computer "subtracts" bone and other tissue from the image, thereby improving visualization of blood vessels. Physicians elect to use a specific MRA or CA technique based upon clinical information from each patient.

B. Nationally Covered MRI and MRA Indications

1. MRI

Although several uses of MRI are still considered investigational and some uses are clearly contraindicated (see subsection C), MRI is considered medically efficacious for a number of uses. Use the following descriptions as general guidelines or examples of what may be considered covered rather than as a restrictive list of specific covered indications. Coverage is limited to MRI units that have received FDA premarket approval, and such units must be operated within the parameters specified by the approval. In addition, the services must be reasonable and necessary for the diagnosis or treatment of the specific patient involved.

a. Effective November 22, 1985, MRI is useful in examining the head, central nervous system, and spine. Multiple sclerosis can be diagnosed with MRI and the contents of the posterior fossa are visible. The inherent tissue contrast resolution of MRI makes it an appropriate standard diagnostic modality for general neuroradiology.

b. Effective November 22, 1985, MRI can assist in the differential diagnosis of mediastinal and retroperitoneal masses, including abnormalities of the large vessels such as aneurysms and dissection. When a clinical need exists to visualize the parenchyma of solid organs to detect anatomic disruption or neoplasia, this can be accomplished in the liver, urogenital system, adrenals, and pelvic organs without the use of radiological contrast materials. When MRI is considered reasonable and necessary, the use of paramagnetic contrast materials may be covered as part of the study. MRI may also be used to detect and stage pelvic and retroperitoneal neoplasms and to evaluate disorders of cancellous bone and soft tissues. It may also be used in the detection of pericardial thickening. Primary and secondary bone neoplasm and aseptic necrosis can be detected at an early stage and monitored with MRI. Patients with metallic prostheses, especially of the hip, can be imaged in order to detect the early stages of infection of the bone to which the prosthesis is attached.

c. Effective March 22, 1994, MRI may also be covered to diagnose disc disease without regard to whether radiological imaging has been tried first to diagnose the problem.

d. Effective March 4, 1991, MRI with gating devices and surface coils, and gating devices that eliminate distorted images caused by cardiac and respiratory movement cycles are now considered state of the art techniques and may be covered. Surface and other specialty coils may also be covered, as they are used routinely for high resolution imaging where small limited regions of the body are studied. They produce high signal-to-noise ratios resulting in images of enhanced anatomic detail.

Currently covered indications include using MRA for specific conditions to evaluate flow in internal carotid vessels of the head and neck, peripheral arteries of lower extremities, abdomen and pelvis, and the chest. Coverage is limited to MRA units that have received FDA premarket approval, and such units must be operated within the parameters specified by the approval. In addition, the services must be reasonable and necessary for the diagnosis or treatment of the specific patient involved.

a. Head and Neck
Effective April 15, 2003, studies have proven that MRA is effective for evaluating flow in internal carotid vessels of the head and neck. However, not all potential applications of MRA have been shown to be reasonable and necessary. All of the following criteria must apply in order for Medicare to provide coverage for MRA of the head and neck:

- MRA is used to evaluate the carotid arteries, the circle of Willis, the anterior, middle or posterior cerebral arteries, the vertebral or basilar arteries or the venous sinuses;
- MRA is performed on patients with conditions of the head and neck for which surgery is anticipated and may be found to be appropriate based on the MRA. These conditions include, but are not limited to, tumor, aneurysms, vascular malformations, vascular occlusion or thrombosis. Within this broad category of disorders, medical necessity is the underlying determinant of the need for an MRA in specific diseases. The medical records should clearly justify and demonstrate the existence of medical necessity; and
- MRA and CA are not expected to be performed on the same patient for diagnostic purposes prior to the application of anticipated therapy. Only one of these tests will be covered routinely unless the physician can demonstrate the medical need to perform both tests.

b. Peripheral Arteries of Lower Extremities
Effective April 15, 2003, studies have proven that MRA of peripheral arteries is useful in determining the presence and extent of peripheral vascular disease in lower extremities. This procedure is non-invasive and has been shown to find occult vessels in some patients for which those vessels were not apparent when CA was performed. Medicare will cover either MRA or CA to evaluate peripheral arteries of the lower extremities. However, both MRA and CA may be useful in some cases, such as:

- A patient has had CA and this test was unable to identify a viable run-off vessel for bypass. When exploratory surgery is not believed to be a reasonable medical course of action for this patient, MRA may be performed to identify the viable runoff vessel; or
- A patient has had MRA, but the results are inconclusive.

c. Abdomen and Pelvis

i. Pre-operative Evaluation of Patients Undergoing Elective Abdominal Aortic Aneurysm (AAA) Repair

Effective July 1, 1999, MRA is covered for pre-operative evaluation of patients undergoing elective AAA repair if the scientific evidence reveals MRA is considered comparable to CA in determining the extent of AAA, as well as in evaluating aortoiliac occlusion disease and renal artery pathology that may be necessary in the surgical planning of AAA repair. These studies also reveal that MRA could provide a net benefit to the patient. If preoperative CA is avoided, then patients are not exposed to the risks associated with invasive procedures, contrast media, end-organ damage, or arterial injury.

ii. Imaging the Renal Arteries and the Aortoiliac Arteries in the Absence of AAA or Aortic Dissection

Effective July 1, 2003, MRA coverage is expanded to include imaging the renal arteries and the aortoiliac arteries in the absence of AAA or aortic dissection. MRA should be obtained in those circumstances in which using MRA is expected to avoid obtaining CA, when physician history, physical examination, and standard assessment tools provide insufficient information for patient management, and obtaining an MRA has a high probability of positively affecting patient management. However, CA may be ordered after obtaining the results of an MRA in those rare instances where medical necessity is demonstrated.

d. Chest

i. Diagnosis of Pulmonary Embolism

Current scientific data has shown that diagnostic pulmonary MRAs are improving due to recent developments such as faster imaging capabilities and gadolinium-enhancement. However, these advances in MRA are not significant enough to warrant replacement of pulmonary angiography in the diagnosis of pulmonary embolism for patients who have no contraindication to receiving intravenous iodinated contrast material. Patients who are allergic to iodinated contrast material face a high risk of developing complications if they undergo pulmonary angiography or computed tomography angiography. Therefore, Medicare will cover MRA of the chest for diagnosing a suspected pulmonary embolism when it is contraindicated for the patient to receive intravascular iodinated contrast material.

ii. Evaluation of Thoracic Aortic Dissection and Aneurysm

Studies have shown that MRA of the chest has a high level of diagnostic accuracy for pre-operative and post-operative evaluation of aortic dissection of aneurysm. Depending on the clinical presentation, MRA may be used as an alternative to other non-invasive imaging technologies, such as transesophageal echocardiography and CT. Generally, Medicare will provide coverage only for MRA or for CA when used as a diagnostic test. However, if both MRA and CA of the chest are used, the physician must demonstrate the medical need for performing these tests.

While the intent of this policy is to provide reimbursement for either MRA or CA, CMS is also allowing flexibility for physicians to make appropriate decisions concerning the use of these tests based on the needs of individual patients. CMS anticipates, however, low utilization of the combined use of MRA and CA. As a result, CMS encourages contractors to monitor the use of these tests and, where indicated, require evidence of the need to perform both MRA and CA.

C. Contraindications and Nationally Non-Covered Indications

1. Contraindications

The MRI is not covered when the following patient-specific contraindications are present:

MRI is not covered for patients with cardiac pacemakers or with metallic clips on vascular aneurysms unless the Medicare beneficiary meets the provisions of the following exceptions:

Effective July 7, 2011, the contraindications will not apply to pacemakers when used according to the FDA-approved labeling in an MRI environment, or

Effective February 24, 2011, CMS believes that the evidence is promising although not yet convincing that MRI will improve patient health outcomes if certain safeguards are in place to ensure that the exposure of the device to an MRI environment adversely affects neither the interpretation of the MRI result nor the proper functioning of the implanted device itself. We believe that specific precautions (as listed below) could maximize benefits of MRI exposure for beneficiaries enrolled in clinical trials designed to assess the utility and safety of MRI exposure. Therefore, CMS determines that MRI will be covered by Medicare when provided in a clinical study under section 1862(a)(1)(E) (consistent with section 1142 of the Act) through the Coverage with Study Participation (CSP) form of Coverage with Evidence Development (CED) if the study meets the criteria in each of the three paragraphs below:

The approved prospective clinical study of MRI must, with appropriate methodology, address one or more aspects of the following questions:

1. Do results of MRI in implanted permanent pacemaker (PM)/implantable cardioverter defibrillator (ICD) beneficiaries with implanted cardiac devices affect physician decision making related to:
   a. Clinical management strategy (e.g., in oncology, toward palliative or curative care)?
   b. Planning of treatment interventions?; or
   c. Prevention of unneeded diagnostic studies or interventions, or preventable exposures?
2. Do results of MRI in PM/ICD beneficiaries with implanted cardiac devices affect patient outcomes related to:
   a. Survival?
   b. Quality of life?; or
   c. Adverse events during and after MR scanning?

In addition, the prospective clinical study of MRI must include safety criteria for all participants. Such required safety measures for such studies, as further explained in guidance documents from professional societies must include, but are not limited to:

1. MRI should be done on a case-by-case and site-by-site basis.
2. MRI scan sequences, field intensity, and field(s) of exposure should be selected to minimize risk to the patient while gaining needed diagnostic information for diagnosis or for managing therapy.
3. MRI scanning should be done only if the site is staffed with individuals with the appropriate radiology and cardiology knowledge and expertise on hand.
4. Implanted device patients who are candidates for recruitment for an MRI clinical study should be advised that life-threatening arrhythmias might occur during MRI and serious device malfunction might occur, requiring replacement of the device.
5. Radiology and cardiology personnel and a fully stocked crash cart should be readily available throughout the procedure in case a significant arrhythmia develops during the examination that does not terminate with the cessation of the MRI study. The cardiologist should be familiar with the patient's arrhythmia history and the implanted device. A programmer that can be used to adjust the device as necessary should be readily available.
6. All such patients should be actively monitored for cardiac and respiratory function throughout the examination. At a minimum, ECG and pulse oximetry should be used. Visual and verbal contact with the patient must be maintained throughout the MRI scan. The patient should be instructed to alert the MRI staff on hand to any unusual sensations, pains, or to any problems.
7. At the conclusion of the examination, the cardiologist should examine the device to confirm that the function is consistent with its pre-examination state.
8. Follow-up should include a check of the patient's device at a time remote (1–6 weeks) after the scan to confirm appropriate function.
9. If the implanted device manufacturer has indicated additional safety precautions appropriate for safe MRI performance, these must be included in the study protocol.

   The clinical study must adhere to the following standards of scientific integrity and relevance to the Medicare population:

   a. The principal purpose of the research study is to test whether a particular intervention potentially improves the participants' health outcomes.
   b. The research study is well supported by available scientific and medical information or it is intended to clarify or establish the health outcomes of interventions already in common clinical use.
   c. The research study does not unjustifiably duplicate existing studies.
   d. The research study design is appropriate to answer the research question being asked in the study.
   e. The research study is sponsored by an organization or individual capable of executing the proposed study successfully.
   f. The research study is in compliance with all applicable Federal regulations concerning the protection of human subjects found at 45 CFR Part 46. If a study is regulated by the FDA, it must be in compliance with 21 CFR Parts 50 and 56.
   g. All aspects of the research study are conducted according to appropriate standards of scientific integrity (see http://www.icmje.org).
   h. The research study has a written protocol that clearly addresses, or incorporates by reference, the standards listed here as Medicare requirements for CED coverage.
   i. The clinical research study is not designed to exclusively test toxicity or disease pathophysiology in healthy individuals. Trials of all medical technologies measuring therapeutic outcomes as one of the objectives meet this standard only if the disease or condition being studied is life threatening as defined in 21 CFR §312.81(a) and the patient has no other viable treatment options.
   j. The clinical research study is registered on the ClinicalTrials.gov website by the principal sponsor/investigator prior to the enrollment of the first study subject.
   k. The research study protocol specifies the method and timing of public release of all pre-specified outcomes to be measured, including release of outcomes if outcomes are negative or study is terminated early. The results must be made public within 24 months of the end of data collection. If a report is planned to be published in a peer reviewed journal, then that initial release may be an abstract that meets the requirements of the International Committee of Medical Journal Editors (http://www.icmje.org). However, a full report of the outcomes must be made public no later than three (3) years after the end of data collection.
   l. The research study protocol must explicitly discuss subpopulations affected by the treatment under investigation, particularly traditionally underrepresented groups in clinical studies, how the inclusion and exclusion criteria effect enrollment of these populations, and a plan for the retention and reporting of said populations in the trial. If the inclusion and exclusion criteria are expected to have a negative effect on the recruitment or retention of underrepresented populations, the protocol must discuss why these criteria are necessary.
   m. The research study protocol explicitly discusses how the results are or are not expected to be generalizable to the Medicare population to infer whether Medicare patients may benefit from the intervention. Separate discussions in the protocol may be necessary for populations eligible for Medicare due to age, disability, or Medicaid eligibility.

   Consistent with section 1142 of the Act, the Agency for Healthcare Research and Quality (AHRQ) supports clinical research studies that CMS determines meet the above-listed standards and address the above-listed research questions.

   - MRI during a viable pregnancy is also contraindicated at this time.
   - The danger inherent in bringing ferromagnetic materials within range of MRI units generally constrains the use of MRI on acutely ill patients requiring life support systems and monitoring devices that employ ferromagnetic materials.
   - In addition, the long imaging time and the enclosed position of the patient may result in claustrophobia, making patients who have a history of claustrophobia unsuitable candidates for MRI procedures.

2. Nationally Non-Covered Indications

CMS has determined that MRI of cortical bone and calcifications, and procedures involving spatial resolution of bone and calcifications, are not considered reasonable and necessary indications within the meaning of section 1862(a)(1)(A) of the Act, and are therefore non-covered.

D. Other

Effective June 3, 2010, all other uses of MRI or MRA for which CMS has not specifically indicated coverage or non-coverage continue to be eligible for coverage through individual local contractor discretion.

(This NCD last reviewed July 2011.)

100-3, 220.2.1

Magnetic Resonance Spectroscopy

(Rev. 21, Issued: 09-10-04, Effective: 09-10-04, Implementation: 09-10-04)

A. General

Magnetic Resonance Spectroscopy (MRS) is an application of magnetic resonance imaging (MRI). It is a non-invasive diagnostic test that uses strong magnetic fields to measure and analyze the chemical composition of human tissues. On March 22, 1994, CMS considered MRS an investigational procedure and issued a national noncoverage determination for all indications of MRS.

B. Nationally Covered Indications

Not applicable.

C. Nationally Noncovered Indications

After thorough review and reconsideration of the existing national noncoverage determination for MRS, as well as the available evidence for the use of MRS as a diagnostic tool for distinguishing indeterminate brain lesions, and/or as an aid in conducting brain biopsies, CMS has determined that the evidence is not adequate to conclude that MRS is reasonable and necessary within the meaning of section 1862(a)(1)(A) of the Social Security Act, for use in the diagnosis of brain tumors. Therefore, CMS reaffirms its current national noncoverage determination for all indications of MRS.

D. Other

Not applicable.

(This NCD last reviewed September 2004.)

100-3, 220.4 - Mammograms

(Rev. 1, 10-03-03) CIM 50-21

A diagnostic mammography is a radiologic procedure furnished to a man or woman with signs and symptoms of breast disease, or a personal history of breast cancer, or a personal history of biopsy – proven benign breast disease, and includes a physician's interpretation of the results of the procedure. A diagnostic mammography is a covered service if it is ordered by a doctor of medicine or osteopathy as defined in §1861 (r) (1) of the Act. A screening mammography is a radiologic procedure furnished to a woman without signs or symptoms of breast disease, for the purpose of early detection of breast cancer, and includes a physician's interpretation of the results of the procedure. A screening mammography has limitations as it must be, at a minimum a two-view exposure (cranio- caudal and a medial lateral oblique view) of each breast. Payment may not be made for a screening mammography performed on a woman under age 35. Payment may be made for only one screening mammography performed on a woman over age 34, but under age 40. For an asymptomatic woman over age 39, payment may be made for a screening mammography performed after at least 11 months have passed following the month in which the last screening mammography was performed.

A radiological mammogram is a covered diagnostic test under the following conditions:

- A patient has distinct signs and symptoms for which a mammogram is indicated;
- A patient has a history of breast cancer; or
- A patient is asymptomatic but, on the basis of the patient's history and other factors the physician considers significant, the physician's judgment is that a mammogram is appropriate.

Use of mammograms in routine screening of: (1) asymptomatic women aged 50 and over, and (2) asymptomatic women aged 40 or over whose mothers or sisters have had the disease, is considered medically appropriate, but would not be covered for Medicare purposes.

Cross-reference:

The Medicare Benefit Policy Manual, Chapter 15, "Covered Medical and Other Health Services," §80.

The Medicare Benefit Policy Manual, Chapter 1, "Inpatient Hospital Services," §50

100-3, 220.5

Ultrasound Diagnostic Procedures

A. General

Ultrasound diagnostic procedures utilizing low energy sound waves are being widely employed to determine the composition and contours of nearly all body tissues except bone and air-filled spaces. This technique permits noninvasive visualization of even the deepest structures in the body. The use of the ultrasound technique is sufficiently developed that it can be considered essential to good patient care in diagnosing a wide variety of conditions.

Ultrasound diagnostic procedures are listed below and are divided into two categories. Medicare coverage is extended to the procedures listed in Category I. Periodic claims review by the intermediary's medical consultants should be conducted to ensure that the techniques are medically appropriate and the general indications specified in these categories are met. Techniques in Category II are considered experimental and should not be covered at this time.

Indications and Limitations of Coverage

B. Nationally Covered Indications

Category I - (Clinically effective, usually part of initial patient evaluation, may be an adjunct to radiologic and nuclear medicine diagnostic technique)

- Echoencephalography, (Diencephalic Midline) (A-Mode).
- Echoencephalography, Complete (Diencephalic Midline and Ventricular Size).
- Ocular and Orbital Echography (A-Mode).
- Covered procedures include efforts to determine the suitability of aphakic patients for implantation of an artificial lens (pseudophakoi) following cataract surgery.
- Ocular and Orbital Sonography (B-Mode).
- Echocardiography, Pericardial Effusion (M-Mode).
- Pericardiocentesis, by Ultrasonic Guidance.
- Echocardiography, Cardiac Valve(s) (M-Mode).
- Echocardiography, Complete (M-Mode).
- Echocardiography, limited (e.g., follow-up or limited study) (M-Mode).
- Pleural Effusion Echography.
- Thoracentesis, by Ultrasonic Guidance.
- Abdominal Sonography, complete survey study (B-Scan).
- Abdominal Sonography, limited (e.g., follow-up or limited study) (B-Scan).
- Abdominal Sonography is not synonymous with ultrasound examination of individual organs.
- Renal Cyst Aspiration, by Ultrasonic Guidance.
- Renal Biopsy, by Ultrasonic Guidance.
- Pancreas Sonography (B-Scan).
- Pancreatic Sonography has proven effective in diagnosing pseudocysts.
- Spleen Sonography (B-Scan).
- Abdominal Aorta Echography (A-Mode).
- Abdominal Aorta Sonography (B-Scan).
- Retroperitoneal Sonography (B-Scan).
- Retroperitoneal Sonography does not include planning of fields for radiation therapy.
- Urinary Bladder Sonography (B-Scan).
- Urinary bladder Sonography does not include staging of bladder tumors.
- Pregnancy Diagnosis Sonography (B-Scan).
- Fetal Age Determination (Biparietal Diameter) Sonography (B-Scan).
- Fetal Growth Rate Sonography (B-Scan).
- Placenta Localization Sonography (B-Scan).
- Pregnancy Sonography, Complete (B-Scan).
- Molar Pregnancy Diagnosis Sonography (B-Scan).
- Ectopic Pregnancy Diagnosis Sonography (B-Scan).
- Passive Testing (Antepartum Monitoring of Fetal Heart Rate In the Resting Fetus).
- Intrauterine Contraceptive Device Sonography (B-Scan).
- Pelvic Mass Diagnosis Sonography (B-Scan).
- Amniocentesis, by Ultrasonic Guidance.
- Arterial Flow Study, Peripheral (Doppler).
- Venous Flow Study, Peripheral (Doppler).
- Arterial Aneurysm, Peripheral (B-Scan).
- Radiation Therapy Planning Sonography (B-Scan).
- Thyroid Echography (A-Mode).
- Thyroid Sonography (B-Scan).
- Breast Echography (A-Mode).
- Breast Sonography (B-Scan).
- Hepatic Sonography (B-Scan).
- Gallbladder Sonography.
- Renal Sonography.
- Two-Dimensional Echocardiography (B-Mode).
- Monitoring of cardiac output(Esophageal Doppler) for ventilated patients in the ICU and operative patients with a need for intra-operative fluid optimization

C. Nationally Non-Covered Indications

Category II - (Clinical reliability and efficacy not proven):

- B-Scan for atherosclerotic narrowing of peripheral arteries.

D. Other

Uses for ultrasound diagnostic procedures not listed in Category I or II above are left to local contractor discretion. In view of the rapid changes in the field of ultrasound diagnosis, uses for ultrasound diagnostic procedures other than those listed under Categories I and II should be carefully reviewed before payment. Medical justification may be required.

(This NCD last reviewed June 2007.)

100-3, 220.6

Positron Emission Tomography (PET) Scans

Item/Service Description Positron Emission Tomography (PET) is a minimally invasive diagnostic imaging procedure used to evaluate metabolism in normal tissue as well as in diseased tissues in conditions such as cancer, ischemic heart disease, and some neurologic disorders. A radiopharmaceutical is injected into the patient that gives off sub-atomic particles, known as positrons, as it decays. PET uses a positron camera (tomograph) to measure the decay of the radiopharmaceutical. The rate of decay provides biochemical information on the metabolism of the tissue being studied. (This NCD last reviewed March 2009.)

100-3, 220.6.1

PET for Perfusion of the Heart

Indications and Limitations of Coverage

1. Rubidium 82 (Effective March 14, 1995)
   Effective for services performed on or after March 14, 1995, PET scans performed at rest or with pharmacological stress used for noninvasive imaging of the perfusion of the heart for the diagnosis and management of patients with known or suspected coronary artery disease using the FDA-approved radiopharmaceutical Rubidium 82 (Rb 82) are covered, provided the requirements below are met:

   The PET scan, whether at rest alone, or rest with stress, is performed in place of, but not in addition to, a single photon emission computed tomography (SPECT); or

   The PET scan, whether at rest alone or rest with stress, is used following a SPECT that was found to be inconclusive. In these cases, the PET scan must have been considered necessary in order to determine what medical or surgical intervention is required to treat the patient. (For purposes of this requirement, an inconclusive test is a test(s) whose results are equivocal, technically uninterpretable, or discordant with a patient's other clinical data and must be documented in the beneficiary's file.)

   For any PET scan for which Medicare payment is claimed for dates of services prior to July 1, 2001, the claimant must submit additional specified information on the claim form (including proper codes and/or modifiers), to indicate the results of the PET scan. The claimant must also include information on whether the PET scan was performed after an inconclusive noninvasive cardiac test. The information submitted with respect to the previous noninvasive cardiac test must specify the type of test performed prior to the PET scan and whether it was inconclusive or unsatisfactory. These explanations are in the form of special G codes used for billing PET scans using Rb 82. Beginning July 1, 2001, claims should be submitted with the appropriate codes.
2. Ammonia N-13 (Effective October 1, 2003)
   Effective for services performed on or after October 1, 2003, PET scans performed at rest or with pharmacological stress used for noninvasive imaging of the perfusion of the heart for the diagnosis and management of patients with known or suspected coronary artery disease using the FDA-approved radiopharmaceutical ammonia N-13 are covered, provided the requirements below are met:

   The PET scan, whether at rest alone, or rest with stress, is performed in place of, but not in addition to, a SPECT; or

   The PET scan, whether at rest alone or rest with stress, is used following a SPECT that was found to be inconclusive. In these cases, the PET scan must have been considered necessary in order to determine what medical or surgical intervention is required to treat the patient. (For purposes of this requirement, an inconclusive test is a test whose results are equivocal, technically uninterpretable, or discordant with a patient's other clinical data and must be documented in the beneficiary's file.)

   (This NCD last reviewed March 2005.)

100-3, 220.6.8

PET (FDG) for Myocardial Viability

1. FDG PET is covered for the determination of myocardial viability following an inconclusive single photon emission computed tomography (SPECT) test from July 1, 2001, through September 30, 2002. Only full ring PET scanners are covered from July 1, 2001, through December 31, 2001. However, as of January 1, 2002, full and partial ring scanners are covered.
2. Beginning October 1, 2002, Medicare covers FDG PET for the determination of myocardial viability as a primary or initial diagnostic study prior to revascularization, or following an inconclusive SPECT. Studies performed by full and partial ring scanners are covered.

Limitations

In the event a patient receives a SPECT test with inconclusive results, a PET scan may be covered. However, if a patient receives a FDG PET study with inconclusive results, a follow up SPECT test is not covered.

Documentation that these conditions are met should be maintained by the referring physician in the beneficiary's medical record, as is normal business practice.

(This NCD last reviewed September 2002.)

100-3, 220.6.9

FDG PET for Refractory Seizures (Effective July 1, 2001)

Beginning July 1, 2001, Medicare covers FDG PET for pre-surgical evaluation for the purpose of localization of a focus of refractory seizure activity.

Limitations: Covered only for pre-surgical evaluation.

Documentation that these conditions are met should be maintained by the referring physician in the beneficiary's medical record, as is normal business practice.

(This NCD last reviewed June 2001.)

100-3, 220.6.10

PET (FDG) for Breast Cancer

220.6.10 - FDG PET for Breast Cancer (Effective October 1, 2002) (Replaced with Section 220.6.17)

100-3, 220.6.11

PET (FDG) for Thyroid Cancer

220.6.11 - FDG PET for Thyroid Cancer (Various Effective Dates Below) (Replaced with Section 220.6.17)

100-3, 220.6.12

PET (FDG) for Soft Tissue Sarcoma

220.6.12 - FDG PET for Soft Tissue Sarcoma (Various Effective Dates Below) (Replaced with Section 220.6.17)

100-3, 220.6.13

PET (FDG) for Dementia and Neurodegenerative Diseases

A. General

Medicare covers FDG PET scans for either the differential diagnosis of fronto-temporal dementia (FTD) and Alzheimer's disease (AD) under specific requirements; OR, its use in a Centers for Medicare & Medicaid Services (CMS)-approved practical clinical trial focused on the utility of FDG PET in the diagnosis or treatment of dementing neurodegenerative diseases. Specific requirements for each indication are clarified below:

B. Nationally Covered Indications

1. FDG PET Requirements for Coverage in the Differential Diagnosis of AD and FTD

An FDG PET scan is considered reasonable and necessary in patients with a recent diagnosis of dementia and documented cognitive decline of at least 6 months, who meet diagnostic criteria for both AD and FTD. These patients have been evaluated for specific alternate neurodegenerative diseases or other causative factors, but the cause of the clinical symptoms remains uncertain.

The following additional conditions must be met before an FDG PET scan will be covered:

a. The patient's onset, clinical presentation, or course of cognitive impairment is such that FTD is suspected as an alternative neurodegenerative cause of the cognitive decline. Specifically, symptoms such as social disinhibition, awkwardness, difficulties with language, or loss of executive function are more prominent early in the course of FTD than the memory loss typical of AD;

b. The patient has had a comprehensive clinical evaluation (as defined by the American Academy of Neurology (AAN)) encompassing a medical history from the patient and a well-acquainted informant (including assessment of activities of daily living), physical and mental status examination (including formal documentation of cognitive decline occurring over at least 6 months) aided by cognitive scales or neuropsychological testing, laboratory tests, and structural imaging such as magnetic resonance imaging (MRI) or computed tomography (CT);

c. The evaluation of the patient has been conducted by a physician experienced in the diagnosis and assessment of dementia;

d. The evaluation of the patient did not clearly determine a specific neurodegenerative disease or other cause for the clinical symptoms, and information available through FDG PET is reasonably expected to help clarify the diagnosis between FTD and AD and help guide future treatment;

e. The FDG PET scan is performed in a facility that has all the accreditation necessary to operate nuclear medicine equipment. The reading of the scan should be done by an expert in nuclear medicine, radiology, neurology, or psychiatry, with experience interpreting such scans in the presence of dementia;

f. A brain single photon emission computed tomography (SPECT) or FDG PET scan has not been obtained for the same indication. (The indication can be considered to be different in patients who exhibit important changes in scope or severity of cognitive decline, and meet all other qualifying criteria listed above and below (including the judgment that the likely diagnosis remains uncertain). The results of a prior SPECT or FDG PET scan must have been inconclusive or, in the case of SPECT, difficult to interpret due to immature or inadequate technology. In these instances, an FDG PET scan may be covered after 1 year has passed from the time the first SPECT or FDG PET scan was performed.)

g The referring and billing provider(s) have documented the appropriate evaluation of the Medicare beneficiary. Providers should establish the medical necessity of an FDG PET scan by ensuring that the following information has been collected and is maintained in the beneficiary medical record:

- Date of onset of symptoms;
- Diagnosis of clinical syndrome (normal aging; mild cognitive impairment (MCI);
- mild, moderate or severe dementia);
- Mini mental status exam (MMSE) or similar test score;

- Presumptive cause (possible, probable, uncertain AD);
- Any neuropsychological testing performed;
- Results of any structural imaging (MRI or CT) performed;
- Relevant laboratory tests (B12, thyroid hormone); and,
- Number and name of prescribed medications.

The billing provider must furnish a copy of the FDG PET scan result for use by CMS and its contractors upon request. These verification requirements are consistent with federal requirements set forth in 42 Code of Federal Regulations section 410.32 generally for diagnostic x-ray tests, diagnostic laboratory tests, and other tests. In summary, section 410.32 requires the billing physician and the referring physician to maintain information in the medical record of each patient to demonstrate medical necessity [410.32(d) (2)] and submit the information demonstrating medical necessity to CMS and/or its agents upon request [410.32(d)(3)(I)] (OMB number 0938-0685).

2. FDG PET Requirements for Coverage in the Context of a CMS-approved Practical Clinical Trial Utilizing a Specific Protocol to Demonstrate the Utility of FDG PET in the Diagnosis, and Treatment of Neurodegenerative Dementing Diseases An FDG PET scan is considered reasonable and necessary in patients with MCI or early dementia (in clinical circumstances other than those specified in subparagraph 1) only in the context of an approved clinical trial that contains patient safeguards and protections to ensure proper administration, use and evaluation of the FDG PET scan.

   The clinical trial must compare patients who do and do not receive an FDG PET scan and have as its goal to monitor, evaluate, and improve clinical outcomes. In addition, it must meet the following basic criteria:

   a. Written protocol on file;
   b. Institutional Review Board review and approval;
   c. Scientific review and approval by two or more qualified individuals who are not part of the research team; and,
   d. Certification that investigators have not been disqualified.

C. Nationally Non-Covered Indications

All other uses of FDG PET for patients with a presumptive diagnosis of dementia-causing neurodegenerative disease (e.g., possible or probable AD, clinically typical FTD, dementia of Lewy bodies, or Creutzfeld-Jacob disease) for which CMS has not specifically indicated coverage continue to be non-covered.

D. Other

Not applicable.

(This NCD last reviewed September 2004.)

100-3, 220.6.14

PET (FDG) for Brain, Cervical, Ovarian, Pancreatic, Small Cell Lung, and Testicular Cancers

See section 220.6.17

100-3, 220.6.17

Positron Emission Tomography (FDG) for Oncologic Conditions

A. General

FDG (2-[F18] fluoro-2-deoxy-D-glucose) Positron Emission Tomography (PET) is a minimally-invasive diagnostic imaging procedure used to evaluate glucose metabolism in normal tissue as well as in diseased tissues in conditions such as cancer, ischemic heart disease, and some neurologic disorders. FDG is an injected radionuclide (or radiopharmaceutical) that emits sub-atomic particles, known as positrons, as it decays. FDG PET uses a positron camera (tomograph) to measure the decay of FDG. The rate of FDG decay provides biochemical information on glucose metabolism in the tissue being studied. As malignancies can cause abnormalities of metabolism and blood flow, FDG PET evaluation may indicate the probable presence or absence of a malignancy based upon observed differences in biologic activity compared to adjacent tissues.

The Centers for Medicare and Medicaid Services (CMS) was asked by the National Oncologic PET Registry (NOPR) to reconsider section 220.6 of the National Coverage Determinations (NCD) Manual to end the prospective data collection requirements under Coverage with Evidence Development (CED) across all oncologic indications of FDG PET imaging. The CMS received public input indicating that the current coverage framework of prospective data collection under CED be ended for all oncologic uses of FDG PET imaging.

1. Framework

   Effective for claims with dates of service on and after June 11, 2013, CMS is adopting a coverage framework that ends the prospective data collection requirements by NOPR under CED for all oncologic uses of FDG PET imaging. CMS is making this change for all NCDs that address coverage of FDG PET for oncologic uses addressed in this decision. This decision does not change coverage for any use of PET imaging using radiopharmaceuticals NaF-18 (fluorine-18 labeled sodium fluoride), ammonia N-13, or rubidium-82 (Rb-82).

2. Initial Anti-Tumor Treatment Strategy

   CMS continues to believe that the evidence is adequate to determine that the results of FDG PET imaging are useful in determining the appropriate initial anti-tumor treatment strategy for beneficiaries with suspected cancer and improve health outcomes and thus are reasonable and necessary under Sec.1862(a)(1)(A) of the Social Security Act (the Act).

   Therefore, CMS continues to nationally cover one FDG PET study for beneficiaries who have cancers that are biopsy proven or strongly suspected based on other diagnostic testing when the beneficiary's treating physician determines that the FDG PET study is needed to determine the location and/or extent of the tumor for the following therapeutic purposes related to the initial anti-tumor treatment strategy:

   To determine whether or not the beneficiary is an appropriate candidate for an invasive diagnostic or therapeutic procedure; or

   To determine the optimal anatomic location for an invasive procedure; or

   To determine the anatomic extent of tumor when the recommended anti-tumor treatment reasonably depends on the extent of the tumor.

   See the table at the end of this section for a synopsis of all nationally covered and non-covered oncologic uses of FDG PET imaging.

B.1. Initial Anti-Tumor Treatment Strategy Nationally Covered Indications

a. CMS continues to nationally cover FDG PET imaging for the initial anti-tumor treatment strategy for male and female breast cancer only when used in staging distant metastasis.

b. CMS continues to nationally cover FDG PET to determine initial anti-tumor treatment strategy for melanoma other than for the evaluation of regional lymph nodes.

c. CMS continues to nationally cover FDG PET imaging for the detection of pre-treatment metastasis (i.e., staging) in newly diagnosed cervical cancers.

d. **C.1 Initial Anti-Tumor Treatment Strategy Nationally Non-Covered Indications**

   a. CMS continues to nationally non-cover initial anti-tumor treatment strategy in Medicare beneficiaries who have adenocarcinoma of the prostate.

   b. CMS continues to nationally non-cover FDG PET imaging for diagnosis of breast cancer and initial staging of axillary nodes.

   c. CMS continues to nationally non-cover FDG PET imaging for initial anti-tumor treatment strategy for the evaluation of regional lymph nodes in melanoma.

   d. CMS continues to nationally non-cover FDG PET imaging for the diagnosis of cervical cancer related to initial anti-tumor treatment strategy.

3. Subsequent Anti-Tumor Treatment Strategy

B.2. Subsequent Anti-Tumor Treatment Strategy Nationally Covered Indications

Three FDG PET scans are nationally covered when used to guide subsequent management of anti-tumor treatment strategy after completion of initial anti-cancer therapy. Coverage of more than three FDG PET scans to guide subsequent management of anti-tumor treatment strategy after completion of initial anti-cancer therapy shall be determined by the local Medicare Administrative Contractors.

4. Synopsis of Coverage of FDG PET for Oncologic Conditions

   Effective for claims with dates of service on and after June 11, 2013, the chart below summarizes national FDG PET coverage for oncologic conditions:

FDG PET for Cancers Tumor Type	Initial Treatment Strategy (formerly "diagnosis" & "staging")	Subsequent Treatment Strategy (formerly "restaging" & "monitoring response to treatment"
Colorectal	Cover	Cover
Esophagus	Cover	Cover
Head & Neck (not Thyroid, CNS)	Cover	Cover
Lymphoma	Cover	Cover
Non-Small Cell Lung	Cover	Cover
Ovary	Cover	Cover
Brain	Cover	Cover
Cervix	Cover w/exception*	Cover
Small Cell Lung	Cover	Cover
Soft Tissue Sarcoma	Cover	Cover
Pancreas	Cover	Cover
Testes	Cover	Cover
Prostate	Non-cover	Cover

FDG PET for Cancers Tumor Type	Initial Treatment Strategy (formerly "diagnosis" & "staging")	Subsequent Treatment Strategy (formerly "restaging" & "monitoring response to treatment"
Thyroid	Cover	Cover
Breast (male and female)	Cover w/exception*	Cover
Melanoma	Cover w/exception*	Cover
All Other Solid Tumors	Cover	Cover
Myeloma	Cover	Cover
All other cancers not listed	Cover	Cover

*Cervix: Nationally non-covered for the initial diagnosis of cervical cancer related to initial anti-tumor treatment strategy. All other indications for initial anti-tumor treatment strategy for cervical cancer are nationally covered.

*Breast: Nationally non-covered for initial diagnosis and/or staging of axillary lymph nodes. Nationally covered for initial staging of metastatic disease. All other indications for initial anti-tumor treatment strategy for breast cancer are nationally covered.

*Melanoma: Nationally non-covered for initial staging of regional lymph nodes. All other indications for initial anti-tumor treatment strategy for melanoma are nationally covered.

D. Other

N/A

100-3, 220.6.19

Positron Emission Tomography NaF-18 (NaF-18 PET) to Identify Bone Metastasis of Cancer (Effective February 26, 2010)

A. General

Positron Emission Tomography (PET) is a non-invasive, diagnostic imaging procedure that assesses the level of metabolic activity and perfusion in various organ systems of the body. A positron camera (tomograph) is used to produce cross-sectional tomographic images, which are obtained from positron-emitting radioactive tracer substances (radiopharmaceuticals) such as

F-18 sodium fluoride. NaF-18 PET has been recognized as an excellent technique for imaging areas of altered osteogenic activity in bone. The clinical value of detecting and assessing the initial extent of metastatic cancer in bone is attested by a number of professional guidelines for oncology. Imaging to detect bone metastases is also recommended when a patient, following completion of initial treatment, is symptomatic with bone pain suspicious for metastases from a known primary tumor.

B. Nationally Covered Indications

Effective February 26, 2010, the Centers for Medicare & Medicaid Services (CMS) will cover NaF-18 PET imaging when the beneficiary's treating physician determines that the NaF-18 PET study is needed to inform to inform the initial antitumor treatment strategy or to guide subsequent antitumor treatment strategy after the completion of initial treatment, and when the beneficiary is enrolled in, and the NaF-18 PET provider is participating in, the following type of prospective clinical study:

A NaF-18 PET clinical study that is designed to collect additional information at the time of the scan to assist in initial antitumor treatment planning or to guide subsequent treatment strategy by the identification, location and quantification of bone metastases in beneficiaries in whom bone metastases are strongly suspected based on clinical symptoms or the results of other diagnostic studies. Qualifying clinical studies must ensure that specific hypotheses are addressed; appropriate data elements are collected; hospitals and providers are qualified to provide the PET scan and interpret the results; participating hospitals and providers accurately report data on all enrolled patients not included in other qualifying trials through adequate auditing mechanisms; and all patient confidentiality, privacy, and other Federal laws must be followed.

The clinical studies for which Medicare will provide coverage must answer one or more of the following questions:

Prospectively, in Medicare beneficiaries whose treating physician determines that the NaF-18 PET study results are needed to inform the initial antitumor treatment strategy or to guide subsequent antitumor treatment strategy after the completion of initial treatment, does the addition of NaF-18 PET imaging lead to:

A change in patient management to more appropriate palliative care; or A change in patient management to more appropriate curative care; or Improved quality of life; or Improved survival?

The study must adhere to the following standards of scientific integrity and relevance to the Medicare population:

a. The principal purpose of the research study is to test whether a particular intervention potentially improves the participants' health outcomes.

b. The research study is well-supported by available scientific and medical information or it is intended to clarify or establish the health outcomes of interventions already in common clinical use.

c. The research study does not unjustifiably duplicate existing studies.

d. The research study design is appropriate to answer the research question being asked in the study.

e. The research study is sponsored by an organization or individual capable of executing the proposed study successfully.

f. The research study is in compliance with all applicable Federal regulations concerning the protection of human subjects found in the Code of Federal Regulations (CFR) at 45 CFR Part 46. If a study is regulated by the Food and Drug Administration (FDA), it also must be in compliance with 21 CFR Parts 50 and 56.

g. All aspects of the research study are conducted according to the appropriate standards of scientific integrity.

h. The research study has a written protocol that clearly addresses, or incorporates by reference, the Medicare standards.

i. The clinical research study is not designed to exclusively test toxicity or disease pathophysiology in healthy individuals. Trials of all medical technologies measuring therapeutic outcomes as one of the objectives meet this standard only if the disease or condition being studied is life-threatening as defined in 21 CFR Sec.312.81(a) and the patient has no other viable treatment options.

j. The clinical research study is registered on the www.ClinicalTrials.gov Web site by the principal sponsor/investigator prior to the enrollment of the first study subject.

k. The research study protocol specifies the method and timing of public release of all pre-specified outcomes to be measured including release of outcomes if outcomes are negative or study is terminated early. The results must be made public within 24 months of the end of data collection. If a report is planned to be published in a peer-reviewed journal, then that initial release may be an abstract that meets the requirements of the International Committee of Medical Journal Editors. However, a full report of the outcomes must be made public no later than three (3) years after the end of data collection.

l. The research study protocol must explicitly discuss subpopulations affected by the treatment under investigation, particularly traditionally underrepresented groups in clinical studies, how the inclusion and exclusion criteria affect enrollment of these populations, and a plan for the retention and reporting of said populations on the trial. If the inclusion and exclusion criteria are expected to have a negative effect on the recruitment or retention of underrepresented populations, the protocol must discuss why these criteria are necessary.

m. The research study protocol explicitly discusses how the results are or are not expected to be generalizable to the Medicare population to infer whether Medicare patients may benefit from the intervention. Separate discussions in the protocol may be necessary for populations eligible for Medicare due to age, disability or Medicaid eligibility.

Consistent with section 1142 of the Social Security Act (the Act), the Agency for Healthcare Research and Quality (AHRQ) supports clinical research studies that the Centers for Medicare and Medicaid Services (CMS) determines meet the above-listed standards and address the above-listed research questions.

C. Nationally Non-Covered Indications

Effective February 26, 2010, CMS determines that the evidence is not sufficient to determine that the results of NaF-18 PET imaging to identify bone metastases improve health outcomes of beneficiaries with cancer and is not reasonable and necessary under Sec.1862(a)(1)(A) of the Act unless it is to inform initial antitumor treatment strategy or to guide subsequent antitumor treatment strategy after completion of initial treatment, and then only under CED. All other uses and clinical indications of NaF-18 PET are nationally non-covered.

D. Other

The only radiopharmaceutical diagnostic imaging agents covered by Medicare for PET cancer imaging are 2-[F-18] Fluoro-D-Glucose (FDG) and NaF-18 (sodium fluoride-18). All other PET radiopharmaceutical diagnostic imaging agents are non-covered for this indication.

(This NCD was last reviewed in February 2010.)

100-3, 220.6.20

Beta Amyloid Positron Emission Tomography in Dementia and Neurodegenerative Disease

A. The Centers for Medicare & Medicaid Services (CMS) has determined that the evidence is insufficient to conclude that the use of positron emission tomography (PET) beta amyloid (also referred to as amyloid-beta (Aß)) imaging is reasonable and necessary for the diagnosis or treatment of illness or injury or to improve the functioning of a malformed body member for Medicare beneficiaries with dementia or neurodegenerative disease, and thus PET Aß imaging is not covered under §1862(a)(1)(A) of the Social Security Act (" the Act").

B. However, there is sufficient evidence that the use of PET Aß imaging is promising in two scenarios: (1) to exclude Alzheimer's disease (AD) in narrowly defined and clinically difficult differential diagnoses, such as AD versus frontotemporal dementia (FTD); and (2) to enrich clinical trials seeking better treatments or prevention strategies for AD, by allowing for selection of patients on the basis of biological as well as clinical and epidemiological factors.

Therefore, we will cover one PET Aß scan per patient through coverage with evidence development (CED), under §1862(a)(1)(E) of the Act, in clinical studies that meet the criteria in each of the paragraphs below.

Clinical study objectives must be to (1) develop better treatments or prevention strategies for AD, or, as a strategy to identify subpopulations at risk for developing AD, or (2) resolve clinically difficult differential diagnoses (e.g., frontotemporal dementia (FTD) versus AD) where the use of PET Aß imaging appears to improve health outcomes. These may include short term outcomes related to changes in management as well as longer term dementia outcomes.

Clinical studies must be approved by CMS, involve subjects from appropriate populations, and be comparative and longitudinal. Where appropriate, studies should be prospective, randomized, and use postmortem diagnosis as the endpoint. Radiopharmaceuticals used in the PET Aß scans must be FDA approved. Approved studies must address one or more aspects of the following questions. For Medicare beneficiaries with cognitive impairment suspicious for AD, or who may be at risk for developing AD:

1. Do the results of PET Aß imaging lead to improved health outcomes? Meaningful health outcomes of interest include: avoidance of futile treatment or tests; improving, or slowing the decline of, quality of life; and survival.
2. Are there specific subpopulations, patient characteristics or differential diagnoses that are predictive of improved health outcomes in patients whose management is guided by the PET Aß imaging?
3. Does using PET Aß imaging in guiding patient management, to enrich clinical trials seeking better treatments or prevention strategies for AD, by selecting patients on the basis of biological as well as clinical and epidemiological factors, lead to improved health outcomes?

Any clinical study undertaken pursuant to this national coverage determination (NCD) must adhere to the timeframe designated in the approved clinical study protocol. Any approved clinical study must also adhere to the following standards of scientific integrity and relevance to the Medicare population.

a. The principal purpose of the research study is to test whether a particular intervention potentially improves the participants' health outcomes.
b. The research study is well supported by available scientific and medical information or it is intended to clarify or establish the health outcomes of interventions already in common clinical use.
c. The research study does not unjustifiably duplicate existing studies.
d. The research study design is appropriate to answer the research question being asked in the study.
e. The research study is sponsored by an organization or individual capable of executing the proposed study successfully.
f. The research study is in compliance with all applicable Federal regulations concerning the protection of human subjects found at 45 CFR Part 46. If a study is regulated by the Food and Drug Administration (FDA), it must be in compliance with 21 CFR parts 50 and 56.
g. All aspects of the research study are conducted according to appropriate standards of scientific integrity (see http://www.icmje.org).
h. The research study has a written protocol that clearly addresses, or incorporates by reference, the standards listed here as Medicare requirements.
i. The clinical research study is not designed to exclusively test toxicity or disease pathophysiology in healthy individuals. Trials of all medical technologies measuring therapeutic outcomes as one of the objectives meet this standard only if the disease or condition being studied is life threatening as defined in 21 CFR §312.81(a) and the patient has no other viable treatment options.
j. The clinical research study is registered on the ClinicalTrials.gov website by the principal sponsor/investigator prior to the enrollment of the first study subject.
k. The research study protocol specifies the method and timing of public release of all pre-specified outcomes to be measured including release of outcomes if outcomes are negative or the study is terminated early. The results must be made public within 24 months of the end of data collection. If a report is planned to be published in a peer reviewed journal, then that initial release may be an abstract that meets the requirements of the International Committee of Medical Journal Editors (http://www.icmje.org). However a full report of the outcomes must be made public no later than three (3) years after the end of data collection.
l. The research study protocol must explicitly discuss subpopulations affected by the treatment under investigation, particularly traditionally underrepresented groups in clinical studies, how the inclusion and exclusion criteria effect enrollment of these populations, and a plan for the retention and reporting of said populations on the trial. If the inclusion and exclusion criteria are expected to have a negative effect on the recruitment or retention of underrepresented populations, the protocol must discuss why these criteria are necessary.
m. The research study protocol explicitly discusses how the results are or are not expected to be generalizable to the Medicare population to infer whether Medicare patients may benefit from the intervention. Separate discussions in the protocol may be necessary for populations eligible for Medicare due to age, disability or Medicaid eligibility.

Consistent with §1142 of the Act, the Agency for Healthcare Research and Quality (AHRQ) supports clinical research studies that CMS determines meet the above-listed standards and address the above-listed research questions.

All other uses are noncovered.

100-3, 220.7

Xenon Scan

Program payment may be made for this diagnostic procedure which involves perfusion lung imaging with 133 xenon. However, review for evidence of abuse which might include absence of reasonable indications, inappropriate sequence, or excessive number or kinds of procedures used in the care of individual patients.

100-3, 220.8

Nuclear Radiology Procedure

Nuclear radiology procedures, including nuclear examinations performed with mobile radiological equipment, are covered if reasonable and necessary for the individual patient. Although these procedures may not be widely used, they are generally accepted. Review claims for these procedures for evidence of abuse which might absence of reasonable indications, inappropriate sequence, or excessive number or kinds of procedures used in the care of individual patients.

100-3, 220.12

Single Photon Emission Computed Tomography (SPECT)

Frequency limitations: Contractor discretion.

In the case of myocardial viability, FDG PET may be used following a SPECT that was found to be inconclusive. However, SPECT may not be used following an inconclusive FDG PET performed to evaluate myocardial viability.

100-3, 220.13

Percutaneous Image-Guided Breast Biopsy

Percutaneous image-guided breast biopsy is a method of obtaining a breast biopsy through a percutaneous incision by employing image guidance systems. Image guidance systems may be either ultrasound or stereotactic.

The Breast Imaging Reporting and Data System (or BIRADS system) employed by the American College of Radiology provides a standardized lexicon with which radiologists may report their interpretation of a mammogram. The BIRADS grading of mammograms is as follows: Grade I-Negative, Grade II-Benign finding, Grade III-Probably benign, Grade IV-Suspicious abnormality, and Grade V-Highly suggestive of malignant neoplasm.

A. Nonpalpable Breast Lesions.

Effective January 1, 2003, Medicare covers percutaneous image-guided breast biopsy using stereotactic or ultrasound imaging for a radiographic abnormality that is nonpalpable and is graded as a BIRADS III, IV, or V.

B. Palpable Breast Lesions.

Effective January 1, 2003, Medicare covers percutaneous image guided breast biopsy using stereotactic or ultrasound imaging for palpable lesions that are difficult to biopsy using palpation alone. Contractors have the discretion to decide what types of palpable lesions are difficult to biopsy using palpation.

100-3, 230.1

Treatment of Kidney Stones

In addition to the traditional surgical/endoscopic techniques for the treatment of kidney stones, the following lithotripsy techniques are also covered for services rendered on or after March I5, I985.

Extracorporeal Shock Wave Lithotripsy.--Extracorporeal Shock Wave Lithotripsy (ESWL) is a non-invasive method of treating kidney stones using a device called a lithotriptor. The lithotriptor uses shock waves generated outside of the body to break up upper urinary tract stones. It focuses the shock waves specifically on stones under X-ray visualization, pulverizing them by repeated shocks. ESWL is covered under Medicare for use in the treatment of upper urinary tract kidney stones.

Percutaneous Lithotripsy.--Percutaneous lithotripsy (or nephrolithotomy) is an invasive method of treating kidney stones by using ultrasound, electrohydraulic or mechanical lithotripsy. A probe is inserted through an incision in the skin directly over the kidney and applied to the stone. A form of lithotripsy is then used to fragment the stone. Mechanical or electrohydraulic lithotripsy may be used as an alternative or adjunct to ultrasonic lithotripsy. Percutaneous lithotripsy of kidney stones by ultrasound or by the related techniques of electrohydraulic or mechanical lithotripsy is covered under Medicare.

The following is covered for services rendered on or after January 16, 1988.

Transurethral Ureteroscopic Lithotripsy.--Transurethral ureteroscopic lithotripsy is a method of fragmenting and removing ureteral and renal stones through a cystoscope. The cystoscope is inserted through the urethra into the bladder. Catheters are passed through the scope into the opening where the ureters enter the bladder. Instruments passed through this opening into the ureters are used to manipulate and ultimately disintegrate stones, using either mechanical crushing, transcystoscopic electrohydraulic shock waves, ultrasound or laser. Transurethral ureteroscopic lithotripsy for the treatment of urinary tract stones of the kidney or ureter is covered under Medicare.

100-3, 230.2

Uroflowmetric Evaluations

Uroflowmetric evaluations (also referred to as urodynamic voiding or urodynamic flow studies) are covered under Medicare for diagnosing various urological dysfunctions, including bladder outlet obstructions.

100-3, 230.3

Sterilization

Payment may be made only where sterilization is a necessary part of the treatment of an illness or injury, e.g., removal of a uterus because of a tumor, removal of diseased ovaries (bilateral oophorectomy), or bilateral orchidectomy in a case of cancer of the prostate. Deny claims when the pathological evidence of the necessity to perform any such procedures to treat an illness or injury is absent; and

Sterilization of a mentally retarded beneficiary is covered if it is a necessary part of the treatment of an illness or injury.

Monitor such surgeries closely and obtain the information needed to determine whether in fact the surgery was performed as a means of treating an illness or injury or only to achieve sterilization.

B - Noncovered Conditions

Elective hysterectomy, tubal ligation, and vasectomy, if the stated reason for these procedures is sterilization;

A sterilization that is performed because a physician believes another pregnancy would endanger the overall general health of the woman is not considered to be reasonable and necessary for the diagnosis or treatment of illness or injury within the meaning of Sec.1862(a)(1) of the Act. The same conclusion would apply where the sterilization is performed only as a measure to prevent the possible development of, or effect on, a mental condition should the individual become pregnant; and

Sterilization of a mentally retarded person where the purpose is to prevent conception, rather than the treatment of an illness or injury.

100-3, 230.4

Diagnosis and Treatment of Impotence

Program payment may be made for diagnosis and treatment of sexual impotence.

100-3, 230.6

Vabra Aspirator

Program payment cannot be made for the aspirator or the related diagnostic services when furnished in connection with the examination of an asymptomatic patient. Payment for routine physical checkups is precluded under the statute (Sec.1862(a)(7) of the Act).

100-3, 230.9

Cryosurgery of Prostate

Cryosurgery of the prostate as a salvage therapy is not covered for any services performed prior to June 30, 2001.

Salvage Cryosurgery of Prostate After Radiation Failure. Salvage cryosurgery of the prostate for recurrent cancer is medically necessary and appropriate only for those patients with localized disease who:

1. Have failed a trial of radiation therapy as their primary treatment; and
2. Meet one of the following conditions: Stage T2B or below, Gleason score <9, PSA <8 ng/mL.

Cryosurgery as salvage therapy is therefore not covered under Medicare after failure of other therapies as the primary treatment. Cryosurgery as salvage is only covered after the failure of a trial of radiation therapy, under the conditions noted above.

100-3, 230.10

Incontinence Control Devices

A - Mechanical/Hydraulic Incontinence Control Devices

Mechanical/hydraulic incontinence control devices are accepted as safe and effective in the management of urinary incontinence in patients with permanent anatomic and neurologic dysfunctions of the bladder. This class of devices achieves control of urination by compression of the urethra. The materials used and the success rate may vary somewhat from device to device. Such a device is covered when its use is reasonable and necessary for the individual patient.

B - Collagen Implant

A collagen implant, which is injected into the submucosal tissues of the urethra and/or the bladder neck and into tissues adjacent to the urethra, is a prosthetic device used in the treatment of stress urinary incontinence resulting from intrinsic sphincter deficiency (ISD). ISD is a cause of stress urinary incontinence in which the urethral sphincter is unable to contract and generate sufficient resistance in the bladder, especially during stress maneuvers.

Prior to collagen implant therapy, a skin test for collagen sensitivity must be administered and evaluated over a 4 week period.

In male patients, the evaluation must include a complete history and physical examination and a simple cystometrogram to determine that the bladder fills and stores properly. The patient then is asked to stand upright with a full bladder and to cough or otherwise exert abdominal pressure on his bladder. If the patient leaks, the diagnosis of ISD is established.

In female patients, the evaluation must include a complete history and physical examination (including a pelvic exam) and a simple cystometrogram to rule out abnormalities of bladder compliance and abnormalities of urethral support. Following that determination, an abdominal leak point pressure (ALLP) test is performed. Leak point pressure, stated in cm H2O, is defined as the intra-abdominal pressure at which leakage occurs from the bladder (around a catheter) when the bladder has been filled with a minimum of 150 cc fluid. If the patient has an ALLP of less than 100 cm H2O, the diagnosis of ISD is established.

To use a collagen implant, physicians must have urology training in the use of a cystoscope and must complete a collagen implant training program.

Coverage of a collagen implant, and the procedure to inject it, is limited to the following types of patients with stress urinary incontinence due to ISD:

- Male or female patients with congenital sphincter weakness secondary to conditions such as myelomeningocele or epispadias;
- Male or female patients with acquired sphincter weakness secondary to spinal cord lesions;
- Male patients following trauma, including prostatectomy and/or radiation; and
- Female patients without urethral hypermobility and with abdominal leak point pressures of 100 cm H2O or less.

Patients whose incontinence does not improve with 5 injection procedures (5 separate treatment sessions) are considered treatment failures, and no further treatment of urinary incontinence by collagen implant is covered. Patients who have a reoccurrence of incontinence following successful treatment with collagen implants in the past (e.g., 6-12 months previously) may benefit from additional treatment sessions. Coverage of additional sessions may be allowed but must be supported by medical justification.

100-3, 230.12

Dimethyl Sulfoxide (DMSO)

The Food and Drug Administration has determined that the only purpose for which DMSO is safe and effective for humans is in the treatment of the bladder condition, interstitial cystitis. Therefore, the use of DMSO for all other indications is not considered to be reasonable and necessary. Payment may be made for its use only when reasonable and necessary for a patient in the treatment of interstitial cystitis.

100-3, 230.14

Ultrafiltration Monitor

Covered:

Ultrafiltration and ultrafiltration monitoring as a component of hemodialysis has an established and critical role in maintaining the well-being of ESRD patients and is a covered service. The Ultrafiltration Monitor is covered under the Medicare program when it is used to calculate fluid rates for those recipients who present difficult fluid management problems. Determine the medical necessity of this device on a case-by-case basis.

Not Covered:

Ultrafiltration, independent of conventional dialysis, is considered experimental, and technology exclusively designed for this purpose is not covered under Medicare.

100-3, 240.3

Heat Treatment, including the Use of Diathermy and Ultrasound for Pulmonary Conditions

There is no physiological rationale or valid scientific documentation of effectiveness of diathermy or ultrasound heat treatments for asthma, bronchitis, or any other pulmonary condition and for such purpose this treatment cannot be considered reasonable and necessary within the meaning of section 1862(a)(1) of the Act.

100-3, 240.4.1

Sleep Testing for Obstructive Sleep Apnea (OSA) (Effective March 3, 2009)

A. General

Obstructive sleep apnea (OSA) is the collapse of the oropharyngeal walls and the obstruction of airflow occurring during sleep. Diagnostic tests for OSA have historically been classified into four types. The most comprehensive is designated Type I attended facility based polysomnography (PSG), which is considered the reference standard for diagnosing OSA. Attended facility based polysomnogram is a comprehensive diagnostic sleep test including at least electroencephalography (EEG), electro-oculography (EOG), electromyography (EMG), heart rate or electrocardiography (ECG), airflow, breathing/respiratory effort, and arterial oxygen saturation (SaO2) furnished in a sleep laboratory facility in which a technologist supervises the recording during sleep time and has the ability to intervene if needed. Overnight PSG is the conventional diagnostic test for OSA. The American Thoracic Society and the American Academy of Sleep Medicine have recommended supervised PSG in the sleep laboratory over 2 nights for the diagnosis of OSA and the initiation of continuous positive airway pressure (CPAP).

Three categories of portable monitors (used both in attended and unattended settings) have been developed for the diagnosis of OSA. Type II monitors have a minimum of 7 channels (e.g., EEG, EOG, EMG, ECG-heart rate, airflow, breathing/respiratory effort, SaO2)-this type of device monitors sleep staging, so AHI can be calculated). Type III monitors have a minimum of 4 monitored channels including ventilation or airflow (at least two channels of respiratory movement or respiratory movement and airflow), heart rate or ECG, and oxygen saturation. Type IV devices may measure one, two, three or more parameters but do not meet all the criteria of a higher category device. Some monitors use an actigraphy algorithm to identify periods of sleep and wakefulness.

B. Nationally Covered Indications

Effective for claims with dates of service on and after March 3, 2009, the Centers for Medicare & Medicaid Services finds that the evidence is sufficient to determine that the results of the sleep tests identified below can be used by a beneficiary's treating physician to diagnose OSA, that the use of such sleep testing technologies demonstrates improved health outcomes in Medicare beneficiaries who have OSA and receive the appropriate treatment, and that these tests are thus reasonable and necessary under section 1862(a)(1)(A) of the Social Security Act.

1. Type I PSG is covered when used to aid the diagnosis of OSA in beneficiaries who have clinical signs and symptoms indicative of OSA if performed attended in a sleep lab facility.
2. Type II or Type III sleep testing devices are covered when used to aid the diagnosis of OSA in beneficiaries who have clinical signs and symptoms indicative of OSA if performed unattended in or out of a sleep lab facility or attended in a sleep lab facility.
3. Type IV sleep testing devices measuring three or more channels, one of which is airflow, are covered when used to aid the diagnosis of OSA in beneficiaries who have signs and symptoms indicative of OSA if performed unattended in or out of a sleep lab facility or attended in a sleep lab facility.
4. Sleep testing devices measuring three or more channels that include actigraphy, oximetry, and peripheral arterial tone, are covered when used to aid the diagnosis of OSA in beneficiaries who have signs and symptoms indicative of OSA if performed unattended in or out of a sleep lab facility or attended in a sleep lab facility.

C. Nationally Non-Covered Indications

Effective for claims with dates of services on and after March 3, 2009, other diagnostic sleep tests for the diagnosis of OSA, other than those noted above for prescribing CPAP, are not sufficient for the coverage of CPAP and are not covered.

D. Other

N/A

(This NCD last reviewed March 2009.)

100-3, 240.6

Transvenous (Catheter) Pulmonary Embolectomy

It is not covered under Medicare because it is still experimental.

100-3, 240.7

Postural Drainage Procedures and Pulmonary Exercises

In most cases, postural drainage procedures and pulmonary exercises can be carried out safely and effectively by nursing personnel. However, in some cases patients may have acute or severe pulmonary conditions involving complex situations in which these procedures or exercises require the knowledge and skills of a physical therapist or a respiratory therapist. Therefore, if the attending physician determines as part of his/her plan of treatment that for the safe and effective administration of such services the procedures or exercises in question need to be performed by a physical therapist, the services of such a therapist constitute covered physical therapy when provided as an inpatient hospital service, extended care service, home health service, or outpatient physical therapy service.

NOTE: Physical therapy furnished in the outpatient department of a hospital is covered under the outpatient physical therapy benefit.

If the attending physician determines that the services should be performed by a respiratory therapist, the services of such a therapist constitute covered respiratory therapy when provided as an inpatient hospital service, outpatient hospital service, or extended care service, assuming that such services are furnished to the skilled nursing facility by a hospital with which the facility has a transfer agreement. Since the services of a respiratory therapist are not covered under the home health benefit, payment may not be made under the home health benefit for visits by a respiratory therapist to a patient's home to provide such services. Postural drainage procedures and pulmonary exercises are also covered when furnished by a physical therapist or a respiratory therapist as incident to a physician's professional service.

100-3, 250.1

Treatment of Psoriasis

Psoriasis is a chronic skin disease, for which several conventional methods of treatment have been recognized as covered. These include topical application of steroids or other drugs; ultraviolet light (actinotherapy); and coal tar alone or in combination with ultraviolet B light (Goeckerman treatment).

A newer treatment for psoriasis uses a psoralen derivative drug in combination with ultraviolet A light, known as PUVA. PUVA therapy is covered for treatment of intractable, disabling psoriasis, but only after the psoriasis has not responded to more conventional treatment. The contractor should document this before paying for PUVA therapy.

In addition, reimbursement for PUVA therapy should be limited to amounts paid for other types of photochemotherapy; ordinarily, payment should not be allowed for more than 30 days of treatment, unless improvement is documented.

100-3, 250.3

Intravenous Immune Globulin for the Treatment of Autoimmune Mucocutaneous Blistering Diseases

Effective October 1, 2002, IVIg is covered for the treatment of biopsy-proven (1) Pemphigus Vulgaris, (2) Pemphigus Foliaceus, (3) Bullous Pemphigoid, (4) Mucous Membrane Pemphigoid (a.k.a., Cicatricial Pemphigoid), and (5) Epidermolysis Bullosa Acquisita for the following patient subpopulations:

- Patients who have failed conventional therapy. Contractors have the discretion to define what constitutes failure of conventional therapy;
- Patients in whom conventional therapy is otherwise contraindicated. Contractors have the discretion to define what constitutes contraindications to conventional therapy; or
- Patients with rapidly progressive disease in whom a clinical response could not be affected quickly enough using conventional agents. In such situations IVIg therapy would be given along with conventional treatment(s) and the IVIg would be used only until the conventional therapy could take effect.

In addition, IVIg for the treatment of autoimmune mucocutaneous blistering diseases must be used only for short-term therapy and not as a maintenance therapy. Contractors have the discretion to decide what constitutes short-term therapy.

100-3, 250.4

Treatment of Actinic Keratosis (AKs)

Actinic keratoses (AKs), also known as solar keratoses, are common, sun-induced skin lesions that are confined to the epidermis and have the potential to become a skin cancer.

Various options exist for treating AKs. Clinicians should select an appropriate treatment based on the patient's medical history, the lesion's characteristics, and on the patient's preference for a specific treatment. Commonly performed treatments for AKs include cryosurgery with liquid nitrogen, topical drug therapy, and curettage. Less commonly performed treatments for AK include dermabrasion, excision, chemical peels, laser therapy, and photodynamic therapy (PDT). An alternative approach to treating AKs is to observe the lesions over time and remove them only if they exhibit specific clinical features suggesting possible transformation to invasive squamous cell carcinoma (SCC).

Effective for services performed on and after November 26, 2001, Medicare covers the destruction of actinic keratoses without restrictions based on lesion or patient characteristics.

100-3, 260.1

Adult Liver Transplantation

A. General

Liver transplantation, which is in situ replacement of a patient's liver with a donor liver, in certain circumstances, may be an accepted treatment for patients with end-stage liver disease due to a variety of causes. The procedure is used in selected patients as a treatment for malignancies, including primary liver tumors and certain metastatic tumors, which are typically rare but lethal with very limited treatment options. It has also been used in the treatment of patients with extrahepatic perihilar malignancies. Examples of malignancies include extrahepatic unresectable cholangiocarcinoma (CCA), liver metastases due to a neuroendocrine tumor (NET), and, hemangioendothelioma (HAE). Despite potential short- and long-term complications, transplantation may offer the only chance of cure for selected patients while providing meaningful palliation for some others.

B. Nationally Covered Indications

Effective July 15, 1996, adult liver transplantation when performed on beneficiaries with end- stage liver disease other than hepatitis B or malignancies is covered under Medicare when performed in a facility which is approved by the Centers for Medicare & Medicaid Services (CMS) as meeting institutional coverage criteria.

Effective December 10, 1999, adult liver transplantation when performed on beneficiaries with end-stage liver disease other than malignancies is covered under Medicare when performed in a facility which is approved by CMS as meeting institutional coverage criteria.

Effective September 1, 2001, Medicare covers adult liver transplantation for hepatocellular carcinoma when the following conditions are met:

- The patient is not a candidate for subtotal liver resection;
- The patient's tumor(s) is less than or equal to 5 cm in diameter;
- There is no macrovascular involvement;
- There is no identifiable extrahepatic spread of tumor to surrounding lymph nodes, lungs, abdominal organs or bone; and,
- The transplant is furnished in a facility that is approved by CMS as meeting institutional coverage criteria for liver transplants (see 65 FR 15006).

Effective June 21, 2012, Medicare Adminstrative Contractors acting within their respective jurisdictions may determine coverage of adult liver transplantation for the following malignancies: (1) extrahepatic unresectable cholangiocarcinoma (CCA); (2) liver metastases due to a neuroendocrine tumor (NET); and, (3) hemangioendothelioma (HAE).

1. Follow-Up Care

   Follow-up care or re-transplantation required as a result of a covered liver transplant is covered, provided such services are otherwise reasonable and necessary. Follow-up care is also covered for patients who have been discharged from a hospital after receiving non-covered liver transplant. Coverage for follow-up care is for items and services that are reasonable and necessary as determined by Medicare guidelines.

2. Immunosuppressive Drugs

   See the Medicare Benefit Policy Manual, Chapter 15, "Covered Medical and Other Health Services," section 50.5.1 and the Medicare Claims Processing Manual, Chapter 17, "Drugs and Biologicals," section 80.3.

C. Nationally Non-Covered Indications

Adult liver transplantation for other malignancies remains excluded from coverage.

D. Other

Coverage of adult liver transplantation is effective as of the date of the facility's approval, but for applications received before July 13, 1991, can be effective as early as March 8, 1990. (See 56 FR 15006 dated April 12, 1991.)

(This NCD last reviewed June 2012.)

100-3, 260.2

Pediatric Liver Transplantation

Liver transplantation is covered for children (under age 18) with extrahepatic biliary atresia or any other form of end stage liver disease, except that coverage is not provided for children with a malignancy extending beyond the margins of the liver or those with persistent viremia.

Liver transplantation is covered for Medicare beneficiaries when performed in a pediatric hospital that performs pediatric liver transplants if the hospital submits an application which CMS approves documenting that:

The hospital's pediatric liver transplant program is operated jointly by the hospital and another facility that has been found by CMS to meet the institutional coverage criteria in the "Federal Register" notice of April 12, 1991;

- The unified program shares the same transplant surgeons and quality assurance program (including oversight committee, patient protocol, and patient selection criteria); and
- The hospital is able to provide the specialized facilities, services, and personnel that are required by pediatric liver transplant patients.

100-3, 260.3

Pancreas Transplants

B. Nationally Covered Indications

Effective for services performed on or after July 1, 1999, whole organ pancreas transplantation is nationally covered by Medicare when performed simultaneous with or after a kidney transplant. If the pancreas transplant occurs after the kidney transplant, immunosuppressive therapy begins with the date of discharge from the inpatient stay for the pancreas transplant.

Effective for services performed on or after April 26, 2006, pancreas transplants alone (PA) are reasonable and necessary for Medicare beneficiaries in the following limited circumstances:

1. PA will be limited to those facilities that are Medicare-approved for kidney transplantation. (Approved centers can be found at http://www.cms.hhs.gov/ESRDGeneralInformation/02_Data.asp#TopOfPage
2. Patients must have a diagnosis of type I diabetes:
   - Patient with diabetes must be beta cell autoantibody positive; or
   - Patient must demonstrate insulinopenia defined as a fasting C-peptide level that is less than or equal to 110% of the lower limit of normal of the laboratory's measurement method. Fasting C-peptide levels will only be considered valid with a concurrently obtained fasting glucose <225 mg/dL;
3. Patients must have a history of medically-uncontrollable labile (brittle) insulin-dependent diabetes mellitus with documented recurrent, severe, acutely life-threatening metabolic complications that require hospitalization. Aforementioned complications include frequent hypoglycemia unawareness or recurring severe ketoacidosis, or recurring severe hypoglycemic attacks;
4. Patients must have been optimally and intensively managed by an endocrinologist for at least 12 months with the most medically-recognized advanced insulin formulations and delivery systems;
5. Patients must have the emotional and mental capacity to understand the significant risks associated with surgery and to effectively manage the lifelong need for immunosuppression; and,
6. Patients must otherwise be a suitable candidate for transplantation.

C. Nationally Non-Covered Indications

The following procedure is not considered reasonable and necessary within the meaning of section 1862(a)(1)(A) of the Social Security Act:

1. Transplantation of partial pancreatic tissue or islet cells (except in the context of a clinical trial (see section 260.3.1 of the National Coverage Determinations Manual).

D. Other

Not applicable.

(This NCD last reviewed April 2006.)

100-3, 260.5

Intestinal and Multi-Visceral Transplantation (Effective May 11, 2006)

(Rev. 58, Issued: 05-26-06; Effective: 05-11-06; Implementation: 06-26-06)

A. General

Medicare covers intestinal and multi-visceral transplantation for the purpose of restoring intestinal function in patients with irreversible intestinal failure. Intestinal failure is defined as the loss of absorptive capacity of the small bowel secondary to severe primary gastrointestinal disease or surgically induced short bowel syndrome. It may be associated with both mortality and profound morbidity. Multi-visceral transplantation includes organs in the digestive system (stomach, duodenum, pancreas, liver and intestine).

The evidence supports the fact that aged patients generally do not survive as well as younger patients receiving intestinal transplantation. Nonetheless, some older patients who are free from other contraindications have received the procedure and are progressing well, as evidenced by the United Network for Organ Sharing (UNOS) data. Thus, it is not appropriate to include specific exclusions from coverage, such as an age limitation, in the national coverage policy.

B. Nationally Covered Indications

Effective for services performed on or after April 1, 2001, this procedure is covered only when performed for patients who have failed total parenteral nutrition (TPN) and only when performed in centers that meet approval criteria.

1. Failed TPN

   The TPN delivers nutrients intravenously, avoiding the need for absorption through the small bowel. TPN failure includes the following:

   - Impending or overt liver failure due to TPN induced liver injury. The clinical manifestations include elevated serum bilirubin and/or liver enzymes, splenomegaly, thrombocytopenia, gastroesophageal varices, coagulopathy, stomal bleeding or hepatic fibrosis/cirrhosis.
   - Thrombosis of the major central venous channels; jugular, subclavian, and femoral veins. Thrombosis of two or more of these vessels is considered a life threatening complication and failure of TPN therapy. The sequelae of central venous thrombosis are lack of access for TPN infusion, fatal sepsis due to infected thrombi, pulmonary embolism, Superior Vena Cava syndrome, or chronic venous insufficiency.
   - Frequent line infection and sepsis. The development of two or more episodes of systemic sepsis secondary to line infection per year that requires hospitalization indicates failure of TPN therapy. A single episode of line related fungemia, septic shock and/or Acute Respiratory Distress Syndrome are considered indicators of TPN failure.
   - Frequent episodes of severe dehydration despite intravenous fluid supplement in addition to TPN. Under certain medical conditions such as secretory diarrhea and non-constructable gastrointestinal tract, the loss of the gastrointestinal and pancreatobiliary secretions exceeds the maximum intravenous infusion rates that can be tolerated by the cardiopulmonary system. Frequent episodes of dehydration are deleterious to all body organs particularly kidneys and the central nervous system with the development of multiple kidney stones, renal failure, and permanent brain damage.

2. Approved Transplant Facilities

   Intestinal transplantation is covered by Medicare if performed in an approved facility. The criteria for approval of centers will be based on a volume of 10 intestinal transplants per year with a 1-year actuarial survival of 65 percent using the Kaplan-Meier technique.

C. Nationally Non-covered Indications

All other indications remain non-covered.

D. Other

NA.

(This NCD last reviewed May 2006.)

100-3, 260.7

Lymphocyte Immune Globulin, Anti-Thymocyte Globulin (Equine)

The FDA has approved one lymphocyte immune globulin preparation for marketing, lymphocyte immune globulin, anti-thymocyte globulin (equine). This drug is indicated for the management of allograft rejection episodes in renal transplantation. It is covered under Medicare when used for this purpose. Other forms of lymphocyte globulin preparation which the FDA approves for this indication in the future may be covered under Medicare.

100-3, 260.9

Heart Transplants

A. General

Cardiac transplantation is covered under Medicare when performed in a facility which is approved by Medicare as meeting institutional coverage criteria. (See CMS Ruling 87-1.)

B. Exceptions

In certain limited cases, exceptions to the criteria may be warranted if there is justification and if the facility ensures our objectives of safety and efficacy. Under no circumstances will exceptions be made for facilities whose transplant programs have been in existence for less than two years, and applications from consortia will not be approved.

Although consortium arrangements will not be approved for payment of Medicare heart transplants, consideration will be given to applications from heart transplant facilities that consist of more than one hospital where all of the following conditions exist:

- The hospitals are under the common control or have a formal affiliation arrangement with each other under the auspices of an organization such as a university or a legally-constituted medical research institute; and
- The hospitals share resources by routinely using the same personnel or services in their transplant programs. The sharing of resources must be supported by the submission of operative notes or other information that documents the routine use of the same personnel and services in all of the individual hospitals. At a minimum, shared resources means:
- The individual members of the transplant team, consisting of the cardiac transplant surgeons, cardiologists and pathologists, must practice in all the hospitals and it can be documented that they otherwise function as members of the transplant team;
- The same organ procurement organization, immunology, and tissue-typing services must be used by all the hospitals;
- The hospitals submit, in the manner required (Kaplan-Meier method) their individual and pooled experience and survival data; and
- The hospitals otherwise meet the remaining Medicare criteria for heart transplant facilities; that is, the criteria regarding patient selection, patient management, program commitment, etc.

C. Pediatric Hospitals

Cardiac transplantation is covered for Medicare beneficiaries when performed in a pediatric hospital that performs pediatric heart transplants if the hospital submits an application which CMS approves as documenting that:

- The hospital's pediatric heart transplant program is operated jointly by the hospital and another facility that has been found by CMS to meet the institutional coverage criteria in CMS Ruling 87-1;
- The unified program shares the same transplant surgeons and quality assurance program (including oversight committee, patient protocol, and patient selection criteria); and
- The hospital is able to provide the specialized facilities, services, and personnel that are required by pediatric heart transplant patients.

D. Follow Up Care

Follow-up care required as a result of a covered heart transplant is covered, provided such services are otherwise reasonable and necessary. Follow-up care is also covered for patients who have been discharged from a hospital after receiving a noncovered heart transplant. Coverage for follow-up care would be for items and services that are reasonable and necessary, as determined by Medicare guidelines. (See the Medicare Benefit Policy Manual, Chapter 16, "General Exclusions from Coverage," Sec.180.)

E. Immunosuppressive Drugs

See the Medicare Claims Processing Manual, Chapter 17, "Drugs and Biologicals," Sec.80.3.1, and Chapter 8, "Outpatient ESRD Hospital, Independent Facility, and Physician/Supplier Claims," Sec.120.1.

F. Artificial Hearts

Medicare does not cover the use of artificial hearts as a permanent replacement for a human heart or as a temporary life-support system until a human heart becomes available for transplant (often referred to as a "bridge to transplant"). Medicare does cover a ventricular assist device (VAD) when used in conjunction with specific criteria listed in Sec.20.9 of the NCD Manual.

100-3, 270.1

Electrical Stimulation (ES) and Electromagnetic Therapy for the Treatment of Wounds

A. Nationally Covered Indications

The use of ES and electromagnetic therapy for the treatment of wounds are considered adjunctive therapies, and will only be covered for chronic Stage III or Stage IV pressure ulcers, arterial ulcers, diabetic ulcers, and venous stasis ulcers. Chronic ulcers are defined as ulcers that have not healed within 30 days of occurrence. ES or electromagnetic therapy will be covered only after appropriate standard wound therapy has been tried for at least 30 days and there are no measurable signs of improved healing. This 30-day period may begin while the wound is acute.

Standard wound care includes: optimization of nutritional status, debridement by any means to remove devitalized tissue, maintenance of a clean, moist bed of granulation tissue with appropriate moist dressings, and necessary treatment to resolve any infection that may be present. Standard wound care based on the specific type of wound includes: frequent repositioning of a patient with pressure ulcers (usually every 2 hours), offloading of pressure and good glucose control for diabetic ulcers, establishment of adequate circulation for arterial ulcers, and the use of a compression system for patients with venous ulcers.

Measurable signs of improved healing include: a decrease in wound size (either surface area or volume), decrease in amount of exudates, and decrease in amount of necrotic tissue. ES or electromagnetic therapy must be discontinued when the wound demonstrates 100% epitheliliazed wound bed.

ES and electromagnetic therapy services can only be covered when performed by a physician, physical therapist, or incident to a physician service. Evaluation of the wound is an integral part of wound therapy. When a physician, physical therapist, or a clinician incident to a physician, performs ES or electromagnetic therapy, the practitioner must evaluate the wound and contact the treating physician if the wound worsens. If ES or electromagnetic therapy is being used, wounds must be evaluated at least monthly by the treating physician.

B. Nationally Noncovered Indications

1. ES and electromagnetic therapy will not be covered as an initial treatment modality.
2. Continued treatment with ES or electromagnetic therapy is not covered if measurable signs of healing have not been demonstrated within any 30-day period of treatment.
3. Unsupervised use of ES or electromagnetic therapy for wound therapy will not be covered, as this use has not been found to be medically reasonable and necessary.

C. Other

All other uses of ES and electromagnetic therapy not otherwise specified for the treatment of wounds remain at local contractor discretion.

(This NCD last reviewed March 2004.)

100-3, 270.2

Noncontact Normothermic Wound Therapy (NNWT)

There is insufficient scientific or clinical evidence to consider this device as reasonable and necessary for the treatment of wounds within the meaning of Sec.1862(a)(1)(A) of the Social Security Act and will not be covered by Medicare.

100-3, 270.3

Blood-Derived Products for Chronic Non-Healing Wounds - (Various Effective Dates Below) (270.3)

(Rev. 83, Issued: 05-02-08, Effective: 03-19-08, Implementation: 06-02-08)

A. General

Wound healing is a dynamic, interactive process that involves multiple cells and proteins. There are three progressive stages of normal wound healing, and the typical wound healing duration is about 4 weeks. While cutaneous wounds are a disruption of the normal, anatomic structure and function of the skin, subcutaneous wounds involve tissue below the skin's surface. Wounds are categorized as either acute, in where the normal wound healing stages are not yet completed but it is presumed they will be, resulting in orderly and timely wound repair, or chronic, in where a wound has failed to progress through the normal wound healing stages and repair itself within a sufficient time period.

Platelet-rich plasma (PRP) is produced in an autologous or homologous manner. Autologous PRP is comprised of blood from the patient who will ultimately receive the PRP. Alternatively, homologous PRP is derived from blood from multiple donors.

Blood is donated by the patient and centrifuged to produce an autologous gel for treatment of chronic, non-healing cutaneous wounds that persists for 30 days or longer and fail to properly complete the healing process. Autologous blood derived products for chronic, non-healing wounds includes both: (1) platelet derived growth factor (PDGF) products (such as Procuren), and (2) PRP.

The PRP is different from previous products in that it contains whole cells including white cells, red cells, plasma, platelets, fibrinogen, stem cells, macrophages, and fibroblasts.

The PRP is used by physicians in clinical settings in treating chronic, non-healing wounds, open, cutaneous wounds, soft tissue, and bone. Alternatively, PDGF does not contain cells and was previously marketed as a product to be used by patients at home.

B. Nationally Covered Indications

Not applicable.

C. Nationally Non-Covered Indications

1. Effective December 28, 1992, the Centers for Medicare & Medicaid Services (CMS) issued a national non-coverage determination for platelet-derived wound-healing formulas intended to treat patients with chronic, non-healing wounds. This decision was based on a lack of sufficient published data to determine safety and efficacy, and a public health service technology assessment.
2. Effective July 23, 2004, upon reconsideration, the clinical effectiveness of autologous PDGF products continues to not be adequately proven in scientific literature. As the evidence is insufficient to conclude that autologous PDGF in a platelet-poor plasma is reasonable and necessary, it remains non-covered for treatment of chronic, non- healing cutaneous wounds. Also, the clinical evidence does not support a benefit in the application of autologous PRP for the treatment of chronic, non-healing, cutaneous wounds. Therefore, CMS determines it is not reasonable and necessary and is nationally non-covered.
3. Effective April 27, 2006, coverage for treatments utilizing becaplermin, a non-autologous growth factor for chronic, non-healing subcutaneous wounds, remains nationally non-covered under Part B based on section 1861(s)(2)(A) and (B) of the Social Security Act because this product is usually administered by the patient.
4. Effective March 19, 2008, upon reconsideration, the evidence is not adequate to conclude that autologous PRP is reasonable and necessary and remains non-covered for the treatment of chronic non-healing, cutaneous wounds. Additionally, upon reconsideration, the evidence is not adequate to conclude that autologous PRP is reasonable and necessary for the treatment of acute surgical wounds when the autologous PRP is applied directly to the closed incision, or for dehiscent wounds.

D. Other

In accordance with section 310.1 of the *National Coverage Determinations Manual,* the routine costs in Federally sponsored or approved clinical trials assessing the efficacy of autologous PRP in treating chronic, non-healing cutaneous wounds are covered by Medicare.

(This NCD last reviewed March 2008.)

100-3, 270.4

Treatment of Decubitus Ulcers

An accepted procedure for healing decubitus ulcers is to remove dead tissue from the lesions and to keep them clean to promote the growth of new tissue. This may be accomplished by hydrotherapy (whirlpool) treatments. Hydrotherapy (whirlpool) treatment for decubitus ulcers is a covered service under Medicare for patients when treatment is reasonable and necessary. Some other methods of treating decubitus ulcers, the safety and effectiveness of which have not been established, are not covered under the Medicare program. Some examples of these types of treatments are: ultraviolet light, low intensity direct current, topical application of oxygen, and topical dressings with Balsam of Peru in castor oil.

100-3, 270.5

Porcine Skin and Gradient Pressure Dressings

Porcine (pig) skin dressings are covered, if reasonable and necessary for the individual patient as an occlusive dressing for burns, donor sites of a homograft, and decubiti and other ulcers.

100-3, 280.13

Transcutaneous Electrical Nerve Stimulators (TENS)

(Rev. 1, 10-03-03)

CIM 60-20

The TENS is a type of electrical nerve stimulator that is employed to treat chronic intractable pain. This stimulator is attached to the surface of the patient's skin over the peripheral nerve to be stimulated. It may be applied in a variety of settings (in the patient's home, a physician's office, or in an outpatient clinic). Payment for TENS may be made under the durable medical equipment benefit. (See §160.13 for an explanation of coverage of medically necessary supplies for the effective use of TENS and §10.2 for an explanation of coverage of TENS for acute post-operative pain.)

100-3, 280.14

Infusion Pumps

B. Nationally Covered Indications

The following indications for treatment using infusion pumps are covered under Medicare:

1. External Infusion Pumps

a. Iron Poisoning (Effective for Services Performed On or After September 26, 1984)

   When used in the administration of deferoxamine for the treatment of acute iron poisoning and iron overload, only external infusion pumps are covered.

b. Thromboembolic Disease (Effective for Services Performed On or After September 26, 1984)

   When used in the administration of heparin for the treatment of thromboembolic disease and/or pulmonary embolism, only external infusion pumps used in an institutional setting are covered.

c. Chemotherapy for Liver Cancer (Effective for Services Performed On or After January 29, 1985)

   The external chemotherapy infusion pump is covered when used in the treatment of primary hepatocellular carcinoma or colorectal cancer where this disease is unresectable; OR, where the patient refuses surgical excision of the tumor.

d. Morphine for Intractable Cancer Pain (Effective for Services Performed On or After April 22, 1985)

   Morphine infusion via an external infusion pump is covered when used in the treatment of intractable pain caused by cancer (in either an inpatient or outpatient setting, including a hospice).

e. Continuous Subcutaneous Insulin Infusion (CSII) Pumps (Effective for Services Performed On or after December 17, 2004)

   Continuous subcutaneous insulin infusion (CSII) and related drugs/supplies are covered as medically reasonable and necessary in the home setting for the treatment of diabetic patients who: (1) either meet the updated fasting C-Peptide testing requirement, or, are beta cell autoantibody positive; and, (2) satisfy the remaining criteria for insulin pump therapy as described below. Patients must meet either Criterion A or B as follows:

   Criterion A: The patient has completed a comprehensive diabetes education program, and has been on a program of multiple daily injections of insulin (i.e., at least 3 injections per day), with frequent self-adjustments of insulin doses for at least 6 months prior to initiation of the insulin pump, and has documented frequency of glucose self-testing an average of at least 4 times per day during the 2 months prior to initiation of the insulin pump, and meets one or more of the following criteria while on the multiple daily injection regimen:

   - Glycosylated hemoglobin level (HbAlc) > 7.0 percent;
   - History of recurring hypoglycemia;
   - Wide fluctuations in blood glucose before mealtime;
   - Dawn phenomenon with fasting blood sugars frequently exceeding 200 mg/dl; or,
   - History of severe glycemic excursions.

   Criterion B: The patient with diabetes has been on a pump prior to enrollment in Medicare and has documented frequency of glucose self-testing an average of at least 4 times per day during the month prior to Medicare enrollment.

   General CSII Criteria

   In addition to meeting Criterion A or B above, the following general requirements must be met:

   The patient with diabetes must be insulinopenic per the updated fasting C-peptide testing requirement, or, as an alternative, must be beta cell autoantibody positive.

   Updated fasting C-peptide testing requirement:

   - Insulinopenia is defined as a fasting C-peptide level that is less than or equal to 110% of the lower limit of normal of the laboratory's measurement method.
   - For patients with renal insufficiency and creatinine clearance (actual or calculated from age, gender, weight, and serum creatinine) <50 ml/minute, insulinopenia is defined as a fasting C-peptide level that is less than or equal to 200% of the lower limit of normal of the laboratory's measurement method.
   - Fasting C-peptide levels will only be considered valid with a concurrently obtained fasting glucose <225 mg/dL.
   - Levels only need to be documented once in the medical records.

   Continued coverage of the insulin pump would require that the patient be seen and evaluated by the treating physician at least every 3 months.

   The pump must be ordered by and follow-up care of the patient must be managed by a physician who manages multiple patients with CSII and who works closely with a team including nurses, diabetes educators, and dietitians who are knowledgeable in the use of CSII.

Other Uses of CSII

The CMS will continue to allow coverage of all other uses of CSII in accordance with the Category B investigational device exemption (IDE) clinical trials regulation (42 CFR 405.201) or as a routine cost under the clinical trials policy (Medicare National Coverage Determinations (NCD) Manual 310.1).

f. Other Uses

Other uses of external infusion pumps are covered if the contractor's medical staff verifies the appropriateness of the therapy and the prescribed pump for the individual patient.

NOTE: Payment may also be made for drugs necessary for the effective use of a covered external infusion pump as long as the drug being used with the pump is itself reasonable and necessary for the patient's treatment.

2. Implantable Infusion Pumps

a. Chemotherapy for Liver Cancer (Effective for Services Performed On or After September 26, 1984)

The implantable infusion pump is covered for intra-arterial infusion of 5-FUdR for the treatment of liver cancer for patients with primary hepatocellular carcinoma or Duke's Class D colorectal cancer, in whom the metastases are limited to the liver, and where: (1) the disease is unresectable, or (2) the patient refuses surgical excision of the tumor.

b. Anti-Spasmodic Drugs for Severe Spasticity

An implantable infusion pump is covered when used to administer anti-spasmodic drugs intrathecally (e.g., baclofen) to treat chronic intractable spasticity in patients who have proven unresponsive to less invasive medical therapy as determined by the following criteria:

As indicated by at least a 6-week trial, the patient cannot be maintained on noninvasive methods of spasm control, such as oral anti-spasmodic drugs, either because these methods fail to control adequately the spasticity or produce intolerable side effects, and prior to pump implantation, the patient must have responded favorably to a trial intrathecal dose of the anti-spasmodic drug.

c. Opioid Drugs for Treatment of Chronic Intractable Pain

An implantable infusion pump is covered when used to administer opioid drugs (e.g., morphine) intrathecally or epidurally for treatment of severe chronic intractable pain of malignant or nonmalignant origin in patients who have a life expectancy of at least 3 months, and who have proven unresponsive to less invasive medical therapy as determined by the following criteria:

The patient's history must indicate that he/she would not respond adequately to noninvasive methods of pain control, such as systemic opioids (including attempts to eliminate physical and behavioral abnormalities which may cause an exaggerated reaction to pain); and a preliminary trial of intraspinal opioid drug administration must be undertaken with a temporary intrathecal/epidural catheter to substantiate adequately acceptable pain relief and degree of side effects (including effects on the activities of daily living) and patient acceptance.

d. Coverage of Other Uses of Implanted Infusion Pumps

Determinations may be made on coverage of other uses of implanted infusion pumps if the contractor's medical staff verifies that:

- The drug is reasonable and necessary for the treatment of the individual patient;
- It is medically necessary that the drug be administered by an implanted infusion pump; and,
- The Food and Drug Administration (FDA)-approved labeling for the pump must specify that the drug being administered and the purpose for which it is administered is an indicated use for the pump.

e. Implantation of Infusion Pump Is Contraindicated

The implantation of an infusion pump is contraindicated in the following patients:

- With a known allergy or hypersensitivity to the drug being used (e.g., oral baclofen, morphine, etc.);
- Who have an infection;
- Whose body size is insufficient to support the weight and bulk of the device; and,
- With other implanted programmable devices since crosstalk between devices may inadvertently change the prescription.

NOTE: Payment may also be made for drugs necessary for the effective use of an implantable infusion pump as long as the drug being used with the pump is itself reasonable and necessary for the patient's treatment.

C. Nationally Noncovered Indications

The following indications for treatment using infusion pumps are not covered under Medicare:

1. External Infusion Pumps

a. Vancomycin (Effective for Services Beginning On or After September 1, 1996)

Medicare coverage of vancomycin as a durable medical equipment infusion pump benefit is not covered. There is insufficient evidence to support the necessity of using an external infusion pump, instead of a disposable elastomeric pump or the gravity drip method, to administer vancomycin in a safe and appropriate manner.

2. Implantable Infusion Pump

a. Thromboembolic Disease (Effective for Services Performed On or After September 26, 1984)

According to the Public Health Service, there is insufficient published clinical data to support the safety and effectiveness of the heparin implantable pump. Therefore, the use of an implantable infusion pump for infusion of heparin in the treatment of recurrent thromboembolic disease is not covered.

b. Diabetes

An implanted infusion pump for the infusion of insulin to treat diabetes is not covered. The data does not demonstrate that the pump provides effective administration of insulin.

D. Other

Not applicable.

(This NCD last reviewed January 2005.)

100-3, 300.1

Obsolete or Unreliable Diagnostic Tests

CIM 50-34

A. Diagnostic Tests

Do not routinely pay for the following diagnostic tests because they are obsolete and have been replaced by more advanced procedures. The listed tests may be paid for only if the medical need for the procedure is satisfactorily justified by the physician who performs it. When the services are subject to the Quality Improvement Organization (QIO) Review, the QIO is responsible for determining that satisfactory medical justification exists. When the services are not subject to QIO review, the intermediary or carrier is responsible for determining that satisfactory medical justification exists. This includes:

- Amylase, blood isoenzymes, electrophoretic,
- Chromium, blood,
- Guanase, blood,
- Zinc sulphate turbidity, blood,
- Skin test, cat scratch fever,
- Skin test, lymphopathia venereum,
- Circulation time, one test,
- Cephalin flocculation,
- Congo red, blood,
- Hormones, adrenocorticotropin quantitative animal tests,
- Hormones, adrenocorticotropin quantitative bioassay,
- Thymol turbidity, blood,
- Skin test, actinomycosis,
- Skin test, brucellosis,
- Skin test, psittacosis,
- Skin test, trichinosis,
- Calcium, feces, 24-hour quantitative,
- Starch, feces, screening,
- Chymotrypsin, duodenal contents,
- Gastric analysis, pepsin,
- Gastric analysis, tubeless,
- Calcium saturation clotting time,
- Capillary fragility test (Rumpel-Leede),
- Colloidal gold,
- Bendien's test for cancer and tuberculosis,
- Bolen's test for cancer,
- Rehfuss test for gastric acidity, and
- Serum seromucoid assay for cancer and other diseases.

B. Cardiovascular Tests

Do not pay for the following phonocardiography and vectorcardiography diagnostic tests because they have been determined to be outmoded and of little clinical value. They include:

- Phonocardiogram with or without ECG lead; with supervision during recording with interpretation and report (when equipment is supplied by the physician),
- Phonocardiogram; tracing only, without interpretation and report (e.g., when equipment is supplied by the hospital, clinic),
- Phonocardiogram; interpretation and report,

- Phonocardiogram with ECG lead, with indirect carotid artery and/or jugular vein tracing, and/or apex cardiogram; with interpretation and report,
- Phonocardiogram; without interpretation and report,
- Phonocardiogram; interpretation and report only,
- Intracardiac,
- Vectorcardiogram (VCG), with or without ECG; with interpretation and report,
- Vectorcardiogram; tracing only, without interpretation and report, and
- Vectorcardiogram; interpretation and report only.

100-4, 1, 30.3.5

Effect of Assignment Upon Purchase of Cataract Glasses From Participating Physician or Supplier on Claims Submitted to Carriers

B3-3045.4

A pair of cataract glasses is comprised of two distinct products: a professional product (the prescribed lenses) and a retail commercial product (the frames). The frames serve not only as a holder of lenses but also as an article of personal apparel. As such, they are usually selected on the basis of personal taste and style. Although Medicare will pay only for standard frames, most patients want deluxe frames. Participating physicians and suppliers cannot profitably furnish such deluxe frames unless they can make an extra (noncovered) charge for the frames even though they accept assignment.

Therefore, a participating physician or supplier (whether an ophthalmologist, optometrist, or optician) who accepts assignment on cataract glasses with deluxe frames may charge the Medicare patient the difference between his/her usual charge to private pay patients for glasses with standard frames and his/her usual charge to such patients for glasses with deluxe frames, in addition to the applicable deductible and coinsurance on glasses with standard frames, if all of the following requirements are met:

A. The participating physician or supplier has standard frames available, offers them for saleto the patient, and issues and ABN to the patient that explains the price and other differences between standard and deluxe frames. Refer to Chapter 30.

B. The participating physician or supplier obtains from the patient (or his/her representative) and keeps on file the following signed and dated statement:

Name of Patient   Medicare Claim Number

Having been informed that an extra charge is being made by the physician or supplier for deluxe frames, that this extra charge is not covered by Medicare, and that standard frames are available for purchase from the physician or supplier at no extra charge, I have chosen to purchase deluxe frames.

Signature   Date

C. The participating physician or supplier itemizes on his/her claim his/her actual charge for the lenses, his/her actual charge for the standard frames, and his/her actual extra charge for the deluxe frames (charge differential). Once the assigned claim for deluxe frames has been processed, the carrier will follow the ABN instructions as described in Sec.60.

100-4, 3, 10.4

Payment of Nonphysician Services for Inpatients

All items and nonphysician services furnished to inpatients must be furnished directly by the hospital or billed through the hospital under arrangements. This provision applies to all hospitals, regardless of whether they are subject to PPS.

Other Medical Items, Supplies, and Services the following medical items, supplies, and services furnished to inpatients are covered under Part A. Consequently, they are covered by the prospective payment rate or reimbursed as reasonable costs under Part A to hospitals excluded from PPS.

- Laboratory services (excluding anatomic pathology services and certain clinical pathology services);
- Pacemakers and other prosthetic devices including lenses, and artificial limbs, knees, and hips;
- Radiology services including computed tomography (CT) scans furnished to inpatients by a physician's office, other hospital, or radiology clinic;
- Total parenteral nutrition (TPN) services; and
- Transportation, including transportation by ambulance, to and from another hospital or freestanding facility to receive specialized diagnostic or therapeutic services not available at the facility where the patient is an inpatient.

The hospital must include the cost of these services in the appropriate ancillary service cost center, i.e., in the cost of the diagnostic or therapeutic service. It must not show them separately under revenue code 0540.

EXCEPTIONS

- Pneumococcal Vaccine -is payable under Part B only and is billed by the hospital on the Form CMS-1450.
- Ambulance Service For purposes of this section "hospital inpatient" means beneficiary who has been formally admitted it does not include a beneficiary who is in the process of being transferred from one hospital to another. Where the patient is transferred from one hospital to another, and is admitted as an inpatient to the second, the ambulance service is payable under only Part B. If transportation is by a hospital owned and operated ambulance, the hospital bills separately on Form CMS-1450 as appropriate. Similarly, if the hospital arranges for the ambulance transportation with an ambulance operator, including paying the ambulance operator, it bills separately. However, if the hospital does not assume any financial responsibility, the billing is to the carrier by the ambulance operator or beneficiary, as appropriate, if an ambulance is used for the transportation of a hospital inpatient to another facility for diagnostic tests or special treatment the ambulance trip is considered part of the DRG, and not separately billable, if the resident hospital is under PPS.
- Part B Inpatient Services Where Part A benefits are not payable, payment maybe made to the hospital under Part B for certain medical and other health services. See Chapter 4 for a description of Part B inpatient services.
- Anesthetist Services "Incident to" Physician Services-If a physician's practice was to employ anesthetists and to bill on a reasonable charge basis for these services and that practice was in effect as of the last day of the hospital's most recent 12-month cost reporting period ending before September 30, 1983, the physician may continue that practice through cost reporting periods beginning October 1, 1984. However, if the physician chooses to continue this practice, the hospital may not add costs of the anesthetist's service to its base period costs for purposes of its transition payment rates. If it is the existing or new practice of the physician to employ certified registered nurse anesthetists (CRNAs) and other qualified anesthetists and include charges for their services in the physician bills for anesthesiology services for the hospital's cost report periods beginning on or after October 1, 1984, and before October 1, 1987, the physician may continue to do so.

B. Exceptions/Waivers

These provisions were waived before cost reporting periods beginning on or after October1, 1986, under certain circumstances. The basic criteria for waiver was that services furnished by outside suppliers are so extensive that a sudden change in billing practices would threaten the stability of patient care. Specific criteria for waiver and processing procedures are in Sec.2804 of the Provider Reimbursement Manual (CMS Pub. 15-1).

100-4, 3, 20.1.2.8

Special Outlier Payments for Burn Cases

For discharges occurring on or after April 1, 1988, the additional payment amount for the DRGs related to burn cases, which are identified in the most recent annual notice of prospective payment rates is computed using the same methodology (as stated above in section 20.1.2.3) except that the payment is made using a marginal cost factor of 90 percent instead of 80 percent.

100-4, 3, 20.7.3

Payment for Blood Clotting Factor Administered to Hemophilia Patients

Section 6011 of Public Law (P.L.) 101-239 amended Sec.1886(a)(4) of the Social Security Act (the Act) to provide that prospective payment system (PPS) hospitals receive anadditional payment for the costs of administering blood clotting factor to Medicare hemophiliacs who are hospital inpatients. Section 6011(b) of P.L. 101.239 specified that the payment be based on a predetermined price per unit of clotting factor multiplied by the number of units provided. This add-on payment originally was effective for blood clotting factors furnished on or after June 19, 1990, and before December 19, 1991. Section 13505 of P. L. 103-66 amended Sec.6011 (d) of P.L. 101-239 to extend the period covered by the add-on payment for blood clotting factors administered to Medicare inpatients with hemophilia through September 30, 1994. Section 4452 of P.L. 105-33 amended Sec.6011(d) of P.L. 101-239 to reinstate the add-on payment for the costs of administering blood clotting factor to Medicare beneficiaries who have hemophilia and who are hospital inpatients for discharges occurring on or after October 1, 1998.

Local carriers shall process non-institutional blood clotting factor claims.

The FIs shall process institutional blood clotting factor claims payable under either Part A or Part B.

A. Inpatient Bills

Under the Inpatient Prospective Payment System (PPS), hospitals receive a special add-on payment for the costs of furnishing blood clotting factors to Medicare beneficiaries with hemophilia, admitted as inpatients of PPS hospitals. The clotting factor add-on payment is calculated using the number of units (as defined in the HCPCS code long descriptor) billed by the provider under special instructions for units of service.

The PPS Pricer software does not calculate the payment amount. The Fiscal Intermediary Standard System (FISS) calculates the payment amount and subtracts the charges from those submitted to Pricer so that the clotting factor charges are not included in cost outlier computations.

Blood clotting factors not paid on a cost or PPS basis are priced as a drug/biological under the Medicare Part B Drug Pricing File effective for the specific date of service. As of January 1, 2005, the average sales price (ASP) plus 6 percent shall be used.

If a beneficiary is in a covered Part A stay in a PPS hospital, the clotting factors are paid in addition to the DRG/HIPPS payment (For FY 2004, this payment is based on 95 percent of average wholesale price.) For a SNF subject to SNF/PPS, the payment is bundled into the SNF/PPS rate.

For SNF inpatient Part A, there is no add-on payment for blood clotting factors.

The codes for blood-clotting factors are found on the Medicare Part B Drug Pricing File. This file is distributed on a quarterly basis.

For discharges occurring on or after October 1, 2000, and before December 31, 2005, report HCPCS Q0187 based on 1 billing unit per 1.2 mg. Effective January 1, 2006, HCPCS code J7189 replaces Q0187 and is defined as 1 billing unit per 1 microgram (mcg).

The examples below include the HCPCS code and indicate the dosage amount specified in the descriptor of that code. Facilities use the units field as a multiplier to arrive at the dosage amount.

EXAMPLE 1

HCPCS	Drug	Dosage
J7189	Factor VIIa	1 mcg

Actual dosage: 13,365 mcg

On the bill, the facility shows J7189 and 13,365 in the units field (13,365 mcg divided by 1 mcg = 13,365 units).

NOTE: The process for dealing with one international unit (IU) is the same as the process of dealing with one microgram.

EXAMPLE 2

HCPCS	Drug	Dosage
J9355	Trastuzumab	10 mg

Actual dosage: 140 mg

On the bill, the facility shows J9355 and 14 in the units field (140 mg divided by 10mg = 14 units).

When the dosage amount is greater than the amount indicated for the HCPCS code, the facility rounds up to determine units. When the dosage amount is less than the amount indicated for the HCPCS code, use 1 as the unit of measure.

EXAMPLE 3

HCPCS	Drug	Dosage
J3100	Tenecteplase	50 mg

Actual Dosage: 40 mg

The provider would bill for 1 unit, even though less than 1 full unit was furnished.

At times, the facility provides less than the amount provided in a single use vial and there is waste, i.e.; some drugs may be available only in packaged amounts that exceed the needs of an individual patient. Once the drug is reconstituted in the hospital's pharmacy, it may have a limited shelf life. Since an individual patient may receive less than the fully reconstituted amount, we encourage hospitals to schedule patients in such a way that the hospital can use the drug most efficiently. However, if the hospital must discard the remainder of a vial after administering part of it to a Medicare patient, the provider may bill for the amount of drug discarded plus the amount administered.

Example 1:

Drug X is available only in a 100-unit size. A hospital schedules three Medicare patients to receive drug X on the same day within the designated shelf life of the product. An appropriate hospital staff member administers 30 units to each patient. The remaining 10 units are billed to Medicare on the account of the last patient. Therefore, 30 units are billed on behalf of the first patient seen and 30 units are billed on behalf of the second patient seen. Forty units are billed on behalf of the last patient seen because the hospital had to discard 10 units at that point.

Example 2:

An appropriate hospital staff member must administer 30 units of drug X to a Medicare patient, and it is not practical to schedule another patient who requires the same drug. For example, the hospital has only one patient who requires drug X, or the hospital sees the patient for the first time and did not know the patient's condition. The hospital bills for 100 units on behalf of the patient, and Medicare pays for 100 units.

When the number of units of blood clotting factor administered to hemophiliac inpatients exceeds 99,999, the hospital reports the excess as a second line for revenue code 0636 and repeats the HCPCS code. One hundred thousand fifty (100,050) units are reported on one line as 99,999, and another line shows 1,051.

Revenue Code 0636 is used. It requires HCPCS. Some other inpatient drugs continue to be billed without HCPCS codes under pharmacy.

No changes in beneficiary notices are required. Coverage is applicable to hospital Part A claims only. Coverage is also applicable to inpatient Part B services in SNFs and all types of hospitals, including CAHs. Separate payment is not made to SNFs for beneficiaries in an inpatient Part A stay.

B. FI Action

The FI is responsible for the following:

- It accepts HCPCS codes for inpatient services;
- It edits to require HCPCS codes with Revenue Code 0636. Multiple iterations of the revenue code are possible with the same or different HCPCS codes. It does not edit units except to ensure a numeric value;
- It reduces charges forwarded to Pricer by the charges for hemophilia clotting factors in revenue code 0636. It retains the charges and revenue and HCPCS codes for CWF; and
- It modifies data entry screens to accept HCPCS codes for hospital (including CAH) swing bed, and SNF inpatient claims (bill types 11X, 12X, 18x, 21x and, 22x).

The September 1, 1993, IPPS final rule (58 FR 46304) states that payment will be made for the blood clotting factor only if an ICD-9-CM diagnosis code for hemophilia is included on the bill.

Since inpatient blood-clotting factors are covered only for beneficiaries with hemophilia, the FI must ensure that one of the following hemophilia diagnosis codes is listed on the bill before payment is made:

286.0 Congenital factor VIII disorder

286.1 Congenital factor IX disorder

286.2 Congenital factor IX disorder

286.3 Congenital deficiency of other clotting factor

286.4 von Willebrands' disease

Effective for discharges on or after August 1, 2001, payment may also be made if one of the following diagnosis codes is reported:

286.5 Hemorrhagic disorder due to circulating anticoagulants

286.7 Acquired coagulation factor deficiency

C. Part A Remittance Advice

1. X12.835 Ver. 003030M
   For remittance reporting PIP and/or non-PIP payments, the Hemophilia Add on will be reported in a claims level 2-090-CAS segment (CAS is the element identifier) exhibiting an "OA" Group Code and adjustment reason code "97" (payment is included in the allowance for the basic service/ procedure) followed by the associated dollar amount (POSITIVE) and units of service. For this version of the 835, "OA" group coded line level CAS segments are informational and are not included in the balancing routine. The Hemophilia Add On amount will always be included in the 2-010-CLP04 Claim Payment Amount.

   For remittance reporting PIP payments, the Hemophilia Add On will also be reported in the provider level adjustment (element identifier PLB) segment with the provider level adjustment reason code "CA" (Manual claims adjustment) followed by the associated dollar amount (NEGATIVE).

   NOTE: A data maintenance request will be submitted to ANSI ASC X12 for a new PLB adjustment reason code specifically for PIP payment Hemophilia Add On situations for future use. However, continue to use adjustment reason code "CA" until further notice.

   The FIs enter MA103 (Hemophilia Add On) in an open MIA (element identifier) remark code data element. This will alert the provider that the reason code 97 and PLB code "CA" adjustments are related to the Hemophilia Add On.

2. X12.835 Ver. 003051
   For remittances reporting PIP and/or non-PIP payments, Hemophilia Add On information will be reported in the claim level 2-062-AMT and 2-064-QTY segments. The 2-062-AMTO1 element will carry a "ZK" (Federal Medicare claim MANDATE - Category 1) qualifier code followed by the total claim level Hemophilia Add On amount (POSITIVE). The 2-064QTY01 element will carry a "FL" (Units) qualifier code followed by the number of units approved for the Hemophilia Add On for the claim. The Hemophilia Add On amount will always be included in the 2-010-CLP04 Claim Payment Amount.

   NOTE: A data maintenance request will be submitted to ANSI ASC X12 for a new AMT qualifier code specifically for the Hemophilia Add On for future use. However, continue to use adjustment reason code "ZK" until further notice.

   For remittances reporting PIP payments, the Hemophilia Add On will be reported in the provider level adjustment PLB segment with the provider level adjustment reason "ZZ" followed by the associated dollar amount (NEGATIVE).

   NOTE: A data maintenance request will be submitted to ANSI ASC X12 for a new PLB, adjustment reason code specifically for the Hemophilia Add On for future use. However, continue to use PLB adjustment reason code "ZZ" until further notice. The FIs enter MA103 (Hemophilia Add On) in an open MIA remark code data element. This will alert the provider that the ZK, FL and ZZ entries are related to the Hemophilia Add On. (Effective with version 4010 of the 835, report ZK in lieu of FL in the QTY segment.)

3. Standard Hard Copy Remittance Advice
   For paper remittances reporting non-PIP payments involving Hemophilia Add On, add a "Hemophilia Add On" category to the end of the "Pass Thru Amounts" listings in the "Summary" section of the paper remittance. Enter the total of the

Hemophilia Add On amounts due for the claims covered by this remittance next to the Hemophilia Add On heading.

The FIs add the Remark Code "MA103" (Hemophilia Add On) to the remittance advice under the REM column for those claims that qualify for Hemophilia Add On payments.

This will be the full extent of Hemophilia Add On reporting on paper remittance notices; providers wishing more detailed information must subscribe to the Medicare Part A specifications for the ANSI ASC X12N 835, where additional information is available.

See chapter 22, for detailed instructions and definitions.

100-4, 3, 40.2.2

Charges to Beneficiaries for Part A Services

The hospital submits a bill even where the patient is responsible for a deductible which covers the entire amount of the charges for non-PPS hospitals, or in PPS hospitals, where the DRG payment amount will be less than the deductible.

A hospital receiving payment for a covered hospital stay (or PPS hospital that includes at least one covered day, or one treated as covered under guarantee of payment or limitation on liability) may charge the beneficiary, or other person, for items and services furnished during the stay only as described in subsections A through H. If limitation of liability applies, a beneficiary's liability for payment is governed by the limitation on liability notification rules in Chapter 30 of this manual. For related notices for inpatient hospitals, see CMS Transmittal 594, Change Request 3903, dated June 24, 2005.

A. Deductible and Coinsurance

The hospital may charge the beneficiary or other person for applicable deductible and coinsurance amounts. The deductible is satisfied only by charges for covered services. The FI deducts the deductible and coinsurance first from the PPS payment. Where the deductible exceeds the PPS amount, the excess will be applied to a subsequent payment to the hospital. (See Chapter 3 of the Medicare General Information, Eligibility, and Entitlement Manual for specific policies.)

B. Blood Deductible

The Part A blood deductible provision applies to whole blood and red blood cells, and reporting of the number of pints is applicable to both PPS and non-PPS hospitals. (See Chapter 3 of the Medicare General Information, Eligibility, and Entitlement Manual for specific policies.) Hospitals shall report charges for red blood cells using revenue code 381, and charges for whole blood using revenue code 382.

C. Inpatient Care No Longer Required

The hospital may charge for services that are not reasonable and necessary or that constitute custodial care. Notification may be required under limitation of liability. See CMS Transmittal 594, Change Request3903, dated June 24, 2005, section V. of the attachment, for specific notification requirements. Note this transmittal will be placed in Chapter 30 of this manual at a future point. Chapter 1, section 150 of this manual also contains related billing information in addition to that provided below.

In general, after proper notification has occurred, and assuming an expedited decision is received from a Quality Improvement Organization (QIO), the following entries are required on the bill the hospital prepares:

- Occurrence code 3l (and date) to indicate the date the hospital notified the patient in accordance with the first bullet above;
- Occurrence span code 76 (and dates) to indicate the period of noncovered care for which it is charging the beneficiary;
- Occurrence span code 77 (and dates) to indicate the period of noncovered care for which the provider is liable, when it is aware of this prior to billing; and
- Value code 3l (and amount) to indicate the amount of charges it may bill the beneficiary for days for which inpatient care was no longer required. They are included as noncovered charges on the bill.

D. Change in the Beneficiary's Condition

If the beneficiary remains in the hospital after receiving notice as described in subsection C, and the hospital, the physician who concurred in the hospital's determination, or the QIO, subsequently determines that the beneficiary again requires inpatient hospital care, the hospital may not charge the beneficiary or other person for services furnished after the beneficiary again required inpatient hospital care until proper notification occurs (see subsection C).

If a patient who needs only a SNF level of care remains in the hospital after the SNF bed becomes available, and the bed ceases to be available, the hospital may continue to charge the beneficiary. It need not provide the beneficiary with another notice when the patient chose not to be discharged to the SNF bed.

E. Admission Denied

If the entire hospital admission is determined to be not reasonable or necessary, limitation of liability may apply. See 2005 CMS transmittal 594, section V. of the attachment, for specific notification requirements.

NOTE: This transmittal will be placed in Chapter 30 of this manual at a future point.

In such cases the following entries are required on the bill:

- Occurrence code 3l (and date) to indicate the date the hospital notified the beneficiary.
- Occurrence span code 76 (and dates) to indicate the period of noncovered care for which the hospital is charging the beneficiary.
- Occurrence span code 77 (and dates) to indicate any period of noncovered care for which the provider is liable (e.g., the period between issuing the notice and the time it may charge the beneficiary) when the provider is aware of this prior to billing.
- Value code 3l (and amount) to indicate the amount of charges the hospital may bill the beneficiary for hospitalization that was not necessary or reasonable. They are included as noncovered charges on the bill.

F. Procedures, Studies and Courses of Treatment That Are Not Reasonable or Necessary

If diagnostic procedures, studies, therapeutic studies and courses of treatment are excluded from coverage as not reasonable and necessary (even though the beneficiary requires inpatient hospital care) the hospital may charge the beneficiary or other person for the services or care according the procedures given in CMS Transmittal 594, Change Request3903, dated June 24, 2005.

The following bill entries apply to these circumstances:

- Occurrence code 32 (and date) to indicate the date the hospital provided the notice to the beneficiary.
- Value code 3l (and amount) to indicate the amount of such charges to be billed to the beneficiary. They are included as noncovered charges on the bill.

G. Nonentitlement Days and Days after Benefits Exhausted

If a hospital stay exceeds the day outlier threshold, the hospital may charge for some, or all, of the days on which the patient is not entitled to Medicare Part A, or after the Part A benefits are exhausted (i.e., the hospital may charge its customary charges for services furnished on those days). It may charge the beneficiary for the lesser of:

- The number of days on which the patient was not entitled to benefits or after the benefits were exhausted; or
- The number of outlier days. (Day outliers were discontinued at the end of FY 1997.)

If the number of outlier days exceeds the number of days on which the patient was not entitled to benefits, or after benefits were exhausted, the hospital may charge for all days on which the patient was not entitled to benefits or after benefits were exhausted. If the number of days on which the beneficiary was not entitled to benefits, or after benefits were exhausted, exceeds the number of outlier days, the hospital determines the days for which it may charge by starting with the last day of the stay (i.e., the day before the day of discharge) and identifying and counting off in reverse order, days on which the patient was not entitled to benefits or after the benefits were exhausted, until the number of days counted off equals the number of outlier days. The days counted off are the days for which the hospital may charge.

H. Contractual Exclusions

In addition to receiving the basic prospective payment, the hospital may charge the beneficiary for any services that are excluded from coverage for reasons other than, or in addition to, absence of medical necessity, provision of custodial care, non-entitlement to Part A, or exhaustion of benefits. For example, it may charge for most cosmetic and dental surgery.

I. Private Room Care

Payment for medically necessary private room care is included in the prospective payment. Where the beneficiary requests private room accommodations, the hospital must inform the beneficiary of the additional charge. (See the Medicare Benefit Policy Manual, Chapter 1.) When the beneficiary accepts the liability, the hospital will supply the service, and bill the beneficiary directly. If the beneficiary believes the private room was medically necessary, the beneficiary has a right to a determination and may initiate a Part A appeal.

J. Deluxe Item or Service

Where a beneficiary requests a deluxe item or service, i.e., an item or service which is more expensive than is medically required for the beneficiary's condition, the hospital may collect the additional charge if it informs the beneficiary of the additional charge. That charge is the difference between the customary charge for the item or service most commonly furnished by the hospital to private pay patients with the beneficiary's condition, and the charge for the more expensive item or service requested. If the beneficiary believes that the more expensive item or service was medically necessary, the beneficiary has a right to a determination and may initiate a Part A appeal.

K. Inpatient Acute Care Hospital Admission Followed By a Death or Discharge Prior To Room Assignment

A patient of an acute care hospital is considered an inpatient upon issuance of written doctor's orders to that effect. If a patient either dies or is discharged prior to being assigned and/or occupying a room, a hospital may enter an appropriate room and board charge on the claim. If a patient leaves of their own volition prior to being assigned and/or occupying a room, a hospital may enter an appropriate room and board charge on the claim as well as a patient status code 07 which indicates they left against medical advice. A hospital is not required to enter a room and board charge, but failure to do so may have a minimal impact on future DRG weight calculations.

100-4, 3, 90.1

Kidney Transplant - General

A3-3612, HO-E414

A major treatment for patients with ESRD is kidney transplantation. This involves removing a kidney, usually from a living relative of the patient or from an unrelated person who has died, and surgically placing the kidney into the patient. After the beneficiary receives a kidney transplant, Medicare pays the transplant hospital for the

transplant and appropriate standard acquisition charges. Special provisions apply to payment. For the list of approved Medicare certified transplant facilities, refer to the following Web site:
http://www.cms.hhs.gov/CertificationandComplianc/20_Transplant.asp#TopOfPage

A transplant hospital may acquire cadaver kidneys by:

- Excising kidneys from cadavers in its own hospital; and
- Arrangements with a freestanding organ procurement organization (OPO) that provides cadaver kidneys to any transplant hospital or by a hospital based OPO.

A transplant hospital that is also a certified organ procurement organization may acquire cadaver kidneys by:

- Having its organ procurement team excise kidneys from cadavers in other hospitals;
- Arrangements with participating community hospitals, whether they excise kidneys on a regular or irregular basis; and
- Arrangements with an organ procurement organization that services the transplant hospital as a member of a network.

When the transplant hospital also excises the cadaver kidney, the cost of the procedure is included in its kidney acquisition costs and is considered in arriving at its standard cadaver kidney acquisition charge. When the transplant hospital excises a kidney to provide another hospital, it may use its standard cadaver kidney acquisition charge or its standard detailed departmental charges to bill that hospital.

When the excising hospital is not a transplant hospital, it bills its customary charges for services used in excising the cadaver kidney to the transplant hospital or organ procurement agency.

If the transplanting hospital's organ procurement team excises the cadaver kidney at another hospital, the cost of operating such a team is included in the transplanting hospital's kidney acquisition costs, along with the reasonable charges billed by the other hospital of its services.

100-4, 3, 90.1.1

The Standard Kidney Acquisition Charge

(Rev. 2008, Issued: 07-30-10, Effective: 01-01-11, Implementation: 01-03-11)

There are two basic standard charges that must be developed by transplant hospitals from costs expected to be incurred in the acquisition of kidneys:

- The standard charge for acquiring a live donor kidney; and
- The standard charge for acquiring a cadaver kidney.

The standard charge is not a charge representing the acquisition cost of a specific kidney; rather, it is a charge that reflects the average cost associated with each type of kidney acquisition.

When the transplant hospital bills the program for the transplant, it shows its standard kidney acquisition charge on a separate line on the billing form.

Acquisition services are billed from the excising hospital to the transplant hospital. A billing form is not submitted from the excising hospital to the FI. The transplant hospital keeps an itemized statement that identifies the services furnished, the charges, the person receiving the service (donor/recipient), and whether this is a potential transplant donor or recipient. These charges are reflected in the transplant hospital's kidney acquisition cost center and are used in determining the hospital's standard charge for acquiring a live donor's kidney or a cadaver's kidney. The standard charge is not a charge representing the acquisition cost of a specific kidney. Rather, it is a charge that reflects the average cost associated with each type of kidney acquisition. Also, it is an all-inclusive charge for all services required in acquisition of a kidney, i.e., tissue typing, post-operative evaluation.

A. Billing For Blood And Tissue Typing of the Transplant Recipient Whether or Not Medicare Entitlement Is Established

Tissue typing and pre-transplant evaluation can be reflected only through the kidney acquisition charge of the hospital where the transplant will take place. The transplant hospital includes in its kidney acquisition cost center the reasonable charges it pays to the independent laboratory or other hospital which typed the potential transplant recipient, either before or after his entitlement. It also includes reasonable charges paid for physician tissue typing services, applicable to live donors and recipients (during the pre-entitlement period and after entitlement, but prior to hospital admission for transplantation).

B. Billing for Blood and Tissue Typing and Other Pre-Transplant Evaluation of Live Donors

The entitlement date of the beneficiary who will receive the transplant is not a consideration in reimbursing for the services to donors, since no bill is submitted directly to Medicare. All charges for services to donors prior to admission into the hospital for excision are "billed" indirectly to Medicare through the live donor acquisition charge of transplanting hospitals.

C. Billing Donor And Recipient Pre-Transplant Services (Performed by Transplant Hospitals or Other Providers) to the Kidney Acquisition Cost Center

The transplant hospital prepares an itemized statement of the services rendered for submittal to its cost accounting department. Regular Medicare billing forms are not necessary for this purpose, since no bills are submitted to the FI at this point.

The itemized statement should contain information that identifies the person receiving the service (donor/recipient), the health care insurance number, the service rendered and the charge for the service, as well as a statement as to whether this is a potential transplant donor or recipient. If it is a potential donor, the provider must identify the prospective recipient.

EXAMPLE:

Mary Jones
Health care insurance number
200 Adams St.
Anywhere, MS

Transplant donor evaluation services for recipient:

John Jones
Health care insurance number
200 Adams St.
Anywhere, MS

Services performed in a hospital other than the potential transplant hospital or by an independent laboratory are billed by that facility to the potential transplant hospital. This holds true regardless of where in the United States the service is performed. For example, if the donor services are performed in a Florida hospital and the transplant is to take place in a California hospital, the Florida hospital bills the California hospital (as described in above). The Florida hospital is paid by the California hospital, which recoups the monies through the kidney acquisition cost center.

D. Billing for Cadaveric Donor Services

Normally, various tests are performed to determine the type and suitability of a cadaver kidney. Such tests may be performed by the excising hospital (which may also be a transplant hospital) or an independent laboratory. When the excising-only hospital performs the tests, it includes the related charges on its bill to the transplant hospital or to the organ procurement agency.

When the tests are performed by the transplant hospital, it uses the related costs in establishing the standard charge for acquiring the cadaver kidney. The transplant hospital includes the costs and charges in the appropriate departments for final cost settlement purposes.

When the tests are performed by an independent laboratory for the excising-only hospital or the transplant hospital, the laboratory bills the hospital that engages its services or the organ procurement agency. The excising-only hospital includes such charges in its charges to the transplant hospital, which then includes the charges in developing its standard charge for acquiring the cadaver kidney. It is the transplant hospitals' responsibility to assure that the independent laboratory does not bill both hospitals.

The cost of these services cannot be billed directly to the program, since such tests and other procedures performed on a cadaver are not identifiable to a specific patient.

E. Billing For Physicians' Services Prior to Transplantation

Physicians' services applicable to kidney excisions involving live donors and recipients (during the pre-entitlement period and after entitlement, but prior to entrance into the hospital for transplantation) as well as all physicians' services applicable to cadavers are considered Part A hospital services (kidney acquisition costs).

F. Billing for Physicians' Services After Transplantation

All physicians' services rendered to the living donor and all physicians' services rendered to the transplant recipient are billed to the Medicare program in the same manner as all Medicare Part B services are billed. All donor physicians' services must be billed to the account of the recipient (i.e., the recipient's Medicare number). Modifier Q3 (Live Kidney Donor and Related Services) appears on the claim. For services performed on or after January 1, 2011 CWF shall allow Edit 5211 to be overridden at the contractor level. Also, contractors shall override Edit 5211 when this modifier appears on claims for donor services it receives when the recipient is deceased (See Publication 100-02, Chapter 11, Section 80.4).

NOTE: For institutional claims which do not require modifiers, contractors may manually override the CWF edit as necessary.

G. Billing For Physicians' Renal Transplantation Services

To ensure proper payment when submitting a Part B bill for the renal surgeon's services to the recipient, the appropriate HCPCS codes must be submitted, including HCPCS codes for concurrent surgery, as applicable.

The bill must include all living donor physicians' services, e.g., Revenue Center code 081X.

100-4, 3, 90.1.2

Billing for Kidney Transplant and Acquisition Services

Applicable standard kidney acquisition charges are identified separately in FL 42 by revenue code 0811 (Living Donor Kidney Acquisition) or 0812 (Cadaver Donor Kidney Acquisition). Where interim bills are submitted, the standard acquisition charge appears on the billing form for the period during which the transplant took place. This charge is in addition to the hospital's charges for services rendered directly to the Medicare recipient.

The contractor deducts kidney acquisition charges for PPS hospitals for processing through Pricer. These costs, incurred by approved kidney transplant hospitals, are not included in the prospective payment DRG 302 (kidney transplant). They are paid on a reasonable cost basis. Interim payment is paid as a "pass through" item. (See the Provider Reimbursement Manual, Part 1, Sec.2802 B.8.) The contractor includes kidney acquisition charges under the appropriate revenue code in CWF.

Bill Review Procedures
The Medicare Code Editor (MCE) creates a Limited Coverage edit for procedure code 55.69 (kidney transplant). Where this procedure code is identified by MCE, the contractor checks the provider number to determine if the provider is an approved transplant center, and checks the effective approval date. The contractor shall also determine if the facility is certified for adults and/or pediatric transplants dependent upon the patient's age. If payment is appropriate (i.e., the center is approved and the service is on or after the approval date) it overrides the limited coverage edit.

100-4, 3, 90.2

Heart Transplants

A3-3613, HO-416

Cardiac transplantation is covered under Medicare when performed in a facility which is approved by Medicare as meeting institutional coverage criteria. On April 6, 1987, CMS Ruling 87-1, "Criteria for Medicare Coverage of Heart Transplants" was published in the "Federal Register." For Medicare coverage purposes, heart transplants are medically reasonable and necessary when performed in facilities that meet these criteria. If a hospital wishes to bill Medicare for heart transplants, it must submit an application and documentation, showing its ongoing compliance with each criterion.

If a contractor has any questions concerning the effective or approval dates of its hospitals, it should contact its RO.

For a complete list of approved transplant centers, visit: http://www.cms.hhs.gov/CertificationandComplianc/20_Transplant.asp#TopOfPage

A. Effective Dates
The effective date of coverage for heart transplants performed at facilities applying after July 6, 1987, is the date the facility receives approval as a heart transplant facility. Coverage is effective for discharges October 17, 1986 for facilities that would have qualified and that applied by July 6, 1987. All transplant hospitals will be recertified under the final rule, Federal Register / Vol. 72, No. 61 / Friday, March 30, 2007, / Rules and Regulations.

The CMS informs each hospital of its effective date in an approval letter.

B. Drugs
Medicare Part B covers immunosuppressive drugs following a covered transplant in an approved facility.

C. Noncovered Transplants
Medicare will not cover transplants or re-transplants in facilities that have not been approved as meeting the facility criteria. If a beneficiary is admitted for and receives a heart transplant from a hospital that is not approved, physicians' services, and inpatient services associated with the transplantation procedure are not covered.

If a beneficiary received a heart transplant from a hospital while it was not an approved facility and later requires services as a result of the noncovered transplant, the services are covered when they are reasonable and necessary in all other respects.

D. Charges for Heart Acquisition Services
The excising hospital bills the OPO, who in turn bills the transplant (implant) hospital for applicable services. It should not submit a bill to its contractor. The transplant hospital must keep an itemized statement that identifies the services rendered, the charges, the person receiving the service (donor/recipient), and whether this person is a potential transplant donor or recipient. These charges are reflected in the transplant hospital's heart acquisition cost center and are used in determining its standard charge for acquiring a donor's heart. The standard charge is not a charge representing the acquisition cost of a specific heart; rather, it reflects the average cost associated with each type of heart acquisition. Also, it is an all inclusive charge for all services required in acquisition of a heart, i.e., tissue typing, post-operative evaluation, etc.

Acquisition charges shall be billed on a 081X revenue code. Such charges are not considered for the IPPS outlier calculation when billed for a heart transplant.

E. Bill Review Procedures
The contractor takes the following actions to process heart transplant bills. It may accomplish them manually or modify its MCE and Grouper interface programs to handle the processing.

1. Change in MCE Interface
   The MCE creates a Limited Coverage edit for procedure code 37.51 (heart transplant). Where this procedure code is identified by MCE, the contractor checks the provider number to determine if the provider is an approved transplant center, and checks the effective approval date. The contractor shall also determine if the facility is certified for adults and/or pediatric transplants dependent upon the patient's age. If payment is appropriate (i.e., the center is approved and the service is on or after the approval date) it overrides the limited coverage edit.
2. Handling Heart Transplant Billings From Nonapproved Hospitals
   Where a heart transplant and covered services are provided by a nonapproved hospital, the bill data processed through Grouper and Pricer must exclude transplant procedure codes and related charges.

100-4, 3, 90.2.1

Artificial Hearts and Related Devices

Effective for discharges before May 1, 2008, Medicare does not cover the use of artificial hearts, either as a permanent replacement for a human heart or as a temporary life-support system until a human heart becomes available for transplant (often referred to a "bridge to transplant").

Medicare does cover a Ventricular Assist Device (VAD). A VAD is used to assist a damaged or weakened heart in pumping blood. VADs are used as a bridge to a heart transplant, for support of blood circulation postcardiotomy or destination therapy. Refer to the NCD Manual, section 20.9 for coverage criteria.

The MCE creates a Limited Coverage edit for procedure code 37.66. This procedure code has limited coverage due to the stringent conditions that must be met by hospitals. Where this procedure code is identified by MCE, the FI shall determine if coverage criteria is met and override the MCE if appropriate.

Effective for discharges on or after May 1, 2008, the use of artificial hearts will be covered by Medicare under Coverage with Evidence Development when beneficiaries are enrolled in a clinical study that meets all of the criteria listed in Pub. 100-03, Medicare NCD Manual, section 20.9.

100-4, 3, 90.3

Stem Cell Transplantation

Stem cell transplantation is a process in which stem cells are harvested from either a patient's or donor's bone marrow or peripheral blood for intravenous infusion. Autologous stem cell transplants (AuSCT) must be used to effect hematopoietic reconstitution following severely myelotoxic doses of chemotherapy (HDCT) and/or radiotherapy used to treat various malignancies. Allogeneic stem cell transplant may also be used to restore function in recipients having an inherited or acquired deficiency or defect.

Bone marrow and peripheral blood stem cell transplantation is a process which includes mobilization, harvesting, and transplant of bone marrow or peripheral blood stem cells and the administration of high dose chemotherapy or radiotherapy prior to the actual transplant. When bone marrow or peripheral blood stem cell transplantation is covered, all necessary steps are included in coverage. When bone marrow or peripheral blood stem cell transplantation is non-covered, none of the steps are covered.

Allogeneic and autologous stem cell transplants are covered under Medicare for specific diagnoses. Effective October 1, 1990, these cases were assigned to MS-DRG 009, Bone Marrow Transplant.

The FI's Medicare Code Editor (MCE) will edit stem cell transplant procedure codes 4101, 4102, 4103, 4104, 4105, 4107, 4108, and 4109 against diagnosis codes to determine which cases meet specified coverage criteria. Cases with a diagnosis code for a covered condition will pass (as covered) the MCE noncovered procedure edit. When a stem cell transplant case is selected for review based on the random selection of beneficiaries, the QIO will review the case on a post-payment basis to assure proper coverage decisions.

Procedure code 41.00 (bone marrow transplant, not otherwise specified) will be classified as noncovered and the claim will be returned to the hospital for a more specific procedure code.

The A/B MACs or the FI may choose to review if data analysis deems it a priority.

100-4, 3, 90.3.1

Allogeneic Stem Cell Transplantation

A. General
Allogeneic stem cell transplantation (ICD-9-CM Procedure Codes 41.02, 41.03, 41.05, and 41.08, CPT-4 Code 38240) is a procedure in which a portion of a healthy donor's stem cells are obtained and prepared for intravenous infusion to restore normal hematopoietic function in recipients having an inherited or acquired hematopoietic deficiency or defect. See Pub. 100-03, National Coverage Determinations Manual, chapter 1, section 110.8.1, for more information.

Expenses incurred by a donor are a covered benefit to the recipient/beneficiary but, except for physician services, are not paid separately. Services to the donor include physician services, hospital care in connection with screening the stem cell, and ordinary follow-up care.

B. Covered Conditions

1. Effective for services performed on or after August 1, 1978:
   - For the treatment of leukemia, leukemia in remission (ICD-9-CM codes 204.00 through 208.91), or aplastic anemia (ICD-9-CM codes 284.0 through 284.9) when it is reasonable and necessary; and
2. Effective for services performed on or after June 3, 1985:
   - For the treatment of severe combined immunodeficiency disease (SCID) (ICD-9-CM code 279.2), and for the treatment of Wiskott-Aldrich syndrome (ICD-9-CM 279.12).

C. Non-Covered Conditions

3. Effective for services performed on or after May 24, 1996:
   - Allogeneic stem cell transplantation is not covered as treatment for multiple myeloma (ICD-9-CM codes 203.00 and 203.01).

4. Effective for services performed on or after August 4, 2010:

The Centers for Medicare & Medicaid Services (CMS) issued an NCD stating that it believes the evidence does not demonstrate that the use of allogeneic hematopoietic stem cell transplantation (HSCT) improves health outcomes in Medicare beneficiaries with Myelodysplastic Syndrome (MDS). Therefore, allogeneic HSCT for MDS is not reasonable and necessary under §1862(a)(1)(A) of the Social Security Act (the Act).

However, allogeneic HSCT for MDS is reasonable and necessary under §1862(a)(1)(E) of the Act and therefore covered by Medicare ONLY if provided pursuant to a Medicare-approved clinical study under Coverage with Evidence Development (CED). These services are covered in both the inpatient and outpatient hospital setting. Refer to Pub. 100-03, NCD Manual, chapter 1, section 110.8.1, for further information about this policy, and Pub. 100-04, MCP Manual, chapter 32, section 90.6, for information on CED.

NOTE: Coverage for conditions other than these specifically designated as covered or non-covered in the CP or NCD Manuals are left to local Medicare contractor discretion.

100-4, 3, 90.3.2

Autologous Stem Cell Transplantation (AuSCT)

A. General

Autologous stem cell transplantation (AuSCT) (ICD-9-CM procedure code 41.01, 41.04, 41.07, and 41.09 and CPT-4 code 38241) is a technique for restoring stem cells using the patient's own previously stored cells. AuSCT must be used to effect hematopoietic reconstitution following severely myelotoxic doses of chemotherapy (high dose chemotherapy (HDCT)) and/or radiotherapy used to treat various malignancies.

B. Covered Conditions

1. Effective for services performed on or after April 28, 1989:

- Acute leukemia in remission (ICD-9-CM codes 204.01, lymphoid; 205.01, myeloid; 206.01, monocytic; 207.01, acute erythremia and erythroleukemia; and 208.01 unspecified cell type) patients who have a high probability of relapse and who have no human leucocyte antigens (HLA)-matched;
- Resistant non-Hodgkin's lymphomas (ICD-9-CM codes 200.00-200.08, 200.10-200.18, 200.20-200.28, 200.80-200.88, 202.00-202.08, 202.80-202.88, and 202.90-202.98) or those presenting with poor prognostic features following an initial response;
- Recurrent or refractory neuroblastoma (see ICD-9-CM Neoplasm by site, malignant); or
- Advanced Hodgkin's disease (ICD-9-CM codes 201.00-201.98) patients who have failed conventional therapy and have no HLA-matched donor.

2. Effective for services performed on or after October 1, 2000:

- Durie-Salmon Stage II or III that fit the following requirement: Newly diagnosed or responsive multiple myeloma (ICD-9-CM codes 203.00 and 238.6). This includes those patients with previously untreated disease, those with at least a partial response to prior chemotherapy (defined as a 50% decrease either in measurable paraprotein [serum and/or urine] or in bone marrow infiltration, sustained for at least 1 month), and those in responsive relapse, and adequate cardiac, renal, pulmonary, and hepatic function.

3. Effective for services performed on or after March 15, 2005, when recognized clinical risk factors are employed to select patients for transplantation, high-dose melphalan (HDM), together with AuSCT, in treating Medicare beneficiaries of any age group with primary amyloid light-chain (AL) amyloidosis who meet the following criteria:

    1. Amyloid deposition in 2 or fewer organs; and,
    2. Cardiac left ventricular ejection fraction (EF) of 45% or greater.

C. Noncovered Conditions

Insufficient data exist to establish definite conclusions regarding the efficacy of autologous stem cell transplantation for the following conditions:

- Acute leukemia not in remission (ICD-9-CM codes 204.00, 205.00, 206.00, 207.00 and 208.00);
- Chronic granulocytic leukemia (ICD-9-CM codes 205.10 and 205.11);
- Solid tumors (other than neuroblastoma) (ICD-9-CM codes 140.0-199.1);
- Multiple myeloma (ICD-9-CM code 203.00 and 238.6), through September 30, 2000.
- Tandem transplantation (multiple rounds of autologous stem cell transplantation) for patients with multiple myeloma (ICD-9-CM code 203.00 and 238.6)
- Non-primary (AL) amyloidosis (ICD-9-CM code 277.3), effective October 1, 2000; or
- Primary (AL) amyloidosis (ICD-9-CM code 277.3) for Medicare beneficiaries age 64 or older, effective October 1, 2000, through March 14, 2005.

NOTE: Coverage for conditions other than these specifically designated as covered or non-covered is left to the FI's discretion.

100-4, 3, 90.3.3

Billing for Stem Cell Transplantation

(Rev. 1882, Issued: 12-21-09; Effective Date: 01-01-10; Implementation Date: 01-04-10)

A. Billing for Allogeneic Stem Cell Transplants

1. Definition of Acquisition Charges for Allogeneic Stem Cell Transplants

    Acquisition charges for allogeneic stem cell transplants include, but are not limited to, charges for the costs of the following services:

    - National Marrow Donor Program fees, if applicable, for stem cells from an unrelated donor;
    - Tissue typing of donor and recipient;
    - Donor evaluation;
    - Physician pre-admission/pre-procedure donor evaluation services;
    - Costs associated with harvesting procedure (e.g., general routine and special care services, procedure/operating room and other ancillary services, apheresis services, etc.);
    - Post-operative/post-procedure evaluation of donor; and
    - Preparation and processing of stem cells.

    Payment for these acquisition services is included in the MS-DRG payment for the allogeneic stem cell transplant when the transplant occurs in the inpatient setting, and in the OPPS APC payment for the allogeneic stem cell transplant when the transplant occurs in the outpatient setting. The Medicare contractor does not make separate payment for these acquisition services, because hospitals may bill and receive payment only for services provided to the Medicare beneficiary who is the recipient of the stem cell transplant and whose illness is being treated with the stem cell transplant. Unlike the acquisition costs of solid organs for transplant (e.g., hearts and kidneys), which are paid on a reasonable cost basis, acquisition costs for allogeneic stem cells are included in prospective payment.

    Acquisition charges for stem cell transplants apply only to allogeneic transplants, for which stem cells are obtained from a donor (other than the recipient himself or herself). Acquisition charges do not apply to autologous transplants (transplanted stem cells are obtained from the recipient himself or herself), because autologous transplants involve services provided to the beneficiary only (and not to a donor), for which the hospital may bill and receive payment (see Pub. 100-04, chapter 4, §231.10 and paragraph B of this section for information regarding billing for autologous stem cell transplants).

2. Billing for Acquisition Services

    The hospital bills and shows acquisition charges for allogeneic stem cell transplants based on the status of the patient (i.e., inpatient or outpatient) when the transplant is furnished. See Pub. 100-04, chapter 4, ?231.11 for instructions regarding billing for acquisition services for allogeneic stem cell transplants that are performed in the outpatient setting.

    When the allogeneic stem cell transplant occurs in the inpatient setting, the hospital identifies stem cell acquisition charges for allogeneic bone marrow/stem cell transplants separately in FL 42 of Form CMS-1450 (or electronic equivalent) by using revenue code 0819 (Other Organ Acquisition). Revenue code 0819 charges should include all services required to acquire stem cells from a donor, as defined above.

    On the recipient's transplant bill, the hospital reports the acquisition charges, cost report days, and utilization days for the donor's hospital stay (if applicable) and/or charges for other encounters in which the stem cells were obtained from the donor. The donor is covered for medically necessary inpatient hospital days of care or outpatient care provided in connection with the allogeneic stem cell transplant under Part A. Expenses incurred for complications are paid only if they are directly and immediately attributable to the stem cell donation procedure. The hospital reports the acquisition charges on the billing form for the recipient, as described in the first paragraph of this section. It does not charge the donor's days of care against the recipient's utilization record. For cost reporting purposes, it includes the covered donor days and charges as Medicare days and charges.

    The transplant hospital keeps an itemized statement that identifies the services furnished, the charges, the person receiving the service (donor/recipient), and whether this is a potential transplant donor or recipient. These charges will be reflected in the transplant hospital's stem cell/bone marrow acquisition cost center. For allogeneic stem cell acquisition services in cases that do not result in transplant, due to death of the intended recipient or other causes, hospitals include the costs associated with the acquisition services on the Medicare cost report.

    The hospital shows charges for the transplant itself in revenue center code 0362 or another appropriate cost center. Selection of the cost center is up to the hospital.

B. Billing for Autologous Stem Cell Transplants

The hospital bills and shows all charges for autologous stem cell harvesting, processing, and transplant procedures based on the status of the patient (i.e., inpatient or outpatient) when the services are furnished. It shows charges for the actual transplant, described by the appropriate ICD-9-CM procedure or CPT codes, in revenue center code 0362 or another appropriate cost center.

The CPT codes describing autologous stem cell harvesting procedures may be billed and are separately payable under the OPPS when provided in the hospital outpatient setting of care. Autologous harvesting procedures are distinct from the acquisition services described in Pub. 100-04, chapter 4, ?231.11 and section A. above for allogeneic stem cell transplants, which include services provided when stem cells are obtained from a donor and not from the patient undergoing the stem cell transplant.The CPT codes describing autologous stem cell processing procedures also may be billed and are separately payable under the OPPS when provided to hospital outpatients.

Payment for autologous stem cell harvesting procedures performed in the hospital inpatient setting of care, with transplant also occurring in the inpatient setting of care, is included in the MS-DRG payment for the autologous stem cell transplant.

100-4, 3, 90.4

Liver Transplants

A. Background

For Medicare coverage purposes, liver transplants are considered medically reasonable and necessary for specified conditions when performed in facilities that meet specific criteria.

To review the current list of approved Liver Transplant Centers, see http://www.cms.hhs.gov/CertificationandComplianc/20_Transplant.asp#TopOfPage

100-4, 3, 90.4.1

Standard Liver Acquisition Charge

A3-3615.1, A3-3615.3

Each transplant facility must develop a standard charge for acquiring a cadaver liver from costs it expects to incur in the acquisition of livers.

This standard charge is not a charge that represents the acquisition cost of a specific liver. Rather, it is a charge that reflects the average cost associated with a liver acquisition.

Services associated with liver acquisition are billed from the organ procurement organization or, in some cases, the excising hospital to the transplant hospital. The excising hospital does not submit a billing form to the FI. The transplant hospital keeps an itemized statement that identifies the services furnished, the charges, the person receiving the service (donor/recipient), and the potential transplant donor. These charges are reflected in the transplant hospital's liver acquisition cost center and are used in determining the hospital's standard charge for acquiring a cadaver's liver. The standard charge is not a charge representing the acquisition cost of a specific liver. Rather, it is a charge that reflects the average cost associated with liver acquisition. Also, it is an all inclusive charge for all services required in acquisition of a liver, e.g., tissue typing, transportation of organ, and surgeons' retrieval fees.

100-4, 3, 90.4.2

Billing for Liver Transplant and Acquisition Services

Form CMS-1450 or its electronic equivalent is completed in accordance with instructions in chapter 25 for the beneficiary who receives a covered liver transplant. Applicable standard liver acquisition charges are identified separately in FL 42 by revenue code 0817 (Donor-Liver). Where interim bills are submitted, the standard acquisition charge appears on the billing form for the period during which the transplant took place. This charge is in addition to the hospital's charge for services furnished directly to the Medicare recipient.

The contractor deducts liver acquisition charges for IPPS hospitals prior to processing through Pricer. Costs of liver acquisition incurred by approved liver transplant facilities are not included in prospective payment DRG 480 (Liver Transplant). They are paid on a reasonable cost basis. This item is a "pass-through" cost for which interim payments are made. (See the Provider Reimbursement Manual, Part 1, Sec.2802 B.8.) The contractor includes liver acquisition charges under revenue code 0817 in the HUIP record that it sends to CWF and the QIO.

A. Bill Review Procedures

The contractor takes the following actions to process liver transplant bills.

1. Operative Report
   The contractor requires the operative report with all claims for liver transplants, or sends a development request to the hospital for each liver transplant with a diagnosis code for a covered condition.
2. MCE Interface
   Code 50.51 (Auxiliary liver transplant) is always a non-covered procedure. However, the MCE contains a limited coverage edit for procedure code 50.59 (liver transplant). Where procedure code 50.59 is identified by the MCE, the contractor shall check the provider number and effective date to determine if the provider is an approved liver transplant facility at the time of the transplant, and the contractor shall also determine if the facility is certified for adults and/or pediatric transplants dependent upon the patient's age. If yes, the claim is suspended for review of the operative report to determine whether the beneficiary has at least one of the covered conditions when the diagnosis code is for a covered condition. If payment is appropriate (i.e., the facility is approved, the service is furnished on or after the approval date, and the beneficiary has a covered condition), the contractor sends the claim to Grouper and Pricer.

   If none of the diagnoses codes are for a covered condition, or if the provider is not an approved liver transplant facility, the contractor denies the claim.

   NOTE: Some non-covered conditions are included in the covered diagnostic codes. (The diagnostic codes are broader than the covered conditions. For example, primary biliary cirrhosis is a covered condition, secondary biliary cirrhosis is not a covered condition. Both primary and secondary biliary cirrhosis have the same diagnosis code ICD 9 571.6) Do not pay for noncovered conditions.
3. Grouper
   If the bill shows a discharge date before March 8, 1990, the liver transplant procedure is not covered. If the discharge date is March 8, 1990 or later, the contractor processes the bill through Grouper and Pricer. If the discharge date is after March 7, 1990, and before October 1, 1990, Grouper assigned CMS DRG 191 or 192. The contractor sent the bill to Pricer with review code 08. Pricer would then overlay CMS DRG 191 or 192 with CMS DRG 480 and the weights and thresholds for CMS DRG 480 to price the bill. If the discharge date is after September 30, 1990, Grouper assigns CMS DRG 480 and Pricer is able to price without using review code 08. If the discharge date is after September 30, 2007, Grouper assigns MS-DRG 005 or 006 (Liver transplant with MCC or Intestinal Transplant or Liver transplant without MCC, respectively) and Pricer is able to price without using review code 08.
4. Liver Transplant Billing From Non-approved Hospitals
   Where a liver transplant and covered services are provided by a non-approved hospital, the bill data processed through Grouper and Pricer must exclude transplant procedure codes and related charges.

   When CMS approves a hospital to furnish liver transplant services, it informs the hospital of the effective date in the approval letter. The contractor will receive a copy of the letter.

100-4, 3, 90.5

Pancreas Transplants Kidney Transplants

A. Background

Effective July 1, 1999, Medicare covered pancreas transplantation when performed simultaneously with or following a kidney transplant (ICD-9-CM procedure code 55.69). Pancreas transplantation is performed to induce an insulin independent, euglycemic state in diabetic patients. The procedure is generally limited to those patients with severe secondary complications of diabetes including kidney failure. However, pancreas transplantation is sometimes performed on patients with labile diabetes and hypoglycemic unawareness.

Medicare has had a policy of not covering pancreas transplantation. The Office of Health Technology Assessment performed an assessment on pancreas-kidney transplantation in 1994. They found reasonable graft survival outcomes for patients receiving either simultaneous pancreas-kidney (SPK) transplantation or pancreas after kidney (PAK) transplantation. For a list of facilities approved to perform SPK or PAK, refer to the following Web site: http://www.cms.hhs.gov/Certificationand Complianc/20_Transplant.asp#TopOfPage

B. Billing for Pancreas Transplants

There are no special provisions related to managed care participants. Managed care plans are required to provide all Medicare covered services. Medicare does not restrict which hospitals or physicians may perform pancreas transplantation.

The transplant procedure and revenue code 0360 for the operating room are paid under these codes. Procedures must be reported using the current ICD-9-CM procedure codes for pancreas and kidney transplants. Providers must place at least one of the following transplant procedure codes on the claim:

52.80 Transplant of pancreas

52.82 Homotransplant of pancreas

The Medicare Code Editor (MCE) has been updated to include 52.80 and 52.82 as limited coverage procedures. The contractor must determine if the facility is approved for the transplant and certified for either pediatric or adult transplants dependent upon the age of the patient.

Effective October 1, 2000, ICD-9-CM code 52.83 was moved in the MCE to non-covered. The contractor must override any deny edit on claims that came in with 52.82 prior to October 1, 2000 and adjust, as 52.82 is the correct code.

If the discharge date is July 1, 1999, or later; the contractor processes the bill through Grouper and Pricer.

Pancreas transplantation is reasonable and necessary for the following diagnosis codes. However, since this is not an all-inclusive list, the contractor is permitted to determine if any additional diagnosis codes will be covered for this procedure.

Diabetes Diagnosis Codes

250.00 Diabetes mellitus without mention of complication, type II (non-insulin dependent) (NIDDM) (adult onset) or unspecified type, not stated as uncontrolled.

250.01 Diabetes mellitus without mention of complication, type I (insulin dependent) (IDDM) (juvenile), not stated as uncontrolled.

250.02 Diabetes mellitus without mention of complication, type II (non-insulin dependent) (NIDDM) (adult onset) or unspecified type, uncontrolled.

250.03 Diabetes mellitus without mention of complication, type I (insulin dependent) (IDDM) (juvenile), uncontrolled.

250.1X Diabetes with ketoacidosis

250.2X Diabetes with hyperosmolarity

250.3X Diabetes with coma

250.4X Diabetes with renal manifestations

250.5X Diabetes with ophthalmic manifestations

250.6X Diabetes with neurological manifestations

250.7X Diabetes with peripheral circulatory disorders

250.8X Diabetes with other specified manifestations

250.9X Diabetes with unspecified complication

NOTE: X=0-3

Hypertensive Renal Diagnosis Codes:

403.01 Malignant hypertensive renal disease, with renal failure

403.11 Benign hypertensive renal disease, with renal failure

403.91 Unspecified hypertensive renal disease, with renal failure

404.02 Malignant hypertensive heart and renal disease, with renal failure

404.03 Malignant hypertensive heart and renal disease, with congestive heart failure or renal failure

404.12 Benign hypertensive heart and renal disease, with renal failure

404.13 Benign hypertensive heart and renal disease, with congestive heart failure or renal failure

404.92 Unspecified hypertensive heart and renal disease, with renal failure

404.93 Unspecified hypertensive heart and renal disease, with congestive heart failure or renal failure

585.1-585.6, 585.9 Chronic Renal Failure Code

NOTE: If a patient had a kidney transplant that was successful, the patient no longer has chronic kidney failure, therefore it would be inappropriate for the provider to bill 585.1 - 585.6, 585.9 on such a patient. In these cases one of the following V-codes should be present on the claim or in the beneficiary's history.

The provider uses the following V-codes only when a kidney transplant was performed before the pancreas transplant:

V42.0 Organ or tissue replaced by transplant kidney

V43.89 Organ tissue replaced by other means, kidney or pancreas

NOTE: If a kidney and pancreas transplants are performed simultaneously, the claim should contain a diabetes diagnosis code and a renal failure code or one of the hypertensive renal failure diagnosis codes. The claim should also contain two transplant procedure codes. If the claim is for a pancreas transplant only, the claim should contain a diabetes diagnosis code and a V-code to indicate a previous kidney transplant. If the V-code is not on the claim for the pancreas transplant, the contractor will search the beneficiary's claim history for a V-code.

C. Drugs

If the pancreas transplant occurs after the kidney transplant, immunosuppressive therapy will begin with the date of discharge from the inpatient stay for the pancreas transplant.

D. Charges for Pancreas Acquisition Services

A separate organ acquisition cost center has been established for pancreas transplantation. The Medicare cost report will include a separate line to account for pancreas transplantation costs. The 42 CFR 412.2(e)(4) was changed to include pancreas in the list of organ acquisition costs that are paid on a reasonable cost basis.

Acquisition costs for pancreas transplantation as well as kidney transplants will occur in Revenue Center 081X. The contractor overrides any claims that suspend due to repetition of revenue code 081X on the same claim if the patient had a simultaneous kidney/pancreas transplant. It pays for acquisition costs for both kidney and pancreas organs if transplants are performed simultaneously. It will not pay for more than two organ acquisitions on the same claim.

E. Medicare Summary Notices (MSN) and Remittance Advice Messages

If the provider submits a claim for simultaneous pancreas kidney transplantation or pancreas transplantation following a kidney transplant, and omits one of the appropriate diagnosis/procedure codes, the contractor rejects the claim, using the following MSN:

- MSN 16.32, "Medicare does not pay separately for this service."
- Use the following Remittance Advice Message:
- Claim adjustment reason code B15, "Claim/service denied/reduced because this procedure or service is not paid separately."
- If a claim is denied because no evidence of a prior kidney transplant is presented, use the following MSN message:
- MSN 15.4, "The information provided does not support the need for this service or item."

The contractor uses the following Remittance Advice Message:

- Claim adjustment reason code 50, "These are non-covered services because this is not deemed a 'medical necessity' by the payer."

To further clarify the situation, the contractor should also use new claim level remark code MA 126, "Pancreas transplant not covered unless kidney transplant performed."

100-4, 3, 90.5.1

90.5.1 – Pancreas Transplants Alone (PA)

(Rev. 1815; Issued: 09-09-09; Effective Date: Discharges on or after October 1, 2009; Implementation Date: 10-05-09)

A. General

Pancreas transplantation is performed to induce an insulin-independent, euglycemic state in diabetic patients. The procedure is generally limited to those patients with severe secondary complications of diabetes, including kidney failure. However, pancreas transplantation is sometimes performed on patients with labile diabetes and hypoglycemic unawareness. Medicare has had a long-standing policy of not covering pancreas transplantation, as the safety and effectiveness of the procedure had not been demonstrated. The Office of Health Technology Assessment performed an assessment of pancreas-kidney transplantation in 1994. It found reasonable graft survival outcomes for patients receiving either simultaneous pancreas-kidney transplantation or pancreas-after kidney transplantation.

B. Nationally Covered Indications

CMS determines that whole organ pancreas transplantation will be nationally covered by Medicare when performed simultaneous with or after a kidney transplant. If the pancreas transplant occurs after the kidney transplant, immunosuppressive therapy will begin with the date of discharge from the inpatient stay for the pancreas transplant.

C. Billing and Claims Processing

Contractors shall pay for Pancreas Transplantation Alone (PA) effective for services on or after April 26, 2006 when performed in those facilities that are Medicare-approved for kidney transplantation. Approved facilities are located at the following address: http://www.cms.hhs.gov/CertificationandComplianc/20_Transplant.asp#TopOfPage Contractors who receive claims for PA services that were performed in an unapproved facility, should reject such claims. Contractors should use the following messages upon the reject or denial:

Medicare Summary Notice MSN Message - MSN code 16.2 (This service cannot be paid when provided in this location/facility)

- Remittance Advice Message - Claim Adjustment Reason Code 58 (Payment adjusted because treatment was deemed by the payer to have been rendered in an inappropriate or invalid place of service)

Payment will be made for a PA service performed in an approved facility, and which meets the coverage guidelines mentioned above for beneficiaries with type I diabetes.

All-Inclusive List of Covered ICD-9 CM Diagnosis Codes for PA

(**NOTE:** "X" = 1 and 3 only)

250.0X	Diabetes mellitus without mention of complication, type I (insulin dependent) (IDDM) (juvenile), not stated as uncontrolled.
250.1X	Diabetes with ketoacidosis
250.2X	Diabetes with hyperosmolarity
250.3X	Diabetes with coma
250.4X	Diabetes with renal manifestations
250.5X	Diabetes with ophthalmic manifestations
250.6X	Diabetes with neurological manifestations
250.7X	Diabetes with peripheral circulatory disorders
250.8X	Diabetes with other specified manifestations
250.9X	Diabetes with unspecified complication

Procedure Codes

ICD-9 CM

52.80 - Transplant of pancreas

52.82 - Homotransplant of pancreas

Contractors who receive claims for PA that are not billed using the covered diagnosis/procedure codes listed above shall reject such claims. The MCE edits to ensure that the transplant is covered based on the diagnosis. The MCE also considers 52.80 and 52.82 as limited coverage dependent upon whether the facility is approved to perform the transplant and is certified for the age of the patient. Contractors should use the following messages upon the reject or denial:

Medicare Summary Notice MSN Message - MSN code 15.4 (The information provided does not support the need for this service or item)

Remittance Advice Message - Claim Adjustment Reason Code 50 (These are non-covered services because this is not deemed a 'medical necessity' by the payer).

Contractors shall hold the provider liable for denied\rejected claims unless the hospital issues a Hospital Issued Notice of Non-coverage (HINN) or a physician issues an Advanced Beneficiary Notice (ABN) for Part-B for physician services.

D. Charges for Pancreas Alone Acquisition Services
A separate organ acquisition cost center has been established for pancreas transplantation. The Medicare cost report will include a separate line to account for pancreas transplantation costs. The 42 CFR 412.2(e)(4) was changed to include PA in the list of organ acquisition costs that are paid on a reasonable cost basis.

Acquisition costs for PA transplantation are billed in Revenue Code 081X. The contractor removes acquisition charges prior tsending the claims tPricer so such charges are not included in the outlier calculation.

100-4, 3, 90.6

Intestinal and Multi-Visceral Transplants

A. Background
Effective for services on or after April 1, 2001, Medicare covers intestinal and multi-visceral transplantation for the purpose of restoring intestinal function in patients with irreversible intestinal failure. Intestinal failure is defined as the loss of absorptive capacity of the small bowel secondary to severe primary gastrointestinal disease or surgically induced short bowel syndrome. Intestinal failure prevents oral nutrition and may be associated with both mortality and profound morbidity. Multi-Visceral transplantation includes organs in the digestive system (stomach, duodenum, liver, and intestine). See Sec.260.5 of the National Coverage Determinations Manual for further information.

B. Approved Transplant Facilities
Medicare will cover intestinal transplantation if performed in an approved facility. The approved facilities are located at:
http://www.cms.hhs.gov/CertificationandComplianc/20_Transplant.asp#TopOfPage

C. Billing
ICD-9-CM procedure code 46.97 is effective for discharges on or after April 1, 2001. The Medicare Code Editor (MCE) lists this code as a limited coverage procedure. The contractor shall override the MCE when this procedure code is listed and the coverage criteria are met in an approved transplant facility, and also determine if the facility is certified for adults and/or pediatric transplants dependent upon the patient's age.

For this procedure where the provider is approved as transplant facility and certified for the adult and/or pediatric population, and the service is performed on or after the transplant approval date, the contractor must suspend the claim for clerical review of the operative report to determine whether the beneficiary has at least one of the covered conditions listed when the diagnosis code is for a covered condition.

This review is not part of the contractor's medical review workload. Instead, the contractor should complete this review as part of its claims processing workload.

Charges for ICD-9-CM procedure code 46.97 should be billed under revenue code 0360, Operating Room Services.

For discharge dates on or after October 1, 2001, acquisition charges are billed under revenue code 081X, Organ Acquisition. For discharge dates between April 1, 2001, and September 30, 2001, hospitals were to report the acquisition charges on the claim, but there was no interim pass-through payment made for these costs.

Bill the procedure used to obtain the donor's organ on the same claim, using appropriate ICD-9-CM procedure codes.

The 11X bill type should be used when billing for intestinal transplants.

Immunosuppressive therapy for intestinal transplantation is covered and should be billed consistent with other organ transplants under the current rules.

There is no specific ICD-9-CM diagnosis code for intestinal failure. Diagnosis codes exist to capture the causes of intestinal failure. Some examples of intestinal failure include, but are not limited to:

- Volvulus 560.2,
- Volvulus gastroschisis 756.79, other [congenital] anomalies of abdominal wall,
- Volvulus gastroschisis 569.89, other specified disorders of intestine,
- Necrotizing enterocolitis 777.5, necrotizing enterocolitis in fetus or newborn,
- Necrotizing enterocolitis 014.8, other tuberculosis of intestines, peritoneum, and mesenteric,
- Necrotizing enterocolitis and splanchnic vascular thrombosis 557.0, acute vascular insufficiency of intestine,
- Inflammatory bowel disease 569.9, unspecified disorder of intestine,
- Radiation enteritis 777.5, necrotizing enterocolitis in fetus or newborn, and
- Radiation enteritis 558.1.

D. Acquisition Costs
A separate organ acquisition cost center was established for acquisition costs incurred on or after October 1, 2001. The Medicare Cost Report will include a separate line to account for these transplantation costs.

For intestinal and multi-visceral transplants performed between April 1, 2001, and October 1, 2001, the DRG payment was payment in full for all hospital services related to this procedure.

E. Medicare Summary Notices (MSN), Remittance Advice Messages, and Notice of Utilization Notices (NOU)
If an intestinal transplant is billed by an unapproved facility after April 1, 2001, the contractor shall deny the claim and use MSN message 21.6, "This item or service is not covered when performed, referred, or ordered by this provider;" 21.18, "This item or service is not covered when performed or ordered by this provider;" or, 16.2, "This service cannot be paid when provided in this location/facility;" and Remittance Advice Message, Claim Adjustment Reason Code 52, "The referring/prescribing/ rendering provider is not eligible to refer/prescribe/order/perform the service billed."

100-4, 3,100.1

Billing for Abortion Services

Effective October 1, 1998, abortions are not covered under the Medicare program except for instances where the pregnancy is a result of an act of rape or incest; or the woman suffers from a physical disorder, physical injury, or physical illness, including a life endangering physical condition caused by the pregnancy itself that would, as certified by a physician, place the woman in danger of death unless an abortion is performed.

A. "G" Modifier
The "G7" modifier is defined as "the pregnancy resulted from rape or incest, or pregnancy certified by physician as life threatening."

Beginning July 1, 1999, providers should bill for abortion services using the new Modifier G7. This modifier can be used on claims with dates of services October 1, 1998, and after. CWF will be able to recognize the modifier beginning July 1, 1999.

B. FI Billing Instructions

1. Hospital Inpatient Billing
   Hospitals will bill the FI on Form CMS-1450 using bill type 11X. Medicare will pay only when condition codes:

   AA Abortion Performed due to Rape

   AB Abortion Performed due to Incest

   AD Abortion Performed due to life endangering physical condition

   in FLs 18-28 of UB04 along with an appropriate ICD-9-CM principal diagnosis code that will group to DRG 770 (Abortion W D&C, Aspiration Curettage Or Hysterotomy) or with an appropriate ICD-9-CM principal diagnosis code and one of the four appropriate ICD-9-CM/ ICD-10-CM operating room procedure codes listed below that will group to DRG 779 (Abortion W/O D&C).

ICD-9-CM	ICD-10-CM
69.01	10A07ZZ Abortion of Products of Conception, Via Natural or Artificial Opening 10A08ZZ Abortion of Products of Conception, Via Natural or Artificial Opening Endoscopic
69.02	10D17ZZ Extraction of Products of Conception, Retained, Via Natural or Artificial Opening 10D18ZZ Extraction of Products of Conception, Retained, Via Natural or Artificial Opening Endoscopic
69.51	10A07ZZ Abortion of Products of Conception, Via Natural or Artificial Opening 10A08ZZ Abortion of Products of Conception, Via Natural or Artificial Opening Endoscopic
74.91	10A00ZZ Abortion of Products of Conception, Open Approach 10A03ZZ Abortion of Products of Conception, Percutaneous Approach 10A04ZZ Abortion of Products of Conception, Percutaneous Endoscopic Approach

   Providers must use ICD-9-CM codes 69.01 and 69.02 or the related 1CD-10-CM codes to describe exactly the procedure or service performed.

   The FI must manually review claims with the above ICD-9-CM/ICD-10-CM procedure codes to verify that all of the above conditions are met.

2. Outpatient Billing
   Hospitals will bill the FI on Form CMS-1450 using bill type 13X, 83X and 85X. Medicare will pay only if one of the following CPT codes is used with the "G7" modifier.

59840	59851	59856	59841
59852	59857	59850	59855
59866			

C. Common Working File (CWF) Edits
For hospital outpatient claims, CWF will bypass its edits for a managed care beneficiary who is having an abortion outside their plan and the claim is submitted with the "G7" modifier and one of the above CPT codes.

For hospital inpatient claims, CWF will bypass its edits for a managed care beneficiary who is having an abortion outside their plan and the claim is submitted with one of the above ICD-9-CM procedure codes.

D. Medicare Summary Notices (MSN)/Explanation of Your Medicare Benefits Remittance Advice Message
If a claim is submitted with one of the above CPT procedure codes but no "G7" modifier, the claim is denied. The FI states on the MSN the following message:

This service was denied because Medicare covers this service only under certain circumstances." (MSN Message 21.21).

For the remittance advice the FI uses existing American National Standard Institute (ANSI) X12-835 claim adjustment reason code B5, "Claim/service denied/reduced because coverage guidelines were not met or were exceeded."

100-4, 3, 100.2

Payment for CRNA or AA Services

A3-3660.9

Anesthesia services furnished on or after January 1, 1990, at a qualified rural hospital by a hospital employed or contracted CRNA or AA can be paid on a reasonable cost basis. The FI determines the hospital's qualification using the following criteria.

The hospital must be located in a rural area (as defined for PPS purposes) to be considered. A rural hospital that qualified and was paid on a reasonable cost basis for CRNA or AA services during calendar year 1989 could continue to be paid on a reasonable cost basis for these services furnished during calendar year 1990 if it could establish before January 1, 1990, that it did not provide more than 500 surgical procedures, both inpatient and outpatient, requiring anesthesia services during 1989.

A rural hospital that was not paid on a reasonable cost basis for CRNA or AA services during calendar year 1989 could be paid on a reasonable cost basis for these services furnished during calendar year 1990 if it established before January 1, 1990, that:

As of January 1, 1988, it employed or contracted with a CRNA or AA (but not more than one full-time equivalent CRNA or AA); and

In both 1987 and 1989, it had a volume of 500 or fewer surgical procedures, including inpatient and outpatient procedures, requiring anesthesia services.

Each CRNA or AA employed by, or under contract with the hospital, must agree in writing not to bill on a fee schedule basis for services furnished at the hospital. A rural hospital can qualify and continue to be paid on a reasonable cost basis for qualified CRNA or AA services for a calendar year beyond 1990 if it could establish before January 1 of that year that it did not provide more than 500 surgical procedures, both inpatient and outpatient, requiring anesthesia services during the preceding year. For a calendar year beyond 1990, it must make its election after September 30, but before January 1. The FI determines the number of anesthetics by annualizing the number of surgical procedures for the 9-month period ending September 30.

A rural hospital that first elects reasonable cost payment for CRNA services for a calendar year after 1990 must demonstrate that:

It had a volume of 500 or fewer surgical procedures, including inpatient and outpatient, requiring anesthesia services in the preceding year; and

It meets the criteria that would have been met by a rural hospital first electing reasonable cost in calendar year 1990.

To prevent duplicate payments, the FI informs carriers of the names of CRNAs or AAs, the hospitals with which they have agreements, and the effective dates of the agreements. If the CRNA or AA bills Part B for anesthesia services furnished prior to the hospital's election of reasonable cost payments, the carrier must recover the overpayment from the CRNA or AA.

100-4, 3, 100.6

Inpatient Renal Services

HO-E400

Section 405.103I of Subpart J of Regulation 5 stipulates that only approved hospitals may bill for ESRD services. Hence, to allow hospitals to bill and be reimbursed for inpatient dialysis services furnished under arrangements, both facilities participating in the arrangement must meet the conditions of 405.2120 and 405.2160 of Subpart U of Regulation 5. In order for renal dialysis facilities to have a written arrangement with each other to provide inpatient dialysis care both facilities must meet the minimum utilization rate requirement, i.e., two dialysis stations with a performance capacity of at least four dialysis treatments per week.

Dialysis may be billed by an SNF as a service if: (a) it is provided by a hospital with which the facility has a transfer agreement in effect, and that hospital is approved to provide staff-assisted dialysis for the Medicare program; or (b) it is furnished directly by an SNF meeting all nonhospital maintenance dialysis facility requirements, including minimum utilization requirements. (See 1861(h)(6), 1861(h)(7), title XVIII.)

100-4, 3, 100.7

Lung Volume Reduction Surgery

Lung Volume Reduction Surgery (LVRS) (also known as reduction pneumoplasty, lung shaving, or lung contouring) is an invasive surgical procedure to reduce the volume of a hyperinflated lung in order to allow the underlying compressed lung to expand, and thus, establish improved respiratory function.

Effective for discharges on or after January 1, 2004, Medicare will cover LVRS under certain conditions as described in 240 of Pub. 100-03, "National Coverage Determinations".

The Medicare Code Editor (MCE) creates a Limited Coverage edit for procedure code 32.22. This procedure code has limited coverage due to the stringent conditions that must be met by hospitals. Where this procedure code is identified by MCE, the FI shall determine if coverage criteria is met and override the MCE if appropriate.

The LVRS can only be performed in the facilities listed on the following Web site: www.cms.hhs.gov/coverage/lvrsfacility.pdf

Medicare previously only covered LVRS as part of the National Emphysema Treatment Trial (NETT). The study was limited to 18 hospitals, and patients were randomized into two arms, either medical management and LVRS or medical management. The study was conducted by The National Heart, Lung, and Blood Institute of the National Institutes of Health and coordinated by Johns Hopkins University (JHU). Hospital claims for patients in the NETT were identified by the presence of Condition Code EY. The JHU instructed hospitals of the correct billing procedures for billing claims under the NETT.

100-4, 4, 10.2.2

Cardiac Resynchronization Therapy

Effective for services furnished on or after January 1, 2012, cardiac resynchronization therapy involving an implantable cardioverter defibrillator (CRT-D) will be recognized as a single, composite service combining implantable cardioverter defibrillator procedures (described by CPT code 33249 (Insertion or repositioning of electrode lead(s) for single or dual chamber pacing cardioverter-defibrillator and insertion of pulse generator)) and pacing electrode insertion procedures (described by CPT code 33225 (Insertion of pacing electrode, cardiac venous system, for left ventricular pacing, at time of insertion of pacing cardioverter-defibrillator or pacemaker pulse generator (including upgrade to dual chamber system))) when performed on the same date of service. When these procedures appear on the same claim but with different dates of service, or appear on the claim without the other procedure, the standard APC assignment for each service will continue to be applied.

Medicare will make a single payment for those procedures that qualify for composite service payment, as well as any packaged services furnished on the same date of service. Because CPT codes 33225 and 33249 may be treated as a composite service for payment purposes, CMS is assigning them status indicator "Q3" (Codes that may be paid through a composite APC) in Addendum B.

Hospitals will continue to use the same CPT codes to report CRT-D procedures, and the I/OCE will evaluate every claim received to determine if payment as a composite service is appropriate. Specifically, the I/OCE will determine whether payment will be made through a single, composite payment when the procedures are done on the same date of service, or through the standard APC payment methodology when they are done on different dates of service.

- CMS is also implementing claims processing edits that will return to providers incorrectly coded claims on which a pacing electrode insertion procedure described by CPT code 33225 is billed without one of the following CPT codes for insertion of an implantable cardioverter defibrillator or pacemaker:
- 33206 (Insertion or replacement of permanent pacemaker with transvenous electrode(s); atrial);
- 33207 (Insertion or replacement of permanent pacemaker with transvenous electrode(s); ventricular);
- 33208 (Insertion or replacement of permanent pacemaker with transvenous electrode(s); atrial and ventricular);
- 33212 (Insertion or replacement of pacemaker pulse generator only; single chamber, atrial or ventricular);
- 33213 (Insertion or replacement of pacemaker pulse generator only; dual chamber, atrial or ventricular);
- 33214 (Upgrade of implanted pacemaker system, conversion of single chamber system to dual chamber system (includes removal of previously placed pulse generator, testing of existing lead, insertion of new lead, insertion of new pulse generator));
- 33216 (Insertion of a single transvenous electrode, permanent pacemaker or cardioverter-defibrillator);
- 33217 (Insertion of 2 transvenous electrodes, permanent pacemaker or cardioverter-defibrillator);
- 33221(Insertion of pacemaker pulse generator only; with existing multiple leads);
- 33222 (Revision or relocation of skin pocket for pacemaker);
- 33230 (Insertion of pacing cardioverter-defibrillator pulse generator only; with existing dual leads);
- 33231 (Insertion of pacing cardioverter-defibrillator pulse generator only; with existing multiple leads)
- 33233 (Removal of permanent pacemaker pulse generator); 33234 (Removal of transvenous pacemaker electrode(s); single lead system, atrial or ventricular);
- 33235 (Removal of transvenous pacemaker electrode(s); dual lead system, atrial or ventricular);
- 33240 (Insertion of single or dual chamber pacing cardioverter-defibrillator pulse generator); or
- 33249 (Insertion or repositioning of electrode lead(s) for single or dual chamber pacing cardioverter-defibrillator and insertion of pulse generator).

100-4, 4,10.4

Packaging

Under the OPPS, packaged services are items and services that are considered to be an integral part of another service that is paid under the OPPS. No separate payment is made for packaged services, because the cost of these items and services is included in the APC payment for the service of which they are an integral part. For example, routine supplies, anesthesia, recovery room use, and most drugs are considered to be an integral part of a surgical procedure so payment for these items is packaged into the APC payment for the surgical procedure.

A. Packaging for Claims Resulting in APC Payments

If a claim contains services that result in an APC payment but also contains packaged services, separate payment for the packaged services is not made since payment is included in the APC. However, charges related to the packaged services are used for outlier and Transitional Corridor Payments (TOPs) as well as for future rate setting.

Therefore, it is extremely important that hospitals report all HCPCS codes and all charges for all services they furnish, whether payment for the services is made separately paid or is packaged.

B. Packaging for Claims Resulting in No APC Payments

If the claim contains only services payable under cost reimbursement, such as corneal tissue, and services that would be packaged services if an APC were payable, then the packaged services are not separately payable. In addition, these charges for the packaged services are not used to calculate TOPs.

If the claim contains only services payable under a fee schedule, such as clinical diagnostic laboratory tests, and also contains services that would be packaged services if an APC were payable, the packaged services are not separately payable. In addition, the charges are not used to calculate TOPs.

If a claim contains services payable under cost reimbursement, services payable under a fee schedule, and services that would be packaged services if an APC were payable, the packaged services are not separately payable. In addition, the charges are not used to calculate TOPs payments.

C. Packaging Types Under the OPPS

1. Unconditionally packaged services are services for which separate payment is never made because the payment for the service is always packaged into the payment for other services. Unconditionally packaged services are identified in the OPPS Addendum B with status indictor of N. See the OPPS Web site at http://www.cms.hhs.gov/HospitalOutpatientPPS/ for the most recent Addendum B (HCPCS codes with status indicators). In general, the charges for unconditionally packaged services are used to calculate outlier and TOPS payments when they appear on a claim with a service that is separately paid under the OPPS because the packaged service is considered to be part of the package of services for which payment is being made through the APC payment for the separately paid service.
2. STVX-packaged services are services for which separate payment is made only if there is no service with status indicator S, T, V or X reported with the same date of service on the same claim. If a claim includes a service that is assigned status indicator S, T, V, or X reported on the same date of service as the STVXpackaged service, the payment for the STVX-packaged service is packaged into the payment for the service(s) with status indicator S, T, V or X and no separate payment is made for the STVX-packaged service. STVX-packaged services are assigned status indicator Q. See the OPPS Webpage at http://www.cms.hhs.gov/HospitalOutpatientPPS/ for identification of STVXpackaged codes.
3. T-packaged services are services for which separate payment is made only if there is no service with status indicator T reported with the same date of service on the same claim. When there is a claim that includes a service that is assigned status indicator T reported on the same date of service as the T-packaged service, the payment for the T-packaged service is packaged into the payment for the service(s) with status indicator T and no separate payment is made for the T-packaged service. T-packaged services are assigned status indicator Q. See the OPPS Web site at http://www.cms.hhs.gov/HospitalOutpatientPPS/ for identification of T-packaged codes.
4. A service that is assigned to a composite APC is a major component of a single episode of care. The hospital receives one payment through a composite APC for multiple major separately identifiable services. Services mapped to composite APCs are assigned status indicator Q. See the discussion of composite APCs in section 10.2.1.

100-4, 4, 61.4.1

Billing for Brachytherapy Sources - General

Brachytherapy sources (e.g., brachytherapy devices or seeds, solutions) are paid separately from the services to administer and deliver brachytherapy in the OPPS, per section 1833(t)(2)(H) of the Act, reflecting the number, isotope, and radioactive intensity of devices furnished, as well as stranded versus non-stranded configurations of sources. Therefore, providers must bill for brachytherapy sources in addition to the brachytherapy services with which the sources are applied, in order to receive payment for the sources. The list of separately payable sources is found in Addendum B of the most recent OPPS annual update published in the Federal Register, as well as in the recurring update notifications of the current year for billing purposes. New sources meeting the OPPS definition of a brachytherapy source may be added for payment beginning any quarter, and the new source codes and descriptors are announced in the recurring update notifications. Each unit of a billable source is identified by the unit measurement in the respective source's long descriptor. Seed-like sources are generally billed and paid "per source" based on the number of units of the source HCPCS code reported, including the billing of the number of sources within a stranded configuration of sources. Providers therefore must bill the number of units of a source used with the brachytherapy service rendered.

100-4, 4, 61.4.2

Definition of Brachytherapy Source for Separate Payment

Brachytherapy sources eligible for separate billing and payment must be radioactive sources, meaning that the source contains a radioactive isotope. Separate brachytherapy source payments reflect the number, isotope, and radioactive intensity of sources furnished to patients, as well as stranded and non-stranded configurations.

100-4, 4, 61.4.3

Billing of Brachytherapy Sources Ordered for a Specific Patient

A hospital may report and charge Medicare and the Medicare beneficiary for all brachytherapy sources that are ordered by the physician for a specific patient, acquired by the hospital, and used in the care of the patient. Specifically, brachytherapy sources prescribed by the physician in accordance with high quality clinical care, acquired by the hospital, and actually implanted in the patient may be reported and charged. In the case where most, but not all, prescribed sources are implanted in the patient, CMS will consider the relatively few brachytherapy sources that were ordered but not implanted due to specific clinical considerations to be used in the care of the patient and billable to Medicare under the following circumstances. The hospital may charge for all sources if they were specifically acquired by the hospital for the particular patient according to a physician's prescription for the sources that was consistent with standard clinical practice and high quality brachytherapy treatment, in order to ensure that the clinically appropriate number of sources was available for the implantation procedure, and they were not implanted in any other patient. Those sources that were not implanted must have been disposed of in accordance with all appropriate requirements for their handling.

In general, the number of sources used in the care of the patient but not implanted would not be expected to constitute more than a small fraction of the sources actually implanted in the patient. Under these circumstances, the beneficiary is liable for the copayment for all the sources billed to Medicare.

100-4, 4, 61.4.4

Billing for Brachytherapy Source Supervision, Handling and Loading Costs

Providers should report charges related to supervision, handling, and loading of radiation sources, including brachytherapy sources, in one of two ways:

1. Report the charge separately using CPT code 77790 (Supervision, handling, loading of radiation source), in addition to reporting the associated HCPCS procedure code(s) for application of the radiation source;
2. Include the supervision, handling, and/or loading charges as part of the charge reported with the HCPCS procedure code(s) for application of the radiation source.

Do not bill a separate charge for brachytherapy source storage costs. These costs are treated as part of the department's overhead costs.

100-4, 4, 160

Clinic and Emergency Visits

CMS has acknowledged from the beginning of the OPPS that CMS believes that CPT Evaluation and Management (E/M) codes were designed to reflect the activities of physicians and do not describe well the range and mix of services provided by hospitals during visits of clinic and emergency department patients. While awaiting the development of a national set of facility-specific codes and guidelines, providers should continue to apply their current internal guidelines to the existing CPT codes. Each hospital's internal guidelines should follow the intent of the CPT code descriptors, in that the guidelines should be designed to reasonably relate the intensity of hospital resources to the different levels of effort represented by the codes. Hospitals should ensure that their guidelines accurately reflect resource distinctions between the five levels of codes.

Effective January 1, 2007, CMS is distinguishing between two types of emergency departments: Type A emergency departments and Type B emergency departments.

A Type A emergency department is defined as an emergency department that is available 24 hours a day, 7 days a week and is either licensed by the State in which it is located under applicable State law as an emergency room or emergency department or it is held out to the public (by name, posted signs, advertising, or other means) as a place that provides care for emergency medical conditions on an urgent basis without requiring a previously scheduled appointment.

A Type B emergency department is defined as an emergency department that meets the definition of a "dedicated emergency department" as defined in 42 CFR 489.24 under the EMTALA regulations. It must meet at least one of the following requirements:

(1) It is licensed by the State in which it is located under applicable State law as an emergency room or emergency department;

(2) It is held out to the public (by name, posted signs, advertising, or other means) as a place that provides care for emergency medical conditions on an urgent basis without requiring a previously scheduled appointment; or

(3) During the calendar year immediately preceding the calendar year in which a determination under 42 CFR 489.24 is being made, based on a representative sample of patient visits that occurred during that calendar year, it provides at least one-third of all of its outpatient visits for the treatment of emergency medical conditions on an urgent basis without requiring a previously scheduled appointment.

Hospitals must bill for visits provided in Type A emergency departments using CPT emergency department E/M codes. Hospitals must bill for visits provided in Type B emergency departments using the G-codes that describe visits provided in Type B emergency departments.

Hospitals that will be billing the new Type B ED visit codes may need to update their internal guidelines to report these codes.

Emergency department and clinic visits are paid in some cases separately and in other cases as part of a composite APC payment. See section 10.2.1 of this chapter for further details.

100-4, 4, 160.1

Critical Care Services

Beginning January 1, 2007, critical care services will be paid at two levels, depending on the presence or absence of trauma activation. Providers will receive one payment rate for critical care without trauma activation and will receive additional payment when critical care is associated with trauma activation.

To determine whether trauma activation occurs, follow the National Uniform Billing Committee (NUBC) guidelines in the Claims Processing Manual, Pub 100-04, Chapter 25, Sec.75.4 related to the reporting of the trauma revenue codes in the 68x series. The revenue code series 68x can be used only by trauma centers/hospitals as licensed or designated by the state or local government authority authorized to do so, or as verified by the American College of Surgeons. Different subcategory revenue codes are reported by designated Level 1-4 hospital trauma centers. Only patients for whom there has been prehospital notification based on triage information from prehospital caregivers, who meet either local, state or American College of Surgeons field triage criteria, or are delivered by inter-hospital transfers, and are given the appropriate team response can be billed a trauma activation charge.

When critical care services are provided without trauma activation, the hospital may bill CPT code 99291, Critical care, evaluation and management of the critically ill or critically injured patient; first 30-74 minutes (and 99292, if appropriate). If trauma activation occurs under the circumstances described by the NUBC guidelines that would permit reporting a charge under 68x, the hospital may also bill one unit of code G0390, which describes trauma activation associated with hospital critical care services. Revenue code 68x must be reported on the same date of service. The OCE will edit to ensure that G0390 appears with revenue code 68x on the same date of service and that only one unit of G0390 is billed. CMS believes that trauma activation is a one-time occurrence in association with critical care services, and therefore, CMS will only pay for one unit of G0390 per day.

The CPT code 99291 is defined by CPT as the first 30-74 minutes of critical care. This 30 minute minimum has always applied under the OPPS. The CPT code 99292, Critical care, evaluation and management of the critically ill or critically injured patient; each additional 30 minutes, remains a packaged service under the OPPS, so that hospitals do not have the ongoing administrative burden of reporting precisely the time for each critical service provided. As the CPT guidelines indicate, hospitals that provide less than 30 minutes of critical care should bill for a visit, typically an emergency department visit, at a level consistent with their own internal guidelines.

Under the OPPS, the time that can be reported as critical care is the time spent by a physician and/or hospital staff engaged in active face-to-face critical care of a critically ill or critically injured patient. If the physician and hospital staff or multiple hospital staff members are simultaneously engaged in this active face-to-face care, the time involved can only be counted once.

- In CY 2007 hospitals may continue to report a charge with RC 68x without any HCPCS code when trauma team activation occurs. In order to receive additional payment when critical care services are associated with trauma activation, the hospital must report G0390 on the same date of service as RC 68x, in addition to CPT code 99291 (or 99292, if appropriate.)
- In CY 2007 hospitals should continue to report 99291 (and 99292 as appropriate) for critical care services furnished without trauma team activation. CPT 99291 maps to APC 0617 (Critical Care). (CPT 99292 is packaged and not paid separately, but should be reported if provided.)

Critical care services are paid in some cases separately and in other cases as part of a composite APC payment. See Section 10.2.1 of this chapter for further details.

100-4, 4, 180.3

Unlisted Service or Procedure

This section does not apply to OPPS hospitals.

There may be services or procedures performed that are not found in HCPCS. These are typically services that are rarely provided, unusual, variable, or new. A number of specific code numbers have been designated for reporting unlisted procedures. When an unlisted procedure code is used, a report describing the service is submitted with the claim. Pertinent information includes a definition or description of the nature, extent, and need for the procedure and the time, effort, and equipment necessary to provide the service.

When an FI receives a claim with an unlisted procedure code, it reviews it to verify that there is no existing code that adequately describes the procedure. If it determines that an adequately descriptive code is contained in HCPCS, it advises the hospital of the proper code and processes the claim. If it determines that no existing code is sufficiently descriptive, it pays the claim using the unlisted procedure code. If the frequency of the procedure warrants assignment of a local code, the FI forwards a copy and the operative report to the RO HCPCS coordinator for a code determination. When it receives a determination, the FI informs the hospital of the correct code for future reporting. Local codes are not accepted under OPPS and line items for local codes are no longer paid on cost.

NOTE: If the claim is submitted via EMC or identified after the bill has been processed, an operative report, the provider number, revenue codes, and charges are sufficient.

The "Unlisted Procedures" and codes for surgery are:

HCPCS code	Unlisted Procedure
15999	Unlisted procedure, excision pressure ulcer
17999	Unlisted procedure, skin, mucous membrane and subcutaneous tissue
19499	Unlisted procedure, breast
20999	Unlisted procedure, musculoskeletal system, general
21299	Unlisted craniofacial and maxillofacial procedures
21499	Unlisted orthopedic procedure, head
21899	Unlisted procedure, neck or thorax
22899	Unlisted procedure, spine
22999	Unlisted procedure, abdomen, musculoskeletal system
23929	Unlisted procedure, shoulder
24999	Unlisted procedure, humerus or elbow
25999	Unlisted procedure, forearm or wrist
26989	Unlisted procedure, hands or fingers
27299	Unlisted procedure, pelvis or hip joint
27599	Unlisted procedure, femur or knee
27899	Unlisted procedure, leg or ankle
28899	Unlisted procedure, foot or toes
29799	Unlisted procedure, casting or strapping
29909	Unlisted procedure, arthroscopy
30999	Unlisted procedure, nose
31299	Unlisted procedure, accessory sinuses
31599	Unlisted procedure, larynx
31899	Unlisted procedure, trachea, bronchi
32999	Unlisted procedure, lungs, and pleura
33999	Unlisted procedure, cardiac surgery
36299	Unlisted procedure, vascular injection
37799	Unlisted procedure, vascular surgery
38999	Unlisted procedure, hemic or lymphatic system
39499	Unlisted procedure, mediastinum
39599	Unlisted procedure, diaphragm
40799	Unlisted procedure, lips
40899	Unlisted procedure, vestibule of mouth
41599	Unlisted procedure, tongue, floor of mouth
41899	Unlisted procedure, dentoalveolar structures
42299	Unlisted procedure, palate, uvula
42699	Unlisted procedure, salivary glands or ducts
42999	Unlisted procedure, pharynx, adenoids, or tonsils
43499	Unlisted procedure, esophag
43999	Unlisted procedure, stomach
44799	Unlisted procedure, intestine
44899	Unlisted procedure, Meckel's diverticulum and the mesentery
45999	Unlisted procedure, rectum
46999	Unlisted procedure, anus
47399	Unlisted procedure, liver
47999	Unlisted procedure, biliary tract

HCPCS code	Unlisted Procedure
48999	Unlisted procedure, pancreas
49999	Unlisted procedure, abdomen, peritoneum, and omentum
53899	Unlisted procedure, urinary system
55899	Unlisted procedure, male genital system
56399	Unlisted procedure, laparoscopy, hysteroscopy
58999	Unlisted procedure, female genital system non-obstetrical
59899	Unlisted procedure, maternity care and delivery
60699	Unlisted procedure, endocrine system
64999	Unlisted procedure, nervous system
66999	Unlisted procedure, anterior segment of eye
67299	Unlisted procedure, posterior segment
67399	Unlisted procedure, ocular muscle
67599	Unlisted procedure, orbit
67999	Unlisted procedure, eyelids
68399	Unlisted procedure, conjunctiva
68899	Unlisted procedure, lacrimal system
69399	Unlisted procedure, external ear
69799	Unlisted procedure, middle ear
69949	Unlisted procedure, inner ear
69979	Unlisted procedure, temporal bone, middle fossa approach

100-4, 3,190.7.3

190.7.3 - Electroconvulsive Therapy (ECT) Payment

(Rev. 1543; Issued: 06-27-08; Effective Date: 07-01-08; Implementation Date: 07-07-08)

IPFs receive an additional payment for each ECT treatment furnished during the IPF stay. The ECT base rate is based on the median hospital cost used to calculate the calendar year 2005 Outpatient Prospective Payment System amount for ECT and is updated annually by the market basket and wage budget neutrality factor. The ECT base rate is adjusted by the wage index and any applicable COLA factor.

In order to receive the payment, an IPF must report revenue code 0901 along with the number of units of ECT on the claim. The units should reflect the number of ECT treatments provided to the patient during the IPF stay. In addition, IPFs must include the ICD-9-CM procedure code for ECT (94.27) in the procedure code field and use the date of the last ECT treatment the patient received during their IPF stay.

It is important to note that since ECT treatment is a specialized procedure, not all providers are equipped to provide the treatment. Therefore, many patients who need ECT treatment during their IPF stay must be referred to other providers to receive the ECT treatments, and then return to the IPF. In accordance with 42 CFR 412.404(d)(3), in these cases where the IPF is not able to furnish necessary treatment directly, the IPF would furnish ECT under arrangements with another provider. While a patient is an inpatient of the IPF, the IPF is responsible for all services furnished, including those furnished under arrangements by another provider. As a result, the IPF claim for these cases should reflect the services furnished under arrangements by other providers.

100-4, 3,190.10.4

190.10.4 - Reporting ECT Treatments

(Rev. 1101, Issued: 11-03-06, Effective: 01-01-05, Implementation: 12-04-06)

IPFs must report on their claims under Revenue Code 0901, along with the total number of ECT treatments provided to the patient during their IPF stay listed under "Service Units." Providers will code ICD-9-CM procedure code 94.27 in the procedure code field and for the procedure date will use the date of the last ECT treatment the patient received during their IPF stay.

100-4, 4, 200.2

Hospital Dialysis Services For Patients with and without End Stage Renal Disease (ESRD)

Effective with claims with dates of service on or after August 1, 2000, hospital-based End Stage Renal Disease (ESRD) facilities must submit services covered under the ESRD benefit in 42 CFR 413.174 (maintenance dialysis and those items and services directly related to dialysis such as drugs, supplies) on a separate claim from services not covered under the ESRD benefit. Items and services not covered under the ESRD benefit must be billed by the hospital using the hospital bill type and be paid under the Outpatient Prospective Payment System (OPPS) (or to a CAH at reasonable cost). Services covered under the ESRD benefit in 42 CFR 413.174 must be billed on the ESRD bill type and must be paid under the ESRD PPS. This requirement is necessary to properly pay only unrelated ESRD services (those not covered under the ESRD benefit) under OPPS (or to a CAH at reasonable cost).

Medicare does not allow payment for routine or related dialysis treatments, which are covered and paid under the ESRD PPS, when furnished to ESRD patients in the outpatient department of a hospital. However, in certain medical situations in which the ESRD outpatient cannot obtain her or his regularly scheduled dialysis treatment at a certified ESRD facility, the OPPS rule for 2003 allows payment for non-routine dialysis treatments (which are not covered under the ESRD benefit) furnished to ESRD outpatients in the outpatient department of a hospital. Payment for unscheduled dialysis furnished to ESRD outpatients and paid under the OPPS is limited to the following circumstances:

- Dialysis performed following or in connection with a dialysis-related procedure such as vascular access procedure or blood transfusions;
- Dialysis performed following treatment for an unrelated medical emergency; e.g., if a patient goes to the emergency room for chest pains and misses a regularly scheduled dialysis treatment that cannot be rescheduled, CMS allows the hospital to provide and bill Medicare for the dialysis treatment; or
- Emergency dialysis for ESRD patients who would otherwise have to be admitted as inpatients in order for the hospital to receive payment.

In these situations, non-ESRD certified hospital outpatient facilities are to bill Medicare using the Healthcare Common Procedure Coding System (HCPCS) code G0257 (Unscheduled or emergency dialysis treatment for an ESRD patient in a hospital outpatient department that is not certified as an ESRD facility).

HCPCS code G0257 may only be reported on type of bill 13X (hospital outpatient service) or type of bill 85X (critical access hospital) because HCPCS code G0257 only reports services for hospital outpatients with ESRD and only these bill types are used to report services to hospital outpatients. Effective for services on and after October 1, 2012, claims containing HCPCS code G0257 will be returned to the provider for correction if G0257 is reported with a type of bill other than 13X or 85X (such as a 12x inpatient claim).

HCPCS code 90935 (Hemodialysis procedure with single physician evaluation) may be reported and paid only if one of the following two conditions is met:

1) The patient is a hospital inpatient with or without ESRD and has no coverage under Part A, but has Part B coverage. The charge for hemodialysis is a charge for the use of a prosthetic device. See Benefits Policy Manual 100-02 Chapter 15 section 120. A. The service must be reported on a type of bill 12X or type of bill 85X. See the Benefits Policy Manual 100-02 Chapter 6 section 10 (Medical and Other Health Services Furnished to Inpatients of Participating Hospitals) for the criteria that must be met for services to be paid when a hospital inpatient has Part B coverage but does not have coverage under Part A; or
2) A hospital outpatient does not have ESRD and is receiving hemodialysis in the hospital outpatient department. The service is reported on a type of bill 13X or type of bill 85X. CPT code 90945 (Dialysis procedure other than hemodialysis (e.g. peritoneal dialysis, hemofiltration, or other continuous replacement therapies)), with single physician evaluation, may be reported by a hospital paid under the OPPS or CAH method I or method II on type of bill 12X, 13X or 85X.

100-4, 4, 200.3.1

Billing for IMRT Planning and Delivery

Effective for services furnished on or after April 1, 2002, HCPCS codes G0174 (IMRT delivery) and G0178 (IMRT planning) are no longer valid codes. HCPCS code G0174 has been replaced with CPT codes 77418 and 0073T for IMRT delivery and HCPCS code G0178 with CPT code 77301. Therefore, hospitals must use CPT codes 77418 or 0073T for IMRT delivery and CPT code 77301 for IMRT planning. Any of the CPT codes 77401 through 77416 or 77418 may be reported on the same day as long as the services are furnished at separate treatment sessions. In these cases, modifier -59 must be appended to the appropriate codes. Additionally, in the context of billing 77301, regardless of the same or different dates of service, CPT codes 77014, 77280-77295, 77305-77321, 77331, 77336, and 77370 may only be billed in addition to 77301 if they are not provided as part of developing the IMRT treatment plan.

77301 Intensity modulated radiotherapy plan, including dose-volume histograms for target and critical structure partial tolerance specifications

77418 Intensity modulated treatment delivery, single or multiple fields/arcs, via narrow spatially and temporally modulated beams, binary, dynamic MLC, per treatment session

0073T Compensator-based beam modulation treatment delivery of inverse planned treatment using three or more high resolution (milled or cast) compensator convergent beam modulated fields, per treatment session

100-4, 4, 200.3.2

Additional Billing Instructions for IMRT Planning

Payment for the services identified by CPT codes 77014, 77280-77295, 77305-77321, 77331, 77336, and 77370 is included in the APC payment for IMRT planning when these services are performed as part of developing an IMRT plan that is reported using CPT code 77301. Under those circumstances, these codes should not be billed in addition to CPT code 77301 for IMRT planning.

100-4, 4, 200.3.3

Billing for Multi-Source Photon (Cobalt 60-Based) Stereotactic Radiosurgery (SRS) Planning and Delivery

Effective for services furnished on or after January 1, 2006, hospitals must bill for multisource photon (cobalt 60-based) SRS planning using existing CPT codes that most accurately describe the service furnished, and HCPCS code G0243 for the delivery. For CY 2007, HCPCS code G0243 is no longer be reportable under the hospital OPPS because the code has been deleted and replaced with CPT code 77371, effective January 1, 2007.

77371 Radiation treatment delivery, stereotactic radiosurgery (SRS) (complete course of treatment of cerebral lesion[s] consisting of 1 session); multisource Cobalt 60 based.

Payment for CPT code 20660 is included in CPT code 77371; therefore, hospitals should not report 20660 separately.

100-4, 4, 200.4

Billing for Amniotic Membrane

Hospitals should report HCPCS code V2790 (Amniotic membrane for surgical reconstruction, per procedure) to report amniotic membrane tissue when the tissue is used. A specific procedure code associated with use of amniotic membrane tissue is CPT code 65780 (Ocular surface reconstruction; amniotic membrane transplantation).

Payment for the amniotic membrane tissue is packaged into payment for CPT code 65780 or other procedures with which the amniotic membrane is used.

100-4, 4, 200.5

Billing and Payment for Cardiac Rehabilitation Services

The National Coverage Determination for cardiac rehabilitation programs requires that programs must be comprehensive and to be comprehensive they must include a medical evaluation, a program to modify cardiac risk factors (e.g., nutritional counseling), prescribed exercise, education, and counseling. See the National Coverage Determination (NCD) Manual, Pub. 100-03, section 20.10, for more information. A cardiac rehabilitation session may include more than one aspect of the comprehensive program. For CY 2008, hospitals will continue to use CPT code 93797 (Physician services for outpatient cardiac rehabilitation, without continuous ECG monitoring (per session)) and CPT code 93798 (Physician services for outpatient cardiac rehabilitation, with continuous ECG monitoring (per session)) to report cardiac rehabilitation services.

However, effective for dates of service on or after January 1, 2008, hospitals may report more than one unit of HCPCS code 93797 or 97398 for a date of service if more than one cardiac rehabilitation session lasting at least 1 hour each is provided on the same day.

In order to report more than one session for a given date of service, each session must last a minimum of 60 minutes. For example, if the cardiac rehabilitation services provided on a given day total 1 hour and 50 minutes, then only one session should be billed to report the cardiac rehabilitation services provided on that day.

100-4, 4, 200.6

Billing and Payment for Alcohol and/or Substance Abuse Assessment and Intervention Services

For CY 2008, the CPT Editorial Panel has created two new Category I CPT codes for reporting alcohol and/or substance abuse screening and intervention services. They are CPT code 99408 (Alcohol and/or substance (other than tobacco) abuse structured screening (e.g., AUDIT, DAST), and brief intervention (SBI) services; 15 to 30 minutes); and CPT code 99409 (Alcohol and/or substance (other than tobacco) abuse structured screening (e.g., AUDIT, DAST), and brief intervention (SBI) services; greater than 30 minutes). However, screening services are not covered by Medicare without specific statutory authority, such as has been provided for mammography, diabetes, and colorectal cancer screening. Therefore, beginning January 1, 2008, the OPPS recognizes two parallel G-codes (HCPCS codes G0396 and G0397) to allow for appropriate reporting and payment of alcohol and substance abuse structured assessment and intervention services that are not provided as screening services, but that are performed in the context of the diagnosis or treatment of illness or injury.

Contractors shall make payment under the OPPS for HCPCS code G0396 (Alcohol and/or substance (other than tobacco) abuse structured assessment (e.g., AUDIT, DAST) and brief intervention, 15 to 30 minutes) and HCPCS code G0397, (Alcohol and/or substance(other than tobacco) abuse structured assessment (e.g., AUDIT, DAST) and intervention greater than 30 minutes), only when reasonable and necessary (i.e., when the service is provided to evaluate patients with signs/symptoms of illness or injury) as per section 1862(a)(1)(A) of the Act.

HCPCS codes G0396 and G0397 are to be used for structured alcohol and/or substance (other than tobacco) abuse assessment and intervention services that are distinct from other clinic and emergency department visit services performed during the same encounter. Hospital resources expended performing services described by HCPCS codes G0396 and G0397 may not be counted as resources for determining the level of a visit service and vice versa (i.e., hospitals may not double count the same facility resources in order to reach a higher level clinic or emergency department visit). However, alcohol and/or substance structured assessment or intervention services lasting less than 15 minutes should not be reported using these HCPCS codes, but the hospital resources expended should be included in determining the level of the visit service reported.

100-4, 4, 200.7.1

Cardiac Echocardiography Without Contrast

Hospitals are instructed to bill for echocardiograms without contrast in accordance with the CPT code descriptors and guidelines associated with the applicable Level I CPT code(s) (93303-93350).

Billing for "Sometimes Therapy" Services that May be Paid as Non-Therapy Services for Hospital Outpatients

Section 1834(k) of the Act, as added by Section 4541 of the BBA, allows payment at 80 percent of the lesser of the actual charge for the services or the applicable fee schedule amount for all outpatient therapy services; that is, physical therapy services, speech-language pathology services, and occupational therapy services. As provided under Section 1834(k)(5) of the Act, a therapy code list was created based on a uniform coding system (that is, the HCPCS) to identify and track these outpatient therapy services paid under the Medicare Physician Fee Schedule (MPFS).

The list of therapy codes, along with their respective designation, can be found on the CMS Website, specifically at http://www.cms.hhs.gov/TherapyServices/05_Annual_Therapy_Update.asp#TopOfPage. Two of the designations that are used for therapy services are: "always therapy" and "sometimes therapy." An "always therapy" service must be performed by a qualified therapist under a certified therapy plan of care, and a "sometimes therapy" service may be performed by an individual outside of a certified therapy plan of care.

Under the OPPS, separate payment is provided for certain services designated as "sometimes therapy" services if these services are furnished to hospital outpatients as a non-therapy service, that is, without a certified therapy plan of care. Specifically, to be paid under the OPPS for a non-therapy service, hospitals SHOULD NOT append the therapy modifier GP (physical therapy), GO (occupational therapy), or GN (speech language pathology), or report a therapy revenue code 042x, 043x, or 044x in association with the "sometimes therapy" codes listed in the table below.

To receive payment under the MPFS, when "sometimes therapy" services are performed by a qualified therapist under a certified therapy plan of care, providers should append the appropriate therapy modifier GP, GO, or GN, and report the charges under an appropriate therapy revenue code, specifically 042x, 043x, or 044x. This instruction does not apply to claims for "sometimes therapy" codes furnished as therapy services in the hospital outpatient department and paid under the MPFS.

Effective January 1, 2010, CPT code 92520 (Laryngeal function studies (i.e., aerodynamic testing and acoustic testing)), is newly designated as a "sometimes therapy" service under the MPFS. CPT code 92520 is not a new code, however, its "sometimes therapy" designation is new and effective January 1, 2010. Under the OPPS, hospitals will receive separate payment when they bill CPT code 92520 as a non-therapy service.

The list of HCPCS codes designated as "sometimes therapy" services that may be paid as non-therapy services when furnished to hospital outpatients as of January 1, 2010, is displayed in the table below.

Services Designated as "Sometimes Therapy" that May be Paid as Non-Therapy Services for Hospital Outpatients as of January 1, 2010

HCPCS Code	Long Descriptor
92520	Laryngeal function studies (i.e., aerodynamic testing and acoustic testing)
97597	Removal of devitalized tissue from wound(s), selective debridement, without anesthesia (e.g., high pressure waterjet with/without suction, sharp selective debridement with scissors, scalpel and forceps), with or without topical application(s), wound assessment, and instruction(s) for ongoing care, may include use of a whirlpool, per session; total wound(s) surface area less than or equal to 20 square centimeters
97598	Removal of devitalized tissue from wound(s), selective debridement, without anesthesia (e.g., high pressure waterjet with/without suction, sharp selective debridement with scissors, scalpel and forceps), with or without topical application(s), wound assessment, and instruction(s) for ongoing care, may include use of a whirlpool, per session; total wound(s) surface area greater than 20 square centimeters
97602	Removal of devitalized tissue from wound(s), non-selective debridement, without anesthesia (e.g., wet-to-moist dressings, enzymatic, abrasion), including topical application(s), wound assessment, and instruction(s) for ongoing care, per session
97605	Negative pressure wound therapy (e.g., vacuum assisted drainage collection), including topical application(s), wound assessment, and instruction(s) for ongoing care, per session; total wound(s) surface area less than or equal to 50 square centimeters

HCPCS Code	Long Descriptor
97606	Negative pressure wound therapy (eg., vacuum assisted drainage collection), including topical application(s), wound assessment, and instruction(s) for ongoing care, per session; total wound(s) surface area greater than 50 square centimeters
0183T	Low frequency, non-contact, non-thermal ultrasound, including topical application(s), when performed, wound assessment, and instruction(s) for ongoing care, per day

100-4, 4, 230.2

Coding and Payment for Drug Administration

A. Overview

Drug administration services furnished under the Hospital Outpatient Prospective Payment System (OPPS) during CY 2005 were reported using CPT codes 90780, 90781, and 96400-96459.

Effective January 1, 2006, some of these CPT codes were replaced with more detailed CPT codes incorporating specific procedural concepts, as defined and described by the CPT manual, such as initial, concurrent, and sequential.

Hospitals are instructed to use the full set of CPT codes, including those codes referencing concepts of initial, concurrent, and sequential, to bill for drug administration services furnished in the hospital outpatient department beginning January 1, 2007. In addition, hospitals are instructed to continue billing the HCPCS codes that most accurately describe the service(s) provided.

Hospitals are reminded to bill a separate Evaluation and Management code (with modifier 25) only if a significant, separately identifiable E/M service is performed in the same encounter with OPPS drug administration services.

B. Billing for Infusions and Injections

Beginning in CY 2007, hospitals were instructed to use the full set of drug administration CPT codes (90760-90779; 96401-96549), (96413-96523 beginning in CY 2008) (96360-96549 beginning in CY 2009) when billing for drug administration services provided in the hospital outpatient department. In addition, hospitals are to continue to bill HCPCS code C8957 (Intravenous infusion for therapy/diagnosis; initiation of prolonged infusion (more than 8 hours), requiring use of portable or implantable pump) when appropriate. Hospitals are expected to report all drug administration CPT codes in a manner consistent with their descriptors, CPT instructions, and correct coding principles. Hospitals should note the conceptual changes between CY 2006 drug administration codes effective under the OPPS and the CPT codes in effect beginning January 1, 2007, in order to ensure accurate billing under the OPPS. Hospitals should report all HCPCS codes that describe the drug administration services provided, regardless of whether or not those services are separately paid or their payment is packaged.

Medicare's general policy regarding physician supervision within hospital outpatient departments meets the physician supervision requirements for use of CPT codes 90760-90779, 96401-96549, (96413-96523 beginning in CY 2008). (Reference: Pub.100-02, Medicare Benefit Policy Manual, Chapter 6, §20.4.)

Drug administration services are to be reported with a line item date of service on the day they are provided. In addition, only one initial drug administration service is to be reported per vascular access site per encounter, including during an encounter where observation services span more than 1 calendar day.

C. Payments For Drug Administration Services

For CY 2007, OPPS drug administration APCs were restructured, resulting in a six-level hierarchy where active HCPCS codes have been assigned according to their clinical coherence and resource use. Contrary to the CY 2006 payment structure that bundled payment for several instances of a type of service (non-chemotherapy, chemotherapy by infusion, non-infusion chemotherapy) into a per-encounter APC payment, structure introduced in CY 2007 provides a separate APC payment for each reported unit of a separately payable HCPCS code.

Hospitals should note that the transition to the full set of CPT drug administration codes provides for conceptual differences when reporting, such as those noted below.

- In CY 2006, hospitals were instructed to bill for the first hour (and any additional hours) by each type of infusion service (non-chemotherapy, chemotherapy by infusion, non-infusion chemotherapy). Beginning in CY 2007, the first hour concept no longer exists. CPT codes in CY 2007 and beyond allow for only one initial service per encounter, for each vascular access site, no matter how many types of infusion services are provided; however, hospitals will receive an APC payment for the initial service and separate APC payment(s) for additional hours of infusion or other drug administration services provided that are separately payable.
- In CY 2006, hospitals providing infusion services of different types (non-chemotherapy, chemotherapy by infusion, non-infusion chemotherapy) received payment for the associated per-encounter infusion APC even if these infusions occurred during the same time period. Beginning in CY 2007, hospitals should report only one initial drug administration service, including infusion services, per encounter for each distinct vascular access site, with other services through the same vascular access site being reported via the sequential, concurrent or additional hour codes. Although new CPT guidance has been issued for reporting initial drug administration services, Medicare contractors shall continue to follow the guidance given in this manual.

(**NOTE:** This list above provides a brief overview of a limited number of the conceptual changes between CY 2006 OPPS drug administration codes and CY 2007 OPPS drug administration codes - this list is not comprehensive and does not include all items hospitals will need to consider during this transition)

For APC payment rates, refer to the most current quarterly version of Addendum B on the CMS Web site at http://www.cms.hhs.gov/HospitalOutpatientPPS/.

D. Infusions Started Outside the Hospital

Hospitals may receive Medicare beneficiaries for outpatient services who are in the process of receiving an infusion at their time of arrival at the hospital (e.g., a patient who arrives via ambulance with an ongoing intravenous infusion initiated by paramedics during transport). Hospitals are reminded to bill for all services provided using the HCPCS code(s) that most accurately describe the service(s) they provided. This includes hospitals reporting an initial hour of infusion, even if the hospital did not initiate the infusion, and additional HCPCS codes for additional or sequential infusion services if needed.

100-4, 4, 231

Coding and Payment for Drug Administration

A. Overview

Drug administration services furnished under the Hospital Outpatient Prospective Payment System (OPPS) during CY 2005 were reported using CPT codes 90780, 90781, and 96400-96459.

Effective January 1, 2006, some of these CPT codes were replaced with more detailed CPT codes incorporating specific procedural concepts, as defined and described by the CPT manual, such as initial, concurrent, and sequential.

Hospitals are instructed to use the full set of CPT codes, including those codes referencing concepts of initial, concurrent, and sequential, to bill for drug administration services furnished in the hospital outpatient department beginning January 1, 2007. In addition, hospitals are instructed to continue billing the HCPCS codes that most accurately describe the service(s) provided.

Hospitals are reminded to bill a separate Evaluation and Management code (with modifier 25) only if a significant, separately identifiable E/M service is performed in the same encounter with OPPS drug administration services.

B. Billing for Infusions and Injections

In CY 2007, hospitals are instructed to use the full set of drug administration CPT codes (90760-90779; 96401-96549) when billing for drug administration services provided in the hospital outpatient department. In addition, hospitals are to continue to bill HCPCS code C8957 (Intravenous infusion for therapy/diagnosis; initiation of prolonged infusion (more than 8 hours), requiring use of portable or implantable pump) when appropriate.

Hospitals are expected to report all drug administration CPT codes in a manner consistent with their descriptors, CPT instructions, and correct coding principles. Hospitals should note the conceptual changes between CY 2006 drug administration codes effective under the OPPS and the CY 2007 CPT codes in order to ensure accurate billing under the OPPS.

Medicare's general policy regarding physician supervision within hospital outpatient departments meets the physician supervision requirements for use of CPT codes 90760- 90779, 96401-96549. (Reference: Medicare Benefit Policy Manual, Pub.100-02, Chapter 6, Sec.20.4.1.) C. Payments For Drug Administration Services For CY 2007, OPPS drug administration APCs have been restructured resulting in a sixlevel hierarchy where active HCPCS codes have been assigned according to their clinical coherence and resource use. Contrary to the CY 2006 payment structure that bundled payment for several instances of a type of service (non-chemotherapy, chemotherapy by infusion, non-infusion chemotherapy) into a per-encounter APC payment, the CY 2007 structure provides a separate APC payment for each reported unit of a separately payable HCPCS code.

Hospitals should note that the transition to the full set of CPT drug administration codes provides for conceptual differences when reporting, such as those noted below.

In CY 2006, hospitals were instructed to bill for the first hour (and any additional hours) by each type of infusion service (non-chemotherapy, chemotherapy by infusion, non-infusion chemotherapy). In CY 2007, the first hour concept no longer exists. CY 2007 CPT codes allow for only one initial service per encounter, for each vascular access site, no matter how many types of infusion services are provided; however, hospitals will receive an APC payment for the initial service and separate APC payment(s) for additional hours of infusion or other drug administration services provided that are separately payable .

In CY 2006, hospitals providing infusion services of different types (nonchemotherapy, chemotherapy by infusion, non-infusion chemotherapy) received payment for the associated per-encounter infusion APC even if these infusions occurred during the same time period. In CY 2007, CPT instructions allow reporting of only one initial drug administration service, including infusion services, per encounter for each distinct vascular access site, with other services through the same vascular access site being reported via the sequential, concurrent or additional hour codes.

NOTE: This list provides a brief overview of a limited number of the conceptual changes between CY 2006 OPPS drug administration codes and CY 2007 OPPS drug administration codes - this list is not comprehensive and does not include all items hospitals will need to consider during this transition) For CY 2007 APC payment rates, refer to Addendum B on the CMS Web site at http://www.cms.hhs.gov/HospitalOutpatientPPS/.

D. Infusions Started Outside the Hospital

Hospitals may receive Medicare beneficiaries for outpatient services who are in the process of receiving an infusion at their time of arrival at the hospital (e.g. a patient who arrives via ambulance with an ongoing intravenous infusion initiated by paramedics during transport). Hospitals are reminded to bill for all services provided using the HCPCS code(s) that most accurately describe the service(s) they provided. This includes hospitals reporting an initial hour of infusion, even if the hospital did not initiate the infusion, and additional HCPCS codes for additional or sequential infusion services if needed.

100-4, 4, 231.4

Billing for Split Unit of Blood

HCPCS code P9011 was created to identify situations where one unit of blood or a blood product is split and some portion of the unit is transfused to one patient and the other portions are transfused to other patients or to the same patient at other times. When a patient receives a transfusion of a split unit of blood or blood product, OPPS providers should bill P9011 for the blood product transfused, as well as CPT 86985 (Splitting, blood products) for each splitting procedure performed to prepare the blood product for a specific patient.

Providers should bill split units of packed red cells and whole blood using Revenue Code 389 (Other blood), and should not use Revenue Codes 381 (Packed red cells) or 382 (Whole blood). Providers should bill split units of other blood products using the applicable revenue codes for the blood product type, such as 383 (Plasma) or 384 (Platelets), rather than 389. Reporting revenue codes according to these specifications will ensure the Medicare beneficiary's blood deductible is applied correctly.

EXAMPLE: OPPS provider splits off a 100cc aliquot from a 250 cc unit of leukocytereduced red blood cells for a transfusion to Patient X. The hospital then splits off an 80cc aliquot of the remaining unit for a transfusion to Patient Y. At a later time, the remaining 70cc from the unit is transfused to Patient Z.

In billing for the services for Patient X and Patient Y, the OPPS provider should report the charges by billing P9011 and 86985 in addition to the CPT code for the transfusion service, because a specific splitting service was required to prepare a split unit for transfusion to each of those patients. However, the OPPS provider should report only P9011 and the CPT code for the transfusion service for Patient Z because no additional splitting was necessary to prepare the split unit for transfusion to Patient Z. The OPPS provider should bill Revenue Code 0389 for each split unit of the leukocyte-reduced red blood cells that was transfused.

100-4, 4, 231.9

Billing for Pheresis and Apheresis Services

Apheresis/pheresis services are billed on a per visit basis and not on a per unit basis. OPPS providers should report the charge for an Evaluation and Management (E&M) visit only if there is a separately identifiable E&M service performed which extends beyond the evaluation and management portion of a typical apheresis/pheresis service. If the OPPS provider is billing an E&M visit code in addition to the apheresis/pheresis service, it may be appropriate to use the HCPCS modifier -25.

100-4, 4, 231.11

Billing for Allogeneic Stem Cell Transplants

1. Definition of Acquisition Charges for Allogeneic Stem Cell Transplants

Acquisition charges for allogeneic stem cell transplants include, but are not limited to, charges for the costs of the following services:

National Marrow Donor Program fees, if applicable, for stem cells from an unrelated donor;

Tissue typing of donor and recipient;

Donor evaluation;

Physician pre-procedure donor evaluation services;

Costs associated with harvesting procedure (e.g., general routine and special care services, procedure/operating room and other ancillary services, apheresis services, etc.);

Post-operative/post-procedure evaluation of donor; and

Preparation and processing of stem cells.

Payment for these acquisition services is included in the OPPS APC payment for the allogeneic stem cell transplant when the transplant occurs in the hospital outpatient setting, and in the MS-DRG payment for the allogeneic stem cell transplant when the transplant occurs in the inpatient setting. The Medicare contractor does not make separate payment for these acquisition services, because hospitals may bill and receive payment only for services provided to the Medicare beneficiary who is the recipient of the stem cell transplant and whose illness is being treated with the stem cell transplant. Unlike the acquisition costs of solid organs for transplant (e.g., hearts and kidneys), which are paid on a reasonable cost basis, acquisition costs for allogeneic stem cells are included in prospective payment. Recurring update notifications describing changes to and billing instructions for various payment policies implemented in the OPPS are issues annually.

Acquisition charges for stem cell transplants apply only to allogeneic transplants, for which stem cells are obtained from a donor (other than the recipient himself or herself). Acquisition charges do not apply to autologous transplants (transplanted stem cells are obtained from the recipient himself or herself), because autologous transplants involve services provided to the beneficiary only (and not to a donor), for which the hospital may bill and receive payment (see Pub. 100-04, chapter 3, Sec.90.3.3 and Sec.231.10 of this chapter for information regarding billing for autologous stem cell transplants).

2. Billing for Acquisition Services

The hospital bills and shows acquisition charges for allogeneic stem cell transplants based on the status of the patient (i.e., inpatient or outpatient) when the transplant is furnished. See Pub. 100-04, chapter 3, Sec.90.3.3 for instructions regarding billing for acquisition services for allogeneic stem cell transplants that are performed in the inpatient setting.

When the allogeneic stem cell transplant occurs in the outpatient setting, the hospital identifies stem cell acquisition charges for allogeneic bone marrow/stem cell transplants separately in FL 42 of Form CMS-1450 (or electronic equivalent) by using revenue code 0819 (Other Organ Acquisition). Revenue code 0819 charges should include all services required to acquire stem cells from a donor, as defined above, and should be reported on the same date of service as the transplant procedure in order to be appropriately packaged for payment purposes.

The transplant hospital keeps an itemized statement that identifies the services furnished, the charges, the person receiving the service (donor/recipient), and whether this is a potential transplant donor or recipient. These charges will be reflected in the transplant hospital's stem cell/bone marrow acquisition cost center. For allogeneic stem cell acquisition services in cases that do not result in transplant, due to death of the intended recipient or other causes, hospitals include the costs associated with the acquisition services on the Medicare cost report.

In the case of an allogeneic transplant in the hospital outpatient setting, the hospital reports the transplant itself with the appropriate CPT code, and a charge under revenue center code 0362 or another appropriate cost center. Selection of the cost center is up to the hospital.

100-4, 4, 240

Inpatient Part B Hospital Services

Inpatient Part B services which are paid under OPPS include:

- Diagnostic x-ray tests, and other diagnostic tests (excluding clinical diagnostic laboratory tests);
- X-ray, radium, and radioactive isotope therapy, including materials and services of technicians;
- Surgical dressings applied during an encounter at the hospital and splints, casts, and other devices used for reduction of fractures and dislocations (splints and casts, etc., include dental splints);
- Implantable prosthetic devices;
- Hepatitis B vaccine and its administration, and certain preventive screening services (pelvic exams, screening sigmoidoscopies, screening colonoscopies, bone mass measurements, and prostate screening.)
- Bone Mass measurements;
- Prostate screening;
- Immunosuppressive drugs;
- Oral anti-cancer drugs;
- Oral drug prescribed for use as an acute anti-emetic used as part of an anti-cancer chemotherapeutic regimen; and
- Epoetin Alfa (EPO)

When a hospital that is not paid under the OPPS furnishes an implantable prosthetic device that meets the criteria for coverage in Medicare Benefits Policy Manual, Pub.100-02, Chapter 6, Sec.10 to an inpatient who has coverage under Part B, payment for the implantable prosthetic device is made under the payment mechanism that applies to other hospital outpatient services (e.g. reasonable cost, all inclusive rate, waiver).

When a hospital that is paid under the OPPS furnishes an implantable prosthetic device to an inpatient who has coverage under Part B, but who does not have coverage of inpatient services on the date that the implanted prosthetic device is furnished, the hospital should report new HCPCS code, C9899, Implanted Prosthetic Device, Payable Only for Inpatients who do not Have Inpatient Coverage, that will be effective for services furnished on or after January 1, 2009. This code may be reported only on claims with TOB 12X when the prosthetic device is implanted on a day on which the beneficiary does not have coverage of the hospital inpatient services he or she is receiving. The line containing this new code will be rejected if it is reported on a claim that is not a TOB 12X or if it is reported with a line item date of service on which the beneficiary has coverage of inpatient hospital services. By reporting C9899, the hospital is reporting that all of the criteria for payment under Part B are met as specified in the Medicare Benefits Policy Manual, Pub.100-02, Chapter 6, Sec.10, and that the item meets all Medicare criteria for coverage as an implantable prosthetic device as defined in that section.

Medicare contractors shall first determine that the item furnished meets the Medicare criteria for coverage as an implantable prosthetic device as specified in the Medicare Benefits Policy Manual, Pub. 100-02, Chapter 6, Sec.10. If the item does not meet the criteria for coverage as an implantable prosthetic device, the contractor shall deny payment on the basis that the item is outside the scope of the benefits for which there is coverage for Part B inpatients. The beneficiary is liable for the charges for the noncovered item when the item does not meet the criteria for coverage as an implanted prosthetic device as specified in the Medicare Benefits Policy Manual, Pub.100-02, Chapter 6, Sec.10.

If the contractor determines that the device is covered, the contractor shall determine if the device has pass through status under the OPPS. If so, the contractor shall establish the payment amount for the device at the product of the charge for the device and the hospital specific cost to charge ratio. Where the device does not have pass through status under the OPPS, the contractor shall establish the payment amount for the device at the amount for a comparable device in the DMEPOS fee schedule where there is such an amount. Payment under the DMEPOS fee schedule is made at the lesser of charges or the fee schedule amount and therefore if there is a fee for the specific item on the DMEPOS fee schedule, the payment amount for the item will be set at the lesser of the actual charges or the DMEPOS fee schedule amount. Where the item does not have pass through payment status and where there is no amount for a comparable device in the DMEPOS fee schedule, the contractor shall establish a payment amount that is specific to the particular implanted prosthetic device for the applicable calendar year. This amount (less applicable unpaid deductible and coinsurance) will be paid for that specific device for services furnished in the applicable calendar year unless the actual charge for the item is less than the established amount). Where the actual charge is less than the established amount, the contractor will pay the actual charge for the item (less applicable unpaid deductible and coinsurance).

In setting a contractor established payment rate for the specific device, the contractor takes into account the cost information available at the time the payment rate is established. This information may include, but is not limited to, the amount of device cost that would be removed from an applicable APC payment for implantation of the device if the provider received a device without cost or a full credit for the cost of the device.

If the contractor chooses to use this amount, see www.cms.hhs.gov/HospitalOutpatientPPS/ for the amount of reduction to the APC payment that would apply in these cases. From the OPPS webpage, select "Device, Radiolabeled Product, and Procedure Edits" from the list on the left side of the page. Open the file "Procedure to Device edits" to determine the HCPCS code that best describes the procedure in which the device would be used. Then identify the APC to which that procedure code maps from the most recent Addenda B on the OPPS webpage and open the file "FB/FC Modifier Procedures and Devices". Select the applicable year's file of APCs subject to full and partial credit reductions (for example: CY 2008 APCs Subject to Full and Partial Credit Reduction Policy"). Select the "Full offset reduction amount" that pertains to the APC that is most applicable to the device described by C9899. It would be reasonable to set this amount as a payment for a device furnished to a Part B inpatient.

For example, if C9899 is reporting insertion of a single chamber pacemaker (C1786 or equivalent narrative description on the claim in "remarks") the file of procedure to device edits shows that a single chamber pacemaker is the dominant device for APC 0090 (APC 0089 is for insertion of both pacemaker and electrodes and therefore would not apply if electrodes are not also billed). The table of offset reduction amounts for CY 2008 shows that the estimated cost of a single chamber pacemaker for APC 0090 is $4881.77. It would therefore be reasonable for the contractor/MAC to set the payment rate for a single chamber pacemaker furnished to a Part B inpatient to $4881.77. In this case the coinsurance would be $936.75 (20 percent of $4881.77, which is less than the inpatient deductible).

The beneficiary coinsurance is 20 percent of the payment amount for the device (i.e. the pass through payment amount, the DMEPOS fee schedule amount, the contractor established amount, or the actual charge if less than the DMEPOS fee schedule amount or the contractor established amount for the specific device), not to exceed the Medicare inpatient deductible that is applicable to the year in which the implanted prosthetic device is furnished.

Inpatient Part B services paid under other payment methods include:

- Clinical diagnostic laboratory tests, prosthetic devices other than implantable ones and other than dental which replace all or part of an internal body organ (including contiguous tissue), or all or part of the function of a permanently inoperative or malfunctioning internal body organ, including replacement or repairs of such devices;
- Leg, arm, back and neck braces; trusses and artificial legs; arms and eyes including adjustments, repairs, and replacements required because of breakage, wear, loss, or a change in the patient's physical condition; take home surgical dressings; outpatient physical therapy; outpatient occupational therapy; and outpatient speech-language pathology services;
- Ambulance services;
- Screening pap smears, screening colorectal tests, and screening mammography;
- Influenza virus vaccine and its administration, pneumococcal vaccine and its administration;
- Diabetes self-management training;
- Hemophilia clotting factors for hemophilia patients competent to use these factors without supervision).

See Chapter 6 of the Medicare Benefit Policy Manual for a discussion of the circumstances under which the above services may be covered as Part B Inpatient services.

100-4, 4, 250.16

Multiple Procedure Payment Reduction (MPPR) on Certain Diagnostic Imaging Procedures Rendered by Physicians

Diagnostic imaging procedures rendered by a physician that has reassigned their billing rights to a Method II CAH are payable by Medicare when the procedures are eligible and billed on type of bill 85x with revenue code (RC) 096x, 097x and/or 098x.

The MPPR on diagnostic imaging applies when multiple services are furnished by the same physician to the same patient in the same session on the same day. Full payment is made for each service with the highest payment under the MPFS and payment is made at 75 percent for each subsequent service.

100-4, 4, 250.3.2

Physician Rendering Anesthesia in a Hospital Outpatient Setting

When a medically necessary anesthesia service is furnished within a HPSA area by a physician, a HPSA bonus is payable. In addition to using the PC/TC indicator on the CORF extract of the MPFS Summary File to identify HPSA services, pay physicians the HPSA bonus when CPT codes 00100 through 01999 are billed with the following modifiers: QY, QK, AA, or GC and "QB" or "QU" in revenue code 963. Modifier QB or QU must be submitted to receive payment of the HPSA bonus for claims with dates of service prior to January 01, 2006. Effective for claims with dates of service on or after January 01, 2006, the modifier AQ, physician providing a service in a health professional shortage area, may be required to receive the HPSA bonus. Refer to 250.2.2 of this chapter for more information on when modifier AQ is required.

The modifiers signify that a physician performed an anesthesia service. Using the Anesthesia File (See Section above) the physician service will be 115 percent times the payment amount to be paid to a CAH on Method II payment plus 10 percent HPSA bonus payment.

Anesthesiology modifiers:

AA = anesthesia services performed personally by anesthesiologist.

GC =service performed, in part, by a resident under the direction of a teaching physician.

QK = medical direction of two, three, or four concurrent anesthesia procedures involving qualified individuals.

QY = medical direction of one CRNA by an anesthesiologist.

Modifiers AA and GC result in physician payment at 80% of the allowed amount.
Modifiers QK and QY result in physician payment at 50% of the allowed amount.

Data elements needed to calculate payment:

HCPCS plus Modifier,

Base Units,

Time units, based on standard 15 minute intervals,

Locality specific anesthesia Conversion factor, and

Allowed amount minus applicable deductions and coinsurance amount.

Formula 1: Calculate payment for a physician performing anesthesia alone

HCPCS = xxxxx
Modifier = AA
Base Units = 4

Anesthesia Time is 60 minutes. Anesthesia time units = 4 (60/15)
Sum of Base Units plus Time Units = 4 + 4 = 8
Locality specific Anesthesia conversion factor = $17.00 (varies by localities)
Coinsurance = 20%

Example 1: Physician personally performs the anesthesia case

Base Units plus time units - 4+4=8
Total units multiplied by the anesthesia conversion factor times .80
8 x $17= ($136.00 - (deductible*) x .80 = $108.80

Payment amount times 115 percent for the CAH method II payment.

$108.80 x 1.15 = $125.12 (Payment amount)

$125.12 x .10 = $12.51 (HPSA bonus payment)

*Assume the Part B deductible has already been met for the calendar year

Formula 2: Calculate the payment for the physician's medical direction service when the physician directs two concurrent cases involving CRNAs. The medical direction allowance is 50% of the allowance for the anesthesia service personally performed by the physician.

HCPCS = xxxxx
Modifier = QK
Base Units = 4
Time Units 60/15=4

Sum of base units plus time units = 8
Locality specific anesthesia conversion factor = $17(varies by localities)
Coinsurance = 20 %

(Allowed amount adjusted for applicable deductions and coinsurance and to reflect payment percentage for medical direction).

Example 2: Physician medically directs two concurrent cases involving CRNAs

Base units plus time - 4+4=8
Total units multiplied by the anesthesia conversion factor times. 50 equal allowed amount minus any remaining deductible
8 x $17 = $136 x .50 = $68.00 -(deductible*) = $68.00

Allowed amount Times 80 percent times 1.15
$68.00 x .80 = $54.40 x 1.15 = 62.56 (Payment amount)
$62.56 x .10 = $6.26 (HPSA bonus payment)

*Assume the deductible has already been met for the calendar year.

100-4, 4, 260.5

260.5 - Line Item Date of Service Reporting for Partial Hospitalization

(Rev. 3019, Issued: 08-07-14, Effective: 01-01-12, ICD-10: Upon Implementation of ICD- 10, Implementation: 09-08-14, ICD-10: Upon Implementation of ICD- 10)

Hospitals other than CAHs are required to report line item dates of service per revenue code line for partial hospitalization claims. Where services are provided on more than one day included in the billing period, the date of service must be identified. Each service (revenue code) provided must be repeated on a separate line item along with the specific date the service was provided for every occurrence. See examples below of reporting line item dates of service. These examples are for group therapy services provided twice during a billing period.

For the claims, report as follows:

Revenue Code	HCPCS	Dates of Service	Units	Total Charges
0915	G0176	20090505	1	$80.00
0915	G0176	20090529	2	$160.00

NOTE: Information regarding the Form CMS-1450 form locators that correspond with these fields is found in Chapter 25 of this manual. See the ASC X12 837 Institutional Claim Implementation Guide for related guidelines for the electronic claim.

The A/B MAC (A) must return to the hospital (RTP) claims where a line item date of service is not entered for each HCPCS code reported, or if the line item dates of service reported are outside of the statement covers period. Line item date of service reporting is effective for claims with dates of service on or after June 5, 2000.

100-4, 4, 290.5.1

Billing and Payment for Observation Services Beginning January 1, 2008

Observation services are reported using HCPCS code G0378 (Hospital observation service, per hour). Beginning January 1, 2008, HCPCS code G0378 for hourly observation services is assigned status indicator N, signifying that its payment is always packaged. No separate payment is made for observation services reported with HCPCS code G0378, and APC 0339 is deleted as of January 1, 2008. In most circumstances, observation services are supportive and ancillary to the other services provided to a patient. Beginning January 1, 2014, in certain circumstances when observation care is billed in conjunction with a clinic visit, high level Type A emergency department visit (Level 4 or 5), high level Type B emergency department visit (Level 5), critical care services, or a direct referral as an integral part of a patient's extended encounter of care, payment may be made for the entire extended care encounter through APC 8009 (Extended Assessment and Management Composite) when certain criteria are met. Prior to January 1, 2014, in certain circumstances when observation care was billed in conjunction with a high level clinic visit (Level 5), high level Type A emergency department visit (Level 4 or 5), high level Type B emergency department visit (Level 5), critical care services, or a direct referral as an integral part of a patient's extended encounter of care, payment could be made for the entire extended care encounter through one of two composite APCs (APCs 8002 and 8003) when certain criteria were met. APCs 8002 and 8003 are deleted as of January 1, 2014. For information about payment for extended assessment and management composite APC, see §10.2.1 (Composite APCs) of this chapter.

There is no limitation on diagnosis for payment of APC 8009; however, composite APC payment will not be made when observation services are reported in association with a surgical procedure (T status procedure) or the hours of observation care reported are less than 8. The I/OCE evaluates every claim received to determine if payment through a composite APC is appropriate. If payment through a composite APC is inappropriate, the I/OCE, in conjunction with the Pricer, determines the appropriate status indicator, APC, and payment for every code on a claim.

All of the following requirements must be met in order for a hospital to receive an APC payment for an extended assessment and management composite APC:

1. Observation Time
   a. Observation time must be documented in the medical record.
   b. Hospital billing for observation services begins at the clock time documented in the patient's medical record, which coincides with the time that observation services are initiated in accordance with a physician's order for observation services.
   c. A beneficiary's time receiving observation services (and hospital billing) ends when all clinical or medical interventions have been completed, including follow-up care furnished by hospital staff and physicians that may take place after a physician has ordered the patient be released or admitted as an inpatient.
   d. The number of units reported with HCPCS code G0378 must equal or exceed 8 hours.
2. Additional Hospital Services
   a. The claim for observation services must include one of the following services in addition to the reported observation services. The additional services listed below must have a line item date of service on the same day or the day before the date reported for observation:
      - A Type A or B emergency department visit (CPT codes 99284 or 99285 or HCPCS code G0384); or
      - A clinic visit (CPT code 99205 or 99215); or
      - Critical care (CPT code 99291); or
      - Direct referral for observation care reported with HCPCS code G0379 (APC 0604) must be reported on the same date of service as the date reported for observation services.
   b. No procedure with a T status indicator can be reported on the same day or day before observation care is provided.
3. Physician Evaluation
   a. The beneficiary must be in the care of a physician during the period of observation, as documented in the medical record by outpatient registration, discharge, and other appropriate progress notes that are timed, written, and signed by the physician.
   b. he medical record must include documentation that the physician explicitly assessed patient risk to determine that the beneficiary would benefit from observation care.

Criteria 1 and 3 related to observation care beginning and ending time and physician evaluation apply regardless of whether the hospital believes that the criteria will be met for payment of the extended encounter through extended assessment and management composite payment.

Only visits, critical care and observation services that are billed on a 13X bill type may be considered for a composite APC payment.

Non-repetitive services provided on the same day as either direct referral for observation care or observation services must be reported on the same claim because the OCE claim-by-claim logic cannot function properly unless all services related to the episode of observation care, including hospital clinic visits, emergency department visits, critical care services, and T status procedures, are reported on the same claim. Additional guidance can be found in chapter 1, section 50.2.2 of this manual.

If a claim for services provided during an extended assessment and management encounter including observation care does not meet all of the requirements listed above, then the usual APC logic will apply to separately payable items and services on the claim; the special logic for direct admission will apply, and payment for the observation care will be packaged into payments for other separately payable services provided to the beneficiary in the same encounter.

100-4, 4, 300

Medical Nutrition Therapy (MNT) Services

Section 105 of the Medicare, Medicaid, and SCHIP Benefits Improvement and Protection Act of 2000 (BIPA) permits Medicare coverage of Medical Nutrition Therapy (MNT) services when furnished by a registered dietitian or nutrition professional meeting certain requirements. The benefit is available for beneficiaries with diabetes or renal disease, when referral is made by a physician as defined in §1861(r)(l) of the Act. It also allows registered dietitians and nutrition professionals to receive direct Medicare reimbursement for the first time. The effective date of this provision is January 1, 2002.

The benefit consists of an initial visit for an assessment; follow-up visits for interventions; and reassessments as necessary during the 12-month period beginning with the initial assessment ("episode of care") to assure compliance with the dietary plan. Effective October 1, 2002, basic coverage of MNT for the first year a beneficiary receives MNT with either a diagnosis of renal disease or diabetes as defined at 42 CFR, 410.130 is 3 hours. Also effective October 1, 2002, basic coverage in subsequent years for renal disease is 2 hours.

For the purposes of this benefit, renal disease means chronic renal insufficiency or the medical condition of a beneficiary who has been discharged from the hospital after a successful renal transplant within the last 36 months. Chronic renal insufficiency means a reduction in renal function not severe enough to require dialysis or transplantation (glomerular filtration rate (GFR) 13-50 ml/min/1.73m^2). Effective January 1, 2004, CMS updated the definition of diabetes to be as follows: Diabetes is defined as diabetes mellitus, a condition of abnormal glucose metabolism diagnosed using the following criteria: a fasting blood sugar greater than or equal to 126 mg/dL on two different occasions; a 2 hour post-glucose challenge greater than or equal to 200 mg/dL on 2 different occasions; or a random glucose test over 200 mg/dL for a person with symptoms of uncontrolled diabetes.

The MNT benefit is a completely separate benefit from the diabetes self-management training (DSMT) benefit. CMS had originally planned to limit how much of both benefits a beneficiary might receive in the same time period. However, the national coverage decision, published May 1, 2002, allows a beneficiary to receive the full amount of both benefits in the same period. Therefore, a beneficiary can receive the full 10 hours of initial DSMT and the full 3 hours of MNT. However, providers are not allowed to bill for both DSMT and MNT on the same date of service for the same beneficiary.

100-4, 4, 300.6

Common Working File (CWF) Edits

The CWF edit will allow 3 hours of therapy for MNT in the initial calendar year. The edit will allow more than 3 hours of therapy if there is a change in the beneficiary's medical condition, diagnosis, or treatment regimen and this change must be documented in the beneficiary's medical record. Two new G codes have been created for use when a beneficiary receives a second referral in a calendar year that allows the beneficiary to receive more than 3 hours of therapy. Another edit will allow 2 hours of follow up MNT with another referral in subsequent years.

Advance Beneficiary Notice (ABN)

The beneficiary is liable for services denied over the limited number of hours with referrals for MNT. An ABN should be issued in these situations. In absence of evidence of a valid ABN, the provider will be held liable.

An ABN should not be issued for Medicare-covered services such as those provided by hospital dietitians or nutrition professionals who are qualified to render the service in their state but who have not obtained Medicare provider numbers.

Duplicate Edits

Although beneficiaries are allowed to receive training and therapy during the same time period Diabetes Self-Management and Training (DSMT) and Medical Nutrition Therapy (MNT) services may not be provided on the same day to the same beneficiary. Effective April 1, 2010 CWF shall implement a new duplicate crossover edit to identify and prevent claims for DSMT/MNT services from being billed with the same dates of services for the same beneficiaries submitted from institutional providers and from a professional provider.

100-4, 4, 320.1

HCPCS Coding for OIVIT

HCPCS code G9147, effective with the April IOCE and MPFSDB updates, is to be used on claims with dates of service on and after December 23, 2009, billing for non-covered OIVIT and any services comprising an OIVIT regimen.

NOTE: HCPCS codes 99199 or 94681(with or without diabetes related conditions 250.00-250.93) are not to be used on claims billing for non-covered OIVIT and any services comprising an OIVIT regimen when furnished pursuant to an OIVIT regimen. Claims billing for HCPCS codes 99199 and 94681 for non-covered OIVIT are to be returned to provider/returned as unprocessable.

100-4, 4, 320.2

Outpatient Intravenous Insulin Treatment (OIVIT)

Effective for claims with dates of service on and after December 23, 2009, the Centers for Medicare and Medicaid Services (CMS) determines that the evidence does not support a conclusion that OIVIT improves health outcomes in Medicare beneficiaries. Therefore, CMS has determined that OIVIT is not reasonable and necessary for any indication under section 1862(a)(1)(A) of the Social Security Act. Services comprising an OIVIT regimen are nationally non-covered under Medicare when furnished pursuant to an OIVIT regimen.

See Pub. 100-03, Medicare National Coverage Determinations Manual, Section 40.7, Outpatient Intravenous Insulin Treatment (Effective December 23, 2009), for general information and coverage indications.

100-4, 5, 10

Part B Outpatient Rehabilitation and Comprehensive Outpatient Rehabilitation Facility (CORF) Services - General

Language in this section is defined or described in Pub. 100-02, chapter 15, sections 220 and 230.

Section 4541(a)(2) of the Balanced Budget Act (BBA) (P.L. 105-33), which added §1834(k)(5) to the Social Security Act (the Act), required that all claims for outpatient rehabilitation services and comprehensive outpatient rehabilitation facility (CORF) services, be reported using a uniform coding system. The CMS chose HCPCS (Healthcare Common Procedure Coding System) as the coding system to be used for the reporting of these services. This coding requirement is effective for all claims for outpatient rehabilitation services and CORF services submitted on or after April 1, 1998.

The BBA also required payment under a prospective payment system for outpatient rehabilitation services including CORF services. Effective for claims with dates of service on or after January 1, 1999, the Medicare Physician Fee Schedule (MPFS) became the method of payment for outpatient therapy services furnished by:

Comprehensive outpatient rehabilitation facilities (CORFs);

Outpatient physical therapy providers (OPTs);

Other rehabilitation facilities (ORFs);

Hospitals (to outpatients and inpatients who are not in a covered Part A stay);

Skilled nursing facilities (SNFs) (to residents not in a covered Part A stay and to nonresidents who receive outpatient rehabilitation services from the SNF); and

Home health agencies (HHAs) (to individuals who are not homebound or otherwise are not receiving services under a home health plan of care (POC)).

NOTE: No provider or supplier other than the SNF will be paid for therapy services during the time the beneficiary is in a covered SNF Part A stay. For information regarding SNF consolidated billing see chapter 6, section 10 of this manual.

Similarly, under the HH prospective payment system, HHAs are responsible to provide, either directly or under arrangements, all outpatient rehabilitation therapy services to beneficiaries receiving services under a home health POC. No other provider or supplier will be paid for these services during the time the beneficiary is in a covered Part A stay. For information regarding HH consolidated billing see chapter10, section 20 of this manual.

Section 143 of the Medicare Improvements for Patients and Provider's Act of 2008 (MIPPA) authorizes the Centers for Medicare & Medicaid Services (CMS) to enroll speech-language pathologists (SLP) as suppliers of Medicare services and for SLPs to begin billing Medicare for outpatient speech-language pathology services furnished in private practice beginning July 1, 2009. Enrollment will allow SLPs in private practice to bill Medicare and receive direct payment for their services. Previously, the Medicare program could only pay SLP services if an institution, physician or nonphysician practitioner billed them.

In Chapter 23, as part of the CY 2009 Medicare Physician Fee Schedule Database, the descriptor for PC/TC indicator "7", as applied to certain HCPCS/CPT codes, is described as specific to the services of privately practicing therapists. Payment may not be made if the service is provided to either a hospital outpatient or a hospital inpatient by a physical therapist, occupational therapist, or speech-language pathologist in private practice.

The MPFS is used as a method of payment for outpatient rehabilitation services furnished under arrangement with any of these providers.

In addition, the MPFS is used as the payment system for CORF services identified by the HCPCS codes in §20. Assignment is mandatory.

The Medicare allowed charge for the services is the lower of the actual charge or the MPFS amount. The Medicare payment for the services is 80 percent of the allowed charge after the Part B deductible is met. Coinsurance is made at 20 percent of the lower of the actual charge or the MPFS amount. The general coinsurance rule (20 percent of the actual charges) does not apply when making payment under the MPFS. This is a final payment.

The MPFS does not apply to outpatient rehabilitation services furnished by critical access hospitals (CAHs). CAHs are to be paid on a reasonable cost basis.

Contractors process outpatient rehabilitation claims from hospitals, including CAHs, SNFs, HHAs, CORFs, outpatient rehabilitation agencies, and outpatient physical therapy providers for which they have received a tie in notice from the RO. These provider types submit their claims to the contractors using the 837 Institutional electronic claim format or the UB-04 paper form when permissible. Contractors also process claims from physicians, certain nonphysician practitioners (NPPs), therapists in private practices (TPPs), (which are limited to physical and occupational therapists, and speech-language pathologists in private practices), and physician-directed clinics that bill for services furnished incident to a physician's service (see Pub. 100-02, Medicare Benefit Policy Manual, chapter 15, for a definition of "incident to"). These provider types submit their claims to the contractor using the 837 Professional electronic claim format or the CMS-1500 paper form when permissible.

There are different fee rates for nonfacility and facility services. Chapter 23 describes the differences in these two rates. (See fields 28 and 29 of the record therein described). Facility rates apply to professional services performed in a facility other than the professional's office. Nonfacility rates apply when the service is performed in the professional's office. The nonfacility rate (that is paid when the provider performs the services in its own facility) accommodates overhead and indirect expenses the provider incurs by operating its own facility. Thus it is somewhat higher than the facility rate.

Contractors pay the nonfacility rate on institutional claims for services performed in the provider's facility. Contractors may pay professional claims using the facility or nonfacility rate depending upon where the service is performed (place of service on the claim), and the provider specialty.

Contractors pay the codes in §20 under the MPFS on professional claims regardless of whether they may be considered rehabilitation services. However, contractors must use this list for institutional claims to determine whether to pay under outpatient rehabilitation rules or whether payment rules for other types of service may apply, e.g., OPPS for hospitals, reasonable costs for CAHs.

Note that because a service is considered an outpatient rehabilitation service does not automatically imply payment for that service. Additional criteria, including coverage, plan of care and physician certification must also be met. These criteria are described in Pub. 100-02, Medicare Benefit Policy Manual, chapters 1 and 15.

Payment for rehabilitation services provided to Part A inpatients of hospitals or SNFs is included in the respective PPS rate. Also, for SNFs (but not hospitals), if the beneficiary has Part B, but not Part A coverage (e.g., Part A benefits are exhausted), the SNF must bill for any rehabilitation service.

Payment for rehabilitation therapy services provided by home health agencies under a home health plan of care is included in the home health PPS rate. HHAs may submit bill type 34X and be paid under the MPFS if there are no home health services billed under a home health plan of care at the same time, and there is a valid rehabilitation POC (e.g., the patient is not homebound).

An institutional employer (other than a SNF) of the TPPs, or physician performing outpatient services, (e.g., hospital, CORF, etc.), or a clinic billing on behalf of the physician or therapist may bill the contractor on a professional claim.

The MPFS is the basis of payment for outpatient rehabilitation services furnished by TPPs, physicians, and certain nonphysician practitioners or for diagnostic tests provided incident to the services of such physicians or nonphysician practitioners. (See Pub. 100-02, Medicare Benefit Policy Manual, chapter 15, for a definition of "incident to, therapist, therapy and related instructions.") Such services are billed to the contractor on the professional claim format. Assignment is mandatory.

The following table identifies the provider and supplier types, and identifies which claim format they may use to submit bills to the contractor. "Provider/Supplier Service" Type

Format	Bill Type	Comment
Inpatient hospital Part A Institutional	11X	Included in PPS
Inpatient SNF Part A Institutional	21X	Included in PPS
Inpatient hospital Part B Institutional	12X	Hospitals may obtain services under arrangements and bill, or rendering provider may bill.
Inpatient SNF Part B (audiology tests are not included) Institutional	22X	SNF must provide and bill, or obtain under arrangements and bill.
Outpatient hospital Institutional	13X	Hospital may provide and bill or obtain under arrangements and bill, or rendering provider may bill.
Outpatient SNF Institutional	23X	SNF must provide and bill or obtain under arrangements and bill.
HHA billing for services rendered under a Part A or Part B home health plan of care. Institutional	32X	Service is included in PPS rate. CMS determines whether payment is from Part A or Part B trust fund.
HHA billing for services not rendered under a Part A or Part B home health plan of care, but rendered under a therapy plan of care. Institutional	34X	Service not under home health plan of care.
Other Rehabilitation Facility (ORF) Institutional	74X	Paid MPFS for outpatient rehabilitation services effective January 1, 1999, and all other services except drugs effective July 1, 2000. Starting April 1, 2002, drugs are paid 95% of the AWP. For claims with dates of service on or after July 1, 2003, drugs and biologicals do not apply in an OPT setting. Therefore, FIs are to advise their OPTs not to bill for them.
Comprehensive Outpatient Rehabilitation Facility (CORF) Institutional	75X	Paid MPFS for outpatient rehabilitation services effective January 1, 1999, and all other services except drugs effective July 1, 2000. Starting April 1, 2002, drugs are paid 95% of the AWP.
Physician, NPPs, TPPs, (service in hospital or SNF) Professional	See Chapter 26 for place of service, and type of service coding.	Payment may not be made for therapy services to Part A Inpatients of hospitals or SNFs, or for Part B SNF residents. Otherwise, suppliers bill to the contractor using the professional claim format. Note that services of a physician/ NPP/TPP employee of a facility may be billed by the facility to a contractor.
Physician/NPP/TPPs office, independent clinic or patient's home Professional	See Chapter 26 for place of service, and type of service coding.	Paid via Physician fee schedule.

Format	Bill Type	Comment
Critical Access Hospital - inpatient Part A Institutional	11X	Rehabilitation services are paid at cost.
Critical Access Hospital - inpatient Part B Institutional	85X	Rehabilitation services are paid at cost.
Critical Access Hospital – outpatient Part B Institutional	85X	Rehabilitation services are paid at cost.

Complete Claim form completion requirements are contained in chapters 25 and 26.

For a list of the outpatient rehabilitation HCPCS codes see §20.

If a contractor receives an institutional claim for one of these HCPCS codes with dates of service on or after July 1, 2003, that does not appear on the supplemental file it currently uses to pay the therapy claims, it contacts its professional claims area to obtain the non-facility price in order to pay the claim.

NOTE: The list of codes in §20 contains commonly utilized codes for outpatient rehabilitation services. Contractors may consider other codes on institutional claims for payment under the MPFS as outpatient rehabilitation services to the extent that such codes are determined to be medically reasonable and necessary and could be performed within the scope of practice of the therapist providing the service.

100-4, 5, 10.2

The Financial Limitation Legislation

A. Legislation on Limitations

The dollar amount of the limitations (caps) on outpatient therapy services is established by statute. The updated amount of the caps is released annually via Recurring Update Notifications and posted on the CMS Website www.cms.gov/TherapyServices, on contractor Websites, and on each beneficiary's Medicare Summary Notice. Medicare contractors shall publish the financial limitation amount in educational articles. It is also available at 1-800-Medicare.

Section 4541(a)(2) of the Balanced Budget Act (BBA) (P.L. 105-33) of 1997, which added §1834(k)(5) to the Act, required payment under a prospective payment system (PPS) for outpatient rehabilitation services (except those furnished by or under arrangements with a hospital). Outpatient rehabilitation services include the following services:

- Physical therapy
- Speech-language pathology; and
- Occupational therapy.

Section 4541(c) of the BBA required application of financial limitations to all outpatient rehabilitation services (except those furnished by or under arrangements with a hospital).

In 1999, an annual per beneficiary limit of $1,500 was applied, including all outpatient physical therapy services and speech-language pathology services. A separate limit applied to all occupational therapy services. The limits were based on incurred expenses and included applicable deductible and coinsurance. The BBA provided that the limits be indexed by the Medicare Economic Index (MEI) each year beginning in 2002.

Since the limitations apply to outpatient services, they do not apply to skilled nursing facility (SNF) residents in a covered Part A stay, including patients occupying swing beds. Rehabilitation services are included within the global Part A per diem payment that the SNF receives under the prospective payment system (PPS) for the covered stay. Also, limitations do not apply to any therapy services covered under prospective payment systems for home health or inpatient hospitals, including critical access hospitals.

The limitation is based on therapy services the Medicare beneficiary receives, not the type of practitioner who provides the service. Physical therapists, speech-language pathologists, and occupational therapists, as well as physicians and certain nonphysician practitioners, could render a therapy service.

B. Moratoria and Exceptions for Therapy Claims

Since the creation of therapy caps, Congress has enacted several moratoria. The Deficit Reduction Act of 2005 directed CMS to develop exceptions to therapy caps for calendar year 2006 and the exceptions have been extended periodically. The cap exception for therapy services billed by outpatient hospitals was part of the original legislation and applies as long as caps are in effect. Exceptions to caps based on the medical necessity of the service are in effect only when Congress legislates the exceptions.

100-4, 5, 10.6

Functional Reporting

A. General

Section 3005(g) of the Middle Class Tax Relief and Jobs Creation Act (MCTRJCA) amended Section 1833(g) of the Act to require a claims-based data collection system for outpatient therapy services, including physical therapy (PT), occupational therapy

(OT) and speech-language pathology (SLP) services. 42 CFR 410.59, 410.60, 410.61, 410.62 and 410.105 implement this requirement. The system will collect data on beneficiary function during the course of therapy services in order to better understand beneficiary conditions, outcomes, and expenditures.

Beneficiary unction information is reported using 42 nonpayable functional G-codes and seven severity/complexity modifiers on claims for PT, OT, and SLP services. Functional reporting on one functional limitation at a time is required periodically throughout an entire PT, OT, or SLP therapy episode of care.

The nonpayable G-codes and severity modifiers provide information about the beneficiary's functional status at the outset of the therapy episode of care, including projected goal status, at specified points during treatment, and at the time of discharge. These G-codes, along with the associated modifiers, are required at specified intervals on all claims for outpatient therapy services - not just those over the cap.

B. Application of New Coding Requirements

This functional data reporting and collection system is effective for therapy services with dates of service on and after January 1, 2013. A testing period will be in effect from January 1, 2013, until July 1, 2013, to allow providers and practitioners to use the new coding requirements to assure that systems work. Claims for therapy services furnished on and after July 1, 2013, that do not contain the required functional G-code/modifier information will be returned or rejected, as applicable.

C. Services Affected

These requirements apply to all claims for services furnished under the Medicare Part B outpatient therapy benefit and the PT, OT, and SLP services furnished under the CORF benefit. They also apply to the therapy services furnished personally by and incident to the service of a physician or a nonphysician practitioner (NPP), including a nurse practitioner (NP), a certified nurse specialist (CNS), or a physician assistant (PA), as applicable.

D. Providers and Practitioners Affected.

The functional reporting requirements apply to the therapy services furnished by the following providers: hospitals, CAHs, SNFs, CORFs, rehabilitation agencies, and HHAs (when the beneficiary is not under a home health plan of care). It applies to the following practitioners: physical therapists, occupational therapists, and speech-language pathologists in private practice (TPPs), physicians, and NPPs as noted above. The term "clinician" is applied to these practitioners throughout this manual section. (See definition section of Pub. 100-02, chapter 15, section 220.)

E. Function-related G-codes

There are 42 functional G-codes, 14 sets of three codes each. Six of the G-code sets are generally for PT and OT functional limitations and eight sets of G-codes are for SLP functional limitations.

The following G-codes are for functional limitations typically seen in beneficiaries receiving PT or OT services. The first four of these sets describe categories of functional limitations and the final two sets describe "other" functional limitations, which are to be used for functional limitations not described by one of the four categories.

NONPAYABLE G-CODES FOR FUNCTIONAL LIMITATIONS

	LONG DESCRIPTOR	SHORT DESCRIPTOR
Mobility G-code Set		
G8978	Mobility: walking & moving around functional limitation, current status, at therapy episode outset and at reporting intervals	Mobility current status
G8979	Mobility: walking & moving around functional limitation, projected goal status, at therapy episode outset, at reporting intervals, and at discharge or to end reporting	Mobility goal status
G8980	Mobility: walking & moving around functional limitation, discharge status, at discharge from therapy or to end reporting	Mobility D/C status
Changing & Maintaining Body Position G-code Set		
G8981	Changing & maintaining body position functional limitation, current status, at therapy episode outset and at reporting intervals	Body pos current status
G8982	Changing & maintaining body position functional limitation, projected goal status, at therapy episode outset, at reporting intervals, and at discharge or to end reporting	Body pos goal status
G8983	Changing & maintaining body position functional limitation, discharge status, at discharge from therapy or to end reporting	Body pos D/C status
Carrying, Moving & Handling Objects G-code Set		
G8984	Carrying, moving & handling objects functional limitation, current status, at therapy episode outset and at reporting intervals	Carry current status
G8985	Carrying, moving & handling objects functional limitation, projected goal status, at therapy episode outset, at reporting intervals, and at discharge or to end reporting	Carry goal status
G8986	Carrying, moving & handling objects functional limitation, discharge status, at discharge from therapy or to end reporting	Carry D/C status
Self Care G-code Set		
G8987	Self care functional limitation, current status, at therapy episode outset and at reporting intervals	Self care current status
G8988	Self care functional limitation, projected goal status, at therapy episode outset, at reporting intervals, and at discharge or to end reporting	Self care goal status
G8989	Self care functional limitation, discharge status, at discharge from therapy or to end reporting	Self care D/C status

The following "other PT/OT" functional G-codes are used to report:

- a beneficiary's functional limitation that is not defined by one of the above four categories;
- a beneficiary whose therapy services are not intended to treat a functional limitation;
- or a beneficiary's functional limitation when an overall, composite or other score from a functional assessment too is used and it does not clearly represent a functional limitation defined by one of the above four code sets.

	LONG DESCRIPTOR	SHORT DESCRIPTOR
Other PT/OT Primary G-code Set		
G8990	Other physical or occupational therapy primary functional limitation, current status, at therapy episode outset and at reporting intervals	Other PT/OT current status
G8991	Other physical or occupational therapy primary functional limitation, projected goal status, at therapy episode outset, at reporting intervals, and at discharge or to end reporting	Other PT/OT goal status
G8992	Other physical or occupational therapy primary functional limitation, discharge status, at discharge from therapy or to end reporting	Other PT/OT D/C status
Other PT/OT Subsequent G-code Set		
G8993	Other physical or occupational therapy subsequent functional limitation, current status, at therapy episode outset and at reporting intervals	Sub PT/OT current status
G8994	Other physical or occupational therapy subsequent functional limitation, projected goal status, at therapy episode outset, at reporting intervals, and at discharge or to end reporting	Sub PT/OT goal status

The following G-codes are for functional limitations typically seen in beneficiaries receiving SLP services. Seven are for specific functional communication measures, which are modeled after the National Outcomes Measurement System (NOMS), and one is for any "other" measure not described by one of the other seven.

	LONG DESCRIPTOR	SHORT DESCRIPTOR
Swallowing G-code Set		
G8996	Swallowing functional limitation, current status, at therapy episode outset and at reporting intervals	Swallow current status
G8997	Swallowing functional limitation, projected goal status, at therapy episode outset, at reporting intervals, and at discharge or to end reporting	Swallow goal status
G8998	Swallowing functional limitation, discharge status, at discharge from therapy or to end reporting	Swallow D/C status
Motor Speech G-code Set (Note: These codes are not sequentially numbered)		
G8999	Motor speech functional limitation, current status, at therapy episode outset and at reporting intervals	Motor speech current status
G9186	Motor speech functional limitation, projected goal status at therapy episode outset, at reporting intervals, and at discharge or to end reporting	Motor speech goal status

	LONG DESCRIPTOR	SHORT DESCRIPTOR
G9158	Motor speech functional limitation, discharge status, at discharge from therapy or to end reporting	Motor speech D/C status
Spoken Language Comprehension G-code Set		
G9159	Spoken language comprehension functional limitation, current status, at therapy episode outset and at reporting intervals	Lang comp current status
G9160	Spoken language comprehension functional limitation, projected goal status, at therapy episode outset, at reporting intervals, and at discharge or to end reporting	Lang comp goal status
G9161	Spoken language comprehension functional limitation, discharge status, at discharge from therapy or to end reporting	Lang comp D/C status
Spoken Language Expressive G-code Set		
G9162	Spoken language expression functional limitation, current status, at therapy episode outset and at reporting intervals	Lang express current status
G9163	Spoken language expression functional limitation, projected goal status, at therapy episode outset, at reporting intervals, and at discharge or to end reporting	Lang press goal status
G9164	Spoken language expression functional limitation, discharge status, at discharge from therapy or to end reporting	Lang express D/C status
Attention G-code Set		
G9165	Attention functional limitation, current status, at therapy episode outset and at reporting intervals	Atten current status
G9166	Attention functional limitation, projected goal status, at therapy episode outset, at reporting intervals, and at discharge or to end reporting	Atten goal status
G9167	Attention functional limitation, discharge status, at discharge from therapy or to end reporting	Atten D/C status
Memory G-code Set		
G9168	Memory functional limitation, current status, at therapy episode outset and at reporting intervals	Memory current status
G9169	Memory functional limitation, projected goal status, at therapy episode outset, at reporting intervals, and at discharge or to end reporting	Memory goal status
G9170	Memory functional limitation, discharge status, at discharge from therapy or to end reporting	Memory D/C status
Voice G-code Set		
G9171	Voice functional limitation, current status, at therapy episode outset and at reporting intervals	Voice current status
G9172	Voice functional limitation, projected goal status, at therapy episode outset, at reporting intervals, and at discharge or to end reporting	Voice goal status
G9173	Voice functional limitation, discharge status, at discharge from therapy or to end reporting	Voice D/C status

The following "other SLP" G-code set is used to report:

- on one of the other eight NOMS-defined functional measures not described by the above code sets; or
- to report an overall, composite or other score from assessment tool that does not clearly represent one of the above seven categorical SLP functional measures.

	LONG DESCRIPTOR	SHORT DESCRIPTOR
Other Speech Language Pathology G-code Set		
G9174	Other speech language pathology functional limitation, current status, at therapy episode outset and at reporting intervals	Speech lang current status
G9175	Other speech language pathology functional limitation, projected goal status, at therapy episode outset, at reporting intervals, and at discharge or to end reporting	Speech lang goal status
G9176	Other speech language pathology functional limitation, discharge status, at discharge from therapy or to end reporting	Speech lang D/C status

F. Severity/Complexity Modifiers

For each nonpayable functional G-code, one of the modifiers listed below must be used to report the severity/complexity for that functional limitation.

Modifier	Impairment Limitation Restriction
• CH	• 0 percent impaired, limited or restricted
• CI	• At least 1 percent but less than 20 percent impaired, limited or restricted
• CJ	• At least 20 percent but less than 40 percent impaired, limited or restricted
• CK	• At least 40 percent but less than 60 percent impaired, limited or restricted
• CL	• At least 60 percent but less than 80 percent impaired, limited or restricted
• CM	• At least 80 percent but less than 100 percent impaired, limited or restricted
• CN	• 100 percent impaired, limited or restricted

The severity modifiers reflect the beneficiary's percentage of functional impairment as determined by the clinician furnishing the therapy services.

G. Required Reporting of Functional G-codes and Severity Modifiers

The functional G-codes and severity modifiers listed above are used in the required reporting on therapy claims at certain specified points during therapy episodes of care. Claims containing these functional G-codes must also contain another billable and separately payable (non-bundled) service. Only one functional limitation shall be reported at a given time for each related therapy plan of care (POC).

Functional reporting using the G-codes and corresponding severity modifiers is required reporting on specified therapy claims. Specifically, they are required on claims:

- At the outset of a therapy episode of care (i.e., on the claim for the date of service (DOS) of the initial therapy service);
- At least once every 10 treatment days, which corresponds with the progress reporting period;
- When an evaluative procedure, including a re-evaluative one, (HCPCS/CPT codes 92506, 92597, 92607, 92608, 92610, 92611, 92612, 92614, 92616, 96105, 96125, 97001, 97002, 97003, 97004) is furnished and billed;
- At the time of discharge from the therapy episode of care – (i.e., on the date services related to the discharge [progress] report are furnished); and
- At the time reporting of a particular functional limitation is ended in cases where the need for further therapy is necessary.
- At the time reporting is begun for a new or different functional limitation within the same episode of care (i.e., after the reporting of the prior functional limitation is ended)

Functional reporting is required on claims throughout the entire episode of care. When the beneficiary has reached his or her goal or progress has been maximized on the initially selected functional limitation, but the need for treatment continues, reporting is required for a second functional limitation using another set of G-codes. In these situations two or more functional limitations will be reported for a beneficiary during the therapy episode of care. Thus, reporting on more than one functional limitation may be required for some beneficiaries but not simultaneously.

When the beneficiary stops coming to therapy prior to discharge, the clinician should report the functional information on the last claim. If the clinician is unaware that the beneficiary is not returning for therapy until after the last claim is submitted, the clinician cannot report the discharge status.

When functional reporting is required on a claim for therapy services, two G-codes will generally be required.

Two exceptions exist:

1. Therapy services under more than one therapy POC. Claims may contain more than two nonpayable functional G-codes when in cases where a beneficiary receives therapy services under multiple POCs (PT, OT, and/or SLP) from the same therapy provider.
2. One-Time Therapy Visit. When a beneficiary is seen and future therapy services are either not medically indicated or are going to be furnished by another provider, the clinician reports on the claim for the DOS of the visit, all three G-codes in the appropriate code set (current status, goal status and discharge status), along with corresponding severity modifiers.

Each reported functional G-code must also contain the following line of service information:

- Functional severity modifier

- Therapy modifier indicating the related discipline/POC -- GP, GO or GN -- for PT, OT, and SLP services, respectively
- Date of the related therapy service
- Nominal charge, e.g., a penny, for institutional claims submitted to the FIs and A/MACs. For professional claims, a zero charge is acceptable for the service line. If provider billing software requires an amount for professional claims, a nominal charge, e.g., a penny, may be included. Note: The KX modifier is not required on the claim line for nonpayable G-codes, but would be required with the procedure code for medically necessary therapy services furnished once the beneficiary's annual cap has been reached.

The following example demonstrates how the G-codes and modifiers are used. In this example, the clinician determines that the beneficiary's mobility restriction is the most clinically relevant functional limitation and selects the Mobility G-code set (G8978 – G8980) to represent the beneficiary's functional limitation. The clinician also determines the severity/complexity of the beneficiary's functional limitation and selects the appropriate modifier. In this example, the clinician determines that the beneficiary has a 75 percent mobility restriction for which the CL modifier is applicable. The clinician expects that at the end of therapy the beneficiaries will have only a 15 percent mobility restriction for which the CI modifier is applicable. When the beneficiary attains the mobility goal, therapy continues to be medically necessary to address a functional limitation for which there is no categorical G-code. The clinician reports this using (G8990 – G8992).

At the outset of therapy. On the DOS for which the initial evaluative procedure is furnished or the initial treatment day of a therapy POC, the claim for the service will also include two G-codes as shown below.

- G8978-CL to report the functional limitation (Mobility with current mobility limitation of "at least 60 percent but less than 80 percent impaired, limited or restricted")
- G8979-CI to report the projected goal for a mobility restriction of "at least 1 percent but less than 20 percent impaired, limited or restricted."

At the end of each progress reporting period. On the claim for the DOS when the services related to the progress report (which must be done at least once each 10 treatment days) are furnished, the clinician will report the same two G-codes but the modifier for the current status may be different.

- G8978 with the appropriate modifier are reported to show the beneficiary's current status as of this DOS. So if the beneficiary has made no progress, this claim will include G8978-CL. If the beneficiary made progress and now has a mobility restriction of 65 percent CL would still be the appropriate modifier for 65 percent, and G8978-CL would be reported in this case. If the beneficiary now has a mobility restriction of 45 percent, G8978-CK would be reported.
- G8979-CI would be reported to show the projected goal. This severity modifier would not change unless the clinician adjusts the beneficiary's goal. This step is repeated as necessary and clinically appropriate, adjusting the current status modifier used as the beneficiary progresses through therapy.

At the time the beneficiary is discharged from the therapy episode. The final claim for therapy episode will include two G-codes.

- G8979-CI would be reported to show the projected goal. G8980-CI would be reported if the beneficiary attained the 15 percent mobility goal. Alternatively, if the beneficiary's mobility restriction only reached 25 percent; G8980-CJ would be reported.

To end reporting of one functional limitation. As noted above, functional reporting is required to continue throughout the entire episode of care. Accordingly, when further therapy is medically necessary after the beneficiary attains the goal for the first reported functional limitation, the clinician would end reporting of the first functional limitation by using the same G-codes and modifiers that would be used at the time of discharge. Using the mobility example, to end reporting of the mobility functional limitation, G8979-CI and G8980-CI would be reported on the same DOS that coincides with end of that progress reporting period.

To begin reporting of a second functional limitation. At the time reporting is begun for a new and different functional limitation, within the same episode of care (i.e., after the reporting of the prior functional limitation is ended). Reporting on the second functional limitation, however, is not begun until the DOS of the next treatment day -- which is day one of the new progress reporting period. When the next functional limitation to be reported is NOT defined by one of the other three PT/OT categorical codes, the G-code set (G8990 - G8992) for the "other PT/OT primary" functional limitation is used, rather than the G-code set for the "other PT/OT subsequent" because it is the first reported "other PT/OT" functional limitation. This reporting begins on the DOS of the first treatment day following the mobility "discharge" reporting, which is counted as the initial service for the "other PT/OT primary" functional limitation and the first treatment day of the new progress reporting period. In this case, G8990 and G8991, along with the corresponding modifiers, are reported on the claim for therapy services.

The table below illustrates when reporting is required using this example and what G-codes would be used.

Example of Required Reporting

Key: Reporting Period (RP)	Begin RP #1 for Mobility at Episode Outset	End RP#1 for Mobility at Progress Report	Mobility RP #2 Begins Next Treatment Day	End RP #2 for Mobility at Progress Report	Mobility RP #3 Begins Next Treatment Day	D/C or End Reporting for Mobility	Begin RP #1 for Other PT/OT Primary
Mobility: Walking & Moving Around							
G8978 – Current Status	X	X		X			
G 8979 – Goal Status	X	X		X		X	
G8980 – Discharge Status						X	
Other PT/OT Primary							
G8990 – Current Status							X
G8991 – Goal Status							X
G8992 – Discharge Status							
No Functional Reporting Required			X		X		

H. Required Tracking and Documentation of Functional G-codes and Severity Modifiers

The clinician who furnishes the services must not only report the functional information on the therapy claim, but, he/she must track and document the G-codes and severity modifiers used for this reporting in the beneficiary's medical record of therapy services.

For details related to the documentation requirements, refer to Pub. 100-02, Medicare Benefit Policy Manual, chapter 15, section 220.3, subsection F - MCTRJCA-required Functional Reporting. For coverage rules related to MCTRJCA and therapy goals, refer to Pub. 100-02: a) for outpatient therapy services, see chapter 15, section 220.1.2 B and b) for instructions specific to PT, OT, and SLP services in the CORF, see chapter 12, section 10.

100-4, 5, 20

HCPCS Coding Requirement

A. Uniform Coding

Section 1834(k)(5) of the Act requires that all claims for outpatient rehabilitation therapy services and all comprehensive outpatient rehabilitation facility (CORF) services be reported using a uniform coding system. The current Healthcare Common Procedure Coding System/Current Procedural Terminology is used for the reporting of these services. The uniform coding requirement in the Act is specific to payment for all CORF services and outpatient rehabilitation therapy services - including physical therapy, occupational therapy, and speech-language pathology - that is provided and billed to Medicare contractors. The Medicare physician fee schedule (MPFS) is used to make payment for these therapy services at the nonfacility rate.

Effective for claims submitted on or after April 1, 1998, providers that had not previously reported HCPCS/CPT for outpatient rehabilitation and CORF services began using HCPCS to report these services. This requirement does not apply to outpatient rehabilitation services provided by:

- Critical access hospitals, which are paid on a cost basis, not MPFS;
- RHCs, and FQHCs for which therapy is included in the all-inclusive rate; or
- Providers that do not furnish therapy services.

The following "providers of services" must bill the FI for outpatient rehabilitation services using HCPCS codes:

- Hospitals (to outpatients and inpatients who are not in a covered Part A1 stay);
- Skilled nursing facilities (SNFs) (to residents not in a covered Part A1 stay and to nonresidents who receive outpatient rehabilitation services from the SNF);
- Home health agencies (HHAs) (to individuals who are not homebound or otherwise are not receiving services under a home health plan of care2 (POC) (See 60.4.1, Definition of Homebound Patient Under the Medicare Home Health (HH) Benefit.);
- Comprehensive outpatient rehabilitation facilities (CORFs); and
- Providers of outpatient physical therapy and speech-language pathology services (OPTs), also known as rehabilitation agencies (previously termed outpatient physical therapy facilities in this instruction).

Note 1. The requirements for hospitals and SNFs apply to inpatient Part B and outpatient services only. Inpatient Part A services are bundled into the respective prospective payment system payment; no separate payment is made.

Note 2. For HHAs, HCPCS/CPT coding for outpatient rehabilitation services is required only when the HHA provides such service to individuals that are not homebound and, therefore, not under a home health plan of care.

The following practitioners must bill the carriers for outpatient rehabilitation therapy services using HCPCS/CPT codes:

- Physical therapists in private practice (PTPPs),
- Occupational therapists in private practice (OTPPs),
- Speech-language pathologists in private practice (SLPPs),
- Physicians, including MDs, DOs, podiatrists and optometrists, and
- Certain nonphysician practitioners (NPPs), acting within their State scope of practice, e.g., nurse practitioners and clinical nurse specialists.

Providers billing to intermediaries shall report:

- The date the therapy plan of care was either established or last reviewed (see Sec.220.1.3B) in Occurrence Code 17, 29, or 30.
- The first day of treatment in Occurrence Code 35, 44, or 45.

B. Applicable Outpatient Rehabilitation HCPCS Codes

The CMS identifies the codes listed at: http://www.cms.hhs.gov/TherapyServices/05_Annual_Therapy_Update.asp#TopOfPage as therapy services, regardless of the presence of a financial limitation. Therapy services include only physical therapy, occupational therapy and speech-language pathology services. Therapist means only a physical therapist, occupational therapist or speech-language pathologist. Therapy modifiers are GP for physical therapy, GO for occupational therapy, and GN for speech-language pathology.

When in effect, any financial limitation will also apply to services represented unless otherwise noted on the therapy page on the CMS Web site.

C. Additional HCPCS Codes

Some HCPCS/CPT codes that are not on the list of therapy services should not be billed with a modifier. For example, outpatient non-rehabilitation HCPCS codes G0237, G0238, and G0239 should be billed without therapy modifiers. These HCPCS codes describe services for the improvement of respiratory function and may represent either "incident to" services or respiratory therapy services that may be appropriately billed in the CORF setting. When the services described by these G-codes are provided by physical therapists (PTs) or occupational therapists (OTs) treating respiratory conditions, they are considered therapy services and must meet the other conditions for physical and occupational therapy. The PT or OT would use the appropriate HCPCS/CPT code(s) in the 97000–97799 series and the corresponding therapy modifier, GP or GO, must be used.

Another example of codes that are not on the list of therapy services and should not be billed with a therapy modifier includes the following HCPCS codes: 95860, 95861, 95863, 95864, 95867, 95869, 95870, 95900, 95903, 95904, and 95934. These services represent diagnostic services – not therapy services; they must be appropriately billed and shall not include therapy modifiers.

Other codes not on the therapy code list, and not paid under another fee schedule, are appropriately billed with therapy modifiers when the services are furnished by therapists or provided under a therapy plan of care and where the services are covered and appropriately delivered (e.g., the therapist is qualified to provide the service). One example of non-listed codes where a therapy modifier is indicated regards the provision of services described in the CPT code series, 29000 through 29590, for the application of casts and strapping. Some of these codes previously appeared on the therapy code list, but were deleted because we determined that they represented services that are most often performed outside a therapy plan of care. However, when these services are provided by therapists or as an integral part of a therapy plan of care, the CPT code must be accompanied with the appropriate therapy modifier.

NOTE: The above lists of HCPCS/CPT codes are intended to facilitate the contractor's ability to pay claims under the MPFS. It is not intended to be an exhaustive list of covered services, imply applicability to provider settings, and does not assure coverage of these services.

100-4, 5, 20.2

Reporting of Service Units With HCPCS

A. General

Effective with claims submitted on or after April 1, 1998, providers billing on Form CMS-1450 were required to report the number of units for outpatient rehabilitation services based on the procedure or service, e.g., based on the HCPCS code reported instead of the revenue code. This was already in effect for billing on the Form CMS-1500, and CORFs were required to report their full range of CORF services on the Form CMS-1450. These unit-reporting requirements continue with the standards required for electronically submitting health care claims under the Health Insurance Portability and Accountability Act of 1996 (HIPAA) - the currently adopted version of the ASC X12 837 transaction standards and implementation guides. The Administrative Simplification Compliance Act mandates that claims be sent to Medicare electronically unless certain exceptions are met.

B. Timed and Untimed Codes

When reporting service units for HCPCS codes where the procedure is not defined by a specific timeframe ("untimed" HCPCS), the provider enters "1" in the field labeled units. For untimed codes, units are reported based on the number of times the procedure is performed, as described in the HCPCS code definition (often once per day).

EXAMPLE: A beneficiary received a speech-language pathology evaluation represented by HCPCS "untimed" code 92521. Regardless of the number of minutes spent providing this service only one unit of service is appropriately billed on the same day.

Several CPT codes used for therapy modalities, procedures, and tests and measurements specify that the direct (one on one) time spent in patient contact is 15 minutes. Providers report procedure codes for services delivered on any single calendar day using CPT codes and the appropriate number of 15 minute units of service.

EXAMPLE: A beneficiary received occupational therapy (HCPCS "timed" code 97530 which is defined in 15 minute units) for a total of 60 minutes. The provider would then report revenue code 043X and 4 units.

C. Counting Minutes for Timed Codes in 15 Minute Units

When only one service is provided in a day, providers should not bill for services performed for less than 8 minutes. For any single timed CPT code in the same day measured in 15 minute units, providers bill a single 15-minute unit for treatment greater than or equal to 8 minutes through and including 22 minutes. If the duration of a single modality or procedure in a day is greater than or equal to 23 minutes through and including 37 minutes, then 2 units should be billed. Time intervals for 1 through 8 units are as follows:

Units	Number of Minutes
1 unit:	≥ 8 minutes through 22 minutes
2 units:	≥ 23 minutes through 37 minutes
3 units:	≥ 38 minutes through 52 minutes
4 units:	≥ 53 minutes through 67 minutes
5 units:	≥ 68 minutes through 82 minutes
6 units:	≥ 83 minutes through 97 minutes
7 units:	≥ 98 minutes through 112 minutes
8 units:	≥ 113 minutes through 127 minutes

The pattern remains the same for treatment times in excess of 2 hours.

If a service represented by a 15 minute timed code is performed in a single day for at least 15 minutes, that service shall be billed for at least one unit. If the service is performed for at least 30 minutes, that service shall be billed for at least two units, etc. It is not appropriate to count all minutes of treatment in a day toward the units for one code if other services were performed for more than 15 minutes. See examples 2 and 3 below.

When more than one service represented by 15 minute timed codes is performed in a single day, the total number of minutes of service (as noted on the chart above) determines the number of timed units billed. See example 1 below.

If any 15 minute timed service that is performed for 7 minutes or less than 7 minutes on the same day as another 15 minute timed service that was also performed for 7 minutes or less and the total time of the two is 8 minutes or greater than 8 minutes, then bill one unit for the service performed for the most minutes. This is correct because the total time is greater than the minimum time for one unit. The same logic is applied when three or more different services are provided for 7 minutes or less than 7 minutes. See example 5 below.

The expectation (based on the work values for these codes) is that a provider's direct patient contact time for each unit will average 15 minutes in length. If a provider has a consistent practice of billing less than 15 minutes for a unit, these situations should be highlighted for review.

If more than one 15 minute timed CPT code is billed during a single calendar day, then the total number of timed units that can be billed is constrained by the total treatment minutes for that day. See all examples below.

Pub. 100-02, Medicare Benefit Policy Manual, Chapter 15, Section 220.3B, Documentation Requirements for Therapy Services, indicates that the amount of time for each specific intervention/modality provided to the patient is not required to be documented in the Treatment Note. However, the total number of timed minutes must be documented. These examples indicate how to count the appropriate number of units for the total therapy minutes provided.

Example 1 –

24 minutes of neuromuscular reeducation, code 97112,

23 minutes of therapeutic exercise, code 97110,

Total timed code treatment time was 47 minutes.

See the chart above. The 47 minutes falls within the range for 3 units = 38 to 52 minutes.

Appropriate billing for 47 minutes is only 3 timed units. Each of the codes is performed for more than 15 minutes, so each shall be billed for at least 1 unit. The correct coding is 2 units of code 97112 and one unit of code 97110, assigning more timed units to the service that took the most time.

Example 2 –

20 minutes of neuromuscular reeducation (97112)

20 minutes therapeutic exercise (97110),

40 Total timed code minutes.

Appropriate billing for 40 minutes is 3 units. Each service was done at least 15 minutes and should be billed for at least one unit, but the total allows 3 units. Since the time for each service is the same, choose either code for 2 units and bill the other for 1 unit. Do not bill 3 units for either one of the codes.

Example 3 –

33 minutes of therapeutic exercise (97110),

7 minutes of manual therapy (97140),

40 Total timed minutes

Appropriate billing for 40 minutes is for 3 units. Bill 2 units of 97110 and 1 unit of 97140. Count the first 30 minutes of 97110 as two full units. Compare the remaining time for 97110 (33-30 = 3 minutes) to the time spent on 97140 (7 minutes) and bill the larger, which is 97140.

Example 4 –

18 minutes of therapeutic exercise (97110),

13 minutes of manual therapy (97140),

10 minutes of gait training (97116),

8 minutes of ultrasound (97035),

49 Total timed minutes

Appropriate billing is for 3 units. Bill the procedures you spent the most time providing. Bill 1 unit each of 97110, 97116, and 97140. You are unable to bill for the ultrasound because the total time of timed units that can be billed is constrained by the total timed code treatment minutes (i.e., you may not bill 4 units for less than 53 minutes regardless of how many services were performed). You would still document the ultrasound in the treatment notes.

Example 5 –

7 minutes of neuromuscular reeducation (97112)

7 minutes therapeutic exercise (97110)

7 minutes manual therapy (97140)

21 Total timed minutes

Appropriate billing is for one unit. The qualified professional (See definition in Pub. 100-02, chapter 15, section 220) shall select one appropriate CPT code (97112, 97110, 97140) to bill since each unit was performed for the same amount of time and only one unit is allowed.

NOTE: The above schedule of times is intended to provide assistance in rounding time into 15-minute increments. It does not imply that any minute until the eighth should be excluded from the total count. The total minutes of active treatment counted for all 15 minute timed codes includes all direct treatment time for the timed codes. Total treatment minutes-- including minutes spent providing services represented by untimed codes-- are also documented. For documentation in the medical record of the services provided see Pub. 100-02, chapter 15, section 220.3.

D. Specific Limits for HCPCS

The Deficit Reduction Act of 2005, section 5107 requires the implementation of clinically appropriate code edits to eliminate improper payments for outpatient therapy services. The following codes may be billed, when covered, only at or below the number of units indicated on the chart per treatment day. When higher amounts of units are billed than those indicated in the table below, the units on the claim line that exceed the limit shall be denied as medically unnecessary (according to 1862(a)(1)(A)). Denied claims may be appealed and an ABN is appropriate to notify the beneficiary of liability.

This chart does not include all of the codes identified as therapy codes; refer to section 20 of this chapter for further detail on these and other therapy codes. For example, therapy codes called "always therapy" must always be accompanied by therapy modifiers identifying the type of therapy plan of care under which the service is provided.

Use the chart in the following manner:

The codes that are allowed one unit for "Allowed Units" in the chart below may be billed no more than once per provider, per discipline, per date of service, per patient.

The codes allowed 0 units in the column for "Allowed Units", may not be billed under a plan of care indicated by the discipline in that column. Some codes may be billed by one discipline (e.g., PT) and not by others (e.g., OT or SLP).

When physicians/NPPs bill always therapy codes they must follow the policies of the type of therapy they are providing e.g., utilize a plan of care, bill with the appropriate therapy modifier (GP, GO, GN), bill the allowed units on the chart below for PT, OT or SLP depending on the plan. A physician/NPP shall not bill an "always therapy" code unless the service is provided under a therapy plan of care. Therefore, NA stands for "Not Applicable" in the chart below.

When a "sometimes therapy" code is billed by a physician/NPP, but as a medical service, and not under a therapy plan of care, the therapy modifier shall not be used, but the number of units billed must not exceed the number of units indicated in the chart below per patient, per provider/supplier, per day.

HCPCS	Code Description	Timed or Untimed	PT Allowed units	OT Allowed units	SLP Allowed units	Physician/NPP NOT under Therapy POC
92521	Evaluation of speech fluency	Untimed	0	0	1	NA
92522	Evaluation of speech sound production	Untimed	0	0	1	NA
92523	Evaluation of language comprehension and expression	Untimed	0	0	1	NA
92524	Behavioral and qualitative analysis of voice and resonance	Untimed	0	0	1	NA
92597	Oral speech device	Untimed	0	1	1	NA
92607	Ex for speech device rx, 1 hr	Timed	0	1	1	NA
92611	Motion fluroscopy/swallow	Untimed	0	1	1	1
92612	Endoscope swallow test (fees)	Untimed	0	1	1	1
92614	Laryngoscopic sensory test	Untimed	0	1	1	1
92616	Fees w/laryngeal sense test	Untimed	0	1	1	1
95833	Limb muscle testing, manual	Untimed	1	1	0	1
95834	Limb muscle testing, manual	Untimed	1	1	0	1
96110	Developmental test, lim	Untimed	1	1	1	1
96111	Developmental test, extend	Untimed	1	1	1	1
97001	PT evaluation	Untimed	1	0	0	NA
97002	PT re-evaluation	Untimed	1	0	0	NA
97003	OT evaluation	Untimed	0	1	0	NA
9704	OT re-evaluation	Untimed	0	1	0	NA

100-4, 5, 20.4

Coding Guidance for Certain CPT Codes - All Claims

The following provides guidance about the use of codes 96105, 97026, 97150, 97545, 97546, and G0128.

CPT Codes 96105, 97545, and 97546.

Providers report code 96105, assessment of aphasia with interpretation and report in 1-hour units. This code represents formal evaluation of aphasia with an instrument such as the Boston Diagnostic Aphasia Examination. If this formal assessment is performed during treatment, it is typically performed only once during treatment and its medical necessity should be documented. If the test is repeated during treatment, the medical necessity of the repeat administration of the test must also be documented. It is common practice for regular assessment of a patient's progress in therapy to be documented in the chart, and this may be done using test items taken from the formal examinations. This is considered to be part of the treatment and should not be billed as 96105 unless a full, formal assessment is completed.

Other timed physical medicine codes are 97545 and 97546. The interval for code 97545 is 2 hours and for code 97546, 1 hour. These are specialized codes to be used in the context of rehabilitating a worker to return to a job. The expectation is that the entire time period specified in the codes 97545 or 97546 would be the treatment period, since a shorter period of treatment could be coded with another code such as codes 97110, 97112, or 97537. (Codes 97545 and 97546 were developed for reporting services to persons in the worker's compensation program, thus we do not expect to see them reported for Medicare patients except under very unusual circumstances. Further, we would not expect to see code 97546 without also seeing code 97545 on the same claim. Code 97546, when used, is used in conjunction with 97545.)

- CPT Code 97026

Effective for services performed on or after October 24, 2006, the Centers for Medicare & Medicaid Services announce a NCD stating the use of infrared and/or near-infrared light and/or heat, including monochromatic infrared energy (MIRE), is non-covered for the treatment, including symptoms such as pain arising from these conditions, of diabetic and/or non-diabetic peripheral sensory neuropathy, wounds and/or ulcers of the skin and/or subcutaneous tissues in Medicare beneficiaries. Further coverage guidelines can be found in the National Coverage Determination Manual (Publication 100-03), section 270.6.

Contractors shall deny claims with CPT 97026 (infrared therapy incident to or as a PT/OT benefit) and HCPCS E0221 or A4639, if the claim contains any of the following ICD-9 codes: 250.60-250.63 354.4, 354.5, 354.9 355.1-355.4 355.6-355.9 356.0, 356.2-356.4, 356.8-356.9 357.0-357.7 674.10, 674.12, 674.14, 674.20, 674.22, 674.24 707.00-707.07, 707.09-707.15, 707.19 870.0-879.9 880.00-887.7 890.0-897.7 998.31-998.32

Contractors can use the following messages when denying the service:

- Medicare Summary Notice # 21.11 "This service was not covered by Medicare at the time you received it."
- Reason Claim Adjustment Code #50 "These are noncovered services because this is not deemed a medical necessity by the payer."

Advanced Beneficiary Notice (ABN):

Physicians, physical therapists, occupational therapists, outpatient rehabilitation facilities (ORFs), comprehensive outpatient rehabilitation facilities (CORFs), home health agencies (HHA), and hospital outpatient departments are liable if the service is performed, unless the beneficiary signs an ABN.

Similarly, DME suppliers and HHA are liable for the devices when they are supplied, unless the beneficiary signs an ABN.

100-4, 5, 100.10

Group Therapy Services (Code 97150)

Policies for group therapy services for CORF are the same as group therapy services for other Part B outpatient services. See Pub 100-02, chapter 15, section 230.

100-4, 8, 50.3

Required Information for In-Facility Claims Paid Under the Composite Rate and the ESRD PPS

The electronic form required for billing ESRD claims is the ANSI X12N 837 Institutional claim transaction. Since the data structure of the 837 transaction is difficult to express in narrative form and to provide assistance to small providers excepted from the electronic claim requirement, the instructions below are given relative to the UB-04 (Form CMS-1450) hardcopy form. A table to crosswalk UB-04 form locators to the 837 transaction is found in Chapter 25, §100.

Type of Bill

Acceptable codes for Medicare are:

721 - Admit Through Discharge Claim - This code is used for a bill encompassing an entire course of outpatient treatment for which the provider expects payment from the payer.

722 - Interim - First Claim - This code is used for the first of an expected series of payment bills for the same course of treatment.

723 - Interim - Continuing Claim - This code is used when a payment bill for the same course of treatment is submitted and further bills are expected to be submitted later.

724 - Interim - Last Claim - This code is used for a payment bill which is the last of a series for this course of treatment. The "Through" date of this bill (FL 6) is the discharge date for this course of treatment.

727 - Replacement of Prior Claim - This code is used when the provider wants to correct (other than late charges) a previously submitted bill. The previously submitted bill needs to be resubmitted in its entirety, changing only the items that need correction. This is the code used for the corrected or "new" bill.

728 - Void/Cancel of a Prior Claim - This code indicates this bill is a cancel-only adjustment of an incorrect bill previously submitted. Cancel-only adjustments should be used only in cases of incorrect provider identification numbers, incorrect HICNs, duplicate payments and some OIG recoveries. For incorrect provider numbers or HICNs, a corrected bill is also submitted using a code 721.

Statement Covers Period (From-Through) - Hospital-based and independent renal dialysis facilities:

The beginning and ending service dates of the period included on this bill. Note: ESRD services are subject to the monthly billing requirements for repetitive services.

Condition Codes

Hospital-based and independent renal facilities complete these items. Note that one of the codes 71-76 is applicable for every bill. Special Program Indicator codes A0-A9 are not required.

Condition Code Structure (only codes affecting Medicare payment/processing are shown).

02 - Condition is Employment Related - Providers enter this code if the patient alleges that the medical condition causing this episode of care is due to environment/events resulting from employment.

04 - **Information Only Bill**- Providers enter this code to indicate the patient is a member of a Medicare Advantage plan.

59 - Non-Primary ESRD Facility – Providers enter this code to indicate that ESRD beneficiary received non-scheduled or emergency dialysis services at a facility other than his/her primary ESRD dialysis facility.

71 - Full Care in Unit - Providers enter this code to indicate the billing is for a patient who received staff-assisted dialysis services in a hospital or renal dialysis facility.

72 - Self-Care in Unit - Providers enter this code to indicate the billing is for a patient who managed his own dialysis in a hospital or renal dialysis facility.

73 - Self-Care in Training - Providers enter this code to indicate the billing is for special dialysis services where a patient and his/her helper (if necessary) were learning to perform dialysis.

76 - Back-up In-facility Dialysis - Providers enter this code to indicate the billing is for a home dialysis patient who received back-up dialysis in a facility.

H3 - Reoccurrence of GI Bleed comorbid category

H4 - Reoccurrence of Pneumonia comorbid category

H5 - Reoccurrence of Pericarditis comorbid Category

Occurrence Codes and Dates

Codes(s) and associated date(s) defining specific events(s) relating to this billing period are shown. Event codes are two alpha-numeric digits, and dates are shown as six numeric digits (MM-DD-YY). When occurrence codes 01-04 and 24 are entered, make sure the entry includes the appropriate value code, if there is another payer involved.

Occurrence and occurrence span codes are mutually exclusive. Occurrence codes have values from 01 through 69 and A0 through L9. Occurrence span codes have values from 70 through 99 and M0 through Z9.

24 - Date Insurance Denied - Code indicates the date of receipt of a denial of coverage by a higher priority payer.

33 - First Day of Medicare Coordination Period for ESRD Beneficiaries Covered by an EGHP - Code indicates the first day of the Medicare coordination period during which Medicare benefits are payable under an EGHP. This is required only for ESRD beneficiaries.

51 - Date of last Kt/V reading. For in-center hemodialysis patients, this is the date of the last reading taken during the billing period. For peritoneal dialysis patients and home hemodialysis patients, this date may be before the current billing period but should be within 4 months of the claim date of service.

Occurrence Span Code and Dates

Code(s) and associated beginning and ending dates(s) defining a specific event relating to this billing period are shown. Event codes are two alpha-numeric digits and dates are shown numerically as MM-DD-YY.

74 - Noncovered Level of Care - This code is used for repetitive Part B services to show a period of inpatient hospital care or of outpatient surgery during the billing period. Use of this code will not be necessary for ESRD claims with dates of service on or after April 1, 2007 due to the requirement of ESRD line item billing.

Document Control Number (DCN)

Required for all provider types on adjustment requests. (Bill Type/FL=XX7). All providers requesting an adjustment to a previous processed claim insert the DCN of the claims to be adjusted.

Value Codes and Amounts

Code(s) and related dollar amount(s) identify monetary data that are necessary for the processing of this claim. The codes are two alphanumeric digits and each value allows up to nine numeric digits (0000000.00). Negative amounts are not allowed. Whole numbers or non-dollar amounts are right justified to the left of the dollars and cents delimiter. Some values are reported as cents, so refer to specific codes for instructions. If more than one value code is shown for a billing period, show the codes in ascending alphanumeric sequence.

Value Code Structure (Only codes used to bill Medicare are shown.):

06 - Medicare Blood Deductible - Code indicates the amount the patient paid for un-replaced deductible blood.

13 - ESRD Beneficiary in the 30- Month Coordination Period With an EGHP - Code indicates that the amount shown is that portion of a higher priority EGHP payment on behalf of an ESRD beneficiary that applies to covered Medicare charges on this bill. If the provider enters six zeros (0000.00) in the amount field, it is claiming a conditional payment because the EGHP has denied coverage or there has been a substantial delay in its payment. Where the provider received no payment or a reduced payment because of failure to file a proper claim, this is the amount that would have been payable had it filed a proper claim.

17 - Not submitted by the provider. The Medicare shared system will display this payer only code on the claim when an outlier payment is being made. The value is the total claim outlier payment.

19 - Not submitted by the provider. The Medicare shared system will display this payer only code on the claim for low volume providers to identify the amount of the low volume adjustment being included in the provider's reimbursement.

37 - Pints of Blood Furnished - Code indicates the total number of pints of blood or units of packed red cells furnished, whether or not replaced. Blood is reported only in terms of complete pints rounded upwards, e.g., 1 1/4 pints is shown as 2 pints. This entry serves a basis for counting pints towards the blood deductible. Hospital-based and independent renal facilities must complete this item.

38 - Blood Deductible Pints - Code indicates the number of un-replaced deductible pints of blood supplied. If all deductible pints furnished have been replaced, no entry is made. Hospital-based and independent renal facilities must complete this item.

39 - Pints of Blood Replaced - Code indicates the total number of pints of blood donated on the patient's behalf. Where one pint is donated, one pint is replaced. If arrangements have been made for replacement, pints are shown as replaced. Where the provider charges only for the blood processing and administration, i.e., it does not charge a "replacement deposit fee" for un-replaced pints, the blood is considered replaced for purposes of this item. In such cases, all blood charges are shown under the 039x revenue code series, Blood Administration. Hospital-based and independent renal facilities must complete this item.

44 - Amount Provider Agreed To Accept From Primary Payer When This Amount is Less Than Charges But Higher than Payment Received - Code indicates the amount shown is the amount the provider was obligated or required to accept from a primary

payer as payment in full when that amount is less than the charges but higher than amount actually received. A Medicare secondary payment is due.

47 - Any Liability Insurance - Code indicates amount shown is that portion from a higher priority liability insurance made on behalf of a Medicare beneficiary that the provider is applying to Medicare covered services on this bill. If six zeros (0000.00) are entered in the amount field, the provider is claiming conditional payment because there has been substantial delay in the other payer's payment.

48 - Hemoglobin Reading - Code indicates the most recent hemoglobin reading taken before the start of this billing period. This is usually reported in three positions with a decimal. Use the right of the delimiter for the third digit. The blood sample for the hemoglobin reading must be obtained before the dialysis treatment.

49 - Hematocrit Reading - Code indicates the most recent hematocrit reading taken before the start of this billing period. This is usually reported in two positions (a percentage) to the left of the dollar/cents delimiter. If the reading is provided with a decimal, use the position to the right of the delimiter for the third digit. The blood sample for the hemoglobin reading must be obtained before the dialysis treatment.

67 - Peritoneal Dialysis - The number of hours of peritoneal dialysis provided during the billing period. Count only the hours spent in the home. Exclude travel time. Report amount in whole units right-justified to the left of the dollar/cents delimiter. (Round to the nearest whole hour.)

Reporting value code 67 will not be required for claims with dates of service on or after April 1, 2007.

68 - Erythropoietin Units - Code indicates the number of units of administered EPO relating to the billing period and reported in whole units to the left of the dollar/cents delimiter. NOTE: The total amount of EPO injected during the billing period is reported. If there were 12 doses injected, the sum of the units administered for the 12 doses is reported as the value to the left of the dollar/cents delimiter.

Medicare no longer requires value code 68 for claims with dates of service on or after January 1, 2008.

71 - Funding of ESRD Networks - Code indicates the amount of Medicare payment reduction to help fund the ESRD networks. This amount is calculated by the FI and forwarded to CWF. (See §120 for discussion of ESRD networks).

79 - Not submitted by the provider. The Medicare shared system will display this payer only code on the claim. The value represents the dollar amount for Medicare allowed payments applicable for the calculation in determining an outlier payment.

A8 - Weight of Patient – Code indicates the weight of the patient in kilograms. The weight of the patient should be measured after the last dialysis session of the month.

A9 - Height of Patient – Code indicates the height of the patient in centimeters. The height of the patient should be measured during the last dialysis session of the month. This height is as the patient presents.

D5 - Result of last Kt/V reading. For in-center hemodialysis patients this is the last reading taken during the billing period. For peritoneal dialysis patients and home hemodialysis this may be before the current billing period but should be within 4 months of the claim date of service.

Revenue Codes

The revenue code for the appropriate treatment modality under the composite rate is billed (e.g., 0821 for hemodialysis). Services included in the composite rate and related charges must not be shown on the bill separately. Hospitals must maintain a log of these charges in their records for cost apportionment purposes.

Services which are provided but which are not included in the composite rate may be billed as described in sections that address those specific services.

082X - Hemodialysis - Outpatient or Home Dialysis - A waste removal process performed in an outpatient or home setting, necessary when the body's own kidneys have failed. Waste is removed directly from the blood. Detailed revenue coding is required. Therefore, services may not be summed at the zero level.

0 - General Classification	HEMO/OP OR HOME
1 - Hemodialysis/Composite or other rate	HEMO/COMPOSITE
2 - Home Supplies	HEMO/HOME/SUPPL
3 - Home Equipment	HEMO/HOME/EQUIP
4 - Maintenance 100%	HEMO/HOME/100%
5 - Support Services	HEMO/HOME/SUPSERV
9 - Other Hemodialysis Outpatient	HEMO/HOME/OTHER

083X - Peritoneal Dialysis - Outpatient or Home - A waste removal process performed in an outpatient or home setting, necessary when the body's own kidneys have failed. Waste is removed indirectly by instilling a special solution into the abdomen using the peritoneal membrane as a filter.

0 - General Classification	PERITONEAL/OP OR HOME
1 - Peritoneal/Composite or other rate	PERTNL/COMPOSITE
2 - Home Supplies	PERTNL/HOME/SUPPL
3 - Home Equipment	PERTNL/HOME/EQUIP
4 - Maintenance 100%	PERTNL/HOME/100%
5 - Support Services	PERTNL/HOME/SUPSERV
9 -Other Peritoneal Dialysis	PERTNL/HOME/OTHER

084X - Continuous Ambulatory Peritoneal Dialysis (CAPD) - Outpatient - A continuous dialysis process performed in an outpatient or home setting, which uses the patient's peritoneal membrane as a dialyzer.

0 - General Classification	CAPD/OP OR HOME
1 - CAPD/Composite or other rate	CAPD/COMPOSITE
2 - Home Supplies	CAPD/HOME/SUPPL
3 - Home Equipment	CAPD/HOME/EQUIP
4 - Maintenance 100%	CAPD/HOME/100%
5 - Support Services	CAPD/HOME/SUPSERV
9 -Other CAPD Dialysis	CAPD/HOME/OTHER

085X - Continuous Cycling Peritoneal Dialysis (CCPD) - Outpatient. - A continuous dialysis process performed in an outpatient or home setting, which uses the patient's peritoneal membrane as a dialyzer.

0 - General Classification	CCPD/OP OR HOME
1 - CCPD/Composite or other rate	CCPD/COMPOSITE
2 - Home Supplies	CCPD/HOME/SUPPL
3 - Home Equipment	CCPD/HOME/EQUIP
4 - Maintenance 100%	CCPD/HOME/100%
5 - Support Services	CCPD/HOME/SUPSERV
9 - Other CCPD Dialysis	CCPD/HOME/OTHER

088X - Miscellaneous Dialysis – Charges for Dialysis services not identified elsewhere.

0 - General Classification	DAILY/MISC
1 - Ultrafiltration	DAILY/ULTRAFILT
2 - Home dialysis aid visit	HOME DIALYSIS AID VISIT
9 - Other misc Dialysis	DAILY/MISC/OTHER

HCPCS/Rates

All hemodialysis claims must include HCPCS 90999 on the line reporting revenue code 082x.

Modifiers

Modifiers are required with ESRD Billing for reporting the adequacy of dialysis and the vascular access. For information on modifiers required for these quality measures see 50.9 of this chapter.

For information on reporting modifiers applicable to the Erythropoietin Stimulating Agents refer to section 60.4 of this chapter.

Route of administration modifiers required are JA, JB and JE.

For information on reporting the AY modifier for services not related to the treatment of ESRD, see sections 60.2.1.1 – Separately Billable ESRD Drugs and 60.1 - Lab Services.

Service Date

Report the line item date of service for each dialysis session and each separately payable item or service.

Service Units

Hospital-based and independent renal facilities must complete this item. The entries quantify services by revenue category, e.g., number of dialysis treatments. Units are defined as follows:

0634 - Erythropoietin (EPO) - Administrations, i.e., the number of times an injection of less than 10,000 units of EPO was administered. For claims with dates of service on or after January 1, 2008, facilities use the units field as a multiplier of the dosage description in the HCPCS to arrive at the dosage amount per administration.

0635 - Erythropoietin (EPO) - Administrations, i.e., the number of times an injection of 10,000 units or more of EPO was administered. For claims with dates of service on or after January 1, 2008, facilities use the units field as a multiplier of the dosage description in the HCPCS to arrive at the dosage amount per administration.

082X - (Hemodialysis) – Sessions

083X - (Peritoneal) – Sessions

084X - (CAPD) - Days covered by the bill

085X - (CCPD) - Days covered by the bill

Effective April 1, 2007, the implementation of ESRD line item billing requires that each dialysis session be billed on a separate line. As a result, claims with dates of service on or after April 1, 2007 should not report units greater than 1 for each dialysis revenue code line billed on the claim.

Total Charges

Hospital-based and independent renal facilities must complete this item. Hospital-based facilities must show their customary charges that correspond to the appropriate revenue code. They must not enter their composite or the EPO` rate as their charge. Independent facilities may enter their composite and/or EPO rates.

Neither revenue codes nor charges for services included in the composite rate may be billed separately (see §90.3 for a description). Hospitals must maintain a log of these charges in their records for cost apportionment purposes.

Services which are provided but which are not included in the composite rate may be billed as described in sections that address those specific services.

The last revenue code entered in as 000l represents the total of all charges billed.

Principal Diagnosis Code

Hospital-based and independent renal facilities must complete this item and it should include a diagnosis of end stage renal disease.

Other Diagnosis Code(s)

For claims with dates of service on or after January 1, 2011 renal dialysis facilities report the appropriate diagnosis code(s) for co-morbidity conditions eligible for an adjustment.

NOTE: Information regarding the form locator numbers that correspond to these data element names and a table to crosswalk UB-04 form locators to the 837 transaction is found in Chapter 25.

100-4, 8, 50.9

Coding for Adequacy of Dialysis, Vascular Access and Infection

A. Reporting the Urea Reduction Ratio(URR) for ESRD Hemodialysis Claims

All hemodialysis claims must indicate the most recent Urea Reduction Ratio (URR) for the dialysis patient. Code all claims using HCPCS code 90999 along with the appropriate G modifier listed in section B.

Claims for dialysis treatments must include the adequacy of hemodialysis data as measured by URR. Dialysis facilities must monitor the adequacy of dialysis treatments monthly for facility patients. Home hemodialysis and peritoneal dialysis patients may be monitored less frequently, but not less than quarterly. If a home hemodialysis patient is not monitored during a month, the last, most recent URR for the dialysis patient must be reported.

HCPCS code 90999 (unlisted dialysis procedure, inpatient or outpatient) must be reported in field location 44 for all bill types 72X. The appropriate G-modifier in field location 44 (HCPCS/RATES) is used, for patients that received seven or more dialysis treatments in a month. Continue to report revenue codes 0820, 0821, 0825, and 0829 in field location 43.

G1 - Most recent URR of less than 60%

G2 - Most recent URR of 60% to 64.9%

G3 - Most recent URR of 65% to 69.9%

G4 - Most recent URR of 70% to 74.9%

G5 - Most recent URR of 75% or greater

For patients that have received dialysis 6 days or less in a month, facilities use the following modifier:

G6 - ESRD patient for whom less than seven dialysis sessions have been provided in a month.

For services beginning January 1, 2003, and after, if the modifier is not present, FIs must return the claim to the provider for the appropriate modifier. Effective April, 2007 due to the requirement of line item billing, at least one revenue code line for hemodialysis on the claim must contain one of the URR modifiers shown above. The URR modifier is not required on every hemodialysis line on the claim.

The techniques to be used to draw the pre- and post-dialysis blood urea Nitrogen samples are listed in the National Kidney Foundation Dialysis Outcomes Quality Initiative Clinical Practice Guidelines for Hemodialysis Adequacy, Guideline 8, Acceptable Methods for BUN sampling, New York, National Kidney Foundation, 2000, pp.53-60.

B. Reporting the Vascular Access for ESRD Hemodialysis Claims

ESRD claims for hemodialysis with dates of service on or after July 1, 2010 must indicate the type of vascular access used for the delivery of the hemodialysis at the last hemodialysis session of the month. One of the following codes is required to be reported on the latest line item date of service billing for hemodialysis revenue code 0821. It may be reported on all revenue code 0821 lines at the discretion of the provider.

NOTE: Modifier V5 must be entered if a vascular catheter is present even if it is not being used for the delivery of the hemodialysis. In this instance 2 modifiers should be entered, V5 for the vascular catheter and either V6 or V7 for the access that is being used for the delivery of hemodialysis.

Modifier V5 - Any Vascular Catheter (alone or with any other vascular access),

Modifier V6 - Arteriovenous Graft (or other Vascular Access not including a vascular catheter in use with two needles)

Modifier V7 - Arteriovenous Fistula Only (in use with two needles)

C. Reporting the Kt/V for ALL ESRD Claims

All ESRD claims with dates of service on or after July 1, 2010 must indicate the applicable Kt/V reading for the dialysis patient. The reading result and the date of the reading must be reported on the claim using the following claim codes:

Value Code D5 – Result of last Kt/V reading. For in-center hemodialysis patients this is the last reading taken during the billing period. For peritoneal dialysis patients and home hemodialysis this may be before the current billing period but should be within 4 months of the claim date of service.

- **Hemodialysis:** For in-center and home-hemodialysis patients prescribed for three or fewer treatments per week, the last Kt/V obtained during the month must be reported. Facilities must report single pool Kt/V using the preferred National Quality Forum (NQF) endorsed methods for deriving the single pool Kt/V value: Daugirdas II or Urea Kinetic Modeling (UKM). The reported Kt/V should not include residual renal function.

A value of 8.88 shall be entered on the claim if the situation exists that a patient is prescribed and receiving greater than three hemodialysis treatments per week for a medically justified and documented clinical need. The 8.88 value is not to be used for patients who are receiving "extra" treatments for a temporary clinical need (e.g. fluid overload). A medical justification must be submitted for patients receiving greater than 13 treatments per month.

- **Peritoneal Dialysis:** When measured the delivered weekly total Kt/V (dialytic and residual) should be reported.

This code is effective and required on all ESRD claims with dates of service on or after July 1, 2010. In the event that no Kt/V reading was performed providers must report the D5 with a value of 9.99.

Occurrence Code 51 – Date of last Kt/V reading. For in-center hemodialysis patients, this is the date of the last reading taken during the billing period. For peritoneal dialysis patients and home hemodialysis patients, this date may be before the current billing period but should be within 4 months of the claim date of service. This code is effective for ESRD claims with dates of service on or after July 1, 2010. This code not required when reporting value code D5 with a value of 9.99 indicating no Kt/V reading is available for reporting or value 8.88 to indicate the patient is prescribed and receiving greater than 3 hemodialysis treatments per week for a medically justified and documented clinical need.

D. Reporting of Infection for ALL ESRD Claims

All ESRD claims with dates of service on or after July 1, 2010 must indicate on the claim if an infection was present at the time of treatment. Claims must report on each dialysis revenue code line one of the following codes:

Modifier V8: Dialysis access-related infection present (documented and treated) during the billing month. Reportable dialysis access-related infection is limited to peritonitis for peritoneal dialysis patients or bacteremia for hemodialysis patients. Facilities must report any peritonitis related to a peritoneal dialysis catheter, and any bacteremia related to hemodialysis access (including arteriovenous fistula, arteriovenous graft, or vascular catheter) if identified during the billing month. For individuals that receive different modalities of dialysis during the billing month and an infection is identified, the V8 code should only be indicated on the claim for the patient's primary dialysis modality at the time the infection was first suspected. Non-access related infections should not be coded as V8. If no dialysis-access related infection is present during the billing month by this definition, providers should instead report modifier V9.

Modifier V9: No dialysis-access related infection, as defined for modifier V8, present during the billing month. Dialysis access-related infection, defined as peritonitis for peritoneal dialysis patients or bacteremia for hemodialysis patients must be reported using modifier V8. Providers must report any peritonitis related to a peritoneal dialysis catheter, and any bacteremia related to hemodialysis access (including arteriovenous fistula, arteriovenous graft, or vascular catheter) using modifier V8.

ESRD facilities may report the HCPCS 90999 Unlisted Dialysis Procedure Inpatient or Outpatient to report the above modifiers.

Effective April 1, 2012, the infection modifiers are terminated and reporting on the claim is no longer required.

100-4, 8, 60.6

Vaccines Furnished to ESRD Patients

The Medicare program covers hepatitis B, influenza virus and Pneumococcal pneumonia virus (PPV) vaccines and their administration when furnished to eligible beneficiaries in accordance with coverage rules. Payment may be made for both the vaccine and the administration. The costs associated with the syringe and supplies are included in the administration fee: HCPCS code A4657 should not be billed for these vaccines.

Vaccines and their administration are reported using separate codes. See Chapter 18 of this manual for the codes required for billing vaccines and the administration of the vaccine.

Payment for vaccine administration (PPV, Influenza Virus, and Hepatitis B Virus) to freestanding RDFs is based on the Medicare Physician Fee Schedule (MPFS) according to the rate in the MPFS associated with code 90782 for services provided prior to March 1, 2003 and code 90471 for services provided March 1, 2005 and later and on reasonable cost for provider-based RDFs.

Vaccines remain separately payable under the ESRD PPS.

100-4, 8, 140

Monthly Capitation Payment Method for Physicians' Services Furnished to Patients on Maintenance Dialysis

Physicians and practitioners managing patients on dialysis (center based) are paid a monthly capitation payment (MCP) for most outpatient dialysis-related physician services furnished to a Medicare end stage renal disease (ESRD) beneficiary. The payment amount varies based on the number of visits provided within each month and the age of the ESRD beneficiary. Physicians and practitioners managing ESRD patients who dialyze at home are paid a single monthly rate based on the age of the ESRD beneficiary, regardless of the number of face-to-face physician or practitioner visits. The MCP is reported once per month for services performed in an outpatient setting that are related to the patients' ESRD.

Physicians and practitioners may receive payment for managing patients on dialysis for less than a full month of care in specific circumstances as discussed in section 140.2. Payment for ESRD related services, less than a full month, is made on a per diem bases.

Payment for ESRD-related services is made at 80 percent of the Medicare approved amount (lesser of the actual charge or applicable Medicare fee schedule amount) after the beneficiary's Part B deductible is met. The beneficiary is responsible for the Part B deductible and the 20 percent coinsurance for physician and practitioner ESRD-related services.

A. Services Included in Monthly Capitation Payment

The following physician services are included in the MCP:

- Assessment of the need for a specified diet and the need for nutritional supplementation for the control of chronic renal failure. Specification of the quantity of total protein, high biologic protein, sodium, potassium, and amount of fluids to be allowed during a given time period. For diabetic patients with chronic renal failure, the prescription usually specifies the number of calories in the diet.
- Assessment of which mode(s) of chronic dialysis (types of hemodialysis or peritoneal dialysis) are suitable for a given patient and recommendation of the type(s) of therapy for a given patient.
- Assessment and determination of which type of dialysis access is best suited for a given patient and arrangement for creation of dialysis access.
- Assessment of whether the patient meets preliminary criteria as a renal transplant candidate and presentation of this assessment to the patient and family.
- Prescription of the parameters of intradialytic management. For chronic hemodialysis therapies, this includes the type of dialysis access, the type and amount of anticoagulant to be employed, blood flow rates, dialysate flow rate, ultrafiltration rate, dialysate temperature, type of dialysate (acetate versus bicarbonate) and composition of the electrolytes in the dialysate, size of hemodialyzer (surface area) and composition of the dialyzer membrane (conventional versus high flux), duration and frequency of treatments, the type and frequency of measuring indices of clearance, and intradialytic medications to be administered. For chronic peritoneal dialysis therapies, this includes the type of peritoneal dialysis, the volume of dialysate, concentration of dextrose in the dialysate, electrolyte composition of the dialysate, duration of each exchange, and addition of medication to the dialysate, such as heparin, and the type and frequency of measuring indices of clearance. For diabetics, the quantity of insulin to be added to each exchange is prescribed.
- Assessment of whether the patient has significant renal failure-related anemia, determination of the etiology(ies) for the anemia based on diagnostic tests, and prescription of therapy for correction of the anemia, such as vitamins, oral or parenteral iron, and hormonal therapy such as erythropoietin.
- Assessment of whether the patient has hyperparathyroidism and/or renal osteodystrophy secondary to chronic renal failure and prescription of appropriate therapy, such as calcium and phosphate binders for control of hyperphosphatemia. Based upon assessment of parahormone levels, serum calcium levels, and evaluation for the presence of metabolic bone disease, the physician determines whether oral or parenteral therapy with vitamin D or its analogs is indicated and prescribes the appropriate therapy. Based upon assessment and diagnosis of bone disease, the physician may prescribe specific chelation therapy with deferoxamine and the use of hemoperfusion for removal of aluminum and the chelation.
- Assessment of whether the patient has dialysis-related arthropathy or neuropathy and adjustment of the patient's prescription accordingly. Referral of the patient for any additional needed specialist evaluation and management of these endorgan problems.
- Assessment of whether the patient has fluid overload resulting from renal failure and establishment of an estimated "ideal (dry) weight." The physician determines the need for fluid removal independent of the dialysis prescription and implements these measures when indicated.
- Determination of the need for and prescription of antihypertensive medications and their timing relative to dialysis when the patient is hypertensive in spite of correction of fluid overload.
- Periodic review of the dialysis records to ascertain whether the patient is receiving the prescribed amount of dialysis and ordering of indices of clearance, such as urea kinetics, in order to ascertain whether the dialysis prescription is producing adequate dialysis. If the indices of clearance suggest that the prescription requires alteration, the physician orders changes in the hemodialysis prescription, such as blood flow rate, dialyzer surface area, dialysis frequency, and/or dialysis duration (length of treatment). For peritoneal dialysis patients, the physician may order changes in the volume of dialysate, dextrose concentration of the dialysate, and duration of the exchanges.
- Periodic visits (at least one per month) to the patient during dialysis to ascertain whether the dialysis is working well and whether the patient is tolerating the procedure well (physiologically and psychologically). During these visits, the physician determines whether alteration in any aspect of a given patient's prescription is indicated, such as changes in the estimate of the patient's dry weight. Review of the treatment with the nurse or technician performing the therapy is also included. The frequency of these visits will vary depending upon the patient's medical status, complicating conditions, and other determinants.
- Performance of periodic physical assessments, based upon the patient's clinical stability, in order to determine the necessity for alterations in various aspects of the patient's prescription. Similarly, the physician reviews the results of periodic laboratory testing in order to determine the need for alterations in the patient's prescription, such as changes in the amount and timing of phosphate binders or dose of erythropoietin.
- Periodic assessment of the adequacy and function of the patient's dialysis access appropriate tests and antibiotic therapy.
- Interpretations of the following tests:
  - Bone mineral density studies (CPT codes 76070, 76075, 78350, and 78351);
  - Noninvasive vascular diagnostic studies of hemodialysis access (CPT codes 93925, 93926, 93930, 93931, and 93990);
  - Nerve conduction studies (CPT codes 95900, 95903, 95904, 95925, 95926, 95927, 95934, 95935, and 95936);
  - Electromyography studies (CPT codes 95860, 95861, 95863, 95864, 95867, 95867, 95869, and 95872).
- Periodic review and update of the patient's short-term and long-term care plans with staff.
- Coordination and direction of the care of patients by other professional staff, such as dieticians and social workers.
- Certification of the need for items and services such as durable medical equipment and home health care services. Care plan oversight services described by CPT code 99375 are included in the MCP and may not be separately reported.

B. Services Excluded from Monthly Capitation Payment

The following physician services furnished to the physician's ESRD patients are excluded from the MCP and should be paid in accordance with the physician fee schedule:

1. Administration of hepatitis B vaccine.
2. Surgical services such as:
   - Temporary or permanent hemodialysis catheter placement;
   - Temporary or permanent peritoneal dialysis catheter placement;
   - Repair of existing dialysis accesses;
   - Placement of catheter(s) for thrombolytic therapy;
   - Thrombolytic therapy (systemic, regional, or access catheter only; hemodialysis or peritoneal dialysis);
   - Thrombectomy of clotted cannula;
   - Arthrocentesis;
   - Bone marrow aspiration; and
   - Bone marrow biopsy.
3. Interpretation of tests that have a professional component such as:
   - Electrocardiograms (12 lead, Holter monitor, stress tests, etc.);
   - Echocardiograms;
   - 24-hour blood pressure monitor;
   - Biopsies; and
   - Spirometry and complete pulmonary function tests.
4. Complete evaluation for renal transplantation. While the physician assessment of whether the patient meets preliminary criteria as a renal transplant candidate is included under the MCP, the complete evaluation for renal transplantation is excluded from the MCP
5. Evaluation of potential living transplant donors.
6. The training of patients to perform home hemodialysis, self hemodialysis, and the various forms of self peritoneal dialysis.
7. Non-renal related physician's services. These services may be furnished by the physician providing renal care or by another physician. They may not be incidental to services furnished during a dialysis session or office visit necessitated by the renal condition. The physician must provide documentation that the illness is not related to the renal condition and that the added visits are required. The contractor's medical staff determines whether additional reimbursement is warranted for treatment of the unrelated illness. For example, the medical management of diabetes mellitus that is not related to the dialysis or furnished during a dialysis session is excluded.
8. Covered physician services furnished to hospital inpatients.
9. All physician services that antedate the initiation of outpatient dialysis.
10. Covered physician services furnished by another physician when the patient is not available to receive the outpatient services as usual; for example, when the patient is traveling out of tow

100-4, 8, 140.1

Payment for ESRD-Related Services Under the Monthly Capitation Payment (Center Based Patients)

Physicians and practitioners managing center based patients on dialysis are paid a monthly rate for most outpatient dialysis-related physician services furnished to a Medicare ESRD beneficiary. The payment amount varies based on the number of visits provided within each month and the age of the ESRD beneficiary. Under this methodology, separate codes are billed for providing one visit per month, two to three visits per month and four or more visits per month. The lowest payment amount applies when a physician provides one visit per month; a higher payment is provided for two to three visits per month. To receive the highest payment amount, a physician or practitioner would have to provide at least four ESRD-related visits per month. The MCP is reported once per month for services performed in an outpatient setting that are related to the patients' ESRD.

The physician or practitioner who provides the complete assessment, establishes the patient's plan of care, and provides the ongoing management is the physician or practitioner who submits the bill for the monthly service.

a. Month defined.

For purposes of billing for physician and practitioner ESRD related services, the term 'month' means a calendar month. The first month the beneficiary begins dialysis treatments is the date the dialysis treatments begin through the end of the calendar month. Thereafter, the term 'month' refers to a calendar month.

b. Determination of the age of beneficiary.

The beneficiary's age at the end of the month is the age of the patient for determining the appropriate age related ESRD-related services code.

c. Qualifying Visits Under the MCP

- General policy.

Visits must be furnished face-to-face by a physician, clinical nurse specialist, nurse practitioner, or physician's assistant.

- Visits furnished by another physician or practitioner (who is not the MCP physician or practitioner).

The MCP physician or practitioner may use other physicians or qualified nonphysician practitioners to provide some of the visits during the month. The MCP physician or practitioner does not have to be present when these other physicians or practitioners provide visits. In this instance, the rules are consistent with the requirements for hospital split/shared evaluation and management visits. The non-MCP physician or practitioner must be a partner, an employee of the same group practice, or an employee of the MCP physician or practitioner. For example, the physician or practitioner furnishing visits under the MCP may be either a W-2 employee or 1099 independent contractor.

When another physician is used to furnish some of the visits during the month, the physician who provides the complete assessment, establishes the patient's plan of care, and provides the ongoing management should bill for the MCP service.

If the nonphysician practitioner is the practitioner who performs the complete assessment and establishes the plan of care, then the MCP service should be billed under the PIN of the clinical nurse specialist, nurse practitioner, or physician assistant.

- Residents, interns and fellows.

Patient visits by residents, interns and fellows enrolled in an approved Medicare graduate medical education (GME) program may be counted towards the MCP visits if the teaching MCP physician is present during the visit.

- Patients designated/admitted as hospital observation status.

ESRD-related visits furnished to patients in hospital observation status that occur on or after January 1, 2005, should be counted for purposes of billing the MCP codes. Visits furnished to patients in hospital observation status are included when submitting MCP claims for ESRD-related services.

- ESRD-related visits furnished to beneficiaries residing in a SNF.

ESRD-related visits furnished to beneficiaries residing in a SNF should be counted for purposes of billing the MCP codes.

- SNF residents admitted as an inpatient.

Inpatient visits are not counted for purposes of the MCP service. If the beneficiary residing in a SNF is admitted to the hospital as an inpatient, the appropriate inpatient visit code should be billed.

- ESRD Related Visits as a Telehealth Service

ESRD-related services with 2 or 3 visits per month and ESRD-related services with 4 or more visits per month may be furnished as a telehealth service. However, at least one visit per month is required in person to examine the vascular access site. A clinical examination of the vascular access site must be furnished face-to-face (not as a telehealth service) by a physician, nurse practitioner or physician's assistant. For more information on how ESRD-related visits may be furnished as a Medicare telehealth service and for general Medicare telehealth policy see Pub. 100-02, Medicare Benefit Policy manual, chapter 15, section 270. For claims processing instructions see Pub. 100-04, Medicare Claims Processing manual chapter 12, section 190.

100-4, 8, 140.1.1

Payment for Managing Patients on Home Dialysis

Physicians and practitioners managing ESRD patients who dialyze at home are paid a single monthly rate based on the age of the beneficiary. The MCP physician (or practitioner) must furnish at least one face-to-face patient visit per month for the home dialysis MCP service. Documentation by the MCP physician (or practitioner) should support at least one face-to-face encounter per month with the home dialysis patient. Medicare contractors may waive the requirement for a monthly face-to-face visit for the home dialysis MCP service on a case by case basis, for example, when the nephrologist's notes indicate that the physician actively and adequately managed the care of the home dialysis patient throughout the month. The management of home dialysis patients who remain a home dialysis patient the entire month should be coded using the ESRD-related services for home dialysis patients HCPCS codes.

When another physician is used to furnish some of the visits during the month, the physician who provides the complete assessment, establishes the patient's plan of care, and provides the ongoing management should bill for the MCP service.

If the nonphysician practitioner is the practitioner who performs the complete assessment and establishes the plan of care, then the MCP service should be billed under the PIN of the clinical nurse specialist, nurse practitioner, or physician assistant.

Residents, interns and fellows. Patient visits by residents, interns and fellows enrolled in an approved Medicare graduate medical education (GME) program may be counted towards the MCP visits if the teaching MCP physician is present during the visit.

a. Month defined.

For purposes of billing for physician and practitioner ESRD related services, the term 'month' means a calendar month. The first month the beneficiary begins dialysis treatments is the date the dialysis treatments begin through the end of the calendar month. Thereafter, the term 'month' refers to a calendar month.

b. Qualifying Visits under the MCP

General policy. Visits must be furnished face-to-face by a physician, clinical nurse specialist, nurse practitioner, or physician's assistant.

Visits furnished by another physician or practitioner (who is not the MCP physician or practitioner). The MCP physician or practitioner may use other physicians or qualified nonphysician practitioners to provide the visit(s) during the month. The MCP physician or practitioner does not have to be present when these other physicians or practitioners provide visit(s). The non-MCP physician or practitioner must be a partner, an employee of the same group practice, or an employee of the MCP physician or practitioner. For example, the physician or practitioner furnishing visits under the MCP may be either a W-2 employee or 1099 independent contractor.

100-4, 9, 182

Medical Nutrition Therapy (MNT) Services

A - FQHCs

Previously, MNT type services were considered incident to services under the FQHC benefit, if all relevant program requirements were met. Therefore, separate all-inclusive encounter rate payment could not be made for the provision of MNT services. With passage of DRA, effective January 1, 2006, FQHCs are eligible for a separate payment under Part B for these services provided they meet all program requirements. Payment is made at the all-inclusive encounter rate to the FQHC. This payment can be in addition to payment for any other qualifying visit on the same date of service as the beneficiary received qualifying MNT services.

For FQHCs to qualify for a separate visit payment for MNT services, the services must be a one-on-one face-to-face encounter. Group sessions don't constitute a billable visit for any FQHC services. Rather, the cost of group sessions is included in the calculation of the all-inclusive FQHC visit rate. To receive payment for MNT services, the MNT services must be billed on TOB 73X with the appropriate individual MNT HCPCS code (codes 97802, 97803, or G0270) and with the appropriate site of service revenue code in the 052X revenue code series. This payment can be in addition to payment for any other qualifying visit on the same date of service as the beneficiary received qualifying MNT services as long as the claim for MNT services contain the appropriate coding specified above.

NOTE: MNT is not a qualifying visit on the same day that DSMT is provided.

Additional information on MNT can be found in Chapter 4, section 300 of this manual.

Group services (HCPCS 97804 or G0271) do not meet the criteria for a separate qualifying encounter. All line items billed on TOB 73x with HCPCS code 97804 or G0271 will be denied.

B - RHCs

Separate payment to RHCs for these practitioners/services continues to be precluded as these services are not within the scope of Medicare-covered RHC benefits. All line items billed on TOB 71x with HCPCS codes for MNT services will be denied.

100-4, 11, 10

Overview

Medicare beneficiaries entitled to hospital insurance (Part A) who have terminal illnesses and a life expectancy of six months or less have the option of electing hospice benefits in lieu of standard Medicare coverage for treatment and management of their terminal condition. Only care provided by a Medicare certified hospice is covered under the hospice benefit provisions.

Hospice care is available for two 90-day periods and an unlimited number of 60-day periods during the remainder of the hospice patient's lifetime. However, a beneficiary may voluntarily terminate his hospice election period. Election/termination dates are retained on CWF.

When hospice coverage is elected, the beneficiary waives all rights to Medicare Part B payments for services that are related to the treatment and management of his/her terminal illness during any period his/her hospice benefit election is in force, except for professional services of an attending physician, which may include a nurse practitioner. If the attending physician, who may be a nurse practitioner, is an employee of the designated hospice, he or she may not receive compensation from the hospice for those services under Part B. These physician professional services are billed to Medicare Part A by the hospice.

To be covered, hospice services must be reasonable and necessary for the palliation or management of the terminal illness and related conditions. The individual must elect hospice care and a certification that the individual is terminally ill must be completed by the patient's attending physician (if there is one), and the Medical Director (or the physician member of the Interdisciplinary Group (IDG)). Nurse practitioners serving as the attending physician may not certify or re-certify the terminal illness. A plan of care must be established before services are provided. To be covered, services must be consistent with the plan of care. Certification of terminal illness is based on the physician's or medical director's clinical judgment regarding the normal course of an individual's illness. It should be noted that predicting life expectancy is not always exact.

See the Medicare Benefit Policy Manual, Chapter 9, for additional general information about the Hospice benefit.

See Chapter 29 of this manual for information on the appeals process that should be followed when an entity is dissatisfied with the determination made on a claim.

See Chapter 9 of the Medicare Benefit Policy Manual for hospice eligibility requirements and election of hospice care.

100-4, 11, 10.1

Hospice Pre-Election Evaluation and Counseling Services

Effective January 1, 2005, Medicare allows payment to a hospice for specified hospice pre-election evaluation and counseling services when furnished by a physician who is either the medical director of or employee of the hospice.

Medicare covers a one- time only payment on behalf of a beneficiary who is terminally ill, (defined as having a prognosis of 6 months or less if the disease follows its normal course), has no previous hospice elections, and has not previously received hospice pre-election evaluation and counseling services.

HCPCS code G0337 "Hospice Pre-Election Evaluation and Counseling Services" is used to designate that these services have been provided by the medical director or a physician employed by the hospice. Hospice agencies bill their Medicare contractor with home health and hospice jurisdiction directly using HCPCS G0337 with Revenue Code 0657. No other revenue codes may appear on the claim.

Claims for "Hospice Pre-Election and Counseling Services", HCPCS code G0337, are not subject to the editing usually required on hospice claims to match the claim to an established hospice period. Further, contractors do not apply payments for hospice pre-election evaluation and counseling consultation services to the overall hospice cap amount.

Medicare must ensure that this counseling service occurs only one time per beneficiary by imposing safeguards to detect and prevent duplicate billing for similar services. If "new patient" physician services (HCPCS codes 99201-99205) are submitted by a Medicare contractor to CWF for payment authorization but HCPCS code G0337 (Hospice Pre-Election Evaluation and Counseling Services) has already been approved for a hospice claim for the same beneficiary, for the same date of service, by the same physician, the physician service will be rejected by CWF and the service shall be denied as a duplicate. Medicare contractors use the following messages in this case:

MSN messages: 16.8: "Payment is included in another service received on the same day" and

16.45: "You cannot be billed separately for this item or service. You do not have to pay this amount."

Claim adjustment reason code (CARC) 97: "The benefit for this service is included in the payment/allowance for another service/procedure that has already been adjudicated."

Remittance advice remark code (RARC) M86:

Likewise, if a "new patient" claim for HCPCS codes 99201-99205 has been approved and subsequently, a hospice claim is submitted to CWF for payment authorization for HCPCS code G0337, (for same beneficiary, same date of service, same physician), CWF shall reject the claim and the contractor shall deny the bill and use the messages above.

HCPCS code G0337 is only payable when billed on a hospice claim. Contractors shall not make payment for HCPCS code G0337 on professional claims. Contractors shall deny line items on professional claims for HCPCS code G0337 and use the following messages:

MSN message 17.9: "Medicare (Part A/Part B) pays for this service. The provider must bill the correct Medicare contractor."

CARC 109: "Claim not covered by this payer/contractor. You must send the claim to the correct payer/contractor."

100-4, 11, 40.1.3

Independent Attending Physician Services

When hospice coverage is elected, the beneficiary waives all rights to Medicare Part B payments for professional services that are related to the treatment and management of his/her terminal illness during any period his/her hospice benefit election is in force, except for professional services of an independent attending physician, who is not an employee of the designated hospice nor receives compensation from the hospice for those services. For purposes of administering the hospice benefit provisions, an "attending physician" means an individual who:

- Is a doctor of medicine or osteopathy or
- A nurse practitioner (for professional services related to the terminal illness that are furnished on or after December 8, 2003); and
- Is identified by the individual, at the time he/she elects hospice coverage, as having the most significant role in the determination and delivery of their medical care.

Hospices should reiterate with patients that they must not see independent physicians for care related to their terminal illness other than their independent attending physician unless the hospice arranges it.

Even though a beneficiary elects hospice coverage, he/she may designate and use an independent attending physician, who is not employed by nor receives compensation from the hospice for professional services furnished, in addition to the services of hospice-employed physicians. The professional services of an independent attending physician, who may be a nurse practitioner as defined in Chapter 9, that are reasonable and necessary for the treatment and management of a hospice patient's terminal illness are not considered Medicare Part A hospice services.

Where the service is related to the hospice patient's terminal illness but was furnished by someone other than the designated "attending physician" [or a physician substituting for the attending physician]) the physician or other provider must look to the hospice for payment.

Professional services related to the hospice patient's terminal condition that were furnished by an independent attending physician, who may be a nurse practitioner, are billed to the Medicare contractor through Medicare Part B. When the independent attending physician furnishes a terminal illness related service that includes both a professional and technical component (e.g., x-rays), he/she bills the professional component of such services to the carrier and looks to the hospice for payment for the technical component. Likewise, the independent attending physician, who may be a nurse practitioner, would look to the hospice for payment for terminal illness related services furnished that have no professional component (e.g., clinical lab tests). The remainder of this section explains this in greater detail.

When a Medicare beneficiary elects hospice coverage he/she may designate an attending physician, who may be a nurse practitioner, not employed by the hospice, in addition to receiving care from hospice-employed physicians. The professional services of a non-hospice affiliated attending physician for the treatment and management of a hospice patient's terminal illness are not considered Medicare Part A "hospice services." These independent attending physician services are billed through Medicare Part B to the Medicare contractor, provided they were not furnished under a payment arrangement with the hospice. The independent attending physician codes services with the GV modifier "Attending physician not employed or paid under agreement by the patient's hospice provider" when billing his/her professional services furnished for the treatment and management of a hospice patient's terminal condition. The Medicare contractor makes payment to the independent attending physician or beneficiary, as appropriate, based on the payment and deductible rules applicable to each covered service.

Payments for the services of an independent attending physician are not counted in determining whether the hospice cap amount has been exceeded because Part B services provided by an independent attending physician are not part of the hospice's care.

Services provided by an independent attending physician who may be a nurse practitioner must be coordinated with any direct care services provided by hospice physicians.

Only the direct professional services of an independent attending physician, who may be a nurse practitioner, to a patient may be billed; the costs for services such as lab or x-rays are not to be included in the bill.

If another physician covers for a hospice patient's designated attending physician, the services of the substituting physician are billed by the designated attending physician under the reciprocal or locum tenens billing instructions. In such instances, the attending physician bills using the GV modifier in conjunction with either the Q5 or Q6 modifier.

When services related to a hospice patient's terminal condition are furnished under a payment arrangement with the hospice by the designated attending physician who may be a nurse practitioner (i.e., by a non-independent physician/nurse practitioner), the physician must look to the hospice for payment. In this situation the physicians' services are Part A hospice services and are billed by the hospice to its Medicare contractor.

Medicare contractors must process and pay for covered, medically necessary Part B services that physicians furnish to patients after their hospice benefits are revoked even if the patient remains under the care of the hospice. Such services are billed without the GV or GW modifiers. Make payment based on applicable Medicare payment and deductible rules for each covered service even if the beneficiary continues to be treated by the hospice after hospice benefits are revoked.

The CWF response contains the periods of hospice entitlement. This information is a permanent part of the notice and is furnished on all CWF replies and automatic notices. Medicare contractor use the CWF reply for validating dates of hospice coverage and to research, examine and adjudicate services coded with the GV or GW modifiers.

100-4, 11, 40.1.3.1

Care Plan Oversight

Care plan oversight (CPO) exists where there is physician supervision of patients under care of hospices that require complex and multidisciplinary care modalities involving regular physician development and/or revision of care plans. Implicit in the concept of CPO is the expectation that the physician has coordinated an aspect of the patient's care with the hospice during the month for which CPO services were billed.

For a physician or NP employed by or under arrangement with a hospice agency, CPO functions are incorporated and are part of the hospice per diem payment and as such may not be separately billed.

For information on separately billable CPO services by the attending physician or nurse practitioner see Chapter 12, 180 of this manual.

100-4, 11, 40.2

Processing Professional Claims for Hospice Beneficiaries

Professional services of attending physicians, who may be nurse practitioners, furnished to hospice beneficiaries are coded with modifier GV. Attending physician not employed or paid under arrangement by the patient's hospice provider. This modifier must be retained and reported to CWF.

Local Part B carriers shall presume that hospice benefits are not involved unless the biller codes services on the claim to indicate that the patient is a hospice enrollee (e.g. the GV modifier is billed by the attending physician, who may be a nurse practitioner, or the GW modifier is billed for services unrelated to the terminal illness) or the trailer information on the CWF reply shows a hospice election. The carrier shall use the hospice enrollment trailer information on the CWF reply to examine and validate the claim information.

For beneficiaries enrolled in hospice, carriers shall deny any services furnished on or after January 1, 2002, that are submitted without either the GV or GW modifier. For services furnished to a hospice patient prior to January 1, 2002, the attending physician is to include an attestation statement that is the written equivalent of the GV modifier and carriers are responsible for determining whether or not a service is related to the patient's terminal condition.

Deny claims for all other services related to the terminal illness furnished by individuals or entities other than the designated attending physician, who may be a nurse practitioner.

Such claims include bills for any DME, supplies or independently practicing speech-language pathologists or physical therapists that are related to the terminal condition.

These services are included in the hospice rate and paid through the FI.

See §110 for MSN and Remittance Advice (RA) coding.

100-4, 12, 30

Correct Coding Policy

B3-15068

The Correct Coding Initiative was developed to promote national correct coding methodologies and to control improper coding leading to inappropriate payment in Part B claims. Refer to Chapter 23 for additional information on the initiative.

The principles for the correct coding policy are:

The service represents the standard of care in accomplishing the overall procedure;

The service is necessary to successfully accomplish the comprehensive procedure.

Failure to perform the service may compromise the success of the procedure; and

The service does not represent a separately identifiable procedure unrelated to the comprehensive procedure planned.

For a detailed description of the correct coding policy, refer to http://www.cms.hhs.gov/medlearn/ncci.asp.

The CMS as well as many third party payers have adopted the HCPCS/CPT coding system for use by physicians and others to describe services rendered. The system contains three levels of codes. Level I contains the American Medical Association's Current Procedural Terminology (CPT) numeric codes. Level II contains alpha-numeric codes primarily for items and services not included in CPT. Level III contains carrier specific codes that are not included in either Level I or Level II. For a list of CPT and HCPCS codes refer to the CMS Web site.

The following general coding policies encompass coding principles that are to be applied in the review of Medicare claims. They are the basis for the correct coding edits that are installed in the claims processing systems effective January 1, 1996.

A. Coding Based on Standards of Medical/Surgical Practice

All services integral to accomplishing a procedure are considered bundled into that procedure and, therefore, are considered a component part of the comprehensive code. Many of these generic activities are common to virtually all procedures and, on other occasions, some are integral to only a certain group of procedures, but are still essential to accomplish these particular procedures. Accordingly, it is inappropriate to separately report these services based on standard medical and surgical principles.

Because many services are unique to individual CPT coding sections, the rationale for rebundling is described in that particular section of the detailed coding narratives that are transmitted to carriers periodically.

B. CPT Procedure Code Definition

The format of the CPT manual includes descriptions of procedures, which are, in order to conserve space, not listed in their entirety for all procedures. The partial description is indented under the main entry. The main entry then encompasses the portion of the description preceding the semicolon. The main entry applies to and is a part of all indented entries, which follow with their codes.

In the course of other procedure descriptions, the code definition specifies other procedures that are included in this comprehensive code. In addition, a code description may define a rebundling relationship where one code is a part of another based on the language used in the descriptor.

C. CPT Coding Manual Instruction/Guideline

Each of the six major subsections include guidelines that are unique to that section.

These directions are not all inclusive of nor limited to, definitions of terms, modifiers, unlisted procedures or services, special or written reports, details about reporting separate, and multiple or starred procedures and qualifying circumstances.

D. Coding Services Supplemental to Principal Procedure (Add-On Codes) Code

Generally, these are identified with the statement "list separately in addition to code for primary procedure" in parentheses, and other times the supplemental code is used only with certain primary codes, which are parenthetically identified. The reason for these CPT codes is to enable physicians and others to separately identify a service that is performed in certain situations as an additional service. Incidental services that are necessary to accomplish the primary procedure (e.g., lysis of adhesions in the course of an open cholecystectomy) are not separately billed.

E. Separate Procedures

The narrative for many CPT codes includes a parenthetical statement that the procedure represents a "separate procedure."

The inclusion of this statement indicates that the procedure, while possible to perform separately, is generally included in a more comprehensive procedure, and the service is not to be billed when a related, more comprehensive, service is performed. The "separate procedure" designation is used with codes in the surgery (CPT codes 10000-69999), radiology (CPT codes 70000-79999), and medicine (CPT codes 90000-99199) sections.

When a related procedure from the same section, subsection, category, or subcategory is performed, a code with the designation of "separate procedure" is not to be billed with the primary procedure.

F. Designation of Sex

Many procedure codes have a sex designation within their narrative. These codes are not billed with codes having an opposite sex designation because this would reflect a conflict in sex classification either by the definition of the code descriptions themselves, or by the fact that the performance of these procedures on the same beneficiary would be anatomically impossible.

G. Family of Codes

In a family of codes, there are two or more component codes that are not billed separately because they are included in a more comprehensive code as members of the code family.

Comprehensive codes include certain services that are separately identifiable by other component codes. The component codes as members of the comprehensive code family represent parts of the procedure that should not be listed separately when the complete procedure is done. However, the component codes are considered individually if performed independently of the complete procedure and if not all the services listed in the comprehensive codes were rendered to make up the total service.

H. Most Extensive Procedures

When procedures are performed together that are basically the same or performed on the same site but are qualified by an increased level of complexity, the less extensive procedure is bundled into the more extensive procedure.

I. Sequential Procedures

An initial approach to a procedure may be followed at the same encounter by a second, usually more invasive approach. There may be separate CPT codes describing each service. The second procedure is usually performed because the initial approach was unsuccessful in accomplishing the medically necessary service. These procedures are considered "sequential procedures." Only the CPT code for one of the services, generally the more invasive service, should be billed.

J. With/Without Procedures

In the CPT manual, there are various procedures that have been separated into two codes with the definitional difference being "with" versus "without" (e.g., with and without contrast). Both procedure codes cannot be billed. When done together, the "without" procedure is bundled into the "with" procedure.

K. Laboratory Panels

When components of a specific organ or disease oriented laboratory panel (e.g., codes 80061 and 80059) or automated multi-channel tests (e.g., codes 80002 - 80019) are billed separately, they must be bundled into the comprehensive panel or automated multichannel test code as appropriate that includes the multiple component tests. The individual tests that make up a panel or can be performed on an automated multi-channel test analyzer are not to be separately billed.

L Mutually Exclusive Procedures

There are numerous procedure codes that are not billed together because they are mutually exclusive of each other. Mutually exclusive codes are those codes that cannot reasonably be done in the same session.

An example of a mutually exclusive situation is when the repair of the organ can be performed by two different methods. One repair method must be chosen to repair the organ and must be billed. Another example is the billing of an "initial" service and a subsequent" service. It is contradictory for a service to be classified as an initial and a subsequent service at the same time.

CPT codes which are mutually exclusive of one another based either on the CPT definition or the medical impossibility/improbability that the procedures could be performed at the same session can be identified as code pairs. These codes are not necessarily linked to one another with one code narrative describing a more comprehensive procedure compared to the component code, but can be identified as code pairs which should not be billed together.

M. Use of Modifiers

When certain component codes or mutually exclusive codes are appropriately furnished, such as later on the same day or on a different digit or limb, it is appropriate that these services be reported using a HCPCS code modifier. Such modifiers are modifiers E1 -E4, FA, F1 - F9, TA, T1 - T9, LT, RT, LC, LD, RC, -58, -78, -79, and -94.

Modifier -59 is not appropriate to use with weekly radiation therapy management codes (77427) or with evaluation and management services codes (99201 - 99499).

Application of these modifiers prevent erroneous denials of claims for several procedures performed on different anatomical sites, on different sides of the body, or at different sessions on the same date of service. The medical record must reflect that the modifier is being used appropriately to describe separate services.

100-4, 12, 30.1

Digestive System (Codes 40000 - 49999)

B3-15100

A. Upper Gastrointestinal Endoscopy Including Endoscopic Ultrasound (EUS) (Code 43259)

If the person performing the original diagnostic endoscopy has access to the EUS and the clinical situation requires an EUS, the EUS may be done at the same time. The procedure, diagnostic and EUS, is reported under the same code, CPT 43259. This code conforms to CPT guidelines for the indented codes. The service represented by the indented code, in this case code 43259 for EUS, includes the service represented by the unintended code preceding the list of indented codes. Therefore, when a diagnostic examination of the upper gastrointestinal tract "including esophagus, stomach, and either the duodenum or jejunum as appropriate," includes the use of endoscopic ultrasonography, the service is reported by a single code, namely 43259.

Interpretation, whether by a radiologist or endoscopist, is reported under CPT code 76975-26. These codes may both be reported on the same day.

B. Incomplete Colonoscopies (Codes 45330 and 45378)

An incomplete colonoscopy, e.g., the inability to extend beyond the splenic flexure, is billed and paid using colonoscopy code 45378 with modifier "-53." The Medicare physician fee schedule database has specific values for code 45378-53. These values are the same as for code 45330, sigmoidoscopy, as failure to extend beyond the splenic flexure means that a sigmoidoscopy rather than a colonoscopy has been performed.

However, code 45378-53 should be used when an incomplete colonoscopy has been done because other MPFSDB indicators are different for codes 45378 and 45330.

100-4, 12, 30.2

Urinary and Male Genital Systems (Codes 50010 - 55899)

B3-15200

A. Cystourethroscopy With Ureteral Catheterization (Code 52005)

Code 52005 has a zero in the bilateral field (payment adjustment for bilateral procedure does not apply) because the basic procedure is an examination of the bladder and urethra (cystourethroscopy), which are not paired organs. The work RVUs assigned take into account that it may be necessary to examine and catheterize one or both ureters. No additional payment is made when the procedure is billed with bilateral modifier "-50." Neither is any additional payment made when both ureters are examined and code 52005 is billed with multiple surgery modifier "-51." It is inappropriate to bill code 52005 twice, once by itself and once with modifier "-51," when both ureters are examined.

B. Cystourethroscopy With Fulgration and/or Resection of Tumors (Codes 52234, 52235, and 52240)

The descriptors for codes 52234 through 52240 include the language "tumor(s)." This means that regardless of the number of tumors removed, only one unit of a single code can be billed on a given date of service. It is inconsistent to allow payment for removal of a small (code 52234) and a large (code 52240) tumor using two codes when only one code is allowed for the removal of more than one large tumor. For these three codes only one unit may be billed for any of these codes, only one of the codes may be billed, and the billed code reflects the size of the largest tumor removed.

100-4, 12, 30.3

Audiology Services

Section 1861(ll)(3)of the Social Security Act (the Act) defines "audiology services" as such hearing and balance assessment services furnished by a qualified audiologist as the audiologist is legally authorized to perform under State law (or the State regulatory mechanism provided by State law), as would otherwise by covered if furnished by a physician. In this section, these hearing and balance assessment services are termed "audiology services," regardless of whether they are furnished by an audiologist, physician, nonphysician practitioner (NPP), or hospital.

Because audiology services are diagnostic tests, when furnished in an office or hospital outpatient department, they must be furnished by or under the appropriate level of supervision of a physician as established in 42 CFR 410.32(b)(1) and 410.28(e). If not personally furnished by a physician, audiologist, or NPP, audiology services must be performed under direct physician supervision. As specified in 42 CFR 410.32(b)(2)(ii) or (v), respectively, these services are excepted from physician supervision when they are personally furnished by a qualified audiologist or performed by a nurse practitioner or clinical nurse specialist authorized to perform the tests under applicable State laws.

References to technicians apply also to other qualified clinical staff. See Pub. 100-02, chapter 15, section 80.3.D.

A - Correct Reporting

1. General. Contact the contractor for guidance if the CPT codebook changes the description of codes mentioned in this section.

   Other policies concerning audiological services are found in Pub. 100-02, chapter 15, section 80.3.

   See chapter 26 of this manual for place of service and type of service coding.

   Section 4541(a)(2) of the Balanced Budget Act (BBA) (P.L. 105-33), which added section 1834(k)(5) to (the Act), required that all claims for certain audiology services be reported using a uniform coding system. CMS chose HCPCS (Healthcare Common Procedure Coding System) as the coding system for the reporting of these services. This coding requirement is effective for all claims for audiology services submitted on or after April 1, 1998.

   The BBA also required payment under a prospective payment system for audiology services. Effective for claims with dates of service on or after January 1, 1999, the Medicare Physician Fee Schedule (MPFS) became the method of payment for audiology services furnished in the office setting and for the associated professional services furnished in physician's office and hospital outpatient settings.

2. Use of the NPI. For audiologists who are enrolled and bill independently for services they render, the audiologist's NPI is required on all claims they submit. For example, in offices and private practice settings, an enrolled audiologist shall use his or her own NPI in the rendering loop to bill under the MPFS for the services the audiologist furnished. If an enrolled audiologist furnishing services to hospital outpatients reassigns his/her benefits to the hospital, the hospital may bill the carrier or Medicare administrative contractor for the professional services of the audiologist under the MPFS using the NPI of the audiologist. If an audiologist is employed by a hospital but is not enrolled in Medicare, the only payment for a hospital outpatient audiology service that can be made is the payment to the hospital for its facility services under the hospital Outpatient Prospective Payment System (OPPS) or other applicable hospital payment system. No payment can be made under the MPFS for professional services of an audiologist who is not enrolled.

   Audiologists must be enrolled and use their NPI on claims for services they render in office settings on or after October 1, 2008 (for additional information about enrollment, refer to Pub. 100-08, Medicare Program Integrity Manual, chapter 15). Before October 1, 2008, the services of audiologists who were not yet enrolled in Medicare were billed by a physician or group who employed the audiologist. Audiologists shall use the billing instructions in the Medicare manuals; for example, see this manual, chapter 1, section 30.

   See the most recent MPFS for pricing and physician supervision levels for audiology services: http://www.cms.hhs.gov/PFSlookup/01_Overview.asp#TopOfPage. The NPI of the supervising physician shall be used to bill audiology services when supervision is appropriate.

The most recent OPPS pricing for audiology services is available in Addendum B at: http://www.cms.gov/HospitalOutpatientPPS/AU/list.asp#TopOfPage.

B. Billing for Audiology Services

See the CMS Web site at http://www.cms.gov/PhysicianFeeSched/50_Audiology.asp for a listing of all CPT codes for audiology services. For information concerning codes that are not on the list, and which codes may be billed when furnished by technicians, contractors shall provide guidance. The Physician Fee Schedule at http://www.cms.gov/PFSlookup/01_Overview.asp#TopOfPage allows you to search pricing amounts, various payment policy indicators, RVUs, and GPCIs.

Audiology services may not be billed when the place of service is a comprehensive outpatient rehabilitation facility (CORF) or a rehabilitation agency.

Audiology services may be furnished and billed by audiologists and, when these services are furnished by an audiologist, no physician supervision is required.

The interpretation and report shall be written in the medical record by the audiologist, physician, or NPP who personally furnished any audiology service, or by the physician who supervised the service. Technicians shall not interpret audiology services, but may record objective test results of those services they may furnish under direct physician supervision.

Payment for the interpretation and report of the services is included in payment for all audiology services, and specifically in the professional component if the audiology service has a professional component/technical component split.

1. Billing under the MPFS for Audiology Services Outside the Facility Setting

   The individuals who furnish audiology services in all settings must be qualified to furnish those services. The qualifications of the individual performing the services must be consistent with the number, type and complexity of the tests, the abilities of the individual, and the patient's ability to interact to produce valid and reliable results. The physician who supervises and bills for the service is responsible for assuring the qualifications of the technician, if applicable are appropriate to the test.

   a. Professional Skills.

      When a professional personally furnishes an audiology service, that individual must interact with the patient to provide professional skills and be directly involved in decision-making and clinical judgment during the test.

      The skills required when professionals furnish audiology services for payment under the MPFS are masters or doctoral level skills that involve clinical judgment or assessment and specialized knowledge and ability including, but not limited to, knowledge of anatomy and physiology, neurology, psychology, physics, psychometrics, and interpersonal communication. The interactions of these knowledge bases are required to attain the clinical expertise for audiology tests. Also required are skills to administer valid and reliable tests safely, especially when they involve stimulating the auditory nerve and testing complex brain functions.

      Diagnostic audiology services also require skills and judgment to administer and modify tests, to make informed interpretations about the causes and implications of the test results in the context of the history and presenting complaints, and to provide both objective results and professional knowledge to the patient and to the ordering physician.

      Examples include, but are not limited to:

      Comparison or consideration of the anatomical or physiological implications of test results or patient responsiveness to stimuli during the test; Development and modification of the test battery and test protocols; Clinical judgment, assessment, evaluation, and decision-making; Interpretation and reporting observations, in addition to the objective data, that may influence interpretation of the test outcomes; Tests related to implantation of auditory prosthetic devices, central auditory processing, contralateral masking; and/or

      Tests to identify central auditory processing disorders, tinnitus, or nonorganic hearing loss. Audiology codes may be billed under the MPFS by audiologists, physicians, and NPPs using their own NPI in the rendering loop when those professionals personally furnish the test. Physicians and NPPs may not bill for these codes when an audiologist has furnished the service.

   b. Technician Skills.

      There may be subtests, or parts of a battery of tests, that may be appropriately furnished by an educated and experienced technician using a specific protocol under the direction of a supervising physician. These services are identified by local contractor determination as services that do not require professional skills. They may be furnished by a qualified technician under the direct supervision of a physician, but not under the supervision of an audiologist or an NPP. The supervising physician is responsible for rendering and documenting all clinical judgment and for the appropriate provision of the service by the technician.

      A technician may not perform any part of a service that requires professional skills. A technician also may not perform a global service. For example, a technician may not interpret test results or engage in clinical decision-making.

   c. Professional Component (PC)/Technical Component (TC) Split Codes.

      The PC of a PC/TC split code may be billed by the audiologist, physician, or NPP who personally furnishes the service. (Note this is also true in the facility setting.) A physician or NPP may bill for the PC when the physician or NPP furnish the PC and an (unsupervised) audiologist furnishes and bills for the TC. The PC may not be billed if a technician furnishes the service. A physician or NPP may not bill for a PC service furnished by an audiologist. The TC of a PC/TC split code may be billed by the audiologist, physician, or NPP who personally furnishes the service. Physicians may bill the TC for services furnished by technicians when the technician furnishes the service under the direct supervision of that physician. Audiologists and NPPs may not bill for the TC of the service when a technician furnishes the service, even if the technician is supervised by the NPP or audiologist. The "global" service is billed when both the PC and TC of a service are personally furnished by the same audiologist, physician, or NPP. The global service may also be billed by a physician, but not an audiologist or NPP, when a technician furnishes the TC of the service under direct physician supervision and that physician furnishes the PC, including the interpretation and report. d. Tests that are Not Described by Specific CPT Codes. Tests that have no appropriate CPT code may be reported under CPT code 92700 (Unlisted otorhinolaryngological service or procedure).

   e. Tests that are Contractor-Priced. For codes valued by contractors, the contractor determines whether and how much, if applicable, to pay for the service. The contractor sets the requirements for personnel furnishing the tests.

2. Billing for Audiology Services Furnished to Hospital Outpatients.

   All codes may be reported for audiology services furnished in the hospital outpatient setting and, in such cases, the code represents the facility service for the diagnostic test. All audiology services furnished to hospital outpatients must be billed and paid to the hospital under the OPPS or other applicable hospital payment system. The hospital bills its fiscal intermediary or Medicare administrative contractor (A/B MAC) and is paid for the facility resources required to furnish the services, regardless of whether the service is furnished by a physician, NPP, audiologist, or technician.

   Physicians, NPPs, and audiologists cannot bill and be paid for the TC of PC/TC split codes when these services are furnished to hospital outpatients. The associated professional services (represented by the PC or the CPT code for the audiology test which has no PC/TC split) of an enrolled audiologist, physician, or NPP who has reassigned benefits may be billed by the hospital to the carrier or A/B MAC, as appropriate. Alternatively, if the physician, NPP, or audiologist has not assigned benefits, the professional would bill his/her carrier or A/B MAC for the professional services furnished.

   The appropriate revenue code for reporting audiology services is 0470 (Audiology; General Classification). Providers are required to report a line-item date of service per revenue code line for audiology services.

3. Billing for Audiology Services Furnished to Skilled Nursing Facility (SNF) Patients.

   Payment for the facility resources (including the TC of PC/TC split codes) of audiology services provided to Part A inpatients of SNFs is included in the PPS rate. For SNFs, if the beneficiary has Part B but not Part A coverage (e.g., Part A benefits are exhausted), the SNF may elect to bill for audiology services but is not required to do so. As explained in Pub. 100-04, chapter 7, section 40.1, since audiology services furnished during a noncovered SNF stay are not bundled with speech-language pathology services, payment can be made either to the SNF or to the audiology service provider/supplier.

   Audiologists, physicians, and NPPs enrolled in Medicare may bill directly for services rendered to Medicare beneficiaries who are in a SNF stay that is not covered by Part A but who have Part B eligibility. Payment is made based on the MPFS, whether on an institutional or professional claim. For beneficiaries in a noncovered SNF stay, audiology services are payable under Part B when billed by the SNF on an institutional claim as type of bill 22X, or when billed directly by the provider or supplier of the service (the audiologist, physician, or NPP who personally furnishes the test) on a professional claim. For PC/TC split codes, the SNF may elect to bill for the TC of the test on an institutional claim but is not required to bill for the service.

C - Implant Processing

Payment for diagnostic testing of implants, such as cochlear, osseointegrated or brainstem implants, including programming or reprogramming following implantation surgery is not included in the global fee for the surgery.

The diagnostic analysis of a cochlear implant shall be billed using CPT codes 92601 through 92604.

Osseointegrated prosthetic devices should be billed and paid for under provisions of the applicable payment system. For example, payment may differ depending upon whether the device is furnished on an inpatient or outpatient basis, and by a hospital subject to the OPPS, or by a Critical Access Hospital, physician's clinic, or a Federally Qualified Health Center.

D - Aural Rehabilitation Services

General policy for evaluation and treatment of conditions related to the auditory system.

For evaluation of auditory processing disorders and speech-reading or lip-reading by a speech-language pathologist, use the untimed code 92506 with "1" as the unit of service, regardless of the duration of the service on a given day. This "always therapy" evaluation code must be provided by speech-language pathologists according to the policies in Pub. 100-02, chapter 15, sections 220 and 230. The codes 92620 and 92621 are diagnostic audiological tests and may not be used for SLP services.

For treatment of auditory processing disorders or auditory rehabilitation/auditory training (including speech-reading or lip-reading), 92507, and 92508 are used to report a single encounter with "1" as the unit of service, regardless of the duration of the service on a given day. These codes always represent SLP services. See Pub. 100-02, chapter 15, sections 220 and 230 for SLP policies. These SLP evaluation and treatment services are not covered when performed or billed by audiologists, even if they are supervised by physicians or qualified NPPs.

For evaluation of auditory rehabilitation to instruct the use of residual hearing provided by an implant or hearing aid related to hearing loss, the timed codes 92626 and 92627 are used. These are not "always therapy" codes. Evaluation of auditory rehabilitation shall be appropriately provided and billed by an audiologist or speech-language pathologist. Also, these services may be provided incident to a physician's or qualified NPP's service by a speech-language pathologist, or personally by a physician or qualified NPP within their scope of practice. Evaluation of auditory rehabilitation is a covered diagnostic test when performed and billed by an audiologist and is an SLP evaluation service covered under the SLP benefit when performed by a speech-language pathologist.

General policies for post implant services.

The services of a speech-language pathologist may be covered for SLP services provided after implantation of auditory devices. For example, a speech-language pathologist may provide evaluation and treatment of speech, language, cognition, voice, and auditory processing using code 92506 and 92507. Use 92626 and 92627 for auditory (aural) rehabilitation evaluation following cochlear implantation or for other hearing impairments.

For diagnostic testing of cochlear implants, audiologists use codes 92601, 92602, 92603 and 92604. These services may not be provided by speech-language pathologists or others, with the exception of physicians and NPPs who may personally provide the services that are within their scope of practice.

100-4, 12, 30.4

Cardiovascular System (Codes 92950-93799)

A. Echocardiography Contrast Agents

Effective October 1, 2000, physicians may separately bill for contrast agents used in echocardiography. Physicians should use HCPCS Code A9700 (Supply of Injectable Contrast Material for Use in Echocardiography, per study). The type of service code is 9. This code will be carrier-priced.

B. Electronic Analyses of Implantable Cardioverter-defibrillators and Pacemakers

The CPT codes 93731, 93734, 93741 and 93743 are used to report electronic analyses of single or dual chamber pacemakers and single or dual chamber implantable cardioverterdefibrillators. In the office, a physician uses a device called a programmer to obtain information about the status and performance of the device and to evaluate the patient's cardiac rhythm and response to the implanted device.

Advances in information technology now enable physicians to evaluate patients with implanted cardiac devices without requiring the patient to be present in the physician's office. Using a manufacturer's specific monitor/transmitter, a patient can send complete device data and specific cardiac data to a distant receiving station or secure Internet server. The electronic analysis of cardiac device data that is remotely obtained provides immediate and long-term data on the device and clinical data on the patient's cardiac functioning equivalent to that obtained during an in-office evaluation. Physicians should report the electronic analysis of an implanted cardiac device using remotely obtained data as described above with CPT code 93731, 93734, 93741 or 93743, depending on the type of cardiac device implanted in the patient.

100-4, 12, 30.5

Payment for Codes for Chemotherapy Administration and Nonchemotherapy Injections and Infusions

A. General

Codes for Chemotherapy administration and nonchemotherapy injections and infusions include the following three categories of codes in the American Medical Association's Current Procedural Terminology (CPT):

1. Hydration;
2. Therapeutic, prophylactic, and diagnostic injections and infusions (excluding chemotherapy); and
3. Chemotherapy administration.

Physician work related to hydration, injection, and infusion services involves the affirmation of the treatment plan and the supervision (pursuant to incident to requirements) of nonphysician clinical staff.

B. Hydration

The hydration codes are used to report a hydration IV infusion which consists of a prepackaged fluid and /or electrolytes (e.g. normal saline, D5-1/2 normal saline +30 mg EqKC1/liter) but are not used to report infusion of drugs or other substances.

C. Therapeutic, prophylactic, and diagnostic injections and infusions (excluding chemotherapy)

A therapeutic, prophylactic, or diagnostic IV infusion or injection, other than hydration, is for the administration of substances/drugs. The fluid used to administer the drug (s) is incidental hydration and is not separately payable.

If performed to facilitate the infusion or injection or hydration, the following services and items are included and are not separately billable:

1. Use of local anesthesia;
2. IV start;
3. Access to indwelling IV, subcutaneous catheter or port;
4. Flush at conclusion of infusion; and
5. Standard tubing, syringes and supplies.

Payment for the above is included in the payment for the chemotherapy administration or nonchemotherapy injection and infusion service.

If a significant separately identifiable evaluation and management service is performed, the appropriate E & M code should be reported utilizing modifier 25 in addition to the chemotherapy administration or nonchemotherapy injection and infusion service. For an evaluation and management service provided on the same day, a different diagnosis is not required.

The CPT 2006 includes a parenthetical remark immediately following CPT code 90772 (Therapeutic, prophylactic or diagnostic injection; (specify substance or drug); subcutaneous or intramuscular.) It states, "Do not report 90772 for injections given without direct supervision. To report, use 99211." This coding guideline does not apply to Medicare patients. If the RN, LPN or other auxiliary personnel furnishes the injection in the office and the physician is not present in the office to meet the supervision requirement, which is one of the requirements for coverage of an incident to service, then the injection is not covered. The physician would also not report 99211 as this would not be covered as an incident to service.

D. Chemotherapy Administration

Chemotherapy administration codes apply to parenteral administration of nonradionuclide anti-neoplastic drugs; and also to anti-neoplastic agents provided for treatment of noncancer diagnoses (e.g., cyclophosphamide for auto-immune conditions) or to substances such as monoclonal antibody agents, and other biologic response modifiers. The following drugs are commonly considered to fall under the category of monoclonal antibodies: infliximab, rituximab, alemtuzumb, gemtuzumab, and trastuzumab. Drugs commonly considered to fall under the category of hormonal antineoplastics include leuprolide acetate and goserelin acetate. The drugs cited are not intended to be a complete list of drugs that may be administered using the chemotherapy administration codes. Local carriers may provide additional guidance as to which drugs may be considered to be chemotherapy drugs under Medicare.

The administration of anti-anemia drugs and anti-emetic drugs by injection or infusion for cancer patients is not considered chemotherapy administration.

If performed to facilitate the chemotherapy infusion or injection, the following services and items are included and are not separately billable:

1. Use of local anesthesia;
2. IV access;
3. Access to indwelling IV, subcutaneous catheter or port;
4. Flush at conclusion of infusion;
5. Standard tubing, syringes and supplies; and
6. Preparation of chemotherapy agent(s).

Payment for the above is included in the payment for the chemotherapy administration service.

If a significant separately identifiable evaluation and management service is performed, the appropriate E & M code should be reported utilizing modifier 25 in addition to the chemotherapy code. For an evaluation and management service provided on the same day, a different diagnosis is not required.

E. Coding Rules for Chemotherapy Administration and Nonchemotherapy Injections and Infusion Services

Instruct physicians to follow the CPT coding instructions to report chemotherapy administration and nonchemotherapy injections and infusion services with the exception listed in subsection C for CPT code 90772. The physician should be aware of the following specific rules.

When administering multiple infusions, injections or combinations, the physician should report only one "initial" service code unless protocol requires that two separate IV sites must be used. The initial code is the code that best describes the key or primary reason for the encounter and should always be reported irrespective of the order in which the infusions or injections occur. If an injection or infusion is of a subsequent or concurrent nature, even if it is the first such service within that group of services, then a subsequent or concurrent code should be reported. For example, the first IV push given subsequent to an initial one-hour infusion is reported using a subsequent IV push code.

If more than one "initial" service code is billed per day, the carrier shall deny the second initial service code unless the patient has to come back for a separately identifiable service on the same day or has two IV lines per protocol. For these separately identifiable services, instruct the physician to report with modifier 59.

The CPT includes a code for a concurrent infusion in addition to an intravenous infusion for therapy, prophylaxis or diagnosis. Allow only one concurrent infusion per patient per encounter. Do not allow payment for the concurrent infusion billed with modifier 59 unless it is provided during a second encounter on the same day with the patient and is documented in the medical record.

For chemotherapy administration and therapeutic, prophylactic and diagnostic injections and infusions, an intravenous or intra-arterial push is defined as: 1.) an injection in which the healthcare professional is continuously present to administer the substance/drug and observe the patient; or 2.) an infusion of 15 minutes or less.

The physician may report the infusion code for "each additional hour" only if the infusion interval is greater than 30 minutes beyond the 1 hour increment. For example if the patient receives an infusion of a single drug that lasts 1 hour and 45 minutes, the physician would report the "initial" code up to 1 hour and the add-on code for the additional 45 minutes.

Several chemotherapy administration and nonchemotherapy injection and infusion service codes have the following parenthetical descriptor included as a part of the CPT code, "List separately in addition to code for primary procedure." Each of these codes has a physician fee schedule indicator of "ZZZ" meaning this service is allowed if billed with another chemotherapy administration or nonchemotherapy injection and infusion service code.

Do not interpret this parenthetical descriptor to mean that the add-on code can be billed only if it is listed with another drug administration primary code. For example, code 90761 will be ordinarily billed with code 90760. However, there may be instances when only the add-on code, 90761, is billed because an "initial" code from another section in the drug administration codes, instead of 90760, is billed as the primary code.

Pay for code 96523, "Irrigation of implanted venous access device for drug delivery systems," if it is the only service provided that day. If there is a visit or other chemotherapy administration or nonchemotherapy injection or infusion service provided on the same day, payment for 96523 is included in the payment for the other service.

F. Chemotherapy Administration (or Nonchemotherapy Injection and Infusion) and Evaluation and Management Services Furnished on the Same Day

For services furnished on or after January 1, 2004, do not allow payment for CPT code 99211, with or without modifier 25, if it is billed with a nonchemotherapy drug infusion code or a chemotherapy administration code. Apply this policy to code 99211 when it is billed with a diagnostic or therapeutic injection code on or after January 1, 2005.

Physicians providing a chemotherapy administration service or a nonchemotherapy drug infusion service and evaluation and management services, other than CPT code 99211, on the same day must bill in accordance with 30.6.6 using modifier 25. The carriers pay for evaluation and management services provided on the same day as the chemotherapy administration services or a nonchemotherapy injection or infusion service if the evaluation and management service meets the requirements of section 30.6.6 even though the underlying codes do not have global periods. If a chemotherapy service and a significant separately identifiable evaluation and management service are provided on the same day, a different diagnosis is not required.

In 2005, the Medicare physician fee schedule status database indicators for therapeutic and diagnostic injections were changed from T to A. Thus, beginning in 2005, the policy on evaluation and management services, other than 99211, that is applicable to a chemotherapy or a nonchemotherapy injection or infusion service applies equally to these codes.

100-4, 12, 30.6.1

Selection of Level of Evaluation and Management Service

A. Use of CPT Codes

Advise physicians to use CPT codes (level 1 of HCPCS) to code physician services, including evaluation and management services. Medicare will pay for E/M services for specific non-physician practitioners (i.e., nurse practitioner (NP), clinical nurse specialist (CNS) and certified nurse midwife (CNM)) whose Medicare benefit permits them to bill these services. A physician assistant (PA) may also provide a physician service, however, the physician collaboration and general supervision rules as well as all billing rules apply to all the above non-physician practitioners. The service provided must be medically necessary and the service must be within the scope of practice for a non-physician practitioner in the State in which he/she practices. Do not pay for CPT evaluation and management codes billed by physical therapists in independent practice or by occupational therapists in independent practice.

Medical necessity of a service is the overarching criterion for payment in addition to the individual requirements of a CPT code. It would not be medically necessary or appropriate to bill a higher level of evaluation and management service when a lower level of service is warranted. The volume of documentation should not be the primary influence upon which a specific level of service is billed. Documentation should support the level of service reported. The service should be documented during, or as soon as practicable after it is provided in order to maintain an accurate medical record.

B. Selection of Level Of Evaluation and Management Service

Instruct physicians to select the code for the service based upon the content of the service. The duration of the visit is an ancillary factor and does not control the level of the service to be billed unless more than 50 percent of the face-to-face time (for non-inpatient services) or more than 50 percent of the floor time (for inpatient services) is spent providing counseling or coordination of care as described in subsection C.

Any physician or non-physician practitioner (NPP) authorized to bill Medicare services will be paid by the carrier at the appropriate physician fee schedule amount based on the rendering UPIN/PIN.

"Incident to" Medicare Part B payment policy is applicable for office visits when the requirements for "incident to" are met (refer to sections 60.1, 60.2, and 60.3, chapter 15 in IOM 100-02).

SPLIT/SHARED E/M SERVICE

Office/Clinic Setting

In the office/clinic setting when the physician performs the E/M service the service must be reported using the physician's UPIN/PIN. When an E/M service is a shared/split encounter between a physician and a non-physician practitioner (NP, PA, CNS or CNM), the service is considered to have been performed "incident to" if the requirements for "incident to" are met and the patient is an established patient. If "incident to" requirements are not met for the shared/split E/M service, the service must be billed under the NPP's UPIN/PIN, and payment will be made at the appropriate physician fee schedule payment.

Hospital Inpatient/Outpatient/Emergency Department Setting

When a hospital inpatient/hospital outpatient or emergency department E/M is shared between a physician and an NPP from the same group practice and the physician provides any face-to-face portion of the E/M encounter with the patient, the service may be billed under either the physician's or the NPP's UPIN/PIN number. However, if there was no face-to-face encounter between the patient and the physician (e.g., even if the physician participated in the service by only reviewing the patient's medical record) then the service may only be billed under the NPP's UPIN/PIN. Payment will be made at the appropriate physician fee schedule rate based on the UPIN/PIN entered on the claim.

EXAMPLES OF SHARED VISITS

1. If the NPP sees a hospital inpatient in the morning and the physician follows with a later face-to-face visit with the patient on the same day, the physician or the NPP may report the service.
2. In an office setting the NPP performs a portion of an E/M encounter and the physician completes the E/M service. If the "incident to" requirements are met, the physician reports the service. If the "incident to" requirements are not met, the service must be reported using the NPP's UPIN/PIN.

In the rare circumstance when a physician (or NPP) provides a service that does not reflect a CPT code description, the service must be reported as an unlisted service with CPT code 99499. A description of the service provided must accompany the claim. The carrier has the discretion to value the service when the service does not meet the full terms of a CPT code description (e.g., only a history is performed). The carrier also determines the payment based on the applicable percentage of the physician fee schedule depending on whether the claim is paid at the physician rate or the non-physician practitioner rate. CPT modifier -52 (reduced services) must not be used with an evaluation and management service. Medicare does not recognize modifier -52 for this purpose.

C. Selection Of Level Of Evaluation and Management Service Based On Duration Of Coordination Of Care and/or Counseling

Advise physicians that when counseling and/or coordination of care dominates (more than 50 percent) the face-to-face physician/patient encounter or the floor time (in the case of inpatient services), time is the key or controlling factor in selecting the level of service. In general, to bill an E/M code, the physician must complete at least 2 out of 3 criteria applicable to the type/level of service provided. However, the physician may document time spent with the patient in conjunction with the medical decision-making involved and a description of the coordination of care or counseling provided. Documentation must be in sufficient detail to support the claim.

EXAMPLE: A cancer patient has had all preliminary studies completed and a medical decision to implement chemotherapy. At an office visit the physician discusses the treatment options and subsequent lifestyle effects of treatment the patient may encounter or is experiencing. The physician need not complete a history and physical examination in order to select the level of service. The time spent in counseling/coordination of care and medical decision-making will determine the level of service billed.

The code selection is based on the total time of the face-to-face encounter or floor time, not just the counseling time. The medical record must be documented in sufficient detail to justify the selection of the specific code if time is the basis for selection of the code.

In the office and other outpatient setting, counseling and/or coordination of care must be provided in the presence of the patient if the time spent providing those services is used to determine the level of service reported. Face-to-face time refers to the time with the physician only. Counseling by other staff is not considered to be part of the face-to-face physician/patient encounter time. Therefore, the time spent by the other staff is not considered in selecting the appropriate level of service. The code used depends upon the physician service provided.

In an inpatient setting, the counseling and/or coordination of care must be provided at the bedside or on the patient's hospital floor or unit that is associated with an individual patient. Time spent counseling the patient or coordinating the patient's care after the patient has left the office or the physician has left the patient's floor or begun to care for another patient on the floor is not considered when selecting the level of service to be reported.

The duration of counseling or coordination of care that is provided face-to-face or on the floor may be estimated but that estimate, along with the total duration of the visit, must be recorded when time is used for the selection of the level of a service that involves predominantly coordination of care or counseling.

D. Use of Highest Levels of Evaluation and Management Codes

Contractors must advise physicians that to bill the highest levels of visit codes, the services furnished must meet the definition of the code (e.g., to bill a Level 5 new patient visit, the history must meet CPT's definition of a comprehensive history).

The comprehensive history must include a review of all the systems and a complete past (medical and surgical) family and social history obtained at that visit. In the case of an established patient, it is acceptable for a physician to review the existing record and update it to reflect only changes in the patient's medical, family, and social history from the last encounter, but the physician must review the entire history for it to be considered a comprehensive history.

The comprehensive examination may be a complete single system exam such as cardiac, respiratory, psychiatric, or a complete multi-system examination.

100-4, 12, 30.6.1.1

Initial Preventive Physical Examination (IPPE) and Annual Wellness Visit (AWV)

A. Definitions

1. Initial Preventive Physical Examination (IPPE)

   The initial preventive physical examination (IPPE), or "Welcome to Medicare Visit" (WMV) is a preventive evaluation and management service (E/M), allowed by Section 611 of the Medicare Prescription Drug Improvement and Modernization Act (MMA) of 2003, that includes:

   (1) review of the individual's medical and social history with attention to modifiable risk factors for disease detection,

   (2) review of the individual's potential (risk factors) for depression or other mood disorders,

   (3) review of the individual's functional ability and level of safety,

   (4) a physical examination to include measurement of the individual's height, weight, blood pressure, a visual acuity screen, and other factors as deemed appropriate by the examining physician or qualified nonphysician practitioner (NPP),

   (5) performance and interpretation of an electrocardiogram (EKG),

   (6) education, counseling, and referral, as deemed appropriate, based on the results of the review and evaluation services described in the previous 5 elements, and,

   (7) education, counseling, and referral including a brief written plan (e.g., a checklist or alternative) provided to the individual for obtaining the appropriate screening and other preventive services.

   Effective January 1, 2007, Section 5112 of the Deficit Reduction Act of 2005 allows for one ultrasound screening for Abdominal Aortic Aneurysm (AAA), HCPCS code G0389, as a result of a referral from an IPPE. This service is not subject to the Part B annual deductible. For AAA physician/practitioner billing, correct coding, and payment policy, refer to chapter 18, §110, of this manual.

   Effective January 1, 2009, Section 101 (b) of the Medicare Improvement for Patients and Providers Act (MIPPA) of 2008 requires the addition of the measurement of an individual's body mass index and, upon an individual's consent, end-of-life planning, to the IPPE. Also, effective January 1, 2009, MIPPA removes the screening electrocardiogram (EKG) as a mandatory service of the IPPE. MIPPA requires that there be education, counseling, and referral for an EKG, as appropriate. This is a once-in-a-lifetime screening EKG as a result of a referral from an IPPE.

   The MIPPA of 2008 allows for possible future payment for additional preventive services not otherwise described in Title XVIII of the Social Security Act (the Act) that identify medical conditions or risk factors for eligible individuals if the Secretary determines through the national coverage determination (NCD) process (as defined in Section 1869(f)(1)(B) of the Act) that they are: (1) reasonable and necessary for the prevention or early detection of illness or disability, (2) recommended with a grade of A or B by the United States Preventive Services Task Force (USPSTF), and, (3) appropriate for individuals entitled to benefits under Part A or enrolled under Part B, or both. MIPPA requires that there be education, counseling, and referral for additional preventive services, as appropriate, under the IPPE, if the Secretary determines in the future that such services are covered.

2. Annual Wellness Visit (AWV)

   Effective January 1, 2011, Section 4103 of the Affordable Care Act (ACA), allows for a preventive physical examination, called the annual wellness visit (AWV), and includes personal prevention plan services (PPPS). The AWV is a new annual Medicare preventive physical examination, available for eligible beneficiaries, and identified by new HCPCS codes G0438 (Annual wellness visit, including PPPS, first visit) and G0439 (Annual wellness visit, including PPPS, subsequent visit). Definitions relative to the AWV are included at Pub. 100-02, Medicare Benefit Policy Manual, chapter 15, section 280.5.

   First AWV services providing PPPS (HCPCS G0438) are a 'one time' allowed Medicare benefit and include the following key elements furnished to an eligible beneficiary by a health professional:

   - Establishment of the individual's medical/family history,
   - Measurement of the individual's height, weight, body mass index (or waist circumference, if appropriate), blood pressure (BP), and other routine measurements as deemed appropriate, based on the individual's medical and family history,
   - Establishment of a list of current providers and suppliers that are regularly involved in providing medical care to the individual,
   - Detection of any cognitive impairment that the individual may have,
   - Review of an individual's potential risk factors for depression , including current or past experiences with depression or other mood disorders, based on the use of an appropriate screening instrument for persons without a current diagnosis of depression, which the health professional may select from various available standardized screening tests designed for this purpose and recognized by national professional medical organizations,
   - Review of the individual's functional ability and level of safety, based on direct observation of the individual, or the use of appropriate screening questions or a screening questionnaire, which the health professional may select from various available screening questions or standardized questionnaires designed for this purpose and recognized by national professional medical organizations,
   - Establishment of a written screening schedule for the individual, such as a checklist for the next 5 to 10 years, as appropriate, based on recommendations of the USPSTF and Advisory Committee of Immunizations Practices (ACIP), the individual's health status, screening history, and age-appropriate preventive services covered by Medicare,
   - Establishment of a list of risk factors and conditions of which primary, secondary, or tertiary interventions are recommended or underway for the individual, including any mental health conditions or any such risk factors or conditions that have been identified through an IPPE, and a list of treatment options and their associated risks and benefits,
   - Provision of personalized health advice to the individual and a referral, as appropriate, to health education or preventive counseling services or programs aimed at reducing identified risk factors and improving self-management or community-based lifestyle interventions to reduce health risks and promote self-management and wellness, including weight loss, physical activity, smoking cessation, fall prevention, and nutrition, and,
   - Any other element(s) determined appropriate by the Secretary through the NCD process.

   Subsequent AWV services providing PPPS (HCPCS G0439) include the following key elements furnished to an eligible beneficiary by a health professional:

   - Update to the individual's medical /family history,
   - Measurements of an individual's weight (or waist circumference), BP, and other routine measurements as deemed appropriate, based on the individual's medical and family history,
   - Update to the list of the individual's current medical providers and suppliers that are regularly involved in providing medical care to the individual as that list was developed for the first AWV providing PPPS,
   - Detection of any cognitive impairment that the individual may have,
   - Update to the individual's written screening schedule as developed at the first AWV providing PPPS,
   - Update to the individual's list of risk factors and conditions for which primary, secondary, or tertiary interventions are recommended or are underway for the individual, as that list was developed at the first AWV providing PPPS,
   - Furnish appropriate personalized health advice to the individual and a referral, as appropriate, to health education or preventive counseling services or programs, and,
   - Any other element determined appropriate by the Secretary through the NCD process.

   Preventive services are separately covered under Medicare Part B. See chapter 18 of this manual.

B. Who May Perform

The IPPE and the AWV may be performed by a doctor of medicine or osteopathy as defined in Section 1861(r) (1) of the Act, by a qualified NPP (nurse practitioner, physician assistant or clinical nurse specialist), or for the AWV, by a health professional (a medical professional including a health educator, registered dietitian, nutrition professional, or other licensed practitioner) or a team of such medical professionals who are working under the direct supervision of a physician. The contractor pays the appropriate physician fee schedule amount based on the rendering National Provider Identification (NPI) number.

C. Eligibility

1. IPPE

   As a result of the MMA 2003, Medicare will pay for one IPPE per beneficiary per lifetime. A beneficiary is eligible when he/she first enrolls in Medicare Part B. For beneficiaries enrolled on or after January 1, 2005, beneficiaries must have received their IPPE within the first 6 months of Medicare coverage. The MIPPA extends the eligibility period for an IPPE to 12 months effective January 1, 2009.

   Beneficiaries in their first 12 months of Part B coverage will continue to be eligible for only the IPPE. Medicare continues to pay for only one IPPE per beneficiary per lifetime.

2. AWV

As a result of the ACA, effective January 1, 2011, Medicare will pay for an AWV for a beneficiary who is no longer within 12 months after the effective date of his/her first Medicare Part B coverage period, and he/she has not received either an IPPE or an

AWV providing PPPS within the past 12 months. Medicare pays for only one first AWV (HCPCS G0438), per beneficiary per lifetime, and all subsequent wellness visits must be billed as a subsequent AWV (HCPCS G0439).

Beneficiaries in their first 12 months of Part B coverage will continue to be eligible for only the IPPE (see 30.6.1.1.A.1).

D. Deductible and Coinsurance

1. IPPE

The Medicare deductible and coinsurance apply for the IPPE provided before January 1, 2009.

The Medicare deductible is waived effective for the IPPE provided on or after January 1, 2009. However, the applicable coinsurance continues to apply for the IPPE provided on or after January 1, 2009.

As a result of the ACA, effective for the IPPE provided on or after January 1, 2011, the Medicare deductible and coinsurance (for HCPCS code G0402 only) are waived.

2. AWV

As a result of the ACA, effective January 1, 2011, the Medicare deductible and coinsurance for the AWV (HCPCS G0438 and G0439) are waived.

E. The EKG Component of the IPPE

Under the MMA of 2003, if the physician or qualified NPP is not able to perform both the examination and the screening EKG, an arrangement may be made to ensure that another physician or entity performs the screening EKG and reports the EKG separately using the appropriate HCPCS G code(s) identified in F.1. of this section. When the screening EKG is performed, the primary physician or qualified NPP shall document the results of the screening EKG into the beneficiary's medical record to complete and bill for the IPPE benefit.

NOTE: Both components of the IPPE (the examination and the screening EKG) must be performed before the claims can be submitted by the physician, qualified NPP, and/or entity.

MIPPA 2008 changes the once-in-a-lifetime screening EKG from a mandated service to a service that may be performed, as appropriate, with a referral from an IPPE. When an EKG is furnished with the IPPE, the deductible and coinsurance will continue to apply for EKG services only.

F. HCPCS Codes Used to Bill the IPPE or AWV

1. HCPCS Codes Used to Bill the IPPE

For IPPE and EKG services provided prior to January 1, 2009, the physician or qualified NPP shall bill HCPCS code G0344 for the physical examination performed face-to-face, and HCPCS code G0366 for performing a screening EKG that includes both the interpretation and report. If the primary physician or qualified NPP performs only the examination, he/she shall bill HCPCS code G0344 only. The physician or entity that performs the screening EKG that includes both the interpretation and report shall bill HCPCS code G0366. The physician or entity that performs the screening EKG tracing only (without interpretation and report) shall bill HCPCS code G0367. The physician or entity that performs the interpretation and report only (without the EKG tracing) shall bill HCPCS code G0368. Medicare will pay for a screening EKG only as part of the IPPE. HCPCS codes G0344, G0366, G0367 and G0368 will not be billable codes effective on or after January 1, 2009.

Effective for a beneficiary who has the IPPE on or after January 1, 2009, and within his/her 12-month enrollment period of Medicare Part B, the IPPE and screening EKG services are billable with the appropriate HCPCS G code(s).

The physician or qualified NPP shall bill HCPCS code G0402 for the physical examination performed face-to-face with the patient.

The physician or entity shall bill HCPCS code G0403 for performing the complete screening EKG that includes the tracing, interpretation and report.

The physician or entity that performs the screening EKG tracing only (without interpretation and report) shall bill HCPCS code G0404.

The physician or entity that performs the screening EKG interpretation and report only, (without the EKG tracing) shall bill HCPCS code G0405.

2. HCPCS Codes Used to Bill the AWV

For the first AWV provided on or after January 1, 2011, the health professional shall bill HCPCS G0438 (Annual wellness visit, including PPPS, first visit). This is a once per beneficiary per lifetime allowable Medicare benefit.

All subsequent AWVs shall be billed with HCPCS G0439 (Annual Wellness Visit, including PPPS, subsequent visit). In the event that a beneficiary selects a new health professional to complete a subsequent AWV, the new health professional will continue to bill the subsequent AWV with HCPCS G0439.

NOTE: For an IPPE or AWV performed during the global period of surgery refer to chapter 12, §30.6.6 of this manual for reporting instructions.

G. Documentation for the IPPE or AWV

The physician and qualified NPP, or for AWV the health professional, shall use the appropriate screening tools typically used in routine physician practice. Physicians, qualified NPPs, and medical professionals are required to use the 1995 and 1997 E/M documentation guidelines to document the medical record with the appropriate clinical information. (http://www.cms.hhs.gov/MLNEdWebGuide/25_EMDOC.asp). All referrals and a written medical plan must be included in this documentation.

H. Reporting a Medically Necessary E/M Service Furnished During the Same Encounter as an IPPE or AWV

When the physician or qualified NPP, or for AWV the health professional, provides a significant, separately identifiable medically necessary E/M service in addition to the IPPE or an AWV, CPT codes 99201–99215 may be reported depending on the clinical appropriateness of the circumstances. CPT Modifier ,Äì25 shall be appended to the medically necessary E/M service identifying this service as a significant, separately identifiable service from the IPPE or AWV code reported (HCPCS code G0344 or G0402, whichever applies based on the date the IPPE is performed, or HCPCS code G0438 or G0439 whichever AWV code applies).

NOTE: Some of the components of a medically necessary E/M service (e.g., a portion of history or physical exam portion) may have been part of the IPPE or AWV and should not be included when determining the most appropriate level of E/M service to be billed for the medically necessary, separately identifiable, E/M service.

100-4, 12, 30.6.2

Billing for Medically Necessary Visit on Same Occasion as Preventive Medicine Service

See Chapter 18 for payment for covered preventive services.

When a physician furnishes a Medicare beneficiary a covered visit at the same place and on the same occasion as a noncovered preventive medicine service (CPT codes 99381- 99397), consider the covered visit to be provided in lieu of a part of the preventive medicine service of equal value to the visit. A preventive medicine service (CPT codes 99381-99397) is a noncovered service. The physician may charge the beneficiary, as a charge for the noncovered remainder of the service, the amount by which the physician's current established charge for the preventive medicine service exceeds his/her current established charge for the covered visit. Pay for the covered visit based on the lesser of the fee schedule amount or the physician's actual charge for the visit. The physician is not required to give the beneficiary written advance notice of noncoverage of the part of the visit that constitutes a routine preventive visit. However, the physician is responsible for notifying the patient in advance of his/her liability for the charges for services that are not medically necessary to treat the illness or injury.

There could be covered and noncovered procedures performed during this encounter (e.g., screening x-ray, EKG, lab tests.). These are considered individually. Those procedures which are for screening for asymptomatic conditions are considered noncovered and, therefore, no payment is made. Those procedures ordered to diagnose or monitor a symptom, medical condition, or treatment are evaluated for medical necessity and, if covered, are paid.

100-4, 12, 30.6.4

Evaluation and Management (E/M) Services Furnished Incident to Physician's Service by Nonphysician Practitioners

When evaluation and management services are furnished incident to a physician's service by a nonphysician practitioner, the physician may bill the CPT code that describes the evaluation and management service furnished.

When evaluation and management services are furnished incident to a physician's service by a nonphysician employee of the physician, not as part of a physician service, the physician bills code 99211 for the service.

A physician is not precluded from billing under the "incident to" provision for services provided by employees whose services cannot be paid for directly under the Medicare program. Employees of the physician may provide services incident to the physician's service, but the physician alone is permitted to bill Medicare.

Services provided by employees as "incident to" are covered when they meet all the requirements for incident to and are medically necessary for the individual needs of the patient.

100-4, 12, 30.6.7

Payment for Office or Other Outpatient Evaluation and Management (E/M) Visits (Codes 99201 - 99215)

A Definition of New Patient for Selection of E/M Visit Code

Interpret the phrase "new patient" to mean a patient who has not received any professional services, i.e., E/M service or other face-to-face service (e.g., surgical procedure) from the physician or physician group practice (same physician specialty) within the previous 3 years. For example, if a professional component of a previous procedure is billed in a 3 year time period, e.g., a lab interpretation is billed and no E/M service or other face-to-face service with the patient is performed, then this patient remains a new patient for the initial visit. An interpretation of a diagnostic test, reading an x-ray or EKG etc., in the absence of an E/M service or other face-to-face service with the patient does not affect the designation of a new patient.

B. Office/Outpatient E/M Visits Provided on Same Day for Unrelated Problems

As for all other E/M services except where specifically noted, carriers may not pay two E/M office visits billed by a physician (or physician of the same specialty from the same group practice) for the same beneficiary on the same day unless the physician documents that the visits were for unrelated problems in the office or outpatient setting which could not be provided during the same encounter (e.g., office visit for blood pressure medication evaluation, followed five hours later by a visit for evaluation of leg pain following an accident).

C. Office/Outpatient or Emergency Department E/M Visit on Day of Admission to Nursing Facility
Carriers may not pay a physician for an emergency department visit or an office visit and a comprehensive nursing facility assessment on the same day. Bundle E/M visits on the same date provided in sites other than the nursing facility into the initial nursing facility care code when performed on the same date as the nursing facility admission by the same physician.

D. Drug Administration Services and E/M Visits Billed on Same Day of Service
Carriers must advise physicians that CPT code 99211 cannot be paid if it is billed with a drug administration service such as a chemotherapy or nonchemotherapy drug infusion code (effective January 1, 2004). This drug administration policy was expanded in the Physician Fee Schedule Final Rule, November 15, 2004, to also include a therapeutic or diagnostic injection code (effective January 1, 2005). Therefore, when a medically necessary, significant and separately identifiable E/M service (which meets a higher complexity level than CPT code 99211) is performed, in addition to one of these drug administration services, the appropriate E/M CPT code should be reported with modifier -25. Documentation should support the level of E/M service billed. For an E/M service provided on the same day, a different diagnosis is not required.

100-4, 12, 30.6.8

Payment for Hospital Observation Services (Codes 99217-99220) and Observation or Inpatient Care Services (Including Admission and Discharge Services – (Codes 99234-99236))

A. Who May Bill Observation Care Codes
Observation care is a well-defined set of specific, clinically appropriate services, which include ongoing short term treatment, assessment, and reassessment, that are furnished while a decision is being made regarding whether patients will require further treatment as hospital inpatients or if they are able to be discharged from the hospital. Observation services are commonly ordered for patients who present to the emergency department and who then require a significant period of treatment or monitoring in order to make a decision concerning their admission or discharge.

In only rare and exceptional cases do reasonable and necessary outpatient observation services span more than 48 hours. In the majority of cases, the decision whether to discharge a patient from the hospital following resolution of the reason for the observation care or to admit the patient as an inpatient can be made in less than 48 hours, usually in less than 24 hours.

Contractors pay for initial observation care billed by only the physician who ordered hospital outpatient observation services and was responsible for the patient during his/her observation care. A physician who does not have inpatient admitting privileges but who is authorized to furnish hospital outpatient observation services may bill these codes.

For a physician to bill observation care codes, there must be a medical observation record for the patient which contains dated and timed physician's orders regarding the observation services the patient is to receive, nursing notes, and progress notes prepared by the physician while the patient received observation services. This record must be in addition to any record prepared as a result of an emergency department or outpatient clinic encounter.

Payment for an initial observation care code is for all the care rendered by the ordering physician on the date the patient's observation services began. All other physicians who furnish consultations or additional evaluations or services while the patient is receiving hospital outpatient observation services must bill the appropriate outpatient service codes.

For example, if an internist orders observation services and asks another physician to additionally evaluate the patient, only the internist may bill the initial and subsequent observation care codes. The other physician who evaluates the patient must bill the new or established office or other outpatient visit codes as appropriate.

For information regarding hospital billing of observation services, see Chapter 4, §290.

B. Physician Billing for Observation Care Following Initiation of Observation Services
Similar to initial observation codes, payment for a subsequent observation care code is for all the care rendered by the treating physician on the day(s) other than the initial or discharge date. All other physicians who furnish consultations or additional evaluations or services while the patient is receiving hospital outpatient observation services must bill the appropriate outpatient service codes.

When a patient receives observation care for less than 8 hours on the same calendar date, the Initial Observation Care, from CPT code range 99218–99220, shall be reported by the physician. The Observation Care Discharge Service, CPT code 99217, shall not be reported for this scenario.

When a patient is admitted for observation care and then is discharged on a different calendar date, the physician shall report Initial Observation Care, from CPT code range 99218–99220, and CPT observation care discharge CPT code 99217. On the rare occasion when a patient remains in observation care for 3 days, the physician shall report an initial observation care code (99218-99220) for the first day of observation care, a subsequent observation care code (99224-99226) for the second day of observation care, and an observation care discharge CPT code 99217 for the observation care on the discharge date. When observation care continues beyond 3 days, the physician shall report a subsequent observation care code (99224-99226) for each day between the first day of observation care and the discharge date.

When a patient receives observation care for a minimum of 8 hours, but less than 24 hours, and is discharged on the same calendar date, Observation or Inpatient Care Services (Including Admission and Discharge Services) from CPT code range 99234–99236 shall be reported. The observation discharge, CPT code 99217, cannot also be reported for this scenario.

C. Documentation Requirements for Billing Observation or Inpatient Care Services (Including Admission and Discharge Services)
The physician shall satisfy the E/M documentation guidelines for furnishing observation care or inpatient hospital care. In addition to meeting the documentation requirements for history, examination, and medical decision making, documentation in the medical record shall include:

- Documentation stating the stay for observation care or inpatient hospital care involves 8 hours, but less than 24 hours;
- Documentation identifying the billing physician was present and personally performed the services; and
- Documentation identifying the order for observation services, progress notes, and discharge notes were written by the billing physician.

In the rare circumstance when a patient receives observation services for more than 2 calendar dates, the physician shall bill observation services furnished on day(s) other than the initial or discharge date using subsequent observation care codes. The physician may not use the subsequent hospital care codes since the patient is not an inpatient of the hospital.

D. Admission to Inpatient Status Following Observation Care
If the same physician who ordered hospital outpatient observation services also admits the patient to inpatient status before the end of the date on which the patient began receiving hospital outpatient observation services, pay only an initial hospital visit for the evaluation and management services provided on that date. Medicare payment for the initial hospital visit includes all services provided to the patient on the date of admission by that physician, regardless of the site of service. The physician may not bill an initial or subsequent observation care code for services on the date that he or she admits the patient to inpatient status. If the patient is admitted to inpatient status from hospital outpatient observation care subsequent to the date of initiation of observation services, the physician must bill an initial hospital visit for the services provided on that date. The physician may not bill the hospital observation discharge management code (code 99217) or an outpatient/office visit for the care provided while the patient received hospital outpatient observation services on the date of admission to inpatient status.

E. Hospital Observation Services During Global Surgical Period
The global surgical fee includes payment for hospital observation (codes 99217, 99218, 99219, 99220, 99224, 99225, 99226, 99234, 99235, and 99236) services unless the criteria for use of CPT modifiers "-24," "-25," or "-57" are met. Contractors must pay for these services in addition to the global surgical fee only if both of the following requirements are met:

- The hospital observation service meets the criteria needed to justify billing it with CPT modifiers "-24," "-25," or "-57" (decision for major surgery); and
- The hospital observation service furnished by the surgeon meets all of the criteria for the hospital observation code billed.

Examples of the decision for surgery during a hospital observation period are:

- An emergency department physician orders hospital outpatient observation services for a patient with a head injury. A neurosurgeon is called in to evaluate the need for surgery while the patient is receiving observation services and decides that the patient requires surgery. The surgeon would bill a new or established office or other outpatient visit code as appropriate with the "-57" modifier to indicate that the decision for surgery was made during the evaluation. The surgeon must bill the office or other outpatient visit code because the patient receiving hospital outpatient observation services is not an inpatient of the hospital. Only the physician who ordered hospital outpatient observation services may bill for observation care.
- A neurosurgeon orders hospital outpatient observation services for a patient with a head injury. During the observation period, the surgeon makes the decision for surgery. The surgeon would bill the appropriate level of hospital observation code with the "-57" modifier to indicate that the decision for surgery was made while the surgeon was providing hospital observation care.

Examples of hospital observation services during the postoperative period of a surgery are:

- A surgeon orders hospital outpatient observation services for a patient with abdominal pain from a kidney stone on the 80th day following a TURP (performed by that surgeon). The surgeon decides that the patient does not require surgery. The surgeon would bill the observation code with CPT modifier "-24" and documentation to support that the observation services are unrelated to the surgery.
- A surgeon orders hospital outpatient observation services for a patient with abdominal pain on the 80th day following a TURP (performed by that surgeon). While the patient is receiving hospital outpatient observation services, the surgeon decides that the patient requires kidney surgery. The surgeon would bill

the observation code with HCPCS modifier "-57" to indicate that the decision for surgery was made while the patient was receiving hospital outpatient observation services. The subsequent surgical procedure would be reported with modifier "-79."

- A surgeon orders hospital outpatient observation services for a patient with abdominal pain on the 20th day following a resection of the colon (performed by that surgeon). The surgeon determines that the patient requires no further colon surgery and discharges the patient. The surgeon may not bill for the observation services furnished during the global period because they were related to the previous surgery.

An example of a billable hospital observation service on the same day as a procedure is when a physician repairs a laceration of the scalp in the emergency department for a patient with a head injury and then subsequently orders hospital outpatient observation services for that patient. The physician would bill the observation code with a CPT modifier 25 and the procedure code.

100-4, 12, 30.6.9

Payment for Inpatient Hospital Visits - General (Codes 99221 - 99239)

A. Hospital Visit and Critical Care on Same Day

When a hospital inpatient or office/outpatient evaluation and management service (E/M) are furnished on a calendar date at which time the patient does not require critical care and the patient subsequently requires critical care both the critical Care Services (CPT codes 99291 and 99292) and the previous E/M service may be paid on the same date of service. Hospital emergency department services are not paid for the same date as critical care services when provided by the same physician to the same patient.

During critical care management of a patient those services that do not meet the level of critical care shall be reported using an inpatient hospital care service with CPT Subsequent Hospital Care using a code from CPT code range 99231–99233.

Both Initial Hospital Care (CPT codes 99221–99223) and Subsequent Hospital Care codes are "per diem" services and may be reported only once per day by the same physician or physicians of the same specialty from the same group practice.

Physicians and qualified nonphysician practitioners (NPPs) are advised to retain documentation for discretionary contractor review should claims be questioned for both hospital care and critical care claims. The retained documentation shall support claims for critical care when the same physician or physicians of the same specialty in a group practice report critical care services for the same patient on the same calendar date as other E/M services.

B. Two Hospital Visits Same Day

Contractors pay a physician for only one hospital visit per day for the same patient, whether the problems seen during the encounters are related or not. The inpatient hospital visit descriptors contain the phrase "per day" which means that the code and the payment established for the code represent all services provided on that date. The physician should select a code that reflects all services provided during the date of the service.

C. Hospital Visits Same Day But by Different Physicians

In a hospital inpatient situation involving one physician covering for another, if physician A sees the patient in the morning and physician B, who is covering for A, sees the same patient in the evening, contractors do not pay physician B for the second visit. The hospital visit descriptors include the phrase "per day" meaning care for the day.

If the physicians are each responsible for a different aspect of the patient's care, pay both visits if the physicians are in different specialties and the visits are billed with different diagnoses. There are circumstances where concurrent care may be billed by physicians of the same specialty.

D. Visits to Patients in Swing Beds

If the inpatient care is being billed by the hospital as inpatient hospital care, the hospital care codes apply. If the inpatient care is being billed by the hospital as nursing facility care, then the nursing facility codes apply.

100-4, 12, 30.6.9.1

Payment for Initial Hospital Care Services (Codes 99221–99223 and Observation or Inpatient Care Services (Including Admission and Discharge Services) (Codes 99234–99236)

A. Initial Hospital Care From Emergency Room

Contractors pay for an initial hospital care service if a physician sees a patient in the emergency room and decides to admit the person to the hospital. They do not pay for both E/M services. Also, they do not pay for an emergency department visit by the same physician on the same date of service. When the patient is admitted to the hospital via another site of service (e.g., hospital emergency department, physician's office, nursing facility), all services provided by the physician in conjunction with that admission are considered part of the initial hospital care when performed on the same date as the admission.

B. Initial Hospital Care on Day Following Visit

Contractors pay both visits if a patient is seen in the office on one date and admitted to the hospital on the next date, even if fewer than 24 hours has elapsed between the visit and the admission.

C. Initial Hospital Care and Discharge on Same Day

When the patient is admitted to inpatient hospital care for less than 8 hours on the same date, then Initial Hospital Care, from CPT code range 99221–99223, shall be reported by the physician. The Hospital Discharge Day Management service, CPT codes 99238 or 99239, shall not be reported for this scenario.

When a patient is admitted to inpatient initial hospital care and then discharged on a different calendar date, the physician shall report an Initial Hospital Care from CPT code range 99221–99223 and a Hospital Discharge Day Management service, CPT code 99238 or 99239.

When a patient has been admitted to inpatient hospital care for a minimum of 8 hours but less than 24 hours and discharged on the same calendar date, Observation or Inpatient Hospital Care Services (Including Admission and Discharge Services), from CPT code range 99234–99236, shall be reported.

D. Documentation Requirements for Billing Observation or Inpatient Care Services (Including Admission and Discharge Services)

The physician shall satisfy the E/M documentation guidelines for admission to and discharge from inpatient observation or hospital care. In addition to meeting the documentation requirements for history, examination and medical decision making documentation in the medical record shall include:

- Documentation stating the stay for hospital treatment or observation care status involves 8 hours but less than 24 hours;
- Documentation identifying the billing physician was present and personally performed the services; and
- Documentation identifying the admission and discharge notes were written by the billing physician.

E. Physician Services Involving Transfer From One Hospital to Another; Transfer Within Facility to Prospective Payment System (PPS) Exempt Unit of Hospital; Transfer From One Facility to Another Separate Entity Under Same Ownership and/or Part of Same Complex; or Transfer From One Department to Another Within Single Facility

Physicians may bill both the hospital discharge management code and an initial hospital care code when the discharge and admission do not occur on the same day if the transfer is between:

- Different hospitals;
- Different facilities under common ownership which do not have merged records; or
- Between the acute care hospital and a PPS exempt unit within the same hospital when there are no merged records.

In all other transfer circumstances, the physician should bill only the appropriate level of subsequent hospital care for the date of transfer.

F. Initial Hospital Care Service History and Physical That Is Less Than Comprehensive

When a physician performs a visit that meets the definition of a Level 5 office visit several days prior to an admission and on the day of admission performs less than a comprehensive history and physical, he or she should report the office visit that reflects the services furnished and also report the lowest level initial hospital care code (i.e., code 99221) for the initial hospital admission. Contractors pay the office visit as billed and the Level 1 initial hospital care code.

Physicians who provide an initial visit to a patient during inpatient hospital care that meets the minimum key component work and/or medical necessity requirements shall report an initial hospital care code (99221-99223). The principal physician of record shall append modifier "-AI" (Principal Physician of Record) to the claim for the initial hospital care code. This modifier will identify the physician who oversees the patient's care from all other physicians who may be furnishing specialty care.

Physicians may bill initial hospital care service codes (99221-99223), for services that were reported with CPT consultation codes (99241–99255) prior to January 1, 2010, when the furnished service and documentation meet the minimum key component work and/or medical necessity requirements. Physicians must meet all the requirements of the initial hospital care codes, including "a detailed or comprehensive history" and "a detailed or comprehensive examination" to report CPT code 99221, which are greater than the requirements for consultation codes 99251 and 99252.

Subsequent hospital care CPT codes 99231 and 99232, respectively, require "a problem focused interval history" and "an expanded problem focused interval history." An E/M service that could be described by CPT consultation code 99251 or 99252 could potentially meet the component work and medical necessity requirements to report 99231 or 99232. Physicians may report a subsequent hospital care CPT code for services that were reported as CPT consultation codes (99241–99255) prior to January 1, 2010, where the medical record appropriately demonstrates that the work and medical necessity requirements are met for reporting a subsequent hospital care code (under the level selected), even though the reported code is for the provider's first E/M service to the inpatient during the hospital stay.

Reporting CPT code 99499 (Unlisted evaluation and management service) should be limited to cases where there is no other specific E/M code payable by Medicare that describes that service.

Reporting CPT code 99499 requires submission of medical records and contractor manual medical review of the service prior to payment. Contractors shall expect reporting under these circumstances to be unusual.

G. Initial Hospital Care Visits by Two Different M.D.s or D.O.s When They Are Involved in Same Admission
In the inpatient hospital setting all physicians (and qualified nonphysician practitioners where permitted) who perform an initial evaluation may bill the initial hospital care codes (99221–99223) or nursing facility care codes (99304–99306). Contractors consider only one M.D. or D.O. to be the principal physician of record (sometimes referred to as the admitting physician.) The principal physician of record is identified in Medicare as the physician who oversees the patient's care from other physicians who may be furnishing specialty care. Only the principal physician of record shall append modifier "-AI" (Principal Physician of Record) in addition to the E/M code. Follow-up visits in the facility setting shall be billed as subsequent hospital care visits and subsequent nursing facility care visits.

100-4, 12, 30.6.9.2

Subsequent Hospital Visit and Hospital Discharge Day Management (Codes 99231 - 99239)

A. Subsequent Hospital Visits During the Global Surgery Period
(Refer to Secs.40-40.4 on global surgery)

The Medicare physician fee schedule payment amount for surgical procedures includes all services (e.g., evaluation and management visits) that are part of the global surgery payment; therefore, contractors shall not pay more than that amount when a bill is fragmented for staged procedures.

B. Hospital Discharge Day Management Service
Hospital Discharge Day Management Services, CPT code 99238 or 99239 is a face-to-face evaluation and management (E/M) service between the attending physician and the patient. The E/M discharge day management visit shall be reported for the date of the actual visit by the physician or qualified nonphysician practitioner even if the patient is discharged from the facility on a different calendar date. Only one hospital discharge day management service is payable per patient per hospital stay.

Only the attending physician of record reports the discharge day management service. Physicians or qualified nonphysician practitioners, other than the attending physician, who have been managing concurrent health care problems not primarily managed by the attending physician, and who are not acting on behalf of the attending physician, shall use Subsequent Hospital Care (CPT code range 99231 - 99233) for a final visit.

Medicare pays for the paperwork of patient discharge day management through the pre- and post- service work of an E/M service.

C. Subsequent Hospital Visit and Discharge Management on Same Day
Pay only the hospital discharge management code on the day of discharge (unless it is also the day of admission, in which case, refer to Sec.30.6.9.1 C for the policy on Observation or Inpatient Care Services (Including Admission and Discharge Services CPT Codes 99234 - 99236). Contractors do not pay both a subsequent hospital visit in addition to hospital discharge day management service on the same day by the same physician. Instruct physicians that they may not bill for both a hospital visit and hospital discharge management for the same date of service.

D. Hospital Discharge Management (CPT Codes 99238 and 99239) and Nursing Facility Admission Code When Patient Is Discharged From Hospital and Admitted to Nursing Facility on Same Day
Contractors pay the hospital discharge code (codes 99238 or 99239) in addition to a nursing facility admission code when they are billed by the same physician with the same date of service.

If a surgeon is admitting the patient to the nursing facility due to a condition that is not as a result of the surgery during the postoperative period of a service with the global surgical period, he/she bills for the nursing facility admission and care with a modifier "-24" and provides documentation that the service is unrelated to the surgery (e.g., return of an elderly patient to the nursing facility in which he/she has resided for five years following discharge from the hospital for cholecystectomy).

Contractors do not pay for a nursing facility admission by a surgeon in the postoperative period of a procedure with a global surgical period if the patient's admission to the nursing facility is to receive post operative care related to the surgery (e.g., admission to a nursing facility to receive physical therapy following a hip replacement). Payment for the nursing facility admission and subsequent nursing facility services are included in the global fee and cannot be paid separately.

E. Hospital Discharge Management and Death Pronouncement
Only the physician who personally performs the pronouncement of death shall bill for the face-to-face Hospital Discharge Day Management Service, CPT code 99238 or 99239. The date of the pronouncement shall reflect the calendar date of service on the day it was performed even if the paperwork is delayed to a subsequent date.

100-4, 12, 30.6.10

Consultation Services

Consultation Services versus Other Evaluation and Management (E/M) Visits
Effective January 1, 2010, the consultation codes are no longer recognized for Medicare Part B payment. Physicians shall code patient evaluation and management visits with E/M codes that represent where the visit occurs and that identify the complexity of the visit performed.

In the inpatient hospital setting and the nursing facility setting, physicians (and qualified nonphysician practitioners where permitted) may bill the most appropriate initial hospital care code (99221-99223), subsequent hospital care code (99231 and 99232), initial nursing facility care code (99304-99306), or subsequent nursing facility care code (99307-99310) that reflects the services the physician or practitioner furnished. Subsequent hospital care codes could potentially meet the component work and medical necessity requirements to be reported for an E/M service that could be described by CPT consultation code 99251 or 99252. Contractors shall not find fault in cases where the medical record appropriately demonstrates that the work and medical necessity requirements are met for reporting a subsequent hospital care code (under the level selected), even though the reported code is for the provider's first E/M service to the inpatient during the hospital stay. Unlisted evaluation and management service (code 99499) shall only be reported for consultation services when an E/M service that could be described by codes 99251 or 99252 is furnished, and there is no other specific E/M code payable by Medicare that describes that service. Reporting code 99499 requires submission of medical records and contractor manual medical review of the service prior to payment. CMS expects reporting under these circumstances to be unusual. T he principal physician of record is identified in Medicare as the physician who oversees the patient's care from other physicians who may be furnishing specialty care. The principal physician of record shall append modifier "-AI" (Principal Physician of Record), in addition to the E/M code. Follow-up visits in the facility setting shall be billed as subsequent hospital care visits and subsequent nursing facility care visits.

In the CAH setting, those CAHs that use method II shall bill the appropriate new or established visit code for those physician and non-physician practitioners who have reassigned their billing rights, depending on the relationship status between the physician and patient.

In the office or other outpatient setting where an evaluation is performed, physicians and qualified nonphysician practitioners shall use the CPT codes (99201–99215) depending on the complexity of the visit and whether the patient is a new or established patient to that physician. All physicians and qualified nonphysician practitioners shall follow the E/M documentation guidelines for all E/M services. These rules are applicable for Medicare secondary payer claims as well as for claims in which Medicare is the primary payer.

100-4, 12, 30.6.11

Emergency Department Visits (Codes 99281 - 99288)

A. Use of Emergency Department Codes by Physicians Not Assigned to Emergency Department
Any physician seeing a patient registered in the emergency department may use emergency department visit codes (for services matching the code description). It is not required that the physician be assigned to the emergency department.

B. Use of Emergency Department Codes In Office
Emergency department coding is not appropriate if the site of service is an office or outpatient setting or any sight of service other than an emergency department. The emergency department codes should only be used if the patient is seen in the emergency department and the services described by the HCPCS code definition are provided. The emergency department is defined as an organized hospital-based facility for the provision of unscheduled or episodic services to patients who present for immediate medical attention.

C. Use of Emergency Department Codes to Bill Nonemergency Services
Services in the emergency department may not be emergencies. However the codes (99281 - 99288) are payable if the described services are provided.

However, if the physician asks the patient to meet him or her in the emergency department as an alternative to the physician's office and the patient is not registered as a patient in the emergency department, the physician should bill the appropriate office/outpatient visit codes. Normally a lower level emergency department code would be reported for a nonemergency condition.

D. Emergency Department or Office/Outpatient Visits on Same Day As Nursing Facility Admission
Emergency department visit provided on the same day as a comprehensive nursing facility assessment are not paid. Payment for evaluation and management services on the same date provided in sites other than the nursing facility are included in the payment for initial nursing facility care when performed on the same date as the nursing facility admission.

E. Physician Billing for Emergency Department Services Provided to Patient by Both Patient's Personal Physician and Emergency Department Physician
If a physician advises his/her own patient to go to an emergency department (ED) of a hospital for care and the physician subsequently is asked by the ED physician to come to the hospital to evaluate the patient and to advise the ED physician as to whether the patient should be admitted to the hospital or be sent home, the physicians should bill as follows:

If the patient is admitted to the hospital by the patient's personal physician, then the patient's regular physician should bill only the appropriate level of the initial hospital care (codes 99221 - 99223) because all evaluation and management services provided by that physician in conjunction with that admission are considered part of the initial hospital care when performed on the same date as the admission. The ED physician who saw the patient in the emergency department should bill the appropriate level of the ED codes.

If the ED physician, based on the advice of the patient's personal physician who came to the emergency department to see the patient, sends the patient home, then the ED physician should bill the appropriate level of emergency department service. The patient's personal physician should also bill the level of emergency department code that describes the service he or she provided in the emergency department. If the patient's personal physician does not come to the hospital to see the patient, but only advises the emergency department physician by telephone, then the patient's personal physician may not bill.

F. Emergency Department Physician Requests Another Physician to See the Patient in Emergency Department or Office/Outpatient Setting

If the emergency department physician requests that another physician evaluate a given patient, the other physician should bill an emergency department visit code. If the patient is admitted to the hospital by the second physician performing the evaluation, he or she should bill an initial hospital care code and not an emergency department visit code.

100-4, 12, 30.6.12

Critical Care Visits and Neonatal Intensive Care (Codes 99291 - 99292)

CRITICAL CARE SERVICES (CODES 99291-99292)

A. Use of Critical Care Codes

Pay for services reported with CPT codes 99291 and 99292 when all the criteria for critical care and critical care services are met. Critical care is defined as the direct delivery by a physician(s) medical care for a critically ill or critically injured patient. A critical illness or injury acutely impairs one or more vital organ systems such that there is a high probability of imminent or life threatening deterioration in the patient's condition.

Critical care involves high complexity decision making to assess, manipulate, and support vital system functions(s) to treat single or multiple vital organ system failure and/or to prevent further life threatening deterioration of the patient's condition.

Examples of vital organ system failure include, but are not limited to: central nervous system failure, circulatory failure, shock, renal, hepatic, metabolic, and/or respiratory failure. Although critical care typically requires interpretation of multiple physiologic parameters and/or application of advanced technology(s), critical care may be provided in life threatening situations when these elements are not present.

Providing medical care to a critically ill, injured, or post-operative patient qualifies as a critical care service only if both the illness or injury and the treatment being provided meet the above requirements.

Critical care is usually, but not always, given in a critical care area such as a coronary care unit, intensive care unit, respiratory care unit, or the emergency department. However, payment may be made for critical care services provided in any location as long as the care provided meets the definition of critical care.

Consult the American Medical Association (AMA) CPT Manual for the applicable codes and guidance for critical care services provided to neonates, infants and children.

B. Critical Care Services and Medical Necessity

Critical care services must be medically necessary and reasonable. Services provided that do not meet critical care services or services provided for a patient who is not critically ill or injured in accordance with the above definitions and criteria but who happens to be in a critical care, intensive care, or other specialized care unit should be reported using another appropriate E/M code (e.g., subsequent hospital care, CPT codes 99231 - 99233).

As described in Section A, critical care services encompass both treatment of "vital organ failure" and "prevention of further life threatening deterioration of the patient's condition." Therefore, although critical care may be delivered in a moment of crisis or upon being called to the patient's bedside emergently, this is not a requirement for providing critical care service. The treatment and management of the patient's condition, while not necessarily emergent, shall be required, based on the threat of imminent deterioration (i.e., the patient shall be critically ill or injured at the time of the physician's visit).

Chronic Illness and Critical Care:

Examples of patients whose medical condition may not warrant critical care services:

1. Daily management of a patient on chronic ventilator therapy does not meet the criteria for critical care unless the critical care is separately identifiable from the chronic long term management of the ventilator dependence.
2. Management of dialysis or care related to dialysis for a patient receiving ESRD hemodialysis does not meet the criteria for critical care unless the critical care is separately identifiable from the chronic long term management of the dialysis dependence (refer to Chapter 8, Sec.160.4). When a separately identifiable condition (e.g., management of seizures or pericardial tamponade related to renal failure) is being managed, it may be billed as critical care if critical care requirements are met. Modifier -25 should be appended to the critical care code when applicable in this situation.

Examples of patients whose medical condition may warrant critical care services:

1. An 81 year old male patient is admitted to the intensive care unit following abdominal aortic aneurysm resection. Two days after surgery he requires fluids and pressors to maintain adequate perfusion and arterial pressures. He remains ventilator dependent.
2. A 67 year old female patient is 3 days status post mitral valve repair. She develops petechiae, hypotension and hypoxia requiring respiratory and circulatory support.
3. A 70 year old admitted for right lower lobe pneumococcal pneumonia with a history of COPD becomes hypoxic and hypotensive 2 days after admission.
4. A 68 year old admitted for an acute anterior wall myocardial infarction continues to have symptomatic ventricular tachycardia that is marginally responsive to antiarrhythmic therapy.

Examples of patients who may not satisfy Medicare medical necessity criteria, or do not meet critical care criteria or who do not have a critical care illness or injury and therefore not eligible for critical care payment:

1. Patients admitted to a critical care unit because no other hospital beds were available;
2. Patients admitted to a critical care unit for close nursing observation and/or frequent monitoring of vital signs (e.g., drug toxicity or overdose); and
3. Patients admitted to a critical care unit because hospital rules require certain treatments (e.g., insulin infusions) to be administered in the critical care unit.

Providing medical care to a critically ill patient should not be automatically deemed to be a critical care service for the sole reason that the patient is critically ill or injured. While more than one physician may provide critical care services to a patient during the critical care episode of an illness or injury each physician must be managing one or more critical illness(es) or injury(ies) in whole or in part.

> EXAMPLE: A dermatologist evaluates and treats a rash on an ICU patient who is maintained on a ventilator and nitroglycerine infusion that are being managed by an intensivist. The dermatologist should not report a service for critical care.

C. Critical Care Services and Full Attention of the Physician

The duration of critical care services to be reported is the time the physician spent evaluating, providing care and managing the critically ill or injured patient's care. That time must be spent at the immediate bedside or elsewhere on the floor or unit so long as the physician is immediately available to the patient.

For example, time spent reviewing laboratory test results or discussing the critically ill patient's care with other medical staff in the unit or at the nursing station on the floor may be reported as critical care, even when it does not occur at the bedside, if this time represents the physician's full attention to the management of the critically ill/injured patient.

For any given period of time spent providing critical care services, the physician must devote his or her full attention to the patient and, therefore, cannot provide services to any other patient during the same period of time.

D. Critical Care Services and Qualified Non-Physician Practitioners (NPP)

Critical care services may be provided by qualified NPPs and reported for payment under the NPP's National Provider Identifier (NPI) when the services meet the definition and requirements of critical care services in Sections A and B. The provision of critical care services must be within the scope of practice and licensure requirements for the State in which the qualified NPP practices and provides the service(s). Collaboration, physician supervision and billing requirements must also be met. A physician assistant shall meet the general physician supervision requirements.

E. Critical Care Services and Physician Time

Critical care is a time- based service, and for each date and encounter entry, the physician's progress note(s) shall document the total time that critical care services were provided. More than one physician can provide critical care at another time and be paid if the service meets critical care, is medically necessary and is not duplicative care. Concurrent care by more than one physician (generally representing different physician specialties) is payable if these requirements are met (refer to the Medicare Benefit Policy Manual, Pub. 100-02, Chapter 15, Sec.30 for concurrent care policy discussion).

The CPT critical care codes 99291 and 99292 are used to report the total duration of time spent by a physician providing critical care services to a critically ill or critically injured patient, even if the time spent by the physician on that date is not continuous. Non-continuous time for medically necessary critical care services may be aggregated. Reporting CPT code 99291 is a prerequisite to reporting CPT code 99292. Physicians of the same specialty within the same group practice bill and are paid as though they were a single physician (Sec.30.6.5).

1. Off the Unit/Floor
   Time spent in activities (excluding those identified previously in Section C) that occur outside of the unit or off the floor (i.e., telephone calls, whether taken at home, in the office, or elsewhere in the hospital) may not be reported as critical care because the physician is not immediately available to the patient. This time is regarded as pre- and post service work bundled in evaluation and management services.
2. Split/Shared Service
   A split/shared E/M service performed by a physician and a qualified NPP of the same group practice (or employed by the same employer) cannot be reported as

a critical care service. Critical care services are reflective of the care and management of a critically ill or critically injured patient by an individual physician or qualified non-physician practitioner for the specified reportable period of time.

Unlike other E/M services where a split/shared service is allowed the critical care service reported shall reflect the evaluation, treatment and management of a patient by an individual physician or qualified non-physician practitioner and shall not be representative of a combined service between a physician and a qualified NPP.

When CPT code time requirements for both 99291 and 99292 and critical care criteria are met for a medically necessary visit by a qualified NPP the service shall be billed using the appropriate individual NPI number. Medically necessary visit(s) that do not meet these requirements shall be reported as subsequent hospital care services.

3. Unbundled Procedures
Time involved performing procedures that are not bundled into critical care (i.e., billed and paid separately) may not be included and counted toward critical care time. The physician's progress note(s) in the medical record should document that time involved in the performance of separately billable procedures was not counted toward critical care time.

4. Family Counseling/Discussions
Critical care CPT codes 99291 and 99292 include pre and post service work. Routine daily updates or reports to family members and or surrogates are considered part of this service. However, time involved with family members or other surrogate decision makers, whether to obtain a history or to discuss treatment options (as described in CPT), may be counted toward critical care time when these specific criteria are met:

   a) The patient is unable or incompetent to participate in giving a history and/or making treatment decisions, and

   b) The discussion is necessary for determining treatment decisions.

   For family discussions, the physician should document:

   a. The patient is unable or incompetent to participate in giving history and/or making treatment decisions

   b. The necessity to have the discussion (e.g., "no other source was available to obtain a history" or "because the patient was deteriorating so rapidly I needed to immediately discuss treatment options with the family",

   c. Medically necessary treatment decisions for which the discussion was needed, and

   d. A summary in the medical record that supports the medical necessity of the discussion
   All other family discussions, no matter how lengthy, may not be additionally counted towards critical care. Telephone calls to family members and or surrogate decision-makers may be counted towards critical care time, but only if they meet the same criteria as described in the aforementioned paragraph.

5. Inappropriate Use of Time for Payment of Critical Care Services.
Time involved in activities that do not directly contribute to the treatment of the critically ill or injured patient may not be counted towards the critical care time, even when they are performed in the critical care unit at a patient's bedside (e.g., review of literature, and teaching sessions with physician residents whether conducted on hospital rounds or in other venues).

F. Hours and Days of Critical Care that May Be Billed
Critical care service is a time-based service provided on an hourly or fraction of an hour basis. Payment should not be restricted to a fixed number of hours, a fixed number of physicians, or a fixed number of days, on a per patient basis, for medically necessary critical care services. Time counted towards critical care services may be continuous or intermittent and aggregated in time increments (e.g., 50 minutes of continuous clock time or (5) 10 minute blocks of time spread over a given calendar date). Only one physician may bill for critical care services during any one single period of time even if more than one physician is providing care to a critically ill patient.

For Medicare Part B physician services paid under the physician fee schedule, critical care is not a service that is paid on a "shift" basis or a "per day" basis. Documentation may be requested for any claim to determine medical necessity. Examples of critical care billing that may require further review could include: claims from several physicians submitting multiple units of critical care for a single patient, and submitting claims for more than 12 hours of critical care time by a physician for one or more patients on the same given calendar date. Physicians assigned to a critical care unit (e.g., hospitalist, intensivist, etc.) may not report critical care for patients based on a "per shift" basis.

The CPT code 99291 is used to report the first 30 - 74 minutes of critical care on a given calendar date of service. It should only be used once per calendar date per patient by the same physician or physician group of the same specialty. CPT code 99292 is used to report additional block(s) of time, of up to 30 minutes each beyond the first 74 minutes of critical care (See table below). Critical care of less than 30 minutes total duration on a given calendar date is not reported separately using the critical care codes. This service should be reported using another appropriate E/M code such as subsequent hospital care.

Clinical Example of Correct Billing of Time:
A patient arrives in the emergency department in cardiac arrest. The emergency department physician provides 40 minutes of critical care services. A cardiologist is called to the ED and assumes responsibility for the patient, providing 35 minutes of critical care services. The patient stabilizes and is transferred to the CCU. In this instance, the ED physician provided 40 minutes of critical care services and reports only the critical care code (CPT code 99291) and not also emergency department services. The cardiologist may report the 35 minutes of critical care services (also CPT code 99291) provided in the ED. Additional critical care services by the cardiologist in the CCU may be reported on the same calendar date using 99292 or another appropriate E/M code depending on the clock time involved.

G. Counting of Units of Critical Care Services
The CPT code 99291 (critical care, first hour) is used to report the services of a physician providing full attention to a critically ill or critically injured patient from 30-74 minutes on a given date. Only one unit of CPT code 99291 may be billed by a physician for a patient on a given date. Physicians of the same specialty within the same group practice bill and are paid as though they were a single physician and would not each report CPT 99291on the same date of service.

The following illustrates the correct reporting of critical care services:

Total Duration of Critical Care	Code(s)
Less than 30 minutes	99232 or 99233 or other appropriate E/M code
30-74 minutes	99291 x 1
75-104 minutes	99291 x 1 and 99292 x 1
105-134 minutes	99291 x 1 and 99292 x 2
135-164 minutes	99291 x 1 and 99292 x 3
165-194 minutes	99291 x 1 and 99292 x 4
194 minutes or longer	99291 - 99292 as appropriate (per the above illustrations)

H. Critical Care Services and Other Evaluation and Management Services Provided on Same Day
When critical care services are required upon the patient's presentation to the hospital emergency department, only critical care codes 99291 - 99292 may be reported. An emergency department visit code may not also be reported.

When critical care services are provided on a date where an inpatient hospital or office/outpatient evaluation and management service was furnished earlier on the same date at which time the patient did not require critical care, both the critical care and the previous evaluation and management service may be paid. Hospital emergency department services are not payable for the same calendar date as critical care services when provided by the same physician to the same patient.

Physicians are advised to submit documentation to support a claim when critical care is additionally reported on the same calendar date as when other evaluation and management services are provided to a patient by the same physician or physicians of the same specialty in a group practice.

I. Critical Care Services Provided by Physicians in Group Practice(s)
Medically necessary critical care services provided on the same calendar date to the same patient by physicians representing different medical specialties that are not duplicative services are payable. The medical specialists may be from the same group practice or from different group practices.

Critically ill or critically injured patients may require the care of more than one physician medical specialty. Concurrent critical care services provided by each physician must be medically necessary and not provided during the same instance of time. Medical record documentation must support the medical necessity of critical care services provided by each physician (or qualified NPP). Each physician must accurately report the service(s) he/she provided to the patient in accordance with any applicable global surgery rules or concurrent care rules. (Refer to Medicare Claims Processing Manual, Pub. 100-04, Chapter 12, Sec.40, and the Medicare Benefit Policy Manual, Pub. 100-02, Chapter 15, Sec.30.)

CPT Code 99291
The initial critical care time, billed as CPT code 99291, must be met by a single physician or qualified NPP. This may be performed in a single period of time or be cumulative by the same physician on the same calendar date. A history or physical exam performed by one group partner for another group partner in order for the second group partner to make a medical decision would not represent critical care services.

CPT Code 99292
Subsequent critical care visits performed on the same calendar date are reported using CPT code 99292. The service may represent aggregate time met by a single physician or physicians in the same group practice with the same medical specialty in order to meet the duration of minutes required for CPT code 99292. The aggregated critical care visits must be medically necessary and each aggregated visit must meet the definition of critical care in order to combine the times.

Physicians in the same group practice who have the same specialty may not each report CPT initial critical care code 99291 for critical care services to the same patient on the same calendar date. Medicare payment policy states that physicians in the same group practice who are in the same specialty must bill and be paid as though each were the single physician. (Refer to the Medicare Claims Processing Manual, Pub. 100-04, Chapter 12, Sec.30.6.) Physician specialty means the self-designated primary specialty by which the physician bills Medicare and is known to the contractor that adjudicates the claims. Physicians in the same group practice who have different medical specialties may bill and be paid without regard to their membership in the same group. For example, if a cardiologist and an endocrinologist are group partners and the critical care services of each are medically necessary and not duplicative, the critical care services may be reported by each regardless of their group practice relationship.

Two or more physicians in the same group practice who have different specialties and who provide critical care to a critically ill or critically injured patient may not in all cases each report the initial critical care code (CPT 99291) on the same date. When the group physicians are providing care that is unique to his/her individual medical specialty and managing at least one of the patient's critical illness(es) or critical injury(ies) then the initial critical care service may be payable to each.

However, if a physician or qualified NPP within a group provides "staff coverage" or "follow-up" for each other after the first hour of critical care services was provided on the same calendar date by the previous group clinician (physician or qualified NPP), the subsequent visits by the "covering" physician or qualified NPP in the group shall be billed using CPT critical care add-on code 99292. The appropriate individual NPI number shall be reported on the claim. The services will be paid at the specific physician fee schedule rate for the individual clinician (physician or qualified NPP) billing the service.

Clinical Examples of Critical Care Services

1. Drs. Smith and Jones, pulmonary specialists, share a group practice. On Tuesday Dr. Smith provides critical care services to Mrs. Benson who is comatose and has been in the intensive care unit for 4 days following a motor vehicle accident. She has multiple organ dysfunction including cerebral hematoma, flail chest and pulmonary contusion. Later on the same calendar date Dr. Jones covers for Dr. Smith and provides critical care services. Medically necessary critical care services provided at the different time periods may be reported by both Drs. Smith and Jones. Dr. Smith would report CPT code 99291 for the initial visit and Dr. Jones, as part of the same group practice would report CPT code 99292 on the same calendar date if the appropriate time requirements are met.
2. Mr. Marks, a 79 year old comes to the emergency room with vague joint pains and lethargy. The ED physician evaluates Mr. Marks and phones his primary care physician to discuss his medical evaluation. His primary care physician visits the ER and admits Mr. Marks to the observation unit for monitoring, and diagnostic and laboratory tests. In observation Mr. Marks has a cardiac arrest. His primary care physician provides 50 minutes of critical care services. Mr. Marks' is admitted to the intensive care unit. On the same calendar day Mr. Marks' condition deteriorates and he requires intermittent critical care services. In this scenario the ED physician should report an emergency department visit and the primary care physician should report both an initial hospital visit and critical care services.

J. Critical Care Services and Other Procedures Provided on the Same Day by the Same Physician as Critical Care Codes 99291- 99292

The following services when performed on the day a physician bills for critical care are included in the critical care service and should not be reported separately:

- The interpretation of cardiac output measurements (CPT 93561, 93562);
- Chest x-rays, professional component (CPT 71010, 71015, 71020);
- Blood draw for specimen (CPT 36415);
- Blood gases, and information data stored in computers (e.g., ECGs, blood pressures, hematologic data-CPT 99090);
- Gastric intubation (CPT 43752, 91105);
- Pulse oximetry (CPT 94760, 94761, 94762);
- Temporary transcutaneous pacing (CPT 92953);
- Ventilator management (CPT 94002 - 94004, 94660, 94662); and
- Vascular access procedures (CPT 36000, 36410, 36415, 36591, 36600).

No other procedure codes are bundled into the critical care services. Therefore, other medically necessary procedure codes may be billed separately.

K. Global Surgery

Critical care services shall not be paid on the same calendar date the physician also reports a procedure code with a global surgical period unless the critical care is billed with CPT modifier -25 to indicate that the critical care is a significant, separately identifiable evaluation and management service that is above and beyond the usual pre and post operative care associated with the procedure that is performed.

Services such as endotracheal intubation (CPT code 31500) and the insertion and placement of a flow directed catheter e.g., Swan-Ganz (CPT code 93503) are not bundled into the critical care codes. Therefore, separate payment may be made for critical care in addition to these services if the critical care was a significant, separately identifiable service and it was reported with modifier -25. The time spent performing the pre, intra, and post procedure work of these unbundled services, e.g., endotracheal intubation, shall be excluded from the determination of the time spent providing critical care.

This policy applies to any procedure with a 0, 10 or 90 day global period including cardiopulmonary resuscitation (CPT code 92950). CPR has a global period of 0 days and is not bundled into critical care codes. Therefore, critical care may be billed in addition to CPR if critical care was a significant, separately identifiable service and it was reported with modifier -25. The time spent performing CPR shall be excluded from the determination of the time spent providing critical care. In this instance it must be the physician who performs the resuscitation who bills for this service. Members of a code team must not each bill Medicare Part B for this service.

When postoperative critical care services (for procedures with a global surgical period) are provided by a physician other than the surgeon, no modifier is required unless all surgical postoperative care has been officially transferred from the surgeon to the physician performing the critical care services. In this situation, CPT modifiers "-54" (surgical care only) and "-55"(postoperative management only) must be used by the surgeon and intensivist who are submitting claims. Medical record documentation by the surgeon and the physician who assumes a transfer (e.g., intensivist) is required to support claims for services when CPT modifiers -54 and -55 are used indicating the transfer of care from the surgeon to the intensivist. Critical care services must meet all the conditions previously described in this manual section.

L. Critical Care Services Provided During Preoperative Portion and Postoperative Portion of Global Period of Procedure with 90 Day Global Period in Trauma and Burn Cases

Preoperative

Preoperative critical care may be paid in addition to a global fee if the patient is critically ill and requires the full attention of the physician, and the critical care is unrelated to the specific anatomic injury or general surgical procedure performed. Such patients may meet the definition of being critically ill and criteria for conditions where there is a high probability of imminent or life threatening deterioration in the patient's condition.

Preoperatively, in order for these services to be paid, two reporting requirements must be met. Codes 99291 - 99292 and modifier -25 (significant, separately identifiable evaluation and management services by the same physician on the day of the procedure) must be used, and documentation identifying that the critical care was unrelated to the specific anatomic injury or general surgical procedure performed shall be submitted. An ICD-9-CM code in the range 800.0 through 959.9 (except 930.0 - 939.9), which clearly indicates that the critical care was unrelated to the surgery, is acceptable documentation.

Postoperative

Postoperatively, in order for critical care services to be paid, two reporting requirements must be met. Codes 99291 - 99292 and modifier -24 (unrelated evaluation and management service by the same physician during a postoperative period) must be used, and documentation that the critical care was unrelated to the specific anatomic injury or general surgical procedure performed must be submitted. An ICD-9-CM code in the range 800.0 through 959.9 (except 930.0 - 939.9), which clearly indicates that the critical care was unrelated to the surgery, is acceptable documentation.

Medicare policy allows separate payment to the surgeon for postoperative critical care services during the surgical global period when the patient has suffered trauma or burns. When the surgeon provides critical care services during the global period, for reasons unrelated to the surgery, these are separately payable as well.

M. Teaching Physician Criteria

In order for the teaching physician to bill for critical care services the teaching physician must meet the requirements for critical care described in the preceding sections. For CPT codes determined on the basis of time, such as critical care, the teaching physician must be present for the entire period of time for which the claim is submitted. For example, payment will be made for 35 minutes of critical care services only if the teaching physician is present for the full 35 minutes. (See IOM, Pub 100-04, Chapter12, Sec. 100.1.4)

1. Teaching
   Time spent teaching may not be counted towards critical care time. Time spent by the resident, in the absence of the teaching physician, cannot be billed by the teaching physician as critical care or other time-based services. Only time spent by the resident and teaching physician together with the patient or the teaching physician alone with the patient can be counted toward critical care time.
2. Documentation
   A combination of the teaching physician's documentation and the resident's documentation may support critical care services. Provided that all requirements for critical care services are met, the teaching physician documentation may tie into the resident's documentation. The teaching physician may refer to the resident's documentation for specific patient history, physical findings and medical assessment. However, the teaching physician medical record documentation must provide substantive information including: (1) the time the teaching physician spent providing critical care, (2) that the patient was critically ill during the time the teaching physician saw the patient, (3) what made the patient critically ill, and (4) the nature of the treatment and management provided by the teaching physician. The medical review criteria are the same for the teaching physician as for all physicians. (See the Medicare Claims Processing, Pub. 100-04, Chapter 12, Sec.100.1.1 for teaching physician documentation guidance.)

Unacceptable Example of Documentation:

"I came and saw (the patient) and agree with (the resident)".

Acceptable Example of Documentation:

"Patient developed hypotension and hypoxia; I spent 45 minutes while the patient was in this condition, providing fluids, pressor drugs, and oxygen. I reviewed the resident's documentation and I agree with the resident's assessment and plan of care."

N. Ventilator Management

Medicare recognizes the ventilator codes (CPT codes 94002 - 94004, 94660 and 94662) as physician services payable under the physician fee schedule. Medicare Part B under the physician fee schedule does not pay for ventilator management services in addition to an evaluation and management service (e.g., critical care services, CPT codes 99291 - 99292) on the same day for the patient even when the evaluation and management service is billed with CPT modifier -2

100-4, 12, 30.6.13

Nursing Facility Services

A. Visits to Perform the Initial Comprehensive Assessment and Annual Assessments

The distinction made between the delegation of physician visits and tasks in a skilled nursing facility (SNF) and in a nursing facility (NF) is based on the Medicare Statute. Section 1819 (b) (6) (A) of the Social Security Act (the Act) governs SNFs while section 1919 (b) (6) (A) of the Act governs NFs. For further information refer to Medlearn Matters article number SE0418 at www.cms.hhs.gov/medlearn/matters.

The federally mandated visits in a SNF and NF must be performed by the physician except as otherwise permitted (42 CFR 483.40 (c) (4) and (f)). The principal physician of record must append the modifier "-AI", (Principal Physician of Record), to the initial nursing facility care code. This modifier will identify the physician who oversees the patient's care from other physicians who may be furnishing specialty care. All other physicians or qualified NPPs who perform an initial evaluation in the NF or SNF may bill the initial nursing facility care code. The initial federally mandated visit is defined in S&C-04-08 (see www.cms.hhs.gov/medlearn/matters) as the initial comprehensive visit during which the physician completes a thorough assessment, develops a plan of care, and writes or verifies admitting orders for the nursing facility resident. For Survey and Certification requirements, a visit must occur no later than 30 days after admission.

Further, per the Long Term Care regulations at 42 CFR 483.40 (c) (4) and (e) (2), in a SNF the physician may not delegate a task that the physician must personally perform. Therefore, as stated in S&C-04-08 the physician may not delegate the initial federally mandated comprehensive visit in a SNF.

The only exception, as to who performs the initial visit, relates to the NF setting. In the NF setting, a qualified NPP (i.e., a nurse practitioner (NP), physician assistant (PA), or a clinical nurse specialist (CNS)), who is not employed by the facility, may perform the initial visit when the State law permits. The evaluation and management (E/M) visit shall be within the State scope of practice and licensure requirements where the E/M visit is performed and the requirements for physician collaboration and physician supervision shall be met.

Under Medicare Part B payment policy, other medically necessary E/M visits may be performed and reported prior to and after the initial visit, if the medical needs of the patient require an E/M visit. A qualified NPP may perform medically necessary E/M visits prior to and after the initial visit if all the requirements for collaboration, general physician supervision, licensure, and billing are met.

The CPT Nursing Facility Services codes shall be used with place of service (POS) 31 (SNF) if the patient is in a Part A SNF stay. They shall be used with POS 32 (nursing facility) if the patient does not have Part A SNF benefits or if the patient is in a NF or in a non-covered SNF stay (e.g., there was no preceding 3-day hospital stay). The CPT Nursing Facility code definition also includes POS 54 (Intermediate Care Facility/Mentally Retarded) and POS 56 (Psychiatric Residential Treatment Center). For further guidance on POS codes and associated CPT codes refer to §30.6.14.

Effective January 1, 2006, the Initial Nursing Facility Care codes 99301,Äì 99303 are deleted.

Beginning January 1, 2006, the new CPT codes, Initial Nursing Facility Care, per day, (99304–99306) shall be used to report the initial federally mandated visit. Only a physician may report these codes for an initial federally mandated visit performed in a SNF or NF (with the exception of the qualified NPP in the NF setting who is not employed by the facility and when State law permits, as explained above).

A readmission to a SNF or NF shall have the same payment policy requirements as an initial admission in both the SNF and NF settings.

A physician who is employed by the SNF/NF may perform the E/M visits and bill independently to Medicare Part B for payment. An NPP who is employed by the SNF or NF may perform and bill Medicare Part B directly for those services where it is permitted as discussed above. The employer of the PA shall always report the visits performed by the PA. A physician, NP or CNS has the option to bill Medicare directly or to reassign payment for his/her professional service to the facility.

As with all E/M visits for Medicare Part B payment policy, the E/M documentation guidelines apply.

Medically Necessary Visits

Qualified NPPs may perform medically necessary E/M visits prior to and after the physician's initial federally mandated visit in both the SNF and NF. Medically necessary E/M visits for the diagnosis or treatment of an illness or injury or to improve the functioning of a malformed body member are payable under the physician fee schedule under Medicare Part B. A physician or NPP may bill the most appropriate initial nursing facility care code (CPT codes 99304-99306) or subsequent nursing facility care code (CPT codes 99307-99310), even if the E/M service is provided prior to the initial federally mandated visit.

SNF Setting--Place of Service Code 31

Following the initial federally mandated visit by the physician, the physician may delegate alternate federally mandated physician visits to a qualified NPP who meets collaboration and physician supervision requirements and is licensed as such by the State and performing within the scope of practice in that State.

NF Setting--Place of Service Code 32

Per the regulations at 42 CFR 483.40 (f), a qualified NPP, who meets the collaboration and physician supervision requirements, the State scope of practice and licensure requirements, and who is not employed by the NF, may at the option of the State, perform the initial federally mandated visit in a NF, and may perform any other federally mandated physician visit in a NF in addition to performing other medically necessary E/M visits.

Questions pertaining to writing orders or certification and recertification issues in the SNF and NF settings shall be addressed to the appropriate State Survey and Certification Agency departments for clarification.

B. Visits to Comply With Federal Regulations (42 CFR 483.40 (c) (1)) in the SNF and NF

Payment is made under the physician fee schedule by Medicare Part B for federally mandated visits. Following the initial federally mandated visit by the physician or qualified NPP where permitted, payment shall be made for federally mandated visits that monitor and evaluate residents at least once every 30 days for the first 90 days after admission and at least once every 60 days thereafter.

Effective January 1, 2006, the Subsequent Nursing Facility Care, per day, codes 99311,Äì 99313 are deleted.

Beginning January 1, 2006, the new CPT codes, Subsequent Nursing Facility Care, per day, (99307–99310) shall be used to report federally mandated physician E/M visits and medically necessary E/M visits.

Carriers shall not pay for more than one E/M visit performed by the physician or qualified NPP for the same patient on the same date of service. The Nursing Facility Services codes represent a "per day" service.

The federally mandated E/M visit may serve also as a medically necessary E/M visit if the situation arises (i.e., the patient has health problems that need attention on the day the scheduled mandated physician E/M visit occurs). The physician/qualified NPP shall bill only one E/M visit.

Beginning January 1, 2006, the new CPT code, Other Nursing Facility Service (99318), may be used to report an annual nursing facility assessment visit on the required schedule of visits on an annual basis. For Medicare Part B payment policy, an annual nursing facility assessment visit code may substitute as meeting one of the federally mandated physician visits if the code requirements for CPT code 99318 are fully met and in lieu of reporting a Subsequent Nursing Facility Care, per day, service (codes 99307–99310). It shall not be performed in addition to the required number of federally mandated physician visits. The new CPT annual assessment code does not represent a new benefit service for Medicare Part B physician services.

Qualified NPPs, whether employed or not by the SNF, may perform alternating federally mandated physician visits, at the option of the physician, after the initial federally mandated visit by the physician in a SNF.

Qualified NPPs in the NF setting, who are not employed by the NF and who are working in collaboration with a physician, may perform federally mandated physician visits, at the option of the State.

Medicare Part B payment policy does not pay for additional E/M visits that may be required by State law for a facility admission or for other additional visits to satisfy facility or other administrative purposes. E/M visits, prior to and after the initial federally mandated physician visit, that are reasonable and medically necessary to meet the medical needs of the individual patient (unrelated to any State requirement or administrative purpose) are payable under Medicare Part B.

C. Visits by Qualified Nonphysician Practitioners

All E/M visits shall be within the State scope of practice and licensure requirements where the visit is performed and all the requirements for physician collaboration and physician supervision shall be met when performed and reported by qualified NPPs. General physician supervision and employer billing requirements shall be met for PA services in addition to the PA meeting the State scope of practice and licensure requirements where the E/M visit is performed.

Medically Necessary Visits

Qualified NPPs may perform medically necessary E/M visits prior to and after the physician's initial visit in both the SNF and NF. Medically necessary E/M visits for the diagnosis or treatment of an illness or injury or to improve the functioning of a malformed body member are payable under the physician fee schedule under Medicare Part B. A physician or NPP may bill the most appropriate initial nursing facility care code (CPT codes 99304-99306) or subsequent nursing facility care code (CPT codes 99307-99310), even if the E/M service is provided prior to the initial federally mandated visit.

SNF Setting--Place of Service Code 31

Following the initial federally mandated visit by the physician, the physician may delegate alternate federally mandated physician visits to a qualified NPP who meets collaboration and physician supervision requirements and is licensed as such by the State and performing within the scope of practice in that State.

NF Setting--Place of Service Code 32

Per the regulations at 42 CFR 483.40 (f), a qualified NPP, who meets the collaboration and physician supervision requirements, the State scope of practice and licensure requirements, and who is not employed by the NF, may at the option of the State, perform the initial federally mandated visit in a NF, and may perform any other federally mandated physician visit in a NF in addition to performing other medically necessary E/M visits.

Questions pertaining to writing orders or certification and recertification issues in the SNF and NF settings shall be addressed to the appropriate State Survey and Certification Agency departments for clarification.

D. Medically Complex Care

Payment is made for E/M visits to patients in a SNF who are receiving services for medically complex care upon discharge from an acute care facility when the visits are reasonable and medically necessary and documented in the medical record. Physicians and qualified NPPs shall report initial nursing facility care codes for their first visit with the patient. The principal physician of record must append the modifier "-AI" (Principal Physician of Record), to the initial nursing facility care code when billed to identify the physician who oversees the patient's care from other physicians who may be furnishing specialty care. Follow-up visits shall be billed as subsequent nursing facility care visits.

E. Incident to Services

Where a physician establishes an office in a SNF/NF, the "incident to" services and requirements are confined to this discrete part of the facility designated as his/her office. "Incident to" E/M visits, provided in a facility setting, are not payable under the Physician Fee Schedule for Medicare Part B. Thus, visits performed outside the designated "office" area in the SNF/NF would be subject to the coverage and payment rules applicable to the SNF/NF setting and shall not be reported using the CPT codes for office or other outpatient visits or use place of service code 11.

F. Use of the Prolonged Services Codes and Other Time-Related Services

Beginning January 1, 2008, typical/average time units for E/M visits in the SNF/NF settings are reestablished. Medically necessary prolonged services for E/M visits (codes 99356 and 99357) in a SNF or NF may be billed with the Nursing Facility Services in the code ranges (99304–99306, 99307–99310 and 99318).

Counseling and Coordination of Care Visits

With the reestablishment of typical/average time units, medically necessary E/M visits for counseling and coordination of care, for Nursing Facility Services in the code ranges (99304–99306, 99307–99310 and 99318) that are time-based services, may be billed with the appropriate prolonged services codes (99356 and 99357).

G. Multiple Visits

The complexity level of an E/M visit and the CPT code billed must be a covered and medically necessary visit for each patient (refer to §§1862 (a)(1)(A) of the Act). Claims for an unreasonable number of daily E/M visits by the same physician to multiple patients at a facility within a 24-hour period may result in medical review to determine medical necessity for the visits. The E/M visit (Nursing Facility Services) represents a "per day" service per patient as defined by the CPT code. The medical record must be personally documented by the physician or qualified NPP who performed the E/M visit and the documentation shall support the specific level of E/M visit to each individual patient.

H. Split/Shared E/M Visit

A split/shared E/M visit cannot be reported in the SNF/NF setting. A split/shared E/M visit is defined by Medicare Part B payment policy as a medically necessary encounter with a patient where the physician and a qualified NPP each personally perform a substantive portion of an E/M visit face-to-face with the same patient on the same date of service. A substantive portion of an E/M visit involves all or some portion of the history, exam or medical decision making key components of an E/M service. The physician and the qualified NPP must be in the same group practice or be employed by the same employer. The split/shared E/M visit applies only to selected E/M visits and settings (i.e., hospital inpatient, hospital outpatient, hospital observation, emergency department, hospital discharge, office and non facility clinic visits, and prolonged visits associated with these E/M visit codes). The split/shared E/M policy does not apply to critical care services or procedures.

I. SNF/NF Discharge Day Management Service

Medicare Part B payment policy requires a face-to-face visit with the patient provided by the physician or the qualified NPP to meet the SNF/NF discharge day management service as defined by the CPT code. The E/M discharge day management visit shall be reported for the date of the actual visit by the physician or qualified NPP even if the patient is discharged from the facility on a different calendar date. The CPT codes 99315–99316 shall be reported for this visit. The Discharge Day Management Service may be reported using CPT code 99315 or 99316, depending on the code requirement, for a patient who has expired, but only if the physician or qualified NPP personally performed the death pronouncement.

100-4, 12, 30.6.14

Home Care and Domiciliary Care Visits (Codes 99324- 99350)

Physician Visits to Patients Residing in Various Places of Service

The American Medical Association's Current Procedural Terminology (CPT) 2006 new patient codes 99324 - 99328 and established patient codes 99334 - 99337(new codes beginning January 2006), for Domiciliary, Rest Home (e.g., Boarding Home), or Custodial Care Services, are used to report evaluation and management (E/M) services to residents residing in a facility which provides room, board, and other personal assistance services, generally on a long-term basis. These CPT codes are used to report E/M services in facilities assigned places of service (POS) codes 13 (Assisted Living Facility), 14 (Group Home), 33 (Custodial Care Facility) and 55 (Residential Substance Abuse Facility). Assisted living facilities may also be known as adult living facilities.

Physicians and qualified nonphysician practitioners (NPPs) furnishing E/M services to residents in a living arrangement described by one of the POS listed above must use the level of service code in the CPT code range 99324 - 99337 to report the service they provide. The CPT codes 99321 - 99333 for Domiciliary, Rest Home (e.g., Boarding Home), or Custodial Care Services are deleted beginning January, 2006.

Beginning in 2006, reasonable and medically necessary, face-to-face, prolonged services, represented by CPT codes 99354 - 99355, may be reported with the appropriate companion E/M codes when a physician or qualified NPP, provides a prolonged service involving direct (face-to-face) patient contact that is beyond the usual E/M visit service for a Domiciliary, Rest Home (e.g., Boarding Home) or Custodial Care Service. All the requirements for prolonged services at Sec.30.6.15.1 must be met.

The CPT codes 99341 through 99350, Home Services codes, are used to report E/M services furnished to a patient residing in his or her own private residence (e.g., private home, apartment, town home) and not residing in any type of congregate/shared facility living arrangement including assisted living facilities and group homes. The Home Services codes apply only to the specific 2-digit POS 12 (Home). Home Services codes may not be used for billing E/M services provided in settings other than in the private residence of an individual as described above.

Beginning in 2006, E/M services provided to patients residing in a Skilled Nursing Facility (SNF) or a Nursing Facility (NF) must be reported using the appropriate CPT level of service code within the range identified for Initial Nursing Facility Care (new CPT codes 99304 - 99306) and Subsequent Nursing Facility Care (new CPT codes 99307 - 99310). Use the CPT code, Other Nursing Facility Services (new CPT code 99318), for an annual nursing facility assessment. Use CPT codes 99315 - 99316 for SNF/NF discharge services. The CPT codes 99301 - 99303 and 99311 - 99313 are deleted beginning January, 2006. The Home Services codes should not be used for these places of service.

The CPT SNF/NF code definition includes intermediate care facilities (ICFs) and long term care facilities (LTCFs). These codes are limited to the specific 2-digit POS 31 (SNF), 32 (Nursing Facility), 54 (Intermediate Care Facility/Mentally Retarded) and 56 (Psychiatric Residential Treatment Center).

The CPT nursing facility codes should be used with POS 31 (SNF) if the patient is in a Part A SNF stay and POS 32 (nursing facility) if the patient does not have Part A SNF benefits. There is no longer a different payment amount for a Part A or Part B benefit period in these POS settings.

100-4, 12, 30.6.14.1

Home Services (Codes 99341 - 99350)

B3-15515, B3-15066

A. Requirement for Physician Presence

Home services codes 99341-99350 are paid when they are billed to report evaluation and management services provided in a private residence. A home visit cannot be billed by a physician unless the physician was actually present in the beneficiary's home.

B. Homebound Status

Under the home health benefit the beneficiary must be confined to the home for services to be covered. For home services provided by a physician using these codes, the beneficiary does not need to be confined to the home. The medical record must document the medical necessity of the home visit made in lieu of an office or outpatient visit.

C. Fee Schedule Payment for Services to Homebound Patients under General Supervision

Payment may be made in some medically underserved areas where there is a lack of medical personnel and home health services for injections, EKGs, and venipunctures that are performed for homebound patients under general physician supervision by nurses and paramedical employees of physicians or physician-directed clinics. Section 10 provides additional information on the provision of services to homebound Medicare patients.

100-4, 12, 30.6.15.1

Prolonged Services With Direct Face-to-Face Patient Contact Service (Codes 99354-99357) (ZZZ codes)

A. Definition

Prolonged physician services (CPT code 99354) in the office or other outpatient setting with direct face-to-face patient contact which require 1 hour beyond the usual service are payable when billed on the same day by the same physician or qualified nonphysician practitioner (NPP) as the companion evaluation and management codes. The time for usual service refers to the typical/average time units associated with the companion evaluation and management service as noted in the CPT code. Each additional 30 minutes of direct face-to-face patient contact following the first hour of prolonged services may be reported by CPT code 99355.

Prolonged physician services (code 99356) in the inpatient setting, with direct face-to-face patient contact which require 1 hour beyond the usual service are payable when they are billed on the same day by the same physician or qualified NPP as the companion evaluation and management codes. Each additional 30 minutes of direct face-to-face patient contact following the first hour of prolonged services may be reported by CPT code 99357.

Prolonged service of less than 30 minutes total duration on a given date is not separately reported because the work involved is included in the total work of the evaluation and management codes.

Code 99355 or 99357 may be used to report each additional 30 minutes beyond the first hour of prolonged services, based on the place of service. These codes may be used to report the final 15–30 minutes of prolonged service on a given date, if not otherwise billed. Prolonged service of less than 15 minutes beyond the first hour or less than 15 minutes beyond the final 30 minutes is not reported separately.

B. Required Companion Codes

The companion evaluation and management codes for 99354 are the Office or Other Outpatient visit codes (99201 - 99205, 99212–99215), the Domiciliary, Rest Home, or Custodial Care Services codes (99324–99328, 99334–99337), the Home Services codes (99341 - 99345, 99347–99350);

The companion codes for 99355 are 99354 and one of the evaluation and management codes required for 99354 to be used;

The companion evaluation and management codes for 99356 are the Initial Hospital Care codes and Subsequent Hospital Care codes (99221 - 99223, 99231–99233); Nursing Facility Services codes (99304 -99318); or

The companion codes for 99357 are 99356 and one of the evaluation and management codes required for 99356 to be used.

Prolonged services codes 99354–99357 are not paid unless they are accompanied by the companion codes as indicated.

C. Requirement for Physician Presence

Physicians may count only the duration of direct face-to-face contact between the physician and the patient (whether the service was continuous or not) beyond the typical/average time of the visit code billed to determine whether prolonged services can be billed and to determine the prolonged services codes that are allowable. In the case of prolonged office services, time spent by office staff with the patient, or time the patient remains unaccompanied in the office cannot be billed. In the case of prolonged hospital services, time spent reviewing charts or discussion of a patient with house medical staff and not with direct face-to-face contact with the patient, or waiting for test results, for changes in the patient's condition, for end of a therapy, or for use of facilities cannot be billed as prolonged services.

D. Documentation

Documentation is not required to accompany the bill for prolonged services unless the physician has been selected for medical review. Documentation is required in the medical record about the duration and content of the medically necessary evaluation and management service and prolonged services billed. The medical record must be appropriately and sufficiently documented by the physician or qualified NPP to show that the physician or qualified NPP personally furnished the direct face-to-face time with the patient specified in the CPT code definitions. The start and end times of the visit shall be documented in the medical record along with the date of service.

E. Use of the Codes

Prolonged services codes can be billed only if the total duration of the physician or qualified NPP direct face-to-face service (including the visit) equals or exceeds the threshold time for the evaluation and management service the physician or qualified NPP provided (typical/average time associated with the CPT E/M code plus 30 minutes). If the total duration of direct face-to-face time does not equal or exceed the threshold time for the level of evaluation and management service the physician or qualified NPP provided, the physician or qualified NPP may not bill for prolonged services.

F. Threshold Times for Codes 99354 and 99355 (Office or Other Outpatient Setting)

If the total direct face-to-face time equals or exceeds the threshold time for code 99354, but is less than the threshold time for code 99355, the physician should bill the evaluation and management visit code and code 99354. No more than one unit of 99354 is acceptable. If the total direct face-to-face time equals or exceeds the threshold time for code 99355 by no more than 29 minutes, the physician should bill the visit code 99354 and one unit of code 99355. One additional unit of code 99355 is billed for each additional increment of 30 minutes extended duration. Contractors use the following threshold times to determine if the prolonged services codes 99354 and/or 99355 can be billed with the office or other outpatient settings including domiciliary, rest home, or custodial care services and home services codes.

Threshold Time for Prolonged Visit Codes 99354 and/or 99355 Billed with Office/Outpatient and Consultation Codes

Code	Typical Time for Code	Threshold Time to Bill Code 99354	Threshold Time to Bill Codes 99354 and 99355
99201	10	40	85
99202	20	50	95
99203	30	60	105
99204	45	75	120
99205	60	90	135
99212	10	40	85
99213	15	45	90
99214	25	55	100
99215	40	70	115
99324	20	50	95
99325	30	60	105
99326	45	75	120
99327	60	90	135
99328	75	105	150
99334	15	45	90
99335	25	55	100
99336	40	70	115
99337	60	90	135
99341	20	50	95
99342	30	60	105
99343	45	75	120
99344	60	90	135
99345	75	105	150
99347	15	45	90
99348	25	55	100
99349	40	70	115
99350	60	90	135

G. Threshold Times for Codes 99356 and 99357

(Inpatient Setting) If the total direct face-to-face time equals or exceeds the threshold time for code 99356, but is less than the threshold time for code 99357, the physician should bill the visit and code 99356. Contractors do not accept more than one unit of code 99356. If the total direct face-to-face time equals or exceeds the threshold time for code 99356 by no more than 29 minutes, the physician bills the visit code 99356 and one unit of code 99357. One additional unit of code 99357 is billed for each additional increment of 30 minutes extended duration. Contractors use the following threshold times to determine if the prolonged services codes 99356 and/or 99357 can be billed with the inpatient setting codes.

Threshold Time for Prolonged Visit Codes 99356 and/or 99357 Billed with Inpatient Setting Codes

Code	Typical Time for Code	Threshold Time to Bill Code 99356	Threshold Time to Bill Codes 99356 and 99357
99221	30	60	105
99222	50	80	125
99223	70	100	145
99231	15	45	90
99232	25	55	100
99233	35	65	110
99304	25	55	100
99305	35	65	110
99306	45	75	120
99307	10	40	85
99308	15	45	90
99309	25	55	100
99310	35	65	110
99318	30	60	10

Add 30 minutes to the threshold time for billing codes 99356 and 99357 to get the threshold time for billing code 99356 and two units of 99357.

H. Prolonged Services Associated With Evaluation and Management Services Based on Counseling and/or Coordination of Care (Time-Based)

When an evaluation and management service is dominated by counseling and/or coordination of care (the counseling and/or coordination of care represents more than 50% of the total time with the patient) in a face-to-face encounter between the physician or qualified NPP and the patient in the office/clinic or the floor time (in the scenario of an inpatient service), then the evaluation and management code is selected based on the typical/average time associated with the code levels. The time approximation must meet or exceed the specific CPT code billed (determined by the typical/average time associated with the evaluation and management code) and should not be "rounded" to the next higher level.

In those evaluation and management services in which the code level is selected based on time, prolonged services may only be reported with the highest code level in that family of codes as the companion code.

I. Examples of Billable Prolonged Services

EXAMPLE 1

A physician performed a visit that met the definition of an office visit code 99213 and the total duration of the direct face-to-face services (including the visit) was 65 minutes. The physician bills code 99213 and one unit of code 99354.

EXAMPLE 2

A physician performed a visit that met the definition of a domiciliary, rest home care visit code 99327 and the total duration of the direct face-to-face contact (including the visit) was 140 minutes. The physician bills codes 99327, 99354, and one unit of code 99355.

EXAMPLE 3

A physician performed an office visit to an established patient that was predominantly counseling, spending 75 minutes (direct face-to-face) with the patient. The physician should report CPT code 99215 and one unit of code 99354.

J. Examples of Nonbillable Prolonged Services

EXAMPLE 1

A physician performed a visit that met the definition of visit code 99212 and the total duration of the direct face-to-face contact (including the visit) was 35 minutes. The physician cannot bill prolonged services because the total duration of direct face-to-face service did not meet the threshold time for billing prolonged services.

EXAMPLE 2

A physician performed a visit that met the definition of code 99213 and, while the patient was in the office receiving treatment for 4 hours, the total duration of the direct face-to-face service of the physician was 40 minutes. The physician cannot bill prolonged services because the total duration of direct face-to-face service did not meet the threshold time for billing prolonged services.

EXAMPLE 3

A physician provided a subsequent office visit that was predominantly counseling, spending 60 minutes (face-to-face) with the patient. The physician cannot code 99214, which has a typical time of 25 minutes, and one unit of code 99354. The physician must bill the highest level code in the code family (99215 which has 40 minutes typical/average time units associated with it). The additional time spent beyond this code is 20 minutes and does not meet the threshold time for billing prolonged services.

100-4, 12, 30.6.15.2

Prolonged Services Without Face to Face Service (Codes 99358 - 99359)

Contractors may not pay prolonged services codes 99358 and 99359, which do not require any direct patient face-to-face contact (e.g., telephone calls). Payment for these services is included in the payment for direct face-to-face services that physicians bill. The physician cannot bill the patient for these services since they are Medicare covered services and payment is included in the payment for other billable services.

100-4, 12, 30.6.15.3

Physician Standby Service (Code 99360)

Standby services are not payable to physicians. Physicians may not bill Medicare or beneficiaries for standby services. Payment for standby services is included in the Part A payment to the facility. Such services are a part of hospital costs to provide quality care.

If hospitals pay physicians for standby services, such services are part of hospital costs to provide quality care.

100-4, 12, 30.6.16

Case Management Services (Codes 99362 and 99371 - 99373)

A. Team Conferences

Team conferences (codes 99361-99362) may not be paid separately. Payment for these services is included in the payment for the services to which they relate.

B. Telephone Calls

Telephone calls (codes 99371-99373) may not be paid separately. Payment for telephone calls is included in payment for billable services (e.g., visit, surgery, diagnostic procedure results).

100-4, 12, 40.2

Billing Requirements for Global Surgeries

To ensure the proper identification of services that are, or are not, included in the global package, the following procedures apply.

A. Procedure Codes and Modifiers

Use of the modifiers in this section apply to both major procedures with a 90-day postoperative period and minor procedures with a 10-day postoperative period (and/or a zero day postoperative period in the case of modifiers "-22" and "-25").

1. Physicians Who Furnish the Entire Global Surgical Package
   Physicians who perform the surgery and furnish all of the usual pre-and postoperative work bill for the global package by entering the appropriate CPT code for the surgical procedure only. Billing is not allowed for visits or other services that are included in the global package.
2. Physicians in Group Practice
   When different physicians in a group practice participate in the care of the patient, the group bills for the entire global package if the physicians reassign benefits to the group. The physician who performs the surgery is shown as the performing physician. (For dates of service prior to January 1, 1994, however, where a new physician furnishes the entire postoperative care, the group billed for the surgical care and the postoperative care as separate line items with the appropriate modifiers.)
3. Physicians Who Furnish Part of a Global Surgical Package
   Where physicians agree on the transfer of care during the global period, the following modifiers are used:
   - "-54" for surgical care only; or
   - "-55" for postoperative management only.

   Both the bill for the surgical care only and the bill for the postoperative care only, will contain the same date of service and the same surgical procedure code, with the services distinguished by the use of the appropriate modifier.

   Providers need not specify on the claim that care has been transferred. However, the date on which care was relinquished or assumed, as applicable, must be shown on the claim. This should be indicated in the remarks field/free text segment on the claim form/format. Both the surgeon and the physician providing the postoperative care must keep a copy of the written transfer agreement in the beneficiary's medical record.

   Where a transfer of postoperative care occurs, the receiving physician cannot bill for any part of the global services until he/she has provided at least one service. Once the physician has seen the patient, that physician may bill for the period beginning with the date on which he/she assumes care of the patient.

   EXCEPTIONS:
   - Where a transfer of care does not occur, occasional post-discharge services of a physician other than the surgeon are reported by the appropriate evaluation and management code. No modifiers are necessary on the claim.
   - If the transfer of care occurs immediately after surgery, the physician other than the surgeon who provides the in-hospital postoperative care bills using subsequent hospital care codes for the inpatient hospital care and the surgical code with the "-55" modifier for the post-discharge care. The surgeon bills the surgery code with the "-54" modifier.
   - Physicians who provide follow-up services for minor procedures performed in emergency departments bill the appropriate level of office visit code. The physician who performs the emergency room service bills for the surgical procedure without a modifier.
   - If the services of a physician other than the surgeon are required during a postoperative period for an underlying condition or medical complication, the other physician reports the appropriate evaluation and management code. No modifiers are necessary on the claim. An example is a cardiologist who manages underlying cardiovascular conditions of a patient.
4. Evaluation and Management Service Resulting in the Initial Decision to Perform Surgery
   Evaluation and management services on the day before major surgery or on the day of major surgery that result in the initial decision to perform the surgery are not included in the global surgery payment for the major surgery and, therefore, may be billed and paid separately.

   In addition to the CPT evaluation and management code, modifier "-57" (decision for surgery) is used to identify a visit which results in the initial decision to perform surgery. (Modifier "-QI" was used for dates of service prior to January 1, 1994.)

   If evaluation and management services occur on the day of surgery, the physician bills using modifier "-57," not "-25." The "-57" modifier is not used with minor surgeries because the global period for minor surgeries does not include the day prior to the surgery. Moreover, where the decision to perform the minor procedure is typically done immediately before the service, it is considered a routine preoperative service and a visit or consultation is not billed in addition to the procedure.
5. Return Trips to the Operating Room During the Postoperative Period
   When treatment for complications requires a return trip to the operating room, physicians must bill the CPT code that describes the procedure(s) performed during the return trip. If no such code exists, use the unspecified procedure code in the correct series, i.e., 47999 or 64999. The procedure code for the original surgery is not used except when the identical procedure is repeated.

   In addition to the CPT code, physicians use CPT modifier "-78" for these return trips (return to the operating room for a related procedure during a postoperative period.)

   The physician may also need to indicate that another procedure was performed during the postoperative period of the initial procedure. When this subsequent procedure is related to the first procedure and requires the use of the operating room, this circumstance may be reported by adding the modifier "-78" to the related procedure.

   NOTE: The CPT definition for this modifier does not limit its use to treatment for complications.
6. Staged or Related Procedures
   Modifier "-58" was established to facilitate billing of staged or related surgical procedures done during the postoperative period of the first procedure. This

modifier is not used to report the treatment of a problem that requires a return to the operating room.

The physician may need to indicate that the performance of a procedure or service during the postoperative period was:

a. Planned prospectively or at the time of the original procedure;

b. More extensive than the original procedure; or

c. For therapy following a diagnostic surgical procedure.

These circumstances may be reported by adding modifier "-58" to the staged procedure. A new postoperative period begins when the next procedure in the series is billed.

7. Unrelated Procedures or Visits During the Postoperative Period
Two CPT modifiers were established to simplify billing for visits and other procedures which are furnished during the postoperative period of a surgical procedure, but which are not included in the payment for the surgical procedure.

Modifier "-79": Reports an unrelated procedure by the same physician during a postoperative period. The physician may need to indicate that the performance of a procedure or service during a postoperative period was unrelated to the original procedure.

A new postoperative period begins when the unrelated procedure is billed.

Modifier "-24": Reports an unrelated evaluation and management service by same physician during a postoperative period. The physician may need to indicate that an evaluation and management service was performed during the postoperative period of an unrelated procedure. This circumstance is reported by adding the modifier "-24" to the appropriate level of evaluation and management service.

Services submitted with the "-24" modifier must be sufficiently documented to establish that the visit was unrelated to the surgery. An ICD-9-CM code that clearly indicates that the reason for the encounter was unrelated to the surgery is acceptable documentation.

A physician who is responsible for postoperative care and has reported and been paid using modifier "-55" also uses modifier "-24" to report any unrelated visits.

8. Significant Evaluation and Management on the Day of a Procedure
Modifier "-25" is used to facilitate billing of evaluation and management services on the day of a procedure for which separate payment may be made.

It is used to report a significant, separately identifiable evaluation and management service by same physician on the day of a procedure. The physician may need to indicate that on the day a procedure or service that is identified with a CPT code was performed, the patient's condition required a significant, separately identifiable evaluation and management service above and beyond the usual preoperative and postoperative care associated with the procedure or service that was performed. This circumstance may be reported by adding the modifier "-25" to the appropriate level of evaluation and management service.

Claims containing evaluation and management codes with modifier "-25" are not subject to prepayment review except in the following situations:

- Effective January 1, 1995, all evaluation and management services provided on the same day as inpatient dialysis are denied without review with the exception of CPT Codes 99221-9223, 99251-99255, and 99238. These codes may be billed with modifier "-25" and reviewed for possible allowance if the evaluation and management service is unrelated to the treatment of ESRD and was not, and could not, have been provided during the dialysis treatment;
- When preoperative critical care codes are being billed for within a global surgical period; and
- When carriers have conducted a specific medical review process and determined, after reviewing the data, that an individual or group have high statistics in terms of the use of modifier "-25," have done a case-by-case review of the records to verify that the use of modifier "-25" was inappropriate, and have educated the individual or group as to the proper use of this modifier.

9. Critical Care
Critical care services provided during a global surgical period for a seriously injured or burned patient are not considered related to a surgical procedure and may be paid separately under the following circumstances.

Preoperative and postoperative critical care may be paid in addition to a global fee if:

- The patient is critically ill and requires the constant attendance of the physician; and
- The critical care is above and beyond, and, in most instances, unrelated to the specific anatomic injury or general surgical procedure performed.

Such patients are potentially unstable or have conditions that could pose a significant threat to life or risk of prolonged impairment.

In order for these services to be paid, two reporting requirements must be met:

- Codes 99291/99292 and modifier "-25" (for preoperative care) or "-24" (for postoperative care) must be used; and
- Documentation that the critical care was unrelated to the specific anatomic injury or general surgical procedure performed must be submitted. An ICD-9-CM code in the range 800.0 through 959.9 (except 930-939), which clearly indicates that the critical care was unrelated to the surgery, is acceptable documentation.

10. Unusual Circumstances
Surgeries for which services performed are significantly greater than usually required may be billed with the "-22" modifier added to the CPT code for the procedure. Surgeries for which services performed are significantly less than usually required may be billed with the "-52" modifier. The biller must provide:

- A concise statement about how the service differs from the usual; and
- An operative report with the claim.

Modifier "-22" should only be reported with procedure codes that have a global period of 0, 10, or 90 days. There is no such restriction on the use of modifier "-52."

B. Date(s) of Service
Physicians, who bill for the entire global surgical package or for only a portion of the care, must enter the date on which the surgical procedure was performed in the "From/To" date of service field. This will enable carriers to relate all appropriate billings to the correct surgery. Physicians who share postoperative management with another physician must submit additional information showing when they assumed and relinquished responsibility for the postoperative care. If the physician who performed the surgery relinquishes care at the time of discharge, he or she need only show the date of surgery when billing with modifier "-54."

However, if the surgeon also cares for the patient for some period following discharge, the surgeon must show the date of surgery and the date on which postoperative care was relinquished to another physician. The physician providing the remaining postoperative care must show the date care was assumed. This information should be shown in Item 19 on the paper Form CMS-1500, in the narrative portion of the HA0 record on the National Standard Format, and in the NTE segment for ANSI X12N electronic claims.

C. Care Provided in Different Payment Localities
If portions of the global period are provided in different payment localities, the services should be billed to the carriers servicing each applicable payment locality. For example, if the surgery is performed in one state and the postoperative care is provided in another state, the surgery is billed with modifier "-54" to the carrier servicing the payment locality where the surgery was performed and the postoperative care is billed with modifier "-55" to the carrier servicing the payment locality where the postoperative care was performed. This is true whether the services were performed by the same physician/group or different physicians/groups.

D. Health Professional Shortage Area (HPSA) Payments for Services Which are Subject to the Global Surgery Rules
HPSA bonus payments may be made for global surgeries when the services are provided in HPSAs. The following are guidelines for the appropriate billing procedures:

- If the entire global package is provided in a HPSA, physicians should bill for the appropriate global surgical code with the applicable HPSA modifier.
- If only a portion of the global package is provided in a HPSA, the physician should bill using a HPSA modifier for the portion which is provided in the HPSA.

EXAMPLE

The surgical portion of the global service is provided in a non-HPSA and the postoperative portion is provided in a HPSA. The surgical portion should be billed with the "-54" modifier and no HPSA modifier. The postoperative portion should be billed with the "-55" modifier and the appropriate HPSA modifier. The 10 percent bonus will be paid on the appropriate postoperative portion only. If a claim is submitted with a global surgical code and a HPSA modifier, the carrier assumes that the entire global service was provided in a HPSA in the absence of evidence otherwise.

NOTE: The sum of the payments made for the surgical and postoperative services provided in different localities will not equal the global amount in either of the localities because of geographic adjustments made through the Geographic Practice Cost Indices.

100-4,12,40.3

40.3 - Claims Review for Global Surgeries

(Rev. 2997, Issued: 07-25-14, Effective: Upon implementation of ICD-10; 01-01-2012 - ASC X12, Implementation: 08-25-2014 - ASC X12; Upon Implementation of ICD-10)

A. Relationship to Correct Coding Initiative (CCI)
The CCI policy and computer edits allow A/B MACs (B) to detect instances of fragmented billing for certain intra-operative services and other services furnished on the same day as the surgery that are considered to be components of the surgical procedure and, therefore, included in the global surgical fee. When both correct coding and global surgery edits apply to the same claim, A/B MACs (B) first apply the correct coding edits, then, apply the global surgery edits to the correctly coded services.

B. Prepayment Edits to Detect Separate Billing of Services Included in the Global Package
In addition to the correct coding edits, A/B MACs (B) must be capable of detecting certain other services included in the payment for a major or minor surgery or for an endoscopy. On a prepayment basis, A/B MACs (B) identify the services that meet the following conditions:

- Preoperative services that are submitted on the same claim or on a subsequent claim as a surgical procedure; or
- Same day or postoperative services that are submitted on the same claim or on a subsequent claim as a surgical procedure or endoscopy;

  and -
- Services that were furnished within the prescribed global period of the surgical procedure;
- Services that are billed without modifier "-78," "-79," "-24," "25," or "-57" or are billed with modifier "-24" but without the required documentation; and
- Services that are billed with the same provider or group number as the surgical procedure or endoscopy. Also, edit for any visits billed separately during the postoperative period without modifier "-24" by a physician who billed for the postoperative care only with modifier "-55."

A/B MACs (B) use the following evaluation and management codes in establishing edits for visits included in the global package. CPT codes 99241, 99242, 99243, 99244,99245, 99251, 99252, 99253, 99254, 99255, 99271, 99272, 99273, 99274, and 99275 have been transferred from the excluded category and are now included in the global surgery edits.

Evaluation and Management Codes for A/B MAC (B) Edits

92012	92014	99211	99212	99213	99214	99215
99217	99218	99219	99220	99221	99222	99223
99231	99232	99233	99234	99235	99236	99238
99239	99241	99242	99243	99244	99245	99251
99252	99253	99254	99255	99261	99262	99263
99271	99272	99273	99274	99275	99291	99292
99301	99302	99303	99311	99312	99313	99315
99316	99331	99332	99333	99347	99348	99349
99350	99374	99375	99377	99378		

NOTE: In order for codes 99291 or 99292 to be paid for services furnished during the preoperative or postoperative period, modifier "-25" or "-24," respectively, must be used to indicate that the critical care was unrelated to the specific anatomic injury or general surgical procedure performed.

If a surgeon is admitting a patient ta nursing facility for a condition not related to the global surgical procedure, the physician should bill for the nursing facility admission and care with a "-24" modifier and appropriate documentation. If a surgeon is admitting a patient ta nursing facility and the patient's admission to that facility relates to the global surgical procedure, the nursing facility admission and any services related to the global surgical procedure are included in the global surgery fee.

C. Exclusions from Prepayment Edits

A/B MACs (B) exclude the following services from the prepayment audit process and allow separate payment if all usual requirements are met:

Services listed in §40.1.B; and

Services billed with the modifier "-25," "-57," "-58," "-78," or "-79."

Exceptions

See §§40.2.A.8, 40.2.A.9, and 40.4.A for instances where prepayment review is required for modifier "-25." In addition, prepayment review is necessary for CPT codes 90935,90937, 90945, and 90947 when a visit and modifier "-25" are billed with these services.

Exclude the following codes from the prepayment edits required in §40.3.B.

92002	92004	99201	99202	99203	99204	99205
99281	99282	99283	99284	99285	99321	99322
99323	99341	99342	99343	99344	99345	

100-4, 12, 40.6

Claims for Multiple Surgeries

B3-4826, B3-15038, B3-15056

A. General

Multiple surgeries are separate procedures performed by a single physician or physicians in the same group practice on the same patient at the same operative session or on the same day for which separate payment may be allowed. Co-surgeons, surgical teams, or assistants-at-surgery may participate in performing multiple surgeries on the same patient on the same day.

Multiple surgeries are distinguished from procedures that are components of or incidental to a primary procedure. These intra-operative services, incidental surgeries, or components of more major surgeries are not separately billable. See Chapter 23 for a description of mandatory edits to prevent separate payment for those procedures. Major surgical procedures are determined based on the MFSDB approved amount and not on the submitted amount from the providers. The major surgery, as based on the MFSDB, may or may not be the one with the larger submitted amount.

Also, see subsection D below for a description of the standard payment policy on multiple surgeries. However, these standard payment rules are not appropriate for certain procedures. Field 21 of the MFSDB indicates whether the standard payment policy rules apply to a multiple surgery, or whether special payment rules apply. Site of service payment adjustments (codes with an indicator of "1" in Field 27 of the MFSDB) should be applied before multiple surgery payment adjustments.

B. Billing Instructions

The following procedures apply when billing for multiple surgeries by the same physician on the same day.

- Report the more major surgical procedure without the multiple procedures modifier "-51."
- Report additional surgical procedures performed by the surgeon on the same day with modifier "-51."

There may be instances in which two or more physicians each perform distinctly different, unrelated surgeries on the same patient on the same day (e.g., in some multiple trauma cases). When this occurs, the payment adjustment rules for multiple surgeries may not be appropriate. In such cases, the physician does not use modifier "-51" unless one of the surgeons individually performs multiple surgeries.

C. Carrier Claims Processing System Requirements

Carriers must be able to:

1. Identify multiple surgeries by both of the following methods:
   - The presence on the claim form or electronic submission of the "-51" modifier; and
   - The billing of more than one separately payable surgical procedure by the same physician performed on the same patient on the same day, whether on different lines or with a number greater than 1 in the units column on the claim form or inappropriately billed with modifier "-78" (i.e., after the global period has expired);
2. Access Field 34 of the MFSDB to determine the Medicare fee schedule payment amount for each surgery;
3. Access Field 21 for each procedure of the MFSDB to determine if the payment rules for multiple surgeries apply to any of the multiple surgeries billed on the same day;
4. If Field 21 for any of the multiple procedures contains an indicator of "0," the multiple surgery rules do not apply to that procedure. Base payment on the lower of the billed amount or the fee schedule amount (Field 34 or 35) for each code unless other payment adjustment rules apply;
5. For dates of service prior to January 1, 1995, if Field 21 contains an indicator of "1," the standard rules for pricing multiple surgeries apply (see items 6-8 below);
6. Rank the surgeries subject to the standard multiple surgery rules (indicator "1") in descending order by the Medicare fee schedule amount;
7. Base payment for each ranked procedure on the lower of the billed amount, or:
   - 100 percent of the fee schedule amount (Field 34 or 35) for the highest valued procedure;
   - 50 percent of the fee schedule amount for the second highest valued procedure; and
   - 25 percent of the fee schedule amount for the third through the fifth highest valued procedures;
8. If more than five procedures are billed, pay for the first five according to the rules listed in 5, 6, and 7 above and suspend the sixth and subsequent procedures for manual review and payment, if appropriate, "by report." Payment determined on a "by report" basis for these codes should never be lower than 25 percent of the full payment amount;
9. For dates of service on or after January 1, 1995, new standard rules for pricing multiple surgeries apply. If Field 21 contains an indicator of "2," these new standard rules apply (see items 10-12 below);
10. Rank the surgeries subject to the multiple surgery rules (indicator "2") in descending order by the Medicare fee schedule amount;
11. Base payment for each ranked procedure (indicator "2") on the lower of the billed amount:
    - 100 percent of the fee schedule amount (Field 34 or 35) for the highest valued procedure; and
    - 50 percent of the fee schedule amount for the second through the fifth highest valued procedures; or
12. If more than five procedures with an indicator of "2" are billed, pay for the first five according to the rules listed in 9, 10, and 11 above and suspend the sixth and subsequent procedures for manual review and payment, if appropriate, "by report." Payment determined on a "by report" basis for these codes should never be lower than 50 percent of the full payment amount. Pay by the unit for services that are already reduced (e.g., 17003). Pay for 17340 only once per session, regardless of how many lesions were destroyed;

    NOTE: For dates of service prior to January 1, 1995, the multiple surgery indicator of "2" indicated that special dermatology rules applied. The payment rules for these codes have not changed. The rules were expanded, however, to all codes that previously had a multiple surgery indicator of "1." For dates of service prior to January 1, 1995, if a dermatological procedure with an indicator of "2" was billed with the "-51" modifier with other procedures that are not dermatological procedures (procedures with an indicator of "1" in Field 21), the standard multiple surgery rules applied. Pay no less than 50 percent for the dermatological procedures with an indicator of "2." See 40.6.C.6-8 for required actions.

13. If Field 21 contains an indicator of "3," and multiple endoscopies are billed, the special rules for multiple endoscopic procedures apply. Pay the full value of the highest valued endoscopy, plus the difference between the next highest and the base endoscopy. Access Field 31A of the MFSDB to determine the base endoscopy.

    EXAMPLE

    In the course of performing a fiber optic colonoscopy (CPT code 45378), a physician performs a biopsy on a lesion (code 45380) and removes a polyp (code 45385) from a different part of the colon. The physician bills for codes 45380 and 45385. The value of codes 45380 and 45385 have the value of the diagnostic colonoscopy (45378) built in.

    Rather than paying 100 percent for the highest valued procedure (45385) and 50 percent for the next (45380), pay the full value of the higher valued endoscopy (45385), plus the difference between the next highest endoscopy (45380) and the base endoscopy (45378).

    Carriers assume the following fee schedule amounts for these codes:

    45378 - $255.40

    45380 - $285.98

    45385 - $374.56

    Pay the full value of 45385 ($374.56), plus the difference between 45380 and 45378 ($30.58), for a total of $405.14.

    NOTE: If an endoscopic procedure with an indicator of "3" is billed with the "-51" modifier with other procedures that are not endoscopies (procedures with an indicator of "1" in Field 21), the standard multiple surgery rules apply. See 40.6.C.6-8 for required actions.

14. Apply the following rules where endoscopies are performed on the same day as unrelated endoscopies or other surgical procedures:
    - Two unrelated endoscopies (e.g., 46606 and 43217): Apply the usual multiple surgery rules;
    - Two sets of unrelated endoscopies (e.g., 43202 and 43217; 46606 and 46608): Apply the special endoscopy rules to each series and then apply the multiple surgery rules. Consider the total payment for each set of endoscopies as one service;
    - Two related endoscopies and a third, unrelated procedure: Apply the special endoscopic rules to the related endoscopies, and, then apply the multiple surgery rules. Consider the total payment for the related endoscopies as one service and the unrelated endoscopy as another service.
15. If two or more multiple surgeries are of equal value, rank them in descending dollar order billed and base payment on the percentages listed above (i.e., 100 percent for the first billed procedure, 50 percent for the second, etc.);
16. If any of the multiple surgeries are bilateral surgeries, consider the bilateral procedure at 150 percent as one payment amount, rank this with the remaining procedures, and apply the appropriate multiple surgery reductions. See 40.7 for bilateral surgery payment instructions.);
17. Round all adjusted payment amounts to the nearest cent;
18. If some of the surgeries are subject to special rules while others are subject to the standard rules, automate pricing to the extent possible. If necessary, price manually;
19. In cases of multiple interventional radiological procedures, both the radiology code and the primary surgical code are paid at 100 percent of the fee schedule amount. The subsequent surgical procedures are paid at the standard multiple surgical percentages (50 percent, 50 percent, 50 percent and 50 percent);
20. Apply the requirements in 40 on global surgeries to multiple surgeries;
21. Retain the "-51" modifier in history for any multiple surgeries paid at less than the full global amount; and
22. Follow the instructions on adjudicating surgery claims submitted with the "-22" modifier. Review documentation to determine if full payment should be made for those distinctly different, unrelated surgeries performed by different physicians on the same day.

D. Ranking of Same Day Multiple Surgeries When One Surgery Has a "-22" Modifier and Additional Payment is Allowed

B3-4826

If the patient returns to the operating room after the initial operative session on the same day as a result of complications from the original surgery, the complications rules apply to each procedure required to treat the complications from the original surgery. The multiple surgery rules would not apply.

However, if the patient is returned to the operating room during the postoperative period of the original surgery, not on the same day of the original surgery, for multiple procedures that are required as a result of complications from the original surgery, the complications rules would apply. The multiple surgery rules would also not apply.

Multiple surgeries are defined as separate procedures performed by a single physician or physicians in the same group practice on the same patient at the same operative session or on the same day for which separate payment may be allowed. Co-surgeons, surgical teams, or assistants-at-surgery may participate in performing multiple surgeries on the same patient on the same day.

Multiple surgeries are distinguished from procedures that are components of or incidental to a primary procedure. These intra-operative services, incidental surgeries, or components of more major surgeries are not separately billable. See Chapter 23 for a description of mandatory edits to prevent separate payment for those procedures.

100-4, 12, 40.7

Claims for Bilateral Surgeries

B3-4827, B3-15040

A. General

Bilateral surgeries are procedures performed on both sides of the body during the same operative session or on the same day.

The terminology for some procedure codes includes the terms "bilateral" (e.g., code 27395; Lengthening of the hamstring tendon; multiple, bilateral.) or "unilateral or bilateral" (e.g., code 52290; cystourethroscopy; with ureteral meatotomy, unilateral or bilateral). The payment adjustment rules for bilateral surgeries do not apply to procedures identified by CPT as "bilateral" or "unilateral or bilateral" since the fee schedule reflects any additional work required for bilateral surgeries.

Field 22 of the MFSDB indicates whether the payment adjustment rules apply to a surgical procedure.

B. Billing Instructions for Bilateral Surgeries

If a procedure is not identified by its terminology as a bilateral procedure (or unilateral or bilateral), physicians must report the procedure with modifier "-50." They report such procedures as a single line item. (NOTE: This differs from the CPT coding guidelines which indicate that bilateral procedures should be billed as two line items.)

If a procedure is identified by the terminology as bilateral (or unilateral or bilateral), as in codes 27395 and 52290, physicians do not report the procedure with modifier "-50."

C. Claims Processing System Requirements

Carriers must be able to:

1. Identify bilateral surgeries by the presence on the claim form or electronic submission of the "-50" modifier or of the same code on separate lines reported once with modifier "-LT" and once with modifier "-RT";
2. Access Field 34 or 35 of the MFSDB to determine the Medicare payment amount;
3. Access Field 22 of the MFSDB:
    - If Field 22 contains an indicator of "0," "2," or "3," the payment adjustment rules for bilateral surgeries do not apply. Base payment on the lower of the billed amount or 100 percent of the fee schedule amount (Field 34 or 35) unless other payment adjustment rules apply.

      NOTE: Some codes which have a bilateral indicator of "0" in the MFSDB may be performed more than once on a given day. These are services that would never be considered bilateral and thus should not be billed with modifier "-50." Where such a code is billed on multiple line tems or with more than 1 in the units field and carriers have determined that the code may be reported more than once, bypass the "0" bilateral indicator and refer to the multiple surgery field for pricing;
    - If Field 22 contains an indicator of "1," the standard adjustment rules apply. Base payment on the lower of the billed amount or 150 percent of the fee schedule amount (Field 34 or 35). (Multiply the payment amount in Field 34 or 35 for the surgery by 150 percent and round to the nearest cent.)
4. Apply the requirements 40 - 40.4 on global surgeries to bilateral surgeries; and
5. Retain the "-50" modifier in history for any bilateral surgeries paid at the adjusted amount.

   (NOTE: The "-50" modifier is not retained for surgeries which are bilateral by definition such as code 27395.)

100-4, 12, 40.8

Claims for Co-Surgeons and Team Surgeons

B3-4828, B3-15046

A. General

Under some circumstances, the individual skills of two or more surgeons are required to perform surgery on the same patient during the same operative session. This may be required because of the complex nature of the procedure(s) and/or the patient's condition.

In these cases, the additional physicians are not acting as assistants-at-surgery.

B. Billing Instructions

The following billing procedures apply when billing for a surgical procedure or procedures that required the use of two surgeons or a team of surgeons:

- If two surgeons (each in a different specialty) are required to perform a specific procedure, each surgeon bills for the procedure with a modifier "-62." Co-surgery also refers to surgical procedures involving two surgeons performing the parts of the procedure simultaneously, i.e., heart transplant or bilateral knee replacements. Documentation of the medical necessity for two surgeons is required for certain services identified in the MFSDB. (See 40.8.C.5.);
- If a team of surgeons (more than 2 surgeons of different specialties) is required to perform a specific procedure, each surgeon bills for the procedure with a modifier "-66." Field 25 of the MFSDB identifies certain services submitted with a "-66" modifier which must be sufficiently documented to establish that a team was medically necessary. All claims for team surgeons must contain sufficient information to allow pricing "by report."
- If surgeons of different specialties are each performing a different procedure (with specific CPT codes), neither co-surgery nor multiple surgery rules apply (even if the procedures are performed through the same incision). If one of the surgeons performs multiple procedures, the multiple procedure rules apply to that surgeon's services. (See 40.6 for multiple surgery payment rules.)

For co-surgeons (modifier 62), the fee schedule amount applicable to the payment for each co-surgeon is 62.5 percent of the global surgery fee schedule amount. Team surgery (modifier 66) is paid for on a "By Report" basis.

C. Claims Processing System Requirements

Carriers must be able to:

1. Identify a surgical procedure performed by two surgeons or a team of surgeons by the presence on the claim form or electronic submission of the "-62" or "-66" modifier;
2. Access Field 34 or 35 of the MFSDB to determine the fee schedule payment amount for the surgery;
3. Access Field 24 or 25, as appropriate, of the MFSDB. These fields provide guidance on whether two or team surgeons are generally required for the surgical procedure;
4. If the surgery is billed with a "-62" or "-66" modifier and Field 24 or 25 contains an indicator of "0," payment adjustment rules for two or team surgeons do not apply:
   - Carriers pay the first bill submitted, and base payment on the lower of the billed amount or 100 percent of the fee schedule amount (Field 34 or 35) unless other payment adjustment rules apply;
   - Carriers deny bills received subsequently from other physicians and use the appropriate MSN message in 40.8.D. As these are medical necessity denials, the instructions in the Program Integrity Manual regarding denial of unassigned claims for medical necessity are applied;
5. If the surgery is billed with a "-62" modifier and Field 24 contains an indicator of "1," suspend the claim for manual review of any documentation submitted with the claim. If the documentation supports the need for co-surgeons, base payment for each physician on the lower of the billed amount or 62.5 percent of the fee schedule amount (Field 34 or 35);
6. If the surgery is billed with a "-62" modifier and Field 24 contains an indicator of "2," payment rules for two surgeons apply. Carriers base payment for each physician on the lower of the billed amount or 62.5 percent of the fee schedule amount (Field 34 or 35);
7. If the surgery is billed with a "-66" modifier and Field 25 contains an indicator of "1," carriers suspend the claim for manual review. If carriers determine that team surgeons were medically necessary, each physician is paid on a "by report" basis;
8. If the surgery is billed with a "-66" modifier and Field 25 contains an indicator of "2," carriers pay "by report";

   NOTE: A Medicare fee may have been established for some surgical procedures that are billed with the "-66" modifier. In these cases, all physicians on the team must agree on the percentage of the Medicare payment amount each is to receive.If carriers receive a bill with a "-66" modifier after carriers have paid one surgeon the full Medicare payment amount (on a bill without the modifier), deny the subsequent claim.
9. Apply the rules global surgical packages to each of the physicians participating in a co- or team surgery; and
10. Retain the "-62" and "-66" modifiers in history for any co- or team surgeries.

D. Beneficiary Liability on Denied Claims for Assistant, Co- surgeon and Team Surgeons

MSN message 23.10 which states "Medicare does not pay for a surgical assistant for this kind of surgery," was established for denial of claims for assistant surgeons. Where such payment is denied because the procedure is subject to the statutory restriction against payment for assistants-at-surgery. Carriers include the following statement in the MSN:

> "You cannot be charged for this service." (Unnumbered add-on message.)

Carriers use Group Code CO on the remittance advice to the physician to signify that the beneficiary may not be billed for the denied service and that the physician could be subject to penalties if a bill is issued to the beneficiary.

If Field 23 of the MFSDB contains an indicator of "0" or "1" (assistant-at-surgery may not be paid) for procedures CMS has determined that an assistant surgeon is not generally medically necessary.

For those procedures with an indicator of "0," the limitation on liability provisions described in Chapter 30 apply to assigned claims. Therefore, carriers include the appropriate limitation of liability language from Chapter 21. For unassigned claims, apply the rules in the Program Integrity Manual concerning denial for medical necessity.

Where payment may not be made for a co- or team surgeon, use the following MSN message (MSN message number 15.13):

> Medicare does not pay for team surgeons for this procedure.

Where payment may not be made for a two surgeons, use the following MSN message (MSN message number 15.12):

> Medicare does not pay for two surgeons for this procedure.

Also see limitation of liability remittance notice REF remark codes M25, M26, and M27.

Use the following message on the remittance notice:

> Multiple physicians/assistants are not covered in this case. (Reason code 54.)

100-4, 12, 50

Payment for Anesthesiology Services

A. General Payment Rule

The fee schedule amount for physician anesthesia services furnished on or after January 1, 1992 is, with the exceptions noted, based on allowable base and time units multiplied by an anesthesia conversion factor specific to that locality. The base unit for each anesthesia procedure is communicated to the Part B Contractors by means of the HCPCS file released annually. The public can access the base units on the CMS homepage through the anesthesiologist's center. The way in which time units are calculated is described in Sec.50.G. CMS releases the conversion factor annually.

B. Payment at Personally Performed Rate

The Part B Contractor must determine the fee schedule payment, recognizing the base unit for the anesthesia code and one time unit per 15 minutes of anesthesia time if: The physician personally performed the entire anesthesia service alone; The physician is involved with one anesthesia case with a resident, the physician is a teaching physician as defined in Sec.100, and the service is furnished on or after January 1, 1996; The physician is involved in the training of physician residents in a single anesthesia case, two concurrent anesthesia cases involving residents or a single anesthesia case involving a resident that is concurrent to another case paid under the medical direction rules. The physician meets the teaching physician criteria in Sec.100.1.4 and the service is furnished on or after January 1, 2010; The physician is continuously involved in a single case involving a student nurse anesthetist; The physician is continuously involved in one anesthesia case involving a CRNA (or AA) and the service was furnished prior to January 1, 1998. If the physician is involved with a single case with a CRNA (or AA) and the service was furnished on or after January 1, 1998, carriers may pay the physician service and the CRNA (or AA) service in accordance with the medical direction payment policy; or The physician and the CRNA (or AA) are involved in one anesthesia case and the services of each are found to be medically necessary. Documentation must be submitted by both the CRNA and the physician to support payment of the full fee for each of the two providers. The physician reports the "AA" modifier and the CRNA reports the "QZ" modifier for a nonmedically directed case.

C. Payment at the Medically Directed Rate

The Part B Contractor determines payment for the physician's medical direction service furnished on or after January 1, 1998, on the basis of 50 percent of the allowance for the service performed by the physician alone. Medical direction occurs if the physician medically directs qualified individuals in two, three, or four concurrent cases and the physician performs the following activities.

Performs a pre-anesthetic examination and evaluation; Prescribes the anesthesia plan; Personally participates in the most demanding procedures in the anesthesia plan, including induction and emergence; Ensures that any procedures in the anesthesia plan that he or she does not perform are performed by a qualified anesthetist; Monitors the course of anesthesia administration at frequent intervals; Remains physically present and available for immediate diagnosis and treatment of emergencies; and Provides indicated-post-anesthesia care.

Prior to January 1, 1999, the physician was required to participate in the most demanding procedures of the anesthesia plan, including induction and emergence.

For medical direction services furnished on or after January 1, 1999, the physician must participate only in the most demanding procedures of the anesthesia plan, including, if applicable, induction and emergence. Also for medical direction services furnished on or after January 1, 1999, the physician must document in the medical record that he or she performed the pre-anesthetic examination and evaluation. Physicians must also document that they provided indicated post-anesthesia care, were present during some portion of the anesthesia monitoring, and were present during the most demanding procedures, including induction and emergence, where indicated.

For services furnished on or after January 1, 1994, the physician can medically direct two, three, or four concurrent procedures involving qualified individuals, all of whom could be CRNAs, AAs, interns, residents or combinations of these individuals. The medical direction rules apply to cases involving student nurse anesthetists if the physician directs two concurrent cases, each of which involves a student nurse anesthetist, or the physician directs one case involving a student nurse anesthetist and another involving a CRNA, AA, intern or resident.

For services furnished on or after January 1, 2010, the medical direction rules do not apply to a single resident case that is concurrent to another anesthesia case paid under the medical direction rules or to two concurrent anesthesia cases involving residents.

If anesthesiologists are in a group practice, one physician member may provide the pre-anesthesia examination and evaluation while another fulfills the other criteria. Similarly, one physician member of the group may provide post-anesthesia care while another member of the group furnishes the other component parts of the anesthesia service. However, the medical record must indicate that the services were furnished by physicians and identify the physicians who furnished them.

A physician who is concurrently directing the administration of anesthesia to not more than four surgical patients cannot ordinarily be involved in furnishing additional services to other patients. However, addressing an emergency of short duration in the immediate area, administering an epidural or caudal anesthetic to ease labor pain, or periodic, rather than continuous, monitoring of an obstetrical patient does not substantially diminish the scope of control exercised by the physician in directing the administration of anesthesia to surgical patients. It does not constitute a separate service for the purpose of determining whether the medical direction criteria are met. Further, while directing concurrent anesthesia procedures, a physician may receive patients entering the operating suite for the next surgery, check or discharge patients in the recovery room, or handle scheduling matters without affecting fee schedule payment.

However, if the physician leaves the immediate area of the operating suite for other than short durations or devotes extensive time to an emergency case or is otherwise not available to respond to the immediate needs of the surgical patients, the physician's services to the surgical patients are supervisory in nature. Carriers may not make payment under the fee schedule.

See Sec.50.J for a definition of concurrent anesthesia procedures.

D. Payment at Medically Supervised Rate

The Part B Contractor may allow only three base units per procedure when the anesthesiologist is involved in furnishing more than four procedures concurrently or is performing other services while directing the concurrent procedures. An additional time unit may be recognized if the physician can document he or she was present at induction.

E. Billing and Payment for Multiple Anesthesia Procedures

Physicians bill for the anesthesia services associated with multiple bilateral surgeries by reporting the anesthesia procedure with the highest base unit value with the multiple procedure modifier "-51." They report the total time for all procedures in the line item with the highest base unit value.

If the same anesthesia CPT code applies to two or more of the surgical procedures, billers enter the anesthesia code with the "-51" modifier and the number of surgeries to which the modified CPT code applies.

Payment can be made under the fee schedule for anesthesia services associated with multiple surgical procedures or multiple bilateral procedures. Payment is determined based on the base unit of the anesthesia procedure with the highest base unit value and time units based on the actual anesthesia time of the multiple procedures. See Sec.Sec.40.6-40.7 for a definition and appropriate billing and claims processing instructions for multiple and bilateral surgeries. F.

F. Payment for Medical and Surgical Services Furnished in Addition to Anesthesia Procedure

Payment may be made under the fee schedule for specific medical and surgical services furnished by the anesthesiologist as long as these services are reasonable and medically necessary or provided that other rebundling provisions (see Sec.30 and Chapter 23) do not preclude separate payment. These services may be furnished in conjunction with the anesthesia procedure to the patient or may be furnished as single services, e.g., during the day of or the day before the anesthesia service. These services include the insertion of a Swan Ganz catheter, the insertion of central venous pressure lines, emergency intubation, and critical care visits.

G. Anesthesia Time and Calculation of Anesthesia Time Units

Anesthesia time is defined as the period during which an anesthesia practitioner is present with the patient. It starts when the anesthesia practitioner begins to prepare the patient for anesthesia services in the operating room or an equivalent area and ends when the anesthesia practitioner is no longer furnishing anesthesia services to the patient, that is, when the patient may be placed safely under postoperative care. Anesthesia time is a continuous time period from the start of anesthesia to the end of an anesthesia service. In counting anesthesia time for services furnished on or after January 1, 2000, the anesthesia practitioner can add blocks of time around an interruption in anesthesia time as long as the anesthesia practitioner is furnishing continuous anesthesia care within the time periods around the interruption.

Actual anesthesia time in minutes is reported on the claim. For anesthesia services furnished on or after January 1, 1994, the A/B MAC computes time units by dividing reported anesthesia time by 15 minutes. Round the time unit to one decimal place. The A/B MAC does not recognize time units for CPT codes 01995 or 01996.

For purposes of this section, anesthesia practitioner means a physician who performs the anesthesia service alone, a CRNA who is not medically directed, or a CRNA or AA, who is medically directed. The physician who medically directs the CRNA or AA would ordinarily report the same time as the CRNA or AA reports for the CRNA service.

H. Base Unit Reduction for Concurrent Medically Directed Procedures

If the physician medically directs concurrent medically directed procedures prior to January 1, 1994, reduce the number of base units for each concurrent procedure as follows.

For two concurrent procedures, the base unit on each procedure is reduced 10 percent.

For three concurrent procedures, the base unit on each procedure is reduced 25 percent.

For four concurrent procedures, the base on each concurrent procedure is reduced 40 percent.

If the physician medically directs concurrent procedures prior to January 1, 1994, and any of the concurrent procedures are cataract or iridectomy anesthesia, reduce the base units for each cataract or iridectomy procedure by 10 percent.

I. Monitored Anesthesia Care

The Part B Contractor pays for reasonable and medically necessary monitored anesthesia care services on the same basis as other anesthesia services. Anesthesiologists use modifier QS to report monitored anesthesia care cases. Monitored anesthesia care involves the intra-operative monitoring by a physician or qualified individual under the medical direction of a physician or of the patient's vital physiological signs in anticipation of the need for administration of general anesthesia or of the development of adverse physiological patient reaction to the surgical procedure. It also includes the performance of a pre-anesthetic examination and evaluation, prescription of the anesthesia care required, administration of any necessary oral or parenteral medications (e.g., atropine, demerol, valium) and provision of indicated postoperative anesthesia care.

Payment is made under the fee schedule using the payment rules in subsection B if the physician personally performs the monitored anesthesia care case or under the rules in subsection C if the physician medically directs four or fewer concurrent cases and monitored anesthesia care represents one or more of these concurrent cases.

J. Definition of Concurrent Medically Directed Anesthesia Procedures

Concurrency is defined with regard to the maximum number of procedures that the physician is medically directing within the context of a single procedure and whether these other procedures overlap each other. Concurrency is not dependent on each of the cases involving a Medicare patient. For example, if an anesthesiologist directs three concurrent procedures, two of which involve non-Medicare patients and the remaining a Medicare patient, this represents three concurrent cases. The following example illustrates this concept and guides physicians in determining how many procedures they are directing.

EXAMPLE Procedures A through E are medically directed procedures involving CRNAs and furnished between January 1, 1992 and December 31, 1997 (1998 concurrent instructions can be found in subsection C.) The starting and ending times for each procedure represent the periods during which anesthesia time is counted. Assume that none of the procedures were cataract or iridectomy anesthesia.

Procedure A begins at 8:00 a.m. and lasts until 8:20 a.m.

Procedure B begins at 8:10 a.m. and lasts until 8:45 a.m.

Procedure C begins at 8:30 a.m. and lasts until 9:15 a.m.

Procedure D begins at 9:00 a.m. and lasts until 12:00 noon.

Procedure E begins at 9:10 a.m. and lasts until 9:55 a.m.

Procedure	Number of Concurrent Medically Directed Procedures	Base Unit Reduction Percentage
A	2	10%
B	2	0%
C	3	25%
D	3	25%
E	3	25%

From 8:00 a.m. to 8:20 a.m., the length of procedure A, the anesthesiologist medically directed two concurrent procedures, A and B.

From 8:10 a.m. to 8:45 a.m., the length of procedure B, the anesthesiologist medically directed two concurrent procedures. From 8:10 to 8:20 a.m., the anesthesiologist medically directed procedures A and B. From 8:20 to 8:30 a.m., the anesthesiologist medically directed only procedure B. From 8:30 to 8:45 a.m., the anesthesiologist medically directed procedures B and C. Thus, during procedure B, the anesthesiologist medically directed, at most, two concurrent procedures.

From 8:30 a.m. to 9:15 a.m., the length of procedure C, the anesthesiologist medically directed three concurrent procedures. From 8:30 to 8:45 a.m., the anesthesiologist medically directed procedures B and C. From 8:45 to 9:00 a.m., the anesthesiologist medically directed procedure C. From 9:00 to 9:10 a.m., the anesthesiologist medically directed procedures C and D. From 9:10 to 9:15 a.m., the anesthesiologist medically directed procedures C, D and E. Thus, during procedure C, the anesthesiologist medically directed, at most, three concurrent procedures.

The same analysis shows that during procedure D or E, the anesthesiologist medically directed, at most, three concurrent procedures.

K. Anesthesia Claims Modifiers

Physicians report the appropriate anesthesia modifier to denote whether the service was personally performed, medically directed, or medically supervised.

Specific anesthesia modifiers include:

AA - Anesthesia Services performed personally by the anesthesiologist;
AD - Medical Supervision by a physician; more than 4 concurrent anesthesia procedures;
G8 - Monitored anesthesia care (MAC) for deep complex complicated, or markedly invasive surgical procedures;
G9 - Monitored anesthesia care for patient who has a history of severe cardio-pulmonary condition;
QK - Medical direction of two, three or four concurrent anesthesia procedures involving qualified individuals;
QS - Monitored anesthesia care service;
QX - CRNA service; with medical direction by a physician;
QY - Medical direction of one certified registered nurse anesthetist by an anesthesiologist;
QZ - CRNA service: without medical direction by a physician; and
GC - these services have been performed by a resident under the direction of a teaching physician.

The GC modifier is reported by the teaching physician to indicate he/she rendered the service in compliance with the teaching physician requirements in Sec.100.1.2. One of the payment modifiers must be used in conjunction with the GC modifier.

The QS modifier is for informational purposes. Providers must report actual anesthesia time on the claim.

The Part B Contractor must determine payment for anesthesia in accordance with these instructions. They must be able to determine the uniform base unit that is assigned to the anesthesia code and apply the appropriate reduction where the anesthesia procedure is medically directed. They must also be able to determine the number of anesthesia time units from actual anesthesia time reported on the claim. The Part B Contractor must multiply allowable units by the anesthesia-specific conversion factor used to determine fee schedule payment for the payment area.

L. Anesthesia and Medical/Surgical Service Provided by the Same Physician

Anesthesia services range in complexity. The continuum of anesthesia services, from least intense to most intense in complexity is as follows: local or topical anesthesia, moderate (conscious) sedation, regional anesthesia and general anesthesia. Prior to 2006, Medicare did not recognize separate payment if the same physician provided the medical or surgical procedure and the anesthesia needed for the procedure.

Moderate sedation is a drug induced depression of consciousness during which the patient responds purposefully to verbal commands, either alone or accompanied by light tactile stimulation. Moderate sedation does not include minimal sedation, deep sedation or monitored anesthesia care. In 2006, the CPT added new codes 99143 to 99150 for moderate or conscious sedation. The moderate (conscious) sedation codes are carrier priced under the Medicare physician fee schedule.

The CPT codes 99143 to 99145 describe moderate sedation provided by the same physician performing the diagnostic or therapeutic service that the sedation supports, requiring the presence of an independent trained observer to assist in the monitoring of the patient's level of consciousness and physiological status. The physician can bill the conscious sedation codes 99143 to 99145 as long as the procedure with it is billed is not listed in Appendix G of CPT. CPT codes 99148 to 99150 describe moderate sedation provided by a physician other than the health care professional performing the diagnostic or therapeutic service that the sedation supports.

The CPT includes Appendix G, Summary of CPT Codes That Include Moderate (Conscious) Sedation. This appendix lists those procedures for which moderate (conscious) sedation is an inherent part of the procedure itself. CPT coding guidelines instruct practices not to report CPT codes 99143 to 99145 in conjunction with codes listed in Appendix G. The National Correct Coding Initiative has established edits that bundle CPT codes 99143 and 99144 into the procedures listed in Appendix G.

In the unusual event when a second physician other than the health care professional performing the diagnostic or therapeutic services provides moderate sedation in the facility setting for the procedures listed in Appendix G, the second physician can bill 99148 to 99150. The term, facility, includes those places of service listed in Chapter 23 Addendum -- field 29. However, when these services are performed by the second physician in the nonfacility setting, CPT codes 99148 to 99150 are not to be reported.

If the anesthesiologist or CRNA provides anesthesia for diagnostic or therapeutic nerve blocks or injections and a different provider performs the block or injection, then the anesthesiologist or CRNA may report the anesthesia service using CPT code 01991. The service must meet the criteria for monitored anesthesia care. If the anesthesiologist or CRNA provides both the anesthesia service and the block or injection, then the anesthesiologist or CRNA may report the anesthesia service using the conscious sedation code and the injection or block. However, the anesthesia service must meet the requirements for conscious sedation and if a lower level complexity anesthesia service is provided, then the conscious sedation code should not be reported.

If the physician performing the medical or surgical procedure also provides a level of anesthesia lower in intensity than moderate or conscious sedation, such as a local or topical anesthesia, then the conscious sedation code should not be reported and no payment should be allowed by the carrier. There is no CPT code for the performance of local anesthesia and as payment for this service is considered in the payment for the underlying medical or surgical service.

100-4, 12, 60

Payment for Pathology Services

B3-15020, AB-01-47 (CR1499)

A. General Payment Rule

Payment may be made under the fee schedule for the professional component of physician laboratory or physician pathology services furnished to hospital inpatients or outpatients by hospital physicians or by independent laboratories, if they qualify as the reassignee for the physician service.. Payment may be made under the fee schedule, as noted below, for the technical component (TC) of pathology services furnished by an independent laboratory to hospital inpatients or outpatients. Payment may be made under the fee schedule for the technical component of physician pathology services furnished by an independent laboratory, or a hospital if it is acting as an independent laboratory, to non-hospital patients. The Medicare physician fee schedule identifies those physician laboratory or physician pathology services that have a technical component service.

CMS published a final regulation in 1999 that would no longer allow independent laboratories to bill under the physician fee schedule for the TC of physician pathology services. The implementation of this regulation was delayed by Section 542 of the Benefits and Improvement and Protection Act of 2000 (BIPA). Section 542 allows the Medicare carrier to continue to pay for the TC of physician pathology services when an independent laboratory furnishes this service to an inpatient or outpatient of a covered hospital. This provision is applicable to TC services furnished in 2001, 2002, 2003, 2004, 2005 or 2006.

For this provision, a covered hospital is a hospital that had an arrangement with an independent laboratory that was in effect as of July 22, 1999, under which a laboratory furnished the TC of physician pathology services to fee-for-service Medicare beneficiaries who were hospital inpatients or outpatients, and submitted claims for payment for the TC to a carrier. The TC could have been submitted separately or combined with the professional component and reported as a combined service.

The term, fee-for-service Medicare beneficiary, means an individual who:

- Is entitled to benefits under Part A or enrolled under Part B of title XVIII or both; and
- Is not enrolled in any of the following: A Medicare + Choice plan under Part C of such title; a plan offered by an eligible organization under 1876 of the Social Security Act; a program of all-inclusive care for the elderly under 1894; or a social health maintenance organization demonstration project established under Section 4108 of the Omnibus Budget Reconciliation Act of 1987.

In implementing Section 542, the carriers should consider as independent laboratories those entities that it has previously recognized as independent laboratories. An independent laboratory that has acquired another independent laboratory that had an arrangement of July 22, 1999, with a covered hospital, can bill the TC of physician pathology services for that hospital's inpatients and outpatients under the physician fee schedule.

An independent laboratory that furnishes the TC of physician pathology services to inpatients or outpatients of a hospital that is not a covered hospital may not bill the carrier for the TC of physician pathology services during the time 542 is in effect.

If the arrangement between the independent laboratory and the covered hospital limited the provision of TC physician pathology services to certain situations or at particular times, then the independent laboratory can bill the carrier only for these limited services.

The carrier shall require independent laboratories that had an arrangement, on or prior to July 22, 1999 with a covered hospital, to bill for the technical component of physician pathology services to provide a copy of this agreement, or other documentation substantiating that an arrangement was in effect between the hospital and the independent laboratory as of this date. The independent laboratory must submit this documentation for each covered hospital that the independent laboratory services.

See Chapter 16 for additional instruction on laboratory services including clinical diagnostic laboratory services.

Physician laboratory and pathology services are limited to:

- Surgical pathology services;
- Specific cytopathology, hematology and blood banking services that have been identified to require performance by a physician and are listed below;
- Clinical consultation services that meet the requirements in subsection D below;
- and
- Clinical laboratory interpretation services that meet the requirements and which are specifically listed in subsection E below.

B. Surgical Pathology Services

Surgical pathology services include the gross and microscopic examination of organ tissue performed by a physician, except for autopsies, which are not covered by Medicare. Surgical pathology services paid under the physician fee schedule are reported under the following CPT codes:

88300, 88302, 88304, 88305, 88307, 88309, 88311, 88312, 88313, 88314, 88318, 88319, 88321, 88323, 88325, 88329, 88331, 88332, 88342, 88346, 88347, 88348, 88349, 88355, 88356, 88358, 88361, 88362, 88365, 88380.

Depending upon circumstances and the billing entity, the carriers may pay professional component, technical component or both.

C. Specific Hematology, Cytopathology and Blood Banking Services

Cytopathology services include the examination of cells from fluids, washings, brushings or smears, but generally excluding hematology. Examining cervical and vaginal smears are the most common service in cytopathology. Cervical and vaginal smears do not require interpretation by a physician unless the results are or appear to be abnormal. In such cases, a physician personally conducts a separate microscopic evaluation to determine the nature of an abnormality. This microscopic evaluation ordinarily does require performance by a physician. When medically necessary and when furnished by a physician, it is paid under the fee schedule.

These codes include 88104, 88106, 88107, 88108, 88112, 88125, 88141, 88160, 88161, 88162, 88172, 88173, 88180, 88182.

For services furnished prior to January 1, 1999, carriers pay separately under the physician fee schedule for the interpretation of an abnormal pap smear furnished to a hospital inpatient by a physician. They must pay under the clinical laboratory fee schedule for pap smears furnished in all other situations. This policy also applies to screening pap smears requiring a physician interpretation. For services furnished on or after January 1, 1999, carriers allow separate payment for a physician's interpretation of a pap smear to any patient (i.e., hospital or non-hospital) as long as: (1) the laboratory's screening personnel suspect an abnormality; and (2) the physician reviews and interprets the pap smear.

This policy also applies to screening pap smears requiring a physician interpretation and described in the National Coverage Determination Manual and Chapter 18. These services are reported under codes P3000 or P3001.

Physician hematology services include microscopic evaluation of bone marrow aspirations and biopsies. It also includes those limited number of peripheral blood smears which need to be referred to a physician to evaluate the nature of an apparent abnormality identified by the technologist. These codes include 85060, 38220, 85097, and 38221.

Carriers pay the professional component for the interpretation of an abnormal blood smear (code 85060) furnished to a hospital inpatient by a hospital physician or an independent laboratory.

For the other listed hematology codes, payment may be made for the professional component if the service is furnished to a patient by a hospital physician or independent laboratory. In addition, payment may be made for these services furnished to patients by an independent laboratory.

Codes 38220 and 85097 represent professional-only component services and have no technical component values.

Blood banking services of hematologists and pathologists are paid under the physician fee schedule when analyses are performed on donor and/or patient blood to determine compatible donor units for transfusion where cross matching is difficult or where contamination with transmissible disease of donor is suspected.

The blood banking codes are 86077, 86078, and 86079 and represent professional component only services. These codes do not have a technical component.

D. Clinical Consultation Services

Clinical consultations are paid under the physician fee schedule only if they:

- Are requested by the patient's attending physician;
- Relate to a test result that lies outside the clinically significant normal or expected range in view of the condition of the patient;
- Result in a written narrative report included in the patient's medical record; and
- Require the exercise of medical judgment by the consultant physician.

Clinical consultations are professional component services only. There is no technical component. The clinical consultation codes are 80500 and 80502.

Routine conversations held between a laboratory director and an attending physician about test orders or results do not qualify as consultations unless all four requirements are met. Laboratory personnel, including the director, may from time to time contact attending physicians to report test results or to suggest additional testing or be contacted by attending physicians on similar matters. These contacts do not constitute clinical consultations. However, if in the course of such a contact, the attending physician requests a consultation from the pathologist, and if that consultation meets the other criteria and is properly documented, it is paid under the fee schedule.

EXAMPLE: A pathologist telephones a surgeon about a patient's suitability for surgery based on the results of clinical laboratory test results. During the course of their conversation, the surgeon ask the pathologist whether, based on test results, patient history and medical records, the patient is a candidate for surgery. The surgeon's request requires the pathologist to render a medical judgment and provide a consultation. The athologist follows up his/her oral advice with a written report and the surgeon notes in the patient's medical record that he/she requested a consultation. This consultation is paid under the fee schedule.

In any case, if the information could ordinarily be furnished by a nonphysician laboratory specialist, the service of the physician is not a consultation payable under the fee schedule.

See the Program Integrity Manual for guidelines for related data analysis to identify inappropriate patterns of billing for consultations.

E. Clinical Laboratory Interpretation Services

Only clinical laboratory interpretation services listed below and which meet the criteria in subsections D.1, D.3, and D.4 for clinical consultations and, as a result, are billable under the fee schedule. These services are reported under the clinical laboratory code with modifier 26. These services can be paid under the physician fee schedule if they are furnished to a patient by a hospital pathologist or an independent laboratory. Note that a hospital's standing order policy can be used as a substitute for the individual request by the patient's attending physician. Carriers are not allowed to revise CMS's list to accommodate local medical practice. The CMS periodically reviews this list and adds or deletes clinical laboratory codes as warranted.

Clinical Laboratory Interpretation Services

Code	Definition
83020	Hemoglobin; electrophoresis
83912	Nucleic acid probe, with electrophoresis, with examination and report
84165	Protein, total, serum; electrophoretic fractionation and quantitation
84181	Protein; Western Blot with interpretation and report, blood or other body fluid
84182	Protein; Western Blot, with interpretation and report, blood or other body fluid, immunological probe for band identification; each
85390	Fibrinolysin; screening
85576	Platelet; aggregation (in vitro), any agent
86255	Fluorescent antibody; screen
86256	Fluorescent antibody; titer
86320	Immunoelectrophoresis; serum, each specimen
86325	Immunoelectrophoresis; other fluids (e.g.urine) with concentration, each specimen
86327	Immunoelectrophoresis; crossed (2 dimensional assay)
86334	Immunofixation electrophoresis
87164	Dark field examination, any source (e.g. penile, vaginal, oral, skin); includes specimen collection
87207	Smear, primary source, with interpretation; special stain for inclusion bodies or intracellular parasites (e.g. malaria, kala azar, herpes)
88371	Protein analysis of tissue by Western Blot, with interpretation and report.
88372	Protein analysis of tissue by Western Blot, immunological probe for band identification, each
89060	Crystal identification by light microscopy with or without polarizing lens analysis, any body fluid (except urine)

100-4, 12, 80.3

Unusual Travel (CPT Code 99082)

B3-15026

In general, travel has been incorporated in the MPFSDB individual fees and is thus not separately payable. Carriers must pay separately for unusual travel (CPT code 99082) only when the physician submits documentation to demonstrate that the travel was very unusual.

100-4, 12, 90.3

Physicians' Services Performed in Ambulatory Surgical Centers (ASC)

B3-2265, B3-2265.4

See Chapter 14, for a description of services that may be billed by an ASC and services separately billed by physicians.

The ASC payment does not include the professional services of the physician. These are billed separately by the physician. Physicians' services include the services of anesthesiologists administering or supervising the administration of anesthesia to ASC patients and the patients' recovery from the anesthesia. The term physicians' services also includes any routine pre- or postoperative services, such as office visits, consultations, diagnostic tests, removal of stitches, changing of dressings, and other services which the individual physician usually performs.

The physician must enter the place of service code (POS) 24 on the claim to show that the procedure was performed in an ASC.

The carrier pays the "facility" fee from the MPFSDB to the physician. The facility fee is for services done in a facility other than the physician's office and is less then the nonfacility fee for services performed in the physician's office.

100-4, 12, 100

Teaching Physician Services

Definitions

For purposes of this section, the following definitions apply.

Resident -An individual who participates in an approved graduate medical education (GME) program or a physician who is not in an approved GME program but who is authorized to practice only in a hospital setting. The term includes interns and fellows in GME programs recognized as approved for purposes of direct GME payments made by the FI. Receiving a staff or faculty appointment or participating in a fellowship does not by itself alter the status of "resident". Additionally, this status remains unaffected regardless of whether a hospital includes the physician in its full time equivalency count of residents.

Student- An individual who participates in an accredited educational program (e.g., a medical school) that is not an approved GME program. A student is never considered to be an intern or a resident. Medicare does not pay for any service furnished by a student. See 100.1.1B for a discussion concerning E/M service documentation performed by students.

Teaching Physician -A physician (other than another resident) who involves residents in the care of his or her patients.

Direct Medical and Surgical Services -Services to individual beneficiaries that are either personally furnished by a physician or furnished by a resident under the supervision of a physician in a teaching hospital making the reasonable cost election for physician services furnished in teaching hospitals. All payments for such services are made by the FI for the hospital.

Teaching Hospital -A hospital engaged in an approved GME residency program in medicine, osteopathy, dentistry, or podiatry.

Teaching Setting -Any provider, hospital-based provider, or nonprovider setting in which Medicare payment for the services of residents is made by the FI under the direct graduate medical education payment methodology or freestanding SNF or HHA in which such payments are made on a reasonable cost basis.

Critical or Key Portion- That part (or parts) of a service that the teaching physician determines is (are) a critical or key portion(s). For purposes of this section, these terms are interchangeable.

Documentation- Notes recorded in the patient's medical records by a resident, and/or teaching physician or others as outlined in the specific situations below regarding the service furnished. Documentation may be dictated and typed or hand-written, or computer-generated and typed or handwritten. Documentation must be dated and include a legible signature or identity. Pursuant to 42 CFR 415.172 (b), documentation must identify, at a minimum, the service furnished, the participation of the teaching physician in providing the service, and whether the teaching physician was physically present.

In the context of an electronic medical record, the term 'macro' means a command in a computer or dictation application that automatically generates predetermined text that is not edited by the user.

When using an electronic medical record, it is acceptable for the teaching physician to use a macro as the required personal documentation if the teaching physician adds it personally in a secured (password protected) system. In addition to the teaching physician's macro, either the resident or the teaching physician must provide customized information that is sufficient to support a medical necessity determination. The note in the electronic medical record must sufficiently describe the specific services furnished to the specific patient on the specific date. It is insufficient documentation if both the resident and the teaching physician use macros only.

Physically Present- The teaching physician is located in the same room (or partitioned or curtained area, if the room is subdivided to accommodate multiple patients) as the patient and/or performs a face-to-face service.

100-4, 12, 100.1.1

Evaluation and Management (E/M) Services

A. General Documentation Instructions and Common Scenarios

Evaluation and Management (E/M) Services -- For a given encounter, the selection of the appropriate level of E/M service should be determined according to the code definitions in the American Medical Association's Current Procedural Terminology (CPT) and any applicable documentation guidelines.

For purposes of payment, E/M services billed by teaching physicians require that they personally document at least the following:

- That they performed the service or were physically present during the key or critical portions of the service when performed by the resident; and
- The participation of the teaching physician in the management of the patient.

When assigning codes to services billed by teaching physicians, reviewers will combine the documentation of both the resident and the teaching physician.

Documentation by the resident of the presence and participation of the teaching physician is not sufficient to establish the presence and participation of the teaching physician.

On medical review, the combined entries into the medical record by the teaching physician and the resident constitute the documentation for the service and together must support the medical necessity of the service.

Following are four common scenarios for teaching physicians providing E/M services:

Scenario 1:

The teaching physician personally performs all the required elements of an E/M service without a resident. In this scenario the resident may or may not have performed the E/M service independently.

In the absence of a note by a resident, the teaching physician must document as he/she would document an E/M service in a nonteaching setting.

Where a resident has written notes, the teaching physician's note may reference the resident's note. The teaching physician must document that he/she performed the critical or key portion(s) of the service, and that he/she was directly involved in the management of the patient. For payment, the composite of the teaching physician's entry and the resident's entry together must support the medical necessity of the billed service and the level of the service billed by the teaching physician.

Scenario 2:

The resident performs the elements required for an E/M service in the presence of, or jointly with, the teaching physician and the resident documents the service. In this case, the teaching physician must document that he/she was present during the performance of the critical or key portion(s) of the service and that he/she was directly involved in the

management of the patient. The teaching physician's note should reference the resident's note. For payment, the composite of the teaching physician's entry and the resident's entry together must support the medical necessity and the level of the service billed by the teaching physician.

Scenario 3:

The resident performs some or all of the required elements of the service in the absence of the teaching physician and documents his/her service. The teaching physician independently performs the critical or key portion(s) of the service with or without the resident present and, as appropriate, discusses the case with the resident. In this instance, the teaching physician must document that he/she personally saw the patient, personally performed critical or key portions of the service, and participated in the management of the patient. The teaching physician's note should reference the resident's note. For payment, the composite of the teaching physician's entry and the resident's entry together must support the medical necessity of the billed service and the level of the service billed by the teaching physician.

Scenario 4:

When a medical resident admits a patient to a hospital late at night and the teaching physician does not see the patient until later, including the next calendar day:

- The teaching physician must document that he/she personally saw the patient and participated in the management of the patient. The teaching physician may reference the resident's note in lieu of re-documenting the history of present illness, exam, medical decision-making, review of systems and/or past family/social history provided that the patient's condition has not changed, and the teaching physician agrees with the resident's note.
- The teaching physician's note must reflect changes in the patient's condition and clinical course that require that the resident's note be amended with further information to address the patient's condition and course at the time the patient is seen personally by the teaching physician.
- The teaching physician's bill must reflect the date of service he/she saw the patient and his/her personal work of obtaining a history, performing a physical, and participating in medical decision-making regardless of whether the combination of the teaching physician's and resident's documentation satisfies criteria for a higher level of service. For payment, the composite of the teaching physician's entry and the resident's entry together must support the medical necessity of the billed service and the level of the service billed by the teaching physician.

Following are examples of minimally acceptable documentation for each of these scenarios:

Scenario 1:

Admitting Note: "I performed a history and physical examination of the patient and discussed his management with the resident. I reviewed the resident's note and agree with the documented findings and plan of care."

Follow-up Visit: "Hospital Day #3. I saw and evaluated the patient. I agree with the findings and the plan of care as documented in the resident's note."

Follow-up Visit: "Hospital Day #5. I saw and examined the patient. I agree with the resident's note except the heart murmur is louder, so I will obtain an echo to evaluate."

(**NOTE:** In this scenario if there are no resident notes, the teaching physician must document as he/she would document an E/M service in a non-teaching setting.)

Scenario 2:

Initial or Follow-up Visit: "I was present with the resident during the history and exam. I discussed the case with the resident and agree with the findings and plan as documented in the resident's note."

Follow-up Visit: "I saw the patient with the resident and agree with the resident's findings and plan."

Scenarios 3 and 4:

Initial Visit: "I saw and evaluated the patient. I reviewed the resident's note and agree, except that picture is more consistent with pericarditis than myocardial ischemia. Will begin NSAIDs."

Initial or Follow-up Visit: "I saw and evaluated the patient. Discussed with resident and agree with resident's findings and plan as documented in the resident's note."

Follow-up Visit: "See resident's note for details. I saw and evaluated the patient and agree with the resident's finding and plans as written."

Follow-up Visit: "I saw and evaluated the patient. Agree with resident's note but lower extremities are weaker, now 3/5; MRI of L/S Spine today."

Following are examples of unacceptable documentation:

"Agree with above.", followed by legible countersignature or identity;

"Rounded, Reviewed, Agree.", followed by legible countersignature or identity;

"Discussed with resident. Agree.", followed by legible countersignature or identity;

"Seen and agree.", followed by legible countersignature or identity;

"Patient seen and evaluated.", followed by legible countersignature or identity; and

A legible countersignature or identity alone.

Such documentation is not acceptable, because the documentation does not make it possible to determine whether the teaching physician was present, evaluated the patient, and/or had any involvement with the plan of care.

B. E/M Service Documentation Provided By Students

Any contribution and participation of a student to the performance of a billable service (other than the review of systems and/or past family/social history which are not separately billable, but are taken as part of an E/M service) must be performed in the physical presence of a teaching physician or physical presence of a resident in a service meeting the requirements set forth in this section for teaching physician billing.

Students may document services in the medical record. However, the documentation of an E/M service by a student that may be referred to by the teaching physician is limited to documentation related to the review of systems and/or past family/social history. The teaching physician may not refer to a student's documentation of physical exam findings or medical decision making in his or her personal note. If the medical student documents E/M services, the teaching physician must verify and redocument the history of present illness as well as perform and redocument the physical exam and medical decision making activities of the service.

C. Exception for E/M Services Furnished in Certain Primary Care Centers

Teaching physicians providing E/M services with a GME program granted a primary care exception may bill Medicare for lower and mid-level E/M services provided by residents. For the E/M codes listed below, teaching physicians may submit claims for services furnished by residents in the absence of a teaching physician:

New Patient	Established Patient
99201	99211
99202	99212
99203	99213

Effective January 1, 2005, the following code is included under the primary care exception: HCPCS code G0402 (Initial preventive physical examination; face-to-face visit services limited to new beneficiary during the first 12 months of Medicare enrollment).

Effective January 1, 2011, the following codes are included under the primary care exception: HCPCS codes G0438 (Annual wellness visit, including personal preventive plan service, first visit) and G0439 (Annual wellness visit, including personal preventive plan service, subsequent visit).

If a service other than those listed above needs to be furnished, then the general teaching physician policy set forth in §100.1 applies. For this exception to apply, a center must attest in writing that all the following conditions are met for a particular residency program. Prior approval is not necessary, but centers exercising the primary care exception must maintain records demonstrating that they qualify for the exception.

The services must be furnished in a center located in the outpatient department of a hospital or another ambulatory care entity in which the time spent by residents in patient care activities is included in determining direct GME payments to a teaching hospital by the hospital's FI. This requirement is not met when the resident is assigned to a physician's office away from the center or makes home visits. In the case of a nonhospital entity, verify with the FI that the entity meets the requirements of a written agreement between the hospital and the entity set forth at 42 CFR 413.78(e)(3)(ii).

Under this exception, residents providing the billable patient care service without the physical presence of a teaching physician must have completed at least 6 months of a GME approved residency program. Centers must maintain information under the provisions at 42 CFR 413.79(a)(6).

Teaching physicians submitting claims under this exception may not supervise more than four residents at any given time and must direct the care from such proximity as to constitute immediate availability. Teaching physicians may include residents with less than 6 months in a GME approved residency program in the mix of four residents under the teaching physician's supervision. However, the teaching physician must be physically present for the critical or key portions of services furnished by the residents with less than 6 months in a GME approved residency program. That is, the primary care exception does not apply in the case of residents with less than 6 months in a GME approved residency program.

Teaching physicians submitting claims under this exception must:

- Not have other responsibilities (including the supervision of other personnel) at the time the service was provided by the resident;
- Have the primary medical responsibility for patients cared for by the residents;
- Ensure that the care provided was reasonable and necessary;
- Review the care provided by the resident during or immediately after each visit. This must include a review of the patient's medical history, the resident's findings on physical examination, the patient's diagnosis, and treatment plan (i.e., record of tests and therapies); and
- Document the extent of his/her own participation in the review and direction of the services furnished to each patient.

Patients under this exception should consider the center to be their primary location for health care services. The residents must be expected to generally provide care to the same group of established patients during their residency training. The types of services furnished by residents under this exception include:

- Acute care for undifferentiated problems or chronic care for ongoing conditions including chronic mental illness;
- Coordination of care furnished by other physicians and providers; and,
- Comprehensive care not limited by organ system or diagnosis.

Residency programs most likely qualifying for this exception include family practice, general internal medicine, geriatric medicine, pediatrics, and obstetrics/gynecology.

Certain GME programs in psychiatry may qualify in special situations such as when the program furnishes comprehensive care for chronically mentally ill patients. These would be centers in which the range of services the residents are trained to furnish, and actually do furnish, include comprehensive medical care as well as psychiatric care. For example, antibiotics are being prescribed as well as psychotropic drugs.

100-4, 12, 110.3

Outpatient Mental Health Limitation

In general, payment for covered PA services is made at 80 percent of the lesser of the actual charge or 85 percent of what a physician is paid under the Medicare Physician Fee Schedule. The contractor must apply the outpatient mental health treatment limitation (the limitation) to all covered mental health therapeutic services furnished by PAs.

Refer to §210 below for a complete discussion of the limitation.

100-4, 12, 140

Certified Registered Nurse Anesthetist (CRNA) Services

B3-16003, B3-16003 A, B3-3040.4, B3-4172 Section 9320 of OBRA 1986 provides for payment under a fee schedule to certified registered nurse anesthetists (CRNAs) and anesthesia assistants (AAs). CRNAs and AAs may bill Medicare directly for their services or have payment made to an employer or an entity under which they have a contract. This could be a hospital, physician or ASC. This provision is effective for services rendered on or after January 1, 1989. Anesthesia services are subject to the usual Part B coinsurance and deductible and when furnished on or after January 1, 1992 by a qualified nurse anesthetist and are paid at the lesser of the actual charge, the physician fee schedule, or the CRNA fee schedule. Payment for CRNA services is made only on an assignment basis.

100-4, 12, 140.1

Qualified Nonphysician Anesthetists

For payment purposes, qualified nonphysician anesthetists include both CRNAs and AAs. Thus, the term qualified nonphysician anesthetist will be used to refer to both CRNAs and AAs unless it is necessary to separately discuss these provider groups.

An AA is a person who:

- Is permitted by State law to administer anesthesia; and who
- Has successfully completed a six-year program for AAs of which two years consist of specialized academic and clinical training in anesthesia.

In contrast, a CRNA is a registered nurse who is licensed by the State in which the nurse practices and who:

- Is currently certified by the Council on Certification of Nurse Anesthetists or the Council on Recertification of Nurse Anesthetists, or
- Has graduated within the past 18 months from a nurse anesthesia program that meets the standards of the Council of Accreditation of Nurse Anesthesia Educational Programs and is awaiting initial certification.

100-4, 12, 140.2

Entity or Individual to Whom CRNA Fee Schedule is Payable

B3-16003.C, B3-4830.A

Payment for the services of a CRNA may be made to the CRNA who furnished the anesthesia services or to a hospital, physician, group practice, or ASC with which the CRNA has an employment or contractual relationship.

100-4, 12, 140.3

Anesthesia Fee Schedule Payment for Qualified Nonphysician Anesthetists

Pay for the services of a qualified nonphysician anesthetist only on an assignment basis. The assignment agreed to by the qualified nonphysician anesthetist is binding upon any other person or entity claiming payment for the service. Except for deductible and coinsurance amounts, any person who knowingly and willfully presents or causes to be presented to a Medicare beneficiary a bill or request for payment for services of a qualified nonphysician anesthetist for which payment may be made on an assignment-related basis is subject to civil monetary penalties.

Services furnished by qualified nonphysician anesthetists are subject to the Part B deductible and coinsurance. If the Part B deductible has been satisfied, the fee schedule for anesthesia services prior to January 1, 1996, is the least of 80 percent of:

- The actual charge;
- The applicable CRNA conversion factor multiplied by the sum of allowable base and time units; or
- The applicable locality participating anesthesiologist's conversion factor multiplied by the sum of allowable base and time units.

For services furnished on or after January 1, 1996, the fee schedule for anesthesia services furnished by qualified nonphysician anesthetists is the least of 80 percent of:

- The actual charge;
- The applicable locality anesthesia conversion factor multiplied by the sum of allowable base and time units.

100-4, 12, 140.3.2

Anesthesia Time and Calculation of Anesthesia Time Units

B3-15018.G Anesthesia time means the time during which a CRNA is present with the patient. It starts when the CRNA begins to prepare the patient for anesthesia services in the operating room or an equivalent area and ends when the CRNA is no longer furnishing anesthesia services to the patient, that is, when the patient may be placed safely under postoperative care. Anesthesia time is a continuous time period from the start of anesthesia to the end of an anesthesia service. In counting anesthesia time for services furnished on or after January 1, 2000, the CRNA can add blocks of time around an interruption in anesthesia time as long as the CRNA is furnishing continuous anesthesia care within the time periods around the interruption.

100-4, 12, 140.3.3

Billing Modifiers

The following modifiers are used when billing for anesthesia services:

- QX - Qualified nonphysician anesthetist with medical direction by a physician.
- QZ - CRNA without medical direction by a physician.
- QS - Monitored anesthesiology care services (can be billed by a qualified nonphysician anesthetist or a physician).
- QY - Medical direction of one qualified nonphysician anesthetist by an anesthesiologist. This modifier is effective for anesthesia services furnished by a qualified nonphysician anesthetist on or after January 1, 1998.

100-4, 12, 140.3.4

General Billing Instructions

Claims for reimbursement for qualified nonphysician anesthetist services should be completed in accord with existing billing instructions for anesthesiologists with the following additions.

- If an employer-physician furnishes concurrent medical direction for a procedure involving CRNAs and the medical direction service is unassigned, the physician should bill on an assigned basis on a separate claim for the qualified nonphysician anesthetist service. If the physician is participating or takes assignment, both services should be billed on one claim but as separate line items.
- All claims forms must have the provider billing number of the CRNA, AA and/or the employer of the qualified nonphysician anesthetist performing the service in either block 24.H of the Form CMS-1500 and/or block 31 as applicable. Verify that the billing number is valid before making payment.

Payments should be calculated in accordance with Medicare payment rules in §140.3. Contractors must institute all necessary payment edits to assure that duplicate payments are not made to physicians for CRNA or AA services or to a CRNA or AA directly for bills submitted on their behalf by qualified billers.

CRNAs are identified on the provider file by specialty code 43. AAs are identified on the provider file by specialty code 32.

100-4, 12, 140.4.1

An Anesthesiologist and Qualified Nonphysician Anesthetist Work Together

Contractors will distribute educational releases and use other established means to ensure that anesthesiologists understand the requirements for medical direction of qualified nonphysician anesthetists.

Contractors will perform reviews of payments for anesthesiology services to identify situations in which an excessive number of concurrent anesthesiology services may have been performed. They will use peer practice and their experience in developing review criteria. They will also periodically review a sample of claims for medical direction of four or fewer concurrent anesthesia procedures. During this process physicians may be requested to submit documentation of the names of procedures performed and the names of the anesthetists directed.

Physicians who cannot supply the necessary documentation for the sample claims must submit documentation with all subsequent claims before payment will be made.

100-4, 12, 140.4.2

Qualified Nonphysician Anesthetist and an Anesthesiologist in a Single Anesthesia Procedure

Where a single anesthesia procedure involves both a physician medical direction service and the service of the medically directed qualified nonphysician anesthetist, and the service is furnished on or after January 1, 1998, the payment amount for the service of each is 50 percent of the allowance otherwise recognized had

the service been furnished by the anesthesiologist alone. The modifier to be used for current procedure identification is QX.

Beginning on or after January 1, 1998, where the qualified nonphysician anesthetist and the anesthesiologist are involved in a single anesthesia case, and the physician is performing medical direction, the service is billed in accordance with the following procedures:

- For the single medically directed service, the physician will use the modifier "QY" (MEDICAL DIRECTION OF ONE QUALIFIED NONPHYSICIAN ANESTHETIST BY AN ANESTHESIOLOGIST). This modifier is effective for claims for dates of service on or after January 1, 1998, and
- For the anesthesia service furnished by the medically directed qualified nonphysician anesthetist, the qualified nonphysician anesthetist will use the current modifier "QX."

In unusual circumstances when it is medically necessary for both the **CRNA** and the anesthesiologist to be completely and fully involved during a procedure, full payment for the services of each provider is allowed. The physician would report using the "AA" modifier and the **CRNA** would use "QZ," or the modifier for a nonmedically directed case.

Documentation must be submitted by each provider to support payment of the full fee.

100-4, 12, 140.4.3

Payment for Medical or Surgical Services Furnished by CRNAs

Payment shall be made for reasonable and necessary medical or surgical services furnished by CRNAs if they are legally authorized to perform these services in the state in which services are furnished. Payment is determined under the physician fee schedule on the basis of the national physician fee schedule conversion factor, the geographic adjustment factor, and the resource-based relative value units for the medical or surgical service.

100-4, 12, 140.4.4

Conversion Factors for Anesthesia Services of Qualified Nonphysician Anesthetists Furnished on or After January 1, 1992

Conversion factors used to determine fee schedule payments for anesthesia services furnished by qualified nonphysician anesthetists on or after January 1, 1992, are determined based on a statutory methodology.

For example, for anesthesia services furnished by a medically directed qualified nonphysician anesthetist in 1994, the medically directed allowance is 60 percent of the allowance that would be recognized for the anesthesia service if the physician personally performed the service without an assistant, i.e., alone. For subsequent years, the medically directed allowance is the following percent of the personally performed allowance.

Services furnished in 1995	57.5 percent
Services furnished in 1996	55.0 percent
Services furnished in 1997	52.5 percent
Services furnished in 1998 and after	50.0 percent

100-4, 12, 150

Clinical Social Worker (CSW) Services

B3-2152, B3-17000 See Medicare Benefit Policy Manual, Chapter 15, for coverage requirements.

Assignment of benefits is required.

Payment is at 75 percent of the physician fee schedule.

CSWs are identified on the provider file by specialty code 80 and provider type 56.

Medicare applies the outpatient mental health limitation to all covered therapeutic services furnished by qualified CSWs. Refer to 210, below, for a discussion of the outpatient mental health limitation. The modifier "AJ" must be applied on CSN services.

100-4, 12, 160

Independent Psychologist Services

B3-2150, B3-2070.2 See the Medicare Benefit Policy Manual, Chapter 15, for coverage requirements.

There are a number of types of psychologists. Educational psychologists engage in identifying and treating education-related issues. In contrast, counseling psychologists provide services that include a broader realm including phobias, familial issues, etc.

Psychometrists are psychologists who have been trained to administer and interpret tests.

However, clinical psychologists are defined as a provider of diagnostic and therapeutic services. Because of the differences in services provided, services provided by psychologists who do not provide clinical services are subject to different billing guidelines. One service often provided by nonclinical psychologist is diagnostic testing.

NOTE: Diagnostic psychological testing services performed by persons who meet these requirements are covered as other diagnostic tests. When, however, the psychologist is not practicing independently, but is on the staff of an institution, agency, or clinic, that entity bills for the diagnostic services.

Expenses for such testing are not subject to the payment limitation on treatment for mental, psychoneurotic, and personality disorders. Independent psychologists are not required by law to accept assignment when performing psychological tests. However, regardless of whether the psychologist accepts assignment, he or she must report on the claim form the name and address of the physician who ordered the test.

100-4, 12, 160.1

Payment

Diagnostic testing services are not subject to the outpatient mental health limitation. Refer to §210, below, for a discussion of the outpatient mental health limitation.

The diagnostic testing services performed by a psychologist (who is not a clinical psychologist) practicing independently of an institution, agency, or physician's office are covered as other diagnostic tests if a physician orders such testing. Medicare covers this type of testing as an outpatient service if furnished by any psychologist who is licensed or certified to practice psychology in the State or jurisdiction where he or she is furnishing services or, if the jurisdiction does not issue licenses, if provided by any practicing psychologist. (It is CMS' understanding that all States, the District of Columbia, and Puerto Ricolicense psychologists, but that some trust territories do not. Examples of psychologists, other than clinical psychologists, whose services are covered under this provision include, but are not limited to, educational psychologists and counseling psychologists.)

To determine whether the diagnostic psychological testing services of a particular independent psychologist are covered under Part B in States which have statutory licensure or certification, carriers must secure from the appropriate State agency a current listing of psychologists holding the required credentials. In States or territories which lack statutory licensing and certification, carriers must check individual qualifications as claims are submitted. Possible reference sources are the national directory of membership of the American Psychological Association, which provides data about the educational background of individuals and indicates which members are board-certified, and records and directories of the State or territorial psychological association. If qualification is dependent on a doctoral degree from a currently accredited program, carriers must verify the date of accreditation of the school involved, since such accreditation is not retroactive. If the reference sources listed above do not provide enough information (e.g., the psychologist is not a member of the association), carriers must contact the psychologist personally for the required information. Carriers may wish to maintain a continuing list of psychologists whose qualifications have been verified.

Medicare excludes expenses for diagnostic testing from the payment limitation on treatment for mental/psychoneurotic/personality disorders.

Carriers must identify the independent psychologist's choice whether or not to accept assignment when performing psychological tests.

Carriers must accept an independent psychologist claim only if the psychologist reports the name/UPIN of the physician who ordered a test.

Carriers pay nonparticipating independent psychologists at 95 percent of the physician fee schedule allowed amount. Carriers pay participating independent psychologists at 100 percent of the physician fee schedule allowed amount.

Independent psychologists are identified on the provider file by specialty code 62 and provider type 35.

100-4, 12, 170

Clinical Psychologist Services

B3-2150 See Medicare Benefit Policy Manual, Chapter 15, for general coverage requirements.

Direct payment may be made under Part B for professional services. However, services furnished incident to the professional services of CPs to hospital patients remain bundled.

Therefore, payment must continue to be made to the hospital (by the FI) for such "incident to" services.

100-4, 12, 170.1

Payment

B3-2150, B3-17001.1 All covered therapeutic services furnished by qualified CPs are subject to the outpatient mental health services limitation (i.e., only 62 1/2 percent of expenses for these services are considered incurred expenses for Medicare purposes). The limitation does not apply to diagnostic services. Refer to 210 below for a discussion of the outpatient mental health limitation.

Payment for the services of CPs is made on the basis of a fee schedule or the actual charge, whichever is less, and only on the basis of assignment.

CPs are identified by specialty code 68 and provider type 27. Modifier "AH" is required on CP services.

100-4, 12, 180

Care Plan Oversight Services

The Medicare Benefit Policy Manual, Chapter 15, contains requirements for coverage for medical and other health services including those of physicians and non-physician practitioners.

Care plan oversight (CPO) is the physician supervision of a patient receiving complex and/or multidisciplinary care as part of Medicare-covered services provided by a participating home health agency or Medicare approved hospice.

CPO services require complex or multidisciplinary care modalities involving:

- Regular physician development and/or revision of care plans;
- Review of subsequent reports of patient status;
- Review of related laboratory and other studies;
- Communication with other health professionals not employed in the same practice who are involved in the patient's care;
- Integration of new information into the medical treatment plan; and/or
- Adjustment of medical therapy.

The CPO services require recurrent physician supervision of a patient involving 30 or more minutes of the physician's time per month. Services not countable toward the 30 minutes threshold that must be provided in order to bill for CPO include, but are not limited to:

- Time associated with discussions with the patient, his or her family or friends to adjust medication or treatment;
- Time spent by staff getting or filing charts;
- Travel time; and/or
- Physician's time spent telephoning prescriptions into the pharmacist unless the telephone conversation involves discussions of pharmaceutical therapies.

Implicit in the concept of CPO is the expectation that the physician has coordinated an aspect of the patient's care with the home health agency or hospice during the month for which CPO services were billed. The physician who bills for CPO must be the same physician who signs the plan of care.

Nurse practitioners, physician assistants, and clinical nurse specialists, practicing within the scope of State law, may bill for care plan oversight. These non-physician practitioners must have been providing ongoing care for the beneficiary through evaluation and management services. These non-physician practitioners may not bill for CPO if they have been involved only with the delivery of the Medicare-covered home health or hospice service.

A. Home Health CPO

Non-physician practitioners can perform CPO only if the physician signing the plan of care provides regular ongoing care under the same plan of care as does the NPP billing for CPO and either:

- The physician and NPP are part of the same group practice; or
- If the NPP is a nurse practitioner or clinical nurse specialist, the physician signing the plan of care also has a collaborative agreement with the NPP; or
- If the NPP is a physician assistant, the physician signing the plan of care is also the physician who provides general supervision of physician assistant services for the practice.

Billing may be made for care plan oversight services furnished by an NPP when:

- The NPP providing the care plan oversight has seen and examined the patient;

- The NPP providing care plan oversight is not functioning as a consultant whose participation is limited to a single medical condition rather than multidisciplinary coordination of care; and
- The NPP providing care plan oversight integrates his or her care with that of the physician who signed the plan of care.

NPPs may not certify the beneficiary for home health care.

B. Hospice CPO
The attending physician or nurse practitioner (who has been designated as the attending physician) may bill for hospice CPO when they are acting as an "attending physician".

An "attending physician" is one who has been identified by the individual, at the time he/she elects hospice coverage, as having the most significant role in the determination and delivery of their medical care. They are not employed nor paid by the hospice. The care plan oversight services are billed using Form CMS-1500 or electronic equivalent.

For additional information on hospice CPO, see Chapter 11, 40.1.3.1 of this manual.

100-4, 12, 180.1

Care Plan Oversight Billing Requirements

A. Codes for Which Separate Payment May Be Made
Effective January 1, 1995, separate payment may be made for CPO oversight services for 30 minutes or more if the requirements specified in the Medicare Benefits Policy Manual, Chapter 15 are met.

Providers billing for CPO must submit the claim with no other services billed on that claim and may bill only after the end of the month in which the CPO services were rendered. CPO services may not be billed across calendar months and should be submitted (and paid) only for one unit of service.

Physicians may bill and be paid separately for CPO services only if all the criteria in the Medicare Benefit Policy Manual, Chapter 15 are met.

B. Physician Certification and Recertification of Home Health Plans of Care
Effective 2001, two new HCPCS codes for the certification and recertification and development of plans of care for Medicare-covered home health services were created.

See the Medicare General Information, Eligibility, and Entitlement Manual, Pub. 100-01, Chapter 4, "Physician Certification and Recertification of Services," 10-60, and the Medicare Benefit Policy Manual, Pub. 100-02, Chapter 7, "Home Health Services", 30.

The home health agency certification code can be billed only when the patient has not received Medicare-covered home health services for at least 60 days. The home health agency recertification code is used after a patient has received services for at least 60 days (or one certification period) when the physician signs the certification after the initial certification period. The home health agency recertification code will be reported only once every 60 days, except in the rare situation when the patient starts a new episode before 60 days elapses and requires a new plan of care to start a new episode.

C. Provider Number of Home Health Agency (HHA) or Hospice
For claims for CPO submitted on or after January 1, 1997, physicians must enter on the Medicare claim form the 6-character Medicare provider number of the HHA or hospice providing Medicare-covered services to the beneficiary for the period during which CPO services was furnished and for which the physician signed the plan of care. Physicians are responsible for obtaining the HHA or hospice Medicare provider numbers.

Additionally, physicians should provide their UPIN to the HHA or hospice furnishing services to their patient.

NOTE: There is currently no place on the HIPAA standard ASC X12N 837 professional format to specifically include the HHA or hospice provider number required for a care plan oversight claim. For this reason, the requirement to include the HHA or hospice provider number on a care plan oversight claim is temporarily waived until a new version of this electronic standard format is adopted under HIPAA and includes a place to provide the HHA and hospice provider numbers for care plan oversight claims.

100-4, 12, 190.3

List of Medicare Telehealth Services

The use of a telecommunications system may substitute for an in-person encounter for professional consultations, office visits, office psychiatry services, and a limited number of other physician fee schedule (PFS) services. The various services and corresponding current procedure terminology (CPT) or Healthcare Common Procedure Coding System (HCPCS) codes are listed below.

- Consultations (CPT codes 99241 - 99275) - Effective October 1, 2001—December 31, 2005;
- Consultations (CPT codes 99241 - 99255) - Effective January 1, 2006—December 31, 2009;
- Telehealth consultations, emergency department or initial inpatient (HCPCS codes G0425–G0427) - Effective January 1, 2010;
- Follow-up inpatient telehealth consultations (HCPCS codes G0406, G0407, and G0408) - Effective January 1, 2009;
- Office or other outpatient visits (CPT codes 99201 - 99215);
- Subsequent hospital care services, with the limitation of one telehealth visit every 3 days (CPT codes 99231, 99232, and 99233)—Effective January 1, 2011;
- Subsequent nursing facility care services, with the limitation of one telehealth visit every 30 days (CPT codes 99307, 99308, 99309, and 99310)—Effective January 1, 2011;
- Pharmacologic management (CPT code 90862)—Effective March 1, 2003 – December 31, 2012; – Effective March 1, 2003 – December 31, 2012; (HCPCS code G0459) – Effective January 1, 2013;
- Individual psychotherapy (CPT codes 90804 - 90809); Psychiatric diagnostic interview examination (CPT code 90801) – Effective March 1, 2003 – December 31, 2012;
- Individual psychotherapy (CPT codes 90832–90834, 90836–90838); Psychiatric diagnostic interview examination (CPT codes 90791 – 90792) – Effective January 1, 2013.
- Neurobehavioral status exam (CPT code 96116) - Effective January 1, 2008;
- End Stage Renal Disease (ESRD) related services (HCPCS codes G0308, G0309, G0311, G0312, G0314, G0315, G0317, and G0318)—Effective January 1, 2005–December 31, 2008;
- End Stage Renal Disease (ESRD) related services (CPT codes 90951, 90952, 90954, 90955, 90957, 90958, 90960, and 90961) – Effective January 1, 2009;
- Individual and group medical nutrition therapy (HCPCS codes G0270, 97802, 97803, and 97804) – Individual effective January 1, 2006; group effective January 1, 2011;
- Individual and group health and behavior assessment and intervention (CPT codes 96150 – 96154) – Individual effective January 1, 2010; group effective January 1, 2011.
- Individual and group kidney disease education (KDE) services (HCPCS codes G0420 and G0421) – Effective January 1, 2011; and
- Individual and group diabetes self-management training (DSMT) services, with a minimum of 1 hour of in-person instruction to be furnished in the initial year training period to ensure effective injection training (HCPCS codes G0108 and G0109) - Effective January 1, 2011.
- Smoking Cessation Services (CPT codes 99406 and 99407and HCPCS codes G0436 and G0437) – Effective January 1, 2012.
- Alcohol and/or substance (other than tobacco) abuse structured assessment and intervention services (HCPCS codes G0396 and G0397) – Effective January 1, 2013.
- Annual alcohol misuse screening (HCPCS code G0442) – Effective January 1, 2013.
- Brief face-to-face behavioral counseling for alcohol misuse (HCPCS code G0443) – Effective January 1, 2013.
- Annual Depression Screening (HCPCS code G0444) – Effective January 1, 2013.
- High-intensity behavioral counseling to prevent sexually transmitted infections (HCPCS code G0445) – Effective January 1, 2013.
- Annual, face-to-face Intensive behavioral therapy for cardiovascular disease (HCPCS code G0446) – Effective January 1, 2013.
- Face-to-face behavioral counseling for obesity (HCPCS code G0447) – Effective January 1, 2013.
- Transitional Care Management Services (CPT codes 99495-99496) – Effective January 1, 2014.

NOTE: Beginning January 1, 2010, CMS eliminated the use of all consultation codes, except for inpatient telehealth consultation G-codes. CMS no longer recognizes office/outpatient or inpatient consultation CPT codes for payment of office/outpatient or inpatient visits. Instead, physicians and practitioners are instructed to bill a new or established patient office/outpatient visit CPT code or appropriate hospital or nursing facility care code, as appropriate to the particular patient, for all office/outpatient or inpatient visits.

100-4, 12, 190.7

Contractor Editing of Telehealth Claims

Medicare telehealth services (as listed in section 190.3) are billed with either the "GT" or "GQ" modifier. The contractor shall approve covered telehealth services if the physician or practitioner is licensed under State law to provide the service. Contractors must familiarize themselves with licensure provisions of States for which they process claims and disallow telehealth services furnished by physicians or practitioners who are not authorized to furnish the applicable telehealth service under State law. For example, if a nurse practitioner is not licensed to provide individual psychotherapy under State law, he or she would not be permitted to receive payment for individual psychotherapy under Medicare. The contractor shall install edits to ensure that only properly licensed physicians and practitioners are paid for covered telehealth services.

If a contractor receives claims for professional telehealth services coded with the "GQ" modifier (representing "via asynchronous telecommunications system"), it shall approve/pay for these services only if the physician or practitioner is affiliated with a Federal telemedicine demonstration conducted in Alaska or Hawaii. The contractor may require the physician or practitioner at the distant site to document his or her participation in a Federal telemedicine demonstration program conducted in Alaska or Hawaii prior to paying for telehealth services provided via asynchronous, store and forward technologies.

If a contractor denies telehealth services because the physician or practitioner may not bill for them, the contractor uses MSN message 21.18: "This item or service is not covered when performed or ordered by this practitioner." The contractor uses remittance advice message 52 when denying the claim based upon MSN message 21.18.

If a service is billed with one of the telehealth modifiers and the procedure code is not designated as a covered telehealth service, the contractor denies the service using MSN message 9.4: "This item or service was denied because information required to make payment was incorrect." The remittance advice message depends on what is incorrect, e.g., B18 if procedure code or modifier is incorrect, 125 for submission billing errors, 4-12 for difference inconsistencies. The contractor uses B18 as the explanation for the denial of the claim.

The only claims from institutional facilities that FIs shall pay for telehealth services at the distant site, except for MNT services, are for physician or practitioner services when the distant site is located in a CAH that has elected Method II, and the physician or practitioner has reassigned his/her benefits to the CAH. The CAH bills its regular FI for the professional services provided at the distant site via a telecommunications system, in any of the revenue codes 096x, 097x or 098x. All requirements for billing distant site telehealth services apply.

Claims from hospitals or CAHs for MNT services are submitted to the hospital's or CAH's regular FI. Payment is based on the non-facility amount on the Medicare Physician Fee Schedule for the particular HCPCS codes.

100-4, 12, 200

Allergy Testing and Immunotherapy

B3-15050

A. Allergy Testing

The MPFSDB fee amounts for allergy testing services billed under codes 95004-95078 are established for single tests. Therefore, the number of tests must be shown on the claim.

EXAMPLE: If a physician performs 25 percutaneous tests (scratch, puncture, or prick) with allergenic extract, the physician must bill code 95004 and specify 25 in the units field of Form CMS-1500 (paper claims or electronic format). To compute payment, the Medicare carrier multiplies the payment for one test (i.e., the payment listed in the fee schedule) by the quantity listed in the units field.

B. Allergy Immunotherapy

For services rendered on or after January 1, 1995, all antigen/allergy immunotherapy services are paid for under the Medicare physician fee schedule. Prior to that date, only the antigen injection services, i.e., only codes 95115 and 95117, were paid for under the fee schedule. Codes representing antigens and their preparation and single codes representing both the antigens and their injection were paid for under the Medicare reasonable charge system. A legislative change brought all of these services under the fee schedule at the beginning of 1995 and the following policies are effective as of January 1, 1995:

1. CPT codes 95120 through 95134 are not valid for Medicare. Codes 95120 through 95134 represent complete services, i.e., services that include both the injection service as well as the antigen and its preparation.
2. Separate coding for injection only codes (i.e., codes 95115 and 95117) and/or the codes representing antigens and their preparation (i.e., codes 95144 through 95170) must be used.

   If both services are provided both codes are billed.

   This includes allergists who provide both services through the use of treatment boards.
3. If a physician bills both an injection code plus either codes 95165 or 95144, carriers pay the appropriate injection code (i.e., code 95115 or code 95117) plus the code 95165 rate. When a provider bills for codes 95115 or 95117 plus code 95144, carriers change 95144 to 95165 and pay accordingly. Code 95144 (single dose vials of antigen) should be billed only if the physician providing the antigen is providing it to be injected by some other entity. Single dose vials, which should be used only as a means of insuring proper dosage amounts for injections, are more costly than multiple dose vials (i.e., code 95165) and therefore their payment rate is higher. Allergists who prepare antigens are assumed to be able to administer proper doses from the less costly multiple dose vials. Thus, regardless of whether they use or bill for single or multiple dose vials at the same time that they are billing for an injection service, they are paid at the multiple dose vial rate.
4. The fee schedule amounts for the antigen codes (95144 through 95170) are for a single dose. When billing those codes, physicians are to specify the number of doses provided. When making payment, carriers multiply the fee schedule amount by the number of doses specified in the units field.
5. If a patient's doses are adjusted, e.g., because of patient reaction, and the antigen provided is actually more or fewer doses than originally anticipated, the physician is to make no change in the number of doses for which he or she bills. The number of doses anticipated at the time of the antigen preparation is the number of doses to be billed. This is consistent with the notes on page 30 of the Spring 1994 issue of the American Medical Association's CPT Assistant. Those notes indicate that the antigen codes mean that the physician is to identify the number of doses "prospectively planned to be provided." The physician is to "identify the number of doses scheduled when the vial is provided." This means that in cases where the patient actually gets more doses than originally anticipated (because dose amounts were decreased during treatment) and in cases where the patient gets fewer doses (because dose amounts were increased), no change is to be made in the billing. In the first case, carriers are not to pay more because the number of doses provided in the original vial(s) increased. In the second case, carriers are not to seek recoupment (if carriers have already made payment) because the number of doses is less than originally planned. This is the case for both venom and nonvenom antigen codes.
6. Venom Doses and Catch-Up Billing - Venom doses are prepared in separate vials and not mixed together - except in the case of the three vespid mix (white and yellow hornets and yellow jackets). A dose of code 95146 (the two-venom code) means getting some of two venoms. Similarly, a dose of code 95147 means getting some of three venoms; a dose of code 95148 means getting some of four venoms; and a dose of 95149 means getting some of five venoms. Some amount of each of the venoms must be provided. Questions arise when the administration of these venoms does not remain synchronized because of dosage adjustments due to patient reaction. For example, a physician prepares ten doses of code 95148 (the four venom code) in two vials - one containing 10 doses of three vespid mix and another containing 10 doses of wasp venom. Because of dose adjustment, the three vespid mix doses last longer, i.e., they last for 15 doses. Consequently, questions arise regarding the amount of "replacement" wasp venom antigen that should be prepared and how it should be billed. Medicare pricing amounts have savings built into the use of the higher venom codes. Therefore, if a patient is in two venom, three venom, four venom or five venom therapy, the carrier objective is to pay at the highest venom level possible. This means that, to the greatest extent possible, code 95146 is to be billed for a patient in two venom therapy, code 95147 is to be billed for a patient in three venom therapy, code 95148 is to be billed for a patient in four venom therapy, and code 95149 is to be billed for a patient in five venom therapy. Thus, physicians are to be instructed that the venom antigen preparation, after dose adjustment, must be done in a manner that, as soon as possible, synchronizes the preparation back to the highest venom code possible. In the above example, the physician should prepare and bill for only 5 doses of "replacement" wasp venom - billing five doses of code 95145 (the one venom code). This will permit the physician to get back to preparing the four venoms at one time and therefore billing the doses of the "cheaper" four venom code. Use of a code below the venom treatment number for the particular patient should occur only for the purpose of "catching up."
7. Code 95165 Doses. - Code 95165 represents preparation of vials of non-venom antigens. As in the case of venoms, some non-venom antigens cannot be mixed together, i.e., they must be prepared in separate vials. An example of this is mold and pollen. Therefore, some patients will be injected at one time from one vial - containing in one mixture all of the appropriate antigens - while other patients will be injected at one time from more than one vial. In establishing the practice expense component for mixing a multidose vial of antigens, we observed that the most common practice was to prepare a 10 cc vial; we also observed that the most common use was to remove aliquots with a volume of 1 cc. Our PE computations were based on those facts. Therefore, a physician's removing 10 1cc aliquot doses captures the entire PE component for the service.

   This does not mean that the physician must remove 1 cc aliquot doses from a multidose vial. It means that the practice expenses payable for the preparation of a 10cc vial remain the same irrespective of the size or number of aliquots removed from the vial. Therefore, a physician may not bill this vial preparation code for more than 10 doses per vial; paying more than 10 doses per multidose vial would significantly overpay the practice expense component attributable to this service. (Note that this code does not include the injection of antigen(s); injection of antigen(s) is separately billable.) When a multidose vial contains less than 10cc, physicians should bill Medicare for the number of 1 cc aliquots that may be removed from the vial. That is, a physician may bill Medicare up to a maximum of 10 doses per multidose vial, but should bill Medicare for fewer than 10 doses per vial when there is less than 10cc in the vial.

   If it is medically necessary, physicians may bill Medicare for preparation of more than one multidose vial.

   EXAMPLES:

   (1) If a 10cc multidose vial is filled to 6cc with antigen, the physician may bill Medicare for 6 doses since six 1cc aliquots may be removed from the vial.

   (2) If a 5cc multidose vial is filled completely, the physician may bill Medicare for 5 doses for this vial.

   (3) If a physician removes ¬¾ cc aliquots from a 10cc multidose vial for a total of 20 doses from one vial, he/she may only bill Medicare for 10 doses. Billing for more than 10 doses would mean that Medicare is overpaying for the practice expense of making the vial.

   (4) If a physician prepares two 10cc multidose vials, he/she may bill Medicare for 20 doses. However, he/she may remove aliquots of any amount from those vials. For example, the physician may remove ¬¾ aliquots from one vial, and 1cc aliquots from the other vial, but may bill no more than a total of 20 doses.

   (5) If a physician prepares a 20cc multidose vial, he/she may bill Medicare for 20 doses, since the practice expense is calculated based on the physician's removing 1cc aliquots from a vial. If a physician removes 2cc aliquots from this vial, thus getting only 10 doses, he/she may nonetheless bill Medicare for 20

doses because the PE for 20 doses reflects the actual practice expense of preparing the vial.

(6) If a physician prepares a 5cc multidose vial, he may bill Medicare for 5 doses, based on the way that the practice expense component is calculated. However, if the physician removes ten ¬¾ cc aliquots from the vial, he/she may still bill only 5 doses because the practice expense of preparing the vial is the same, without regard to the number of additional doses that are removed from the vial.

C. Allergy Shots and Visit Services on the Same Day

At the outset of the physician fee schedule, the question was posed as to whether visits should be billed on the same day as an allergy injection (CPT codes 95115-95117), since these codes have status indicators of A rather than T. Visits should not be billed with allergy injection services 95115 or 95117 unless the visit represents another separately identifiable service. This language parallels CPT editorial language that accompanies the allergen immunotherapy codes, which include codes 9515 and 95117. Prior to January 1, 1995, you appeared to be enforcing this policy through three (3) different means:

- Advising physician to use modifier 25 with the visit service;
- Denying payment for the visit unless documentation has been provided; and
- Paying for both the visit and the allergy shot if both are billed for.

For services rendered on or after January 1, 1995, you are to enforce the requirement that visits not be billed and paid for on the same day as an allergy injection through the following means. Effective for services rendered on or after that date, the global surgery policies will apply to all codes in the allergen immunotherapy series, including the allergy shot codes 95115 and 95117. To accomplish this, CMS changed the global surgery indicator for allergen immunotherapy codes from XXX, which meant that the global surgery concept did not apply to those codes, to 000, which means that the global surgery concept applies, but that there are no days in the postoperative global period.

Now that the global surgery policies apply to these services, you are to rely on the use of modifier 25 as the only means through which you can make payment for visit services provided on the same day as allergen immunotherapy services. In order for a physician to receive payment for a visit service provided on the same day that the physician also provides a service in the allergen immunotherapy series (i.e., any service in the series from 95115 through 95199), the physician is to bill a modifier 25 with the visit code, indicating that the patient's condition required a significant, separately identifiable visit service above and beyond the allergen immunotherapy service provided.

D. Reasonable Supply of Antigens

See CMS Manual System, Internet Only Manual, Medicare Benefits Policy Manual, CMS Pub. 100-02 Chapter 15, section 50.4.4, regarding the coverage of antigens, including what constitutes a reasonable supply of antige

100-4, 12, 210

Outpatient Mental Health Limitation

B3-2470

Regardless of the actual expenses a beneficiary incurs in connection with the treatment of mental, psychoneurotic, and personality disorders while the beneficiary is not an inpatient of a hospital at the time such expenses are incurred, the amount of those expenses that may be recognized for Part B deductible and payment purposes is limited to 62.5 percent of the Medicare approved amount for those services. This limitation is called the outpatient mental health treatment limitation (the limitation). The 62.5 percent limitation has been in place since the inception of the Medicare Part B program and it will remain effective at this percentage amount until January 1, 2010. However, effective January 1, 2010, through January 1, 2014, the limitation will be phased out as follows:

- January 1, 2010 – December 31, 2011, the limitation percentage is 68.75%. (Medicare pays 55% and the patient pays 45%).
- January 1, 2012 – December 31, 2012, the limitation percentage is 75%. (Medicare pays 60% and the patient pays 40%).
- January 1, 2013 – December 31, 2013, the limitation percentage is 81.25%. (Medicare pays 65% and the patient pays 35%).
- January 1, 2014 – onward, the limitation percentage is 100%. (Medicare pays 80% and the patient pays 20%).

For additional details concerning computation of the limitation, please see the examples under section 210.1 E.

100-4, 12, 210.1

Application of Limitation

A. Status of Patient

The limitation is applicable to expenses incurred in connection with the treatment of an individual who is not an inpatient of a hospital. Thus, the limitation applies to mental health services furnished to a person in a physician's office, in the patient's home, in a

skilled nursing facility, as an outpatient, and so forth. The term "hospital" in this context means an institution, which is primarily engaged in providing to inpatients, by or under the supervision of a physician(s):

- Diagnostic and therapeutic services for medical diagnosis, treatment and care of injured, disabled, or sick persons;
- Rehabilitation services for injured, disabled, or sick persons; or
- Psychiatric services for the diagnosis and treatment of mentally ill patients.

B. Disorders Subject to the Limitation

The term "mental, psychoneurotic, and personality disorders" is defined as the specific psychiatric diagnoses described in the International Classification of Diseases, 9th Revision (ICD-9), under the code range 290-319.

When the treatment services rendered are both for a psychiatric diagnosis as defined in the ICD-9 and one or more nonpsychiatric conditions, separate the expenses for the psychiatric aspects of treatment from the expenses for the nonpsychiatric aspects of treatment. However, in any case in which the psychiatric treatment component is not readily distinguishable from the nonpsychiatric treatment component, all of the expenses are allocated to whichever component constitutes the primary diagnosis.

1. Diagnosis Clearly Meets Definition - If the primary diagnosis reported for a particular service is the same as or equivalent to a condition described in the ICD-9 under the code range 290-319 that represents mental, psychoneurotic and personality disorders, the expense for the service is subject to the limitation except as described in subsection D.
2. Diagnosis Does Not Clearly Meet Definition - When it is not clear whether the primary diagnosis reported meets the definition of mental, psychoneurotic, and personality disorders, it may be necessary to contact the practitioner to clarify the diagnosis. In deciding whether contact is necessary in a given case, give consideration to such factors as the type of services rendered, the diagnosis, and the individual's previous utilization history.

C. Services Subject to the Limitation

Medicare Contractors must apply the limitation to claims for professional services that represent mental health treatment furnished to individuals who are not hospital inpatients by physicians, clinical psychologists, clinical social workers, nurse practitioners, clinical nurse specialists and physician assistants. Items and supplies furnished by physicians or other mental health practitioners in connection with treatment are also subject to the limitation.

Generally, Medicare Contractors must apply the limitation only to treatment services. However, diagnostic psychological and neuropsychological testing services performed to evaluate a patient's progress during treatment are considered part of treatment and are subject to the limitation.

D. Services Not Subject to the Limitation

1. Diagnosis of Alzheimer's Disease or Related Disorder - When the primary diagnosis reported for a particular service is Alzheimer's Disease or an Alzheimer's related disorder, Medicare Contractors must look to the nature of the service that has been rendered in determining whether it is subject to the limitation. Alzheimer's disease is coded 331.0 in the "International Classification of Diseases, 9th Revision", which is outside the code range 290-319 that represents mental, psychoneurotic and personality disorders. Additionally, Alzheimer's related disorders are identified by contractors under ICD-9 codes that are within the 290-319 code range (290.XX or others as contractors determine appropriate) or outside the 290-319 code range as determined appropriate by contractors. When the primary treatment rendered to a patient with a diagnosis of Alzheimer's disease or a related disorder is psychotherapy, it is subject to the limitation. However, typically, treatment provided to a patient with a diagnosis of Alzheimer's Disease or a related disorder represents medical management of the patient's condition (such as described under CPT code 90862 or any successor code) and is not subject to the limitation. CPT code 90862 describes pharmacologic management, including prescription, use, and review of medication with no more than minimal medical psychotherapy.
2. Brief Office Visits for Monitoring or Changing Drug Prescriptions - Brief office visits for the sole purpose of monitoring or changing drug prescriptions used in the treatment of mental, psychoneurotic and personality disorders are not subject to the limitation. These visits are reported using HCPCS code M0064 or any successor code (brief office visit for the sole purpose of monitoring or changing drug prescriptions used in the treatment of mental, psychoneurotic, and personality disorders). Claims where the diagnosis reported is a mental, psychoneurotic, or personality disorder (other than a diagnosis specified in subsection A) are subject to the limitation except for the procedure identified by HCPCS code M0064 or any successor code.
3. Diagnostic Services ?edicare Contractors do not apply the limitation to psychiatric diagnostic evaluations and diagnostic psychological and neuropsychological tests performed to establish or confirm the patient's diagnosis. Diagnostic services include psychiatric diagnostic evaluations billed under CPT codes 90801 or 90802 (or any successor codes) and, psychological and neuropsychological tests billed under CPT code range 96101-96118 (or any successor code range).

   An initial visit to a practitioner for professional services often combines diagnostic evaluation and the start of therapy. Such a visit is neither solely diagnostic nor solely therapeutic. Therefore, contractors must deem the initial visit to be diagnostic so that the limitation does not apply. Separating diagnostic and therapeutic components of a visit is not administratively feasible, unless the practitioner already has separately identified them on the bill. Determining the entire visit to be therapeutic is not justifiable since some diagnostic work must be done before even a tentative diagnosis can be made and certainly before therapy can be instituted. Moreover, the patient should not be disadvantaged because therapeutic as well as diagnostic services were provided in the initial visit. In the rare cases where a practitioner's diagnostic services take more than one visit, Medicare contractors must not apply the limitation to the additional visits. However, it is expected such cases are few. Therefore, when a practitioner bills for more than one visit for professional diagnostic services, Medicare contractors may find it necessary to request documentation to justify the reason for more than one diagnostic visit.

4. Partial Hospitalization Services Not Directly Provided by a Physician or a Practitioner - The limitation does not apply to partial hospitalization services that are not directly provided by a physician, clinical psychologist, nurse practitioner, clinical nurse specialist or a physician assistant. Partial hospitalization services are billed by hospital outpatient departments and community mental health centers (CMHCs) to Medicare Contractors. However, services furnished by physicians, clinical psychologists, nurse practitioners, clinical nurse specialists, and physician assistants to partial hospitalization patients are billed separately from the partial hospitalization program of services. Accordingly, these professional's mental health services to partial hospitalization patients are paid under the physician fee schedule by Medicare Contractors and may be subject to the limitation. (See chapter 4, section 260.1C).

E. Computation of Limitation

Medicare Contractors determine the Medicare approved payment amount for services subject to the limitation. They:

- Multiply the approved amount by the limitation percentage amount;
- Subtract any unsatisfied deductible; and,
- Multiply the remainder by 0.8 to obtain the amount of Medicare payment.

The beneficiary is responsible for the difference between the amount paid by Medicare and the full Medicare approved amount.

The following examples illustrate the application of the limitation in various circumstances as it is gradually reduced under section 102 of the Medicare Improvements for Patients and Providers Act (MIPPA). Please note that although the calendar year 2009 Part B deductible of $135 is used under these examples, the actual deductible amount for calendar year 2010 and future years is unknown and will be subject to change.

Example #1: In 2010, a clinical psychologist submits a claim for $200 for outpatient treatment of a patient's mental disorder. The Medicare-approved amount is $180. Since clinical psychologists must accept assignment, the patient is not liable for the $20 in excess charges. The patient previously satisfied the $135 annual Part B deductible. The limitation reduces the amount of incurred expenses to 68 ? percent of the approved amount. Medicare pays 80 percent of the remaining incurred expenses. The Medicare payment and patient liability are computed as follows:

1. Actual charges	$200.00
2. Medicare-approved amount	$180.00
3. Medicare incurred expenses (0.6875 x line 2)	$123.75
4. Unmet deductible	$0.00
5. Remainder after subtracting deductible (line 3 minus line 4)	$123.75
6. Medicare payment (0.80 x line 5)	$99.00
7. Patient liability (line 2 minus line 6)	$81.00

Example #2: In 2012, a clinical social worker submits a claim for $135 for outpatient treatment of a patient's mental disorder. The Medicare-approved amount is $120. Since clinical social workers must accept assignment, the patient is not liable for the $15 in excess charges. The limitation reduces the amount of incurred expenses to 75 percent of the approved amount. The patient previously satisfied $70 of the $135 annual Part B deductible, leaving $65 unmet. The Medicare payment and patient liability are computed as follows:

1. Actual charges	$135.00
2. Medicare-approved amount	$120.00
3. Medicare incurred expenses (0.75 x line 2)	$90.00
4. Unmet deductible	$65.00
5. Remainder after subtracting deductible (line 3 minus line 4)	$25.00
6. Medicare payment (0.80 x line 5)	$20.00
7. Patient liability (line 2 minus line 6)	$100.00

Example #3: In calendar year 2013, a physician who does not accept assignment submits a claim for $780 for services in connection with the treatment of a mental disorder that did not require inpatient hospitalization. The Medicare-approved amount is $750. Because the physician does not accept assignment, the patient is liable for the $30 in excess charges. The patient has not satisfied any of the $135 Part B annual deductible. The Medicare payment and patient liability are computed as follows:

1. Actual charges	$780.00
2. Medicare-approved amount	$750.00
3. Medicare incurred expenses (0.8125 x line 2)	$609.38
4. Unmet deductible	$135.00
5. Remainder after subtracting deductible (line 3 minus line 4)	$474.38
6. Medicare payment (0.80 x line 5)	$379.50
7. Patient liability (line 1 minus line 6)	$400.50

Example #4: A patient's Part B expenses during calendar year 2014 are for a physician's services in connection with the treatment of a mental disorder that initially required inpatient hospitalization, with subsequent physician services furnished on an outpatient basis. The patient has not satisfied any of the $135 Part B deductible. The physician accepts assignment and submits a claim for $780. The Medicare-approved amount is $750. Since the limitation will be completely phased out as of January 1, 2014, the entire $750 Medicare-approved amount is recognized as the total incurred expenses because such expenses are no longer reduced. Also, there is no longer any distinction between mental health services the patient receives as an inpatient or outpatient. The Medicare payment and patient liability are computed as follows:

1. Actual charges	$780.00
2. Medicare-approved amount	$750.00
3. Medicare incurred expenses (1.00 x line 2)	$750.00
4. Unmet deductible	$135.00
5. Remainder after subtracting deductible (line 3 minus line 4)	$615.00
6. Medicare payment (0.80 x line 5)	$492.00
Beneficiary liability (line 2 minus line 6)	$258.00

100-4, 12, 230

Primary Care Incentive Payment Program (PCIP)

Section 5501(a) of the Affordable Care Act revises Section 1833 of the Social Security Act (the Act) by adding a new paragraph, (x), "Incentive Payments for Primary Care Services." Section 1833(x) of the Act states that in the case of primary care services furnished on or after January 1, 2011, and before January 1, 2016, there shall be a 10 percent incentive payment for such services under Part B when furnished by a primary care practitioner.

Information regarding Primary Care Incentive Payment Program (PCIP) payments made to critical access hospitals (CAHs) paid under the optional method can be found in Pub. 100-04, Chapter 4, §250.12 of this manual.

100-4, 12, 230.1

Definition of Primary Care Practitioners and Primary Care Services

Primary care practitioners are defined as:

1. A physician who has a primary specialty designation of family medicine, internal medicine, geriatric medicine, or pediatric medicine for whom primary care services accounted for at least 60 percent of the allowed charges under Part B for the practitioner in a prior period as determined appropriate by the Secretary; or
2. A nurse practitioner, clinical nurse specialist, or physician assistant for whom primary care services accounted for at least 60 percent of the allowed charges under Part B for the practitioner in a prior period as determined appropriate by the Secretary.

Primary care services are defined as HCPCS Codes:

1. 99201 through 99215 for new and established patient office or outpatient evaluation and management (E/M) visits;
2. 99304 through 99340 for initial, subsequent, discharge, and other nursing facility E/M services; new and established patient domiciliary, rest home or custodial care E/M services; and domiciliary, rest home or home care plan oversight services; and
3. 99341 through 99350 for new and established patient home E/M visits.

Practitioner Identification

Eligible practitioners will be identified on claims by the National Provider Identifier (NPI) number of the rendering practitioner. If the claim is submitted by a practitioner's group practice, the rendering practitioner's NPI must be included on the line-item for the primary care service and reflect an eligible HCPCS as identified. In order to be eligible for the PCIP, physician assistants, clinical nurse specialists, and nurse practitioners must be billing for their services under their own NPI and not furnishing services incident to physicians' services. Regardless of the specialty area in which they may be practicing, the specific nonphysician practitioners are eligible for the PCIP based on their profession and historical percentage of allowed charges as primary care services that equals or exceeds the 60 percent threshold.

Beginning in calendar year (CY) 2011, primary care practitioners will be identified based on their primary specialty of enrollment in Medicare and percentage of allowed charges for primary care services that equals or exceeds the 60 percent threshold from Medicare claims data 2 years prior to the bonus payment year.

Eligible practitioners for PCIP payments in a given calendar year (CY) will be listed by eligible NPI in the Primary Care Incentive Payment Program Eligibility File, available after January 31, of the payment year on their Medicare contractor's website. Practitioners should contact their contractor with any questions regarding their eligibility for the PCIP.

100-4, 12, 230.2

Coordination with Other Payments

Section 5501(a)(3) of the Affordable Care Act provides payment under the PCIP as an additional payment amount for specified primary care services without regard to any additional payment for the service under Section 1833(m) of the Act. Therefore, an eligible primary care physician furnishing a primary care service in a health professional shortage area (HPSA) may receive both a HPSA physician bonus payment (as described in the Medicare Claims Processing Manual, Pub. 100-04, Chapter 12, §90.4) under the HPSA physician bonus program and a PCIP incentive payment under the new program beginning in CY 2011.

100-4, 12, 230.3

Claims Processing and Payment

A. General Overview

Incentive payments will be made on a quarterly basis and shall be equal to 10 percent of the amount paid for such services under the Medicare Physician Fee Schedule (PFS) for those services furnished during the bonus payment year. For information on PCIP payments to CAHs paid under the optional method, see the Medicare Claims Processing Manual, Pub. 100-04, Chapter 4, §250.12.

On an annual basis Medicare contractors shall receive a Primary Care Incentive Payment Program Eligibility File that they shall post to their website. The file will list the NPIs of all practitioners who are eligible to receive PCIP payments for the upcoming CY.

B. Method of Payment

- Calculate and pay qualifying primary care practitioners an additional 10 percent incentive payment;
- Calculate the payment based on the amount actually paid for the services, not the Medicare approved amounts;
- Combine the PCIP incentive payments, when appropriate, with other incentive payments, including the HPSA physician bonus payment, and the HPSA Surgical Incentive Payment Program (HSIP) payment;
- Provide a special remittance form that is forwarded with the incentive payment so that physicians and practitioners can identify which type of incentive payment (HPSA physician and/or PCIP) was paid for which services.
- Practitioners should contact their contractor with any questions regarding PCIP payments.

C. Changes for Contractor Systems

The Medicare Carrier System, (MCS), Common Working File (CWF) and the National Claims History (NCH) shall be modified to accept a new PCIP indicator on the claim line. Once the type of incentive payment has been identified by the shared systems, the shared system shall modify their systems to set the indicator on the claim line as follows:

1 = HPSA;

2 = PSA;

3 = HPSA and PSA;

4 = HSIP;

5 = HPSA and HSIP;

6 = PCIP;

7 = HPSA and PCIP; and

Space = Not Applicable.

The contractor shared system shall send the HIGLAS 810 invoice for incentive payment invoices, including the new PCIP payment. The contractor shall also combine the provider's HPSA physician bonus, physician scarcity (PSA) bonus (if it should become available at a later date), HSIP payment and/or PCIP payment invoice per provider. The contractor shall receive the HIGLAS 835 payment file from HIGLAS showing a single incentive payment per provider.

100-4, 13, 10

ICD-9-CM Coding for Diagnostic Tests

The ICD-9-CM Coding Guidelines for Outpatient Services (hospital-based and physician office) have instructed physicians to report diagnoses based on test results. Instructions and examples for coding specialists, contractors, physicians, hospitals, and other health care providers to use in determining the use of ICD-9-CM codes for coding diagnostic test results is found in Chapter 23.

100-4, 13, 30

Computerized Axial Tomography (CT) Procedures

Carriers do not reduce or deny payment for medically necessary multiple CT scans of different areas of the body that are performed on the same day.

The TC RVUs for CT procedures that specify "with contrast" include payment for high osmolar contrast media. When separate payment is made for low osmolar contrast media under the conditions set forth in 30.1.1, reduce payment for the contrast media as set forth in 30.1.2.

100-4, 13, 40

Magnetic Resonance Imaging (MRI) Procedures

Effective September 28, 2009

The Centers for Medicare & Medicaid Services (CMS) finds that the non-coverage of magnetic resonance imaging (MRI) for blood flow determination is no longer supported by the available evidence. CMS is removing the phrase "blood flow measurement" and local Medicare contractors will have the discretion to cover (or not cover).

Consult Publication (Pub.) 100-03, National Coverage Determinations (NCD) Manual, chapter 1, section 220.2, for specific coverage and non-coverage indications associated with MRI and MRA (Magnetic Resonance Angiography).

Prior to January 1, 2007

Carriers do not make additional payments for three or more MRI sequences. The relative value units (RVUs) reflect payment levels for two sequences.

The technical component (TC) RVUs for MRI procedures that specify "with contrast" include payment for paramagnetic contrast media. Carriers do not make separate payment under code A4647.

A diagnostic technique has been developed under which an MRI of the brain or spine is first performed without contrast material, then another MRI is performed with a standard (0.1mmol/kg) dose of contrast material and, based on the need to achieve a better image, a third MRI is performed with an additional double dosage (0.2mmol/kg) of contrast material. When the high-dose contrast technique is utilized, carriers:

- Do not pay separately for the contrast material used in the second MRI procedure;
- Pay for the contrast material given for the third MRI procedure through supply code Q9952, the replacement code for A4643, when billed with Current Procedural Terminology (CPT) codes 70553, 72156, 72157, and 72158;
- Do not pay for the third MRI procedure. For example, in the case of an MRI of the brain, if CPT code 70553 (without contrast material, followed by with contrast material(s) and further sequences) is billed, make no payment for CPT code 70551 (without contrast material(s)), the additional procedure given for the purpose of administering the double dosage, furnished during the same session. Medicare does not pay for the third procedure (as distinguished from the contrast material) because the CPT definition of code 70553 includes all further sequences; and
- Do not apply the payment criteria for low osmolar contrast media in §30.1.2 to billings for code Q9952, the replacement code for A4643.

Effective January 1, 2007

With the implementation for calendar year 2007 of a bottom-up methodology, which utilizes the direct inputs to determine the practice expense (PE) relative value units (RVUs), the cost of the contrast media is not included in the PE RVUs. Therefore, a separate payment for the contrast media used in various imaging procedures is paid. In addition to the CPT code representing the imaging procedure, separately bill the appropriate HCPCS "Q" code (Q9945–Q9954; Q9958-Q9964) for the contrast medium utilized in performing the service.

Effective February 24, 2011

Medicare will allow for coverage of MRI for beneficiaries with implanted PMs or cardioverter defibrillators (ICDs) for use in an MRI environment in a Medicare-approved clinical study as described in section 220.C.1 of the NCD manual.

Effective July 7, 2011

Medicare will allow for coverage of MRI for beneficiaries with implanted pacemakers (PMs) when the PMs are used according to the Food and Drug Administration (FDA)-approved labeling for use in an MRI environment as described in section 220.2.C.1 of the NCD Manual.

100-4, 13, 40.1.1

Magnetic Resonance Angiography (MRA) Coverage Summary

Section 1861(s)(2)(C) of the Social Security Act provides for coverage of diagnostic testing. Coverage of magnetic resonance angiography (MRA) of the head and neck, and MRA of the peripheral vessels of the lower extremities is limited as described in Publication (Pub.) 100-03, the Medicare National Coverage Determinations (NCD) Manual. This instruction has been revised as of July 1, 2003, based on a determination that coverage is reasonable and necessary in additional circumstances. Under that instruction, MRA is generally covered only to the extent that it is used as a substitute for contrast angiography, except to the extent that there are documented circumstances consistent with that instruction that demonstrates the medical necessity of both tests. Prior to June 3, 2010, there was no coverage of MRA outside of the indications and circumstances described in that instruction.

Effective for claims with dates of service on or after June 3, 2010, contractors have the discretion to cover or not cover all indications of MRA (and magnetic resonance imaging (MRI)) that are not specifically nationally covered or nationally non-covered as stated in section 220.2 of the NCD Manual.

Because the status codes for HCPCS codes 71555, 71555-TC, 71555-26, 74185, 74185-TC, and 74185-26 were changed in the Medicare Physician Fee Schedule Database from 'N' to 'R' on April 1, 1998, any MRA claims with those HCPCS codes with dates of service between April 1, 1998, and June 30, 1999, are to be processed according to the contractor's discretionary authority to determine payment in the absence of national policy.

Effective for claims with dates of service on or after February 24, 2011, Medicare will provide coverage for MRIs for beneficiaries with implanted cardiac pacemakers or implantable cardioverter defibrillators if the beneficiary is enrolled in an approved clinical study under the Coverage with Study Participation form of Coverage with Evidence Development that meets specific criteria per Pub. 100-03, the NCD Manual, chapter 1, section 220.2.C.1

100-4, 13, 40.1.2

HCPCS Coding Requirements

Providers must report HCPCS codes when submitting claims for MRA of the chest, abdomen, head, neck or peripheral vessels of lower extremities. The following HCPCS codes should be used to report these services:

MRA of head	70544, 70544-26, 70544-TC
MRA of head	70545, 70545-26, 70545-TC
MRA of head	70546, 70546-26, 70546-TC
MRA of neck	70547, 70547-26, 70547-TC
MRA of neck	70548, 70548-26, 70548-TC
MRA of neck	70549, 70549-26, 70549-TC
MRA of chest	71555, 71555-26, 71555-TC
MRA of pelvis	72198, 72198-26, 72198-TC
MRA of abdomen (dates of service on or after July 1, 2003) – see below.	74185, 74185-26, 74185-TC
MRA of peripheral vessels of lower extremities	73725, 73725-26, 73725-TC

100-4, 13, 60

Positron Emission Tomography (PET) Scans – General Information

(Rev. 1833; Issued: 10-16-09; Effective Date: 04-03-09; Implementation Date: 10-30-09)

Positron emission tomography (PET) is a noninvasive imaging procedure that assesses perfusion and the level of metabolic activity in various organ systems of the human body. A positron camera (tomograph) is used to produce cross-sectional tomographic images which are obtained by detecting radioactivity from a radioactive tracer substance (radiopharmaceutical) that emits a radioactive tracer substance (radiopharmaceutical FDG) such as 2 –[F-18] flouro-D-glucose FDG, that is administered intravenously to the patient.

The Medicare National Coverage Determinations (NCD) Manual, chapter 1, §220.6, contains additional coverage instructions to indicate the conditions under which a PET scan is performed.

A. Definitions

For all uses of PET, excluding Rubidium 82 for perfusion of the heart, myocardial viability and refractory seizures, the following definitions apply:

- **Diagnosis:** PET is covered only in clinical situations in which the PET results may assist in avoiding an invasive diagnostic procedure, or in which the PET results may assist in determining the optimal anatomical location to perform an invasive diagnostic procedure. In general, for most solid tumors, a tissue diagnosis is made prior to the performance of PET scanning. PET scans following a tissue diagnosis are generally performed for the purpose of staging, rather than diagnosis. Therefore, the use of PET in the diagnosis of lymphoma, esophageal and colorectal cancers, as well as in melanoma, should be rare. PET is not covered for other diagnostic uses, and is not covered for screening (testing of patients without specific signs and symptoms of disease).
- **Staging:** PET is covered in clinical situations in which (1) (a) the stage of the cancer remains in doubt after completion of a standard diagnostic workup, including conventional imaging (computed tomography, magnetic resonance imaging, or ultrasound) or, (b) the use of PET would also be considered reasonable and necessary if it could potentially replace one or more conventional imaging studies when it is expected that conventional study information is insufficient for the clinical management of the patient and, (2) clinical management of the patient would differ depending on the stage of the cancer identified.

NOTE: Effective for services on or after April 3, 2009, the terms "diagnosis" and "staging" will be replaced with "Initial Treatment Strategy." For further information on this new term, refer to Pub. 100-03, NCD Manual, section 220.6.17.

- **Restaging:** PET will be covered for restaging: (1) after the completion of treatment for the purpose of detecting residual disease, (2) for detecting suspected recurrence, or metastasis, (3) to determine the extent of a known recurrence, or (4) if it could potentially replace one or more conventional imaging studies when it is expected that conventional study information is to determine the extent of a known recurrence, or if study information is insufficient for the clinical management of the patient. Restaging applies to testing after a course of treatment is completed and is covered subject to the conditions above.
- **Monitoring:** Use of PET to monitor tumor response to treatment during the planned course of therapy (i.e., when a change in therapy is anticipated).

NOTE: Effective for services on or after April 3, 2009, the terms "restaging" and "monitoring" will be replaced with "Subsequent Treatment Strategy." For further information on this new term, refer to Pub. 100-03, NCD Manual, section 220.6.17.

B. Limitations

For staging and restaging: PET is covered in either/or both of the following circumstances:

- The stage of the cancer remains in doubt after completion of a standard diagnostic workup, including conventional imaging (computed tomography, magnetic resonance imaging, or ultrasound); and/or
- The clinical management of the patient would differ depending on the stage of the cancer identified. PET will be covered for restaging after the completion of treatment for the purpose of detecting residual disease, for detecting suspected recurrence, or to determine the extent of a known recurrence. Use of PET would also be considered reasonable and necessary if it could potentially replace one or more conventional imaging studies when it is expected that conventional study information is insufficient for the clinical management of the patient.

The PET is not covered for other diagnostic uses, and is not covered for screening (testing of patients without specific symptoms). Use of PET to monitor tumor response during the planned course of therapy (i.e., when no change in therapy is being contemplated) is not covered.

100-4, 13, 60.1

Billing Instructions

A. Billing and Payment Instructions or Responsibilities for Carriers

Claims for PET scan services must be billed on Form-CMS 1500 or the electronic equivalent with the appropriate HCPCS or CPT code and diagnosis codes to the local carrier. Effective for claims received on or after July 1, 2001, PET modifiers were discontinued and are no longer a claims processing requirement for PET scan claims. Therefore, July 1, 2001, and after the MSN messages regarding the use of PET modifiers can be discontinued. The type of service (TOS) for the new PET scan procedure codes is TOS 4, Diagnostic Radiology. Payment is based on the Medicare Physician Fee Schedule.

B. Billing and Payment Instructions or Responsibilities for FIs

Claims for PET scan procedures must be billed to the FI on Form CMS-1450 (UB-92) or the electronic equivalent with the appropriate diagnosis and HCPCS "G" code or CPT code to indicate the conditions under which a PET scan was done. These codes represent the technical component costs associated with these procedures when furnished to hospital and SNF outpatients. They are paid as follows:

- under OPPS for hospitals subject to OPPS
- under current payment methodologies for hospitals not subject to OPPS
- on a reasonable cost basis for critical access hospitals.
- on a reasonable cost basis for skilled nursing facilities.

Institutional providers bill these codes under Revenue Code 0404 (PET Scan).

Medicare contractors shall pay claims submitted for services provided by a critical access hospital (CAH) as follows: Method I technical services are paid at 101% of reasonable cost; Method II technical services are paid at 101% of reasonable cost, and professional services are paid at 115% of the Medicare Physician Fee Schedule Data Base.

C. Frequency

In the absence of national frequency limitations, for all indications covered on and after July 1, 2001, contractors can, if necessary, develop frequency limitations on any or all covered PET scan services.

D. Post-Payment Review for PET Scans

As with any claim, but particularly in view of the limitations on this coverage, Medicare may decide to conduct post-payment reviews to determine that the use of PET scans is consistent with coverage instructions. Pet scanning facilities must keep patient record information on file for each Medicare patient for whom a PET scan claim is made. These medical records can be used in any post-payment reviews and must include the information necessary to substantiate the need for the PET scan. These records must include standard information (e.g., age, sex, and height) along with sufficient patient histories to allow determination that the steps required in the coverage instructions were followed. Such information must include, but is not limited to, the date, place and results of previous diagnostic tests (e.g., cytopathology and surgical pathology reports, CT), as well as the results and reports of the PET scan(s) performed at the center. If available, such records should include the prognosis derived from the PET scan, together with information regarding the physician or institution to which the patient proceeded following the scan for treatment or evaluation. The ordering physician is responsible for forwarding appropriate clinical data to the PET scan facility.

Effective for claims received on or after July 1, 2001, CMS no longer requires paper documentation to be submitted up front with PET scan claims. Contractors shall be aware and advise providers of the specific documentation requirements for PET scans for dementia and neurodegenerative diseases. This information is outlined in section 60.12. Documentation requirements such as physician referral and medical necessity determination are to be maintained by the provider as part of the beneficiary's medical record. This information must be made available to the carrier or FI upon request of additional documentation to determine appropriate payment of an individual claim.

100-4, 13, 60.2

Use of Gamma Cameras and Full Ring and Partial Ring PET Scanners for PET Scans

See the Medicare NCD Manual, Section 220.6, concerning 2-[F-18] Fluoro-D-Glucose (FDG) PET scanners and details about coverage.

On July 1, 2001, HCPCS codes G0210 - G0230 were added to allow billing for all currently covered indications for FDG PET. Although the codes do not indicate the type of PET scanner, these codes were used until January 1, 2002, by providers to bill for services in a manner consistent with the coverage policy.

Effective January 1, 2002, HCPCS codes G0210 - G0230 were updated with new descriptors to properly reflect the type of PET scanner used. In addition, four new HCPCS codes became effective for dates of service on and after January 1, 2002, (G0231, G0232, G0233, G0234) for covered conditions that may be billed if a gamma camera is used for the PET scan. For services performed from January 1, 2002, through January 27, 2005, providers should bill using the revised HCPCS codes G0210 - G0234.

Beginning January 28, 2005 providers should bill using the appropriate CPT code.

100-4, 13, 60.3

PET Scan Qualifying Conditions and HCPCS Code Chart

Below is a summary of all covered PET scan conditions, with effective dates.

NOTE: The G codes below except those a # can be used to bill for PET Scan services through January 27, 2005. Effective for dates of service on or after January 28, 2005, providers must bill for PET Scan services using the appropriate CPT codes. See section 60.3.1. The G codes with a # can continue to be used for billing after January 28, 2005 and these remain non-covered by Medicare. (NOTE: PET Scanners must be FDA-approved.)

Conditions	Coverage Effective Date	****HCPCS/ CPT
*Myocardial perfusion imaging (following previous PET G0030-G0047) single study, rest or stress (exercise and/or pharmacologic)	3/14/95	G0030
*Myocardial perfusion imaging (following previous PET G0030-G0047) multiple studies, rest or stress (exercise and/or pharmacologic)	3/14/95	G0031
*Myocardial perfusion imaging (following rest SPECT, 78464); single study, rest or stress (exercise and/or pharmacologic)	'3/14/95	G0032
*Myocardial perfusion imaging (following rest SPECT 78464); multiple studies, rest or stress (exercise and/or pharmacologic)	3/14/95	G0033
*Myocardial perfusion (following stress SPECT 78465); single study, rest or stress (exercise and/or pharmacologic)	3/14/95	G0034
*Myocardial Perfusion Imaging (following stress SPECT 78465); multiple studies, rest or stress (exercise and/or pharmacologic)	3/14/95	G0035
*Myocardial Perfusion Imaging (following coronary angiography 93510-93529); single study, rest or stress (exercise and/or pharmacologic)	3/14/95	G0036
*Myocardial Perfusion Imaging, (following coronary angiography), 93510-93529); multiple studies, rest or stress (exercise and/or pharmacologic)	3/14/95	G0037
*Myocardial Perfusion Imaging (following stress planar myocardial perfusion, 78460), single study, rest or stress (exercise and/or pharmacologic)	3/14/95	G0038
*Myocardial Perfusion Imaging (following stress planar myocardial perfusion, 78460); multiple studies, rest or stress (exercise and/or pharmacologic)	3/14/95	G0039
*Myocardial Perfusion Imaging (following stress echocardiogram 93350); single study, rest or stress (exercise and/or pharmacologic)	3/14/95	G0040
*Myocardial Perfusion Imaging (following stress echocardiogram, 93350); multiple studies, rest or stress (exercise and/or pharmacologic)	3/14/95	G0041
*Myocardial Perfusion Imaging (following stress nuclear ventriculogram 78481 or 78483); single study, rest or stress (exercise and/or pharmacologic)	3/14/95	G0042

* Carriers must report A4641 for the tracer Rubidium 82 when used with PET scan codes G0030 through G0047 for services performed on or before January 27, 2005

** Not FDG PET

*** For dates of service October 1, 2003, through December 31, 2003, use temporary code Q4078 for billing this radiopharmaceutical.

Conditions	Coverage Effective Date	****HCPCS/ CPT
*Myocardial Perfusion Imaging (following stress nuclear ventriculogram 78481 or 78483); multiple studies, rest or stress (exercise and/or pharmacologic)	3/14/95	G0043
*Myocardial Perfusion Imaging (following stress ECG, 93000); single study, rest or stress (exercise and/or pharmacologic)	3/14/95	G0044
*Myocardial perfusion (following stress ECG, 93000), multiple studies; rest or stress (exercise and/or pharmacologic)	3/14/95	G0045
*Myocardial perfusion (following stress ECG, 93015), single study; rest or stress (exercise and/or pharmacologic)	3/14/95	G0046
*Myocardial perfusion (following stress ECG, 93015); multiple studies, rest or stress (exercise and/or pharmacologic)	3/14/95	G0047
PET imaging regional or whole body; single pulmonary nodule	1/1/98	G0125
Lung cancer, non-small cell (PET imaging whole body) Diagnosis, Initial Staging, Restaging	7/1/01	G0210 G0211 G0212
Colorectal cancer (PET imaging whole body) Diagnosis, Initial Staging, Restaging	7/1/01	G0213 G0214 G0215
Melanoma (PET imaging whole body) Diagnosis, Initial Staging, Restaging	7/1/01	G0216 G0217 G0218
Melanoma for non-covered indications	7/1/01	G0219
Lymphoma (PET imaging whole body) Diagnosis, Initial Staging, Restaging	7/1/01	G0220 G0221 G0222
Head and neck cancer; excluding thyroid and CNS cancers (PET imaging whole body or regional) Diagnosis, Initial Staging, Restaging	7/1/01	G0223 G0224 G0225
Esophageal cancer (PET imaging whole body) Diagnosis, Initial Staging, Restaging	7/1/01	G0226 G0227 G0228
Metabolic brain imaging for pre-surgical evaluation of refractory seizures	7/1/01	G0229
Metabolic assessment for myocardial viability following inconclusive SPECT study	7/1/01	G0230
Recurrence of colorectal or colorectal metastatic cancer (PET whole body, gamma cameras only)	1/1/02	G0231
Staging and characterization of lymphoma (PET whole body, gamma cameras only)	1/1/02	G0232
Recurrence of melanoma or melanoma metastatic cancer (PET whole body, gamma cameras only)	1/1/02	G0233
Regional or whole body, for solitary pulmonary nodule following CT, or for initial staging of nonsmall cell lung cancer (gamma cameras only)	1/1/02	G0234
Non-Covered Service PET imaging, any site not otherwise specified	1/28/05	G0235
Non-Covered Service Initial diagnosis of breast cancer and/or surgical planning for breast cancer (e.g., initial staging of axillary lymph nodes), not covered (full- and partialring PET scanners only)	10/1/02	G0252
Breast cancer, staging/restaging of local regional recurrence or distant metastases, i.e., staging/restaging after or prior to course of treatment (full- and partial-ring PET scanners only)	10/1/02	G0253
Breast cancer, evaluation of responses to treatment, performed during course of treatment (full- and partial-ring PET scanners only)	10/1/02	G0254
Myocardial imaging, positron emission tomography (PET), metabolic evaluation)	10/1/02	78459

* Carriers must report A4641 for the tracer Rubidium 82 when used with PET scan codes G0030 through G0047 for services performed on or before January 27, 2005

** Not FDG PET

*** For dates of service October 1, 2003, through December 31, 2003, use temporary code Q4078 for billing this radiopharmaceutical.

Conditions	Coverage Effective Date	****HCPCS/ CPT
Restaging or previously treated thyroid cancer of follicular cell origin following negative I-131 whole body scan (full- and partial-ring PET scanner only)	10/1/03	G0296
Tracer Rubidium**82 (Supply of Radiopharmaceutical Diagnostic Imaging Agent) (This is only billed through Outpatient Perspective Payment System, OPPS.) (Carriers must use HCPCS Code A4641).	10/1/03	Q3000
Supply of Radiopharmaceutical Diagnostic Imaging Agent, Ammonia N-13	01/1/04	A9526
PET imaging, brain imaging for the differential diagnosis of Alzheimer's disease with aberrant features vs. fronto-temporal dementia	09/15/04	Appropriate CPT Code from section 60.3.1
PET Cervical Cancer Staging as adjunct to conventional imaging, other staging, diagnosis, restaging, monitoring	1/28/05	Appropriate CPT Code from section 60.3.1

* Carriers must report A4641 for the tracer Rubidium 82 when used with PET scan codes G0030 through G0047 for services performed on or before January 27, 2005

** Not FDG PET

*** For dates of service October 1, 2003, through December 31, 2003, use temporary code Q4078 for billing this radiopharmaceutical.

100-4, 13, 60.3.1

Appropriate CPT Codes Effective for PET Scans for Services Performed on or After January 28, 2005

NOTE: All PET scan services require the use of a radiopharmaceutical diagnostic imaging agent (tracer). The applicable tracer code should be billed when billing for a PET scan service. See section 60.3.2 below for applicable tracer codes.

CPT Code	Description
78459	Myocardial imaging, positron emission tomography (PET), metabolic evaluation
78491	Myocardial imaging, positron emission tomography (PET), perfusion, single study at rest or stress
78492	Myocardial imaging, positron emission tomography (PET), perfusion, multiple studies at rest and/or stress
78608	Brain imaging, positron emission tomography (PET); metabolic evaluation
78811	Tumor imaging, positron emission tomography (PET); limited area (eg, chest, head/neck)
78812	Tumor imaging, positron emission tomography (PET); skull base to mid-thigh
78813	Tumor imaging, positron emission tomography (PET); whole body
78814	Tumor imaging, positron emission tomography (PET) with concurrently acquired computed tomography (CT) for attenuation correction and anatomical localization; limited area (eg, chest, head/neck)
78815	Tumor imaging, positron emission tomography (PET) with concurrently acquired computed tomography (CT) for attenuation correction and anatomical localization; skull base to mid-thigh
78816	Tumor imaging, positron emission tomography (PET) with concurrently acquired computed tomography (CT) for attenuation correction and anatomical localization; whole body

100-4, 13, 60.3.2

Tracer Codes Required for PET Scans

The following tracer codes are applicable only to CPT 78491 and 78492. They can not be reported with any other code.

Institutional providers billing the fiscal intermediary

HCPCS	Description
*A9555	Rubidium Rb-82, Diagnostic, Per study dose, Up To 60 Millicuries
*Q3000 (Deleted effective 12/31/05)	Supply of Radiopharmaceutical Diagnostic Imaging Agent, Rubidium Rb-82, per dose
A9526	Nitrogen N-13 Ammonia, Diagnostic, Per study dose, Up To 40 Millicuries

NOTE: For claims with dates of service prior to 1/01/06, providers report Q3000 for supply of radiopharmaceutical diagnostic imaging agent, Rubidium Rb-82. For claims with dates of service 1/01/06 and later, providers report A9555 for radiopharmaceutical diagnostic imaging agent, Rubidium Rb-82 in place of Q3000.

Physicians / practitioners billing the carrier:

*A4641	Supply of Radiopharmaceutical Diagnostic Imaging Agent, Not Otherwise Classified
A9526	Nitrogen N-13 Ammonia, Diagnostic, Per study dose, Up To 40 Millicuries
A9555	Rubidium Rb-82, Diagnostic, Per study dose, Up To 60 Millicuries

***NOTE:** Effective January 1, 2008, tracer code A4641 is not applicable for PET Scans.

The following tracer codes are applicable only to CPT 78459, 78608, 78811-78816. They can not be reported with any other code:

Institutional providers billing the fiscal intermediary:

* A9552	Fluorodeoxyglucose F18, FDG, Diagnostic, Per study dose, Up to 45 Millicuries
* C1775 (Deleted effective 12/31/05)	Supply of Radiopharmaceutical Diagnostic Imaging Agent, Fluorodeoxyglucose F18, (2-Deoxy-2-18F Fluoro-D-Glucose), Per dose (4-40 Mci/Ml)
**A4641	Supply of Radiopharmaceutical Diagnostic Imaging Agent, Not Otherwise Classified
A9580	Sodium Fluoride F-18, Diagnostic, per study dose, up to 30 Millicuries

NOTE: For claims with dates of service prior to 1/01/06, OPPS hospitals report C1775 for supply of radiopharmaceutical diagnostic imaging agent, Fluorodeoxyglucose F18. For claims with dates of service January 1, 2006 and later, providers report A9552 for radiopharmaceutical diagnostic imaging agent, Fluorodeoxyglucose F18 in place of C1775.

** **NOTE:** Effective January 1, 2008, tracer code A4641 is not applicable for PET Scans.

*****NOTE:** Effective for claims with dates of service February 26, 2010 and later, tracer code

A9580 is applicable for PET Scans.	Physicians / practitioners billing the carrier:
A9552	Fluorodeoxyglucose F18, FDG, Diagnostic, Per study dose, Up to 45 Millicuries
*A4641	Supply of Radiopharmaceutical Diagnostic Imaging Agent, Not Otherwise Classified
A9580	Sodium Fluoride F-18, Diagnostic, per study dose, up to 30 Millicuries

***NOTE:** Effective January 1, 2008, tracer code A4641 is not applicable for PET Scans.

*****NOTE:** Effective for claims with dates of service February 26, 2010 and later, tracer code

A9580 is applicable for PET Scans.	Positron Emission Tomography Reference Table CPT

CPT	Short Descriptor	Tracer/ Code	or	Tracer/ Code	Comment
78459	Myocardial imaging, positron emission tomography (PET), metabolic imaging	FDG A9552	--	--	N/A
78491	Myocardial imaging, positron emission tomography (PET), perfusion; single study at rest or stress	N-13 A9526	or	Rb-82 A9555	N/A
78492	Myocardial imaging, positron emission tomography (PET), perfusion; multiple studies at rest and/or stress	N-13 A9526	or	Rb-82 A9555	N/A

CPT	Short Descriptor	Tracer/ Code	or	Tracer/ Code	Comment
78608	Brain imaging, positron emission tomography (PET); metabolic evaluation	FDG A9552	--	--	Covered indications: Alzheimer's disease/dementias, intractable seizures Note: This code is also covered for dedicated PET brain tumor imaging.
78609	Brain imaging, positron emission tomography (PET); perfusion evaluation	--	--	--	Nationally noncovered
78811	Positron emission tomography (PET) imaging; limited area (e.g, chest, head/neck)	FDG A9552	or	NaF-18 A9580	NaF-18 PET is covered only to identify bone metastasis of cancer.

100-4, 13, 60.4

PET Scans for Imaging of the Perfusion of the Heart Using Rubidium 82 (Rb 82)(Rev. 223, Issued: 07-02-04) (Effective/Implementation: Not Applicable)

For dates of service on or after March 14, 1995, Medicare covers one PET scan for imaging of the perfusion of the heart using Rubidium 82 (Rb 82), provided that the following conditions are met:

- The PET is done at a PET imaging center with a PET scanner that has been approved by the FDA;
- The PET scan is a rest alone or rest with pharmacologic stress PET scan, used for noninvasive imaging of the perfusion of the heart for the diagnosis and management of patients with known or suspected coronary artery disease, using Rb 82; and
- Either the PET scan is used in place of, but not in addition to, a single photon emission computed tomography (SPECT) or the PET scan is used following a SPECT that was found inconclusive.

100-4, 13, 60.9

Coverage of PET Scans for Myocardial Viability

FDG PET is covered for the determination of myocardial viability following an inconclusive single photon computed tomography test (SPECT) from July 1, 2001, through September 30, 2002. Only full ring scanners are covered as the scanning medium for this service from July 1, 2001, through December 31, 2001. However, as of January 1, 2002, full and partial ring scanners are covered for myocardial viability following an inconclusive SPECT.

Beginning October 1, 2002, Medicare will cover FDG PET for the determination of myocardial viability as a primary or initial diagnostic study prior to revascularization, and will continue to cover FDG PET when used as a follow-up to an inconclusive SPECT.

However, if a patient received a FDG PET study with inconclusive results, a follow-up SPECT is not covered. FDA full and partial ring PET scanners are covered. In the event that a patient receives a SPECT with inconclusive results, a PET scan may be performed and covered by Medicare. However, a SPECT is not covered following a FDG PET with inconclusive results. See the Medicare National Coverage Determinations Manual, Section 220.6 for specific frequency limitations for Myocardial Viability following an inconclusive SPECT.

Documentation that these conditions are met should be maintained by the referring provider as part of the beneficiary's medical record.

HCPCS Code for PET Scan for Myocardial Viability

78459 Myocardial imaging, positron emission tomography (PET), metabolic evaluation

100-4, 13, 60.11

Coverage of PET Scans for Perfusion of the Heart Using Ammonia N-13

Effective for service performed on or after October 1, 2003, PET scans performed at rest or with pharmacological stress used for noninvasive imaging of the perfusion of the heart for the diagnosis and management of patients with known or suspected coronary artery disease using the FDA-approved radiopharmaceutical ammonia N-13 are covered, provided the following requirements are met.

100-4, 13, 60.12

Coverage for PET Scans for Dementia and Neurodegenerative Diseases

Effective for dates of service on or after September 15, 2004, Medicare will cover FDG PET scans for a differential diagnosis of fronto-temporal dementia (FTD) and Alzheimer's disease OR; its use in a CMS-approved practical clinical trial focused on the utility of FDG-PET in the diagnosis or treatment of dementing neurodegenerative diseases. Refer to Pub. 100-03, NCD Manual, section 220.6.13, for complete coverage conditions and clinical trial requirements and section 60.15 of this manual for claims processing information.

A. Carrier and FI Billing Requirements for PET Scan Claims for FDG-PET for the Differential Diagnosis of Fronto-temporal Dementia and Alzheimer's Disease:

- CPT Code for PET Scans for Dementia and Neurodegenerative Diseases

  Contractors shall advise providers to use the appropriate CPT code from section 60.3.1 for dementia and neurodegenerative diseases for services performed on or after January 28, 2005.
- Diagnosis Codes for PET Scans for Dementia and Neurodegenerative Diseases

  The contractor shall ensure one of the following appropriate diagnosis codes is present on claims for PET Scans for AD:

  - 290.0, 290.10 - 290.13, 290.20 - 290, 21, 290.3, 331.0, 331.11, 331.19, 331.2, 331.9, 780.93

  Medicare contractors shall use an appropriate Medicare Summary Notice (MSN) message such as 16.48, "Medicare does not pay for this item or service for this condition" to deny claims when submitted with an appropriate CPT code from section 60.3.1 and with a diagnosis code other than the range of codes listed above. Also, contractors shall use an appropriate Remittance Advice (RA) such as 11, "The diagnosis is inconsistent with the procedure."

  Medicare contractors shall instruct providers to issue an Advanced Beneficiary Notice to beneficiaries advising them of potential financial liability prior to delivering the service if one of the appropriate diagnosis codes will not be present on the claim.
- Provider Documentation Required with the PET Scan Claim

  Medicare contractors shall inform providers to ensure the conditions mentioned in the NCD Manual, section 220.6.13, have been met. The information must also be maintained in the beneficiary's medical record:

  - Date of onset of symptoms;
  - Diagnosis of clinical syndrome (normal aging, mild cognitive impairment or MCI: mild, moderate, or severe dementia);
  - Mini mental status exam (MMSE) or similar test score;
  - Presumptive cause (possible, probably, uncertain AD);
  - Any neuropsychological testing performed;
  - Results of any structural imaging (MRI, CT) performed;
  - Relevant laboratory tests (B12, thyroid hormone); and,
  - Number and name of prescribed medications.

B. Billing Requirements for Beta Amyloid Positron Emission Tomography (PET) in Dementia and Neurodegenerative Disease:

Effective for claims with dates of service on and after September 27, 2013, Medicare will only allow coverage with evidence development (CED) for Positron Emission Tomography (PET) beta amyloid (also referred to as amyloid-beta (Aβ)) imaging (HCPCS A9586)or (HCPCS A9599) (one PET Aβ scan per patient).

Note: Please note that effective January 1, 2014 the following code A9599 will be updated in the IOCE and HCPCS update. This code will be contractor priced.

Medicare Summary Notices, Remittance Advice Remark Codes, and Claim Adjustment Reason Codes

Effective for dates of service on or after September 27, 2013, contractors shall return as unprocessable/return to provider claims for PET Aβ imaging, through CED during a clinical trial, not containing the following:

- Condition code 30, (FI only)
- Modifier Q0 and/or modifier Q1 as appropriate
- ICD-9 dx code V70.7/ICD-10 dx code Z00.6 (on either the primary/secondary position)
- A PET HCPCS code (78811 or 78814)
- At least, one Dx code from the table below,

ICD-9 Codes Corresponding	ICD-10 Codes
290.0 Senile dementia, uncomplicated	F03.90 Unspecified dementia without behavioral disturbance
290.10 Presenile dementia, uncomplicated	F03.90 Unspecified dementia without behavioral disturbance
290.11 Presenile dementia with delirium	F03.90 Unspecified dementia without behavioral disturbance

ICD-9 Codes Corresponding	ICD-10 Codes
290.12 Presenile dementia with delusional features	F03.90Unspecified dementia without behavioral disturbance
290.13 Presenile dementia with depressive features	F03.90Unspecified dementia without behavioral disturbance
290.20 Senile dementia with delusional features	F03.90Unspecified dementia without behavioral disturbance
290.21 Senile dementia with depressive features	F03.90Unspecified dementia without behavioral disturbance
290.3 Senile dementia with delirium	F03.90Unspecified dementia without behavioral disturbance
290.40 Vascular dementia, uncomplicated	F01.50Vascular dementia without behavioral disturbance
290.41 Vascular dementia with delirium	F01.51Vascular dementia with behavioral disturbance
290.42 Vascular dementia with delusions	F01.51Vascular dementia with behavioral disturbance
290.43 Vascular dementia with depressed mood	F01.51Vascular dementia with behavioral disturbance
294.10 Dementia in conditions classified elsewhere without behavioral disturbance	F02.80 Dementia in other diseases classified elsewhere without behavioral disturbance
294.11 Dementia in conditions classified elsewhere with behavioral disturbance	F02.81 Dementia in other diseases classified elsewhere with behavioral disturbance
294.20 Dementia, unspecified, without behavioral disturbance	F03.90 Unspecified dementia without behavioral disturbance
294.21 Dementia, unspecified, with behavioral disturbance	F03.91 Unspecified dementia with behavioral disturbance
331.11 Pick's Disease	G31.01 Pick's disease
331.19 Other Frontotemporal dementia	G31.09 Other frontotemporal dementia
331.6 Corticobasal degeneration	G31.85 Corticobasal degeneration
331.82 Dementia with Lewy Bodies	G31.83 Dementia with Lewy bodies
331.83 Mild cognitive impairment, so stated	G31.84 Mild cognitive impairment, so stated
780.93 Memory Loss	R41.1 Anterograde amnesia R41.2 Retrograde amnesia R41.3 Other amnesia (Amnesia NOS, Memory loss NOS)
V70.7 Examination for normal comparison or control in clinical	Z00.6Encounter for examination for normal comparison and control in clinical research program

and

• Aβ HCPCS code A9586 or A9599

Contractors shall return as unprocessable claims for PET Aβ imaging using the following messages:

- Claim Adjustment Reason Code 4 – the procedure code is inconsistent with the modifier used or a required modifier is missing.

NOTE: Refer to the 835 Healthcare Policy Identification Segment (loop 2110 Service Payment Information REF), if present.

- Remittance Advice Remark Code N517 - Resubmit a new claim with the requested information.
- Remittance Advice Remark Code N519 - Invalid combination of HCPCS modifiers.

Contractors shall line-item deny claims for PET Aβ , HCPCS code A9586 or A9599 , where a previous PET Aβ, HCPCS code A9586 or A9599 is paid in history using the following messages:

- CARC 149: "Lifetime benefit maximum has been reached for this service/benefit category."
- RARC N587: "Policy benefits have been exhausted".
- MSN 20.12: "This service was denied because Medicare only covers this service once a lifetime."
- Spanish Version: "Este servicio fue negado porque Medicare sólo cubre este servicio una vez en la vida."
- Group Code: PR, if a claim is received with a GA modifier
- Group Code: CO, if a claim is received with a GZ modifier

100-4, 13, 60.13

Billing Requirements for PET Scans for Specific Indications of Cervical Cancer for Services Performed on or After January 28, 2005

Contractors shall accept claims for these services with the appropriate CPT code listed in section 60.3.1. Refer to Pub. 100-03, section 220.6.17, for complete coverage guidelines for this new PET oncology indication. The implementation date for these CPT codes will be April 18, 2005. Also see section 60.17, of this chapter for further claims processing instructions for cervical cancer indications.

100-4, 13, 60.15

Billing Requirements for CMS - Approved Clinical Trials and Coverage With Evidence Development Claims for PET Scans for Neurodegenerative Diseases, Previously Specified Cancer Indications, and All Other Cancer Indications Not Previously Specified

(Rev. 2932, Issued: 04-18-14, Effective: 06-11-13, Implementation: 05-19-14 - MAC Non-Shared System Edits; July 7, 2014 - CWF development/testing, FISS requirement development; October 6, 2014 - CWF, FISS, MCS Shared System Edits)

Parts A and B Medicare Administrative Contractors (MACs)

Effective for services on or after January 28, 2005, contractors shall accept and pay for claims for Positron Emission Tomography (PET) scans for lung cancer, esophageal cancer, colorectal cancer, lymphoma, melanoma, head & neck cancer, breast cancer, thyroid cancer, soft tissue sarcoma, brain cancer, ovarian cancer, pancreatic cancer, small cell lung cancer, and testicular cancer, as well as for neurodegenerative diseases and all other cancer indications not previously mentioned in this chapter, if these scans were performed as part of a Centers for Medicare & Medicaid (CMS)-approved clinical trial. (See Pub. 100-03, National Coverage Determinations (NCD) Manual, sections 220.6.13 and 220.6.17.)

Contractors shall also be aware that PET scans for all cancers not previously specified at Pub. 100-03, NCD Manual, section 220.6.17, remain nationally non-covered unless performed in conjunction with a CMS-approved clinical trial.

Effective for dates of service on or after June 11, 2013, Medicare has ended the coverage with evidence development (CED) requirement for FDG (2-[F18] fluoro-2-deoxy-D-glucose) PET and PET/computed tomography (CT) and PET/magnetic resonance imaging (MRI) for all oncologic indications contained in section 220.6.17 of the NCD Manual. Modifier -Q0 (Investigational clinical service provided in a clinical research study that is in an approved clinical research study) or -Q1 (routine clinical service provided in a clinical research study that is in an approved clinical research study) is no longer mandatory for these services when performed on or after June 11, 2013.

Part B MACs Only

Part B MACs shall pay claims for PET scans for beneficiaries participating in a CMS-approved clinical trial submitted with an appropriate current procedural terminology (CPT) code from section 60.3.1 of this chapter and modifier -Q0/-Q1 for services performed on or after January 1, 2008, through June 10, 2013. (NOTE: Modifier -QR (Item or service provided in a Medicare specified study) and -QA (FDA investigational device exemption) were replaced by modifier -Q0 effective January 1, 2008.) Modifier -QV (item or service provided as routine care in a Medicare qualifying clinical trial) was replaced by modifier -Q1 effective January 1, 2008.) Beginning with services performed on or after June 11, 2013, modifier -Q0/-Q1 is no longer required for PET FDG services.

Part A MACs Only

In order to pay claims for PET scans on behalf of beneficiaries participating in a CMS-approved clinical trial, Part A MACs require providers to submit claims with ICD-9/ICD-10 code V70.7/Z00.6 in the primary/secondary diagnosis position on the CMS-1450 (UB-04), or the electronic equivalent, with the appropriate principal diagnosis code and an appropriate CPT code from section 60.3.1. Effective for PET scan claims for dates of service on or after January 28, 2005, through December 31, 2007, FIs shall accept claims with the –QR, -QV, or -QA modifier on other than inpatient claims. Effective for services on or after January 1, 2008, through June 10, 2013, modifier -Q0 replaced the -QR and –QA modifier, modifier –Q1 replaced the –QV modifier. Modifier -Q0/-Q1 is no longer required for services performed on or after June 11, 2013.

100-4, 13, 60.16

Billing and Coverage Changes for PET Scans Effective for Services on or After April 3, 2009

(Rev. 2932, Issued: 04-18- 14, Effective: 06-11-13, Implementation: 05-19-14- MAC Non-Shared System Edits; July 7, 2014 - CWF development/testing, FISS requirement development; October 6, 2014 - CWF, FISS, MCS Shared System Edits)

A. Summary of Changes

Effective for services on or after April 3, 2009, Medicare will not cover the use of FDG PET imaging to determine initial treatment strategy in patients with adenocarcinoma of the prostate.

Medicare will also not cover FDG PET imaging for subsequent treatment strategy for tumor types other than breast, cervical, colorectal, esophagus, head and neck (non-CNS/thyroid), lymphoma, melanoma, myeloma, non-small cell lung, and ovarian, unless the FDG PET is provided under the coverage with evidence development (CED) paradigm (billed with modifier -Q0/-Q1, see section 60.15 of this chapter).

Medicare will cover FDG PET imaging for initial treatment strategy for myeloma.

Effective for services performed on or after June 11, 2013, Medicare has ended the CED requirement for FDG PET and PET/CT and PET/MRI for all oncologic indications contained in section 220.6.17 of the NCD Manual. Effective for services on or after June 11, 2013, the -Q0/Q1 modifier is no longer required.

Beginning with services performed on or after June 11, 2013, contractors shall pay for up to three (3) FDG PET scans when used to guide subsequent management of anti-tumor treatment strategy (modifier –PS) after completion of initial anti-cancer therapy (modifier –PI) for the exact same cancer diagnosis.

Coverage of any additional FDG PET scans (that is, beyond 3) used to guide subsequent management of anti-tumor treatment strategy after completion of initial anti-tumor therapy for the same cancer diagnosis will be determined by the local MACs. Claims will include the –KX modifier indicating the coverage criteria is met for coverage of four or more FDG PET scans for subsequent treatment strategy for the same cancer diagnosis under this NCD.

A different cancer diagnosis whether submitted with a –PI or a –PS modifier will begin the count of one initial and three subsequent FDG PET scans not requiring the –KX modifier and four or more FDG PET scans for subsequent treatment strategy for the same cancer diagnosis requiring the –KX modifier.

NOTE: The presence or absence of an initial treatment strategy claim in a beneficiary's record does not impact the frequency criteria for subsequent treatment strategy claims for the same cancer diagnosis.

NOTE: Providers please refer to Attachment A of the CR for a list of appropriate diagnosis codes.

For further information regarding the changes in coverage, refer to Pub.100-03, NCD Manual, section 220.6.17.

B. Modifiers for PET Scans

Effective for claims with dates of service on or after April 3, 2009, the following modifiers have been created for use to inform for the initial treatment strategy of biopsy-proven or strongly suspected tumors or subsequent treatment strategy of cancerous tumors:

PI -Positron Emission Tomography (PET) or PET/Computed Tomography (CT) to inform the initial treatment strategy of tumors that are biopsy proven or strongly suspected of being cancerous based on other diagnostic testing.

Short descriptor: PET tumor init tx strat

PS - Positron Emission Tomography (PET) or PET/Computed Tomography (CT) to inform the subsequent treatment strategy of cancerous tumors when the beneficiary's treatment physician determines that the PET study is needed to inform subsequent anti-tumor strategy.

Short descriptor: PS - PET tumor subsq tx strategy

C. Billing for A/B MACs

Effective for claims with dates of service on or after April 3, 2009, contractors shall accept FDG PET claims billed to inform initial treatment strategy with the following CPT codes AND modifier –PI: 78608, 78811, 78812, 78813, 78814, 78815, 78816.

Effective for claims with dates of service on or after April 3, 2009, contractors shall accept FDG PET claims with modifier –PS for the subsequent treatment strategy for solid tumors using a CPT code above AND a cancer diagnosis code.

Contractors shall also accept FDG PET claims billed to inform initial treatment strategy or subsequent treatment strategy when performed under CED with one of the PET or PET/CT CPT codes above AND modifier -PI OR modifier -PS AND a cancer diagnosis code AND modifier -Q0/Q1. Effective for services performed on or after June 11, 2013, the CED requirement has ended and modifier -Q0/-Q1, along with condition code 30 (institutional claims only), or V70.7 (both institutional and practitioner claims) are no longer required

D. Medicare Summary Notices, Remittance Advice Remark Codes, and Claim Adjustment Reason Codes

Effective for dates of service on or after April 3, 2009, contractors shall return as unprocessable/return to provider claims that do not include the -PI modifier with one of the PET/PET/CT CPT codes listed in subsection C. above when billing for the initial treatment strategy for solid tumors in accordance with Pub.100-03, NCD Manual, section 220.6.17.

In addition, contractors shall return as unprocessable/return to provider claims that do not include the -PS modifier with one of the CPT codes listed in subsection C. above when billing for the subsequent treatment strategy for solid tumors in accordance with Pub.100-03, NCD Manual, section 220.6.17.

The following messages apply:

- Claim Adjustment Reason Code (CARC) 4 – the procedure code is inconsistent with the modifier used or a required modifier is missing.
- Remittance Advice Remark Code (RARC) MA-130 - Your claim contains incomplete and/or invalid information, and no appeal rights are afforded because the claim is unprocessable. Submit a new claim with the complete/correct information.
- RARC M16 - Alert: See our Web site, mailings, or bulletins for more details concerning this policy/procedure/decision.

Also, effective for claims with dates of service on or after April 3, 2009, through June 10, 2013, contractors shall return as unprocessable/return to provider FDG PET claims billed to inform initial treatment strategy or subsequent treatment strategy when performed under CED without one of the PET/PET/CT CPT codes listed in subsection C. above AND modifier -PI OR modifier -PS AND a cancer diagnosis code AND modifier -Q0/-Q1.

The following messages apply to return as unprocessable claims:

- CARC 4 – the procedure code is inconsistent with the modifier used or a required modifier is missing.
- RARC MA-130 - Your claim contains incomplete and/or invalid information, and no appeal rights are afforded because the claim is unprocessable. Submit a new claim with the complete/correct information.
- RARC M16 - Alert: See our Web site, mailings, or bulletins for more details concerning this policy/procedure/decision.

Effective April 3, 2009, contractors shall deny claims with ICD-9/ICD-10 diagnosis code 185/C61 for FDG PET imaging for the initial treatment strategy of patients with adenocarcinoma of the prostate.

For dates of service prior to June 11, 2013, contractors shall also deny claims for FDG PET imaging for subsequent treatment strategy for tumor types other than breast, cervical, colorectal, esophagus, head and neck (non-CNS/thyroid), lymphoma, melanoma, myeloma, non-small cell lung, and ovarian, unless the FDG PET is provided under CED (submitted with the -Q0/Q1 modifier) and use the following messages:

- Medicare Summary Notice 15.4 - Medicare does not support the need for this service or item
- CARC 50 - These are non-covered services because this is not deemed a 'medical necessity' by the payer.
- Contractors shall use Group Code CO (Contractual Obligation)

If the service is submitted with a -GA modifier indicating there is a signed Advance Beneficiary Notice (ABN) on file, the liability falls to the beneficiary. However, if the service is submitted with a -GZ modifier indicating no ABN was provided, the liability falls to the provider.

Effective for dates of service on or after June 11, 2013, contractors shall use the following messages when denying claims in excess of three for PET FDG scans for subsequent treatment strategy when the –KX modifier is not included, identified by CPT codes 78608, 78811, 78812, 78813, 78814, 78815, or 78816, modifier –PS, HCPCS A9552, and the same cancer diagnosis code.

CARC 96: "Non-Covered Charge(s). Note: Refer to the 835 Healthcare Policy Identification Segment (loop 2110 Service Payment Information REF), if present."

RARC N435: "Exceeds number/frequency approved/allowed within time period without support documentation."

MSN 23.17: "Medicare won't cover these services because they are not considered medically necessary."

Spanish Version: "Medicare no cubrirá estos servicios porque no son considerados necesarios por razones médicas."

Contractors shall use Group Code PR assigning financial liability to the beneficiary, if a claim is received with a GA modifier indicating a signed ABN is on file.

Contractors shall use Group Code CO assigning financial liability to the provider, if a claim is received with a GZ modifier indicating no signed ABN is on file.

100-4, 13, 60.17

Billing and Coverage Changes for PET Scans for Cervical Cancer Effective for Services on or After November 10, 2009

A. Billing Changes for A/B MACs, FIs, and Carriers

Effective for claims with dates of service on or after November 10, 2009, contractors shall accept FDG PET oncologic claims billed to inform initial treatment strategy; specifically for staging in beneficiaries who have biopsy-proven cervical cancer when the beneficiary's treating physician determines the FDG PET study is needed to determine the location and/or extent of the tumor as specified in Pub 100-03, section 220.6.17.

EXCEPTION: CMS continues to non-cover FDG PET for initial diagnosis of cervical cancer related to initial treatment strategy.

NOTE: Effective for claims with dates of service on and after November 10, 2009, the -Q0 modifier is no longer necessary for FDG PET for cervical cancer.

B. Medicare Summary Notices, Remittance Advice Remark Codes, and Claim Adjustment Reason Codes

Additionally, contractors shall return as unprocessable /return to provider for FDG PET for cervical cancer for initial treatment strategy billed without the following: one of the PET/PET/ CT CPT codes listed in 60.16 C above AND modifier -PI AND an ICD-9 cervical cancer diagnosis code.

Use the following messages:

- Claim Adjustment Reason Code 4 - the procedure code is inconsistent with the modifier used or a required modifier is missing.
- Remittance Advice Remark Code MA-130 - Your claim contains incomplete and/or invalid information, and no appeal rights are afforded because the claim is unprocessable. Submit a new claim with the complete/correct information.
- Remittance Advice Remark Code M16 - Alert: See our Web site, mailings, or bulletins for more details concerning this policy/procedure/decision.

100-4, 13, 60.18

Billing and Coverage Changes for PET (NaF-18) Scans to Identify Bone Metastasis of Cancer Effective for Claims With Dates of Services on or After February 26, 2010

A. Billing Changes for A/B MACs, FIs, and Carriers

Effective for claims with dates of service on and after February 26, 2010, contractors shall pay for NaF-18 PET oncologic claims to inform of initial treatment strategy (PI) or subsequent treatment strategy (PS) for suspected or biopsy proven bone metastasis ONLY in the context of a clinical study and as specified in Pub. 100-03, section 220.6. All other claims for NaF-18 PET oncology claims remain non-covered.

B. Medicare Summary Notices, Remittance Advice Remark Codes, and Claim Adjustment Reason Codes

Effective for claims with dates of service on or after February 26, 2010, contractors shall return as unprocessable NaF-18 PET oncologic claims billed with modifier TC or globally (for FIs modifier TC or globally does not apply) and HCPCS A9580 to inform the initial treatment strategy or subsequent treatment strategy for bone metastasis that do not include ALL of the following:

- PI or –PS modifier AND
- PET or PET/CT CPT code (78811, 78812, 78813, 78814, 78815, 78816) AND
- ICD-9 cancer diagnosis code AND
- Q0 modifier–Investigational clinical service provided in a clinical research study, are present on the claim.

NOTE: For institutional claims, continue to include diagnosis code V70.7 and condition code 30 to denote a clinical study.

Use the following messages:

- Claim Adjustment Reason Code 4–The procedure code is inconsistent with the modifier used or a required modifier is missing. Note: Refer to the 835 Healthcare Policy Identification Segment (loop 2110 Service Payment Information REF), if present.
- Remittance Advice Remark Code MA-130 - Your claim contains incomplete and/or invalid information, and no appeal rights are afforded because the claim is unprocessable. Submit a new claim with the complete/correct information.
- Remittance Advice Remark Code M16 - Alert: See our Web site, mailings, or bulletins for more details concerning this policy/procedure/decision.
- Claim Adjustment Reason Code 167–This (these) diagnosis(es) is (are) not covered.

Effective for claims with dates of service on or after February 26, 2010, contractors shall accept PET oncologic claims billed with modifier 26 and modifier KX to inform the initial treatment strategy or strategy or subsequent treatment strategy for bone metastasis that include the following:

- PI or –PS modifier AND
- PET or PET/CT CPT code (78811, 78812, 78813, 78814, 78815, 78816) AND
- ICD-9 cancer diagnosis code AND
- Q0 modifier–Investigational clinical service provided in a clinical research study, are present on the claim.

NOTE: If modifier KX is present on the professional component service, Contractors shall process the service as PET NaF-18 rather than PET with FDG.

Contractors shall also return as unprocessable NaF-18 PET oncologic professional component claims (i.e., claims billed with modifiers 26 and KX) to inform the initial treatment strategy or strategy or subsequent treatment strategy for bone metastasis billed with HCPCS A9580 and use the following message:

Claim Adjustment Reason Code 97–The benefit for this service is included in the payment/allowance for another service/procedure that has already been adjudicated.

NOTE: Refer to the 835 Healthcare Policy identification Segment (loop 2110 Service Payment Information REF), if present.

100-4,13,60.3.2

Tracer Codes Required for PET Scans

The following tracer codes are applicable only to CPT 78491 and 78492. They can not be reported with any other code.

Institutional providers billing the fiscal intermediary

HCPCS	Description
*A9555	Rubidium Rb-82, Diagnostic, Per study dose, Up To 60 Millicuries
* Q3000 (Deleted effective 12/31/05)	Supply of Radiopharmaceutical Diagnostic Imaging Agent, Rubidium Rb-82, per dose
A9526	Nitrogen N-13 Ammonia, D Diagnostic, Per study dose, Up To 40 Millicuries

NOTE: For claims with dates of service prior to 1/01/06, providers report Q3000 for supply of radiopharmaceutical diagnostic imaging agent, Rubidium Rb-82. For claims with dates of service 1/01/06 and later, providers report A9555 for radiopharmaceutical diagnostic imaging agent, Rubidium Rb-82 in place of Q3000.

Physicians / practitioners billing the carrier:

*A4641 Supply of Radiopharmaceutical Diagnostic Imaging Agent, Not Otherwise Classified

A9526 Nitrogen N-13 Ammonia, Diagnostic, Per study dose, Up To 40 Millicuries

A9555 Rubidium Rb-82, Diagnostic, Per study dose, Up To 60 Millicuries

***NOTE:** Effective January 1, 2008, tracer code A4641 is not applicable for PET Scans.

The following tracer codes are applicable only to CPT 78459, 78608, 78811-78816. They can not be reported with any other code:

Institutional providers billing the fiscal intermediary:

* A9552 Fluorodeoxyglucose F18, FDG, Diagnostic, Per study dose, Up to 45 Millicuries

* C1775 (Deleted effective 12/31/05) Supply of Radiopharmaceutical Diagnostic Imaging Agent, Fluorodeoxyglucose F18, (2-Deoxy-2-18F Fluoro-D-Glucose), Per dose (4-40 Mci/Ml)

**A4641 Supply of Radiopharmaceutical Diagnostic Imaging Agent, Not Otherwise Classified

A9580 Sodium Fluoride F-18, Diagnostic, per study dose, up to 30 Millicuries

NOTE: For claims with dates of service prior to 1/01/06, OPPS hospitals report C1775 for supply of radiopharmaceutical diagnostic imaging agent, Fluorodeoxyglucose F18. For claims with dates of service January 1, 2006 and later, providers report A9552 for radiopharmaceutical diagnostic imaging agent, Fluorodeoxyglucose F18 in place of C1775.

** **NOTE:** Effective January 1, 2008, tracer code A4641 is not applicable for PET Scans.

*****NOTE:** Effective for claims with dates of service February 26, 2010 and later, tracer code A9580 is applicable for PET Scans.

Physicians / practitioners billing the carrier:

A9552 Fluorodeoxyglucose F18, FDG, Diagnostic, Per study dose, Up to 45 Millicuries

*A4641Supply of Radiopharmaceutical Diagnostic Imaging Agent, Not Otherwise Classified

A9580 Sodium Fluoride F-18, Diagnostic, per study dose, up to 30 Millicuries

***NOTE:** Effective January 1, 2008, tracer code A4641 is not applicable for PET Scans.

*****NOTE:** Effective for claims with dates of service February 26, 2010 and later, tracer code A9580 is applicable for PET Scans.

100-4, 13, 70.1

Weekly Radiation Therapy Management (CPT 77419 - 77430)

Carriers must pay for a physician's weekly treatment management services under code 77427. Billing entities must indicate on each claim the number of fractions for which payment is sought.

A weekly unit of treatment management is equal to five fractions or treatment sessions.

A week for the purpose of making payments under these codes is comprised of five fractions regardless of the actual time period in which the services are furnished. It is not necessary that the radiation therapist personally examine the patient during each fraction for the weekly treatment management code to be payable. Multiple fractions representing two or more treatment sessions furnished on the same day may be counted as long as there has been a distinct break in therapy sessions, and the fractions are of the character usually furnished on different days. If, at the final billing of the treatment course, there are three or four fractions beyond a multiple of five, those three or four fractions are paid for as a week. If there are one or two fractions beyond a multiple of five, payment for these services is considered as having been made through prior payments.

EXAMPLE:

18 fractions = 4 weekly services

62 fractions = 12 weekly services

8 fractions = 2 weekly services

6 fractions = 1 weekly service

If billings have occurred which indicate that the treatment course has ended (and, therefore, the number of residual fractions has been determined), but treatments resume, adjust carrier payments for the additional services consistent with the above policy.

EXAMPLE:

8 fractions = payment for 2 weeks

2 additional fractions are furnished by the same physician. No additional Medicare payment is made for the 2 additional fractions.

A. SNF Treatment Management Delivery Services

A SNF may not bill weekly treatment management services for its outpatients (codes 77419, 77420, 77425, 77430, and 77431). Instead, the SNF should bill for radiation treatment delivery (codes 77401 - 77404, 77406 - 77409, 77411 - 77414, and 77416).

Also, SNFs bill for therapeutic radiology port film (code 77417), which was previously a part of the weekly services. They enter the number of services in the units field.

100-4, 13, 70.3

Radiation Treatment Delivery (CPT 77401 - 77417)

Carriers pay for these TC services on a daily basis under CPT codes 77401-77416 for radiation treatment delivery. They do not use local codes and RVUs in paying for the TC of radiation oncology services. Multiple treatment sessions on the same day are payable as long as there has been a distinct break in therapy services, and the individual sessions are of the character usually furnished on different days. Carriers pay for CPT code 77417 (Therapeutic radiology port film(s)) on a weekly (five fractions) basis.

100-4, 13, 70.4

Clinical Brachytherapy (CPT Codes 77750 - 77799)

Carriers must apply the bundled services policy to procedures in this family of codes other than CPT code 77776. For procedures furnished in settings in which TC payments are made, carriers must pay separately for the expendable source associated with these procedures under CPT code 79900 except in the case of remote after-loading high intensity brachytherapy procedures (CPT codes 77781-77784). In the four codes cited, the expendable source is included in the RVUs for the TC of the procedures.

100-4, 13, 70.5

Radiation Physics Services (CPT Codes 77300 - 77399)

Carriers pay for the PC and TC of CPT codes 77300-77334 and 77399 on the same basis as they pay for radiologic services generally. For professional component billings in all settings, carriers presume that the radiologist participated in the provision of the service, e.g., reviewed/validated the physicist's calculation. CPT codes 77336 and 77370 are technical services only codes that are payable by carriers in settings in which only technical component is are payable.

100-4, 13, 80.1

Physician Presence

Radiologic supervision and interpretation (S&I) codes are used to describe the personal supervision of the performance of the radiologic portion of a procedure by one or more physicians and the interpretation of the findings. In order to bill for the supervision aspect of the procedure, the physician must be present during its performance. This kind of personal supervision of the performance of the procedure is a service to an individual beneficiary and differs from the type of general supervision of the radiologic procedures performed in a hospital for which FIs pay the costs as physician services to the hospital. The interpretation of the procedure may be performed later by another physician. In situations in which a cardiologist, for example, bills for the supervision (the "S") of the S&I code, and a radiologist bills for the interpretation (the "I") of the code, both physicians should use a "-52" modifier indicating a reduced service, e.g., only one of supervision and/or interpretation. Payment for the fragmented S&I code is no more than if a single physician furnished both aspects of the procedure.

100-4, 13, 80.2

Multiple Procedure Reduction

Carriers make no multiple procedure reductions in the S&I or primary non-radiologic codes in these types of procedures, or in any procedure codes for which the descriptor and RVUs reflect a multiple service reduction. For additional procedure codes that do not reflect such a reduction, carriers apply the multiple procedure reductions.

100-4, 13, 140

Bone Mass Measurements (BMMs)

Sections H1861(s)(15)H and H(rr)(1)H of the Social Security Act (the Act) (as added by 4106 of the Balanced Budget Act (BBA) of 1997) standardize Medicare coverage of medically necessary bone mass measurements by providing for uniform coverage under Medicare Part B. This coverage is effective for claims with dates of service furnished on or after July 1, l998.

Effective for dates of service on and after January 1, 2007, the CY 2007 Physician Fee Schedule final rule expanded the number of beneficiaries qualifying for BMM by reducing the dosage requirement for glucocorticoid (steroid) therapy from 7.5 mg of prednisone per day to 5.0 mg. It also changed the definition of BMM by removing coverage for a single-photon absorptiometry as it is not considered reasonable and necessary under section 1862 (a)(1)(A) of the Act. Finally, it required that in the case of monitoring and confirmatory baseline BMMs, they be performed with a dual-energy xray absorptiometry (axial) test.

Conditions of Coverage for BMMs are located in Pub.100-02, Medicare Benefit Policy Manual, chapter 15.

100-4, 13, 140.1

Payment Methodology and HCPCS Coding

Carriers pay for BMM procedures based on the Medicare physician fee schedule. Claims from physicians, other practitioners, or suppliers where assignment was not taken are subject to the Medicare limiting charge.

The FIs pay for BMM procedures under the current payment methodologies for radiology services according to the type of provider.

Do not pay BMM procedure claims for dual photon absorptiometry, CPT procedure code 78351.

Deductible and coinsurance apply.

Any of the following CPT procedure codes may be used when billing for BMMs through December 31, 2006. All of these codes are bone densitometry measurements except code 76977, which is bone sonometry measurements. CPT procedure codes are applicable to billing FIs and carriers.

76070 76071 76075 76076 76078 76977 78350 G0130

Effective for dates of services on and after January 1, 2007, the following changes apply to BMM:

- New 2007 CPT bone mass procedure codes have been assigned for BMM. The following codes will replace current codes, however the CPT descriptors for the services remain the same:

  77078 replaces 76070

  77079 replaces 76071

  77080 replaces 76075

  77081 replaces 76076

  77083 replaces 76078
- Certain BMM tests are covered when used to screen patients for osteoporosis subject to the frequency standards described in chapter 15, section 80.5.5 of the Medicare Benefit Policy Manual.
  - Contractors will pay claims for screening tests when coded as follows:
    - Contains CPT procedure code 77078, 77079, 77080, 77081, 77083, 76977 or G0130, and
    - Contains a valid ICD-9-CM diagnosis code indicating the reason for the test is postmenopausal female, vertebral fracture, hyperparathyroidism, or steroid therapy. Contractors are to maintain local lists of valid codes for the benefit's screening categories.
  - Contractors will deny claims for screening tests when coded as follows:
    - Contains CPT procedure code 77078, 77079, 77081, 77083, 76977 or G0130, but
    - Does not contain a valid ICD-9-CM diagnosis code from the local lists of valid ICD-9-CM diagnosis codes maintained by the contractor for the benefit's screening categories indicating the reason for the test is postmenopausal female, vertebral fracture, hyperparathyroidism, or steroid therapy.
- Dual-energy x-ray absorptiometry (axial) tests are covered when used to monitor FDA-approved osteoporosis drug therapy subject to the 2-year frequency standards described in chapter 15, section 80.5.5 of the Medicare Benefit Policy Manual.
  - Contractors will pay claims for monitoring tests when coded as follows:
    - Contains CPT procedure code 77080, and
    - Contains 733.00, 733.01, 733.02, 733.03, 733.09, 733.90, or 255.0 as the ICD-9-CM diagnosis code.

- Contractors will deny claims for monitoring tests when coded as follows:
  - Contains CPT procedure code 77078, 77079, 77081, 77083, 76977 or G0130, and
  - Contains 733.00, 733.01, 733.02, 733.03, 733.09, 733.90, or 255.0 as the ICD-9-CM diagnosis code, but
  - Does not contain a valid ICD-9-CM diagnosis code from the local lists of valid ICD-9-CM diagnosis codes maintained by the contractor for the benefit's screening categories indicating the reason for the test is postmenopausal female, vertebral fracture, hyperparathyroidism, or steroid therapy.
- Single photon absorptiometry tests are not covered. Contractors will deny CPT procedure code 78350.

The FIs are billed using the ANSI X12N 837 I or hardcopy Form CMS-1450. The appropriate bill types are: 12X, 13X, 22X, 23X, 34X, 71X (Provider-based and independent), 72X, 73X (Provider-based and freestanding), 83X, and 85X. Effective April 1, 2006, type of bill 14X is for non-patient laboratory specimens and is no longer applicable for bone mass measurements. Information regarding the claim form locators that correspond to the HCPCS/CPT code or Type of Bill and a table to crosswalk its CMS-1450 form locators to the 837 transaction are found in Chapter 25.

Providers must report HCPCS codes for bone mass measurements under revenue code 320 with number of units and line item dates of service per revenue code line for each bone mass measurement reported.

Carriers are billed for bone mass measurement procedures using the ANSI X12N 837 P or hardcopy Form CMS-1500.

100-4, 14, 10

General

Payment is made under Part B for certain surgical procedures that are furnished in ASCs and are approved for being furnished in an ASC. These procedures are those that generally do not exceed 90 minutes in length and do not require more than four hours recovery or convalescent time.

To be paid under this provision, a facility must be certified as meeting the requirements for an ASC and must enter into a written agreement with the Centers for Medicare & Medicaid Services (CMS). The certification process is described in the State Operations Manual.

Medicare will not pay an ASC for those procedures that require more than an ASC level of care, or for minor procedures that are normally performed in a physician's office.

The CMS publishes updates to the list of procedures for which an ASC may be paid each year. The complete list of procedures is available through the Public Use files (PUF) at http://www.cms.hhs.gov/researchers/. This includes applicable codes, payment groups, and payment amounts for each ASC group before adjustments for regional wage variations. Applicable wage indices are also published via program memorandum.

ASCs must accept Medicare's payment for such procedures as payment in full for the facility service with respect to those services defined as ASC facility services. The physician and anesthesiologist may bill and be paid for the professional component of the service also.

Certain other services may be performed in an ASC facility, billed by the appropriate certified provider/supplier, or in certain cases by the ASC facility itself, and paid outside of the facility rate.

100-4, 14, 40.3

Payment for Intraocular Lens (IOL)

Prior to January 1, 2008, payment for facility services furnished by an ASC for IOL insertion during or subsequent to cataract surgery includes an allowance for the lens. The procedures that include insertion of an IOL are: Payment Group 6: CPT-4 Codes 66985 and 66986 Payment Group 8: CPT-4 Codes 66982, 66983 and 66984 Physicians or suppliers are not paid for an IOL furnished to a beneficiary in an ASC after July 1, 1988. Separate claims for IOLs furnished to ASC patients beginning March 12, 1990 are denied. Also, effective March 12, 1990, procedures 66983 and 66984 are treated as single procedures for payment purposes.

Beginning January 1, 2008, the Medicare payment for the IOL is included in the Medicare ASC payment for the associated surgical procedure. Consequently, no separate payment for the IOL is made, except for a payment adjustment for NTIOLs established according to the process outlined in 42 CFR 416.185. ASCs should not report separate charges for conventional IOLs because their payment is included in the Medicare payment for the associated surgical procedure. The ASC payment system logic that excluded $150 for IOLs for purposes of the multiple surgery reduction in cases of cataract surgery prior to January 1, 2008 no longer applies, effective for dates of service on or after January 1, 2008.

Effective for dates of service on and after February 27, 2006, through February 26, 2011, Medicare pays an additional $50 for specified Category 3 NTIOLs that are provided in association with a covered ASC surgical procedure. The list of Category 3 NTIOLS is available at:
http://www.cms.hhs.gov/ASCPayment/08_NTIOLs.asp#TopOfPage.

ASCs should use HCPCS code Q1003 to bill for a Category 3 NTIOL. HCPCS code Q1003, along with one of the approved surgical procedure codes (CPT codes 66982, 66983, 66984, 66985, 66986) are to be used on all NTIOL Category 3 claims associated with reduced spherical aberration from February 27, 2006, through February 26, 2011. The payment adjustment for the NTIOL is subject to beneficiary coinsurance but is not wage-adjusted.

Any subsequent IOL recognized by CMS as having the same characteristics as the first NTIOL recognized by CMS for a payment adjustment as a Category III NTIOL (those of reduced spherical aberration) will receive the same adjustment for the remainder of the 5-year period established by the first recognized IOL.

100-4, 14, 40.6

Payment for Extracorporeal Shock Wave Lithotripsy (ESWL)

A ninth ASC payment group was established in a "Federal Register" notice (56 FR 67666) published December 31, 1991. The ninth payment group amount ($1,150) was assigned to only one procedure, CPT code 50590, extracorporeal shock wave lithotripsy (ESWL). However, a court order issued March 12, 1992, has stayed the Group 9 payment rate until the Secretary publishes all information relevant to the setting of the ESWL rate, receives comments, and publishes a subsequent final notice. This has not yet been completed.

In a previous instruction (Medicare Carrier's Manual Transmittal 1435), CMS advised carriers to make payment to ASCs for ESWL services furnished after January 29, 1992, and through the date when the ASC received notice from the carrier of the court order staying the Group 9 payment rate. This was a temporary measure to avoid penalizing ASCs that furnished ESWL services in accordance with the December 31, 1991, "Federal Register" notice and that could not have been expected to know that the March 12, 1992, court order set aside the ESWL provisions of that notice. Carriers did not make Medicare payment for ESWL as an ASC procedure when such services were furnished after the date that the carrier advised an ASC of the court order.

However carriers were instructed to retain all ASC claims for ESWL with a service date after January 29, 1992, and before the date when they were notified about the court order. It may be necessary to retrieve these clams for further action at some later date.

Beginning January 1, 2008 with the revised ASC payment system, contractors may pay for any of the ESWL services that are included on the ASC list of covered surgical procedures.

100-4, 14, 40.8

Payment When a Device is Furnished With No Cost or With Full or Partial Credit Beginning January 1, 2008

Contractors pay ASCs a reduced amount for certain specified procedures when a specified device is furnished without cost or for which either a partial or full credit is received (e.g., device recall). For specified procedure codes that include payment for a device, ASCs are required to include modifier -FB on the procedure code when a specified device is furnished without cost or for which full credit is received. If the ASC receives a partial credit of 50 percent or more of the cost of a specified device, the ASC is required to include modifier -FC on the procedure code if the procedure is on the list of specified procedures to which the -FC reduction applies. A single procedure code should not be submitted with both modifiers -FB and -FC. The pricing determination related to modifiers -FB and -FC is made prior to the application of multiple procedure payment reductions. Contractors adjust beneficiary coinsurance to reflect the reduced payment amount. Tables listing the procedures and devices to which the payment adjustments apply, and the full and partial adjustment amounts, are available on the CMS Web site.

In order to report that the receipt of a partial credit of 50 percent or more of the cost of a device, ASCs have the option of either: 1) Submitting the claim for the procedure to their Medicare contractor after the procedure's performance but prior to manufacturer acknowledgement of credit for a specified device, and subsequently contacting the contractor regarding a claims adjustment once the credit determination is made; or 2) holding the claim for the procedure until a determination is made by the manufacturer on the partial credit and submitting the claim with modifier -FC appended to the implantation procedure HCPCS code if the partial credit is 50 percent or more of the cost of the device. If choosing the first billing option, to request a claims adjustment once the credit determination is made, ASCs should keep in mind that the initial Medicare payment for the procedure involving the device is conditional and subject to adjustment.

100-4, 14, 40.9

Payment and Coding for Presbyopia Correcting IOLs (P-C IOLs) and Astigmatism Correcting IOLs (A-C IOLs)

(CMS payment policies and recognition of P-C IOLs and A-C IOLs are contained in Transmittal 636 (CR3927) and Transmittal 1228 (CR5527) respectively.

Effective for dates of service on and after January 1, 2008, when inserting an approved A-C IOL in an ASC concurrent with cataract extraction, HCPCS code V2787 (Astigmatism-correcting function of intraocular lens) should be billed to report the non-covered charges for the A-C IOL functionality of the inserted intraocular lens. Additionally, note that HCPCS code V2788 (Presbyopia-correcting function of intraocular lens) is no longer valid to report non-covered charges associated with the A-C IOL. However, this code continues to be valid to report non-covered charges for a

P-C IOL. The payment for the conventional lens portion of the A-C IOL and P-C IOL continues to be bundled with the ASC procedure payment.

Effective for services on and after January 1, 2010, ASCs are to bill for insertion of a Category 3 new technology intraocular lens (NTIOL) that is also an approved A-C IOL or P-C IOL, concurrent with cataract extraction, using three separate codes. ASCs shall use HCPCS code V2787 or V2788, as appropriate, to report charges associated with the non-covered functionality of the A-C IOL or P-C IOL, the appropriate HCPCS code 66982 (Extracapsular cataract removal with insertion of intraocular lens prosthesis (one stage procedure), manual or mechanical technique (e.g., irrigation and aspiration or phacoemulsification), complex, requiring devices or techniques not generally used in routine cataract surgery (e.g., iris expansion device, suture support for intraocular lens, or primary posterior capsulorrhexis) or performed on patients in the amblyogenic developmental stage); 66983 (Intracapsular cataract extraction with insertion of intraocular lens prosthesis (1 stage procedure)); or 66984 (Extracapsular cataract removal with insertion of intraocular lens prosthesis (1 stage procedure), manual or mechanical technique (e.g., irrigation and aspiration or phacoemulsification)), to report the covered cataract extraction and insertion procedure; and Q1003 (New technology, intraocular lens, category 3 (reduced spherical aberration) as defined in Federal Register notice, Vol. 65, dated May 3, 2000) to report the covered NTIOL aspect of the lens on claims for insertion of an A-C IOL or P-C IOL that is also designated as an NTIOL. Listings of the CMS-approved Category 3 NTIOLs, A-C IOLs, and P-C IOLs are available on the CMS web site.

100-4, 16, 40.6.1

Automated Multi-Channel Chemistry (AMCC) Tests for ESRD Beneficiaries - FIs

Effective January 1, 2011

Section 153b of the MIPPA requires that all ESRD-related laboratory tests must be reported by the ESRD facility whether provided directly or under arrangements with an independent laboratory. When laboratory services are billed by providers other than the ESRD facility and the laboratory test furnished is designated as a laboratory test that is included in the ESRD PPS (ESRD-related), the claim will be rejected or denied. In the event that an ESRD-related laboratory test was furnished to an ESRD beneficiary for reasons other than for the treatment of ESRD, the provider may submit a claim for separate payment using modifier AY. The AY modifier serves as an attestation that the item or service is medically necessary for the dialysis patient but is not being used for the treatment of ESRD. The items and services subject to consolidated billing located at http://www.cms.gov/ESRDPayment/50_Consolidated_Billing.asp#TopOfPage includes the list of ESRD-related laboratory tests that are routinely performed for the treatment of ESRD.

For services provided on or after January 1, 2011, the 50/50 rule no longer applies to independent laboratory claims for AMCC tests furnished to ESRD beneficiaries. The 50/50 rule modifiers (CD, CE, and CF) are sunsetted for independent laboratories effective for dates of service on and after January 1, 2011. However, the 50/50 rule modifiers are still required for use by ESRD facilities that are receiving the transitional blended payment amount (the transition ends in CY 2014). Information regarding the ESRD PPS transition can be found in Publication 100-04, Chapter 8, section 20.1.

Effective for dates of service on and after January 1, 2012, contractors shall allow organ disease panel codes (i.e., HCPCS codes 80047, 80048, 80051, 80053, 80061, 80069, and 80076) to be billed by independent laboratories for AMCC panel tests furnished to ESRD eligible beneficiaries if:

- The beneficiary is not receiving dialysis treatment for any reason (e.g., post-transplant beneficiaries), or
- The test is not related to the treatment of ESRD, in which case the supplier would append modifier "AY".

Contractors shall make payment for organ disease panels according to the Clinical Laboratory Fee Schedule and shall apply the normal ESRD PPS editing rules for independent laboratory claims described in Transmittal 2134, issued January 14, 2011. The aforementioned organ disease panel codes will be added to the list of bundled ESRD PPS laboratory tests in January 2012.

Prior to January 1, 2011

For claims with dates of service prior to January 1, 2011, Medicare will apply the following rules to Automated Multi-Channel Chemistry (AMCC) tests for ESRD beneficiaries:

- Payment is at the lowest rate for tests performed by the same provider, for the same beneficiary, for the same date of service.
- The facility/laboratory must identify, for a particular date of service, the AMCC tests ordered that are included in the composite rate and those that are not included. See Publication 100-02, Chapter 11, Section 30.2.2 for the chart detailing the composite rate tests for Hemodialysis, Intermittent Peritoneal Dialysis (IPD), Continuous Cycling Peritoneal Dialysis (CCPD), and Hemofiltration as well as a second chart detailing the composite rate tests for Continuous Ambulatory Peritoneal Dialysis (CAPD).
- If 50 percent or more of the covered tests are included under the composite rate payment, then all submitted tests are included within the composite payment. In this case, no separate payment in addition to the composite rate is made for any of the separately billable tests.
- If less than 50 percent of the covered tests are composite rate tests, all AMCC tests submitted for that Date of Service (DOS) for that beneficiary are separately payable.
- A noncomposite rate test is defined as any test separately payable outside of the composite rate or beyond the normal frequency covered under the composite rate that is reasonable and necessary.
- For carrier processed claims, all chemistries ordered for beneficiaries with chronic dialysis for ESRD must be billed individually and must be rejected when billed as a panel.

(See section 100.6UH for details regarding pricing modifiers.)

Implementation of this Policy:

ESRD facilities when ordering an ESRD-related AMCC must specify for each test within the AMCC whether the test:

a. Is part of the composite rate and not separately payable;
b. Is a composite rate test but is, on the date of the order, beyond the frequency covered under the composite rate and thus separately payable; or
c. Is not part of the ESRD composite rate and thus separately payable.

Laboratories must:

a. Identify which tests, if any, are not included within the ESRD facility composite rate payment
b. Identify which tests ordered for chronic dialysis for ESRD as follows:
    1) Modifier CD: AMCC Test has been ordered by an ESRD facility or MCP physician that is part of the composite rate and is not separately billable.
    2) Modifier CE: AMCC Test has been ordered by an ESRD facility or MCP physician that is a composite rate test but is beyond the normal frequency covered under the rate and is separately reimbursable based on medical necessity.
    3) Modifier CF: AMCC Test has been ordered by an ESRD facility or MCP physician that is not part of the composite rate and is separately billable.
c. Bill all tests ordered for a chronic dialysis ESRD beneficiary individually and not as a panel.

The shared system must calculate the number of AMCC tests provided for any given date of service. Sum all AMCC tests with a CD modifier and divide the sum of all tests with a CD, CE, and CF modifier for the same beneficiary and provider for any given date of service.

If the result of the calculation for a date of service is 50 percent or greater, do not pay for the tests.

If the result of the calculation for a date of service is less than 50 percent, pay for all of the tests.

For FI processed claims, all tests for a date of service must be billed on the monthly ESRD bill. Providers that submit claims to a FI must send in an adjustment if they identify additional tests that have not been billed.

Carrier standard systems shall adjust the previous claim when the incoming claim for a date of service is compared to a claim on history and the action is adjust payment. Carrier standard systems shall spread the payment amount over each line item on both claims (the claim on history and the incoming claim).

The organ and disease oriented panels (80048, 80051, 80053, and 80076) are subject to the 50 percent rule. However, clinical diagnostic laboratories shall not bill these services as panels, they must be billed individually. Laboratory tests that are not covered under the composite rate and that are furnished to CAPD end stage renal disease (ESRD) patients dialyzing at home are billed in the same way as any other test furnished home patients.

FI Business Requirements for ESRD Reimbursement of AMCC Tests:

Requirement #	Requirements	Responsibility
1.1	The FI shared system must RTP a claim for AMCC tests when a claim for that date of service has already been submitted.	Shared system
1.2	Based upon the presence of the CD, CE and CF payment modifiers, identify the AMCC tests ordered that are included and not included in the composite rate payment.	Shared System
1.3	Based upon the determination of requirement 1.2, if 50 percent or more of the covered tests are included under the composite rate, no separate payment is made.	Shared System
1.4	Based upon the determination of requirement 1.2, if less than 50 percent are covered tests included under the composite rate, all AMCC tests for that date of service are payable.	Shared System

Requirement #	Requirements	Responsibility
1.5	Effective for claims with dates of service on or after January 1, 2006, include any line items with a modifier 91 used in conjunction with the "CD," "CE," or "CF" modifier in the calculation of the 50/50 rule.	Shared System
1.6	FIs must return any claims for additional tests for any date of service within the billing period when the provider has already submitted a claim. Instruct the provider to adjust the first claim.	FI or Shared System
1.7	After the calculation of the 50/50 rule, services used to determine the payment amount may never exceed 22. Effective for claims with dates of service on or after January 1, 2006, accept all valid line items submitted for the date of service and pay a maximum of the ATP 22 rate.	Shared System

Carrier Business Requirements for ESRD Reimbursement of AMCC Tests:

Requirement #	Requirements	Responsibility
1	The standard systems shall calculate payment at the lowest rate for these automated tests even if reported on separate claims for services performed by the same provider, for the same beneficiary, for the same date of service.	Standard Systems
2	Standard Systems shall identify the AMCC tests ordered that are included and are not included in the composite rate payment based upon the presence of the "CD," "CE" and "CF" modifiers.	Standard Systems
3	Based upon the determination of requirement 2 if 50 percent or more of the covered services are included under the composite rate payment, Standard Systems shall indicate that no separate payment is provided for the services submitted for that date of service.	Standard Systems
4	Based upon the determination of requirement 2 if less than 50 percent are covered services included under the composite rate, Standard Systems shall indicate that all AMCC tests for that date of service are payable under the 50/50 rule.	Standard Systems
5	Effective for claims with dates of service on or after January 1, 2006, include any line items with a modifier 91 used in conjunction with the "CD," "CE," or "CF" modifier in the calculation of the 50/50 rule.	Standard Systems
6	Standard Systems shall adjust the previous claim when the incoming claim is compared to the claim on history and the action is to deny the previous claim. Spread the payment amount over each line item on both claims (the adjusted claim and the incoming claim).	Standard Systems
7	Standard Systems shall spread the adjustment across the incoming claim unless the adjusted amount would exceed the submitted amount of the services on the claim.	Standard System
8	After the calculation of the 50/50 rule, services used to determine the payment amount may never exceed 22. Accept all valid line items for the date of service and pay a maximum of the ATP 22 rate.	Standard Systems

Examples of the Application of the 50/50 Rule

The following examples are to illustrate how claims should be paid. The percentages in the action section represent the number of composite rate tests over the total tests. If this percentage is 50 percent or greater, no payment should be made for the claim.

Example 1:
Provider Name: Jones Hospital
DOS 2/1/02

Claim/Services
82040 Mod CD
82310 Mod CD
82374 Mod CD
82435 Mod CD
82947 Mod CF
84295 Mod CF
82040 Mod CD (Returned as duplicate)
84075 Mod CE
82310 Mod CE
84155 Mod CE

ACTION: 9 services total, 2 non-composite rate tests, 3 composite rate tests beyond the frequency, 4 composite rate tests; 4/9 = 44.4%<50% pay at ATP 09

Example 2:
Provider Name: Bon Secours Renal Facility
DOS 2/15/02

Claim/Services
82040 Mod CE and Mod 91
84450 Mod CE
82310 Mod CE
82247 Mod CF
82465 No modifier present

100-4, 16, 60.1.4

Coding Requirements for Specimen Collection

The following HCPCS codes and terminology must be used:

- 36415 – Collection of venous blood by venipuncture.
- P96l5 – Catheterization for collection of specimen(s).

The allowed amount for specimen collection in each of the above circumstances is included in the laboratory fee schedule distributed annually by CMS.

100-4, 16, 70.8

Certificate of Waiver

Effective September 1, 1992, all laboratory testing sites (except as provided in 42 CFR 493.3(b)) must have either a CLIA certificate of waiver, certificate for provider-performed microscopy procedures, certificate of registration, certificate of compliance, or certificate of accreditation to legally perform clinical laboratory testing on specimens from individuals in the United States.

The Food and Drug Administration approves CLIA waived tests on a flow basis. The CMS identifies CLIA waived tests by providing an updated list of waived tests to the Medicare contractors on a quarterly basis via a Recurring Update Notification. To be recognized as a waived test, some CLIA waived tests have unique HCPCS procedure codes and some must have a QW modifier included with the HCPCS code.

For a list of specific HCPCS codes subject to CLIA see

http://www.cms.hhs.gov/CLIA/downloads/waivetbl.pdf

100-4, 17, 20.5.7

Injection Services

Where the sole purpose of an office visit was for the patient to receive an injection, payment may be made only for the injection service (if it is covered). Conversely, injection services (codes 90782, 90783, 90784, 90788, and 90799) included in the Medicare Physician Fee Schedule (MPFS) are not paid for separately, if the physician is paid for any other physician fee schedule service furnished at the same time. Pay separately for those injection services only if no other physician fee schedule service is being paid. However, pay separately for cancer chemotherapy injections (CPT codes 96400-96549) in addition to the visit furnished on the same day. In either case, the drug is separately payable. All injection claims must include the specific name of the drug and dosage. Identification of the drug enables you to pay for the services.

100-4, 18, 1.2

Table of Preventive and Screening Services

(Rev. 2693, Issued: 05-02-13, Effective: 11-20-12, for code 906661: 01-01-13 – For codes 90653, 90672, 90685, 90686, 90687, 90688, 90739, and Q2033, Implementation: 10-07-13)

Service	CPT/ HCPCS	Long Descriptor	USPSTF Rating	Coins / Deductible
Initial Preventive Physical Examination, IPPE	G0402	Initial preventive physical examination; face to face visits, services limited to new beneficiary during the first 12 months of Medicare enrollment	*Not Rated	WAIVED
	G0403	Electrocardiogram, routine ECG with 12 leads; performed as a screening for the initial preventive physical examination with interpretation and report		Not Waived
	G0404	Electrocardiogram, routine ECG with 12 leads; tracing only, without interpretation and report, performed as a screening for the initial preventive physical examination		Not Waived
	G0405	Electrocardiogram, routine ECG with 12 leads; interpretation and report only, performed as a screening for the initial preventive physical examination		Not Waived
Ultrasound Screening for Abdominal Aortic Aneurysm (AAA)	G0389	Ultrasound, B-scan and /or real time with image documentation; for abdominal aortic aneurysm (AAA) ultrasound screening	B	WAIVED
Cardiovascular Disease Screening	80061	Lipid panel	A	WAIVED
	82465	Cholesterol, serum or whole blood, total		WAIVED
	83718	Lipoprotein, direct measurement; high density cholesterol (hdl cholesterol)		WAIVED
	84478	Triglycerides		WAIVED
Diabetes Screening Tests	82947	Glucose; quantitative, blood (except reagent strip)	B	WAIVED
	82950	Glucose; post glucose dose (includes glucose)		WAIVED
	82951	Glucose; tolerance test (gtt), three specimens (includes glucose)	*Not Rated	WAIVED
Diabetes Self Management Training Services (DSMT)	G0108	Diabetes outpatient self-management training services, individual, per 30 minutes	*Not Rated	Not Waived
	G0109	Diabetes outpatient self-management training services, group session (2 or more), per 30 minutes		Not Waived

Service	CPT/ HCPCS	Long Descriptor	USPSTF Rating	Coins / Deductible
Medical Nutrition Therapy (MNT) Services	97802	Medical nutrition therapy; initial assessment and intervention, individual, face-to-face with the patient, each 15 minutes	B	WAIVED
	97803	Medical nutrition therapy; re-assessment and intervention, individual, face-to-face with the patient, each 15 minutes		WAIVED
	97804	Medical nutrition therapy; group (2 or more individual(s)), each 30 minutes		WAIVED
	G0270	Medical nutrition therapy; reassessment and subsequent intervention(s) following second referral in same year for change in diagnosis, medical condition or treatment regimen (including additional hours needed for renal disease), individual, face to face with the patient, each 15 minutes		WAIVED
	G0271	Medical nutrition therapy, reassessment and subsequent intervention(s) following second referral in same year for change in diagnosis, medical condition, or treatment regimen (including additional hours needed for renal disease), group (2 or more individuals), each 30 minutes		WAIVED

Service	CPT/ HCPCS	Long Descriptor	USPSTF Rating	Coins / Deductible
Screening Pap Test	G0123	Screening cytopathology, cervical or vaginal (any reporting system), collected in preservative fluid, automated thin layer preparation, screening by cytotechnologist under physician supervision	A	WAIVED
	G0124	Screening cytopathology, cervical or vaginal (any reporting system), collected in preservative fluid, automated thin layer preparation, requiring interpretation by physician		WAIVED
	G0141	Screening cytopathology smears, cervical or vaginal, performed by automated system, with manual rescreening, requiring interpretation by physician		WAIVED
	G0143	Screening cytopathology, cervical or vaginal (any reporting system), collected in preservative fluid, automated thin layer preparation, with manual screening and rescreening by cytotechnologist under physician supervision		WAIVED
	G0144	Screening cytopathology, cervical or vaginal (any reporting system), collected in preservative fluid, automated thin layer preparation, with screening by automated system, under physician supervision		WAIVED
	G0145	Screening cytopathology, cervical or vaginal (any reporting system), collected in preservative fluid, automated thin layer preparation, with screening by automated system and manual rescreening under physician supervision		WAIVED
	G0147	Screening cytopathology smears, cervical or vaginal, performed by automated system under physician supervision		WAIVED
	G0148	Screening cytopathology smears, cervical or vaginal, performed by automated system with manual rescreening		WAIVED
	P3000	Screening papanicolaou smear, cervical or vaginal, up to three smears, by technician under physician supervision		WAIVED
	P3001	Screening papanicolaou smear, cervical or vaginal, up to three smears, requiring interpretation by physician		WAIVED
	Q0091	Screening papanicolaou smear; obtaining, preparing and conveyance of cervical or vaginal smear to laboratory		WAIVED

Service	CPT/ HCPCS	Long Descriptor	USPSTF Rating	Coins / Deductible
Screening Pelvic Exam	G0101	Cervical or vaginal cancer screening; pelvic and clinical breast examination	A	WAIVED
Screening Mammography	77052	Computer-aided detection (computer algorithm analysis of digital image data for lesion detection) with further physician review for interpretation, with or without digitization of film radiographic images; screening mammography (list separately in addition to code for primary procedure)	B	WAIVED
	77057	Screening mammography, bilateral (2-view film study of each breast)		WAIVED
	G0202	Screening mammography, producing direct digital image, bilateral, all views		WAIVED
Bone Mass Measurement	G0130	Single energy x-ray absorptiometry (sexa) bone density study, one or more sites; appendicular skeleton (peripheral) (e.g., radius, wrist, heel)	B	WAIVED
	77078	Computed tomography, bone mineral density study, 1 or more sites; axial skeleton (e.g., hips, pelvis, spine)		WAIVED
	77079	Computed tomography, bone mineral density study, 1 or more sites; appendicular skeleton (peripheral) (e.g., radius, wrist, heel)		WAIVED
	77080	Dual-energy x-ray absorptiometry (dxa), bone density study, 1 or more sites; axial skeleton (e.g., hips, pelvis, spine)		WAIVED
	77081	Dual-energy x-ray absorptiometry (dxa), bone density study, 1 or more sites; appendicular skeleton (peripheral) (e.g., radius, wrist, heel)		WAIVED
	77083	Radiographic absorptiometry (e.g., photo densitometry, radiogrammetry), 1 or more sites		WAIVED
	76977	Ultrasound bone density measurement and interpretation, peripheral site(s), any method		WAIVED

Service	CPT/ HCPCS	Long Descriptor	USPSTF Rating	Coins / Deductible
Colorectal Cancer Screening	G0104	Colorectal cancer screening; flexible sigmoidoscopy	A	WAIVED
	G0105	Colorectal cancer screening; colonoscopy on individual at high risk		WAIVED
	G0106	Colorectal cancer screening; alternative to G0104, screening sigmoidoscopy, barium enema	*Not Rated	Coins. Applies & Ded. is waived
	G0120	Colorectal cancer screening; alternative to G0105, screening colonoscopy, barium enema.	A	Coins. Applies & Ded. is waived
	G0121	Colorectal cancer screening; colonoscopy on individual not meeting criteria for high risk		WAIVED
	82270	Blood, occult, by peroxidase activity (e.g., guaiac), qualitative; feces, consecutive		WAIVED
	G0328	Colorectal cancer screening; fecal occult blood test, immunoassay, 1-3 simultaneous		WAIVED
Prostate Cancer Screening	G0102	Prostate cancer screening; digital rectal examination	D	Not Waived
	G0103	Prostate cancer screening; prostate specific antigen test (PSA)		WAIVED
Glaucoma Screening	G0117	Glaucoma screening for high risk patients furnished by an optometrist or ophthalmologist	I	Not Waived
	G0118	Glaucoma screening for high risk patient furnished under the direct supervision of an optometrist or ophthalmologist		Not Waived
Influenza Virus Vaccine	90653	Influenza virus vaccine, inactivated, subunit, adjuvanted, for intramuscular use	B	WAIVED
	90654	Influenza virus vaccine, split virus, preservative free, for intradermal use, for adults ages 18-64		WAIVED
	90655	Influenza virus vaccine, split virus, preservative free, when administered to children 6-35 months of age, for intramuscular use		WAIVED
	90656	Influenza virus vaccine, split virus, preservative free, when administered to individuals 3 years and older, for intramuscular use		WAIVED
	90657	Influenza virus vaccine, split virus, when administered to children 6-35 months of age, for intramuscular use		WAIVED
	90660	Influenza virus vaccine, live, for intranasal use		WAIVED
	90661	Influenza virus vaccine, derived from cell cultures, subunit, preservative and antibiotic free, for intramuscular use		WAIVED
Influenza Virus Vaccine (continued)	90662	Influenza virus vaccine, split virus, preservative free, enhanced immunogenicity via increased antigen content, for intramuscular use	B	WAIVED
	90672	Influenza virus vaccine, live, quadrivalent, for intranasal use		WAIVED
	90673	Influenza virus vaccine, trivalent, derived from recombinant DNA (RIV3), hemagglutinin (HA) protein only, preservative and antibiotic free, for intramuscular use		WAIVED
	90685	Influenza virus vaccine, quadrivalent, split virus, preservative free, when administered to children 6-35 months of age, for intramuscular use		WAIVED
	90686	Influenza virus vaccine, quadrivalent, split virus, preservative free, when administered to individuals 3 years of age and older, for intramuscular use		WAIVED
	90687	Influenza virus vaccine, quadrivalent, split virus, when administered to children 6-35 months of age, for intramuscular use		WAIVED
	90688	Influenza virus vaccine, quadrivalent, split virus, when administered to individuals 3 years of age and older, for intramuscular use		WAIVED
	Q2034	Influenza virus vaccine, split virus, for intramuscular use (Agriflu)		WAIVED
	Q2035	Influenza virus vaccine, split virus, when administered to individuals 3 years of age and older, for intramuscular use (afluria)		WAIVED
	Q2036	Influenza virus vaccine, split virus, when administered to individuals 3 years of age and older, for intramuscular use (flulaval)		WAIVED
	Q2037	Influenza virus vaccine, split virus when administered to individuals 3 years of age and older, for intramuscular use (fluvirin)		WAIVED
	Q2038	Influenza virus vaccine, split virus, when administered to individuals 3 years of age and older, for intramuscular use (fluzone)		WAIVED
	Q2039	Influenza virus vaccine, split virus, when administered to individuals 3 years of age and older, for intramuscular use (not otherwise specified)		WAIVED

Service	CPT/ HCPCS	Long Descriptor	USPSTF Rating	Coins / Deductible
Influenza Virus Vaccine (continued)	G0008	Administration of influenza virus vaccine	B	WAIVED
	G9141	Influenza A (H1N1) immunization administration (includes the physician counseling the patient/family)		WAIVED
	G9142	Influenza A (H1N1) Vaccine, any route of administration		WAIVED
Pneumococcal Vaccine	90669	Pneumococcal conjugate vaccine, polyvalent, when administered to children younger than 5 years, for intramuscular use	B	WAIVED
	90670	Pneumococcal conjugate vaccine, 13 valent, for intramuscular use.		WAIVED
	90732	Pneumococcal polysaccharide vaccine, 23-valent, adult or immunosuppressed patient dosage, when administered to individuals 2 years or older, for subcutaneous or intramuscular use		WAIVED
	G0009	Administration of pneumococcal vaccine		WAIVED
Hepatitis B Vaccine	90739	Hepatitis B vaccine, adult dosage (2 dose schedule), for intramuscular use	A	WAIVED
	90740	Hepatitis B vaccine, dialysis or immunosuppressed patient dosage (3 dose schedule), for intramuscular use		WAIVED
	90743	Hepatitis B vaccine, adolescent (2 dose schedule), for intramuscular use		WAIVED
	90744	Hepatitis B vaccine, pediatric/adolescent dosage (3 dose schedule), for intramuscular use		WAIVED
	90746	Hepatitis B vaccine, adult dosage, for intramuscular use		WAIVED
	90747	Hepatitis B vaccine, dialysis or immunosuppressed patient dosage (4 dose schedule), for intramuscular use		WAIVED
	G0010	Administration of hepatitis B vaccine		WAIVED
HIV Screening	G0432	Infectious agent antigen detection by enzyme immunoassay (EIA) technique, qualitative or semi-qualitative, multiple-step method, HIV-1 or HIV-2, screening	A	WAIVED
	G0433	Infectious agent antigen detection by enzyme-linked immunosorbent assay (ELISA) technique, antibody, HIV-1 or HIV-2, screening		WAIVED
	G0435	Infectious agent antigen detection by rapid antibody test of oral mucosa transudate, HIV-1 or HIV-2 , screening		WAIVED
Smoking Cessation	G0436	Smoking and tobacco cessation counseling visit for the asymptomatic patient; intermediate, greater than 3 minutes, up to 10 minutes	A	WAIVED
	G0437	Smoking and tobacco cessation counseling visit for the asymptomatic patient intensive, greater than 10 minutes		WAIVED
Annual Wellness Visit	G0438	Annual wellness visit, including PPPS, first visit	*Not Rated	WAIVED
	G0439	Annual wellness visit, including PPPS, subsequent visit		WAIVED

100-4, 18, 10.1.2

Influenza Virus Vaccine

Effective for services furnished on or after May 11, 1993, the influenza virus vaccine and its administration is covered when furnished in compliance with any applicable State law. Typically, this vaccine is administrated once a flu season. Medicare does not require for coverage purposes that a doctor of medicine or osteopathy order the vaccine. Therefore, the beneficiary may receive the vaccine upon request without a physician's order and without physician supervision. Since there is no yearly limit, contractors determine whether such services are reasonable and allow payment if appropriate.

See Pub. 100-02, Medicare Benefit Policy Manual, Chapter 15, Section 50.4.4.2 for additional coverage requirements for influenza virus vaccine.

100-4,18, 10.2.1

Healthcare Common Procedure Coding System (HCPCS) and Diagnosis Codes

Vaccines and their administration are reported using separate codes. The following codes are for reporting the vaccines only.

HCPCS	Definition
90653	Influenza virus vaccine, inactivated, subunit, adjuvanted, for intramuscular use
90654	Influenza virus vaccine, split virus, preservative-free, for intradermal use, for adults ages 18 – 64;
90655	Influenza virus vaccine, split virus, preservative free, for children 6-35 months of age, for intramuscular use;
90656	Influenza virus vaccine, split virus, preservative free, for use in individuals 3 years and above, for intramuscular use;
90657	Influenza virus vaccine, split virus, for children 6-35 months of age, for intramuscular use;
90660	Influenza virus vaccine, live, for intranasal use;
90661	Influenza virus vaccine, derived from cell cultures, subunit, preservative and antibiotic free, for intramuscular use
90662	Influenza virus vaccine, split virus, preservative free, enhanced immunogenicity via increased antigen content, for intramuscular use
90669	Pneumococcal conjugate vaccine, polyvalent, for children under 5 years, for intramuscular use
90670	Pneumococcal conjugate vaccine, 13 valent, for intramuscular use
90672	Influenza virus vaccine, live, quadrivalent, for intranasal use
90673	Influenza virus vaccine, trivalent, derived from recombinant DNA (RIV3), hemagglutinin (HA) protein only, preservative and antibiotic free, for intramuscular use
90685	Influenza virus vaccine, quadrivalent, split virus, preservative free, when administered to children 6-35 months of age, for intramuscular use
90686	Influenza virus vaccine, quadrivalent, split virus, preservative free, when administered to individuals 3 years of age and older, for intramuscular use

HCPCS	Definition
90687	Influenza virus vaccine, quadrivalent, split virus, when administered to children 6-35 months of age, for intramuscular use
90688	Influenza virus vaccine, quadrivalent, split virus, when administered to individuals 3 years of age and older, for intramuscular use
90732	Pneumococcal polysaccharide vaccine, 23-valent, adult or immunosuppressed patient dosage, for use in individuals 2 years or older, for subcutaneous or intramuscular use;
90739	Hepatitis B vaccine, adult dosage (2 dose schedule), for intramuscular use
90740	Hepatitis B vaccine, dialysis or immunosuppressed patient dosage (3 dose schedule), for intramuscular use;
90743	Hepatitis B vaccine, adolescent (2 dose schedule), for intramuscular use;
90744	Hepatitis B vaccine, pediatric/adolescent dosage (3 dose schedule), for intramuscular use;
90746	Hepatitis B vaccine, adult dosage, for intramuscular use; and
90747	Hepatitis B vaccine, dialysis or immunosuppressed patient dosage (4 dose schedule), for intramuscular use.

The following codes are for reporting administration of the vaccines only. The administration of the vaccines is billed using:

HCPCS	Definition
G0008	Administration of influenza virus vaccine;
G0009	Administration of pneumococcal vaccine; and
*G0010	Administration of hepatitis B vaccine.
*90471	Immunization administration. (For OPPS hospitals billing for the hepatitis B vaccine administration)
*90472	Each additional vaccine. (For OPPS hospitals billing for the hepatitis B vaccine administration)

* NOTE: For claims with dates of service prior to January 1, 2006, OPPS and non-OPPS hospitals report G0010 for hepatitis B vaccine administration. For claims with dates of service January 1, 2006 until December 31, 2010, OPPS hospitals report 90471 or 90472 for hepatitis B vaccine administration as appropriate in place of G0010. Beginning January 1, 2011, providers should report G0010 for billing under the OPPS rather than 90471 or 90472 to ensure correct waiver of coinsurance and deductible for the administration of hepatitis B vaccine.

One of the following diagnosis codes must be reported as appropriate. If the sole purpose for the visit is to receive a vaccine or if a vaccine is the only service billed on a claim the applicable following diagnosis code may be used.

Diagnosis Code	Description
V03.82	Pneumococcus
V04.81**	Influenza
V06.6***	Pneumococcus and Influenza
V05.3	Hepatitis B

**Effective for influenza virus claims with dates of service October 1, 2003 and later.

***Effective October 1, 2006, providers may report diagnosis code V06.6 on claims for pneumococcus and/or influenza virus vaccines when the purpose of the visit was to receive both vaccines.

If a diagnosis code for pneumococcus, hepatitis B, or influenza virus vaccination is not reported on a claim, contractors may not enter the diagnosis on the claim. Contractors must follow current resolution processes for claims with missing diagnosis codes.

If the diagnosis code and the narrative description are correct, but the HCPCS code is incorrect, the carrier or intermediary may correct the HCPCS code and pay the claim. For example, if the reported diagnosis code is V04.81 and the narrative description (if annotated on the claim) says "flu shot" but the HCPCS code is incorrect, contractors may change the HCPCS code and pay for the flu vaccine. Effective October 1, 2006, carriers/AB MACs should follow the instructions in Pub. 100-04, Chapter 1, Section 80.3.2.1.1 (Carrier Data Element Requirements) for claims submitted without a HCPCS code.

Claims for hepatitis B vaccinations must report the I.D. Number of the referring physician. In addition, if a doctor of medicine or osteopathy does not order the influenza virus vaccine, the intermediary claims require:

- UPIN code SLF000 to be reported on claims submitted prior to May 23, 2008, when Medicare began accepting NPIs, only
- The provider's own NPI to be reported in the NPI field for the attending physician on claims submitted on or after May 23, 2008, when NPI requirements were implemented.

100-4, 18, 10.2.2.1

FI/AB MAC Payment for Pneumococcal Pneumonia Virus, Influenza Virus, and Hepatitis B Virus Vaccines and Their Administration

Payment for Vaccines

Payment for all of these vaccines is on a reasonable cost basis for hospitals, home health agencies (HHAs), skilled nursing facilities (SNFs), critical access hospitals (CAHs), and hospital-based renal dialysis facilities (RDFs). Payment for comprehensive outpatient rehabilitation facilities (CORFs), Indian Health Service hospitals (IHS), IHS CAHs and independent RDFs is based on 95 percent of the average wholesale price (AWP). Section 10.2.4 of this chapter contains information on payment of these vaccines when provided by RDFs or hospices. See Sec.10.2.2.2 for payment to independent and provider- based Rural Health Centers and Federally Qualified Health Clinics.

Payment for these vaccines is as follows:

Facility	Type of Bill	Payment
Hospitals, other than Indian Health Service (IHS) Hospitals and Critical Access Hospitals (CAHs)	12x, 13x	Reasonable cost
IHS Hospitals	12x, 13x, 83x	95% of AWP
IHS CAHs	85x	95% of AWP
CAHs	85x	Reasonable cost
Method I and Method II		
Skilled Nursing Facilities	22x, 23x	Reasonable cost
Home Health Agencies	34x	Reasonable cost
Comprehensive Outpatient Rehabilitation Facilities	75x	95% of the AWP
Independent Renal Dialysis Facilities	72x	95% of the AWP
Hospital-based Renal Dialysis Facilities	72x	Reasonable cost

Payment for Vaccine Administration

Payment for the administration of Influenza Virus and PPV vaccines is as follows:

Facility	Type of Bill	Payment
Hospitals, other than IHS Hospitals and CAHs	12x, 13x	Outpatient Prospective Payment System (OPPS) for hospitals subject to OPPS
		Reasonable cost for hospitals not subject to OPPS
IHS Hospitals	12x, 13x, 83x	MPFS as indicated in guidelines below.
IHS CAHs	85x	MPFS as indicated in guidelines below.
CAHs	85x	Reasonable cost
Method I and II		
Skilled Nursing Facilities	22x, 23x	MPFS as indicated in the guidelines below
Home Health Agencies	34x	OPPS
Comprehensive Outpatient Rehabilitation Facilities	75x	MPFS as indicated in the guidelines below

Facility	Type of Bill	Payment
Independent RDFs	72x	MPFS as indicated in the guidelines below
Hospital-based RDFs	72x	Reasonable cost

Guidelines for pricing PPV and Influenza vaccine administration under the MPFS.

Make reimbursement based on the rate in the MPFS associated with the CPT code 90782 or 90471 as follows:

HCPCS code	Effective prior to March 1, 2003	Effective on and after March 1, 2003
G0008	90782	90471
G0009	90782	90471

See Sec.10.2.2.2 for payment to independent and provider based Rural Health Centers and Federally Qualified Health Clinics.

Payment for the administration of Hepatitis B vaccine is as follows:

Facility	Type of Bill	Payment
Hospitals other than IHS hospitals and CAHs	12x, 13x	Outpatient Prospective Payment System (OPPS) for hospitals subject to OPPS
		Reasonable cost for hospitals not subject to OPPS
IHS Hospitals	12x, 13x, 83x	MPFS as indicated in the guidelines below
CAHs	85x	Reasonable cost
Method I and II		
IHS CAHs	85x	MPFS as indicated in guidelines below.
Skilled Nursing Facilities	22x, 23x	MPFS as indicated in the chart below
Home Health Agencies	34x	OPPS
Comprehensive Outpatient Rehabilitation Facilities	75x	MPFS as indicated in the guidelines below
Independent RDFs	72x	MPFS as indicated in the chart below
Hospital-based RDFs	72x	Reasonable cost

Guidelines for pricing Hepatitis B vaccine administration under the MPFS.

Make reimbursement based on the rate in the MPFS associated with the CPT code 90782 or 90471 as follows:

HCPCS code	Effective prior to March 1, 2003	Effective on and after March 1, 2003
G0010	90782	90471

See Sec.10.2.2.2 for payment to independent and provider based Rural Health Centers and Federally Qualified Health Clinics.

100-4, 18, 10.4

CWF Edits

In order to prevent duplicate payments for influenza virus and pneumococcal vaccination claims by the local contractor/AB MAC and the centralized billing contractor, effective for claims received on or after July 1, 2002, CWF has implemented a number of edits.

NOTE: 90659 was discontinued December 31, 2003.

CWF returns information in Trailer 13 information from the history claim. The following fields are returned to the contractor:

- Trailer Code;
- Contractor Number;
- Document Control Number;
- First Service Date;
- Last Service Date;
- Provider, Physician, Supplier Number;
- Claim Type; Procedure code;
- Alert Code (where applicable); and,
- More history (where applicable.)

100-4, 18, 10.4.1

CWF Edits on FI/AB MAC Claims

In order to prevent duplicate payment by the same FI/AB MAC, CWF edits by line item on the FI/AB MAC number, the beneficiary Health Insurance Claim (HIC) number, and the date of service, the influenza virus procedure codes 90653, 90654, 90655, 90656, 90657, 90660, 90661, 90662, 90672, 90673, 90685, 90686, 90687, or 90688 and the pneumococcal procedure codes 90669, 90670, or 90732, and the administration codes G0008 or G0009.

If CWF receives a claim with either HCPCS codes 90653, 90654, 90655, 90656, 90657, 90660, 90661, 90662, 90672, 90673, 90685, 90686, 90687, or 90688 and it already has on record a claim with the same HIC number, same FI/AB MAC number, same date of service, and any one of those HCPCS codes, the second claim submitted to CWF rejects.

If CWF receives a claim with HCPCS codes 90669, 90670, or 90732 and it already has on record a claim with the same HIC number, same FI/AB MAC number, same date of service, and the same HCPCS code, the second claim submitted to CWF rejects when all four items match.

If CWF receives a claim with HCPCS administration codes G0008 or G0009 and it already has on record a claim with the same HIC number, same FI/AB MAC number, same date of service, and same procedure code, CWF rejects the second claim submitted when all four items match.

CWF returns to the FI/AB MAC a reject code "7262" for this edit. FIs/AB MACs must deny the second claim and use the same messages they currently use for the denial of duplicate claims.

100-4, 18, 10.4.2

CWF Edits on Carrier/AB MAC Claims

In order to prevent duplicate payment by the same carrier/AB MAC, CWF will edit by line item on the carrier/AB MAC number, the HIC number, the date of service, the influenza virus procedure codes 90653, 90654, 90655, 90656, 90657, 90660, 90661, 90662, 90672, 90673, 90685, 90686, 90687, or 90688; the pneumococcal procedure codes 90669, 90670, or 90732; and the administration code G0008 or G0009.

If CWF receives a claim with either HCPCS codes 90653, 90654, 90655, 90656, 90657, 90660, 90661, 90662, 90672, 90673, 90685, 90686, 90687, or 90688 and it already has on record a claim with the same HIC number, same carrier/AB MAC number, same date of service, and any one of those HCPCS codes, the second claim submitted to CWF will reject.

If CWF receives a claim with HCPCS codes 90669, 90670, or 90732 and it already has on record a claim with the same HIC number, same carrier/AB MAC number, same date of service, and the same HCPCS code, the second claim submitted to CWF will reject when all four items match.

If CWF receives a claim with HCPCS administration codes G0008 or G0009 and it already has on record a claim with the same HIC number, same carrier/AB MAC number, same date of service, and same procedure code, CWF will reject the second claim submitted.

CWF will return to the carrier/AB MAC a specific reject code for this edit. Carriers/AB MACs must deny the second claim and use the same messages they currently use for the denial of duplicate claims.

In order to prevent duplicate payment by the centralized billing contractor and local carrier/AB MAC, CWF will edit by line item for carrier number, same HIC number, same date of service, the influenza virus procedure codes 90653, 90654, 90655, 90656, 90657, 90660, 90661, 90662, 90672, 90673, 90685, 90686, 90687, or 90688; the pneumococcal procedure codes 90669, 90670, or 90732; and the administration code G0008 or G0009.

If CWF receives a claim with either HCPCS codes 90653, 90654, 90655, 90656, 90657, 90660, 90661, 90662, 90672, 90673, 90685, 90686, 90687, or 90688 and it already has on record a claim with a different carrier/AB MAC number, but same HIC number, same date of service, and any one of those same HCPCS codes, the second claim submitted to CWF will reject.

If CWF receives a claim with HCPCS codes 90669, 90670, or 90732 and it already has on record a claim with the same HIC number, different carrier/AB MAC number, same date of service, and the same HCPCS code, the second claim submitted to CWF will reject.

If CWF receives a claim with HCPCS administration codes G0008 or G0009 and it already has on record a claim with a different carrier/AB MAC number, but the same HIC number, same date of service, and same procedure code, CWF will reject the second claim submitted.

CWF will return a specific reject code for this edit. Carriers/AB MACs must deny the second claim. For the second edit, the reject code should automatically trigger the following Medicare Summary Notice (MSN) and Remittance Advice (RA) messages.

MSN: 7.2 – "This is a duplicate of a claim processed by another contractor. You should receive a Medicare Summary Notice from them."

Claim adjustment reason code 18 – duplicate claim or service

100-4, 18, 10.4.3

CWF A/B Crossover Edits for FI/AB MAC and Carrier/AB MAC Claims

When CWF receives a claim from the carrier/AB MAC, it will review Part B outpatient claims history to verify that a duplicate claim has not already been posted.

CWF will edit on the beneficiary HIC number; the date of service; the influenza virus procedure codes 90653, 90654, 90655, 90656, 90657, 90660, 90661, 90662, 90672, 90673, 90685, 90686, 90687, or 90688; the pneumococcal procedure codes 90669, 90670, or 90732; and the administration code G0008 or G0009.

CWF will return a specific reject code for this edit. Contractors must deny the second claim and use the same messages they currently use for the denial of duplicate claims.

100-4, 18, 20

Mammography Services (Screening and Diagnostic)

A. Screening Mammography

Beginning January 1, 1991, Medicare provides Part B coverage of screening mammographies for women. Screening mammographies are radiologic procedures for early detection of breast cancer and include a physician's interpretation of the results. A doctor's prescription or referral is not necessary for the procedure to be covered.

Whether payment can be made is determined by a woman's age and statutory frequency parameter. See Pub. 100-02, Medicare Benefit Policy Manual, chapter 15, section 280.3 for additional coverage information for a screening mammography.

Section 4101 of the Balanced Budget Act (BBA) of 1997 provides for annual screening mammographies for women over age 39 and waives the Part B deductible. Coverage applies as follows:

Age Groups	Screening Period
Under age 35	No payment allowed for screening mammography.
35-39	Baseline (pay for only one screening mammography performed on a woman between her 35thand 40thbirthday)
Over age 39	Annual (11 full months have elapsed following the month of last screening

NOTE: Count months between screening mammographies beginning the month after the date of the examination. For example, if Mrs. Smith received a screening mammography examination in January 2005, begin counting the next month (February 2005) until 11 months have elapsed. Payment can be made for another screening mammography in January 2006.

B. Diagnostic Mammography

A diagnostic mammography is a radiological mammogram and is a covered diagnostic test under the following conditions:

- A patient has distinct signs and symptoms for which a mammogram is indicated;
- A patient has a history of breast cancer; or
- A patient is asymptomatic, but based on the patient's history and other factors the physician considers significant, the physician's judgment is that a mammogram is appropriate.
- Beginning January 1, 2005, Medicare Prescription Drug, Improvement, and Modernization Act (MMA) of 2003, Sec. 644, Public Law 108-173 has changed the way Medicare pays for diagnostic mammography. Medicare will pay based on the MPFS in lieu of OPPS or the lower of the actual change.

100-4, 18, 20.4

Billing Requirements - FI/A/B MAC Claims

Contractors use the weekly-updated MQSA file to verify that the billing facility is certified by the FDA to perform mammography services, and has the appropriate certification to perform the type of mammogram billed (film and/or digital). (See Sec.20.1.) FIs/A/B MACs use the provider number submitted on the claim to identify the facility and use the MQSA data file to verify the facility's certification(s). FIs/A/B MACs complete the following activities in processing mammography claims:

- If the provider number on the claim does not correspond with a certified mammography facility on the MQSA file, then intermediaries/A/B MACs deny the claim.
- When a film mammography HCPCS code is on a claim, the claim is checked for a "1" film indicator.
- If a film mammography HCPCS code comes in on a claim and the facility is certified for film mammography, the claim is paid if all other relevant Medicare criteria are met.
- If a film mammography HCPCS code is on a claim and the facility is certified for digital mammography only, the claim is denied.
- When a digital mammography HCPCS code is on a claim, the claim is checked for "2" digital indicator.
- If a digital mammography HCPCS code is on a claim and the facility is certified for digital mammography, the claim is paid if all other relevant Medicare criteria are met.
- If a digital mammography HCPCS code is on a claim and the facility is certified for film mammography only, the claim is denied.

NOTE: The Common Working File (CWF) no longer receives the mammography file for editing purposes.

Except as provided in the following sections for RHCs and FQHCs, the following procedures apply to billing for screening mammographies: The technical component portion of the screening mammography is billed on Form CMS-1450 under bill type 12X, 13X, 14X**, 22X, 23X or 85X using revenue code 0403 and HCPCS code 77057* (76092*).

The technical component portion of the diagnostic mammography is billed on Form CMS-1450 under bill type 12X, 13X, 14X**, 22X, 23X or 85X using revenue code 0401 and HCPCS code 77055* (76090*), 77056* (76091*), G0204 and G0206.

Separate bills are required for claims for screening mammographies with dates of service prior to January 1, 2002. Providers include on the bill only charges for the screening mammography. Separate bills are not required for claims for screening mammographies with dates of service on or after January 1, 2002.

See separate instructions below for rural health clinics (RHCs) and federally qualified health centers (FQHCs).

* For claims with dates of service prior to January 1, 2007, providers report CPT codes 76090, 76091, and 76092. For claims with dates of service January 1, 2007 and later, providers report CPT codes 77055, 77056, and 77057 respectively.

** For claims with dates of service April 1, 2005 and later, hospitals bill for all mammography services under the 13X type of bill or for dates of service April 1, 2007 and later, 12X or 13X as appropriate. The 14X type of bill is no longer applicable. Appropriate bill types for providers other than hospitals are 22X, 23X, and 85X.

In cases where screening mammography services are self-referred and as a result an attending physician NPI is not available, the provider shall duplicate their facility NPI in the attending physician identifier field on the claim.

100-4, 18, 20.5

Carrier Processing Requirements

Contractors use the weekly-updated file to verify that the billing facility is certified by the FDA to perform mammography services, and has the appropriate certification to perform the type of mammogram billed (film and/or digital). Carriers/B MACs match the FDA assigned, 6-digit mammography certification number on the claim to the FDA mammography certification number appearing on the file for the billing facility. Carriers/B MACs complete the following activities in processing mammography claims:

- If the claim does not contain the facility's 6-digit certification number, or if a 6-digit certification number is not reported in item 32 of the Form CMS-1500 for paper claims, or in the 2400 loop (REF 02 segment, where 01=EW segment) of the ASC X12N 837 professional claim format, version 4010A1, for electronic claims, then carriers/B MACs return the claim as unprocessable.
- If the claim contains a 6-digit certification number that is reported in the proper field or segment (as specified in the previous bullet) but such number does not correspond to the number specified in the MQSA file for the facility, then carriers/B MACs deny the claim.
- When a film mammography HCPCS code is on a claim, the claim is checked for a "1" film indicator.
- If a film mammography HCPCS code comes in on a claim and the facility is certified for film mammography, the claim is paid if all other relevant Medicare criteria are met.
- If a film mammography HCPCS code is on a claim and the facility is certified for digital mammography only, the claim is denied.
- When a digital mammography HCPCS code is on a claim, the claim is checked for "2" digital indicator.
- If a digital mammography HCPCS code is on a claim and the facility is certified for digital mammography, the claim is paid if all other relevant Medicare criteria are met.
- If a digital mammography HCPCS code is on a claim and the facility is certified for film mammography only, the claim is denied.
- Process the claim to the point of payment based on the information provided on the claim and in carrier claims history.
- Identify the claim as a screening mammography claim by the CPT-4 code listed in field 24D and the diagnosis code(s) listed in field 21 of Form CMS-1500.
- Assign physician specialty code 45 to facilities that are certified to perform only screening mammography.
- Ensure that entities that bill globally for screening mammography contain a blank in modifier modifier position #1.

- Ensure that entities that bill for the technical component use only HCPCS modifier "-TC."
- Ensure that physicians who bill the professional component separately use HCPCS modifier "-26."
- Send the mammography modifier to CWF in the first modifier position on the claim. If more than one modifier is necessary, e.g., if the service was performed in a rural Health Manpower Shortage Area (HMSA) facility, instruct providers to bill the mammography modifier in modifier position 1 and the rural (or other) modifier in modifier position 2.
- Ensure all those who are qualified include the 6-digit FDA-assigned certification number of the screening center in field 32 of Form CMS-1500 and in the REF02 segment (where 01 = EW segment) of the 2400 loop for the ASC X12N 837 professional claim format, version 4010A1. Carriers/B MACs retain this number in their provider files.
- Waive Part B deductible and apply coinsurance for a screening mammography.
- Add diagnosis code V76.12 if a claim comes in for screening mammography without a diagnosis and the carrier file data shows this is appropriate. If there are other diagnoses on the claim, but not code V76.12, add it. (Do not change or overlay code V76.12 but ADD it.) At a minimum, edit for age, frequency, and place of service (POS).
- After May 23, 2008, accept the screening mammography facility's NPI number in place of the attending/referring physician NPI number for self-referred mammography claims.
- When a mammography claim contains services subject to the anti-markup payment limitation and the service was acquired from another billing jurisdiction, the provider must submit their own NPI with the name, address, and zip code of the performing physician/supplier.
- Refer to Pub. 100-04, chapter 1, section 10.1.1.1., for claims processing instructions for payment jurisdiction on Form CMS-1500 and electronic form ANSI X12 837P.

NOTE: Beginning October 1, 2003, carriers/B MACs are no longer permitted to add the ICD-9 code for a screening mammography when the screening mammography claim has no diagnosis code. Screening mammography claims with no diagnosis code must be returned as unprocessable for assigned claims. For unassigned claims, deny the claim.

Carrier Provider Education

- Educate providers that when a screening mammography turns to a diagnostic mammography on the same day for the same beneficiary, add the "-GG" modifier to the diagnostic code and bill both codes on the same claim. Both services are reimbursable by Medicare.
- Educate providers that they cannot bill an add-on code without also billing for the appropriate mammography code. If just the add-on code is billed, the service will be denied. Both the add-on code and the appropriate mammography code should be on the same claim.
- Educate providers to submit their own NPI in place of an attending/referring physician NPI in cases where screening mammography services are self-referred.

100-4, 18, 60.1

Payment

Payment (contractor) is under the MPFS except as follows:

- Fecal occult blood tests (82270* (G0107*) and G0328) are paid under the clinical diagnostic lab fee schedule except reasonable cost is paid to all non-OPPS hospitals, including CAHs, but not IHS hospitals billing on TOB 83x. IHS hospitals billing on TOB 83x are paid the ASC payment amount. Other IHS hospitals (billing on TOB 13x) are paid the OMB approved AIR, or the facility specific per visit amount as applicable. Deductible and coinsurance do not apply for these tests. See section A below for payment to Maryland waiver on TOB 13X. Payment from all hospitals for non-patient laboratory specimens on TOB 14X will be based on the clinical diagnostic fee schedule, including CAHs and Maryland waiver hospitals
- Flexible sigmoidoscopy (code G0104) is paid under OPPS for hospital outpatient departments and on a reasonable cost basis for CAHs; or current payment methodologies for hospitals not subject to OPPS.
- Colonoscopies (G0105 and G0121) and barium enemas (G0106 and G0120) are paid under OPPS for hospital outpatient departments and on a reasonable costs basis for CAHs or current payment methodologies for hospitals not subject to OPPS. Also colonoscopies may be done in an Ambulatory Surgical Center (ASC) and when done in an ASC the ASC rate applies. The ASC rate is the same for diagnostic and screening colonoscopies. The ASC rate is paid to IHS hospitals when the service is billed on TOB 83x.

Prior to January 1, 2007, deductible and coinsurance apply to HCPCS codes G0104, G0105, G0106, G0120, and G0121. Beginning with services provided on or after January 1, 2007, Section 5113 of the Deficit Reduction Act of 2005 waives the requirement of the annual Part B deductible for these screening services. Coinsurance still applies. Coinsurance and deductible applies to the diagnostic colorectal service codes listed below.

The following screening codes must be paid at rates consistent with the diagnostic codes indicated.

Screening Code	Diagnostic Code
G0104	45330
G0105 and G0121	45378
G0106 and G0120	74280

A. Special Payment Instructions for TOB 13X Maryland Waiver Hospitals

For hospitals in Maryland under the jurisdiction of the Health Services Cost Review Commission, screening colorectal services HCPCS codes G0104, G0105, G0106, 82270* (G0107*), G0120, G0121 and G0328 are paid according to the terms of the waiver, that is 94% of submitted charges minus any unmet existing deductible, co-insurance and non-covered charges. Maryland Hospitals bill TOB 13X for outpatient colorectal cancer screenings.

B. Special Payment Instructions for Non-Patient Laboratory Specimen (TOB 14X) for all hospitals

Payment for colorectal cancer screenings (82270* (G0107*) and G0328) to a hospital for a non-patient laboratory specimen (TOB 14X), is the lesser of the actual charge, the fee schedule amount, or the National Limitation Amount (NLA), (including CAHs and Maryland Waiver hospitals). Part B deductible and coinsurance do not apply.

*NOTE: For claims with dates of service prior to January 1, 2007, physicians, suppliers, and providers report HCPCS code G0107. Effective January 1, 2007, code G0107 is discontinued and replaced with CPT code 82270.

100-4, 18, 60.2

HCPCS Codes, Frequency Requirements, and Age Requirements (If Applicable)

Effective for services furnished on or after January 1, 1998, the following codes are used for colorectal cancer screening services:

- 82270* (G0107*) - Colorectal cancer screening; fecal-occult blood tests, 1-3 simultaneous determinations;
- G0104 - Colorectal cancer screening; flexible sigmoidoscopy;
- G0105 - Colorectal cancer screening; colonoscopy on individual at high risk;
- G0106 - Colorectal cancer screening; barium enema; as an alternative to G0104, screening sigmoidoscopy;
- G0120 - Colorectal cancer screening; barium enema; as an alternative to G0105, screening colonoscopy.

Effective for services furnished on or after July 1, 2001, the following codes are used for colorectal cancer screening services:

- G0121 - Colorectal cancer screening; colonoscopy on individual not meeting criteria for high risk. Note that the description for this code has been revised to remove the term "noncovered."
- G0122 - Colorectal cancer screening; barium enema (noncovered).

Effective for services furnished on or after January 1, 2004, the following code is used for colorectal cancer screening services as an alternative to 82270* (G0107*):

- G0328 - Colorectal cancer screening; immunoassay, fecal-occult blood test, 1-3 simultaneous determinations

*NOTE: For claims with dates of service prior to January 1, 2007, physicians, suppliers, and providers report HCPCS code G0107. Effective January 1, 2007, code G0107 is discontinued and replaced with CPT code 82270.

G0104 - Colorectal Cancer Screening; Flexible Sigmoidoscopy

Screening flexible sigmoidoscopies (code G0104) may be paid for beneficiaries who have attained age 50, when performed by a doctor of medicine or osteopathy at the frequencies noted below.

For claims with dates of service on or after January 1, 2002, contractors pay for screening flexible sigmoidoscopies (code G0104) for beneficiaries who have attained age 50 when these services were performed by a doctor of medicine or osteopathy, or by a physician assistant, nurse practitioner, or clinical nurse specialist (as defined in Sec.1861(aa)(5) of the Act and in the Code of Federal Regulations at42 CFR 410.74, 410.75, and410.76) at the frequencies noted above. For claims with dates of service prior to January 1, 2002, contractors pay for these services under the conditions noted only when a doctor of medicine or osteopathy performs them.

For services furnished from January 1, 1998, through June 30, 2001, inclusive:

- Once every 48 months (i.e., at least 47 months have passed following the month in which the last covered screening flexible sigmoidoscopy was done).

For services furnished on or after July 1, 2001:

- Once every 48 months as calculated above unless the beneficiary does not meet the criteria for high risk of developing colorectal cancer (refer to Sec.60.3 of this chapter) and he/she has had a screening colonoscopy (code G0121) within the preceding 10 years. If such a beneficiary has had a screening colonoscopy within the preceding 10 years, then he or she can have covered a screening flexible sigmoidoscopy only after at least 119 months have passed following the month that he/she received the screening colonoscopy (code G0121).

NOTE: If during the course of a screening flexible sigmoidoscopy a lesion or growth is detected which results in a biopsy or removal of the growth; the appropriate diagnostic procedure classified as a flexible sigmoidoscopy with biopsy or removal should be billed and paid rather than code G0104.

G0105 - Colorectal Cancer Screening; Colonoscopy on Individual at High Risk
Screening colonoscopies (code G0105) may be paid when performed by a doctor of medicine or osteopathy at a frequency of once every 24 months for beneficiaries at high risk for developing colorectal cancer (i.e., at least 23 months have passed following the month in which the last covered G0105 screening colonoscopy was performed). Refer to Sec.60.3of this chapter for the criteria to use in determining whether or not an individual is at high risk for developing colorectal cancer.

NOTE: If during the course of the screening colonoscopy, a lesion or growth is detected which results in a biopsy or removal of the growth, the appropriate diagnostic procedure classified as a colonoscopy with biopsy or removal should be billed and paid rather than code G0105.

A. Colonoscopy Cannot be Completed Because of Extenuating Circumstances

1. FIs
   When a covered colonoscopy is attempted but cannot be completed because of extenuating circumstances, Medicare will pay for the interrupted colonoscopy as long as the coverage conditions are met for the incomplete procedure. However, the frequency standards associated with screening colonoscopies will not be applied by CWF. When a covered colonoscopy is next attempted and completed, Medicare will pay for that colonoscopy according to its payment methodology for this procedure as long as coverage conditions are met, and the frequency standards will be applied by CWF. This policy is applied to both screening and diagnostic colonoscopies.

   When submitting a facility claim for the interrupted colonoscopy, providers are to suffix the colonoscopy HCPCS codes with a modifier of "-73" or "-74" as appropriate to indicate that the procedure was interrupted. Payment for covered incomplete screening colonoscopies shall be consistent with payment methodologies currently in place for complete screening colonoscopies, including those contained in42 CFR 419.44(b). In situations where a critical access hospital (CAH) has elected payment Method II for CAH patients, payment shall be consistent with payment methodologies currently in place as outlined in Chapter 3. As such, instruct CAHs that elect Method II payment to use modifier "-53" to identify an incomplete screening colonoscopy (physician professional service(s) billed in revenue code 096X, 097X, and/or 098X). Such CAHs will also bill the technical or facility component of the interrupted colonoscopy in revenue code 075X (or other appropriate revenue code) using the "-73" or "-74" modifier as appropriate.

   Note that Medicare would expect the provider to maintain adequate information in the patient's medical record in case it is needed by the contractor to document the incomplete procedure.

2. Carriers
   When a covered colonoscopy is attempted but cannot be completed because of extenuating circumstances (see Chapter 12), Medicare will pay for the interrupted colonoscopy at a rate consistent with that of a flexible sigmoidoscopy as long as coverage conditions are met for the incomplete procedure. When a covered colonoscopy is next attempted and completed, Medicare will pay for that colonoscopy according to its payment methodology for this procedure as long as coverage conditions are met. This policy is applied to both screening and diagnostic colonoscopies.

   When submitting a claim for the interrupted colonoscopy, professional providers are to suffix the colonoscopy code with a modifier of "-53" to indicate that the procedure was interrupted. When submitting a claim for the facility fee associated with this procedure, Ambulatory Surgical Centers (ASCs) are to suffix the colonoscopy code with "-73" or "-74" as appropriate. Payment for covered screening colonoscopies, including that for the associated ASC facility fee when applicable, shall be consistent with payment for diagnostic colonoscopies, whether the procedure is complete or incomplete.

   Note that Medicare would expect the provider to maintain adequate information in the patient's medical record in case it is needed by the contractor to document the incomplete procedure.

G0106 - Colorectal Cancer Screening; Barium Enema; as an Alternative to G0104, Screening Sigmoidoscopy
Screening barium enema examinations may be paid as an alternative to a screening sigmoidoscopy (code G0104). The same frequency parameters for screening sigmoidoscopies (see those codes above) apply. In the case of an individual aged 50 or over, payment may be made for a screening barium enema examination (code G0106) performed after at least 47 months have passed following the month in which the last screening barium enema or screening flexible sigmoidoscopy was performed. For example, the beneficiary received a screening barium enema examination as an alternative to a screening flexible sigmoidoscopy in January 1999. Start counts beginning February 1999. The beneficiary is eligible for another screening barium enema in January 2003. The screening barium enema must be ordered in writing after a determination that the test is the appropriate screening test. Generally, it is expected that this will be a screening double contrast enema unless the individual is unable to withstand such an exam. This means that in the case of a particular individual, the attending physician must determine that the estimated screening potential for the barium enema is equal to or greater than the screening potential that has been estimated for a screening flexible sigmoidoscopy for the same individual. The screening single contrast barium enema also requires a written order from the beneficiary's attending physician in the same manner as described above for the screening double contrast barium enema examination.

82270* (G0107*) - Colorectal Cancer Screening; Fecal-Occult Blood Test, 1-3 Simultaneous Determinations
Effective for services furnished on or after January 1, 1998, screening FOBT (code 82270* (G0107*) may be paid for beneficiaries who have attained age 50, and at a frequency of once every 12 months (i.e., at least 11 months have passed following the month in which the last covered screening FOBT was performed). This screening FOBT means a guaiac-based test for peroxidase activity, in which the beneficiary completes it by taking samples from two different sites of three consecutive stools. This screening requires a written order from the beneficiary's attending physician. (The term "attending physician" is defined to mean a doctor of medicine or osteopathy (as defined in Sec.1861(r)(1)of the Act) who is fully knowledgeable about the beneficiary's medical condition, and who would be responsible for using the results of any examination performed in the overall management of the beneficiary's specific medical problem.)

Effective for services furnished on or after January 1, 2004, payment may be made for a immunoassay-based FOBT (G0328, described below) as an alternative to the guaiacbased FOBT, 82270* (G0107*). Medicare will pay for only one covered FOBT per year, either 82270* (G0107*) or G0328, but not both.

*NOTE: For claims with dates of service prior to January 1, 2007, physicians, suppliers, and providers report HCPCS code G0107. Effective January 1, 2007, code G0107 is discontinued and replaced with CPT code 82270.

G0328 - Colorectal Cancer Screening; Immunoassay, Fecal-Occult Blood Test, 1-3 Simultaneous Determinations
Effective for services furnished on or after January 1, 2004, screening FOBT, (code G0328) may be paid as an alternative to 82270* (G0107*) for beneficiaries who have attained age 50. Medicare will pay for a covered FOBT (either 82270* (G0107*) or G0328, but not both) at a frequency of once every 12 months (i.e., at least 11 months have passed following the month in which the last covered screening FOBT was performed). Screening FOBT, immunoassay, includes the use of a spatula to collect the appropriate number of samples or the use of a special brush for the collection of samples, as determined by the individual manufacturer's instructions. This screening requires a written order from the beneficiary's attending physician. (The term "attending physician" is defined to mean a doctor of medicine or osteopathy (as defined in Sec.1861(r)(1) of the Act) who is fully knowledgeable about the beneficiary's medical condition, and who would be responsible for using the results of any examination performed in the overall management of the beneficiary's specific medical problem.)

G0120 - Colorectal Cancer Screening; Barium Enema; as an Alternative to or G0105, Screening Colonoscopy
Screening barium enema examinations may be paid as an alternative to a screening colonoscopy (code G0105) examination. The same frequency parameters for screening colonoscopies (see those codes above) apply. In the case of an individual who is at high risk for colorectal cancer, payment may be made for a screening barium enema examination (code G0120) performed after at least 23 months have passed following the month in which the last screening barium enema or the last screening colonoscopy was performed. For example, a beneficiary at high risk for developing colorectal cancer received a screening barium enema examination (code G0120) as an alternative to a screening colonoscopy (code G0105) in January 2000. Start counts beginning February 2000. The beneficiary is eligible for another screening barium enema examination (code G0120) in January 2002. The screening barium enema must be ordered in writing after a determination that the test is the appropriate screening test. Generally, it is expected that this will be a screening double contrast enema unless the individual is unable to withstand such an exam. This means that in the case of a particular individual, the attending physician must determine that the estimated screening potential for the barium enema is equal to or greater than the screening potential that has been estimated for a screening colonoscopy, for the same individual. The screening single contrast barium enema also requires a written order from the beneficiary's attending physician in the same manner as described above for the screening double contrast barium enema examination.

G0121 - Colorectal Screening; Colonoscopy on Individual Not Meeting Criteria for High Risk - Applicable On and After July 1, 2001
Effective for services furnished on or after July 1, 2001, screening colonoscopies (code G0121) performed on individuals not meeting the criteria for being at high risk for developing colorectal cancer (refer to Sec.60.3 of this chapter) may be paid under the following conditions:

- At a frequency of once every 10 years (i.e., at least 119 months have passed following the month in which the last covered G0121 screening colonoscopy was performed.)
- If the individual would otherwise qualify to have covered a G0121 screening colonoscopy based on the above but has had a covered screening flexible sigmoidoscopy (code G0104), then he or she may have covered a G0121 screening colonoscopy only after at least 47 months have passed following the month in which the last covered G0104 flexible sigmoidoscopy was performed.

NOTE: If during the course of the screening colonoscopy, a lesion or growth is detected which results in a biopsy or removal of the growth, the appropriate diagnostic procedure classified as a colonoscopy with biopsy or removal should be billed and paid rather than code G0121.

G0122 - Colorectal Cancer Screening; Barium Enema
The code is not covered by Medicare.

100-4, 18, 60.6

Billing Requirements for Claims Submitted to FIs

(Follow the general bill review instructions in Chapter 25. Hospitals use the ANSI X12N 837I to bill the FI or on the hardcopy Form CMS-1450. Hospitals bill revenue codes and HCPCS codes as follows:

Screening Test/Procedure	Revenue Code	HCPCS Code	TOB
Fecal Occult blood test	030X	82270*** (G0107***), G0328	12X, 13X, 14X**, 22X, 23X, 83X, 85X
Barium enema	032X	G0106, G0120, G0122	12X, 13X, 22X, 23X, 85X****
Flexible Sigmoidoscopy	*	G0104	12X, 13X, 22X, 23X, 83X, 85X****
Colonoscopy-high risk	*	G0105, G0121	12X, 13X, 22X, 23X, 83X, 85X****

* The appropriate revenue code when reporting any other surgical procedure.

** 14X is only applicable for non-patient laboratory specimens.

*** For claims with dates of service prior to January 1, 2007, physicians, suppliers, and providers report HCPCS code G0107. Effective January 1, 2007, code G0107, is discontinued and replaced with CPT code 82270.

**** CAHs that elect Method II bill revenue code 096X, 097X, and/or 098X for professional services and 075X (or other appropriate revenue code) for the technical or facility component.

Special Billing Instructions for Hospital Inpatients

When these tests/procedures are provided to inpatients of a hospital or when Part A benefits have been exhausted, they are covered under this benefit. However, the provider bills on bill type 12X using the discharge date of the hospital stay to avoid editing in the Common Working File (CWF) as a result of the hospital bundling rules.

100-4, 18, 80.2

A/B Medicare Administrative Contractor (MAC) and Contractor Billing Requirements

Effective for dates of service on and after January 1, 2005, through December 31, 2008, contractors shall recognize the HCPCS codes G0344, G0366, G0367, and G0368 shown above in §80.1 for an IPPE. The type of service (TOS) for each of these codes is as follows:

G0344: TOS = 1

G0366: TOS = 5

G0367: TOS = 5

G0368: TOS = 5

Contractors shall pay physicians or qualified nonphysician practitioners for only one IPPE performed not later than 6 months after the date the individual's first coverage begins under Medicare Part B, but only if that coverage period begins on or after January 1, 2005.

Effective for dates of service on and after January 1, 2009, contractors shall recognize the HCPCS codes G0402, G0403, G0404, and G0405 shown above in §80.1 for an IPPE. The TOS for each of these codes is as follows:

G0402: TOS = 1

G0403: TOS = 5

G0404: TOS = 5

G0405: TOS = 5

Under the MIPPA of 2008, contractors shall pay physicians or qualified nonphysician practitioners for only one IPPE performed not later than 12 months after the date the individual's first coverage begins under Medicare Part B only if that coverage period begins on or after January 1, 2009.

Contractors shall allow payment for a medically necessary Evaluation and Management (E/M) service at the same visit as the IPPE when it is clinically appropriate. Physicians and qualified nonphysician practitioners shall use CPT codes 99201-99215 to report an E/M with CPT modifier 25 to indicate that the E/M is a significant, separately identifiable service from the IPPE code reported (G0344 or G0402, whichever applies based on the date the IPPE is performed). Refer to chapter 12, § 30.6.1.1, of this manual for the physician/practitioner billing correct coding and payment policy regarding E/M services.

If the EKG performed as a component of the IPPE is not performed by the primary physician or qualified NPP during the IPPE visit, another physician or entity may perform and/or interpret the EKG. The referring physician or qualified NPP needs to make sure that the performing physician or entity bills the appropriate G code for the screening EKG, and not a CPT code in the 93000 series. Both the IPPE and the EKG should be billed in order for the beneficiary to receive the complete IPPE service. Effective for dates of service on and after January 1, 2009, the screening EKG is optional and is no longer a mandated service of an IPPE if performed as a result of a referral from an IPPE.

Should the same physician or NPP need to perform an additional medically necessary EKG in the 93000 series on the same day as the IPPE, report the appropriate EKG CPT code(s) with modifier 59, indicating that the EKG is a distinct procedural service.

Physicians or qualified nonphysician practitioners shall bill the contractor the appropriate HCPCS codes for IPPE on the Form CMS-1500 claim or an approved electronic format. The HCPCS codes for an IPPE and screening EKG are paid under the Medicare Physician Fee Schedule (MPFS). The appropriate deductible and coinsurance applies to codes G0344, G0366, G0367, G0368, G0403, G0404, and G0405. The deductible is waived for code G0402 but the coinsurance still applies.

100-4, 18, 150

Counseling to Prevent Tobacco Use

Effective for claims with dates of service on and after August 25, 2010, the Centers for Medicare & Medicaid Services (CMS) will cover counseling to prevent tobacco use services for outpatient and hospitalized Medicare beneficiaries:

1. Who use tobacco, regardless of whether they have signs or symptoms of tobacco-related disease;
2. Who are competent and alert at the time that counseling is provided; and,
3. Whose counseling is furnished by a qualified physician or other Medicare-recognized practitioner. These individuals who do not have signs or symptoms of tobacco-related disease will be covered under Medicare Part B when the above conditions of coverage are met, subject to certain frequency and other limitations.

Conditions of Medicare Part A and Medicare Part B coverage for counseling to prevent tobacco use are located in the Medicare National Coverage Determinations (NCD) Manual, Publication 100-3, chapter 1, section 210.4.1.

100-4, 18, 150.1

Healthcare Common Procedure Coding System (HCPCS) and Diagnosis Coding

The CMS has created two new G codes for billing for tobacco cessation counseling services to prevent tobacco use for those individuals who use tobacco but do not have signs or symptoms of tobacco-related disease. These are in addition to the two CPT codes 99406 and 99407 that currently are used for smoking and tobacco-use cessation counseling for symptomatic individuals.

The following HCPCS codes should be reported when billing for counseling to prevent tobacco use effective January 1, 2011:

G0436 Smoking and tobacco cessation counseling visit for the asymptomatic patient; intermediate, greater than 3 minutes, up to 10 minutes

Short descriptor: Tobacco-use counsel 3-10 min

G0437 Smoking and tobacco cessation counseling visit for the asymptomatic patient; intensive, greater than 10 minutes

Short descriptor: Tobacco-use counsel >10min

NOTE: The above G codes will not be active in contractors' systems until January 1, 2011. Therefore, contractors shall advise non-outpatient perspective payment system (OPPS) providers to use unlisted code 99199 to bill for counseling to prevent tobacco use and tobacco-related disease services during the interim period of August 25, 2010, through December 31, 2010.

On January 3, 2011, contractor's systems will accept the new G codes for services performed on or after August 25, 2010.

Two new C codes have been created for facilities paid under OPPS when billing for counseling to prevent tobacco use and tobacco-related disease services during the interim period of August 25, 2010, through December 31, 2010:

C9801 Smoking and tobacco cessation counseling visit for the asymptomatic patient, intermediate, greater than 3 minutes, up to 10 minutes

Short descriptor: Tobacco-use counsel 3-10 min

C9802 Smoking and tobacco cessation counseling visit for the asymptomatic patient, intensive, greater than 10 minutes

Short descriptor: Tobacco-use counsel >10min

Claims for smoking and tobacco use cessation counseling services G0436 and G0437 shall be submitted with diagnosis code V15.82, history of tobacco use, or 305.1, non-dependent tobacco use disorder.

Contractors shall allow payment for a medically necessary E/M service on the same day as the smoking and tobacco-use cessation counseling service when it is clinically appropriate. Physicians and qualified non-physician practitioners shall use an appropriate HCPCS code to report an E/M service with modifier -25 to indicate that the E/M service is a separately identifiable service from G0436 or G0437.

100-4, 18, 150.2

Carrier Billing Requirements

Carriers shall pay for counseling to prevent tobacco use services billed with code G0436 or G0437 for dates of service on or after January 1, 2011. Carriers shall pay for counseling services billed with code 99199 for dates of service performed on or after August 25, 2010 through December 31, 2010. The type of service (TOS) for each of the new codes is 1.

Carriers pay for counseling services billed based on the Medicare Physician Fee Schedule (MPFS). Deductible and coinsurance apply for services performed on August 25, 2010, through December 31, 2010. For claims with dates of service on and after January 1, 2011, coinsurance and deductible do not apply on G0436 and G0437.

Physicians or qualified non-physician practitioners shall bill the carrier for counseling to prevent tobacco use services on Form CMS-1500 or an approved electronic format.

NOTE: The above G codes will not be active in contractors' systems until January 1, 2011. Therefore, contractors shall advise providers to use unlisted code 99199 to bill for counseling to prevent tobacco use services during the interim period of August 25, 2010, through December 31, 2010.

100-4, 18, 150.2.1

Fiscal Intermediary (FI) Billing Requirements

The FIs shall pay for counseling to prevent tobacco use services with codes G0436 and G0437 for dates of service on or after January 1, 2011. FIs shall pay for counseling services billed with code 99199 for dates of service performed on or after August 25, 2010, through December 31, 2010. For facilities paid under OPPS, FIs shall pay for counseling services billed with codes C9801 and C9802 for dates of service performed on or after August 25, 2010, through December 31, 2010.

Claims for counseling to prevent tobacco use services should be submitted on Form CMS-1450 or its electronic equivalent.

The applicable bill types are 12X, 13X, 22X, 23X, 34X, 71X, 77X, and 85X.

Payment for outpatient services is as follows:

Type of Facility	Method of Payment
Rural Health Centers (RHCs) TOB 71X/Federally Qualified Health Centers (FQHCs)TOB 77X	All-inclusive rate (AIR) for the encounter
Hospitals TOBs 12X and 13X	OPPS for hospitals subject to OPPS MPFS for hospitals not subject to OPPS
Indian Health Services (IHS) Hospitals TOB 13X	AIR for the encounter
Skilled Nursing Facilities (SNFs) TOBs 22X and 23X	Medicare Physician Fee Schedule (MPFS)
Home Health Agencies (HHAs) TOB 34X	MPFS
Critical Access Hospitals (CAHs) TOB 85X	Method I: Technical services are paid at 101% of reasonable cost. Method II: technical services are paid at 101% of reasonable cost, and Professional services are paid at 115% of the MPFS Data Base
IHS CAHs TOB 85X	Based on specific rate
Maryland Hospitals	Payment is based according to the Health Services Cost Review Commission (HSCRC). That is 94% of submitted charges subject to any unmet deductible, coinsurance, and non-covered charges policies.

100-4, 18, 150.4

Common Working File (CWF)

The Common Working File (CWF) shall edit for the frequency of service limitations of counseling to prevent tobacco use sessions and smoking and tobacco-use cessation counseling services (G0436, G0437, 99406, 99407) rendered to a beneficiary for a combined total of 8 sessions within a 12-month period. The beneficiary may receive another 8 sessions during a second or subsequent year after 11 full months have passed since the first Medicare covered counseling session was performed. To start the count for the second or subsequent 12-month period, begin with the month after the month in which the first Medicare covered counseling session was performed and count until 11 full months have elapsed.

By entering the beneficiary's health insurance claim number (HICN), providers have the capability to view the number of sessions a beneficiary has received for this service via inquiry through CWF.

100-4, 18, 170.1

Healthcare Common Procedure Coding System (HCPCS) Codes for Screening for STIs and HIBC to Prevent STIs

Effective for claims with dates of service on and after November 8, 2011, the claims processing instructions for payment of screening tests for STI will apply to the following HCPCS codes:

- Chlamydia: 86631, 86632, 87110, 87270, 87320, 87490, 87491, 87810, 87800 (used for combined chlamydia and gonorrhea testing)
- Gonorrhea: 87590, 87591, 87850, 87800 (used for combined chlamydia and gonorrhea testing)
- Syphilis: 86592, 86593, 86780
- Hepatitis B: (hepatitis B surface antigen): 87340, 87341

Effective for claims with dates of service on and after November 8, 2011, implemented with the January 2, 2012, IOCE, the following HCPCS code is to be billed for HIBC to prevent STIs:

- G0445 – high-intensity behavioral counseling to prevent sexually transmitted infections, face-to-face, individual, includes: education, skills training, and guidance on how to change sexual behavior, performed semi-annually, 30 minutes.

100-4,18,170.2

Diagnosis Code Reporting

A claim that is submitted for screening chlamydia, gonorrhea, syphilis, and/or hepatitis B shall be submitted with one or more of the following diagnosis codes in the header and pointed to the line item:

a. For claims for screening for chlamydia, gonorrhea, and syphilis in women at increased risk who are not pregnant use the following diagnosis codes:
   - V74.5—Screening, bacterial—sexually transmitted; and
   - V69.8—Other problems related to lifestyle as secondary (This diagnosis code is used to indicate high/increased risk for STIs).

b. For claims for screening for syphilis in men at increased risk use the following diagnosis codes:
   - V74.5—Screening, bacterial—sexually transmitted; and
   - V69.8—Other problems related to lifestyle as secondary.

c. For claims for screening for chlamydia and gonorrhea in pregnant women at increased risk for STIs use the following diagnosis codes:
   - V74.5—Screening, bacterial—sexually transmitted; and
   - V69.8—Other problems related to lifestyle, and,
   - V22.0—Supervision of normal first pregnancy, or
   - V22.1—Supervision of other normal pregnancy, or,
   - V23.9—Supervision of unspecified high-risk pregnancy.

d. For claims for screening for syphilis in pregnant women use the following diagnosis codes:
   - V74.5—Screening, bacterial—sexually transmitted; and
   - V22.0—Supervision of normal first pregnancy, or,
   - V22.1—Supervision of other normal pregnancy, or,
   - V23.9—Supervision of unspecified high-risk pregnancy.

e. For claims for screening for syphilis in pregnant women at increased risk for STIs use the following diagnosis codes:
   - V74.5—Screening, bacterial—sexually transmitted; and
   - V69.8—Other problems related to lifestyle, and,
   - V22.0—Supervision of normal first pregnancy, or
   - V22.1—Supervision of other normal pregnancy, or,
   - V23.9—Supervision of unspecified high-risk pregnancy.

f. For claims for screening for hepatitis B in pregnant women use the following diagnosis codes:
   - V73.89—Screening, disease or disorder, viral, specified type NEC; and
   - V22.0—Supervision of normal first pregnancy, or,
   - V22.1—Supervision of other normal pregnancy, or,
   - V23.9—Supervision of unspecified high-risk pregnancy.

g. For claims for screening for hepatitis B in pregnant women at increased risk for STIs use the following diagnosis codes:
   - V73.89—Screening, disease or disorder, viral, specified type NEC; and
   - V 69.8—Other problems related to lifestyle, and,
   - V22.0—Supervision of normal first pregnancy, or,
   - V22.1—Supervision of other normal pregnancy, or,
   - V23.9—Supervision of unspecified high-risk pregnancy.

ICD-10 Diagnosis Coding:

Contractors shall note the appropriate ICD-10 code(s) that are listed below for future implementation. Contractors shall track the ICD-10 codes and ensure that the updated edit is turned on as part of the ICD-10 implementation effective October 1, 2013.

ICD-10	Description
Z113	Encounter for screening for infections with a predominantly sexual mode of transmission
Z1159	Encounter for screening for other viral diseases
Z7289	Other problems related to lifestyle
Z3400	Encounter for supervision of normal first pregnancy, unspecified trimester
Z3480	Encounter for supervision of other normal pregnancy, unspecified trimester
O0990	Supervision of high risk pregnancy, unspecified, unspecified trimester

100-4,18,170.3

Billing Requirements

Effective for dates of service November 8, 2011, and later, contractors shall recognize HCPCS code G0445 for HIBC. Medicare shall cover up to two occurrences of G0445 when billed for HIBC to prevent STIs. A claim that is submitted with HCPCS code G0445 for HIBC shall be submitted with ICD-9 diagnosis code V69.8.

Medicare contractors shall pay for screening for chlamydia, gonorrhea, and syphilis (As indicated by the presence of ICD-9 diagnosis code V74.5); and/or hepatitis B (as indicated by the presence of ICD-9 diagnosis code V73.89) as follows:

- One annual occurrence of screening for chlamydia, gonorrhea, and syphilis (i.e., 1 per 12-month period) in women at increased risk who are not pregnant,
- One annual occurrence of screening for syphilis (i.e., 1 per 12-month period) in men at increased risk,
- Up to two occurrences per pregnancy of screening for chlamydia and gonorrhea in pregnant women who are at increased risk for STIs and continued increased risk for the second screening,
- One occurrence per pregnancy of screening for syphilis in pregnant women,
- Up to an additional two occurrences per pregnancy of screening for syphilis in pregnant women if the beneficiary is at continued increased risk for STIs,
- One occurrence per pregnancy of screening for hepatitis B in pregnant women, and,
- One additional occurrence per pregnancy of screening for hepatitis B in pregnant women who are at continued increased risk for STIs.

100-4,18,170.4

Types of Bill (TOBs) and Revenue Codes

The applicable types of bill (TOBs) for HIBC screening, HCPCS code G0445, are: 13X, 71X, 77X, and 85X.

On institutional claims, TOBs 71X and 77X, use revenue code 052X to ensure coinsurance and deductible are not applied.

Critical access hospitals (CAHs) electing the optional method of payment for outpatient services report this service under revenue codes 096X, 097X, or 098X.

100-4,18,170.5

Specialty Codes and Place of Service (POS)

Medicare provides coverage for screening for chlamydia, gonorrhea, syphilis, and/or hepatitis B and HIBC to prevent STIs only when ordered by a primary care practitioner (physician or non-physician) with any of the following specialty codes:

- 01—General Practice
- 08—Family Practice
- 11—Internal Medicine
- 16—Obstetrics/Gynecology
- 37—Pediatric Medicine
- 38—Geriatric Medicine
- 42—Certified Nurse Midwife
- 50—Nurse Practitioner
- 89—Certified Clinical Nurse Specialist
- 97—Physician Assistant

Medicare provides coverage for HIBC to prevent STIs only when provided by a primary care practitioner (physician or non-physician) with any of the specialty codes identified above.

Medicare provides coverage for HIBC to prevent STIs only when the POS billed is 11, 22, 49, or 71.

100-4, 20, 100.2.2

Evidence of Medical Necessity for Parenteral and Enteral Nutrition (PEN) Therapy

The PEN coverage is determined by information provided by the treating physician and the PEN supplier. A completed certification of medical necessity (CMN) must accompany and support initial claims for PEN to establish whether coverage criteria are met and to ensure that the PEN therapy provided is consistent with the attending or ordering physician's prescription.

Contractors ensure that the CMN contains pertinent information from the treating physician. Uniform specific medical data facilitate the review and promote consistency in coverage determinations and timelier claims processing.The medical and prescription information on a PEN CMN can be most appropriately completed by the treating physician or from information in the patient's records by an employee of the physician for the physician's review and signature.

Although PEN suppliers sometimes may assist in providing the PEN services, they cannot complete the CMN since they do not have the same access to patient information needed to properly enter medical or prescription information. Contractors use appropriate professional relations issuances, training sessions, and meetings to ensure that all persons and PEN suppliers are aware of this limitation of their role. When properly completed, the PEN CMN includes the elements of a prescription as well as other data needed to determine whether Medicare coverage is possible. This practice will facilitate prompt delivery of PEN services and timely submittal of the related claim.

100-4, 32, 10.1

Ambulatory Blood Pressure Monitoring (ABPM) Billing Requirements

A. Coding Applicable to A/B MACs (A and B)

Effective April 1, 2002, a National Coverage Decision was made to allow for Medicare coverage of ABPM for those beneficiaries with suspected "white coat hypertension" (WCH). ABPM involves the use of a non-invasive device, which is used to measure blood pressure in 24-hour cycles. These 24-hour measurements are stored in the device and are later interpreted by a physician. Suspected "WCH" is defined as: (1) Clinic/office blood pressure >140/90 mm Hg on at least three separate clinic/office visits with two separate measurements made at each visit; (2) At least two documented separate blood pressure measurements taken outside the clinic/office which are < 140/90 mm Hg; and (3) No evidence of end-organ damage. ABPM is not covered for any other uses. Coverage policy can be found in Medicare National Coverage Determinations Manual, Chapter 1, Section 20.19. (http://www.cms.hhs.gov/manuals/103_cov_determ/ncd103index.asp).

The ABPM must be performed for at least 24 hours to meet coverage criteria. Payment is not allowed for institutionalized beneficiaries, such as those receiving Medicare covered skilled nursing in a facility. In the rare circumstance that ABPM needs to be performed more than once for a beneficiary, the qualifying criteria described above must be met for each subsequent ABPM test.

Effective dates for applicable Common Procedure Coding System (HCPCS) codes for ABPM for suspected WCH and their covered effective dates are as follows:

HCPCS	Definition	Effective Date
93784	ABPM, utilizing a system such as magnetic tape and/or computer disk, for 24 hours or longer; including recording, scanning analysis, interpretation and report.	04/01/2002
93786	ABPM, utilizing a system such as magnetic tape and/or computer disk, for 24 hours or longer; recording only.	04/01/2002
93788	ABPM, utilizing a system such as magnetic tape and/or computer disk, for 24 hours or longer; scanning analysis with report.	01/01/2004

HCPCS Definition Effective Date

93790	ABPM, utilizing a system such as magnetic tape and/or computer disk, for 24 hours or longer; physician review with interpretation and report.	04/01/2002

In addition, one of the following diagnosis codes must be present:

	Diagnosis Code	Description
If ICD-9-CM is applicable	796.2	Elevated blood pressure reading without diagnosis of hypertension.
If ICD-10-CM is applicable	R03.0	Elevated blood pressure reading without diagnosis of hypertension

B. A/B MAC (A) Billing Instructions

The applicable types of bills acceptable when billing for ABPM services are 13X, 23X, 71X, 73X, 75X, and 85X. Chapter 25 of this manual provides general billing instructions that must be followed for bills submitted to A/B MACs (A). The A/B MACs (A) pay for hospital outpatient ABPM services billed on a 13X type of bill with HCPCS

93786 and/or 93788 as follows: (1) Outpatient Prospective Payment System (OPPS) hospitals pay based on the Ambulatory Payment Classification (APC); (2) non-OPPS hospitals (Indian Health Services Hospitals, Hospitals that provide Part B services only, and hospitals located in American Samoa, Guam, Saipan and the Virgin Islands) pay based on reasonable cost, except for Maryland Hospitals which are paid based on a percentage of cost. Effective 4/1/06, type of bill 14X is for non-patient laboratory specimens and is no longer applicable for ABPM.

The A/B MACs (A) pay for comprehensive outpatient rehabilitation facility (CORF) ABPM services billed on a 75x type of bill with HCPCS code 93786 and/or 93788 based on the Medicare Physician Fee Schedule (MPFS) amount for that HCPCS code.

The A/B MACs (A) pay for ABPM services for critical access hospitals (CAHs) billed on a 85x type of bill as follows: (1) for CAHs that elected the Standard Method and billed HCPCS code 93786 and/or 93788, pay based on reasonable cost for that HCPCS code; and (2) for CAHs that elected the Optional Method and billed any combination of HCPCS codes 93786, 93788 and 93790 pay based on reasonable cost for HCPCS 93786 and 93788 and pay 115% of the MPFS amount for HCPCS 93790.

The A/B MACs (A) pay for ABPM services for skilled nursing facility (SNF) outpatients billed on a 23x type of bill with HCPCS code 93786 and/or 93788, based on the MPFS.

The A/B MACs (A) accept independent and provider-based rural health clinic (RHC) bills for visits under the all-inclusive rate when the RHC bills on a 71x type of bill with revenue code 052x for providing the professional component of ABPM services. The A/B MACs (A) should not make a separate payment to a RHC for the professional component of ABPM services in addition to the all-inclusive rate. RHCs are not required to use ABPM HCPCS codes for professional services covered under the all-inclusive rate.

The A/B MACs (A) accept free-standing and provider-based federally qualified health center (FQHC) bills for visits under the all-inclusive rate when the FQHC bills on a 73x type of bill with revenue code 052x for providing the professional component of ABPM services.

The A/B MACs (A) should not make a separate payment to a FQHC for the professional component of ABPM services in addition to the all-inclusive rate. FQHCs are not required to use ABPM HCPCS codes for professional services covered under the all-inclusive rate.

The A/B MACs (A) pay provider-based RHCs/FQHCs for the technical component of ABPM services when billed under the base provider's number using the above requirements for that particular base provider type, i.e., a OPPS hospital based RHC would be paid for the ABPM technical component services under the OPPS using the APC for code 93786 and/or 93788 when billed on a 13x type of bill.

Independent and free-standing RHC/FQHC practitioners are only paid for providing the technical component of ABPM services when billed to the A/B MAC (B) following the MAC's instructions.

C. A/B MAC (B) Claims

A/B MACs (B) pay for ABPM services billed with ICD-9-CM diagnosis code 796.2 (if ICD-9 is applicable) or, if ICD-10 is applicable, ICD-10-CM diagnosis code R03.0 and HCPCS codes 93784 or for any combination of 93786, 93788 and 93790, based on the MPFS for the specific HCPCS code billed.

D. Coinsurance and Deductible

The A/B MACs (A and B) shall apply coinsurance and deductible to payments for ABPM services except for services billed to the A/B MAC (A) by FQHCs. For FQHCs only co-insurance applies.

100-4, 32, 12

Smoking and Tobacco-Use Cessation Counseling Services

Background: Effective for services furnished on or after March 22, 2005, a National Coverage Determination (NCD) provides for coverage of smoking and tobacco-use cessation counseling services. Conditions of Medicare Part A and Medicare Part B coverage for smoking and tobacco-use cessation counseling services are located in the Medicare National Coverage Determinations Manual, Publication 100-3, section 210.4.

100 4, 32, 12.1

HCPCS and Diagnosis Coding

The following HCPCS codes should be reported when billing for smoking and tobacco- use cessation counseling services:

99406 Smoking and tobacco-use cessation counseling visit; intermediate, greater than 3 minutes up to 10 minutes

99407 Smoking and tobacco-use cessation counseling visit; intensive, greater than 10 minutes

Note the above codes are payable for dates of service on or after January 1, 2008. Codes G0375 and G0376, below, are not valid or payable for dates of service on or after January 1, 2008.

G0375 Smoking and tobacco-use cessation counseling visit; intermediate, greater than 3 minutes up to 10 minutes

Short Descriptor: Smoke/Tobacco counseling 3-10

G0376 Smoking and tobacco-use cessation counseling visit; intensive, greater than 10 minutes

Short Descriptor: Smoke/Tobacco counseling greater than 10

NOTE: The above G codes will NOT be active in contractors' systems until July 5, 2005. Therefore, contractors shall advise providers to use unlisted code 99199 to bill for smoking and tobacco- use cessation counseling services during the interim period of March 22, 2005, through July 4, 2005, and received prior to July 5, 2005.

On July 5, 2005, contractors' systems will accept the new G codes for services performed on and after March 22, 2005.

Contractors shall allow payment for a medically necessary E/M service on the same day as the smoking and tobacco-use cessation counseling service when it is clinically appropriate. Physicians and qualified non-physician practitioners shall use an appropriate HCPCS code, such as HCPCS 99201- 99215, to report an E/M service with modifier 25 to indicate that the E/M service is a separately identifiable service from G0375 or G0376.

Contractors shall only pay for 8 Smoking and Tobacco-Use Cessation Counseling sessions in a 12-month period. The beneficiary may receive another 8 sessions during a second or subsequent year after 11 full months have passed since the first Medicare covered cessation session was performed. To start the count for the second or subsequent 12-month period, begin with the month after the month in which the first Medicare covered cessation session was performed and count until 11 full months have elapsed.

Claims for smoking and tobacco use cessation counseling services shall be submitted with an appropriate diagnosis code. Diagnosis codes should reflect: the condition the patient has that is adversely affected by tobacco use or the condition the patient is being treated for with a therapeutic agent whose metabolism or dosing is affected by tobacco use.

NOTE: This decision does not modify existing coverage for minimal cessation counseling (defined as 3 minutes or less in duration) which is already considered to be covered as part of each Evaluation and Management (E/M) visit and is not separately billable.

100-4, 32, 12.2

A/B MAC (B) Billing Requirements

A/B MACs (B) shall pay for counseling services billed with codes 99406 and 99407 for dates of service on or after January 1, 2008. A/B MACs (B) shall pay for counseling services billed with codes G0375 and G0376 for dates of service performed on and after March 22, 2005 through Dec. 31, 2007. The type of service (TOS) for each of the new codes is 1.

A/B MACs (B) pay for counseling services billed based on the Medicare Physician Fee Schedule (MPFS). Deductible and coinsurance apply. Claims from physicians or other providers where assignment was not taken are subject to the Medicare limiting charge, which means that charges to the beneficiary may be no more than 115 percent of the allowed amount.

Physicians or qualified non-physician practitioners shall bill the A/B MAC (B) for smoking and tobacco-use cessation counseling services using the ASC X12 837 professional claim format or the Form CMS-1500.

100-4, 32, 12.3

A/B MAC (A) Billing Requirements

The A/B MACs (A) shall pay for Smoking and Tobacco-Use Cessation Counseling services with codes 99406 and 99407 for dates of service on or after January 1, 2008. A/B MACs (A) shall pay for counseling services billed with codes G0375 and G0376 for dates of service performed on or after March 22, 2005 through December 31, 2007.

A. Claims for Smoking and Tobacco-Use Cessation Counseling Services should be submitted using the ASC X12 837 institutional claim format or Form CMS-1450. The applicable bill types are 12X, 13X, 22X, 23X, 34X, 71X, 73X, 83X, and 85X. Effective 4/1/06, type of bill 14X is for non-patient laboratory specimens and is no longer applicable for Smoking and Tobacco-Use Cessation Counseling services.

Applicable revenue codes are as follows:

Provider Type	Revenue Code
Rural Health Centers (RHCs)/Federally Qualified Health Centers (FQHCs)	052X
Indian Health Services (IHS)	0510
Critical Access Hospitals (CAHs) Method II	096X, 097X, 098X
All Other Providers	0942

NOTE: When these services are provided by a clinical nurse specialist in the RHC/FQHC setting, they are considered "incident to" and do not constitute a billable visit.

Payment for outpatient services is as follows:

Type of Facility	Method of Payment
Rural Health Centers (RHCs)/Federally Qualified Health Centers (FQHCs)	All-inclusive rate (AIR) for the encounter
Indian Health Service (IHS)/Tribally owned or operated hospitals and hospital- based facilities	All-inclusive rate (AIR)
IHS/Tribally owned or operated non-hospital-based facilities	Medicare Physician Fee Schedule (MPFS)

Type of Facility	Method of Payment
IHS/Tribally owned or operated Critical Access Hospitals (CAHs)	Facility Specific Visit Rate
Hospitals subject to the Outpatient Prospective Payment System (OPPS)	Ambulatory Payment Classification (APC)
Hospitals not subject to OPPS	Payment is made under current methodologies
Skilled Nursing Facilities (SNFs) NOTE: Included in Part A PPS for skilled patients.	Medicare Physician Fee Schedule (MPFS)
Home Health Agencies (HHAs)	Medicare Physician Fee Schedule (MPFS)
Critical Access Hospitals (CAHs)	Method I: Technical services are paid at 101% of reasonable cost. Method II: technical services are paid at 101% of reasonable cost, and Professional services are paid at 115% of the MMPFS Data Base
Maryland Hospitals	Payment is based according to the Health Services Cost Review Commission (HSCRC). That is 94% of submitted charges subject to any unmet deductible, coinsurance, and non-covered charges policies.

NOTE: Inpatient claims submitted with Smoking and Tobacco-Use Cessation Counseling Services are processed under the current payment methodologies.

100-4, 32, 30.1

Billing Requirements for HBO Therapy for the Treatment of Diabetic Wounds of the Lower Extremities

Hyperbaric Oxygen Therapy is a modality in which the entire body is exposed to oxygen under increased atmospheric pressure. Effective April 1, 2003, a National Coverage Decision expanded the use of HBO therapy to include coverage for the treatment of diabetic wounds of the lower extremities. For specific coverage criteria for HBO Therapy, refer to the National Coverage Determinations Manual, chapter 1, section 20.29.

NOTE: Topical application of oxygen does not meet the definition of HBO therapy as stated above. Also, its clinical efficacy has not been established. Therefore, no Medicare reimbursement may be made for the topical application of oxygen.

I. Billing Requirements for A/B MACs (A)
Claims for HBO therapy should be submitted using the ASC X12 837 institutional claim format or, in rare cases, on Form CMS-1450.

a. Applicable Bill Types
The applicable hospital bill types are 11X, 13X and 85X.

b. Procedural Coding

99183 Physician attendance and supervision of hyperbaric oxygen therapy, per session.

C1300 Hyperbaric oxygen under pressure, full body chamber, per 30-minute interval.

NOTE: Code C1300 is not available for use other than in a hospital outpatient department. In skilled nursing facilities (SNFs), HBO therapy is part of the SNF PPS payment for beneficiaries in covered Part A stays.

For hospital inpatients and critical access hospitals (CAHs) not electing Method I, HBO therapy is reported under revenue code 940 without any HCPCS code. For inpatient services, if ICD-9-is applicable, show ICD-9-CM procedure code 93.59. If ICD-10 is applicable, show ICD-10-PCS code 5A05121.

For CAHs electing Method I, HBO therapy is reported under revenue code 940 along with HCPCS code 99183.

c. Payment Requirements for A/B MACs (A)
Payment is as follows:

A/B MACs (A) payment is allowed for HBO therapy for diabetic wounds of the lower extremities when performed as a physician service in a hospital outpatient setting and for inpatients. Payment is allowed for claims with valid diagnosis codes as shown above with dates of service on or after April 1, 2003. Those claims with invalid codes should be denied as not medically necessary.

For hospitals, payment will be based upon the Ambulatory Payment Classification (APC) or the inpatient Diagnosis Related Group (DRG). Deductible and coinsurance apply.

Payment to Critical Access Hospitals (electing Method I) is made under cost reimbursement. For Critical Access Hospitals electing Method II, the technical component is paid under cost reimbursement and the professional component is paid under the Physician Fee Schedule.

NOTE: Information regarding the form locator numbers that correspond to these data element names and a table to crosswalk UB-04 form locators to the 837 transaction is found in Chapter 25.

II. A/B MAC (B) Billing Requirements
Claims for this service should be submitted using the ASC X12 837 professional claim format or Form CMS-1500.

The following HCPCS code applies:

- 99183 - Physician attendance and supervision of hyperbaric oxygen therapy, per session.

a. Payment Requirements for A/B MACs (B)
Payment and pricing information will occur through updates to the Medicare Physician Fee Schedule Database (MPFSDB). Pay for this service on the basis of the MPFSDB. Deductible and coinsurance apply. Claims from physicians or other practitioners where assignment was not taken, are subject to the Medicare limiting charge.

III. Medicare Summary Notices (MSNs)
Use the following MSN Messages where appropriate:

In situations where the claim is being denied on the basis that the condition does not meet our coverage requirements, use one of the following MSN Messages:

"Medicare does not pay for this item or service for this condition." (MSN Message 16.48)

The Spanish version of the MSN message should read:

"Medicare no paga por este articulo o servicio para esta afeccion."

In situations where, based on the above utilization policy, medical review of the claim results in a determination that the service is not medically necessary, use the following MSN message:

"The information provided does not support the need for this service or item." (MSN Message 15.4)

The Spanish version of the MSN message should read:

"La informacion proporcionada no confirma la necesidad para este servicio o articulo."

IV. Remittance Advice Notices
Use appropriate existing remittance advice remark codes and claim adjustment reason codes at the line level to express the specific reason if you deny payment for HBO therapy for the treatment of diabetic wounds of lower extremities.

100-4, 32, 40

Sacral Nerve Stimulation

A sacral nerve stimulator is a pulse generator that transmits electrical impulses to the sacral nerves through an implanted wire. These impulses cause the bladder muscles to contract, which gives the patient ability to void more properly.

100-4, 32, 40.1

Coverage Requirements

Effective January 1, 2002, sacral nerve stimulation is covered for the treatment of urinary urge incontinence, urgency-frequency syndrome and urinary retention. Sacral nerve stimulation involves both a temporary test stimulation to determine if an implantable stimulator would be effective and a permanent implantation in appropriate candidates. Both the test and the permanent implantation are covered.

The following limitations for coverage apply to all indications:

- Patient must be refractory to conventional therapy (documented behavioral, pharmacologic and/or surgical corrective therapy) and be an appropriate surgical candidate such that implantation with anesthesia can occur.
- Patients with stress incontinence, urinary obstruction, and specific neurologic diseases (e.g., diabetes with peripheral nerve involvement) that are associated with secondary manifestations of the above three indications are excluded.
- Patient must have had a successful test stimulation in order to support subsequent implantation. Before a patient is eligible for permanent implantation, he/she must demonstrate a 50% or greater improvement through test stimulation. Improvement is measured through voiding diaries.
- Patient must be able to demonstrate adequate ability to record voiding diary data such that clinical results of the implant procedure can be properly evaluated.

100-4, 32, 40.2.2

Payment Requirements for Test Procedures (HCPCS Codes 64585, 64590 and 64595)

Payment is as follows:

- Hospital outpatient departments ?OPPS
- Critical access hospital (CAH) - Reasonable cost
- Comprehensive outpatient rehabilitation facility - Medicare physician fee schedule (MPFS)
- Rural health clinics/federally qualified health centers (RHCs/FQHCs) - All inclusive rate, professional component only. The technical component is outside the scope of the RHC/FQHC benefit. Therefore, the provider of that technical service bills their A/B MAC (B) using the ASC X12 837 professional claim format or Form CMS-1500 and payment is made under the MPFS. For provider-based RHCs/FQHCs payment for the technical component is made as indicated above based on the type of provider the RHC/FQHC is based with.

Deductible and coinsurance apply.

100-4, 32, 50

Deep Brain Stimulation for Essential Tremor and Parkinson's Disease

Deep brain stimulation (DBS) refers to high-frequency electrical stimulation of anatomic regions deep within the brain utilizing neurosurgically implanted electrodes. These DBS electrodes are stereotactically placed within targeted nuclei on one (unilateral) or both (bilateral) sides of the brain. There are currently three targets for DBS -- the thalamic ventralis intermedius nucleus (VIM), subthalamic nucleus (STN) and globus pallidus interna (GPi).

Essential tremor (ET) is a progressive, disabling tremor most often affecting the hands. ET may also affect the head, voice and legs. The precise pathogenesis of ET is unknown. While it may start at any age, ET usually peaks within the second and sixth decades. Beta-adrenergic blockers and anticonvulsant medications are usually the first line treatments for reducing the severity of tremor. Many patients, however, do not adequately respond or cannot tolerate these medications. In these medically refractory ET patients, thalamic VIM DBS may be helpful for symptomatic relief of tremor.

Parkinson's disease (PD) is an age-related progressive neurodegenerative disorder involving the loss of dopaminergic cells in the substantia nigra of the midbrain. The disease is characterized by tremor, rigidity, bradykinesia and progressive postural instability. Dopaminergic medication is typically used as a first line treatment for reducing the primary symptoms of PD. However, after prolonged use, medication can become less effective and can produce significant adverse events such as dyskinesias and other motor function complications. For patients who become unresponsive to medical treatments and/or have intolerable side effects from medications, DBS for symptom relief may be considered.

100-4, 32, 60.4.1

Allowable Covered Diagnosis Codes

For services furnished on or after July 1, 2002, the applicable ICD-9-CM diagnosis code for this benefit is V43.3, organ or tissue replaced by other means; heart valve.

For services furnished on or after March 19, 2008, the applicable ICD-9-CM diagnosis codes for this benefit are:

- V43.3 (organ or tissue replaced by other means; heart valve),
- 289.81 (primary hypercoagulable state),
- 451.0-451.9 (includes 451.11, 451.19, 451.2, 451.80-451.84, 451.89) (phlebitis & thrombophlebitis),
- 453.0-453.3 (other venous embolism & thrombosis),
- 453.40-453.49 (includes 453.40-453.42, 453.8-453.9) (venous embolism and thrombosis of the deep vessels of the lower extremity, and other specified veins/unspecified sites)
- 415.11-415.12, 415.19 (pulmonary embolism & infarction) or,
- 427.31 (atrial fibrillation (established) (paroxysmal)).

100-4, 32, 60.5.2

Applicable Diagnosis Codes for Carriers

For services furnished on or after July 1, 2002, the applicable ICD-9-CM diagnosis code for this benefit is V43.3, organ or tissue replaced by other means; heart valve.

For services furnished on or after March 19, 2008, the applicable ICD-9-CM diagnosis codes for this benefit are:

- V43.3 (organ or tissue replaced by other means; heart valve),
- 289.81 (primary hypercoagulable state),
- 451.0-451.9 (includes 451.11, 451.19, 451.2, 451.80-451.84, 451.89) (phlebitis & thrombophlebitis),
- 453.0-453.3 (other venous embolism & thrombosis),
- 453.40-453.49 (includes 453.40-453.42, 453.8-453.9) (venous embolism and thrombosis of the deep vessels of the lower extremity, and other specified veins/unspecified sites)
- 415.11-415.12, 415.19 (pulmonary embolism & infarction) or,
- 427.31 (atrial fibrillation (established) (paroxysmal)).

100-4, 32, 60.12

Coverage for PET Scans for Dementia and Neurodegenerative DiseasesCoverage for PET Scans for Dementia and Neurodegenerative Diseases

Effective for dates of service on or after September 15, 2004, Medicare will cover FDG PET scans for a differential diagnosis of fronto-temporal dementia (FTD) and Alzheimer's disease OR; its use in a CMS-approved practical clinical trial focused on the utility of FDG-PET in the diagnosis or treatment of dementing neurodegenerative diseases. Refer to Pub. 100-03, NCD Manual, section 220.6.13, for complete coverage conditions and clinical trial requirements and section 60.15 of this manual for claims processing information.

A. Carrier and FI Billing Requirements for PET Scan Claims for FDG-PET for the Differential Diagnosis of Fronto-temporal Dementia and Alzheimer's Disease:

- **CPT Code for PET Scans for Dementia and Neurodegenerative Diseases**

  Contractors shall advise providers to use the appropriate CPT code from section 60.3.1 for dementia and neurodegenerative diseases for services performed on or after January 28, 2005.

- **Diagnosis Codes for PET Scans for Dementia and Neurodegenerative Diseases**

  The contractor shall ensure one of the following appropriate diagnosis codes is present on claims for PET Scans for AD:

  - 290.0, 290.10 - 290.13, 290.20 - 290, 21, 290.3, 331.0, 331.11, 331.19, 331.2, 331.9, 780.93

  Medicare contractors shall use an appropriate Medicare Summary Notice (MSN) message such as 16.48, "Medicare does not pay for this item or service for this condition" to deny claims when submitted with an appropriate CPT code from section 60.3.1 and with a diagnosis code other than the range of codes listed above. Also, contractors shall use an appropriate Remittance Advice (RA) such as 11, "The diagnosis is inconsistent with the procedure."

  Medicare contractors shall instruct providers to issue an Advanced Beneficiary Notice to beneficiaries advising them of potential financial liability prior to delivering the service if one of the appropriate diagnosis codes will not be present on the claim.

- **Provider Documentation Required with the PET Scan Claim**

  Medicare contractors shall inform providers to ensure the conditions mentioned in the NCD Manual, section 220.6.13, have been met. The information must also be maintained in the beneficiary's medical record:

  - Date of onset of symptoms;
  - Diagnosis of clinical syndrome (normal aging, mild cognitive impairment or MCI: mild, moderate, or severe dementia);
  - Mini mental status exam (MMSE) or similar test score;
  - Presumptive cause (possible, probably, uncertain AD);
  - Any neuropsychological testing performed;
  - Results of any structural imaging (MRI, CT) performed;
  - Relevant laboratory tests (B12, thyroid hormone); and,
  - Number and name of prescribed medications.

B. Billing Requirements for Beta Amyloid Positron Emission Tomography (PET) in Dementia and Neurodegenerative Disease:

Effective for claims with dates of service on and after September 27, 2013, Medicare will only allow coverage with evidence development (CED) for Positron Emission Tomography (PET) beta amyloid (also referred to as amyloid-beta (Aß)) imaging (HCPCS A9586)or (HCPCS A9599) (one PET Aß scan per patient).

Note: Please note that effective January 1, 2014 the following code A9599 will be updated in the IOCE and HCPCS update. This code will be contractor priced.

Medicare Summary Notices, Remittance Advice Remark Codes, and Claim Adjustment Reason Codes

Effective for dates of service on or after September 27, 2013, contractors shall **return as unprocessable/return to provider** claims for PET Aß imaging, through CED during a clinical trial, not containing the following:

- Condition code 30, (FI only)
- Modifier Q0 and/or modifier Q1 as appropriate
- ICD-9 dx code V70.7/ICD-10 dx code Z00.6 (on either the primary/secondary position)
- A PET HCPCS code (78811 or 78814)
- At least, one Dx code from the table below

ICD-9 Codes	Corresponding ICD-10 Codes
290.0 Senile dementia, uncomplicated	F03.90 Unspecified dementia without behavioral disturbance
290.10 Presenile dementia, uncomplicated	F03.90 Unspecified dementia without behavioral disturbance
290.11 Presenile dementia with delirium	F03.90 Unspecified dementia without behavioral disturbance
290.12 Presenile dementia with delusional features	F03.90 Unspecified dementia without behavioral disturbance
290.13 Presenile dementia with depressive features	F03.90 Unspecified dementia without behavioral disturbance
290.20 Senile dementia with delusional features	F03.90 Unspecified dementia without behavioral disturbance
290.21 Senile dementia with depressive features	F03.90 Unspecified dementia without behavioral disturbance
290.3 Senile dementia with delirium	F03.90 Unspecified dementia without behavioral disturbance

ICD-9 Codes	Corresponding ICD-10 Codes
290.40 Vascular dementia, uncomplicated	F01.50 Vascular dementia without behavioral disturbance
290.41 Vascular dementia with delirium	F01.51 Vascular dementia with behavioral disturbance
290.42 Vascular dementia with delusions	F01.51 Vascular dementia with behavioral disturbance
290.43 Vascular dementia with depressed mood	F01.51 Vascular dementia with behavioral disturbance
294.10 Dementia in conditions classified elsewhere without behavioral disturbance	F02.80 Dementia in other diseases classified elsewhere without behavioral disturbance
294.11 Dementia in conditions classified elsewhere with behavioral disturbance	F02.81 Dementia in other diseases classified elsewhere with behavioral disturbance
294.20 Dementia, unspecified, without behavioral disturbance	F03.90 Unspecified dementia without behavioral disturbance
294.21 Dementia, unspecified, with behavioral disturbance	F03.91 Unspecified dementia with behavioral disturbance
331.11 Pick's Disease	G31.01 Pick's disease
331.19 Other Frontotemporal dementia	G31.09 Other frontotemporal dementia
331.6 Corticobasal degeneration	G31.85 Corticobasal degeneration
331.82 Dementia with Lewy Bodies	G31.83 Dementia with Lewy bodies
331.83 Mild cognitive impairment, so stated	G31.84 Mild cognitive impairment, so stated
780.93 Memory Loss	R41.1 Anterograde amnesia R41.2 Retrograde amnesia R41.3 Other amnesia (Amnesia NOS, Memory loss NOS)
V70.7 Examination for normal comparison or control in clinical	Z00.6 Encounter for examination for normal comparison and control in clinical research program

and

- Aß HCPCS code A9586 or A9599

Contractors shall return as unprocessable claims for PET Aß imaging using the following messages:

- Claim Adjustment Reason Code 4 ?the procedure code is inconsistent with the modifier used or a required modifier is missing.

  Note: Refer to the 835 Healthcare Policy Identification Segment (loop 2110 Service Payment Information REF), if present.
- Remittance Advice Remark Code N517 - Resubmit a new claim with the requested information.
- Remittance Advice Remark Code N519 - Invalid combination of HCPCS modifiers.

Contractors shall line-item deny claims for PET Aß, HCPCS code A9586 or A9599, where a previous PET Aß, HCPCS code A9586 or A9599 is paid in history using the following messages:

- CARC 149: "Lifetime benefit maximum has been reached for this service/benefit category"
- RARC N587: "Policy benefits have been exhausted"
- MSN 20.12: "This service was denied because Medicare only covers this service once a lifetime."
- Spanish Version: "Este servicio fue negado porque Medicare sólo cubre este servicio una vez en la vida."
- Group Code: PR, if a claim is received with a GA modifier
- Group Code: CO, if a claim is received with a GZ modifier

100-4, 32, 80.8

CWF Utilization Edits

Edit 1 - Should CWF receive a claim from an FI for G0245 or G0246 and a second claim from a contractor for either G0245 or G0246 (or vice versa) and they are different dates of service and less than 6 months apart, the second claim will reject. CWF will edit to allow G0245 or G0246 to be paid no more than every 6 months for a particular beneficiary, regardless of who furnished the service. If G0245 has been paid, regardless of whether it was posted as a facility or professional claim, it must be 6 months before G0245 can be paid again or G0246 can be paid. If G0246 has been paid, regardless of whether it was posted as a facility or professional claim, it must be 6 months before G0246 can be paid again or G0245 can be paid. CWF will not impose limits on how many times each code can be paid for a beneficiary as long as there has been 6 months between each service.

The CWF will return a specific reject code for this edit to the contractors and FIs that will be identified in the CWF documentation. Based on the CWF reject code, the contractors and FIs must deny the claims and return the following messages:

> MSN 18.4 -- This service is being denied because it has not been __ months since your last examination of this kind (NOTE: Insert 6 as the appropriate number of months.)

RA claim adjustment reason code 96 - Non-covered charges, along with remark code M86 - Service denied because payment already made for same/similar procedure within set time frame.

Edit 2 - The CWF will edit to allow G0247 to pay only if either G0245 or G0246 has been submitted and accepted as payable on the same date of service. CWF will return a specific reject code for this edit to the contractors and FIs that will be identified in the CWF documentation. Based on this reject code, contractors and FIs will deny the claims and return the following messages:

> MSN 21.21 - This service was denied because Medicare only covers this service under certain circumstances.
>
> RA claim adjustment reason code 107 - The related or qualifying claim/service was not identified on this claim.

Edit 3 - Once a beneficiary's condition has progressed to the point where routine foot care becomes a covered service, payment will no longer be made for LOPS evaluation and management services. Those services would be considered to be included in the regular exams and treatments afforded to the beneficiary on a routine basis. The physician or provider must then just bill the routine foot care codes, per Pub 100-02, Chapter 15, Sec.290.

The CWF will edit to reject LOPS codes G0245, G0246, and/or G0247 when on the beneficiary's record it shows that one of the following routine foot care codes were billed and paid within the prior 6 months: 11055, 11056, 11057, 11719, 11720, and/or 11721.

The CWF will return a specific reject code for this edit to the contractors and FIs that will be identified in the CWF documentation. Based on the CWF reject code, the contractors and FIs must deny the claims and return the following messages:

> MSN 21.21 - This service was denied because Medicare only covers this service under certain circumstances.

The RA claim adjustment reason code 96 - Non-covered charges, along with remark code M86 - Service denied because payment already made for same/similar procedure within set time frame.

100-4, 32, 90

Stem Cell Transplantation

Stem cell transplantation is a process in which stem cells are harvested from either a patient's or donor's bone marrow or peripheral blood for intravenous infusion. Autologous stem cell transplantation (AuSCT) must be used to effect hematopoietic reconstitution following severely myelotoxic doses of chemotherapy (HDCT) and/or radiotherapy used to treat various malignancies. Allogeneic stem cell transplant may also be used to restore function in recipients having an inherited or acquired deficiency or defect.

Bone marrow and peripheral blood stem cell transplantation is a process which includes mobilization, harvesting, and transplant of bone marrow or peripheral blood stem cells and the administration of high dose chemotherapy or radiotherapy prior to the actual transplant. When bone marrow or peripheral blood stem cell transplantation is covered, all necessary steps are included in coverage. When bone marrow or peripheral blood stem cell transplantation is non-covered, none of the steps are covered.

Allogeneic and autologous stem cell transplants are covered under Medicare for specific diagnoses. See Pub. 100-03, National Coverage Determinations Manual, section 110.8.1, for a complete description of covered and noncovered conditions. For Part A hospital inpatient claims processing instructions, refer to Pub. 100-04, Chapter 3, section 90.3. The following sections contain claims processing instructions for all other claims.

100-4,32,90.2

90.2 - HCPCS and Diagnosis Coding – ICD-9-CM Applicable

(Rev. 2998, Issued: 07-25-14, Effective: Upon implementation of ICD-10; 01-01-12 - ASC X12, Implementation: 08-25-2014 - ASC X12; Upon Implementation of ICD-10)

Allogeneic Stem Cell Transplantation

- Effective for services performed on or after August 1, 1978:
  - For the treatment of leukemia or leukemia in remission, providers shall use

ICD-9-CM codes 204.00 through 208.91 and HCPCS code 38240.

  - For the treatment of aplastic anemia, providers shall use ICD-9-CM codes 284.0 through 284.9 and HCPCS code 38240.
- Effective for services performed on or after June 3, 1985:
  - For the treatment of severe combined immunodeficiency disease, providers shall use ICD-9-CM code 279.2 and HCPCS code 38240.
  - For the treatment of Wiskott-Aldrich syndrome, providers shall use ICD-9-CM code 279.12 and HCPCS code 38240.
- Effective for services performed on or after May 24, 1996:

- Allogeneic stem cell transplantation, HCPCS code 38240 is not covered as treatment for the diagnosis of multiple myeloma ICD-9-CM codes 203.00 or 203.01.

Autologous Stem Cell Transplantation.--Is covered under the following circumstances effective for services performed on or after April 28, 1989:

- For the treatment of patients with acute leukemia in remission who have a high probability of relapse and who have no human leucocyte antigens (HLA) matched, providers shall use ICD-9-CM code 204.01 lymphoid; ICD-9-CM code 205.01 myeloid; ICD-9-CM code 206.01 monocytic; or ICD-9-CM code 207.01 acute erythremia and erythroleukemia; or ICD-9-CM code 208.01 unspecified cell type and HCPCS code 38241.
- For the treatment of resistant non-Hodgkin's lymphomas for those patients presenting with poor prognostic features following an initial response, providers shall use ICD-9-CM codes 200.00 - 200.08, 200.10-200.18, 200.20-200.28, 200.80-200.88, 202.00-202.08, 202.80-202.88 or 202.90-202.98 and HCPCS code 38241.
- For the treatment of recurrent or refractory neuroblastoma, providers shall use ICD-9-CM codes Neoplasm by site, malignant, the appropriate HCPCS code and HCPCS code 38241.
- For the treatment of advanced Hodgkin's disease for patients whhave failed conventional therapy and have no HLA-matched donor, providers shall use ICD-9-CM codes 201.00 - 201.98 and HCPCS code 38241.

Autologous Stem Cell Transplantation.--Is covered under the following circumstances effective for services furnished on or after October 1, 2000:

- For the treatment of multiple myeloma (only for beneficiaries whare less than age 78, have Durie-Salmon stage II or III newly diagnosed or responsive multiple myeloma, and have adequate cardiac, renal, pulmonary and hepatic functioning), providers shall use ICD- 9-CM code 203.00 or 238.6 and HCPCS code 38241.
- For the treatment of recurrent or refractory neuroblastoma, providers shall use appropriate code (see ICD-9-CM neoplasm by site, malignant) and HCPCS code 38241.
- Effective for services performed on or after March 15, 2005, when recognized clinical risk factors are employed to select patients for transplantation, high-dose melphalan (HDM) together with autologous stem cell transplantation (HDM/AuSCT) is reasonable and necessary for Medicare beneficiaries of any age group for the treatment of primary amyloid light chain (AL) amyloidosis, ICD-9-CM code 277.3 who meet the following criteria:
- Amyloid deposition in 2 or fewer organs; and,
- Cardiac left ventricular ejection fraction (EF) greater than 45%.

100-4,32,90.3

90.3 - Non-Covered Conditions

(Rev. 2998, Issued: 07-25-14, Effective: Upon implementation of ICD-10; 01-01-12 - ASC X12, Implementation: 08-25-2014 - ASC X12; Upon Implementation of ICD-10)

Autologous stem cell transplantation is not covered for the following conditions:

- Acute leukemia not in remission (If ICD-9-CM is applicable, ICD-9-CM codes 204.00, 205.00, 206.00, 207.00 and 208.00) or (If ICD-10-CM is applicable, ICD-10-CM codes C91.00, C92.00, C93.00, C94.00, and C95.00)
- Chronic granulocytic leukemia (ICD-9-CM codes 205.10 and 205.11 if ICD-9-CM is applicable) or (if ICD-10-CM is applicable, ICD-10-CM codes C92.10 and C92.11);
- Solid tumors (other than neuroblastoma) (ICD-9-CM codes 140.0 through 199.1 if ICD-9-CM is applicable or if ICD-10-CM is applicable, iCD-10-CM codes C00.0 – C80.2 and D00.0 – D09.9.)
- Effective for services rendered on or after May 24, 1996 through September 30, 2000, multiple myeloma (ICD-9-CM code 203.00 and 203.01 if ICD-9-CM is applicable or if ICD-10-CM is applicable, ICD-10-CM codes C90.00 and D47.Z9);
- Effective for services on or after October 1, 2000, through March 14, 2005, for Medicare beneficiaries age 64 or older, all forms of amyloidosis, primary and non-primary
- Effective for services on or after 10/01/00, for all Medicare beneficiaries, non-primary amyloidosis

ICD-9-CM	Description	ICD-10-CM	Description
277.30	Amyloidosis, unspecified	E85.9	Amyloidosis, unspecified
277.31	Familial Mediterranean fever	E85.0	Non-neuropathic heredofamilial amyloidosis
277.39	Other amyloidosis	E85.1	Neuropathic heredofamilial amyloidosis
277.39	Other amyloidosis	E85.2	Heredofamilial amyloidosis, unspecified
277.39	Other amyloidosis	E85.3	Secondary systemic amyloidosis
277.39	Other amyloidosis	E85.4	Organ-limited amyloidosis
277.39	Other amyloidosis	E85.8	Other amyloidosis

NOTE: Coverage for conditions other than those specifically designated as covered in 90.2 or 90.2.1 or specifically designated as non-covered in this section will be at the discretion of the individual A/B MAC (B).

100-4,32,90.4

90.4 - Edits

(Rev. 2998, Issued: 07-25-14, Effective: Upon implementation of ICD-10; 01-01-12 - ASC X12, Implementation: 08-25-2014 - ASC X12; Upon Implementation of ICD-10)

NOTE: Coverage for conditions other than those specifically designated as covered in 80.2 or specifically designated as non-covered in this section will be at the discretion of the individual A/B MAC (B).

- Appropriate diagnosis to procedure code edits should be implemented for the non-covered conditions and services in 90.2 90.2.1, and 90.3 as applicable
- As the ICD-9-CM code 277.3 for amyloidosis does not differentiate between primary and non-primary, A/B MACs (B) should perform prepay reviews on all claims with a diagnosis of ICD-9-CM code 277.3 and a HCPCS procedure code of 38241 to determine whether payment is appropriate.

If ICD-10-CM is applicable, the applicable ICD-10 CM codes are: E85.0, E85.1, E85.2, E85.3, E85.4, E85.8, and E85.9.

100-4,32,90.6

90.6 - Clinical Trials for Allogeneic Hematopoietic Stem Cell Transplantation (HSCT) for Myelodysplastic Syndrome (MDS)

(Rev. 2998, Issued: 07-25-14, Effective: Upon implementation of ICD-10; 01-01-12 - ASC X12, Implementation: 08-25-2014 - ASC X12; Upon Implementation of ICD-10)

A.Background

- Myelodysplastic Syndrome (MDS) refers ta group of diverse blood disorders in which the bone marrow does not produce enough healthy, functioning blood cells.These disorders are varied with regard to clinical characteristics, cytologic and pathologic features, and cytogenetics.

On August 4, 2010, the Centers for Medicare & Medicaid Services (CMS) issued a national coverage determination (NCD) stating that CMS believes that the evidence does not demonstrate that the use of allogeneic hematopoietic stem cell transplantation (HSCT) improves health outcomes in Medicare beneficiaries with MDS.Therefore, allogeneic HSCT for MDS is not reasonable and necessary under §1862(a)(1)(A) of the Social

- Security Act (the Act).However, allogeneic HSCT for MDS is reasonable and necessary under §1862(a)(1)(E) of the Act and therefore covered by Medicare ONLY if provided pursuant ta Medicare-approved clinical study under Coverage with Evidence Development (CED). Refer tPub.100-03, National Coverage Determinations Manual, Chapter 1, section 110.8.1, for more information about this policy, and Pub. 100-04, Medicare Claims Processing Manual, Chapter 3, section 90.3.1, for information on CED.

B.Adjudication Requirements

Payable Conditions.For claims with dates of service on and after August 4, 2010, contractors shall pay for claims for HSCT for MDS when the service was provided

100-4, 32, 100

Billing Requirements for Expanded Coverage of Cochlear Implantation

Effective for dates of services on and after April 4, 2005, the Centers for Medicare & Medicaid Services (CMS) has expanded the coverage for cochlear implantation to cover moderate-to-profound hearing loss in individuals with hearing test scores equal to or less than 40% correct in the best aided listening condition on tape-recorded tests of open-set sentence recognition and who demonstrate limited benefit from amplification. (See Publication 100-03, chapter 1, section 50.3, for specific coverage criteria).

In addition CMS is covering cochlear implantation for individuals with open-set sentence recognition test scores of greater than 40% to less than or equal to 60% correct but only when the provider is participating in, and patients are enrolled in, either:

A Food and Drug Administration (FDA)-approved category B investigational device exemption (IDE) clinical trial; or

A trial under the CMS clinical trial policy (see Pub. 100-03, section 310.1); or

A prospective, controlled comparative trial approved by CMS as consistent with the evidentiary requirements for national coverage analyses and meeting specific quality standards.

100-4, 32, 120.2

Coding and General Billing Requirements

Physicians and hospitals must report one of the following Current Procedural Terminology (CPT) codes on the claim:

66982 Extracapsular cataract removal with insertion of intraocular lens prosthesis (one stage procedure), manual or mechanical technique (e.g., irrigation and aspiration or phacoemulsification), complex requiring devices or techniques not generally used in routine cataract surgery (e.g., iris expansion device, suture support for intraocular lens, or primary posterior capsulorrhexis) or performed on patients in the amblyogenic development stage.

66983 Intracapsular cataract with insertion of intraocular lens prosthesis (one stage procedure)

66984 Extracapsular cataract removal with insertion of intraocular lens prosthesis (one stage procedure), manual or mechanical technique (e.g., irrigation and aspiration or phacoemulsification)

66985 Insertion of intraocular lens prosthesis (secondary implant), not associated with concurrent cataract extraction

66986 Exchange of intraocular lens

In addition, physicians inserting a P-C IOL or A-C IOL in an office setting may bill code V2632 (posterior chamber intraocular lens) for the IOL. Medicare will make payment for the lens based on reasonable cost for a conventional IOL. Place of Service (POS) = 11.

Effective for dates of service on and after January 1, 2006, physician, hospitals and ASCs may also bill the non-covered charges related to the P-C function of the IOL using HCPCS code V2788. Effective for dates of service on and after January 22, 2007 through January 1, 2008, non-covered charges related to A-C function of the IOL can be billed using HCPCS code V2788. The type of service indicator for the non-covered billed charges is Q. (The type of service is applied by the Medicare carrier and not the provider). Effective for A-C IOL insertion services on or after January 1, 2008, physicians, hospitals and ASCs should use V2787 rather than V2788 to report any additional charges that accrue.

When denying the non-payable charges submitted with V2787 or V2788, contractors shall use an appropriate Medical Summary Notice (MSN) such as 16.10 (Medicare does not pay for this item or service) and an appropriate claim adjustment reason code such as 96 (non-covered charges) for claims submitted with the non-payable charges.

Hospitals and physicians may use the proper CPT code(s) to bill Medicare for evaluation and management services usually associated with services following cataract extraction surgery, if appropriate.

A - Applicable Bill Types

The hospital applicable bill types are 12X, 13X, 83X and 85X.

B - Other Special Requirements for Hospitals

Hospitals shall continue to pay CAHs method 2 claims under current payment methodologies for conditional IOLs.

100-4, 32, 130

External Counterpulsation (ECP) Therapy

Commonly referred to as enhanced external counterpulsation, is a non-invasive outpatient treatment for coronary artery disease refractory medical and/or surgical therapy. Effective for dates of service July 1, 1999, and after, Medicare will cover ECP when its use is in patients with stable angina (Class III or Class IV, Canadian Cardiovascular Society Classification or equivalent classification) who, in the opinion of a cardiologist or cardiothoracic surgeon, are not readily amenable to surgical intervention, such as PTCA or cardiac bypass, because:

- Their condition is inoperable, or at high risk of operative complications or post-operative failure;
- Their coronary anatomy is not readily amenable to such procedures; or
- They have co-morbid states that create excessive risk.

(Refer to Publication 100-03, section 20.20 for further coverage criteria.)

100-4, 32, 130.1

Billing and Payment Requirements

Effective for dates of service on or after January 1, 2000, use HCPCS code G0166 (External counterpulsation, per session) to report ECP services. The codes for external cardiac assist (92971), ECG rhythm strip and report (93040 or 93041), pulse oximetry (94760 or 94761) and plethysmography (93922 or 93923) or other monitoring tests for examining the effects of this treatment are not clinically necessary with this service and should not be paid on the same day, unless they occur in a clinical setting not connected with the delivery of the ECP. Daily evaluation and management service, e.g., 99201-99205, 99211-99215, 99217-99220, 99241-99245, cannot be billed with the ECP treatments. Any evaluation and management service must be justified with adequate documentation of the medical necessity of the visit. Deductible and coinsurance apply.

100-4, 32, 140.2

Cardiac Rehabilitation Program Services Furnished On or After January 1, 2010

As specified at 42 CFR 410.49, Medicare covers cardiac rehabilitation items and services for patients who have experienced one or more of the following:

- An acute myocardial infarction within the preceding 12 months; or
- A coronary artery bypass surgery; or
- Current stable angina pectoris; or
- Heart valve repair or replacement; or
- Percutaneous transluminal coronary angioplasty (PTCA) or coronary stenting; or
- A heart or heart-lung transplant; or
- A stable, chronic heart failure defined as patients with left ventricular ejection fraction of 35% or less and New York Heart Association (NYHA) class II to IV symptoms despite being on optimal heart failure therapy for at least 6 weeks (effective February 18, 2014).

Cardiac rehabilitation programs must include the following components:

- Physician-prescribed exercise each day cardiac rehabilitation items and services are furnished;
- Cardiac risk factor modification, including education, counseling, and behavioral intervention at least once during the program, tailored to patients' individual needs;
- Psychosocial assessment;
- Outcomes assessment; and
- An individualized treatment plan detailing how components are utilized for each patient.

Cardiac rehabilitation items and services must be furnished in a physician's office or a hospital outpatient setting. All settings must have a physician immediately available and accessible for medical consultations and emergencies at all time items and services are being furnished under the program. This provision is satisfied if the physician meets the requirements for the direct supervision of physician's office services as specified at 42 CFR 410.26 and for hospital outpatient therapeutic services as specified at 42 CFR 410.27.

As specified at 42 CFR 410.49(f)(1), cardiac rehabilitation program sessions are limited to a maximum of 2 1-hour sessions per day for up to 36 sessions over up to 36 weeks, with the option for an additional 36 sessions over an extended period of time if approved by the Medicare contractor.

100-4, 32, 140.2.1

Coding Requirements for Cardiac Rehabilitation Services Furnished On or After January 1, 2010

The following are the applicable CPT codes for cardiac rehabilitation services: 93797 - Physician services for outpatient cardiac rehabilitation; without continuous ECG monitoring (per session) and 93798 - Physician services for outpatient cardiac rehabilitation; with continuous ECG monitoring (per session) Effective for dates of service on or after January 1, 2010, hospitals and practitioners may report a maximum of 2 1-hour sessions per day. In order to report one session of cardiac rehabilitation services in a day, the duration of treatment must be at least 31 minutes. Two sessions of cardiac rehabilitation services may only be reported in the same day if the duration of treatment is at least 91 minutes. In other words, the first session would account for 60 minutes and the second session would account for at least 31 minutes if two sessions are reported. If several shorter periods of cardiac rehabilitation services are furnished on a given day, the minutes of service during those periods must be added together for reporting in 1-hour session increments.

Example: If the patient receives 20 minutes of cardiac rehabilitation services in the day, no cardiac rehabilitation session may be reported because less than 31 minutes of services were furnished.

Example: If a patient receives 20 minutes of cardiac rehabilitation services in the morning and 35 minutes of cardiac rehabilitation services in the afternoon of a single day, the hospital or practitioner would report 1 session of cardiac rehabilitation services under 1 unit of the appropriate CPT code for the total duration of 55 minutes of cardiac rehabilitation services on that day.

Example: If the patient receives 70 minutes of cardiac rehabilitation services in the morning and 25 minutes of cardiac rehabilitation services in the afternoon of a single day, the hospital or practitioner would report two sessions of cardiac rehabilitation services under the appropriate CPT code(s) because the total duration of cardiac rehabilitation services on that day of 95 minutes exceeds 90 minutes.

Example: If the patient receives 70 minutes of cardiac rehabilitation services in the morning and 85 minutes of cardiac rehabilitation services in the afternoon of a single day, the hospital or practitioner would report two sessions of cardiac rehabilitation services under the appropriate CPT code(s) for the total duration of cardiac rehabilitation services of 155 minutes. A maximum of two sessions per day may be reported, regardless of the total duration of cardiac rehabilitation services.

100-4, 32, 140.2.2.1

Correct Place of Service (POS) Code for CR and ICR Services on Professional Claims

Effective for claims with dates of service on and after January 1, 2010, place of service (POS) code 11 shall be used for CR and ICR services provided in a physician's office and POS 22 shall be used for services provided in a hospital outpatient setting. All other POS codes shall be denied. Contractors shall adjust their prepayment procedure edits as appropriate.

The following messages shall be used when contractors deny CR and ICR claims for POS:

Claim Adjustment Reason Code (CARC) 171 – Payment is denied when performed/billed by this type of provider in this type of facility.

NOTE: Refer to the 832 Healthcare Policy Identification Segment (loop 2110 Service payment Information REF), if present.

Remittance Advice Remark Code (RARC) N428 - Service/procedure not covered when performed in this place of service.

Medicare Summary Notice (MSN) 21.25 - This service was denied because Medicare only covers this service in certain settings.

Group Code PR (Patient Responsibility) - Where a claim is received with the GA modifier indicating that a signed ABN is on file.

Group Code CO (Contractor Responsibility) - Where a claim is received with the GZ modifier indicating that no signed ABN is on file.

100-4,32,140.2.2.2

140.2.2.2 – Requirements for CR and ICR Services on Institutional Claims

(Rev. 2989, Issued: 07-18-14, Effective: 02-18-14, Implementation: 08-18-14)

Effective for claims with dates of service on and after January 1, 2010, contractors shall pay for CR and ICR services when submitted on Types of Bill (TOBs) 13X and 85X only. All other TOBs shall be denied.

The following messages shall be used when contractors deny CR and ICR claims for TOBs 13X and 85X:

Claim Adjustment Reason Code (CARC) 171 – Payment is denied when performed/billed by this type of provider in this type of facility.

Remittance Advice Remark Code (RARC) N428 - Service/procedure not covered when performed in this place of service.

Medicare Summary Notice (MSN) 21.25 - This service was denied because Medicare only covers this service in certain settings.

Group Code PR (Patient Responsibility) – Where a claim is received with the GA modifier indicating that a signed ABN is on file.

Group Code CO (Contractor Responsibility) – Where a claim is received with the GZ modifier indicating that no signed ABN is on file.

100-4,32,140.2.2.4

140.2.2.4 – Edits for CR Services Exceeding 36 Sessions

(Rev. 2989, Issued: 07-18-14, Effective: 02-18-14, Implementation: 08-18-14)

Effective for claims with dates of service on or after January 1, 2010, contractors shall deny all claims with HCPCS 93797 and 93798 (both professional and institutional claims) that exceed 36 CR sessions when a KX modifier is not included on the claim line.

The following messages shall be used when contractors deny CR claims that exceed 36 sessions, when a KX modifier is not included on the claim line:

Claim Adjustment Reason Code (CARC) 119 – Benefit maximum for this period or occurrences has been reached.

RARC N435 - Exceeds number/frequency approved/allowed within time period without support documentation.

MSN 23.17- Medicare won't cover these services because they are not considered medically necessary.

Spanish Version - Medicare no cubrirá estos servicios porque no son considerados necesarios por razones médicas.

Group Code PR (Patient Responsibility) – Where a claim is received with the GA modifier indicating that a signed ABN is on file.

Group Code CO (Contractor Responsibility) – Where a claim is received with the GZ modifier indicating that no signed ABN is on file.

Contractors shall not research and adjust CR claims paid for more than 36 sessions processed prior to the implementation of CWF edits. However, contractors may adjust claims brought to their attention.

100-4, 32, 140.3

Intensive Cardiac Rehabilitation Program Services Furnished On or After January 1, 2010

As specified at 42 CFR 410.49, Medicare covers intensive cardiac rehabilitation items and services for patients who have experienced one or more of the following:

- An acute myocardial infarction within the preceding 12 months; or
- A coronary artery bypass surgery; or
- Current stable angina pectoris; or
- Heart valve repair or replacement; or
- Percutaneous transluminal coronary angioplasty (PTCA) or coronary stenting; or
- A heart or heart-lung transplant.

Intensive cardiac rehabilitation programs must include the following components:

- Physician-prescribed exercise each day cardiac rehabilitation items and services are furnished;
- Cardiac risk factor modification, including education, counseling, and behavioral intervention at least once during the program, tailored to patients' individual needs;
- Psychosocial assessment;
- Outcomes assessment; and
- An individualized treatment plan detailing how components are utilized for each patient.

Intensive cardiac rehabilitation programs must be approved by Medicare. In order to be approved, a program must demonstrate through peer-reviewed published research that it has accomplished one or more of the following for its patients:

- Positively affected the progression of coronary heart disease;
- Reduced the need for coronary bypass surgery; and
- Reduced the need for percutaneous coronary interventions.

An intensive cardiac rehabilitation program must also demonstrate through peer-reviewed published research that it accomplished a statistically significant reduction in 5 or more of the following measures for patients from their levels before cardiac rehabilitation services to after cardiac rehabilitation services:

- Low density lipoprotein;
- Triglycerides;
- Body mass index;
- Systolic blood pressure;
- Diastolic blood pressure; and
- The need for cholesterol, blood pressure, and diabetes medications.

Intensive cardiac rehabilitation items and services must be furnished in a physician's office or a hospital outpatient setting. All settings must have a physician immediately available and accessible for medical consultations and emergencies at all time items and services are being furnished under the program. This provision is satisfied if the physician meets the requirements for direct supervision of physician office services as specified at 42 CFR 410.26 and for hospital outpatient therapeutic services as specified at 42 CFR 410.27.

As specified at 42 CFR 410.49(f)(2), intensive cardiac rehabilitation program sessions are limited to 72 1-hour sessions, up to 6 sessions per day, over a period of up to 18 weeks.

100-4, 32, 150.1

General

Bariatric Surgery for Treatment of Co-Morbid Conditions Related to Morbid Obesity

Effective for services on or after February 21, 2006, Medicare has determined that the following bariatric surgery procedures are reasonable and necessary under certain conditions for the treatment of morbid obesity. The patient must have a body-mass index (BMI) ≥35, have at least one co-morbidity related to obesity, and have been previously unsuccessful with medical treatment for obesity. This medical information must be documented in the patient's medical record. In addition, the procedure must be performed at an approved facility. A list of approved facilities may be found at http://www.cms.gov/Medicare/Medicare-General-Information/MedicareApproved Facilitie/Bariatric-Surgery.html

Effective for services performed on and after February 12, 2009, Medicare has determined that Type 2 diabetes mellitus is a co-morbidity for purposes of processing bariatric surgery claims.

Effective for dates of service on and after September 24, 2013, the Centers for Medicare & Medicaid Services (CMS) has removed the certified facility requirements for Bariatric Surgery for Treatment of Co-Morbid Conditions Related to Morbid Obesity.

Please note the additional national coverage determinations related to bariatric surgery will be consolidated and subsumed into Publication 100-03, Chapter 1, section 100.1. These include sections 40.5, 100.8, 100.11 and 100.14.

- Open Roux-en-Y gastric bypass (RYGBP)
- Laparoscopic Roux-en-Y gastric bypass (RYGBP)
- Laparoscopic adjustable gastric banding (LAGB)
- Open biliopancreatic diversion with duodenal switch (BPD/DS) or gastric reduction duodenal switch (BPD/GRDS)
- Laparoscopic biliopancreatic diversion with duodenal switch (BPD/DS) or gastric reduction duodenal switch (BPD/GRDS)
- Laparoscopic sleeve gastrectomy (LSG) (Effective June 27, 2012, covered at Medicare Administrative Contractor (MAC) discretion.

100-4, 32, 150.2

HCPCS Procedure Codes for Bariatric Surgery

A. Covered HCPCS Procedure Codes

For services on or after February 21, 2006, the following HCPCS procedure codes are covered for bariatric surgery:

43770 - Laparoscopy, surgical, gastric restrictive procedure; placement of adjustable gastric band (gastric band and subcutaneous port components).

43644 - Laparoscopy, surgical, gastric restrictive procedure; with gastric bypass and Roux-en-Y gastroenterostomy (roux limb 150 cm or less).

43645 - Laparoscopy with gastric bypass and small intestine reconstruction to limit absorption. (Do not report 43645 in conjunction with 49320, 43847.)

43845 - Gastric restrictive procedure with partial gastrectomy, pylorus-preserving duodenoileostomy and ileoieostomy (50 to 100 cm common channel) to limit absorption (biliopancreatic diversion with duodenal switch).

43846 - Gastric restrictive procedure, with gastric bypass for morbid obesity; with short limb (150 cm or less Roux-en-Y gastroenterostomy. (For greater than 150 cm, use 43847.) (For laparoscopic procedure, use 43644.)

43847 - With small intestine reconstruction to limit absorption.

43775 - Laparoscopy, surgical, gastric restrictive procedure; longitudinal gastrectomy (i.e., sleeve gastrectomy) (Effective June 27, 2012, covered at contractor's discretion.)

B. Noncovered HCPCS Procedure Codes

For services on or after February 21, 2006, the following HCPCS procedure codes are non-covered for bariatric surgery:

43842 - Gastric restrictive procedure, without gastric bypass, for morbid obesity; vertical banded gastroplasty.

NOC code 43999 used to bill for:

Laparoscopic vertical banded gastroplasty

Open sleeve gastrectomy

Laparoscopic sleeve gastrectomy (for contractor non-covered instances)

Open adjustable gastric banding

100-4, 32, 150.5

ICD-9 Diagnosis Codes for BMI Greater Than or Equal to 35

The following ICD-9 diagnosis codes identify BMI ≥35:

V85.35 - Body Mass Index 35.0-35.9, adult

V85.36 - Body Mass Index 36.0-36.9, adult

V85.37 - Body Mass Index 37.0-37.9, adult

V85.38 - Body Mass Index 38.0-38.9, adult

V85.39 - Body Mass Index 39.0-39.9, adult

V85.41 - Body Mass Index 40.0-44.9, adult

V85.42 - Body Mass Index 45.0-49.9, adult

V85.43 - Body Mass Index 50.0-59.9, adult

V85.44 - Body Mass Index 60.0-69.9, adult

V85.45 - Body Mass Index 70.0 and over, adult

The following ICD-10 diagnosis codes identify BMI ≥35:

Z6835 - Body Mass Index 35.0-35.9, adult

Z6836 - Body Mass Index 36.0-36.9, adult.

Z6837 - Body Mass Index 37.0-37.9, adult

Z6838 - Body Mass Index 38.0-38.9, adult

Z6839 - Body Mass Index 39.0-39.9, adult

Z6841 - Body Mass Index 40.0-44.9, adult

Z6842 - Body Mass Index 45.0-49.9, adult

Z6843 - Body Mass Index 50.0-59.9, adult

Z6844 - Body Mass Index 60.0-69.9, adult

Z6845 - Body Mass Index 70.0 and over, adult

100-4, 32,150.6

150.6 - Claims Guidance for Payment

(Rev. 2841, Issued: 12-23-13, Effective: 09-24-13, Implementation: 12-17-13)

Covered Bariatric Surgery Procedures for Treatment of Co-Morbid Conditions Related to Morbid Obesity

Contractors shall process covered bariatric surgery claims as follows:

1. Identify bariatric surgery claims.

   Contractors identify inpatient bariatric surgery claims by the presence of ICD-9/ICD-10 diagnosis code 278.01/E66.01as the primary diagnosis (for morbid obesity) and one of the covered ICD-9/ICD-10 procedure codes listed in §150.3.

   Contractors identify practitioner bariatric surgery claims by the presence of ICD-9/ICD-10 diagnosis code 278.01/E66.01 as the primary diagnosis (for morbid obesity) and one of the covered HCPCS procedure codes listed in §150.2.

2. Perform facility certification validation for all bariatric surgery claims on a pre-pay basis up to and including date of service September 23, 2013.

   A list of approved facilities are found at the link noted in section 150.1, section A, above.

3. Review bariatric surgery claims data and determine whether a pre- or post-pay sample of bariatric surgery claims need further review to assure that the beneficiary has a BMI ≥35 (V85.35-V85.45/Z68.35-Z68.45) (see ICD-10 equivalents above in section 150.5), and at least one co-morbidity related to obesity

   The A/B MAC medical director may define the appropriate method for addressing the obesity-related co-morbid requirement.

   Effective for dates of service on and after September 24, 2013, CMS has removed the certified facility requirements for Bariatric Surgery for Treatment of Co-Morbid Conditions Related to Morbid Obesity.

NOTE: If ICD-9/IC. D-10 diagnosis code 278.01/E66.01 is present, but a covered procedure code (listed in §150.2 or §150.3) is/are not present, the claim is not for bariatric surgery and should be processed under normal procedures.

100-4, 32, 160.2

Post-Approval Study Coverage

Effective October 12, 2004, Medicare covers PTA of the carotid artery concurrent with the placement of an FDA-approved carotid stent and an FDA-approved or -cleared embolic protection device (effective December 9, 2009) for an FDA-approved indication when furnished in accordance with FDA-approved protocols governing post-approval studies. Billing post-approval studies is similar to normal Category B IDE billing procedures, except that under post-approval coverage, providers must bill the Pre-Market Approval (PMA) number assigned to the stent system by the FDA. PMA numbers are like typical IDE Numbers in that they have six-digits, but they begin with a "P" (i.e., P123456) instead of a "G."

100-4, 32,160.2.1

160.2.1 – Carotid Artery Stenting (CAS) for Post-Approval Studies

(Rev. 2998, Issued: 07-25-14, Effective: Upon implementation of ICD-10; 01-01-12 - ASC X12, Implementation: 08-25-2014 - ASC X12; Upon Implementation of ICD-10)

A. Background

As the post-approval studies began to end, CMS received requests to extend coverage for the post-approval studies. CMS has reviewed the extension requests and has determined that patients participating in post-approval extension studies are also included in the currently covered population of patients participating in FDA-approved post-approval studies.

B. Policy

To grant approval for post-approval studies, the FDA reviews each study protocol. Once approval is granted, the FDA issues a formal approval letter to the study sponsor. Extensions of post-approval studies are not subject to approval by the FDA because they surpass the post-approval study requirements identified in the conditions of approval for post-approval studies. Since the FDA cannot approve these extension studies, individual Post-Market Approval (PMA) numbers cannot be issued to separately identify each study. Currently, in order to receive reimbursement for procedures performed as part of a carotid artery stenting post-approval study, providers must include the FDA-issued PMA number on each claim to indicate participation in a specific study.

CMS has determined that all extension studies must be reviewed by the FDA. The FDA will issue an acknowledgement letter stating that the extension study is scientifically valid and will generate clinically relevant post-market data. Upon receipt of this letter and review of the extension study protocol, CMS will issue a letter to the study sponsor indicating that the study under review will be covered by Medicare. Since an individual PMA number cannot be assigned by the FDA to each extension study, these studies will use the PMA number assigned to the original FDA-approved post-approval study (i.e., CAPTURE 2 shall use the PMA number assigned to CAPTURE 1).

C. Billing

In order to receive Medicare coverage for patients participating in post-approval extension studies, providers shall submit both the FDA acknowledgement letter and the CMS letter providing coverage for the extension study to their contractor. Additionally, providers shall submit any other materials contractors would require for FDA-approved post- approval studies.

In response, contractors will issue a letter assigning an effective date for each facility's participation in the extension study. Providers may bill for procedures performed in the extension study for dates of service on and after the assigned effective date. Providers billing A/B MACs (A) must bill using the most current ICD-9 CM if ICD-9-CM is applicable, or, if ICD-10-CM is applicable, ICD-10-PCS codes 037G34Z, 037G3DZ, 037G3ZZ, 037G44Z, 037G4DZ, 037G4ZZ, 03CG3ZZ, 057L3DZ, 057L4DZ & 05CL3ZZ procedure codes may be used.

100-4, 32,161

161 - Intracranial Percutaneous Transluminal Angioplasty (PTA) With Stenting

(Rev. 2998, Issued: 07-25-14, Effective: Upon implementation of ICD-10; 01-01-12 - ASC X12, Implementation: 08-25-2014 - ASC X12; Upon Implementation of ICD-10)

A. Background

In the past, PTA to treat obstructive lesions of the cerebral arteries was non-covered by Medicare because the safety and efficacy of the procedure had not been established. This national coverage determination (NCD) meant that the procedure was also non-covered for beneficiaries participating in Food and Drug Administration (FDA)-approved investigational device exemption (IDE) clinical trials.

B. Policy

On February 9, 2006, a request for reconsideration of this NCD initiated a national coverage analysis. CMS reviewed the evidence and determined that intracranial PTA with stenting is reasonable and necessary under §1862(a)(1)(A) of the Social Security Act for the treatment of cerebral vessels (as specified in *The National Coverage Determinations Manual*, Chapter 1, part 1, section 20.7) only when furnished in accordance with FDA- approved protocols governing Category B IDE clinical trials. All other indications for intracranial PTA with stenting remain non-covered.

C. Billing

Providers of covered intracranial PTA with stenting shall use Category B IDE billing requirements, as listed above in section 68.4. In addition to these requirements, providers must bill the appropriate procedure and diagnosis codes for the date of service to receive payment. That is, under Part A, providers must bill intracranial PTA using ICD-9-CM procedure codes 00.62 and 00.65, if ICD-9-CM is applicable, or, if ICD-10-PCS is applicable, ICD-10-PCS procedure codes 037G34Z, 037G3DZ, 037G3ZZ, 037G44Z,037G4DZ, 037G4ZZ, 03CG3ZZ, 057L3DZ, 057L4DZ and 05CL3ZZ. ICD-9-CM diagnosis code 437.0 or ICD-10-CM diagnosis code 167.2applies, depending on the date of service.

Under Part B, providers must bill HCPCS procedure code 37799. If ICD-9-CM is applicable, ICD-9-CM diagnosis code 437.0 or if ICD-10-CM is applicable,ICD-10-CM diagnosis code 167.2applies.

NOTE: ICD- codes are subject to modification. Providers must always ensure they are using the latest and most appropriate codes.

100-4, 32, 170.1

General

Effective for services performed from May 16, 2006 through August 13, 2007, the Centers for Medicare & Medicaid Services (CMS) made the decision that lumbar artificial disc replacement (LADR) with the CharitéTM lumbar artificial disc is non-covered for Medicare beneficiaries over 60 years of age. See Pub. 100-03, Medicare National Coverage Determinations Manual, section 150.10, for more information about the non-covered determination.

Effective for services performed on or after August 14, 2007, CMS made the decision that LADR with any lumbar artificial disc is non-covered for Medicare beneficiaries over 60 years of age, (i.e. on or after a beneficiary's 61st birthday).

For Medicare beneficiaries 60 years of age and younger, there is no national coverage determination for LADR, leaving such determinations to continue to be made by the local contractors.

100-4, 32, 170.2

Carrier Billing Requirements

Effective for services performed on or after May 16, 2006 through December 31, 2006, carriers shall deny claims, for Medicare beneficiaries over 60 years of age, submitted with the following Category III Codes:

0091T Single interspace, lumbar; and

0092T Each additional interspace (List separately in addition to code for primary procedure.)

Effective for services performed on or after January 1, 2007 through August 13, 2007, for Medicare beneficiaries over 60 years of age, LADR with the CharitéTM lumbar artificial disc, carriers shall deny claims submitted with the following codes:

22857 Total disc arthroplasty (artificial disc), anterior approach, including discectomy to prepare interspace (other than for decompression), lumbar, single interspace; and

0163T Total disc arthroplasty (artificial disc), anterior approach, including discectomy to prepare interspace (other than for decompression), lumbar, each additional interspace.

Carriers shall continue to follow their normal claims processing criteria for IDEs for LADR performed with an implant eligible under the IDE criteria.

For dates of service May 16, 2006 through August 13, 2007, Medicare coverage under the investigational device exemption (IDE) for LADR with a disc other than the CharitéTM lumbar disc in eligible clinical trials is not impacted.

Effective for services performed on or after August 14, 2007, carriers shall deny claims for LADR surgery, for Medicare beneficiaries over 60 years of age, (i.e. on or after a beneficiary's 61st birthday) submitted with the following codes:

22857 Total disc arthroplasty (artificial disc), anterior approach, including discectomy to prepare interspace (other than for decompression), lumbar, single interspace; and

0163T Total disc arthroplasty (artificial disc), anterior approach, including discectomy to prepare interspace (other than for decompression), lumbar, each additional interspace.

100-4, 32, 180.1

Coverage Requirements

Medicare covers cryosurgery of the prostate gland effective for claims with dates of service on or after July 1, 1999. The coverage is for:

1. Primary treatment of patients with clinically localized prostate cancer, Stages T1 - T3 (diagnosis code is 185 - malignant neoplasm of prostate).
2. Salvage therapy (effective for claims with dates of service on or after July 1, 2001 for patients:
   a. Having recurrent, localized prostate cancer;
   b. Failing a trial of radiation therapy as their primary treatment; and
   c. Meeting one of these conditions: State T2B or below; Gleason score less than 9 or; PSA less than 8 ng/ml.

100-4, 32, 180.2

Billing Requirements

Claims for cryosurgery for the prostate gland are to be submitted on the ANSI X12 ASC 837, or, in exceptional circumstances, on a hard copy Form CMS - 1450. This procedure can be rendered in an inpatient or outpatient hospital setting (types of bill (TOBs) 11x 13x, 83x, and 85x).

The A/B MAC (A) will look for the following when processing claims with cryosurgery services:

- If ICD-9-CM is applicable, ICD-9 CM diagnosis code 185 or
- If ICD-10-CM is applicable, ICD-10 CM diagnosis code C61 must be on all cryosurgical claims;
- For outpatient claims HCPCS 55873 and revenue codes 0360, 0361, or 0369 Cryosurgery ablation of localized prostate cancer, stages T1- T3 (includes ultrasonic guidance for interstitial cryosurgery probe placement, postoperative irrigations and aspiration of sloughing tissue included) must be on all outpatient claims; and
- For inpatient claims correct procedure codes are:
  - If ICD-9-CM is applicable, ICD-9-CM procedure code 60.62 (perineal prostatectomy- the definition includes cryoablation of prostate, cryostatectomy of prostate, and radical cryosurgical ablation of prostate)
  - If ICD-10 is applicable,ICD-10-PCS procedure code 0V500ZZ (Destruction of Prostate, Open Approach), or 0V503ZZ (Destruction of Prostate, Percutaneous Approach), or 0V504ZZ (Destruction of Prostate, Percutaneous Endoscopic Approach).

100-4, 32, 190

Billing Requirements for Extracorporeal Photopheresis

Effective for dates of services on and after December 19, 2006, Medicare has expanded coverage for extracorporeal photopheresis for patients with acute cardiac allograft rejection whose disease is refractory to standard immunosuppresive drug treatment and patients with chronic graft versus host disease whose disease is refractory to standard immunosuppresive drug treatment. (See Pub. 100-03, chapter 1, section 110.4, for complete coverage guidelines).

Effective for claims with dates of service on or after April 30, 2012, CMS has expanded coverage for extracorporeal photopheresis for the treatment of BOS following lung allograft transplantation only when extracorporeal photopheresis is provided under a clinical research study that meets specific requirements to assess the effect of extracorporeal photopheresis for the treatment of bronchialitis obliterans syndrome (BOS) following lung allograft transplantation. Further coverage criteria is outlined in Publication 100-03, Section 110.4 of the NCD.

100-4, 32, 190.2

Healthcare Common Procedural Coding System (HCPCS), Applicable Diagnosis Codes and Procedure Code

The following HCPCS procedure code is used for billing extracorporeal photopheresis

- 36522 - Photopheresis, extracorporeal

The following are the applicable ICD-9-CM diagnosis codes for the new expanded coverage:

- 996.83 - Complications of transplanted heart, or
- 996.85 - Complications of transplanted bone marrow

Effective for services for BOS following lung allograft transplantation the following is a list of applicable ICD-9-CM diagnosis codes:

- 996.84 – Complications of transplanted lung
- 491.9 – Unspecified chronic bronchitis
- 491.20 – Obstructive chronic bronchitis without exacerbation
- 491.21 – Obstructive chronic bronchitis with (acute) exacerbation
- 496 – Chronic airway obstruction, not elsewhere classified

The following is the applicable ICD-9-CM procedure code for the new expanded coverage:

- 99.88 - Therapeutic photopheresis.

If ICD-10 is applicable, use the ICD-10-CM diagnosis codes

ICD9 CODE	LONG DESCRIPTION	ICD10 CODE	I10 Description
491.20	Obstructive chronic bronchitis without exacerbation	J44.9	Chronic obstructive pulmonary disease, unspecified
491.21	Obstructive chronic bronchitis with (acute) exacerbation	J44.1	Chronic obstructive pulmonary disease with (acute) exacerbation
491.9	Unspecified chronic bronchitis	J42	Unspecified chronic bronchitis
496	Chronic airway obstruction, not elsewhere classified	J44.9	Chronic obstructive pulmonary disease, unspecified
996.84	Complications of transplanted lung	T86.810	Lung transplant rejection
996.84	Complications of transplanted lung	T86.811	Lung transplant failure
996.84	Complications of transplanted lung	T86.812	Lung transplant infection (not recommended for ECP coverage)
996.84	Complications of transplanted lung	T86.818	Other complications of lung transplant
996.84	Complications of transplanted lung	T86.819	Unspecified complication of lung transplant
V70.7	Examination of participant in clinical trial	Z00.6	Encounter for examination for normal comparison and control in clinical research program (needed for CED)

NOTE: Contractors shall edit for an appropriate oncological and autoimmune disorder diagnosis for payment of extracorporeal photopheresis according to the National Coverage Determination

Effective for claims with dates of service on or after April 30, 2012, in addition to HCPCS 36522, the following ICD-9-CM/ICD-10-CM codes are applicable for extracorporeal photopheresis for the treatment of BOS following lung allograft transplantation only with ECP is provided under a clinical research study as outlined in Section 190 above:

A reference listing of ICD-9 CM and ICD-10-CM diagnosis coding and descriptions is listed above.

Providers must also report modifier Q0 - (Investigational clinical service provided in a clinical research study that is in an approved research study) on these claims. Providers must use ICD-9-CM diagnosis code V70.7 if ICD-9 is applicable and condition code 30 (A/B MACs (A) only) for these claims. If ICD-10 is applicable, providers must use ICD-10-CM diagnosis code Z00.6.

100-4, 32, 190.3

Medicare Summary Notices (MSNs), Remittance Advice Remark Codes (RAs) and Claim Adjustment Reason Code

Contractors shall continue to use the appropriate existing messages that they have in place when denying claims submitted that do not meet the Medicare coverage criteria for extracorporeal photopheresis.

Contractors shall deny claims when the service is not rendered to an inpatient or outpatient of a hospital, including critical access hospitals (CAHs) using the following codes:

- Claim Adjustment Reason code: 58—"Claim/service denied/reduced because treatment was deemed by payer to have been rendered in an inappropriate or invalid place of service."
- MSN 16.2—"This service cannot be paid when provided in this location/facility." Spanish translation: "Este servicio no se puede pagar cuando es suministrado en esta sitio/facilidad." (Include either MSN 36.1 or 36.2 dependant on liablity.)
- RA MA 30—"Missing/incomplete/invalid type of bill." (FIs and A/MACs only)
- Group Code—CO (Contractual Obligations) or PR (Patient Responsibility) dependant on liability. Contractors shall return to provider/ return as unprocessable claims for BOS containing HCPCS procedure code 36522 along with one of the following ICD-9-CM diagnosis codes: 996.84, 491.9, 491.20, 491.21, and 496 but is missing Diagnosis code V70.7 (as secondary diagnosis, Institutional only), Condition code 30 Institutional claims only), Clinical trial modifier Q0. Use the following messages:
- CARC 4—The procedure code is inconsistent with the modifier used or a required modifier is missing. Note: Refer to the 835 Healthcare Policy Identification Segment (loop 2110 Service Payment Information REF), if present.
- RARC MA 130—Your claim contains incomplete and/or invalid information, and no appeal rights are afforded because the claim is unprocessable. Please submit a new claim with the complete/correct information.
- RARC M16—Alert: Please see our web site, mailings, or bulletins for more details concerning this policy/procedure/decision.

100-4, 32, 220.1

220.1 - General

Effective for services on or after September 29, 2008, the Center for Medicare & Medicaid Services (CMS) made the decision that Thermal Intradiscal Procedures (TIPS) are not reasonable and necessary for the treatment of low back pain. Therefore, TIPs are non-covered. Refer to Pub.100-03, Medicare National Coverage Determination (NCD) Manual Chapter 1, Part 2, Section 150.11, for further information on the NCD.

100-4, 32, 220.2

220.2 - Contractors, A/B Medicare Administrative Contractors (MACs)

The following Healthcare Common Procedure Coding System (HCPCS) codes will be nationally non-covered by Medicare effective for dates of service on and after September 29, 2008: 22526: Percutaneous intradiscal electrothermal annuloplasty, unilateral or bilateral including fluoroscopic guidance; single level 22527: Percutaneous intradiscal electrothermal annuloplasty, unilateral or bilateral including fluoroscopic guidance; one or more additional levels 0062T: Percutaneous intradiscal annuloplasty, any method except electrothermal, unilateral or bilateral including fluoroscopic guidance; single level 0063T: Percutaneous intradiscal annuloplasty, any method except electrothermal, unilateral or bilateral including fluoroscopic guidance; one or more additional levels NOTE: The change to add the non-covered indicator for the above HCPCS codes will be part of the January 2009 Medicare Physician Fee Schedule Update. The change to the status indicator to non-cover the above HCPCS will be part of the January Integrated Outpatient Code Editor (IOCE) update.

Claims submitted with the non-covered HCPCS codes on or after September 29, 2008, will be denied by Medicare contractors

100-4, 32, 270

Claims Processing for Implantable Automatic Defibrillators

Coverage Requirements- The implantable automatic defibrillator is an electronic device designed to detect and treat life threatening tachyarrhythmias. The device consists of a pulse generator and electrodes for sensing and defibrillating.

See Sec.20.4 -Medicare National Coverage Determinations (NCD) Manual for the complete list of covered indications.

100-4, 32, 270.1

Coding Requirements for Implantable Automatic Defibrillators

The following are the applicable HCPCS procedure codes for implantable automatic defibrillators:

33240- (Insertion of single or dual chamber pacing cardioverter-defibrillator pulse generator)

33241(Subcutaneous removal of single or dual chamber pacing cardioverter-defibrillator pulse generator)

33243 (Removal of single or dual chamber pacing cardioverter-defibrillator electrode(s); by thoracotomy)

33244 (Removal of single or dual chamber pacing cardioverter-defibrillator electrodes by thoracotomy)

33249- (Insertion or repositioning of electrode leads(s) for single or dual chamber pacing cardioverter-defibrillator and insertion of pulse generator)

For inpatient hospitals claims, if ICD-9 CM is applicable use procedure code 37.94. If ICD-10-PCS is applicable the following applies.

More than one ICD-10-PCS code (a cluster) is required. There are two possible clusters:

FIRST CLUSTER: Use 1 code from the first list and one code from the second list.

Cluster 1 first list:

0JH608Z Insertion of Defibrillator Generator into Chest Subcutaneous Tissue and Fascia, Open Approach

0JH638Z Insertion of Defibrillator Generator into Chest Subcutaneous Tissue and Fascia, Percutaneous Approach

0JH808Z Insertion of Defibrillator Generator into Abdomen Subcutaneous Tissue and Fascia, Open Approach

0JH838Z Insertion of Defibrillator Generator into Abdomen Subcutaneous Tissue and Fascia, Percutaneous Approach

Cluster 1 second list:

02H60KZ Insertion of Defibrillator Lead into Right Atrium, Open Approach

02H63KZ Insertion of Defibrillator Lead into Right Atrium, Percutaneous Approach

02H64KZ Insertion of Defibrillator Lead into Right Atrium, Percutaneous Endoscopic Approach

02H70KZ Insertion of Defibrillator Lead into Left Atrium, Open Approach

02H73KZ Insertion of Defibrillator Lead into Left Atrium, Percutaneous Approach

02H74KZ Insertion of Defibrillator Lead into Left Atrium, Percutaneous Endoscopic Approach

02HK0KZ Insertion of Defibrillator Lead into Right Ventricle, Open Approach

02HK3KZ Insertion of Defibrillator Lead into Right Ventricle, Percutaneous Approach

02HK4KZ Insertion of Defibrillator Lead into Right Ventricle, Percutaneous Endoscopic Approach

02HL0KZ Insertion of Defibrillator Lead into Left Ventricle, Open Approach

02HL3KZ Insertion of Defibrillator Lead into Left Ventricle, Percutaneous Approach

02HL4KZ Insertion of Defibrillator Lead into Left Ventricle, Percutaneous Endoscopic Approach

SECOND CLUSTER:

Use 1 code from 1st list & 1 code from the 4th list; also add one code from each of the 2nd & 3rd lists if doing a replacement instead of initial insertion.

Cluster 2 first list:

0JH608Z Insertion of Defibrillator Generator into Chest Subcutaneous Tissue and Fascia, Open Approach

0JH638Z Insertion of Defibrillator Generator into Chest Subcutaneous Tissue and Fascia, Percutaneous Approach

0JH808Z Insertion of Defibrillator Generator into Abdomen Subcutaneous Tissue and Fascia, Open Approach

0JH838Z Insertion of Defibrillator Generator into Abdomen Subcutaneous Tissue and Fascia, Percutaneous Approach

Cluster 2 second list:

0JPT0PZ Removal of Cardiac Rhythm Related Device from Trunk Subcutaneous Tissue and Fascia, Open Approach

0JPT3PZ Removal of Cardiac Rhythm Related Device from Trunk Subcutaneous Tissue and Fascia, Percutaneous Approach

Cluster 2 third list:

02PA0MZ Removal of Cardiac Lead from Heart, Open Approach

02PA3MZ Removal of Cardiac Lead from Heart, Percutaneous Approach

02PA4MZ Removal of Cardiac Lead from Heart, Percutaneous Endoscopic Approach

02PAXMZ Removal of Cardiac Lead from Heart, External Approach

Cluster 2 fourth list:

02H60KZ Insertion of Defibrillator Lead into Right Atrium, Open Approach

02H63KZ Insertion of Defibrillator Lead into Right Atrium, Percutaneous Approach

02H64KZ Insertion of Defibrillator Lead into Right Atrium, Percutaneous Endoscopic Approach

02H70KZ Insertion of Defibrillator Lead into Left Atrium, Open Approach

02H73KZ Insertion of Defibrillator Lead into Left Atrium, Percutaneous Approach

02H74KZ Insertion of Defibrillator Lead into Left Atrium, Percutaneous Endoscopic Approach

02HK0KZ Insertion of Defibrillator Lead into Right Ventricle, Open Approach

02HK3KZ Insertion of Defibrillator Lead into Right Ventricle, Percutaneous Approach

02HK4KZ Insertion of Defibrillator Lead into Right Ventricle, Percutaneous Endoscopic Approach

02HL0KZ Insertion of Defibrillator Lead into Left Ventricle, Open Approach

02HL3KZ Insertion of Defibrillator Lead into Left Ventricle, Percutaneous Approach

02HL4KZ Insertion of Defibrillator Lead into Left Ventricle, Percutaneous Endoscopic Approach

100-4, 32, 270.2

Billing Requirements for Patients Enrolled in a Data Collection System

Effective for dates of service on or after April 1, 2005, Medicare required that patients receiving a defibrillator for the primary prevention of sudden cardiac arrest be enrolled in a qualifying data collection system. Providers shall use modifier Q0 to identify patients whose data is being submitted to a data collection system.

The following ICD-9 diagnosis codes identify non-primary prevention (secondary prevention) patient or replacement implantations (e.g. due to recalled devices):

If ICD-9-CM is applicable, select from the following diagnosis codes:

427.1 Ventricular tachycardia

427.41 Ventricular fibrillation

427.42 Ventricular flutter

427.5 Cardiac arrest

427.9 Cardiac dysrhythmia, unspecified

V12.53 Personal history of sudden cardiac arrest

996.04 Mechanical complication of cardiac device, implant, and graft, due to automatic implantable cardiac defibrillator

V53.32 Fitting and adjustment of other device, automatic implantable cardiac defibrillator

If ICD-10-CM is applicable, select from the following list:

I47.0 Re-entry Ventricular Arrhythmia

I47.2 Ventricular Tachycardiaselect

I49.3 Ventricular Premature depolarization

I49.01 Ventricular Fibrillation

I49.02 Ventricular Flutter

I46.2 Cardiac arrest due to underlying cardiac condition

I46.8 Cardiac arrest due to other underlying condition

I46.9 Cardiac arrest, cause unspecified

I49.9 Cardiac arrhythmia, unspecified

T82.110A Breakdown (mechanical) of cardiac electrode, initial encounter

T82.111A Breakdown (mechanical) of cardiac pulse generator (battery), initial encounter

T82.118A Breakdown (mechanical) of other cardiac electronic device, initial encounter

T82.119A Breakdown (mechanical) of unspecified cardiac electronic device, initial encounter

T82.120A Displacement of cardiac electrode, initial encounter

T82.121A Displacement of cardiac pulse generator (battery), initial encounter

T82.128A Displacement of other cardiac electronic device, initial encounter

T82.129A Displacement of unspecified cardiac electronic device, initial encounter

T82.190A Other mechanical complication of cardiac electrode, initial encounter

T82.191A Other mechanical complication of cardiac pulse generator (battery), initial encounter

T82.198A Other mechanical complication of other cardiac electronic device, initial encounter

T82.199A Other mechanical complication of unspecified cardiac device, initial encounter

Z86.74 Personal history of sudden cardiac arrest

Z45.02 Encounter for adjustment and management of automatic implantable cardiac defibrillator

When any of the above codes appear on a claim, the Q0 modifier is not required. The Q0 modifier may be appended to claims for secondary prevention indications when data is being entered into a qualifying data collection system.

100-4, 32, 290.1.1

Coding Requirements for TAVR Services Furnished on or After January 1, 2013

Beginning January 1, 2013, the following are the applicable Current Procedural Terminology (CPT) codes for TAVR:

33361 Transcatheter aortic valve replacement (TAVR/TAVI) with prosthetic valve; percutaneous femoral artery approach

33362 Transcatheter aortic valve replacement (TAVR/TAVI) with prosthetic valve; open femoral approach

33363 Transcatheter aortic valve replacement (TAVR/TAVI) with prosthetic valve; open axillary artery approach

33364 Transcatheter aortic valve replacement (TAVR/TAVI) with prosthetic valve; open iliac artery approach

33365 Transcatheter aortic valve replacement (TAVR/TAVI) with prosthetic valve; transaortic approach (e.g., median sternotomy, mediastinotomy)

0318T Transcatheter aortic valve replacement (TAVR/TAVI) with prosthetic valve; transapical approach (e.g., left thoracotomy)

Beginning January 1, 2014, temporary CPT code 0318T above is retired. TAVR claims with dates of service on and after January 1, 2014 shall instead use permanent CPT code:

33366 Transcatheter aortic valve replacement (TAVR/TAVI) with prosthetic valve; transapical exposure (e.g., left thoracotomy)

100-4, 32, 290.2

Claims Processing Requirements for TAVR Services on Professional Claims

(Rev. 2737, Issued: 07-11-13, Effective: 07-01-13, Implementation: 10-07-13)

Effective for claims with dates of service on and after May 1, 2012, place of service (POS) code 21 shall be used for transcatheter aortic valve replacement (TAVR) services. All other POS codes shall be denied.

The following messages shall be used when Medicare contractors deny TAVR claims for POS:

Claim Adjustment Reason Code (CARC) 58: "Treatment was deemed by the payer to have been rendered in an inappropriate or invalid place of service.

NOTE: Refer to the 835 Healthcare Policy Identification Segment (loop 2110 Service Payment Information REF), if present."

Remittance advice remark code (RARC) N428: "Not covered when performed in this place of service."

Medicare Summary Notice (MSN) 21.25: "This service was denied because Medicare only covers this service in certain settings."

Spanish Version: "El servicio fue denegado porque Medicare solamente lo cubre en ciertas situaciones."

Professional Claims Modifier - 62

For claims processed on or after July 1, 2013, contractors shall pay claim lines with 0256T, 0257T, 0258T, 0259T, 33361, 33362, 33363, 33364, 33365 & 0318T only when billed with modifier -62. Claim lines billed without modifier 62 shall be returned as unprocessable.

Beginning January 1, 2014, temporary CPT code 0318T above is retired. TAVR claims with dates of service on and after January 1, 2014 shall instead use permanent CPT code 33366.

The following messages shall be used when Medicare contractors return TAVR claims billed without modifier -62 as unprocessable:

CARC 4: "The procedure code is inconsistent with the modifier used or a required modifier is missing. Note: Refer to the 835 Healthcare Policy Identification Segment (loop 2110 Service Payment Information REF), if present."

RARC N29: "Missing documentation/orders/notes/summary/report/chart."

RARC MA130: "Your claim contains incomplete and/or invalid information, and no appeal rights are afforded because the claim is unprocessable. Please submit a new claim with the complete/correct information."

Professional Claims Modifier - Q0

For claims processed on or after July 1, 2013, contractors shall pay claim lines for 0256T, 0257T, 0258T, 0259T, 33361, 33362, 33363, 33364, 33365 & 0318T when billed with modifier Q0. Claim lines billed without modifier Q0 shall be returned as unprocessable.

Beginning January 1, 2014, temporary CPT code 0318T above is retired. TAVR claims with dates of service on and after January 1, 2014 shall instead use permanent CPT code 33366.

The following messages shall be used when Medicare contractors return TAVR claims billed without modifier Q0 as unprocessable:

CARC 4: "The procedure code is inconsistent with the modifier used or a required modifier is missing. Note: Refer to the 835 Healthcare Policy Identification Segment (loop 2110 Service Payment Information REF), if present."

RARC N29: "Missing documentation/orders/notes/summary/report/chart."

RARC MA130: "Your claim contains incomplete and/or invalid information, and no appeal rights are afforded because the claim is unprocessable. Please submit a new claim with the complete/correct information."

For claims processed on or after July 1, 2013, contractors shall pay claim lines for 0256T, 0257T, 0258T, 0259T, 33361, 33362, 33363, 33364, 33365 & 0318T when billed with secondary diagnosis code V70.7 (ICD-10=Z00.6). Claim lines billed without secondary diagnosis code V70.7 (ICD-10=Z00.6) shall be returned as unprocessable.

Beginning January 1, 2014, temporary CPT code 0318T above is retired. TAVR claims with dates of service on and after January 1, 2014 shall instead use permanent CPT code 33366.

The following messages shall be used when Medicare contractors return TAVR claims billed without secondary diagnosis code V70.7 (ICD-10=Z00.6) as unprocessable:

CARC 16: "Claim/service lacks information which is needed for adjudication. At least one Remark Code must be provided (may be comprised of either the NCPDP Reject Reason Code, or Remittance Advice Remark Code that is not an ALERT.)"

RARC M76: "Missing/incomplete/invalid diagnosis or condition"

RARC MA130: "Your claim contains incomplete and/or invalid information, and no appeal rights are afforded because the claim is unprocessable. Please submit a new claim with the complete/correct information."

Professional Claims 8-digit Clinical Trial Number

For claims processed on or after July 1, 2013, contractors shall pay claim lines for 0256T, 0257T, 0258T, 0259T, 33361, 33362, 33363, 33364, 33365 & 0318T when billed with the numeric, 8-digit clinical trial registry number preceded by the two alpha characters "CT" when placed in Field 19 of paper Form CMS-1500, or when entered without the "CT" prefix in the electronic 837P in Loop 2300REF02(REF01=P4). Claim lines billed without an 8-digit clinical trial registry number shall be returned as unprocessable.

Beginning January 1, 2014, temporary CPT code 0318T above is retired. TAVR claims with dates of service on and after January 1, 2014 shall instead use permanent CPT code 33366.

The following messages shall be used when Medicare contractors return TAVR claims billed without an 8-digit clinical trial registry number as unprocessable:

CARC 16: "Claim/service lacks information which is needed for adjudication. At least one Remark Code must be provided (may be comprised of either NCPDP Reject Reason Code, or Remittance Advice Remark Code that is not an ALERT.)"

RARC MA50: "Missing/incomplete/invalid Investigational Device Exemption number for FDA-approved clinical trial services."

RARC MA130: "Your claim contains incomplete and/or invalid information, and no appeal rights are afforded because the claim is unprocessable. Please submit a new claim with the complete/correct information."

NOTE: Clinical trial registry numbers for TAVR are listed on our website: (http://www.cms.gov/Medicare/Coverage/Coverage-with-Evidence-Development/Transcatheter-Aortic-Valve-Replacement-TAVR-.html).

100-4, 32, 290.3

Claims Processing Requirements for TAVR Services on Inpatient Hospital Claims

(Rev. 2737, Issued: 07-11-13, Effective: 07-01-13, Implementation: 10-07-13)

Inpatient hospitals shall bill for TAVR on an 11X TOB effective for discharges on or after May 1, 2012. Refer to Section 69 of this chapter for further guidance on billing under CED.

Inpatient hospital discharges for TAVR shall be covered when billed with:

- V70.7 and Condition Code 30.
- An 8-digit clinical trial registry number listed on the CMS website (effective July 1, 2013)

Inpatient hospital discharges for TAVR shall be rejected when billed without:

- V70.7 and Condition Code 30.
- An 8-digit clinical trial registry number listed on the CMS website (effective July 1, 2013)

Claims billed by hospitals not participating in the trial/registry, shall be rejected with the following message:

CARC: 50 -These are non-covered services because this is not deemed a "medical necessity" by the payer.

RARC N386 - This decision was based on a National Coverage Determination (NCD). An NCD provides a coverage determination as to whether a particular item or service is covered. A copy of this policy is available at http://www.cms.hhs.gov/mcd/search.asp. If you do not have web access, you may contact the contractor to request a copy of the NCD.

Group Code – Contractual Obligation (CO)

MSN 16.77 – This service/item was not covered because it was not provided as part of a qualifying trial/study. Este servicio/artículo no fue cubierto porque no estaba incluido como parte de un ensayo clínico/estudio calificado.)

100-4, 32, 290.4

Claims Processing Requirements for TAVR Services for Medicare Advantage (MA) Plan Participants

MA plans are responsible for payment of TAVR services for MA plan participants. Medicare coverage for TAVR is included under section 310.1 of the NCD Manual (Routine Costs in Clinical Trials).

100-4, 32, 300

Billing Requirements for Ocular Photodynamic Therapy (OPT) with Verteporfin

Ocular Photodynamic Therapy (OPT) is used in the treatment of ophthalmologic diseases; specifically, for age-related macular degeneration (AMD), a common eye disease among the elderly. OPT involves the infusion of an intravenous photosensitizing drug called Verteporfin, followed by exposure to a laser. For complete Medical coverage guidelines, see National Coverage Determinations (NCD) Manual (Pub 100-03) § 80.2 through 80.3.1.

100-4, 32, 300.1

Coding Requirements for OPT with Verteporfin

The following are applicable Current Procedural Terminology (CPT) codes for OPT with Verteporfin:

67221- Destruction of localized lesion of choroid (e.g. choroidal neovascularization); photodynamic therapy (includes intravenous infusion)

67225- Destruction of localized lesion of choroid (e.g. choroidal neovascularization); photodynamic therapy, second eye, at single session (List separately in addition to code for primary eye treatment)

The following are applicable Healthcare Common Procedure Coding System (HCPCS) code for OPT with Verteporfin:

J3396- Injection, Verteporfin, 0.1 mg

100-4, 32, 300.2

Claims Processing Requirements for OPT with Verteporfin Services on Professional Claims and Outpatient Facility Claims

OPT with Verteporfin is a covered service when billed with ICD-9-CM code 362.52 (Exudative Senile Macular Degeneration of Retina (Wet)) or ICD-10-CM code H35.32 (Exudative Age-related Macular Degeneration).

Coverage is denied when billed with either ICD-9-CM code 362.50 (Macular Degeneration (Senile), Unspecified) or 362.51 (Non-exudative Senile Macular Degeneration) or their equivalent ICD-10-CM code H35.30 (Unspecified Macular Degeneration) or H35.31 (Non-exudative Age-Related Macular Degeneration).

OPT with Verteporfin for other ocular indications are eligible for local coverage determinations through individual contractor discretion.

Payment for OPT service (CPT code 67221/67225) must be billed on the same claim as the drug (J3396) for the same date of service.

Claims for OPT with Verteporfin for dates of service prior to April 3, 2013 are covered at the initial visit as determined by a fluorescein angiogram (FA) CPT code 92235 . Subsequent follow-up visits also require a FA prior to treatment.

For claims with dates of service on or after April 3, 2013, contractors shall accept and process claims for subsequent follow-up visits with either a FA, CPT code 92235, or optical coherence tomography (OCT), CPT codes 92133 or 92134, prior to treatment.

Regardless of the date of service of the claim, the FA or OCT is not required to be submitted on the claim for OPT and can be maintained in the patient's file for audit purposes.

100-4, 32, 310.1

Coding Requirements for Transesophageal Doppler Cardiac Monitoring Furnished Before January 1, 2013

Prior to January 1, 2013, the applicable HCPCS code for Transesophageal Doppler cardiac monitoring is:

HCPCS 76999 (billed with modifier -26) when performed in a hospital setting for ventilated patients in the ICU or for operative patients with a need for intra-operative fluid optimization.

If globally billed using code 76999, it shall be returned as unprocessable to the provider using a claim adjustment reason code (CARC) such as:

CARC 58: "Treatment was deemed by the payer to have been rendered in an inappropriate or invalid place of service. Note: Refer to the 835 Healthcare Policy Identification Segment (loop 2110 Service Payment Information REF), if present."

HCPCS 76999 (billed with modifier -TC) shall be denied when performed in a hospital setting for ventilated patients in the ICU or for operative patients with a need for intra-operative fluid optimization with a message such as:

CARC 58: "Treatment was deemed by the payer to have been rendered in an inappropriate or invalid place of service. Note: Refer to the 835 Healthcare Policy Identification Segment (loop 2110 Service Payment Information REF), if present."

RARC M77: "Missing/incomplete/invalid place of service."

MSN 17.9: "Medicare (Part A/Part B) pays for this service. The provider must bill the correct Medicare contractor." (English version) or "Este servicio es pagado por Medicare (Parte A/Parte B). El proveedor debe enviar la facture al contratista de Medicare correcto."(Spanish version).

HCPCS 76999 (billed globally or with -26 or -TC) when performed in an ASC setting for operative patients with a need for intra-operative fluid optimization, ultrasound diagnostic procedures are covered when performed by an entity other than the ASC.

100-4, 32, 320.1

320.1 – Cardiac Pacemakers: Single and Dual Chamber Policy

(Rev. 2872, Issued: 02-06-14, Effective: 08-13-13, Implementation: 07-07-14)

On August 13, 2013, the Centers for Medicare & Medicaid Services (CMS) issued a National Coverage Determination (NCD). In this NCD, CMS concluded that implanted permanent cardiac pacemakers, single chamber or dual chamber, are reasonable and necessary for the treatment of non-reversible symptomatic bradycardia due to sinus node dysfunction and second and/or third degree atrioventricular block. Symptoms of bradycardia are symptoms that can be directly attributable to a heart rate less than 60 beats per minute (for example: syncope, seizures, congestive heart failure, dizziness, or confusion). See Pub. 100-03, chapter 1, section 20.83 of the Medicare NCD Manual.

NOTE: Medicare Administrative Contractors (MACs) will determine coverage under section 1862(a)(1)(A) of the Social Security Act for any other indications for the implantation and use of single chamber or dual chamber cardiac pacemakers that are not specifically addressed in this NCD.

100-4, 32, 320.2

Cardiac Pacemaker Healthcare Common Procedure Coding System (HCPCS) and Current Procedural Terminology (CPT) Codes

Professional claims

Effective for claims with dates of service on or after August 13, 2013, MACs shall pay for implanted permanent cardiac pacemakers, single chamber or dual chamber, for one of the following CPT codes:

- 33206 - Insertion or replacement of permanent pacemaker with transvenous electrode(s)—atrial
- 33207 - Insertion or replacement of permanent pacemaker with transvenous electrode(s)—ventricular
- 33208 - Insertion or replacement of permanent pacemaker with transvenous electrode(s)—atrial and ventricular Institutional claims

Effective for claims with dates of service on or after August 13, 2013, MACs shall pay for implanted permanent cardiac pacemakers, single chamber or dual chamber, for the following HCPCS codes:

- C1785 - Pacemaker, dual chamber, rate-responsive (implantable)
- C1786 - Pacemaker, single chamber, rate-responsive (implantable)
- C2619 - Pacemaker, dual chamber, nonrate-responsive (implantable)
- C2620 - Pacemaker, single chamber, nonrate-responsive (implantable)
- 33206 - Insertion or replacement of permanent pacemaker with transvenous electrode(s)-atrial
- 33207 - Insertion or replacement of permanent pacemaker with transvenous electrode(s)-ventricular
- 33208 - Insertion or replacement of permanent pacemaker with transvenous electrode(s)-atrialand ventricular

100-4, 32, 320.3

320.3 – Cardiac Pacemaker Covered ICD-9/ICD-10 Diagnosis Codes

(Rev. 2872, Issued: 02-06-14, Effective: 08-13-13, Implementation: 07-07-14)

Professional claims

For claims with dates of service on and after August 13, 2013, for implanted permanent cardiac pacemakers, single chamber or dual chamber, claims submitted with one of the following CPT codes: 33206, 33207, or 33208, and contains at least one of the following ICD-9/ICD-10 diagnosis codes are covered:

- 426.0 Atrioventricular block, complete/ I44.2 Atrioventricular block, complete
- 426.12 Mobitz (type) II atrioventricular block/ I44.1 Atrioventricular block, second degree
- 426.13 Other second degree atrioventricular block/ I44.1 Atrioventricular block, second degree
- 427.81 Sinoatrial node dysfunction/ I49.5 Sick sinus syndrome
- 746.86 Congenital heart block/ Q24.6 – Congenital heart block

The following diagnosis codes can be covered at contractor discretion if submitted with at least one of the CPT codes and diagnosis codes listed above:

- 426.10 Atrioventricular block, unspecified/ I44.30 Unspecified atrioventricular block
- 426.4 Right bundle branch block/ I45.10 Unspecified right bundle-branch block / I45.19 Other right bundle branch block
- 427.0 Paroxysmal supraventricular tachycardia/ I47.1 Supraventricular tachycardia

Institutional claims

For claims with dates of service on and after August 13, 2013, for implanted permanent cardiac pacemakers, single chamber or dual chamber, using HCPCS codes: C1785, C1786, C2619, C2620, 33206, 33207, or 33208, the following ICD-9 diagnosis codes are covered (see ICD-10 translations below):

- 37.81 Initial insertion of single chamber device, not specified as rate responsive
- 37.82 Initial insertion of single chamber device, rate responsive
- 37.83 Initial insertion of single chamber device
- 426.0 Atrioventricular block, complete
- 426.12 Mobitz (type) II atrioventricular block
- 426.13 Other second degree atrioventricular block
- 427.81 Sinoatrial node dysfunction
- 746.86 Congenital heart block

The following diagnosis codes can be covered at contractor discretion if submitted with at least one of the CPT codes and diagnosis codes listed above:

- 426.10 Atrioventricular block, unspecified/ I44.30 Unspecified atrioventricular block
- 426.4 Right bundle branch block/ I45.10 Unspecified right bundle-branch block / I45.19 Other right bundle branch block

- 427.0 Paroxysmal supraventricular tachycardia/ I47.1 Supraventricular tachycardia

Contractors shall note the appropriate ICD-10 diagnosis code(s) that are listed below for future implementation. Contractors shall track the ICD-10 codes and ensure that the updated edit is turned on as part of the ICD-10 implementation effective October 1, 2014.

ICD-9-CM Codes	ICD-10-CM Codes
37.81 Initial insertion of single-chamber device, not specified as rate responsive	**0JH604Z** Insertion of Pacemaker, Single Chamber into Chest Subcutaneous Tissue and Fascia, Open Approach
	0JH634Z Insertion of Pacemaker, Single Chamber into Chest Subcutaneous Tissue and Fascia, Percutaneous Approach
	0JH804Z Insertion of Pacemaker, Single Chamber into Abdomen Subcutaneous Tissue and Fascia, Open Approach
	0JH834Z Insertion of Pacemaker, Single Chamber into Abdomen Subcutaneous Tissue and Fascia, Percutaneous Approach
37.82 Initial insertion of single-chamber device, rate responsive	**0JH605Z** Insertion of Pacemaker, Single Chamber Rate Responsive into Chest Subcutaneous Tissue and Fascia, Open Approach
	0JH635Z Insertion of Pacemaker, Single Chamber Rate Responsive into Chest Subcutaneous Tissue and Fascia, Percutaneous Approach
	0JH805Z Insertion of Pacemaker, Single Chamber Rate Responsive into Abdomen Subcutaneous Tissue and Fascia, Open Approach
	0JH835Z Insertion of Pacemaker, Single Chamber Rate Responsive into Abdomen Subcutaneous Tissue and Fascia, Percutaneous Approach
37.83 Initial insertion of dual-chamber device	**0JH606Z** Insertion of Pacemaker, Dual Chamber into Chest Subcutaneous Tissue and Fascia, Open Approach
	0JH636Z Insertion of Pacemaker, Dual Chamber into Chest Subcutaneous Tissue and Fascia, Percutaneous Approach
	0JH806Z Insertion of Pacemaker, Dual Chamber into Abdomen Subcutaneous Tissue and Fascia, Open Approach
	0JH836Z Insertion of Pacemaker, Dual Chamber into Abdomen Subcutaneous Tissue and Fascia, Percutaneous Approach
426.0 Atrioventricular block, complete	**I44.2** Atrioventricular block, complete
426.12 Mobitz (type) II atrioventricular block	**I44.1** Atrioventricular block, second degree
426.13 Other second degree atrioventricular block	**I44.1** Atrioventricular block, second degree
427.81 Sinoatrial node dysfunction	**I49.5** Sick sinus syndrome
746.86 Congenital heart block	**Q24.6** Congenital heart block

100-4, 32, 320.4

Cardiac Pacemaker Claims Require the KX Modifier

Contractors shall pay for implanted permanent cardiac pacemakers, single chamber or dual chamber claims containing HCPCS and/or CPT codes listed in section 320.2, when submitted with the -KX modifier.

NOTE: MACs shall accept the inclusion of the -KX modifier on the claim line(s) as an attestation by the practitioner and/or provider of the service that coverage criteria has been met; i.e., documentation is on file verifying the patient has non-reversible symptomatic bradycardia (symptoms of bradycardia are symptoms that can be directly attributable to a heart rate less than 60 beats per minute (for example: syncope, seizures, congestive heart failure, dizziness, or confusion).

100-4, 32, 320.5

Cardiac Pacemaker Claims Without the KX Modifier

Professional claims

Contractors shall return claims lines for implanted permanent cardiac pacemakers, single chamber or dual chamber, containing one of the following CPT codes: 33206, 33207, or 33208, as unprocessable when the -KX modifier is not present. Contractors shall use the following messages:

CARC 4 - The procedure code is inconsistent with the modifier used or a required modifier is missing

RARC N517 - Resubmit a new claim with the requested information.

Institutional claims

Contractors shall return to providers claims for implanted permanent cardiac pacemakers, single chamber or dual chamber, when the -KX modifier is not present on the claim.

100-4, 32, 320.6

Cardiac Pacemaker Non Covered ICD-9/ICD-10 Diagnosis Codes

For claims with dates of service on and after August 13, 2013, for implanted permanent cardiac pacemakers, single chamber or dual chamber, using one of the following HCPCS and/or CPT codes: C1785, C1786, C2619,C2620, 33206, 33207, or 33208, and at least one of the following ICD-9-CM/ICD-10-CM diagnosis codes, are not covered:

- 426.10 Atrioventricular block, unspecified/ I44.30 Unspecified atrioventricular block
- 426.11 First degree atrioventricular block/ I44.0 Atrioventricular block first degree
- 426.4 Right bundle branch block/ I45.10 Unspecified right bundle-branch block / I45.19 Other right bundle branch block
- 427.0 Paroxysmal supraventricular tachycardia/ I47.1 Supraventricular tachycardia
- 427.31 Atrial fibrillation/ I48.1 Persistent atrial fibrillation/ I48.2 Chronic atrial fibrillation
- 427.32 Atrial flutter/ I48.3 Typical atrial flutter/ I48.4 Atypical atrial flutter
- 427.89 Other specified cardiac dysrhythmias, Other/ I49.8 Other specified cardiac arrhythmias780.2 Syncope and collapse/ R55 Syncope and collapse

The following diagnosis codes are not covered if they are not submitted with at least one of the CPT codes and diagnosis codes listed in section 320.3:

- 426.10 Atrioventricular block, unspecified/ I44.30 Unspecified atrioventricular block
- 426.4 Right bundle branch block/ I45.10 Unspecified right bundle-branch block / I45.19 Other right bundle branch block
- 427.0 Paroxysmal supraventricular tachycardia/ I47.1 Supraventricular tachycardia

100-4, 32, 330

Percutaneous Image-guided Lumbar Decompression (PILD) for Lumbar Spinal Stenosis (LSS)

PILD is a posterior decompression of the lumbar spine performed under indirect image guidance without any direct visualization of the surgical area. This is a procedure proposed as a treatment for symptomatic LSS unresponsive to conservative therapy. This procedure is generally described as a non-invasive procedure using specially designed instruments to percutaneously remove a portion of the lamina and debulk the ligamentum flavum. The procedure is performed under x-ray guidance (e.g., fluoroscopic, CT) with the assistance of contrast media to identify and monitor the compressed area via epidurogram. For complete Medical coverage guidelines, see National Coverage Determinations (NCD) Manual (Pub 100-03) ? 150.13

100-4, 32, 330.1

Claims Processing Requirements for Percutaneous Image-guided Lumbar Decompression (PILD) for Lumbar Spinal Stenosis (LSS) on Professional Claims

For claims with dates of service on or after January 9, 2014, PILD, procedure code 0275T, is a covered service only when billed as part of a clinical trial approved by CMS, when billed for the ICD-9 diagnosis of 724.01-724.03 or the ICD-10 diagnosis of M48.05-M48.07, when billed in places of service 22 (Outpatient) or 24 (Ambulatory Surgical Center), when billed along with V70.7 (ICD-9) or Z00.6 (ICD-10) in either the primary/secondary positions, and when billed with modifier Q0.

Additionally, per Transmittal 2805 (Change Request 8401), issued October 30, 2013, all claims for clinical trials must contain the 8 digit clinical trial identifier number.

The following message(s) shall be used to notify providers of return situations that may occur:

Professional Claims 8-digit Clinical Trial Number

For claims with dates of service on or after January 9, 2014, contractors shall pay for PILD only when billed with the numeric, 8-digit clinical trial identifier number preceded by the two alpha characters "CT" when placed in Field 19 of paper Form CMS-1500, or when entered without the "CT" prefix in the electronic 837P in Loop 2300 REF02 (REF01=P4). Claims for PILD which are billed without an 8-digit clinical trial identifier number shall be returned as unprocessable.

The following messages shall be used when Medicare contractors return PILD claims billed without an 8-digit clinical trial identifier number as unprocessable: Claims Adjustment Reason Code 16: "Claim/service lacks information or has submission/billing error(s) which is needed for adjudication"

Remittance Advice Remark Code N721: "This service is only covered when performed as part of a clinical trial."

Remittance Advice Remark Code MA50: "Missing/incomplete/invalid Investigational Device Exemption number or Clinical Trial number."

Remittance Advice Remark Code N704: "Alert: You may not appeal this decision but can resubmit this claim/service with corrected information if warranted."

Professional Claims Place of Service — 22 or 24

For claims with dates of service on or after January 9, 2014, contractors shall pay for PILD only when billed in place of service 22 or 24. Claims for PILD which are billed in any other place of service shall be returned as unprocessable.

The following messages shall be used when Medicare contractors return PILD claims not billed in place of service 22 or 24:

Claims Adjustment Reason Code 58: "Treatment was deemed by the payer to have been rendered in an inappropriate or invalid place of service."

Remittance Advice Remark Code N704: "Alert: You may not appeal this decision but can resubmit this claim/service with corrected information if warranted."

Professional Claims Modifier — Q0

For claims with dates of service on or after January 9, 2014, contractors shall pay for PILD only when billed with modifier Q0. Claims for PILD which are billed without modifier Q0 shall be returned as unprocessable.

The following messages shall be used when Medicare contractors return PILD claims billed without modifier Q0 as unprocessable:

Claims Adjustment Reason Code 4: "The procedure code is inconsistent with the modifier used or a required modifier is missing."

Remittance Advice Remark Code N657: "This should be billed with the appropriate code for these services."

Remittance Advice Remark Code N704: "Alert: You may not appeal this decision but can resubmit this claim/service with corrected information if warranted."

Non-covered Diagnosis

For claims with dates of service on or after January 9, 2014, contractors shall pay for PILD only when billed with the ICD-9 diagnosis of 724.01-724.03 or the ICD-10 diagnosis of M48.05-M48.07.

The following messages shall be used when Medicare contractors return PILD claims, billed without the covered diagnosis, as unprocessable:

Claims Adjustment Reason Code B22: "This payment is adjusted based on the diagnosis."

Remittance Advice Remark Code N704: "Alert: You may not appeal this decision but can resubmit this claim/service with corrected information if warranted."

Clinical Trial Diagnosis

For claims with dates of service on or after January 9, 2014, contractors shall pay for PILD only when billed with the ICD-9 diagnosis of V70.7 (ICD-9) or Z00.6 (ICD-10) in either the primary or secondary positions.

The following messages shall be used when Medicare contractors return PILD claims, billed without the clinical trial diagnosis, as unprocessable:

Claims Adjustment Reason Code B22: "This payment is adjusted based on the diagnosis."

Remittance Advice Remark Code N704: "Alert: You may not appeal this decision but can resubmit this claim/service with corrected information if warranted."

100-4, 32, 330.2

Claims Processing Requirements for PILD for Outpatient Facilities

Hospital Outpatient facilities shall bill for PILD for percutaneous image-guided lumbar decompression (PILD,) procedure code 0275T for lumbar spinal stenosis (LSS) on a 13X or 85X TOB, effective on or after January 9, 2014. Refer to Section 69 of this chapter for further guidance on billing under CED.

Hospital outpatient procedures for PILD shall be covered when billed with:

- ICD-9 V70.7 (ICD-10 Z00.6) and Condition Code 30.
- Modifier Q0—An 8-digit clinical trial identifier number listed on the CMS Coverage with Evidence Development website Hospital outpatient procedures for PILD shall be rejected when billed without:
- ICD-9 V70.7 (ICD-10 Z00.6) and Condition Code 30.
- Modifier Q0—An 8-digit clinical trial identifier number listed on the CMS Coverage with Evidence Development website

Claims billed by hospitals not participating in the trial /registry, shall be rejected with the following message:

CARC: 50 -These are non-covered services because this is not deemed a "medical necessity" by the payer.

RARC N386 - This decision was based on a National Coverage Determination (NCD). An NCD provides a coverage determination as to whether a particular item or service is covered. A copy of this policy is available at http://www.cms.hhs.gov/mcd/search.asp. If you do not have web access, you may contact the contractor to request a copy of the NCD.

Group Code—Contractual Obligation (CO)

MSN 16.77 ?This service/item was not covered because it was not provided as part of a qualifying trial/study. (Este servicio/art?ulo no fue cubierto porque no estaba incluido como parte de un ensayo cl?ico/estudio calificado.)

100-5, 5, 40.7

Billing for Biofeedback Training for the Treatment of Urinary Incontinence

Medicare covered biofeedback training for the treatment of urinary incontinence may be provided by physical therapists in facility settings. For information regarding the coverage of this service, see the Medicare National Coverage Determinations Manual, Chapter 1, Section 30.1.1. Medicare pays for this service under the Medicare Physician Fee Schedule.

Providers bill this service on one of the types of bill listed in section 40.2 using revenue code 042X and one of the following HCPCS codes:

- 90901 - Biofeedback training by any modality
- 90911 - Biofeedback training, perineal muscles, anorectal or urethral sphincter, including EMG and/or manometry

100-8, 15, 4.2.8

Cardiac Rehabilitation (CR) and Intensive Cardiac Rehabilitation (ICR)

A. General Background Information

Effective January 1, 2010, Medicare Part B covers Cardiac Rehabilitation (CR) and Intensive Cardiac Rehabilitation (ICR) program services for beneficiaries who have experienced one or more of the following:

- An acute myocardial infarction within the preceding 12 months;
- A coronary artery bypass surgery;
- Current stable angina pectoris;
- Heart valve repair or replacement;
- Percutaneous transluminal coronary angioplasty or coronary stenting;
- A heart or heart-lung transplant; or,
- A stable, chronic heart failure defined as patients with left ventricular ejection fraction of 35% or less and New York Heart Association (NYHA) class II to IV symptoms despite being on optimal heart failure therapy for at least 6 weeks (effective February 18, 2014).

ICR programs must be approved by the Centers for Medicare & Medicaid Services (CMS) through the national coverage determination (NCD) process and must meet certain criteria for approval. Individual sites wishing to provide ICR services via an approved ICR program must enroll with their local Medicare Administrative Contractor (MAC) as an ICR program supplier.

B. ICR Enrollment

In order to enroll as an ICR site, a supplier must complete a Form CMS-855B, with the supplier type of "Other" selected. MACs shall verify that the ICR program is approved by CMS through the NCD process. A list of approved ICR programs will be identified through the NCD listings, the CMS Web site and the Federal Register. MACs shall use one of these options to verify that the ICR program has met CMS approval.

ICR suppliers shall be enrolled using specialty code 31. ICR suppliers must separately enroll each of their practice locations. Therefore, each enrolling ICR supplier can only have one practice location on its CMS-855B enrollment application and shall receive its own Provider Transaction Account Number. MACs shall only accept and process reassignments (855R's) to ICR suppliers for physicians defined in 1861(r)(1) of the Social Security Act.

C. Additional Information

For more information on ICR suppliers, refer to:

- 42 CFR §410.49
- Pub. 100-04, Medicare Claims Processing Manual, chapter 32, section 140
- Pub. 100-02, Medicare Benefit Policy Manual, chapter 15, section 232
- Pub. 100-03, National Coverage Determinations Manual, chapter 1, part 1, section 20.10

Appendix H — Glossary

-centesis. Puncture, as with a needle, trocar, or aspirator; often done for withdrawing fluid from a cavity.

-ectomy. Excision, removal.

-orrhaphy. Suturing.

-ostomy. Indicates a surgically created artificial opening.

-otomy. Making an incision or opening.

-plasty. Indicates surgically formed or molded.

abdominal lymphadenectomy. Surgical removal of the abdominal lymph nodes grouping, with or without para-aortic and vena cava nodes.

ablation. Removal or destruction of a body part or tissue or its function. Ablation may be performed by surgical means, hormones, drugs, radiofrequency, heat, chemical application, or other methods.

abnormal alleles. Form of gene that includes disease-related variations.

absorbable sutures. Strands prepared from collagen or a synthetic polymer and capable of being absorbed by tissue over time. Examples include surgical gut and collagen sutures; or synthetics like polydioxanone (PDS), polyglactin 910 (Vicryl), poliglecaprone 25 (Monocryl), polyglyconate (Maxon), and polyglycolic acid (Dexon).

acetabuloplasty. Surgical repair or reconstruction of the large cup-shaped socket in the hipbone (acetabulum) with which the head of the femur articulates.

Achilles tendon. Tendon attached to the back of the heel bone (calcaneus) that flexes the foot downward.

acromioclavicular joint. Junction between the clavicle and the scapula. The acromion is the projection from the back of the scapula that forms the highest point of the shoulder and connects with the clavicle. Trauma or injury to the acromioclavicular joint is often referred to as a dislocation of the shoulder. This is not correct, however, as a dislocation of the shoulder is a disruption of the glenohumeral joint.

acromionectomy. Surgical treatment for acromioclavicular arthritis in which the distal portion of the acromion process is removed.

acromioplasty. Repair of the part of the shoulder blade that connects to the deltoid muscles and clavicle.

actigraphy. Science of monitoring activity levels, particularly during sleep. In most cases, the patient wears a wristband that records motion while sleeping. The data are recorded, analyzed, and interpreted to study sleep/wake patterns and circadian rhythms.

air conduction. Transportation of sound from the air, through the external auditory canal, to the tympanic membrane and ossicular chain. Air conduction hearing is tested by presenting an acoustic stimulus through earphones or a loudspeaker to the ear.

air puff device. Instrument that measures intraocular pressure by evaluating the force of a reflected amount of air blown against the cornea.

alleles. Form of gene usually arising from a mutation responsible for a hereditary variation.

allogeneic collection. Collection of blood or blood components from one person for the use of another. Allogeneic collection was formerly termed homologous collection.

allograft. Graft from one individual to another of the same species.

amniocentesis. Surgical puncture through the abdominal wall, with a specialized needle and under ultrasonic guidance, into the interior of the pregnant uterus and directly into the amniotic sac to collect fluid for diagnostic analysis or therapeutic reduction of fluid levels.

anastomosis. Surgically created connection between ducts, blood vessels, or bowel segments to allow flow from one to the other.

anesthesia time. Time period factored into anesthesia procedures beginning with the anesthesiologist preparing the patient for surgery and ending when the patient is turned over to the recovery department.

Angelman syndrome. Early childhood emergence of a pattern of interrupted development, stiff, jerky gait, absence or impairment of speech, excessive laughter, and seizures.

angioplasty. Reconstruction or repair of a diseased or damaged blood vessel.

annuloplasty. Surgical plicaton of weakened tissue of the heart, to improve its muscular function. Annuli are thick, fibrous rings and one is found surrounding each of the cardiac chambers. The atrial and ventricular muscle fibers attach to the annuli. In annuloplasty, weakened annuli may be surgically plicated, or tucked, to improve muscular functions.

anorectal anometry. Measurement of pressure generated by anal sphincter to diagnose incontinence.

anterior chamber lenses. Lenses inserted into the anterior chamber following intracapsular cataract extraction.

applanation tonometer. Instrument that measures intraocular pressure by recording the force required to flatten an area of the cornea.

appropriateness of care. Proper setting of medical care that best meets the patient's care or diagnosis, as defined by a health care plan or other legal entity.

aqueous humor. Fluid within the anterior and posterior chambers of the eye that is continually replenished as it diffuses out into the blood. When the flow of aqueous is blocked, a build-up of fluid in the eye causes increased intraocular pressure and leads to glaucoma and blindness.

arteriogram. Radiograph of arteries.

arteriovenous fistula. Connecting passage between an artery and a vein.

arteriovenous malformation. Connecting passage between an artery and a vein.

arthrotomy. Surgical incision into a joint that may include exploration, drainage, or removal of a foreign body.

ASA. American Society of Anesthesiologists. National organization for anesthesiology that maintains and publishes the guidelines and relative values for anesthesia coding.

aspirate. To withdraw fluid or air from a body cavity by suction.

assay. A chemical analysis of a substance to establish the presence and strength of its components. A therapeutic drug assay is used to determine if a drug is within the expected therapeutic range for a patient.

atrial septal defect. Cardiac anomaly consisting of a patent opening in the atrial septum due to a fusion failure, classified as ostium secundum type, ostium primum defect, or endocardial cushion defect.

attended surveillance. Ability of a technician at a remote surveillance center or location to respond immediately to patient transmissions regarding rhythm or device alerts as they are produced and received at the remote location. These transmissions may originate from wearable or implanted therapy or monitoring devices.

auricle. External ear, which is a single elastic cartilage covered in skin and normal adnexal features (hair follicles, sweat glands, and sebaceous glands), shaped to channel sound waves into the acoustic meatus.

autogenous transplant. Tissue, such as bone, that is harvested from the patient and used for transplantation back into the same patient.

autograft. Any tissue harvested from one anatomical site of a person and grafted to another anatomical site of the same person. Most commonly, blood vessels, skin, tendons, fascia, and bone are used as autografts.

AVF. Arteriovenous fistula.

AVM. Arteriovenous malformation. Clusters of abnormal blood vessels that grow in the brain comprised of a blood vessel "nidus" or nest through which arteries and veins connect directly without going through the capillaries. As time passes, the nidus may enlarge resulting in the formation of a mass that may bleed. AVMs are more prone to bleeding in patients ages 10 to 55. Once older than age 55, the possibility of bleeding is reduced dramatically.

backbench preparation. Procedures performed on a donor organ following procurement to prepare the organ for transplant into the recipient. Excess fat and other tissue may be removed, the organ may be perfused, and vital arteries may be sized, repaired, or modified to fit the patient. These procedures are done on a back table in the operating room before transplantation can begin.

Bartholin's gland. Mucous-producing gland found in the vestibular bulbs on either side of the vaginal orifice and connected to the mucosal membrane at the opening by a duct.

Bartholin's gland abscess. Pocket of pus and surrounding cellulitis caused by infection of the Bartholin's gland and causing localized swelling and pain in the posterior labia majora that may extend into the lower vagina.

basic value. Relative weighted value based upon the usual anesthesia services and the relative work or cost of the specific anesthesia service assigned to each anesthesia-specific procedure code.

Berman locator. Small, sensitive tool used to detect the location of a metallic foreign body in the eye.

bifurcated. Having two branches or divisions, such as the left pulmonary veins that split off from the left atrium to carry oxygenated blood away from the heart.

biopsy. Tissue or fluid removed for diagnostic purposes through analysis of the cells in the biopsy material.

Blalock-Hanlon procedure. Excision of a segment of the right atrium, creating an atrial septal defect.

Blalock-Taussig procedure. Anastomosis of the left subclavian artery to the left pulmonary artery or the right subclavian artery to the right pulmonary artery in order to shunt some of the blood flow from the systemic to the pulmonary circulation.

blepharochalasis. Loss of elasticity and relaxation of skin of the eyelid, thickened or indurated skin on the eyelid associated with recurrent episodes of edema, and intracellular atrophy.

blepharoplasty. Plastic surgery of the eyelids to remove excess fat and redundant skin weighting down the lid. The eyelid is pulled tight and sutured to support sagging muscles.

blepharoptosis. Droop or displacement of the upper eyelid, caused by paralysis, muscle problems, or outside mechanical forces.

blepharorrhaphy. Suture of a portion or all of the opposing eyelids to shorten the palpebral fissure or close it entirely.

bone conduction. Transportation of sound through the bones of the skull to the inner ear.

bone mass measurement. Radiologic or radioisotopic procedure or other procedure approved by the FDA for identifying bone mass, detecting bone loss, or determining bone quality. The procedure includes a physician's interpretation of the results. Qualifying individuals must be an estrogen-deficient woman at clinical risk for osteoporosis with vertebral abnormalities.

brachytherapy. Form of radiation therapy in which radioactive pellets or seeds are implanted directly into the tissue being treated to deliver their dose of radiation in a more directed fashion. Brachytherapy provides radiation to the prescribed body area while minimizing exposure to normal tissue.

breakpoint. Point at which a chromosome breaks.

Bristow procedure. Anterior capsulorrhaphy prevents chronic separation of the shoulder. In this procedure, the bone block is affixed to the anterior glenoid rim with a screw.

buccal mucosa. Tissue from the mucous membrane on the inside of the cheek.

bundle of His. Bundle of modified cardiac fibers that begins at the atrioventricular node and passes through the right atrioventricular fibrous ring to the interventricular septum, where it divides into two branches. Bundle of His recordings are taken for intracardiac electrograms.

Caldwell-Luc operation. Intraoral antrostomy approach into the maxillary sinus for the removal of tooth roots or tissue, or for packing the sinus to reduce zygomatic fractures by creating a window above the teeth in the canine fossa area.

canthorrhaphy. Suturing of the palpebral fissure, the juncture between the eyelids, at either end of the eye.

canthotomy. Horizontal incision at the canthus (junction of upper and lower eyelids) to divide the outer canthus and enlarge lid margin separation.

cardio-. Relating to the heart.

cardiopulmonary bypass. Venous blood is diverted to a heart-lung machine, which mechanically pumps and oxygenates the blood temporarily so the heart can be bypassed while an open procedure on the heart or coronary arteries is performed. During bypass, the lungs are deflated and immobile.

cardioverter-defibrillator. Device that uses both low energy cardioversion or defibrillating shocks and antitachycardia pacing to treat ventricular tachycardia or ventricular fibrillation.

care plan oversight services. Physician's ongoing review and revision of a patient's care plan involving complex or multidisciplinary care modalities.

case management services. Physician case management is a process of involving direct patient care as well as coordinating and controlling access to the patient or initiating and/or supervising other necessary health care services.

cataract extraction. Surgical removal of the cataract or cloudy lens. Anterior chamber lenses are inserted in conjunction with intracapsular cataract extraction and posterior chamber lenses are inserted in conjunction with extracapsular cataract extraction.

catheter. Flexible tube inserted into an area of the body for introducing or withdrawing fluid.

Centers for Medicare and Medicaid Services. Federal agency that oversees the administration of the public health programs such as Medicare, Medicaid, and State Children's Insurance Program.

certified nurse midwife. Registered nurse who has successfully completed a program of study and clinical experience or has been certified by a recognized organization for the care of pregnant or delivering patients.

CFR. Code of Federal Regulations.

CHAMPUS. Civilian Health and Medical Program of the Uniformed Services. See Tricare.

CHAMPVA. Civilian Health and Medical Program of the Veteran's Administration.

chemodenervation. Chemical destruction of nerves. A substance, for example, Botox, is used to temporarily inhibit the transfer of chemicals at the presynaptic membrane, blocking the neuromuscular junctions.

chemoembolization. Administration of chemotherapeutic agents directly to a tumor in combination with the percutaneous administration of an occlusive substance into a vessel to deprive the tumor of its blood supply. This ensures a prolonged level of therapy directed at the tumor. Chemoembolization is primarily being used for cancers of the liver and endocrine system.

chemosurgery. Application of chemical agents to destroy tissue, originally referring to the in situ chemical fixation of premalignant or malignant lesions to facilitate surgical excision.

Chiari osteotomy. Top of the femur is altered to correct a dislocated hip caused by congenital conditions or cerebral palsy. Plate and screws are often used.

chimera. Organ or anatomic structure consisting of tissues of diverse genetic constitution.

choanal atresia. Congenital, membranous, or bony closure of one or both posterior nostrils due to failure of the embryonic bucconasal membrane to rupture and open up the nasal passageway.

chondromalacia. Condition in which the articular cartilage softens, seen in various body sites but most often in the patella, and may be congenital or acquired.

chorionic villus sampling. Aspiration of a placental sample through a catheter, under ultrasonic guidance. The specialized needle is placed transvaginally through the cervix or transabdominally into the uterine cavity.

chronic pain management services. Distinct services frequently performed by anesthesiologists who have additional training in pain management procedures. Pain management services include initial and subsequent evaluation and management (E/M) services, trigger point injections, spine and spinal cord injections, and nerve blocks.

cineplastic amputation. Amputation in which muscles and tendons of the remaining portion of the extremity are arranged so that they may be utilized for motor functions. Following this type of amputation, a specially constructed prosthetic device allows the individual to execute more complex movements because the muscles and tendons are able to communicate independent movements to the device.

circadian. Relating to a cyclic, 24-hour period.

clinical social worker. Individual who possesses a master's or doctor's degree in social work and, after obtaining the degree, has performed at least two years of supervised clinical social work. A clinical social worker must be licensed by the state or, in the case of states without licensure, must completed at least two years or 3,000 hours of post-master's degree supervised clinical social work practice under the supervision of a master's level social worker.

clinical staff. Someone who works for, or under, the direction of a physician or qualified health care professional and does not bill services separately. The person may be licensed or regulated to help the physician perform specific duties.

clonal. Originating from one cell.

CMS. Centers for Medicare and Medicaid Services. Federal agency that administers the public health programs.

CO2 laser. Carbon dioxide laser that emits an invisible beam and vaporizes water-rich tissue. The vapor is suctioned from the site.

codons. Series of three adjoining bases in one polynucleotide chain of a DNA or RNA molecule that provides the codes for a specific amino acid.

cognitive. Being aware by drawing from knowledge, such as judgment, reason, perception, and memory.

colostomy. Artificial surgical opening anywhere along the length of the colon to the skin surface for the diversion of feces.

commissurotomy. Surgical division or disruption of any two parts that are joined to form a commissure in order to increase the opening. The procedure most often refers to opening the adherent leaflet bands of fibrous tissue in a stenosed mitral valve.

common variants. Nucleotide sequence differences associated with abnormal gene function. Tests are usually performed in a single series of laboratory testing (in a single, typically multiplex, assay arrangement or using more than one assay to include all variants to be examined). Variants are representative of a mutation that mainly causes a single disease, such as cystic fibrosis. Other uncommon variants could provide additional information. Tests may be performed based on society recommendations and guidelines.

community mental health center. Facility providing outpatient mental health day treatment, assessments, and education as appropriate to community members.

computerized corneal topography. Digital imaging and analysis by computer of the shape of the corneal.

conjunctiva. Mucous membrane lining of the eyelids and covering of the exposed, anterior sclera.

conjunctivodacryocystostomy. Surgical connection of the lacrimal sac directly to the conjunctival sac.

conjunctivorhinostomy. Correction of an obstruction of the lacrimal canal achieved by suturing the posterior flaps and removing any lacrimal obstruction, preserving the conjunctiva.

constitutional. Cells containing genetic code that may be passed down to future generations. May also be referred to as germline.

consultation. Advice or opinion regarding diagnosis and treatment or determination to accept transfer of care of a patient rendered by a medical professional at the request of the primary care provider.

continuous positive airway pressure device. Pressurized device used to maintain the patient's airway for spontaneous or mechanically aided breathing. Often used for patients with mild to moderate sleep apnea.

core needle biopsy. Large-bore biopsy needle inserted into a mass and a core of tissue is removed for diagnostic study.

corpectomy. Removal of the body of a bone, such as a vertebra.

costochondral. Pertaining to the ribs and the scapula.

CPT. Current Procedural Terminology. Definitive procedural coding system developed by the American Medical Association that lists descriptive terms and identifying codes to provide a uniform language that describes medical, surgical, and diagnostic services for nationwide communication among physicians, patients, and third parties, used to report professional and outpatient services.

craniosynostosis. Congenital condition in which one or more of the cranial sutures fuse prematurely, creating a deformed or aberrant head shape.

craterization. Excision of a portion of bone creating a crater-like depression to facilitate drainage from infected areas of bone.

cricoid. Circular cartilage around the trachea.

CRNA. Certified registered nurse anesthetist. Nurse trained and specializing in the administration of anesthesia.

cryolathe. Tool used for reshaping a button of corneal tissue.

cryosurgery. Application of intense cold, usually produced using liquid nitrogen, to locally freeze diseased or unwanted tissue and induce tissue necrosis without causing harm to adjacent tissue.

CT. Computed tomography.

cutdown. Small, incised opening in the skin to expose a blood vessel, especially over a vein (venous cutdown) to allow venipuncture and permit a needle or cannula to be inserted for the withdrawal of blood or administration of fluids.

cytogenetic studies. Procedures in CPT that are related to the branch of genetics that studies cellular (cyto) structure and function as it relates to heredity (genetics). White blood cells, specifically T-lymphocytes, are the most commonly used specimen for chromosome analysis.

cytogenomic. Chromosomic evaluation using molecular methods.

dacryocystotome. Instrument used for incising the lacrimal duct strictures.

debride. To remove all foreign objects and devitalized or infected tissue from a burn or wound to prevent infection and promote healing.

definitive drug testing. Drug tests used to further analyze or confirm the presence or absence of specific drugs or classes of drugs used by the patient. These tests are able to provide more conclusive information regarding the concentration of the drug and their metabolites. May be used for medical, workplace, or legal purposes.

definitive identification. Identification of microorganisms using additional tests to specify the genus or species (e.g., slide cultures or biochemical panels).

Department of Health and Human Services. Cabinet department that oversees the operating divisions of the federal government responsible for health and welfare. HHS oversees the Centers for Medicare and Medicaid Services, Food and Drug Administration, Public Health Service, and other such entities.

Department of Justice. Attorneys from the DOJ and the United States Attorney's Office have, under the memorandum of understanding, the same direct access to contractor data and records as the OIG and the Federal Bureau of Investigation (FBI). DOJ is responsible for prosecution of fraud and civil or criminal cases presented.

dermis. Skin layer found under the epidermis that contains a papillary upper layer and the deep reticular layer of collagen, vascular bed, and nerves.

dermis graft. Skin graft that has been separated from the epidermal tissue and the underlying subcutaneous fat, used primarily as a substitute for fascia grafts in plastic surgery.

desensitization. 1) Administration of extracts of allergens periodically to build immunity in the patient. 2) Application of medication to decrease the symptoms, usually pain, associated with a dental condition or disease.

destruction. Ablation or eradication of a structure or tissue.

diabetes outpatient self-management training services. Educational and training services furnished by a certified provider in an outpatient setting. The physician managing the individual's diabetic condition must certify that the services are needed under a comprehensive plan of care and provide the patient with the skills and knowledge necessary for therapeutic program compliance (including skills related to the self-administration of injectable drugs). The provider must meet applicable standards established by the National Diabetes Advisory or be recognized by an organization that represents individuals with diabetes as meeting standards for furnishing the services.

diagnostic procedures. Procedure performed on a patient to obtain information to assess the medical condition of the patient or to identify a disease and to determine the nature and severity of an illness or injury.

diaphragm. 1) Muscular wall separating the thorax and its structures from the abdomen. 2) Flexible disk inserted into the vagina and against the cervix as a method of birth control.

diaphysectomy. Surgical removal of a portion of the shaft of a long bone, often done to facilitate drainage from infected bone.

diathermy. Applying heat to body tissues by various methods for therapeutic treatment or surgical purposes to coagulate and seal tissue.

dilation. Artificial increase in the diameter of an opening or lumen made by medication or by instrumentation.

dissect. Cut apart or separate tissue for surgical purposes or for visual or microscopic study.

DNA. Deoxyribonucleic acid (DNA) is the chemical containing the genetic information necessary to produce and propagate living organisms. Molecules are comprised of two twisting, paired strands, called a double helix.

DNA marker. Specific gene sequence within a chromosome indicating the inheritance of a certain trait.

dorsal. Pertaining to the back or posterior aspect.

drugs and biologicals. Drugs and biologicals included - or approved for inclusion - in the United States Pharmacopoeia, the National Formulary, the United States Homeopathic Pharmacopoeia, in New Drugs or Accepted Dental Remedies, or approved by the pharmacy and drug therapeutics committee of the medical staff of the hospital. Also included are medically accepted and FDA approved drugs used in an anticancer chemotherapeutic regimen. The carrier determines medical acceptance based on supportive clinical evidence.

dual-lead device. Implantable cardiac device (pacemaker or implantable cardioverter-defibrillator [ICD]) in which pacing and sensing components are placed in only two chambers of the heart.

duplex scan. Noninvasive vascular diagnostic technique that uses ultrasonic scanning to identify the pattern and direction of blood flow within arteries or veins displayed in real time images. Duplex scanning combines B-mode two-dimensional pictures of the vessel structure with spectra and/or color flow Doppler mapping or imaging of the blood as it moves through the vessels.

duplication/deletion (DUP/DEL). Term used in molecular testing which examines genomic regions to determine if there are extra chromosomes (duplication) or missing chromosomes (deletions). Normal gene dosage is two copies per cell except for the sex chromosomes which have one per cell.

DuToit staple capsulorrhaphy. Reattachment of the capsule of the shoulder and glenoid labrum to the glenoid lip using staples to anchor the avulsed capsule and glenoid labrum.

Dx. Diagnosis.

DXA. Dual energy x-ray absorptiometry. Radiological technique for bone density measurement using a two-dimensional projection system in which two x-ray beams with different levels of energy are pulsed alternately and the results are given in two scores, reported as standard deviations from peak bone mass density.

dynamic mutation. Unstable or changing polynucleotides resulting in repeats related to genes that can undergo disease-producing increases or decreases in the repeats that differ within tissues or over generations.

ECMO. Extracorporeal membrane oxygenation.

ectropion. Drooping of the lower eyelid away from the eye or outward turning or eversion of the edge of the eyelid, exposing the palpebral conjunctiva and causing irritation.

Eden-Hybinette procedure. Anterior shoulder repair using an anterior bone block to augment the bony anterior glenoid lip.

EDTA. Drug used to inhibit damage to the cornea by collagenase. EDTA is especially effective in alkali burns as it neutralizes soluble alkali, including lye.

effusion. Escape of fluid from within a body cavity.

electrocardiographic rhythm derived. Analysis of data obtained from readings of the heart's electrical activation, including heart rate and rhythm, variability of heart rate, ST analysis, and T-wave alternans. Other data may also be assessed when warranted.

electrocautery. Division or cutting of tissue using high-frequency electrical current to produce heat, which destroys cells.

electrode array. Electronic device containing more than one contact whose function can be adjusted during programming services. Electrodes are specialized for a particular electrochemical reaction that acts as a medium between a body surface and another instrument.

electromyography. Test that measures muscle response to nerve stimulation determining if muscle weakness is present and if it is related to the muscles themselves or a problem with the nerves that supply the muscles.

electrooculogram (EOG). Record of electrical activity associated with eye movements.

electrophysiologic studies. Electrical stimulation and monitoring to diagnose heart conduction abnormalities that predispose patients to bradyarrhythmias and to determine a patient's chance for developing ventricular and supraventricular tachyarrhythmias.

emergency. Serious medical condition or symptom (including severe pain) resulting from injury, sickness, or mental illness that arises suddenly and requires immediate care and treatment, generally received within 24 hours of onset, to avoid jeopardy to the life, limb, or health of a covered person.

empyema. Accumulation of pus within the respiratory, or pleural, cavity.

EMTALA. Emergency Medical Treatment and Active Labor Act.

endarterectomy. Removal of the thickened, endothelial lining of a diseased or damaged artery.

endomicroscopy. Diagnostic technology that allows for the examination of tissue at the cellular level during endoscopy. The technology decreases the need for biopsy with histological examination for some types of lesions.

endovascular embolization. Procedure whereby vessels are occluded by a variety of therapeutic substances for the treatment of abnormal blood vessels by inhibiting the flow of blood to a tumor, arteriovenous malformations, lymphatic malformation, and to prevent or stop hemorrhage.

entropion. Inversion of the eyelid, turning the edge in toward the eyeball and causing irritation from contact of the lashes with the surface of the eye.

enucleation. Removal of a growth or organ cleanly so as to extract it in one piece.

epidermis. Outermost, nonvascular layer of skin that contains four to five differentiated layers depending on its body location: stratum corneum, lucidum, granulosum, spinosum, and basale.

epiphysiodesis. Surgical fusion of an epiphysis performed to prematurely stop further bone growth.

escharotomy. Surgical incision into the scab or crust resulting from a severe burn in order to relieve constriction and allow blood flow to the distal unburned tissue.

established patient. 1) Patient who has received professional services in a face-to-face setting within the last three years from the same physician/qualified health care professional or another physician/qualified health care professional of the exact same specialty and subspecialty who belongs to the same group practice. 2) For OPPS hospitals, patient who has been registered as an inpatient or outpatient in a hospital's provider-based clinic or emergency department within the past three years.

evacuation. Removal or purging of waste material.

evaluation and management codes. Assessment and management of a patient's health care.

evaluation and management service components. Key components of history, examination, and medical decision making that are key to selecting the correct E/M codes. Other non-key components include counseling, coordination of care, nature of presenting problem, and time.

event recorder. Portable, ambulatory heart monitor worn by the patient that makes electrocardiographic recordings of the length and frequency of aberrant cardiac rhythm to help diagnose heart conditions and to assess pacemaker functioning or programming.

exenteration. Surgical removal of the entire contents of a body cavity, such as the pelvis or orbit.

exon. One of multiple nucleic acid sequences used to encode information for a gene polypeptide or protein. Exons are separated from other exons by non-protein-coding sequences known as introns.

extended care services. Items and services provided to an inpatient of a skilled nursing facility, including nursing care, physical or occupational therapy, speech pathology, drugs and supplies, and medical social services.

external electrical capacitor device. External electrical stimulation device designed to promote bone healing. This device may also promote neural regeneration, revascularization, epiphyseal growth, and ligament maturation.

external pulsating electromagnetic field. External stimulation device designed to promote bone healing. This device may also promote neural regeneration, revascularization, epiphyseal growth, and ligament maturation.

extracorporeal. Located or taking place outside the body.

Eyre-Brook capsulorrhaphy. Reattachment of the capsule of the shoulder and glenoid labrum to the glenoid lip.

False Claims Act. Governs civil actions for filing false claims. Liability under this act pertains to any person who knowingly presents or causes to be presented a false or fraudulent claim to the government for payment or approval.

fascia. Fibrous sheet or band of tissue that envelops organs, muscles, and groupings of muscles.

fasciectomy. Excision of fascia or strips of fascial tissue.

fasciotomy. Incision or transection of fascial tissue.

fat graft. Graft composed of fatty tissue completely freed from surrounding tissue that is used primarily to fill in depressions.

FDA. Food and Drug Administration. Federal agency responsible for protecting public health by substantiating the safety, efficacy, and security of human and veterinary drugs, biological products, medical devices, national food supply, cosmetics, and items that give off radiation.

filtered speech test. Test most commonly used to identify central auditory dysfunction in which the patient is presented monosyllabic words that are low pass filtered, allowing only the parts of each word below a certain pitch to be presented. A score is given on the number of correct responses. This may be a subset of a standard battery of tests provided during a single encounter.

fissure. Deep furrow, groove, or cleft in tissue structures.

fistulization. Creation of a communication between two structures that were not previously connected.

flexor digitorum profundus tendon. Tendon originating in the proximal forearm and extending to the index finger and wrist. A thickened FDP sheath, usually caused by age, illness, or injury, can fill the carpal canal and lead to impingement of the median nerve.

fluoroscopy. Radiology technique that allows visual examination of part of the body or a function of an organ using a device that projects an x-ray image on a fluorescent screen.

focal length. Distance between the object in focus and the lens.

focused medical review. Process of targeting and directing medical review efforts on Medicare claims where the greatest risk of inappropriate program payment exists. The goal is to reduce the number of noncovered claims or unnecessary services. CMS analyzes national data such as internal billing, utilization, and payment data and provides its findings to the FI. Local medical review policies are developed identifying aberrances, abuse, and overutilized services. Providers are responsible for knowing national Medicare coverage and billing guidelines and local medical review policies, and for determining whether the services provided to Medicare beneficiaries are covered by Medicare.

fragile X syndrome. Intellectual disabilities, enlarged testes, big jaw, high forehead, and long ears in males. In females, fragile X presents with mild intellectual disabilities and heterozygous sexual structures. In some families, males have shown no symptoms but carry the gene.

free flap. Tissue that is completely detached from the donor site and transplanted to the recipient site, receiving its blood supply from capillary ingrowth at the recipient site.

free microvascular flap. Tissue that is completely detached from the donor site following careful dissection and preservation of the blood vessels, then attached to the recipient site with the transferred blood vessels anastomosed to the vessels in the recipient bed.

fulguration. Destruction of living tissue by using sparks from a high-frequency electric current.

gas tamponade. Absorbable gas may be injected to force the retina against the choroid. Common gases include room air, short-acting sulfahexafluoride, intermediate-acting perfluoroethane, or long-acting perfluorooctane.

Gaucher disease. Genetic metabolic disorder in which fat deposits may accumulate in the spleen, liver, lungs, bone marrow, and brain.

gene. Basic unit of heredity that contains nucleic acid. Genes are arranged in different and unique sequences or strings that determine the gene's function. Human genes usually include multiple protein coding regions such as exons separated by introns which are nonprotein coding sections.

genome. The complete set of DNA of an organism. Each cell in the human body is comprised of a complete copy of the approximately 3 billion DNA base pairs that constitute the human genome.

HCPCS. Healthcare Common Procedure Coding System.

HCPCS Level I. Healthcare Common Procedure Coding System Level I. Numeric coding system used by physicians, facility outpatient departments, and ambulatory surgery centers (ASC) to code ambulatory, laboratory, radiology, and other diagnostic services for Medicare billing. This coding system contains only the American Medical Association's Physicians' Current Procedural Terminology (CPT) codes. The AMA updates codes annually.

HCPCS Level II. Healthcare Common Procedure Coding System Level II. National coding system, developed by CMS, that contains alphanumeric codes for physician and nonphysician services not included in the CPT coding system. HCPCS Level II covers such things as ambulance services, durable medical equipment, and orthotic and prosthetic devices.

HCPCS modifiers. Two-character code (AA-ZZ) that identifies circumstances that alter or enhance the description of a service or supply. They are recognized by carriers nationally and are updated annually by CMS.

Hct. Hematocrit.

health care provider. Entity that administers diagnostic and therapeutic services.

hemilaminectomy. Excision of a portion of the vertebral lamina.

hemodialysis. Cleansing of wastes and contaminating elements from the blood by virtue of different diffusion rates through a semipermeable membrane, which separates blood from a filtration solution that diffuses other elements out of the blood.

hemoperitoneum. Effusion of blood into the peritoneal cavity, the space between the continuous membrane lining the abdominopelvic walls and encasing the visceral organs.

heterograft. Surgical graft of tissue from one animal species to a different animal species. A common type of heterograft is porcine (pig) tissue, used for temporary wound closure.

heterotopic transplant. Tissue transplanted from a different anatomical site for usage as is natural for that tissue, for example, buccal mucosa to a conjunctival site.

HGNC. HUGO gene nomenclature committee.

HGVS. Human genome variation society.

Hickman catheter. Central venous catheter used for long-term delivery of medications, such as antibiotics, nutritional substances, or chemotherapeutic agents.

HLA. Human leukocyte antigen.

home health services. Services furnished to patients in their homes under the care of physicians. These services include part-time or intermittent skilled nursing care, physical therapy, medical social services, medical supplies, and some rehabilitation equipment. Home health supplies and services must be prescribed by a physician, and the beneficiary must be confined at home in order for Medicare to pay the benefits in full.

homograft. Graft from one individual to another of the same species.

hospice care. Items and services provided to a terminally ill individual by a hospice program under a written plan established and periodically reviewed by the individual's attending physician and by the medical director: Nursing care provided by or under the supervision of a registered professional nurse; Physical or occupational therapy or speech-language pathology services; Medical social services under the direction of a physician; Services of a home health aide who has successfully completed a training program; Medical supplies (including drugs and biologicals) and the use of medical appliances; Physicians' services; Short-term inpatient care (including both respite care and procedures necessary for pain control and acute and chronic symptom management) in an inpatient facility on an intermittent basis and not consecutively over longer than five days; Counseling (including dietary counseling) with respect to care of the terminally ill individual and adjustment to his death; Any item or service which is specified in the plan and for which payment may be made.

hospital. Institution that provides, under the supervision of physicians, diagnostic, therapeutic, and rehabilitation services for medical diagnosis, treatment, and care of patients. Hospitals receiving federal funds must maintain clinical records on all patients, provide 24-hour nursing services, and have a discharge planning process in place. The term "hospital" also includes religious nonmedical health care institutions and facilities of 50 beds or less located in rural areas.

HUGO. Human genome organization

IA. Intra-arterial.

ICD. Implantable cardioverter defibrillator.

ICD-10-CM. International Classification of Diseases, 10th Revision, Clinical Modification. Clinical modification of the alphanumeric classification of diseases used by the World Health Organization, already in use in much of the world, and used for mortality reporting in the United States. The implementation date for ICD-10-CM diagnostic coding system to replace ICD-9-CM in the United States is October 1, 2015.

ICD-10-PCS. International Classification of Diseases, 10th Revision, Procedure Coding System. Beginning October 1, 2015, inpatient hospital services and surgical procedures must be coded using ICD-10-PCS codes, replacing the current ICD-9-CM, Volume 3 for procedures.

ICM. Implantable cardiovascular monitor.

ileostomy. Artificial surgical opening that brings the end of the ileum out through the abdominal wall to the skin surface for the diversion of feces through a stoma.

iliopsoas tendon. Fibrous tissue that connects muscle to bone in the pelvic region, common to the iliacus and psoas major.

ILR. Implantable loop recorder.

IM. 1) Infectious mononucleosis. 2) Internal medicine. 3) Intramuscular.

immunotherapy. Therapeutic use of serum or gamma globulin.

implant. Material or device inserted or placed within the body for therapeutic, reconstructive, or diagnostic purposes.

implantable cardiovascular monitor. Implantable electronic device that stores cardiovascular physiologic data such as intracardiac pressure waveforms collected from internal sensors or data such as weight and blood pressure collected from external sensors. The information stored in these devices is used as an aid in managing patients with heart failure and other cardiac conditions that are non-rhythm related. The data may be transmitted via local telemetry or remotely to a surveillance technician or an internet-based file server.

implantable cardioverter-defibrillator. Implantable electronic cardiac device used to control rhythm abnormalities such as tachycardia, fibrillation, or bradycardia by producing high- or low-energy stimulation and pacemaker functions. It may also have the capability to provide the functions of an implantable loop recorder or implantable cardiovascular monitor.

implantable loop recorder. Implantable electronic cardiac device that constantly monitors and records electrocardiographic rhythm. It may be triggered by the patient when a symptomatic episode occurs or activated automatically by rapid or slow heart rates. This may be the sole purpose of the device or it may be a component of another cardiac device, such as a pacemaker or implantable cardioverter-defibrillator. The data can be transmitted via local telemetry or remotely to a surveillance technician or an internet-based file server.

implantable venous access device. Catheter implanted for continuous access to the venous system for long-term parenteral feeding or for the administration of fluids or medications.

IMRT. Intensity modulated radiation therapy. External beam radiation therapy delivery using computer planning to specify the target dose and to modulate the radiation intensity, usually as a treatment for a malignancy. The delivery system approaches the patient from multiple angles, minimizing damage to normal tissue.

in situ. Located in the natural position or contained within the origin site, not spread into neighboring tissue.

incontinence. Inability to control urination or defecation.

infundibulectomy. Excision of the anterosuperior portion of the right ventricle of the heart.

internal direct current stimulator. Electrostimulation device placed directly into the surgical site designed to promote bone regeneration by encouraging cellular healing response in bone and ligaments.

interrogation device evaluation. Assessment of an implantable cardiac device (pacemaker, cardioverter-defibrillator, cardiovascular monitor, or loop recorder) in which collected data about the patient's heart rate and rhythm, battery and pulse generator function, and any leads or sensors present, are retrieved and evaluated. Determinations regarding device programming and appropriate treatment settings are made based on the findings. CPT provides required components for evaluation of the various types of devices.

intramedullary implants. Nail, rod, or pin placed into the intramedullary canal at the fracture site. Intramedullary implants not only provide a method of aligning the fracture, they also act as a splint and may reduce fracture pain. Implants may be rigid or flexible. Rigid implants are preferred for prophylactic treatment of diseased bone, while flexible implants are preferred for traumatic injuries.

intraocular lens. Artificial lens implanted into the eye to replace a damaged natural lens or cataract.

intravenous. Within a vein or veins.

introducer. Instrument, such as a catheter, needle, or tube, through which another instrument or device is introduced into the body.

intron. Nonprotein section of a gene that separates exons in human genes. Contains vital sequences that allow splicing of exons to produce a functional protein from a gene. Sometimes referred to as intervening sequences (IVS).

IP. 1) Interphalangeal. 2) Intraperitoneal.

irrigation. To wash out or cleanse a body cavity, wound, or tissue with water or other fluid.

Kayser-Fleischer ring. Condition found in Wilson's disease in which deposits of copper cause a pigmented ring around the cornea's outer border in the deep epithelial layers.

keratoprosthesis. Surgical procedure in which the physician creates a new anterior chamber with a plastic optical implant to replace a severely damaged cornea that cannot be repaired.

keratotomy. Surgical incision of the cornea.

krypton laser. Laser light energy that uses ionized krypton by electric current as the active source, has a radiation beam between the visible yellow-red spectrum, and is effective in photocoagulation of retinal bleeding, macular lesions, and vessel aberrations of the choroid.

lacrimal. Tear-producing gland or ducts that provides lubrication and flushing of the eyes and nasal cavities.

lacrimal punctum. Opening of the lacrimal papilla of the eyelid through which tears flow to the canaliculi to the lacrimal sac.

lacrimotome. Knife for cutting the lacrimal sac or duct.

lacrimotomy. Incision of the lacrimal sac or duct.

laparotomy. Incision through the flank or abdomen for therapeutic or diagnostic purposes.

laryngoscopy. Examination of the hypopharynx, larynx, and tongue base with an endoscope.

larynx. Musculocartilaginous structure between the trachea and the pharynx that functions as the valve preventing food and other particles from entering the respiratory tract, as well as the voice mechanism. Also called the voicebox, the larynx is composed of three single cartilages: cricoid, epiglottis, and thyroid; and three paired cartilages: arytenoid, corniculate, and cuneiform.

laser surgery. Use of concentrated, sharply defined light beams to cut, cauterize, coagulate, seal, or vaporize tissue.

LEEP. Loop electrode excision procedure. Biopsy specimen or cone shaped wedge of cervical tissue is removed using a hot cautery wire loop with an electrical current running through it.

levonorgestrel. Drug inhibiting ovulation and preventing sperm from penetrating cervical mucus. It is delivered subcutaneously in polysiloxone capsules. The capsules can be effective for up to five years, and provide a cumulative pregnancy rate of less than 2 percent. The capsules are not biodegradable, and therefore must be removed. Removal is more difficult than insertion of levonorgestrel capsules because fibrosis develops around the capsules. Normal hormonal activity and a return to fertility begins immediately upon removal.

ligament. Band or sheet of fibrous tissue that connects the articular surfaces of bones or supports visceral organs.

ligation. Tying off a blood vessel or duct with a suture or a soft, thin wire.

lymphadenectomy. Dissection of lymph nodes free from the vessels and removal for examination by frozen section in a separate procedure to detect early-stage metastases.

lysis. Destruction, breakdown, dissolution, or decomposition of cells or substances by a specific catalyzing agent.

Magnuson-Stack procedure. Treatment for recurrent anterior dislocation of the shoulder that involves tightening and realigning the subscapularis tendon.

maintenance of wakefulness test. Attended study determining the patient's ability to stay awake.

Manchester operation. Preservation of the uterus following prolapse by amputating the vaginal portion of the cervix, shortening the cardinal ligaments, and performing a colpoperineorrhaphy posteriorly.

mapping. Multidimensional depiction of a tachycardia that identifies its site of origin and its electrical conduction pathway after tachycardia has been induced. The recording is made from multiple catheter sites within the heart, obtaining electrograms simultaneously or sequentially.

marsupialization. Creation of a pouch in surgical treatment of a cyst in which one wall is resected and the remaining cut edges are sutured to adjacent tissue creating an open pouch of the previously enclosed cyst.

mastectomy. Surgical removal of one or both breasts.

McDonald procedure. Polyester tape is placed around the cervix with a running stitch to assist in the prevention of pre-term delivery. Tape is removed at term for vaginal delivery.

MCP. Metacarpophalangeal.

medial. Middle or midline.

medical review. Review by a Medicare administrative contractor, carrier, and/or quality improvement organization (QIO) of services and items provided by physicians, other health care practitioners, and providers of health care services under Medicare. The review determines if the items and services are reasonable and necessary and meet Medicare coverage requirements, whether the quality meets professionally recognized standards of health care, and whether the services are medically appropriate in an inpatient, outpatient, or other setting as supported by documentation.

Medicare contractor. Medicare Part A fiscal intermediary, Medicare Part B carrier, Medicare administrative contractor (MAC), or a durable medical equipment Medicare administrative contractor (DME MAC).

Medicare physician fee schedule. List of payments Medicare allows by procedure or service. Payments may vary through geographic adjustments. The MPFS is based on the resource-based relative value scale (RBRVS). A national total relative value unit (RVU) is given to each procedure (HCPCS Level I CPT, Level II national codes). Each total RVU has three components: physician work, practice expense, and malpractice insurance.

metabolite. Chemical compound resulting from the natural process of metabolism. In drug testing, the metabolite of the drug may endure in a higher concentration or for a longer duration than the initial (parent) drug.

methylation. Mechanism used to regulate genes and protect DNA from some types of cleavage.

microarray. Small surface onto which multiple specific nucleic acid sequences can be attached to be used for analysis. Microarray may also be known as a gene chip or DNA chip. Tests can be run on the sequences for any variants that may be present.

mitral valve. Valve with two cusps that is between the left atrium and left ventricle of the heart.

moderate sedation. Medically controlled state of depressed consciousness, with or without analgesia, while maintaining the patient's airway, protective reflexes, and ability to respond to stimulation or verbal commands.

Mohs micrographic surgery. Special technique used to treat complex or ill-defined skin cancer and requires a single physician to provide two distinct services. The first service is surgical and involves the destruction of the lesion by a combination of chemosurgery and excision. The second service is that of a pathologist and includes mapping, color coding of specimens, microscopic examination of specimens, and complete histopathologic preparation.

monitored anesthesia care. Sedation, with or without analgesia, used to achieve a medically controlled state of depressed consciousness while maintaining the patient's airway, protective reflexes, and ability to respond to stimulation or verbal commands. In dental conscious sedation, the patient is rendered free of fear, apprehension, and anxiety through the use of pharmacological agents.

monoclonal. Relating to a single clone of cells.

multiple sleep latency test (MSLT). Attended study to determine the tendency of the patient to fall asleep.

multiple-lead device. Implantable cardiac device (pacemaker or implantable cardioverter-defibrillator [ICD]) in which pacing and sensing components are placed in at least three chambers of the heart.

Mustard procedure. Corrective measure for transposition of great vessels involves an intra-atrial baffle made of pericardial tissue or synthetic material. The baffle is secured between pulmonary veins and mitral valve and between mitral and tricuspid valves. The baffle directs systemic venous flow into the left ventricle and lungs and pulmonary venous flow into the right ventricle and aorta.

mutation. Alteration in gene function that results in changes to a gene or chromosome. Can cause deficits or disease that can be inherited, can have beneficial effects, or result in no noticeable change.

mutation scanning. Process normally used on multiple polymerase chain reaction (PCR) amplicons to determine DNA sequence variants by differences in characteristics compared to normal. Specific DNA variants can then be studied further.

myasthenia gravis. Autoimmune neuromuscular disorder caused by antibodies to the acetylcholine receptors at the neuromuscular junction, interfering with proper binding of the neurotransmitter from the neuron to the target muscle, causing muscle weakness, fatigue, and exhaustion, without pain or atrophy.

myotomy. Surgical cutting of a muscle to gain access to underlying tissues or for therapeutic reasons.

myringotomy. Incision in the eardrum done to prevent spontaneous rupture precipitated by fluid pressure build-up behind the tympanic membrane and to prevent stagnant infection and erosion of the ossicles.

nasal polyp. Fleshy outgrowth projecting from the mucous membrane of the nose or nasal sinus cavity that may obstruct ventilation or affect the sense of smell.

nasal sinus. Air-filled cavities in the cranial bones lined with mucous membrane and continuous with the nasal cavity, draining fluids through the nose.

nasogastric tube. Long, hollow, cylindrical catheter made of soft rubber or plastic that is inserted through the nose down into the stomach, and is used for feeding, instilling medication, or withdrawing gastric contents.

nasolacrimal punctum. Opening of the lacrimal duct near the nose.

nasopharynx. Membranous passage above the level of the soft palate.

Nd:YAG laser. Laser light energy that uses an yttrium, aluminum, and garnet crystal doped with neodymium ions as the active source, has a radiation beam nearing the infrared spectrum, and is effective in photocoagulation, photoablation, cataract extraction, and lysis of vitreous strands.

nebulizer. Latin for mist, a device that converts liquid into a fine spray and is commonly used to deliver medicine to the upper respiratory, bronchial, and lung areas.

nerve conduction study. Diagnostic test performed to assess muscle or nerve damage. Nerves are stimulated with electric shocks along the course of the muscle. Sensors are utilized to measure and record nerve functions, including conduction and velocity.

neurectomy. Excision of all or a portion of a nerve.

neuromuscular junction. Nerve synapse at the meeting point between the terminal end of a nerve (motor neuron) and a muscle fiber.

neuropsychological testing. Evaluation of a patient's behavioral abilities wherein a physician or other health care professional administers a series of tests in thinking, reasoning, and judgment.

new patient. Patient who is receiving face-to-face care from a provider/qualified health care professional or another physician/qualified health care professional of the exact same specialty and subspecialty who belongs to the same group practice for the first time in three years. For OPPS hospitals, a patient who has not been registered as an inpatient or outpatient, including off-campus provider based clinic or emergency department, within the past three years.

Niemann-Pick syndrome. Accumulation of phospholipid in histiocytes in the bone marrow, liver, lymph nodes, and spleen, cerebral involvement, and red macular spots similar to Tay-Sachs disease. Most commonly found in Jewish infants.

Nissen fundoplasty. Surgical repair technique that involves the fundus of the stomach being wrapped around the lower end of the esophagus to treat reflux esophagitis.

nonabsorbable sutures. Strands of natural or synthetic material that resist absorption into living tissue and are removed once healing is under way. Nonabsorbable sutures are commonly used to close skin wounds and repair tendons or collagenous tissue.

obturator. Prosthesis used to close an acquired or congenital opening in the palate that aids in speech and chewing.

obturator nerve. Lumbar plexus nerve with anterior and posterior divisions that innervate the adductor muscles (e.g., adductor longus, adductor brevis) of the leg and the skin over the medial area of the thigh or a sacral plexus nerve with anterior and posterior divisions that innervate the superior gemellus muscles.

occult blood test. Chemical or microscopic test to determine the presence of blood in a specimen.

ocular implant. Implant inside muscular cone.

oophorectomy. Surgical removal of all or part of one or both ovaries, either as open procedure or laparoscopically. Menstruation and childbearing ability continues when one ovary is removed.

orthosis. Derived from a Greek word meaning "to make straight," it is an artificial appliance that supports, aligns, or corrects an anatomical deformity or improves the use of a moveable body part. Unlike a prosthesis, an orthotic device is always functional in nature.

osteo-. Having to do with bone.

osteogenesis stimulator. Device used to stimulate the growth of bone by electrical impulses or ultrasound.

osteotomy. Surgical cutting of a bone.

ostomy. Artificial (surgical) opening in the body used for drainage or for delivery of medications or nutrients.

pacemaker. Implantable cardiac device that controls the heart's rhythm and maintains regular beats by artificial electric discharges. This device consists of the pulse generator with a battery and the electrodes, or leads, which are placed in single or dual chambers of the heart, usually transvenously.

palmaris longus tendon. Tendon located in the hand that flexes the wrist joint.

paratenon graft. Graft composed of the fatty tissue found between a tendon and its sheath.

passive mobilization. Pressure, movement, or pulling of a limb or body part utilizing an apparatus or device.

pedicle flap. Full-thickness skin and subcutaneous tissue for grafting that remains partially attached to the donor site by a pedicle or stem in which the blood vessels supplying the flap remain intact.

Pemberton osteotomy. Osteotomy is performed to position triradiate cartilage as a hinge for rotating the acetabular roof in cases of dysplasia of the hip in children.

penetrance. Being formed by, or pertaining to, a single clone.

percutaneous intradiscal electrothermal annuloplasty. Procedure corrects tears in the vertebral annulus by applying heat to the collagen disc walls percutaneously through a catheter. The heat contracts and thickens the wall, which may contract and close any annular tears.

percutaneous skeletal fixation. Treatment that is neither open nor closed and the injury site is not directly visualized. Fixation devices (pins, screws) are placed through the skin to stabilize the dislocation using x-ray guidance.

pericardium. Thin and slippery case in which the heart lies that is lined with fluid so that the heart is free to pulse and move as it beats.

peripheral arterial tonometry (PAT)**.** Pulsatile volume changes in a digit are measured to determine activity in the sympathetic nervous system for respiratory analysis.

peritoneal. Space between the lining of the abdominal wall, or parietal peritoneum, and the surface layer of the abdominal organs, or visceral peritoneum. It contains a thin, watery fluid that keeps the peritoneal surfaces moist.

peritoneal dialysis. Dialysis that filters waste from blood inside the body using the peritoneum, the natural lining of the abdomen, as the semipermeable membrane across which ultrafiltration is accomplished. A special catheter is inserted into the abdomen and a dialysis solution is drained into the abdomen. This solution extracts fluids and wastes, which are then discarded when the fluid is drained. Various forms of peritoneal dialysis include CAPD, CCPD, and NIDP.

peritoneal effusion. Persistent escape of fluid within the peritoneal cavity.

pessary. Device placed in the vagina to support and reposition a prolapsing or retropositioned uterus, rectum, or vagina.

phenotype. Physical expression of a trait or characteristic as determined by an individual's genetic makeup or genotype.

photocoagulation. Application of an intense laser beam of light to disrupt tissue and condense protein material to a residual mass, used especially for treating ocular conditions.

physical status modifiers. Alphanumeric modifier used to identify the patient's health status as it affects the work related to providing the anesthesia service.

physical therapy modality. Therapeutic agent or regimen applied or used to provide appropriate treatment of the musculoskeletal system.

physician. Legally authorized practitioners including a doctor of medicine or osteopathy, a doctor of dental surgery or of dental medicine, a doctor of podiatric medicine, a doctor of optometry, and a chiropractor only with respect to treatment by means of manual manipulation of the spine (to correct a subluxation).

PICC. Peripherally inserted central catheter. PICC is inserted into one of the large veins of the arm and threaded through the vein until the tip sits in a large vein just above the heart.

PKR. Photorefractive therapy. Procedure involving the removal of the surface layer of the cornea (epithelium) by gentle scraping and use of a computer-controlled excimer laser to reshape the stroma.

pleurodesis. Injection of a sclerosing agent into the pleural space for creating adhesions between the parietal and the visceral pleura to treat a collapsed lung caused by air trapped in the pleural cavity, or severe cases of pleural effusion.

plication. Surgical technique involving folding, tucking, or pleating to reduce the size of a hollow structure or organ.

polyclonal. Containing one or more cells.

polymorphism. Genetic variation in the same species that does not harm the gene function or create disease.

polypeptide. Chain of amino acids held together by covalent bonds. Proteins are made up of amino acids.

polysomnography. Test involving monitoring of respiratory, cardiac, muscle, brain, and ocular function during sleep.

Potts-Smith-Gibson procedure. Side-to-side anastomosis of the aorta and left pulmonary artery creating a shunt that enlarges as the child grows.

Prader-Willi syndrome. Rounded face, almond-shaped eyes, strabismus, low forehead, hypogonadism, hypotonia, intellectual disabilities, and an insatiable appetite.

presumptive drug testing. Drug screening tests to identify the presence or (not) of drugs in a patient's system. Tests are usually able to identify low concentrations of the drug. May be used for medical, workplace, or legal purposes.

presumptive identification. Identification of microorganisms using media growth, colony morphology, gram stains, or up to three specific tests (e.g., catalase, indole, oxidase, urease).

professional component. Portion of a charge for health care services that represents the physician's (or other practitioner's) work in providing the service, including interpretation and report of the procedure. This component of the service usually is charged for and billed separately from the inpatient hospital charges.

profunda. Denotes a part of a structure that is deeper from the surface of the body than the rest of the structure.

prolonged physician services. Extended pre- or post-service care provided to a patient whose condition requires services beyond the usual.

prostate. Male gland surrounding the bladder neck and urethra that secretes a substance into the seminal fluid.

prosthetic. Device that replaces all or part of an internal body organ or body part, or that replaces part of the function of a permanently inoperable or malfunctioning internal body organ or body part.

provider of services. Institution, individual, or organization that provides health care.

proximal. Located closest to a specified reference point, usually the midline.

psychiatric hospital. Specialized institution that provides, under the supervision of physicians, services for the diagnosis and treatment of mentally ill persons.

pterygium. Benign, wedge-shaped, conjunctival thickening that advances from the inner corner of the eye toward the cornea.

pterygomaxillary fossa. Wide depression on the external surface of the maxilla above and to the side of the canine tooth socket.

pulmonary artery banding. Surgical constriction of the pulmonary artery to prevent irreversible pulmonary vascular obstructive changes and overflow into the left ventricle.

Putti-Platt procedure. Realignment of the subscapularis tendon to treat recurrent anterior dislocation, thereby partially eliminating external rotation. The anterior capsule is also tightened and reinforced.

pyloroplasty. Enlargement and reconstruction of the lower portion of the stomach opening into the duodenum performed after vagotomy to speed gastric emptying and treat duodenal ulcers.

qualified health care professional. Educated, licensed or certified, and regulated professional operating under a specified scope of practice to provide patient services that are separate and distinct from other clinical staff. Services may be billed independently or under the facility's services.

RAC. Recovery audit contractor. National program using CMS-affiliated contractors to review claims prior to payment as well as for payments on claims already processed, including overpayments and underpayments.

radiation therapy simulation. Radiation therapy simulation. Procedure by which the specific body area to be treated with radiation is defined and marked. A CT scan is performed to define the body contours and these images are used to create a plan customized treatment for the patient, targeting the area to be treated while sparing adjacent tissue. The center of the area to be treated is marked and an immobilization device (e.g., cradle, mold) is created to make sure the patient is in the same position each time for treatment. Complexity of treatment depends on the number of treatment areas and the use of tools to isolate the area of treatment.

radioactive substances. Materials used in the diagnosis and treatment of disease that emit high-speed particles and energy-containing rays.

radiology services. Services that include diagnostic and therapeutic radiology, nuclear medicine, CT scan procedures, magnetic resonance imaging services, ultrasound, and other imaging procedures.

radiotherapy afterloading. Part of the radiation therapy process in which the chemotherapy agent is actually instilled into the tumor area subsequent to surgery and placement of an expandable catheter into the void remaining after tumor excision. The specialized catheter remains in place and the patient may come in for multiple treatments with radioisotope placed to treat the margin of tissue surrounding the excision. After the radiotherapy is completed, the patient returns to have the catheter emptied and removed. This is a new therapy in breast cancer treatment.

Rashkind procedure. Transvenous balloon atrial septectomy or septostomy performed by cardiac catheterization. A balloon catheter is inserted into the heart either to create or enlarge an opening in the interatrial septal wall.

repair. Surgical closure of a wound. The wound may be a result of injury/trauma or it may be a surgically created defect. Repairs are divided into three categories: simple, intermediate, and complex. Simple repair is performed when the wound is superficial and only requires simple, one layer, primary suturing. Intermediate repair is performed for wounds and lacerations in which one or more of the deeper layers of subcutaneous tissue and non-muscle fascia are repaired in addition to the skin and subcutaneous tissue. Complex repair includes repair of wounds requiring more than layered closure.

respiratory airflow (ventilation). Assessment of air movement during inhalation and exhalation as measured by nasal pressure sensors and thermistor.

respiratory analysis. Assessment of components of respiration obtained by other methods such as airflow or peripheral arterial tone.

respiratory effort. Measurement of diaphragm and/or intercostal muscle for airflow using transducers to estimate thoracic and abdominal motion.

respiratory movement. Measurement of chest and abdomen movement during respiration.

ribbons. In oncology, small plastic tubes containing radioactive sources for interstitial placement that may be cut into specific lengths tailored to the size of the area receiving ionizing radiation treatment.

Ridell sinusotomy. Frontal sinus tissue is destroyed to eliminate tumors.

RNA. Ribonucleic acid.

rural health clinic. Clinic in an area where there is a shortage of health services staffed by a nurse practitioner, physician assistant, or certified nurse midwife under physician direction that provides routine diagnostic services, including clinical laboratory services, drugs, and biologicals and that has prompt access to additional diagnostic services from facilities meeting federal requirements.

Salter osteotomy. Innominate bone of the hip is cut, removed, and repositioned to repair a congenital dislocation, subluxation, or deformity.

saucerization. Creation of a shallow, saucer-like depression in the bone to facilitate drainage of infected areas.

Schiotz tonometer. Instrument that measures intraocular pressure by recording the depth of an indentation on the cornea by a plunger of known weight.

screening mammography. Radiologic images taken of the female breast for the early detection of breast cancer.

screening pap smear. Diagnostic laboratory test consisting of a routine exfoliative cytology test (Papanicolaou test) provided to a woman for the early detection of cervical or vaginal cancer. The exam includes a clinical breast examination and a physician's interpretation of the results.

seeds. Small (1 mm or less) sources of radioactive material that are permanently placed directly into tumors.

senning procedure. Flaps of intra-atrial septum and right atrial wall are used to create two interatrial channels to divert the systemic and pulmonary venous circulation.

sensitivity tests. Number of methods of applying selective suspected allergens to the skin or mucous.

sensorineural conduction. Transportation of sound from the cochlea to the acoustic nerve and central auditory pathway to the brain.

sentinel lymph node. First node to which lymph drainage and metastasis from a cancer can occur.

separate procedures. Services commonly carried out as a fundamental part of a total service and, as such, do not usually warrant separate identification. These services are identified in CPT with the parenthetical phrase (separate procedure) at the end of the description and are payable only when performed alone.

septectomy. 1) Surgical removal of all or part of the nasal septum. 2) Submucosal resection of the nasal septum.

Shirodkar procedure. Treatment of an incompetent cervical os by placing nonabsorbent suture material in purse-string sutures as a cerclage to support the cervix.

short tandem repeat (STR). Short sequences of a DNA pattern that are repeated. Can be used as genetic markers for human identity testing.

sialodochoplasty. Surgical repair of a salivary gland duct.

single-lead device. Implantable cardiac device (pacemaker or implantable cardioverter-defibrillator [ICD]) in which pacing and sensing components are placed in only one chamber of the heart.

single-nucleotide polymorphism (SNP). Single nucleotide (A, T, C, or G that is different in a DNA sequence. This difference occurs at a significant frequency in the population.

sinus of Valsalva. Any of three sinuses corresponding to the individual cusps of the aortic valve, located in the most proximal part of the aorta just above the cusps. These structures are contained within the pericardium and appear as distinct but subtle outpouchings or dilations of the aortic wall between each of the semilunar cusps of the valve.

sleep apnea. Intermittent cessation of breathing during sleep that may cause hypoxemia and pulmonary arterial hypertension.

sleep latency. Time period between lying down in bed and the onset of sleep.

sleep staging. Determination of the separate levels of sleep according to physiological measurements.

somatic. 1) Pertaining to the body or trunk. 2) In genetics acquired or occurring after birth.

speculoscopy. Viewing the cervix utilizing a magnifier and a special wavelength of light, allowing detection of abnormalities that may not be discovered on a routine Pap smear.

speech-language pathology services. Speech, language, and related function assessment and rehabilitation service furnished by a qualified speech-language pathologist. Audiology services include hearing and balance assessment services furnished by a qualified audiologist. A qualified speech pathologist and audiologist must have a master's or doctoral degree in their respective fields and be licensed to serve in the state. Speech pathologists and audiologists practicing in states without licensure must complete 350 hours of supervised clinical work and perform at least nine months of supervised full-time service after earning their degrees.

sphincteroplasty. Surgical repair done to correct, augment, or improve the muscular function of a sphincter, such as the anus or intestines.

spirometry. Measurement of the lungs' breathing capacity.

splint. Brace or support. 1) dynamic splint: brace that permits movement of an anatomical structure such as a hand, wrist, foot, or other part of the body after surgery or injury. 2) static splint: brace that prevents movement and maintains support and position for an anatomical structure after surgery or injury.

stent. Tube to provide support in a body cavity or lumen.

stereotactic radiosurgery. Delivery of externally-generated ionizing radiation to specific targets for destruction or inactivation. Most often utilized in the treatment of brain or spinal tumors, high-resolution stereotactic imaging is used to identify the target and then deliver the treatment. Computer-assisted planning may also be employed. Simple and complex cranial lesions and spinal lesions are typically treated in a single planning and treatment session, although a maximum of five sessions may be required. No incision is made for stereotactic radiosurgery procedures.

stereotaxis. Three-dimensional method for precisely locating structures.

Stoffel rhizotomy. Nerve roots are sectioned to relieve pain or spastic paralysis.

strabismus. Misalignment of the eyes due to an imbalance in extraocular muscles.

surgical package. Normal, uncomplicated performance of specific surgical services, with the assumption that, on average, all surgical procedures of a given type are similar with respect to skill level, duration, and length of normal follow-up care.

symblepharopterygium. Adhesion in which the eyelid is adhered to the eyeball by a band that resembles a pterygium.

sympathectomy. Surgical interruption or transection of a sympathetic nervous system pathway.

tarso-. 1) Relating to the foot. 2) Relating to the margin of the eyelid.

tarsocheiloplasty. Plastic operation upon the edge of the eyelid for the treatment of trichiasis.

tarsorrhaphy. Suture of a portion or all of the opposing eyelids together for the purpose of shortening the palpebral fissure or closing it entirely.

technical component. Portion of a health care service that identifies the provision of the equipment, supplies, technical personnel, and costs attendant to the performance of the procedure other than the professional services.

tendon. Fibrous tissue that connects muscle to bone, consisting primarily of collagen and containing little vasculature.

tendon allograft. Allografts are tissues obtained from another individual of the same species. Tendon allografts are usually obtained from cadavers and frozen or freeze dried for later use in soft tissue repairs where the physician elects not to obtain an autogenous graft (a graft obtained from the individual on whom the surgery is being performed).

tendon suture material. Tendons are composed of fibrous tissue consisting primarily of collagen and containing few cells or blood vessels. This tissue heals more slowly than tissues with more vascularization. Because of this, tendons are usually repaired with nonabsorbable suture material. Examples include surgical silk, surgical cotton, linen, stainless steel, surgical nylon, polyester fiber, polybutester (Novafil), polyethylene (Dermalene), and polypropylene (Prolene, Surilene).

tendon transplant. Replacement of a tendon with another tendon.

tenon's capsule. Connective tissue that forms the capsule enclosing the posterior eyeball, extending from the conjunctival fornix and continuous with the muscular fascia of the eye.

tenonectomy. Excision of a portion of a tendon to make it shorter.

tenotomy. Cutting into a tendon.

TENS. Transcutaneous electrical nerve stimulator. TENS is applied by placing electrode pads over the area to be stimulated and connecting the electrodes to a transmitter box, which sends a current through the skin to sensory nerve fibers to help decrease pain in that nerve distribution.

tensilon. Edrophonium chloride. Agent used for evaluation and treatment of myasthenia gravis.

terminally ill. Individual whose medical prognosis for life expectancy is six months or less.

tetralogy of Fallot. Specific combination of congenital cardiac defects: obstruction of the right ventricular outflow tract with pulmonary stenosis, interventricular septal defect, malposition of the aorta, overriding the interventricular septum and receiving blood from both the venous and arterial systems, and enlargement of the right ventricle.

therapeutic services. Services performed for treatment of a specific diagnosis. These services include performance of the procedure, various incidental elements, and normal, related follow-up care.

thoracentesis. Surgical puncture of the chest cavity with a specialized needle or hollow tubing to aspirate fluid from within the pleural space for diagnostic or therapeutic reasons.

thoracic lymphadenectomy. Procedure to cut out the lymph nodes near the lungs, around the heart, and behind the trachea.

thoracostomy. Creation of an opening in the chest wall for drainage.

thyroglossal duct. Embryonic duct at the front of the neck, which becomes the pyramidal lobe of the thyroid gland with obliteration of the remaining duct, but may form a cyst or sinus in adulthood if it persists.

total disc arthroplasty with artificial disc. Removal of an intravertebral disc and its replacement with an implant. The implant is an artificial disc consisting of two metal plates with a weight-bearing surface of polyethylene between the plates. The plates are anchored to the vertebral immediately above and below the affected disc.

total shoulder replacement. Prosthetic replacement of the entire shoulder joint, including the humeral head and the glenoid fossa.

trabeculae carneae cordis. Bands of muscular tissue that line the walls of the ventricles in the heart.

trabeculectomy. Surgical incision between the anterior portion of the eye and the canal of Schlemm to drain the aqueous humor.

tracheostomy. Formation of a tracheal opening on the neck surface with tube insertion to allow for respiration in cases of obstruction or decreased patency. A tracheostomy may be planned or performed on an emergency basis for temporary or long-term use.

tracheotomy. Formation of a tracheal opening on the neck surface with tube insertion to allow for respiration in cases of obstruction or decreased patency. A tracheotomy may be planned or performed on an emergency basis for temporary or long-term use.

traction. Drawing out or holding tension on an area by applying a direct therapeutic pulling force.

transcranial magnetic stimulation. Application of electromagnetic energy to the brain through a coil placed on the scalp. The procedure stimulates cortical neurons and is intended to activate and normalize their processes.

transcription. Process by which messenger RNA is synthesized from a DNA template resulting in the transfer of genetic information from the DNA molecule to the messenger RNA.

translocation. Disconnection of all or part of a chromosome that reattaches to another position in the DNA sequence of the same or another chromosome. Often results in a reciprocal exchange of DNA sequences between two differently numbered chromosomes. May or may not result in a clinically significant loss of DNA.

trephine. 1) Specialized round saw for cutting circular holes in bone, especially the skull. 2) Instrument that removes small disc-shaped buttons of corneal tissue for transplanting.

tricuspid atresia. Congenital absence of the valve that may occur with other defects, such as atrial septal defect, pulmonary atresia, and transposition of great vessels.

turbinates. Scroll or shell-shaped elevations from the wall of the nasal cavity, the inferior turbinate being a separate bone, while the superior and middle turbinates are of the ethmoid bone.

tympanic membrane. Thin, sensitive membrane across the entrance to the middle ear that vibrates in response to sound waves, allowing the waves to be transmitted via the ossicular chain to the internal ear.

tympanoplasty. Surgical repair of the structures of the middle ear, including the eardrum and the three small bones, or ossicles.

unlisted procedure. Procedural descriptions used when the overall procedure and outcome of the procedure are not adequately described by an existing procedure code. Such codes are used as a last resort and only when there is not a more appropriate procedure code.

ureterorrhaphy. Surgical repair using sutures to close an open wound or injury of the ureter.

vagotomy. Division of the vagus nerves, interrupting impulses resulting in lower gastric acid production and hastening gastric emptying. Used in the treatment of chronic gastric, pyloric, and duodenal ulcers that can cause severe pain and difficulties in eating and sleeping.

variant. Nucleotide deviation from the normal sequence of a region. Variations are usually either substitutions or deletions. Substitution variations are the result of one nucleotide taking the place of another. A deletion occurs when one or more nucleotides are left out. In some cases, several in a reasonably close proximity on the same chromosome in a DNA strand. These variations result in amino acid changes in the protein made by the gene. However, the term variant does not itself imply a functional change. Intron variations are usually described in one of two ways: 1) the changed nucleotide is defined by a plus or a minus sign indicating the position relative to the first or last nucleotide to the intron, or 2) the second variant description is indicated relative to the last nucleotide of the preceding exon or first nucleotide of the following exon.

vasectomy. Surgical procedure involving the removal of all or part of the vas deferens, usually performed for sterilization or in conjunction with a prostatectomy.

ventricular assist device. Temporary measure used to support the heart by substituting for left and/or right heart function. The device replaces the work of the left and/or right ventricle when a patient has a damaged or weakened heart. A left ventricular assist device (VAD) helps the heart pump blood through the rest of the body. A right VAD helps the heart pump blood to the lungs to become oxygenated again. Catheters are inserted to circulate the blood through external tubing to a pump machine located outside of the body and back to the correct artery.

ventricular septal defect. Congenital cardiac anomaly resulting in a continual opening in the septum between the ventricles that, in severe cases, causes oxygenated blood to flow back into the lungs, resulting in pulmonary hypertension.

vertebral interspace. Non-bony space between two adjacent vertebral bodies that contains the cushioning intervertebral disk.

volar. Palm of the hand (palmar) or sole of the foot (plantar).

Waterston procedure. Type of aortopulmonary shunting done to increase pulmonary blood flow where the ascending aorta is anastomosed to the right pulmonary artery.

Wharton's ducts. Salivary ducts below the mandible.

wick catheter. Device used to monitor interstitial fluid pressure, and sometimes used intraoperatively during fasciotomy procedures to evaluate the effectiveness of the decompression.

xenograft. Tissue that is nonhuman and harvested from one species and grafted to another. Pigskin is the most common xenograft for human skin and is applied to a wound as a temporary closure until a permanent option is performed.

z-plasty. Plastic surgery technique used primarily to release tension or elongate contractured scar tissue in which a Z-shaped incision is made with the middle line of the Z crossing the area of greatest tension. The triangular flaps are then rotated so that they cross the incision line in the opposite direction, creating a reversed Z.

ZPIC. Zone Program Integrity Contractor. CMS contractor that replaced the existing Program Safeguard Contractors (PSC). Contractors are responsible for ensuring the integrity of all Medicare-related claims under Parts A and B (hospital, skilled nursing, home health, provider, and durable medical equipment claims), Part C (Medicare Advantage health plans), Part D (prescription drug plans), and coordination of Medicare-Medicaid data matches (Medi-Medi).

Appendix I — Listing of Sensory, Motor, and Mixed Nerves

This list contains the sensory, motor, and mixed nerves assigned to each nerve conduction study to improve coding accuracy. Each nerve makes up one single unit of service.

Motor Nerves Assigned to Codes 95900 and 95907-95913.

I. Upper extremity, cervical plexus, and brachial plexus motor nerves
   A. Axillary motor nerve to the deltoid
   B. Long thoracic motor nerve to the serratus anterior
   C. Median nerve
      1. Median motor nerve to the abductor pollicis brevis
      2. Median motor nerve, anterior interosseous branch, to the flexor pollicis longus
      3. Median motor nerve, anterior interosseous branch, to the pronator quadratus
      4. Median motor nerve to the first lumbrical
      5. Median motor nerve to the second lumbrical
   D. Musculocutaneous motor nerve to the biceps brachii
   E. Radial nerve
      1. Radial motor nerve to the extensor carpi ulnaris
      2. Radial motor nerve to the extensor digitorum communis
      3. Radial motor nerve to the extensor indicis proprius
      4. Radial motor nerve to the brachioradialis
   F. Suprascapular nerve
      1. Suprascapular motor nerve to the supraspinatus
      2. Suprascapular motor nerve to the infraspinatus
   G. Thoracodorsal motor nerve to the latissimus dorsi
   H. Ulnar nerve
      1. Ulnar motor nerve to the abductor digiti minimi
      2. Ulnar motor nerve to the palmar interosseous
      3. Ulnar motor nerve to the first dorsal interosseous
      4. Ulnar motor nerve to the flexor carpi ulnaris
   I. Other

II. Lower extremity motor nerves
   A. Femoral motor nerve to the quadriceps
      1. Femoral motor nerve to vastus medialis
      2. Femoral motor nerve to vastus lateralis
      3. Femoral motor nerve to vastus intermedialis
      4. Femoral motor nerve to rectus femoris
   B. Ilioinguinal motor nerve
   C. Peroneal (fibular) nerve
      1. Peroneal motor nerve to the extensor digitorum brevis
      2. Peroneal motor nerve to the peroneus brevis
      3. Peroneal motor nerve to the peroneus longus
      4. Peroneal motor nerve to the tibialis anterior
   D. Plantar motor nerve
   E. Sciatic nerve
   F. Tibial nerve
      1. Tibial motor nerve, inferior calcaneal branch, to the abductor digiti minimi
      2. Tibial motor nerve, medial plantar branch, to the abductor hallucis
      3. Tibial motor nerve, lateral plantar branch, to the flexor digiti minimi brevis
   G. Other

III. Cranial nerves and trunk
   A. Cranial nerve VII (facial motor nerve)
      1. Facial nerve to the frontalis
      2. Facial nerve to the nasalis
      3. Facial nerve to the orbicularis oculi
      4. Facial nerve to the orbicularis oris
   B. Cranial nerve XI (spinal accessory motor nerve)
   C. Cranial nerve XII (hypoglossal motor nerve)
   D. Intercostal motor nerve
   E. Phrenic motor nerve to the diaphragm
   F. Recurrent laryngeal nerve
   G. Other

IV. Nerve Roots
   A. Cervical nerve root stimulation
      1. Cervical level 5 (C5)
      2. Cervical level 6 (C6)
      3. Cervical level 7 (C7)
      4. Cervical level 8 (C8)
   B. Thoracic nerve root stimulation
      1. Thoracic level 1 (T1)
      2. Thoracic level 2 (T2)
      3. Thoracic level 3 (T3)
      4. Thoracic level 4 (T4)
      5. Thoracic level 5 (T5)
      6. Thoracic level 6 (T6)
      7. Thoracic level 7 (T7)
      8. Thoracic level 8 (T8)
      9. Thoracic level 9 (T9)
      10. Thoracic level 10 (T10)
      11. Thoracic level 11 (T11)
      12. Thoracic level 12 (T12)
   C. Lumbar nerve root stimulation
      1. Lumbar level 1 (L1)
      2. Lumbar level 2 (L2)
      3. Lumbar level 3 (L3)
      4. Lumbar level 4 (L4)
      5. Lumbar level 5 (L5)
   D. Sacral nerve root stimulation
      1. Sacral level 1 (S1)
      2. Sacral level 2 (S2)
      3. Sacral level 3 (S3)
      4. Sacral level 4 (S4)

Sensory and Mixed Nerves Assigned to Codes 95907–95913

I. Upper extremity sensory and mixed nerves
   A. Lateral antebrachial cutaneous sensory nerve
   B. Medial antebrachial cutaneous sensory nerve
   C. Medial brachial cutaneous sensory nerve
   D. Median nerve
      1. Median sensory nerve to the first digit
      2. Median sensory nerve to the second digit
      3. Median sensory nerve to the third digit
      4. Median sensory nerve to the fourth digit
      5. Median palmar cutaneous sensory nerve
      6. Median palmar mixed nerve
   E. Posterior antebrachial cutaneous sensory nerve
   F. Radial sensory nerve
      1. Radial sensory nerve to the base of the thumb
      2. Radial sensory nerve to digit 1
   G. Ulnar nerve
      1. Ulnar dorsal cutaneous sensory nerve
      2. Ulnar sensory nerve to the fourth digit
      3. Ulnar sensory nerve to the fifth digit
      4. Ulnar palmar mixed nerve
   H. Intercostal sensory nerve
   I. Other

II. Lower extremity sensory and mixed nerves
   A. Lateral femoral cutaneous sensory nerve
   B. Medical calcaneal sensory nerve
   C. Medial femoral cutaneous sensory nerve
   D. Peroneal nerve
      1. Deep peroneal sensory nerve
      2. Superficial peroneal sensory nerve, medial dorsal cutaneous branch
      3. Superficial peroneal sensory nerve, intermediate dorsal cutaneous branch
   E. Posterior femoral cutaneous sensory nerve
   F. Saphenous nerve
      1. Saphenous sensory nerve (distal technique)
      2. Saphenous sensory nerve (proximal technique)
   G. Sural nerve
      1. Sural sensory nerve, lateral dorsal cutaneous branch
      2. Sural sensory nerve
   H. Tibial sensory nerve (digital nerve to toe 1)
   I. Tibial sensory nerve (medial plantar nerve)
   J. Tibial sensory nerve (lateral plantar nerve)
   K. Other

III. Head and trunk sensory nerves
   A. Dorsal nerve of the penis
   B. Greater auricular nerve
   C. Ophthalmic branch of the trigeminal nerve
   D. Pudendal sensory nerve
   E. Suprascapular sensory nerves
   F. Other

In the following table, the reasonable maximum number of studies per diagnostic category is listed that allows for a physician or other qualified health care professional to obtain a diagnosis for 90 percent of patients with that same final diagnosis. The numbers denote the suggested number of studies, although the decision is up to the provider.

Type of Study/Maximum Number of Studies

Indication	Limbs Studied by Needle EMG (95860–95864, 95867–95870, 95885–95887)	Nerve Conduction Studies (Total nerves studied, 95907-95913)	Neuromuscular Junction Testing (Repetitive Stimulation 95937)
Carpal Tunnel (Unilateral)	1	7	—
Carpal Tunnel (Bilateral)	2	10	—
Radiculopathy	2	7	—
Mononeuropathy	1	8	—
Polyneuropathy/Mononeuropathy Multiplex	3	10	—
Myopathy	2	4	2
Motor Neuronopathy (e.g., ALS)	4	6	2
Plexopathy	2	12	—
Neuromuscular Junction	2	4	3
Tarsal Tunnel Syndrome (Unilateral)	1	8	—
Tarsal Tunnel Syndrome (Bilateral)	2	11	—
Weakness, Fatigue, Cramps, or Twitching (Focal)	2	7	2
Weakness, Fatigue, Cramps, or Twitching (General)	4	8	2
Pain, Numbness, or Tingling (Unilateral)	1	9	—
Pain, Numbness, or Tingling (Bilateral)	2	12	—

Appendix J — Vascular Families

This table assumes that the starting point is catheterization of the aorta. This categorization would not be accurate, for instance, if a femoral or carotid artery were catheterized with the blood's flow. The names of the arteries appearing in bold face type in the following table indicate those arteries that are most often the subject of arteriographic procedures.

First Order	Second Order Branch	Third Order Branch	Beyond Third Order Branches
Innominate	**Right Common Carotid**	**Right Internal Carotid**	Right Ophthalmic Right Posterior Communicating Right Middle Cerebral Right Anterior Cerebral
		Right External Carotid	Right Superior Thyroid Right Ascending Pharyngeal Right Facial Right Lingual Right Occipital Right Posterior Auricular Right Superficial Temporal Right Internal Maxillary Right Middle Meningeal
	Right Subclavian and Axillary	**Right Vertebral**	Basilar
		Right Internal Thoracic (Internal Mammary)	
		Right Thyrocervical Trunk	Right Inferior Thyroid Right Surascapular Right Transverse Cervical
		Right Costocervical Trunk	Right Highest Intercostal Right Deep Cervical
		Right Lateral Thoracic	
		Right Thoracromial	
		Right Humeral Circumflex (A/P)	
		Right Subscapular	Right Circumflex Scapular
		Right Brachial	
		Right Deep Brachial	Right Ulnar Right Radial Right Interosseous Right Deep Palmar Arch Right Superficial Palmar Arch Right Metacarpals and Digitals
Left Common Carotid	**Left Internal Carotid**	Left Ophthalmic Left Posterior Communicating Left Middle Cerebral Left Anterior Cerebral	
	Left External Carotid	Left Superior Thyroid Left Ascending Pharyngeal Left Facial Left Lingual Left Occipital Left Posterior Auricular Left Superficial Temporal	
		Left Internal Maxillary	Left Middle Meningeal

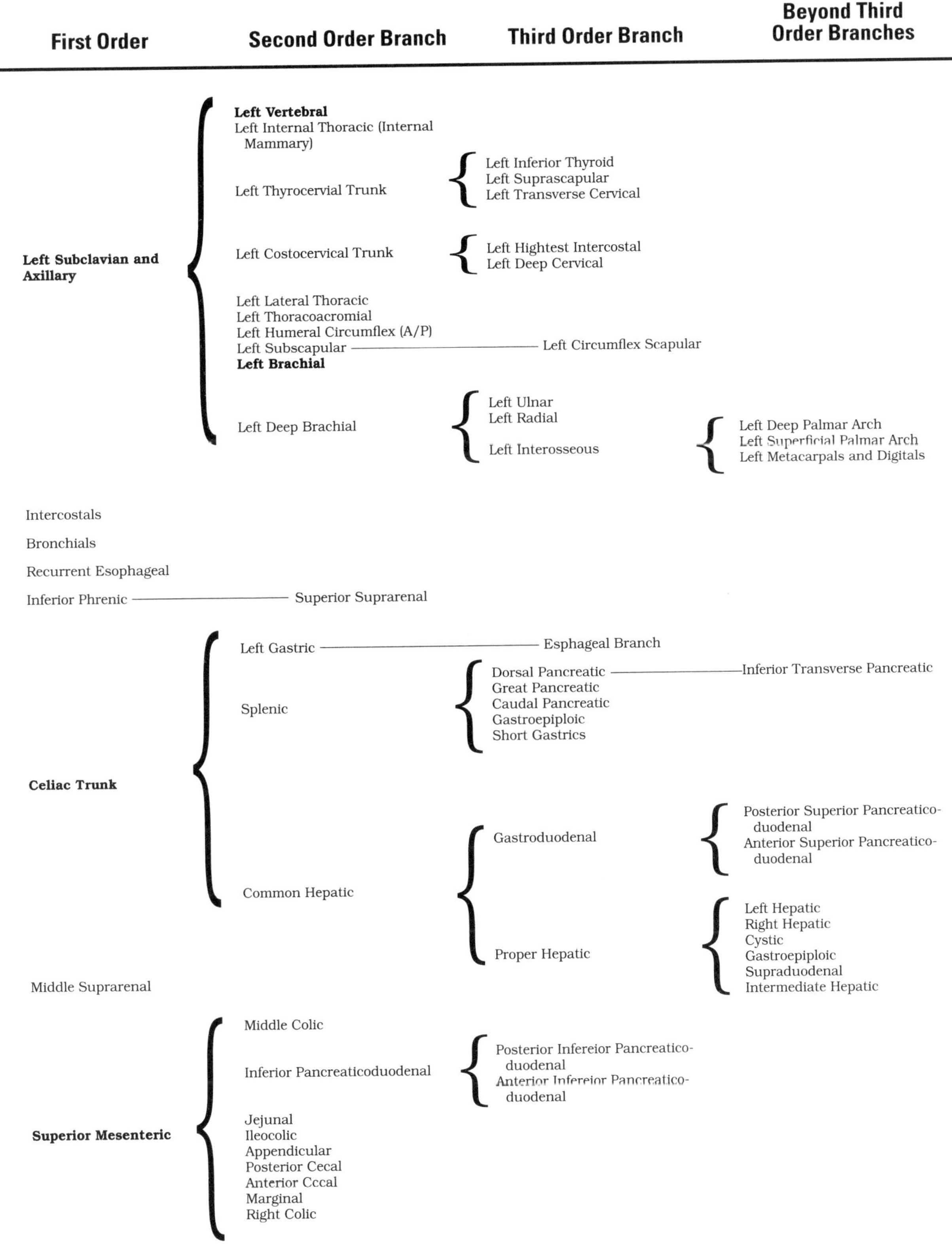
First Order
Second Order Branch
Third Order Branch
Beyond Third Order Branches
Left Subclavian and Axillary
Left Vertebral
Left Internal Thoracic (Internal Mammary)
Left Thyrocervial Trunk
Left Inferior Thyroid
Left Suprascapular
Left Transverse Cervical
Left Costocervical Trunk
Left Hightest Intercostal
Left Deep Cervical
Left Lateral Thoracic
Left Thoracoacromial
Left Humeral Circumflex (A/P)
Left Subscapular
Left Circumflex Scapular
Left Brachial
Left Deep Brachial
Left Ulnar
Left Radial
Left Interosseous
Left Deep Palmar Arch
Left Superficial Palmar Arch
Left Metacarpals and Digitals
Intercostals
Bronchials
Recurrent Esophageal
Inferior Phrenic
Superior Suprarenal
Celiac Trunk
Left Gastric
Esphageal Branch
Splenic
Dorsal Pancreatic
Inferior Transverse Pancreatic
Great Pancreatic
Caudal Pancreatic
Gastroepiploic
Short Gastrics
Common Hepatic
Gastroduodenal
Posterior Superior Pancreatico-duodenal
Anterior Superior Pancreatico-duodenal
Proper Hepatic
Left Hepatic
Right Hepatic
Cystic
Gastroepiploic
Supraduodenal
Intermediate Hepatic
Middle Suprarenal
Superior Mesenteric
Middle Colic
Inferior Pancreaticoduodenal
Posterior Infereior Pancreatico-duodenal
Anterior Infereior Pancreatico-duodenal
Jejunal
Ileocolic
Appendicular
Posterior Cecal
Anterior Cccal
Marginal
Right Colic

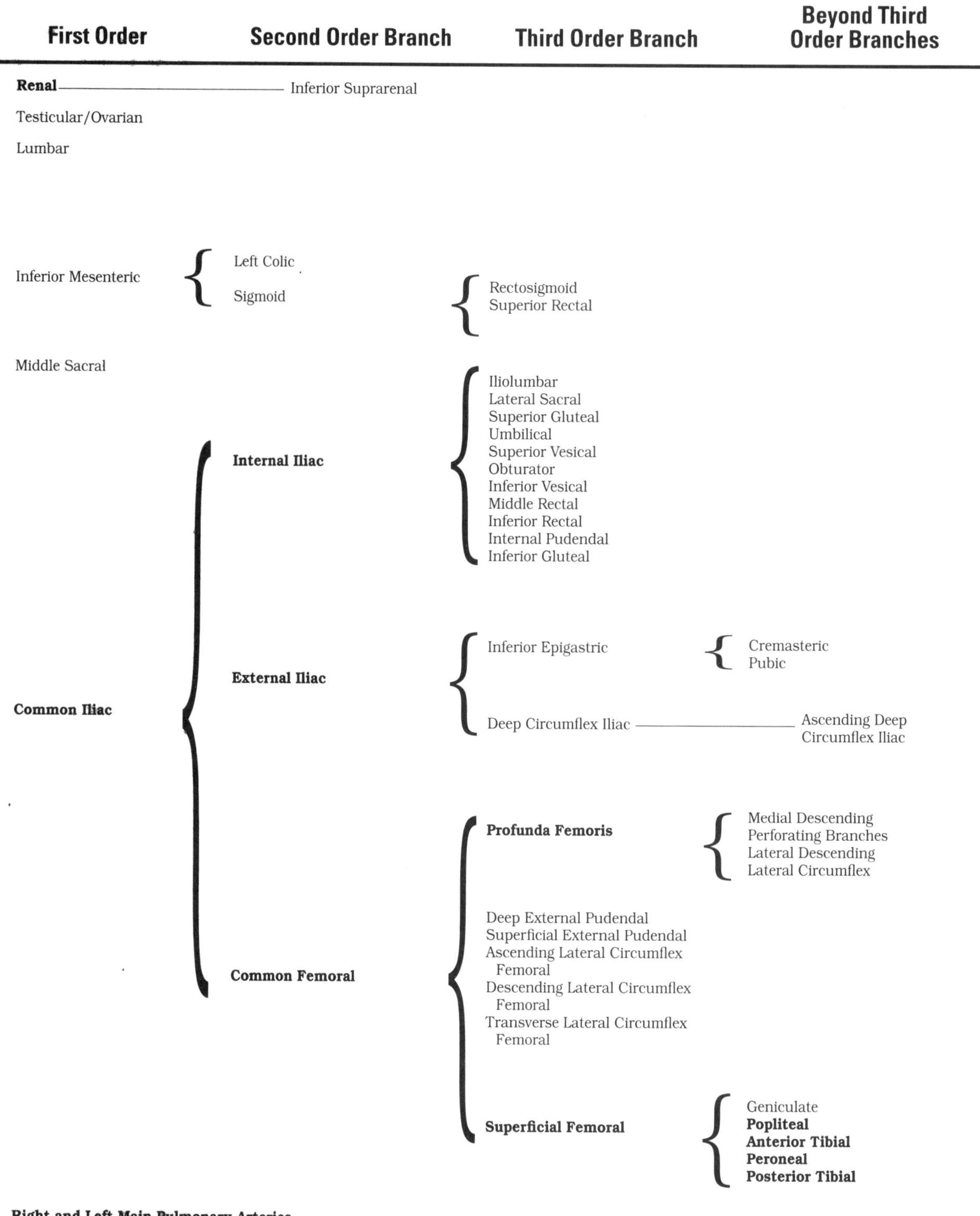

Reference: Kadir S. *Atlas of Normal and Variant Angiographic Anatomy*. Philadelphia, Pa: WB Saunders Co; 1991

Appendix K — Physician Quality Reporting System (PQRS)

Numerator	Associated Diagnostic Denominator	Associated Procedure Denominator	Associated Modifiers
0509F, 1091F	788.38-788.31, 788.37-307.6, 788.33, 788.35-625.6, 788.39-788.30, 788.34, 788.36	99201-99205, 99212-99215, 99324-99337, 99341-99350, G0402	8P
0513F	585.3-585.4, 585.5	99201-99205, 99212-99215, 99304-99310, 99324-99337, 99341-99350	8P
0517F, 3284F	365.70-365.71, 365.74-365.10, 365.11	99201-99205, 99212-99215, 99307-99310, 99324-99337, 92002-92014	8P
0518F	N/A	99201-99215, 99304-99310, 99324-99337, 99341-99350, 97001-97004, 1100F, G0402, G0438	1P, 8P
0520F	162.4-157.0, 198.1-157.8, 196.2-162.2, 198.4-157.2, 196.8, 197.1-162.5, 197.2-196.6, 198.2-157.4, 196.3, 197.7, 198.81-196.0, 198.7-162.9, 196.9-157.3, 196.5, 197.3-157.1, 197.4, 198.6, 198.89-162.3, 198.82-157.9, 197.8-162.0, 197.6, 198.5-196.1, 197.0, 197.5	77295	8P
0521F, 1125F	201.60-200.84, 202.25-202.13, 237.1, 238.0-162.4, 172.4-157.0, 174.1, 190.9, 195.3, 201.14, 201.26, 201.90, 202.06-201.46, 202.80-148.2, 201.94, 207.20-202.68, 202.83-148.8, 202.22, 236.0-145.0, 204.20-160.3, 176.2, 190.7, 198.1, 201.02, 201.07, 201.20, 201.93-200.04, 204.21-140.5, 170.3-156.1, 198.0, 201.92, 202.02, 204.81-147.2, 158.9, 200.00, 201.75, 202.50, 202.85-200.16, 200.21, 200.83, 208.81-188.8, 202.34-170.0, 203.80-153.1, 153.5, 153.9, 172.9, 191.7, 194.6, 201.95, 205.00, 205.91-154.8, 200.08, 200.32, 200.40, 200.54, 200.57, 200.68, 200.72, 209.03, 209.25-208.22, 209.33-173.11, 173.19, 173.40, 173.49, 173.90, 202.65, 239.0-146.1, 204.10-153.6, 157.8, 160.5, 174.8, 194.8, 200.03, 202.01, 207.10-141.4, 237.72-161.9, 194.9, 201.01, 206.11-186.9, 202.33-140.0, 140.6, 235.5, 236.6-155.1, 176.9, 182.8, 196.2, 201.12, 201.24-149.8, 194.1, 201.56, 202.66-187.8, 188.2, 188.6, 189.3, 202.21-142.1, 170.9, 239.5-184.0, 201.76, 202.20, 202.35-141.9, 200.27-142.8, 238.4-152.0, 181, 201.03, 201.21, 205.11, 206.90-202.94, 203.81-159.9, 207.01, 238.76-200.34, 200.37, 200.46, 200.70, 202.76, 202.78, 209.02, 209.10, 209.20, 209.27-204.12, 206.22-204.82, 207.22, 209.73, 209.79-173.00, 173.09, 173.20, 173.50, 173.80, 173.89, 200.17-188.1, 189.2-142.9, 238.6-170.8, 171.6, 191.3, 194.0, 198.4, 201.10, 201.96, 205.01, 205.30, 206.10-202.07, 202.53-171.4, 172.1, 203.00, 204.00-152.3, 157.2, 159.8, 175.0, 196.8, 197.1, 201.16, 201.28, 207.00-140.8, 239.6-146.3, 159.0, 174.2, 201.08-200.13, 200.18-149.1, 150.9, 236.99-235.4, 236.4-162.5, 165.8, 202.93-151.8, 153.7, 176.8, 207.11-201.71, 202.84-140.4, 175.9, 202.63-188.4, 202.40, 237.9-161.3, 170.6, 171.9-144.8, 145.5, 203.01-176.3, 192.2, 197.2, 200.07, 201.17, 201.54-191.9, 201.91, 238.79-200.33, 200.35, 200.47, 200.51-200.52, 200.60, 200.62-200.64, 200.67, 209.14, 209.17-203.12, 207.82-205.12, 205.82-173.10, 173.30, 173.62, 173.92-173.99, 202.51-149.0, 150.1, 150.8, 161.8-151.6, 153.2, 160.0, 183.9, 185, 204.80, 204.91, 208.80-155.2, 192.1, 201.66-200.25, 200.82-149.9, 151.0, 151.5, 202.17-163.9, 239.7-144.1, 153.4, 174.4, 195.0, 200.06, 201.77, 202.04, 205.90, 208.10, 237.2-143.9, 238.1, 239.2-152.2, 155.0, 160.8, 196.6-146.0, 182.1, 195.2, 198.2, 202.58-140.1, 202.97-154.3, 157.4, 174.0, 184.2, 190.8, 196.3, 197.7, 198.81, 201.40, 206.21-200.81, 202.28, 236.2-161.1, 208.11, 238.72-200.36, 200.50, 200.65-200.66, 200.71, 200.76-200.77, 202.71, 209.01, 209.13, 209.22-204.02, 204.22, 205.02, 206.02, 208.82, 209.71-173.12, 173.39, 173.52, 173.70, 201.42, 202.47,	99201-99205, 99212-99215, 51720, 77427-77435, 77470, 96401-96549, 0521F	8P

Numerator	Associated Diagnostic Denominator	Associated Procedure Denominator	Associated Modifiers
0521F, 1125F (continued)	202.81-187.7, 202.30-141.5, 202.91-152.1, 184.3, 190.1, 191.8, 192.3, 196.0, 201.22, 208.20-150.4, 202.31, 238.8-146.9, 174.9, 201.45, 201.58-189.0, 189.4-142.2, 237.71, 238.9-161.2, 170.5, 202.88-191.6, 192.0, 194.4, 198.7, 205.21, 206.01-151.3, 202.24, 235.9-201.50, 201.61, 202.48-147.8, 151.4, 202.32, 237.70-171.7, 172.0-145.3, 204.11-176.1, 183.3, 191.4, 194.3, 202.08, 239.1, 239.3-151.9, 156.2, 201.72-188.0, 189.8-143.1, 235.1, 236.1-158.8, 184.9, 190.0, 200.02-150.0, 238.5-165.9, 194.5, 238.71-200.45, 200.74, 202.74-199.2, 209.16, 209.23, 209.30-203.02, 206.12, 209.74-173.22, 173.31-173.32, 173.51, 201.55, 201.68, 202.55-187.1, 188.5, 188.9, 189.9-148.1, 202.42-140.3, 235.8-144.9, 180.0, 201.05, 208.01-172.5, 202.87-160.1, 201.70, 202.62, 208.91-150.3, 202.27, 237.4-162.9, 164.8-154.2, 184.1, 190.3, 201.51, 202.92-154.1, 191.5, 206.91-148.3, 202.15-153.3, 154.0, 174.3, 180.1, 182.0, 184.4, 190.2, 190.6, 192.8, 200.05, 201.00, 201.15, 201.27, 201.98-191.1, 202.10, 206.80-202.18, 236.90-145.1, 146.5, 160.4, 174.6, 196.9, 199.1, 201.13, 204.90, 205.80, 207.21-200.20, 202.41-157.3, 200.30, 200.41, 200.61, 200.75, 200.78, 209.11-205.22, 208.92-203.82, 208.02, 209.32, 209.72, 239.81-173.02, 173.41, 173.59, 173.60, 173.71-173.72, 173.82, 202.86-200.88, 202.14-143.8, 236.91-171.2, 239.4-145.2, 146.7, 156.0, 196.5, 197.3, 201.74, 202.12-164.0, 180.8, 187.4, 188.7-147.9, 202.44-141.2, 141.8, 143.0, 171.8-145.9, 153.0, 153.8, 160.9	99201-99205, 99212-99215, 51720, 77427-77435, 77470, 96401-96549, 0521F	8P
0528F	V76.51	44388, 45378, G0121	1P, 8P
0529F	V12.72	44388-44389, 44392-44394, 45355-45378, 45380-45381, 45383-45385, G0105	1P, 3P, 8P
0540F, 3455F	714.0, 714.2, 714.1	99201-99205, 99212-99215, 99341-99350, G0402	1P, 8P
0556F	411.1-410.72, 414.9-411.0, 413.1-410.32, 410.82-410.31, 413.9-410.01, 410.22, 410.92, 414.02, 414.3-411.81, 414.04-410.00, 410.20, 410.60, 410.81, 410.91, 414.06-410.02, 410.52, 410.70-410.12, V45.81-410.71, 410.90, 411.89, 414.2-410.10, 412-410.42, 414.8-410.11, 410.40, 413.0-410.41, 410.51, 414.03-410.30, 410.80-410.62, V45.82-410.21, 414.00-410.50, 414.07	99201-99205, 99212-99215, 99304-99310, 99324-99337, 99341-99350	8P
0557F	411.1-410.72, 414.9-411.0, 413.1-410.32, 410.82-410.31, 413.9-410.01, 410.22, 410.92, 414.02, 414.3-411.81, 414.04-410.00, 410.20, 410.60, 410.81, 410.91, 414.06-410.02, 410.52, 410.70-410.12, V45.81-410.71, 410.90, 411.89, 414.2-410.10, 412-410.42, 414.8-410.11, 410.40, 413.0-410.41, 410.51, 414.03-410.30, 410.80-410.62, V45.82-410.21, 414.00-410.50, 414.07	99201-99205, 99212-99215, 99304-99310, 99324-99337, 99341-99350, 1010F	1P, 2P, 3P, 8P
0575F, 3502F, 4290F, 4293F	042	99201-99205, 99212-99215	8P
1006F, 1007F	715.16, 715.30, 715.97-715.28, 715.32-715.10, 715.96-715.14, 715.26-715.09, 715.23-715.24, 715.36, 715.90-715.00, 715.12, 715.34-715.17, 715.80-715.15, 715.94-715.18, 715.35-715.11, 715.38, 715.98-715.13, 715.91-715.21, 715.92-715.04, 715.93-715.33, 715.37, 715.89, 715.22	99201-99205, 99212-99215	8P
1010F	411.1-410.72, 414.9-411.0, 413.1-410.32, 410.82-410.31, 413.9-410.01, 410.22, 410.92, 414.02, 414.3-411.81, 414.04-410.00, 410.20, 410.60, 410.81, 410.91, 414.06-410.02, 410.52, 410.70-410.12, V45.81-410.71, 410.90, 411.89, 414.2-410.10, 412-410.42, 414.8-410.11, 410.40, 413.0-410.41, 410.51, 414.03-410.30, 410.80-410.62, V45.82-410.21, 414.00-410.50, 414.07	99201-99205, 99212-99215, 99304-99310, 99324-99337, 99341-99350, 1010F	8P
1011F, 1012F, G0911, G0912, G8787, G8788	411.1-410.72, 414.9-411.0, 413.1-410.32, 410.82-410.31, 413.9-410.01, 410.22, 410.92, 414.02, 414.3-411.81, 414.04-410.00, 410.20, 410.60, 410.81, 410.91, 414.06-410.02, 410.52, 410.70-410.12, V45.81-410.71, 410.90, 411.89, 414.2-410.10, 412-410.42, 414.8-410.11, 410.40, 413.0-410.41, 410.51, 414.03-410.30, 410.80-410.62, V45.82-410.21, 414.00-410.50, 414.07	99201-99205, 99212-99215, 99304-99310, 99324-99337, 99341-99350, 1010F	N/A

Appendix K — Physician Quality Reporting System (PQRS)

Numerator	Associated Diagnostic Denominator	Associated Procedure Denominator	Associated Modifiers
1031F, 4000F, 4001F	493.92-493.01, 493.22, 493.81, 493.90-493.02, 493.11-493.00, 493.10, 493.12, 493.21, 493.82	99201-99205, 99212-99220, 99341-99350	8P
1032F, 1033F, G8751	493.92-493.01, 493.22, 493.81, 493.90-493.02, 493.11-493.00, 493.10, 493.12, 493.21, 493.82	99201-99205, 99212-99220, 99341-99350	N/A
1036F	N/A	99201-99205, 99212-99215, 99406-99407, 90791-90832, 90834, 90837, 90839, 90845, 92002-92014, 96150-96152, 97003-97004, G0438	N/A
1038F, 1039F, 4144F	493.92-493.01, 493.22, 493.81, 493.90-493.02, 493.11-493.00, 493.10, 493.12, 493.21, 493.82	99201-99205, 99212-99215, 99341-99350, 1038F	N/A
1040F, 3085F	296.33-296.21, 296.23-296.24, 296.30-296.20, 296.22	99201-99205, 99212-99215, 99281-99285, 90791-90832, 90834, 90837, 90839, 90845	8P
1090F	N/A	99201-99205, 99212-99215, 99324-99337, 99341-99350, G0402	1P, 8P
1100F	N/A	99201-99215, 99304-99310, 99324-99337, 99341-99350, 97001-97004, 1100F, G0402, G0438	N/A
1101F	N/A	99201-99215, 99304-99310, 99324-99337, 99341-99350, 97001-97004, G0402, G0438	8P
1110F	N/A	99201-99215, 99324-99337, 99341-99350, 90791-90832, 90834, 90837, 90839, 90845, G0402, G0438	N/A
1111F	N/A	99201-99215, 99324-99337, 99341-99350, 90791-90832, 90834, 90837, 90839, 90845, G0402, G0438	8P
1116F	380.11, 380.22-380.10, 380.13	99201-99205, 99212-99215, 99281-99285	1P, 8P
1119F, 1121F	070.51, 070.54	99201-99205, 99212-99215, 1119F, G9202	N/A
1123F	N/A	99201-99205, 99212-99215, 99218-99220, 99221-99236, 99291, 99304-99310, 99324-99337, 99341-99350, G0402	8P
1124F	N/A	99201-99205, 99212-99215, 99218-99220, 99221-99236, 99291, 99304-99310, 99324-99337, 99341-99350, G0402	N/A
1126F	201.60-200.84, 202.25-202.13, 237.1, 238.0-162.4, 172.4-157.0, 174.1, 190.9, 195.3, 201.14, 201.26, 201.90, 202.06-201.46, 202.80-148.2, 201.94, 207.20-202.68, 202.83-148.8, 202.22, 236.0-145.0, 204.20-160.3, 176.2, 190.7, 198.1, 201.02, 201.07, 201.20, 201.93-200.04, 204.21-140.5, 170.3-156.1, 198.0, 201.92, 202.02, 204.81-147.2, 158.9, 200.00, 201.75, 202.50, 202.85-200.16, 200.21, 200.83, 208.81-188.8, 202.34-170.0, 203.80-153.1, 153.5, 153.9, 172.9, 191.7, 194.6, 201.95, 205.00, 205.91-154.8, 200.08, 200.32, 200.40, 200.54, 200.57, 200.68, 200.72, 209.03, 209.25-208.22, 209.33-173.11, 173.19, 173.40, 173.49, 173.90, 202.65, 239.0-146.1, 204.10-153.6, 157.8, 160.5, 174.8, 194.8, 200.03, 202.01, 207.10-141.4, 237.72-161.9, 194.9, 201.01, 206.11-186.9, 202.33-140.0, 140.6, 235.5, 236.6-155.1, 176.9, 182.8, 196.2, 201.12, 201.24-149.8, 194.1, 201.56, 202.66-187.8, 188.2, 188.6, 189.3, 202.21-142.1, 170.9, 239.5-184.0, 201.76, 202.20, 202.35-141.9, 200.27-142.8, 238.4-152.0, 181, 201.03, 201.21, 205.11, 206.90-202.94, 203.81-159.9, 207.01, 238.76-200.34, 200.37, 200.46, 200.70, 202.76, 202.78, 209.02, 209.10, 209.20, 209.27-204.12, 206.22-204.82, 207.22, 209.73, 209.79-173.00, 173.09, 173.20, 173.50, 173.80, 173.89, 200.17-188.1, 189.2-142.9, 238.6-170.8, 171.6, 191.3, 194.0, 198.4, 201.10, 201.96, 205.01, 205.30, 206.10-202.07, 202.53-171.4, 172.1, 203.00, 204.00-152.3, 157.2, 159.8, 175.0, 196.8, 197.1, 201.16, 201.28, 207.00-140.8, 239.6-146.3, 159.0, 174.2, 201.08-200.13, 200.18-149.1, 150.9, 236.99-235.4, 236.4-162.5, 165.8, 202.93-151.8, 153.7, 176.8, 207.11-201.71, 202.84-140.4, 175.9, 202.63-188.4, 202.40, 237.9-161.3, 170.6, 171.9-144.8, 145.5, 203.01-176.3, 192.2, 197.2, 200.07, 201.17, 201.54-191.9, 201.91, 238.79-200.33, 200.35, 200.47, 200.51-200.52, 200.60, 200.62-200.64, 200.67, 209.14, 209.17-203.12, 207.82-205.12, 205.82-173.10, 173.30, 173.62, 173.92-173.99, 202.51-149.0, 150.1, 150.8, 161.8-151.6, 153.2, 160.0, 183.9, 185, 204.80, 204.91, 208.80-155.2, 192.1, 201.66-200.25, 200.82-149.9, 151.0, 151.5,	99201-99205, 99212-99215, 51720, 77427-77435, 77470, 96401-96549	N/A

Numerator	Associated Diagnostic Denominator	Associated Procedure Denominator	Associated Modifiers
1126F (continued)	202.17-163.9, 239.7-144.1, 153.4, 174.4, 195.0, 200.06, 201.77, 202.04, 205.90, 208.10, 237.2-143.9, 238.1, 239.2-152.2, 155.0, 160.8, 196.6-146.0, 182.1, 195.2, 198.2, 202.58-140.1, 202.97-154.3, 157.4, 174.0, 184.2, 190.8, 196.3, 197.7, 198.81, 201.40, 206.21-200.81, 202.28, 236.2-161.1, 208.11, 238.72-200.36, 200.50, 200.65-200.66, 200.71, 200.76-200.77, 202.71, 209.01, 209.13, 209.22-204.02, 204.22, 205.02, 206.02, 208.82, 209.71-173.12, 173.39, 173.52, 173.70, 201.42, 202.47, 202.81-187.7, 202.30-141.5, 202.91-152.1, 184.3, 190.1, 191.8, 192.3, 196.0, 201.22, 208.20-150.4, 202.31, 238.8-146.9, 174.9, 201.45, 201.58-189.0, 189.4-142.2, 237.71, 238.9-161.2, 170.5, 202.88-191.6, 192.0, 194.4, 198.7, 205.21, 206.01-151.3, 202.24, 235.9-201.50, 201.61, 202.48-147.8, 151.4, 202.32, 237.70-171.7, 172.0-145.3, 204.11-176.1, 183.3, 191.4, 194.3, 202.08, 239.1, 239.3-151.9, 156.2, 201.72-188.0, 189.8-143.1, 235.1, 236.1-158.8, 184.9, 190.0, 200.02-150.0, 238.5-165.9, 194.5, 238.71-200.45, 200.74, 202.74-199.2, 209.16, 209.23, 209.30-203.02, 206.12, 209.74-173.22, 173.31-173.32, 173.51, 201.55, 201.68, 202.55-187.1, 188.5, 188.9, 189.9-148.1, 202.42-140.3, 235.8-144.9, 180.0, 201.05, 208.01-172.5, 202.87-160.1, 201.70, 202.62, 208.91-150.3, 202.27, 237.4-162.9, 164.8-154.2, 184.1, 190.3, 201.51, 202.92-154.1, 191.5, 206.91-148.3, 202.15-153.3, 154.0, 174.3, 180.1, 182.0, 184.4, 190.2, 190.6, 192.8, 200.05, 201.00, 201.15, 201.27, 201.98-191.1, 202.10, 206.80-202.18, 236.90-145.1, 146.5, 160.4, 174.6, 196.9, 199.1, 201.13, 204.90, 205.80, 207.21-200.20, 202.41-157.3, 200.30, 200.41, 200.61, 200.75, 200.78, 209.11-205.22, 208.92-203.82, 208.02, 209.32, 209.72, 239.81-173.02, 173.41, 173.59, 173.60, 173.71-173.72, 173.82, 202.86-200.88, 202.14-143.8, 236.91-171.2, 239.4-145.2, 146.7, 156.0, 196.5, 197.3, 201.74, 202.12-164.0, 180.8, 187.4, 188.7-147.9, 202.44-141.2, 141.8, 143.0, 171.8-145.9, 153.0, 153.8, 160.9	99201-99205, 99212-99215, 51720, 77427-77435, 77470, 96401-96549	N/A
1170F, 3470F, 3475F, 4194F	714.0, 714.2, 714.1	99201-99205, 99212-99215, 99341-99350, G0402	8P
1200F	345.51-345.00, 345.70-345.61, 345.91-345.50, 345.90-345.10, 345.41-345.11, 345.40	99201-99205, 99212-99215, 99304-99309	1P, 2P, 8P
1205F	345.51-345.00, 345.70-345.61, 345.91-345.50, 345.90-345.10, 345.41-345.11, 345.40	99201-99205, 99212-99215, 99304-99309	8P
1220F	304.00, 304.30-304.02, 304.72, 305.01-304.01, 305.32-304.62, 305.90, 305.92-304.41, 305.80-303.91, 305.60-303.90, 304.50, 305.41-304.51, 305.81-303.92, 304.52, 305.72-305.52, 305.62-305.50, 305.71-304.81, 304.91, 305.30-304.21, 305.22-304.11, 305.20, 305.91-304.70, 305.70-304.80, 304.90-304.10, 304.40, 304.71-304.22, 305.61, 305.82-304.31, 305.42-304.12, 304.32, 304.20	99201-99205, 99212-99215, 90791-90832, 90834, 90837, 90839, 90845, 96150-96152	1P, 8P
1460F, 1461F, 4510F	410.72, 413.1-410.32, 410.82-410.31, 413.9-410.01, 410.22, 410.92-122.9, 410.00, 410.20, 410.60, 410.81, 410.91-410.02, 410.52, 410.70-122.2, 410.71, 410.90-410.10, 412-122.8, 410.42-122.0, 410.11, 410.40, 413.0-410.41, 410.51-410.30, 410.80-122.1, 410.62-410.21, 410.50	99201-99205, 99212-99215, 99387, 99395-99396, 33361-33365, 33400-33430, 33463-33496, 33510-33536, 33572-33602, 33935, 33945, 33999, 35500, 35600, 92920, 92924, 92928, 92933, 92937, 92941-92943, 1460F, G0438	N/A
2000F	250.01, 250.41-250.33, 250.52-250.51, 362.03-250.53, 250.62-250.02, 250.20, 250.80-250.30, 362.01-250.42, 250.93-250.70, 250.72-250.32, 250.50-250.00, 648.04-250.40, 250.92, 362.06-250.13, 648.02-250.71, 250.73, 648.00-250.31, 648.03-250.22, 366.41, 648.01-250.82, 362.05-250.12, 362.07-250.63, 357.2-250.10, 250.83-250.03, 362.04	99201-99205, 99212-99215, 99304-99310, 99324-99337, 99341-99350, 97802-97804	8P
2010F	483.0, 485, 487.0-482.30, 482.84-482.40, 482.42-481, 482.2, 486-482.31, 482.82-482.1, 483.8-482.0, 482.89-482.32, 482.81, 482.83	99201-99205, 99212-99215, 99221-99223, 99281-99285, 99291, 99324-99337, 99341-99350	8P

Numerator	Associated Diagnostic Denominator	Associated Procedure Denominator	Associated Modifiers
2014F	483.0, 485, 487.0-482.30, 482.84-482.40, 482.42-481, 482.2, 486-482.31, 482.82-482.1, 483.8-482.0, 482.89-482.32, 482.81, 482.83	99201-99205, 99212-99215, 99281-99285, 99291, 99324-99337, 99341-99350	8P
2015F, 2016F	493.92-493.01, 493.22, 493.81, 493.90-493.02, 493.11-493.00, 493.10, 493.12, 493.21, 493.82	99201-99205, 99212-99215, 99341-99350	8P
2019F	362.51-362.50, 362.52	99201-99205, 99212-99215, 99304-99310, 99324-99337, 92002-92014	1P, 2P, 8P
2021F, 5010F	362.03-362.01, 362.06-362.02, 362.04	99201-99205, 99212-99215, 99304-99310, 99324-99337, 92002-92014	1P, 2P, 8P
2022F, 2024F, 2026F	250.01, 250.41-250.33, 250.52-250.51, 362.03-250.53, 250.62-250.02, 250.20, 250.80-250.30, 362.01-250.42, 250.93-250.70, 250.72-250.32, 250.50-250.00, 648.04-250.40, 250.92, 362.06-250.13, 648.02-250.71, 250.73, 648.00-250.31, 648.03-250.22, 366.41, 648.01-250.82, 362.05-250.12, 362.07-250.63, 357.2-250.10, 250.83-250.03, 362.04	99201-99220, 99221-99233, 99238-99239, 99281-99285, 99291, 99304-99337, 99341-99350, 99455-99456, 92002-92014, 97802-97804, G0402, G0438	8P
2027F	365.70-365.71, 365.74-365.10, 365.11	99201-99205, 99212-99215, 99304-99310, 99324-99337, 92002-92014	1P, 8P
2028F	250.01, 250.41-250.33, 250.52-250.51, 362.03 250.53, 250.62-250.02, 250.20, 250.80-250.30, 362.01-250.42, 250.93-250.70, 250.72-250.32, 250.50-250.00, 648.04-250.40, 250.92, 362.06-250.13, 648.02-250.71, 250.73, 648.00-250.31, 648.03-250.22, 366.41, 648.01-250.82, 362.05-250.12, 362.07-250.63, 357.2-250.10, 250.83-250.03, 362.04	99201-99220, 99221-99233, 99238-99239, 99281-99285, 99291, 99304-99337, 99341-99350, 99455-99456, 97802-97804, G0402, G0438	1P, 8P
3014F	N/A	99201-99205, 99212-99215, G0402	1P, 8P
3016F	N/A	99201-99205, 99212-99215, 90791-90832, 90834, 90837, 90839, 90845, 96150-96152, 97003-97004, 97802-97804, 98960-98962, G0270, G0271	1P, 8P
3017F	N/A	99201-99205, 99212-99215, 99304-99310, 99324-99337, G0402	1P, 8P
3021F	404.13, 428.23, 428.41-404.91, 428.40-404.93, 428.31-402.11, 428.21, 428.42-402.91, 428.22, 428.43-404.01, 428.32, 428.9-428.0, 428.20, 428.33-402.01, 404.03	99201-99205, 99212-99215, 99238-99239, 99304-99310, 99324-99337, 99341-99350, 3021F	8P
3022F	404.13, 428.23, 428.41-404.91, 428.40-404.93, 428.31-402.11, 428.21, 428.42-402.91, 428.22, 428.43-404.01, 428.32, 428.9-428.0, 428.20, 428.33-402.01, 404.03	99201-99205, 99212-99215, 99238-99239, 99304-99310, 99324-99337, 99341-99350, 3021F	N/A
3023F, 4025F	496-491.21, 492.0-491.0, 493.20-491.1, 491.20	99201-99205, 99212-99215	1P, 2P, 3P, 8P
3025F	496-491.21, 492.0-491.0, 493.20-491.1, 491.20	99201-99205, 99212-99215	8P
3027F, G8924, G8925, G8926	496-491.21, 492.0-491.0, 493.20-491.1, 491.20	99201-99205, 99212-99215	N/A
3028F	483.0, 485, 487.0-482.30, 482.84-482.40, 482.42-481, 482.2, 486-482.31, 482.82-482.1, 483.8-482.0, 482.89-482.32, 482.81, 482.83	99201-99205, 99212-99215, 99281-99285, 99291, 99324-99337, 99341-99350	1P, 2P, 3P, 8P
3038F	N/A	32440-32488, 32503-32505, 32663, 32666, 32669-32672	1P, 8P
3044F	404.13-250.01, 250.41, 428.23-250.33, 250.52-250.51, 428.41-250.53, 404.91, 428.40-250.61, 404.93-250.02, 428.31-250.20, 402.11-250.30, 362.01-250.42, 428.21, 428.42-250.93, 428.22, 428.43-250.70, 250.72-250.32, 250.50-250.00, 428.30, 648.04-250.40, 250.92, 362.06-250.13, 648.02-250.71, 250.73, 648.00-362.02, 404.11-250.31, 404.01, 648.03-250.22, 366.41, 648.01-250.82, 362.05-250.43, 428.32-250.21, 428.9-250.12, 362.07, 428.0-250.63, 428.20-250.10, 428.33-250.83, 428.1-250.03, 362.04	99201-99220, 99221-99233, 99238-99239, 99281-99285, 99291, 99304-99337, 99341-99350, 99455-99456, 97802-97804, G0402-G0270, G0439-G0271, G8923	N/A
3045F, 3049F, 3050F	250.01, 250.41-250.33, 250.52-250.51, 362.03-250.53, 250.62-250.02, 250.20, 250.80-250.30, 362.01-250.42, 250.93-250.70, 250.72-250.32, 250.50-250.00, 648.04-250.40, 250.92, 362.06-250.13, 648.02-250.71, 250.73, 648.00-250.31, 648.03-250.22, 366.41, 648.01-250.82, 362.05-250.12, 362.07-250.63, 357.2-250.10, 250.83-250.03, 362.04	99201-99220, 99221-99233, 99238-99239, 99281-99285, 99291, 99304-99337, 99341-99350, 99455-99456, 97802-97804, G0402-G0270, G0271	N/A

Numerator	Associated Diagnostic Denominator	Associated Procedure Denominator	Associated Modifiers
3046F, 3048F	250.01, 250.41-250.33, 250.52-250.51, 362.03-250.53, 250.62-250.02, 250.20, 250.80-250.30, 362.01-250.42, 250.93-250.70, 250.72-250.32, 250.50-250.00, 648.04-250.40, 250.92, 362.06-250.13, 648.02-250.71, 250.73, 648.00-250.31, 648.03-250.22, 366.41, 648.01-250.82, 362.05-250.12, 362.07-250.63, 357.2-250.10, 250.83-250.03, 362.04	99201-99220, 99221-99233, 99238-99239, 99281-99285, 99291, 99304-99337, 99341-99350, 99455-99456, 97802-97804, G0402-G0270, G0271	8P
3060F, 3061F, 3062F	250.01, 250.41-250.33, 250.52-250.51, 362.03-250.53, 250.62-250.02, 250.20, 250.80-250.30, 362.01-250.42, 250.93-250.70, 250.72-250.32, 250.50-250.00, 648.04-250.40, 250.92, 362.06-250.13, 648.02-250.71, 250.73, 648.00-250.31, 648.03-250.22, 366.41, 648.01-250.82, 362.05-250.12, 362.07-250.63, 357.2-250.10, 250.83-250.03, 362.04	99201-99219, 99221-99233, 99238-99239, 99281-99285, 99291, 99304-99337, 99341-99350, 99455-99456, 97802-97804, G0402, G0438	8P
3066F, G8506	250.01, 250.41-250.33, 250.52-250.51, 362.03-250.53, 250.62-250.02, 250.20, 250.80-250.30, 362.01-250.42, 250.93-250.70, 250.72-250.32, 250.50-250.00, 648.04-250.40, 250.92, 362.06-250.13, 648.02-250.71, 250.73, 648.00-250.31, 648.03-250.22, 366.41, 648.01-250.82, 362.05-250.12, 362.07-250.63, 357.2-250.10, 250.83-250.03, 362.04	99201-99219, 99221-99233, 99238-99239, 99281-99285, 99291, 99304-99337, 99341-99350, 99455-99456, 97802-97804, G0402, G0438	N/A
3072F	250.01, 250.41-250.33, 250.52-250.51, 362.03-250.53, 250.62-250.02, 250.20, 250.80-250.30, 362.01-250.42, 250.93-250.70, 250.72-250.32, 250.50-250.00, 648.04-250.40, 250.92, 362.06-250.13, 648.02-250.71, 250.73, 648.00-250.31, 648.03-250.22, 366.41, 648.01-250.82, 362.05-250.12, 362.07-250.63, 357.2-250.10, 250.83-250.03, 362.04	99201-99220, 99221-99233, 99238-99239, 99281-99285, 99291, 99304-99337, 99341-99350, 99455-99456, 92002-92014, 97802-97804, G0402, G0438	N/A
3074F, 3075F, 3077F, 3078F, 3079F, 3080F, G8919, G8920, G8921, G8922	250.01, 250.41-250.33, 250.52-250.51, 362.03-250.53, 250.62-250.02, 250.20, 250.80-250.30, 362.01-250.42, 250.93-250.70, 250.72-250.32, 250.50-250.00, 648.04-250.40, 250.92, 362.06-250.13, 648.02-250.71, 250.73, 648.00-250.31, 648.03-250.22, 366.41, 648.01-250.82, 362.05-250.12, 362.07-250.63, 357.2-250.10, 250.83-250.03, 362.04	99201-99205, 99212-99215, 99304-99310, 99324-99337, 99341-99350, 97802-97804	N/A
3092F, G8930, G8931, G8932, G8933	296.33-296.21, 296.23-296.24, 296.30-296.20, 296.22	99201-99205, 99212-99215, 99281-99285, 90791-90832, 90834, 90837, 90839, 90845	N/A
3095F, 3096F	805.07, 820.11-805.12, 820.00-805.01, 805.14, 805.3, 820.19-733.03, 813.53-805.05, 813.54-733.13, 805.6-733.02, 733.14, 813.41-733.19, 820.09, 820.8-805.08, 820.10-805.00, 813.46-733.01, 805.03, 820.13, 820.32-813.50, 820.30-805.02, 805.15, 820.02, 820.20-805.8, 820.01-733.09, 820.03-813.40, 813.52-733.12, 820.31-733.00, 805.2, 805.7, 820.12, 820.22, 820.9-805.4, 813.47-805.13, 805.17, 805.16	99201-99205, 99212-99215, 99238-99239, 22305-22327, 22520-22521, 22523-22524, 25600-25609, 27230-27248, G0402	1P, 2P, 3P, 8P
3100F	N/A	36222-36224, 70498, 70547-70549, 93880-93882	8P
3110F	368.2, 434.11, 435.8, 784.51-435.9, 781.3-433.81, 784.59-432.0, 433.11, 781.4-432.1, 780.02-386.2, 434.91, 782.0-432.9, 433.21-433.01, 435.2-431, 784.3-430, 433.91, 437.7-368.12, 435.0	70450-70470, 70551-70553, 0042T	8P
3111F, 3112F	368.2, 434.11, 435.8, 784.51-435.9, 781.3-433.81, 784.59-432.0, 433.11, 781.4-432.1, 780.02-386.2, 434.91, 782.0-432.9, 433.21-433.01, 435.2-431, 784.3-430, 433.91, 437.7-368.12, 435.0	70450-70470, 70551-70553, 0042T	N/A
3120F	413.1, 786.50-413.9, 786.59-413.0, 786.52	99281-99285, 99291	1P, 2P, 8P
3125F	530.85	88305	1P, 8P
3155F	207.20-205.00, 207.22-204.00, 207.00, 238.72-204.02, 205.02, 206.02, 207.02, 206.00	99201-99205, 99212-99215	1P, 2P, 3P, 8P
3160F	238.75	99201-99205, 99212-99215	3P, 8P
3170F	204.10, 204.12	99201-99205, 99212-99215	1P, 2P, 3P, 8P
3210F	462-034.0, 463	99201-99205, 99212-99220, 99281-99285, G0402	1P, 8P
3215F, 3216F	070.51, 070.54	99201-99205, 99212-99215	N/A
3218F	070.54	99201-99205, 99212-99215, G9205	1P, 8P
3220F	070.54	99201-99205, 99212-99215, G8461	1P, 2P, 8P

Numerator	Associated Diagnostic Denominator	Associated Procedure Denominator	Associated Modifiers
3250F	174.1, 174.8, 175.0-174.2, 175.9-174.0, 174.9-174.3, 174.5	88307-88309	N/A
3260F	174.1, 174.8, 175.0-174.2, 175.9-174.0, 174.9-174.3, 174.5	88307-88309	1P, 8P
3265F	070.51, 070.54	99201-99205, 99212-99215, 1119F, G9202	1P, 2P, 8P
3266F	070.54	99201-99205, 99212-99215, G9206	8P
3267F	185	88309	1P, 8P
3269F	185	55810-55815, 55840-55845, 55866, 55873-55876, 77427, 77776-77778, 77787	1P, 3P
3270F, 3271F, 3272F, 3273F, 3274F	185	55810-55815, 55840-55845, 55866, 55873-55876, 77427, 77776-77778, 77787	N/A
3285F	365.70-365.71, 365.74-365.10, 365.11	99201-99205, 99212-99215, 99307-99310, 99324-99337, 92002-92014	N/A
3288F	N/A	99201-99215, 99304-99310, 99324-99337, 99341-99350, 97001-97004, G0402, G0438	1P, 8P
3300F	201.60, 202.25-162.4, 172.4-157.0, 174.1, 201.14, 201.26, 201.90, 202.06-201.46, 202.80-148.2, 201.94, 202.83-148.8, 202.22-145.0, 160.3, 201.02, 201.07, 201.20, 201.93-140.5, 170.3-156.1, 201.92, 202.02-147.2, 158.9, 201.75, 202.85-153.1, 153.5, 153.9, 172.9, 201.95-154.8, 200.32, 200.40, 200.54, 200.57, 200.68, 200.72, 209.03, 209.25, 209.33-173.11, 173.19, 173.40, 173.49, 173.90-146.1, 153.6, 157.8, 174.8, 202.01-141.4, 161.9, 201.01-140.0, 140.6, 172.7-155.1, 182.8, 201.12, 201.24, 201.56-188.2, 188.6, 189.3, 202.21-142.1, 170.9, 184.0, 201.76, 202.20-141.9, V10.06-142.8, 162.2-152.0, 181, 201.03, 201.21-200.34, 200.37, 200.46, 200.70, 202.76, 202.78, 209.02, 209.10, 209.20, 209.27-173.00, 173.09, 173.20, 173.50, 173.80, 173.89, 188.1, 189.2-142.9, 170.8, 171.6, 201.10, 201.96, 202.07-171.4, 172.1-152.3, 157.2, 175.0, 201.16, 201.28-140.8, 146.3, 174.2, 201.08-150.9, 162.5-151.8, 153.7, 201.71, 202.84-140.4, 175.9, 188.4-161.3, 170.6, 171.9-144.8, 145.5, 201.17, 201.54, 201.91-200.33, 200.35, 200.47, 200.51-200.52, 200.60, 200.62-200.64, 200.67, 209.14, 209.17-173.10, 173.30, 173.62, 173.92-150.1, 150.8, 161.8-151.6, 153.2, 160.0, 185-155.2, 201.66-151.0, 151.5, 202.17-144.1, 153.4, 174.4, 201.77, 202.04-143.9, 172.6-152.2, 155.0, 164.3-146.0, 182.1-140.1, 154.3, 157.4, 174.0, 184.2, 201.40, 202.28-161.1, 200.36, 200.50, 200.65-200.66, 200.71, 200.76-200.77, 202.71, 209.01, 209.13, 209.22-173.12, 173.39, 173.52, 173.70, 201.42, 202.81-141.5, 152.1, 184.3, 190.1, 201.22, V10.3-146.9, 174.9, 201.45, 201.58-142.2, 161.2, 170.5, 202.88-151.3, 202.24-201.50, 201.61-147.8, 151.4, 171.7, 172.0-145.3, 202.08-151.9, 156.2, 201.72-143.1, 172.3-150.0, 200.43-200.45, 200.74, 202.74-202.75, 209.16, 209.23, 209.30-173.22, 173.31-173.32, 173.51, 201.55, 201.68-187.1, 188.5, 188.9-140.3, 170.2-144.9, 180.0, 201.05-172.5, 202.87-150.3, 202.27-162.9, 164.8-154.2, 184.1, 190.3, 201.51-148.3, 202.15-153.3, 154.0, 174.3, 180.1, 182.0, 190.2, 201.00, 201.15, 201.27, 201.98, 202.10, 202.18-145.1, 146.5, 174.6, 201.13-157.3, 200.30, 200.41, 200.61, 200.75, 200.78, 209.11, 209.32-173.02, 173.41, 173.59, 173.60, 173.71-173.72, 173.82, 202.86-143.8, 171.2-145.2, 146.7, 156.0, 201.74, 202.12-164.0, 180.8, 188.7-141.2, 141.8, 143.0, 171.8-145.9, 153.0, 153.8, 193-162.8, 170.7, 202.00, 202.82-187.3, 202.26-145.8, 146.2, 146.8, 157.1, 201.06, 201.11, 201.23-162.3, 201.04-140.9, 141.3, 171.0, 172.8-147.0, 183.0, 201.25-141.1, 172.2, 200.31, 200.48, 200.55-200.56, 200.73, 209.00, 209.15, 209.21, 209.31, 209.36-173.21, 173.61, 173.79, 173.81, 201.64-142.0, 163.0-145.6, 147.1, 152.9, 183.2, 201.18, 202.16-157.9, 201.73-201.52, 201.62-145.4, 146.4, 158.0, 180.9-147.3, 201.43, 201.65-141.0, 141.6, 163.8, 164.2-144.0, 160.2, V10.05-201.47, 201.53, 201.63, 201.67-148.0, 150.5, 202.23-152.8, 179, 202.05, 202.11-146.6, 174.5,	99201-99205, 99212-99215, 77261-77263	N/A

Numerator	Associated Diagnostic Denominator	Associated Procedure Denominator	Associated Modifiers
3300F (continued)	202.03-200.38, 200.42, 200.53, 200.58, 202.70, 202.72-202.73, 202.77, 209.12, 209.24, 209.26, 209.29, 209.35-173.01, 173.29, 173.42, 173.69, 173.91	99201-99205, 99212-99215, 77261-77263	N/A
3301F	201.60, 202.25-162.4, 172.4-157.0, 174.1, 201.14, 201.26, 201.90, 202.06-201.46, 202.80-148.2, 201.94, 202.83-148.8, 202.22-145.0, 160.3, 201.02, 201.07, 201.20, 201.93-140.5, 170.3-156.1, 201.92, 202.02-147.2, 158.9, 201.75, 202.85-153.1, 153.5, 153.9, 172.9, 201.95-154.8, 200.32, 200.40, 200.54, 200.57, 200.68, 200.72, 209.03, 209.25, 209.33-173.11, 173.19, 173.40, 173.49, 173.90-146.1, 153.6, 157.8, 174.8, 202.01-141.4, 161.9, 201.01-140.0, 140.6, 172.7-155.1, 182.8, 201.12, 201.24, 201.56-188.2, 188.6, 189.3, 202.21-142.1, 170.9, 184.0, 201.76, 202.20-141.9, V10.06-142.8, 162.2-152.0, 181, 201.03, 201.21-200.34, 200.37, 200.46, 200.70, 202.76, 202.78, 209.02, 209.10, 209.20, 209.27-173.00, 173.09, 173.20, 173.50, 173.80, 173.89, 188.1, 189.2-142.9, 170.8, 171.6, 201.10, 201.96, 202.07-171.4, 172.1-152.3, 157.2, 175.0, 201.16, 201.28-140.8, 146.3, 174.2, 201.08-150.9, 162.5-151.8, 153.7, 201.71, 202.84-140.4, 175.9, 188.4-161.3, 170.6, 171.9-144.8, 145.5, 201.17, 201.54, 201.91-200.33, 200.35, 200.47, 200.51-200.52, 200.60, 200.62-200.64, 200.67, 209.14, 209.17-173.10, 173.30, 173.62, 173.92-150.1, 150.8, 161.8-151.6, 153.2, 160.0, 185-155.2, 201.66-151.0, 151.5, 202.17-144.1, 153.4, 174.4, 201.77, 202.04-143.9, 172.6-152.2, 155.0, 164.3-146.0, 182.1-140.1, 154.3, 157.4, 174.0, 184.2, 201.40, 202.28-161.1, 200.36, 200.50, 200.65-200.66, 200.71, 200.76-200.77, 202.71, 209.01, 209.13, 209.22-173.12, 173.39, 173.52, 173.70, 201.42, 202.81-141.5, 152.1, 184.3, 190.1, 201.22, V10.3-146.9, 174.9, 201.45, 201.58-142.2, 161.2, 170.5, 202.88-151.3, 202.24-201.50, 201.61-147.8, 151.4, 171.7, 172.0-145.3, 202.08-151.9, 156.2, 201.72-143.1, 172.3-150.0, 200.43-200.45, 200.74, 202.74-202.75, 209.16, 209.23, 209.30-173.22, 173.31-173.32, 173.51, 201.55, 201.68-187.1, 188.5, 188.9-140.3, 170.2-144.9, 180.0, 201.05-172.5, 202.87-150.3, 202.27-162.9, 164.8-154.2, 184.1, 190.3, 201.51-148.3, 202.15-153.3, 154.0, 174.3, 180.1, 182.0, 190.2, 201.00, 201.15, 201.27, 201.98, 202.10, 202.18-145.1, 146.5, 174.6, 201.13-157.3, 200.30, 200.41, 200.61, 200.75, 200.78, 209.11, 209.32-173.02, 173.41, 173.59, 173.60, 173.71-173.72, 173.82, 202.86-143.8, 171.2-145.2, 146.7, 156.0, 201.74, 202.12-164.0, 180.8, 188.7-141.2, 141.8, 143.0, 171.8-145.9, 153.0, 153.8, 193-162.8, 170.7, 202.00, 202.82-187.3, 202.26-145.8, 146.2, 146.8, 157.1, 201.06,201.11, 201.23-162.3, 201.04-140.9, 141.3, 171.0, 172.8-147.0, 183.0, 201.25-141.1, 172.2, 200.31, 200.48, 200.55-200.56, 200.73, 209.00, 209.15, 209.21, 209.31, 209.36-173.21, 173.61, 173.79, 173.81, 201.64-142.0, 163.0-145.6, 147.1, 152.9, 183.2, 201.18, 202.16-157.9, 201.73-201.52, 201.62-145.4, 146.4, 158.0, 180.9-147.3, 201.43, 201.65-141.0, 141.6, 163.8, 164.2-144.0, 160.2, V10.05-201.47, 201.53, 201.63, 201.67-148.0, 150.5, 202.23-152.8, 179, 202.05, 202.11-146.6, 174.5, 202.03-200.38, 200.42, 200.53, 200.58, 202.70, 202.72-202.73, 202.77, 209.12, 209.24, 209.26, 209.29, 209.35-173.01, 173.29, 173.42, 173.69, 173.91	99201-99205, 99212-99215, 77261-77263	8P
3315F, 3372F, 3374F, 3376F, 3378F, 3380F	174.1, 174.8-174.2, 174.4-174.0, 174.9-174.3, 174.5	99201-99205, 99212-99215	N/A
3316F, 3370F	174.1, 174.8-174.2, 174.4-174.0, 174.9-174.3, 174.5	99201-99205, 99212-99215	8P
3319F	172.4, 172.9-172.7, V10.82-172.1, 172.6-172.0, 172.3, 172.5, 172.2	99201-99205, 99212-99215, G8749, G8944	1P, 3P
3320F, G8749, G8750, G8944	172.4, 172.9-172.7, V10.82-172.1, 172.6-172.0, 172.3, 172.5, 172.2	99201-99205, 99212-99215, G8749, G8944	N/A
3323F	162.4-162.2, 162.5-150.8, 151.0-150.3, 150.5	32440-32488, 32503-32507, 32663, 32666-32673, 43107-43124	1P, 8P

Numerator	Associated Diagnostic Denominator	Associated Procedure Denominator	Associated Modifiers
3328F	162.4-150.9, 162.5-150.1, 150.8, 151.0-150.3, 162.9-150.2, 150.5	32440-32488, 32503-32507, 32663, 32666-32671, 43107-43124	8P
3340F, 3341F, 3342F, 3343F, 3344F, 3345F, 3350F	V76.11	77057, G0202	N/A
3382F	153.1, 153.9-153.2, 153.4-153.0, 153.8	99201-99205, 99212-99215	8P
3384F, 3386F, 3388F, 3390F, G8927, G8928, G8929	153.1, 153.9-153.2, 153.4-153.0, 153.8	99201-99205, 99212-99215	N/A
3394F	174.1, 174.8, 175.0-174.2, 175.9-174.0, 174.9-174.3, 174.5	88360-88361	8P
3395F	174.1, 174.8, 175.0-174.2, 175.9-174.0, 174.9-174.3, 174.5	88360-88361	N/A
3471F, 3472F, 3476F, 4192F, 4193F, 4195F, 4196F	714.0, 714.2, 714.1	99201-99205, 99212-99215, 99341-99350, G0402	N/A
3490F, 3492F, 3493F, 3503F, 4270F, 4271F	042	99201-99205, 99212-99215	N/A
3494F, 3500F	042	99201-99205, 99212-99215, G0402	8P
3495F, 3496F, G9214, G9215, G9216, G9217, G9218, G9219, G9220, G9221, G9222, G9223, G9228, G9229, G9230, G9242, G9243, G9244, G9245	042	99201-99205, 99212-99215, G0402	N/A
3511F	042	99201-99205, 99212-99215, G0402	2P, 8P
3512F	042	99201-99205, 99212-99215	2P, 8P
3570F	N/A	78300-78320	3P, 8P
4004F	N/A	99201-99205, 99212-99215, 99406-99407, 90791-90832, 90834, 90837, 90839, 90845, 92002-92014, 96150-96152, 97003-97004, G0438	1P, 8P
4005F	733.03-733.01, 733.00	99201-99205, 99212-99215, G0402	1P, 2P, 3P, 8P
4008F	411.1-410.72, 414.9-411.0, 413.1-410.32, 410.82-410.31, 413.9-410.01, 410.22, 410.92, 414.02, 414.3-411.81, 414.04-410.00, 410.20, 410.60, 410.81, 410.91, 414.06-410.02, 410.52, 410.70-410.12, V45.81-410.71, 410.90, 411.89, 414.2-410.10, 412-410.42, 414.8-410.11, 410.40, 413.0-410.41, 410.51, 414.03-410.30, 410.80-410.62, V45.82-410.21, 414.00-410.50, 414.07	99201-99205, 99212-99215, 99304-99310, 99324-99337, 99341-99350, 33140, 33510-33523, 33533-33536, 92920, 92924, 92928, 92933, 92937, 92941-92943, G8694	1P, 2P, 3P, 8P
4010F	404.13, 428.23, 428.41-404.91, 428.40-404.93, 428.31-402.11, 428.21, 428.42-402.91, 428.22, 428.43-404.01, 428.32, 428.9-428.0, 428.20, 428.33-402.01, 404.03	99201-99205, 99212-99215, 99238-99239, 99304-99310, 99324-99337, 99341-99350, 3021F	1P, 2P, 3P, 8P
4013F, 4086F	411.1-410.72, 414.9-411.0, 413.1-410.32, 410.82-410.31, 413.9-410.01, 410.22, 410.92, 414.02, 414.3-411.81, 414.04-410.00, 410.20, 410.60, 410.81, 410.91, 414.06-410.02, 410.52, 410.70-410.12, V45.81-410.71, 410.90, 411.89, 414.2-410.10, 412-410.42, 414.8-410.11, 410.40, 413.0-410.41, 410.51, 414.03-410.30, 410.80-410.62, V45.82-410.21, 414.00-410.50, 414.07	99201-99205, 99212-99215, 99304-99310, 99324-99337, 99341-99350	1P, 2P, 3P, 8P
4040F	N/A	99201-99215, 99218-99220, 99324-99337, 99341-99350, 99356-99357, G0402	1P, 8P

Numerator	Associated Diagnostic Denominator	Associated Procedure Denominator	Associated Modifiers
4041F	N/A	15732-15738, 15830-15837, 19260-19272, 19300-19380, 21627, 21632, 21740, 21750, 21805, 21825, 22325, 22524, 22551, 22554, 22558, 22586, 22600, 22612, 22630, 22800-22804, 23470-23474, 23616, 24363, 24370-24371, 27080, 27125-27138, 27158, 27202-27218, 27235-27236, 27244-27245, 27269, 27280-27282, 27440-27447, 27702-27704, 27758-27759, 27766, 27769, 27792, 27814, 27880-27888, 28192-28193, 28293, 28415-28420, 28445, 28465, 28485, 28505, 28525, 28531, 28555, 28585, 28615, 28645, 28675-28737, 31400-31420, 31760-31775, 31786, 31805, 32096-32150, 32215-32320, 32440-32501, 32505-32507, 32800-32815, 32900-32940, 33020-33202, 33250-33251, 33256, 33261, 33300-33322, 33332-33366, 33400-33411, 33413, 33416, 33422-33465, 33475, 33496, 33510-33572, 33877-33883, 33886-33891, 34051, 34800-34805, 34812, 34820-34825, 34830-34834, 34900, 35011-35021, 35081-35103, 35131, 35141-35152, 35206, 35211-35216, 35241-35246, 35266-35276, 35301, 35311, 35363-35372, 35460, 35512, 35521-35526, 35533, 35537-35558, 35565-35587, 35601-35671, 36830, 37224-37231, 37616-37617, 38100-38101, 38115-38120, 38381, 38571-38572, 38700-38780, 39000-39220, 39501, 39540-39561, 43020-43135, 43279-43282, 43300-43337, 43340-43425, 43496, 43500-43634, 43640-43645, 43651-43653, 43770-43880, 43886-43888, 44005-44010, 44020-44021, 44050-44100, 44120, 44125-44127, 44130-44136, 44140-44202, 44204-44212, 44227, 44300-44346, 44602-44700, 44800-44850, 44900, 44950-44970, 45000, 45020, 45110-45172, 45395-45402, 45540-45825, 47100-47130, 47140-47142, 47350, 47370-47371, 47380-47381, 47400-47480, 47560-47570, 47600-47900, 48000-48160, 48500-48548, 48554-48556, 49000-49060, 49203-49250, 49320-49323, 49505-49507, 49568, 50320, 50340-50380, 57267, 58150-58294, 58951, 58953-58956, 60200-60281, 60500-60650, 61154, 61312-61313, 61315, 61510-61512, 61518, 61548, 61697, 61700, 61750-61751, 61867, 62223, 62230, 63015, 63020-63030, 63042, 63045, 63047, 63056, 63075, 63081, 63267, 63276, 64746, 0236T	1P, 8P
4042F, 4046F	N/A	15732-15738, 15830-15837, 19260-19272, 19300-19380, 21346-21348, 21422-21423, 21432-21436, 21454-21470, 21627, 21632, 21740, 21750, 21805, 21825, 22325, 22524, 22551, 22554, 22558, 22586, 22600, 22612, 22630, 22800-22804, 23470-23474, 23616, 24363, 24370-24371, 27080, 27125-27138, 27158, 27202-27218, 27235-27236, 27244-27245, 27269, 27280-27282, 27440-27447, 27702-27704, 27758-27759, 27766, 27769, 27792, 27814, 27880-27888, 28192-28193, 28293, 28415-28420, 28445, 28465, 28485, 28505, 28525, 28531, 28555, 28585, 28615, 28645, 28675-28737, 31360-31420, 31760-31775, 31786, 31805, 32096-32150, 32215-32320, 32440-32501, 32505-32507, 32800-32815, 32900-32940, 33020-33050, 33202-33208, 33212-33213, 33214-33233, 33234-33240, 33241, 33243-33249, 33254-33255, 33300, 33310, 33320-33322, 33361-33364, 33877-33883, 33886-33891, 34051, 34800-34805, 34812, 34820-34825, 34830-34834, 34900, 35011-35021, 35081-35103, 35131, 35141-35152, 35206, 35211-35216, 35241-35246, 35266-35276, 35301, 35311, 35363-35372, 35460, 35512, 35521-35526, 35533, 35537-35558, 35565-35587, 35601-35671, 36830, 37224-37231, 37616-37617, 38100-38101, 38115-38120, 38381, 38571-38572, 38700-38780, 39000-39220, 39501, 39540-39561, 41130-41155, 43020-43135, 43279-43282, 43300-43337, 43340-43425, 43496, 43500-43634, 43640-43645, 43651-43653, 43770-43880, 43886-43888, 44005-44010, 44020-44120, 44125-44127, 44130-44136, 44140-44202, 44204-44212, 44227, 44300-44346, 44602-44700, 44800-44850, 44900, 44950-44970, 45000, 45020, 45108-45190, 45395-45402, 45500-45825, 47100-47130, 47140-47142, 47350, 47370-47371,	N/A

Numerator	Associated Diagnostic Denominator	Associated Procedure Denominator	Associated Modifiers
4042F, 4046F (continued)	N/A	47380-47381, 47400-47480, 47560-47570, 47600-47900, 48000-48160, 48500-48548, 48554-48556, 49000-49060, 49203-49250, 49320-49323, 49505-49507, 49568, 50320, 50340-50380, 51597, 57267, 58150-58294, 58951, 58953-58956, 60200-60281, 60500-60505, 60520-60650, 61154, 61312-61313, 61315, 61510-61512, 61518, 61520, 61526-61530, 61548, 61591, 61595-61596, 61598, 61606, 61616-61619, 61697, 61700, 61750-61751, 61867, 62223, 62230, 63015, 63020-63030, 63042, 63045, 63047, 63056, 63075, 63081, 63267, 63276, 64746, 69720, 69930, 69955-69970, 0236T	N/A
4043F	N/A	33120-33141, 33250-33251, 33256, 33261, 33305, 33315, 33332-33335, 33365-33366, 33400-33411, 33413, 33416, 33422-33465, 33475, 33496, 33510-33572	1P, 8P
4044F	N/A	15734, 15830-15837, 19260-19272, 19300-19330, 19342-19380, 21346-21348, 21422-21423, 21432-21436, 21454-21470, 21627, 21632, 21740, 21750, 21805, 21825, 22551, 22554, 22558, 22600, 22612, 22630, 27080, 27125-27138, 27158, 27202-27218, 27235-27236, 27244-27245, 27269, 27280-27282, 27440-27447, 27880-27888, 31360-31395, 31760-31775, 31786, 31805, 32096-32150, 32215-32320, 32440-32501, 32505-32507, 32800-32815, 32900-32940, 33020-33050, 33300, 33310, 33320, 33361-33366, 33877-33883, 33886-33891, 34051, 34800-34805, 34812, 34820-34825, 34830-34834, 34900, 35011-35021, 35081-35103, 35131, 35141-35152, 35206, 35211-35216, 35241-35246, 35266-35276, 35301, 35311, 35363-35372, 35460, 35512, 35521-35526, 35533, 35537-35558, 35565-35587, 35601-35671, 36830, 37224-37231, 37616-37617, 38100-38101, 38115-38120, 38381, 38571-38572, 38700-38780, 39000-39220, 39501-39561, 41130-41155, 43020-43135, 43279-43282, 43300-43337, 43340-43425, 43496, 43500-43634, 43640-43645, 43651-43653, 43770-43774, 43800-43830, 43832-43880, 43886-43888, 44005-44010, 44020-44055, 44110-44127, 44130, 44140-44202, 44204-44212, 44227, 44300-44346, 44602-44700, 44800-44850, 44900, 44950-44970, 45000, 45020-45190, 45395-45402, 45500-45505, 45540-45825, 46715-46762, 47010, 47015-47130, 47135-47142, 47300-47371, 47380-47382, 47400-47480, 47500-47505, 47560-47570, 47600-47900, 48000-48160, 48500-48548, 48554-48556, 49000-49060, 49203-49323, 49505-49507, 49560-49570, 50020, 50220-50240, 50320, 50340-50380, 50543, 50545-50548, 50715-50728, 50760-50820, 50947-50948, 51550-51597, 51800-51820, 51900-51925, 51960, 55810-55845, 55866, 56630-56640, 57267, 58150-58294, 58951, 58953-58956, 60200-60281, 60500-60505, 60520-60650, 61312-61313, 61315, 61510-61512, 61518, 61520, 61526-61530, 61548, 61591, 61595-61596, 61598, 61606, 61616-61619, 61697, 61700, 62230, 63015, 63020, 63045, 63047, 63056, 63075, 63081, 63267, 63276, 64746, 69720, 69955-69970, 0236T	1P, 8P
4045F	483.0, 485, 487.0-482.30, 482.84-482.40, 482.42-481, 482.2, 486-482.31, 482.82-482.1, 483.8-482.0, 482.89-482.32, 482.81, 482.83	99201-99205, 99212-99215, 99221-99223, 99281-99285, 99291, 99324-99337, 99341-99350	1P, 2P, 3P, 8P
4047F	N/A	00100-00103, 00120, 00140, 00145-00147, 00160-00322, 00350-00406, 00450-00500, 00528-00634, 00670-00700, 00730, 00750-00802, 00820-00832, 00840, 00844-00870, 00880-00944, 01120, 01140-01150, 01170-01190, 01202-01215, 01230-01320, 01360, 01382, 01392-01404, 01430-01444, 01464-01486, 01500-01610, 01622-01670, 01710-01716, 01732-01810, 01829-01852, 01924-01926, 01951-01953, 01961-01966, 01968-01969	8P

Numerator	Associated Diagnostic Denominator	Associated Procedure Denominator	Associated Modifiers
4048F	N/A	00100-00103, 00120, 00140, 00145-00147, 00160-00322, 00350-00406, 00450-00500, 00528-00634, 00670-00700, 00730, 00750-00802, 00820-00832, 00840, 00844-00870, 00880-00944, 01120, 01140-01150, 01170-01190, 01202-01215, 01230-01320, 01360, 01382, 01392-01404, 01430-01444, 01464-01486, 01500-01610, 01622-01670, 01710-01716, 01732-01810, 01829-01852, 01924-01926, 01951-01953, 01961-01966, 01968-01969	1P, 8P
4049F	N/A	15732-15738, 15830-15837, 19260-19272, 19300-19380, 21346-21348, 21422-21423, 21432-21436, 21454-21470, 21627, 21632, 21740, 21750, 21805, 21825, 22325, 22524, 22551, 22554, 22558, 22586, 22600, 22612, 22630, 22800-22804, 23470-23474, 23616, 24363, 24370-24371, 27080, 27125-27138, 27158, 27202-27218, 27235-27236, 27244-27245, 27269, 27280-27282, 27440-27447, 27702-27704, 27758-27759, 27766, 27769, 27792, 27814, 27880-27888, 28192-28193, 28293, 28415-28420, 28445, 28465, 28485, 28505, 28525, 28531, 28555, 28585, 28615, 28645, 28675-28737, 31360-31420, 31760-31775, 31786, 31805, 32096-32150, 32215-32320, 32440-32501, 32505-32507, 32800-32815, 32900-32940, 33020-33050, 33202-33208, 33212-33213, 33214-33233, 33234-33240, 33241, 33243-33249, 33254-33255, 33300, 33310, 33320-33322, 33361-33364, 33877-33883, 33886-33891, 34051, 34800-34805, 34812, 34820-34825, 34830-34834, 34900, 35011-35021, 35081-35103, 35131, 35141-35152, 35206, 35211-35216, 35241-35246, 35266-35276, 35301, 35311, 35363-35372, 35460, 35512, 35521-35526, 35533, 35537-35558, 35565-35587, 35601-35671, 36830, 37224-37231, 37616-37617, 38100-38101, 38115-38120, 38381, 38571-38572, 38700-38780, 39000-39220, 39501, 39540-39561, 41130-41155, 43020-43135, 43279-43282, 43300-43337, 43340-43425, 43496, 43500-43634, 43640-43645, 43651-43653, 43770-43880, 43886-43888, 44005-44010, 44020-44120, 44125-44127, 44130-44136, 44140-44202, 44204-44212, 44227, 44300-44346, 44602-44700, 44800-44850, 44900, 44950-44970, 45000, 45020, 45108-45190, 45395-45402, 45500-45825, 47100-47130, 47140-47142, 47350, 47370-47371, 47380-47381, 47400-47480, 47560-47570, 47600-47900, 48000-48160, 48500-48548, 48554-48556, 49000-49060, 49203-49250, 49320-49323, 49505-49507, 49568, 50320, 50340-50380, 51597, 57267, 58150-58294, 58951, 58953-58956, 60200-60281, 60500-60505, 60520-60650, 61154, 61312-61313, 61315, 61510-61512, 61518, 61520, 61526-61530, 61548, 61591, 61595-61596, 61598, 61606, 61616-61619, 61697, 61700, 61750-61751, 61867, 62223, 62230, 63015, 63020-63030, 63042, 63045, 63047, 63056, 63075, 63081, 63267, 63276, 64746, 69720, 69930, 69955-69970, 0236T	1P, 8P
4050F	404.13, 404.91, 404.93-404.12, 404.90-403.01, 403.10, 404.02-401.9, 402.91, 404.00, 404.10-401.1, 404.92-402.00, 404.11-402.90, 403.90-403.00, 403.91-402.01, 404.03-401.0, 403.11	99201-99205, 99212-99215, 99304-99310, 99324-99337, 99341-99350	8P
4070F	434.11-432.0, 433.11-432.1, 434.91-432.9, 433.21-433.01, 433.31-430, 433.91	99221-99233, 99291	1P, 2P, 8P
4075F	434.11, 435.8-433.81, 585.6-427.31, 435.3-434.91, V56.0-433.01, 435.2-433.31, 433.91, 435.0	99221-99233, 99238-99239, 90957-90962, 90966, 90970, G9240	1P, 2P, 8P
4084F	410.31-410.00, 410.20, 410.60, 410.81, 410.91-410.71, 410.90-410.11, 410.40-410.41, 410.51-410.30, 410.80-410.21, 410.50	99281-99285, 99291	1P, 2P, 8P
4090F, 4095F	238.75	99201-99205, 99212-99215	N/A
4100F	203.00, 203.02	99201-99205, 99212-99215	1P, 2P, 8P
4110F	N/A	33510-33523, 33533-33536	1P, 8P
4115F	N/A	00562, 00566-00567, 33510-33536	1P, 8P
4120F	466.0	99201-99205, 99212-99220, 99281-99285, G0402	1P
4124F	466.0	99201-99205, 99212-99220, 99281-99285, G0402	N/A

Numerator	Associated Diagnostic Denominator	Associated Procedure Denominator	Associated Modifiers
4130F	380.11, 380.22-380.10, 380.13	99201-99205, 99212-99215, 99281-99285	1P, 2P, 8P
4131F	380.11, 380.22-380.10, 380.13	99201-99205, 99212-99215, 99281-99285	1P
4132F	380.11, 380.22-380.10, 380.13	99201-99205, 99212-99215, 99281-99285	N/A
4140F	493.92-493.01, 493.22, 493.81, 493.90-493.02, 493.11-493.00, 493.10, 493.12, 493.21, 493.82	99201-99205, 99212-99215, 99341-99350, 1038F	2P, 8P
4145F	404.13, 405.99-404.91, 404.93-404.12, 404.90-403.01, 403.10, 404.02, 405.11-401.9, 402.91, 404.00, 404.10, 405.91-401.1, 404.92, 405.09-402.00, 404.11, 405.01-404.01, 405.19-402.90, 403.90-403.00, 403.91-402.01, 404.03-401.0, 403.11	99201-99205, 99212-99215, 99304-99310, 99324-99337, 99341-99350	1P, 2P, 3P, 8P
4148F, 4149F	070.51, 070.54	99201-99205, 99212-99215	1P, 2P, 8P
4150F, 4151F, G9203, G9204	070.54	99201-99205, 99212-99215, G9205	N/A
4153F	070.54	99201-99205, 99212-99215	1P, 2P, 3P, 8P
4158F	070.51, 070.54	99201-99205, 99212-99215	8P
4159F	070.54	99201-99205, 99212-99215	1P, 8P
4164F	185	77427	1P, 2P, 8P
4165F	198.1-198.0, 198.4-185, 198.2-197.7, 198.81-197.4, 198.6, 198.89-197.6, 198.5 197.0, 197.5	77427	8P
4171F, 4172F, G0908, G0909, G0910, G8725, G8726, G8728	585.5	99201-99205, 99212-99215, 99304-99310, 99324-99337, 99341-99350	N/A
4175F	364.22-360.00, 940.4-362.81, 365.24, 377.52, 379.07-363.63, 365.14-362.72, 363.00, 363.05, 365.63-362.55, 379.09-371.62, 377.39-360.14, 363.32, 363.56, 365.81, 377.31, 377.51, 940.0, 940.9-365.20, 371.02-363.54, 365.43, 371.53-362.51, 377.11, 377.33, 379.04, 871.2, 950.0-362.03, 362.22, 363.55-361.00, 362.82, 366.33, 871.3-363.13, 365.82, 871.6, 940.5-364.04, 368.02, 369.15-363.52, 365.13-363.04, 365.51, 950.2-362.89, 377.30-360.03, 362.41, 365.59, 377.13-360.20, 363.35-363.03, 365.60, 371.70-362.53, 365.62, 369.04, 369.10-360.23, 371.01, 371.44, 371.72, 377.41, 950.3-364.00, 364.23, 369.03, 371.00, 371.04, 371.21-361.07, 362.76, 365.61, 377.14-369.14, 871.0-360.24, 362.01, 363.20, 363.30-362.85, 363.06-362.71, 871.7-362.25, 365.21-363.31, 363.51, 379.11-360.02, 362.16, 377.15, 871.4-362.21, 363.43, 364.3-362.12, 363.10, 363.14, 365.31-361.06, 362.06, 363.21, 370.03, 371.54, 377.12, 377.34-362.70, 371.22-361.03, 362.84, 371.51, 371.56, 371.61-362.35, 362.50, 940.1-362.18, 369.08-362.83, 371.55, 371.71, 379.12-365.83, 377.54, 950.9-362.24, 369.06, 369.13-360.13, 360.29, 362.02, 363.61, 365.22, 365.89, 921.3-369.12, 371.52-360.19, 363.33, 363.57, 365.42, 379.51-363.08, 365.23, 365.41-362.57, 369.01-361.04, 371.58-362.05, 362.20, 362.23, 362.26, 364.03, 371.03-361.05, 363.07, 363.11-362.42, 362.52, 364.01-360.11, 365.52, 377.53-360.01, 360.21, 363.62-362.54, 379.06-371.57, 940.2-369.05, 369.11, 369.18, 371.23-362.73, 363.01-362.56, 377.16-362.75, 363.15-362.07, 362.27, 364.10-360.04, 371.20-362.74, 365.32, 365.65, 379.05, 950.1-363.53, 377.10, 377.32-361.02, 365.44-361.01, 363.12, 371.50, 371.60-364.02, 364.21-360.12, 365.64, 371.73-362.32, 362.04	66840-66984	8P
4177F	362.51-362.50, 362.52	99201-99205, 99212-99215, 99307-99310, 99324-99337, 92002-92014	8P
4179F	174.1, 174.8-174.2, 174.4-174.0, 174.9-174.3, 174.5	99201-99205, 99212-99215	1P, 2P, 3P, 8P
4180F	153.1, 153.9-153.2, 153.4-153.0, 153.8	99201-99205, 99212-99215	1P, 2P, 3P, 8P
4187F	714.0, 714.2, 714.1	99201-99205, 99212-99215, 99341-99350, G0402, G0438	1P, 8P
4200F, 4201F	198.1-198.0, 198.4-185, 198.2-197.7, 198.81-197.4, 198.6, 198.89-197.6, 198.5-197.0, 197.5	77427	N/A

Numerator	Associated Diagnostic Denominator	Associated Procedure Denominator	Associated Modifiers
4250F	N/A	00100-00560, 00566, 00580-01860, 01924-01952, 01961-01966, 01968-01969	1P, 8P
4255F, 4256F	N/A	00100-00560, 00566, 00580-01860, 01924-01952, 01961-01966, 01968-01969	N/A
4260F, 4265F	707.13-707.06, 707.09, 707.14-459.11, 707.12, 707.9-459.13, 707.15-707.01, 707.07-454.2, 707.05, 707.8-707.00, 707.02, 707.11-459.33, 707.04-454.0, 707.03	99201-99205, 99212-99215, 99304-99310, 99324-99337, 99341-99350, 97001-97002	1P
4261F, 4266F	707.13-707.06, 707.09, 707.14-459.11, 707.12, 707.9-459.13, 707.15-707.01, 707.07-454.2, 707.05, 707.8-707.00, 707.02, 707.11-459.33, 707.04-454.0, 707.03	99201-99205, 99212-99215, 99304-99310, 99324-99337, 99341-99350, 97001-97002	N/A
4267F	707.13-459.11, 707.12, 707.19-459.13, 707.15-454.2, 454.0	99201-99205, 99212-99215, 99304-99310, 99324-99337, 99341-99350, 29580-29581	1P, 2P, 3P, 8P
4276F	V23.5-V08, V23.82-V22.0, V23.7-079.53, V22.1, V23.1, V23.81-V23.49, V23.84-V23.0, V23.89-V22.2, V23.83-042, V23.2, V23.42-V23.3, V23.87	99201-99205, 99212-99215	8P
4280F	042	99201-99205, 99212-99215, G0402	1P, 8P
4320F	303.91-303.90, 303.92	99201-99205, 99212-99215, 90791-90832, 90834, 90837, 90839, 90845, 96150-96152	8P
4340F	345.51-345.00, 345.70-345.61, 345.91-345.50, 345.90-345.10, 345.41-345.11, 345.40	99201-99205, 99212-99215, 99304-99309	1P, 8P
4500F	410.72, 413.1-410.32, 410.82-410.31, 413.9-410.01, 410.22, 410.92-122.9, 410.00, 410.20, 410.60, 410.81, 410.91-410.02, 410.52, 410.70-122.2, 410.71, 410.90-410.10, 412-122.8, 410.42-122.0, 410.11, 410.40, 413.0-410.41, 410.51-410.30, 410.80-122.1, 410.62-410.21, 410.50	99201-99205, 99212-99215, 99387, 99395-99396, 33361-33365, 33400-33430, 33463-33496, 33510-33536, 33572-33602, 33935, 33945, 33999, 35500, 35600, 92920, 92924, 92928, 92933, 92937, 92941-92943, 1460F, G0438	1P, 2P, 3P, 8P
5015F	805.07, 820.11-805.12, 820.00-805.01, 805.14, 805.3, 820.19-733.03, 813.53-805.05, 813.54-733.13, 808.1-733.02, 808.0-733.14, 813.41-733.19, 820.09, 820.8-805.08, 820.10-805.00, 813.46-733.01, 805.03, 820.13, 820.32-813.50, 820.30-805.02, 805.15, 820.02, 820.20-805.8, 820.01-733.09, 820.03-813.40, 813.52-733.12, 820.31-733.00, 805.2, 805.7, 820.12, 820.22, 820.9-805.4, 813.47-805.13, 805.17, 805.16	99201-99205, 99212-99215, 99238-99239, 22305-22327, 22520-22521, 22523-22524, 25600-25609, 27230-27248, G0402	1P, 2P, 8P
5050F	172.4, 172.9-172.1, 172.6-172.0, 172.3, 172.5, 172.2	99201-99205, 99212-99215, 11600-11646, 14000-14302, 17311, 17313	2P, 3P, 8P
6010F	434.11-432.0, 433.11-432.1, 434.91-432.9, 433.21-433.01, 433.31-430, 433.91	99218-99220, 99221-99239, 99281-99285, 99291	1P, 2P, 8P
6015F, 6020F	434.11-432.0, 433.11-432.1, 434.91-432.9, 433.21-433.01, 433.31-430, 433.91	99218-99220, 99221-99239, 99281-99285, 99291	N/A
6030F	N/A	36555-36571, 36578-36585, 93503	1P, 8P
6045F	N/A	25606, 25651, 26608, 26650, 26676, 26706, 26727, 27096, 27235, 27244-27245, 27509, 27756, 27759, 28406, 28436, 28456, 28476, 36147, 36221-36226, 36251-36254, 36598, 37182-37184, 37187-37188, 37211-37214, 37210, 37217-37232, 37234-37236, 37238, 37241-37244, 43260-43265, 43267-43269, 43271-43272, 43275-43278, 43752, 44500, 49440-49465, 50382-50389, 50590, 61623, 62263-62264, 62280-62282, 63610, 64610, 64620, 70010-70015, 70170, 70332, 70370-70373, 70390, 71023, 71034, 72240-72291, 72295, 73040, 73085, 73115, 73525, 73580, 73615, 74190-74260, 74270-74300, 74305-74363, 74425-74485, 74740-74742, 75600-75630, 75658-75756, 75791-75810, 75825-75902, 75952-75962, 75966, 75970-75984, 76000-76001, 76080, 76120, 76496, 76499, 77001-77003, 92611, 93565-93568, 0075T, 0080T, 0234T-0235T, 0238T, G0106, G0120	8P

Numerator	Associated Diagnostic Denominator	Associated Procedure Denominator	Associated Modifiers
65235, 65800, 65810, 65815, 65860, 65880, 65900, 65920, 66030, 66250, 66820, 66825, 66830, 66986, 67005, 67010, 67015, 67025, 67028, 67030, 67031, 67101, 67105, 67107, 67108, 67110, 67112, 67141, 67145, 67250, 67255, G8627, G8628	364.22-360.32, 940.4-360.30, 364.63, 365.14, 365.63-364.71, 365.81, 940.0, 940.9-743.30, 871.5-365.20, 371.02, 371.53, 871.2, 950.0-364.89, 376.52-366.33, 871.3-364.76, 365.82, 871.6, 940.5-364.04, 365.13, 365.51, 950.2-364.64, 364.73, 365.59, 367.0-360.20, 364.60, 365.60-364.77, 365.62-364.42, 371.01, 371.44-364.72, 743.36, 950.3-364.00, 364.23, 371.00, 371.04, 371.21-365.61, 871.0, 871.7-364.82, 365.21, 366.22, 379.32-364.05, 743.31-364.61, 871.4-362.21, 364.3, 365.31-364.70, 370.03, 371.54-371.22, 371.51, 371.56, 940.1-360.33, 371.55-360.31, 365.83, 366.21, 950.9-365.22, 365.89, 921.3-360.34, 379.34-364.62, 365.23, 366.23, 371.58, 379.42-364.03, 371.03-360.11, 365.52-360.21, 364.75, 371.57, 940.2-371.23, 376.50-364.10, 371.20-364.74, 365.32, 365.65, 950.1-365.15, 371.50-366.11, 379.33-364.02, 364.21-360.12, 365.64, 940.3-365.11, 366.20	66840-66984, 67036-67043	N/A
67036, 67039, 67041, 67042, 67043	364.22-360.32, 940.4-360.30, 364.63, 365.14, 365.63-364.71, 365.81, 940.0, 940.9-743.30, 871.5-365.20, 371.02, 371.53, 871.2, 950.0-364.89, 376.52-366.33, 871.3-364.76, 365.82, 871.6, 940.5-364.04, 365.13, 365.51, 950.2-364.64, 364.73, 365.59, 367.0-360.20, 364.60, 365.60-364.77, 365.62-364.42, 371.01, 371.44-364.72, 743.36, 950.3-364.00, 364.23, 371.00, 371.04, 371.21-365.61, 871.0, 871.7-364.82, 365.21, 366.22, 379.32-364.05, 743.31-364.61, 871.4-362.21, 364.3, 365.31-364.70, 370.03, 371.54-371.22, 371.51, 371.56, 940.1-360.33, 371.55-360.31, 365.83, 366.21, 950.9-365.22, 365.89, 921.3-360.34, 379.34-364.62, 365.23, 366.23, 371.58, 379.42-364.03, 371.03-360.11, 365.52-360.21, 364.75, 371.57, 940.2-371.23, 376.50-364.10, 371.20-364.74, 365.32, 365.65, 950.1-365.15, 371.50-366.11, 379.33-364.02, 364.21-360.12, 365.64, 940.3-365.11, 366.20	66840-66984, 67036-67043	55 or 56, 56
7010F	172.4, 172.9-172.7, V10.82-172.1, 172.6-172.0, 172.3, 172.5, 172.2	99201-99205, 99212-99215	3P, 8P
7025F	V76.11	77057, G0202	8P
9006F, 9007F	N/A	35301, 37215, 9006F-9007F	N/A
G0101	N/A	99201-99205, 99212-99215, 99218-99223, 99234-99236, 99281-99285, 99304-99310, 99318-99337, 99340-99350, 99495-99496, 90791-90832, 90834, 90837, 90839, 90845, 90880, 90956-90960, 90962, 90965-90966, 92002-92014, 92506-92508, 92526, 92541-92545, 92547-92548, 92552-92555, 92557, 92561-92582, 92584-92586, 92587-92588, 92601-92604, 92610-92612, 92620-92627, 92640, 96116-96118, 96150-96152, 97001-97004, 97110, 97140, 97532, 97750, 97802-97804, 98940-98942, 98960-98962, G0108-D7140, G0402-G0270, G0444-G0101, G0439-G0438, G0447-D7210, G0271	N/A
G0105	V12.72	44388-44389, 44392-44394, 45355-45378, 45380-45381, 45383-45385, G0105	N/A

Numerator	Associated Diagnostic Denominator	Associated Procedure Denominator	Associated Modifiers
G0106, G0120, G0275, G0278	N/A	25606, 25651, 26608, 26650, 26676, 26706, 26727, 27096, 27235, 27244-27245, 27509, 27756, 27759, 28406, 28436, 28456, 28476, 36147, 36221-36226, 36251-36254, 36598, 37182-37184, 37187-37188, 37211-37214, 37210, 37217-37232, 37234-37236, 37238, 37241-37244, 43260-43265, 43267-43269, 43271-43272, 43275-43278, 43752, 44500, 49440-49465, 50382-50389, 50590, 61623, 62263-62264, 62280-62282, 63610, 64610, 64620, 70010-70015, 70170, 70332, 70370-70373, 70390, 71023, 71034, 72240-72291, 72295, 73040, 73085, 73115, 73525, 73580, 73615, 74190-74260, 74270-74300, 74305-74363, 74425-74485, 74740-74742, 75600-75630, 75658-75756, 75791-75810, 75825-75902, 75952-75962, 75966, 75970-75984, 76000-76001, 76080, 76120, 76496, 76499, 77001-77003, 92611, 93565-93568, 0075T, 0080T, 0234T-0235T, 0238T, G0106, G0120	N/A
G0108	N/A	99201-99205, 99212-99215, 99221-99223, 99324-99337, 99341-99350, 99495-99496, 90791-90832, 90834, 90837, 90839, 90956-90960, 90962, 90965-90966, 92002-92014, 92506-92508, 92526, 92541-92545, 92547-92548, 92552-92555, 92557, 92561-92582, 92584-92586, 92587-92588, 92601-92604, 92610-92612, 92620-92627, 92640, 96116, 96150-96152, 97001-97004, 97110, 97140, 97532, 97750, 97802-97804, 98940-98942, 98960-98962, G0108-D7140, G0402-G0101, G0439-G0438, G0447-D7210, G0271	N/A
G0109, G0442, G0443, G0445, G0446, G8954	N/A	99201-99205, 99212-99215, 90791-90832, 90834, 90837, 90839, 92002-92014, 92506-92508, 92526, 92541-92544, 92548, 92552-92555, 92557, 92561-92582, 92584-92586, 92587-92588, 92601-92604, 92610-92612, 92620-92627, 92640, 96150-96152, 97001-97004, 97532, 97750, 97802-97804, 98940-98942, D7210	N/A
G0121	V76.51-V16.0, V18.51	44388, 45378, 45380-45381, 45383-45385, G0121	N/A
G0202	V76.11	77057, G0202	TC
G0270	250.01, 250.41-250.33, 250.52-250.51, 362.03-250.53, 250.62-250.02, 250.20, 250.80-250.30, 362.01-250.42, 250.93-250.70, 250.72-250.32, 250.50-250.00, 648.04-250.40, 250.92, 362.06-250.13, 648.02-250.71, 250.73, 648.00-250.31, 648.03-250.22, 366.41, 648.01-250.82, 362.05-250.12, 362.07-250.63, 357.2-250.10, 250.83-250.03, 362.04	99201-99220, 99221-99233, 99238-99239, 99281-99285, 99291, 99304-99337, 99341-99350, 99455-99456, 99495-99496, 90791-90832, 90834, 90837, 90839, 90845, 90956-90960, 90962, 90965-90966, 92002-92014, 92506-92508, 92526, 92541-92545, 92547-92548, 92552-92555, 92557, 92561-92582, 92584-92586, 92587-92588, 92601-92604, 92610-92612, 92620-92627, 92640, 96116, 96150-96152, 97001-97004, 97110, 97140, 97532, 97750, 97802-97804, 98940-98942, 98960-98962, G0108-D7140, G0402-G0101, G0439-G0438, G0447-D7210, G0271	N/A
G0271	250.01, 250.41-250.33, 250.52-250.51, 362.03-250.53, 250.62-250.02, 250.20, 250.80-250.30, 362.01-250.42, 250.93-250.70, 250.72-250.32, 250.50-250.00, 648.04-250.40, 250.92, 362.06-250.13, 648.02-250.71, 250.73, 648.00-250.31, 648.03-250.22, 366.41, 648.01-250.82, 362.05-250.12, 362.07-250.63, 357.2-250.10, 250.83-250.03, 362.04	99201-99220, 99221-99233, 99238-99239, 99281-99285, 99291, 99304-99337, 99341-99350, 99455-99456, 90791-90832, 90834, 90837, 90839, 90845, 92002-92014, 92506-92508, 92526, 92541-92544, 92548, 92552-92555, 92557, 92561-92582, 92584-92586, 92587-92588, 92601-92604, 92610-92612, 92620-92627, 92640, 96150-96152, 97001-97004, 97532, 97750, 97802-97804, 98940-98942, 98960-98962, G0108-D7140, G0402-G0101, G0439-G0438, G0447-D7210, G0271	N/A

Numerator	Associated Diagnostic Denominator	Associated Procedure Denominator	Associated Modifiers
G0402	296.33, 433.20, 714.0, 805.07, V23.5-250.01, 411.1, 440.21-250.41, 410.72, 820.11-411.0, 413.1-410.32, 434.11-250.33, 250.52, 805.12, 820.00-250.51, 805.11-250.81, 410.31-309.1, 462, 465.9-445.02, 805.01, 805.14, 805.3, 820.19-250.53, 733.03-410.01, 410.22, 445.89, 813.53, V08-296.34, 440.20-250.62, V23.82-250.61, 445.81, V22.0-250.60, V23.7-410.92, 440.31-250.02, 813.42-414.02, 434.01, 813.54-414.3, 444.01-411.81, 414.04-079.53, 250.20, 414.01, 433.81, 466.0, 813.45-714.2, 733.13, 808.1-805.6, V22.1-250.80, 733.15-250.30, 410.00, 410.20, 444.21, 733.02, 808.0-250.42, 410.60, 788.31-296.21, 440.4-250.93, 410.81, 788.37-250.70, 410.91, 440.30-250.32, 250.50-250.00, 433.00, 433.11, 648.04, 813.41-805.04, V23.1, V23.81-250.40, 296.23, 410.02, 410.52, 410.70, 733.19-250.92, 410.12-309.0, 444.81, 445.01, 820.09, V23.49-444.1, 820.8-362.06, 401.1-250.13, 307.6, 434.10, 648.02, 813.43, V23.84-296.24, 788.33, 788.35, V23.41-410.71, 805.08-410.90, 411.89-250.71, 433.10, 820.10, V23.0, V23.89-250.73, 648.00-434.91, 696.0, V22.2, V23.83-440.22, 805.00-414.2, 813.46-042, 429.2, 733.01-410.10, 444.22, 805.03, 820.13-412, 434.90, 820.32-250.31, 813.50, 820.30-410.42, 414.8, 648.03, 788.39, 805.02, 805.15, 820.02, 820.20-034.0, 250.91-250.22, 433.01-410.11, 410.40-366.41, 648.01, V23.2-250.82, 362.05, V23.42-250.43, 300.4, 433.31-410.41, 410.51, 813.51-696.1, 805.8, 820.01, V23.3-250.21, 296.25, 788.30-714.81, 733.09, 820.03-296.31, 813.40, 813.52-733.12, 820.31-250.11, 296.20, 296.32, 465.8, 733.00, 805.2, 805.7, 820.12,	99201-99239, 99281-99285, 99291, 99304-99337, 99340-99350, 99356-99357, 99455-99456, 99495-99496, 22305-22327, 22520-22521, 22523-22524, 25600-25609, 27230-27248, 33140, 33510-33523, 33533-33536, 90791-90832, 90834, 90837, 90839, 90845, 90849-90863, 90880, 90956-90960, 90962, 90965-90966, 92002-92014, 92506-92508, 92526, 92541-92545, 92547-92548, 92552-92555, 92557, 92561-92582, 92584-92586, 92587-92588, 92601-92604, 92610-92612, 92620-92627, 92640, 92920, 92924, 92928, 92933, 92937, 92941-92943, 96116-96118, 96150-96152, 97001-97004, 97110, 97140, 97532, 97750, 97802-97804, 98940-98942, 98960-98962, 99078, 1100F, G0108-D7140, G8711-G0270, G0444-G0101, G0439-G0438, G0447-D7210, G0271	N/A
G0402 (continued)	820.22, 820.9-250.12, 410.30, 410.80, 805.4, V23.9-362.07, 813.47-296.22, 433.91-410.62, 444.89-250.90, 410.61, 805.13-250.63, 357.2, 434.00, 465.0, 805.17, 820.21-250.10, 410.21, 414.00-250.83, 463, 813.44-714.1, 805.5-250.03, 444.9, 805.16-298.0, 433.30-410.50, 788.36-362.04, V23.87	99201-99239, 99281-99285, 99291, 99304-99337, 99340-99350, 99356-99357, 99455-99456, 99495-99496, 22305-22327, 22520-22521, 22523-22524, 25600-25609, 27230-27248, 33140, 33510-33523, 33533-33536, 90791-90832, 90834, 90837, 90839, 90845, 90849-90863, 90880, 90956-90960, 90962, 90965-90966, 92002-92014, 92506-92508, 92526, 92541-92545, 92547-92548, 92552-92555, 92557, 92561-92582, 92584-92586, 92587-92588, 92601-92604, 92610-92612, 92620-92627, 92640, 92920, 92924, 92928, 92933, 92937, 92941-92943, 96116-96118, 96150-96152, 97001-97004, 97110, 97140, 97532, 97750, 97802-97804, 98940-98942, 98960-98962, 99078, 1100F, G0108-D7140, G8711-G0270, G0444-G0101, G0439-G0438, G0447-D7210, G0271	N/A
G0438	714.0-250.01, 250.41, 410.72, 413.1-368.2, 410.32, 434.11, 435.8-250.33, 250.52-250.51, 362.03, 784.51-250.81, 410.31-250.53, 413.9-410.01, 410.22, 435.9-250.61, 781.3-250.60, 410.92-250.02, 434.01-122.9, 433.81, 714.2-250.80, 401.9-250.30, 410.00, 410.20-250.42, 410.60, 784.59-250.93, 410.81-250.70, 432.0-250.32, 250.50-250.00, 433.11, 648.04, 781.4-250.40, 410.02, 410.52, 410.70-250.92, 410.12, 432.1, 780.02-362.06, 401.1-250.13, 435.3, 648.02-122.2, 410.71, 410.90-250.71, 386.2-250.73, 648.00-434.91, 782.0-362.02, 432.9-410.10, 412-122.8, 433.21-410.42, 648.03-122.0, 433.01-410.11, 410.40, 435.2-366.41, 648.01-250.82, 362.05, 413.0-250.43, 433.31-410.41, 410.51-250.21, 714.81-250.11, 784.3-250.12, 410.30, 410.80-122.1, 430, 433.91-410.62, 437.7-250.90, 410.61-250.63, 357.2, 435.1-250.10, 410.21-250.83, 435.0, 714.1-250.03, 401.0, 362.04	99201-99239, 99281-99285, 99291, 99304-99337, 99340-99350, 99387, 99395-99396, 99406-99407, 99455-99456, 99495-99496, 33361-33365, 33400-33430, 33463-33496, 33510-33536, 33572-33602, 33935, 33945, 33999, 35500, 35600, 70450-70470, 70551-70553, 90653, 90655-90657, 90660-90668, 90791-90832, 90834, 90837, 90839, 90845, 90880, 90945-90999, 92002-92014, 92506-92508, 92526, 92541-92545, 92547-92548, 92552-92555, 92557, 92561-92582, 92584-92586, 92587-92588, 92601-92604, 92610-92612, 92620-92627, 92640, 92920, 92924, 92928, 92933, 92937, 92941-92943, 96116-96118, 96150-96152, 97001-97004, 97110, 97140, 97532, 97750, 97802-97804, 98940-98942, 98960-98962, 1100F, 1460F, 0042T, G0108, Q2037-D7140, G0402, Q2039-G0270, G0444-G0101, G0439, Q2038-G0438, Q2035-D7210, G0271	N/A

Numerator	Associated Diagnostic Denominator	Associated Procedure Denominator	Associated Modifiers
G0439	714.0-250.01, 250.41, 410.72, 413.1-410.32, 410.82-250.33, 250.52-250.51, 362.03-250.81, 410.31-250.53, 413.9-410.01, 410.22-250.60, 410.92-250.02, 250.20-122.9, 714.2-250.80, 401.9-250.30, 410.00, 410.20-250.42, 410.60-250.93, 410.81-250.70, 410.91-250.32, 250.50-250.00, 648.04-250.40, 410.02, 410.52, 410.70-250.92, 410.12-362.06, 401.1-250.13, 648.02-122.2, 410.71, 410.90-250.71, 250.73, 648.00-362.02, 410.10, 412-122.8, 410.42, 648.03-122.0, 410.11, 410.40-366.41, 648.01-250.82, 362.05, 413.0-250.43, 410.41, 410.51-250.21, 714.81-250.12, 410.30, 410.80-122.1, 410.62-250.90, 410.61-250.63, 357.2-250.10, 410.21-250.83, 714.1-250.03, 401.0, 362.04	99201-99239, 99281-99285, 99291, 99304-99337, 99340-99350, 99387, 99395-99396, 99406-99407, 99455-99456, 99495-99496, 33361-33365, 33400-33430, 33463-33496, 33510-33536, 33572-33602, 33935, 33945, 33999, 35500, 35600, 90653, 90655-90657, 90660-90668, 90791-90832, 90834, 90837, 90839, 90845, 90880, 90945-90999, 92002-92014, 92506-92508, 92526, 92541-92545, 92547-92548, 92552-92555, 92557, 92561-92582, 92584-92586, 92587-92588, 92601-92604, 92610-92612, 92620-92627, 92640, 92920, 92924, 92928, 92933, 92937, 92941-92943, 96116-96118, 96150-96152, 97001-97004, 97110, 97140, 97532, 97750, 97802-97804, 98940-98942, 98960-98962, 1100F, 1460F, G0108, Q2037-D7140, G0402, Q2039-G0270, G0444-G0101, G0439, Q2038-G0438, Q2035-D7210, G0271	N/A
G0444, G8431, G8432, G8433, G8510, G8511, G8940	N/A	99201-99205, 99212-99215, 90791-90832, 90834, 90837, 90839, 92557, 92567-92568, 92625-92626, 96116-96118, 96150-96151, 97003, G0402, G0444-G0101, G0438	N/A
G0447	N/A	99201-99205, 99212-99215, 90791-90832, 90834, 90837, 90839, 92002-92014, 92506-92508, 92526, 92541-92544, 92548, 92552-92555, 92557, 92561-92582, 92584-92586, 92587-92588, 92601-92604, 92610-92612, 92620-92627, 92640, 96150-96152, 97001-97004, 97532, 97750, 97802-97804, 98940-98942, 98960, G0108-D7140, G0402-G0101, G0439-G0438, G0447-D7210, G0271	N/A
G0913, G0914, G0915, G0916, G0917, G0918	N/A	66840-66940, 66983-66984	N/A
G0919, G8482, G8483, G8484	N/A	99201-99205, 99212-99215, 99304-99316, 99324-99337, 99341-99350, 90653, 90655-90657, 90660-90668, 90945-90999, Q2037, Q2039-G0439, Q2038-G0438, Q2036	N/A
G8126, G8127, G8128	296.33, 309.1-296.21, 296.23, 309.0-296.24, 296.30, 300.4-296.25, 296.31-296.20, 296.32-296.22, 298.0	99201-99205, 99212-99215, 99341-99350, 90791-90832, 90834, 90837, 90839, 90845, 90849-90863, 99078, G0402	N/A
G8395, G8396, G8923	404.13, 428.23, 428.41-404.91, 428.40-404.93, 428.31-402.11, 428.21, 428.42-402.91, 428.22, 428.43-404.01, 428.32, 428.9-428.0, 428.20, 428.33-402.01, 404.03	99201-99205, 99212-99215, 99238-99239, 99304-99310, 99324-99337, 99341-99350, G8923	N/A
G8397, G8398	362.03-362.01, 362.06-362.02, 362.04	99201-99205, 99212-99215, 99304-99310, 99324-99337, 92002-92014	N/A
G8399, G8400, G8401	N/A	99201-99205, 99212-99215	N/A
G8404, G8405, G8406, G8410, G8415, G8416	250.01, 250.41-250.33, 250.52-250.51, 250.81-250.53, 250.62-250.02, 250.20, 250.80-250.30, 250.42, 250.93-250.70, 250.72-250.32, 250.50-250.00, 250.40, 250.92-250.13, 250.71, 250.73-250.31, 250.91-250.22, 250.82-250.12, 250.90-250.10, 250.03	99201-99205, 99212-99215, 99304-99310, 99324-99337, 99341-99350, 11042, 11043, 11044, 11055-11057, 11719-11730, 11740, 97001-97002, 97597-97598, 97802-97803	N/A
G8417, G8418, G8419, G8420, G8421, G8422, G8938	N/A	99201-99205, 99212-99215, 90791-90832, 90834, 90837, 90839, 96150-96152, 97001, 97003, 97802-97803, 98960, G0108-D7140, G0402-G0101, G0439-G0438, G0447-D7210, G0271	N/A
G8427, G8428, G8430	N/A	99201-99205, 99212-99215, 99221-99223, 99324-99337, 99341-99350, 99495-99496, 90791-90832, 90834, 90837, 90839, 90956-90960, 90962, 90965-90966, 92002-92014, 92507-92508, 92526, 92541-92545, 92547-92548, 92557, 92567-92570, 92585, 92588, 92626, 96116, 96150, 96152, 97001-97004, 97110, 97140, 97532, 97802-97804, 98960-98962, G0108, G0402-G0101, G0438	N/A
G8442, G8509, G8730, G8731, G8732, G8939	N/A	99201-99205, 99212-99215, 90791-90792, 92002-92014, 92507-92508, 92526, 96116-96118, 96150, 97001-97004, 97532, 98940-98942, D7140, G0402-G0101, D7210	N/A
G8447, G8448	N/A	99201-99205, 99212-99215, 92002-92014, 92506-92507, 92526, 92541-92544, 92548, 92552-92555, 92557, 92561-92582, 92584-92586, 92587-92588, 92601-92604, 92610-92612, 92620-92627, 92640, 96150-96152, 97001-97004, 97750, 97802-97804, 98940-98942, D7210	N/A

Numerator	Associated Diagnostic Denominator	Associated Procedure Denominator	Associated Modifiers
G8450, G8451, G8452	404.13, 428.23, 428.41-404.91, 428.40-404.93, 428.31-402.11, 428.21, 428.42-402.91, 428.22, 428.43-404.01, 428.32, 428.9-428.0, 428.20, 428.33-402.01, 404.03	99201-99205, 99212-99215, 99238-99239, 99304-99310, 99324-99337, 99341-99350, 3021F, G8923	N/A
G8458, G8459, G9208	070.54	99201-99205, 99212-99215, G9206	N/A
G8460, G8461, G9209, G9210, G9211	070.54	99201-99205, 99212-99215, G8461	N/A
G8462, G8463	070.54	99201-99205, 99212-99215	N/A
G8464, G8465	185	77427	N/A
G8468, G8469, G8470, G8471, G8472, G8934, G8935, G8936, G8937	411.1-410.72, 414.9-411.0, 413.1-410.32, 410.82-410.31, 413.9-410.01, 410.22, 410.92, 414.02, 414.3-411.81, 414.04-410.00, 410.20, 410.60, 410.81, 410.91, 414.06-410.02, 410.52, 410.70-410.12, V45.81-410.71, 410.90, 411.89, 414.2-410.10, 412-410.42, 414.8-410.11, 410.40, 413.0-410.41, 410.51, 414.03-410.30, 410.80-410.62, V45.82-410.21, 414.00-410.50, 414.07	99201-99205, 99212-99215, 99304-99310, 99324-99337, 99341-99350, G8934	N/A
G8473, G8474, G8475	250.01, 411.1-250.41, 410.72, 414.9 411.0, 413.1-410.32, 410.82-250.33, 250.52 250.51, 250.81, 410.31-250.53, 413.9-410.01, 410.22-250.60, 410.92-250.02, 414.02, 414.3-411.81, 414.04-250.20, 414.01-250.30, 410.00, 410.20-250.42, 410.60-250.93, 410.81-250.70, 410.91-250.32, 250.50-250.00, 414.06-250.40, 410.02, 410.52, 410.70-250.92, 410.12, V45.81-250.13, 414.05-410.71, 410.90, 411.89-250.71, 250.73, 414.2-410.10, 412-250.31, 410.42, 414.8-250.22, 410.11, 410.40-250.82, 413.0-250.43, 410.41, 410.51-250.21, 414.03-250.12, 410.30, 410.80-410.62, V45.82-250.90, 410.61-250.10, 410.21, 414.00-250.03, 410.50, 414.07	99201-99205, 99212-99215, 99304-99310, 99324-99337, 99341-99350	N/A
G8476, G8477, G8478	585.3-585.4, 585.5	99201-99205, 99212-99215, 99304-99310, 99324-99337, 99341-99350	N/A
G8524, G8525, G8526, G9258, G9260, G9261	N/A	35301	N/A
G8530, G8531, G8532	996.73-585.3, 585.5	36818-36821, 36825-36830	N/A
G8535, G8536, G8733, G8734, G8735, G8941	N/A	99201-99205, 99212-99215, 99304-99310, 99318-99337, 99341-99350, 90791-90832, 90834, 90837, 96116, 96150-96151, 97003, 97802-97803, G0402-G0101, G0438	N/A
G8539, G8540, G8541, G8542, G8543, G8942, G9227	N/A	97001-97004, 98940-98942	N/A
G8556, G8557, G8558	380.02, 744.03-380.51, 380.81-380.01, 380.32-380.30, 744.01-380.31, 744.09-380.03, 380.89-380.10, 380.39, 380.00	92550, 92557, 92567-92570, 92575	N/A
G8559, G8560, G8561, G8562, G8563	382.2-382.3, 388.69-382.01, 388.60-382.1, 388.61-381.01, 382.02	92550, 92557, 92567-92570, 92575	N/A
G8564, G8565, G8566, G8567, G8568	389.16-389.05, 389.15, 389.20-389.14, 389.9-389.17, 389.8-389.08, 389.11-389.06, 389.13-389.02, 389.10-389.00, 389.18-389.01, 389.12, 389.21	92550, 92557, 92567-92570, 92575	N/A
G8569, G8570, G8571, G8572, G8573, G8574, G8575, G8576, G8577, G8578, G8579, G8580, G8581, G8582, G8583, G8584, G8585, G8586, G8587	N/A	33510-33536	N/A

Numerator	Associated Diagnostic Denominator	Associated Procedure Denominator	Associated Modifiers
G8588, G8589, G8590, G8591, G8592	433.20-411.1, 440.21-411.0, 413.1, 434.11-410.31, 445.02-413.9, 445.89-440.20, 445.81-414.02, 434.01, 444.01-411.81, 414.04-414.01, 433.81, 444.21-440.23, 440.4-410.81, 410.91, 433.00, 433.11-414.06, 444.81, 445.01-410.71, 411.89, 433.10, 434.91, 440.22-414.2, 440.24-429.2, 444.22-414.8, 433.01-410.11, 413.0, 433.31-410.41, 410.51, 414.03, 444.09-433.91, 444.89-410.61, 434.00-410.21, 414.00, 444.9-433.30, 414.07	99201-99220, 99341-99350, 99455-99456, 33140, 33510-33523, 33533-33536, 92920, 92924, 92928, 92933, 92937, 92941-92943	N/A
G8593, G8594, G8595, G8597, G8598, G8599	433.20-411.1, 440.21-411.0, 413.1, 434.11-410.31, 445.02-410.01, 445.89-440.20, 445.81-414.02, 434.01, 444.01-411.81, 414.04-414.01, 433.81, 444.21-440.23, 440.4-410.81, 410.91, 433.00, 433.11-414.06, 444.81, 445.01-410.71, 411.89, 433.10, 434.91, 440.22-414.2, 440.24-429.2, 444.22-414.8, 433.01-410.11, 413.0, 433.31-410.41, 410.51, 414.03, 444.09-433.91, 444.89-410.61, 434.00-410.21, 414.00, 444.9-433.30, 414.07	99201-99220, 99341-99350, 99455-99456, 33140, 33510-33523, 33533-33536, 92920, 92924, 92928, 92933, 92937, 92941-92943, G0402	N/A
G8600, G8601, G8602	434.11, 436-433.10, 434.91-433.01, 433.31, 433.91, 434.00	99221-99223, 99291	N/A
G8603, G8604, G8605, G8612, G8613, G8614, G8615, G8616, G8617, G8618, G8619, G8620, G8621, G8622, G8623, G8741, G8744, G8745, G8746, G8747	438.32, 438.51, 438.9-438.10, 438.50-438.21, 438.85-438.14, 438.30, 438.41-438.42, 438.89-438.11, 438.52, 438.7-438.22, 438.6, 438.81-438.12, 438.53-438.40, 438.83-438.20, 438.82-438.31, 784.3	92507-92508	N/A
G8606, G8607, G8608, G8609, G8610, G8611, G8742, G8743	438.32, 438.51, 438.9-438.10, 438.50-438.21, 438.85-438.14, 438.30, 438.41-438.42, 438.89-438.11, 438.52, 438.7-438.0, 438.22, 438.6, 438.81-438.12, 438.53-438.40, 438.83-438.20, 438.31	97532	N/A
G8624, G8625, G8626, G8748	787.23-784.51, 787.20, 787.29-438.82, 787.22, 787.24	92526	N/A

Numerator	Associated Diagnostic Denominator	Associated Procedure Denominator	Associated Modifiers
G8629, G8630, G8631, G8632	N/A	15732-15738, 15830-15837, 19260-19272, 19300-19380, 21346-21348, 21422-21423, 21432-21436, 21454-21470, 21627, 21632, 21740, 21750, 21805, 21825, 22325, 22524, 22551, 22554, 22558, 22586, 22600, 22612, 22630, 22800-22804, 23470-23474, 23616, 24363, 24370-24371, 27080, 27125-27138, 27158, 27202, 27235-27236, 27244-27245, 27269, 27280-27282, 27440-27447, 27702-27704, 27758-27759, 27766, 27769, 27792, 27814, 27880-27888, 28192-28193, 28293, 28415-28420, 28445, 28465, 28485, 28505, 28525, 28531, 28555, 28585, 28615, 28645, 28675-28737, 31360-31420, 31760-31775, 31786, 31805, 32096-32150, 32215-32320, 32440-32501, 32505-32507, 32800-32815, 32900-32940, 33020-33208, 33212-33213, 33214-33233, 33234-33240, 33241, 33243-33256, 33261, 33300-33322, 33332-33366, 33400-33411, 33413, 33416, 33422-33465, 33475, 33496, 33510-33572, 33877-33883, 33886-33891, 34051, 34800-34805, 34812, 34820-34825, 34830-34834, 34900, 35011-35021, 35081-35103, 35131, 35141-35152, 35206, 35211-35216, 35241-35246, 35266-35276, 35301, 35311, 35363-35372, 35460, 35512, 35521 35526, 35533, 35537-35558, 35565 35587, 35601-35671, 36830, 37224-37231, 37616-37617, 38100-38101, 38115-38120, 38381, 38571-38572, 38700-38780, 39000-39220, 39501, 39540-39561, 41130-41155, 43020-43135, 43279-43282, 43300-43337, 43340-43425, 43496, 43500-43634, 43640-43645, 43651-43653, 43770-43880, 43886-43888, 44005-44010, 44020-44120, 44125-44127, 44130-44136, 44140-44202, 44204-44212, 44227, 44300-44346, 44602-44700, 44800-44850, 44900, 44950-44970, 45000, 45020-45190, 45395-45402, 45500-45825, 47100-47130, 47135-47142, 47350-47360, 47400-47480, 47560-47570, 47600-47900, 48000-48155, 48500-48548, 48554-48556, 49000-49060, 49203-49250, 49320-49323, 49505-49507, 49568, 50020, 50234-50236, 50320, 50340-50380, 50548, 50727-50728, 50760-50820, 50947-50948, 50951-50980, 51550-51597, 51800-51820, 51900-51925, 51960, 52007, 52204-52265, 52281, 52300-52301, 52310-52315, 52325-52332, 52341-52346, 52352, 52354, 52400-52450, 52601-52649, 53445, 53850-53852, 54400-54417, 54700, 55700-55706, 55801-55845, 55866, 57267, 58150-58294, 58951, 58953-58956, 60200-60281, 60500-60650, 61154, 61312-61313, 61315, 61510-61512, 61518, 61520, 61526-61530, 61548, 61591, 61595-61596, 61598, 61606, 61616-61619, 61697, 61700, 61750-61751, 61867, 62223, 62230, 63015, 63020-63030, 63042, 63045, 63047, 63056, 63075, 63081, 63267, 63276, 64746, 69720, 69930, 69955-69970, 0236T	N/A
G8633, G8634, G8635	805.07, 820.11-805.12, 820.00-805.01, 805.14, 805.3, 820.19-733.03, 813.53-805.05, 813.54-733.13, 805.6-733.02, 733.14, 813.41-733.19, 820.09, 820.8-805.08, 820.10-805.00, 813.46-733.01, 805.03, 820.13, 820.32-813.50, 820.30-805.02, 805.15, 820.02, 820.20-805.8, 820.01-733.09, 820.03-813.40, 813.52-733.12, 820.31-733.00, 805.2, 805.7, 820.12, 820.22, 820.9-805.4, 813.47-805.13, 805.17, 805.16	99201-99205, 99212-99215, 99238-99239, 22305-22327, 22520-22521, 22523-22524, 25600-25609, 27230-27248, G0402	N/A
G8647, G8648, G8649, G8650, G8651, G8652, G8653, G8654, G8655, G8656, G8657, G8658, G8659, G8660, G8661, G8662, G8663, G8664, G8665, G8666, G8667, G8668, G8669, G8670, G8671, G8672, G8673, G8674	N/A	97001-97004	N/A

Numerator	Associated Diagnostic Denominator	Associated Procedure Denominator	Associated Modifiers
G8675, G8676, G8677, G8678, G8679, G8680	404.13, 404.91, 404.93-404.12, 404.90-403.01, 403.10, 404.02-401.9, 402.91, 404.00, 404.10-401.1, 404.92-402.00, 404.11-402.90, 403.90-403.00, 403.91-402.01, 404.03-401.0, 403.11	99201-99205, 99212-99215, 99304-99310, 99324-99337, 99341-99350	N/A
G8682, G8683, G8685	404.13, 428.23, 428.41-404.91, 428.40-404.93, 428.31-402.11, 428.21, 428.42-402.91, 428.22, 428.43-404.01, 428.32, 428.9-428.0, 428.20, 428.33-402.01, 404.03	99221-99233, 99238-99239, 99291	N/A
G8694, G8695, G9188, G9189, G9190, G9191, G9192	411.1-410.72, 414.9-411.0, 413.1-410.32, 410.82-410.31, 413.9-410.01, 410.22, 410.92, 414.02, 414.3-411.81, 414.04-410.00, 410.20, 410.60, 410.81, 410.91, 414.06-410.02, 410.52, 410.70-410.12, V45.81-410.71, 410.90, 411.89, 414.2-410.10, 412-410.42, 414.8-410.11, 410.40, 413.0-410.41, 410.51, 414.03-410.30, 410.80-410.62, V45.82-410.21, 414.00-410.50, 414.07	99201-99205, 99212-99215, 99304-99310, 99324-99337, 99341-99350, 33140, 33510-33523, 33533-33536, 92920, 92924, 92928, 92933, 92937, 92941-92943, G8694	N/A
G8696, G8697, G8698	434.11, 435.8-433.11, 435.3-433.01, 435.2-433.31, 433.91, 435.0	99221-99239	N/A
G8699, G8700, G8701	434.11-432.0, 433.11-432.1, 434.91-432.9, 433.21-433.01, 433.31-430, 433.91	99221-99239	N/A
G8702, G8703	N/A	33120-33141, 33250-33251, 33256, 33261, 33305, 33315, 33332-33335, 33365-33366, 33400-33411, 33413, 33416, 33422-33465, 33475, 33496, 33510-33572	N/A
G8704, G8705, G8706, G8707	780.2	99281-99285, 99291	N/A
G8708, G8709, G8710	465.9-460, 465.0	99201-99205, 99212-99220, 99281-99285, G0402	N/A
G8711, G8712	462-034.0, 463	99201-99205, 99212-99220, 99281-99285, G0402	N/A
G8713, G8714, G8715, G8716, G8717	585.6, V56.0-V56.1, V56.32	90957-90962, 90965-90966, 90969-90970	N/A
G8718, G8720	585.6, V56.8-V56.2, V56.32	90945-90947, 90957-90962, 90965-90966, 90969-90970	N/A
G8721, G8722, G8723, G8724	153.1, 153.5, 153.9, 154.8-153.2, 153.4, 154.1-153.3, 154.0-153.0, 153.8	88309	N/A
G8736, G8737, G8943	411.1-410.72, 414.9-411.0, 413.1-410.32, 410.82-410.31, 413.9-410.01, 410.22, 410.92, 414.02, 414.3-411.81, 414.04-410.00, 410.20, 410.60, 410.81, 410.91, 414.06-410.02, 410.52, 410.70-410.12, V45.81-410.71, 410.90, 411.89, 414.2-410.10, 412-410.42, 414.8-410.11, 410.40, 413.0-410.41, 410.51, 414.03-410.30, 410.80-410.62, V45.82-410.21, 414.00-410.50, 414.07	99201-99205, 99212-99215, 99304-99310, 99324-99337, 99341-99350	N/A
G8738, G8739, G8740	404.13, 428.23, 428.41-404.91, 428.40-404.93, 428.31-402.11, 428.21, 428.42-402.91, 428.22, 428.43-404.01, 428.32, 428.9-428.0, 428.20, 428.33-402.01, 404.03	99201-99205, 99212-99215, 99304-99310, 99324-99337, 99341-99350	N/A
G8752, G8753, G8754, G8755, G8756, G9231	401.0	99201-99215, G0402, G0438	N/A
G8783, G8784, G8785, G8950, G8951, G8952	N/A	99201-99205, 99212-99215, 99218-99226, 99234-99236, 99281-99285, 99304-99310, 99318-99337, 99340-99350, 90791-90832, 90834, 90837, 90839, 90845, 90880, 92002-92014, 96118, 97532, 98940-98942, D7140, G0402-G0101, D7210	N/A
G8790, G8791, G8792, G8793, G8794, G8795, G8796	404.13, 405.99-404.91, 404.93-404.12, 404.90-403.01, 403.10, 404.02, 405.11-401.9, 402.91, 404.00, 404.10, 405.91-401.1, 404.92, 405.09-402.00, 404.11, 405.01-404.01, 405.19-402.90, 403.90-403.00, 403.91-402.01, 404.03-401.0, 403.11	99201-99205, 99212-99215, 99304-99310, 99324-99337, 99341-99350	N/A
G8797	530.85	88305	N/A
G8798	185	88309	N/A
G8799, G8800, G8801	415.19	99281-99285, 99291	N/A

Numerator	Associated Diagnostic Denominator	Associated Procedure Denominator	Associated Modifiers
G8802, G8803, G8805	789.49-789.00, 789.04, 789.46, 789.65-789.05, 789.60-789.31, 789.45, 789.64-789.37, 789.40, 789.66-789.01, 789.34-789.02, 789.33, 789.61-789.36, 789.62-789.42, 789.67-789.03, 789.69-789.06, 789.41-789.07, 789.35-789.09, 789.30, 789.39, 789.32	99281-99285, 99291	N/A
G8806, G8807, G8808	789.00, 789.04, 789.65-641.23, 789.05-641.33, 789.60-640.03, 789.64-640.00, 640.83, 789.63, 789.66-641.10, 641.93-640.80, 641.90-640.93, 641.30, 648.90-641.13, 641.20, 789.67-641.83, 789.03-640.90, 789.69-641.80, 648.93	99281-99285, 99291	N/A
G8809, G8810, G8811	633.91, 636.11, 656.00-634.10, 637.10, 639.1-634.12, 641.23-637.12, 638.1, 641.33, 656.13-640.00, 640.83-633.80, 641.10, 641.93-633.81, 641.90-640.93, 641.30, 656.10-641.13, 641.20, 641.83-637.11, 640.90-632, 656.03-634.11, 636.12	99281-99285, 99291	N/A
G8812, G8813, G8814	N/A	34800-34805, 34825-34826, 34900	N/A
G8815, G8816, G8817	N/A	35556, 35566, 35571, 35583-35587, 35656, 35666-35671	N/A
G8818, G8819, G8820, G8822, G8823, G8824, G8825	N/A	35081, 35102, 9003F-9004F	N/A
G8826, G8828, G8829, G8830, G8831, G8832, G8833	N/A	34800-34805, 9003F-9004F	N/A
G8827, G8945	N/A	34800-34805, 35081, 35102, 9003F-9004F	N/A
G8834, G8835, G8836, G8837, G8838	N/A	35301, 9006F-9007F	N/A
G8856, G8857, G8858	386.11	92540-92550, 92557, 92567-92570, 92575	N/A
G8872, G8873, G8874	174.1, 793.89-611.2, 611.82-174.8, 611.0-217, 611.72, 793.82-175.0, 610.8-174.2, 175.9, 611.83-174.4, 611.5, 611.9-174.0, 198.81, 610.9, 611.3-174.9, 611.6-239.3, 610.1, 793.80-174.3, 610.0, 610.4, 611.1-174.6, 611.89-611.71, 611.81-610.2, 174.5	19125, 19301-19302	N/A
G8875, G8876, G8877, G8946	174.1, 174.8, 175.0-174.2, 175.9-174.0, 198.81-174.3, 174.5	19301-19303, 19307	N/A
G8878, G8879, G8880, G8881, G8882	174.1, 174.8, 175.0-174.2, 175.9-174.0, 174.9-174.3, 174.5	19301-19302, 19307, 38500, 38510-38542, 38740-38745, 38900, G8879	N/A
G8883, G8884, G8885	N/A	99201-99205, 11100, 11755, 19081, 19083, 19085, 19100-19103, 19125, 20200-20251, 21550, 21920-21925, 23065-23066, 23100-23101, 24065-24066, 24100-24101, 25065-25066, 25100-25101, 26100-26110, 27040-27041, 27050-27052, 27323-27324, 27330-27331, 27613-27614, 27620, 28050-28054, 29800, 29805, 29830, 29840, 29860, 29870, 29900, 30100, 31050-31051, 31237, 31510, 31576, 31625, 31628-31629, 31632-31633, 31717, 32096-32100, 32400-32405, 32604-32609, 37200, 37609, 38221, 38500-38530, 38570, 38572, 39400, 40490, 40808, 41100-41108, 42100, 42400-42405, 42800-42806, 43193, 43197-43198, 43202, 43239, 43261, 43605, 44010, 44020, 44025, 44100, 44322, 44361, 44377, 44382, 44386, 44389, 45100, 45305, 45331, 45380, 45392, 46606, 47000-47001, 47100, 47553, 47561, 48100-48102, 49000, 49010, 49180, 49321, 50200-50205, 50555-50557, 50574-50576, 50955-50957, 50974-50976, 52007, 52204, 52224, 52250, 52354, 53200, 54100-54105, 54500-54505, 54800, 54865, 55700-55706, 55812, 55842, 55862, 56605, 56821, 57100-57105, 57421, 57454-57455, 57460, 57500, 57520, 58100, 58558, 58900, 59015, 60100, 60540-60545, 60650, 61140, 61575-61576, 61750-61751, 62269, 63275-63290,	N/A

Numerator	Associated Diagnostic Denominator	Associated Procedure Denominator	Associated Modifiers
G8883, G8884, G8885 (continued)	N/A	63615, 64795, 65410, 67346, 67400, 67415, 67450, 67810, 68100, 68510, 68525, 69100-69105, 75970, 89290-89291, 93505	N/A
G8955, G8956, G8957, G8958	585.6	90951-90959, 90963-90965, 90967-90969	N/A
G8959, G8960, G9232	296.33, 404.13-250.01, 411.1-250.41, 410.72, 414.9-411.0, 413.1-410.32, 434.11-250.33, 250.52-250.51, 428.41-250.81, 410.31-250.53, 404.91, 413.9-410.01, 410.22, 428.40-250.61, 404.93-250.60, 410.92-250.02, 428.31-414.02, 434.01-411.81, 414.04-250.20, 414.01, 433.81-250.30, 410.00, 410.20-250.42, 410.60, 428.21, 428.42-296.21, 585.6-250.93, 410.81, 428.22, 428.43-250.70, 432.0-250.32, 250.50-250.00, 433.11-250.40, 296.23, 410.02, 410.52, 410.70-250.92, 410.12, 432.1, V45.81-250.13, 414.05-296.24, 410.71, 410.90, 411.89-250.71, 250.73, 434.91-296.30, 432.9-404.11, 412-250.31, 404.01, 433.21-410.42, 414.8-250.22, 433.01-410.11, 410.40-250.82, 585.4-250.43, 433.31-410.41, 410.51, 428.32-250.21, 296.31, 431-250.11, 296.20, 296.32-250.12, 410.30, 410.80, 585.5-296.22, 430, 433.91-410.62, 428.0, V45.82-250.90, 410.61-250.63, 428.20-250.10, 410.21, 428.33-250.83, 428.1-250.03, 404.03, 410.50, 414.07	99201-99205, 99212-99215, 90791-90832, 90834, 90837, 90839, 90845	N/A
G8961, G8962, G8963, G8964, G8965, G8966	N/A	75559, 75563, 75571-75574, 78451-78454, 78491-78494, 93350-93351	N/A
G8967, G8968, G8969, G8970, G8971, G8972	427.32	99201-99205, 99212-99215, 99304-99310, 99324-99337, 99341-99350	N/A
G8973, G8974, G8975, G8976	585.6	90945-90959, 90963-90965, 90967-90969	N/A
G9193, G9194, G9195	296.33, 309.1-296.21, 296.23, 309.0-296.24, 296.30, 300.4-296.25, 296.31-296.20, 296.32-296.22, 298.0	99201-99205, 99212-99215, 99341-99350, 90791-90832, 90834, 90837, 90839, 90845, 90849-90853, 99078, G0402	N/A
G9196, G9197, G9198	N/A	15732-15738, 15830-15837, 19260-19272, 19300-19380, 21627, 21632, 21740, 21750, 21805, 21825, 22325, 22524, 22551, 22554, 22558, 22586, 22600, 22612, 22630, 22800-22804, 23470-23474, 23616, 24363, 24370-24371, 27080, 27125-27138, 27158, 27202-27218, 27235-27236, 27244-27245, 27269, 27280-27282, 27440-27447, 27702-27704, 27758-27759, 27766, 27769, 27792, 27814, 27880-27888, 28192-28193, 28293, 28415-28420, 28445, 28465, 28485, 28505, 28525, 28531, 28555, 28585, 28615, 28645, 28675-28737, 31400-31420, 31760-31775, 31786, 31805, 32096-32150, 32215-32320, 32440-32501, 32505-32507, 32800-32815, 32900-32940, 33020-33202, 33250-33251, 33256, 33261, 33300-33322, 33332-33366, 33400-33411, 33413, 33416, 33422-33465, 33475, 33496, 33510-33572, 33877-33883, 33886-33891, 34051, 34800-34805, 34812, 34820-34825, 34830-34834, 34900, 35011-35021, 35081-35103, 35131, 35141-35152, 35206, 35211-35216, 35241-35246, 35266-35276, 35301, 35311, 35363-35372, 35460, 35512, 35521-35526, 35533, 35537-35558, 35565-35587, 35601-35671, 36830, 37224-37231, 37616-37617, 38100-38101, 38115-38120, 38381, 38571-38572, 38700-38780, 39000-39220, 39501, 39540-39561, 43020-43135, 43279-43282, 43300-43337, 43340-43425, 43496, 43500-43634, 43640-43645, 43651-43653, 43770-43880, 43886-43888, 44005-44010, 44020-44021, 44050-44100, 44120, 44125-44127, 44130-44136, 44140-44202, 44204-44212, 44227, 44300-44346, 44602-44700, 44800-44850, 44900, 44950-44970, 45000, 45020, 45110-45172, 45395-45402, 45540-45825, 47100-47130, 47140-47142, 47350, 47370-47371, 47380-47381, 47400-47480, 47560-47570, 47600-47900, 48000-48160, 48500-48548, 48554-48556, 49000-49060, 49203-49250, 49320-49323, 49505-49507, 49568, 50320, 50340-50380, 57267, 58150-58294, 58951,	N/A

Numerator	Associated Diagnostic Denominator	Associated Procedure Denominator	Associated Modifiers
G9196, G9197, G9198 (continued)	N/A	58953-58956, 60200-60281, 60500-60650, 61154, 61312-61313, 61315, 61510-61512, 61518, 61548, 61697, 61700, 61750-61751, 61867, 62223, 62230, 63015, 63020-63030, 63042, 63045, 63047, 63056, 63075, 63081, 63267, 63276, 64746, 0236T	N/A
G9199	805.07, 820.11-434.11, 805.12, 820.00-805.01, 805.14, 805.3, 820.19-733.03, 813.53-434.01, 813.54-433.81, 813.45-733.13, 805.6-733.02, 733.14-432.0, 433.11, 813.41-432.1, 820.09, 820.8-805.08, 820.10-434.91, 805.00, 813.46-432.9, 733.01, 805.03, 820.13, 820.32-813.50, 820.30-433.21, 805.02, 805.15, 820.02, 820.20-433.01, 433.31, 813.51-805.8, 820.01-733.09, 820.03-431, 813.40, 813.52-733.12, 820.31-733.00, 805.2, 805.7, 820.12, 820.22, 820.9-805.4, 813.47-430, 433.91, 805.13, 805.17, 805.16	99201-99205, 99212-99215, 99221-99233, 99238-99239, 99291, 22305-22327, 22520-22521, 22523-22524, 25600-25609, 27230-27248, G0402	N/A
G9200, G9201	434.11-432.0, 433.11-432.1, 434.91-432.9, 433.21-433.01, 433.31-430, 433.91	99221-99233, 99291	N/A
G9207	070.54	99201-99205, 99212-99215, G8461, G9206	N/A
G9224, G9225, G9226	250.01, 250.41-250.33, 250.52-250.51, 362.03-250.53, 250.62-250.02, 250.20, 250.80-250.30, 362.01-250.42, 250.93-250.70, 250.72-250.32, 250.50-250.00, 648.04-250.40, 250.92, 362.06-250.13, 648.02-250.71, 250.73, 648.00-250.31, 648.03-250.22, 366.41, 648.01-250.82, 362.05-250.12, 362.07-250.63, 357.2-250.10, 250.83-250.03, 362.04	99201-99220, 99221-99233, 99238-99239, 99281-99285, 99291, 99304-99337, 99341-99350, 99455-99456, 97802-97804, G0402, G0438	N/A
G9239, G9241	585.6, V56.0	90957-90962, 90966, 90970	N/A
G9240, G9264, G9265, G9266	585.6, V56.0	90957-90962, 90966, 90970, G9240	N/A
G9246, G9247, G9248, G9249	042	99201-99205, 99212-99214, G0402	N/A
G9250, G9251	N/A	99324-99326, 99337, 99377, G0182	N/A
G9252, G9253	V76.51-V16.0, V18.51	45378, 45380-45381, 45383-45385, G0121	N/A
G9254, G9255, G9256, G9257, G9259	N/A	37215, 9006F-9007F	N/A
G9262, G9263	N/A	34800-34802, 9003F-9004F	N/A
G9267, G9268, G9269, G9270	N/A	33216-33220, 33223, 33240, 33241, 33249	N/A
G9271, G9272, G9273, G9274, G9275, G9276, G9277, G9278	433.20-411.1, 440.21-410.72, 433.80-411.0, 413.1-410.32, 434.11-410.31, 445.02-410.01, 410.22, 445.89-440.20, 445.81-410.92, 440.31-414.02, 434.01-414.3, 444.01-411.81, 414.04-414.01, 433.81-410.00, 410.20, 444.21-410.60, 440.4-410.81, 410.91, 440.30-433.00, 433.11-410.02, 410.52, 410.70-410.12, 444.81, 445.01-410.71, 410.90, 411.89, 433.10, 440.32-434.91, 440.22-414.2, 440.24-410.10, 444.22-412, 434.90-410.42, 414.8, 433.01-410.11, 410.40, 413.0, 433.31-410.41, 410.51, 414.03-410.30, 410.80, 444.09-410.62, 444.89-410.61, 434.00-410.21, 414.00, 444.9-410.50, 414.07	99201-99215, 99455-99456, G0402	N/A
G9286, G9287, G9313, G9314, G9315, G9348, G9349, G9350	461.9-461.1, 461.2	99201-99205, 99212-99215, 99281-99285, 99304-99310, 99324-99337, 99341-99350	N/A
G9316, G9317	N/A	10121-11006, 11010-11011, 11042, 11043, 11044, 11401-11446, 11601-11603, 11960, 14301, 15040, 15150, 15155, 15200, 15220, 15240, 15260, 15570-15770, 15830, 15920-15951, 15953-15958, 19020, 19101, 19110, 19120-19125, 19260-19272, 19296-19380, 19499-20150, 20696, 20900-20910, 20922, 20926, 20938, 20955-20956, 20999, 21011-21026, 21034-21049, 21139, 21154, 21235, 21299, 21360, 21395, 21462-21465, 21499-21510, 21555-21600, 21615-21705, 21740-21750, 21805-21810, 21825-22102, 22110-22114, 22206-22207, 22210-22214, 22220-22224, 22318-22327, 22520-22521, 22523-22524, 22532-22533, 22548-22551, 22554-22558, 22586-22612,	N/A

Numerator	Associated Diagnostic Denominator	Associated Procedure Denominator	Associated Modifiers
G9316, G9317 (continued)	N/A	22630, 22800-22830, 22841, 22849-22850, 22852-23044, 23075-23078, 23101, 23106-23140, 23146-23150, 23156-23170, 23180-23220, 23395-23405, 23410-23472, 23480-23485, 23491, 23515, 23530-23532, 23550-23552, 23585, 23615-23616, 23630, 23660, 23670, 23680, 23800-23920, 23929, 23935-24079, 24102-24105, 24116-24125, 24130-24136, 24140-24145, 24149-24152, 24201, 24301, 24310-24330, 24332-24342, 24344-24346, 24358-24361, 24363-24366, 24400, 24430-24435, 24495-24498, 24515-24516, 24538-24546, 24575, 24579, 24586-24587, 24615, 24635, 24665-24666, 24685-24925, 24999-25025, 25040-25085, 25101-25107, 25110-25118, 25120-25125, 25130-25240, 25248, 25260-25270, 25274-25295, 25301-25315, 25320-25332, 25337-25360, 25375-25392, 25400-25420, 25430-25440, 25442-25443, 25445-25449, 25490, 25515, 25525-25526, 25545, 25574-25575, 25607-25609, 25628, 25645, 25652, 25670, 25676, 25685, 25695, 25900-25905, 25909, 25920, 25927, 25999, 26115-26123, 26130, 26145, 26180, 26350-26410, 26415, 26418-26426, 26433-26471, 26477-26478, 26480-26492, 26496-26498, 26500-26502, 26510, 26520-26548, 26561, 26565-26568, 26587, 26591-26593, 26615, 26650-26665, 26676-26686, 26715, 26727-26735, 26746, 26765, 26776-26785, 26952-27001, 27005-27059, 27054-27066, 27070-27087, 27097, 27110, 27120-27170, 27176-27177, 27179-27181, 27187, 27202, 27226-27228, 27235-27238, 27244-27245, 27248, 27253-27254, 27258-27259, 27267, 27269, 27280, 27290-27305, 27307-27310, 27327-27339, 27331-27357, 27360-27365, 27372-27390, 27392, 27403-27472, 27477, 27485-27499, 27506-27507, 27509, 27511-27514, 27519, 27524, 27535-27536, 27540, 27556-27557, 27566, 27580-27612, 27615-27647, 27650-27687, 27695-27709, 27715-27726, 27745, 27756-27759, 27766, 27769, 27784, 27792, 27814, 27822-27823, 27826-27829, 27832, 27846-27848, 27880-27899, 28002-28003, 28043-28047, 28192-28193, 28293, 28415-28420, 28445-28446, 28465, 28485, 28505, 28525, 28531, 28555, 28585, 28615, 28645, 28675-28737, 28800-28825, 29806-29825, 29827-29828, 29834-29835, 29837-29838, 29844, 29846-29847, 29850, 29855, 29862, 29914-29868, 29871-29891, 29893, 29895-29898, 29904-29999, 31300-31367, 31370-31420, 31580, 31587, 31590, 31599, 31611, 31614, 31750-31760, 31775-31800, 31820-31825, 31899-32036, 32100-32200, 32215-32320, 32440-32491, 32503-32505, 32540, 32560, 32650-32666, 32669-32672, 32800-32820, 32900-32940, 32999, 33020-33050, 33300, 33310, 33320, 33875-33883, 33886-33891, 34001-34805, 34812, 34820-34825, 34830-34834, 34900-35021, 35045-35152, 35184, 35189-35236, 35246-35271, 35281-35305, 35311-35372, 35471-35472, 35501-35510, 35512-35571, 35583-35587, 35601-35671, 35691-35695, 35701-35907, 36475, 36478, 36818-36821, 36825-36830, 36838, 37140, 37160-37181, 37215, 37220-37221, 37224-37231, 37500, 37565, 37605, 37607, 37615-37618, 37650-37785, 37799-38101, 38115-38129, 38230, 38305-38382, 38542-38745, 38760-38780, 38999-39599, 40510-40525, 40530-40652, 40800-40801, 40810-40816, 41000-41009, 41016-41018, 41110-41114, 41116-41155, 41599, 41806-41820, 41822-41826, 41830-41850, 42104-42160, 42210, 42300-42305, 42330-42340, 42408-42507, 42665-42725, 42808, 42810-42815, 42821, 42826, 42831, 42836-42845, 42870-42894, 42950-42962, 42972-43135, 43279-43282, 43289-43313, 43320-43337, 43340-43425, 43496, 43500-43634, 43640-43645, 43651-43652, 43659, 43770-43825, 43832-43840, 43843-43880, 43886-44010, 44020-44055, 44110-44120, 44125-44127	N/A
G9352, G9353, G9354	473.0, 473.3-473.1, 473.8-473.2, 473.9	99201-99205, 99212-99215, 99281-99285, 99304-99310, 99324-99337, 99341-99350	N/A

Numerator	Associated Diagnostic Denominator	Associated Procedure Denominator	Associated Modifiers
G9355, G9356, G9361	V27.0	59409, 59514, 59612, 59620	N/A
G9357, G9358	N/A	59430-59510, 59515, 59610, 59614-59618, 59622	N/A
G9359, G9360	714.0, 714.2-696.1, 714.81	99201-99205, 99212-99215, G0402	N/A
	N/A		N/A

Appendix L — Medically Unlikely Edits (MUEs)

The Centers for Medicare & Medicaid Services (CMS) began to publish many of the edits used in the medically unlikely edits (MUE) program for the first time effective October 2008. What follows below is a list of the published CPT codes that have MUEs assigned to them and the number of units allowed with each code. CMS publishes the updates on a quarterly basis. Not all MUEs will be published, however. MUEs intended to detect and discourage any questionable payments will not be published as the agency feels the efficacy of these edits would be compromised.

The quarterly updates will be published on the CMS website at http://www.cms.gov/NationalCorrectCodInitEd/08_MUE.asp.

Professional

CPT	MUE
0001M	1
0002M	1
0003M	1
0019T	1
0042T	1
0051T	1
0052T	1
0053T	1
0054T	2
0055T	2
0058T	1
0059T	1
0071T	1
0072T	1
0073T	2
0075T	1
0076T	2
0092T	1
0095T	1
0098T	1
0099T	2
0100T	2
0101T	1
0102T	2
0103T	1
0106T	4
0107T	4
0108T	4
0109T	4
0110T	4
0111T	1
0123T	2
0126T	1
0159T	2
0163T	2
0164T	4
0165T	4
0169T	1
0171T	1
0172T	3
0174T	1
0175T	1
0178T	1
0179T	1
0180T	1
0181T	1
0182T	3
0184T	1
0190T	2
0191T	2
0195T	1

CPT	MUE
0196T	1
0197T	2
0198T	2
01996	1
0199T	1
0200T	1
0201T	1
0202T	1
0206T	1
0207T	2
0208T	1
0209T	1
0210T	1
0211T	1
0212T	1
0213T	1
0214T	1
0215T	1
0216T	1
0217T	1
0218T	1
0219T	1
0220T	1
0221T	1
0222T	1
0223T	1
0224T	1
0225T	1
0226T	1
0227T	1
0228T	1
0230T	1
0232T	1
0233T	1
0234T	2
0235T	2
0236T	1
0237T	2
0239T	1
0240T	1
0241T	1
0243T	1
0244T	1
0245T	1
0246T	1
0247T	1
0248T	1
0249T	1
0253T	1
0254T	2
0255T	2
0262T	1

CPT	MUE
0263T	1
0264T	1
0265T	1
0266T	1
0267T	1
0268T	1
0269T	1
0270T	1
0271T	1
0272T	1
0273T	1
0274T	1
0275T	1
0278T	1
0281T	1
0282T	1
0283T	1
0284T	1
0285T	1
0286T	1
0287T	2
0288T	1
0289T	2
0290T	1
0291T	1
0292T	1
0293T	1
0294T	1
0295T	1
0296T	1
0297T	1
0298T	1
0299T	1
0300T	1
0301T	1
0302T	1
0303T	1
0304T	1
0305T	1
0306T	1
0307T	1
0308T	1
0309T	1
0310T	1
0311T	1
0312T	1
0313T	1
0314T	1
0315T	1
0316T	1
0317T	1
0319T	1

CPT	MUE
0320T	1
0321T	1
0322T	1
0323T	1
0324T	1
0325T	1
0326T	1
0327T	1
0328T	1
0329T	1
0330T	1
0331T	1
0332T	1
0333T	1
0334T	2
0335T	2
0336T	1
0337T	1
0338T	1
0339T	1
0347T	1
0348T	1
0349T	1
0350T	1
0351T	5
0352T	5
0353T	2
0354T	2
0355T	1
0356T	4
0358T	1
0359T	1
0360T	1
0361T	3
0362T	1
0363T	3
0364T	1
0366T	1
0368T	1
0370T	1
0371T	1
0372T	1
0373T	1
10040	1
10060	1
10061	1
10080	1
10081	1
10180	3
11000	1
11004	1
11005	1

CPT	MUE
11006	1
11008	1
11010	1
11011	1
11012	2
11042	1
11043	1
11044	1
11055	1
11056	1
11057	1
11100	1
11200	1
11201	0
11446	3
11450	1
11451	1
11462	1
11463	1
11470	3
11471	2
11646	3
11719	1
11720	1
11721	1
11730	1
11732	9
11770	1
11771	1
11772	1
11900	1
11901	1
11920	1
11921	1
11922	1
11950	1
11951	1
11952	1
11954	1
11960	3
11970	2
11971	2
11976	1
11980	1
11981	1
11982	1
11983	1
12001	1
12002	1
12004	1
12005	1
12006	1

CPT	MUE
12007	1
12011	1
12013	1
12014	1
12015	1
12016	1
12017	1
12018	1
12020	3
12021	3
12031	1
12032	1
12034	1
12035	1
12036	1
12037	1
12041	1
12042	1
12044	1
12045	1
12046	1
12047	1
12051	1
12052	1
12053	1
12054	1
12055	1
12056	1
12057	1
13100	1
13101	1
13120	1
13121	1
13131	1
13132	1
13151	1
13152	1
13160	3
14301	2
15002	1
15004	1
15040	1
15050	1
15100	1
15110	1
15115	1
15116	2
15120	1
15130	1
15135	1
15150	1
15151	1

CPT	MUE
15152	2
15155	1
15156	1
15200	1
15220	1
15240	1
15260	1
15271	1
15272	3
15273	1
15275	1
15276	3
15277	1
15570	3
15572	2
15574	2
15576	2
15600	2
15610	2
15620	2
15630	2
15650	1
15731	1
15740	3
15750	2
15756	2
15757	3
15758	3
15760	2
15770	2
15775	1
15776	1
15777	1
15780	1
15781	2
15782	2
15783	2
15786	1
15787	3
15788	1
15789	1
15792	1
15793	1
15819	1
15820	1
15821	1
15822	1
15823	1
15824	1
15825	1
15826	1
15828	1

CPT	MUE
15829	1
15830	1
15832	1
15833	1
15834	1
15835	1
15836	1
15837	2
15838	1
15839	2
15840	1
15841	2
15842	2
15845	2
15847	1
15851	1
15852	2
15860	1
15876	1
15877	1
15878	1
15879	1
15920	1
15922	1
15931	1
15933	1
15934	1
15935	1
15936	1
15937	1
15940	2
15941	2
15944	2
15945	2
15946	2
15950	2
15951	2
15952	2
15953	2
15956	2
15958	2
16000	1
16020	1
16025	1
16030	1
16035	1
17000	1
17003	13
17004	1
17106	1
17107	1
17108	1

CPT	MUE
17110	1
17111	1
17264	3
17266	2
17276	3
17286	3
17340	1
17360	1
17380	1
19000	2
19001	5
19020	2
19030	1
19081	1
19083	1
19085	1
19101	3
19110	1
19112	2
19120	1
19125	1
19126	3
19260	2
19271	2
19272	2
19281	1
19283	1
19285	1
19287	1
19296	1
19297	2
19298	1
19300	1
19301	1
19302	1
19303	1
19304	1
19305	1
19306	1
19307	1
19316	1
19318	1
19324	1
19325	1
19328	1
19330	1
19340	1
19342	1
19350	1
19355	1
19357	1
19361	1
19364	1
19366	1
19367	1
19368	1
19369	1
19370	1
19371	1
19380	1
19396	1
20100	2
20102	4
20103	4
20150	2

CPT	MUE
20200	3
20205	4
20206	3
20250	3
20251	3
20526	1
20527	1
20552	1
20553	1
20555	1
20612	2
20615	1
20660	1
20661	1
20662	1
20663	1
20664	1
20665	1
20670	2
20680	2
20692	3
20693	2
20696	2
20697	4
20802	1
20805	1
20808	1
20816	3
20822	3
20824	1
20827	1
20838	1
20900	2
20910	2
20912	1
20920	2
20922	2
20924	4
20926	2
20931	1
20937	1
20938	1
20950	2
20955	1
20956	1
20957	1
20962	1
20969	2
20970	1
20972	2
20973	1
20974	1
20975	1
20979	1
20982	1
20985	2
21010	1
21012	3
21014	3
21015	1
21016	2
21025	2
21026	2
21029	1
21030	1

CPT	MUE
21031	2
21032	1
21034	1
21040	2
21044	1
21045	1
21046	2
21047	2
21048	2
21049	2
21050	1
21060	1
21070	1
21073	1
21076	1
21077	1
21079	1
21080	1
21081	1
21082	1
21083	1
21084	1
21085	1
21086	1
21087	1
21088	1
21100	1
21110	2
21116	1
21120	1
21121	1
21122	1
21123	1
21125	2
21127	2
21137	1
21138	1
21139	1
21141	1
21142	1
21143	1
21145	1
21146	1
21147	1
21150	1
21151	1
21154	1
21155	1
21159	1
21160	1
21172	1
21175	1
21179	1
21180	1
21181	1
21182	1
21183	1
21184	1
21188	1
21193	1
21194	1
21195	1
21196	1
21198	1
21199	1

CPT	MUE
21206	1
21208	1
21209	1
21210	2
21215	2
21230	2
21235	2
21240	1
21242	1
21243	1
21244	1
21245	2
21246	2
21247	1
21255	1
21256	1
21260	1
21261	1
21263	1
21267	1
21268	1
21270	1
21275	1
21280	1
21282	1
21295	1
21296	1
21310	1
21315	1
21320	1
21325	1
21330	1
21335	1
21336	1
21337	1
21338	1
21339	1
21340	1
21343	1
21344	1
21345	1
21346	1
21347	1
21348	1
21355	1
21356	1
21360	1
21365	1
21366	1
21385	1
21386	1
21387	1
21390	1
21395	1
21400	1
21401	1
21406	1
21407	1
21408	1
21421	1
21422	1
21423	1
21431	1
21432	1
21433	1

CPT	MUE
21435	1
21436	1
21440	2
21445	2
21450	1
21451	1
21452	1
21453	1
21454	1
21461	1
21462	1
21465	1
21470	1
21480	1
21485	1
21490	1
21495	1
21497	1
21501	3
21502	1
21510	1
21550	3
21554	3
21556	3
21557	1
21558	1
21610	2
21615	1
21616	1
21620	1
21627	1
21630	1
21632	1
21685	1
21700	1
21705	1
21720	1
21725	1
21740	1
21742	1
21743	1
21750	1
21805	3
21810	1
21820	1
21825	1
21920	3
21925	3
21931	3
21933	3
21935	1
21936	1
22010	2
22015	2
22100	1
22101	1
22102	1
22103	3
22110	1
22112	1
22114	1
22116	3
22206	1
22207	1
22210	1

CPT	MUE
22212	1
22214	1
22216	6
22220	1
22222	1
22224	1
22305	1
22310	1
22315	1
22318	1
22319	1
22325	1
22326	1
22327	1
22328	8
22505	1
22520	1
22521	1
22522	5
22523	1
22524	1
22525	5
22532	1
22533	1
22534	3
22548	1
22551	1
22554	1
22556	1
22558	1
22585	7
22586	1
22590	1
22595	1
22600	1
22610	1
22612	1
22614	15
22630	1
22632	4
22633	1
22634	4
22800	1
22802	1
22804	1
22808	1
22810	1
22812	1
22818	1
22819	1
22830	1
22840	1
22842	1
22843	1
22844	1
22845	1
22846	1
22847	1
22848	1
22849	1
22850	1
22851	9
22852	1
22855	1
22856	1

CPT	MUE
22857	1
22861	1
22862	1
22864	1
22865	1
22900	3
22901	3
22903	3
22904	1
22905	1
23000	1
23020	1
23030	2
23031	2
23035	2
23040	1
23044	1
23065	2
23066	2
23071	3
23073	3
23075	4
23076	2
23077	1
23078	1
23100	1
23101	2
23105	1
23106	1
23107	1
23120	1
23125	1
23130	1
23140	1
23145	1
23146	1
23150	1
23155	1
23156	1
23170	1
23172	1
23174	1
23180	1
23182	1
23184	1
23190	1
23195	1
23200	1
23210	1
23220	1
23330	2
23334	1
23335	1
23350	1
23395	1
23397	1
23400	1
23405	2
23406	1
23410	1
23412	1
23415	1
23420	1
23430	1
23440	1

CPT	MUE
23450	1
23455	1
23460	1
23462	1
23465	1
23466	1
23470	1
23472	1
23473	1
23474	1
23480	1
23485	1
23490	1
23491	1
23500	1
23505	1
23515	1
23520	1
23525	1
23530	1
23532	1
23540	1
23545	1
23550	1
23552	1
23570	1
23575	1
23585	1
23600	1
23605	1
23615	1
23616	1
23620	1
23625	1
23630	1
23650	1
23655	1
23660	1
23665	1
23670	1
23675	1
23680	1
23700	1
23800	1
23802	1
23900	1
23920	1
23921	1
23930	2
23931	2
23935	2
24000	1
24006	1
24065	2
24066	2
24071	3
24073	3
24077	1
24079	1
24100	1
24101	1
24102	1
24105	1
24110	1
24115	1

Appendix L — Medically Unlikely Edits (MUEs) — Professional

CPT	MUE
24116	1
24120	1
24125	1
24126	1
24130	1
24134	1
24136	1
24138	1
24140	1
24145	1
24147	1
24149	1
24150	1
24152	1
24155	1
24160	1
24164	1
24200	3
24201	3
24220	1
24300	1
24301	2
24305	4
24320	2
24330	1
24331	1
24332	1
24340	1
24342	2
24343	1
24344	1
24345	1
24346	1
24357	2
24358	2
24359	2
24360	1
24361	1
24362	1
24363	1
24365	1
24366	1
24370	1
24371	1
24400	1
24410	1
24420	1
24430	1
24435	1
24470	1
24495	1
24498	1
24500	1
24505	1
24515	1
24516	1
24530	1
24535	1
24538	1
24545	1
24546	1
24560	1
24565	1
24566	1
24575	1

CPT	MUE
24576	1
24577	1
24579	1
24582	1
24586	1
24587	1
24600	1
24605	1
24615	1
24620	1
24635	1
24640	1
24650	1
24655	1
24665	1
24666	1
24670	1
24675	1
24685	1
24800	1
24802	1
24900	1
24920	1
24925	1
24930	1
24931	1
24935	1
24940	1
25000	2
25001	1
25020	1
25023	1
25024	1
25025	1
25031	2
25035	2
25040	1
25065	5
25066	3
25071	3
25073	3
25076	5
25077	1
25078	1
25085	1
25100	1
25101	1
25105	1
25107	1
25110	3
25111	1
25112	1
25115	1
25116	1
25119	1
25120	1
25125	1
25126	1
25130	1
25135	1
25136	1
25145	1
25150	1
25151	1
25170	1

CPT	MUE
25210	2
25215	1
25230	1
25240	1
25246	1
25248	3
25250	1
25251	1
25259	1
25275	2
25295	9
25300	1
25301	1
25315	1
25316	1
25320	1
25332	1
25335	1
25337	1
25350	1
25355	1
25360	1
25365	1
25370	1
25375	1
25390	1
25391	1
25392	1
25393	1
25394	1
25400	1
25405	1
25415	1
25420	1
25425	1
25426	1
25430	1
25431	2
25440	1
25441	1
25442	1
25443	1
25444	1
25445	1
25446	1
25449	1
25450	1
25455	1
25490	1
25491	1
25492	1
25500	1
25505	1
25515	1
25520	1
25525	1
25526	1
25530	1
25535	1
25545	1
25560	1
25565	1
25574	1
25575	1
25600	1

CPT	MUE
25605	1
25606	1
25607	1
25608	1
25609	1
25622	1
25624	1
25628	1
25630	1
25635	1
25645	1
25650	1
25651	1
25652	1
25660	1
25670	1
25671	1
25675	1
25676	1
25680	1
25685	1
25690	1
25695	1
25800	1
25805	1
25810	1
25820	1
25825	1
25830	1
25900	1
25905	1
25907	1
25909	1
25915	1
25920	1
25922	1
25924	1
25927	1
25929	1
25931	1
26010	3
26011	3
26025	1
26030	1
26034	2
26035	3
26037	1
26040	1
26045	1
26070	3
26100	2
26105	2
26110	3
26116	2
26117	2
26118	1
26121	1
26123	1
26185	1
26200	2
26205	1
26210	2
26215	2
26230	2
26235	2

CPT	MUE
26236	2
26250	2
26260	1
26262	1
26341	3
26357	3
26358	3
26390	3
26392	3
26416	2
26428	2
26432	2
26433	2
26434	3
26494	1
26496	1
26497	2
26498	1
26508	1
26516	1
26517	1
26518	1
26548	3
26550	1
26551	1
26553	1
26554	1
26555	2
26556	2
26560	2
26561	2
26562	2
26580	1
26641	1
26645	1
26650	1
26665	1
26740	3
26742	3
26746	3
26820	1
26841	1
26842	1
26860	1
26862	1
26990	2
26991	2
26992	2
27000	1
27001	1
27003	1
27005	1
27006	1
27025	1
27027	1
27030	1
27033	1
27035	1
27036	1
27040	2
27041	3
27043	3
27045	3
27048	2
27049	1

CPT	MUE
27050	1
27052	1
27054	1
27057	1
27059	1
27060	1
27062	1
27065	1
27066	1
27067	1
27070	1
27071	1
27075	1
27076	1
27077	1
27078	1
27080	1
27086	2
27087	2
27090	1
27091	1
27093	1
27095	1
27096	1
27097	1
27098	1
27100	1
27105	1
27110	1
27111	1
27120	1
27122	1
27125	1
27130	1
27132	1
27134	1
27137	1
27138	1
27140	1
27146	1
27147	1
27151	1
27156	1
27158	1
27161	1
27165	1
27170	1
27175	1
27176	1
27177	1
27178	1
27179	1
27181	1
27185	1
27187	1
27193	1
27194	1
27200	1
27202	1
27220	1
27222	1
27226	1
27227	1
27228	1
27230	1

CPT	MUE
27232	1
27235	1
27236	1
27238	1
27240	1
27244	1
27245	1
27246	1
27248	1
27250	1
27252	1
27253	1
27254	1
27256	1
27257	1
27258	1
27259	1
27265	1
27266	1
27267	1
27268	1
27269	1
27275	2
27280	1
27282	1
27284	1
27286	1
27290	1
27295	1
27303	2
27305	1
27306	1
27307	1
27310	1
27325	1
27326	1
27329	1
27330	1
27331	1
27332	1
27333	1
27334	1
27335	1
27340	1
27345	1
27347	1
27350	1
27355	1
27356	1
27357	1
27358	1
27360	2
27364	1
27365	1
27370	1
27380	2
27381	2
27385	2
27386	2
27390	1
27391	1
27392	1
27393	1
27394	1
27395	1

CPT	MUE
27396	1
27397	1
27400	1
27403	1
27405	2
27407	2
27409	1
27412	1
27415	1
27416	1
27418	1
27420	1
27422	1
27424	1
27425	1
27427	1
27428	1
27429	1
27430	1
27435	1
27437	1
27438	1
27440	1
27441	1
27442	1
27443	1
27445	1
27446	1
27447	1
27448	1
27450	1
27454	1
27455	1
27457	1
27465	1
27466	1
27468	1
27470	1
27472	1
27475	1
27477	1
27479	1
27485	1
27486	1
27487	1
27488	1
27495	1
27496	1
27497	1
27498	1
27499	1
27500	1
27501	1
27502	1
27503	1
27506	1
27507	1
27508	1
27509	1
27510	1
27511	1
27513	1
27514	1
27516	1
27517	1

CPT	MUE
27519	1
27520	1
27524	1
27530	1
27532	1
27535	1
27536	1
27538	1
27540	1
27550	1
27552	1
27556	1
27557	1
27558	1
27560	1
27562	1
27566	1
27570	1
27580	1
27590	1
27591	1
27592	1
27594	1
27596	1
27598	1
27600	1
27601	1
27602	1
27604	2
27605	1
27606	1
27607	2
27610	1
27612	1
27615	1
27616	1
27620	1
27625	1
27626	1
27630	2
27635	1
27637	1
27638	1
27640	1
27641	1
27645	1
27646	1
27647	1
27648	1
27650	1
27652	1
27654	1
27656	2
27658	2
27659	2
27664	2
27665	2
27675	1
27676	1
27680	3
27681	1
27685	2
27686	2
27687	1
27690	2

CPT	MUE
27691	2
27695	1
27696	1
27698	2
27700	1
27702	1
27703	1
27704	1
27705	1
27707	1
27709	1
27712	1
27715	1
27720	1
27722	1
27724	1
27725	1
27726	1
27727	1
27730	1
27732	1
27734	1
27740	1
27742	1
27745	1
27750	1
27752	1
27756	1
27758	1
27759	1
27760	1
27762	1
27766	1
27767	1
27768	1
27769	1
27780	1
27781	1
27784	1
27786	1
27788	1
27792	1
27808	1
27810	1
27814	1
27816	1
27818	1
27822	1
27823	1
27824	1
27825	1
27826	1
27827	1
27828	1
27829	1
27830	1
27831	1
27832	1
27840	1
27842	1
27846	1
27848	1
27860	1
27870	1
27871	1

CPT	MUE
27880	1
27881	1
27882	1
27884	1
27886	1
27888	1
27889	1
27892	1
27893	1
27894	1
28001	2
28002	3
28003	2
28005	3
28008	2
28035	1
28039	3
28041	3
28046	1
28047	1
28052	2
28054	2
28055	1
28060	1
28062	1
28086	2
28088	2
28090	2
28092	2
28100	1
28102	1
28103	1
28104	2
28106	1
28107	1
28108	2
28110	1
28111	1
28113	1
28114	1
28116	1
28118	1
28119	1
28120	2
28122	4
28124	4
28130	1
28171	1
28173	2
28175	2
28192	2
28193	2
28202	2
28210	2
28220	1
28222	1
28225	1
28226	1
28230	1
28238	1
28240	1
28250	1
28260	1
28261	1
28262	1

CPT	MUE
28264	1
28280	1
28285	4
28286	1
28289	1
28290	1
28292	1
28293	1
28294	1
28296	1
28297	1
28298	1
28299	1
28300	1
28302	1
28304	1
28305	1
28306	1
28307	1
28309	1
28310	1
28315	1
28320	1
28322	2
28340	2
28341	2
28344	1
28360	1
28400	1
28405	1
28406	1
28415	1
28420	1
28430	1
28435	1
28436	1
28445	1
28446	1
28490	1
28495	1
28496	1
28505	1
28530	1
28531	1
28540	1
28545	1
28546	1
28555	1
28570	1
28575	1
28576	1
28585	1
28600	2
28605	2
28630	2
28635	2
28705	1
28715	1
28725	1
28730	1
28735	1
28737	1
28750	1
28755	1
28760	1

CPT	MUE
28800	1
28805	1
28825	10
28890	1
29000	1
29010	1
29015	1
29020	1
29025	1
29035	1
29040	1
29044	1
29046	1
29049	1
29055	1
29058	1
29065	1
29075	1
29085	1
29086	2
29105	1
29125	1
29126	1
29130	3
29131	2
29200	1
29240	1
29260	1
29280	2
29305	1
29325	1
29345	1
29355	1
29358	1
29365	1
29405	1
29425	1
29435	1
29440	1
29445	1
29450	1
29505	1
29515	1
29520	1
29530	1
29540	1
29550	1
29580	1
29581	1
29582	1
29583	1
29584	1
29700	2
29705	1
29710	1
29715	1
29720	1
29730	2
29740	1
29750	1
29800	1
29804	1
29805	1
29806	1
29807	1

CPT	MUE
29819	1
29820	1
29821	1
29822	1
29823	1
29824	1
29825	1
29826	1
29827	1
29828	1
29830	1
29834	1
29835	1
29836	1
29837	1
29838	1
29840	1
29843	1
29844	1
29845	1
29846	1
29847	1
29848	1
29850	1
29851	1
29855	1
29856	1
29860	1
29861	1
29862	1
29863	1
29866	1
29867	1
29868	1
29870	1
29871	1
29873	1
29874	1
29875	1
29876	1
29877	1
29879	1
29880	1
29881	1
29882	1
29883	1
29884	1
29885	1
29886	1
29887	1
29888	1
29889	1
29891	1
29892	1
29893	1
29894	1
29895	1
29897	1
29898	1
29899	1
29900	2
29901	2
29902	2
29904	1
29905	1

CPT	MUE
29906	1
29907	1
29914	1
29915	1
29916	1
30000	1
30020	1
30100	3
30110	1
30115	1
30117	2
30118	2
30120	1
30124	2
30125	1
30130	1
30140	1
30150	1
30160	1
30200	1
30210	1
30220	1
30300	1
30310	1
30320	1
30400	1
30410	1
30420	1
30430	1
30435	1
30450	1
30460	1
30462	1
30465	1
30520	1
30540	1
30545	1
30560	1
30580	2
30600	1
30620	1
30630	1
30801	1
30802	1
30901	1
30903	1
30905	1
30906	1
30915	1
30920	1
30930	1
31000	1
31002	1
31020	1
31030	1
31032	1
31040	1
31050	1
31051	1
31070	1
31075	1
31080	1
31081	1
31084	1
31085	1

CPT	MUE
31086	1
31087	1
31090	1
31200	1
31201	1
31205	1
31225	1
31230	1
31231	1
31233	1
31235	1
31237	1
31238	1
31239	1
31240	1
31254	1
31255	1
31256	1
31267	1
31276	1
31287	1
31288	1
31290	1
31291	1
31292	1
31293	1
31294	1
31295	1
31296	1
31297	1
31300	1
31320	1
31360	1
31365	1
31367	1
31368	1
31370	1
31375	1
31380	1
31382	1
31390	1
31395	1
31400	1
31420	1
31500	2
31502	1
31505	1
31510	1
31511	1
31512	1
31513	1
31515	1
31520	1
31525	1
31526	1
31527	1
31528	1
31529	1
31530	1
31531	1
31535	1
31536	1
31540	1
31541	1
31545	1

Appendix L — Medically Unlikely Edits (MUEs) — Professional

CPT	MUE
31546	1
31560	1
31561	1
31570	1
31571	1
31575	1
31576	1
31577	1
31578	1
31579	1
31580	1
31582	1
31584	1
31587	1
31588	1
31590	1
31595	1
31600	1
31601	1
31603	1
31605	1
31610	1
31611	1
31612	1
31613	1
31614	1
31615	1
31620	1
31622	1
31623	1
31624	1
31625	1
31626	1
31627	1
31628	1
31629	1
31630	1
31631	1
31632	2
31633	2
31634	1
31635	1
31636	1
31637	2
31638	2
31640	1
31641	1
31643	1
31645	1
31646	2
31647	1
31648	1
31660	1
31661	1
31717	1
31720	1
31725	1
31730	1
31750	1
31755	1
31760	1
31766	1
31770	2
31775	1
31780	1

CPT	MUE
31781	1
31785	1
31786	1
31800	1
31805	1
31820	1
31825	1
31830	1
32035	1
32036	1
32096	1
32097	1
32098	1
32100	1
32110	1
32120	1
32124	1
32140	1
32141	1
32150	1
32151	1
32160	1
32200	2
32215	1
32220	1
32225	1
32310	1
32320	1
32400	2
32405	2
32440	1
32442	1
32445	1
32480	1
32482	1
32484	2
32486	1
32488	1
32491	1
32501	1
32503	1
32504	1
32505	1
32506	3
32507	2
32540	1
32550	2
32552	2
32553	1
32554	3
32555	3
32556	3
32557	3
32560	1
32561	1
32562	1
32601	1
32604	1
32606	1
32607	1
32608	1
32609	1
32650	1
32651	1
32652	1

CPT	MUE
32653	1
32654	1
32655	1
32656	1
32658	1
32659	1
32661	1
32662	1
32663	1
32664	1
32665	1
32666	1
32667	3
32668	2
32669	2
32670	1
32671	1
32672	1
32673	1
32674	1
32701	1
32800	1
32810	1
32815	1
32820	1
32850	1
32851	1
32852	1
32853	1
32854	1
32855	1
32856	1
32900	1
32905	1
32906	1
32940	1
32960	1
32997	1
32998	1
33010	1
33011	1
33015	1
33020	1
33025	1
33030	1
33031	1
33050	1
33120	1
33130	1
33140	1
33141	1
33202	1
33203	1
33206	1
33207	1
33208	1
33210	1
33211	1
33212	1
33213	1
33214	1
33215	2
33216	1
33217	1
33218	1

CPT	MUE
33220	1
33221	1
33222	1
33223	1
33224	1
33225	1
33226	1
33227	1
33228	1
33229	1
33230	1
33231	1
33233	1
33234	1
33235	1
33236	1
33237	1
33238	1
33240	1
33241	1
33243	1
33244	1
33249	1
33250	1
33251	1
33254	1
33255	1
33256	1
33257	1
33258	1
33259	1
33261	1
33262	1
33263	1
33264	1
33265	1
33266	1
33282	1
33284	1
33300	1
33305	1
33310	1
33315	1
33320	1
33321	1
33322	1
33330	1
33332	1
33335	1
33361	1
33362	1
33363	1
33364	1
33365	1
33366	1
33367	1
33368	1
33369	1
33400	1
33401	1
33403	1
33404	1
33405	1
33406	1
33410	1

CPT	MUE
33411	1
33412	1
33413	1
33414	1
33415	1
33416	1
33417	1
33420	1
33422	1
33425	1
33426	1
33427	1
33430	1
33460	1
33463	1
33464	1
33465	1
33468	1
33470	1
33471	1
33472	1
33474	1
33475	1
33476	1
33478	1
33496	1
33500	1
33501	1
33502	1
33503	1
33504	1
33505	1
33506	1
33507	1
33508	1
33510	1
33511	1
33512	1
33513	1
33514	1
33516	1
33517	1
33518	1
33519	1
33521	1
33522	1
33523	1
33530	1
33533	1
33534	1
33535	1
33536	1
33542	1
33545	1
33548	1
33572	3
33600	1
33602	1
33606	1
33608	1
33610	1
33611	1
33612	1
33615	1
33617	1

CPT	MUE
33619	1
33620	1
33621	1
33622	1
33641	1
33645	1
33647	1
33660	1
33665	1
33670	1
33675	1
33676	1
33677	1
33681	1
33684	1
33688	1
33690	1
33692	1
33694	1
33697	1
33702	1
33710	1
33720	1
33722	1
33724	1
33726	1
33730	1
33732	1
33735	1
33736	1
33737	1
33750	1
33755	1
33762	1
33764	1
33766	1
33767	1
33768	1
33770	1
33771	1
33774	1
33775	1
33776	1
33777	1
33778	1
33779	1
33780	1
33781	1
33782	1
33783	1
33786	1
33788	1
33800	1
33802	1
33803	1
33813	1
33814	1
33820	1
33822	1
33824	1
33840	1
33845	1
33851	1
33852	1
33853	1

CPT	MUE
33860	1
33863	1
33864	1
33870	1
33875	1
33877	1
33880	1
33881	1
33883	1
33884	3
33886	1
33889	1
33891	1
33910	1
33915	1
33916	1
33917	1
33920	1
33922	1
33924	1
33925	1
33926	1
33930	1
33933	1
33935	1
33940	1
33944	1
33945	1
33960	1
33961	1
33967	1
33968	1
33970	1
33971	1
33973	1
33974	1
33975	1
33976	1
33977	1
33978	1
33979	1
33980	1
33981	1
33982	1
33983	1
33990	1
33991	1
33992	1
33993	1
34001	1
34051	1
34101	1
34111	2
34151	2
34201	1
34203	1
34401	1
34421	1
34451	1
34471	1
34490	1
34501	1
34502	1
34510	2
34520	1

CPT	MUE
34530	1
34800	1
34802	1
34803	1
34804	1
34805	1
34806	1
34808	1
34812	1
34813	1
34820	1
34825	2
34826	4
34830	1
34831	1
34832	1
34833	1
34834	1
34841	1
34842	1
34843	1
34844	1
34845	1
34846	1
34847	1
34848	1
34900	1
35001	1
35002	1
35005	1
35011	1
35013	1
35021	1
35022	1
35045	2
35081	1
35082	1
35091	1
35092	1
35102	1
35103	1
35111	1
35112	1
35121	2
35122	1
35131	1
35132	1
35141	1
35142	1
35151	1
35152	1
35180	2
35182	2
35184	2
35188	2
35189	1
35190	2
35201	2
35206	2
35207	3
35211	3
35216	3
35221	3
35226	3
35231	2

CPT	MUE
35236	2
35241	2
35246	2
35251	2
35256	2
35261	1
35266	2
35271	2
35276	2
35281	2
35286	2
35301	2
35302	1
35303	1
35304	1
35305	1
35306	2
35311	1
35321	1
35331	1
35341	3
35351	1
35355	1
35361	1
35363	1
35371	1
35372	1
35390	1
35400	1
35450	2
35452	1
35458	3
35471	3
35472	1
35500	2
35501	1
35506	1
35508	1
35509	1
35510	1
35511	1
35512	1
35515	1
35516	1
35518	1
35521	1
35522	1
35523	1
35525	1
35526	1
35531	2
35533	1
35535	1
35536	1
35537	1
35538	1
35539	1
35540	1
35556	1
35558	1
35560	1
35563	1
35565	1
35566	1
35570	1

CPT	MUE
35571	2
35572	2
35583	1
35585	2
35587	2
35600	2
35601	1
35606	1
35612	1
35616	1
35621	1
35623	1
35626	3
35631	4
35632	1
35633	1
35634	1
35636	1
35637	1
35638	1
35642	1
35645	1
35646	1
35647	1
35650	1
35654	1
35656	1
35661	1
35663	1
35665	1
35666	2
35671	2
35681	1
35682	1
35683	1
35685	2
35686	1
35691	1
35693	1
35694	1
35695	1
35697	2
35700	2
35701	1
35721	1
35741	1
35761	2
35800	2
35820	2
35840	2
35860	2
35870	1
35875	2
35876	2
35879	2
35881	2
35883	1
35884	1
35901	1
35903	2
35905	1
35907	1
36002	2
36005	2
36010	2

CPT	MUE
36013	2
36014	2
36100	2
36120	2
36160	2
36200	2
36221	1
36222	1
36223	1
36224	1
36225	1
36226	1
36227	1
36251	1
36252	1
36253	1
36254	1
36260	1
36261	1
36262	1
36400	1
36405	1
36406	1
36410	3
36420	2
36425	1
36430	1
36440	1
36450	1
36455	1
36468	1
36469	1
36470	1
36471	1
36475	1
36478	1
36479	2
36481	1
36510	1
36511	1
36512	1
36513	1
36514	1
36515	1
36516	1
36522	1
36555	2
36556	2
36557	2
36558	2
36560	2
36561	2
36563	2
36565	2
36566	2
36568	2
36569	2
36570	2
36571	2
36575	2
36576	2
36578	2
36580	2
36581	2
36582	2

CPT	MUE
36583	2
36584	2
36585	2
36589	2
36590	2
36591	2
36592	1
36593	2
36595	2
36596	2
36597	2
36598	2
36620	3
36625	2
36640	1
36660	1
36680	1
36800	1
36810	1
36815	1
36818	1
36819	1
36820	1
36821	2
36822	1
36823	1
36825	1
36830	2
36831	1
36832	2
36833	1
36835	1
36838	1
36860	2
36861	2
36870	2
37140	1
37145	1
37160	1
37180	1
37181	1
37182	1
37183	1
37184	1
37185	2
37186	2
37187	1
37188	1
37191	1
37192	1
37193	1
37195	1
37197	2
37200	2
37211	1
37212	1
37213	1
37214	1
37215	1
37217	1
37220	2
37221	2
37222	2
37223	2
37224	2

CPT	MUE
37225	2
37226	2
37227	2
37228	2
37229	2
37230	2
37231	2
37232	2
37233	2
37234	2
37235	2
37236	1
37238	1
37250	1
37500	1
37565	1
37600	1
37605	1
37606	1
37607	1
37609	1
37615	2
37616	1
37617	3
37618	2
37619	1
37650	1
37660	1
37700	1
37718	1
37722	1
37735	1
37760	1
37761	1
37765	1
37766	1
37780	1
37785	1
37788	1
37790	1
38100	1
38101	1
38102	1
38115	1
38120	1
38200	1
38205	1
38206	1
38220	1
38221	1
38230	1
38232	1
38240	1
38241	1
38242	1
38243	1
38300	2
38305	2
38308	1
38380	1
38381	1
38382	1
38500	2
38505	3
38510	1

CPT	MUE
38520	1
38525	1
38530	1
38542	1
38550	1
38555	1
38562	1
38564	1
38570	1
38571	1
38572	1
38700	1
38720	1
38724	1
38740	1
38745	1
38746	1
38747	1
38760	1
38765	1
38770	1
38780	1
38790	1
38792	1
38794	1
38900	1
39000	1
39010	1
39200	1
39220	1
39400	1
39501	1
39503	1
39540	1
39541	1
39545	1
39560	1
39561	1
40490	3
40500	2
40510	2
40520	2
40525	2
40527	2
40530	2
40650	2
40652	2
40654	2
40700	1
40701	1
40702	1
40720	1
40761	1
40800	2
40801	2
40804	2
40805	2
40806	2
40808	4
40810	4
40812	4
40814	4
40816	2
40818	2
40819	2

CPT	MUE
40820	5
40830	2
40831	2
40840	1
40842	1
40843	1
40844	1
40845	1
41000	2
41005	2
41006	2
41007	2
41008	2
41009	2
41010	1
41015	2
41016	2
41017	2
41018	2
41019	1
41100	3
41105	3
41108	2
41110	2
41112	2
41113	2
41114	2
41115	1
41116	2
41120	1
41130	1
41135	1
41140	1
41145	1
41150	1
41153	1
41155	1
41250	2
41251	2
41252	2
41500	1
41510	1
41512	1
41520	1
41530	1
41800	2
41805	3
41806	3
41820	4
41821	2
41822	1
41823	1
41825	2
41826	2
41827	2
41828	4
41830	2
41850	2
41870	2
41872	4
41874	4
42000	1
42100	3
42104	3
42106	2

CPT	MUE
42107	2
42120	1
42140	1
42145	1
42160	2
42180	1
42182	1
42200	1
42205	1
42210	1
42215	1
42220	1
42225	1
42226	1
42227	1
42235	1
42260	1
42280	1
42281	1
42300	2
42305	2
42310	2
42320	2
42330	2
42335	2
42340	1
42400	2
42405	2
42408	1
42409	1
42410	1
42415	1
42420	1
42425	1
42426	1
42440	1
42450	2
42500	2
42505	2
42507	1
42508	1
42509	1
42510	1
42550	2
42600	2
42650	2
42660	2
42665	2
42700	2
42720	1
42725	1
42800	3
42804	3
42806	1
42808	2
42809	1
42810	1
42815	1
42820	1
42821	1
42825	1
42826	1
42830	1
42831	1
42835	1

CPT	MUE
42836	1
42842	1
42844	1
42845	1
42860	1
42870	1
42890	1
42892	1
42894	1
42900	1
42950	1
42953	1
42955	1
42960	1
42961	1
42962	1
42970	1
42971	1
42972	1
43020	1
43030	1
43045	1
43100	1
43101	1
43107	1
43108	1
43112	1
43113	1
43116	1
43117	1
43118	1
43121	1
43122	1
43123	1
43124	1
43130	1
43135	1
43191	1
43192	1
43193	1
43194	1
43195	1
43196	1
43197	1
43198	1
43200	1
43201	1
43202	1
43204	1
43205	1
43206	1
43211	1
43212	1
43213	1
43214	1
43215	1
43216	1
43217	1
43220	1
43226	1
43227	1
43229	1
43231	1
43232	1
43233	1

CPT	MUE
43235	1
43236	1
43237	1
43238	1
43239	1
43240	1
43241	1
43242	1
43243	1
43244	1
43245	1
43246	1
43247	1
43248	1
43249	1
43250	1
43251	1
43252	1
43253	1
43254	1
43255	2
43257	1
43259	1
43260	1
43261	1
43262	2
43263	1
43264	1
43265	1
43266	1
43270	1
43273	1
43275	1
43277	3
43278	1
43279	1
43280	1
43281	1
43282	1
43283	1
43300	1
43305	1
43310	1
43312	1
43313	1
43314	1
43320	1
43325	1
43327	1
43328	1
43330	1
43331	1
43332	1
43333	1
43334	1
43335	1
43336	1
43337	1
43338	1
43340	1
43341	1
43350	1
43351	1
43352	1
43360	1

CPT	MUE
43361	1
43400	1
43401	1
43405	1
43410	1
43415	1
43420	1
43425	1
43450	1
43453	1
43460	1
43496	1
43500	1
43501	1
43502	1
43510	1
43520	1
43605	1
43610	2
43611	2
43620	1
43621	1
43622	1
43631	1
43632	1
43633	1
43634	1
43635	1
43640	1
43641	1
43644	1
43645	1
43647	1
43648	1
43651	1
43652	1
43653	1
43752	2
43753	1
43754	1
43755	1
43756	1
43757	1
43760	2
43761	2
43770	1
43771	1
43772	1
43773	1
43774	1
43775	1
43800	1
43810	1
43820	1
43825	1
43830	1
43831	1
43832	1
43840	2
43843	1
43845	1
43846	1
43847	1
43848	1
43850	1

CPT	MUE
43855	1
43860	1
43865	1
43870	1
43880	1
43881	1
43882	1
43886	1
43887	1
43888	1
44005	1
44010	1
44015	1
44020	2
44021	1
44025	1
44050	1
44055	1
44100	1
44110	1
44111	1
44120	1
44121	4
44125	1
44126	1
44127	1
44128	2
44130	3
44132	1
44133	1
44135	1
44136	1
44137	1
44139	1
44140	2
44141	1
44143	1
44144	1
44145	1
44146	1
44147	1
44150	1
44151	1
44155	1
44156	1
44157	1
44158	1
44160	1
44180	1
44186	1
44187	1
44188	1
44202	1
44203	2
44204	2
44205	1
44206	1
44207	1
44208	1
44210	1
44211	1
44212	1
44213	1
44227	1
44300	1

CPT	MUE
44310	2
44312	1
44314	1
44316	1
44320	1
44322	1
44340	1
44345	1
44346	1
44360	1
44361	1
44363	1
44364	1
44365	1
44366	1
44369	1
44370	1
44372	1
44373	1
44376	1
44377	1
44378	1
44379	1
44380	1
44382	1
44383	1
44385	1
44386	1
44388	1
44389	1
44390	1
44391	1
44392	1
44393	1
44394	1
44397	1
44500	1
44602	1
44603	1
44604	1
44605	1
44615	4
44620	2
44625	1
44626	1
44640	2
44650	2
44660	1
44661	1
44680	1
44700	1
44701	1
44705	1
44715	1
44720	2
44721	2
44800	1
44820	1
44850	1
44900	1
44950	1
44955	1
44960	1
44970	1
45000	1

CPT	MUE
45005	1
45020	1
45100	2
45108	1
45110	1
45111	1
45112	1
45113	1
45114	1
45116	1
45119	1
45120	1
45121	1
45123	1
45126	1
45130	1
45135	1
45136	1
45150	1
45160	1
45171	2
45172	2
45190	1
45300	1
45303	1
45305	1
45307	1
45308	1
45309	1
45315	1
45317	1
45320	1
45321	1
45327	1
45330	1
45331	1
45332	1
45333	1
45334	1
45335	1
45337	1
45338	1
45339	1
45340	1
45341	1
45342	1
45345	1
45355	1
45378	1
45379	1
45380	1
45381	1
45382	1
45383	1
45384	1
45385	1
45386	1
45387	1
45391	1
45392	1
45395	1
45397	1
45400	1
45402	1
45500	1

CPT	MUE
45505	1
45520	1
45540	1
45541	1
45550	1
45560	1
45562	1
45563	1
45800	1
45805	1
45820	1
45825	1
45900	1
45905	1
45910	1
45915	1
45990	1
46020	2
46030	1
46040	2
46045	2
46050	2
46060	2
46070	1
46080	1
46083	2
46200	1
46220	1
46221	1
46230	1
46250	1
46255	1
46257	1
46258	1
46260	1
46261	1
46262	1
46270	1
46275	1
46280	1
46285	1
46288	1
46320	2
46500	1
46505	1
46600	1
46604	1
46606	1
46608	1
46610	1
46611	1
46612	1
46614	1
46615	1
46700	1
46705	1
46706	1
46707	1
46710	1
46712	1
46715	1
46716	1
46730	1
46735	1
46740	1

CPT	MUE
46742	1
46744	1
46746	1
46748	1
46750	1
46751	1
46753	1
46754	1
46760	1
46761	1
46762	1
46900	1
46910	1
46916	1
46917	1
46922	1
46924	1
46930	1
46940	1
46942	1
46945	1
46946	1
46947	1
47000	3
47001	3
47010	3
47015	1
47100	3
47120	2
47122	1
47125	1
47130	1
47133	1
47135	1
47136	1
47140	1
47141	1
47142	1
47143	1
47144	1
47145	1
47146	3
47147	2
47300	2
47350	1
47360	1
47361	1
47362	1
47370	1
47371	1
47380	1
47381	1
47382	1
47400	1
47420	1
47425	1
47460	1
47480	1
47490	1
47500	2
47505	2
47510	2
47511	2
47525	3
47530	2

CPT	MUE	CPT	MUE	CPT	MUE	CPT	MUE	CPT	MUE	CPT	MUE	CPT	MUE	CPT	MUE
47550	1	49002	1	49555	1	50360	1	50740	1	51701	2	52318	1	53449	1
47552	1	49010	1	49557	1	50365	1	50750	1	51702	2	52320	1	53450	1
47553	1	49020	2	49560	2	50370	1	50760	1	51703	2	52325	1	53460	1
47554	1	49040	2	49561	2	50380	1	50770	1	51705	1	52327	1	53500	1
47555	1	49060	2	49565	2	50382	1	50780	1	51710	1	52330	1	53502	1
47556	1	49062	1	49566	2	50384	1	50782	1	51715	1	52332	1	53505	1
47560	1	49082	1	49568	2	50385	1	50783	1	51720	1	52334	1	53510	1
47561	1	49083	2	49570	1	50386	1	50785	1	51725	1	52341	1	53515	1
47562	1	49084	1	49572	1	50387	1	50800	1	51726	1	52342	1	53520	1
47563	1	49180	2	49580	1	50389	1	50810	1	51727	1	52343	1	53600	1
47564	1	49203	1	49582	1	50390	2	50815	1	51728	1	52344	1	53601	1
47570	1	49204	1	49585	1	50391	1	50820	1	51729	1	52345	1	53605	1
47600	1	49205	1	49587	1	50392	1	50825	1	51736	1	52346	1	53620	1
47605	1	49215	1	49590	1	50393	1	50830	1	51741	1	52351	1	53621	1
47610	1	49220	1	49600	1	50394	1	50840	1	51784	1	52352	1	53660	1
47612	1	49250	1	49605	1	50395	1	50845	1	51785	1	52353	1	53661	1
47620	1	49255	1	49606	1	50396	1	50860	1	51792	1	52354	1	53665	1
47630	1	49320	1	49610	1	50398	1	50900	1	51797	1	52355	1	53850	1
47700	1	49321	1	49611	1	50400	1	50920	2	51798	1	52356	1	53852	1
47701	1	49322	1	49650	1	50405	1	50930	2	51800	1	52400	1	53855	1
47711	1	49323	1	49651	1	50500	1	50940	1	51820	1	52402	1	53860	1
47712	1	49324	1	49652	2	50520	1	50945	1	51840	1	52450	1	54000	1
47715	1	49325	1	49653	2	50525	1	50947	1	51841	1	52500	1	54001	1
47720	1	49326	1	49654	2	50526	1	50948	1	51845	1	52601	1	54015	1
47721	1	49327	1	49655	2	50540	1	50951	1	51860	1	52630	1	54050	1
47740	1	49400	1	49656	2	50541	1	50953	1	51865	1	52640	1	54055	1
47741	1	49402	1	49657	2	50542	1	50955	1	51880	1	52647	1	54056	1
47760	1	49411	1	49900	1	50543	1	50957	1	51900	1	52648	1	54057	1
47765	1	49412	1	49904	1	50544	1	50961	1	51920	1	52649	1	54060	1
47780	1	49418	1	49905	1	50545	1	50970	1	51925	1	52700	1	54065	1
47785	1	49419	1	49906	1	50546	1	50972	1	51940	1	53000	1	54100	2
47800	1	49421	1	50010	1	50547	1	50974	1	51960	1	53010	1	54105	2
47801	1	49422	1	50020	1	50548	1	50976	1	51980	1	53020	1	54110	1
47802	1	49423	2	50040	1	50551	1	50980	1	51990	1	53025	1	54111	1
47900	1	49424	3	50045	1	50553	1	51020	1	51992	1	53040	1	54112	1
48000	1	49425	1	50060	1	50555	1	51030	1	52000	1	53060	1	54115	1
48001	1	49426	1	50065	1	50557	1	51040	1	52001	1	53080	1	54120	1
48020	1	49427	1	50070	1	50561	1	51045	2	52005	2	53085	1	54125	1
48100	1	49428	1	50075	1	50562	1	51050	1	52007	1	53200	1	54130	1
48102	1	49429	1	50080	1	50570	1	51060	1	52010	1	53210	1	54135	1
48105	1	49435	1	50081	1	50572	1	51065	1	52204	1	53215	1	54150	1
48120	1	49436	1	50100	1	50574	1	51080	1	52214	1	53220	1	54160	1
48140	1	49440	1	50120	1	50575	1	51100	1	52224	1	53230	1	54161	1
48145	1	49441	1	50125	1	50576	1	51101	1	52234	1	53235	1	54162	1
48146	1	49442	1	50130	1	50580	1	51102	1	52235	1	53240	1	54163	1
48148	1	49446	1	50135	1	50590	1	51500	1	52240	1	53250	1	54164	1
48150	1	49450	1	50200	1	50592	1	51520	1	52250	1	53260	1	54200	1
48152	1	49451	1	50205	1	50593	1	51525	1	52260	1	53265	1	54205	1
48153	1	49452	1	50220	1	50600	1	51530	1	52265	1	53270	1	54220	1
48154	1	49460	1	50225	1	50605	1	51535	1	52270	1	53275	1	54230	1
48155	1	49465	1	50230	1	50610	1	51550	1	52275	1	53400	1	54231	1
48400	1	49491	1	50234	1	50620	1	51555	1	52276	1	53405	1	54235	1
48500	1	49492	1	50236	1	50630	1	51565	1	52277	1	53410	1	54240	1
48510	1	49495	1	50240	1	50650	1	51570	1	52281	1	53415	1	54250	1
48520	1	49496	1	50250	1	50660	1	51575	1	52282	1	53420	1	54300	1
48540	1	49500	1	50280	1	50684	1	51580	1	52283	1	53425	1	54304	1
48545	1	49501	1	50290	1	50686	2	51585	1	52285	1	53430	1	54308	1
48547	1	49505	1	50300	1	50688	2	51590	1	52287	1	53431	1	54312	1
48548	1	49507	1	50320	1	50690	2	51595	1	52290	1	53440	1	54316	1
48550	1	49520	1	50323	1	50700	1	51596	1	52300	1	53442	1	54318	1
48551	1	49521	1	50325	1	50715	1	51597	1	52301	1	53444	1	54322	1
48552	2	49525	1	50327	1	50722	1	51600	1	52305	1	53445	1	54324	1
48554	1	49540	1	50328	1	50725	1	51605	1	52310	1	53446	1	54326	1
48556	1	49550	1	50329	1	50727	1	51610	1	52315	2	53447	1	54328	1
49000	1	49553	1	50340	1	50728	1	51700	1	52317	1	53448	1	54332	1

CPT	MUE
54336	1
54340	1
54344	1
54348	1
54352	1
54360	1
54380	1
54385	1
54390	1
54400	1
54401	1
54405	1
54406	1
54408	1
54410	1
54411	1
54415	1
54416	1
54417	1
54420	1
54430	1
54435	1
54440	1
54450	1
54500	1
54505	1
54512	1
54520	1
54522	1
54530	1
54535	1
54550	1
54560	1
54600	1
54620	1
54640	1
54650	1
54660	1
54670	1
54680	1
54690	1
54692	1
54700	1
54800	1
54830	1
54840	1
54860	1
54861	1
54865	1
54900	1
54901	1
55000	1
55040	1
55041	1
55060	1
55100	2
55110	1
55120	1
55150	1
55175	1
55180	1
55200	1
55250	1
55300	1
55400	1

CPT	MUE
55450	1
55500	1
55520	1
55530	1
55535	1
55540	1
55550	1
55600	1
55605	1
55650	1
55680	1
55700	1
55705	1
55706	1
55720	1
55725	1
55801	1
55810	1
55812	1
55815	1
55821	1
55831	1
55840	1
55842	1
55845	1
55860	1
55862	1
55865	1
55866	1
55870	1
55873	1
55875	1
55876	1
55920	1
56405	2
56420	1
56440	1
56441	1
56442	1
56501	1
56515	1
56605	1
56606	6
56620	1
56625	1
56630	1
56631	1
56632	1
56633	1
56634	1
56637	1
56640	1
56700	1
56740	1
56800	1
56805	1
56810	1
56820	1
56821	1
57000	1
57010	1
57020	1
57022	1
57023	1
57061	1

CPT	MUE
57065	1
57100	3
57105	2
57106	1
57107	1
57109	1
57110	1
57111	1
57112	1
57120	1
57130	1
57135	2
57150	1
57155	1
57156	1
57160	1
57170	1
57180	1
57200	1
57210	1
57220	1
57230	1
57240	1
57250	1
57260	1
57265	1
57267	2
57268	1
57270	1
57280	1
57282	1
57283	1
57284	1
57285	1
57287	1
57288	1
57289	1
57291	1
57292	1
57295	1
57296	1
57300	1
57305	1
57307	1
57308	1
57310	1
57311	1
57320	1
57330	1
57335	1
57400	1
57410	1
57415	1
57420	1
57421	1
57423	1
57425	1
57426	1
57452	1
57454	1
57455	1
57456	1
57460	1
57461	1
57500	1

CPT	MUE
57505	1
57510	1
57511	1
57513	1
57520	1
57522	1
57530	1
57531	1
57540	1
57545	1
57550	1
57555	1
57556	1
57558	1
57700	1
57720	1
57800	1
58100	1
58110	1
58120	1
58140	1
58145	1
58146	1
58150	1
58152	1
58180	1
58200	1
58210	1
58240	1
58260	1
58262	1
58263	1
58267	1
58270	1
58275	1
58280	1
58285	1
58290	1
58291	1
58292	1
58293	1
58294	1
58301	1
58321	1
58322	1
58323	1
58340	1
58345	1
58346	1
58350	1
58353	1
58356	1
58400	1
58410	1
58520	1
58540	1
58541	1
58542	1
58543	1
58544	1
58545	1
58546	1
58548	1
58550	1
58552	1

CPT	MUE
58553	1
58554	1
58555	1
58558	1
58559	1
58560	1
58561	1
58562	1
58563	1
58565	1
58570	1
58571	1
58572	1
58573	1
58600	1
58605	1
58611	1
58615	1
58660	1
58661	1
58662	1
58670	1
58671	1
58672	1
58673	1
58700	1
58720	1
58740	1
58750	1
58752	1
58760	1
58770	1
58800	1
58805	1
58820	1
58822	1
58825	1
58900	1
58920	1
58925	1
58940	1
58943	1
58950	1
58951	1
58952	1
58953	1
58954	1
58956	1
58957	1
58958	1
58960	1
58970	1
58974	1
58976	2
59000	1
59001	1
59012	1
59015	1
59020	2
59025	3
59030	4
59050	1
59051	1
59070	2
59072	2

CPT	MUE
59074	1
59076	1
59100	1
59120	1
59121	1
59130	1
59135	1
59136	1
59140	1
59150	1
59151	1
59160	1
59200	1
59300	1
59320	1
59325	1
59350	1
59400	1
59409	2
59410	1
59412	1
59414	1
59425	1
59426	1
59430	1
59510	1
59514	1
59515	1
59525	1
59610	1
59612	2
59614	1
59618	1
59620	1
59622	1
59812	1
59820	1
59821	1
59830	1
59840	1
59841	1
59850	1
59851	1
59852	1
59855	1
59856	1
59857	1
59866	1
59870	1
59871	1
60000	1
60100	3
60200	2
60210	1
60212	1
60220	1
60225	1
60240	1
60252	1
60254	1
60260	1
60270	1
60271	1
60280	1
60281	1

CPT	MUE
60300	2
60500	1
60502	1
60505	1
60512	1
60520	1
60521	1
60522	1
60540	1
60545	1
60600	1
60605	1
60650	1
61000	1
61001	1
61020	2
61026	2
61050	1
61055	1
61070	2
61105	1
61107	1
61108	1
61120	1
61140	1
61150	1
61151	1
61154	1
61156	1
61210	1
61215	1
61250	1
61253	1
61304	1
61305	1
61312	2
61313	2
61314	2
61315	1
61316	1
61320	2
61321	1
61322	1
61323	1
61330	1
61332	1
61333	1
61334	1
61340	1
61343	1
61345	1
61440	1
61450	1
61458	1
61460	1
61470	1
61480	1
61490	1
61500	1
61501	1
61510	1
61512	1
61514	2
61516	1
61517	1

CPT	MUE
61518	1
61519	1
61520	1
61521	1
61522	1
61524	2
61526	1
61530	1
61531	1
61533	2
61534	1
61535	2
61536	1
61537	1
61538	1
61539	1
61540	1
61541	1
61542	1
61543	1
61544	1
61545	1
61546	1
61548	1
61550	1
61552	1
61556	1
61557	1
61558	1
61559	1
61563	2
61564	1
61566	1
61567	1
61570	1
61571	1
61575	1
61576	1
61580	1
61581	1
61582	1
61583	1
61584	1
61585	1
61586	1
61590	1
61591	1
61592	1
61595	1
61596	1
61597	1
61598	1
61600	1
61601	1
61605	1
61606	1
61607	1
61608	1
61609	1
61610	1
61611	1
61612	1
61613	1
61615	1
61616	1

CPT	MUE
61618	2
61619	2
61623	2
61624	2
61626	2
61630	1
61635	2
61680	1
61682	1
61684	1
61686	1
61690	1
61692	1
61697	2
61698	1
61700	2
61702	1
61703	1
61705	1
61708	1
61710	1
61711	1
61720	1
61735	1
61750	2
61751	2
61760	1
61770	1
61781	1
61782	1
61783	1
61790	1
61791	1
61796	1
61797	4
61798	1
61799	4
61800	1
61850	1
61860	1
61863	1
61864	1
61867	1
61868	2
61870	1
61875	1
61880	1
61885	1
61886	1
61888	1
62000	1
62005	1
62010	1
62100	1
62115	1
62116	1
62117	1
62120	1
62121	1
62140	1
62141	1
62142	2
62143	2
62145	2
62146	2

CPT	MUE
62147	1
62148	1
62160	1
62161	1
62162	1
62163	1
62164	1
62165	1
62180	1
62190	1
62192	1
62194	1
62200	1
62201	1
62220	1
62223	1
62225	2
62230	2
62252	2
62256	1
62258	1
62263	1
62264	1
62267	2
62268	1
62269	2
62270	2
62272	1
62273	2
62280	1
62281	1
62282	1
62284	1
62287	1
62290	5
62291	4
62292	1
62294	1
62310	1
62311	1
62318	1
62319	1
62350	1
62351	1
62355	1
62360	1
62361	1
62362	1
62365	1
62367	1
62368	1
62369	1
62370	1
63001	1
63003	1
63005	1
63011	1
63012	1
63015	1
63016	1
63017	1
63020	1
63030	1
63035	4
63040	1

CPT	MUE
63042	1
63043	4
63044	4
63045	1
63046	1
63047	1
63048	5
63050	1
63051	1
63055	1
63056	1
63057	3
63064	1
63066	1
63075	1
63076	3
63077	1
63078	3
63081	1
63082	6
63085	1
63086	2
63087	1
63088	4
63090	1
63091	3
63101	1
63102	1
63103	3
63170	1
63172	1
63173	1
63180	1
63182	1
63185	1
63190	1
63191	1
63194	1
63195	1
63196	1
63197	1
63198	1
63199	1
63200	1
63250	1
63251	1
63252	1
63265	1
63266	1
63267	1
63268	1
63270	1
63271	1
63272	1
63273	1
63275	1
63276	1
63277	1
63278	1
63280	1
63281	1
63282	1
63283	1
63285	1
63286	1

CPT	MUE
63287	1
63290	1
63295	1
63300	1
63301	1
63302	1
63303	1
63304	1
63305	1
63306	1
63307	1
63308	3
63600	2
63610	1
63615	1
63620	1
63621	2
63650	2
63655	1
63661	1
63662	1
63663	1
63664	1
63685	1
63688	1
63700	1
63702	1
63704	1
63706	1
63707	1
63709	1
63710	1
63740	1
63741	1
63744	1
63746	1
64400	4
64402	1
64405	1
64408	1
64410	1
64412	1
64413	1
64415	1
64416	1
64417	1
64418	1
64420	3
64421	3
64425	1
64430	1
64435	1
64445	1
64446	1
64447	1
64448	1
64449	1
64450	10
64455	1
64479	1
64480	4
64483	1
64484	4
64490	1
64491	1

CPT	MUE
64492	1
64493	1
64494	1
64495	1
64505	1
64508	1
64510	1
64517	1
64520	1
64530	1
64550	1
64553	1
64555	2
64561	1
64565	2
64566	1
64568	1
64569	1
64570	1
64575	2
64580	2
64581	2
64585	2
64590	1
64595	1
64600	2
64605	1
64610	1
64611	1
64612	1
64615	1
64616	1
64617	1
64620	5
64630	1
64632	1
64633	1
64635	1
64640	5
64642	1
64643	3
64644	1
64645	3
64646	1
64647	1
64650	1
64653	1
64680	1
64681	1
64702	2
64704	4
64708	3
64712	1
64713	1
64714	1
64716	2
64718	1
64719	1
64721	1
64722	4
64726	2
64727	2
64732	1
64734	1
64736	1

CPT	MUE
64738	1
64740	1
64742	1
64744	1
64746	1
64752	1
64755	1
64760	1
64761	1
64763	1
64766	1
64771	2
64772	2
64774	2
64776	1
64778	1
64782	2
64783	2
64784	3
64786	1
64787	4
64788	5
64790	1
64792	2
64795	2
64802	1
64804	1
64809	1
64818	1
64820	4
64821	1
64822	1
64823	1
64831	1
64832	3
64834	1
64835	1
64836	1
64837	2
64840	1
64856	2
64857	2
64858	1
64859	2
64861	1
64862	1
64864	2
64865	1
64866	1
64868	1
64870	1
64872	1
64874	1
64876	1
64885	1
64886	1
64890	2
64891	2
64892	2
64893	2
64895	2
64896	2
64897	2
64898	2
64901	2

CPT	MUE
64902	1
64905	1
64907	1
64910	3
64911	2
65091	1
65093	1
65101	1
65103	1
65105	1
65110	1
65112	1
65114	1
65125	1
65130	1
65135	1
65140	1
65150	1
65155	1
65175	1
65205	1
65210	1
65220	1
65222	1
65235	1
65260	1
65265	1
65270	1
65272	1
65273	1
65275	1
65280	1
65285	1
65286	1
65290	1
65400	1
65410	1
65420	1
65426	1
65430	1
65435	1
65436	1
65450	1
65600	1
65710	1
65730	1
65750	1
65755	1
65756	1
65757	1
65770	1
65772	1
65775	1
65778	1
65779	1
65780	1
65781	1
65782	1
65800	1
65810	1
65815	1
65820	1
65850	1
65855	1
65860	1

CPT	MUE
65865	1
65870	1
65875	1
65880	1
65900	1
65920	1
65930	1
66020	1
66030	1
66130	1
66150	1
66155	1
66160	1
66165	1
66170	1
66172	1
66174	1
66175	1
66180	1
66183	1
66185	1
66220	1
66225	1
66250	1
66500	1
66505	1
66600	1
66605	1
66625	1
66630	1
66635	1
66680	1
66682	1
66700	1
66710	1
66711	1
66720	1
66740	1
66761	1
66762	1
66770	1
66820	1
66821	1
66825	1
66830	1
66840	1
66850	1
66852	1
66920	1
66930	1
66940	1
66982	1
66983	1
66984	1
66985	1
66986	1
66990	1
67005	1
67010	1
67015	1
67025	1
67027	1
67028	1
67030	1
67031	1

Appendix L — Medically Unlikely Edits (MUEs) — Professional

CPT	MUE
67036	1
67039	1
67040	1
67041	1
67042	1
67043	1
67101	1
67105	1
67107	1
67108	1
67110	1
67112	1
67113	1
67115	1
67120	1
67121	1
67141	1
67145	1
67208	1
67210	1
67218	1
67220	1
67221	1
67225	1
67227	1
67228	1
67229	1
67250	1
67255	1
67311	1
67312	1
67314	1
67316	1
67318	1
67320	2
67331	1
67332	1
67334	1
67335	1
67340	2
67343	1
67345	1
67346	1
67400	1
67405	1
67412	1
67413	1
67414	1
67415	1
67420	1
67430	1
67440	1
67445	1
67450	1
67500	1
67505	1
67515	1
67550	1
67560	1
67570	1
67700	2
67710	1
67715	1
67800	1
67801	1

CPT	MUE
67805	1
67808	1
67810	2
67820	1
67825	1
67830	1
67835	1
67840	4
67850	3
67875	1
67880	1
67882	1
67900	1
67901	1
67902	1
67903	1
67904	1
67906	1
67908	1
67909	1
67911	4
67912	1
67914	1
67915	1
67916	1
67917	1
67921	1
67922	1
67923	1
67924	1
67930	2
67935	2
67938	2
67950	2
67961	4
67966	4
67971	1
67973	1
67974	1
67975	1
68020	1
68040	1
68100	1
68110	1
68115	1
68130	1
68135	1
68200	1
68320	1
68325	1
68326	2
68328	2
68330	1
68335	1
68340	1
68360	1
68362	1
68371	1
68400	1
68420	1
68440	2
68500	1
68505	1
68510	1
68520	1

CPT	MUE
68525	1
68530	1
68540	1
68550	1
68700	1
68705	2
68720	1
68745	1
68750	1
68760	4
68761	4
68770	1
68801	4
68810	1
68811	1
68815	1
68816	1
68840	1
68850	1
69000	1
69005	1
69020	1
69100	3
69105	1
69110	1
69120	1
69140	1
69145	1
69150	1
69155	1
69200	1
69205	1
69210	1
69220	1
69222	1
69300	1
69310	1
69320	1
69400	1
69401	1
69405	1
69420	1
69421	1
69424	1
69433	1
69436	1
69440	1
69450	1
69501	1
69502	1
69505	1
69511	1
69530	1
69535	1
69540	1
69550	1
69552	1
69554	1
69601	1
69602	1
69603	1
69604	1
69605	1
69610	1
69620	1

CPT	MUE
69631	1
69632	1
69633	1
69635	1
69636	1
69637	1
69641	1
69642	1
69643	1
69644	1
69645	1
69646	1
69650	1
69660	1
69661	1
69662	1
69666	1
69667	1
69670	1
69676	1
69700	1
69711	1
69714	1
69715	1
69717	1
69718	1
69720	1
69725	1
69740	1
69745	1
69801	1
69805	1
69806	1
69820	1
69840	1
69905	1
69910	1
69915	1
69930	1
69950	1
69955	1
69960	1
69970	1
69990	1
70010	1
70015	1
70030	2
70100	1
70110	1
70120	2
70130	2
70134	1
70140	1
70150	1
70160	1
70170	2
70190	1
70200	1
70210	1
70220	1
70240	1
70250	1
70260	1
70300	1
70310	1

CPT	MUE
70320	1
70328	1
70330	1
70332	2
70336	1
70350	1
70355	1
70360	1
70370	1
70371	1
70373	1
70380	2
70390	2
70450	3
70460	1
70470	2
70480	1
70481	1
70482	1
70486	1
70487	1
70488	1
70490	1
70491	1
70492	1
70496	1
70498	1
70540	1
70542	1
70543	1
70544	1
70545	1
70546	1
70547	1
70548	1
70549	1
70551	1
70552	1
70553	1
70554	1
70555	1
70557	1
70558	1
70559	1
71015	2
71021	1
71022	1
71023	2
71030	2
71034	1
71035	2
71100	1
71101	1
71110	1
71111	1
71120	1
71130	1
71250	1
71260	1
71270	1
71275	1
71550	1
71551	1
71552	1
71555	1

CPT	MUE
72010	1
72020	4
72040	3
72050	1
72052	1
72069	1
72070	1
72072	1
72074	1
72080	1
72090	1
72100	1
72110	1
72114	1
72120	1
72125	1
72126	1
72127	1
72128	1
72129	1
72130	1
72131	1
72132	1
72133	1
72141	1
72142	1
72146	1
72147	1
72148	1
72149	1
72156	1
72157	1
72158	1
72170	1
72190	1
72191	1
72192	1
72193	1
72194	1
72195	1
72196	1
72197	1
72198	1
72200	1
72202	1
72220	1
72240	1
72255	1
72265	1
72270	1
72275	3
72292	3
73000	2
73010	2
73020	2
73030	2
73040	2
73050	1
73060	2
73070	2
73080	2
73085	2
73090	2
73092	2
73100	2

CPT	MUE
73110	2
73115	2
73120	2
73130	2
73140	2
73200	2
73201	2
73202	2
73206	2
73218	2
73219	2
73220	2
73221	2
73222	2
73223	2
73500	1
73510	2
73520	2
73525	2
73530	2
73540	1
73550	2
73560	2
73562	2
73564	2
73565	1
73580	2
73590	2
73592	2
73600	2
73610	2
73615	2
73620	2
73630	2
73650	2
73660	2
73700	2
73701	2
73702	2
73706	2
73718	2
73719	2
73720	2
73721	4
73722	2
73723	4
73725	2
74000	3
74010	2
74020	2
74022	2
74150	1
74160	1
74170	1
74174	1
74175	1
74176	1
74177	1
74178	1
74181	1
74182	1
74183	1
74185	1
74190	1
74210	1

CPT	MUE
74220	1
74230	1
74235	1
74240	1
74241	1
74245	1
74246	1
74247	1
74249	1
74250	1
74251	1
74260	1
74261	1
74262	1
74270	1
74280	1
74283	1
74290	1
74291	1
74300	1
74301	2
74305	1
74320	1
74327	1
74328	1
74329	1
74330	1
74340	1
74355	1
74360	1
74363	2
74400	1
74410	1
74415	1
74420	2
74425	1
74430	1
74440	1
74445	1
74450	1
74455	1
74470	2
74475	2
74480	2
74485	2
74710	1
74740	1
74742	2
74775	1
75557	1
75559	1
75561	1
75563	1
75565	1
75571	1
75572	1
75573	1
75574	1
75600	1
75605	1
75625	1
75630	1
75635	1
75658	2
75710	1

CPT	MUE
75716	1
75726	3
75731	1
75733	1
75736	2
75741	1
75743	1
75746	1
75756	2
75791	1
75801	1
75803	1
75805	1
75807	1
75809	1
75810	1
75820	1
75822	1
75825	1
75827	1
75831	1
75833	1
75840	1
75842	1
75860	2
75870	1
75872	1
75880	2
75885	1
75887	1
75889	1
75891	1
75896	3
75898	1
75901	1
75902	2
75945	1
75952	1
75953	4
75954	2
75956	1
75957	1
75958	2
75959	1
75962	1
75964	4
75966	1
75968	2
75970	2
75980	1
75982	2
75984	2
75989	2
76000	3
76001	2
76010	2
76080	2
76100	2
76101	1
76102	1
76120	1
76125	1
76376	2
76377	2
76380	1

CPT	MUE
76506	1
76510	2
76511	2
76512	2
76513	2
76514	1
76516	1
76519	2
76529	2
76536	1
76604	1
76645	1
76700	1
76705	2
76770	1
76775	2
76776	1
76800	1
76801	1
76802	3
76805	1
76810	3
76811	1
76812	3
76813	1
76814	3
76815	1
76817	1
76830	1
76831	1
76856	1
76857	1
76870	1
76872	1
76873	1
76881	2
76882	2
76885	1
76886	1
76930	1
76932	1
76936	2
76937	2
76940	1
76942	1
76945	1
76946	1
76948	1
76950	1
76965	2
76970	1
76975	1
76977	1
76998	1
77001	1
77002	1
77003	1
77011	1
77012	1
77013	1
77014	2
77021	1
77022	1
77051	1
77052	1

CPT	MUE
77053	2
77054	2
77055	1
77056	1
77057	1
77058	1
77059	1
77071	1
77072	1
77073	1
77074	1
77075	1
77076	1
77077	1
77078	1
77080	1
77081	1
77082	1
77084	1
77261	1
77262	1
77263	1
77280	2
77285	1
77290	1
77293	1
77295	1
77300	10
77301	1
77305	2
77310	2
77315	2
77321	1
77326	1
77327	1
77328	1
77332	4
77333	4
77336	1
77338	1
77370	1
77371	1
77372	1
77373	1
77401	2
77402	2
77403	2
77404	2
77406	2
77407	2
77408	2
77409	2
77411	2
77412	2
77413	2
77414	2
77416	2
77417	1
77418	2
77421	2
77422	1
77423	1
77424	1
77425	1
77427	1

CPT	MUE
77431	1
77432	1
77435	1
77469	1
77470	1
77520	1
77522	1
77523	1
77525	1
77600	1
77605	1
77610	1
77615	1
77620	1
77750	1
77761	1
77762	1
77763	1
77776	1
77777	1
77778	1
77785	3
77786	3
77787	3
77789	2
77790	2
78012	1
78013	1
78014	1
78015	1
78016	1
78018	1
78020	1
78070	1
78071	1
78072	1
78075	1
78102	1
78103	1
78104	1
78110	1
78111	1
78120	1
78121	1
78122	1
78130	1
78135	1
78140	1
78185	1
78190	1
78191	1
78195	1
78201	1
78202	1
78205	1
78206	1
78215	1
78216	1
78226	1
78227	1
78230	1
78231	1
78232	1
78258	1
78261	1

CPT	MUE
78262	1
78264	1
78267	1
78268	1
78270	1
78271	1
78272	1
78278	2
78282	1
78290	1
78291	1
78300	1
78305	1
78306	1
78315	1
78320	1
78414	1
78428	1
78445	1
78451	1
78452	1
78453	1
78454	1
78456	1
78457	1
78458	1
78459	1
78466	1
78468	1
78469	1
78472	1
78473	1
78481	1
78483	1
78491	1
78492	1
78494	1
78496	1
78579	1
78580	1
78582	1
78597	1
78598	1
78600	1
78601	1
78605	1
78606	2
78607	1
78608	1
78610	1
78630	2
78635	1
78645	1
78647	1
78650	1
78660	1
78700	1
78701	2
78707	1
78708	1
78709	1
78710	1
78725	1
78730	1
78740	1

CPT	MUE
78761	1
78800	1
78801	1
78802	1
78803	1
78804	1
78805	1
78806	1
78807	1
78808	1
78811	1
78812	1
78813	1
78814	1
78815	1
78816	1
79005	1
79101	1
79200	1
79300	1
79403	1
79440	1
79445	1
80047	2
80048	2
80051	2
80053	1
80061	1
80069	1
80074	1
80076	1
80100	0
80101	0
80102	10
80103	2
80104	1
80150	2
80152	2
80154	2
80156	2
80157	2
80158	2
80160	2
80162	2
80164	2
80166	2
80168	2
80170	2
80172	2
80173	2
80174	2
80176	1
80178	2
80182	2
80184	2
80185	2
80186	2
80188	2
80190	2
80192	2
80194	2
80195	2
80197	2
80198	2
80200	2

CPT	MUE
80201	2
80202	2
80299	3
80400	1
80402	1
80406	1
80408	1
80410	1
80412	1
80414	1
80415	1
80416	1
80417	1
80418	1
80420	1
80422	1
80424	1
80426	1
80428	1
80430	1
80432	1
80434	1
80435	1
80436	1
80438	1
80439	1
80440	1
80500	1
80502	1
81000	2
81001	2
81002	2
81003	2
81005	2
81007	1
81015	2
81020	1
81025	1
81050	2
81161	1
81200	1
81201	1
81202	1
81203	1
81205	1
81206	1
81207	1
81208	1
81209	1
81210	1
81211	1
81212	1
81213	1
81214	1
81215	2
81216	1
81217	2
81220	1
81221	1
81222	1
81223	1
81224	1
81225	1
81226	1
81227	1

CPT	MUE
81228	1
81229	1
81235	1
81240	1
81241	1
81242	1
81243	1
81244	1
81245	1
81250	1
81251	1
81252	1
81253	1
81254	1
81255	1
81256	1
81257	1
81260	1
81261	1
81262	1
81263	1
81264	1
81265	1
81266	3
81267	1
81270	1
81275	1
81280	1
81281	1
81282	1
81287	1
81290	1
81291	1
81292	1
81293	1
81294	1
81295	1
81296	1
81297	1
81298	1
81299	1
81300	1
81301	1
81302	1
81303	1
81304	1
81310	1
81315	1
81316	1
81317	1
81318	1
81319	1
81321	1
81322	1
81323	1
81324	1
81325	1
81326	1
81330	1
81331	1
81332	1
81340	1
81341	1
81342	1
81350	1

Appendix L — Medically Unlikely Edits (MUEs) — Professional

CPT	MUE
81355	1
81370	1
81371	1
81372	1
81373	2
81374	3
81375	1
81377	3
81378	1
81379	1
81380	2
81383	3
81400	2
81401	2
81402	1
81403	4
81404	5
81405	2
81406	2
81407	1
81408	2
81500	1
81503	1
81504	1
81506	1
81507	1
81508	1
81509	1
81510	1
81511	1
81512	1
82000	1
82003	2
82009	1
82010	4
82013	1
82016	1
82017	1
82030	1
82040	1
82042	2
82043	1
82044	1
82045	1
82055	2
82075	2
82085	1
82088	2
82101	1
82103	1
82104	1
82105	1
82106	4
82107	1
82108	1
82120	1
82127	2
82128	2
82131	3
82135	1
82136	3
82139	3
82140	2
82143	2
82145	2

CPT	MUE
82150	4
82154	1
82157	1
82160	1
82163	1
82164	1
82172	3
82175	2
82180	1
82190	4
82205	2
82232	2
82239	1
82240	1
82247	2
82248	2
82252	1
82261	1
82270	1
82271	1
82272	1
82274	1
82286	1
82300	1
82306	1
82308	3
82310	2
82330	2
82331	1
82340	1
82355	3
82360	3
82365	3
82370	3
82373	1
82374	2
82375	1
82376	1
82378	1
82379	1
82380	1
82382	1
82383	1
82384	2
82387	1
82390	1
82415	1
82435	2
82436	1
82438	1
82441	1
82465	1
82480	2
82482	1
82485	1
82486	2
82487	2
82488	1
82489	2
82491	4
82492	2
82495	1
82507	1
82520	2
82523	1

CPT	MUE
82525	2
82528	1
82530	2
82540	1
82542	6
82543	2
82544	2
82550	3
82552	3
82553	3
82554	1
82565	2
82570	3
82575	1
82585	1
82595	1
82600	1
82607	1
82608	1
82610	1
82615	1
82626	1
82627	1
82633	1
82634	1
82638	1
82646	1
82649	1
82651	1
82652	1
82654	1
82656	1
82657	3
82658	2
82666	1
82668	1
82670	2
82671	1
82672	1
82677	1
82679	1
82690	1
82693	2
82696	1
82705	1
82710	1
82715	3
82725	1
82726	1
82728	1
82731	1
82735	1
82742	1
82746	1
82747	1
82757	1
82759	1
82760	1
82775	1
82776	1
82777	1
82784	6
82785	1
82787	4
82800	1

CPT	MUE
82805	2
82820	1
82930	1
82941	1
82943	1
82946	1
82950	3
82951	1
82952	3
82953	1
82955	1
82960	1
82963	1
82965	1
82975	1
82977	1
82978	1
82979	1
82980	1
82985	1
83003	5
83008	1
83009	1
83010	1
83012	1
83013	1
83014	1
83015	1
83018	7
83020	2
83021	2
83026	1
83030	1
83033	1
83036	1
83037	1
83045	1
83050	1
83051	1
83055	1
83060	1
83065	1
83068	1
83069	1
83070	1
83071	1
83080	2
83088	1
83090	2
83150	1
83491	1
83497	1
83498	2
83499	1
83500	1
83505	1
83518	2
83525	4
83527	1
83528	1
83540	2
83550	1
83570	1
83582	1
83586	1

CPT	MUE
83593	1
83605	3
83615	2
83625	1
83630	1
83631	1
83632	1
83633	1
83634	1
83655	2
83661	4
83662	4
83663	4
83664	4
83670	1
83690	2
83695	1
83698	1
83700	1
83701	1
83704	1
83718	1
83719	1
83721	1
83727	1
83735	4
83775	1
83785	1
83788	3
83789	4
83805	2
83825	2
83835	2
83840	2
83857	1
83858	1
83861	2
83864	1
83866	1
83872	2
83873	1
83874	2
83876	1
83880	1
83885	2
83887	2
83915	1
83916	2
83918	2
83919	1
83921	2
83925	4
83930	2
83935	2
83937	1
83945	2
83950	1
83951	1
83970	2
83986	2
83987	1
83992	2
83993	1
84022	2
84030	1

CPT	MUE
84035	1
84060	1
84061	1
84066	1
84075	2
84078	1
84080	1
84081	1
84085	1
84087	1
84100	3
84105	1
84106	1
84110	1
84112	1
84119	1
84120	1
84126	1
84127	1
84132	3
84133	2
84134	1
84135	1
84138	1
84140	1
84143	2
84144	1
84145	1
84146	3
84150	2
84152	1
84153	1
84154	1
84155	1
84156	1
84157	3
84160	2
84163	1
84165	1
84166	2
84202	1
84203	1
84206	1
84207	1
84210	1
84220	1
84228	1
84233	2
84234	2
84235	1
84238	3
84252	1
84255	2
84260	1
84270	1
84275	1
84285	1
84295	3
84300	2
84302	1
84305	1
84307	1
84311	2
84315	2
84375	1

CPT	MUE
84376	1
84377	1
84378	2
84379	1
84392	1
84402	1
84403	2
84425	1
84430	1
84431	1
84432	1
84436	1
84437	1
84439	1
84442	1
84443	4
84445	1
84446	1
84449	1
84450	1
84460	1
84466	1
84478	1
84479	1
84480	1
84481	1
84482	1
84484	2
84485	1
84488	1
84490	1
84510	1
84512	1
84520	4
84525	1
84540	2
84545	1
84550	1
84560	2
84577	1
84578	1
84580	1
84583	1
84585	1
84586	1
84588	1
84590	1
84591	1
84597	1
84600	2
84620	1
84630	2
84681	1
84702	2
84703	1
84704	1
84830	1
85002	1
85004	2
85007	1
85008	1
85009	1
85013	2
85014	2
85018	2

CPT	MUE
85025	2
85032	3
85041	2
85044	1
85045	1
85046	1
85048	2
85049	2
85055	1
85060	1
85097	2
85130	1
85170	1
85175	1
85210	2
85220	2
85230	2
85240	2
85244	1
85245	2
85246	2
85247	2
85250	2
85260	2
85270	2
85280	2
85290	2
85291	1
85292	1
85293	1
85300	2
85301	1
85302	1
85303	2
85305	2
85306	2
85307	2
85335	2
85337	1
85345	1
85347	5
85348	1
85360	1
85362	2
85366	1
85370	1
85378	1
85379	2
85380	1
85384	2
85385	1
85390	3
85396	1
85400	1
85410	1
85415	2
85420	2
85421	1
85441	1
85445	1
85460	1
85461	1
85475	1
85525	2
85530	1

CPT	MUE
85536	1
85540	1
85547	1
85549	1
85555	1
85557	1
85597	1
85598	1
85611	2
85612	1
85613	1
85635	1
85651	1
85652	1
85660	1
85670	2
85675	1
85705	1
85732	4
85810	2
86021	1
86022	1
86023	3
86038	1
86039	1
86060	1
86063	1
86077	1
86078	1
86079	1
86140	1
86141	1
86146	3
86147	4
86148	3
86152	1
86153	1
86155	1
86156	1
86157	1
86160	4
86161	3
86162	1
86171	2
86200	1
86215	1
86225	1
86226	1
86243	1
86277	1
86280	1
86294	1
86300	2
86301	1
86304	1
86305	1
86308	1
86309	1
86310	1
86316	3
86320	1
86325	2
86327	1
86332	1
86334	1

CPT	MUE
86335	2
86336	1
86337	1
86340	1
86341	1
86343	1
86344	1
86352	1
86355	1
86357	1
86359	1
86360	1
86361	1
86367	1
86376	2
86378	1
86382	3
86384	1
86386	1
86406	2
86430	2
86431	2
86480	1
86481	1
86485	1
86486	2
86490	1
86510	1
86580	1
86590	1
86592	2
86593	2
86602	3
86603	2
86612	2
86617	2
86618	2
86619	2
86625	2
86628	3
86632	3
86641	2
86644	1
86645	1
86648	2
86651	2
86652	2
86653	2
86654	2
86663	2
86664	2
86665	2
86668	2
86674	3
86677	3
86684	2
86687	2
86688	2
86689	2
86692	2
86694	2
86695	2
86696	2
86698	3
86701	2

CPT	MUE
86702	2
86703	1
86704	1
86705	1
86706	2
86707	1
86708	1
86709	1
86711	2
86713	3
86720	2
86723	2
86727	2
86732	2
86738	2
86741	2
86744	2
86747	2
86750	4
86753	3
86756	2
86759	2
86762	2
86768	5
86771	2
86774	2
86777	2
86778	2
86780	2
86784	2
86787	2
86788	2
86789	2
86793	2
86800	1
86803	1
86804	1
86807	2
86808	1
86812	1
86813	1
86816	1
86817	1
86821	1
86822	1
86825	1
86828	2
86829	2
86830	2
86831	2
86832	2
86833	1
86834	1
86835	1
86850	3
86860	2
86880	4
86885	3
86886	3
86890	1
86891	1
86900	1
86901	1
86904	2
86906	1

CPT	MUE
86921	2
86927	2
86930	2
86932	2
86940	1
86941	1
86945	3
86950	1
86960	1
86965	1
86970	1
86975	2
86976	2
86977	2
86978	1
86985	1
87001	1
87003	1
87040	2
87045	3
87070	3
87073	3
87084	2
87086	3
87103	3
87109	3
87110	2
87116	2
87118	3
87143	2
87158	1
87164	2
87166	2
87168	2
87169	2
87172	1
87176	2
87177	3
87187	3
87197	1
87205	3
87207	3
87220	3
87230	3
87250	3
87253	2
87255	2
87260	1
87265	1
87267	1
87269	1
87270	1
87271	1
87272	1
87273	1
87274	1
87275	1
87276	1
87277	1
87278	1
87279	1
87280	1
87281	1
87283	1
87285	1

CPT	MUE
87290	1
87299	1
87301	1
87305	1
87320	1
87324	1
87327	1
87328	1
87329	1
87332	1
87335	1
87336	1
87337	1
87338	1
87339	1
87340	1
87341	1
87350	1
87380	1
87385	1
87389	1
87390	1
87391	1
87400	2
87420	1
87425	1
87427	2
87430	1
87449	3
87450	2
87451	2
87470	1
87471	1
87472	1
87475	1
87476	1
87477	1
87480	1
87481	1
87482	1
87485	1
87486	1
87487	1
87490	1
87491	1
87492	1
87493	1
87495	1
87496	1
87497	1
87498	1
87500	1
87501	1
87502	1
87503	1
87510	1
87511	1
87512	1
87515	1
87516	1
87517	1
87520	1
87521	1
87522	1
87525	1

CPT	MUE
87526	1
87527	1
87528	1
87529	1
87530	1
87531	1
87532	1
87533	1
87534	1
87535	1
87536	1
87537	1
87538	1
87539	1
87540	1
87541	1
87542	1
87550	1
87551	1
87552	1
87555	1
87556	1
87557	1
87560	1
87561	1
87562	1
87580	1
87581	1
87582	1
87590	1
87591	1
87592	1
87620	1
87621	1
87622	1
87631	1
87632	1
87633	1
87640	1
87641	1
87650	1
87651	1
87652	1
87653	1
87660	1
87661	1
87797	3
87799	3
87800	2
87802	2
87803	3
87804	2
87807	2
87808	1
87810	2
87850	1
87880	2
87900	1
87901	1
87902	1
87903	1
87905	2
87906	2
87910	1
87912	1

CPT	MUE
88104	4
88106	3
88120	2
88121	2
88125	1
88130	1
88140	1
88141	1
88142	1
88143	1
88147	1
88148	1
88150	1
88152	1
88153	1
88154	1
88155	1
88160	4
88161	4
88162	3
88164	1
88165	1
88166	1
88167	1
88172	3
88173	3
88174	1
88175	1
88177	2
88182	2
88184	1
88187	1
88188	1
88189	1
88230	2
88233	3
88239	3
88240	3
88241	3
88245	1
88248	1
88249	1
88261	2
88262	2
88263	1
88264	2
88267	2
88269	2
88273	3
88283	2
88289	1
88291	1
88300	2
88302	2
88309	3
88311	4
88321	1
88323	1
88325	1
88329	4
88331	11
88333	4
88342	0
88343	0
88347	4

CPT	MUE
88348	1
88349	1
88355	1
88356	1
88358	2
88360	6
88361	6
88362	1
88363	1
88371	1
88372	1
88375	1
88380	1
88381	1
88387	3
88388	3
88720	1
88738	1
88740	1
88741	1
89049	1
89050	2
89051	2
89055	2
89060	2
89125	2
89160	1
89190	1
89220	1
89230	1
89250	1
89251	1
89253	1
89254	1
89255	1
89257	1
89258	1
89259	1
89260	1
89261	1
89264	1
89268	1
89272	1
89280	1
89281	1
89290	1
89291	1
89300	1
89310	1
89320	1
89321	1
89322	1
89325	1
89329	1
89330	1
89331	1
89335	1
89342	1
89343	1
89344	1
89346	1
89352	1
89353	1
89354	1
89356	2

Appendix L — Medically Unlikely Edits (MUEs) — Professional

CPT	MUE
90284	1
90296	1
90375	20
90376	20
90385	1
90393	1
90396	1
90460	3
90471	1
90472	4
90473	1
90474	1
90476	1
90477	1
90581	1
90585	1
90586	1
90632	1
90633	1
90634	1
90636	1
90644	1
90645	1
90646	1
90647	1
90648	1
90649	1
90650	1
90653	1
90654	1
90655	1
90656	1
90657	1
90658	1
90660	1
90661	1
90662	1
90664	1
90666	1
90667	1
90668	1
90669	1
90670	1
90672	1
90673	1
90675	1
90676	1
90680	1
90681	1
90685	1
90686	1
90687	1
90688	1
90690	1
90691	1
90692	1
90693	1
90696	1
90698	1
90700	1
90702	1
90703	1
90704	1
90705	1
90706	1

CPT	MUE
90707	1
90708	1
90710	1
90712	1
90713	1
90714	1
90715	1
90716	1
90717	1
90719	1
90720	1
90721	1
90725	1
90727	1
90732	1
90733	1
90734	1
90735	1
90736	1
90738	1
90739	1
90740	1
90743	1
90744	1
90746	1
90747	1
90785	1
90791	1
90792	1
90832	1
90833	1
90834	1
90836	1
90837	1
90838	1
90839	1
90845	1
90846	1
90847	1
90849	1
90853	1
90863	1
90865	1
90867	1
90868	1
90869	1
90870	2
90880	1
90901	1
90911	1
90935	1
90937	1
90940	2
90945	1
90947	1
90951	1
90952	1
90953	1
90954	1
90955	1
90956	1
90957	1
90958	1
90959	1
90960	1

CPT	MUE
90961	1
90962	1
90963	1
90964	1
90965	1
90966	1
90967	1
90968	1
90969	1
90970	1
90989	1
90993	1
90997	1
91010	1
91013	1
91020	1
91022	1
91030	1
91034	1
91035	1
91037	1
91038	1
91040	1
91065	2
91110	1
91111	1
91112	1
91117	1
91120	1
91122	1
91132	1
91133	1
92002	1
92004	1
92012	1
92014	1
92018	1
92019	1
92020	1
92025	1
92060	1
92065	1
92071	2
92072	1
92081	1
92082	1
92083	1
92100	1
92132	1
92133	1
92134	1
92136	2
92140	1
92225	2
92226	2
92227	1
92228	1
92230	2
92235	2
92240	2
92250	1
92260	1
92265	1
92270	1
92275	1

CPT	MUE
92283	1
92284	1
92285	1
92286	1
92287	1
92311	1
92312	1
92313	1
92315	1
92316	1
92317	1
92325	1
92326	2
92502	1
92504	1
92507	1
92508	1
92511	1
92512	1
92516	1
92520	1
92521	1
92522	1
92523	1
92524	1
92526	1
92540	1
92541	1
92542	1
92543	4
92544	1
92545	1
92546	1
92547	1
92548	1
92550	1
92552	1
92553	1
92555	1
92556	1
92557	1
92558	0
92561	1
92562	1
92563	1
92564	1
92565	1
92567	1
92568	1
92570	1
92571	1
92572	1
92575	1
92576	1
92577	1
92579	1
92582	1
92583	1
92584	1
92585	1
92586	1
92587	1
92588	1
92596	1
92601	1

CPT	MUE
92602	1
92603	1
92604	1
92605	0
92609	1
92610	1
92613	1
92615	1
92617	1
92618	0
92620	1
92625	1
92626	1
92920	1
92924	1
92928	1
92933	1
92937	3
92938	3
92941	1
92943	1
92944	1
92950	3
92953	2
92960	2
92961	1
92970	1
92971	1
92973	2
92974	1
92975	1
92977	1
92978	1
92979	2
92986	1
92987	1
92990	1
92992	1
92993	1
92997	1
92998	2
93000	3
93005	3
93015	1
93016	1
93017	1
93018	1
93024	1
93025	1
93040	3
93041	2
93042	3
93224	1
93225	1
93226	1
93227	1
93228	1
93229	1
93268	1
93270	1
93271	1
93272	1
93278	1
93279	1
93280	1

CPT	MUE
93281	1
93282	1
93283	1
93284	1
93285	1
93286	2
93287	2
93288	1
93289	1
93290	1
93291	1
93292	1
93293	1
93294	1
93295	1
93296	1
93297	1
93298	1
93299	1
93303	1
93304	1
93306	1
93307	1
93308	1
93312	1
93313	1
93314	1
93315	1
93316	1
93317	1
93318	1
93320	1
93321	1
93325	1
93350	1
93351	1
93352	1
93451	1
93452	1
93453	1
93454	1
93455	1
93456	1
93457	1
93458	1
93459	1
93460	1
93461	1
93462	1
93463	1
93464	1
93503	2
93505	1
93530	1
93531	1
93532	1
93533	1
93561	1
93562	1
93563	1
93564	1
93565	1
93566	1
93567	1
93568	1

CPT	MUE
93571	1
93572	2
93580	1
93581	1
93582	1
93583	1
93600	1
93602	1
93603	1
93609	1
93610	1
93612	1
93613	1
93615	1
93616	1
93618	1
93619	1
93620	1
93621	1
93622	1
93623	1
93624	1
93631	1
93640	1
93641	1
93642	1
93650	1
93653	1
93654	1
93655	1
93656	1
93657	1
93660	1
93662	1
93701	1
93724	1
93745	1
93750	4
93784	1
93786	1
93788	1
93790	1
93797	2
93798	2
93880	1
93882	1
93886	1
93888	1
93890	1
93892	1
93893	1
93922	1
93923	1
93924	1
93925	1
93926	1
93930	1
93931	1
93965	1
93970	1
93971	1
93975	1
93976	1
93978	1
93979	1

CPT	MUE
93980	1
93981	1
93982	1
93990	2
94002	1
94003	1
94004	1
94010	1
94011	1
94012	1
94013	1
94014	1
94015	1
94016	1
94060	1
94070	1
94200	1
94250	1
94375	1
94400	1
94450	1
94452	1
94453	1
94610	2
94620	1
94621	1
94640	4
94642	1
94644	1
94645	2
94660	1
94662	1
94664	1
94667	1
94669	4
94680	1
94681	1
94690	1
94726	1
94727	1
94728	1
94729	1
94750	1
94760	1
94761	1
94762	1
94770	1
94772	1
94774	1
94775	1
94776	1
94777	1
94780	1
94781	1
95012	2
95018	19
95056	1
95060	1
95065	1
95070	1
95071	1
95076	1
95079	2
95115	1
95117	1

CPT	MUE
95250	1
95251	1
95782	1
95783	1
95800	1
95801	1
95803	1
95805	1
95806	1
95807	1
95808	1
95810	1
95811	1
95812	1
95813	1
95816	1
95819	1
95822	1
95824	1
95827	1
95829	1
95830	1
95831	5
95832	1
95851	3
95852	1
95857	1
95860	1
95861	1
95863	1
95864	1
95865	1
95866	1
95867	1
95868	1
95869	1
95873	1
95874	1
95875	2
95885	4
95886	4
95887	1
95905	2
95907	1
95908	1
95909	1
95910	1
95911	1
95912	1
95913	1
95921	1
95922	1
95923	1
95924	1
95925	1
95926	1
95927	1
95928	1
95929	1
95930	1
95933	1
95938	1
95939	1
95943	1
95950	1

CPT	MUE
95951	1
95953	1
95954	1
95955	1
95956	1
95957	1
95958	1
95961	1
95965	1
95966	1
95967	3
95970	1
95971	1
95972	1
95974	1
95975	2
95978	1
95980	1
95981	1
95982	1
95990	2
95991	2
95992	1
96000	1
96001	1
96002	1
96003	1
96004	1
96020	1
96103	1
96105	3
96120	1
96125	2
96360	1
96365	1
96368	1
96369	1
96370	3
96371	1
96373	2
96374	1
96376	0
96402	2
96405	1
96406	1
96409	1
96413	1
96416	1
96420	2
96422	2
96425	1
96440	1
96446	1
96450	1
96521	2
96522	1
96523	1
96542	1
96567	1
96570	1
96571	3
96900	1
96904	1
96910	1
96912	1

CPT	MUE
96913	1
96920	1
96921	1
96922	1
97012	1
97016	1
97018	1
97022	1
97024	1
97026	1
97028	1
97150	1
97545	1
97546	2
97597	1
97605	1
97606	1
97610	1
98925	1
98926	1
98927	1
98928	1
98929	1
98940	1
98941	1
98942	1
99082	1
99143	2
99144	2
99148	2
99149	2
99170	1
99175	1
99183	1
99191	1
99192	1
99195	2
99201	1
99202	1
99203	1
99204	1
99205	1
99211	1
99212	2
99213	2
99214	2
99215	1
99217	1
99218	1
99219	1
99220	1
99221	1
99222	1
99223	1
99224	1
99225	1
99226	1
99231	1
99232	1
99233	1
99234	1
99235	1
99236	1
99238	1
99239	1

CPT	MUE
99281	1
99282	1
99283	1
99284	1
99285	1
99291	1
99304	1
99305	1
99306	1
99307	1
99308	1
99309	1
99310	1
99315	1
99316	1
99318	1
99324	1
99325	1
99326	1
99327	1
99328	1
99334	1
99335	1
99336	1
99337	1
99341	1
99342	1
99343	1
99344	1
99345	1
99347	1
99348	1
99349	1
99350	1
99354	1
99356	1
99406	1
99407	1
99446	1
99447	1
99448	1
99449	1
99455	1
99456	1
99460	1
99461	1
99462	1
99463	1
99464	1
99465	1
99466	1
99468	1
99469	1
99471	1
99472	1
99475	1
99476	1
99477	1
99478	1
99479	1
99480	1
99481	1
99482	1
99485	1
99487	1

CPT	MUE
99488	1
99495	1
99496	1
99605	0
99606	0
99607	0
A0382	0
A0384	0
A0392	0
A0394	0
A0396	0
A0398	0
A0420	0
A0422	0
A0424	0
A0426	2
A0427	2
A0428	4
A0429	2
A0430	1
A0431	1
A0432	1
A0433	1
A0434	2
A0435	999
A0436	300
A4221	1
A4235	2
A4253	0
A4255	0
A4257	0
A4258	0
A4259	0
A4301	1
A4356	1
A4470	1
A4480	1
A4555	0
A4557	2
A4561	1
A4562	1
A4565	2
A4606	1
A4611	0
A4614	1
A4625	30
A4633	0
A4635	0
A4638	0
A4640	0
A4642	1
A4648	5
A4650	3
A5056	90
A5057	90
A5120	150
A5500	0
A5501	0
A5503	0
A5504	0
A5505	0
A5506	0
A5507	0
A5508	0
A5510	0

CPT	MUE
A5512	0
A5513	0
A6501	2
A6502	2
A6503	2
A6504	4
A6505	4
A6506	4
A6507	4
A6508	4
A6509	2
A6510	2
A6511	2
A6513	0
A6531	0
A6532	0
A6545	0
A7000	0
A7003	0
A7005	0
A7006	0
A7013	0
A7014	0
A7016	0
A7017	0
A7020	0
A7025	0
A7026	0
A7027	0
A7028	0
A7029	0
A7032	0
A7035	0
A7036	0
A7037	0
A7039	0
A7040	2
A7041	2
A7042	2
A7043	10
A7044	0
A7047	0
A7501	0
A7504	0
A7507	0
A7520	0
A7524	0
A7527	0
A9272	0
A9284	0
A9500	3
A9501	3
A9502	3
A9503	1
A9504	1
A9507	1
A9508	2
A9510	1
A9512	30
A9520	1
A9521	2
A9526	2
A9536	1
A9537	1
A9538	1

CPT	MUE
A9539	2
A9540	2
A9541	1
A9542	1
A9543	1
A9544	1
A9545	1
A9546	1
A9547	2
A9550	1
A9551	1
A9552	1
A9553	1
A9554	1
A9555	3
A9556	10
A9557	2
A9559	1
A9560	2
A9561	1
A9562	2
A9566	1
A9567	2
A9569	1
A9570	1
A9571	1
A9579	100
A9580	1
A9582	1
A9583	18
A9584	1
A9585	300
A9586	1
A9599	1
A9600	7
A9604	1
A9700	2
B4083	0
B4149	0
B4153	0
B4157	0
B4160	0
B4164	0
B4176	0
B4189	0
B4199	0
B5200	0
C1722	1
C1749	1
C1767	2
C1772	1
C1785	1
C1813	1
C1820	2
C1830	2
C1840	1
C1841	1
C1886	1
C2616	1
C5271	1
C5272	3
C5273	1
C5274	35
C5275	1
C5276	3

CPT	MUE
C5277	1
C5278	15
C9254	0
C9275	1
C9285	2
C9290	266
C9293	700
C9352	3
C9353	4
C9354	300
C9355	3
C9356	125
C9358	800
C9359	30
C9360	300
C9361	10
C9362	60
C9363	500
C9364	600
C9600	3
C9601	2
C9602	3
C9603	2
C9604	3
C9605	3
C9606	2
C9607	1
C9608	2
C9733	1
C9734	1
C9735	1
C9737	1
C9739	1
C9740	1
E0100	0
E0105	0
E0110	0
E0111	0
E0112	0
E0113	0
E0114	0
E0116	0
E0117	0
E0118	0
E0130	0
E0135	0
E0140	0
E0141	0
E0143	0
E0144	0
E0147	0
E0148	0
E0149	0
E0153	0
E0154	0
E0155	0
E0156	0
E0157	0
E0158	0
E0159	2
E0160	0
E0161	0
E0162	0
E0163	0
E0165	0

Appendix L — Medically Unlikely Edits (MUEs) — Professional

CPT	MUE
E0167	0
E0168	0
E0170	0
E0171	0
E0172	0
E0175	0
E0181	0
E0182	0
E0184	0
E0185	0
E0186	0
E0187	0
E0188	0
E0189	0
E0190	0
E0191	0
E0193	0
E0194	0
E0196	0
E0197	0
E0198	0
E0199	0
E0200	0
E0202	0
E0203	0
E0205	0
E0210	0
E0215	0
E0217	0
E0218	0
E0221	0
E0225	0
E0231	0
E0232	0
E0235	0
E0236	0
E0239	0
E0240	0
E0241	0
E0242	0
E0243	0
E0244	0
E0245	0
E0246	0
E0247	0
E0248	0
E0249	0
E0250	0
E0251	0
E0255	0
E0256	0
E0260	0
E0261	0
E0265	0
E0266	0
E0270	0
E0271	0
E0272	0
E0273	0
E0274	0
E0275	0
E0276	0
E0277	0
E0280	0
E0290	0

CPT	MUE
E0291	0
E0292	0
E0293	0
E0294	0
E0295	0
E0296	0
E0297	0
E0300	0
E0301	0
E0302	0
E0303	0
E0304	0
E0305	0
E0310	0
E0315	0
E0316	0
E0325	0
E0326	0
E0328	0
E0329	0
E0350	0
E0352	0
E0370	0
E0371	0
E0372	0
E0373	0
E0424	0
E0425	0
E0430	0
E0431	0
E0434	0
E0435	0
E0439	0
E0440	0
E0441	0
E0442	0
E0443	0
E0444	0
E0445	0
E0446	0
E0450	0
E0455	0
E0457	0
E0459	0
E0460	0
E0461	0
E0462	0
E0463	0
E0464	0
E0470	0
E0471	0
E0472	0
E0480	0
E0481	0
E0482	0
E0483	0
E0484	0
E0485	0
E0486	0
E0487	0
E0500	0
E0550	0
E0555	0
E0560	0
E0561	0

CPT	MUE
E0562	0
E0565	0
E0570	0
E0572	0
E0574	0
E0575	0
E0580	0
E0585	0
E0600	0
E0601	0
E0602	0
E0603	0
E0604	0
E0605	0
E0606	0
E0607	0
E0610	0
E0615	0
E0616	1
E0617	0
E0618	0
E0619	0
E0620	0
E0621	0
E0625	0
E0627	0
E0628	0
E0629	0
E0630	0
E0635	0
E0636	0
E0637	0
E0638	0
E0639	0
E0640	0
E0641	0
E0642	0
E0650	0
E0651	0
E0652	0
E0655	0
E0656	0
E0657	0
E0660	0
E0665	0
E0666	0
E0667	0
E0668	0
E0669	0
E0670	0
E0671	0
E0672	0
E0673	0
E0675	0
E0676	1
E0691	0
E0692	0
E0693	0
E0694	0
E0700	0
E0705	0
E0710	0
E0720	0
E0730	0
E0731	0

CPT	MUE
E0740	0
E0744	0
E0745	0
E0746	1
E0747	0
E0748	0
E0749	1
E0755	0
E0760	0
E0761	0
E0762	0
E0764	0
E0765	0
E0766	0
E0769	0
E0770	1
E0776	0
E0779	0
E0780	0
E0781	1
E0782	1
E0783	1
E0784	0
E0785	1
E0786	1
E0791	0
E0830	0
E0840	0
E0849	0
E0850	0
E0855	0
E0856	0
E0860	0
E0870	0
E0880	0
E0890	0
E0900	0
E0910	0
E0911	0
E0912	0
E0920	0
E0930	0
E0935	0
E0936	0
E0940	0
E0941	0
E0942	0
E0944	0
E0945	0
E0946	0
E0947	0
E0948	0
E0950	0
E0951	0
E0952	0
E0955	0
E0956	0
E0957	0
E0958	0
E0959	0
E0960	0
E0961	0
E0966	0
E0967	0
E0968	0

CPT	MUE
E0970	0
E0971	0
E0973	0
E0974	0
E0978	0
E0981	0
E0982	0
E0983	0
E0984	0
E0985	0
E0986	0
E0988	0
E0990	0
E0992	0
E0994	0
E0995	0
E1002	0
E1003	0
E1004	0
E1005	0
E1006	0
E1007	0
E1008	0
E1009	0
E1010	0
E1011	0
E1014	0
E1015	0
E1016	0
E1017	0
E1018	0
E1020	0
E1028	0
E1029	0
E1030	0
E1031	0
E1035	0
E1037	0
E1038	0
E1039	0
E1050	0
E1060	0
E1070	0
E1083	0
E1084	0
E1085	0
E1086	0
E1087	0
E1088	0
E1089	0
E1090	0
E1092	0
E1093	0
E1100	0
E1110	0
E1130	0
E1140	0
E1150	0
E1160	0
E1161	0
E1170	0
E1171	0
E1172	0
E1180	0
E1190	0

CPT	MUE
E1195	0
E1200	0
E1220	0
E1221	0
E1222	0
E1223	0
E1224	0
E1225	0
E1226	0
E1228	0
E1229	0
E1230	0
E1231	0
E1232	0
E1233	0
E1234	0
E1235	0
E1236	0
E1237	0
E1238	0
E1240	0
E1250	0
E1260	0
E1270	0
E1280	0
E1285	0
E1290	0
E1295	0
E1300	0
E1310	0
E1352	0
E1353	0
E1354	0
E1355	0
E1356	0
E1357	0
E1358	0
E1372	0
E1390	0
E1391	0
E1392	0
E1405	0
E1406	0
E1500	0
E1510	0
E1520	0
E1530	0
E1540	0
E1550	0
E1560	0
E1570	0
E1575	0
E1580	0
E1590	0
E1592	0
E1594	0
E1600	0
E1610	0
E1615	0
E1620	0
E1625	0
E1630	0
E1632	0
E1634	0
E1635	0

CPT	MUE
E1636	0
E1637	0
E1639	0
E1700	0
E1701	0
E1702	0
E1800	0
E1801	0
E1802	0
E1805	0
E1806	0
E1810	0
E1811	0
E1812	0
E1815	0
E1816	0
E1818	0
E1820	0
E1821	0
E1825	0
E1830	0
E1831	0
E1840	0
E1841	0
E1902	0
E2000	0
E2100	0
E2101	0
E2120	0
E2201	0
E2202	0
E2203	0
E2204	0
E2205	0
E2206	0
E2207	0
E2208	0
E2209	0
E2210	0
E2211	0
E2212	0
E2213	0
E2214	0
E2215	0
E2216	0
E2217	0
E2218	0
E2219	0
E2220	0
E2221	0
E2222	0
E2224	0
E2225	0
E2226	0
E2227	0
E2228	0
E2231	0
E2291	1
E2292	1
E2293	1
E2294	1
E2295	0
E2300	0
E2301	0
E2310	0

CPT	MUE
E2311	0
E2312	0
E2313	0
E2321	0
E2322	0
E2323	0
E2324	0
E2325	0
E2326	0
E2327	0
E2328	0
E2329	0
E2330	0
E2331	0
E2340	0
E2341	0
E2342	0
E2343	0
E2351	0
E2358	0
E2359	0
E2361	0
E2363	0
E2365	0
E2366	0
E2367	0
E2368	0
E2369	0
E2370	0
E2371	0
E2373	0
E2374	0
E2375	0
E2376	0
E2377	0
E2378	0
E2381	0
E2382	0
E2383	0
E2384	0
E2385	0
E2386	0
E2387	0
E2388	0
E2389	0
E2390	0
E2391	0
E2392	0
E2394	0
E2395	0
E2396	0
E2397	0
E2402	0
E2500	0
E2502	0
E2504	0
E2506	0
E2508	0
E2510	0
E2511	0
E2512	0
E2601	0
E2602	0
E2603	0
E2604	0

CPT	MUE
E2605	0
E2606	0
E2607	0
E2608	0
E2609	0
E2611	0
E2612	0
E2613	0
E2614	0
E2615	0
E2616	0
E2617	0
E2619	0
E2620	0
E2621	0
E2622	0
E2623	0
E2624	0
E2625	0
E2626	0
E2627	0
E2628	0
E2629	0
E2630	0
E2631	0
E2632	0
E2633	0
G0008	1
G0009	1
G0010	2
G0027	1
G0101	1
G0102	1
G0103	1
G0104	1
G0105	1
G0106	1
G0117	1
G0118	1
G0120	1
G0121	1
G0123	1
G0124	1
G0127	1
G0128	1
G0130	1
G0141	1
G0143	1
G0144	1
G0145	1
G0147	1
G0148	1
G0166	2
G0168	2
G0173	1

CPT	MUE
G0175	1
G0177	0
G0179	1
G0180	1
G0181	1
G0182	1
G0186	1
G0202	1
G0204	2
G0206	2
G0235	1
G0239	1
G0245	1
G0246	1
G0247	1
G0248	1
G0249	1
G0250	1
G0251	2
G0259	2
G0260	2
G0268	1
G0278	1
G0281	1
G0283	1
G0288	1
G0289	1
G0293	1
G0294	1
G0302	1
G0303	1
G0304	1
G0305	1
G0306	2
G0307	2
G0328	1
G0329	1
G0333	0
G0337	1
G0339	1
G0340	2
G0341	1
G0342	1
G0343	1
G0364	2
G0365	2
G0372	1
G0389	1
G0396	1
G0397	1
G0398	1
G0399	1
G0400	1
G0402	1
G0403	1

CPT	MUE
G0404	1
G0405	1
G0406	1
G0407	1
G0408	1
G0412	1
G0413	1
G0414	1
G0415	1
G0416	1
G0417	1
G0418	1
G0419	1
G0420	2
G0424	2
G0425	1
G0426	1
G0427	1
G0429	1
G0431	1
G0432	1
G0433	1
G0434	1
G0435	1
G0436	1
G0437	1
G0438	1
G0439	1
G0442	1
G0443	1
G0444	1
G0445	1
G0448	1
G0452	1
G0454	1
G0455	1
G0456	1
G0457	1
G0458	1
G0459	1
G0460	1
G0461	9
G0462	60
G0463	0
G3001	1
G9143	1
G9156	1
G9157	1
G9187	1
J0130	6
J0131	400
J0133	1200
J0135	8
J0151	180
J0178	4

CPT	MUE
J0210	4
J0215	30
J0220	1
J0221	300
J0256	3500
J0257	1400
J0275	1
J0278	15
J0280	7
J0289	50
J0300	8
J0348	200
J0350	0
J0360	2
J0364	6
J0456	4
J0475	8
J0485	1500
J0490	160
J0597	250
J0638	150
J0697	4
J0712	120
J0717	400
J0745	2
J0760	4
J0770	5
J0780	4
J0800	3
J0833	3
J0890	0
J0897	120
J0900	1
J0945	4
J1050	1000
J1162	1
J1442	3360
J1446	192
J1556	300
J1557	300
J1561	300
J1568	300
J1569	300
J1572	300
J1725	250
J1744	30
J2212	240
J2265	400
J2507	8
J2995	0
J3010	100
J3060	900
J3285	1
J3465	40
J3489	5

CPT	MUE
J7196	175
J7301	0
J7310	2
J7316	4
J7326	2
J7527	0
J7604	0
J7607	0
J7609	0
J7610	0
J7615	0
J7622	0
J7624	0
J7627	0
J7628	0
J7629	0
J7632	0
J7634	0
J7635	0
J7636	0
J7637	0
J7638	0
J7640	0
J7641	0
J7642	0
J7643	0
J7645	0
J7647	0
J7650	0
J7657	0
J7660	0
J7665	127
J7667	0
J7670	0
J7676	0
J7680	0
J7681	0
J7683	0
J7684	0
J7685	0
J8510	0
J9019	60
J9042	200
J9047	120
J9179	50
J9228	450
J9262	700
J9306	840
J9354	600
J9355	100
J9400	600
K0001	0
K0002	0
K0003	0
K0004	0

CPT	MUE
K0005	0
K0006	0
K0007	0
K0009	0
K0015	0
K0017	0
K0018	0
K0019	0
K0020	0
K0037	0
K0038	0
K0039	0
K0040	0
K0041	0
K0042	0
K0043	0
K0044	0
K0045	0
K0046	0
K0047	0
K0050	0
K0051	0
K0052	0
K0053	0
K0056	0
K0065	0
K0069	0
K0070	0
K0071	0
K0072	0
K0073	0
K0077	0
K0105	0
K0195	0
K0455	0
K0462	0
K0602	0
K0605	0
K0606	0
K0607	0
K0608	0
K0609	0
K0672	0
K0730	0
K0733	0
K0738	0
K0743	0
K0744	0
K0745	0
K0746	0
K0800	0
K0801	0
K0802	0
K0806	0
K0807	0

CPT	MUE
K0808	0
K0812	0
K0813	0
K0814	0
K0815	0
K0816	0
K0820	0
K0821	0
K0822	0
K0823	0
K0824	0
K0825	0
K0826	0
K0827	0
K0828	0
K0829	0
K0830	0
K0831	0
K0835	0
K0836	0
K0837	0
K0838	0
K0839	0
K0840	0
K0841	0
K0842	0
K0843	0
K0848	0
K0849	0
K0850	0
K0851	0
K0852	0
K0853	0
K0854	0
K0855	0
K0856	0
K0857	0
K0858	0
K0859	0
K0860	0
K0861	0
K0862	0
K0863	0
K0864	0
K0868	0
K0869	0
K0870	0
K0871	0
K0877	0
K0878	0
K0879	0
K0880	0
K0884	0
K0885	0
K0886	0

CPT	MUE
K0890	0
K0891	0
K0898	1
K0900	0
L0112	0
L0113	0
L0120	0
L0130	0
L0140	0
L0150	0
L0160	0
L0170	0
L0172	0
L0174	0
L0180	0
L0190	0
L0200	0
L0220	0
L0450	0
L0452	0
L0454	0
L0455	0
L0456	0
L0457	0
L0458	0
L0460	0
L0462	0
L0464	0
L0466	0
L0467	0
L0468	0
L0469	0
L0470	0
L0472	0
L0480	0
L0482	0
L0484	0
L0486	0
L0488	0
L0490	0
L0491	0
L0492	0
L0621	0
L0622	0
L0623	0
L0624	0
L0625	0
L0626	0
L0627	0
L0628	0
L0629	0
L0630	0
L0631	0
L0632	0
L0633	0

CPT	MUE
L0634	0
L0635	0
L0636	0
L0637	0
L0638	0
L0639	0
L0640	0
L0641	0
L0642	0
L0643	0
L0648	0
L0649	0
L0650	0
L0651	0
L0700	0
L0710	0
L0810	0
L0820	0
L0830	0
L0859	0
L0861	0
L0970	0
L0972	0
L0974	0
L0976	0
L0978	0
L0980	0
L0982	0
L0984	0
L1000	0
L1001	0
L1005	0
L1010	0
L1020	0
L1025	0
L1030	0
L1040	0
L1050	0
L1060	0
L1070	0
L1080	0
L1085	0
L1090	0
L1100	0
L1110	0
L1120	0
L1200	0
L1210	0
L1220	0
L1230	0
L1240	0
L1250	0
L1260	0
L1270	0
L1280	0
L1290	0
L1300	0
L1310	0
L1499	1
L1600	0
L1610	0
L1620	0
L1630	0
L1640	0
L1650	0

CPT	MUE
L1652	0
L1660	0
L1680	0
L1685	0
L1686	0
L1690	0
L1700	0
L1710	0
L1720	0
L1730	0
L1755	0
L1810	0
L1812	0
L1820	0
L1830	0
L1831	0
L1832	0
L1833	0
L1834	0
L1836	0
L1840	0
L1843	0
L1844	0
L1845	0
L1846	0
L1847	0
L1848	0
L1850	0
L1860	0
L1900	0
L1902	0
L1904	0
L1906	0
L1907	0
L1910	0
L1920	0
L1930	0
L1932	0
L1940	0
L1945	0
L1950	0
L1951	0
L1960	0
L1970	0
L1971	0
L1980	0
L1990	0
L2000	0
L2005	0
L2010	0
L2020	0
L2030	0
L2034	0
L2035	0
L2036	0
L2037	0
L2038	0
L2040	0
L2050	0
L2060	0
L2070	0
L2080	0
L2090	0
L2106	0
L2108	0

CPT	MUE
L2112	0
L2114	0
L2116	0
L2126	0
L2128	0
L2132	0
L2134	0
L2136	0
L2180	0
L2182	0
L2184	0
L2186	0
L2188	0
L2190	0
L2192	0
L2200	0
L2210	0
L2220	0
L2230	0
L2232	0
L2240	0
L2250	0
L2260	0
L2265	0
L2270	0
L2275	0
L2280	0
L2300	0
L2310	0
L2320	0
L2330	0
L2335	0
L2340	0
L2350	0
L2360	0
L2370	0
L2375	0
L2380	0
L2385	0
L2387	0
L2390	0
L2395	0
L2397	0
L2405	0
L2415	0
L2425	0
L2430	0
L2492	0
L2500	0
L2510	0
L2520	0
L2525	0
L2526	0
L2530	0
L2540	0
L2550	0
L2570	0
L2580	0
L2600	0
L2610	0
L2620	0
L2622	0
L2624	0
L2627	0
L2628	0

CPT	MUE
L2630	0
L2640	0
L2650	0
L2660	0
L2670	0
L2680	0
L2750	0
L2755	0
L2760	0
L2768	0
L2780	0
L2785	0
L2795	0
L2800	0
L2810	0
L2820	0
L2830	0
L3000	0
L3001	0
L3002	0
L3003	0
L3010	0
L3020	0
L3030	0
L3031	0
L3040	0
L3050	0
L3060	0
L3070	0
L3080	0
L3090	0
L3100	0
L3140	0
L3150	0
L3160	0
L3170	0
L3215	0
L3216	0
L3217	0
L3219	0
L3221	0
L3222	0
L3224	0
L3225	0
L3230	0
L3250	0
L3251	0
L3252	0
L3253	0
L3300	0
L3310	0
L3330	0
L3332	0
L3334	0
L3340	0
L3350	0
L3360	0
L3370	0
L3380	0
L3390	0
L3400	0
L3410	0
L3420	0
L3430	0
L3440	0

CPT	MUE
L3450	0
L3455	0
L3460	0
L3465	0
L3470	0
L3480	0
L3485	0
L3500	0
L3510	0
L3520	0
L3530	0
L3540	0
L3550	0
L3560	0
L3570	0
L3580	0
L3590	0
L3595	0
L3600	0
L3610	0
L3620	0
L3630	0
L3640	0
L3650	0
L3660	0
L3670	0
L3671	0
L3674	0
L3675	0
L3677	0
L3678	0
L3702	0
L3710	0
L3720	0
L3730	0
L3740	0
L3760	0
L3762	0
L3763	0
L3764	0
L3765	0
L3766	0
L3806	0
L3807	0
L3808	0
L3809	0
L3900	0
L3901	0
L3904	0
L3905	0
L3906	0
L3908	0
L3912	0
L3913	0
L3915	0
L3916	0
L3917	0
L3918	0
L3919	0
L3921	0
L3923	0
L3924	0
L3925	0
L3927	0
L3929	0

CPT	MUE
L3930	0
L3931	0
L3933	0
L3935	0
L3956	0
L3960	0
L3961	0
L3962	0
L3967	0
L3971	0
L3973	0
L3975	0
L3976	0
L3977	0
L3978	0
L3980	0
L3982	0
L3984	0
L4000	0
L4002	0
L4010	0
L4020	0
L4030	0
L4040	0
L4045	0
L4050	0
L4055	0
L4060	0
L4070	0
L4080	0
L4090	0
L4100	0
L4110	0
L4130	0
L4205	0
L4210	0
L4350	0
L4360	0
L4361	0
L4370	0
L4386	0
L4387	0
L4392	0
L4394	0
L4396	0
L4397	0
L4398	0
L4631	0
L5000	0
L5010	0
L5020	0
L5050	0
L5060	0
L5100	0
L5105	0
L5150	0
L5160	0
L5200	0
L5210	0
L5220	0
L5230	0
L5250	0
L5270	0
L5280	0
L5301	0

CPT	MUE
L5312	0
L5321	0
L5331	0
L5341	0
L5400	0
L5410	0
L5420	0
L5430	0
L5450	0
L5460	0
L5500	0
L5505	0
L5510	0
L5520	0
L5530	0
L5535	0
L5540	0
L5560	0
L5570	0
L5580	0
L5585	0
L5590	0
L5595	0
L5600	0
L5610	0
L5611	0
L5613	0
L5614	0
L5616	0
L5617	0
L5618	0
L5620	0
L5622	0
L5624	0
L5626	0
L5628	0
L5629	0
L5630	0
L5631	0
L5632	0
L5634	0
L5636	0
L5637	0
L5638	0
L5639	0
L5640	0
L5642	0
L5643	0
L5644	0
L5645	0
L5646	0
L5647	0
L5648	0
L5649	0
L5650	0
L5651	0
L5652	0
L5653	0
L5654	0
L5655	0
L5656	0
L5658	0
L5661	0
L5665	0
L5666	0

CPT	MUE
L5668	0
L5670	0
L5671	0
L5672	0
L5673	0
L5676	0
L5677	0
L5678	0
L5679	0
L5680	0
L5681	0
L5682	0
L5683	0
L5684	0
L5685	0
L5686	0
L5688	0
L5690	0
L5692	0
L5694	0
L5695	0
L5696	0
L5697	0
L5698	0
L5699	0
L5700	0
L5701	0
L5702	0
L5703	0
L5704	0
L5705	0
L5706	0
L5707	0
L5710	0
L5711	0
L5712	0
L5714	0
L5716	0
L5718	0
L5722	0
L5724	0
L5726	0
L5728	0
L5780	0
L5781	0
L5782	0
L5785	0
L5790	0
L5795	0
L5810	0
L5811	0
L5812	0
L5814	0
L5816	0
L5818	0
L5822	0
L5824	0
L5826	0
L5828	0
L5830	0
L5840	0
L5845	0
L5848	0
L5850	0
L5855	0

CPT	MUE
L5856	0
L5857	0
L5858	0
L5859	0
L5910	0
L5920	0
L5925	0
L5930	0
L5940	0
L5950	0
L5960	0
L5961	0
L5962	0
L5964	0
L5966	0
L5968	0
L5969	0
L5970	0
L5971	0
L5972	0
L5974	0
L5975	0
L5976	0
L5978	0
L5979	0
L5980	0
L5981	0
L5982	0
L5984	0
L5985	0
L5986	0
L5987	0
L5988	0
L5990	0
L6000	0
L6010	0
L6020	0
L6025	0
L6050	0
L6055	0
L6100	0
L6110	0
L6120	0
L6130	0
L6200	0
L6205	0
L6250	0
L6300	0
L6310	0
L6320	0
L6350	0
L6360	0
L6370	0
L6380	0
L6382	0
L6384	0
L6386	0
L6388	0
L6400	0
L6450	0
L6500	0
L6550	0
L6570	0
L6580	0
L6582	0
L6584	0
L6586	0
L6588	0
L6590	0
L6600	0
L6605	0
L6610	0
L6611	0
L6615	0
L6616	0
L6620	0
L6621	0
L6623	0
L6624	0
L6625	0
L6628	0
L6629	0
L6630	0
L6632	0
L6635	0
L6637	0
L6638	0
L6640	0
L6641	0
L6642	0
L6645	0
L6646	0
L6647	0
L6648	0
L6650	0
L6655	0
L6660	0
L6665	0
L6670	0
L6672	0
L6675	0
L6676	0
L6677	0
L6680	0
L6682	0
L6684	0
L6686	0
L6687	0
L6688	0
L6689	0
L6690	0
L6691	0
L6692	0
L6693	0
L6694	0
L6695	0
L6696	0
L6697	0
L6698	0
L6703	0
L6704	0
L6706	0
L6707	0
L6708	0
L6709	0
L6711	0
L6712	0
L6713	0
L6714	0
L6715	0
L6721	0
L6722	0
L6805	0
L6810	0
L6880	0
L6881	0
L6882	0
L6883	0
L6884	0
L6885	0
L6890	0
L6895	0
L6900	0
L6905	0
L6910	0
L6915	0
L6920	0
L6925	0
L6930	0
L6935	0
L6940	0
L6945	0
L6950	0
L6955	0
L6960	0
L6965	0
L6970	0
L6975	0
L7007	0
L7008	0
L7009	0
L7040	0
L7045	0
L7170	0
L7180	0
L7181	0
L7185	0
L7186	0
L7190	0
L7191	0
L7260	0
L7261	0
L7360	0
L7362	0
L7364	0
L7366	0
L7367	0
L7368	0
L7400	0
L7401	0
L7402	0
L7403	0
L7404	0
L7405	0
L7900	0
L7902	0
L8000	0
L8001	0
L8002	0
L8015	0
L8020	0
L8030	0
L8031	0
L8032	0
L8035	0
L8039	0
L8040	0
L8041	0
L8042	0
L8043	0
L8044	0
L8045	0
L8046	0
L8047	0
L8048	1
L8049	0
L8300	0
L8310	0
L8320	0
L8330	0
L8400	0
L8410	0
L8415	0
L8417	0
L8420	0
L8430	0
L8435	0
L8440	0
L8460	0
L8465	0
L8470	0
L8480	0
L8485	0
L8500	0
L8501	0
L8507	0
L8509	1
L8510	0
L8511	1
L8514	1
L8515	1
L8600	2
L8604	3
L8605	4
L8606	5
L8609	1
L8610	2
L8612	2
L8613	2
L8614	2
L8615	2
L8616	2
L8617	2
L8618	2
L8619	2
L8621	600
L8622	2
L8627	2
L8628	2
L8629	2
L8631	4
L8641	4
L8642	2
L8658	4
L8659	4
L8670	4
L8679	3
L8681	1
L8682	2
L8683	1
L8684	1
L8685	1
L8686	2
L8687	1
L8688	1
L8689	1
L8690	2
L8691	1
L8692	0
L8693	1
L8695	1
M0064	1
P2028	1
P2029	1
P2033	1
P2038	1
P3000	1
P3001	1
P9041	5
P9043	5
P9045	20
P9046	25
P9047	20
P9048	1
P9612	1
P9615	1
Q0035	1
Q0091	1
Q0111	2
Q0112	3
Q0113	2
Q0114	1
Q0115	1
Q0144	0
Q0161	0
Q0478	1
Q0479	1
Q0480	1
Q0481	1
Q0482	1
Q0483	1
Q0484	1
Q0485	1
Q0486	1
Q0487	1
Q0488	1
Q0489	1
Q0490	1
Q0491	1
Q0492	1
Q0493	1
Q0494	1
Q0495	1
Q0497	2
Q0498	1
Q0499	1
Q0501	1
Q0502	1
Q0503	3
Q0504	1
Q0507	1
Q0508	1
Q0509	1
Q0510	0
Q0511	0
Q0512	0
Q0513	0
Q0514	0
Q1004	2
Q1005	2
Q2004	1
Q2028	1470
Q2034	1
Q2035	1
Q2036	1
Q2037	1
Q2038	1
Q2039	1
Q2043	1
Q2050	14
Q2052	1
Q3014	1
Q3027	30
Q3028	0
Q4001	1
Q4002	1
Q4003	2
Q4004	2
Q4025	1
Q4026	1
Q4027	1
Q4028	1
Q4074	3
Q4101	88
Q4102	21
Q4103	0
Q4104	50
Q4105	250
Q4106	76
Q4107	50
Q4108	250
Q4110	250
Q4111	56
Q4112	2
Q4113	4
Q4114	6
Q4115	240
Q4116	192
Q4117	0
Q4118	1000
Q4119	150
Q4120	0
Q4121	78
Q4122	96
Q4123	160
Q4124	140
Q4125	28
Q4126	32
Q4127	100
Q4128	128
Q4129	81
Q4130	100
Q4131	49
Q4132	50
Q4133	113
Q4134	160
Q4135	900
Q4136	900
Q9955	10
R0070	2
R0075	2
V2020	0
V2100	0
V2101	0
V2102	0
V2103	0
V2104	0
V2105	0
V2106	0
V2107	0
V2108	0
V2109	0
V2110	0
V2111	0
V2112	0
V2113	0
V2114	0
V2115	0
V2118	0
V2121	0
V2199	2
V2200	0
V2201	0
V2202	0
V2203	0
V2204	0
V2205	0
V2206	0
V2207	0
V2208	0
V2209	0
V2210	0
V2211	0
V2212	0
V2213	0
V2214	0
V2215	0
V2218	0
V2219	0
V2220	0
V2221	0
V2299	0
V2300	0
V2301	0
V2302	0
V2303	0
V2304	0
V2305	0
V2306	0
V2307	0
V2308	0
V2309	0
V2310	0
V2311	0
V2312	0
V2313	0
V2314	0
V2315	0
V2318	0
V2319	0
V2320	0
V2321	0
V2399	0
V2410	0
V2430	0
V2499	2
V2500	0
V2501	0
V2502	0
V2503	0
V2510	0
V2511	0
V2512	0
V2513	0
V2520	2
V2521	2
V2522	2
V2523	2
V2530	0
V2531	0
V2599	2
V2600	0
V2610	0
V2615	0
V2623	0
V2624	0
V2625	0
V2626	0
V2627	0
V2628	0
V2629	0
V2630	2
V2631	2
V2632	2
V2700	0
V2710	0
V2715	0
V2718	0
V2730	0
V2744	0
V2745	0
V2750	0
V2755	0
V2761	0
V2770	0
V2780	0
V2781	0
V2782	0
V2783	0
V2784	0
V2785	2
V2790	1
V2797	0
V5008	0
V5010	0
V5011	0
V5274	0
V5281	0
V5282	0
V5284	0
V5285	0
V5286	0
V5287	0
V5288	0
V5289	0

OPPS

CPT	MUE
0001M	1
0002M	1
0003M	1
0019T	1
0042T	1
0051T	1
0052T	1
0053T	1
0054T	2
0055T	2
0058T	1
0059T	1
0071T	1
0072T	1
0073T	2
0075T	1
0076T	2
0092T	1
0095T	1
0098T	1
0099T	2
0100T	2
0101T	1
0102T	2
0103T	1
0106T	4
0107T	4
0108T	4
0109T	4
0110T	4
0111T	1
0123T	2
0159T	2
0163T	2
0164T	4
0165T	4
0169T	1
0171T	1
0172T	3
0174T	1
0175T	1
0178T	1
0179T	1
0180T	1
0181T	1
0182T	3
0190T	2
0191T	2
0195T	1
0196T	1
0197T	2
0198T	2
0199T	1
0200T	1
0201T	1
0202T	1
0206T	1
0207T	2
0208T	1
0209T	1
0210T	1
0211T	1
0212T	1

CPT	MUE
0213T	1
0214T	1
0215T	1
0216T	1
0217T	1
0218T	1
0219T	1
0220T	1
0221T	1
0222T	1
0223T	1
0224T	1
0225T	1
0226T	1
0227T	1
0228T	1
0230T	1
0232T	1
0233T	1
0234T	2
0235T	2
0236T	1
0237T	2
0239T	1
0240T	1
0241T	1
0243T	1
0244T	1
0245T	1
0246T	1
0247T	1
0248T	1
0249T	1
0253T	1
0254T	2
0255T	2
0262T	1
0263T	1
0264T	1
0265T	1
0266T	1
0267T	1
0268T	1
0269T	1
0270T	1
0271T	1
0272T	1
0273T	1
0274T	1
0275T	1
0278T	1
0281T	1
0282T	1
0283T	1
0284T	1
0285T	1
0286T	1
0287T	2
0288T	1
0289T	2
0290T	1
0291T	1
0292T	1

CPT	MUE
0293T	1
0294T	1
0295T	1
0296T	1
0297T	1
0298T	1
0299T	1
0300T	1
0301T	1
0302T	1
0303T	1
0304T	1
0305T	1
0306T	1
0307T	1
0308T	1
0309T	1
0310T	1
0311T	1
0312T	1
0313T	1
0314T	1
0315T	1
0316T	1
0317T	1
0319T	1
0320T	1
0321T	1
0322T	1
0323T	1
0324T	1
0325T	1
0326T	1
0327T	1
0328T	1
0329T	1
0330T	1
0331T	1
0332T	1
0333T	1
0334T	2
0335T	2
0336T	1
0337T	1
0338T	1
0339T	1
0347T	1
0348T	1
0349T	1
0350T	1
0351T	5
0352T	5
0353T	2
0354T	2
0355T	1
0356T	4
0358T	1
0359T	1
0360T	1
0361T	3
0362T	1
0363T	3
0364T	1

CPT	MUE
0366T	1
0368T	1
0370T	1
0371T	1
0372T	1
0373T	1
10040	1
10060	1
10061	1
10080	1
10081	1
10180	3
11000	1
11001	2
11004	1
11005	1
11006	1
11008	1
11010	1
11011	1
11012	2
11042	1
11043	1
11044	1
11055	1
11056	1
11057	1
11100	1
11200	1
11201	0
11446	3
11450	1
11451	1
11462	1
11463	1
11470	3
11471	2
11646	3
11719	1
11720	1
11721	1
11730	1
11732	9
11770	1
11771	1
11772	1
11900	1
11901	1
11920	1
11921	1
11922	1
11950	1
11951	1
11952	1
11954	1
11960	3
11970	2
11971	2
11976	1
11980	1
11981	1
11982	1
11983	1

CPT	MUE
12001	1
12002	1
12004	1
12005	1
12006	1
12007	1
12011	1
12013	1
12014	1
12015	1
12016	1
12017	1
12018	1
12020	3
12021	3
12031	1
12032	1
12034	1
12035	1
12036	1
12037	1
12041	1
12042	1
12044	1
12045	1
12046	1
12047	1
12051	1
12052	1
12053	1
12054	1
12055	1
12056	1
12057	1
13100	1
13101	1
13120	1
13121	1
13131	1
13132	1
13151	1
13152	1
13160	3
14301	2
15002	1
15004	1
15005	2
15040	1
15050	1
15100	1
15110	1
15111	2
15115	1
15116	2
15120	1
15130	1
15135	1
15150	1
15151	1
15152	2
15155	1
15156	1
15200	1

CPT	MUE
15220	1
15240	1
15260	1
15271	1
15272	3
15273	1
15275	1
15276	3
15277	1
15570	3
15572	2
15574	2
15576	2
15600	2
15610	2
15620	2
15630	2
15650	1
15731	1
15740	3
15750	2
15756	2
15757	3
15758	3
15760	2
15770	2
15775	1
15776	1
15777	1
15780	1
15781	2
15782	2
15783	2
15786	1
15787	3
15788	1
15789	1
15792	1
15793	1
15819	1
15820	1
15821	1
15822	1
15823	1
15824	1
15825	1
15826	1
15828	1
15829	1
15830	1
15832	1
15833	1
15834	1
15835	1
15836	1
15837	2
15838	1
15839	2
15840	1
15841	2
15842	2
15845	2
15847	1

CPT	MUE
15850	1
15851	1
15852	2
15860	1
15876	1
15877	1
15878	1
15879	1
15920	1
15922	1
15931	1
15933	1
15934	1
15935	1
15936	1
15937	1
15940	2
15941	2
15944	2
15945	2
15946	2
15950	2
15951	2
15952	2
15953	2
15956	2
15958	2
16000	1
16020	1
16025	1
16030	1
17000	1
17003	13
17004	1
17106	1
17107	1
17108	1
17110	1
17111	1
17264	3
17266	2
17276	3
17286	3
17340	1
17360	1
17380	1
19000	2
19001	5
19020	2
19030	1
19081	1
19083	1
19085	1
19101	3
19110	1
19112	2
19120	1
19125	1
19126	3
19260	2
19271	2
19272	2
19281	1

CPT	MUE
19283	1
19285	1
19287	1
19296	1
19297	2
19298	1
19300	1
19301	1
19302	1
19303	1
19304	1
19305	1
19306	1
19307	1
19316	1
19318	1
19324	1
19325	1
19328	1
19330	1
19340	1
19342	1
19350	1
19355	1
19357	1
19361	1
19364	1
19366	1
19367	1
19368	1
19369	1
19370	1
19371	1
19380	1
19396	1
20100	2
20102	4
20103	4
20150	2
20200	3
20205	4
20206	3
20250	3
20251	3
20526	1
20527	1
20552	1
20553	1
20555	1
20612	2
20615	1
20660	1
20661	1
20662	1
20663	1
20664	1
20665	1
20670	2
20680	2
20692	3
20693	2
20696	2
20697	4

CPT	MUE
20802	1
20805	1
20808	1
20816	3
20822	3
20824	1
20827	1
20838	1
20900	2
20910	2
20912	1
20920	2
20922	2
20924	4
20926	2
20931	1
20937	1
20938	1
20950	2
20955	1
20956	1
20957	1
20962	1
20969	2
20970	1
20972	2
20973	1
20974	1
20975	1
20979	1
20982	1
20985	2
21010	1
21012	3
21014	3
21015	1
21016	2
21025	2
21026	2
21029	1
21030	1
21031	2
21032	1
21034	1
21040	2
21044	1
21045	1
21046	2
21047	2
21048	2
21049	2
21050	1
21060	1
21070	1
21073	1
21076	1
21077	1
21079	1
21080	1
21081	1
21082	1
21083	1
21084	1
21085	1
21086	1

CPT	MUE
21087	1
21088	1
21100	1
21110	2
21116	1
21120	1
21121	1
21122	1
21123	1
21125	2
21127	2
21137	1
21138	1
21139	1
21141	1
21142	1
21143	1
21145	1
21146	1
21147	1
21150	1
21151	1
21154	1
21155	1
21159	1
21160	1
21175	1
21179	1
21180	1
21181	1
21182	1
21183	1
21184	1
21188	1
21193	1
21194	1
21195	1
21196	1
21198	1
21199	1
21206	1
21208	1
21209	1
21210	2
21215	2
21230	2
21235	2
21240	1
21242	1
21243	1
21244	1
21245	2
21246	2
21247	1
21255	1
21256	1
21260	1
21261	1
21263	1
21267	1
21268	1
21270	1
21275	1
21280	1
21282	1

CPT	MUE
21295	1
21296	1
21310	1
21315	1
21320	1
21325	1
21330	1
21335	1
21336	1
21337	1
21338	1
21339	1
21340	1
21343	1
21344	1
21345	1
21346	1
21347	1
21348	1
21355	1
21356	1
21360	1
21365	1
21366	1
21385	1
21386	1
21387	1
21390	1
21395	1
21400	1
21401	1
21406	1
21407	1
21408	1
21421	1
21422	1
21423	1
21431	1
21432	1
21433	1
21435	1
21436	1
21440	2
21445	2
21450	1
21451	1
21452	1
21453	1
21454	1
21461	1
21462	1
21465	1
21470	1
21480	1
21485	1
21490	1
21495	1
21497	1
21501	3
21502	1
21510	1
21550	3
21554	3
21556	3
21557	1

CPT	MUE
21558	1
21610	2
21615	1
21616	1
21620	1
21627	1
21630	1
21632	1
21685	1
21700	1
21705	1
21720	1
21725	1
21740	1
21742	1
21743	1
21750	1
21805	3
21810	1
21820	1
21825	1
21920	3
21925	3
21931	3
21933	3
21935	1
21936	1
22010	2
22015	2
22100	1
22101	1
22102	1
22103	3
22110	1
22112	1
22114	1
22116	3
22206	1
22207	1
22210	1
22212	1
22214	1
22216	6
22220	1
22222	1
22224	1
22305	1
22310	1
22315	1
22318	1
22319	1
22325	1
22326	1
22327	1
22328	8
22505	1
22520	1
22521	1
22522	5
22523	1
22524	1
22525	5
22532	1
22533	1
22534	3

CPT	MUE
22548	1
22551	1
22554	1
22556	1
22558	1
22585	7
22586	1
22590	1
22595	1
22600	1
22610	1
22612	1
22614	15
22630	1
22632	4
22633	1
22634	4
22800	1
22802	1
22804	1
22808	1
22810	1
22812	1
22818	1
22819	1
22830	1
22840	1
22842	1
22843	1
22844	1
22845	1
22846	1
22847	1
22848	1
22849	1
22850	1
22851	9
22852	1
22855	1
22856	1
22857	1
22861	1
22862	1
22864	1
22865	1
22900	3
22901	3
22903	3
22904	1
22905	1
23000	1
23020	1
23030	2
23031	2
23035	2
23040	1
23044	1
23065	2
23066	2
23071	3
23073	3
23075	4
23076	2
23077	1
23078	1

CPT	MUE
23100	1
23101	2
23105	1
23106	1
23107	1
23120	1
23125	1
23130	1
23140	1
23145	1
23146	1
23150	1
23155	1
23156	1
23170	1
23172	1
23174	1
23180	1
23182	1
23184	1
23190	1
23195	1
23200	1
23210	1
23220	1
23330	2
23334	1
23335	1
23350	1
23395	1
23397	1
23400	1
23405	2
23406	1
23410	1
23412	1
23415	1
23420	1
23430	1
23440	1
23450	1
23455	1
23460	1
23462	1
23465	1
23466	1
23470	1
23472	1
23473	1
23474	1
23480	1
23485	1
23490	1
23491	1
23500	1
23505	1
23515	1
23520	1
23525	1
23530	1
23532	1
23540	1
23545	1
23550	1
23552	1

CPT	MUE
23570	1
23575	1
23585	1
23600	1
23605	1
23615	1
23616	1
23620	1
23625	1
23630	1
23650	1
23655	1
23660	1
23665	1
23670	1
23675	1
23680	1
23700	1
23800	1
23802	1
23900	1
23920	1
23921	1
23930	2
23931	2
23935	2
24000	1
24006	1
24065	2
24066	2
24071	3
24073	3
24077	1
24079	1
24100	1
24101	1
24102	1
24105	1
24110	1
24115	1
24116	1
24120	1
24125	1
24126	1
24130	1
24134	1
24136	1
24138	1
24140	1
24145	1
24147	1
24149	1
24150	1
24152	1
24155	1
24160	1
24164	1
24200	3
24201	3
24220	1
24300	1
24301	2
24305	4
24320	2
24330	1

CPT	MUE
24331	1
24332	1
24340	1
24342	2
24343	1
24344	1
24345	1
24346	1
24357	2
24358	2
24359	2
24360	1
24361	1
24362	1
24363	1
24365	1
24366	1
24370	1
24371	1
24400	1
24410	1
24420	1
24430	1
24435	1
24470	1
24495	1
24498	1
24500	1
24505	1
24515	1
24516	1
24530	1
24535	1
24538	1
24545	1
24546	1
24560	1
24565	1
24566	1
24575	1
24576	1
24577	1
24579	1
24582	1
24586	1
24587	1
24600	1
24605	1
24615	1
24620	1
24635	1
24640	1
24650	1
24655	1
24665	1
24666	1
24670	1
24675	1
24685	1
24800	1
24802	1
24900	1
24920	1
24925	1
24930	1

CPT	MUE
24931	1
24935	1
24940	1
25000	2
25001	1
25020	1
25023	1
25024	1
25025	1
25031	2
25035	2
25040	1
25065	5
25066	3
25071	3
25073	3
25076	5
25077	1
25078	1
25085	1
25100	1
25101	1
25105	1
25107	1
25110	3
25111	1
25112	1
25115	1
25116	1
25119	1
25120	1
25125	1
25126	1
25130	1
25135	1
25136	1
25145	1
25150	1
25151	1
25170	1
25210	2
25215	1
25230	1
25240	1
25246	1
25248	3
25250	1
25251	1
25259	1
25275	2
25295	9
25300	1
25301	1
25315	1
25316	1
25320	1
25332	1
25335	1
25337	1
25350	1
25355	1
25360	1
25365	1
25370	1
25375	1

CPT	MUE
25390	1
25391	1
25392	1
25393	1
25394	1
25400	1
25405	1
25415	1
25420	1
25425	1
25426	1
25430	1
25431	2
25440	1
25441	1
25442	1
25443	1
25444	1
25445	1
25446	1
25449	1
25450	1
25455	1
25490	1
25491	1
25492	1
25500	1
25505	1
25515	1
25520	1
25525	1
25526	1
25530	1
25535	1
25545	1
25560	1
25565	1
25574	1
25575	1
25600	1
25605	1
25606	1
25607	1
25608	1
25609	1
25622	1
25624	1
25628	1
25630	1
25635	1
25645	1
25650	1
25651	1
25652	1
25660	1
25670	1
25671	1
25675	1
25676	1
25680	1
25685	1
25690	1
25695	1
25800	1
25805	1

CPT	MUE
25810	1
25820	1
25825	1
25830	1
25900	1
25905	1
25907	1
25909	1
25915	1
25920	1
25922	1
25924	1
25927	1
25929	1
25931	1
26010	3
26011	3
26025	1
26030	1
26034	2
26035	3
26037	1
26040	1
26045	1
26070	3
26100	2
26105	2
26110	3
26116	2
26117	2
26118	1
26121	1
26123	1
26185	1
26200	2
26205	1
26210	2
26215	2
26230	2
26235	2
26236	2
26250	2
26260	1
26262	1
26341	3
26357	3
26358	3
26390	3
26392	3
26416	2
26428	2
26432	2
26433	2
26434	3
26494	1
26496	1
26497	2
26498	1
26508	1
26516	1
26517	1
26518	1
26548	3
26550	1
26551	1

CPT	MUE
26553	1
26554	1
26555	2
26556	2
26560	2
26561	2
26562	2
26580	1
26641	1
26645	1
26650	1
26665	1
26740	3
26742	3
26746	3
26820	1
26841	1
26842	1
26860	1
26862	1
26990	2
26991	2
26992	2
27000	1
27001	1
27003	1
27005	1
27006	1
27025	1
27027	1
27030	1
27033	1
27035	1
27036	1
27040	2
27041	3
27043	3
27045	3
27048	2
27049	1
27050	1
27052	1
27054	1
27057	1
27059	1
27060	1
27062	1
27065	1
27066	1
27067	1
27070	1
27071	1
27075	1
27076	1
27077	1
27078	1
27080	1
27086	2
27087	2
27090	1
27091	1
27093	1
27095	1
27096	1
27097	1

CPT	MUE
27098	1
27100	1
27105	1
27110	1
27111	1
27120	1
27122	1
27125	1
27130	1
27132	1
27134	1
27137	1
27138	1
27140	1
27146	1
27147	1
27151	1
27156	1
27158	1
27161	1
27165	1
27170	1
27175	1
27176	1
27177	1
27178	1
27179	1
27181	1
27185	1
27187	1
27193	1
27194	1
27200	1
27202	1
27220	1
27222	1
27226	1
27227	1
27228	1
27230	1
27232	1
27235	1
27236	1
27238	1
27240	1
27244	1
27245	1
27246	1
27248	1
27250	1
27252	1
27253	1
27254	1
27256	1
27257	1
27258	1
27259	1
27265	1
27266	1
27267	1
27268	1
27269	1
27275	2
27280	1
27282	1

CPT	MUE
27284	1
27286	1
27290	1
27295	1
27303	2
27305	1
27306	1
27307	1
27310	1
27325	1
27326	1
27329	1
27330	1
27331	1
27332	1
27333	1
27334	1
27335	1
27340	1
27345	1
27347	1
27350	1
27355	1
27356	1
27357	1
27358	1
27360	2
27364	1
27365	1
27370	1
27380	2
27381	2
27385	2
27386	2
27390	1
27391	1
27392	1
27393	1
27394	1
27395	1
27396	1
27397	1
27400	1
27403	1
27405	2
27407	2
27409	1
27412	1
27415	1
27416	1
27418	1
27420	1
27422	1
27424	1
27425	1
27427	1
27428	1
27429	1
27430	1
27435	1
27437	1
27438	1
27440	1
27441	1
27442	1

CPT	MUE
27443	1
27445	1
27446	1
27447	1
27448	1
27450	1
27454	1
27455	1
27457	1
27465	1
27466	1
27468	1
27470	1
27472	1
27475	1
27477	1
27479	1
27485	1
27486	1
27487	1
27488	1
27495	1
27496	1
27497	1
27498	1
27499	1
27500	1
27501	1
27502	1
27503	1
27506	1
27507	1
27508	1
27509	1
27510	1
27511	1
27513	1
27514	1
27516	1
27517	1
27519	1
27520	1
27524	1
27530	1
27532	1
27535	1
27536	1
27538	1
27540	1
27550	1
27552	1
27556	1
27557	1
27558	1
27560	1
27562	1
27566	1
27570	1
27580	1
27590	1
27591	1
27592	1
27594	1
27596	1
27598	1

CPT	MUE
27600	1
27601	1
27602	1
27604	2
27605	1
27606	1
27607	2
27610	1
27612	1
27615	1
27616	1
27620	1
27625	1
27626	1
27630	2
27635	1
27637	1
27638	1
27640	1
27641	1
27645	1
27646	1
27647	1
27648	1
27650	1
27652	1
27654	1
27656	2
27658	2
27659	2
27664	2
27665	2
27675	1
27676	1
27680	3
27681	1
27685	2
27686	2
27687	1
27690	2
27691	2
27695	1
27696	1
27698	2
27700	1
27702	1
27703	1
27704	1
27705	1
27707	1
27709	1
27712	1
27715	1
27720	1
27722	1
27724	1
27725	1
27726	1
27727	1
27730	1
27732	1
27734	1
27740	1
27742	1
27745	1

CPT	MUE
27750	1
27752	1
27756	1
27758	1
27759	1
27760	1
27762	1
27766	1
27767	1
27768	1
27769	1
27780	1
27781	1
27784	1
27786	1
27788	1
27792	1
27808	1
27810	1
27814	1
27816	1
27818	1
27822	1
27823	1
27824	1
27825	1
27826	1
27827	1
27828	1
27829	1
27830	1
27831	1
27832	1
27840	1
27842	1
27846	1
27848	1
27860	1
27870	1
27871	1
27880	1
27881	1
27882	1
27884	1
27886	1
27888	1
27889	1
27892	1
27893	1
27894	1
28001	2
28002	3
28003	2
28005	3
28008	2
28035	1
28039	3
28041	3
28046	1
28047	1
28052	2
28054	2
28055	1
28060	1
28062	1

CPT	MUE
28086	2
28088	2
28090	2
28092	2
28100	1
28102	1
28103	1
28104	2
28106	1
28107	1
28108	2
28110	1
28111	1
28113	1
28114	1
28116	1
28118	1
28119	1
28120	2
28122	4
28124	4
28130	1
28171	1
28173	2
28175	2
28192	2
28193	2
28202	2
28210	2
28220	1
28222	1
28225	1
28226	1
28230	1
28238	1
28240	1
28250	1
28260	1
28261	1
28262	1
28264	1
28280	1
28285	4
28286	1
28289	1
28290	1
28292	1
28293	1
28294	1
28296	1
28297	1
28298	1
28299	1
28300	1
28302	1
28304	1
28305	1
28306	1
28307	1
28309	1
28310	1
28315	1
28320	1
28322	2
28340	2

CPT	MUE
28341	2
28344	1
28360	1
28400	1
28405	1
28406	1
28415	1
28420	1
28430	1
28435	1
28436	1
28445	1
28446	1
28490	1
28495	1
28496	1
28505	1
28530	1
28531	1
28540	1
28545	1
28546	1
28555	1
28570	1
28575	1
28576	1
28585	1
28600	2
28605	2
28630	2
28635	2
28705	1
28715	1
28725	1
28730	1
28735	1
28737	1
28750	1
28755	1
28760	1
28800	1
28805	1
28825	10
28890	1
29000	1
29010	1
29015	1
29020	1
29025	1
29035	1
29040	1
29044	1
29046	1
29049	1
29055	1
29058	1
29065	1
29075	1
29085	1
29086	2
29105	1
29125	1
29126	1
29130	3
29131	2

CPT	MUE
29200	1
29240	1
29260	1
29280	2
29305	1
29325	1
29345	1
29355	1
29358	1
29365	1
29405	1
29425	1
29435	1
29440	1
29445	1
29450	1
29505	1
29515	1
29520	1
29530	1
29540	1
29550	1
29580	1
29581	1
29582	1
29583	1
29584	1
29700	2
29705	1
29710	1
29715	1
29720	1
29730	2
29740	1
29750	1
29800	1
29804	1
29805	1
29806	1
29807	1
29819	1
29820	1
29821	1
29822	1
29823	1
29824	1
29825	1
29826	1
29827	1
29828	1
29830	1
29834	1
29835	1
29836	1
29837	1
29838	1
29840	1
29843	1
29844	1
29845	1
29846	1
29847	1
29848	1
29850	1
29851	1

CPT	MUE
29855	1
29856	1
29860	1
29861	1
29862	1
29863	1
29866	1
29867	1
29868	1
29870	1
29871	1
29873	1
29874	1
29875	1
29876	1
29877	1
29879	1
29880	1
29881	1
29882	1
29883	1
29884	1
29885	1
29886	1
29887	1
29888	1
29889	1
29891	1
29892	1
29893	1
29894	1
29895	1
29897	1
29898	1
29899	1
29900	2
29901	2
29902	2
29904	1
29905	1
29906	1
29907	1
29914	1
29915	1
29916	1
30000	1
30020	1
30100	3
30110	1
30115	1
30117	2
30118	2
30120	1
30124	2
30125	1
30130	1
30140	1
30150	1
30160	1
30200	1
30210	1
30220	1
30300	1
30310	1
30320	1

CPT	MUE
30400	1
30410	1
30420	1
30430	1
30435	1
30450	1
30460	1
30462	1
30465	1
30520	1
30540	1
30545	1
30560	1
30580	2
30600	1
30620	1
30630	1
30801	1
30802	1
30901	1
30903	1
30905	1
30906	1
30915	1
30920	1
30930	1
31000	1
31002	1
31020	1
31030	1
31032	1
31040	1
31050	1
31051	1
31070	1
31075	1
31080	1
31081	1
31084	1
31085	1
31086	1
31087	1
31090	1
31200	1
31201	1
31205	1
31225	1
31230	1
31231	1
31233	1
31235	1
31237	1
31238	1
31239	1
31240	1
31254	1
31255	1
31256	1
31267	1
31276	1
31287	1
31288	1
31290	1
31291	1
31292	1

CPT	MUE
31293	1
31294	1
31295	1
31296	1
31297	1
31300	1
31320	1
31360	1
31365	1
31367	1
31368	1
31370	1
31375	1
31380	1
31382	1
31390	1
31395	1
31400	1
31420	1
31500	2
31502	1
31505	1
31510	1
31511	1
31512	1
31513	1
31515	1
31520	1
31525	1
31526	1
31527	1
31528	1
31529	1
31530	1
31531	1
31535	1
31536	1
31540	1
31541	1
31545	1
31546	1
31560	1
31561	1
31570	1
31571	1
31575	1
31576	1
31577	1
31578	1
31579	1
31580	1
31582	1
31584	1
31587	1
31588	1
31590	1
31595	1
31600	1
31601	1
31603	1
31605	1
31610	1
31611	1
31612	1
31613	1

CPT	MUE
31614	1
31615	1
31620	1
31622	1
31623	1
31624	1
31625	1
31626	1
31627	1
31628	1
31629	1
31630	1
31631	1
31632	2
31633	2
31634	1
31635	1
31636	1
31637	2
31638	2
31640	1
31641	1
31643	1
31645	1
31646	2
31647	1
31648	1
31660	1
31661	1
31717	1
31720	2
31725	1
31730	1
31750	1
31755	1
31760	1
31766	1
31770	2
31775	1
31780	1
31781	1
31785	1
31786	1
31800	1
31805	1
31820	1
31825	1
31830	1
32035	1
32036	1
32096	1
32097	1
32098	1
32100	1
32110	1
32120	1
32124	1
32140	1
32141	1
32150	1
32151	1
32160	1
32200	2
32215	1
32220	1

Appendix L — Medically Unlikely Edits (MUEs) — OPPS

CPT	MUE
32225	1
32310	1
32320	1
32400	2
32405	2
32440	1
32442	1
32445	1
32480	1
32482	1
32484	2
32486	1
32488	1
32491	1
32501	1
32503	1
32504	1
32505	1
32506	3
32507	2
32540	1
32550	2
32552	2
32553	1
32554	3
32555	3
32556	3
32557	3
32560	1
32561	1
32562	1
32601	1
32604	1
32606	1
32607	1
32608	1
32609	1
32650	1
32651	1
32652	1
32653	1
32654	1
32655	1
32656	1
32658	1
32659	1
32661	1
32662	1
32663	1
32664	1
32665	1
32666	1
32667	3
32668	2
32669	2
32670	1
32671	1
32672	1
32673	1
32674	1
32701	1
32800	1
32810	1
32815	1
32820	1

CPT	MUE
32850	1
32851	1
32852	1
32853	1
32854	1
32855	1
32856	1
32900	1
32905	1
32906	1
32940	1
32960	1
32997	1
32998	1
33010	1
33011	1
33015	1
33020	1
33025	1
33030	1
33031	1
33050	1
33120	1
33130	1
33140	1
33141	1
33202	1
33203	1
33206	1
33207	1
33208	1
33210	1
33211	1
33212	1
33213	1
33214	1
33215	2
33216	1
33217	1
33218	1
33220	1
33221	1
33222	1
33223	1
33224	1
33225	1
33226	1
33227	1
33228	1
33229	1
33230	1
33231	1
33233	1
33234	1
33235	1
33236	1
33237	1
33238	1
33240	1
33241	1
33243	1
33244	1
33249	1
33250	1
33251	1

CPT	MUE
33254	1
33255	1
33256	1
33257	1
33258	1
33259	1
33261	1
33262	1
33263	1
33264	1
33265	1
33266	1
33282	1
33284	1
33300	1
33305	1
33310	1
33315	1
33320	1
33321	1
33322	1
33330	1
33332	1
33335	1
33361	1
33362	1
33363	1
33364	1
33365	1
33366	1
33367	1
33368	1
33369	1
33400	1
33401	1
33403	1
33404	1
33405	1
33406	1
33410	1
33411	1
33412	1
33413	1
33414	1
33415	1
33416	1
33417	1
33420	1
33422	1
33425	1
33426	1
33427	1
33430	1
33460	1
33463	1
33464	1
33465	1
33468	1
33470	1
33471	1
33472	1
33474	1
33475	1
33476	1
33478	1

CPT	MUE
33496	1
33500	1
33501	1
33502	1
33503	1
33504	1
33505	1
33506	1
33507	1
33508	1
33510	1
33511	1
33512	1
33513	1
33514	1
33516	1
33517	1
33518	1
33519	1
33521	1
33522	1
33523	1
33530	1
33533	1
33534	1
33535	1
33536	1
33542	1
33545	1
33548	1
33572	3
33600	1
33602	1
33606	1
33608	1
33610	1
33611	1
33612	1
33615	1
33617	1
33619	1
33620	1
33621	1
33622	1
33641	1
33645	1
33647	1
33660	1
33665	1
33670	1
33675	1
33676	1
33677	1
33681	1
33684	1
33688	1
33690	1
33692	1
33694	1
33697	1
33702	1
33710	1
33720	1
33722	1
33724	1

CPT	MUE
33726	1
33730	1
33732	1
33735	1
33736	1
33737	1
33750	1
33755	1
33762	1
33764	1
33766	1
33767	1
33768	1
33770	1
33771	1
33774	1
33775	1
33776	1
33777	1
33778	1
33779	1
33780	1
33781	1
33782	1
33783	1
33786	1
33788	1
33800	1
33802	1
33803	1
33813	1
33814	1
33820	1
33822	1
33824	1
33840	1
33845	1
33851	1
33852	1
33853	1
33860	1
33863	1
33864	1
33870	1
33875	1
33877	1
33880	1
33881	1
33883	1
33884	3
33886	1
33889	1
33891	1
33910	1
33915	1
33916	1
33917	1
33920	1
33922	1
33924	1
33925	1
33926	1
33930	1
33933	1
33935	1

CPT	MUE
33940	1
33944	1
33945	1
33960	1
33961	1
33967	1
33968	1
33970	1
33971	1
33973	1
33974	1
33975	1
33976	1
33977	1
33978	1
33979	1
33980	1
33981	1
33982	1
33983	1
33990	1
33991	1
33992	1
33993	1
34001	1
34051	1
34101	1
34111	2
34151	2
34201	1
34203	1
34401	1
34421	1
34451	1
34471	1
34490	1
34501	1
34502	1
34510	2
34520	1
34530	1
34800	1
34802	1
34803	1
34804	1
34805	1
34806	1
34808	1
34812	1
34813	1
34820	1
34825	2
34826	4
34830	1
34831	1
34832	1
34833	1
34834	1
34841	1
34842	1
34843	1
34844	1
34845	1
34846	1
34847	1

CPT	MUE
34848	1
34900	1
35001	1
35002	1
35005	1
35011	1
35013	1
35021	1
35022	1
35045	2
35081	1
35082	1
35091	1
35092	1
35102	1
35103	1
35111	1
35112	1
35121	2
35122	1
35131	1
35132	1
35141	1
35142	1
35151	1
35152	1
35180	2
35182	2
35184	2
35188	2
35189	1
35190	2
35201	2
35206	2
35207	3
35211	3
35216	3
35221	3
35226	3
35231	2
35236	2
35241	2
35246	2
35251	2
35256	2
35261	1
35266	2
35271	2
35276	2
35281	2
35286	2
35301	2
35302	1
35303	1
35304	1
35305	1
35306	2
35311	1
35321	1
35331	1
35341	3
35351	1
35355	1
35361	1
35363	1

CPT	MUE
35371	1
35372	1
35390	1
35400	1
35450	2
35452	1
35458	3
35471	3
35472	1
35500	2
35501	1
35506	1
35508	1
35509	1
35510	1
35511	1
35512	1
35515	1
35516	1
35518	1
35521	1
35522	1
35523	1
35525	1
35526	1
35531	2
35533	1
35535	1
35536	1
35537	1
35538	1
35539	1
35540	1
35556	1
35558	1
35560	1
35563	1
35565	1
35566	1
35570	1
35571	2
35572	2
35583	1
35585	2
35587	2
35600	2
35601	1
35606	1
35612	1
35616	1
35621	1
35623	1
35626	3
35631	4
35632	1
35633	1
35634	1
35636	1
35637	1
35638	1
35642	1
35645	1
35646	1
35647	1
35650	1

CPT	MUE
35654	1
35656	1
35661	1
35663	1
35665	1
35666	2
35671	2
35681	1
35682	1
35683	1
35685	2
35686	1
35691	1
35693	1
35694	1
35695	1
35697	2
35700	2
35701	1
35721	1
35741	1
35761	2
35800	2
35820	2
35840	2
35860	2
35870	1
35875	2
35876	2
35879	2
35881	2
35883	1
35884	1
35901	1
35903	2
35905	1
35907	1
36002	2
36005	2
36010	2
36013	2
36014	2
36100	2
36120	2
36160	2
36200	2
36221	1
36222	1
36223	1
36224	1
36225	1
36226	1
36227	1
36251	1
36252	1
36253	1
36254	1
36260	1
36261	1
36262	1
36400	1
36405	1
36406	1
36410	3
36420	2

CPT	MUE
36425	3
36430	1
36440	1
36450	1
36455	1
36468	1
36469	1
36470	1
36471	1
36475	1
36478	1
36479	2
36481	1
36510	1
36511	1
36512	1
36513	1
36514	1
36515	1
36516	1
36522	1
36555	2
36556	2
36557	2
36558	2
36560	2
36561	2
36563	2
36565	2
36566	2
36568	2
36569	3
36570	2
36571	2
36575	2
36576	2
36578	2
36580	2
36581	2
36582	2
36583	2
36584	2
36585	2
36589	2
36590	2
36591	2
36592	1
36593	2
36595	2
36596	2
36597	2
36598	2
36620	3
36625	2
36640	1
36660	1
36680	1
36800	1
36810	1
36815	1
36818	1
36819	1
36820	1
36821	2
36822	1

CPT	MUE
36823	1
36825	1
36830	2
36831	1
36832	2
36833	1
36835	1
36838	1
36860	2
36861	2
36870	2
37140	1
37145	1
37160	1
37180	1
37181	1
37182	1
37183	1
37184	1
37185	2
37186	2
37187	1
37188	1
37191	1
37192	1
37193	1
37195	1
37197	2
37200	2
37211	1
37212	1
37213	1
37214	1
37215	1
37217	1
37220	2
37221	2
37222	2
37223	2
37224	2
37225	2
37226	2
37227	2
37228	2
37229	2
37230	2
37231	2
37232	2
37233	2
37234	2
37235	2
37236	1
37238	1
37250	1
37500	1
37565	1
37600	1
37605	1
37606	1
37607	1
37609	1
37615	2
37616	1
37617	3
37618	2

CPT	MUE
37619	1
37650	1
37660	1
37700	1
37718	1
37722	1
37735	1
37760	1
37761	1
37765	1
37766	1
37780	1
37785	1
37788	1
37790	1
38100	1
38101	1
38102	1
38115	1
38120	1
38200	1
38204	1
38205	1
38206	1
38207	1
38208	1
38209	1
38210	1
38211	1
38212	1
38213	1
38214	1
38215	1
38220	1
38221	1
38230	1
38232	1
38240	1
38241	1
38242	1
38243	1
38300	2
38305	2
38308	1
38380	1
38381	1
38382	1
38500	2
38505	3
38510	1
38520	1
38525	1
38530	1
38542	1
38550	1
38555	1
38562	1
38564	1
38570	1
38571	1
38572	1
38700	1
38720	1
38724	1
38740	1

CPT	MUE
38745	1
38746	1
38747	1
38760	1
38765	1
38770	1
38780	1
38790	1
38792	1
38794	1
38900	1
39000	1
39010	1
39200	1
39220	1
39400	1
39501	1
39503	1
39540	1
39541	1
39545	1
39560	1
39561	1
40490	3
40500	2
40510	2
40520	2
40525	2
40527	2
40530	2
40650	2
40652	2
40654	2
40700	1
40701	1
40702	1
40720	1
40761	1
40800	2
40801	2
40804	2
40805	2
40806	2
40808	4
40810	4
40812	4
40814	4
40816	2
40818	2
40819	2
40820	5
40830	2
40831	2
40840	1
40842	1
40843	1
40844	1
40845	1
41000	2
41005	2
41006	2
41007	2
41008	2
41009	2
41010	1

CPT	MUE
41015	2
41016	2
41017	2
41018	2
41019	1
41100	3
41105	3
41108	2
41110	2
41112	2
41113	2
41114	2
41115	1
41116	2
41120	1
41130	1
41135	1
41140	1
41145	1
41150	1
41153	1
41155	1
41250	2
41251	2
41252	2
41500	1
41510	1
41512	1
41520	1
41530	1
41800	2
41805	3
41806	3
41820	4
41821	2
41822	1
41823	1
41825	2
41826	2
41827	2
41828	4
41830	2
41850	2
41870	2
41872	4
41874	4
42000	1
42100	3
42104	3
42106	2
42107	2
42120	1
42140	1
42145	1
42160	2
42180	1
42182	1
42200	1
42205	1
42210	1
42215	1
42220	1
42225	1
42226	1
42227	1

CPT	MUE
42235	1
42260	1
42280	1
42281	1
42300	2
42305	2
42310	2
42320	2
42330	2
42335	2
42340	1
42400	2
42405	2
42408	1
42409	1
42410	1
42415	1
42420	1
42425	1
42426	1
42440	1
42450	2
42500	2
42505	2
42507	1
42508	1
42509	1
42510	1
42550	2
42600	2
42650	2
42660	2
42665	2
42700	2
42720	1
42725	1
42800	3
42804	3
42806	1
42808	2
42809	1
42810	1
42815	1
42820	1
42821	1
42825	1
42826	1
42830	1
42831	1
42835	1
42836	1
42842	1
42844	1
42845	1
42860	1
42870	1
42890	1
42892	1
42894	1
42900	1
42950	1
42953	1
42955	1
42960	1
42961	1

CPT	MUE
42962	1
42970	1
42971	1
42972	1
43020	1
43030	1
43045	1
43100	1
43101	1
43107	1
43108	1
43112	1
43113	1
43116	1
43117	1
43118	1
43121	1
43122	1
43123	1
43124	1
43130	1
43135	1
43191	1
43192	1
43193	1
43194	1
43195	1
43196	1
43197	1
43198	1
43200	1
43201	1
43202	1
43204	1
43205	1
43206	1
43211	1
43212	1
43213	1
43214	1
43215	1
43216	1
43217	1
43220	1
43226	1
43227	1
43229	1
43231	1
43232	1
43233	1
43235	1
43236	1
43237	1
43238	1
43239	1
43240	1
43241	1
43242	1
43243	1
43244	1
43245	1
43246	1
43247	1
43248	1
43249	1

Appendix L — Medically Unlikely Edits (MUEs) — OPPS

CPT	MUE
43250	1
43251	1
43252	1
43253	1
43254	1
43255	2
43257	1
43259	1
43260	1
43261	1
43262	2
43263	1
43264	1
43265	1
43266	1
43270	1
43273	1
43275	1
43277	3
43278	1
43279	1
43280	1
43282	1
43283	1
43300	1
43305	1
43310	1
43312	1
43313	1
43314	1
43320	1
43325	1
43327	1
43328	1
43330	1
43331	1
43332	1
43333	1
43334	1
43335	1
43336	1
43337	1
43338	1
43340	1
43341	1
43350	1
43351	1
43352	1
43360	1
43361	1
43400	1
43401	1
43405	1
43410	1
43415	1
43420	1
43425	1
43450	1
43453	1
43460	1
43496	1
43500	1
43501	1
43502	1
43510	1

CPT	MUE
43520	1
43605	1
43610	2
43611	2
43620	1
43621	1
43622	1
43631	1
43632	1
43633	1
43634	1
43635	1
43640	1
43641	1
43644	1
43645	1
43647	1
43648	1
43651	1
43652	1
43653	1
43752	2
43753	1
43754	1
43755	1
43756	1
43757	1
43760	2
43761	2
43770	1
43771	1
43772	1
43773	1
43774	1
43775	1
43800	1
43810	1
43820	1
43825	1
43830	1
43831	1
43832	1
43840	2
43843	1
43845	1
43846	1
43847	1
43848	1
43850	1
43855	1
43860	1
43865	1
43870	1
43880	1
43881	1
43882	1
43886	1
43887	1
43888	1
44005	1
44010	1
44015	1
44020	2
44021	1
44025	1

CPT	MUE
44050	1
44055	1
44100	1
44110	1
44111	1
44120	1
44121	4
44125	1
44126	1
44127	1
44128	2
44130	3
44132	1
44133	1
44135	1
44136	1
44137	1
44139	1
44140	2
44141	1
44143	1
44144	1
44145	1
44146	1
44147	1
44150	1
44151	1
44155	1
44156	1
44157	1
44158	1
44160	1
44180	1
44186	1
44187	1
44188	1
44202	1
44203	2
44204	2
44205	1
44206	1
44207	1
44208	1
44210	1
44211	1
44212	1
44213	1
44227	1
44300	1
44310	2
44312	1
44314	1
44316	1
44320	1
44322	1
44340	1
44345	1
44346	1
44360	1
44361	1
44363	1
44364	1
44365	1
44366	1
44369	1

CPT	MUE
44370	1
44372	1
44373	1
44376	1
44377	1
44378	1
44379	1
44380	1
44382	1
44383	1
44385	1
44386	1
44388	1
44389	1
44390	1
44391	1
44392	1
44393	1
44394	1
44397	1
44500	1
44602	1
44603	1
44604	1
44605	1
44615	4
44620	2
44625	1
44626	1
44640	2
44650	2
44660	1
44661	1
44680	1
44700	1
44701	1
44705	1
44715	1
44720	2
44721	2
44800	1
44820	1
44850	1
44900	1
44950	1
44955	1
44960	1
44970	1
45000	1
45005	1
45020	1
45100	2
45108	1
45110	1
45111	1
45112	1
45113	1
45114	1
45116	1
45119	1
45120	1
45121	1
45123	1
45126	1
45130	1

CPT	MUE
45135	1
45136	1
45150	1
45160	1
45171	2
45172	2
45190	1
45300	1
45303	1
45305	1
45307	1
45308	1
45309	1
45315	1
45317	1
45320	1
45321	1
45327	1
45330	1
45331	1
45332	1
45333	1
45334	1
45335	1
45337	1
45338	1
45339	1
45340	1
45341	1
45342	1
45345	1
45355	1
45378	1
45379	1
45380	1
45381	1
45382	1
45383	1
45384	1
45385	1
45386	1
45387	1
45391	1
45392	1
45395	1
45397	1
45400	1
45402	1
45500	1
45505	1
45520	1
45540	1
45541	1
45550	1
45560	1
45562	1
45563	1
45800	1
45805	1
45820	1
45825	1
45900	1
45905	1
45910	1
45915	1

CPT	MUE
45990	1
46020	2
46030	1
46040	2
46045	2
46050	2
46060	2
46070	1
46080	1
46083	2
46200	1
46220	1
46221	1
46230	1
46250	1
46255	1
46257	1
46258	1
46260	1
46261	1
46262	1
46270	1
46275	1
46280	1
46285	1
46288	1
46320	2
46500	1
46505	1
46600	1
46604	1
46606	1
46608	1
46610	1
46611	1
46612	1
46614	1
46615	1
46700	1
46705	1
46706	1
46707	1
46710	1
46712	1
46715	1
46716	1
46730	1
46735	1
46740	1
46742	1
46744	1
46746	1
46748	1
46750	1
46751	1
46753	1
46754	1
46760	1
46761	1
46762	1
46900	1
46910	1
46916	1
46917	1
46922	1

CPT	MUE
46924	1
46930	1
46940	1
46942	1
46945	1
46946	1
46947	1
47000	3
47001	3
47010	3
47015	1
47100	3
47120	2
47122	1
47125	1
47130	1
47133	1
47135	1
47136	1
47140	1
47141	1
47142	1
47143	1
47144	1
47145	1
47146	3
47147	2
47300	2
47350	1
47360	1
47361	1
47362	1
47370	1
47371	1
47380	1
47381	1
47382	1
47400	1
47420	1
47425	1
47460	1
47480	1
47490	1
47500	2
47505	2
47510	2
47511	2
47525	3
47530	2
47550	1
47552	1
47553	1
47554	1
47555	1
47556	1
47560	1
47561	1
47562	1
47563	1
47564	1
47570	1
47600	1
47605	1
47610	1
47612	1

CPT	MUE
47620	1
47630	1
47700	1
47701	1
47711	1
47712	1
47715	1
47720	1
47721	1
47740	1
47741	1
47760	1
47765	1
47780	1
47785	1
47800	1
47801	1
47802	1
47900	1
48000	1
48001	1
48020	1
48100	1
48102	1
48105	1
48120	1
48140	1
48145	1
48146	1
48148	1
48150	1
48152	1
48153	1
48154	1
48155	1
48400	1
48500	1
48510	1
48520	1
48540	1
48545	1
48547	1
48548	1
48550	1
48551	1
48552	2
48554	1
48556	1
49000	1
49002	1
49010	1
49020	2
49040	2
49060	2
49062	1
49082	1
49083	2
49084	1
49180	2
49203	1
49204	1
49205	1
49215	1
49220	1
49250	1

CPT	MUE
49255	1
49320	1
49321	1
49322	1
49323	1
49324	1
49325	1
49326	1
49327	1
49400	1
49402	1
49411	1
49412	1
49418	1
49419	1
49421	1
49422	1
49423	2
49424	3
49425	1
49426	1
49427	1
49428	1
49429	1
49435	1
49436	1
49440	1
49441	1
49442	1
49446	1
49450	1
49451	1
49452	1
49460	1
49465	1
49491	1
49492	1
49495	1
49496	1
49500	1
49501	1
49505	1
49507	1
49520	1
49521	1
49525	1
49540	1
49550	1
49553	1
49555	1
49557	1
49560	2
49561	2
49565	2
49566	2
49568	2
49570	1
49572	1
49580	1
49582	1
49585	1
49587	1
49590	1
49600	1
49605	1

CPT	MUE
49606	1
49610	1
49611	1
49650	1
49651	1
49652	2
49653	2
49654	2
49655	2
49656	2
49657	2
49900	1
49904	1
49905	1
49906	1
50010	1
50020	1
50040	1
50045	1
50060	1
50065	1
50070	1
50075	1
50080	1
50081	1
50100	1
50120	1
50125	1
50130	1
50135	1
50200	1
50205	1
50220	1
50225	1
50230	1
50234	1
50236	1
50240	1
50250	1
50280	1
50290	1
50300	1
50320	1
50323	1
50325	1
50327	1
50328	1
50329	1
50340	1
50360	1
50365	1
50370	1
50380	1
50382	1
50384	1
50385	1
50386	1
50387	1
50389	1
50390	2
50391	1
50392	1
50393	1
50394	1
50395	1

CPT	MUE
50396	1
50398	1
50400	1
50405	1
50500	1
50520	1
50525	1
50526	1
50540	1
50541	1
50542	1
50543	1
50544	1
50545	1
50546	1
50547	1
50548	1
50551	1
50553	1
50555	1
50557	1
50561	1
50562	1
50570	1
50572	1
50574	1
50575	1
50576	1
50580	1
50590	1
50592	1
50593	1
50600	1
50605	1
50610	1
50620	1
50630	1
50650	1
50660	1
50684	1
50686	2
50688	2
50690	2
50700	1
50715	1
50722	1
50725	1
50727	1
50728	1
50740	1
50750	1
50760	1
50770	1
50780	1
50782	1
50783	1
50785	1
50810	1
50815	1
50820	1
50825	1
50830	1
50840	1
50845	1
50860	1

CPT	MUE
50900	1
50920	2
50930	2
50940	1
50945	1
50947	1
50948	1
50951	1
50953	1
50955	1
50957	1
50961	1
50970	1
50972	1
50974	1
50976	1
50980	1
51020	1
51030	1
51040	1
51045	2
51050	1
51060	1
51065	1
51080	1
51100	1
51101	1
51102	1
51500	1
51520	1
51525	1
51530	1
51535	1
51550	1
51555	1
51565	1
51570	1
51575	1
51580	1
51585	1
51590	1
51595	1
51596	1
51597	1
51600	1
51605	1
51610	1
51700	1
51701	2
51702	2
51703	2
51705	2
51710	1
51715	1
51720	1
51725	1
51726	1
51727	1
51728	1
51729	1
51736	1
51741	1
51784	1
51785	1
51792	1

CPT	MUE
51797	1
51798	1
51800	1
51820	1
51840	1
51841	1
51845	1
51860	1
51865	1
51880	1
51900	1
51920	1
51925	1
51940	1
51960	1
51980	1
51990	1
51992	1
52000	1
52001	1
52005	2
52007	1
52010	1
52204	1
52214	1
52224	1
52234	1
52235	1
52240	1
52250	1
52260	1
52265	1
52270	1
52275	1
52276	1
52277	1
52281	1
52282	1
52283	1
52285	1
52287	1
52290	1
52300	1
52301	1
52305	1
52310	1
52315	2
52317	1
52318	1
52320	1
52325	1
52327	1
52330	1
52332	1
52334	1
52341	1
52342	1
52343	1
52344	1
52345	1
52346	1
52351	1
52352	1
52353	1
52354	1

CPT	MUE
52355	1
52356	1
52400	1
52402	1
52450	1
52500	1
52601	1
52630	1
52640	1
52647	1
52648	1
52649	1
52700	1
53000	1
53010	1
53020	1
53025	1
53040	1
53060	1
53080	1
53085	1
53200	1
53210	1
53215	1
53220	1
53230	1
53235	1
53240	1
53250	1
53260	1
53265	1
53270	1
53275	1
53400	1
53405	1
53410	1
53415	1
53420	1
53425	1
53430	1
53431	1
53440	1
53442	1
53444	1
53445	1
53446	1
53447	1
53448	1
53449	1
53450	1
53460	1
53500	1
53502	1
53505	1
53510	1
53515	1
53520	1
53600	1
53601	1
53605	1
53620	1
53621	1
53660	1
53661	1
53665	1

CPT	MUE
53850	1
53852	1
53855	1
53860	1
54000	1
54001	1
54015	1
54050	1
54055	1
54056	1
54057	1
54060	1
54065	1
54100	2
54105	2
54110	1
54111	1
54112	1
54115	1
54120	1
54125	1
54130	1
54135	1
54150	1
54160	1
54161	1
54162	1
54163	1
54164	1
54200	1
54205	1
54220	1
54230	1
54231	1
54235	1
54240	1
54250	1
54300	1
54304	1
54308	1
54312	1
54316	1
54318	1
54322	1
54324	1
54326	1
54328	1
54332	1
54336	1
54340	1
54344	1
54348	1
54352	1
54360	1
54380	1
54385	1
54390	1
54400	1
54401	1
54405	1
54406	1
54408	1
54410	1
54411	1
54415	1

CPT	MUE
54416	1
54417	1
54420	1
54430	1
54435	1
54440	1
54450	1
54500	1
54505	1
54512	1
54520	1
54522	1
54530	1
54535	1
54550	1
54560	1
54600	1
54620	1
54640	1
54650	1
54660	1
54670	1
54680	1
54690	1
54692	1
54700	1
54800	1
54830	1
54840	1
54860	1
54861	1
54865	1
54900	1
54901	1
55000	1
55040	1
55041	1
55060	1
55100	2
55110	1
55120	1
55150	1
55175	1
55180	1
55200	1
55250	1
55300	1
55400	1
55450	1
55500	1
55520	1
55530	1
55535	1
55540	1
55550	1
55600	1
55605	1
55650	1
55680	1
55700	1
55705	1
55706	1
55720	1
55725	1
55801	1

Appendix L — Medically Unlikely Edits (MUEs) — OPPS

CPT	MUE
55810	1
55812	1
55815	1
55821	1
55831	1
55840	1
55842	1
55845	1
55860	1
55862	1
55865	1
55866	1
55870	1
55873	1
55875	1
55876	1
55920	1
56405	2
56420	1
56440	1
56441	1
56442	1
56501	1
56515	1
56605	1
56606	6
56620	1
56625	1
56630	1
56631	1
56632	1
56633	1
56634	1
56637	1
56640	1
56700	1
56740	1
56800	1
56805	1
56810	1
56820	1
56821	1
57000	1
57010	1
57020	1
57022	1
57023	1
57061	1
57065	1
57100	3
57105	2
57106	1
57107	1
57109	1
57110	1
57111	1
57112	1
57120	1
57130	1
57135	2
57150	1
57155	1
57156	1
57160	1
57170	1

CPT	MUE
57180	1
57200	1
57210	1
57220	1
57230	1
57240	1
57250	1
57260	1
57265	1
57267	2
57268	1
57270	1
57280	1
57282	1
57283	1
57284	1
57285	1
57287	1
57288	1
57289	1
57291	1
57292	1
57295	1
57296	1
57300	1
57305	1
57307	1
57308	1
57310	1
57311	1
57320	1
57330	1
57335	1
57400	1
57410	1
57415	1
57420	1
57421	1
57423	1
57425	1
57426	1
57452	1
57454	1
57455	1
57456	1
57460	1
57461	1
57500	1
57505	1
57510	1
57511	1
57513	1
57520	1
57522	1
57530	1
57531	1
57540	1
57545	1
57550	1
57555	1
57556	1
57558	1
57700	1
57720	1
57800	1

CPT	MUE
58100	1
58110	1
58120	1
58140	1
58145	1
58146	1
58150	1
58152	1
58180	1
58200	1
58210	1
58240	1
58260	1
58262	1
58263	1
58267	1
58270	1
58275	1
58280	1
58285	1
58290	1
58291	1
58292	1
58293	1
58294	1
58301	1
58321	1
58322	1
58323	1
58340	1
58345	1
58346	1
58350	1
58353	1
58356	1
58400	1
58410	1
58520	1
58540	1
58541	1
58542	1
58543	1
58544	1
58545	1
58546	1
58548	1
58550	1
58552	1
58553	1
58554	1
58555	1
58558	1
58559	1
58560	1
58561	1
58562	1
58563	1
58565	1
58570	1
58571	1
58572	1
58573	1
58600	1
58605	1
58611	1

CPT	MUE
58615	1
58660	1
58661	1
58662	1
58670	1
58671	1
58672	1
58673	1
58700	1
58720	1
58740	1
58750	1
58752	1
58760	1
58770	1
58800	1
58805	1
58820	1
58822	1
58825	1
58900	1
58920	1
58925	1
58940	1
58943	1
58950	1
58951	1
58952	1
58953	1
58954	1
58956	1
58957	1
58958	1
58960	1
58970	1
58974	1
58976	2
59000	1
59001	1
59012	1
59015	1
59020	2
59025	3
59030	4
59050	1
59051	1
59070	2
59072	2
59074	1
59076	1
59100	1
59120	1
59121	1
59130	1
59135	1
59136	1
59140	1
59150	1
59151	1
59160	1
59200	1
59300	1
59320	1
59325	1
59350	1

CPT	MUE
59400	1
59409	2
59410	1
59412	1
59414	1
59425	1
59426	1
59430	1
59510	1
59514	1
59515	1
59525	1
59610	1
59612	2
59614	1
59618	1
59620	1
59622	1
59812	1
59820	1
59821	1
59830	1
59840	1
59841	1
59850	1
59851	1
59852	1
59855	1
59856	1
59857	1
59866	1
59870	1
59871	1
60000	1
60100	3
60200	2
60210	1
60212	1
60220	1
60225	1
60240	1
60252	1
60254	1
60260	1
60270	1
60271	1
60280	1
60281	1
60300	2
60500	1
60502	1
60505	1
60512	1
60520	1
60521	1
60522	1
60540	1
60545	1
60600	1
60605	1
60650	1
61000	1
61001	1
61020	2
61026	2

CPT	MUE
61050	1
61055	1
61070	2
61105	1
61107	1
61108	1
61120	1
61140	1
61150	1
61151	1
61154	1
61156	1
61210	1
61215	1
61250	1
61253	1
61304	1
61305	1
61312	2
61313	2
61314	2
61315	1
61316	1
61320	2
61321	1
61322	1
61323	1
61330	1
61332	1
61333	1
61334	1
61340	1
61343	1
61345	1
61440	1
61450	1
61458	1
61460	1
61470	1
61480	1
61490	1
61500	1
61501	1
61510	1
61512	1
61514	2
61516	1
61517	1
61518	1
61519	1
61520	1
61521	1
61522	1
61524	2
61526	1
61530	1
61531	1
61533	2
61534	1
61535	2
61536	1
61537	1
61538	1
61539	1
61540	1

CPT	MUE
61541	1
61542	1
61543	1
61544	1
61545	1
61546	1
61548	1
61550	1
61552	1
61556	1
61557	1
61558	1
61559	1
61563	2
61564	1
61566	1
61567	1
61570	1
61571	1
61575	1
61576	1
61580	1
61581	1
61582	1
61583	1
61584	1
61585	1
61586	1
61590	1
61591	1
61592	1
61595	1
61596	1
61597	1
61598	1
61600	1
61601	1
61605	1
61606	1
61607	1
61608	1
61609	1
61610	1
61611	1
61612	1
61613	1
61615	1
61616	1
61618	2
61619	2
61623	2
61624	2
61626	2
61630	1
61635	2
61680	1
61682	1
61684	1
61686	1
61690	1
61692	1
61697	2
61698	1
61700	2
61702	1

CPT	MUE
61703	1
61705	1
61708	1
61710	1
61711	1
61720	1
61735	1
61750	2
61751	2
61760	1
61770	1
61781	1
61782	1
61783	1
61790	1
61791	1
61796	1
61797	4
61798	1
61799	4
61800	1
61850	1
61860	1
61863	1
61864	1
61867	1
61868	2
61870	1
61875	1
61880	1
61885	1
61886	1
61888	1
62000	1
62005	1
62010	1
62100	1
62115	1
62116	1
62117	1
62120	1
62121	1
62140	1
62141	1
62142	2
62143	2
62145	2
62146	2
62147	1
62148	1
62160	1
62161	1
62162	1
62163	1
62164	1
62165	1
62180	1
62190	1
62192	1
62194	1
62200	1
62201	1
62220	1
62223	1
62225	2

CPT	MUE
62230	2
62252	2
62256	1
62258	1
62263	1
62264	1
62267	2
62268	1
62269	2
62270	2
62272	2
62273	2
62280	1
62281	1
62282	1
62284	1
62287	1
62290	5
62291	4
62292	1
62294	1
62310	1
62311	1
62318	1
62319	1
62350	1
62351	1
62355	1
62360	1
62361	1
62362	1
62365	1
62367	1
62368	1
62369	1
62370	1
63001	1
63003	1
63005	1
63011	1
63012	1
63015	1
63016	1
63017	1
63020	1
63030	1
63035	4
63040	1
63042	1
63043	4
63044	4
63045	1
63046	1
63047	1
63048	5
63050	1
63051	1
63055	1
63056	1
63057	3
63064	1
63066	1
63075	1
63076	3
63077	1
63078	3
63081	1
63082	6
63085	1
63086	2
63087	1
63088	4
63090	1
63091	3
63101	1
63102	1
63103	3
63170	1
63172	1
63173	1
63180	1
63182	1
63185	1
63190	1
63191	1
63194	1
63195	1
63196	1
63197	1
63198	1
63199	1
63200	1
63250	1
63251	1
63252	1
63265	1
63266	1
63267	1
63268	1
63270	1
63271	1
63272	1
63273	1
63275	1
63276	1
63277	1
63278	1
63280	1
63281	1
63282	1
63283	1
63285	1
63286	1
63287	1
63290	1
63295	1
63300	1
63301	1
63302	1
63303	1
63304	1
63305	1
63306	1
63307	1
63308	3
63600	2
63610	1
63615	1
63620	1
63621	2
63650	2
63655	1
63661	1
63662	1
63663	1
63664	1
63685	1
63688	1
63700	1
63702	1
63704	1
63706	1
63707	1
63709	1
63710	1
63740	1
63741	1
63744	1
63746	1
64400	4
64402	1
64405	1
64408	1
64410	1
64412	1
64413	1
64415	1
64416	1
64417	1
64418	1
64420	3
64421	3
64425	1
64430	1
64435	1
64445	1
64446	1
64447	1
64448	1
64449	1
64450	10
64455	1
64479	1
64480	4
64483	1
64484	4
64490	1
64491	1
64492	1
64493	1
64494	1
64495	1
64505	1
64508	1
64510	1
64517	1
64520	1
64530	1
64550	1
64553	1
64555	2
64561	1
64565	2
64566	1
64568	1
64569	1
64570	1
64575	2
64580	2
64581	2
64585	2
64590	1
64595	1
64600	2
64605	1
64610	1
64611	1
64612	1
64615	1
64616	1
64617	1
64620	5
64630	1
64632	1
64633	1
64635	1
64640	5
64642	1
64643	3
64644	1
64645	3
64646	1
64647	1
64650	1
64653	1
64680	1
64681	1
64702	2
64704	4
64708	3
64712	1
64713	1
64714	1
64716	2
64718	1
64719	1
64721	1
64722	4
64726	2
64727	2
64732	1
64734	1
64736	1
64738	1
64740	1
64742	1
64744	1
64746	1
64752	1
64755	1
64760	1
64761	1
64763	1
64766	1
64771	2
64772	2
64774	2
64776	1
64778	1
64782	2
64783	2
64784	3
64786	1
64787	4
64788	5
64790	1
64792	2
64795	2
64802	1
64804	1
64809	1
64818	1
64820	4
64821	1
64822	1
64823	1
64831	1
64832	3
64834	1
64835	1
64836	1
64837	2
64840	1
64856	2
64857	2
64858	1
64859	2
64861	1
64862	1
64864	2
64865	1
64866	1
64868	1
64870	1
64872	1
64874	1
64876	1
64885	1
64886	1
64890	2
64891	2
64892	2
64893	2
64895	2
64896	2
64897	2
64898	2
64901	2
64902	1
64905	1
64907	1
64910	3
64911	2
65091	1
65093	1
65101	1
65103	1
65105	1
65110	1
65112	1
65114	1
65125	1
65130	1
65135	1
65140	1
65150	1
65155	1
65175	1
65205	1
65210	1
65220	1
65222	1
65235	1
65260	1
65265	1
65270	1
65272	1
65273	1
65275	1
65280	1
65285	1
65286	1
65290	1
65400	1
65410	1
65420	1
65426	1
65430	1
65435	1
65436	1
65450	1
65600	1
65710	1
65730	1
65750	1
65755	1
65756	1
65757	1
65770	1
65772	1
65775	1
65778	1
65779	1
65780	1
65781	1
65782	1
65800	1
65810	1
65815	1
65820	1
65850	1
65855	1
65860	1
65865	1
65870	1
65875	1
65880	1
65900	1
65920	1
65930	1
66020	1
66030	1
66130	1
66150	1
66155	1
66160	1
66165	1
66170	1
66172	1
66174	1
66175	1
66180	1
66183	1
66185	1
66220	1
66225	1
66250	1
66500	1
66505	1
66600	1
66605	1
66625	1
66630	1
66635	1
66680	1
66682	1
66700	1
66710	1
66711	1
66720	1
66740	1
66761	1
66762	1
66770	1
66820	1
66821	1
66825	1
66830	1
66840	1
66850	1
66852	1
66920	1
66930	1
66940	1
66982	1
66983	1
66984	1
66985	1
66986	1
66990	1
67005	1
67010	1
67015	1
67025	1
67027	1
67028	1
67030	1
67031	1
67036	1
67039	1
67040	1
67041	1
67042	1
67043	1
67101	1
67105	1
67107	1
67108	1
67110	1
67112	1
67113	1
67115	1
67120	1
67121	1
67141	1
67145	1
67208	1
67210	1
67218	1
67220	1
67221	1
67225	1
67227	1
67228	1
67229	1
67250	1
67255	1
67311	1
67312	1
67314	1
67316	1
67318	1
67320	2
67331	1
67332	1
67334	1
67335	1
67340	2
67343	1
67345	1
67346	1
67400	1
67405	1
67412	1
67413	1
67414	1
67415	1
67420	1
67430	1
67440	1
67445	1
67450	1
67500	1
67505	1
67515	1
67550	1
67560	1
67570	1
67700	2
67710	1
67715	1
67800	1
67801	1
67805	1
67808	1
67810	2
67820	1
67825	1
67830	1
67835	1
67840	4
67850	3
67875	1
67880	1
67882	1
67900	1
67901	1
67902	1
67903	1
67904	1

CPT	MUE
67906	1
67908	1
67909	1
67911	4
67912	1
67914	1
67915	1
67916	1
67917	1
67921	1
67922	1
67923	1
67924	1
67930	2
67935	2
67938	2
67950	2
67961	4
67966	4
67971	1
67973	1
67974	1
67975	1
68020	1
68040	1
68100	1
68110	1
68115	1
68130	1
68135	1
68200	1
68320	1
68325	1
68326	2
68328	2
68330	1
68335	1
68340	1
68360	1
68362	1
68371	1
68400	1
68420	1
68440	2
68500	1
68505	1
68510	1
68520	1
68525	1
68530	1
68540	1
68550	1
68700	1
68705	2
68720	1
68745	1
68750	1
68760	4
68761	4
68770	1
68801	4
68810	1
68811	1
68815	1
68816	1

CPT	MUE
68840	1
68850	1
69000	1
69005	1
69020	1
69100	3
69105	1
69110	1
69120	1
69140	1
69145	1
69150	1
69155	1
69200	1
69205	1
69210	1
69220	1
69222	1
69300	1
69310	1
69320	1
69400	1
69401	1
69405	1
69420	1
69421	1
69424	1
69433	1
69436	1
69440	1
69450	1
69501	1
69502	1
69505	1
69511	1
69530	1
69535	1
69540	1
69550	1
69552	1
69554	1
69601	1
69602	1
69603	1
69604	1
69605	1
69610	1
69620	1
69631	1
69632	1
69633	1
69635	1
69636	1
69637	1
69641	1
69642	1
69643	1
69644	1
69645	1
69646	1
69650	1
69660	1
69661	1
69662	1
69666	1

CPT	MUE
69667	1
69670	1
69676	1
69700	1
69711	1
69714	1
69715	1
69717	1
69718	1
69720	1
69725	1
69740	1
69745	1
69801	1
69805	1
69806	1
69820	1
69840	1
69905	1
69910	1
69915	1
69930	1
69950	1
69955	1
69960	1
69970	1
69990	1
70010	1
70015	1
70030	2
70100	1
70110	1
70120	2
70130	2
70134	1
70140	1
70150	1
70160	1
70170	2
70190	1
70200	1
70210	1
70220	1
70240	1
70250	1
70260	1
70300	1
70310	1
70320	1
70328	1
70330	1
70332	2
70336	1
70350	1
70355	1
70360	1
70370	1
70371	1
70373	1
70380	2
70390	2
70450	3
70460	1
70470	2
70480	1

CPT	MUE
70481	1
70482	1
70486	1
70487	1
70488	1
70490	1
70491	1
70492	1
70496	1
70498	1
70540	1
70542	1
70543	1
70544	1
70545	1
70546	1
70547	1
70548	1
70549	1
70551	1
70552	1
70553	1
70554	1
70555	1
70557	1
70558	1
70559	1
71015	2
71021	1
71022	1
71023	2
71030	2
71034	1
71035	2
71100	1
71101	1
71110	1
71111	1
71120	1
71130	1
71250	1
71260	1
71270	1
71275	1
71550	1
71551	1
71552	1
71555	1
72010	1
72020	4
72040	3
72050	1
72052	1
72069	1
72070	1
72072	1
72074	1
72080	1
72090	1
72100	1
72110	1
72114	1
72120	1
72125	1
72126	1

CPT	MUE
72127	1
72128	1
72129	1
72130	1
72131	1
72132	1
72133	1
72141	1
72142	1
72146	1
72147	1
72148	1
72149	1
72156	1
72157	1
72158	1
72170	1
72190	1
72191	1
72192	1
72193	1
72194	1
72195	1
72196	1
72197	1
72198	1
72200	1
72202	1
72220	1
72240	1
72255	1
72265	1
72270	1
72275	3
72292	3
73000	2
73010	2
73020	2
73030	2
73040	2
73050	1
73060	2
73070	2
73080	2
73085	2
73090	2
73092	2
73100	2
73110	2
73115	2
73120	2
73130	2
73140	2
73200	2
73201	2
73202	2
73206	2
73218	2
73219	2
73220	2
73221	2
73222	2
73223	2
73500	1
73510	2

CPT	MUE
73520	2
73525	2
73530	2
73540	1
73550	2
73560	2
73562	2
73564	2
73565	1
73580	2
73590	2
73592	2
73600	2
73610	2
73615	2
73620	2
73630	2
73650	2
73660	2
73700	2
73701	2
73702	2
73706	2
73718	2
73719	2
73720	2
73721	4
73722	2
73723	4
73725	2
74000	3
74010	2
74020	2
74022	2
74150	1
74160	1
74170	1
74174	1
74175	1
74176	1
74177	1
74178	1
74181	1
74182	1
74183	1
74185	1
74190	1
74210	1
74220	1
74230	1
74235	1
74240	1
74241	1
74245	1
74246	1
74247	1
74249	1
74250	1
74251	1
74260	1
74261	1
74262	1
74270	1
74280	1
74283	1

CPT	MUE
74290	1
74291	1
74300	1
74301	2
74305	1
74320	1
74327	1
74328	1
74329	1
74330	1
74340	1
74355	1
74360	1
74363	2
74400	1
74410	1
74415	1
74420	2
74425	1
74430	1
74440	1
74445	1
74450	1
74455	1
74470	2
74475	2
74480	2
74485	2
74710	1
74740	1
74742	2
74775	1
75557	1
75559	1
75561	1
75563	1
75565	1
75571	1
75572	1
75573	1
75574	1
75600	1
75605	1
75625	1
75630	1
75635	1
75658	2
75710	1
75716	1
75726	3
75731	1
75733	1
75736	2
75741	1
75743	1
75746	1
75756	2
75791	1
75801	1
75803	1
75805	1
75807	1
75809	1
75810	1
75820	1

CPT	MUE
75822	1
75825	1
75827	1
75831	1
75833	1
75840	1
75842	1
75860	2
75870	1
75872	1
75880	2
75885	1
75887	1
75889	1
75891	1
75896	3
75898	1
75901	1
75902	2
75945	1
75952	1
75953	4
75954	2
75956	1
75957	1
75958	2
75959	1
75962	1
75964	4
75966	1
75968	2
75970	2
75980	1
75982	2
75984	2
75989	2
76000	3
76001	2
76010	2
76080	2
76100	2
76101	1
76102	1
76120	1
76125	1
76376	2
76377	2
76380	2
76506	1
76510	2
76511	2
76512	2
76513	2
76514	1
76516	1
76519	2
76529	2
76536	1
76604	1
76645	1
76700	1
76705	2
76770	1
76775	2
76776	1

CPT	MUE	CPT	MUE	CPT	MUE	CPT	MUE	CPT	MUE	CPT	MUE	CPT	MUE	CPT	MUE
76800	1	77082	1	77763	1	78428	1	79101	1	80426	1	81260	1	81405	2
76801	1	77084	1	77776	1	78445	1	79200	1	80428	1	81261	1	81406	3
76802	3	77261	1	77777	1	78451	1	79300	1	80430	1	81262	1	81407	1
76805	1	77262	1	77778	1	78452	1	79403	1	80432	1	81263	1	81408	1
76810	3	77263	1	77785	3	78453	1	79440	1	80434	1	81264	1	81500	1
76811	1	77280	2	77786	3	78454	1	79445	1	80435	1	81265	1	81503	1
76812	3	77285	1	77787	3	78456	1	80047	2	80436	1	81266	3	81504	1
76813	1	77290	1	77789	2	78457	1	80048	2	80438	1	81267	1	81506	1
76814	3	77293	1	77790	2	78458	1	80051	4	80439	1	81270	1	81507	1
76815	1	77295	1	78012	1	78459	1	80053	1	80440	1	81275	1	81508	1
76817	1	77300	10	78013	1	78466	1	80061	1	80500	1	81280	1	81509	1
76830	1	77301	1	78014	1	78468	1	80069	1	80502	1	81281	1	81510	1
76831	1	77305	2	78015	1	78469	1	80074	1	81000	2	81282	1	81511	1
76856	1	77310	2	78016	1	78472	1	80076	1	81001	2	81287	1	81512	1
76857	1	77315	2	78018	1	78473	1	80100	0	81002	2	81290	1	82000	1
76870	1	77321	1	78020	1	78481	1	80101	0	81003	2	81291	1	82003	3
76872	1	77326	1	78070	1	78483	1	80102	10	81005	2	81292	1	82009	3
76873	1	77327	1	78071	1	78491	1	80103	2	81007	1	81293	1	82010	4
76881	2	77328	1	78072	1	78492	1	80104	1	81015	2	81294	1	82013	1
76882	2	77332	4	78075	1	78494	1	80150	2	81020	1	81295	1	82016	1
76885	1	77333	4	78102	1	78496	1	80152	2	81025	1	81296	1	82017	1
76886	1	77336	1	78103	1	78579	1	80154	2	81050	2	81297	1	82030	1
76930	1	77338	1	78104	1	78580	1	80156	2	81161	1	81298	1	82040	1
76932	1	77370	1	78110	1	78582	1	80157	2	81200	1	81299	1	82042	2
76936	2	77371	1	78111	1	78597	1	80158	3	81201	1	81300	1	82043	1
76937	2	77372	1	78120	1	78598	1	80160	2	81202	1	81301	1	82044	1
76940	1	77373	1	78121	1	78600	1	80162	2	81203	1	81302	1	82045	1
76942	1	77401	2	78122	1	78601	1	80164	2	81205	1	81303	1	82055	3
76945	1	77402	2	78130	1	78605	1	80166	2	81206	1	81304	1	82075	2
76946	1	77403	2	78135	1	78606	2	80168	2	81207	1	81310	1	82085	1
76948	1	77404	2	78140	1	78607	1	80170	2	81208	1	81315	1	82088	2
76950	1	77406	2	78185	1	78608	1	80172	2	81209	1	81316	1	82101	1
76965	2	77407	2	78190	1	78610	1	80173	2	81210	1	81317	1	82103	1
76970	1	77408	2	78191	1	78630	2	80174	2	81211	1	81318	1	82104	1
76975	1	77409	2	78195	1	78635	1	80176	1	81212	1	81319	1	82105	1
76977	1	77411	2	78201	1	78645	1	80178	2	81213	1	81321	1	82106	4
76998	1	77412	2	78202	1	78647	1	80182	2	81214	1	81322	1	82107	1
77001	2	77413	2	78205	1	78650	1	80184	2	81215	2	81323	1	82108	1
77002	1	77414	2	78206	1	78660	1	80185	2	81216	1	81324	1	82120	1
77003	1	77416	2	78215	1	78700	1	80186	2	81217	2	81325	1	82127	2
77011	1	77417	1	78216	1	78701	2	80188	2	81220	1	81326	1	82128	2
77012	1	77418	2	78226	1	78707	1	80190	2	81221	1	81330	1	82131	3
77013	1	77421	2	78227	1	78708	1	80192	2	81222	1	81331	1	82135	1
77014	2	77422	1	78230	1	78709	1	80194	2	81223	1	81332	1	82136	3
77021	1	77423	1	78231	1	78710	1	80195	2	81224	1	81340	1	82139	3
77022	1	77424	1	78232	1	78725	1	80197	2	81225	1	81341	1	82140	2
77051	1	77425	1	78258	1	78730	1	80198	2	81226	1	81342	1	82143	2
77052	1	77427	1	78261	1	78740	1	80200	2	81227	1	81350	1	82145	2
77053	2	77431	1	78262	1	78761	1	80201	2	81228	1	81355	1	82150	4
77054	2	77432	1	78264	1	78800	1	80202	2	81229	1	81370	1	82154	1
77055	1	77435	1	78267	1	78801	1	80299	3	81235	1	81371	1	82157	1
77056	1	77469	1	78268	1	78802	1	80400	1	81240	1	81372	1	82160	1
77057	1	77470	1	78270	1	78803	1	80402	1	81241	1	81373	2	82163	1
77058	1	77520	1	78271	1	78804	1	80406	1	81242	1	81374	3	82164	1
77059	1	77522	1	78272	1	78805	1	80408	1	81243	1	81375	1	82172	3
77071	1	77523	1	78278	2	78806	1	80410	1	81244	1	81377	3	82175	2
77072	1	77525	1	78282	1	78807	1	80412	1	81245	1	81378	1	82180	1
77073	1	77600	1	78290	1	78808	1	80414	1	81250	1	81379	1	82190	4
77074	1	77605	1	78291	1	78811	1	80415	1	81251	1	81380	2	82205	2
77075	1	77610	1	78300	1	78812	1	80416	1	81252	1	81383	3	82232	2
77076	1	77615	1	78305	1	78813	1	80417	1	81253	1	81400	2	82239	1
77077	1	77620	1	78306	1	78814	1	80418	1	81254	1	81401	3	82240	1
77078	1	77750	1	78315	1	78815	1	80420	1	81255	1	81402	1	82247	2
77080	1	77761	1	78320	1	78816	1	80422	1	81256	1	81403	3	82248	2
77081	1	77762	1	78414	1	79005	1	80424	1	81257	1	81404	3	82252	1

Appendix L — Medically Unlikely Edits (MUEs) — OPPS

CPT	MUE
82261	1
82270	1
82271	3
82272	1
82274	1
82286	1
82300	1
82306	1
82308	3
82310	4
82330	4
82331	1
82340	1
82355	3
82360	3
82365	3
82370	3
82373	1
82374	3
82375	4
82376	2
82378	1
82379	1
82380	1
82382	1
82383	1
82384	2
82387	1
82390	1
82415	1
82435	3
82436	1
82438	1
82441	1
82465	1
82480	2
82482	1
82485	1
82486	2
82487	2
82488	1
82489	2
82491	4
82492	2
82495	1
82507	1
82520	2
82523	1
82525	2
82528	1
82530	2
82540	1
82542	6
82543	2
82544	2
82550	3
82552	3
82553	3
82554	2
82565	3
82570	3
82575	1
82585	1
82595	1
82600	1

CPT	MUE
82607	1
82608	1
82610	1
82615	1
82626	1
82627	1
82633	1
82634	1
82638	1
82646	1
82649	1
82651	1
82652	1
82654	1
82656	1
82657	3
82658	2
82666	1
82668	1
82670	2
82671	1
82672	1
82677	1
82679	1
82690	1
82693	2
82696	1
82705	1
82710	1
82715	3
82725	1
82726	1
82728	1
82731	1
82735	1
82742	1
82746	1
82747	1
82757	1
82759	1
82760	1
82775	1
82776	1
82777	1
82784	6
82785	1
82787	4
82800	2
82820	1
82930	1
82941	1
82943	1
82946	1
82950	3
82951	1
82952	3
82953	1
82955	1
82960	1
82963	1
82965	1
82975	1
82977	1
82978	1
82979	1

CPT	MUE
82980	1
82985	1
83003	5
83008	1
83009	1
83010	1
83012	1
83013	1
83014	1
83015	1
83018	7
83020	2
83021	2
83026	1
83030	1
83033	1
83036	1
83037	1
83045	1
83050	4
83051	1
83055	1
83060	1
83065	1
83068	1
83069	1
83070	1
83071	1
83080	2
83088	1
83090	2
83150	1
83491	1
83497	1
83498	2
83499	1
83500	1
83505	1
83518	2
83525	4
83527	1
83528	1
83540	2
83550	1
83570	1
83582	1
83586	1
83593	1
83605	3
83615	3
83625	1
83630	1
83631	1
83632	1
83633	1
83634	1
83655	2
83661	4
83662	4
83663	4
83664	4
83670	1
83690	2
83695	1
83698	1

CPT	MUE
83700	1
83701	1
83704	1
83718	1
83719	1
83721	1
83727	1
83735	4
83775	1
83785	1
83788	3
83789	4
83805	2
83825	2
83835	2
83840	2
83857	1
83858	1
83861	2
83864	1
83866	1
83872	2
83873	1
83874	4
83876	1
83880	1
83885	2
83887	2
83915	1
83916	2
83918	2
83919	1
83921	2
83925	4
83930	2
83935	2
83937	1
83945	2
83950	1
83951	1
83970	4
83986	2
83987	1
83992	2
83993	1
84022	2
84030	1
84035	1
84060	1
84061	1
84066	1
84075	2
84078	1
84080	1
84081	1
84085	1
84087	1
84100	3
84105	1
84106	1
84110	1
84112	1
84119	1
84120	1
84126	1

CPT	MUE
84127	1
84132	4
84133	2
84134	1
84135	1
84138	1
84140	1
84143	2
84144	1
84145	1
84146	3
84150	2
84152	1
84153	1
84154	1
84155	1
84156	1
84157	3
84160	2
84163	1
84165	1
84166	2
84202	1
84203	1
84206	1
84207	1
84210	1
84220	1
84228	1
84233	2
84234	2
84235	1
84238	3
84252	1
84255	2
84260	1
84270	1
84275	1
84285	1
84295	4
84300	2
84302	3
84305	1
84307	1
84311	2
84315	2
84375	1
84376	1
84377	1
84378	2
84379	1
84392	1
84402	1
84403	2
84425	1
84430	1
84431	1
84432	1
84436	1
84437	1
84439	1
84442	1
84443	4
84445	1
84446	1

CPT	MUE
84449	1
84450	1
84460	1
84466	1
84478	1
84479	1
84480	1
84481	1
84482	1
84484	4
84485	1
84488	1
84490	1
84510	1
84512	3
84520	4
84525	1
84540	2
84545	1
84550	1
84560	2
84577	1
84578	1
84580	1
84583	1
84585	1
84586	1
84588	1
84590	1
84591	1
84597	1
84600	2
84620	1
84630	2
84681	1
84702	2
84703	1
84704	1
84830	1
85002	1
85004	2
85007	1
85008	1
85009	1
85013	2
85014	4
85018	4
85025	2
85032	3
85041	2
85044	1
85045	1
85046	1
85048	2
85049	2
85055	1
85060	1
85097	2
85130	1
85170	1
85175	1
85210	2
85220	2
85230	2
85240	2

CPT	MUE
85244	1
85245	2
85246	2
85247	2
85250	2
85260	2
85270	2
85280	2
85290	2
85291	1
85292	1
85293	1
85300	2
85301	1
85302	1
85303	2
85305	2
85306	2
85307	2
85335	2
85337	1
85345	1
85347	9
85348	4
85360	1
85362	2
85366	1
85370	1
85378	2
85379	2
85380	2
85384	2
85385	1
85390	3
85396	1
85400	1
85410	1
85415	2
85420	2
85421	1
85441	1
85445	1
85460	1
85461	1
85475	1
85525	2
85530	1
85536	1
85540	1
85547	1
85549	1
85555	1
85557	1
85597	1
85598	1
85611	2
85612	1
85613	1
85635	1
85651	1
85652	1
85660	1
85670	2
85675	1
85705	1

CPT	MUE
85732	4
85810	2
86021	1
86022	1
86023	3
86038	1
86039	1
86060	1
86063	1
86077	1
86078	1
86079	1
86140	1
86141	1
86146	3
86147	4
86148	3
86152	1
86153	1
86155	1
86156	1
86157	1
86160	4
86161	3
86162	1
86171	3
86200	1
86215	1
86225	1
86226	1
86243	1
86277	1
86280	1
86294	1
86300	2
86301	1
86304	1
86305	1
86308	1
86309	1
86310	1
86316	3
86320	1
86325	2
86327	1
86332	1
86334	1
86335	2
86336	1
86337	1
86340	1
86341	1
86343	1
86344	1
86352	1
86355	1
86357	1
86359	1
86360	1
86361	1
86367	2
86376	2
86378	1
86382	3
86384	1

CPT	MUE
86386	1
86406	2
86430	2
86431	2
86480	1
86481	1
86485	1
86486	2
86490	1
86510	1
86580	1
86590	1
86592	2
86593	2
86602	3
86603	2
86612	2
86617	2
86618	2
86619	2
86625	2
86628	3
86632	3
86641	2
86644	1
86645	1
86648	2
86651	2
86652	2
86653	2
86654	2
86663	2
86664	2
86665	2
86668	2
86674	3
86677	3
86684	2
86687	2
86688	2
86689	2
86692	2
86694	2
86695	2
86696	2
86698	3
86701	2
86702	2
86703	1
86704	1
86705	1
86706	2
86707	1
86708	1
86709	1
86711	2
86713	3
86720	2
86723	2
86727	2
86732	2
86738	2
86741	2
86744	2
86747	2

CPT	MUE
86750	4
86753	3
86756	2
86759	2
86762	2
86768	5
86771	2
86774	2
86777	2
86778	2
86780	2
86784	2
86787	2
86788	2
86789	2
86793	2
86800	1
86803	1
86804	1
86807	2
86808	1
86812	1
86813	1
86816	1
86817	1
86821	1
86822	1
86825	1
86828	2
86829	2
86830	2
86831	2
86832	2
86833	1
86834	1
86835	1
86850	3
86860	2
86880	4
86885	3
86886	3
86890	2
86891	2
86900	3
86901	3
86906	1
86930	3
86940	3
86941	3
86945	3
86950	1
86960	3
86965	4
86975	2
86976	2
86977	2
87001	1
87003	1
87045	3
87073	3
87084	2
87086	3
87103	3
87109	3
87110	2

CPT	MUE
87118	3
87143	2
87164	2
87166	2
87168	2
87169	2
87172	1
87176	3
87177	3
87187	3
87197	1
87207	3
87220	3
87230	3
87250	3
87253	3
87255	2
87260	1
87265	1
87267	1
87269	1
87270	1
87271	1
87272	1
87273	1
87274	1
87275	1
87276	1
87277	1
87278	1
87279	1
87280	1
87281	1
87283	1
87285	1
87290	1
87299	1
87301	1
87305	1
87320	1
87324	1
87327	1
87328	1
87329	1
87332	1
87335	1
87336	1
87337	1
87338	1
87339	1
87340	1
87341	1
87350	1
87380	1
87385	1
87389	1
87390	1
87391	1
87400	2
87420	1
87425	1
87427	2
87430	1
87449	3
87450	2

CPT	MUE
87451	2
87470	1
87471	1
87472	1
87475	1
87476	1
87477	1
87480	1
87481	1
87482	1
87485	1
87486	1
87487	1
87490	1
87491	1
87492	1
87493	1
87495	1
87496	1
87497	1
87498	1
87500	1
87501	1
87502	1
87503	1
87510	1
87511	1
87512	1
87515	1
87516	1
87517	1
87520	1
87521	1
87522	1
87525	1
87526	1
87527	1
87528	1
87529	1
87530	1
87531	1
87532	1
87533	1
87534	1
87535	1
87536	1
87537	1
87538	1
87539	1
87540	1
87541	1
87542	1
87550	1
87551	1
87552	1
87555	1
87556	1
87557	1
87560	1
87561	1
87562	1
87580	1
87581	1
87582	1
87590	1

CPT	MUE
87591	1
87592	1
87620	1
87621	1
87622	1
87631	1
87632	1
87633	1
87640	1
87641	1
87650	1
87651	1
87652	1
87653	1
87660	1
87661	1
87797	3
87799	3
87800	2
87802	2
87803	3
87804	2
87807	2
87808	1
87810	2
87850	1
87880	2
87900	1
87901	1
87902	1
87903	1
87905	2
87906	2
87910	1
87912	1
88104	4
88106	3
88120	2
88121	2
88125	1
88130	1
88140	1
88141	1
88142	1
88143	1
88147	1
88148	1
88150	1
88152	1
88153	1
88154	1
88155	1
88160	4
88161	4
88162	3
88164	1
88165	1
88166	1
88167	1
88172	3
88173	3
88174	1
88175	1
88177	2
88182	2

CPT	MUE
88184	1
88187	1
88188	1
88189	1
88230	2
88233	2
88239	3
88240	3
88241	3
88245	1
88248	1
88249	1
88261	2
88262	2
88263	1
88264	2
88267	2
88269	2
88273	3
88283	2
88289	1
88291	1
88300	2
88302	2
88309	3
88311	4
88321	1
88323	1
88325	1
88329	4
88331	11
88333	4
88342	0
88343	0
88347	4
88348	1
88349	1
88355	1
88356	1
88358	2
88360	6
88361	6
88362	1
88363	1
88371	1
88372	1
88375	1
88380	1
88381	1
88387	3
88388	3
88720	1
88738	2
88740	1
88741	1
89049	1
89050	2
89051	2
89055	2
89060	2
89125	2
89160	1
89190	1
89220	2
89230	1

CPT	MUE
89240	2
89250	1
89251	1
89253	1
89254	1
89255	1
89257	1
89258	1
89259	1
89260	1
89261	1
89264	1
89268	1
89272	1
89280	1
89281	1
89290	1
89291	1
89300	1
89310	1
89320	1
89321	1
89322	1
89325	1
89329	1
89330	1
89331	1
89335	1
89342	1
89343	1
89344	1
89346	1
89352	1
89353	1
89354	1
89356	2
90284	1
90296	1
90375	20
90376	20
90385	1
90393	1
90396	1
90460	3
90471	1
90472	4
90473	1
90474	1
90476	1
90477	1
90581	1
90585	1
90586	1
90632	1
90633	1
90634	1
90636	1
90644	1
90645	1
90646	1
90647	1
90648	1
90649	1
90650	1
90653	1

CPT	MUE
90655	1
90656	1
90657	1
90658	1
90660	1
90661	1
90664	1
90666	1
90667	1
90668	1
90669	1
90672	1
90673	1
90675	1
90676	1
90680	1
90681	1
90685	1
90686	1
90687	1
90688	1
90690	1
90691	1
90692	1
90693	1
90696	1
90698	1
90700	1
90702	1
90703	1
90704	1
90705	1
90706	1
90707	1
90708	1
90710	1
90712	1
90713	1
90714	1
90715	1
90716	1
90717	1
90719	1
90720	1
90721	1
90725	1
90727	1
90732	1
90733	1
90734	1
90735	1
90736	1
90738	1
90739	1
90740	1
90743	1
90744	1
90746	1
90747	1
90785	2
90791	1
90792	2
90832	2
90833	2
90834	2

CPT	MUE
90836	2
90837	2
90838	2
90839	1
90845	1
90846	2
90847	2
90849	2
90853	5
90863	1
90865	1
90867	1
90868	1
90869	1
90870	2
90880	1
90885	1
90887	1
90889	1
90901	1
90911	1
90935	1
90937	1
90940	2
90945	1
90947	1
90951	1
90952	1
90953	1
90954	1
90955	1
90956	1
90957	1
90958	1
90959	1
90960	1
90961	1
90962	1
90963	1
90964	1
90965	1
90966	1
90967	1
90968	1
90969	1
90970	1
90989	1
90993	1
90997	1
91010	1
91013	1
91020	1
91022	1
91030	1
91034	1
91035	1
91037	1
91038	1
91040	1
91065	2
91110	1
91111	1
91112	1
91117	1
91120	1

CPT	MUE
91122	1
91132	1
91133	1
92002	1
92004	1
92012	1
92014	1
92018	1
92019	1
92020	1
92025	1
92060	1
92065	1
92071	2
92072	1
92081	1
92082	1
92083	1
92100	1
92132	1
92133	1
92134	1
92136	1
92140	1
92225	2
92226	2
92227	1
92228	1
92230	2
92235	2
92240	2
92250	1
92260	1
92265	1
92270	1
92275	1
92283	1
92284	1
92285	1
92286	1
92287	1
92311	1
92312	1
92313	1
92315	1
92316	1
92317	1
92325	1
92326	2
92352	1
92353	1
92354	1
92355	1
92358	1
92371	1
92502	1
92504	1
92507	1
92508	1
92511	1
92512	1
92516	1
92520	1
92521	1
92522	1

CPT	MUE
92523	1
92524	1
92526	1
92531	1
92532	1
92533	4
92534	1
92540	1
92541	1
92542	1
92543	4
92544	1
92545	1
92546	1
92547	1
92548	1
92550	1
92552	1
92553	1
92555	1
92556	1
92557	1
92558	0
92561	1
92562	1
92563	1
92564	1
92565	1
92567	1
92568	1
92570	1
92571	1
92572	1
92575	1
92576	1
92577	1
92579	1
92582	1
92583	1
92584	1
92585	1
92586	1
92587	1
92588	1
92596	1
92601	1
92602	1
92603	1
92604	1
92605	1
92606	1
92609	1
92610	1
92613	1
92615	1
92617	1
92618	1
92620	1
92625	1
92626	1
92920	1
92924	1
92928	1
92933	1
92937	3

CPT	MUE
92938	3
92941	1
92943	1
92944	1
92950	4
92953	2
92960	2
92961	1
92970	1
92971	1
92973	2
92974	1
92975	1
92977	1
92978	1
92979	2
92986	1
92987	1
92990	1
92992	1
92993	1
92997	1
92998	2
93000	3
93005	3
93015	1
93016	1
93017	1
93018	1
93024	1
93025	1
93040	3
93041	3
93042	3
93224	1
93225	1
93226	1
93227	1
93228	1
93229	1
93268	1
93270	1
93271	1
93272	1
93278	1
93279	1
93280	1
93281	1
93282	1
93283	1
93284	1
93285	1
93286	2
93287	2
93288	1
93289	1
93290	1
93291	1
93292	1
93293	1
93294	1
93295	1
93296	1
93297	1
93298	1

CPT	MUE
93299	1
93303	1
93304	1
93306	1
93307	1
93308	1
93312	1
93313	1
93314	1
93315	1
93316	1
93317	1
93318	1
93320	1
93321	1
93325	1
93350	1
93351	1
93352	1
93451	1
93452	1
93453	1
93454	1
93455	1
93456	1
93457	1
93458	1
93459	1
93460	1
93461	1
93462	1
93463	1
93464	1
93503	2
93505	1
93530	1
93531	1
93532	1
93533	1
93561	1
93562	1
93563	1
93564	1
93565	1
93566	1
93567	1
93568	1
93571	1
93572	2
93580	1
93581	1
93582	1
93583	1
93600	1
93602	1
93603	1
93609	1
93610	1
93612	1
93613	1
93615	1
93616	1
93618	1
93619	1
93620	1

CPT	MUE
93621	1
93622	1
93623	1
93624	1
93631	1
93640	1
93641	1
93642	1
93650	1
93653	1
93654	1
93655	1
93656	1
93657	1
93660	1
93662	1
93701	1
93724	1
93740	1
93745	1
93750	1
93770	1
93784	1
93786	1
93788	1
93790	1
93797	2
93798	2
93880	1
93882	1
93886	1
93888	1
93890	1
93892	1
93893	1
93922	1
93923	1
93924	1
93925	1
93926	1
93930	1
93931	1
93965	1
93970	1
93971	1
93975	1
93976	1
93978	1
93979	1
93980	1
93981	1
93982	1
93990	2
94002	1
94003	1
94004	1
94010	1
94011	1
94012	1
94013	1
94014	1
94015	1
94016	1
94060	1
94070	1

CPT	MUE
94150	2
94200	1
94250	1
94375	1
94400	1
94450	1
94452	1
94453	1
94610	2
94620	1
94621	1
94640	10
94642	1
94644	1
94645	2
94660	1
94662	1
94664	1
94667	1
94669	4
94680	1
94681	1
94690	1
94726	1
94727	1
94728	1
94729	1
94750	1
94760	1
94761	1
94762	1
94770	1
94772	1
94774	1
94775	1
94776	1
94777	1
94780	1
94781	1
95012	2
95018	19
95056	1
95060	1
95065	1
95070	1
95071	1
95076	1
95079	2
95115	1
95117	1
95250	1
95251	1
95782	1
95783	1
95800	1
95801	1
95803	1
95805	1
95806	1
95807	1
95808	1
95810	1
95811	1
95812	1
95813	1

CPT	MUE
95816	1
95819	1
95822	1
95824	1
95827	1
95829	1
95830	1
95831	5
95832	1
95851	3
95852	1
95857	1
95860	1
95861	1
95863	1
95864	1
95865	1
95866	1
95867	1
95868	1
95869	1
95873	1
95874	1
95875	2
95885	4
95886	4
95887	1
95905	2
95907	1
95908	1
95909	1
95910	1
95911	1
95912	1
95913	1
95921	1
95922	1
95923	1
95924	1
95925	1
95926	1
95927	1
95928	1
95929	1
95930	1
95933	1
95938	1
95939	1
95943	1
95950	1
95951	1
95953	1
95954	1
95955	1
95956	1
95957	1
95958	1
95961	1
95962	3
95965	1
95966	1
95967	3
95970	1
95971	1
95972	1

CPT	MUE
95974	1
95975	2
95978	1
95980	1
95981	1
95982	1
95990	2
95991	2
95992	1
96000	1
96001	1
96002	1
96003	1
96004	1
96020	1
96103	1
96105	3
96120	1
96125	2
96360	1
96365	1
96368	1
96369	1
96370	3
96371	1
96373	3
96374	1
96376	10
96402	2
96405	1
96406	1
96409	1
96413	1
96416	1
96420	2
96422	2
96425	1
96440	1
96446	1
96450	1
96521	2
96522	1
96523	2
96542	1
96567	1
96570	1
96571	3
96900	1
96902	1
96904	1
96910	1
96912	1
96913	1
96920	1
96921	1
96922	1
97010	1
97012	1
97016	1
97018	1
97022	1
97024	1
97026	1
97028	1
97150	1

CPT	MUE
97545	1
97546	2
97597	1
97602	1
97605	1
97606	1
97610	1
98925	1
98926	1
98927	1
98928	1
98929	1
98940	1
98941	1
98942	1
99002	1
99024	1
99050	1
99051	1
99053	1
99056	1
99058	1
99060	1
99070	1
99071	1
99078	3
99080	1
99082	1
99090	1
99091	1
99100	3
99116	1
99135	1
99140	2
99143	2
99144	2
99148	2
99149	2
99170	1
99175	1
99183	1
99191	1
99192	1
99195	2
99201	1
99202	1
99203	1
99204	1
99205	1
99211	2
99212	2
99213	2
99214	2
99215	2
99217	1
99218	1
99219	1
99220	1
99221	0
99222	0
99223	0
99224	1
99225	1
99226	1
99231	0

CPT	MUE
99232	0
99233	0
99234	1
99235	1
99236	1
99238	0
99239	0
99281	2
99282	2
99283	2
99284	2
99285	2
99288	1
99291	1
99304	1
99305	1
99306	1
99307	1
99308	1
99309	1
99310	1
99315	1
99316	1
99318	1
99324	1
99325	1
99326	1
99327	1
99328	1
99334	1
99335	1
99336	1
99337	1
99339	1
99340	1
99341	1
99342	1
99343	1
99344	1
99345	1
99347	1
99348	1
99349	1
99350	1
99354	1
99356	1
99358	1
99359	1
99363	1
99364	1
99366	3
99367	1
99368	3
99374	1
99377	1
99379	1
99380	1
99406	1
99407	1
99446	1
99447	1
99448	1
99449	1
99455	1
99456	1

CPT	MUE
99460	1
99461	1
99462	1
99463	1
99464	1
99465	1
99466	1
99468	1
99469	1
99471	1
99472	1
99475	1
99476	1
99477	1
99478	1
99479	1
99480	1
99481	1
99482	1
99485	1
99487	1
99488	1
99495	1
99496	1
99605	0
99606	0
99607	0
A0382	0
A0384	0
A0392	0
A0394	0
A0396	0
A0398	0
A0420	0
A0422	0
A0424	0
A0426	2
A0427	2
A0428	4
A0429	2
A0430	1
A0431	1
A0432	1
A0433	1
A0434	2
A0435	999
A0436	300
A4221	0
A4222	0
A4233	0
A4234	0
A4235	0
A4236	0
A4253	0
A4255	0
A4256	0
A4257	0
A4258	0
A4259	0
A4262	4
A4263	4
A4301	1
A4356	1
A4396	3
A4399	2

CPT	MUE
A4463	3
A4470	1
A4480	1
A4555	0
A4557	0
A4561	1
A4562	1
A4565	2
A4595	0
A4604	0
A4605	0
A4606	1
A4611	0
A4612	0
A4613	0
A4614	0
A4618	0
A4623	90
A4624	0
A4625	30
A4628	0
A4633	0
A4635	0
A4636	0
A4637	0
A4638	0
A4640	0
A4642	1
A4648	3
A4650	3
A4670	0
A4932	0
A5056	90
A5057	90
A5102	1
A5120	150
A5500	0
A5501	0
A5503	0
A5504	0
A5505	0
A5506	0
A5507	0
A5508	0
A5510	0
A5512	0
A5513	0
A6501	2
A6502	2
A6503	2
A6504	4
A6505	4
A6506	4
A6507	4
A6508	4
A6509	2
A6510	2
A6511	2
A6513	2
A6545	2
A6550	0
A7000	0
A7001	0
A7002	0
A7003	0

CPT	MUE
A7004	0
A7005	0
A7006	0
A7007	0
A7010	0
A7012	0
A7013	0
A7014	0
A7015	0
A7016	0
A7017	0
A7018	0
A7020	0
A7025	0
A7026	0
A7027	0
A7028	0
A7029	0
A7030	0
A7031	0
A7032	0
A7033	0
A7034	0
A7035	0
A7036	0
A7037	0
A7038	0
A7039	0
A7040	2
A7041	2
A7042	2
A7043	10
A7044	0
A7045	0
A7046	0
A7047	0
A7502	3
A7503	3
A7504	180
A7506	90
A7507	200
A7508	200
A7509	300
A7522	1
A7524	2
A7526	36
A9272	0
A9284	1
A9500	3
A9501	3
A9502	3
A9503	1
A9504	1
A9507	1
A9508	2
A9510	1
A9512	30
A9520	1
A9521	2
A9526	2
A9536	1
A9537	1
A9538	1
A9539	2
A9540	2

CPT	MUE
A9541	1
A9542	1
A9543	1
A9544	1
A9545	1
A9546	1
A9547	2
A9550	1
A9551	1
A9552	1
A9553	1
A9554	1
A9555	3
A9556	10
A9557	2
A9559	1
A9560	2
A9561	1
A9562	2
A9566	1
A9567	2
A9569	1
A9570	1
A9571	1
A9579	100
A9580	1
A9582	1
A9583	18
A9584	1
A9585	300
A9586	1
A9599	1
A9600	7
A9604	1
A9700	2
B4034	0
B4035	0
B4036	0
B4081	0
B4082	0
B4083	0
B4087	1
B4149	0
B4150	0
B4152	0
B4153	0
B4154	0
B4155	0
B4157	0
B4158	0
B4159	0
B4160	0
B4161	0
B4162	0
B4164	0
B4168	0
B4172	0
B4176	0
B4178	0
B4180	0
B4189	0
B4193	0
B4197	0
B4199	0
B4216	0

CPT	MUE
B4220	0
B4222	0
B4224	0
B5000	0
B5100	0
B5200	0
B9000	0
B9002	0
B9004	0
B9006	0
C1721	1
C1722	1
C1731	2
C1732	3
C1733	3
C1749	1
C1750	2
C1751	3
C1752	2
C1753	2
C1754	2
C1755	2
C1756	2
C1758	2
C1759	2
C1764	1
C1767	2
C1768	3
C1770	3
C1771	1
C1772	1
C1773	3
C1777	2
C1779	2
C1780	2
C1782	1
C1783	2
C1784	2
C1785	1
C1786	1
C1787	2
C1788	2
C1789	2
C1813	1
C1814	2
C1815	1
C1816	2
C1817	1
C1818	2
C1820	2
C1830	2
C1840	1
C1841	1
C1878	2
C1880	2
C1881	2
C1882	1
C1886	1
C1888	2
C1891	1
C1895	2
C1896	2
C1897	2
C1898	2
C1899	2

Appendix L — Medically Unlikely Edits (MUEs) — OPPS

CPT	MUE	CPT	MUE	CPT	MUE	CPT	MUE	CPT	MUE	CPT	MUE	CPT	MUE	CPT	MUE
C1900	1	C9359	30	E0181	0	E0297	0	E0575	0	E0748	0	E0981	0	E1222	0
C2614	3	C9360	300	E0182	0	E0300	0	E0580	0	E0749	1	E0982	0	E1223	0
C2615	2	C9361	10	E0184	0	E0301	0	E0585	0	E0755	0	E0983	0	E1224	0
C2616	1	C9362	60	E0185	0	E0302	0	E0600	0	E0760	0	E0984	0	E1225	0
C2619	1	C9363	500	E0186	0	E0303	0	E0601	0	E0761	0	E0985	0	E1226	1
C2620	1	C9364	600	E0187	0	E0304	0	E0602	0	E0762	1	E0986	0	E1228	0
C2621	1	C9600	3	E0188	0	E0305	0	E0603	0	E0764	0	E0988	0	E1229	0
C2622	1	C9601	2	E0189	0	E0310	0	E0604	0	E0765	0	E0990	2	E1230	0
C2626	1	C9602	3	E0190	0	E0315	0	E0605	0	E0766	0	E0992	1	E1231	0
C2627	2	C9603	2	E0191	0	E0316	0	E0606	0	E0769	0	E0994	0	E1232	0
C2631	1	C9604	3	E0193	0	E0325	0	E0607	0	E0770	1	E0995	2	E1233	0
C5271	1	C9605	3	E0194	0	E0326	0	E0610	0	E0776	0	E1002	0	E1234	0
C5272	3	C9606	2	E0196	0	E0328	0	E0615	0	E0779	0	E1003	0	E1235	0
C5273	1	C9607	1	E0197	0	E0329	0	E0616	1	E0780	0	E1004	0	E1236	0
C5274	35	C9608	2	E0198	0	E0350	0	E0617	0	E0781	0	E1005	0	E1237	0
C5275	1	C9724	1	E0199	0	E0352	0	E0618	0	E0782	1	E1006	0	E1238	0
C5276	3	C9725	1	E0200	0	E0370	0	E0619	0	E0783	1	E1007	0	E1239	0
C5277	1	C9726	2	E0202	0	E0371	0	E0620	0	E0784	0	E1008	0	E1240	0
C5278	15	C9727	1	E0203	0	E0372	0	E0621	0	E0785	1	E1009	0	E1250	0
C8900	1	C9728	1	E0205	0	E0373	0	E0625	0	E0786	1	E1010	0	E1260	0
C8901	1	C9733	1	E0210	0	E0424	0	E0627	0	E0791	0	E1011	0	E1270	0
C8902	1	C9734	1	E0215	0	E0425	0	E0628	0	E0830	0	E1014	0	E1280	0
C8903	1	C9735	1	E0217	0	E0430	0	E0629	0	E0840	0	E1015	0	E1285	0
C8904	1	C9737	1	E0218	0	E0431	0	E0630	0	E0849	0	E1016	0	E1290	0
C8905	1	C9739	1	E0221	0	E0433	0	E0635	0	E0850	0	E1017	0	E1295	0
C8906	1	C9740	1	E0225	0	E0434	0	E0636	0	E0855	0	E1018	0	E1300	0
C8907	1	C9800	1	E0231	0	E0435	0	E0637	0	E0856	0	E1020	0	E1310	0
C8908	1	C9898	1	E0232	0	E0439	0	E0638	0	E0860	0	E1028	0	E1352	0
C8909	1	E0100	0	E0235	0	E0440	0	E0639	0	E0870	0	E1029	0	E1353	0
C8910	1	E0105	0	E0236	0	E0441	0	E0640	0	E0880	0	E1030	0	E1354	0
C8911	1	E0110	0	E0239	0	E0442	0	E0641	0	E0890	0	E1031	0	E1355	0
C8912	1	E0111	0	E0240	0	E0443	0	E0642	0	E0900	0	E1035	0	E1356	0
C8913	1	E0112	0	E0241	0	E0444	0	E0650	0	E0910	0	E1036	0	E1357	0
C8914	1	E0113	0	E0242	0	E0445	0	E0651	0	E0911	0	E1037	0	E1358	0
C8918	1	E0114	0	E0243	0	E0446	0	E0652	0	E0912	0	E1038	0	E1372	0
C8919	1	E0116	0	E0244	0	E0450	0	E0655	0	E0920	0	E1039	0	E1390	0
C8920	1	E0117	0	E0245	0	E0455	0	E0656	0	E0930	0	E1050	0	E1391	0
C8921	1	E0118	0	E0246	0	E0457	0	E0657	0	E0935	0	E1060	0	E1392	0
C8922	1	E0130	0	E0247	0	E0459	0	E0660	0	E0936	0	E1070	0	E1405	0
C8923	1	E0135	0	E0248	0	E0460	0	E0665	0	E0940	0	E1083	0	E1406	0
C8924	1	E0140	0	E0249	0	E0461	0	E0666	0	E0941	0	E1084	0	E1500	0
C8925	1	E0141	0	E0250	0	E0462	0	E0667	0	E0942	0	E1085	0	E1510	0
C8926	1	E0143	0	E0251	0	E0463	0	E0668	0	E0944	0	E1086	0	E1520	0
C8927	1	E0144	0	E0255	0	E0464	0	E0669	0	E0945	0	E1087	0	E1530	0
C8928	1	E0147	0	E0256	0	E0470	0	E0670	0	E0946	0	E1088	0	E1540	0
C8929	1	E0148	0	E0260	0	E0471	0	E0671	0	E0947	0	E1089	0	E1550	0
C8930	1	E0149	0	E0261	0	E0472	0	E0672	0	E0948	0	E1090	0	E1560	0
C8931	1	E0153	0	E0265	0	E0480	0	E0673	0	E0950	0	E1092	0	E1570	0
C8932	1	E0154	0	E0266	0	E0481	0	E0675	0	E0951	0	E1093	0	E1575	0
C8933	1	E0155	0	E0270	0	E0482	0	E0676	1	E0952	0	E1100	0	E1580	0
C8934	2	E0156	0	E0271	0	E0483	0	E0691	0	E0955	0	E1110	0	E1590	0
C8935	2	E0157	0	E0272	0	E0484	0	E0692	0	E0956	0	E1130	0	E1592	0
C8936	2	E0158	0	E0273	0	E0485	0	E0693	0	E0957	0	E1140	0	E1594	0
C8957	2	E0159	0	E0274	0	E0486	0	E0694	0	E0958	0	E1150	0	E1600	0
C9254	400	E0160	0	E0275	0	E0487	0	E0700	0	E0959	2	E1160	0	E1610	0
C9275	1	E0161	0	E0276	0	E0500	0	E0705	1	E0960	0	E1161	0	E1615	0
C9285	2	E0162	0	E0277	0	E0550	0	E0710	0	E0961	2	E1170	0	E1620	0
C9290	266	E0163	0	E0280	0	E0555	0	E0720	0	E0966	1	E1171	0	E1625	0
C9293	700	E0165	0	E0290	0	E0560	0	E0730	0	E0967	0	E1172	0	E1630	0
C9352	3	E0167	0	E0291	0	E0561	0	E0731	0	E0968	0	E1180	0	E1632	0
C9353	4	E0168	0	E0292	0	E0562	0	E0740	0	E0970	0	E1190	0	E1634	0
C9354	300	E0170	0	E0293	0	E0565	0	E0744	0	E0971	2	E1195	0	E1635	0
C9355	3	E0171	0	E0294	0	E0570	0	E0745	0	E0973	2	E1200	0	E1636	0
C9356	125	E0172	0	E0295	0	E0572	0	E0746	1	E0974	2	E1220	0	E1637	0
C9358	800	E0175	0	E0296	0	E0574	0	E0747	0	E0978	1	E1221	0	E1639	0

CPT	MUE
E1700	0
E1701	0
E1702	0
E1800	0
E1801	0
E1802	0
E1805	0
E1806	0
E1810	0
E1811	0
E1812	0
E1815	0
E1816	0
E1818	0
E1820	0
E1821	0
E1825	0
E1830	0
E1831	0
E1840	0
E1841	0
E1902	0
E2000	0
E2100	0
E2101	0
E2120	0
E2201	0
E2202	0
E2203	0
E2204	0
E2205	0
E2206	0
E2207	0
E2208	0
E2209	0
E2210	0
E2211	0
E2212	0
E2213	0
E2214	0
E2215	0
E2216	0
E2217	0
E2218	0
E2219	0
E2220	0
E2221	0
E2222	0
E2224	0
E2225	0
E2226	0
E2227	0
E2228	0
E2231	0
E2291	1
E2292	1
E2293	1
E2294	1
E2295	0
E2300	0
E2301	0
E2310	0
E2311	0
E2312	0
E2313	0

CPT	MUE
E2321	0
E2322	0
E2323	0
E2324	0
E2325	0
E2326	0
E2327	0
E2328	0
E2329	0
E2330	0
E2331	0
E2340	0
E2341	0
E2342	0
E2343	0
E2351	0
E2358	0
E2359	0
E2361	0
E2363	0
E2365	0
E2366	0
E2367	0
E2368	0
E2369	0
E2370	0
E2371	0
E2373	0
E2374	0
E2375	0
E2376	0
E2377	0
E2378	0
E2381	0
E2382	0
E2383	0
E2384	0
E2385	0
E2386	0
E2387	0
E2388	0
E2389	0
E2390	0
E2391	0
E2392	0
E2394	0
E2395	0
E2396	0
E2397	0
E2402	0
E2500	0
E2502	0
E2504	0
E2506	0
E2508	0
E2510	0
E2511	0
E2512	0
E2601	0
E2602	0
E2603	0
E2604	0
E2605	0
E2606	0
E2607	0

CPT	MUE
E2608	0
E2609	0
E2611	0
E2612	0
E2613	0
E2614	0
E2615	0
E2616	0
E2617	0
E2619	0
E2620	0
E2621	0
E2622	0
E2623	0
E2624	0
E2625	0
E2626	0
E2627	0
E2628	0
E2629	0
E2630	0
E2631	0
E2632	0
E2633	0
G0008	1
G0009	1
G0010	2
G0027	1
G0101	1
G0102	1
G0103	1
G0104	1
G0105	1
G0106	1
G0117	1
G0118	1
G0120	1
G0121	1
G0123	1
G0124	1
G0127	1
G0128	1
G0129	3
G0130	1
G0141	1
G0143	1
G0144	1
G0145	1
G0147	1
G0148	1
G0166	2
G0168	2
G0173	1
G0175	1
G0176	5
G0177	3
G0179	1
G0180	1
G0181	1
G0182	1
G0186	1
G0202	1
G0204	2
G0206	2
G0235	1

CPT	MUE
G0239	2
G0245	1
G0246	1
G0247	1
G0248	1
G0249	3
G0250	1
G0251	2
G0257	2
G0259	2
G0260	2
G0268	1
G0278	1
G0281	1
G0283	1
G0288	1
G0289	1
G0293	1
G0294	1
G0302	1
G0303	1
G0304	1
G0305	1
G0306	2
G0307	2
G0328	1
G0329	1
G0333	0
G0337	1
G0339	1
G0340	2
G0341	1
G0342	1
G0343	1
G0364	2
G0365	2
G0372	1
G0379	1
G0380	2
G0381	2
G0382	2
G0383	2
G0384	2
G0389	1
G0390	1
G0396	1
G0397	1
G0398	1
G0399	1
G0400	1
G0402	1
G0403	1
G0404	1
G0405	1
G0412	1
G0413	1
G0414	1
G0415	1
G0416	1
G0417	1
G0418	1
G0419	1
G0420	2
G0424	2
G0429	1

CPT	MUE
G0431	1
G0432	1
G0433	1
G0434	1
G0435	1
G0436	1
G0437	1
G0438	1
G0439	1
G0442	1
G0443	1
G0444	1
G0445	1
G0448	1
G0452	1
G0454	1
G0455	1
G0456	1
G0457	1
G0458	1
G0459	0
G0460	1
G0461	9
G0462	60
G0463	6
G3001	1
G9143	1
G9156	1
G9157	1
G9187	0
J0130	6
J0131	400
J0133	1200
J0135	8
J0151	180
J0178	4
J0210	16
J0215	30
J0220	20
J0221	300
J0256	3500
J0257	1400
J0275	1
J0278	15
J0280	10
J0289	115
J0300	8
J0348	200
J0350	0
J0360	6
J0364	6
J0456	4
J0475	8
J0485	1500
J0490	160
J0597	250
J0638	150
J0697	12
J0712	180
J0717	400
J0745	8
J0760	4
J0770	5
J0780	10
J0800	3

CPT	MUE
J0833	3
J0890	0
J0897	120
J0900	1
J0945	4
J1050	1000
J1162	10
J1442	3360
J1446	192
J1556	300
J1557	300
J1561	300
J1568	300
J1569	300
J1572	300
J1725	250
J1744	90
J2212	240
J2265	400
J2507	8
J2995	0
J3010	100
J3060	900
J3285	9
J3465	120
J3489	5
J7196	175
J7301	0
J7310	2
J7316	4
J7326	2
J7527	20
J7604	0
J7607	0
J7609	0
J7610	0
J7615	0
J7622	0
J7624	0
J7627	0
J7628	0
J7629	0
J7632	0
J7634	0
J7635	0
J7636	0
J7637	0
J7638	0
J7640	0
J7641	0
J7642	0
J7643	0
J7645	0
J7647	0
J7650	0
J7657	0
J7660	0
J7665	127
J7667	0
J7670	0
J7676	0
J7680	0
J7681	0
J7683	0
J7684	0

CPT	MUE
J7685	0
J8510	5
J9019	60
J9042	200
J9047	120
J9179	50
J9228	450
J9262	700
J9306	840
J9354	600
J9355	100
J9400	600
K0001	0
K0002	0
K0003	0
K0004	0
K0005	0
K0006	0
K0007	0
K0008	0
K0009	0
K0013	0
K0015	0
K0017	0
K0018	0
K0019	0
K0020	0
K0037	0
K0038	0
K0039	0
K0040	0
K0041	0
K0042	0
K0043	0
K0044	0
K0045	0
K0046	0
K0047	0
K0050	0
K0051	0
K0052	0
K0053	0
K0056	0
K0065	0
K0069	0
K0070	0
K0071	0
K0072	0
K0073	0
K0077	0
K0105	0
K0195	0
K0455	0
K0462	0
K0552	0
K0601	0
K0602	0
K0603	0
K0604	0
K0605	0
K0606	0
K0607	0
K0608	0
K0609	0
K0730	0

CPT	MUE
K0733	0
K0738	0
K0743	0
K0800	0
K0801	0
K0802	0
K0806	0
K0807	0
K0808	0
K0812	0
K0813	0
K0814	0
K0815	0
K0816	0
K0820	0
K0821	0
K0822	0
K0823	0
K0824	0
K0825	0
K0826	0
K0827	0
K0828	0
K0829	0
K0830	0
K0831	0
K0835	0
K0836	0
K0837	0
K0838	0
K0839	0
K0840	0
K0841	0
K0842	0
K0843	0
K0848	0
K0849	0
K0850	0
K0851	0
K0852	0
K0853	0
K0854	0
K0855	0
K0856	0
K0857	0
K0858	0
K0859	0
K0860	0
K0861	0
K0862	0
K0863	0
K0864	0
K0868	0
K0869	0
K0870	0
K0871	0
K0877	0
K0878	0
K0879	0
K0880	0
K0884	0
K0885	0
K0886	0
K0890	0
K0891	0

Appendix L — Medically Unlikely Edits (MUEs) — OPPS

CPT	MUE
K0898	1
K0900	0
L0112	1
L0113	1
L0120	1
L0130	1
L0140	1
L0150	1
L0160	1
L0170	1
L0172	1
L0174	1
L0180	1
L0190	1
L0200	1
L0220	1
L0450	1
L0452	1
L0454	1
L0455	1
L0456	1
L0457	1
L0458	1
L0460	1
L0462	1
L0464	1
L0466	1
L0467	1
L0468	1
L0469	1
L0470	1
L0472	1
L0480	1
L0482	1
L0484	1
L0486	1
L0488	1
L0490	1
L0491	1
L0492	1
L0621	1
L0622	1
L0623	1
L0624	1
L0625	1
L0626	1
L0627	1
L0628	1
L0629	1
L0630	1
L0631	1
L0632	1
L0633	1
L0634	1
L0635	1
L0636	1
L0637	1
L0638	1
L0639	1
L0640	1
L0641	1
L0642	1
L0643	1
L0648	1
L0649	1

CPT	MUE
L0650	1
L0651	1
L0700	1
L0710	1
L0810	1
L0820	1
L0830	1
L0859	1
L0861	1
L0970	1
L0972	1
L0974	1
L0976	1
L0978	2
L0980	1
L0982	1
L0984	3
L1000	1
L1001	1
L1005	1
L1010	2
L1020	2
L1025	1
L1030	1
L1040	1
L1050	1
L1060	1
L1070	2
L1080	2
L1085	1
L1090	1
L1100	2
L1110	2
L1120	3
L1200	1
L1210	2
L1220	1
L1230	1
L1240	1
L1250	2
L1260	1
L1270	3
L1280	2
L1290	2
L1300	1
L1310	1
L1499	1
L1600	1
L1610	1
L1620	1
L1630	1
L1640	1
L1650	1
L1652	1
L1660	1
L1680	1
L1685	1
L1686	1
L1690	1
L1700	1
L1710	1
L1720	2
L1730	1
L1755	2
L1810	2

CPT	MUE
L1812	2
L1820	2
L1830	2
L1831	2
L1832	2
L1833	2
L1834	2
L1836	2
L1840	2
L1843	2
L1844	2
L1845	2
L1846	2
L1847	2
L1848	2
L1850	2
L1860	2
L1900	2
L1902	2
L1904	2
L1906	2
L1907	2
L1910	2
L1920	2
L1930	2
L1932	2
L1940	2
L1945	2
L1950	2
L1951	2
L1960	2
L1970	2
L1971	2
L1980	2
L1990	2
L2000	2
L2005	2
L2010	2
L2020	2
L2030	2
L2034	2
L2035	2
L2036	2
L2037	2
L2038	2
L2040	1
L2050	1
L2060	1
L2070	1
L2080	1
L2090	1
L2106	2
L2108	2
L2112	2
L2114	2
L2116	2
L2126	2
L2128	2
L2132	2
L2134	2
L2136	2
L2180	2
L2182	4
L2184	4
L2186	4

CPT	MUE
L2188	2
L2190	2
L2192	2
L2200	4
L2210	4
L2220	4
L2230	2
L2232	2
L2240	2
L2250	2
L2260	2
L2265	2
L2270	2
L2275	2
L2280	2
L2300	1
L2310	1
L2320	2
L2330	2
L2335	2
L2340	2
L2350	2
L2360	2
L2370	2
L2375	2
L2380	2
L2500	2
L2510	2
L2520	2
L2525	2
L2526	2
L2530	2
L2540	2
L2550	2
L2570	2
L2580	2
L2600	2
L2610	2
L2620	2
L2622	2
L2624	2
L2627	1
L2628	1
L2630	1
L2640	1
L2650	2
L2660	1
L2670	2
L2680	2
L2795	2
L2800	2
L2820	2
L2830	2
L3000	2
L3001	2
L3002	2
L3003	2
L3010	2
L3020	2
L3030	2
L3031	2
L3040	2
L3050	2
L3060	2
L3070	2

CPT	MUE
L3080	2
L3090	2
L3100	2
L3140	1
L3150	1
L3160	2
L3170	2
L3215	0
L3216	0
L3217	0
L3219	0
L3221	0
L3222	0
L3224	2
L3225	2
L3230	2
L3250	2
L3251	2
L3252	2
L3253	2
L3330	2
L3332	2
L3340	2
L3350	2
L3360	2
L3370	2
L3380	2
L3390	2
L3400	2
L3410	2
L3420	2
L3430	2
L3440	2
L3450	2
L3455	2
L3460	2
L3465	2
L3470	2
L3480	2
L3485	2
L3500	2
L3510	2
L3520	2
L3530	2
L3540	2
L3550	2
L3560	2
L3570	2
L3580	2
L3590	2
L3595	2
L3600	2
L3610	2
L3620	2
L3630	2
L3640	1
L3650	1
L3660	1
L3670	1
L3671	1
L3674	1
L3675	1
L3677	1
L3678	1
L3702	2

CPT	MUE
L3710	2
L3720	2
L3730	2
L3740	2
L3760	2
L3762	2
L3763	2
L3764	2
L3765	2
L3766	2
L3806	2
L3807	2
L3808	2
L3809	2
L3900	2
L3901	2
L3904	2
L3905	2
L3906	2
L3908	2
L3912	2
L3913	2
L3915	2
L3916	2
L3917	2
L3918	2
L3919	2
L3921	2
L3923	2
L3924	2
L3925	4
L3927	4
L3929	2
L3930	2
L3931	2
L3933	3
L3935	3
L3960	1
L3961	1
L3962	1
L3967	1
L3971	1
L3973	1
L3975	1
L3976	1
L3977	1
L3978	1
L3980	2
L3982	2
L3984	2
L4000	1
L4010	2
L4020	2
L4030	2
L4040	2
L4045	2
L4050	2
L4055	2
L4060	2
L4070	2
L4080	2
L4100	2
L4130	2
L4350	2
L4360	2

CPT	MUE
L4361	2
L4370	2
L4386	2
L4387	2
L4392	2
L4394	2
L4396	2
L4397	2
L4398	2
L4631	2
L5000	2
L5010	2
L5020	2
L5050	2
L5060	2
L5100	2
L5105	2
L5150	2
L5160	2
L5200	2
L5210	2
L5220	2
L5230	2
L5250	2
L5270	2
L5280	2
L5301	2
L5312	2
L5321	2
L5331	2
L5341	2
L5400	2
L5410	2
L5420	2
L5430	2
L5450	2
L5460	2
L5500	2
L5505	2
L5510	2
L5520	2
L5530	2
L5535	2
L5540	2
L5560	2
L5570	2
L5580	2
L5585	2
L5590	2
L5595	2
L5600	2
L5610	2
L5611	2
L5613	2
L5614	2
L5616	2
L5617	2
L5628	2
L5629	2
L5630	2
L5631	2
L5632	2
L5634	2
L5636	2
L5637	2

CPT	MUE
L5638	2
L5639	2
L5640	2
L5642	2
L5643	2
L5644	2
L5645	2
L5646	2
L5647	2
L5648	2
L5649	2
L5650	2
L5651	2
L5652	2
L5653	2
L5654	2
L5655	2
L5656	2
L5658	2
L5661	2
L5665	2
L5666	2
L5668	2
L5670	2
L5671	2
L5672	2
L5676	2
L5677	2
L5678	2
L5680	2
L5681	2
L5682	2
L5683	2
L5684	2
L5686	2
L5688	2
L5690	2
L5692	2
L5694	2
L5695	2
L5696	2
L5697	2
L5698	2
L5699	2
L5700	2
L5701	2
L5702	2
L5703	2
L5704	2
L5705	2
L5706	2
L5707	2
L5710	2
L5711	2
L5712	2
L5714	2
L5716	2
L5718	2
L5722	2
L5724	2
L5726	2
L5728	2
L5780	2
L5781	2
L5782	2

CPT	MUE
L5785	2
L5790	2
L5795	2
L5810	2
L5811	2
L5812	2
L5814	2
L5816	2
L5818	2
L5822	2
L5824	2
L5826	2
L5828	2
L5830	2
L5840	2
L5845	2
L5848	2
L5850	2
L5855	2
L5856	2
L5857	2
L5858	2
L5859	2
L5910	2
L5920	2
L5925	2
L5930	2
L5940	2
L5950	2
L5960	2
L5961	1
L5962	2
L5964	2
L5966	2
L5968	2
L5969	0
L5970	2
L5971	2
L5972	2
L5973	2
L5974	2
L5975	2
L5976	2
L5978	2
L5979	2
L5980	2
L5981	2
L5982	2
L5984	2
L5985	2
L5986	2
L5987	2
L5988	2
L5990	2
L6000	2
L6010	2
L6020	2
L6025	2
L6050	2
L6055	2
L6100	2
L6110	2
L6120	2
L6130	2
L6200	2

CPT	MUE
L6205	2
L6250	2
L6300	2
L6310	2
L6320	2
L6350	2
L6360	2
L6370	2
L6380	2
L6382	2
L6384	2
L6386	2
L6388	2
L6400	2
L6450	2
L6500	2
L6550	2
L6570	2
L6580	2
L6582	2
L6584	2
L6586	2
L6588	2
L6590	2
L6600	2
L6605	2
L6610	2
L6611	2
L6615	2
L6616	2
L6620	2
L6621	2
L6623	2
L6624	2
L6625	2
L6628	2
L6629	2
L6630	2
L6635	2
L6637	2
L6638	2
L6640	2
L6641	2
L6642	2
L6645	2
L6646	2
L6647	2
L6648	2
L6650	2
L6670	2
L6672	2
L6675	2
L6676	2
L6677	2
L6686	2
L6687	2
L6688	2
L6689	2
L6690	2
L6693	2
L6694	2
L6695	2
L6696	2
L6697	2
L6698	2

CPT	MUE
L6703	2
L6704	2
L6706	2
L6707	2
L6708	2
L6709	2
L6711	2
L6712	2
L6713	2
L6714	2
L6715	4
L6721	2
L6722	2
L6805	2
L6810	2
L6880	2
L6881	2
L6882	2
L6883	2
L6884	2
L6885	2
L6890	2
L6895	2
L6900	2
L6905	2
L6910	2
L6915	2
L6920	2
L6925	2
L6930	2
L6935	2
L6940	2
L6945	2
L6950	2
L6955	2
L6960	2
L6965	2
L6970	2
L6975	2
L7007	2
L7008	2
L7009	2
L7040	2
L7045	2
L7170	2
L7180	2
L7181	2
L7185	2
L7186	2
L7190	2
L7191	2
L7260	2
L7261	2
L7362	1
L7366	1
L7368	1
L7400	2
L7401	2
L7402	2
L7403	2
L7404	2
L7405	2
L7900	1
L7902	1
L8030	2

CPT	MUE
L8031	2
L8032	2
L8035	2
L8039	2
L8040	1
L8041	1
L8042	2
L8043	1
L8044	1
L8045	2
L8046	1
L8047	1
L8048	1
L8300	1
L8310	1
L8320	2
L8330	2
L8500	1
L8501	2
L8507	3
L8509	1
L8510	1
L8511	1
L8514	1
L8515	1
L8600	2
L8604	3
L8605	4
L8606	5
L8609	1
L8610	2
L8612	2
L8613	2
L8614	2
L8615	2
L8616	2
L8617	2
L8618	2
L8619	2
L8621	600
L8622	2
L8627	2
L8628	2
L8629	2
L8631	4
L8641	4
L8642	2
L8658	4
L8659	4
L8670	4
L8679	3
L8681	1
L8682	2
L8683	1
L8684	1
L8685	1
L8686	2
L8687	1
L8688	1
L8689	1
L8690	2
L8691	1
L8692	0
L8693	1
L8695	1

CPT	MUE
M0064	1
P2028	1
P2029	1
P2033	1
P2038	1
P3000	1
P3001	1
P9041	100
P9043	10
P9045	20
P9046	40
P9047	20
P9048	2
P9612	1
P9615	1
Q0035	1
Q0085	2
Q0091	1
Q0111	2
Q0112	3
Q0113	2
Q0114	1
Q0115	1
Q0144	0
Q0161	30
Q0478	1
Q0479	1
Q0480	1
Q0481	1
Q0482	1
Q0483	1
Q0484	1
Q0485	1
Q0486	1
Q0487	1
Q0488	1
Q0489	1
Q0490	1
Q0491	1
Q0492	1
Q0493	1
Q0494	1
Q0495	1
Q0497	2
Q0498	1
Q0499	1
Q0501	1
Q0502	1
Q0503	3
Q0504	1
Q0507	1
Q0508	1
Q0509	1
Q0510	1
Q0511	1
Q0512	4
Q0513	1
Q0514	1
Q1004	2
Q1005	2
Q2004	1
Q2028	1470
Q2034	1
Q2035	1
Q2036	1

CPT	MUE
Q2037	1
Q2038	1
Q2039	1
Q2043	1
Q2050	20
Q2052	1
Q3014	2
Q3027	30
Q3028	0
Q3031	1
Q4001	1
Q4002	1
Q4003	2
Q4004	2
Q4025	1
Q4026	1
Q4027	1
Q4028	1
Q4074	0
Q4101	176
Q4102	140
Q4103	0
Q4104	250
Q4105	250
Q4106	152
Q4107	128
Q4108	250
Q4110	250
Q4111	112
Q4112	2
Q4113	4
Q4114	6
Q4115	240
Q4116	320
Q4117	0
Q4118	1000
Q4119	300
Q4120	0
Q4121	156
Q4122	96
Q4123	160
Q4124	280
Q4125	28
Q4126	0
Q4127	100
Q4128	128
Q4129	81
Q4130	100
Q4131	49
Q4132	50
Q4133	113
Q4134	160
Q4135	900
Q4136	900
Q9955	10
R0070	2
R0075	2
R0076	1
V2020	1
V2101	2
V2102	2
V2104	2
V2105	2
V2106	2
V2107	2

CPT	MUE
V2108	2
V2109	2
V2110	2
V2111	2
V2112	2
V2113	2
V2114	2
V2115	2
V2118	2
V2121	2
V2199	2
V2200	2
V2201	2
V2202	2
V2203	2
V2204	2
V2205	2
V2206	2
V2207	2
V2208	2
V2209	2
V2210	2
V2211	2
V2212	2
V2213	2
V2214	2
V2215	2
V2218	2
V2219	2
V2220	2
V2221	2
V2299	2
V2300	2
V2301	2
V2302	2
V2303	2
V2304	2
V2305	2
V2306	2
V2307	2
V2308	2
V2309	2
V2310	2
V2311	2
V2312	2
V2313	2
V2314	2
V2315	2
V2318	2
V2319	2
V2320	2
V2321	2
V2399	2
V2410	2
V2430	2
V2499	2
V2500	2
V2501	2
V2502	2
V2503	2
V2510	2
V2511	2
V2512	2
V2513	2
V2520	2

CPT	MUE
V2521	2
V2522	2
V2523	2
V2530	2
V2531	2
V2599	2
V2600	1
V2610	1
V2615	2
V2623	2
V2624	2
V2625	2
V2626	2
V2627	2
V2628	2
V2629	2
V2630	2
V2631	2
V2632	2
V2700	2
V2710	2
V2718	2
V2730	2
V2761	2
V2770	2
V2780	2
V2781	2
V2782	2
V2783	2
V2785	2
V2790	1
V2797	1
V5008	0
V5010	0
V5011	0
V5274	0
V5281	0
V5282	0
V5284	0
V5285	0
V5286	0
V5287	0
V5288	0
V5289	0

Appendix L — Medically Unlikely Edits (MUEs) — OPPS

Appendix M — Inpatient Only Procedures

Inpatient Only Procedures—This appendix identifies services with the status indicator C. Medicare will not pay an OPPS hospital or ASC when they are performed on a Medicare patient as an outpatient. Physicians should refer to this list when scheduling Medicare patients for surgical procedures. CMS updates this list quarterly.

00176 Anesth pharyngeal surgery
00192 Anesth facial bone surgery
00211 Anesth cran surg hemotoma
00214 Anesth skull drainage
00215 Anesth skull repair/fract
00452 Anesth surgery of shoulder
00474 Anesth surgery of rib
0051T Implant total heart system
00524 Anesth chest drainage
0052T Replace thrc unit hrt syst
0053T Replace implantable hrt syst
00540 Anesth chest surgery
00542 Anesthesia removal pleura
00546 Anesth lung chest wall surg
00560 Anesth heart surg w/o pump
00561 Anesth heart surg <1 yr
00562 Anesth hrt surg w/pmp age 1+
00567 Anesth cabg w/pump
00580 Anesth heart/lung transplnt
00604 Anesth sitting procedure
00622 Anesth removal of nerves
00632 Anesth removal of nerves
00670 Anesth spine cord surgery
0075T Perq stent/chest vert art
0076T S&i stent/chest vert art
00792 Anesth hemorr/excise liver
00794 Anesth pancreas removal
00796 Anesth for liver transplant
00802 Anesth fat layer removal
00844 Anesth pelvis surgery
00846 Anesth hysterectomy
00848 Anesth pelvic organ surg
00864 Anesth removal of bladder
00865 Anesth removal of prostate
00866 Anesth removal of adrenal
00868 Anesth kidney transplant
00882 Anesth major vein ligation
00904 Anesth perineal surgery
00908 Anesth removal of prostate
0092T Artific disc addl cervical
00932 Anesth amputation of penis
00934 Anesth penis nodes removal
00936 Anesth penis nodes removal
00944 Anesth vaginal hysterectomy
0095T Rmvl artific disc addl crvcl
0098T Rev artific disc addl
01140 Anesth amputation at pelvis
01150 Anesth pelvic tumor surgery
01212 Anesth hip disarticulation
01214 Anesth hip arthroplasty
01232 Anesth amputation of femur
01234 Anesth radical femur surg
01272 Anesth femoral artery surg
01274 Anesth femoral embolectomy
01402 Anesth knee arthroplasty
01404 Anesth amputation at knee
01442 Anesth knee artery surg
01444 Anesth knee artery repair
01486 Anesth ankle replacement
01502 Anesth lwr leg embolectomy
01634 Anesth shoulder joint amput
01636 Anesth forequarter amput
01638 Anesth shoulder replacement
0163T Lumb artif diskectomy addl
0164T Remove lumb artif disc addl
01652 Anesth shoulder vessel surg
01654 Anesth shoulder vessel surg
01656 Anesth arm-leg vessel surg
0165T Revise lumb artif disc addl
0169T Place stereo cath brain
01756 Anesth radical humerus surg
0195T Prescrl fuse w/o instr l5/s1
0196T Prescrl fuse w/o instr l4/l5
01990 Support for organ donor
0202T Post vert arthrplst 1 lumbar
0219T Plmt post facet implt cerv
0220T Plmt post facet implt thor
0235T Trluml perip athrc visceral
0254T Evasc rpr iliac art bifur
0255T Evasc rpr iliac art bifr s&i
0262T Impltj pulm vlv evasc appr
0266T Implt/rpl crtd sns dev total
0281T Laa closure w/implant
0293T Ins lt atrl press monitor
0294T Ins lt atrl mont pres lead
0309T Prescrl fuse w/ instr l4/l5
0312T Laps impltj nstim vagus
0343T Transcath mtral vlve repair
0344T Transcath mtral vlve repair
0345T Transcath mtral vlve repair
11004 Debride genitalia & perineum
11005 Debride abdom wall
11006 Debride genit/per/abdom wall
11008 Remove mesh from abd wall
15756 Free myo/skin flap microvasc
15757 Free skin flap microvasc
15758 Free fascial flap microvasc
16036 Escharotomy addl incision
19271 Revision of chest wall
19272 Extensive chest wall surgery
19305 Mast radical
19306 Mast rad urban type
19361 Breast reconstr w/lat flap
19364 Breast reconstruction
19367 Breast reconstruction
19368 Breast reconstruction
19369 Breast reconstruction
20661 Application of head brace
20664 Application of halo
20802 Replantation arm complete
20805 Replant forearm complete
20808 Replantation hand complete
20816 Replantation digit complete
20824 Replantation thumb complete
20827 Replantation thumb complete
20838 Replantation foot complete
20936 Sp bone agrft local add-on
20937 Sp bone agrft morsel add-on
20938 Sp bone agrft struct add-on
20955 Fibula bone graft microvasc
20956 Iliac bone graft microvasc
20957 Mt bone graft microvasc
20962 Other bone graft microvasc
20969 Bone/skin graft microvasc
20970 Bone/skin graft iliac crest
21045 Extensive jaw surgery
21141 Lefort i-1 piece w/o graft
21142 Lefort i-2 piece w/o graft
21143 Lefort i-3/> piece w/o graft
21145 Lefort i-1 piece w/ graft
21146 Lefort i-2 piece w/ graft
21147 Lefort i-3/> piece w/ graft
21151 Lefort ii w/bone grafts
21154 Lefort iii w/o lefort i
21155 Lefort iii w/ lefort i
21159 Lefort iii w/fhdw/o lefort i
21160 Lefort iii w/fhd w/ lefort i
21179 Reconstruct entire forehead
21180 Reconstruct entire forehead
21182 Reconstruct cranial bone
21183 Reconstruct cranial bone
21184 Reconstruct cranial bone
21188 Reconstruction of midface
21194 Reconst lwr jaw w/graft
21196 Reconst lwr jaw w/fixation
21247 Reconstruct lower jaw bone
21255 Reconstruct lower jaw bone
21268 Revise eye sockets
21343 Open tx dprsd front sinus fx
21344 Open tx compl front sinus fx
21347 Opn tx nasomax fx multple
21348 Opn tx nasomax fx w/graft
21366 Opn tx complx malar w/grft
21422 Treat mouth roof fracture
21423 Treat mouth roof fracture
21431 Treat craniofacial fracture

21432 Treat craniofacial fracture
21433 Treat craniofacial fracture
21435 Treat craniofacial fracture
21436 Treat craniofacial fracture
21510 Drainage of bone lesion
21615 Removal of rib
21616 Removal of rib and nerves
21620 Partial removal of sternum
21627 Sternal debridement
21630 Extensive sternum surgery
21632 Extensive sternum surgery
21705 Revision of neck muscle/rib
21740 Reconstruction of sternum
21750 Repair of sternum separation
21810 Treatment of rib fracture(s)
21825 Treat sternum fracture
22010 I&d p-spine c/t/cerv-thor
22015 I&d abscess p-spine l/s/ls
22110 Remove part of neck vertebra
22112 Remove part thorax vertebra
22114 Remove part lumbar vertebra
22116 Remove extra spine segment
22206 Incis spine 3 column thorac
22207 Incis spine 3 column lumbar
22208 Incis spine 3 column adl seg
22210 Incis 1 vertebral seg cerv
22212 Incis 1 vertebral seg thorac
22214 Incis 1 vertebral seg lumbar
22216 Incis addl spine segment
22220 Incis w/discectomy cervical
22222 Incis w/discectomy thoracic
22224 Incis w/discectomy lumbar
22226 Revise extra spine segment
22318 Treat odontoid fx w/o graft
22319 Treat odontoid fx w/graft
22325 Treat spine fracture
22326 Treat neck spine fracture
22327 Treat thorax spine fracture
22328 Treat each add spine fx
22532 Lat thorax spine fusion
22533 Lat lumbar spine fusion
22534 Lat thor/lumb addl seg
22548 Neck spine fusion
22552 Addl neck spine fusion
22556 Thorax spine fusion
22558 Lumbar spine fusion
22585 Additional spinal fusion
22586 Prescrl fuse w/ instr l5-s1
22590 Spine & skull spinal fusion
22595 Neck spinal fusion
22600 Neck spine fusion
22610 Thorax spine fusion
22630 Lumbar spine fusion
22632 Spine fusion extra segment
22633 Lumbar spine fusion combined
22634 Spine fusion extra segment
22800 Post fusion </6 vert seg
22802 Post fusion 7-12 vert seg
22804 Post fusion 13/> vert seg
22808 Ant fusion 2-3 vert seg
22810 Ant fusion 4-7 vert seg
22812 Ant fusion 8/> vert seg
22818 Kyphectomy 1-2 segments
22819 Kyphectomy 3 or more
22830 Exploration of spinal fusion
22840 Insert spine fixation device
22841 Insert spine fixation device
22842 Insert spine fixation device
22843 Insert spine fixation device
22844 Insert spine fixation device
22845 Insert spine fixation device
22846 Insert spine fixation device
22847 Insert spine fixation device
22848 Insert pelv fixation device
22849 Reinsert spinal fixation
22850 Remove spine fixation device
22852 Remove spine fixation device
22855 Remove spine fixation device
22857 Lumbar artif diskectomy
22861 Revise cerv artific disc
22862 Revise lumbar artif disc
22864 Remove cerv artif disc
22865 Remove lumb artif disc
23200 Resect clavicle tumor
23210 Resect scapula tumor
23220 Resect prox humerus tumor
23335 Shoulder prosthesis removal
23472 Reconstruct shoulder joint
23474 Revis reconst shoulder joint
23900 Amputation of arm & girdle
23920 Amputation at shoulder joint
24900 Amputation of upper arm
24920 Amputation of upper arm
24930 Amputation follow-up surgery
24931 Amputate upper arm & implant
24940 Revision of upper arm
25900 Amputation of forearm
25905 Amputation of forearm
25915 Amputation of forearm
25920 Amputate hand at wrist
25924 Amputation follow-up surgery
25927 Amputation of hand
26551 Great toe-hand transfer
26553 Single transfer toe-hand
26554 Double transfer toe-hand
26556 Toe joint transfer
26992 Drainage of bone lesion
27005 Incision of hip tendon
27025 Incision of hip/thigh fascia
27030 Drainage of hip joint
27036 Excision of hip joint/muscle
27054 Removal of hip joint lining
27070 Part remove hip bone super
27071 Part removal hip bone deep
27075 Resect hip tumor
27076 Resect hip tum incl acetabul
27077 Resect hip tum w/innom bone
27078 Rsect hip tum incl femur
27090 Removal of hip prosthesis
27091 Removal of hip prosthesis
27120 Reconstruction of hip socket
27122 Reconstruction of hip socket
27125 Partial hip replacement
27130 Total hip arthroplasty
27132 Total hip arthroplasty
27134 Revise hip joint replacement
27137 Revise hip joint replacement
27138 Revise hip joint replacement
27140 Transplant femur ridge
27146 Incision of hip bone
27147 Revision of hip bone
27151 Incision of hip bones
27156 Revision of hip bones
27158 Revision of pelvis
27161 Incision of neck of femur
27165 Incision/fixation of femur
27170 Repair/graft femur head/neck
27175 Treat slipped epiphysis
27176 Treat slipped epiphysis
27177 Treat slipped epiphysis
27178 Treat slipped epiphysis
27181 Treat slipped epiphysis
27185 Revision of femur epiphysis
27187 Reinforce hip bones
27222 Treat hip socket fracture
27226 Treat hip wall fracture
27227 Treat hip fracture(s)
27228 Treat hip fracture(s)
27232 Treat thigh fracture
27236 Treat thigh fracture
27240 Treat thigh fracture
27244 Treat thigh fracture
27245 Treat thigh fracture
27248 Treat thigh fracture
27253 Treat hip dislocation
27254 Treat hip dislocation
27258 Treat hip dislocation
27259 Treat hip dislocation
27268 Cltx thigh fx w/mnpj
27269 Optx thigh fx
27280 Fusion of sacroiliac joint
27282 Fusion of pubic bones
27284 Fusion of hip joint
27286 Fusion of hip joint
27290 Amputation of leg at hip
27295 Amputation of leg at hip
27303 Drainage of bone lesion
27365 Resect femur/knee tumor
27445 Revision of knee joint
27447 Total knee arthroplasty
27448 Incision of thigh
27450 Incision of thigh
27454 Realignment of thigh bone
27455 Realignment of knee

27457 Realignment of knee
27465 Shortening of thigh bone
27466 Lengthening of thigh bone
27468 Shorten/lengthen thighs
27470 Repair of thigh
27472 Repair/graft of thigh
27477 Surgery to stop leg growth
27485 Surgery to stop leg growth
27486 Revise/replace knee joint
27487 Revise/replace knee joint
27488 Removal of knee prosthesis
27495 Reinforce thigh
27506 Treatment of thigh fracture
27507 Treatment of thigh fracture
27511 Treatment of thigh fracture
27513 Treatment of thigh fracture
27514 Treatment of thigh fracture
27519 Treat thigh fx growth plate
27535 Treat knee fracture
27536 Treat knee fracture
27540 Treat knee fracture
27556 Treat knee dislocation
27557 Treat knee dislocation
27558 Treat knee dislocation
27580 Fusion of knee
27590 Amputate leg at thigh
27591 Amputate leg at thigh
27592 Amputate leg at thigh
27596 Amputation follow-up surgery
27598 Amputate lower leg at knee
27645 Resect tibia tumor
27646 Resect fibula tumor
27702 Reconstruct ankle joint
27703 Reconstruction ankle joint
27712 Realignment of lower leg
27715 Revision of lower leg
27724 Repair/graft of tibia
27725 Repair of lower leg
27727 Repair of lower leg
27880 Amputation of lower leg
27881 Amputation of lower leg
27882 Amputation of lower leg
27886 Amputation follow-up surgery
27888 Amputation of foot at ankle
28800 Amputation of midfoot
31225 Removal of upper jaw
31230 Removal of upper jaw
31290 Nasal/sinus endoscopy surg
31291 Nasal/sinus endoscopy surg
31360 Removal of larynx
31365 Removal of larynx
31367 Partial removal of larynx
31368 Partial removal of larynx
31370 Partial removal of larynx
31375 Partial removal of larynx
31380 Partial removal of larynx
31382 Partial removal of larynx
31390 Removal of larynx & pharynx
31395 Reconstruct larynx & pharynx
31584 Treat larynx fracture
31587 Revision of larynx
31725 Clearance of airways
31760 Repair of windpipe
31766 Reconstruction of windpipe
31770 Repair/graft of bronchus
31775 Reconstruct bronchus
31780 Reconstruct windpipe
31781 Reconstruct windpipe
31786 Remove windpipe lesion
31800 Repair of windpipe injury
31805 Repair of windpipe injury
32035 Thoracostomy w/rib resection
32036 Thoracostomy w/flap drainage
32096 Open wedge/bx lung infiltr
32097 Open wedge/bx lung nodule
32098 Open biopsy of lung pleura
32100 Exploration of chest
32110 Explore/repair chest
32120 Re-exploration of chest
32124 Explore chest free adhesions
32140 Removal of lung lesion(s)
32141 Remove/treat lung lesions
32150 Removal of lung lesion(s)
32151 Remove lung foreign body
32160 Open chest heart massage
32200 Drain open lung lesion
32215 Treat chest lining
32220 Release of lung
32225 Partial release of lung
32310 Removal of chest lining
32320 Free/remove chest lining
32440 Remove lung pneumonectomy
32442 Sleeve pneumonectomy
32445 Removal of lung extrapleural
32480 Partial removal of lung
32482 Bilobectomy
32484 Segmentectomy
32486 Sleeve lobectomy
32488 Completion pneumonectomy
32491 Lung volume reduction
32501 Repair bronchus add-on
32503 Resect apical lung tumor
32504 Resect apical lung tum/chest
32505 Wedge resect of lung initial
32506 Wedge resect of lung add-on
32507 Wedge resect of lung diag
32540 Removal of lung lesion
32650 Thoracoscopy w/pleurodesis
32651 Thoracoscopy remove cortex
32652 Thoracoscopy rem totl cortex
32653 Thoracoscopy remov fb/fibrin
32654 Thoracoscopy contrl bleeding
32655 Thoracoscopy resect bullae
32656 Thoracoscopy w/pleurectomy
32658 Thoracoscopy w/sac fb remove
32659 Thoracoscopy w/sac drainage
32661 Thoracoscopy w/pericard exc
32662 Thoracoscopy w/mediast exc
32663 Thoracoscopy w/lobectomy
32664 Thoracoscopy w/ th nrv exc
32665 Thoracoscop w/esoph musc exc
32666 Thoracoscopy w/wedge resect
32667 Thoracoscopy w/w resect addl
32668 Thoracoscopy w/w resect diag
32669 Thoracoscopy remove segment
32670 Thoracoscopy bilobectomy
32671 Thoracoscopy pneumonectomy
32672 Thoracoscopy for lvrs
32673 Thoracoscopy w/thymus resect
32674 Thoracoscopy lymph node exc
32800 Repair lung hernia
32810 Close chest after drainage
32815 Close bronchial fistula
32820 Reconstruct injured chest
32850 Donor pneumonectomy
32851 Lung transplant single
32852 Lung transplant with bypass
32853 Lung transplant double
32854 Lung transplant with bypass
32855 Prepare donor lung single
32856 Prepare donor lung double
32900 Removal of rib(s)
32905 Revise & repair chest wall
32906 Revise & repair chest wall
32940 Revision of lung
32997 Total lung lavage
33015 Incision of heart sac
33020 Incision of heart sac
33025 Incision of heart sac
33030 Partial removal of heart sac
33031 Partial removal of heart sac
33050 Resect heart sac lesion
33120 Removal of heart lesion
33130 Removal of heart lesion
33140 Heart revascularize (tmr)
33141 Heart tmr w/other procedure
33202 Insert epicard eltrd open
33203 Insert epicard eltrd endo
33236 Remove electrode/thoracotomy
33237 Remove electrode/thoracotomy
33238 Remove electrode/thoracotomy
33243 Remove eltrd/thoracotomy
33250 Ablate heart dysrhythm focus
33251 Ablate heart dysrhythm focus
33254 Ablate atria lmtd
33255 Ablate atria w/o bypass ext
33256 Ablate atria w/bypass exten
33257 Ablate atria lmtd add-on
33258 Ablate atria x10sv add-on
33259 Ablate atria w/bypass add-on
33261 Ablate heart dysrhythm focus
33265 Ablate atria lmtd endo
33266 Ablate atria x10sv endo
33300 Repair of heart wound

33305 Repair of heart wound
33310 Exploratory heart surgery
33315 Exploratory heart surgery
33320 Repair major blood vessel(s)
33321 Repair major vessel
33322 Repair major blood vessel(s)
33330 Insert major vessel graft
33332 Insert major vessel graft
33335 Insert major vessel graft
33361 Replace aortic valve perq
33362 Replace aortic valve open
33363 Replace aortic valve open
33364 Replace aortic valve open
33365 Replace aortic valve open
33366 Trcath replace aortic valve
33367 Replace aortic valve w/byp
33368 Replace aortic valve w/byp
33369 Replace aortic valve w/byp
33400 Repair of aortic valve
33401 Valvuloplasty open
33403 Valvuloplasty w/cp bypass
33404 Prepare heart-aorta conduit
33405 Replacement of aortic valve
33406 Replacement of aortic valve
33410 Replacement of aortic valve
33411 Replacement of aortic valve
33412 Replacement of aortic valve
33413 Replacement of aortic valve
33414 Repair of aortic valve
33415 Revision subvalvular tissue
33416 Revise ventricle muscle
33417 Repair of aortic valve
33420 Revision of mitral valve
33422 Revision of mitral valve
33425 Repair of mitral valve
33426 Repair of mitral valve
33427 Repair of mitral valve
33430 Replacement of mitral valve
33460 Revision of tricuspid valve
33463 Valvuloplasty tricuspid
33464 Valvuloplasty tricuspid
33465 Replace tricuspid valve
33468 Revision of tricuspid valve
33470 Revision of pulmonary valve
33471 Valvotomy pulmonary valve
33472 Revision of pulmonary valve
33474 Revision of pulmonary valve
33475 Replacement pulmonary valve
33476 Revision of heart chamber
33478 Revision of heart chamber
33496 Repair prosth valve clot
33500 Repair heart vessel fistula
33501 Repair heart vessel fistula
33502 Coronary artery correction
33503 Coronary artery graft
33504 Coronary artery graft
33505 Repair artery w/tunnel
33506 Repair artery translocation
33507 Repair art intramural
33510 Cabg vein single
33511 Cabg vein two
33512 Cabg vein three
33513 Cabg vein four
33514 Cabg vein five
33516 Cabg vein six or more
33517 Cabg artery-vein single
33518 Cabg artery-vein two
33519 Cabg artery-vein three
33521 Cabg artery-vein four
33522 Cabg artery-vein five
33523 Cabg art-vein six or more
33530 Coronary artery bypass/reop
33533 Cabg arterial single
33534 Cabg arterial two
33535 Cabg arterial three
33536 Cabg arterial four or more
33542 Removal of heart lesion
33545 Repair of heart damage
33548 Restore/remodel ventricle
33572 Open coronary endarterectomy
33600 Closure of valve
33602 Closure of valve
33606 Anastomosis/artery-aorta
33608 Repair anomaly w/conduit
33610 Repair by enlargement
33611 Repair double ventricle
33612 Repair double ventricle
33615 Repair modified fontan
33617 Repair single ventricle
33619 Repair single ventricle
33620 Apply r&l pulm art bands
33621 Transthor cath for stent
33622 Redo compl cardiac anomaly
33641 Repair heart septum defect
33645 Revision of heart veins
33647 Repair heart septum defects
33660 Repair of heart defects
33665 Repair of heart defects
33670 Repair of heart chambers
33675 Close mult vsd
33676 Close mult vsd w/resection
33677 Cl mult vsd w/rem pul band
33681 Repair heart septum defect
33684 Repair heart septum defect
33688 Repair heart septum defect
33690 Reinforce pulmonary artery
33692 Repair of heart defects
33694 Repair of heart defects
33697 Repair of heart defects
33702 Repair of heart defects
33710 Repair of heart defects
33720 Repair of heart defect
33722 Repair of heart defect
33724 Repair venous anomaly
33726 Repair pul venous stenosis
33730 Repair heart-vein defect(s)
33732 Repair heart-vein defect
33735 Revision of heart chamber
33736 Revision of heart chamber
33737 Revision of heart chamber
33750 Major vessel shunt
33755 Major vessel shunt
33762 Major vessel shunt
33764 Major vessel shunt & graft
33766 Major vessel shunt
33767 Major vessel shunt
33768 Cavopulmonary shunting
33770 Repair great vessels defect
33771 Repair great vessels defect
33774 Repair great vessels defect
33775 Repair great vessels defect
33776 Repair great vessels defect
33777 Repair great vessels defect
33778 Repair great vessels defect
33779 Repair great vessels defect
33780 Repair great vessels defect
33781 Repair great vessels defect
33782 Nikaidoh proc
33783 Nikaidoh proc w/ostia implt
33786 Repair arterial trunk
33788 Revision of pulmonary artery
33800 Aortic suspension
33802 Repair vessel defect
33803 Repair vessel defect
33813 Repair septal defect
33814 Repair septal defect
33820 Revise major vessel
33822 Revise major vessel
33824 Revise major vessel
33840 Remove aorta constriction
33845 Remove aorta constriction
33851 Remove aorta constriction
33852 Repair septal defect
33853 Repair septal defect
33860 Ascending aortic graft
33863 Ascending aortic graft
33864 Ascending aortic graft
33870 Transverse aortic arch graft
33875 Thoracic aortic graft
33877 Thoracoabdominal graft
33880 Endovasc taa repr incl subcl
33881 Endovasc taa repr w/o subcl
33883 Insert endovasc prosth taa
33884 Endovasc prosth taa add-on
33886 Endovasc prosth delayed
33889 Artery transpose/endovas taa
33891 Car-car bp grft/endovas taa
33910 Remove lung artery emboli
33915 Remove lung artery emboli
33916 Surgery of great vessel
33917 Repair pulmonary artery
33920 Repair pulmonary atresia
33922 Transect pulmonary artery
33924 Remove pulmonary shunt

33925 Rpr pul art unifocal w/o cpb
33926 Repr pul art unifocal w/cpb
33930 Removal of donor heart/lung
33933 Prepare donor heart/lung
33935 Transplantation heart/lung
33940 Removal of donor heart
33944 Prepare donor heart
33945 Transplantation of heart
33960 External circulation assist
33961 External circulation assist
33967 Insert ia percut device
33968 Remove aortic assist device
33970 Aortic circulation assist
33971 Aortic circulation assist
33973 Insert balloon device
33974 Remove intra-aortic balloon
33975 Implant ventricular device
33976 Implant ventricular device
33977 Remove ventricular device
33978 Remove ventricular device
33979 Insert intracorporeal device
33980 Remove intracorporeal device
33981 Replace vad pump ext
33982 Replace vad intra w/o bp
33983 Replace vad intra w/bp
33990 Insert vad artery access
33991 Insert vad art&vein access
33992 Remove vad different session
33993 Reposition vad diff session
34001 Removal of artery clot
34051 Removal of artery clot
34151 Removal of artery clot
34401 Removal of vein clot
34451 Removal of vein clot
34502 Reconstruct vena cava
34800 Endovas aaa repr w/sm tube
34802 Endovas aaa repr w/2-p part
34803 Endovas aaa repr w/3-p part
34804 Endovas aaa repr w/1-p part
34805 Endovas aaa repr w/long tube
34806 Aneurysm press sensor add-on
34808 Endovas iliac a device addon
34812 Xpose for endoprosth femorl
34813 Femoral endovas graft add-on
34820 Xpose for endoprosth iliac
34825 Endovasc extend prosth init
34826 Endovasc exten prosth addl
34830 Open aortic tube prosth repr
34831 Open aortoiliac prosth repr
34832 Open aortofemor prosth repr
34833 Xpose for endoprosth iliac
34834 Xpose endoprosth brachial
34841 Endovasc visc aorta 1 graft
34842 Endovasc visc aorta 2 graft
34843 Endovasc visc aorta 3 graft
34844 Endovasc visc aorta 4 graft
34845 Visc & infraren abd 1 prosth
34846 Visc & infraren abd 2 prosth
34847 Visc & infraren abd 3 prosth
34848 Visc & infraren abd 4+ prost
34900 Endovasc iliac repr w/graft
35001 Repair defect of artery
35002 Repair artery rupture neck
35005 Repair defect of artery
35013 Repair artery rupture arm
35021 Repair defect of artery
35022 Repair artery rupture chest
35081 Repair defect of artery
35082 Repair artery rupture aorta
35091 Repair defect of artery
35092 Repair artery rupture aorta
35102 Repair defect of artery
35103 Repair artery rupture aorta
35111 Repair defect of artery
35112 Repair artery rupture spleen
35121 Repair defect of artery
35122 Repair artery rupture belly
35131 Repair defect of artery
35132 Repair artery rupture groin
35141 Repair defect of artery
35142 Repair artery rupture thigh
35151 Repair defect of artery
35152 Repair ruptd popliteal art
35182 Repair blood vessel lesion
35189 Repair blood vessel lesion
35211 Repair blood vessel lesion
35216 Repair blood vessel lesion
35221 Repair blood vessel lesion
35241 Repair blood vessel lesion
35246 Repair blood vessel lesion
35251 Repair blood vessel lesion
35271 Repair blood vessel lesion
35276 Repair blood vessel lesion
35281 Repair blood vessel lesion
35301 Rechanneling of artery
35302 Rechanneling of artery
35303 Rechanneling of artery
35304 Rechanneling of artery
35305 Rechanneling of artery
35306 Rechanneling of artery
35311 Rechanneling of artery
35331 Rechanneling of artery
35341 Rechanneling of artery
35351 Rechanneling of artery
35355 Rechanneling of artery
35361 Rechanneling of artery
35363 Rechanneling of artery
35371 Rechanneling of artery
35372 Rechanneling of artery
35390 Reoperation carotid add-on
35400 Angioscopy
35450 Repair arterial blockage
35452 Repair arterial blockage
35501 Art byp grft ipsilat carotid
35506 Art byp grft subclav-carotid
35508 Art byp grft carotid-vertbrl
35509 Art byp grft contral carotid
35510 Art byp grft carotid-brchial
35511 Art byp grft subclav-subclav
35512 Art byp grft subclav-brchial
35515 Art byp grft subclav-vertbrl
35516 Art byp grft subclav-axilary
35518 Art byp grft axillary-axilry
35521 Art byp grft axill-femoral
35522 Art byp grft axill-brachial
35523 Art byp grft brchl-ulnr-rdl
35525 Art byp grft brachial-brchl
35526 Art byp grft aor/carot/innom
35531 Art byp grft aorcel/aormesen
35533 Art byp grft axill/fem/fem
35535 Art byp grft hepatorenal
35536 Art byp grft splenorenal
35537 Art byp grft aortoiliac
35538 Art byp grft aortobi-iliac
35539 Art byp grft aortofemoral
35540 Art byp grft aortbifemoral
35556 Art byp grft fem-popliteal
35558 Art byp grft fem-femoral
35560 Art byp grft aortorenal
35563 Art byp grft ilioiliac
35565 Art byp grft iliofemoral
35566 Art byp fem-ant-post tib/prl
35570 Art byp tibial-tib/peroneal
35571 Art byp pop-tibl-prl-other
35583 Vein byp grft fem-popliteal
35585 Vein byp fem-tibial peroneal
35587 Vein byp pop-tibl peroneal
35600 Harvest art for cabg add-on
35601 Art byp common ipsi carotid
35606 Art byp carotid-subclavian
35612 Art byp subclav-subclavian
35616 Art byp subclav-axillary
35621 Art byp axillary-femoral
35623 Art byp axillary-pop-tibial
35626 Art byp aorsubcl/carot/innom
35631 Art byp aor-celiac-msn-renal
35632 Art byp ilio-celiac
35633 Art byp ilio-mesenteric
35634 Art byp iliorenal
35636 Art byp spenorenal
35637 Art byp aortoiliac
35638 Art byp aortobi-iliac
35642 Art byp carotid-vertebral
35645 Art byp subclav-vertebrl
35646 Art byp aortobifemoral
35647 Art byp aortofemoral
35650 Art byp axillary-axillary
35654 Art byp axill-fem-femoral
35656 Art byp femoral-popliteal
35661 Art byp femoral-femoral
35663 Art byp ilioiliac
35665 Art byp iliofemoral
35666 Art byp fem-ant-post tib/prl
35671 Art byp pop-tibl-prl-other

35681 Composite byp grft pros&vein
35682 Composite byp grft 2 veins
35683 Composite byp grft 3/> segmt
35691 Art trnsposj vertbrl carotid
35693 Art trnsposj subclavian
35694 Art trnsposj subclav carotid
35695 Art trnsposj carotid subclav
35697 Reimplant artery each
35700 Reoperation bypass graft
35701 Exploration carotid artery
35721 Exploration femoral artery
35741 Exploration popliteal artery
35800 Explore neck vessels
35820 Explore chest vessels
35840 Explore abdominal vessels
35870 Repair vessel graft defect
35901 Excision graft neck
35905 Excision graft thorax
35907 Excision graft abdomen
36660 Insertion catheter artery
36822 Insertion of cannula(s)
36823 Insertion of cannula(s)
37140 Revision of circulation
37145 Revision of circulation
37160 Revision of circulation
37180 Revision of circulation
37181 Splice spleen/kidney veins
37182 Insert hepatic shunt (tips)
37215 Transcath stent cca w/eps
37217 Stent placemt retro carotid
37616 Ligation of chest artery
37617 Ligation of abdomen artery
37618 Ligation of extremity artery
37660 Revision of major vein
37788 Revascularization penis
38100 Removal of spleen total
38101 Removal of spleen partial
38102 Removal of spleen total
38115 Repair of ruptured spleen
38380 Thoracic duct procedure
38381 Thoracic duct procedure
38382 Thoracic duct procedure
38562 Removal pelvic lymph nodes
38564 Removal abdomen lymph nodes
38724 Removal of lymph nodes neck
38746 Remove thoracic lymph nodes
38747 Remove abdominal lymph nodes
38765 Remove groin lymph nodes
38770 Remove pelvis lymph nodes
38780 Remove abdomen lymph nodes
39000 Exploration of chest
39010 Exploration of chest
39200 Resect mediastinal cyst
39220 Resect mediastinal tumor
39499 Chest procedure
39501 Repair diaphragm laceration
39503 Repair of diaphragm hernia
39540 Repair of diaphragm hernia
39541 Repair of diaphragm hernia
39545 Revision of diaphragm
39560 Resect diaphragm simple
39561 Resect diaphragm complex
39599 Diaphragm surgery procedure
41130 Partial removal of tongue
41135 Tongue and neck surgery
41140 Removal of tongue
41145 Tongue removal neck surgery
41150 Tongue mouth jaw surgery
41153 Tongue mouth neck surgery
41155 Tongue jaw & neck surgery
42426 Excise parotid gland/lesion
42845 Extensive surgery of throat
42894 Revision of pharyngeal walls
42953 Repair throat esophagus
42961 Control throat bleeding
42971 Control nose/throat bleeding
43045 Incision of esophagus
43100 Excision of esophagus lesion
43101 Excision of esophagus lesion
43107 Removal of esophagus
43108 Removal of esophagus
43112 Removal of esophagus
43113 Removal of esophagus
43116 Partial removal of esophagus
43117 Partial removal of esophagus
43118 Partial removal of esophagus
43121 Partial removal of esophagus
43122 Partial removal of esophagus
43123 Partial removal of esophagus
43124 Removal of esophagus
43135 Removal of esophagus pouch
43279 Lap myotomy heller
43282 Lap paraesoph her rpr w/mesh
43283 Lap esoph lengthening
43300 Repair of esophagus
43305 Repair esophagus and fistula
43310 Repair of esophagus
43312 Repair esophagus and fistula
43313 Esophagoplasty congenital
43314 Tracheo-esophagoplasty cong
43320 Fuse esophagus & stomach
43325 Revise esophagus & stomach
43327 Esoph fundoplasty lap
43328 Esoph fundoplasty thor
43330 Esophagomyotomy abdominal
43331 Esophagomyotomy thoracic
43332 Transab esoph hiat hern rpr
43333 Transab esoph hiat hern rpr
43334 Transthor diaphrag hern rpr
43335 Transthor diaphrag hern rpr
43336 Thorabd diaphr hern repair
43337 Thorabd diaphr hern repair
43338 Esoph lengthening
43340 Fuse esophagus & intestine
43341 Fuse esophagus & intestine
43350 Surgical opening esophagus
43351 Surgical opening esophagus
43352 Surgical opening esophagus
43360 Gastrointestinal repair
43361 Gastrointestinal repair
43400 Ligate esophagus veins
43401 Esophagus surgery for veins
43405 Ligate/staple esophagus
43410 Repair esophagus wound
43415 Repair esophagus wound
43425 Repair esophagus opening
43460 Pressure treatment esophagus
43496 Free jejunum flap microvasc
43500 Surgical opening of stomach
43501 Surgical repair of stomach
43502 Surgical repair of stomach
43520 Incision of pyloric muscle
43605 Biopsy of stomach
43610 Excision of stomach lesion
43611 Excision of stomach lesion
43620 Removal of stomach
43621 Removal of stomach
43622 Removal of stomach
43631 Removal of stomach partial
43632 Removal of stomach partial
43633 Removal of stomach partial
43634 Removal of stomach partial
43635 Removal of stomach partial
43640 Vagotomy & pylorus repair
43641 Vagotomy & pylorus repair
43644 Lap gastric bypass/roux-en-y
43645 Lap gastr bypass incl smll i
43771 Lap revise gastr adj device
43772 Lap rmvl gastr adj device
43773 Lap replace gastr adj device
43774 Lap rmvl gastr adj all parts
43775 Lap sleeve gastrectomy
43800 Reconstruction of pylorus
43810 Fusion of stomach and bowel
43820 Fusion of stomach and bowel
43825 Fusion of stomach and bowel
43832 Place gastrostomy tube
43840 Repair of stomach lesion
43843 Gastroplasty w/o v-band
43845 Gastroplasty duodenal switch
43846 Gastric bypass for obesity
43847 Gastric bypass incl small i
43848 Revision gastroplasty
43850 Revise stomach-bowel fusion
43855 Revise stomach-bowel fusion
43860 Revise stomach-bowel fusion
43865 Revise stomach-bowel fusion
43880 Repair stomach-bowel fistula
43881 Impl/redo electrd antrum
43882 Revise/remove electrd antrum
44005 Freeing of bowel adhesion
44010 Incision of small bowel
44015 Insert needle cath bowel
44020 Explore small intestine

44021 Decompress small bowel
44025 Incision of large bowel
44050 Reduce bowel obstruction
44055 Correct malrotation of bowel
44110 Excise intestine lesion(s)
44111 Excision of bowel lesion(s)
44120 Removal of small intestine
44121 Removal of small intestine
44125 Removal of small intestine
44126 Enterectomy w/o taper cong
44127 Enterectomy w/taper cong
44128 Enterectomy cong add-on
44130 Bowel to bowel fusion
44132 Enterectomy cadaver donor
44133 Enterectomy live donor
44135 Intestine transplnt cadaver
44136 Intestine transplant live
44137 Remove intestinal allograft
44139 Mobilization of colon
44140 Partial removal of colon
44141 Partial removal of colon
44143 Partial removal of colon
44144 Partial removal of colon
44145 Partial removal of colon
44146 Partial removal of colon
44147 Partial removal of colon
44150 Removal of colon
44151 Removal of colon/ileostomy
44155 Removal of colon/ileostomy
44156 Removal of colon/ileostomy
44157 Colectomy w/ileoanal anast
44158 Colectomy w/neo-rectum pouch
44160 Removal of colon
44187 Lap ileo/jejuno-stomy
44188 Lap colostomy
44202 Lap enterectomy
44203 Lap resect s/intestine addl
44204 Laparo partial colectomy
44205 Lap colectomy part w/ileum
44206 Lap part colectomy w/stoma
44207 L colectomy/coloproctostomy
44208 L colectomy/coloproctostomy
44210 Laparo total proctocolectomy
44211 Lap colectomy w/proctectomy
44212 Laparo total proctocolectomy
44213 Lap mobil splenic fl add-on
44227 Lap close enterostomy
44300 Open bowel to skin
44310 Ileostomy/jejunostomy
44314 Revision of ileostomy
44316 Devise bowel pouch
44320 Colostomy
44322 Colostomy with biopsies
44345 Revision of colostomy
44346 Revision of colostomy
44602 Suture small intestine
44603 Suture small intestine
44604 Suture large intestine
44605 Repair of bowel lesion
44615 Intestinal stricturoplasty
44620 Repair bowel opening
44625 Repair bowel opening
44626 Repair bowel opening
44640 Repair bowel-skin fistula
44650 Repair bowel fistula
44660 Repair bowel-bladder fistula
44661 Repair bowel-bladder fistula
44680 Surgical revision intestine
44700 Suspend bowel w/prosthesis
44715 Prepare donor intestine
44720 Prep donor intestine/venous
44721 Prep donor intestine/artery
44800 Excision of bowel pouch
44820 Excision of mesentery lesion
44850 Repair of mesentery
44899 Bowel surgery procedure
44900 Drain appendix abscess open
44960 Appendectomy
45110 Removal of rectum
45111 Partial removal of rectum
45112 Removal of rectum
45113 Partial proctectomy
45114 Partial removal of rectum
45116 Partial removal of rectum
45119 Remove rectum w/reservoir
45120 Removal of rectum
45121 Removal of rectum and colon
45123 Partial proctectomy
45126 Pelvic exenteration
45130 Excision of rectal prolapse
45135 Excision of rectal prolapse
45136 Excise ileoanal reservior
45395 Lap removal of rectum
45397 Lap remove rectum w/pouch
45400 Laparoscopic proc
45402 Lap proctopexy w/sig resect
45540 Correct rectal prolapse
45550 Repair rectum/remove sigmoid
45562 Exploration/repair of rectum
45563 Exploration/repair of rectum
45800 Repair rect/bladder fistula
45805 Repair fistula w/colostomy
45820 Repair rectourethral fistula
45825 Repair fistula w/colostomy
46705 Repair of anal stricture
46710 Repr per/vag pouch sngl proc
46712 Repr per/vag pouch dbl proc
46715 Rep perf anoper fistu
46716 Rep perf anoper/vestib fistu
46730 Construction of absent anus
46735 Construction of absent anus
46740 Construction of absent anus
46742 Repair of imperforated anus
46744 Repair of cloacal anomaly
46746 Repair of cloacal anomaly
46748 Repair of cloacal anomaly
46751 Repair of anal sphincter
47010 Open drainage liver lesion
47015 Inject/aspirate liver cyst
47100 Wedge biopsy of liver
47120 Partial removal of liver
47122 Extensive removal of liver
47125 Partial removal of liver
47130 Partial removal of liver
47133 Removal of donor liver
47135 Transplantation of liver
47136 Transplantation of liver
47140 Partial removal donor liver
47141 Partial removal donor liver
47142 Partial removal donor liver
47143 Prep donor liver whole
47144 Prep donor liver 3-segment
47145 Prep donor liver lobe split
47146 Prep donor liver/venous
47147 Prep donor liver/arterial
47300 Surgery for liver lesion
47350 Repair liver wound
47360 Repair liver wound
47361 Repair liver wound
47362 Repair liver wound
47380 Open ablate liver tumor rf
47381 Open ablate liver tumor cryo
47400 Incision of liver duct
47420 Incision of bile duct
47425 Incision of bile duct
47460 Incise bile duct sphincter
47480 Incision of gallbladder
47550 Bile duct endoscopy add-on
47570 Laparo cholecystoenterostomy
47600 Removal of gallbladder
47605 Removal of gallbladder
47610 Removal of gallbladder
47612 Removal of gallbladder
47620 Removal of gallbladder
47700 Exploration of bile ducts
47701 Bile duct revision
47711 Excision of bile duct tumor
47712 Excision of bile duct tumor
47715 Excision of bile duct cyst
47720 Fuse gallbladder & bowel
47721 Fuse upper gi structures
47740 Fuse gallbladder & bowel
47741 Fuse gallbladder & bowel
47760 Fuse bile ducts and bowel
47765 Fuse liver ducts & bowel
47780 Fuse bile ducts and bowel
47785 Fuse bile ducts and bowel
47800 Reconstruction of bile ducts
47801 Placement bile duct support
47802 Fuse liver duct & intestine
47900 Suture bile duct injury
48000 Drainage of abdomen
48001 Placement of drain pancreas
48020 Removal of pancreatic stone

48100 Biopsy of pancreas open
48105 Resect/debride pancreas
48120 Removal of pancreas lesion
48140 Partial removal of pancreas
48145 Partial removal of pancreas
48146 Pancreatectomy
48148 Removal of pancreatic duct
48150 Partial removal of pancreas
48152 Pancreatectomy
48153 Pancreatectomy
48154 Pancreatectomy
48155 Removal of pancreas
48400 Injection intraop add-on
48500 Surgery of pancreatic cyst
48510 Drain pancreatic pseudocyst
48520 Fuse pancreas cyst and bowel
48540 Fuse pancreas cyst and bowel
48545 Pancreatorrhaphy
48547 Duodenal exclusion
48548 Fuse pancreas and bowel
48551 Prep donor pancreas
48552 Prep donor pancreas/venous
48554 Transpl allograft pancreas
48556 Removal allograft pancreas
49000 Exploration of abdomen
49002 Reopening of abdomen
49010 Exploration behind abdomen
49020 Drainage abdom abscess open
49040 Drain open abdom abscess
49060 Drain open retroperi abscess
49062 Drain to peritoneal cavity
49203 Exc abd tum 5 cm or less
49204 Exc abd tum over 5 cm
49205 Exc abd tum over 10 cm
49215 Excise sacral spine tumor
49220 Multiple surgery abdomen
49255 Removal of omentum
49412 Ins device for rt guide open
49425 Insert abdomen-venous drain
49428 Ligation of shunt
49605 Repair umbilical lesion
49606 Repair umbilical lesion
49610 Repair umbilical lesion
49611 Repair umbilical lesion
49900 Repair of abdominal wall
49904 Omental flap extra-abdom
49905 Omental flap intra-abdom
49906 Free omental flap microvasc
50010 Exploration of kidney
50040 Drainage of kidney
50045 Exploration of kidney
50060 Removal of kidney stone
50065 Incision of kidney
50070 Incision of kidney
50075 Removal of kidney stone
50100 Revise kidney blood vessels
50120 Exploration of kidney
50125 Explore and drain kidney
50130 Removal of kidney stone
50135 Exploration of kidney
50205 Renal biopsy open
50220 Remove kidney open
50225 Removal kidney open complex
50230 Removal kidney open radical
50234 Removal of kidney & ureter
50236 Removal of kidney & ureter
50240 Partial removal of kidney
50250 Cryoablate renal mass open
50280 Removal of kidney lesion
50290 Removal of kidney lesion
50300 Remove cadaver donor kidney
50320 Remove kidney living donor
50323 Prep cadaver renal allograft
50325 Prep donor renal graft
50327 Prep renal graft/venous
50328 Prep renal graft/arterial
50329 Prep renal graft/ureteral
50340 Removal of kidney
50360 Transplantation of kidney
50365 Transplantation of kidney
50370 Remove transplanted kidney
50380 Reimplantation of kidney
50400 Revision of kidney/ureter
50405 Revision of kidney/ureter
50500 Repair of kidney wound
50520 Close kidney-skin fistula
50525 Repair renal-abdomen fistula
50526 Repair renal-abdomen fistula
50540 Revision of horseshoe kidney
50545 Laparo radical nephrectomy
50546 Laparoscopic nephrectomy
50547 Laparo removal donor kidney
50548 Laparo remove w/ureter
50600 Exploration of ureter
50605 Insert ureteral support
50610 Removal of ureter stone
50620 Removal of ureter stone
50630 Removal of ureter stone
50650 Removal of ureter
50660 Removal of ureter
50700 Revision of ureter
50715 Release of ureter
50722 Release of ureter
50725 Release/revise ureter
50728 Revise ureter
50740 Fusion of ureter & kidney
50750 Fusion of ureter & kidney
50760 Fusion of ureters
50770 Splicing of ureters
50780 Reimplant ureter in bladder
50782 Reimplant ureter in bladder
50783 Reimplant ureter in bladder
50785 Reimplant ureter in bladder
50800 Implant ureter in bowel
50810 Fusion of ureter & bowel
50815 Urine shunt to intestine
50820 Construct bowel bladder
50825 Construct bowel bladder
50830 Revise urine flow
50840 Replace ureter by bowel
50845 Appendico-vesicostomy
50860 Transplant ureter to skin
50900 Repair of ureter
50920 Closure ureter/skin fistula
50930 Closure ureter/bowel fistula
50940 Release of ureter
51525 Removal of bladder lesion
51530 Removal of bladder lesion
51550 Partial removal of bladder
51555 Partial removal of bladder
51565 Revise bladder & ureter(s)
51570 Removal of bladder
51575 Removal of bladder & nodes
51580 Remove bladder/revise tract
51585 Removal of bladder & nodes
51590 Remove bladder/revise tract
51595 Remove bladder/revise tract
51596 Remove bladder/create pouch
51597 Removal of pelvic structures
51800 Revision of bladder/urethra
51820 Revision of urinary tract
51840 Attach bladder/urethra
51841 Attach bladder/urethra
51865 Repair of bladder wound
51900 Repair bladder/vagina lesion
51920 Close bladder-uterus fistula
51925 Hysterectomy/bladder repair
51940 Correction of bladder defect
51960 Revision of bladder & bowel
51980 Construct bladder opening
53415 Reconstruction of urethra
53448 Remov/replc ur sphinctr comp
54125 Removal of penis
54130 Remove penis & nodes
54135 Remove penis & nodes
54390 Repair penis and bladder
54411 Remov/replc penis pros comp
54417 Remv/replc penis pros compl
54430 Revision of penis
55605 Incise sperm duct pouch
55650 Remove sperm duct pouch
55801 Removal of prostate
55810 Extensive prostate surgery
55812 Extensive prostate surgery
55815 Extensive prostate surgery
55821 Removal of prostate
55831 Removal of prostate
55840 Extensive prostate surgery
55842 Extensive prostate surgery
55845 Extensive prostate surgery
55862 Extensive prostate surgery
55865 Extensive prostate surgery
55866 Laparo radical prostatectomy
56630 Extensive vulva surgery

56631 Extensive vulva surgery
56632 Extensive vulva surgery
56633 Extensive vulva surgery
56634 Extensive vulva surgery
56637 Extensive vulva surgery
56640 Extensive vulva surgery
57110 Remove vagina wall complete
57111 Remove vagina tissue compl
57112 Vaginectomy w/nodes compl
57270 Repair of bowel pouch
57280 Suspension of vagina
57296 Revise vag graft open abd
57305 Repair rectum-vagina fistula
57307 Fistula repair & colostomy
57308 Fistula repair transperine
57311 Repair urethrovaginal lesion
57531 Removal of cervix radical
57540 Removal of residual cervix
57545 Remove cervix/repair pelvis
58140 Myomectomy abdom method
58146 Myomectomy abdom complex
58150 Total hysterectomy
58152 Total hysterectomy
58180 Partial hysterectomy
58200 Extensive hysterectomy
58210 Extensive hysterectomy
58240 Removal of pelvis contents
58267 Vag hyst w/urinary repair
58275 Hysterectomy/revise vagina
58280 Hysterectomy/revise vagina
58285 Extensive hysterectomy
58293 Vag hyst w/uro repair compl
58400 Suspension of uterus
58410 Suspension of uterus
58520 Repair of ruptured uterus
58540 Revision of uterus
58548 Lap radical hyst
58605 Division of fallopian tube
58611 Ligate oviduct(s) add-on
58700 Removal of fallopian tube
58720 Removal of ovary/tube(s)
58740 Adhesiolysis tube ovary
58750 Repair oviduct
58752 Revise ovarian tube(s)
58760 Fimbrioplasty
58822 Drain ovary abscess percut
58825 Transposition ovary(s)
58940 Removal of ovary(s)
58943 Removal of ovary(s)
58950 Resect ovarian malignancy
58951 Resect ovarian malignancy
58952 Resect ovarian malignancy
58953 Tah rad dissect for debulk
58954 Tah rad debulk/lymph remove
58956 Bso omentectomy w/tah
58957 Resect recurrent gyn mal
58958 Resect recur gyn mal w/lym
58960 Exploration of abdomen
59120 Treat ectopic pregnancy
59121 Treat ectopic pregnancy
59130 Treat ectopic pregnancy
59135 Treat ectopic pregnancy
59136 Treat ectopic pregnancy
59140 Treat ectopic pregnancy
59325 Revision of cervix
59350 Repair of uterus
59514 Cesarean delivery only
59525 Remove uterus after cesarean
59620 Attempted vbac delivery only
59830 Treat uterus infection
59850 Abortion
59851 Abortion
59852 Abortion
59855 Abortion
59856 Abortion
59857 Abortion
60254 Extensive thyroid surgery
60270 Removal of thyroid
60505 Explore parathyroid glands
60521 Removal of thymus gland
60522 Removal of thymus gland
60540 Explore adrenal gland
60545 Explore adrenal gland
60600 Remove carotid body lesion
60605 Remove carotid body lesion
60650 Laparoscopy adrenalectomy
61105 Twist drill hole
61107 Drill skull for implantation
61108 Drill skull for drainage
61120 Burr hole for puncture
61140 Pierce skull for biopsy
61150 Pierce skull for drainage
61151 Pierce skull for drainage
61154 Pierce skull & remove clot
61156 Pierce skull for drainage
61210 Pierce skull implant device
61250 Pierce skull & explore
61253 Pierce skull & explore
61304 Open skull for exploration
61305 Open skull for exploration
61312 Open skull for drainage
61313 Open skull for drainage
61314 Open skull for drainage
61315 Open skull for drainage
61316 Implt cran bone flap to abdo
61320 Open skull for drainage
61321 Open skull for drainage
61322 Decompressive craniotomy
61323 Decompressive lobectomy
61332 Explore/biopsy eye socket
61333 Explore orbit/remove lesion
61340 Subtemporal decompression
61343 Incise skull (press relief)
61345 Relieve cranial pressure
61440 Incise skull for surgery
61450 Incise skull for surgery
61458 Incise skull for brain wound
61460 Incise skull for surgery
61470 Incise skull for surgery
61480 Incise skull for surgery
61490 Incise skull for surgery
61500 Removal of skull lesion
61501 Remove infected skull bone
61510 Removal of brain lesion
61512 Remove brain lining lesion
61514 Removal of brain abscess
61516 Removal of brain lesion
61517 Implt brain chemotx add-on
61518 Removal of brain lesion
61519 Remove brain lining lesion
61520 Removal of brain lesion
61521 Removal of brain lesion
61522 Removal of brain abscess
61524 Removal of brain lesion
61526 Removal of brain lesion
61530 Removal of brain lesion
61531 Implant brain electrodes
61533 Implant brain electrodes
61534 Removal of brain lesion
61535 Remove brain electrodes
61536 Removal of brain lesion
61537 Removal of brain tissue
61538 Removal of brain tissue
61539 Removal of brain tissue
61540 Removal of brain tissue
61541 Incision of brain tissue
61542 Removal of brain tissue
61543 Removal of brain tissue
61544 Remove & treat brain lesion
61545 Excision of brain tumor
61546 Removal of pituitary gland
61548 Removal of pituitary gland
61550 Release of skull seams
61552 Release of skull seams
61556 Incise skull/sutures
61557 Incise skull/sutures
61558 Excision of skull/sutures
61559 Excision of skull/sutures
61563 Excision of skull tumor
61564 Excision of skull tumor
61566 Removal of brain tissue
61567 Incision of brain tissue
61570 Remove foreign body brain
61571 Incise skull for brain wound
61575 Skull base/brainstem surgery
61576 Skull base/brainstem surgery
61580 Craniofacial approach skull
61581 Craniofacial approach skull
61582 Craniofacial approach skull
61583 Craniofacial approach skull
61584 Orbitocranial approach/skull
61585 Orbitocranial approach/skull
61586 Resect nasopharynx skull
61590 Infratemporal approach/skull

61591 Infratemporal approach/skull
61592 Orbitocranial approach/skull
61595 Transtemporal approach/skull
61596 Transcochlear approach/skull
61597 Transcondylar approach/skull
61598 Transpetrosal approach/skull
61600 Resect/excise cranial lesion
61601 Resect/excise cranial lesion
61605 Resect/excise cranial lesion
61606 Resect/excise cranial lesion
61607 Resect/excise cranial lesion
61608 Resect/excise cranial lesion
61609 Transect artery sinus
61610 Transect artery sinus
61611 Transect artery sinus
61612 Transect artery sinus
61613 Remove aneurysm sinus
61615 Resect/excise lesion skull
61616 Resect/excise lesion skull
61618 Repair dura
61619 Repair dura
61624 Transcath occlusion cns
61630 Intracranial angioplasty
61635 Intracran angioplsty w/stent
61680 Intracranial vessel surgery
61682 Intracranial vessel surgery
61684 Intracranial vessel surgery
61686 Intracranial vessel surgery
61690 Intracranial vessel surgery
61692 Intracranial vessel surgery
61697 Brain aneurysm repr complx
61698 Brain aneurysm repr complx
61700 Brain aneurysm repr simple
61702 Inner skull vessel surgery
61703 Clamp neck artery
61705 Revise circulation to head
61708 Revise circulation to head
61710 Revise circulation to head
61711 Fusion of skull arteries
61735 Incise skull/brain surgery
61750 Incise skull/brain biopsy
61751 Brain biopsy w/ct/mr guide
61760 Implant brain electrodes
61850 Implant neuroelectrodes
61860 Implant neuroelectrodes
61863 Implant neuroelectrode
61864 Implant neuroelectrde addl
61867 Implant neuroelectrode
61868 Implant neuroelectrde addl
61870 Implant neuroelectrodes
61875 Implant neuroelectrodes
62005 Treat skull fracture
62010 Treatment of head injury
62100 Repair brain fluid leakage
62115 Reduction of skull defect
62116 Reduction of skull defect
62117 Reduction of skull defect
62120 Repair skull cavity lesion
62121 Incise skull repair
62140 Repair of skull defect
62141 Repair of skull defect
62142 Remove skull plate/flap
62143 Replace skull plate/flap
62145 Repair of skull & brain
62146 Repair of skull with graft
62147 Repair of skull with graft
62148 Retr bone flap to fix skull
62161 Dissect brain w/scope
62162 Remove colloid cyst w/scope
62163 Zneuroendoscopy w/fb removal
62164 Remove brain tumor w/scope
62165 Remove pituit tumor w/scope
62180 Establish brain cavity shunt
62190 Establish brain cavity shunt
62192 Establish brain cavity shunt
62200 Establish brain cavity shunt
62201 Brain cavity shunt w/scope
62220 Establish brain cavity shunt
62223 Establish brain cavity shunt
62256 Remove brain cavity shunt
62258 Replace brain cavity shunt
63043 Laminotomy addl cervical
63044 Laminotomy addl lumbar
63050 Cervical laminoplsty 2/> seg
63051 C-laminoplasty w/graft/plate
63077 Spine disk surgery thorax
63078 Spine disk surgery thorax
63081 Remove vert body dcmprn crvl
63082 Remove vertebral body add-on
63085 Remove vert body dcmprn thrc
63086 Remove vertebral body add-on
63087 Remov vertbr dcmprn thrclmbr
63088 Remove vertebral body add-on
63090 Remove vert body dcmprn lmbr
63091 Remove vertebral body add-on
63101 Remove vert body dcmprn thrc
63102 Remove vert body dcmprn lmbr
63103 Remove vertebral body add-on
63170 Incise spinal cord tract(s)
63172 Drainage of spinal cyst
63173 Drainage of spinal cyst
63180 Revise spinal cord ligaments
63182 Revise spinal cord ligaments
63185 Incise spine nrv half segmnt
63190 Incise spine nrv >2 segmnts
63191 Incise spine accessory nerve
63194 Incise spine & cord cervical
63195 Incise spine & cord thoracic
63196 Incise spine&cord 2 trx crvl
63197 Incise spine&cord 2 trx thrc
63198 Incise spin&cord 2 stgs crvl
63199 Incise spin&cord 2 stgs thrc
63200 Release spinal cord lumbar
63250 Revise spinal cord vsls crvl
63251 Revise spinal cord vsls thrc
63252 Revise spine cord vsl thrlmb
63265 Excise intraspinl lesion crv
63266 Excise intrspinl lesion thrc
63267 Excise intrspinl lesion lmbr
63268 Excise intrspinl lesion scrl
63270 Excise intrspinl lesion crvl
63271 Excise intrspinl lesion thrc
63272 Excise intrspinl lesion lmbr
63273 Excise intrspinl lesion scrl
63275 Bx/exc xdrl spine lesn crvl
63276 Bx/exc xdrl spine lesn thrc
63277 Bx/exc xdrl spine lesn lmbr
63278 Bx/exc xdrl spine lesn scrl
63280 Bx/exc idrl spine lesn crvl
63281 Bx/exc idrl spine lesn thrc
63282 Bx/exc idrl spine lesn lmbr
63283 Bx/exc idrl spine lesn scrl
63285 Bx/exc idrl imed lesn cervl
63286 Bx/exc idrl imed lesn thrc
63287 Bx/exc idrl imed lesn thrlmb
63290 Bx/exc xdrl/idrl lsn any lvl
63295 Repair laminectomy defect
63300 Remove vert xdrl body crvcl
63301 Remove vert xdrl body thrc
63302 Remove vert xdrl body thrlmb
63303 Remov vert xdrl bdy lmbr/sac
63304 Remove vert idrl body crvcl
63305 Remove vert idrl body thrc
63306 Remov vert idrl bdy thrclmbr
63307 Remov vert idrl bdy lmbr/sac
63308 Remove vertebral body add-on
63700 Repair of spinal herniation
63702 Repair of spinal herniation
63704 Repair of spinal herniation
63706 Repair of spinal herniation
63707 Repair spinal fluid leakage
63709 Repair spinal fluid leakage
63710 Graft repair of spine defect
63740 Install spinal shunt
64752 Incision of vagus nerve
64755 Incision of stomach nerves
64760 Incision of vagus nerve
64809 Remove sympathetic nerves
64818 Remove sympathetic nerves
64866 Fusion of facial/other nerve
64868 Fusion of facial/other nerve
65273 Repair of eye wound
69155 Extensive ear/neck surgery
69535 Remove part of temporal bone
69554 Remove ear lesion
69950 Incise inner ear nerve
75952 Endovasc repair abdom aorta
75953 Abdom aneurysm endovas rpr
75954 Iliac aneurysm endovas rpr
75956 Xray endovasc thor ao repr
75957 Xray endovasc thor ao repr
75958 Xray place prox ext thor ao
75959 Xray place dist ext thor ao
92970 Cardioassist internal

92971 Cardioassist external
92975 Dissolve clot heart vessel
92992 Revision of heart chamber
92993 Revision of heart chamber
93583 Perq transcath septal reduxn
99190 Special pump services
99191 Special pump services
99192 Special pump services
99356 Prolonged service inpatient
99357 Prolonged service inpatient
99462 Sbsq nb em per day hosp
99468 Neonate crit care initial
99469 Neonate crit care subsq
99471 Ped critical care initial
99472 Ped critical care subsq
99475 Ped crit care age 2-5 init
99476 Ped crit care age 2-5 subsq
99477 Init day hosp neonate care
99478 Ic lbw inf < 1500 gm subsq
99479 Ic lbw inf 1500-2500 g subsq
99480 Ic inf pbw 2501-5000 g subsq
G0341 Percutaneous islet celltrans
G0342 Laparoscopy islet cell trans
G0343 Laparotomy islet cell transp
G0412 Open tx iliac spine uni/bil
G0414 Pelvic ring fx treat int fix
G0415 Open tx post pelvic fxcture

Appendix N — Multianalyte Assays with Algorithmic Analyses

The following is a list of administrative codes for multianalyte assays with algorithmic analysis (MAAA) procedures that are usually exclusive to one single clinical laboratory or manufacturer. These tests use the results from several different assays, including molecular pathology assays, fluorescent in situ hybridization assays, and nonnucleic acid-based assays (e.g., proteins, polypeptides, lipids, and carbohydrates) to perform an algorithmic analysis that is reported as a numeric score or probability. Although the laboratory report may list results of individual component tests of the MAAAs, these assays are not separately reportable.

The following list includes the proprietary name and clinical laboratory/manufacturer, an alphanumeric code, and the code descriptor.

The format for the code descriptor usually includes:

- Type of disease (e.g., oncology, autoimmune, tissue rejection)
- Chemical(s) analyzed (e.g., DNA, RNA, protein, antibody)
- Number of markers (e.g., number of genes, number of proteins)
- Methodology(s) (e.g., microarray, real-time [RT]-PCR, in situ hybridization [ISH], enzyme linked immunosorbent assays [ELISA])
- Number of functional domains (when indicated)
- Type of specimen (e.g., blood, fresh tissue, formalin-fixed paraffin embedded)
- Type of algorithm result (e.g., prognostic, diagnostic)
- Report (e.g., probability index, risk score)

MAAA procedures with a Category I code are noted on the following list and can also be found in code range 81500–81599 in the pathology and laboratory chapter. If a specific MAAA test does not have a Category I code, it is denoted with a four-digit number and the letter M. Use code 81599 if an MAAA test is not included on the following list or in the Category I codes. The codes on the list are exclusive to the assays identified by proprietary name. Report code 81599 also when an analysis is performed that may possibly fall within a specific descriptor but the proprietary name is not included in the list. The list does not contain all MAAA procedures.

Proprietary Name/Clinical Laboratory/Manufacturer	Code	Descriptor
Administrative Codes for Multianalyte Assays with Algorithmic Analyses (MAAA)		
HCV FibroSURE, LabCorp	0001M	Infectious disease, HCV, six biochemical assays (ALT, A2-macroglobulin, apolipoprotein A-1, total bilirubin, GGT, and haptoglobin) utilizing serum, prognostic algorithm reported as scores for fibrosis and necroinflammatory activity in liver
ASH FibroSURE, LabCorp	0002M	Liver disease, 10 biochemical assays (ALT, A2-macroglobulin, apolipoprotein A-1, total bilirubin, GGT, haptoglobin, AST, glucose, total cholesterol, and triglycerides) utilizing serum, prognostic algorithm reported as quantitative scores for fibrosis, steatosis, and alcoholic steatohepatitis (ASH)
NASH FibroSURE, LabCorp	0003M	Liver disease, 10 biochemical assays (ALT, A2-macroglobulin, apolipoprotein A-1, total bilirubin, GGT, haptoglobin, AST, glucose, total cholesterol, and triglycerides) utilizing serum, prognostic algorithm reported as quantitative scores for fibrosis, steatosis, and nonalcoholic steatohepatitis (NASH)
ScoliScore Transgenomic	0004M	Scoliosis, DNA analysis of 53 single nucleotide polymorphisms (SNPs), using saliva, prognostic algorithm reported as a risk score
HeproDX™, GoPath Laboratories, LLC	●0006M	Oncology (hepatic), mRNA expression levels of 161 genes, utilizing fresh hepatocellular carcinoma tumor tissue, with alpha-fetoprotein level, algorithm reported as a risk classifier
NETest (Wren Laboratories, LLC)	●0007M	Oncology (gastrointestinal neuroendocrine tumors), real-time PCR expression analysis of 51 genes, utilizing whole peripheral blood, algorithm reported as a nomogram of tumor disease index
Prosigna Breast Cancer Assay (NanoString Technologies)	●0008M	Oncology (breast), mRNA analysis of 58 genes using hybrid capture, on formalin-fixed paraffin-embedded (FFPE) tissue, prognostic algorithm reported as a risk score
	●0009M	Fetal aneuploidy (trisomy 21, and 18) DNA sequence analysis of selected regions using maternal plasma, algorithm reported as a risk score for each trisomy
	●0010M	Oncology (High-Grade Prostate Cancer), biochemical assay of four proteins (Total PSA, Free PSA, Intact PSA and human kallikrein 2 [hK2]) plus patient age, digital rectal examination status, and no history of positive prostate biopsy, utilizing plasma, prognostic algorithm reported as a probability score
Category I Codes for Multianalyte Assays with Algorithmic Analyses (MAAA)		
Risk of Ovarian Malignancy Algorithm (ROMA), Fujirebio Diagnostics	81500	Oncology (ovarian), biochemical assays of two proteins (CA-125 and HE4), utilizing serum, with menopausal status, algorithm reported as a risk score
OVA1, Vermillion, Inc.	81503	Oncology (ovarian), biochemical assays of five proteins (CA-125, apolipoprotein A1, beta-2 microglobulin, transferrin, and pre-albumin), utilizing serum, algorithm reported as a risk score
Pathwork Tissue of Origin Test, Pathwork Diagnostics	81504	Oncology (tissue of origin), microarray gene expression profiling of >2000 genes, utilizing formalin-fixed paraffin embedded tissue, algorithm reported as tissue similarity scores

Proprietary Name/Clinical Laboratory/Manufacturer	Code	Descriptor
PreDx Diabetes Risk Score, Tethys Clinical Laboratory	81506	Endocrinology (type 2 diabetes), biochemical assays of seven analytes (glucose, HbA1c, insulin, hs-CRP, adiponectin, ferritin, interleukin 2-receptor alpha), utilizing serum or plasma, algorithm reporting a risk score
Harmony Prenatal Test, Ariosa Diagnostics	81507	Fetal aneuploidy (trisomy 21, 18, and 13) DNA sequence analysis of selected regions using maternal plasma, algorithm reported as a risk score for each trisomy
Maternal serum screening procedures are performed by many labs and are not exclusive to a single facility.	81508	Fetal congenital abnormalities, biochemical assays of two proteins (PAPP-A, hCG [any form]), utilizing maternal serum, algorithm reported as a risk score
	81509	Fetal congenital abnormalities, biochemical assays of three proteins (PAPP-A, hCG [any form], DIA), utilizing maternal serum, algorithm reported as a risk score
	81510	Fetal congenital abnormalities, biochemical assays of three analytes (AFP, uE3, hCG (any form)), utilizing maternal serum, algorithm reported as a risk score
	81511	Fetal congenital abnormalities, biochemical assays of four analytes (AFP, uE3, hCG (any form), DIA) utilizing maternal serum, algorithm reported as a risk score (may include additional results from previous biochemical testing)
	81512	Fetal congenital abnormalities, biochemical assays of five analytes (AFP, uE3, total hCG, hyperglycosylated hCG, DIA) utilizing maternal serum, algorithm reported as a risk score
Oncotype DX® (Genomic Health)	●81519	Oncology (breast), mRNA, gene expression profiling by real-time RT-PCR of 21 genes, utilizing formalin-fixed paraffin embedded tissue, algorithm reported as recurrence score
Maternal serum screening procedures are performed by many labs and are not exclusive to a single facility.	81599	Unlisted multianalyte assay with algorithmic analysis